Insall & Scott 膝关节外科学

下卷

第 6 版

人民卫生出版社
·北 京·

图书在版编目（CIP）数据

Insall & Scott 膝关节外科学 = Insall & Scott
Surgery of the Knee，6e：上、下卷：英文 /（美）
W. 诺尔曼·斯考特（W. Norman Scott）主编 . —北京：
人民卫生出版社，2021.10
ISBN 978-7-117-32174-7

Ⅰ. ①I… Ⅱ. ①W… Ⅲ. ①膝关节 – 外科学 – 英文
Ⅳ. ①R687.4

中国版本图书馆 CIP 数据核字（2021）第 201311 号

| 人卫智网 | www.ipmph.com | 医学教育、学术、考试、健康，购书智慧智能综合服务平台 |
| 人卫官网 | www.pmph.com | 人卫官方资讯发布平台 |

图字：01-2021-5355 号

Insall & Scott 膝关节外科学
Insall & Scott Xiguanjie Waikexue
（上、下卷）

主　　编：W. Norman Scott
出版发行：人民卫生出版社（中继线 010-59780011）
地　　址：北京市朝阳区潘家园南里 19 号
邮　　编：100021
E - mail：pmph @ pmph.com
购书热线：010-59787592　010-59787584　010-65264830
印　　刷：廊坊一二〇六印刷厂
经　　销：新华书店
开　　本：889 × 1194　1/16　总印张：147.5
总 字 数：7316 千字
版　　次：2021 年 10 月第 1 版
印　　次：2021 年 11 月第 1 次印刷
标准书号：ISBN 978-7-117-32174-7
定价（上、下卷）：1800.00 元

打击盗版举报电话：**010-59787491**　**E-mail：WQ @ pmph.com**
质量问题联系电话：**010-59787234**　**E-mail：zhiliang @ pmph.com**

Insall & Scott
SURGERY of the KNEE

VOLUME 2

Sixth Edition

EDITOR-IN-CHIEF

W. NORMAN SCOTT, MD, FACS

Clinical Professor of Orthopaedic Surgery
New York University Langone Medical Center
Hospital for Joint Diseases;
Joan C. Edwards School of Medicine
Marshall University
Founding Director
Insall Scott Kelly Institute for Orthopaedic Sports
   Medicine
New York, New York

ASSOCIATE EDITORS

DAVID R. DIDUCH, MS, MD

Alfred R. Shands Professor of Orthopaedic Surgery
Vice Chairman, Department of Orthopaedic Surgery
Head Orthopaedic Team Physician
University of Virginia
Charlottesville, Virginia

ARLEN D. HANSSEN, MD

Professor
Department of Orthopedic Surgery
Mayo Clinic
Rochester, Minnesota

RICHARD IORIO, MD

Dr. William and Susan Jaffe Professor of Orthopaedic Surgery
Chief Division of Adult Reconstructive Surgery
Department of Orthopaedic Surgery
New York University Langone Medical Center
Hospital for Joint Diseases
New York, New York

WILLIAM J. LONG, MD, FRCSC

Director,
Attending Orthopaedic Surgeon
Insall Scott Kelly Institute
St. Francis Hospital
Lenox Hill Hospital
New York, New York

ELSEVIER

Elsevier (Singapore) Pte Ltd.
3 Killiney Road,
#08-01 Winsland House I,
Singapore 239519
Tel: (65) 6349-0200; Fax: (65) 6733-1817

ELSEVIER

This English Reprint of Insall & Scott Surgery of The Knee, 6E by W. Norman Scott was undertaken by People's Medical Publishing House and is published by arrangement with Elsevier (Singapore) Pte Ltd.

Insall & Scott Surgery of The Knee, 6E by W. Norman Scott 由人民卫生出版社进行影印，并根据人民卫生出版社与爱思唯尔（新加坡）私人有公司的协议约定出版。

ISBN: 978-7-117-32174-7

Notice

Practitioners and researchers must always rely on their own experience and knowledge in evaluating and using any information, methods, compounds or experiments described herein. Because of rapid advances in the medical sciences, in particular, independent verification of diagnoses and drug dosages should be made. To the fullest extent of the law, no responsibility is assumed by Elsevier, authors, editors or contributors in relation to the adaptation or for any injury and/or damage to persons or property as a matter of products liability, negligence or otherwise, or from any use or operation of any methods, products, instructions, or ideas contained in the material herein.

Arthur Atchabahian, MD
Professor of Clinical Anesthesiology
Department of Anesthesiology
New York University School of Medicine
New York, New York

Geoffrey S. Baer, MD, PhD
Department of Orthopedic Surgery and
    Rehabilitation
Division of Sports Medicine
University of Wisconsin—Madison
Madison, Wisconsin

Asheesh Bedi, MD
Chief, Sports Medicine and Surgery
Harold and Helen Gehring Professor
Department of Orthopaedic Surgery
University of Michigan
Ann Arbor, Michigan

Jenny T. Bencardino, MD
Attending Radiologist
Department of Radiology
New York University Hospital for Joint
    Diseases
New York, New York

Henry D. Clarke, MD
Consultant, Department of Orthopedics
Professor of Orthopedics
Mayo Clinic
Phoenix, Arizona

David R. Diduch, MD, MS
Alfred R. Shands Professor of Orthopaedic
    Surgery
Vice Chairman, Department of
    Orthopaedic Surgery
Head Orthopaedic Team Physician
University of Virginia
Charlottesville, Virginia

Andrew G. Franks, Jr., BA, MD
Clinical Professor
Internal Medicine (Rheumatology)
New York University School of Medicine
Director
Autoimmune Connective Tissue Disease
    Section
New York University School of Medicine
Attending Rheumatologist
Hospital for Joint Diseases
New York University School of Medicine
New York, New York

George J. Haidukewych, MD
Division of Orthopaedic Trauma and
    Complex Adult Reconstruction
Department of Orthopaedic Surgery
Orlando Regional Medical Center
Orlando, Florida

Arlen D. Hanssen, MD
Professor
Department of Orthopedic Surgery
Mayo Clinic
Rochester, Minnesota

Richard Iorio, MD
Dr. William and Susan Jaffe Professor of
    Orthopaedic Surgery
Chief Division of Adult Reconstructive
    Surgery
Department of Orthopaedic Surgery
New York University Langone Medical
    Center
New York, New York

Mininder S. Kocher, MD, MPH
Professor of Orthopaedic Surgery
Harvard Medical School
Associate Director
Division of Sports Medicine
Boston Children's Hospital
Boston, Massachusettes

Richard D. Komistek, BSME, MSME, PhD
Fred M. Roddy Professor
Biomedical Engineering
Co-Center Director
Center for Musculoskeletal Research
University of Tennessee
Knoxville, Tennessee

William J. Long, BSc, MD, FRCSC
Director,
Attending Orthopaedic Surgeon
Insall Scott Kelly Institute,
St. Franics Hospital,
Lenox Hill Hospital,
Hospital for Joint Diseases
New York, New York

Milad Nazemzadeh, MD
Clinical Assistant
Professor of Anesthesiology
Department of Anesthesiology,
    Perioperative Care, and Pain Medicine
New York University Langone Medical
    Center
New York, New York

Mary I. O'Connor, MD
Director and Professor
Center for Musculoskeletal Care at Yale
    School of Medicine and Yale—New
    Haven Hospital
Yale School of Medicine
New Haven, Connecticut

Susan Craig Scott, MD, FACS
Clinical Assistant Professor
Department of Orthopaedic Surgery
Division of Hand Surgery
NYU Hospital for Joint Diseases
Assistant Attending
Department of Orthopedics
Department of Veterans Affairs
New York Harbor Healthcare System
New York, New York

W. Norman Scott, MD, FACS
Clinical Professor of Orthopaedic Surgery
NYU Hospital for Joint Disease Joan C.
    Edwards School of Medicine
Marshall University Founding Director
Insall Scott Kelly Institute for Orthopaedics
    and Sports Medicine
New York, New York

It's been stated that the "family" is the "smallest unit of society,"
yet it's the most complex. While the commitments can be intimidating the
rewards are awesome!

To my wife, Susan, the pillar of our family, your sacrifices have made us one!
My life has been so enriched because of you. You are where my heart resides!

To our children, Eric, Will, and Kelly, we never stop counting our blessings!
The three of you exude success because of your character, personality,
compassion, and work ethic. "To whom much has been given, much is
required." The three of you have overachieved!

To Nina, Danielle, and Erik, we love the expansion of our family. We have been
blessed by your inclusion in our family and look forward to an incredible
future.

To Ella and Layla, and your cousins to come, you bring joy to our hearts
and your successes in life will be abundant because of your parents!

Thank you ALL!

W. Norman Scott, MD

Matthew P. Abdel, MD
Associate Professor of Orthopedic Surgery
and Senior Associate Consultant
Department of Orthopedic Surgery
Mayo Clinic
Rochester, Minnesota

Aryeh M. Abeles, MD
Associate Clinical Professor
Department of Rheumatology
University of Connecticut
Farmington, Connecticut

Ronald S. Adler, MD, PhD
Professor of Radiology
New York University School of Medicine;
Department of Radiology
Langone Medical Center
New York, New York

Paolo Adravanti, MD
Chief of Orthopedics
Department of Orthopedics
Clinic Città di Parma
Parma, Italy

Vinay K. Aggarwal, MD
Resident Physician
Hospital for Joint Diseases
NYU Langone Medical Center
New York, New York

Eduard Alentorn-Geli, MD, MSc, PhD, FEBOT
Duke Sports Science Institute
Department of Orthopedic Surgery
Duke University
Durham, North Carolina

Azhar A. Ali, MD
Center for Orthopaedic Biomechanics
University of Denver
Denver, Colorado

Sana Ali, MD
Resident in Diagnostic Radiology
Department of Diagnostic Imaging
Maimonides Medical Center
Brooklyn, New York

Hassan Alosh, MD

Aaron Althaus, MD
Fellow
Department of Orthopedic Surgery
Insall Scott Kelly
New York, New York

Annunziato Amendola, MD
Department of Orthopedic Surgery
Division of Sports Medicine
Duke University
Durham, North Carolina

Ned Amendola, MD

Priyadarshi Amit, MS Ortho, DNB Ortho, MRCSEd
Sicot Fellow
Department of Orthopedics and
Traumatology
Fondazione IRCCS Policlinico San Matteo
Università degli Studi di Pavia
Pavia, Italy;
Department of Orthopedics
Max Institute of Medical Sciences
New Delhi, India

Aldo Ampollini, MD
Orthopaedic Surgeon
Department of Orthopaedic Surgery
Clinic Città di Parma
Parma, Italy

Allen F. Anderson, MD
Orthopaedic Surgeon
Tennessee Orthopaedic Alliance/The
Lipscomb Clinic
Nashville, Tennessee

Christian N. Anderson, MD
Orthopaedic Surgeon
Tennessee Orthopaedic Alliance/The
Lipscomb Clinic
Nashville, Tennessee

Thomas P. Andriacchi, MD

Shawn G. Anthony, MD, MBA
Assistant Professor, Sports Medicine
Department of Orthopaedic Surgery
Icahn School of Medicine at Mount Sinai
Mount Sinai Health System
New York, New York

Jason D. Archibald, MD
New England Orthopedic Specialists
Peabody, Massachusetts

Elizabeth A. Arendt, MD
Professor and Vice Chair
Department of Orthopaedic Surgery
University of Minnesota
Minneapolis, Minnesota

Jean Noël Argenson, APHM
Institute for Locomotion
Department of Orthopaedic Surgery
Sainte-Marguerite Hospital;
Professor
Aix-Marseille University
Marseille, France

Yeseniya Aronova, MD
Resident Physician
Department of Anesthesiology,
Perioperative Care, and Pain Medicine
New York University Langone Medical
Center
New York, New York

Arthur Atchabahian, MD
Professor of Clinical Anesthesiology
Anesthesiology
New York University School of Medicine
New York, New York

Matthew S. Austin, MD
Professor
Department of Orthopaedic Surgery
Rothman Institute at Thomas Jefferson
University Hospital
Philadelphia, Pennsylvania

Christophe Aveline, MD
Department of Anesthesia and Surgical
Intensive Care
Private Hospital Sevigne
Cesson Sevigne, France

Bernard R. Bach, Jr., MD
Professor
Orthopaedic Surgery
Division of Sports Medicine
Rush University Medical Center
Chicago, Illinois

Geoffrey S. Baer, MD, PhD
Department of Orthopedic Surgery and
Rehabilitation
Division of Sports Medicine
University of Wisconsin—Madison
Madison, Wisconsin

Giovanni Balato, MD
Department of Public Health
School of Medicine
Federico II University
Naples, Italy

Andrea Baldini, MD, PhD
Institute Director
Department of Orthopaedics—Adult
    Reconstruction
IFCA Institute
Florence, Italy

Mark A. Baldwin, MD
Center for Orthopaedic Biomechanics
University of Denver
Denver, Colorado

Laura W. Bancroft, MD
Chief of MSK Radiology
Department of Radiology
Florida Hospital;
Adjunct Professor
University of Central Florida School of
    Medicine
Orlando, Florida;
Clinical Professor
Florida State University School of Medicine
Tallahassee, Florida

Sue D. Barber-Westin, BS
Director Clinical Studies
Noyes Knee Institute
Cincinnati, Ohio

William L. Bargar, BAAE, MMAE, MD
Medical Director
Joint Replacement Center
Sutter Medical Center Sacramento;
Assistant Clinical Professor
Department of Orthopaedic Surgery
UC Davis
Sacramento, California

Christopher P. Beauchamp, MD
Associate Professor
Department of Orthopaedics
Mayo Medical School
Mayo Clinic
Phoenix, Arizona

John P. Begly, MD
Resident Physician
Orthopaedics
New York University Hospital for Joint
    Diseases
New York, New York

Johan Bellemans, MD, PhD
Professor in Orthopaedics
Department of Orthopaedics and
    Traumatology
ZOL Hospitals
Genk, Belgium

Javier Beltran, MD, FACR
Chairman
Radiology
Maimonides Medical Center
Brooklyn, New York

Luis S. Beltran, MD
Assistant Professor of Radiology
Department of Radiology
New York University Langone Medical
    Center
New York, New York

Francesco Benazzo, MD
Professor of Orthopedics and Traumatology
Department of Orthopedics and
    Traumatology
Fondazione IRCCS
Policlinico San Matteo
Università degli Studi di Pavia
Pavia, Italy

Jenny T. Bencardino, MD
Attending Radiologist
Department of Radiology
New York University Hospital for Joint
    Diseases
New York, New York

Matthew Beran, MD
Attending Physician
Department of Orthopedic Surgery
Nationwide Children's Hospital;
Clinical Assistant Professor
The Ohio State University
Columbus, Ohio

Keith R. Berend, MD

Jeffrey S. Berger, MD, MS
Professor of Medicine and Surgery
Leon H. Charney Division of Cardiology
New York University School of Medicine
New York, New York

Thomas Bernasek, MD

Daniel J. Berry, MD
Past L.Z. Gund Professor and Chairman
Department of Orthopedic Surgery
Mayo Clinic
Rochester, Minnesota

Michael R. Boniello, MD, MS
Eastern Virginia Medical School
Norfolk, Virginia;
Orthopedic Surgery Resident
Cooper Bone and Joint Institute
Camden, New Jersey

Kevin F. Bonner, MD
Orthopedic Surgeon
Jordan-Young Institute
Virginia Beach, Virginia;
Assistant Professor
Department of Surgery
Eastern Virginia Medical School
Norfolk, Virginia

Joseph A. Bosco III, MD
Department of Orthopedic Surgery
New York University Langone Medical
    Center
New York, New York

Jan Boublik, MD, PhD
Department of Anesthesiology,
    Perioperative and Pain Medicine
Stanford University School of Medicine
Stanford, California

Seth Bowman, MD
Department of Orthopaedic Surgery
Medical University of South Carolina
Charleston, South Carolina

Adam C. Brekke, MD
Resident
Department of Orthopaedics and
    Rehabilitation
Vanderbilt University Medical Center
Nashville, Tennessee

Claire L. Brockett, MD
Institute of Medical and Biological
    Engineering
School of Mechanical Engineering
University of Leeds
Leeds, United Kingdom

James A. Brown, MD
Associate Professor and Division Head of
    Adult Reconstruction
Department of Orthopaedic Surgery
University of Virginia
Charlottesville, Virginia

Michael K. Brooks, MD, MPH
Clinical Assistant Professor of Radiology
    SUNY-Stony Brook
Musculoskeletal Radiology and
    InterventionWinthrop University
    Hospital
Mineola, New York

Jarett S. Burak, MD
Assistant Professor of Radiology
Hofstra-Northwell School of Medicine;
Medical Director
Northwell Health Imaging at Syosset
Northwell Health—Department of
    Radiology
Greak Neck, New York

Christopher John Burke, MBChB FRCR
Doctor/Assistant Professor
Department of Radiology
New York University;
Doctor/Assistant Professor
Department of Radiology
New York University, Langone Medical
    Center;
Doctor/Assistant Professor
Department of Radiology
New York University, Hospital for Joint
    Diseases
New York, New York

M. Tyrrell Burrus, MD
Resident Physician
Orthopaedic Surgery
University of Virginia Health System,
Charlottesville, Virginia

Charles Bush-Joseph, MD
Professor
Divsion of Sports Medicine
Department of Orthopaedic Surgery
Rush University Medical Center
Chicago, Illinois

Frank A. Buttacavoli, MD
Orthopedic Surgeon
Orthopedic Care Center
Aventura, Florida

Asokumar Buvanendran, MD, MBBS
Professor
Vice Chair Research & Director of
    Orthopedic Anesthesia
Department of Anesthesiology
Rush University Medical Center
Chicago, Illinois

Matthew G. Cable, MD
Clinical Assistant Professor
Department of Orthopaedics
Section of Musculoskeletal Oncology
Louisiana State University Health Sciences
    Center
New Orleans, Louisiana

Giuseppe Calafiore, MD
Orthopaedic Surgeon
Department of Orthopedics
Clinic Città di Parma
Parma, Italy

Tristan Camus, BSc (Hons), MD, FRCSC
Fellow
Department of Orthopaedic Surgery, Adult
    Reconstruction
New York University Langone Medical
    Center
Insall Scott Kelly
New York, New York

Jourdan M. Cancienne, MD
Resident Physician
Department of Orthopaedic Surgery
University of Virginia Health System
Charlottesville, Virginia

Thomas R. Carter, MD
The Orthopedic Clinic Association, PC
Phoenix, Arizona

Simone Cerciello, MD
Casa di Cura Villa Betania
Rome, Italy;
Marrelli Hospital
Crotone, Italy

Jorge Chahla, MD
Regenerative Sports Medicine Fellow
Center for Translational and Regenerative
    Medicine Research
Steadman Philippon Research Institute
Vail, Colorado

Eric Y. Chang, MD
Assistant Professor
Department of Radiology
VA San Diego Healthcare System;
Assistant Professor
Department of Radiology
University of California, San Diego Medical
    Center
San Diego, California

Anikar Chhabra, MD, MS
Assistant Professor
Department of Orthopedic Surgery
Mayo Clinic Arizona,
Phoenix, Arizona;
Head Team Orthopedic Surgeon
Arizona State University
Tempe, Arizona

Brian Chilelli, MD
Regional Medical Group Orthopaedics
Northwestern Medicine
Warrenville, Illinois

J.H. James Choi, MD
Duke Sports Science Institute
Department of Orthopedic Surgery
Duke University
Durham, North Carolina

Constance R. Chu, MD

Christine B. Chung, MD
Professor of Radiology
University of California School of
    Medicine;
Professor of Radiology
Veterans Affairs Medicine Center
San Diego, California

Michael P. Clare, MD
Director
Foot and Ankle Fellowship
Florida Orthopaedic Institute
Tampa, Florida

Henry D. Clarke, MD
Consultant
Department of Orthopedic Surgery
Mayo Clinic
Phoenix, Arizona;
Professor of Orthopedics
Mayo Clinic College of Medicine
Rochester, Minnesota

David E. Cohen, MD

Brian J. Cole, MD, MBA
Department of Sports Medicine
Rush University Medical Center
Chicago, Illinois

Kristopher D. Collins, MD
Fellow in Adult Reconstruction
Department of Orthopaedic Surgery
ISK Institute
New York, New York

Christopher R. Conley, MD
Consultant
Laboratory Medicine and Pathology
Mayo Clinic
Phoenix, Arizona;
Assistant Professor of Pathology
Mayo Clinic College of Medicine
Rochester, Minnesota

Raelene M. Cowie, MD
Institute of Medical and Biological
    Engineering
School of Mechanical Engineering
University of Leeds
Leeds, United Kingdom

David A. Crawford, MD

Brian M. Culp, MD
Orthopaedic Surgeon
Princeton Orthopaedic Associates
Princeton, New Jersey

John H. Currier, MS
Research Engineer
Thayer School of Engineering at
    Dartmouth College
Hanover, New Hampshire

Fred D. Cushner, MD

Brian P. Dahl, MD
Fellow
Hofmann Arthritis Institute
Salt Lake City, Utah

Diane L. Dahm, MD
Professor of Orthopedics, Mayo Clinic
    College of Medicine
Department of Orthopedic Surgery
Mayo Clinic
Rochester, Minnesota

Timothy A. Damron, MD
Vice-Chairman and David G. Murray
    Endowed Professor of Orthopedic
    Surgery
Department of Orthopedic Surgery
SUNY Upstate Medical University
Syracuse, New York

Chase S. Dean, MD
Steadman Philippon Research Institute
Vail, Colorado

Jospeh P. DeAngelia, MD, MBA
Carl J. Shapiro Department of
    Orthopaedics
Beth Israel Deaconess Medical Center
Boston, Massachusetts

David DeJour, MD
Orthopedic Surgeon
Lyon, France

Craig J. Della Valle, MD
Professor and Chief
Division of Adult Reconstruction
Department of Orthopaedic Surgery
Rush University Medical Center
Chicago, Illinois

Edward M. DelSole, MD
Resident Physician
Department of Orthopaedic Surgery
New York University Langone Medical
    Center/Hospital for Joint Diseases
New York, New York

Douglas A. Dennis, MD
Colorado Joint Replacement;
Adjunct Professor of Bioengineering
Department of Mechanical and Materials
    Engineering
University of Denver
Denver, Colorado;
Adjunct Professor
Department of Biomedical Engineering
University of Tennessee
Knoxville Tennessee;
Assistant Clinical Professor
Department of Orthopaedics
University of Colorado School of Medicine
Aurora, Colorado

Edward J. Derrick, MD

Ajit J. Deshmukh, MD
Assistant Professor
Orthopaedic Surgery
New York University Langone Medical
    Center/New York University Hospital
    for Joint Diseases;
Assistant Chief
Department of Orthopaedics
Surgery
VA New York Harbor Healthcare System
New York, New York

**Ian D. Dickey, MD, P Eng (HON)
FRCSC**
St. Luke's/Presbyterian Hospital
Denver, Colorado

Sorosch Didehvar, MD
Department of Anesthesiology
New York University Langone Medical
    Center
New York, New York

David R. Diduch, MD, MS
Alfred R. Shands Professor of Orthopaedic
    Surgery
Vice Chairman, Department of
    Orthopaedic Surgery
Head Orthopaedic Team Physician
University of Virginia
Charlottesville, Virginia

Lisa V. Doan, MD
Assistant Professor
Department of Anesthesiology,
    Perioperative Care, and Pain Medicine
New York University School of Medicine
New York, New York

Christopher A.F. Dodd, FRCS
Consultant Orthopaedic Surgeon
Nuffield Orthopaedic Centre
Oxford University Hospitals NHS Trust
Oxford, Great Britain

Shawna Dorman, MD
Assistant Professor of Anesthesiology and
    Assistant Director of Ambulatory
    Surgery
Department of Anesthesiology
New York University Langone Hospital for
    Joint Diseases
New York, New York

James C. Dreese, MD

Kostas Economopoulos, MD
The Orthopedic Clinic Association, PC
Phoenix, Arizona

Michele N. Edison, BS, MD
Department of Radiology
Florida Hospital;
Assistant Professor
University of Central Florida College of
    Medicine
Orlando, Florida

Nima Eftekhary, MD
Resident Physician
Orthopaedic Surgery
New York University Hospital for Joint
    Diseases
New York, New York

Brandon J. Erickson, MD
Orthopaedic Surgery Resident
Department of Orthopaedic Surgery
Rush University
Chicago, Illinois

Jean-Pierre Estèbe, MD, PhD
Department of Anesthesiology, Intensive
    Care, and Pain Medicine
University Hospital of Rennes
Rennes, France

Cody L. Evans, BS, MD
Resident Physician
Orthopaedic Surgery
University of Virginia
Charlottesville, Virginia

Gregory C. Fanelli, MD
Orthopaedic Surgeon
GHS Orthopaedics
Danville, Pennsylvania

Jack Farr, MD
OrthoIndy Cartilage Restoration Center
Professor of Orthopaedic Surgery
Indiana University Medical Center
Indianapolis, Indiana

Andrew Feldman, MD
Assistant Professor
Department of Orthopaedic Surgery
New York University Hospital for Joint
    Diseases
New York, New York

Jonathon T. Finoff, MD

John Fisher, MD
Institute of Medical and Biological
    Engineering
School of Mechanical Engineering
University of Leeds
Leeds, United Kingdom

Wolfgang Fitz, MD
Assistant Professor
Orthopedic Surgery
Brigham and Women's and Faulkner
    Hospital, Harvard Medical School
Boston, Massachusetts

Clare K. Fitzpatrick, MD
Center for Orthopaedic Biomechanics
University of Denver
Denver, Colorado

Vincenzo Franceschini, MD
Department of Orthopaedics and
    Traumatology
"Sapienza" University of Rome, ICOT
Latina, Italy

Corinna C. Franklin, MD
Pediatric Orthopaedic Surgeon
Shriners Hospital for Children,
Philadelphia, Pennsylvania

Andrew G. Franks, Jr., BA, MD
Clinical Professor
Department of Internal Medicine
    (Rheumatology)
New York University School of Medicine;
Director
Autoimmune Connective Tissue Disease
    Section
New York University School of Medicine;
Attending Rheumatologist
Hospital for Joint Diseases
New York University School of Medicine
New York, New York

Richard J. Friedman, MD, FRCSC
Department of Orthopaedic Surgery
Medical University of South Carolina
Charleston, South Carolina

Nicole A. Friel, MD

Mark Froimson, MD, MBA
Executive Vice President, Chief Clinical
    Officer
Trinity Health
Livonia, Michigan

**Freddie H. Fu, MD, DSc (Hon),
DPs (Hon)**
Distinguished Service Professor
University of Pittsburgh;
David Silver Professor and Chairman
Department of Orthopaedic Surgery
University of Pittsburgh School of
    Medicine;
Head Team Physician
Departmento of Athletics
University of Pittsburgh
Pittsburgh, Pennsylvania

John P. Fulkerson, MD
Orthopaedic Associates of Hartford
Hartford, Connecticut

Theodore J. Ganley, MD
Associate Professor of Orthopaedic Surgery;
    Director of Sports Medicine
Division of Orthopaedic Surgery
Children's Hospital of Philadelphia
Philadelphia, Pennsylvania

Donald S. Garbuz, MD
Professor and Head
Division of Lower Limb Reconstruction
    and Oncology
Department of Orthopaedics
University of British Columbia
Vancouver, British Columbia, Canada

Christopher Gharibo, MD
Associate Professor of Anesthesiology &
    Orthopedics
New York University School of Medicine
New York, New York

Matteo Ghiara, MD
Department of Orthopedics and
    Traumatology
Fondazione IRCCS Policlinico San Matteo
Università degli Studi di Pavia
Pavia, Italy

Thomas J. Gill, AB, MD
Director
Boston Sports Medicine and Research
    Institute
New England Baptist Hospital
Boston, Massachusetts

Megan M. Gleason, MD
Fellow
Department of Orthopedic Surgery
University of Virginia
Charlottesville, Virginia

Alyssa Reiffel Golas, MD
Resident
Hansjorg Wyss Department of Plastic
    Surgery
New York University Langone Medical
    Center
New York, New York

Gregory Golladay, MD

Andreas H. Gomoll, MD
Associate Professor of Orthopaedic Surgery
Harvard Medical School;
Orthopaedic Surgery
Brigham and Women's Hospital
Boston, Massachusetts

Felix M. Gonzalez, MD

Guillem Gonzalez-Lomas, MD
Assistant Professor
Orthopaedic Surgery
New York University Hospital for Joint
    Diseases
New York, New York

**John A. Grant, MD, PhD, FRCSC, Dip
Sport Med**
Assistant Professor
MedSport, Orthopaedic Surgery
University of Michigan
Ann Arbor, Michigan

Stephen Gregorius, MD
Department of Orthopaedics
University of Utah
Salt Lake City, Utah

Justin Greisberg, MD
Associate Professor
Department of Orthopaedic Surgery
Columbia University
New York, New York

Ulrik Grevstad, MD, PHD
Associate Professor
Anesthesia and Intensive Care
Gentofte Hospital
Copenhagen, Denmark

Trevor Grieco, BS
Graduate Research Assistant
Mechanical, Aerospace, and Biomedical
    Engineering
University of Tennessee
Knoxville, Tennessee

Justin W. Griffin, MD
Sports and Shoulder Surgery Fellow
Department of Orthopaedic Surgery
Rush University Medical Center
Chicago, Illinois

Daniel Guenther, MD

F. Winston Gwathmey, Jr., MD
Assistant Professor
Department of Orthopaedic Surgery
University of Virginia Health System
Charlottesville, Virginia

George J. Haidukewych, MD
Division of Orthopaedic Trauma and
    Complex Adult Reconstruction
Department of Orthopaedic Surgery
Orlando Regional Medical Center
Orlando, Florida

Christopher A. Hajnik, MD

Arielle J. Hall, MD
Research Intern
Sports and Shoulder Service
Hospital for Special Surgery
New York, New York

David A. Halsey, MD
Professor
University of Vermont College of Medicine
    and Rehabilitation
Burlington, Vermont

William R. Hamel, PhD, MS, BS
Professor
IEEE Fellow, ASME Fellow
Department of Mechanical, Aerospace, &
    Biomedical Engineering
The University of Tennessee–Knoxville
Knoxville, Tennessee

Arlen D. Hanssen, MD
Professor
Department of Orthopedic Surgery
Mayo Clinic
Rochester, Minnesota

John M. Hardcastle, MD
Crystal Run Healthcare
Middletown, New York

Christopher D. Harner, MD
Department of Orthopaedic Surgery
University of Texas
Houston, Texas

Joe Hart, PhD, ATC
Associate Professor
Department of Kinesiology
University of Virginia;
Director of Clinical Research
Department of Orthopaedic Surgery
University of Virginia
Charlottesville, Virginia

William L. Healy, MD

Emma Heath, MPhty, BAppSc
North Sydney Orthopaedic and Sports
    Medicine Centre
Sydney, New South Wales, Australia

Petra Heesterbeek, PhD
Research Co-ordinator/Senior Researcher
Orthopedic Research
Sint Maartenskliniek
Nijmegen, The Netherlands

Tarek M. Hegazi, MD

Yonah Heller, MD
Orthopedic Resident
Department of Orthopedics
Northwell Health
New Hyde Park, New York

Shane Hess, MD

Benton E. Heyworth, MD
Assistant Professor of Orthopaedic Surgery
Harvard Medical School
Division of Sports Medicine
Boston Children's Hospital
Boston, Massachusetts

Betina B. Hinckel, MD
Orthopaedic Surgeon
Department Institute of Orthopedics and
    Traumatology
Clinical Hospital
Medical School
University of São Paulo
São Paulo, Brazil

Richard Y. Hinton, MD, MPH
Director, Sports Medicine Fellowship
MedStar Sports Medicine
MedStar Union Memorial Hospital/
    MedStar Washington Hospital Center;
Attending
Department of Orthopaedics
MedStar Union Memorial Hospital
Baltimore, Maryland

Jason P. Hochfelder, MD
Fellow
Adult Reconstruction
Insall Scott Kelly Institute
New York, New York

Aaron A. Hofmann, MD
Director
Center for Precision Joint Replacement
Salt Lake Regional Medical Center
Salt Lake City, Utah

Ginger E. Holt, MD
Department of Orthopaedics and
    Rehabilitation
Vanderbilt Medical Center
Nashville, Tennessee

Mohammed M. Hoque, MD
Radiology Resident, R2
Department of Radiology
Maimonides Medical Center
Brooklyn, New York

Stephen M. Howell, MD
Professor of Biomedical Engineering
Department of Mechanical Engineering
University of California at Davis
Davis, California;
Orthopedic Surgeon
Methodist Hospital
Sacramento, California

Johnny Huard, PhD

Maury L. Hull, BS, MS, PhD
Distinguished Professor
Department of Biomedical Engineering
University of California Davis;
Distinguished Professor
Department of Mechanical Engineering
University of California Davis
Davis, California

Ian D. Hutchinson, MD
Research Fellow
Sports Medicine and Shoulder Service
Hospital for Special Surgery
New York, New York

Lorraine H. Hutzler, BA
Department of Orthopaedic Surgery
NYU Hospital for Joint Diseases
NYU Langone Medical Center
New York, New York

John N. Insall, MD†
Formerly Clinical Professor of Orthopedic
    Surgery
Albert Einstein College of Medicine
Bronx, New York;
Director
Insall Scott Kelly Institute for Orthopedics
    and Sports Medicine
Beth Israel Medical Center
New York, New York

Richard Iorio, MD
Dr. William and Susan Jaffe Professor of
    Orthopaedic Surgery
Chief Division of Adult Reconstructive
    Surgery
Department of Orthopaedic Surgery
New York University Langone Medical
    Center
New York, New York

Sebastián Irarrázaval, MD
Department of Orthopaedic Surgery
Pontificia Universidad Católica de Chile
Santiago, Chile

†Deceased.

Ghislaine M. Isidore, MD
Clinical Assistant Professor of
    Anesthesiology
Anesthesiology, Perioperative Care and Pain
    Medicine
New York University Langone Medical
    Center
New York, New York

Pia Jæger, MD, PhD
Doctor
Department of Anaesthesia, Centre of Head
    and Orthopeadics
Rigshospitalet
Copenhagen, Denmark

Andre M. Jakoi, MD
Fellow
Department of Orthopaedic Surgery
University of Southern California
Los Angeles, California

James G. Jarvis, MD, FRCSC
Associate Professor of Surgery
University of Ottawa;
Division of Orthopaedic Surgery
Children's Hospital of Eastern Ontario
Ottawa, Ontario, Canada

Jason M. Jennings, MD, DPT
Colorado Joint Replacement
Porter Adventist Hospital
Denver, Colorado

Louise M. Jennings, PhD
Associate Professor of Medical Engineering
Institute of Medical and Biological
    Engineering
School of Mechanical Engineering
University of Leeds
Leeds, United Kingdom

William A. Jiranek, MD
Professor and Chief of Adult
    Reconstruction
Dept. of Orthopaedic Surgery
Virginia Commonwealth University School
    of Medicine
Richmond, Virginia

Charles E. Johnston II, MD
Assistant Chief of Staff (Emeritus)
Texas Scottish Rite Hospital for Children;
Professor
Department of Orthopedic Surgery
University of Texas Southwestern Medical
    School
Dallas, Texas

Justin B. Jones, MD
Fellow
Adult Reconstruction
Isall Scott Kelly Institute
New York, New York

V. Karthik Jonna, MD

Daniel J. Kaplan, BA
Research Fellow
Orthopaedic Surgery
New York University Langone Medical
    Center
New York, New York

Jonathan Katz, MD
Department of Orthopaedic Surgery
Medical University of South Carolina
Charleston, South Carolina

Erdan Kayupov, MSE
Research Fellow
Orthopaedic Surgery
Rush University Medical Center
Chicago, Illinois

Saurabh Khakharia, MD

Arif Khan, MD

Harpal S. Khanuja, MD
Associate Professor
Chief of Adult Reconstruction
Department of Orthopaedic Surgery
The Johns Hopkins University;
Chair
Department of Orthopaedic Surgery
Johns Hopkins Bayview Medical Center
Baltimore, Maryland

Nayoung Kim, BS
Rothman Institute
Philadelphia, Pennsylvania

Raymond H. Kim, MD
Colorado Joint Replacement;
Adjunct Associate Professor of
    Bioengineering
Department of Mechanical and Materials
    Engineering
University of Denver
Denver, Colorado;
Clinical Associate Professor
Department of Orthopedic Surgery
Joan C. Edwards School of Medicine at
    Marshall University
Huntington, West Virginia

Sung-Hwan Kim, MD
Assistant Professor
Department of Othopaedic Surgery
Arthroscopy and Joint Research Institute
Yonsei University College of Medicine;
Assistant Professor
Department of Orthopaedic Surgery
Gangnam Severance Hospital
Seoul, Republic of Korea

Sung-Jae Kim, MD, PhD
Emeritus Professor
Department of Orthopaedic Surgery
Yonsei University College of Medicine;
Director
Department of Orthopaedic Surgery
Gangdong Yonsesarang Hospital
Seoul, Republic of Korea

Yair D. Kissin, MD

Kevin Klingele, MD
Chief
Department of Orthopaedic Surgery
Nationwide Children's Hospital
Columbus, Ohio

Kevin R. Knox, MD
Indiana Hand to Shoulder Center
Indianapolis, Indiana

Mininder S. Kocher, MD, MPH
Professor of Orthopaedic Surgery
Harvard Medical School;
Associate Director
Division of Sports Medicine
Boston Children's Hospital
Boston, Massachusettes

**Richard D. Komistek,
BSME, MSME, PhD**
Fred M. Roddy Professor
Biomedical Engineering,
Co-Center Director
Center for Musculoskeletal Research
University of Tennessee
Knoxville, Tennessee

Dennis E. Kramer, MD
Assistant Professor of Orthopaedic Surgery
Orthopedic Center
Boston Childrens Hospital
Boston, Massachusetts

Mark J. Kransdorf, MD
Consultant
Diagnostic Radiology
Mayo Clinic,
Phoenix, Arizona;
Professor of Radiology
Mayo Clinic College of Medicine
Rochester, Minnesota

Tomas J. Kucera, MD

Christopher M. Kuenze, PhD, ATC
Assistant Professor
Department of Kinesiology
Michigan State University
East Lansing, Michigan

Vinícius Canello Kuhn, MD
Orthopedic Surgeon
Instituto de Ortopedia e Traumatologia de
Passo Fundo
Passo Fundo, Brazil

Shinichi Kuriyama, MD
Professor and Chairman
Department of Orthopedic Surgery
Kyoto Univeristy
Kyoto, Japan

Anne Kuwabara, BA
Department of Physical Medicine and
Rehabilitation
The Johns Hopkins University
Baltimore, Maryland

Paul F. Lachiewicz, MD
Consulting Professor
Department of Orthopaedic Surgery
Duke University,
Orthopaedic Surgeon
Veterans Administration Medical Center
Durham, North Carolina;
Orthopaedic Surgeon
Chapel Hill Orthopedics Surgery & Sports
Medicine
Chapel Hill, North Carolina

Michael T. LaCour, BS
Graduate Research Assistant
Mechanical, Aerospace, and Biomedical
Engineering
University of Tennessee
Knoxville, Tennessee

Claudette Lajam, MD
Assistant Professor of Orthopaedic Surgery
Department of Orthopaedics
New York University Langone Medical
Center
New York, New York

Alfredo Lamberti, MD
Orthopaedics, Adult Reconstruction
IFCA Institute
Florence, Italy

Jason E. Lang, MD
Attending Surgeon
Blue Ridge Bone and Joint
Asheville, North Carolina

Joshua R. Langford, MD
Division of Orthopaedic Trauma and
Complex Adult Reconstruction
Department of Orthopaedic Surgery
Orlando Regional Medical Center
Orlando, Florida

Robert F. LaPrade, MD, PhD
The Steadman Clinic;
The Steadman Philippon Research Institute
Vail, Colorado

Nicholas J. Lash, MD
Clinical Fellow
Department of Orthopaedics
University of British Columbia
Vancouver, British Columbia, Canada

Sherlin Lavianlivi, MD
MSK Fellow/Radiologist
Department of Radiology
Maimonides Medical Center
Brooklyn, New York

Gary Lawera, BS, CMPE
Chief Operating Officer
University of Toledo Physicians, LLC
Toledo, Ohio

Peter J. Laz, MD
Center for Orthopaedic Biomechanics
University of Denver
Denver, Colorado

Cheng-Ting Lee, MD
Anesthesiology Resident
Columbia University Medical Center
New York, New York

Gabriel Levi, MD

Richard G. Levine, MD

Dieter Lindskog, MD
Associate Professor
Department of Orthopaedics and
Rehabilitation
Yale University School of Medicine
New Haven, Connecticut

Davidm R. Lionberger, MD

Frank A. Liporace, MD
Division of Orthopaedic Trauma and
Complex Adult Reconstruction
Department of Orthopaedic Surgery
Jersey City Medical Center
Jersey City, New Jersey

Sanford M. Littwin, MD
Associate Professor of Anesthesiology,
Clinical Director Operating Rooms
UPP Department of Anesthesiology
UPMC Presbyterian and Montefiore
Hospitals
Pittsburgh, Pennsylvania

Phillip Locker, MD

Adolph V. Lombardi, MD

William J. Long, BSc, MD, FRCSC
Director,
Attending Orthopaedic Surgeon
Insall Scott Kelly Institute,
St. Francis Hospital, Lenox Hill Hospital,
Hospital for Joint Diseases
New York, New York

Jess H. Lonner, MD
Attending Orthopaedic Surgeon
Rothman Institute;
Associate Professor
Department of Orthopaedic Surgery
Thomas Jefferson University
Philadelphia, Pennsylvania

Walter R. Lowe, MD

Sébastien Lustig, MD, PhD
Albert Trillat Center
Orthopedic Surgery
Lyon North University Hospital
Lyon, France

Thomas Luyckx, MD, PhD
Full Professor of Orthopedics and
Traumatology
Chair, Department of Orthopedics and
Traumatology
Ghent University
Ghent, Belgium

Dana Lycans, MD
Resident
Department of Orthopaedic Surgery
Marshall University
Huntington, West Virginia

Steven Lyons, MD
Florida Orthopedic Institute
Tampa, Florida

Samuel D. Madoff, MD
Department of Radiology
New England Baptist Hospital
Boston, Massachusetts

Robert A. Magnussen, MD, MPH
Associate Professor
Department of Orthopaedics
The Ohio State University
Columbus, Ohio

Suzanne A. Maher, PhD
Associate Scientist,
Associate Director
Department of Biomechanics,
Associate Director
Tissue Engineering Regeneration and
    Repair Program
Hospital for Special Surgery
New York, New York;
Associate Professor of Applied
    Biomechanics in Orthopaedic Surgery,
Adjunct Professor of Biomedical
    Engineering
Department of Biomedical Engineering
Weill Cornell Medical College
Cornell University
Ithica, New York

Mohamed R. Mahfouz, MS, PhD
Professor of Biomedical Engineering
Mechanical Aerospace and Biomedical
    Engineering
University of Tennessee
Knoxville, Tennessee

Amun Makani, MD
Attending Surgeon
Department of Orthopaedic Surgery
Watson Clinic
Lakeland, Florida

Eric C. Makhni, MD
Department of Sports Medicine
Henry Ford Health Center
Detroit, Michigan

Parul R. Maniar, MD
Consultant Ophthalmologist
Nook Clinic, Santacruz (W)
Mumbai, India

**Rajesh N. Maniar, MS, MCh Orth (UK),
DNB**
Head
Department of Orthopaedics & Joint
    Reconstruction
Lilavati Hospital & Research Centre;
Consultant and Joint Replacement Surgeon
Department of Orthopaedics & Joint
    Reconstruction
Breach Candy Hospital
Mumbai, India

Patrick G. Marinello, MD
Resident Orthopaedic Surgery
Cleveland Clinic Foundation
Cleveland, Ohio

Milica Markovic, MD
Assistant Professor
Department of Anesthesiology
Weill Cornell Medical College
New York Presbyterian Hospital
New York, New York

J. Bohannon Mason, MD

Bassam A. Masri, MD, FRCSC
Professor and Chairman
Department of Orthopaedics
University of British Columbia
Vancouver, British Columbia, Canada

Henry Masur, MD
Chief
Critical Care Medicine Department
Clinical Center, National Institutes of
    Health
Bethesda, Maryland

Kevin R. Math, MD
Associate Professor of Radiology
Hospital for Special Surgery
New York, New York

Kenneth B. Mathis, MD

Shuichi Matsuda, MD, PhD
Professor and Chairman
Department of Orthopedic Surgery
Kyoto University
Kyoto, Japan

Tomoyuki Matsumoto, MD, PhD
Assistant Professor
Department of Orthopaedic Surgery
Kobe University Graduate School of
    Medicine
Kobe, Japan

Chan-Nyein Maung, MD
Clinical Instructor of Anesthesiology
Department of Anesthesiology,
    Perioperative Care, and Pain Medicine
New York University Langone Medical
    Center
New York, New York

Kristen E. McClure, MD

Brian J. McGrory, MD, MS
Clinical Professor
Department of Orthopaedic Surgery
Tufts University School of Medicine
Boston, Massachusetts;
Co-Director
Maine Joint Replacement Institute
Portland, Maine

David C. McNabb, MD
Colorado Joint Replacement
Porter Adventist Hospital
Denver, Colorado

Brad Meccia, BS
University of Tennessee, Knoxville
Knoxville, Tennessee

Michael B. Mechlin, MD
Assistant Professor of Radiology
New York University School of Medicine
New York, New York

Patrick A. Meere, MD, CM
Clinical Associate Professor
Orthopaedic Surgery
New York University Langone Hospital for
    Joint Diseases
New York, New York

R. Michael Meneghini, MD
Associate Professor
Orthopaedic Surgery
Indiana University School of Medicine;
Director of Lower Extremity Adult
    Reconstruction Fellowship
Indiana University School of Medicine
Indianapolis, Indiana;
Director of Joint Replacement
IU Health Saxony Hospital
Fishers, Indiana

John J. Mercuri, MD, MA
Chief Resident
Department of Orthopaedic Surgery
Hospital for Joint Diseases
New York University Langone Medical
    Center
New York, New York

Maximilian A. Meyer, MD
Department of Sports Medicine
Rush University Medical Center
Chicago, Illinois

Cory Messerschmidt, MD
Department of Orthopaedic Surgery
Medical University of South Carolina
Charleston, South Carolina

Matthew D. Milewski, MD
Assistant Professor
Department of Orthopaedic Surgery
Connecticut Children's Medical Center—
    Elite Sports Medicine
Farmington, Connecticut

Mark D. Miller, MD
S. Ward Casscells Professor
Department of Orthopaedics
University of Virginia
Charlottesville, Virginia

Patrick J. Milord, MD, MBA
Interventional Pain Management Fellow
Department of Anesthesiology,
    Perioperative Care and Pain Medicine
New York University Langone Medical
    Center
New York, New York

Claude T. Moorman III, MD
Duke Sports Science Institute
Department of Orthopedic Surgery
Duke University
Durham, North Carolina

Vincent M. Moretti, MD
Rothman Institute
Philadelphia, Pennsylvania

William B. Morrison, MD
Professor
Department of Radiology
Thomas Jefferson University
Director
Division of Musculoskeletal and General
    Diagnostic Radiology
Thomas Jefferson University Hospital
Philadelphia, Pennsylvania

James R. Mullen, MD
Orthopedic Resident
Northwell Health
New Hyde Park, NY

Hirotsugu Muratsu, MD
Department of Orthopaedic Surgery
Steel Memorial Hirohata Hospital
Himeji, Japan

David Murray, MD
Professor of Orthopaedic Surgery
Nuffield Department of Orthopaedics
Rheumatology and Musculoskeletal
    Sciences
University of Oxford;
Consultant and Orthopaedic Surgeon
Nuffield Orthopaedic Centre
Oxford University Hospitals NHS Trust
Oxford, Great Britain

Volker Musahl, MD
Associate Professor
Department of Orthopaedic Surgery
University of Pittsburgh
Pittsburgh, Pennsylvania

Zan A. Naseer, BS
New York Medical College
New York, New York

Amit Nathani, MD, MS
Resident
Department of Orthopaedic Surgery
University of Michigan
Ann Arbor, Michigan

Milad Nazemzadeh, MD
Clinical Assistant,
Professor of Anesthesiology
Department of Anesthesiology,
    Perioperative Care, and Pain Medicine
New York University Langone Medical
    Center
New York, New York

Michael D. Neel, MD
Department of Orthopaedic Surgery
St Jude Children's Research Hospital
Memphis, West Virginia

Charles L. Nelson, MD
Chief of Adult Reconstruction
Associate Professor of Orthopaedic Surgery
University of Pennsylvania
Philadelphia, Pennsylvania

Nathan A. Netravali, MD

Michael P. Nett, MD
Orthopedic Surgeon, Coordinator of
    Quality and Clinical Arthroplasty
Department of Orthopedic Surgery
North Shore Long Island Jewish
    Orthopedic Institute @ Southside
    Hospital
Bay Shore, New York

Phillipe Neyret, MD, PhD
Head of Department
Orthopaedic Surgery and Traumatology
Hospices Civils de Lyon—Centre Albert
    Trillat
Lyon, Rhône, France

Jesse Ng, MD
Clinical Assistant Professor of
    Anesthesiology

Carl W. Nissen, MD
Physician
Elite Sports Medicine
Connecticut Children's Medical Center;
Professor
Department of Orthopaedics
University of Connecticut
Farmington, Connecticut

Philip C. Noble, BE, MES, PhD

Frank R. Noyes, MD
President and Medical Director
Noyes Knee Institute
Cincinnati, Ohio

Mary I. O'Connor, MD
Director and Professor
Center for Musculoskeletal Care at Yale
    School of Medicine and Yale—New
    Haven Hospital
Yale School of Medicine
New Haven, Connecticut

Khalid Odeh, BA

Russell M. Odono, MD
Orthopaedic Surgeon
Department of Orthopaedic Surgery
Insall Scott Kelly Institute
New York, New York

Louis Okafor, MD
Department of Orthopaedic Surgery
The Johns Hopkins University
Baltimore, Maryland

Andrew B. Old, AB, MD
Fellow
Orthopaedics and Adult Reconstruction
New York University
New York, New York

Ali Oliashirazi, MD
Chairman
Department of Orthopaedic Surgery
Marshall University
Huntington, West Virginia

Matthieu Ollivier, APHM
Institute for Locomotion
Department of Orthopaedic Surgery
Sainte-Marguerite Hospital;
Professor
Aix-Marseille University
Marseille, France

Mark W. Pagnano, MD
Chairman and Professor of Orthopedic
    Surgery
Department of Orthopedic Surgery
Mayo Clinic
Rochester, Minnesota

Christopher J. Palestro, MD
Professor
Department of Radiology
School of Medicine of Hofstra University
Hempstead, New York;
Chief of Nuclear Medicine & Molecular
    Imaging
New Hyde Park, New York

**Hemant Pandit, FRCS (Orth), D Phil
(Oxon)**
Professor
Nuffield Department of Orthopaedics,
    Rheumatology and Musculoskeletal
    Sciences
University of Oxford
Oxford, Great Britain;
Professor of Orthopaedics and Honorary
    Consultant
University of Leeds
Leeds, Great Britain

Bertrand W. Parcells, MD

Sebastien Parratte, APHM
Institute for Locomotion
Department of Orthopaedic Surgery
Sainte-Marguerite Hospital;
Professor
Aix-Marseille University
Marseille, France

Brian S. Parsley, MD

Javad Parvizi, MD, FRCS
Professor
Department of Orthopaedic Surgery
Rothman Institute of Orthopaedics at
    Thomas Jefferson University
Philadelphia, Pennsylvania

Alopi Patel, MD
Resident
Department of Anesthesiology
Mount Sinai St. Luke's—Roosevelt Hospital
    Center
New York, New York

Hersh Patel, MD

Jay Patel, MD
Hoag Orthopaedic Institute
Irvine, California;
Orthopaedic Specialty Institute
Orange, California

Henrik Bo Pedersen, MD
Director Medical Multimedia
Insall Scott Kelly Institute
New York, New York

Dawn Pedinelli, RN, MBA
Director of Research
Trinity Health
Livonia, Michigan

Vincent D. Pellegrini, Jr., MD
John A. Siegling Professor and Chair
Department of Orthopaedics
Medical University of South Carolina;
Director
Musculoskeletal Integrated Center of
    Clinical Excellence
Medical University of South Carolina;
Adjunct Professor
Department of Bioengineering
Clemson University
Charleston, South Carolina

Kevin I. Perry, MD
Mayo Clinic
Rochester, Minnesota

Catherine N. Petchprapa, MD
Assistant Professor
Department of Radiology
New York University Langone Medical
    Center—Hospital for Joint Diseases
New York, New York

Christopher L. Peters, MD
Professor, George S. Eccles Endowed Chair
Department of Orthopaedics
University of Utah
Salt Lake City, Utah

Lars Peterson, MD,PhD
Professor of Orthopaedics
Institutions for Surgical Sciences,
    Gothenburg University
Gothenburg, Vastra Gotaland, Sweden

Christopher R. Pettis, MD
Clinical Assistant Professor of Radiology
    UCF/FSU
Department of Radiology
Florida Hospital
Orlando, Florida

Michael H. Pillinger, MD
Professor of Medicine and Biochemistry
    and Molecular Pharmacology,
Director, Rheumatology Training,
Director, Masters of Science in Clinical
    Investigation Program,
New York University School of Medicine;
Section Chief
Department of Rheumatology
New York Harbor Health Care System—NY
    Campus
Department of Veterans Affairs
New York, New York

Leo A. Pinczewski, MBBS, FRACS
Associate Professor Department of
    Orthopaedics
Notre Dame University;
Consultant Orthopaedic SurgeonMater
    Hospital;
North Sydney Orthopaedic and Sports
    Medicine Centre
Sydney, New South Wales, Australia

Mark Pinto, MD, MBA
Orthopedic Surgeon
Chelsea Orthopedic Specialists
Chelsea, Michigan;
Medical Director
Perioperative Services
Trinity Health
Livonia, Michigan

William R. Post, MD
Mountaineer Orthopedic Specialists
Morgantown, West Virginia

Ian Power, MD

Jared S. Preston, MD

Peter Pyrko, MD, PhD
Assistant Professor
Department of Orthopedic Surgery
Loma Linda University
Loma Linda, California

Sridhar R. Rachala, MD
Assistant Professor of Orthopaedic Surgery
University at Buffalo
Buffalo, New York

Craig S. Radnay, MD, MPH
Director
Insall Scott Kelly Institute for Orthopaedics
    and Sports Medicine;
Clinical Assistant Professor
Department of Orthopaedic Surgery
New York University/Hospital for Joint
    Diseases
New York, New York;
Attending Physician
Department of Orthopaedic Surgery
St Francis Hospital
Roslyn, New York

Adam Rana, MD
Attending Orthopedic Surgeon
Orthopedic Surgery
Maine Medical Center
Portland, Maine

R. Lor Randall, MD
The L.B. & Olive S. Young Endowed Chair
    for Cancer Research,
Director
Sarcoma Services
Huntsman Cancer Institute, University of
    Utah;
Medical Director
Huntsman Cancer Institute Surgical
    Services,
Professor
Department of Orthopaedics
University of Utah
Salt Lake City, Utah

Amer Rasheed, MD
University of Illinois
Illinois

Parthiv A. Rathod, MD
Assistant Professor
Department of Orthopaedic Surgery
New York University Langone Medical
    Center/Hospital for Joint Diseases;
Chief of Orthopaedics
Woodhull Hospital Center
New York, New York

Robert S. Reiffel, MD
Attending Physician
Department of Surgery/Plastic Surgery
White Plains Hospital
White Plains, New York

Timothy G. Reish, MD, FACS
Associate Professor
Orthopaedic Surgery
New York University Langone Medical
    Center, Hospital For Joint Diseases;
Director
Insall Scott Kelly Institute for Orthopaedics
    and Sports Medicine
New York, New York

Daniel L. Riddle, PT, PhD, FAPTA
Otto D. Payton Professor of Physical
    Therapy
Department of Orthopaedic Surgery and
    Rheumatology
Virginia Commonwealth University
Richmond, Virginia

Samuel P. Robinson, MD
Orthopedic Surgeon
Jordan-Young Institute
Virginia Beach, Virginia

Scott A. Rodeo, MD
Professor of Orthopaedic Surgery
    (Academic Track)
Weill Medical College of Cornell University;
Co-Chief
Emeritus Sports Medicine and Shoulder
    Service
Hospital for Special Surgery;
Attending Orthopaedic Surgeon
Hospital for Special Surgery;
Head Team Physician
New York Giants Football
New York, New York

David Rodriguez-Quintana, MD

Gregory J. Roehrig, MD
Orthopaedic Institute of Central Jersey
Hackensack Meridian Health;
Director of Joint Replacement Program
Jersey Shore University Medical Center
Neptune, New Jersey

Aaron G. Rosenberg, MD
Professor of Surgery
Department of Orthopedic Surgery
Rush Unuiversity Medical College
Chicago, Illinois

Pamela B. Rosenthal, MD

Stefano M.P. Rossi, MD
Clinica Ortopedica e Traumatologica
Fondazione IRCCS
Policlinico San Matteo
Università degli Studi di Pavia
Pavia, Italy

Paul J. Rullkoetter, PhD
Professor
Department of Mechanical & Materials
    Engineering
Center for Orthopaedic Biomechanics
University of Denver
Denver, Colorado

Neda Sadeghi, BS, MD
Resident
Department of Anesthesiology
Mount Sinai St. Lukes Hospital
New York, New York

Paulo R.F. Saggin, MD
Orthopedic Surgeon
Instituto de Ortopedia e Traumatologia de
    Passo Fundo,
Passo Fundo, Brazil

Lucy Salmon, PhD
North Sydney Orthopaedic and Sports
    Medicine Centre
Sydney, New South Wales, Australia

Matthew J. Salzler, MD
Clinical Instructor
Department of Orthopaedics
Tufts Medical Center
Boston, Massachusetts

Thomas L. Sanders, MD
Orthopedic Surgery Resident
Department of Orthopedic Surgery
Mayo Clinic
Rochester, Minnesota

Sarah Sasor, MD
Indiana University Division of Plastic
    Surgery
Indiana

Adam A. Sassoon, MD
Department of Orthopaedics and Sports
    Medicine
University of Washington
Seattle, Washington

Robert C. Schenck, Jr., MD

Kurt F. Scherer, MD

**Oliver S. Schindler, BSc (Hons), PhD,
FMH, MFSEM (UK), FRCSEd, FRCSEng,
FRCS (Orth)**
Consultant Orthopaedic Surgeon
Bristol Arthritis & Sports Injury Clinic
Chesterfield Hospital
Bristol, United Kingdom;
The Manor Hospital
Oxford, United Kingdom;
Exeter Nuffield Hospital
Exeter, Devon, United Kingdom

Jason M. Schon, BS
Research Assistant
BioMedical Engineering
Steadman Philippon Research Institute
Vail, Colorado

Verena M. Schreiber, MD
Cincinnati Children's Hospital Medical
    Center
Division of Pediatric Orthopaedic Surgery
Cincinnati, Ohio

Kelly L. Scott, MD
Resident
Department of Orthopedic Surgery
Mayo Clinic
Phoenix, Arizona

Susan Craig Scott, MD
Clinical Assistant Professor
Department of Orthopaedic Surgery
Hansjorg Wyss Department of Plastic
    Surgery
New York University School of Medicine;
Surgeon
Department of Hand Surgery
NYU Hospital for Joint Diseases;
Assistant Attending
Department of Orthopedics
Bellevue Hospital Center;
Consulting Physician
Departments of Surgery and Orthopedic
    Surgery
Department of Veterans Affairs
New York Harbor Healthcare System
New York, New York

W. Norman Scott, MD, FACS
Clinical Professor of Orthopaedic Surgery
New York University Langone Medical
    Center
Hospital for Joint Diseases;
Joan C. Edwards School of Medicine
Marshall University
Founding Director
Insall Scott Kelly Institute for Orthaepedic
    Sports Medicine
New York, New York

Giles R. Scuderi, MD
Vice President
Orthopedic Service Line
Northwell Health;
Fellowship Director
Adult Knee Reconstruction
Lenox Hill Hospital
New York, New York;
Associate Clinical Professor of Orthopedic
    Surgery
Hofstra Northwell School of Medicine
Hempstead, New York

Elvire Servien, MD, PhD
Professor
Department of Orthopedic Surgery

Erik P. Severson, MD
Minnesota Center for Orthopaedics
Crosby/Aitkin, Minnesota

Nicholas A. Sgaglione, MD
Professor and Chair
Department of Orthopaedic Surgery
Northwell Health,
New Hyde Park, New York

Peter F. Sharkey, MD
Rothman Institute
Philadelphia, Pennsylvania

Adrija Sharma, PhD
Research Assistant Professor
Mechanical Aerospace and Biomedical
    Engineering
University of Tennessee
Knoxville, Tennessee

Kevin G. Shea, MD
Orthopedic Surgeon
Department of Sports Medicine
St. Luke's
Boise, Idaho;
Associate Professor
Department of Orthopaedics
University of Utah
Salt Lake City, Utah

Courtney E. Sherman, MD
Assistant Professor of Orthopedics
Department of Orthopedics
Mayo Clinic Jacksonville
Jacksonville, Florida

Jodi Sherman, MD
Assistant Professor of Anesthesiology
Yale University, School of Medicine
New Haven, Connecticut

Seth L. Sherman, MD
Attending Orthopaedic Surgeon
Department of Orthopaedic Surgery
University of Missouri
Columbia, Missouri

Michael S. Shin, MD

Rafael J. Sierra, MD
Associate Professor of Orthopedics
Department of Orthopedic Surgery
College of Medicine
Mayo Clinic
Rochester, Minnesota

Tushar Singhi, MD
Associate Professor
Department of Orthopedics
Padamshree D Y Patil Medical College
Navi Mumbai, India

David L. Skaggs, MD, MMM
Children's Orthopaedic Center
Children's Hospital Los Angeles
Los Angeles, California

Harris S. Slone, MD
Assistant Professor
Department of Orthopaedics
Medical University of South Carolina
Charleston, South Carolina

James D. Slover, MD, MS
Associate Professor
Adult Reconstruction Division
Department of Orthopaedic Surgery
Hospital for Joint Diseases
New York University Langone Medical
    Center
New York, New York

Nathaniel R. Smilowitz, MD
Professor of Medicine and Surgery
Leon H. Charney Division of Cardiology
New York University School of Medicine
New York, New York

Daniel C. Smith, MD
Adult Reconstruction Fellow
Department of Orthopaedic Surgery
New York University Langone Hospital for
    Joint Diseases
New York, New York

Gideon P. Smith, MD PhD
Director of Connective Tissue Diseases
Department of Dermatology
Mass General Hospital of Harvard University
Boston, Massachusetts

Gary E. Solomon, MD
Associate Professor
Department of Medicine
New York University Langone School of
    Medicine
New York, New York

Jeffrey T. Spang, MD
Assistant Professor
Department of Orthopaedics
University of North Carolina
Chapel Hill, North Carolina

Kurt P. Spindler, BS, MD
Vice Chairman of Research
Director Orthopaedic Clinical Outcomes
Academic Director
Cleveland Clinic Sports Health
Orthopaedic and Rheumatologic Institute
Cleveland Clinic
Cleveland, Ohio;
Adjoint Professor
Department of Orthopaedics
Vanderbilt University Medical Center
Nashville, Tennessee

Bryan D. Springer, MD
Attending Orthopaedic Surgeon
OrthoCarolina Hip and Knee Center
Charlotte, North Carolina

Ryan Stancil, MD
Department of Orthopaedics and Sports
    Medicine
University of Washington
Seattle, Washington

Samuel R.H. Steiner
Department of Orthopedic Surgery and
    Rehabilitation
Division of Sports Medicine
University of Wisconsin—Madison
Madison, Wisconsin

James Bowen Stiehl, MD
Chief of Surgery
St Mary's Hospital
Centralia, Illinois

Jonathan A. Stone, MD
Resident
Department of Orthopedic Surgery
Tufts Medical Center
Boston, Massachusetts

Eric J. Strauss, MD
Assistant Professor
Department of Orthopaedic Surgery
New York University Hospital for Joint
    Diseases
New York, New York

Joseph J. Stuart, MD
Duke Sports Science Institute
Department of Orthopedic Surgery
Duke University
Durham, North Carolina

Nathan Summers, MD

Stephanie J. Swensen, MD
Resident Physician
Department of Orthopaedic Surgery
New York University Hospital for Joint
    Diseases,
New York, New York

Monica Tafur, MD
Joint Department of Medical Imaging
University Health Network
Mount Sinai Hospital and Women's College
    Hospital
Toronto, Ontario, Canada

Timothy Lang Tan, MD
Resident
Department of Orthopaedic Surgery
Rothman Institute
Philadelphia, Pennsylvania

David P. Taormina, MD
New York University Hospital for Joint
    Diseases
New York, New York

Majd Tarabichi, MD
Research Fellow
Department of Research
Rothman Institute
Philadelphia, Pennsylvania

Sam Tarabichi, MD
Director General & Consultant Orthopedic
Surgeon
Burjeel Hospital for Advanced Surgery
Dubai, United Arab Emirates

Dean C. Taylor, MD
Duke Sports Science Institute
Department of Orthopedic Surgery
Duke University
Durham, North Carolina

Kimberly Templeton, MD
Professor of Orthopaedic Surgery
Department of Orthopaedic Surgery
University of Kansas Medical Center
Kansas City, Kansas

Emmanuel Thienpont, MD, MBA
Department of Orthopaedic Surgery
University Hospital Saint Luc
Brussels, Belgium

Nicholas T. Ting, MD
Department of Orthopaedic Surgery
RUSH University Medical Center
Chicago, Illinois

Marc A. Tompkins, MD
Assistant Professor
Department of Orthopaedic Surgery
University of Minnesota
Minneapolis, Minnesota

Gehron Treme, MD
Department of Orthopaedic Surgery
University of New Mexico
Albuquerque, New Mexico

Alfred J. Tria, Jr., MD
Clinical Professor of Orthopaedic Surgery
Department of Orthopaedic Surgery
Robert Wood Johnson Medical School;
Chief of Orthopaedic Surgery
Division of Orthopaedic Surgery
St. Peters University Hospital
New Brunswick, New Jersey

Hans K. Uhthoff, MD, FRCSC
Professor Emeritus
Department of Surgery
University of Ottawa
Ottawa, Ontario, Canada

Uchenna O. Umeh, MD
Assistant Professor of Anesthesiology
Department of Anesthesiology,
    Perioperative Care and Pain Medicine
New York University Langone Medical
    Center
New York, New York

Thomas Parker Vail, MD
James L. Young Professor and Chairman
Department of Orthopaedic Surgery
University of California, San Francisco
San Francisco, California

Douglas W. Van Citters, PhD
Assistant Professor
Thayer School of Engineering at
    Dartmouth College
Hanover, New Hampshire

Geoffrey S. Van Thiel, MD, MBA
OrthoIllinois
Rockford, Illinois

Rishi Vashishta, MD
Resident
Department of Anesthesiology,
    Perioperative Care, and Pain Medicine
New York University Langone Medical
    Center
New York, New York

Haris S. Vasiliadis, MD, PhD
Orthopädie Sonnenhof
Bern, Switzerland;
Molecular Cell Biology and Regenerative
    Medicine
Sahlgrenska Academy, University of
    Gothenburg
Gothenburg, Sweden

Sebastiano Vasta, MD
Department of Orthopaedics and Trauma
    Surgery
University Campus Bio Medico of Rome
Rome, Italy

Jan Victor, MD, PhD
Full Professor of Orthopedics and
    Traumatology
Ghent University;
Chair Department of Orthopedics and
    Traumatology
University Hospital Ghent
Ghent, Belgium

Jonathan M. Vigdorchik, MD
Assistant Professor of Orthopaedic Surgery,
Co-Director of Robotics
New York University Langone Hospital for
    Joint Diseases
New York, New York

Shaleen Vira, MD
Resident Physician
Department of Orthopaedic Surgery
New York University Hospital for Joint
    Diseases
New York, New York

Pramod B. Voleti, MD
Department of Orthopaedic Surgery
Montefiore Medical Center
New York, New York

Brian E. Walczak, MD
Department of Orthopedic Surgery and
    Rehabilitation
Division of Sports Medicine
University of Wisconsin—Madison
Madison, Wisconsin

Andrew Waligora, MD

Andrew Wall, MD

Daniel M. Walz, MD
Assistant Professor
Department of Radiology
Hofstra-North Shore LIJ School of
    Medicine
Great Neck, New York

Lucian C. Warth, MD
Assistant Professor
Department of Orthopaedic Surgery;
Assistant Director of Lower Extremity
    Adult Reconstruction Fellowship
Indiana University School of Medicine
Indianapolis, Indiana

Christopher W. Wasyliw, MD

Jonathan N. Watson, MD
Department of Orthopaedic Surgery
University of Illinois at Chicago
Chicago, Illinois

Nicholas P. Webber, MD
Medical Director
Sarcoma Services and Orthopaedic
    Oncology at Aurora Cancer Care;
Chief of Orthopaedics
Aurora St. Lukes Medical Center
Aurora Healthcare
Milwaukee, Wisconsin

Jennifer Weiss, MD
Southern California Permanente Medical
    Group
Los Angeles Medical Center
Los Angeles, California

Barbara N. Weissman, MD
Vice Chair Emeritus
Professor of Radiology
Harvard Medical School;
Musculoskeletal Radiologist
Brigham and Women's Hospital
Boston, Massachusetts

Jarrett D. Williams, MD
Department of Orthopedic Surgery
New York University Langone Medical
    Center
New York, New York

Riley J. Williams III, MD
Attending Surgeon
Department of Orthopaedic Surgery
Hospital for Special Surgery;
Associate Professor
Department of Orthopaedic Surgery
Weill Medical College of Cornell University
New York, New York

Adam S. Wilson, MD
Resident
Department of Orthopaedic Surgery
University of Virginia
Charlottesville, Virginia

Robert J. Wilson II, BA, MD
Orthopaedic Surgical Resident
Vanderbilt Department of Orthopaedics
    and Rehabilitation
Vanderbilt Orthopaedic Institute
Nashville, Tennessee

Lisa Mouzi Wofford, MD
Assistant Professor
Department of Anesthesiology
Baylor College of Medicine
Houston, Texas

Paul Woods, MD, MS
Senior Vice President
Physician Networks
Trinity Health
Livonia, Michigan

Clint Wooten, MD
Orthopedic Surgeon
Mountain Orthopedic
Bountiful, Utah

Ate Wymenga, MD, PhD
Consultant Orthopedic Surgeon
Department of Orthopedic Surgery
Saint Maartenskliniek
Nijmegen, The Netherlands

John W. Xerogeanes, MD
Department of Orthopaedic Surgery
Emory University
Atlanta, Georgia

Grace Xiong, MD

Zaneb Yaseen, MD

Yi-Meng Yen, MD, PhD, MS
Assistant Professor of Orthopaedic Surgery
Harvard Medical School
Boston Children's Hosptial
Boston, Massachusetts

Richard S. Yoon, MD
Division of Orthopaedic Trauma and
    Complex Adult Reconstruction
Department of Orthopaedic Surgery
Orlando Regional Medical Center
Orlando, Florida

Adam C. Young, MD, BS
Assistant Professor
Director of Acute Pain Service
Department of Anesthesiology
Rush University Medical Center
Chicago, Illinois

Stephen Yu, MD
Adult Reconstruction Research Fellow
Department of Orthopaedic Surgery
New York University Hospital for Joint
    Diseases
New York, New York

Biagio Zampogna, MD
Department of Orthopaedics and Trauma
    Surgery
University Campus Bio Medico of Rome
Rome, Italy

Ian M. Zeller, BS, MS
Graduate Research Assistant
Department of Mechanical, Aerospace and
    Biomedical Engineering
University of Tennessee
Knoxville, Tennessee

Adam C. Zoga, MD
Associate Professor
Department of Radiology
Thomas Jefferson University;
Vice Chair for Clinical Practice
Department of Radiology
Thomas Jefferson University Hospital
Philadelphia, Pennsylvania

FOREWORD

It is fair to say that *the Insall & Scott Surgery of the Knee* series has served as the definitive chronicle to the evolution of modern reconstructive surgery of the knee. So it is with the Sixth Edition of this comprehensive textbook that we, as interested readers, are once again privileged to avail ourselves of this carefully curated knowledge from today's leaders in knee surgery. It is a vibrant time to be a knee surgeon as intellectual excitement permeates our field and opportunities to alleviate pain and improve function for our patients continue to expand.

As an orthopedic community we are indebted to the foresight of John Insall and W. Norman Scott to recognize in the early 1980s the coming sea-change in the efficacy of knee surgery and to initiate the process that captured that collective knowledge in written form. Knee surgery has progressed dramatically over the past four decades from a last-resort option reserved for the markedly disabled to a largely elective surgical option that definitively improves the quality of life for patients with a spectrum of problems involving the bone, cartilage, or ligaments of the knee. Within the field of knee replacement, Dr. Insall helped carefully push the boundaries of patient age and activity that now allow us to successfully treat a wide spectrum of patients with knee arthroplasty. Within the field of ligament reconstruction, Dr. Scott brought to light what was possible at the highest levels of sport after cruciate ligament reconstruction. Together Drs. Insall & Scott shared a vision of improving patient care and advancing the understanding of reconstructive knee surgery for which we all have reaped benefit.

The Sixth Edition continues the long and academically rich history associated with this text that began in 1984. This series was so thoughtfully conceived that every surgeon performing total knee arthroplasty today could improve their fundamental understanding of contemporary knee replacement surgery by reading Dr. Insall's chapter on surgical technique and instrumentation from the First Edition. Subsequent versions of the textbook have preserved the fundamental spirit of the original which was to be at once comprehensive yet still accessible and relevant for the practicing orthopedic surgeon. The editor of the Sixth Edition has wisely chosen from amongst today's experts in contemporary knee surgery and the individual chapters are written in keeping with that spirit of comprehensive yet accessible and relevant. With national and international experts authoring each chapter the depth and breadth of real-world experience is evident throughout each of the chapters in this text.

The Sixth Edition *of Insall & Scott Surgery of the Knee* incorporates a broad international perspective that recognizes the rich contributions that surgeons from around the globe make to the field of knee surgery. Technology has fostered broader connections amongst orthopedic surgeons in disparate parts of the world and has quickened the pace of discovery and translation of new ideas into clinical practice. The Sixth Edition incorporates such technology and includes robust, high-quality illustrations, video demonstrations, and advanced electronic media resources that aid the process of education for the interested reader. The combination of text, illustration, and video material has been carefully balanced and clearly hits the mark for educational excellence.

I invite you to enjoy this textbook as more than just a source for knowledge about knee surgery. Insall & Scott's Surgery of the Knee also captures the energy, enthusiasm, and intellectual curiosity of today's most creative, innovative, and industrious knee surgeons. I hope that excitement is evident to you as a reader and inspires you to continually improve your individual skills and to support our collective-efforts to improve knee surgery for patients in our communities, patients nationwide, and patients world-wide.

Mark W. Pagnano, MD
Professor and Chairman
Department of Orthopaedic Surgery
Mayo Clinic
Rochester, Minnesota

FOREWORD

When the late Dr. John Insall wrote the preface of the First Edition of *Insall & Scott Surgery of the Knee* in 1984, he already had a vision of a comprehensive evolutionary textbook related exclusively to knee pathology and surgery. Some 33 years later this book is now in its Sixth Edition due to the continued efforts and innovations brought by Dr. Insall's original partner and friend Dr. W. Norman Scott. This book is not only covering all aspects of knee surgery such as ligament reconstruction, meniscus disease, cartilage repair, fractures about the knee, and knee arthroplasty, but also is considering the clinical, anatomical, biomechanical, and imaging evaluation of the knee joint. This book is also considering the patient himself in terms of demographic differences, expectations of the surgery, and perioperative management such as postoperative pain control.

The computer world has overwhelmed the field of continuous medical education and the Sixth Edition of *Insall & Scott Surgery of the Knee* has beautifully taken up the challenge of providing, both for the young and committed orthopedic surgeons, an evolving video technique section to maintain the status of the book as current as possible. This Sixth Edition also expands the world-wide contributions from the United States, Europe, and Asia, focusing on all aspects of clinical examinations, MRI imaging, knee anatomy, sports medicine, and reconstructive knee surgical techniques. Dr. Insall's decision in the First Edition was to reach out of the walls of his own hospital in New York City in order to include additional expertise. This Sixth Edition of *Insall & Scott Surgery of the Knee* further expands the horizon across the oceans, East, and West, with more than 20 chapters from International contributors.

Understanding the biomechanics of the knee starts with a correct comprehension of the anatomy and Rayesh Maniar from India describes the features of the Asian knee. The field of articular cartilage repair has now reached the time of maturity, consensus, while controversies will continue to be beneficial in the pursuit of progress. Lars Peterson from Sweden provides an international overview and results with autologous chondrocyte implantation techniques. Dr. Pinczewski from Australia, a pioneer in ACL reconstruction, and Dr. Kim from Korea likewise for PCL reconstruction, demonstrate their own vast experiences. The surgical correction of bony deformity both for the patella-femoral or the tibio-femoral joint has always been a trade-mark of the Lyon school in France, and respectively, Dr. Dejour and Dr. Neyret with their co-authors detail their own specific contribution.

Considering the knee as three separate articulations has led to selective compartmental replacement, a tradition in Europe for several decades. Contributions in that field come from the United Kingdom with Chris Dodd; Italy with Paolo Adravanti and Francesco Benazzo; Belgium with Emmanuel Thienpont; and France with Jean-Noel Argenson, Matthieu Ollivier, and Sebastien Parratte. The last three decades in the field of total knee arthroplasty has been fraught with debates, controversies, and most importantly success. The Sixth Edition of *Insall & Scott Surgery of the Knee* includes PCL retaining or substituting options provided respectively by Ate Wymenga from the Netherlands and Sam Tarabichi from the Middle East. Dr. Schindler from the UK and Dr. Matsumoto from Japan reflect on the debate regarding resurfacing of the patella or not. Both inside and outside the United States we are seeing new interpretations about alignment considerations and surgical options to obtain a mobile and stable knee after the arthroplasty. Johan Bellemans and Jan Victor from Belgium discuss the issues exhaustively. Intraarticular or extraarticular deformities at the time of total knee arthroplasty are world-wide challenges and Shuichi Matsuda from Asia and Andrea Baldini for Europe accurately describe their successful approaches. These surgical techniques are also often applicable to the use of specific technologies such as computer, robotics, or custom guides, and Emmanuel Thienpont details these approaches in an expert fashion.

The Sixth Edition of *Insall & Scott Surgery of the Knee* maintains this book's reputation as "The" reference for knee surgery providing the orthopedic surgeon from the United States, Europe, Middle East, or Asia with a considerable number of principles, details, and experiences covering all aspects of knee pathology, evaluation, and surgical treatments. While the spirit of late Dr. John Insall is still evident in the Sixth Edition of *Insall and Scott Surgery of the Knee,* the considerable and unique contributions of Dr. W. Norman Scott and his section editors in the organization of this book and its video section is now even more evident with the inclusion of so many international innovators and experts throughout the world.

Jean-Noel A. Argenson, MD
Professor and Chairman
Department of Orthopedic Surgery
The Institute for Locomotion, Aix-Marseille University
Marseille, France

It would have been inconceivable 33 years ago when the First Edition of this text book was drafted that the success of knee surgery would lead to a revolutionary approach to health care economics and care delivery. The projected increase of demand for total knee replacement over the next 20 years and the current and projected cost of the procedure have caused the value based health care movement to focus on the treatment of arthritis of the knee. For the first time, *Insall & Scott Surgery of the Knee* has focused an entire section (Economics, Quality, and Payment Paradigms for Total Knee Arthroplasty) on the value based issues facing knee surgeons in the next decade.

Since the passage of the Patient Protection and Affordable Care Act (PPACA) in 2010 and Medicare Access and CHIPS Reauthorization Act (MACRA) in 2015, the Center for Medicare and Medicaid Services (CMS) has been mandated to transform from a passive consumer to an active purchaser of health care. Orthopaedic surgeons are well positioned to provide leadership and detailed analysis of the processes related to the provision of orthopaedic care. Early and active involvement by orthopaedic surgeons in the development and implementation of care improvement processes in bundled payment systems such as the BPCI, CJR and any future initiatives is critical for the efficacy and sustainability of value-based orthopaedic care pathways. Moreover, orthopaedic surgeons need to be involved in all components of health care delivery that impact the care of their patients in order to preserve access and maintain affordability. In the next 5 years, physicians will be individually held accountable for cost and quality measures affecting their patients. The Merit Based Incentive Payment System (MIPS) will change reimbursement from not just a hospital at risk, quality driven model but also to a physician at risk, quality driven model.

The Bundled Payment for Care Initiative (BPCI) was begun in 2013 by CMS. Under the voluntary BPCI program, organizations entered into payment arrangements that include financial and performance accountability for episodes of care. A successful BPCI requires that quality is maintained and that care is delivered at a lower cost. CJR is a mandatory extension of Model 2 BPCI with hospital quality and Patient Reported Outcome Measures (PROM's) reporting requirements in addition to financial performance measures. This requires physicians and hospitals to align their interests and in this context, orthopaedic surgeons must assume a leadership role in cost-containment, surgical safety, and quality assurance so that cost-effective care is provided. Because most orthopaedic surgeons practice independently and are not hospital-employed, models of physician-hospital alignment such as physician-hospital organizations or contracted gainsharing arrangements between practices and hospitals may be necessary for bundled pricing to succeed. Under BPCI, hospitals, surgeons, or third parties can share the rewards, but also assume the risk for the bundle. It is forecast that most TKA cases covered under private and public insurance will be compensated under a bundled, quality driven program within the next 5 years.

For patients, cost savings must be associated with maintenance or improvement in quality metrics. However, the manner in which quality is defined and measured and what processes and outcomes are rewarded can vary. Risk-stratified allowances for nonpreventable complications must be incorporated into bundled pricing agreements to prevent the exclusion of patients with significant comorbidities and the anticipated higher care costs. Bundled pricing depends on economies of scale for success and it may not be appropriate for smaller orthopaedic groups or hospitals, where one costly patient could impact the success of the entire program. Furthermore, significant investment in infrastructure is required to develop programs to improve the quality and coordination of care, to manage quality data, and to distribute payments. Perhaps, smaller groups of surgeons can be joined together under advanced alternative payment models in the future so that all patients can benefit from bundled, value-based care.

In the current unsustainable healthcare environment, hospitals and administrators are facing increased pressure to optimize the value equation by decreasing the risk of complications. The ethical implications of reducing provider (physician and hospital) complication rates following joint replacement is compelling. Additionally, public transparency concerning provider complication rates would help patients make more informed decisions as to where to have their TJA performed. Nevertheless, it is morally incumbent on providers and policy makers to aggressively explore options for lowering cost while maintaining access and improving quality. Patients, physicians, and health care administrators must begin to see themselves acting not just as individuals involved in the decision to undergo TKA, but rather, as part of a system that administers health care within a larger societal context. It is simply unsustainable for surgeons and hospitals to perform elective surgery in higher risk patients with modifiable risk factors without increasing efforts to reduce them. Risk modification is a component of a larger, new era of medicine in which all stakeholders ought to accept some share of responsibility to create a safer, more cost-efficient health system. As TKA surgery shows, true shared decision making which involves patients, their physicians, the hospital, and the payers in a paradigm where interventions are provided only after modifiable risk factors have been addressed, can be an effective tool for delivering high quality, ethical health care at a reasonable price with a minimum of complications. We hope the information provided within the Sixth Edition of *Insall & Scott Surgery of the Knee* will help make this transition easier for all knee surgeons and the patients they care for.

Joseph D. Zuckerman, MD
Richard Iorio, MD
Dr. William and Susan Jaffe Professor of Orthopaedic Surgery
Chief Division of Adult Reconstructive Surgery
Department of Orthopaedic Surgery
New York University Langone Medical Center
Hospital for Joint Diseases
New York, New York

PREFACE

Why write a textbook in 2017? All pertinent information is now at our fingertips, the APP should be sufficient (if it works!) right? Electronic media is all we need or is it? Search engines are often "a mile wide and an inch deep" in detailing medical specifics in general and subspecialty knowledge in particular. Just think of our patients "surfing the net" and becoming fully cognizant of all aspects of knee surgery! Thus the need for a textbook for the lifelong students of the diagnosis and treatment of knee disorders.

Obviously the successes achieved in the field of knee surgery since the 1970s are absolutely incredible. The prefaces for the last five editions of *Insall & Scott Surgery of the Knee* are included in the Sixth Edition to reflect the historical perspective and to illustrate "how far we've (patients and physicians) come." And if we are to continue succeeding we need to learn by past mistakes to minimize the future ones.

Welcome to the Sixth Edition of *Insall & Scott Surgery of the Knee* (and yes we do have a companion electronic version).

The Sixth Edition of *Insall & Scott Surgery of the Knee* has greatly expanded on the Fifth Edition. Reviewing, refreshing and updating the excellent chapters of previous authors were, of course, a must. Almost all of these lead contributors added new authors to assure the viewer would receive the most recent subject information. The Sixth Edition, unlike the Fifth, has two complete volumes, and is accompanied not only by an e-version (at expertconsult.com) but also by an enhanced video section and a glossary. There are 14 sections and more than 78 new chapters!

Dr. Henry Clarke, the section editor for Basic Science has in this section enhanced the multifaceted anatomic perspective. I believe this comprehensive (microscopic, gross, arthroscopic, and radiographic) anatomy section is the best in the knee literature.

Dr. Jenny Bencardino, an orthopedic radiologist has taken over the imaging section of *Insall & Scott Surgery of the Knee* and has added 4 new chapters with the help of 14 expert radiologists. Similarly, Rick Komistek, PhD has updated the excellent Biomechanics section (Section III) with two new chapters.

One of the two largest sections of the Sixth Edition of *Insall & Scott Surgery of the Knee* has been organized and completed by associate editor, David Diduch. David has worked with section editors Asheesh Bedi and Geoff Baer to present 53 chapters spanning the basic science, diagnoses, and treatment of cartilage, ligament, and patella femoral conditions. This is an awesome contribution to the education of the innumerable "sports medicine" students throughout the world.

Dr. Andrew Franks, a renowned Professor of Rheumatology and Dermatology has once again modernized and updated the fundamental aspects of diagnosing and treating the most common systemic arthritic conditions that orthopedists will encounter. Topics such as gout and other crystalline arthropathies, psoriatic arthritis, degenerative arthritis, and rheumatoid arthritis are discussed succinctly. Dr. Franks has also devoted a chapter to arthropathies associated with hemophilia and pigmented villondular synovitis and discussed in detail a subject pertinent to all reconstructive orthopedic surgeons, systemic allergic dermatitis in total knee arthroplasty (TKA).

One of orthopedic surgery's major advances in patient care has been the diminution of postoperative complications and more recently patients' postoperative discomfort. It is for this reason that we have devoted an entire section to anesthesia for knee surgery. Dr. Arthur Atchabahian has put this section, "Anesthesia for Knee Surgery," together by stressing different aspects: preoperative evaluation, perioperative management of inpatient and ambulatory procedures, and a section on peripheral nerve blocks. These chapters are well organized, practical, concise, and essential for successful patient care. The orthopedist needs to be cognizant of these pain modality specifics.

Wound problems are the bane of any orthopedic procedures and we are once again honored to have Drs. Susan Scott and Robert Reiffel discuss prevention and treatment of these situations, which left unrecognized or untreated will destroy any knee arthroplasty.

Under the direction of Dr. George Haidukwych, the discussions and treatments of fractures about the knee have been updated with more recent data supporting alternative treatments. This is especially helpful in the treatment of periprosthetic fractures, an increasing problem due to the abundance of replacements in more active patients.

The overlap of treating pediatric, adolescent, and adult knee conditions is often daunting for the nonpediatric orthopedist. Dr. Min Kocher and his contributors in Section XI skillfully updated the eight chapters on pediatric knee problems; these chapters now allow all orthopedists to be current and to undertake treatments or, if necessary, to refer patients appropriately.

The largest section in the book, Sections XII A and XII B, Joint Replacement and Its Alternatives and Revision Complex Knee Arthroplasty, consists of 59 chapters and to my knowledge, is the most comprehensive compendium of an exhaustive discussion on these topics in one textbook. These sections represent an international approach to knee arthroplasty and the authors are pioneers and active clinicians in this discipline. In particular, Dr. Arlen Hanssen's contributions to the world of knee arthroplasty are legendary, and this section, thankfully, has his fingerprints all over it!

The other contributors in Sections XII A and XII B, too numerous to mention in a Preface, truly comprise the majority of worldwide knee arthroplasty innovators, surgeons, academicians, and teachers to us all. This section is a "must read" for any serious student in the field of knee arthroplasty.

In addition to the obvious importance of design and surgical technique in the world of knee arthroplasty, we as surgeons have continued to strive to make our patients safe, comfortable, happy, and convinced that they experienced both an excellent and cost effective knee arthroplasty procedure.

As section editor, Dr. Rich Iorio has enhanced the Sixth Edition of *Insall & Scott Surgery of the Knee* by discussing in over 20 chapters the present day approach to perioperative and hospital management of our patients in a comprehensive cost effective paradigm. In today's complicated and controversial health care environment, these chapters represent the foundation for the future of cost effective *and* superb care for our patients.

Mary O'Connor has once again assembled an outstanding faculty to discuss "Tumors about the Knee". From evaluation to diagnosis (benign or malignant) and treatment (local, extensive, or even a situation requiring a mega prosthesis) the authors have done an excellent job in providing us with current and practical approaches to treating these tumors.

As mentioned, the Sixth Edition of *Insall & Scott Surgery of the Knee* will once again include an extensive video section. In the Fifth Edition, we had 168 videos which we have now expanded to approximately 236 technique-oriented videos. In addition to this update of pediatric, sports, and knee arthroplasty surgical techniques, we plan to remain current, to add approximately 10-12 videos of both surgical techniques and superb seminars on a monthly basis until the publication of the Seventh Edition of *Insall & Scott Surgery of the Knee*. This approach, I believe, allows the book to never be out of date.

In a similar fashion the glossary of knee prosthesis has been updated and we thank the various companies' voluntary submissions. We requested the companies' cooperation, without any compensation or advertising, and are delighted with their collective enthusiasm. We also have the ability to electronically update our glossary and have invited all companies to take advantage of this educational opportunity.

I would personally like to thank my associate editors, Drs. Diduch and Hanssen; all the section editors and all the contributors, Residents, Fellows, attendings, private practitioners, academicians, and professors. All of us students working together to advance our subspecialty are rewarded when we see our patients' happiness and gratitude.

W. Norman Scott, MD

PREFACE TO THE FIFTH EDITION

There is nothing that "succeeds like success," and for the last five decades the treatment of knee disorders has been a major success story. From the First Edition of *Surgery of the Knee* to the present Fifth Edition, inclusive of approximately 1000 National and International contributors, we have been fortunate to chronicle these tremendous advancements. Although history is often overlooked, we think it is important, so important in fact, that we have included the prefaces for the first four editions of *Surgery of the Knee* to hopefully facilitate the progressive understanding of the anatomic, physiologic, clinical, diagnostic, and therapeutic advances that allow students of the knee to "push the envelope" even further. It requires, however, an understanding of the historical failures in the scientific pursuit of helping our patients if we are to minimize the chances of repeating past mistakes and hopefully avoid future ones. The authors throughout this edition attempt to highlight these potential pitfalls.

The Fifth Edition of *Surgery of the Knee* contains one textbook, a complete e-version, an e-glossary of knee implants, and a video section that we believe is the most comprehensive sports and adult reconstruction video section in any knee textbook. The book has 14 sections, 2 more than the previous edition, and 153 chapters written by almost 200 worldwide contributors. The Fifth Edition will be enhanced by quarterly updates in a video journal format and updates to the glossary of knee replacement designs, past and present, as presented by all the manufacturers who chose to participate. Similar to the quarterly updates, the manufacturers will have the opportunity to update their prosthetic designs to keep the information timely.

In Section 1, Basic Science of Anatomy, Anatomic Aberrations, and Clinical Examination are updated and now include a more detailed video on the examination of the knee. Section 2, Imaging, has been rewritten by an orthopedic radiologist, Dan Walz, and presents the most current diagnostic criteria for knee imaging. Similarly, the Biomechanics section also has a new leader in Rick Komistek, who has assembled a stellar group of contributors.

The Sports Medicine section, almost a third of the book, has been spearheaded by David Diduch. It is a tremendous enhancement to the work of previous editors, and David's work in putting this section together has truly been Herculean! From articular cartilage biology and biomechanics, extensor mechanism issues, meniscal repair, resection, or replacement, isolated or combined cruciate and collateral ligament treatments, the information in the Fifth Edition is truly state of the art. And, of course will remain current via the aforementioned quarterly updates.

Section 7, developed by Andy Franks, pertains to the current concepts regarding the diagnosis of knee arthritis, both inflammatory and noninflammatory.

Sections 8 and 9 include updates on synovium, hemophilia, HIV, and plastic surgery as it relates to wound healing and skin coverage options about the knee.

In Section 10, George Haidukewych, once again, has done an outstanding job of organizing fractures about the knee and periprosthetic fractures, probably one of the major causes for TKR revision today.

Likewise, in Section 11, Min Kocher presents today's state of the art treatment of pediatric knee disorders, which will continue via the quarterly updates.

Section 12, Joint Replacement and Its Alternatives, includes another new feature, the International and National Roundtables Discussions. We believe that this approach really allows the reader to comprehend the international differences and similarities in understanding worldwide controversial areas. Gil Scuderi did an excellent job in organizing these discussions and the 40 other chapters encompassing the totality of the treatment of the arthritic knee. Similar to the other sections, the surgical video techniques enhance the learning experience.

Section 13 includes the extremely controversial orthopedic medical issues such as DVT prophylaxes management and comprehensive pain management protocols associated with knee surgery.

In Section 14, Mary O'Connor once again has her contributors present the latest evidence on treating tumors about the knee. The mega prosthesis chapter, of course, is often apropos to the nontumor arthritic or revision TKR and is necessary reading for the TKR revision surgeon.

A new feature on the e-version, the glossary of implants, is presented in the spirit of helping the practicing physician determine the implant that he or she is evaluating whether in a primary or revision setting. We thank the companies for their cooperation and welcome their updates since the glossary is presented as an e-version which does not require the rigors of print media.

In the last five decades, better understanding of the basic sciences has allowed the knee community to develop much more of a consensus in the treatment of the "sports knee" and the arthritic knee. From a surgical perspective, techniques are continuing to be refined but one has to question whether "better is now the enemy of good?" It is a fine line and the surgical techniques cannot be the sole indication for treatment. For instance, registries in joint replacement are often at odds with published series by experts. Is this an indication, surgical technique, or patient expectation problem? We must be able to address and solve these issues before the publication of the Sixth Edition of *Surgery of the Knee*.

In the 1980s, Dr. Insall penciled an often quoted statement that one should not perform a revision TKR, unless the etiology of the failure was thoroughly understood. If he were with us today, I am sure that he would likewise want us to ascertain the indications for procedures based on a careful analysis of resultant treatments, whether it be nonoperative or operative. Better analysis of patient demographics and expectations, design considerations, biologic advances, and evidence-based results will allow us to better develop the treatment of knee disorders as a science rather than just an art. Physicians specializing in knee disorders must understand the practical consequences of all treatments to truly give our patients the best advice.

Once again, a tremendous "thanks" to all our contributors who join me in hoping that the "knee student" truly gains from studying the text, e-version, videos, and updates in the Fifth Edition of *Surgery of the Knee!*

W. Norman Scott, MD

In 1984, John Insall almost single-handedly wrote the First Edition of *Surgery of the Knee*. There were only 24 contributors to that single volume. In 1993, the Second Edition had 40 contributors and 4 associate editors and consisted of 2 volumes. In 2001, we combined efforts (*The Knee*, Mosby, 1994) to enhance the Third Edition (159 contributors) of *Surgery of the Knee*. Thus in 17 years, 3 Editions were published, and now the Fourth Edition has published less than 5 years later. This shortened publication time reflects our interest in being current and in using the latest technology and leading experts to inform our readers. In this Fourth Edition of *Surgery of the Knee*, we have updated basic chapters and introduced new information utilizing text and visual aids (DVDs), and we are inaugurating a new feature, a companion online e-dition: www.scottkneesurgery.com. The e-dition website will include full text search, hyperlinks to PubMed, an image library, and monthly content updates, to minimize the customary complaint of the "perpetual lag" inherent with textbooks in general. Our goal is to create an interactive current environment for all students of the diagnosis and treatment of knee disorders.

The Fourth Edition of *Surgery of the Knee* has 12 sections, 112 chapters, and 191 international contributors. The DVD sections include (1) a classic video recorded in 1994 (Drs. Insall and Scott) detailing "Exposures, Approaches and Soft Tissue Balancing in Knee Arthroplasty"; (2) interactive anatomic and physical examination recordings, which enhance the material presented in Chapters 1, 2, 3, 5, 6, and 7; and (3) three commonly used minimally invasive surgical techniques for knee arthroplasty.

In Section I, Basic Science, Chapters 1 to 5, the core information presented in the Third Edition is updated. The DVD of the Anatomy Section is interactive with the imaging in Section II, so the reader can see the normal and abnormal findings side by side. Chapter 3, Clinical Examination of the Knee, now, as mentioned, has the added feature of an actual examination on the DVD to enhance the text.

Section III, Biomechanics, has been expanded under the guidance of A. Seth Greenwald, DPhil (Oxon), to include soft tissue and implant considerations that are essential to executing surgical decisions.

With the plethora of Internet information available to patients today, it behooves the knee physician to be absolutely familiar with the various nonoperative and operative alternatives for the treatment of articular cartilage and meniscal disorders (Section IV). Dr. Henry Clarke has done a magnificent job in assembling the innovators in the field. The 18 chapters in this section truly capture the basic science, including the potential of gene therapy, biomechanics, and various treatment options, presented in great detail with the most current results. The section is further highlighted by Dr. Clarke's algorithm for clinical management of articular cartilage injuries.

The advances in the treatment of knee ligament injuries since 1984 are, needless to say, overwhelming. The success achieved today in the treatment of ligament injuries would have been unimaginable 25 years ago. As Section Editor of Section V, Ligament Injuries, Dr. Fred Cushner has assembled most of the people associated with these improvements. The foundations for treatments, controversies, and specific techniques are well chronicled throughout this section. Similarly, Section VI, Patellar and Extensor Mechanism Disorders, represents an updated comprehensive review by Dr. Aglietti and surgical chapters by Drs. Fulkerson and Scuderi.

Sections VII and VIII are "must reads" for all knee clinicians. In addition to discussing the normal and abnormal synovium, we have recruited distinguished authors to discuss the application of current topics of concern to both the patient and clinician, e.g., HIV and hepatitis (Chapter 59), anesthesia for knee surgery (Chapter 60), and an understanding of reflex sympathetic dystrophy (Chapter 61). The orthopaedic knee surgeon must have an absolute awareness of the potential problems inherent in the skin about the knee. In Chapter 63, Soft-Tissue Healing, Drs. Susan Scott and Robert Reiffel give us a foundation for avoiding and treating these potential problems.

Section IX focuses on fractures about the knee and has been organized by Dr. George Haidukewych. These fracture experts have covered all the fractures that occur, including the difficult periprosthetic fractures. Treatment modalities are detailed and reflect the current options with the latest equipment.

Section X, Pediatric Knee, has been reinvigorated with the help of Carl Stanitski. We decided to present the orthopaedic pediatric approach, rather than the sole view-point of the knee physician who treats pediatric injuries. The section is well organized, comprehensive, and, I believe, an improvement over the Third Edition of *Surgery of the Knee*.

The largest section in this two-volume edition is Section XI, Joint Replacement and Its Alternatives. Dr. Gil Scuderi has organized this section of the surgical treatment of the arthritic knee, including osteotomy, unicompartment replacement, patellofemoral arthroplasty, total knee replacement, and the more challenging revision surgery. While establishing the indications and contraindications for techniques, he has been careful to include the identification and management of difficult complications, such as infection, bone defects, extensor mechanism disruption, blood management, and thrombophlebitis. The tremendous success achieved in knee arthroplasty has paralleled the improvements in surgical instrumentation. In this section, several authors have detailed the current concepts of computer and navigation surgery, a truly exciting recent development. In the aforementioned e-dition version of *Surgery of the Knee*, the first several streaming videos will focus on specific techniques. Thus, these chapters provide an excellent foundation for interpreting the subsequent e-version techniques.

Dr. Mary O'Connor has developed Section XII, Tumors about the Knee, in a concise, clinically rational framework for those physicians who do not necessarily treat many of these difficult problems. Chapters 106 to 112 are well written and are truly outstanding contributions to this text.

Surgery of the Knee is a text that includes audiovisual teaching aids and now a monthly means of communicating current information in a timely audiovisual manner. To me, it's very exciting, and I look forward to integrating the contributions of these authors into a rapidly current technology for the benefit of all our patients.

W. Norman Scott, MD

PREFACE TO THE THIRD EDITION

Twenty-five years ago, the adolescent with knee pain unresponsive to immobilization, with subsequent atrophy and increasing disability afterwards, underwent a totally unnecessary arthrotomy and meniscectomy, sometimes preceded by a very inaccurate athrography.

When symptoms persisted, the other meniscus was usually considered the source of discomfort, and the treatment was unsuccessfully repeated. Then, with the evolution of failed arthrotomies, the patella was believed to be the culprit. Unfortunately, there was no nonoperative or operative intervention that was universally successful. Surgically, distal and then proximal realignments were performed on almost all types of "chondromalacia" complaints. Anterior cruciate ligament injuries, if diagnosed, were treated in a spectrum from purposeful neglect to an assortment of combined intra- and extra-articular reconstructions. The recovery from these procedures was truly, in today's perspective, a tribute to the dedication of the patient and therapist and somewhat of a warning to avoid surgery!

Unfortunately, many of these patients' knee disorders led to posttraumatic arthritis unresponsive to most nonsteroidal anti-inflammatory medicines; thus, they were candidates for an osteotomy. Even though the osteotomy would probably not be indicated today, there were no other surgical options. Today, a better understanding of clinical diagnosis, imaging techniques, and rehabilitative modalities has eliminated many unnecessary surgeries. Arthroscopy has revolutionized the diagnosis and treatment of cartilage lesions and ligament disruptions. Total knee arthroplasty, on the other hand, has yielded unparalleled success in alleviating patients' discomfort while eliminating their disability.

This 25-year retrospective view is, I believe, somewhat predictive of how we will perceive the contribution of classic textbooks to continuing medical education. As we enter the digital century, if not millennium, it is increasingly difficult to accept the analog world's perpetual lag of inadequacy of the published word while attempting to enhance education and subsequently new breakthrough treatments for our patients. Thus, we have attempted in this two-volume comprehensive color text to "bridge the gap" between the analog and digital worlds. In combining our two previous textbooks, *Surgery of the Knee* and *The Knee,* we have solicited the contributions of national and international experts recognized worldwide by serious knee students.

This textbook consists of 95 chapters divided into 11 sections. In Basic Science (Section I) we have introduced an interactive CD-ROM combining the anatomic and imaging chapters. While we believe this approach, either by CD or through Internet access, is the future, practical considerations precluded us from presenting the entire book in this format at this time. The CD takes studying, browsing, and researching anatomy and imaging in a new direction. Thanks to Drs. Clarke and Pedersen, the CD contains an extensive collection of medical data pertaining to anatomy, anatomic aberrations, imaging, and surgical exposures. We believe this is truly a breakthrough in understanding comprehensive knee anatomy.

In Biomechanics (Section II), Dr. Michael Freeman has truly enhanced our understanding of the dynamics of knee motion in an extensive MRI-controlled model of knee motion. The remainder of this section reinforces basic principles of knee biomechanics and explains the relationship of the knee to normal and abnormal gait.

Healing articular cartilage defects has enticed orthopaedists since the beginning of our specialty. Today, the enthusiasm seems to be at fever pitch. Thus, we have included many, if not all, of the therapeutic approaches by the recognized international originators of the technique. From Europe to the United States, contributors lay the foundation for what will hopefully be therapeutic success in the year to come.

Although the more than 150 contributors to this edition are too numerous to focus on individually, there are some especially innovative chapters that deserve special attention. Chapter 41, "Revision ACL Surgery: How I Do It," allows the reader to see step-by-step the "pearls" of various experts on how they approach this difficult problem in the operating theater.

With increasing focus on recreational athletics, the problems with the pediatric knee are becoming more manifest. Thus, Chapters 64 to 68 give the reader the opportunity to learn from pediatric orthopaedists on normal growth and development, congenital deformities, physeal fractures, and dealing with ACL injuries in skeletally immature patients.

Almost a quarter of this text is devoted to knee replacement and surgical alternatives. The success of the former necessitates such an approach. Osteotomy, however, must not be forgotten; thanks to Drs. Hanssen and Poilvache, we get both the European and American perspective. The standard issues with knee replacement, designs, technique, thrombophlebitis, skin problems (Section VII), infection, and complications requiring revision surgery are extensively detailed. Just as with revision ACL surgery, there are six sections devoted to revision TKR surgery. The diversity of surgical approaches and "tips" is truly priceless.

It is a true honor to have collaborated with my mentor, partner, and, most importantly, friend in publishing this comprehensive text. Dr. Insall's published works on all aspects of knee surgery are unparalleled. For me to have continued my "residency" under his guidance for the past 2 years has been a gift beyond measure.

On behalf of all the authors, we hope that you, the reader, are stimulated by this text to learn, analyze your observations, challenge thoughtfully, and make a contribution that will ultimately help your patients!

W. Norman Scott, MD

This textbook is larger than before, a change made necessary by the many advances made in knee surgery since the First Edition was published 10 years ago. Radiology of the knee has been revolutionized by computed tomography (CT) and magnetic resonance imaging (MRI), which have added a degree of certainty to the diagnosis of meniscal and some ligament injuries. Clinical acumen and careful examination are, of course, still required, but when these state of the art investigations are available, precise diagnosis will avoid unnecessary surgery. The ligament chapters are completely new, reflecting greater understanding of the pathology of ligament injuries. The classification of these injuries was in disarray in the early 1980s without true recognition of the role of the cruciate ligaments in causing knee instability. Anteromedial and anterolateral instabilities and the tests for their diagnosis were previously discussed without mentioning the anterior cruciate ligament (ACL), and it was still widely believed that the ACL was not an important stabilizer of the knee. Lesions of the posterior cruciate ligament (PCL) were also poorly understood, and the terminology was complexed and confusing. Due to the work of the late John Marshall and his successors, ligament injuries and laxities are today logically classified. The contribution to knee stability of the ACL in particular is universally accepted. It is fitting that Russell Warren, who followed Marshall as the Director of Sports Medicine at The Hospital for Special Surgery, coauthored the chapter on acute ligament injuries.

Arthroscopy was included in the First Edition only to outline general principles. Today such limited treatment is impossible because arthroscopy has become a major part of knee surgery. Norman Scott, who has himself written a text on arthroscopy, has comprehensively described the techniques and advances in this subspecialty.

The chapters on knee arthroplasty are all new. Very little has been carried over except for historical reference. Advances in knee prostheses and especially in surgical instrumentation and technique have made the operation reliable and predictable. A preeminent bioengineer, Peter Walker, has contributed the section on knee prosthesis design. Clement Sledge and C. Lowry Bames have written on PCL retention in knee arthroplasty, and Richard Scott describes the role of unicompartmental replacement. George Galante and Aaron Rosenberg make the case for cementless fixation. However, not all of these innovations have proven successful and new problems such as polyethylene wear have recently become a major clinical issue. Osteolysis caused by polyethylene debris is an even newer complication. The extent and severity of both problems will have to wait the passage of time and further evaluation.

I may have suggested in the earlier preface that I was a "complete" knee surgeon: even if this was once true, it most certainly is not today. I do not believe that one surgeon can be equally expert in all of the conditions that affect even a single joint such as the knee: for example, since 1984 over 500 articles have been published in the three major English language journals on the subject of total knee arthroplasty alone. Therefore, to prepare this edition, I have enlisted the help of four associate editors, all of whom I have trained at some stage of their careers and who have continued to work closely with me. In addition to their editorial functions, they have also contributed material of their own. Paolo Aglietti has revised his previous chapters on fractures of the knee and in this edition provides additional chapters on chronic ligament injuries and the management of the patellofemoral joint. Norman Scott, calling upon his vast experience in athletic injuries, has contributed chapters on arthroscopy and the classification of ligament injuries. Russell Windsor has written on the management of infection, arthrodesis, and soft-tissue disorders. Michael Kelly has revised the chapters on anatomy and physical examination. Between us it is hoped that we covered the material adequately.

Mrs. Martha Moore has labored on this edition as she did on the first one, again earning my profound gratitude. I also thank Ms. Virginia Ferrante and Ms. Elizabeth Roselius for the new illustrations.

John N. Insall, MD

PREFACE TO THE FIRST EDITION

If the 1960s saw a revolution in hip surgery, the knee had its turn during the 1970s. Much has changed and is still changing. Arthroscopic surgery has emerged as a new discipline; knee arthroplasty has become a reliable treatment for gonarthrosis; and concepts in the treatment of ligament injuries have altered radically in the last 10 years. Also, surgeons interested in the knee have separated into three groups, their major involvement being either in arthroscopy, sports medicine, or knee replacement. As one who has dabbled in all of these areas, it is my hope that this book will have some unifying benefit.

However, there is still no unanimity of opinion about how to treat all disorders of the knee joint, and for one who has the temerity to edit a textbook on the subject, there is the certain knowledge that he cannot please everyone. On the other hand, a textbook must have cohesion so that one chapter does not contradict the next. My solution to this dilemma is to present the current opinion and practice at The Hospital for Special Surgery, and, therefore, most of the contributors are past or present members of the staff. Where there are significant areas of controversy, I have also sought other viewpoints, notably on ligament surgery, the place of cruciate ligaments in knee arthroplasty, and the fixation of prosthetic components to bone. I have also reached beyond the walls of my own hospital for additional expertise, and well-known authorities have written chapters on osteochondrosis dissecans, hemophilia, surgical pathology of arthritis, and arthroscopy.

With regard to the chapter on arthroscopy, I foresee that this chapter may be considered too short in an era when arthroscopic surgery and knee surgery are becoming synonymous in the minds of many surgeons. This decision to keep this chapter short was made deliberately for two reasons: (1) Excellent textbooks devoted specifically to the techniques of arthroscopic surgery already exist, and (2) both Doctor McGinty and I felt that, because arthroscopic surgery has not been placed in full perspective, some currently popular arthroscopic techniques may become discredited with time.

I also decided not to include specific details of AO surgical techniques in the fracture chapter as these are also very well described elsewhere.

It would not have been possible to complete this book without the invaluable assistance of my secretary, Mrs. Martha Moore, who has put in as much effort as I and must now know every word and every reference by heart. I also wish to thank Ms. Joelle Pacht for her endless retyping of the manuscript, Miss Dottie Page and the Photographic Department at The Hospital for Special Surgery for their assistance in preparing the photographic material, and Mr. William Thackeray who has done most of the book's illustrations and drawings.

John N. Insall, MD

ACKNOWLEDGMENTS

It would be impossible to undertake a book, especially a two volume e-version with 374 contributors and approximately 237 videos, without the unbelievable help of a dedicated team.

- Dr. Henrik Bo Pedersen has been extensively involved in the Third, Fourth, Fifth and now the Sixth Editions of *Insall & Scott Surgery of the Knee*. His devotion to detail has allowed us to produce "top of the line" photographs and videos that have been a major aspect of our success.
Thank you, Henrik.

- Likewise, Ruth Pupke has been involved since the Third Edition. Her involvement has been immeasurable. Connecting editors, authors and their staff, and the publishers is a never ending task without which it's likely these editions would never have been produced.
Thank you, Ruth.

- For 25 years, Kathleen Lenhardt has been the "hub" of the Insall Scott Kelly (ISK) Fellowship, (now the NYU Langone/ ISK Adult Reconstruction Fellowship). She has also been the person responsible for the organization of the selection process, and coordination of both the involvement of the Insall Travelling Fellowship with the Knee Society and the host medical centers throughout the United States. Her importance to this edition of *Insall & Scott Surgery of the Knee* is especially manifest in the number of ISK Fellows and Insall Travelling Fellows who are significant contributors to the Sixth Edition.
Thank you, Kathy.

- Dina Potaris, last but certainly not least, is the "lynchpin" who kept everything together for the Sixth Edition of *Insall & Scott Surgery of the Knee*. She was the star!
Thanks, Dina.

W. Norman Scott, MD

CONTENTS

ONLINE CONTENTS

View Expertconsult.com for periodic updates.

SECTION VIII

Anesthesia for Knee Surgery

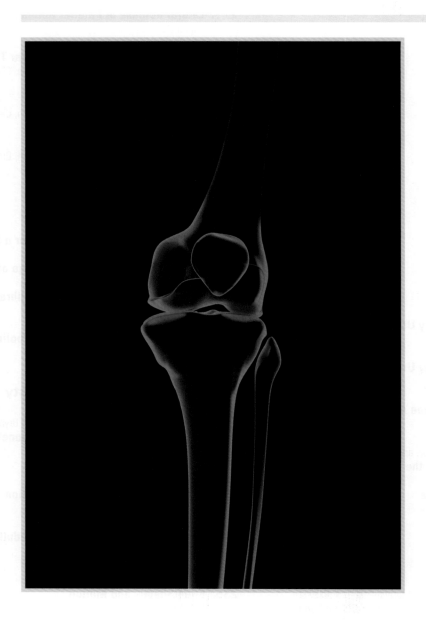

PART III

Preoperative Analgesia: Nerve Blocks

Femoral Nerve Block

Jodi Sherman

INTRODUCTION

Procedures to provide postoperative analgesia should be easy to perform, rapid in onset, facilitate early mobilization, and have minimal side effects. The femoral nerve block is one of the single most helpful and technically straightforward peripheral nerve block procedures and is a key element in multimodal pain control for the knee.

FEMORAL NERVE BLOCK LEVELS

There are several levels along the trajectory of the femoral nerve at which peripheral nerve block procedures are well described. The most common approach to blockade of the femoral nerve is at the level of the femoral triangle, the borders of which are constituted by the inguinal ligament, the sartorius, and the adductor longus muscles. Blockade at this level is itself properly referred to as the "femoral nerve block," also sometimes called perivascular femoral block or "3-in-1" block.[6] Other well-described blockade levels of the femoral nerve include the (posterior) lumbar plexus block or psoas compartment block, the most proximal variant, performed lateral to the spine near the L2-4 nerve roots; the fascia iliaca compartment block, performed near the level of the anterior inferior iliac spine; the adductor canal block, a distal variant performed at the mid-thigh level; and the saphenous nerve block, the most distal approach to femoral nerve blockade. The more proximal approaches (lumbar plexus block, fascia iliaca compartment block, and femoral nerve block) affect both motor and sensory fibers of the femoral nerve. The more distal adductor canal block is predominantly sensory, whereas the most distal saphenous nerve block is only sensory in effect. Different approaches to blockade of the femoral nerve have unique merits and drawbacks.

ANATOMY (Figs. 91.1 and 91.2)

The femoral nerve originates from the L2-4 nerve roots of the lumbar plexus and courses through the psoas muscle. It then passes out between the psoas and iliacus muscles and exits the pelvis into the anterior thigh deep to the inguinal ligament. The femoral nerve continues along the medial thigh via the adductor canal and then provides articular branches to the knee before terminating in the leg as the saphenous nerve.

The femoral nerve block is classically performed at the level of the femoral triangle, just inferior to the inguinal ligament. At this location the femoral nerve fibers are consistently lateral to the common femoral artery, superficial to the iliopsoas muscle, and deep to the fascia iliaca. These structures are easily visualized by ultrasound (US) (Fig. 91.3), making the US-guided femoral nerve block one of the simplest and most expeditious peripheral nerve block procedures to perform. Real-time US visualization of injectate spread around the femoral nerve ensures an exceptionally high femoral nerve block success rate, approaching 100%.[6]

Motor Effects

The femoral nerve provides motor input to the quadriceps muscles—rectus femoris, vastus medialis, vastus lateralis, and vastus intermedius—as well as to the sartorius and pectineus muscles. The femoral nerve block is performed at the level of the femoral triangle, just before the bifurcation of the common femoral artery, and is expected to result in weakness of leg extension. Some lesser weakness of hip flexion may occur; however, it is less common when performed at this level compared with more proximal blockade. Muscle weakness can be reduced through minimizing the dose of local anesthetic (discussed later).

Sensory Effects

The femoral nerve block provides sensory blockade distal to the injection site at the level of the femoral triangle (Figs. 91.4 and 91.5). It affects the anterior thigh down to the medial aspect of the lower leg, ankle, and foot. The femoral nerve block also provides sensory blockade of most of the knee joint itself, making it exceptionally useful for analgesia of the surgical knee. The sciatic nerve innervates the posterior aspects of the knee joint and skin and the obturator nerve a variable portion of the medial knee, and thus complete analgesia is not expected from femoral nerve blockade alone. Because of anatomic and also surgical technical variations, some patients may benefit greatly from the addition of a sciatic nerve block in conjunction with the femoral nerve block (see Chapter 95).

When initially described by Winnie as a 3-in-1 block,[9] it was believed that, because of close proximity of the obturator nerve within the tissue planes of the femoral nerve block injection, obturator nerve blockade would be accomplished. However, this was because of the testing being done on purely sensory criteria and the medial thigh sensation being almost exclusively dependent on the femoral nerve. Moreover, because the femoral nerve also innervates the pectineus muscle, adductor motor power will decrease after a block of the femoral nerve sparing the obturator nerve (see Chapter 96). Capdevila et al.[1] demonstrated an obturator block only in 38% of their patients who received a femoral nerve block.

Older techniques for localizing the femoral nerve include landmarks and fascial "pops" and neurostimulation to obtain a

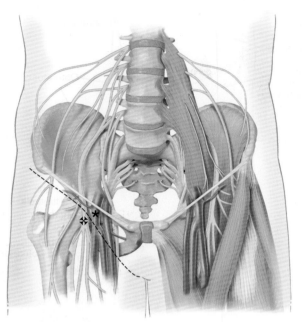

FIG 91.1 Lumbar plexus 74.2 (Anesthesia for Knee Surgery from Insall).

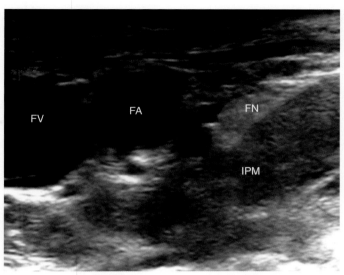

FIG 91.3 Ultrasound image by Jodi Sherman, MD. The left side is lateral. *FA*, Femoral artery; *FN*, femoral nerve; *FV,* femoral vein; *IPM*, iliopsoas muscle.

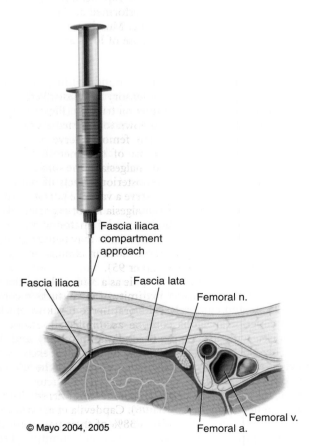

FIG 91.2 Lumbar plexus block 74.3 (Anesthesia for Knee Surgery from Insall).

response of the quadriceps muscle, typically in the rectus femoris with a "patellar tendon" twitch. Because the actual injection was blind, high volumes of local anesthetic (40 mL) were historically required to increase block success rate. Because of spread of local anesthetic within the tissue planes, the lateral cutaneous nerve was often also affected by this block, resulting in sensory blockade of the lateral aspect of the anterior thigh. The current standard approach is the US-guided femoral nerve block, which permits real-time visualization of injection. Much lower volumes of local anesthetic (20 mL) are now required to achieve reliable effects, and thus the lateral femoral cutaneous nerve is less reliably affected by a femoral nerve block.

INDICATIONS AND BENEFITS

The femoral nerve block is a highly reliable, technically simple, key component to multimodal pain management of the surgical knee. Peripheral nerve blocks dramatically reduce opioid requirements and their associated side effects, including sedation, respiratory depression, delirium, nausea, and vomiting. With the femoral nerve block, analgesia facilitates early ambulation and participation in physical therapy. These benefits enable earlier discharge and increased patient satisfaction scores.[2] Depending on the nature of the surgical procedure and patient conditions, different approaches to this block impacting duration of effect are indicated.

Two different management strategies for peripheral nerve blocks are the single-shot injection and the continuous nerve catheter. As the name implies, the single-shot nerve block is a one-time only dose of local anesthetic. Typical effect duration for a single-shot femoral nerve block with a long-acting anesthetic, such as ropivacaine or bupivacaine, is 8 to 10 hours. A continuous femoral nerve block using a perineural catheter may provide continuous analgesia for up to 3 to 7 days, depending on hospital policy on infection prevention, necessitating either catheter removal or replacement. In general, single-shot injections are indicated for minimally invasive procedures typically seen in the ambulatory setting, whereas continuous nerve

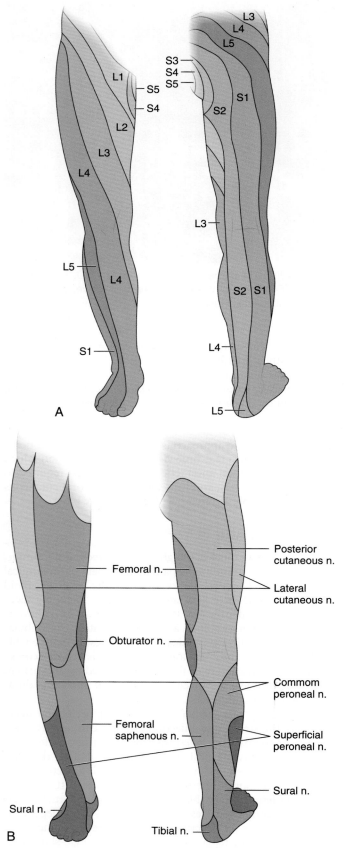

FIG 91.4 A, Cutaneous distribution of the lumbosacral nerves. B, Cutaneous distribution of the peripheral nerves of the lower extremity (Miller's Anesthesia 6th ed.).

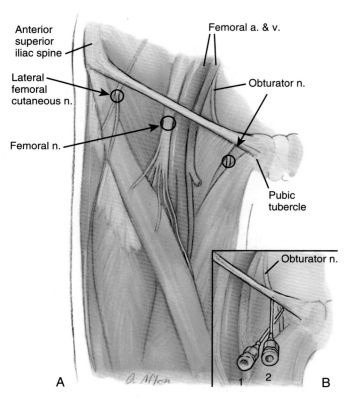

FIG 91.5 A, Anatomic landmarks for lateral femoral cutaneous, femoral, and obturator nerve blocks. B, For an obturator nerve block.

catheters are indicated for more invasive and painful procedures as with trauma patients and total knee arthroplasty. Peripheral nerve catheters are most commonly managed in the in-patient setting; however, home continuous catheter systems exist (see section "Single-Shot vs. Continuous Block later").

The continuous femoral nerve block was until recently considered the gold standard for post-operative analgesia for total knee arthroplasty.[2,3] In 2014, the Cochrane Collaboration reviewed femoral nerve blocks,[2] and included 2710 total knee replacement patients from 45 randomly controlled trials. The authors concluded that for the first 72 hours postoperatively, femoral nerve blocks with or without posterior condylar axis (PCA) opioids were more effective for postsurgical analgesia (both at rest and with movement) than PCA opioid alone, were similar for quality of analgesia to epidurals, and were associated with less nausea/vomiting and higher patient satisfaction compared to PCAs and epidurals. Additionally, continuous blocks provided superior analgesia compared to single-shot femoral nerve blocks, with lower opioid consumption at 24 and 48 hours. The Cochrane Collaboration determined there was insufficient evidence to conclude on comparison to local infiltration or oral analgesia.

Peripheral nerve blocks are best performed pre-incision. Pre-incision nerve blocks reduce intra-operative anesthesia and opioid requirements, along with their associated side effects including respiratory depression, nausea and vomiting. Pre-incision nerve blocks also help to avert acute onset of pain during gaps in analgesia coverage when transitioning from the OR to Post Anesthesia Care Unit (PACU) management. By interrupting efferent conduction pre-incision, nerve blocks also prevent the painful stimulation that primes neural pathways contributing to chronic pain even under general anesthesia. For patients receiving single-shot peripheral nerve blocks, the duration of post-operative analgesia may be significantly reduced when a block is performed pre-incision. For surgeries of long duration, either a pre-incision catheter may be placed or a post-operative single-shot injection can be performed to ensure longer effect duration (see section "Single Shot vs. Continuous Block later"). However, routine postsurgical block placement is not controversial. If expedience is an issue, surgeons are encouraged to work together with anesthesiologists to improve workflow conditions.

CONTRAINDICATIONS AND RISKS

Risks from peripheral nerve blocks are generally quite low and vary according to anatomic location, technique, and patient factors. Risks may include nerve injury, infection, bleeding, and incomplete or failed block. Standard precautions are taken to minimize these risks.

Overall, injuries from peripheral nerve blocks are rare. The American Society of Anesthesiologists Closed Claims Project* database was initiated in 1985 to facilitate targeted improvements in patient safety. Between 1990 and 2010, of the 8954 anesthesia related claims, 189 involved peripheral nerve blocks. Of those, femoral nerve blocks accounted for eight claims.[5] Seven out of eight of the femoral nerve block claims were related to temporary or nondisabling injuries. One femoral nerve block claim was related to a permanent or disabling nerve injury (0.53% of all nerve block related claims and 0.01% of all anesthesia related claims over a 20-year period). None of the peripheral nerve block claims was associated with US-guided technique but rather were associated with electrical stimulation–guided/landmark-based techniques. This suggests that the US-guided peripheral nerve block may be safer; however, it is too soon after the adoption of this new technology to conclude. Although closed claim data have limitations (discussed elsewhere)[5,8] and the lack of total procedure denominator prevents calculation of risk, the femoral nerve block may be considered overall an extremely low-risk procedure.

Fall Risk

Because the femoral nerve block affects motor fibers in addition to sensory fibers, muscle weakness is an expected outcome. There is reasonable concern that motor weakness increases the risk of falls. A review of 190,000 records of total knee replacement patients from 400 hospitals demonstrated an incidence of inpatient falls of 1.6%, associated with morbidity and mortality. This risk was similar whether patients received femoral nerve blocks or not. The study concluded that the peripheral nerve block did not alter the risk of inpatient fall in this already at-risk population.[7] Regardless, vigilance and precautions to prevent falls are essential in all postsurgical knee patients.

Fall risk with the femoral nerve block can be reduced through several strategies, including: reducing total dose of the local anesthetic (concentration and/or rate) to minimize quadriceps weakness; limitation of patient-controlled bolus doses of local

anesthetic; using ambulatory aid devices, such as knee immobilizers, walkers and crutches; and aggressive staff education on femoral nerve block–related muscle weakness and strict attention to fall precautions.[4]

ALTERNATIVES

An alternative approach to blocking the femoral nerve is via the adductor canal block. This block is performed mid-thigh level after some motor branching of the femoral nerve, and therefore the degree of quadriceps motor weakness is expected to be lower than with the femoral nerve block. The adductor canal block may be preferred for patients who will be discharged early from care, namely in the ambulatory setting. However, this block may be less reliable in its analgesic effect than the femoral nerve block, which must be weighed against the benefit of less motor involvement.

Neuraxial local anesthesia is an alternative to the femoral nerve block. However, single-shot spinal analgesic effect on the knee is short lived, lasting approximately 4 hours, although intrathecal opioid can provide some longer-lasting analgesia. Epidural catheters provide excellent intraoperative anesthesia and postoperative analgesia, but there are several drawbacks. Epidurals must be removed early, typically postoperative day 1, for patients on aggressive venous thrombosis prophylaxis, as seen with total knee arthrotomy and trauma patients, although this might be less true now that many surgeons are using aspirin for deep venous thrombosis (DVT) prophylaxis. Epidurals affect bilateral lower extremities, making early ambulation exceptionally difficult unless such low doses of local anesthetic are used as to make the analgesic benefits marginal. Furthermore, indwelling urinary catheters are required with epidurals, increasing the risk of health care–acquired urinary tract infection. Even though complications are rare, because of the location within the vertebral spinal canal and proximity to the spinal cord, bleeding and nerve injury secondary to neuraxial techniques can be devastating. Unless the femoral nerve block is contraindicated or technically impossible (eg, history of femoral artery bypass), it is more desirable than neuraxial techniques for postoperative pain control for the surgical knee—even for bilateral surgery.

The lumbar plexus block is the most proximal approach to femoral nerve blockade, performed at the level of the L2-4 nerve roots. Because of its proximal location, this block affects the hip joint, as well as the knee joint. The lumbar plexus block is superior to the neuraxial approach to postoperative analgesia in that its effects are unilateral, thus making early ambulation possible. Furthermore, urinary catheters are not required with the lumbar plexus block. However the lumbar plexus block is technically much more challenging than either the neuraxial analgesia or the femoral nerve block, has more potential complications, and does not appear to provide better analgesia following knee surgery. Thus the lumbar plexus block is best reserved for analgesia of the hip.

Because the femoral nerve block does not affect the sciatic distribution of the posterior knee, some patients receive insufficient local analgesia effects from this block even with multimodal pain adjuvants. For this reason the sciatic nerve block can be an important addition to the femoral nerve block. Some institutions routinely perform both blocks in combination for major surgery of the knee, whereas others will reserve the sciatic block for "rescue" analgesia only (see section "Sciatic Nerve Block").

---

*http://depts.washington.edu/asaccp/welcome-anesthesia-closed-claims-project-its-registries (accessed August 12, 2015).

Local intra-articular infiltration of the joint is gaining in popularity among orthopedic surgeons. Logistically it is simple for the surgeon to perform this injection intraoperatively, compared with a separate anesthesiologist peripheral nerve block procedure. There is concern that for continuous catheters, the intra-articular block is higher risk compared with a femoral nerve catheter. Although catheter-related infections are rare, an infection of the knee joint is likely to be more devastating than one at the femoral nerve catheter site. The Cochrane Collaboration determined there was insufficient evidence to conclude on comparison of the femoral nerve block with local infiltration for total knee arthoplasty.[2]

Lastly, an alternative approach to the femoral nerve block for postoperative analgesia is no block whatsoever. Patients may rely completely on oral and/or intravenous analgesics. The most important indication for this approach is patient wish to avoid a nerve block. Other indications include technical difficulty, such as history of groin trauma or femoral bypass resulting in distortion of the anatomy.

CONCLUSION

The femoral nerve block is very safe, effective, technically easy to perform expeditiously, highly reliable, and is therefore a core component of multimodal analgesia of the surgical knee. The femoral nerve continuous block was considered the gold standard for total knee arthroplasty, but this is currently debated. Quadriceps muscle weakness is an expected outcome of the femoral nerve block; however, this can be minimized with low dose/concentration of local anesthetic. Muscle weakness may be lessened with a more distal approach to block of the femoral nerve, such as the adductor canal block. The sciatic nerve block may be added to the femoral nerve block for posterior coverage of the knee joint.

KEY REFERENCES

1. Capdevila X, Biboulet P, Bouregba M, et al: Comparison of the three-in-one and fascia iliaca compartment blocks in adults: clinical and radiographic analysis. *Anesth Analg* 86(5):1039–1044, 1998.
2. Chan EY, Fransen M, Parker DA, et al: Femoral nerve blocks for acute postoperative pain after knee replacement surgery. *Cochrane Database Syst Rev* (5):CD009941, 2014.
3. Fischer HB, Simanski CJ, Sharp C, et al: A procedure-specific systematic review and consensus recommendations for postoperative analgesia following total knee arthroplasty. *Anaesthesia* 63:1105–1123, 2008.
4. Ilfeld BM, Duke KB, Donohue MC: The association between lower extremity continuous peripheral nerve blocks and patient falls after knee and hip arthroplasty. *Anesth Analg* 111:1552–1554, 2010.
5. Lee LA, Posner KL, Kent CD, et al: Complications associated with peripheral nerve blocks: lessons from the ASA Closed Claims Project. *Int Anesthesiol Clin* 49:56–67, 2011.
6. Marhofer P, Greher M, Kapral S: Ultrasound guidance in regional anaesthesia. *Br J Anaesth* 94:7–17, 2005.
7. Memtsoudis SG, Danninger T, Rasul R, et al: Inpatient falls after total knee arthroplasty: the role of anesthesia type and peripheral nerve blocks. *Anesthesiology* 120:551–563, 2014.
8. Metzner J, Posner KL, Lam MS, et al: Closed claims' analysis. *Best Pract Res Clin Anaesthesiol* 25:263–276, 2011.
9. Winnie AP, Ramamurthy S, Durrani Z: The inguinal paravascular technic of lumbar plexus anesthesia: the "3-in-1 block". *Anesth Analg* 52(6):989–996, 1973.

92

Adductor Canal Block

Shawna Dorman, Pia Jæger, Ulrik Grevstad

Providing effective analgesia after knee surgery is essential for both patient satisfaction and functional recovery yet remains challenging to accomplish. The femoral nerve block (FNB) is a well-established and effective method of targeting pain control for any procedure involving the knee. However, its effect on quadriceps motor function, fall risk, and delayed rehabilitation[12,19] has been the source of recent discussion. The adductor canal block (ACB) has emerged as a mostly sensory nerve block that can provide analgesia to the knee with significantly less risk of motor weakness.[13,16,23]

ANATOMY

The adductor canal, also known as Hunter canal or the subsartorial canal, is an aponeurotic structure in the middle third of the thigh bounded anterolaterally by the vastus medialis, anteromedially by the vasoadductor membrane (and the sartorius muscle) and posteromedially by the adductor muscles, the adductor longus proximally, and the adductor magnus distally. It contains the femoral artery, the femoral vein, the saphenous nerve, and branches of the femoral nerve, including the nerve to the vastus medialis. The distal part of the adductor canal also contains articular branches from the obturator nerve.[5,11] The saphenous nerve innervates the infrapatellar skin and the anterior knee capsule, whereas the nerve to the vastus medialis provides sensory innervation to the superomedial aspect of the knee and the knee capsule. The posterior branch of the obturator nerve contributes to the innervation of the posterior capsule of the knee joint, as part of a plexus formed with branches of the sciatic nerve. Thus, the sensory changes after an ACB are not limited to the saphenous distribution but include the medial and anterior aspects of the knee from the superior pole of the patella to the proximal tibia. The nerve to the vastus lateralis and vastus intermedius are posterior divisions of the femoral nerve and do not course through the adductor canal. Thus, the only motor branches passing through the canal are those from the vastus medialis nerve. The vastus medialis muscle constitutes one of the four components of the quadriceps femoris muscle. However, studies in healthy volunteers have shown that the ACB reduces quadriceps strength by less than 10% and does not compromise ambulation ability (Fig. 92.1).[16,22]

TECHNIQUE

The ACB is typically performed at the mid-thigh level, using a high-frequency ultrasound probe and a lateral needle entry site. The superficial femoral artery is identified in the short axis view, deep to the sartorius muscle. Between 20 mL and 30 mL of local anesthetic are injected in proximity of the saphenous nerve, lying in the "corner" between the superficial femoral artery, the vastus medialis muscle, and the sartorius muscle. The block can be administered either as a single bolus injection, a continuous infusion, or repeated boluses via a catheter. A long-acting local anesthetic is used because the goal is to provide postoperative analgesia rather than surgical anesthesia. As the ACB is still in its infancy, the optimal administration form, local anesthetic type, concentration, and volume have yet to be determined (Fig. 92.2A and B).

TOTAL KNEE ARTHROPLASTIES

The ACB should not be expected to provide complete analgesia of the knee because the posterior aspect of the knee is primarily innervated by the sciatic nerve, which is not anesthetized by the ACB. Following total knee arthroplasty (TKA), studies have shown that the ACB provides clinically relevant pain relief compared to placebo, both at rest and during mobilization.[6,14,18] When comparing the ACB with the FNB, the analgesic effect seems to be similar.* When compared to local infiltration, the addition of an ACB after TKA has been shown to significantly reduce postoperative pain, improve ambulation on the day of surgery, produce less sleep disturbance on the first night after surgery, and produce a higher rate of discharge home.[1,28] However, this needs to be confirmed in larger, prospective, randomized controlled studies.

In patients undergoing TKA, it has been shown that quadriceps strength was reduced by approximately 80% from the preoperative baseline value in patients receiving a FNB, whereas patients receiving an ACB only had about a 50% reduction.[16,22] In this context, it is important to remember that TKA surgery in itself reduces quadriceps strength by approximately 60%.[8] A recent study accounted for the effect of surgery by collecting postoperative baseline values prior to preforming the ACB. The study showed that the ACB almost doubled the quadriceps strength compared to no ACB, most likely resulting from the analgesic effect of the ACB.[7] Finally, a number of studies have shown that the preservation of strength following an ACB correlates with improved ability to ambulate, both when compared to placebo[1,18,26] and to the FNB.[7]

A common fear associated with peripheral nerve blocks for knee surgery is the risk of falls. This is a relevant concern, and

*References 7, 17, 21, 25, 27, and 28.

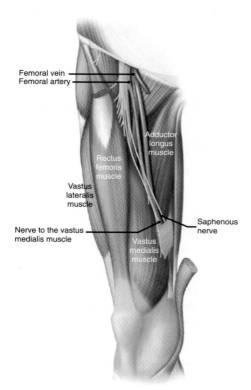

FIG 92.1 Adductor canal anatomy.

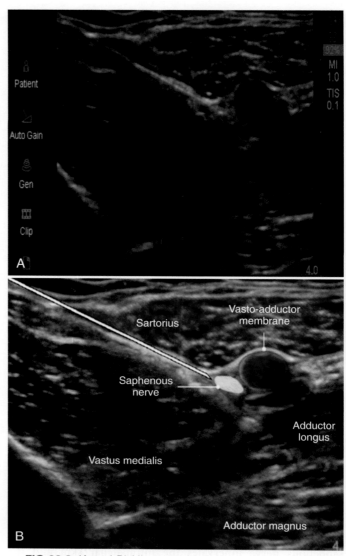

FIG 92.2 (A and B) Ultrasound image of adductor canal.

a large retrospective study found an increased risk of falls associated with blocks involving the femoral nerve,[12] although a recent database analysis on over 190,000 patients who underwent elective TKA failed to show an increased risk of fall in patients who had received peripheral nerve blocks.[24] As impaired quadriceps function increases the risk of falls and the ACB preserves quadriceps function, the ACB may theoretically decrease the fall risk. However, this remains to be established in large clinical studies.

Only one study has been performed, evaluating the ACB for analgesia after revision TKA. The study was a small sample study with low power; therefore no recommendations can be made at this point.[15]

MINOR KNEE SURGERY

The ACB is a technically easy and reliable method for blocking the saphenous nerve and will also result in the block of the infrapatellar nerve and nerve to the vastus medialis, rendering the block useful for any procedure involving the anterior and/or medial aspect of the knee.

The evidence regarding the analgesic effect of an ACB for minor knee surgery is contradictory. This may be a result of low assay sensitivity in some of the studies where pain scores did not exceed mild pain.[2,3] In other studies where pain scores were higher, there was a clinically relevant reduction in pain scores after an ACB compared with placebo.[4,9] Thus, for minor knee surgery, a basic analgesic regimen may be sufficient and the ACB reserved for patients presenting with more than mild pain postoperatively.

COMPLICATIONS

The complications associated with the ACB are the same for any regional anesthetic technique and include block failure, bleeding, infection, local anesthetic toxicity, and nerve injury. However, as the saphenous nerve is purely sensory, any nerve injury may be less clinically significant. One study found the only indication of saphenous nerve injury was in the infrapatellar branch of the saphenous nerve.[10] However, this is a well-described injury that occurs with incision of surgeries on the anterior knee and is more likely related to the surgical procedure than the ACB.[20] Additionally, in skilled hands performing the block with ultrasound, the risk of local anesthetic toxicity is likely low.

CONCLUSION

The ACB is an easy and expedient peripheral nerve block that can be used to decrease postoperative pain after any procedure involving the anterior knee. The block has been found to be noninferior to the traditional FNB in terms of analgesia and has the benefit of limiting or eliminating quadriceps weakness caused by the peripheral nerve block. It is also a very safe block with low risk for complications if performed by a skilled anesthesiologist. The ideal peripheral nerve block would provide effective analgesia, reduce opioid requirements, and promote early mobilization by preserving muscular strength. The ACB, as part of a multimodal pain regimen including opioids, acetaminophen, nonsteroidal antiinflammatory drugs (NSAIDs), and LIA, may be the answer.

The references for this chapter can also be found on www.expertconsult.com.

93

Fascia Iliaca Compartment Block

Jan Boublik

The fascia iliaca compartment block (FICB) represents a relatively "low-risk" alternative to a femoral nerve or a lumbar plexus block for the blockade of the nerves of lumbar plexus. The mechanism behind this block is that the femoral and lateral femoral cutaneous nerves (LFCNs) lie under the fascia iliaca that surrounds the iliopsoas muscle. The distribution of anesthesia and analgesia that is accomplished with the fascia iliaca block (FIB) depends on the extent of the local anesthetic spread and the nerves blocked. Blockade of the femoral nerve results in anesthesia of the anterior and medial thigh (down to and including the knee) and anesthesia of a variable strip of skin on the medial leg and foot through the saphenous nerve, as well as articular branches to both the hip and knee joints. The LFCN confers cutaneous innervation to the anterolateral thigh.

Therefore, a sufficient volume of local anesthetic deposited beneath the fascia iliaca, even if placed some distance from the nerves, has the potential to spread underneath the fascia and reach these nerves.[3] Winnie introduced the concept of the "3-in-1 block": an anterior approach to the lumbar plexus using a simple paravascular inguinal injection to anesthetize the femoral, LFCN of the thigh and obturator nerves.[14] He postulated that the local anesthetic could also spread underneath fascia iliaca proximally toward the lumbosacral plexus by holding pressure distally to the injection site; however, this has not been demonstrated consistently.[11]

The landmark technique involves placement of the needle at the lateral third of the distance from the anterior superior iliac spine and the pubic tubercle, using a "double-pop" technique as the needle passes through fascia lata and fascia iliaca. Capdevila et al.[2] compared the 3-in-1 and FICB techniques in 100 patients undergoing surgeries of the lower extremity and observed complete plexus anesthesia in 38% (3-in-1) and 34% (FICB). Sensory block of the femoral, obturator, genitofemoral, and LFCN nerves was obtained in 90% and 88%, 52% and 38%, 38% and 34%, and 62% and 90% of the patients, respectively. Sensory LFCN blockade was obtained more rapidly for the patients in the FICB group. Concurrent internal and external spread of the local anesthetic solution under the fascia iliaca and between the iliacus and psoas muscles was noted in 62 of the 92 block procedures analyzed radiographically. Isolated external spreads under the fascia iliaca and over the iliacus muscle were noted in 10% of the 3-in-1 and 36% of the FICB patients. However, the lumbar plexus was reached by the local anesthetic in only five radiographs. They concluded that the FICB is more effective, faster, and more consistent than the 3-in-1 block, producing simultaneous blockade of the LFCN and femoral nerves in adults.

Efficacy of the FICB similar to a femoral nerve block (FNB) was confirmed by a study of 98 patients ($n = 47$ FNB and $n = 51$ FICB) undergoing total knee arthroplasty (TKA)[1] that found no significant differences in analgesia use (fentanyl and tramadol) at 12 and 36 hours in pain, nausea, and range of motion at 6 weeks among the groups. There was one case of paresthesia in the femoral nerve area of innervation in the FNB group, and the authors concluded that FICB is as effective as FNB as part of a multimodal anesthetic regimen, consisting of acetaminophen and celecoxib for TKA.

Similarly, Farid et al.[5] found no significant difference in pain scores or opioid between nerve-stimulator located FNB ($n = 11$) and landmark-based FICB ($n = 12$) in 23 adolescents undergoing anterior cruciate ligament reconstruction.

Meanwhile, Gallardo et al.[6] compared postoperative analgesia from a FICB to continuous epidural analgesia in 40 patients following knee arthroplasty ($n = 20$ each). One group received spinal anesthesia plus a FICB with 0.1% bupivacaine at a rate of 10 mL/h, while the second group received combined spinal-epidural anesthesia plus epidural analgesia with 0.1% bupivacaine in continuous infusion at a rate of 8 mL/h. They concluded that FICB and continuous epidural infusion are similarly efficient in providing postoperative analgesia for patients after total knee replacement, with the FICB being associated with a lower incidence of postoperative hemodynamic complications.

However, block success with the landmark technique remains unpredictable because false "pops" can occur, leading to imprecise injection in the wrong fascial plane and block failure. The ultrasound-guided technique is essentially the same; however, monitoring of the needle placement and local anesthetic delivery assures deposition of the local anesthetic into the correct plane. Dolan et al.[4] compared the traditional landmark technique[14] with an ultrasound-guided FICB. They reported a statistically significant increase in the incidence of sensory loss in the medial aspect of the thigh from 60% to 95% ($P = .001$), with complete loss of sensation in the anterior, medial, and lateral aspects of the thigh in 82% of patients using ultrasound and 47% of patients in the landmark group ($P = .001$). Ultrasound-guided FICB resulted in a statistically significant increase in motor block of the femoral (from 63% to 90%; $P = .006$) and obturator (from 22% to 40%; $P = .033$) nerves.

Although deposition of the injectate in the correct plane is of the essence, one has to remember that in the classic FICB technique, the local anesthetic is deposited distal to the inguinal ligament, which may inhibit local anesthetic spread to the more medial branches of the lumbar plexus or to the lumbar plexus itself.

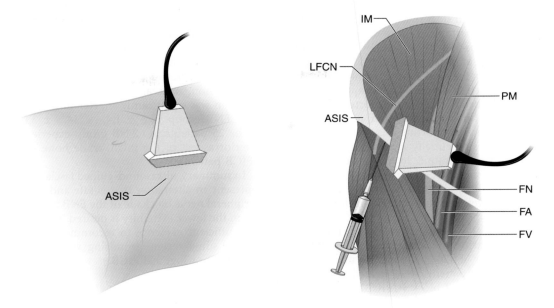

FIG 93.1 Probe and needle position and diagram of dissected iliac fossa showing anatomy for the supra-inguinal FIB. *ASIS,* Anterior superior iliac spine; *FA,* femoral artery; *FN,* femoral nerve; *FV,* femoral vein; *IM,* iliacus muscle; *LFCN,* lateral femoral cutaneous nerve; *PM,* psoas muscle; *U,* umbilicus. (From Hebbard P, Ivanusic J, Sha S: Ultrasound-guided supra-inguinal fascia iliaca block: a cadaveric evaluation of a novel approach. *Anaesthesia* 66(4):300–305, 2011.)

This point was underscored in a study by Shariat et al.[12] that tested whether the administration of a FIB decreases the intensity of postoperative pain compared with sham block in patients after total hip arthroplasty. Thirty-two patients (*n* = 16 in each group) completed the study; all patients received an FIB. There was no difference in pain intensity (NRS-11 = 5.0 ± 0.6 vs. 4.7 ± 0.6, respectively) or in opioid consumption (8.97 ± 1.6 vs. 5.7 ± 1.6 mg morphine, respectively) between the groups at 1 hour or over 24 hours (49.0 ± 29.9 vs. 50.4 ± 34.5 mg, *P* = 0.88), respectively.

However, several letters to the editor[10,13] noted concerns with the technique used regarding a too distal infrainguinal and misdirected injection with too low a volume that led to the inadequate analgesia; specifically, the needle was inserted lateral to medial instead of caudad to cephalad, and a volume of 30 mL instead of 50 mL to 70 mL was used.

To address the issue regarding the optimal point of injection, Hebbard et al.[7] explored injectate spread and nerve involvement in a cadaveric dye-injection model, using a supra-inguinal ultrasound-guided technique that places local anesthetic directly into the iliac fossa. The rational is that by advancing a needle beneath the fascia iliaca from below the inguinal ligament, the needle tip lies superior to the ligament, which may be advantageous as the LFCN leaves the fascia iliaca plane at the inguinal ligament level, as do branches of the femoral nerve to the iliacus muscle and acetabulum that leave the nerve proximal to the inguinal ligament might be anesthetized. In addition, the proximal LFCN and femoral nerve lie close together in the iliac fossa and may be blocked simultaneously by a smaller volume injection. In their study, a linear ultrasound probe was placed over the inguinal ligament, close to the anterior superior iliac spine, and orientated in the parasagittal plane (Fig. 93.1). Initially, the thick white line of the ilium and then the more superficial, hypoechoic iliacus muscle with the fascia iliaca

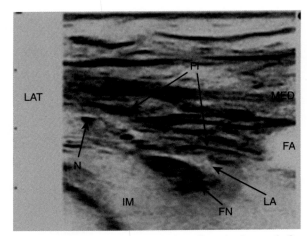

FIG 93.2 Transverse Scan at the Conclusion of Supra-Inguinal Fascia Iliaca Block The needle (N) is lateral to the femoral nerve (FN) which has local anaesthetic (LA) passing over the superficial surface deep to the fascia iliaca (FI). *FA,* Femoral artery; *IM,* iliacus muscle; *LAT,* lateral; *MED,* medial. (From Hebbard P, Ivanusic J, Sha S: Ultrasound-guided supra-inguinal fascia iliaca block: a cadaveric evaluation of a novel approach. *Anaesthesia* 66(4):300–305, 2011.)

covering its surface are identified. The view is enhanced by tilting the transducer more laterally to orientate the fascia more perpendicular to the beam. If the needle is correctly placed, the local anesthetic injectate forms a lens deep to the fascia (Fig. 93.2). In their cadaveric study, they observed extensive spread of dye in the iliac fossa with the femoral nerve stained in all 12 injections. The LFCN was stained bilaterally in five cadavers, but the nerve was absent on both sides in the sixth cadaver. The authors stated that they had performed more than 150 blocks in patients using this approach without complications and conclude that their technique of ultrasound-guided FICB might have the advantage of placing the local anesthetic more directly into the target area than existing described techniques, as well as facilitating convenient catheter placement. Unfortunately, the authors do not provide any further information, nor are there any clinical studies or abstracts supporting this statement.

One interesting case series potentially supporting this statement evaluated the above technique in pediatric patients undergoing hip or femur surgery.[9] Postoperative assessment revealed nerve blockade of the lateral femoral cutaneous, femoral, and obturator nerves, and no requirement for opioid analgesics.

Another study hinting at a potential role[8] is a randomized controlled trial comparing the analgesic efficacy of the ultrasound-guided FNB or FICB in patients undergoing patella fracture surgery. Fifty patients were treated with continuous fascia iliaca compartment block (CFICB) ($n = 25$) or continuous femoral nerve block (CFNB) ($n = 25$). Both groups received a loading of dose of 20 mL of 0.375% ropivacaine followed by an infusion of 0.15% ropivacaine via the catheter at a rate of 5 mL/h for 48 hours. No significant differences in visible analog scales at rest and during movement, fentanyl consumption, nausea, and vomiting were reported. Catheter insertion was significantly shorter in the CFICB compared to the CFNB group (8.3 ± 1.4 vs. 14.5 ± 3.0 minutes). Three of the 25 patients in CFNB group experienced dysesthesia of anterior aspect of the thigh, while none was observed in the CFICB patients.

In summary, ultrasound-guided fascia iliaca nerve block may represent an alternative that is safe and easy to perform when peripheral nerve blockade of the FNB and/or tourniquet coverage in the lower extremity is desired. However, at present there is insufficient evidence to recommend this for knee surgery, despite some recent promising reports for the ultrasound-guided supra-inguinal FICB.

The references for this chapter can also be found on www.expertconsult.com.

94

Psoas Compartment Block

Uchenna O. Umeh

PSOAS COMPARTMENT BLOCK

The psoas compartment block (PCB), also known as the posterior lumbar plexus block, is so named because local anesthetic is placed around the main components of the lumbar plexus as it travels within the psoas major muscle. The compartment lies anterior to the lumbar transverse processes, within the posterior third of the psoas muscle, lateral to the vertebral body and medial to the quadratus lumborum muscle. The block reliably covers the three main branches of the lumbar plexus, the lateral femoral cutaneous, the femoral, and the obturator nerves. The PCB is classically used in patients undergoing total hip arthroplasty or hip fracture surgery. The block can also be used in patients undergoing total knee arthroplasty (TKA) surgery because of its blockade of the femoral nerve, which innervates the anteromedial thigh and the medial portion of the leg via the saphenous nerve, and the obturator nerve, which innervates the medial portion of the medial femoral condyle.

The lumbar plexus is a group of six nerves that supply the lower abdomen and anterolateral thigh. The plexus is formed by the division of the first lumbar nerves (L1-L4) with contributions from the subcostal nerve (T12) in 50% of cases. The ventral rami of the L4, along with the L5 nerve also contribute to the sacral plexus. The nerves of the lumbar plexus include the iliohypogastric (T12-L1), ilioinguinal (L1), genitofemoral (L1-L2), lateral femoral cutaneous (L2-L3), femoral (L2-L4), and obturator (L2-L4) nerves (Fig. 94.1). The femoral and lateral femoral cutaneous (LFC) nerves run in a fascial plane that divides the psoas muscle into an anterior part (two thirds of the muscle mass) and a posterior third.[14] The obturator nerve may also run in this fascial plane, but in 50% of cases it is separated from the other nerves by a muscle fold.[14]

In 1973, Winnie et al. described an anterior approach for blocking the lumbar plexus with a needle insertion point lateral to the femoral artery and 1 cm below the inguinal ligament.[21] The "3-in-1" block they described was supposed to cover the femoral, obturator, and lateral femoral cutaneous nerves because they traveled within the nerve sheath, although we now know that the obturator nerve is almost never blocked by this approach.[11,12] In the article, Winnie mentioned a posterior approach to the lumbar plexus, which he later explained in a 1974 article. Chayen et al. also described a posterior approach to the lumbar plexus in 1976 and coined the term *psoas compartment block*.[4] In their initial study of 100 patients, Chayen et al. reported a 10% block failure with a loss-of-resistance technique. Over the years, many others have modified the technique and approach to the lumbar plexus.[3,9,17] After the development of nerve stimulation, the lumbar plexus block is now placed routinely using a low-intensity current to elicit a quadriceps response. Additionally, ultrasound guidance has provided a novel way to block the lumbar plexus under real-time visualization. The main limitation of ultrasound (US) is the inability to visualize the lumbar plexus clearly within the psoas muscle with the ultrasound machines currently available.

TECHNIQUE

The PCB is considered a "deep" block because the lumbar plexus is typically found at a depth of least 5 to 10 cm from the skin of the back after needle insertion.[3] In obese patients, the depth can be more than 10 cm. The block is typically placed with the patient lying in the lateral decubitus position. The needle insertion point is usually 3 to 5 cm lateral to the midline spinous processes along a line transecting the body at the iliac crest. In 2002, after computed tomography (CT) evaluation of 70 lumbar plexuses, Capdevila et al. suggested a different method of determining the needle insertion point for the PCB. The original Winnie landmark of a line transecting the posterior superior iliac spine (PSIS) proved to be too lateral after review of CT scans. Capdevila's needle insertion point is the junction of the lateral third and medial two thirds of a line between the spinous process of L4, a line parallel to the spinal column passing through the PSIS, and a perpendicular line that crosses about 1 cm above the iliac crests to approximate the L4 spinous process (Fig. 94.2).

Using a nerve stimulator with a starting output of 1.5 mA (frequency 1 Hz, time 0.1 ms), the needle is advanced perpendicular to the skin until contact with the transverse process is made. The needle is pulled back slightly and advanced under the transverse process until a quadriceps femoris muscle twitch is elicited. The nerve stimulator is turned down until quadriceps contractions are still palpable at 0.3 mA to 0.5 mA. After aspiration to ensure that the needle tip is not intravascular or intrathecal, incremental injections of local anesthetic can be made. Lumbar plexus blockade occurs after the spread of local anesthetic within the fascial plane with cephalad spread to the lumbar nerve roots. In 25% of cases, the block of the first sacral root occurs and in 70% of cases, an ilioinguinal/iliohypogastric block is achieved.[14]

Ultrasound guidance may also be used during block placement. This technique involves placing a low-frequency curvilinear probe in the transverse fashion across the patient's back midline at the level of the L4 spinous process or the iliac crests. The main challenges in obtaining adequate views of the anatomy that are relevant for the lumbar plexus block are the depth at which the structures are located and the "acoustic shadow" of

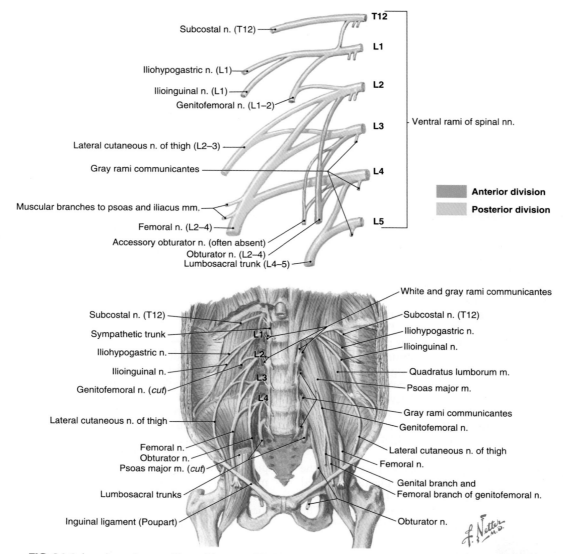

Subcostal n. (T12)

Iliohypogastric n. (L1)

Ilioinguinal n. (L1)
Genitofemoral n. (L1–2)

Lateral cutaneous n. of thigh (L2–3)

Gray rami communicantes

Muscular branches to psoas and iliacus mm.

Femoral n. (L2–4)
Accessory obturator n. (often absent)
Obturator n. (L2–4)
Lumbosacral trunk (L4–5)

T12
L1
L2
L3
L4
L5

Ventral rami of spinal nn.

Anterior division
Posterior division

White and gray rami communicantes

Subcostal n. (T12)
Sympathetic trunk
Iliohypogastric n.
Ilioinguinal n.
Genitofemoral n. (cut)
Lateral cutaneous n. of thigh
Femoral n.
Obturator n.
Psoas major m. (cut)
Lumbosacral trunks
Inguinal ligament (Poupart)

Subcostal n. (T12)
Iliohypogastric n.
Ilioinguinal n.
Quadratus lumborum m.
Psoas major m.
Gray rami communicantes
Genitofemoral n.
Lateral cutaneous n. of thigh
Femoral n.
Genital branch and
Femoral branch of genitofemoral n.
Obturator n.

FIG 94.1 Lumbar plexus. (From Hansen JT: *Netter's clinical anatomy,* ed 2, New York, 2009, Elsevier.)

the transverse processes that overlie the lumbar paravertebral region and obstruct parts of the anatomy.[13] After identification of the L4 spinous processes, the probe is moved left or right (depending on the side of the surgery) over the transverse process. Beneath the transverse process lies the psoas muscle (Fig. 94.3A and B). In most adult patients, it is difficult to visualize the lumbar plexus with the currently available ultrasound machines. In a thin patient or in a child, it may be possible to identify the lumbar plexus as it travels within the posterior third of the psoas muscle. As described by Karmakar et al., to avoid the acoustic shadow of the transverse process, which obscures the plexus, one can place the US probe in a paramedian transverse fashion, in the intertransverse space (between two transverse processes). Once the lumbar plexus (LP) is identified, a stimulating needle connected to a nerve stimulator is used to confirm with femoral nerve stimulation. Once a quadriceps muscle contraction is elicited, the nerve stimulator is decreased below 0.5 mA and the local anesthetic solution is injected after negative aspiration for blood or cerebrospinal fluid (CSF). If the lumbar plexus cannot be identified within the psoas muscle, needle placement is still made under direct ultrasound visualization. The needle is usually advanced in the area approximately 2 cm beyond the transverse process and a quadriceps contraction is used to confirm lumbar plexus stimulation.

COMPLICATIONS

The lumbar plexus block is considered an advanced technique and complications include intrathecal or epidural injection with sympathetic blockade, vascular injury resulting in retroperitoneal bleeding, kidney and other retroperitoneal organ injury from needle puncture, and intravascular injection of local anesthetic resulting in seizure, cardiac arrest, and potentially death. In rare cases, there may be intraperitoneal injection of local anesthetic with the risk of peritonitis (Table 94.1).

The most commonly seen side effect after PCB is epidural or contralateral spread of local anesthetic. The risk factors for this occurrence include a more medial needle insertion point or medially pointed needle, a more cephalad approach (L2-L3), and higher local anesthetic injection pressures (>20 psi).[8] Mannion's comparison of Winnie's approach versus Capdevila's approach to the PCB resulted in 40% contralateral spread of local anesthetic (LA) in the Winnie group compared to 33% contralateral spread in the Capdevila group.[15] A large injected volume of local anesthetic seems to be the most important prognostic factor for epidural or bilateral spread.[7]

Development of a retroperitoneal hematoma is a concerning adverse event after a PCB. The hematoma may develop after a single injection or after removal of an indwelling catheter.[2] Patients on anticoagulants or antiplatelet medications are at a higher risk of developing these complications although spontaneous retroperitoneal hematomas have been described.[6] The current American Society of Regional Anesthesiology (ASRA) guidelines published in 2010 recommend avoiding lumbar plexus blocks, classified as a "deep" plexus blocks, in patients on anticoagulants and antiplatelet medications. In addition, the ASRA recommends avoidance of catheter removal after anticoagulation has been initiated postoperatively.[10] Aspirin therapy is not a contraindication to block placement or catheter removal. Several studies refute the ASRA's conservative recommendations on the removal of block catheters on the anticoagulated patient. Chelly and Schilling published a case series of 3588

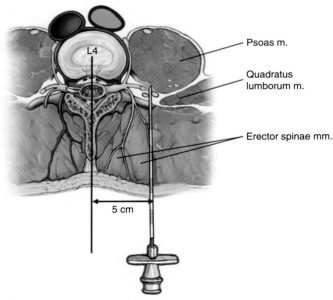

FIG 94.2 Lumbar paravertebral block: cross-sectional view. (From Brown DL: *Atlas of regional anesthesia*, ed 4, Philadelphia, 2010, Saunders [see Fig. 37.6].)

TABLE 94.1 Side Effects and Complications of the Psoas Compartment
Epidural spread
Total spinal anesthesia
Mild hypotension
Plexopathy/neuropathy
Systemic toxicity (CNS/cardiac)
Intraperitoneal injection
Retroperitoneal injection
Renal puncture

CNS, Central nervous system.
Reproduced from de Leeuw MA, Zuurmond WW, Perez RS. The psoas compartment block for hip surgery: the past, present, and future. *Anesthesiol Res Pract* 2011:159541, 2011.

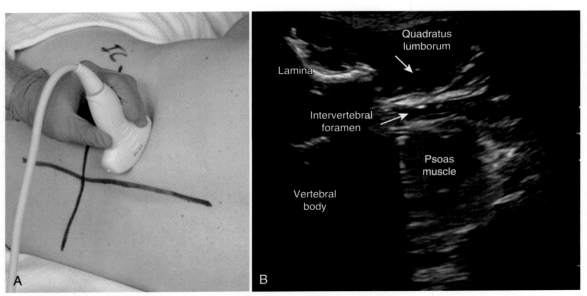

FIG 94.3 (A) Once the acoustic window between the adjacent transverse processes is identified, the lateral aspect of the ultrasound transducer is rocked anteriorly to identify the intervertebral foramen, the lateral margin of the vertebral body, and the psoas muscle. *IC,* Iliac crest. (B) Transverse ultrasound image taken with the curvilinear ultrasound transducer rocked to see around the vertebral body to identify the psoas muscle. (From Waldman SD: *Atlas of interventional pain management,* ed 4, Philadelphia, 2015, Saunders [see Figs. 121.15 and 121.16].)

patients who received single and continuous femoral, sciatic, and lumbar plexus blocks with catheter removal while on anticoagulants such as warfarin, fondaparinux, dalteparin, enoxaparin, and aspirin without a single hemorrhagic complication.[5] The fourth edition of the ASRA guidelines on patients receiving antithrombotic or thromboprophylactic therapy is forthcoming and may reflect some changes based on studies by Chelly and Schilling.

Intravascular injection of local anesthetic is one of the more serious complications of a PCB. Aspiration prior to injection of the local anesthetic and slow and fractionated injections are the best way to prevent this complication. A false negative result may occur resulting in systemic toxicity such as seizures and cardiac arrest. The first line of treatment in such an event is cardiopulmonary resuscitation (CPR) and infusion of intralipid, a 20% fat emulsion that acts as a local anesthetic sink by extracting the lipid-soluble bupivacaine molecules from the aqueous plasma.[19]

CLINICAL EFFICACY

The PCB has been widely used for anesthesia and/or analgesia for total hip arthroplasty surgery or other hip procedures (such as open reduction and internal fixation [ORIF] and hip arthroscopy) with success.[16,20] This technique is not routinely used for knee surgery because the femoral nerve block is more familiar to most anesthesiologists, technically easier to perform, has a lower side-effect profile, and is just as efficacious as the PCB.[12] The advantage of the PCB over a femoral nerve block is that it reliably produces blockade of the entire lumbar plexus including the obturator and the lateral femoral cutaneous nerves.[1] In another study, 10% to 25% of patients may also have a partial epidural or sacral block.[11]

Kaloul et al. compared the PCB to the femoral 3-in-1 block in patients undergoing TKA surgery. Morphine consumption and pain scores were similar between the two groups. Both blocks provided better analgesia than patient-controlled analgesia (PCA) alone after TKA surgery.[12] A possible limitation of the study is the lack of sciatic nerve blockade data because the posterior compartment of the knee contributes to about 20% of pain post TKA. A 2003 study by Jankowski et al. compared PCB versus spinal or general anesthesia in patients having knee arthroscopies. The general anesthesia group reported higher pain scores than the spinal and the PCB group. There was no difference in postoperative visual analogue scale (VAS) pain scores between the spinal and psoas block groups.[11]

In a second study of patients undergoing knee arthroscopies, Atim et al. compared a PCB combined with a sciatic nerve block versus a femoral 3-in-1 block plus a sciatic block. They concluded that although the sciatic-psoas compartment (SPC) group and the sciatic-femoral (SF) group had sufficient anesthesia for the knee arthroscopy, the SPC group had lower opioid requirements than the SF group. More patients from the SF group experienced tourniquet pain and it was hypothesized that insufficient block of the obturator and the lateral femoral cutaneous nerves might have contributed to this finding.

In another study by Raimer et al., 63 patients undergoing TKA were randomly assigned to three groups: one group received continuous PCB and sciatic nerve blocks, the second group received epidural analgesia, and the third group had intravenous PCA pumps. Among the three groups, the group with the sciatic and PCB block and the epidural analgesia group reported lower pain scores than the PCA group on postoperative day (POD) 1. Postoperative opioid consumption was higher in the PCA group, although there was no difference in functional recovery among the three groups.[18]

CONCLUSION

The PCB is a useful technique for patients undergoing surgery of the knee from arthroscopy to replacement. Review of the efficacy and safety for postoperative analgesia has shown it to be superior to opioids for pain relief after surgery. For surgical anesthesia, it was comparable to spinal or epidural anesthesia but better than general anesthesia when comparing intraoperative opioid requirements. When compared to the femoral 3-in-1 block, the PCB was associated with a more consistent block of the obturator and lateral femoral cutaneous nerves, which may be valuable in surgeries where a thigh tourniquet will be used. The main limitations of the PCB are the risk of serious complications and the fact that many physicians may not be trained in the placement of this advanced block technique, making the femoral block the easier alternative. Rapid rehabilitation after surgery and quadriceps-sparing analgesic techniques have also become more important to the orthopedist, in which case an adductor canal block may be preferable to the PCB.

The references for this chapter can also be found on www.expertconsult.com.

95

Sciatic Nerve Block

Jan Boublik

INTRODUCTION

Although first described by Victor Pauchet, a French surgeon, in L'Anesthésie Régionale in 1920,[25] it was his mentee, Seychelles-born surgeon-turned-anesthesiologist Gaston Labat, who popularized this technique with his famous textbook[11] after his arrival in the United States.[6] It remained popular and virtually unchanged until Winnie's modification in 1975.[33]

Beck's anterior approach[3] and Raj's[20] lithotomy approach made valuable contributions to sciatic blockade in the supine patient. Other useful approaches worth noting are the suprasacral, parasacral, and subgluteal approaches described by Bendtsen,[4] Di Benedetto,[7] and Mansour,[15] respectively.

The technical aspects of these nerves blocks are beyond the scope and intent of this chapter. We will focus on the functional anatomy, conceptually discuss the most significant approaches and indications as they pertain to anesthesia for knee surgery, and where available, the functional and clinical outcomes.

FUNCTIONAL ANATOMY

The sciatic nerve originates from the sacral plexus, combining the lumbosacral branch from the last two roots of the lumbar plexus and the anterior branches of the first through third sacral nerves. Shaped like a triangle pointing to the sacral notch, the sciatic nerve is anterior to the piriformis muscle and is covered by the pelvis fascia, separating it from the hypogastric vessels and pelvic organs. The sciatic nerve is the largest peripheral nerve in the body, measuring more than 1 cm in breadth, and is the terminal branch of the seven branches of the plexus.

The sciatic nerve exits the pelvis through the greater sciatic notch below (tibial part) and through or above (peroneal part) the piriformis muscle prior to descending between the greater trochanter of the femur and the ischial tuberosity. The upper course of the sciatic nerve is deep to the gluteus maximus and rests on the ischium. It crosses the external rotators, obturator internus, and gemelli muscles prior to passing the quadratus femoris muscle, which separates it from the hip joint and obturator externus. It is accompanied medially by the posterior cutaneous nerve of the thigh and the inferior gluteal plexus, until it comes to lie posterior to the adductor magnus more distally.

The nerve then runs along the posterior thigh, posteromedial to the femur and sandwiched between the biceps femoris muscle laterally, after being crossed obliquely by its long head, and the semitendinosus and semimembranosus muscles medially. Its course can be approximated by drawing a line on the back of the thigh from the apex of the popliteal fossa to the midpoint of the line between the greater trochanter and ischial tuberosity.

The articular branches of the sciatic nerve arise from the proximal part of the nerve and supply the posterior part of the hip joint capsule, although they can arise directly from the sacral plexus. Meanwhile, the muscular branches innervate the gluteal muscles, the ischial head of the adductor magnus, the semimembranosus and semitendinosus muscles, and the biceps femoris muscle. A common trunk gives rise to the branches innervating the semimembranosus and adductor magnus muscles, while the nerve to the short head of the biceps femoris arises from the common peroneal division, in contrast to the other muscular branches that arise from the tibial division.

Anywhere in the lower third of the femur, most commonly 5 to 12 cm[31] above the popliteal crease, the common perineural sheath containing the common peroneal and tibial nerves divides into individual nerve sheaths to form the respective nerves.

The common peroneal nerve divides into the deep and superficial peroneal nerves after descending around the neck of the fibula. Its major branches in this region innervate the posterior knee joint and the cutaneous branches and contribute to the sural nerve, prior to dividing into its terminal branches, the superficial and deep peroneal nerves.

The larger tibial nerve continues its path vertically prior to dividing into its terminal branches, the medial and lateral plantar nerves, after sending branches to the sural nerve, to the muscles of the calf, and to the ankle joint. It is important to note that, unlike the peroneal nerve, the tibial nerve does have a well-defined perineurium.

Fig. 95.1 illustrates the dermatomes, myotomes, and sclerotomes relevant to the sciatic nerve, its terminal branches, and the innervation of the knee joint.

APPROACHES TO THE SCIATIC NERVE

There are numerous approaches to the sciatic nerve, with the choice dictated by the anesthetic goal and by the clinical conditions, such as the patient's mobility and body habitus, and the skill and preference of the anesthesiologist. For clarity, the approaches are listed from proximal to distal. The following section will then discuss how the different approaches are best logically grouped for optimal conceptual understanding and clinical results.

Most proximally, the sciatic nerve can be blocked in the parasacral region right after it forms from the sacral roots, as described by Mansour.[15] This approach results in the most comprehensive blockade with the characteristics of a plexus

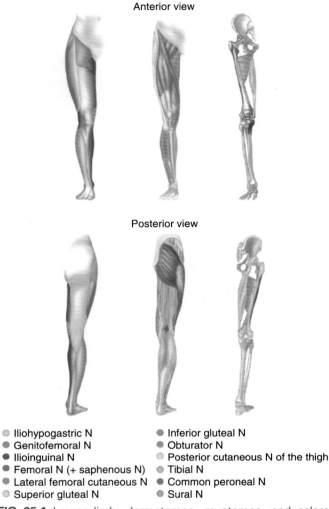

Anterior view

Posterior view

- Iliohypogastric N
- Genitofemoral N
- Ilioinguinal N
- Femoral N (+ saphenous N)
- Lateral femoral cutaneous N
- Superior gluteal N
- Inferior gluteal N
- Obturator N
- Posterior cutaneous N of the thigh
- Tibial N
- Common peroneal N
- Sural N

FIG 95.1 Lower limb; dermatomes, myotomes, and sclerotomes. (Adapted from Jochum D and Delaunay L, with permission from AstraZeneca France.)

block including the posterior cutaneous nerve of the thigh and possibly the obturator nerve. This approach can be easily integrated in an efficient workflow with the neuraxial or lumbar plexus as a single injection or continuous block in a single area requiring only one skin preparation.[17]

A similar option is the parasacral blockade[4] under the piriformis muscle, which has essentially the same benefits and clinical characteristics. Although the subgluteal blockade provides a similar anesthetic effect, it requires additional skin cleansing and repositioning of the patient, and will most often not block the posterior cutaneous nerve of the thigh, more anesthesiologists are familiar with and able to perform this approach.[8]

Anterior blockade of the sciatic nerve is attractive because it can be combined with a femoral or saphenous/adductor canal nerve block without the need to reposition the patient. If combined with a femoral nerve block (FNB), anesthesia can be achieved to pretty much the entire lower extremity (except for the skin on the posterior aspect of the thigh).[14] One of the potential drawbacks of this approach is that it can be severely affected by the patient's body habitus, which can make this

technically complex nerve block difficult to perform. Furthermore, it is not ideally suited for catheter insertion given the perpendicular angle and deep location.

Blockade of the sciatic nerve at the popliteal level provides reliable surgical anesthesia of the posterior aspect of the knee joint and the whole lower leg except for the medial skin innervated by the saphenous nerve. A side effect is the motor blockade of the hamstring muscles because of the cranial extension of the local anesthetic and foot drop because of peroneal blockade, which limits ambulation. In addition, it does not, unlike all the previously mentioned approaches, provide thigh tourniquet coverage if desired and used. It can be performed with remarkable safety posteriorly[21] or laterally with equivalent results.[10] The lateral approach can be performed with the patient supine and does not require extensive repositioning.

It is also possible to selectively block the tibial nerve in the popliteal area, minimizing the risk of foot drop.[22]

Another technique developed by the same group[26,27] is called infiltration of the interspace between the popliteal artery and the capsule of the posterior knee (iPACK). This ultrasound-guided periarticular infiltration (PAI) is performed just above the femoral condyles, deposits the local anesthetic right next to the periarticular branches of the sciatic nerve,[9,26,27] and completely avoids the risk of inadvertent peroneal blockade. The technique also has an anterior component that provides a targeted ultrasound-guided infiltration of the terminal branches of the genicular, saphenous, and obturator nerves supplying the knee joint.

INDICATIONS

Indications for sciatic blockade include lower limb surgery, during which it is most often combined with FNB or lumbar plexus block. It is particularly advantageous in patients in whom general anesthesia would be deleterious, for example, because of multiple medical comorbidities and cognitive issues such as dementia or cerebral vascular disease, or for whom neuraxial anesthesia is, relatively or absolutely, contraindicated. Examples are spinal conditions like severe scoliosis, previous spinal instrumentation, and certain neurologic conditions such as multiple sclerosis.

Examples of knee surgeries for which a sciatic block is used are procedures involving the posterior capsule, most commonly total knee arthroplasty.

Whenever possible, or if no tourniquet coverage is needed, the more distal popliteal fossa sciatic block, selective tibial nerve block or posterior infiltration (by the anesthesiologist or surgeon) are preferable to avoid blockade of the hamstring or biceps muscles and facilitate ambulation.

Contraindications, other than patient (or surgeon) refusal, are few, but include infection at the injection or catheter site, severe coagulopathy, and allergy to local anesthetics. Caution should be exercised with preexisting central and peripheral nerve lesions.

FUNCTIONAL OUTCOMES

Sciatic Nerve

As early as 2005, Pham et al.[19] observed, in a randomized controlled trial (RCT), the benefit of adding a sciatic nerve block (SNB) to the femoral block to improve analgesia after total knee arthroplasty compared to a continuous FNB or continuous blocks of both the femoral and sciatic nerves. During the 36 hours immediately following total knee replacement, the combination of continuous femoral blocks and SNBs improved analgesia and decreased morphine consumption and postoperative nausea and vomiting (PONV).

In a retrospective analysis, Liu et al.[12] reported significantly lower postoperative pain and opioid use in patients with continuous femoral and SNBs ($n = 1329$) than those with opioids alone ($n = 439$) after total knee arthroplasty (TKA). There was no detectable decrease in strength associated with nerve blocks, while a significantly greater proportion of patients with nerve blocks were able to participate in physical therapy on postoperative day 1 (96.4% vs. 57.1%), suggesting that better pain control allowed for an easier start to rehabilitation.

Huebner et al.[5] compared continuous femoral nerve analgesia alone, continuous femoral nerve analgesia combined with single-shot sciatic nerve analgesia, and continuous femoral nerve analgesia combined with continuous sciatic nerve analgesia in a retrospective study of 364 patients. The additional continuous SNB led to lower visual analogue scale (VAS) scores after 8 and 24 hours (mean values, 1.8 and 4.0, respectively) than a continuous femoral block alone (mean values, 2.7 and 4.9). In addition, patients with a continuous SNB had lower VAS scores than those with a single-shot SNB (mean values, 1.9 and 4.5) at 8 and 24 hours. Meperidine consumption in the continuous SNB group was lower (32% of patients) as compared with the two other groups (65%). Consequently, there were fewer opioid side effects per group: 24% of in the continuous SNB group, 52% in the single-shot sciatic nerve group, and 44% in the FNB-alone group. An RCT of 60 patients undergoing TKA with FNB and either single-injection or continuous SNB found that total morphine consumption in the 48-hour period after surgery was significantly lower in the continuous SNB group compared with the single-injection SNB group (4.9 [5.9] vs. 9.7 [9.5] mg, $p = 0.002$), although the difference might not be clinically significant. VAS pain scores at rest were also significantly lower in the continuous SNB group ($p = 0.035$).[24] The combined findings of these two studies suggest, at the very least, an opioid-sparing effect and improved analgesia for a continuous technique.

Morin et al.,[16] in their RCT of 90 patients, sought to evaluate whether a psoas compartment catheter provides better postoperative analgesia than a femoral nerve catheter and whether the psoas compartment catheter is as effective as the combination of a femoral nerve catheter and a sciatic nerve catheter and thus improves functional outcome. The combined femoral nerve and sciatic nerve catheter proved superior to both the femoral catheter alone and a psoas catheter with respect to reduced analgesic requirements after total knee replacement. Postoperative pain scores were the same, and no differences occurred with respect to short-term or long-term functional outcome.

In their prospective blinded randomized trial of 210 patients undergoing TKA, Uesugi et al.[30] reported that both PAI and peripheral nerve blockade (PNB) (femoral and sciatic) provided good patient satisfaction with no significant differences in pain at rest up to 48 hours after surgery. In another RCT,[29] 46 patients scheduled for TKA were randomized into two groups: concomitant administration of femoral and SNB or FNB and PAI. Average pain scores during the first 21 days after surgery were similar in the two groups and remained at a low level. There was no significant difference in the need for adjuvant analgesics,

patient satisfaction level, time to achieve rehabilitation goals, and length of hospital stay. They concluded that PAI offers a potentially safer alternative to SNB as an adjunct to FNB.

Wegener et al.[32] investigated whether reduced postoperative pain after addition of SNB to continuous femoral nerve block for TKA translated into improved long-term outcomes after surgery. Physical function, stiffness, and pain were measured using the Western Ontario and McMaster Universities Osteoarthritis Index (WOMAC), Oxford Knee Score 12-item knee questionnaires, and VAS at rest and during mobilization before TKA and 3 and 12 months after surgery. They did not detect any differences and concluded that improved postoperative pain control did not translate into improved functional outcome or a reduction in chronic pain.

The most comprehensive review on the subject is by Abdallah and Brull,[1] who examined the effects on acute pain and related outcomes of adding SNB to FNB for TKA compared with FNB alone in a total of seven studies: four intermediate-quality randomized and three observational trials with a total of 391 patients. Three of four trials investigating the addition of single-shot SNB and two of three trials investigating continuous SNB reported improved early analgesia at rest and reduced early opioid consumption. Only two trials specifically assessed posterior knee pain. The authors concluded that there was inconclusive evidence in the literature to define the effect of adding SNB to FNB on acute pain and related outcomes compared with FNB alone for TKA and were unable to determine any clinically important analgesic advantages for SNB beyond 24 hours postoperatively.

Liu et al.[13] compared general anesthesia and PNB consisting of lumbar plexus and sciatic nerve blockade. Intraoperative blood pressure and heart rate and recovery in physiologic, emotional (depression and anxiety), nociceptive (pain and nausea), and modified cognitive domains were better with PNB, but those benefits did extend to activities of daily living. Intraoperative drugs and the postoperative sufentanil requirement of the PNB group were lower (all $p < 0.001$). Differences and benefits were greatest early after surgery, with no detectable difference at the end of 1 week.

Meanwhile, Patel et al.[18] performed a retrospective analysis of the safety and efficacy of PNBs compared to epidural anesthesia in 221 consecutive patients undergoing bilateral TKA. They reported that incidences of hypotension, urinary retention, and pruritus were all lower in the PNB group compared the epidural group. Epidural patients also required more blood transfusions and greater volumes of colloids and crystalloids. The authors concluded that PNBs are a safe and effective modality of analgesia for bilateral TKA and provide adequate pain relief with a significant decrease in postoperative complications compared to epidural anesthesia.

Popliteal Nerve

Less information is available on the effects of sciatic nerve blockade at the popliteal level. Abdallah et al.[2] performed a randomized controlled trial comparing proximal, distal (popliteal), and no SNB after TKA. They observed a reduction of about 60% in the number of patients who experienced moderate-to-severe posterior knee pain. Both proximal and distal SNB reduced resting pain in the posterior and anterior knee up to 8 hours postoperatively compared with no SNB. The popliteal technique required shorter procedural time, fewer needle passes, and produced less discomfort.

Safa et al.[23] investigated the value of the popliteal nerve block and an alternative technique of posterior capsule local anesthetic infiltration analgesia. One hundred patients were prospectively randomized into three groups: popliteal nerve block, posterior local anesthetic infiltration, and control. All patients received a femoral nerve block and spinal anesthesia. They observed no differences in pain scores between groups. The popliteal nerve block seemed to provide a brief, clinically insignificant opioid-sparing effect. They concluded that neither SNB nor posterior local anesthetic infiltration provides significant analgesic benefits.

Selective Tibial Nerve Block

A potentially attractive option is selective tibial nerve blockade, as it seems to strike a balance of analgesia, ease of performance, and noninterference with rehabilitation. In their 2012 paper, Sinha et al.[22] randomized 80 patients undergoing TKA to receive a tibial nerve block in the popliteal fossa or an SNB proximal to its bifurcation in combination with a femoral nerve block as part of a multimodal analgesia regimen. A sufficient volume of local anesthetic solution to provide circumferential spread of the target nerve was administered for the block, up to a maximum of 20 mL. A lower volume of ropivacaine 0.5% was used for the tibial nerve block, 8.7 mL (99% CI, 7.9 to 9.4) versus 15.2 mL (99% CI, 14.9 to 15.5), respectively (99% CI for difference between means, 5.6 to 7.3; $p < 0.001$). No patient receiving a tibial nerve block developed complete peroneal motor block compared to 82.5% of patients receiving the SNB ($p < 0.001$). There were no significant differences in the pain scores or opioid consumption between the groups. The authors concluded that selective tibial nerve block performed in the popliteal fossa in close proximity to the popliteal crease avoided complete peroneal motor block and provided similar postoperative analgesia compared to the SNB when combined with a femoral nerve block for patients undergoing TKA.

Periarticular Infiltration

Sinha et al.[26] reported in 2012 that ultrasound-guided iPACK with local anesthetic solution might be an alternative option in controlling posterior knee pain. They postulated that with iPACK only, the terminal branches innervating the posterior knee joint would be blocked and the main trunk of the tibial nerve would be spared. All patients in the study received multimodal analgesia, a femoral nerve block, general anesthesia supplemented with fentanyl and hydromorphone, and either iPACK or a tibial nerve block.

No differences were observed in the pain scores and opioid consumption between groups in their study of fourteen patients. No patient in either group developed a footdrop. They concluded that iPACK provided equivalent analgesia compared to tibial nerve block when combined with FNB and could be an alternative method in controlling posterior knee pain following TKA.[26]

Elliott et al.[9] investigated the role of iPACK within multimodal analgesia, continuous femoral nerve, or adductor canal blockade (ACB) in a retrospective chart review of 45 consecutive patients undergoing primary unilateral TKA. They observed improved ambulation distance for all measurements in the ACB/iPACK group compared to the femoral nerve block group. Time to discharge was greatly improved in ACB/iPACK patients with similar VAS scores and slightly higher opioid consumption. They concluded that the ACB/IPACK technique results in

excellent analgesia with reduced motor weakness, allows timely discharge with excellent patient satisfaction, and might strike a balance of optimal pain control and motor recovery following TKA and regional anesthesia.

Intra-articular Infiltration

For completeness, a brief paragraph addressing the alternative of postoperative intra-articular infusion is provided here. Stathellis et al.[28] randomly assigned 50 patients undergoing TKA to two groups: a group receiving a continuous femoral and single-shot sciatic nerve block (CNFB, $n = 25$) and a group receiving intraoperative PAIs followed by postoperative intra-articular infusion group (PIAC group, $n = 25$). The VAS for pain ($p < 0.001$) and Knee Society scores ($p = 0.05$) were significantly better for the PIAC group and increased rebound pain following CFNB compared to the PIAC group. They did not observe a difference with regard to knee function, but straight leg raise was significantly better following PIAC. There were also two falls in patients with CFNB. The authors concluded that pericapsular injections combined with an intra-articular catheter provide better pain control with no rebound pain and better function, and might decrease the risk of complications related to motor weakness. However, the authors used a high concentration and infusion rate of ropivacaine for the continuous FNB, thus leading to significant motor blockade.

CONCLUSION

Patients often complain of posterior knee pain after knee surgery, even when a femoral or adductor canal block is performed. SNB, whether as a single-shot or continuous technique, is an effective way to control that posterior pain. SNB has an opioid-sparing effect and provides effective analgesia. It does cause weakness of the hamstrings, with the extent depending on exact location of the block and the concentration of the local anesthetic. It may offer analgesia benefits for the first 24 hours,[1] but nonconclusively beyond that.

Newer techniques such as selective tibial nerve block, iPACK, and peri- and intra-articular infiltration may offer comparable analgesia effects without much, if any, motor blockade. However, too little data is available at this point to routinely recommend any technique. These should be offered on an as-needed basis for patients after knee surgery, especially TKA.

KEY REFERENCES

1. Abdallah FW, Brull R: Is sciatic nerve block advantageous when combined with femoral nerve block for postoperative analgesia following total knee arthroplasty? A systematic review. *Reg Anesth Pain Med* 36:493–498, 2011.
5. Benthien JP, Huebner D: Efficacy of continuous catheter analgesia of the sciatic nerve after total knee arthroplasty. *Swiss Med Wkly* 145:w14119, 2015.
12. Liu Q, Chelly JE, Williams JP, et al: Impact of peripheral nerve block with low dose local anesthetics on analgesia and functional outcomes following total knee arthroplasty: a retrospective study. *Pain Med* 16:998–1006, 2015.
16. Morin AM, Kratz CD, Eberhart LH, et al: Postoperative analgesia and functional recovery after total-knee replacement: comparison of a continuous posterior lumbar plexus (psoas compartment) block, a continuous femoral nerve block, and the combination of a continuous femoral and sciatic nerve block. *Reg Anesth Pain Med* 30:434–445, 2005.

19. Pham Dang C, Gautheron E, Guilley J, et al: The value of adding sciatic block to continuous femoral block for analgesia after total knee replacement. *Reg Anesth Pain Med* 30:128–133, 2005.

22. Sinha SK, Abrams JH, Arumugam S, et al: Femoral nerve block with selective tibial nerve block provides effective analgesia without foot drop after total knee arthroplasty: a prospective, randomized, observer-blinded study. *Anesth Analg* 115:202–206, 1980.

23. Safa B, Gollish J, Haslam L, et al: Comparing the effects of single-shot sciatic nerve block versus posterior capsule local anesthetic infiltration on analgesia and functional outcome after total knee arthroplasty: a prospective, randomized, double-blinded, controlled trial. *J Arthroplasty* 29:1149–1153, 2014.

26. Sinha S, Abrams J, Sivasenthil A, et al: Use of ultrasound guided popliteal fossa infiltration to control pain after total knee arthroplasy: a prospective randomized observer-blinded study. American Society of Regional Anesthesia and Pain Medicine, Spring Meeting 2012. Poster A51.

30. Uesugi K, Kitano N, Kikuchi T, et al: Comparison of peripheral nerve block with periarticular injection analgesia after total knee arthroplasty: a randomized, controlled study. *Knee* 21:848–852, 2014.

32. Wegener JT, Wegener JT, van Ooij B, et al: Long-term pain and functional disability after total knee arthroplasty with and without single-injection or continuous sciatic nerve block in addition to continuous femoral nerve block: a prospective, 1-year follow-up of a randomized controlled trial. *Reg Anesth Pain Med* 38:58–63, 2013.

The references for this chapter can also be found on www.expertconsult.com.

96

Obturator Nerve Block

Arthur Atchabahian

The obturator nerve (ON) arises from the lumbar plexus and innervates most of the adductors in the medial compartment of the thigh, an inconstant area of skin on the medial thigh, and part of the medial femur. The posterior lumbar plexus block often includes the ON, but the more commonly used anterior femoral nerve three-in-one block usually fails to block the ON.[2,5] Following knee surgery, ON blockade can be used to supplement femoral and sciatic nerve blocks for analgesia.

The ON is a mixed nerve and contains both motor and sensory nerve fibers. It arises from the L2-L4 branches of the lumbar plexus, although the contribution from L2 is often insignificant or even nonexistent.[4] It descends into the pelvis with the iliac and obturator vessels and passes through the obturator foramen into the thigh. At the level of the obturator foramen, the nerve bifurcates into an anterior and a posterior branch. The anterior branch provides an articular branch to the anterior hip joint and innervates the anterior adductor muscles (pectineus, adductor longus, and adductor brevis). It makes, to a variable degree, a small cutaneous sensory contribution to the medial and inferior aspects of the thigh: in a study by Bouaziz et al., more than 50% of patients (17/30) had no area of cutaneous hypoesthesia after an ON block.[4] The posterior branch innervates the deep adductor muscles (adductor brevis and magnus, obturator externus) and often sends a variable contribution to the medial portions of the knee joint. This minor contribution may be meaningful for analgesia following knee surgery.

Up to 30% of individuals may have a small accessory obturator nerve (AON) that originates from the ventral rami of the L3 and L4 or branches off the ON.[1] This accessory nerve in part contributes to motor innervation of the pectineus muscle and hip joint.

The reduction in adductor power is the best method to test ON blockade. Nonetheless, even with a complete ON block, there is some residual adductor strength because of the pectineus (femoral nerve innervation) and part of the adductor magnus (sciatic nerve innervation) muscles.[4]

Different approaches to ON blockade[14,18] have been suggested since Labat's description in 1928.[10] For knee surgery, a very proximal blockade is not useful. Therefore, we will focus on the approaches located in the proximal thigh, at the level where the nerve has already split into two branches.

Choquet et al.[6] described the neurostimulation-guided inguinal approach, which reduces the risk of complications and is less uncomfortable for the patient than approaches in the groin.[7,13]

The patient is placed in a supine position with the leg slightly abducted and externally rotated. The adductor longus tendon is palpated at the pubic tubercle, as the most peripheral perceptible tendon in the medial region of the thigh. The needle insertion point is located 0.5 caudad to the inguinal crease, midway between the femoral arterial pulse and the inner border of the adductor longus tendon.[6] This approach is performed in two stages. First, a stimulating needle is introduced in a cephalad direction with a 30-degree angle to the skin until adductor muscle (adductor longus or gracilis) contractions are elicited.[14] The adductor longus response of the obturator nerve (anterior branch) is perceived at the anterior part of the inner thigh. Weak contraction of the gracilis, which frequently accompanies the former, forms a narrow muscular band down to the medial part of the knee. When a muscle response is preserved at a current below 0.5 mA, 5 mL of local anesthetic are injected to block the anterior branch of the obturator nerve. The needle is then advanced about 0.5 to 1 cm while redirecting it about 5 degrees laterally. The adductor magnus response is felt in the posterior aspect of the inner thigh and produces noticeable hip adduction. Another 5 mL of local anesthetic is then injected to block the posterior branch. At the inguinal level, the anterior and posterior branches are only divided by the adductor brevis muscle. An injection of a larger volume near a single branch could thus possibly obtain an entire block of both branches by diffusion.

The block can also be performed under ultrasound guidance[17] as a dual-injection technique (Figs. 96.1 and 96.2) targeting each of the two divisions individually, first between the adductor longus (or pectineus, if the block is performed very proximally) and adductor brevis for the anterior branch, and between the adductor brevis and adductor magnus. Sinha et al.[16] demonstrated that the injection under ultrasound guidance of half of the local anesthetic solution between the pectineus and adductor brevis muscles, and half between the adductor brevis and adductor magnus muscles, without attempting to visualize the nerves, leads to a mean muscle strength reduction of 82% in 93% of their population (30 patients scheduled for knee surgery), and thus a fairly complete ON block.

The usefulness of the obturator nerve to provide analgesia after knee surgery is controversial. Literature data is contradictory, and whether an obturator block is added to other analgesic modalities is often a matter of personal preference of the anesthesiologist. It seems to be more common in Europe than in the United States, for example.

- Macalou et al.[11] randomly assigned 90 patients undergoing total knee arthroplasty (TKA) under general anesthesia into three groups: group 1 patients received a femoral nerve block (FNB), group 2 patients a FNB and an ON block, and group 3 patients a placebo FNB. Morphine consumption and pain

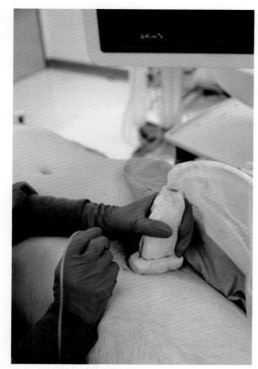

FIG 96.1 External photograph showing an in-plane approach to obturator nerve block in the medial thigh. (From Gray, AT: *Atlas of ultrasound-guided regional anesthesia*, ed 2, Philadelphia, 2012, Saunders, p 172.)

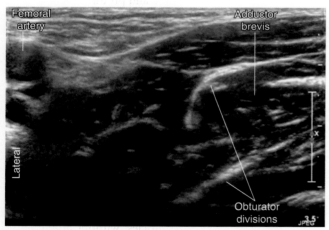

FIG 96.2 Sonogram of the medial thigh showing the divisions of the obturator nerve. The anterior and posterior divisions lie on the anterior and posterior sides of the adductor brevis muscle, medial to the femoral vessels. (From Gray, AT: *Atlas of ultrasound-guided regional anesthesia*, ed 2, Philadelphia, 2012, Saunders, p 172.)

scores were lower for group 2 patients than patients in the other groups (total morphine use in the first 6 hours: 8.1 ± 7.6 mg in group 2, 21.1 ± 8 mg in group 1, 21.8 ± 7.2 mg in group 3; $p < 0.001$). Also, the incidence of postoperative nausea was higher in group 1 and 3 patients (4/30 in group 2, 10/30 in group 1, 13/30 in group 3; $p = 0.01$). This led the

authors to conclude that the addition of an ON block to FNB improves analgesia after TKA.

- Kaloul et al.[8] studied 60 patients undergoing TKA under spinal anesthesia and randomly assigned them to receive a psoas compartment block (PCB), or an FNB, or no block. Morphine consumption over the first 48 hours was reduced in patients who received blocks (72.2 ± 26.6 mg for the control group, 37.3 ± 34.7 mg for the FNB group; $p = 0.0002$, 36.1 ± 25.8 mg for the PCB group; $p < 0.0001$) but no difference was seen between the two blocks. Pain scores at rest, 6, and 24 hours were lower in the FNB and PCB groups compared to the control group ($p < 0.0001$). Thus, despite the fact that motor blockade of the adductors, a surrogate for adequate ON blockade, was more frequent in the PCB group ($p = 0.004$ at 6 hours), there seemed to be no analgesic advantage to ON blockade.
- Kardash et al.[9] randomized 60 patients scheduled for TKA under spinal anesthesia to receive an FNB, an ON block, or a sham block at the end of the procedure. No significant difference was found in pain scores at rest over the first two postoperative days, but pain scores with motion were lower in the FNB group than in the ON block group at recovery room discharge ($p = 0.03$) but not at any other time. Thus, the authors concluded that there was no advantage to ON blockade after TKA. A subsequent article[3] reported the one-year follow-up of these patients. No difference was found among the three groups in terms of Hospital for Special Surgery knee scores or similar subscores such as range of motion, daily function, and resting and dynamic pain.
- McNamee et al.[12] randomized 60 patients undergoing TKA to receive either combined femoral and sciatic blocks, or combined femoral, sciatic, and obturator nerve blocks. While the pain scores were not different between groups, patients who received an obturator nerve block had significantly longer analgesia (mean time to first request for analgesia 257.0 vs. 433.6 min) and required significantly less morphine throughout the study period (mean 83.8 vs. 63.0 mg) ($p < 0.05$ for both outcomes).

ON blockade has also been suggested to enhance analgesia for anterior cruciate ligament (ACL) reconstruction using a hamstring autograft.[15] The authors randomly assigned 41 patients about to undergo ACL reconstruction to receive, as a sole anesthetic, a combination of femoral, lateral femoral cutaneous, and sciatic nerve blocks with or without an ON block. Only 6/21 patients who received an ON block required intraoperative analgesia (25 ± 45 mcg of fentanyl) while all 20 patients who did not get an ON block required fentanyl (130 ± 55 mcg) ($p < 0.0001$ for both number of patients needing analgesics, and dose of fentanyl). However, there was no difference in analgesic requirements postoperatively, which does not support the routine use of ON blockade for that indication.

KEY REFERENCES

4. Bouaziz H, Vial F, Jochum D, et al: An evaluation of the cutaneous distribution after obturator nerve block. *Anesth Analg* 94:445–449, 2002.
6. Choquet O, Capdevila X, Bennourine K, et al: A new inguinal approach for the obturator nerve block: anatomical and randomized clinical studies. *Anesthesiology* 103:1238–1245, 2005.
9. Kardash K, Hickey D, Tessler MJ, et al: Obturator versus femoral nerve block for analgesia after total knee arthroplasty. *Anesth Analg* 105(3):853–858, 2007.

11. Macalou D, Trueck S, Meuret P, et al: Postoperative analgesia after total knee replacement: the effect of an obturator nerve block added to the femoral 3-in-1 nerve block. *Anesth Analg* 99(1):251–254, 2004.

12. McNamee DA, Parks L, Milligan KR: Post-operative analgesia following total knee replacement: an evaluation of the addition of an obturator nerve block to combined femoral and sciatic nerve block. *Acta Anaesthesiol Scand* 46(1):95–99, 2002.

14. Parks CR, Kennedy WF: Obturator nerve block: a simplified approach. *Anesthesiology* 28:775–778, 1967.

15. Sakura S, Hara K, Ota J, et al: Ultrasound-guided peripheral nerve blocks for anterior cruciate ligament reconstruction: effect of obturator nerve block during and after surgery. *J Anesth* 24(3):411–477, 2010.

16. Sinha SK, Abrams JH, Houle TT, et al: Ultrasound-guided obturator nerve block: an interfascial injection approach without nerve stimulation. *Reg Anesth Pain Med* 34:261–264, 2009.

The references for this chapter can also be found on www.expertconsult.com.

97

Continuous Perineural Analgesia for Knee Surgery

Christophe Aveline

During major knee surgery, tissue injury, comorbidities, postoperative pain intensity, neuropsychological consequences, and opioid use affect postoperative function. Other factors such as prior joint damage, bone deformities, and preoperative muscle impairment are likely to worsen functional recovery. Preoperative pain and opioid use increase the risk of chronic pain[12,31,64,76,92] and affect the functional benefit of surgery.[92]

Preoperative and postoperative pain combine inflammatory and neuropathic components involving peripheral and central sensitization.[48,69] Preoperative hyperalgesia is associated with higher postoperative visual analog scale (VAS) scores,[67] morphine consumption,[48] and worse functional rehabilitation scores.[69] An observational study found preoperative mechanical and thermal hyperalgesia in 50% of patients with long-term opioid use, with a 36% increase of morphine consumption on postoperative day (POD) 3.[39]

Continuous nerve blocks (CNBs) using local anesthetics (LA) reduce pain, inflammation and hyperalgesia. A femoral catheter associated with a single-shot sciatic nerve block and maintained for 48 hours significantly decreased inflammation of the knee, VAS scores, and morphine consumption by 50%.[68] In contrast, intravenous (IV) administration of lidocaine, which possesses antiinflammatory and antihyperalgesic effects during visceral surgery, is not effective in reducing VAS scores, mechanical hyperalgesia, and pain thresholds after hip replacement compared with placebo.[67] In animal studies, a sciatic catheter significantly reduced mechanical allodynia and thermal hyperalgesia as well as prostaglandin E_2 levels in the cerebrospinal fluid and the expression of cyclooxygenase-2 in homolateral and contralateral dorsal root ganglion, whereas IV LA had no significant effect.[10] The combined use of continuous posterior lumbar and sciatic catheters during total knee arthroplasty (TKA) for 48 hours significantly reduced the plasma concentration of C-reactive protein on POD1 and POD2 compared with IV morphine, without modification of interleukin-6.[7] The systemic antiinflammatory effect of a CNB is accompanied by a reduction in VAS scores at rest on POD1 and during flexion on POD1 and POD2.[7]

The neuropathic component of pain evaluated by the DN4 score (a ten-item questionnaire effective to detect the neuropathic component of pain) can affect 49% of preoperative patients.[11a,74] Microglia is one of the key components of the interaction between inflammation and neuropathy and is a target of perineural LA infusion.[72] In animals, a sciatic nerve block performed before nerve ligation reduced the elevation of p38, a protein kinase, in microglia, whereas it was ineffective after ligation.[88] Some mitogen-activated protein kinases are overexpressed in patients with long-term use of opioids before surgery, worsening allodynia by adenosine triphosphate and cytokines and amplifying central sensitization.[40]

These clinical and experimental data support using CNBs as part of a multimodal analgesic strategy to optimize analgesic and antihyperalgesic effectiveness. Results of studies favored CNB for TKA compared with oral or IV opioids, with lower mean and maximum VAS scores between POD0 and POD3 and 63% less morphine consumption.[78,91] CNB also reduced the risk of nausea and vomiting with a number needed to treat of four.[91] In a meta-analysis of 19 studies, CNB produced a 15-mg mean reduction in morphine consumption after single-injection nerve block or CNB on POD1, decreased the risk of postoperative nausea and vomiting by 53%, improved knee flexion, and lowered VAS scores at rest and during mobilization.[43] VAS scores at rest and during mobilization within the first 48 hours were also reduced after CNB compared with single-injection block.[91] Femoral catheters allowed a 13-mg reduction in mean morphine consumption on POD1 and 15-mg reduction on POD2 compared with single-injection nerve block.[91]

Intensity and duration of pain relief are better controlled by CNB compared with single-injection nerve block and opioid administration. An elegant experimental study showed that repeated administration of ropivacaine through a sciatic catheter significantly reduced the duration and intensity of hyperalgesia induced by skin incision in the first 2 days, whereas hyperalgesia persisted until POD4 with a single injection of LA and until POD7 with placebo.[70] After IV fentanyl administered before plantar incision, the benefit of a CNB on nociceptive thresholds was seen during the first 2 days, whereas no impact on the intensity and duration of hyperalgesia was observed with placebo.[70] These experimental data offer a clinically relevant way to achieve effective antihyperalgesia, a phenomenon amplified by perioperative opioid use.

POSTERIOR LUMBAR PLEXUS BLOCK

Clinical Data

Clinically, a continuous posterior lumbar catheter and a femoral catheter produced a 48% to 50% reduction in morphine consumption compared with placebo without differences between the two CNBs.[56] The obturator nerve was more frequently blocked with the posterior approach than with the femoral approach, but VAS scores were not affected.[56] A second study compared a continuous posterior lumbar catheter, a femoral catheter, and a combined femoral and sciatic catheter.[73] Opioid consumption was decreased in patients in the combined group compared with patients with posterior or femoral catheters alone (−60% vs −63%), suggesting the superiority of the combination sciatic-femoral nerve block for TKA and the lack of interest of extending to the obturator and cutaneous lateral nerves, although VAS scores were not different between groups. Patients in the combined femoral-sciatic group had more difficulty ambulating than patients in the posterior lumbar or in the femoral groups, indicating the potential pitfall of motor weakness.[73] Comparing a 48-hour continuous posterior lumbar block and a single-injection block (associated in both cases with a sciatic nerve block), no differences were noted in tramadol consumption despite a prolongation of the time to first demand in the CNB group.[29] Finally, a placebo-controlled study compared the posterior lumbar plexus catheter over 48 hours with a single-injection block (both associated with a single-injection sciatic nerve block) with morphine consumption as a primary outcome.[85] Patients in the catheter group required 41% less morphine than patients in the single-injection group and ambulated earlier from POD1.[85] If the posterior lumbar catheter benefits are documented after TKA, CNBs were performed with neurostimulation alone, without anti-hyperalgesic optimization, and associated with a sciatic nerve block.

The evolution of surgical and anesthetic techniques and the need to promote active early rehabilitation have led to less invasive analgesic techniques for TKA, and posterior lumbar plexus block could be an alternative in selected patients. The development of ultrasound guidance is a positive step for the proponents of this technique.

In general, insertion must be done aseptically with preparation of a large cutaneous area, surgical draping, gloves and caps for the operator and assistant, use of a sterile sheath covering the probe completely, and sterile gel. This recommendation is valid for all continuous catheters.

Ultrasound-Guided Posterior Lumbar Plexus Block

Until more recently, most posterior approaches had been performed with neurostimulation alone with surface landmarks at the L3, L4, or L5 levels. Capdevila and colleagues[14] showed that the L4 level described by Winnie and associates[90] using the intersection between the line connecting the iliac crests and the perpendicular line passing through the posterior superior iliac spine parallel to the axis of the spinous processes was too lateral. Computed tomography scan has determined the optimal insertion point at the lateral one-third and medial two-thirds of a line between the L4 spinal process and the line parallel to the spinal processes passing through the posterior spinal iliac spine.[14] After opacification of catheters, 74% of them were shown to be located in the psoas major muscle, and 22% were shown to be between the psoas and quadratus lumborum muscles.[14] One study[4] compared catheters inserted with either a medial or a lateral approach at the L4 level and found a higher frequency of catheters with opacification outside of the psoas muscle laterally, caudally, and around the kidney in a more lateral approach than initially described.[90] The medial edge of the lumbar paravertebral space was constantly opacified with an apical limit at the L1-2 disk level.[66]

The risks associated with posterior lumbar plexus block performed using cutaneous landmarks and neurostimulation are peritoneal puncture, kidney puncture, epidural or intrathecal extension, hematoma, or systemic absorption.[33] The combination of neurostimulation and ultrasound guidance (Figs. 97.1 and 97.2) was assessed to define the deep transverse process and facilitate the identification of the lumbar plexus.[43,59,60]

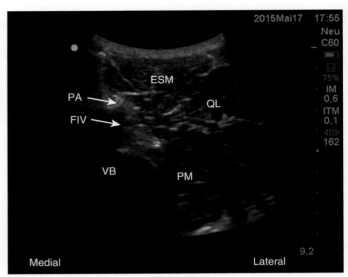

FIG 97.1 Ultrasound scan with a 2- to 5-MHz curved array positioned to obtain a transverse sonogram of the lumbar paravertebral region. *AP,* Articular process; *asterisk,* lumbar plexus; *ESM,* erector spinae muscles; *FIV,* foramen intervertebrale; *PM,* psoas muscle; *QL,* quadratus lumborum muscle; *VB,* vertebral body.

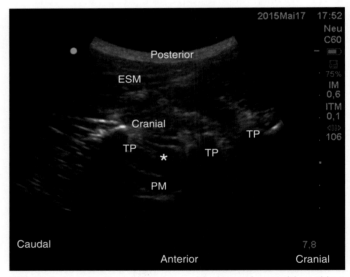

FIG 97.2 Longitudinal sonogram with the probe positioned in a sagittal and paramedian orientation. Transverse processes *(TP)* of L5, L4, and L3 are visualized with, from caudal to cranial. The needle is introduced with an in-plane approach, associated with neurostimulation (see text for description). *,* Location of lumbar plexus; *ESM,* erector spinae muscles.

In both procedures, ultrasound eliminates the issue of using Tuffier's (intercristal) line as a landmark, which can vary from L5-S1 to L3-4. Compared with the puncture site described by Capdevila and colleagues,[14] the puncture is too lateral in 50% of cases to help identify the costiform process, and optimization of the image is obtained after repositioning of the probe more medially by approximately 0.75 cm.[43] It is impossible to identify the transverse processes with ultrasound in only 6% of cases.[43]

FEMORAL CATHETER

Clinical Data

The femoral nerve arises from dorsal divisions of the ventral rami of L2 to L4. Many anatomical variations were described on its disposal within the psoas major muscle, the content of the dorsal divisions and its course.[75] The benefit of continuous femoral blockade was validated in a meta-analysis including more than 1000 patients.[17] VAS scores were reduced at rest and during movement, and IV morphine requirements decreased by 15 mg within the first 48 hours postoperatively.[8] The risk of postoperative nausea and vomiting was also reduced by 53% compared with opioids.[17] Femoral catheters were more effective than single-injection nerve blocks in decreasing VAS scores at rest and during mobilization and opioid requirements, with a mean reduction of 14 mg.[17] The two main questions for femoral catheters concern the ultrasound-guided optimization of catheter position and the risk of quadriceps weakness.

Clinical data did not find a decisive advantage of ultrasound guidance compared with neurostimulation for the effectiveness of CNB.[20] The benefit of ultrasound guidance demonstrated for single-injection blocks compared with surface landmarks or neurostimulation[2,8] cannot be transposed directly to catheters. However, ultrasound-guided femoral catheters allowed the reduction of LA by 30% compared with neurostimulation.[6] This constitutes an option to decrease quadriceps dysfunction associated with CNBs, although quadriceps dysfunction is also due to other factors such as the surgery itself and the use of a tourniquet. One study showed that only 23% of femoral catheters inserted with neurostimulation are correctly positioned, whereas 33% are located under the fascia of the psoas muscle and 37% are located below the iliacus muscle.[13] The sensory and motor block success rate in the last two positions was low, 52% and 27%, whereas it reached 91% when the catheter was correctly located.[13]

Stimulating catheters do not reduce LA use,[38] time to sensory and motor block,[25] or postoperative morphine consumption.[2] The success rate of neurostimulation is influenced by several factors such as length of catheter in contact with the nerve, surface landmarks used, anatomic variations,[4,86] minimal stimulus intensity, and choice of normal saline or 5% dextrose in water.[77] Ultrasound improves the quality of the block, reduces the risk of vascular puncture and systemic toxicity,[2,8,82] and enhances optimization of catheter's tip position in contact with the nerve under the iliac fascia.[20]

Catheters can be inserted using a long-axis view of the femoral nerve with a cephalad orientation (Figs. 97.3 and 97.4), using a short-axis view of the femoral nerve (Fig. 97.5), or more often perpendicular to the nerve with a lateral-to-medial orientation (Figs. 97.6 and 97.7). The approach using a long-axis view is more difficult and increases the procedure time.[36] Comparing an in-plane and an out-of-plane approach in a short-axis view, the maximum intensity of pain (primary outcome) as well as LA use did not differ.[30] However, satisfaction evaluated with pain during catheter insertion was higher among patients in the out-of-plane group than in the in-plane group.[30] The out-of-plane approach (see Fig. 97.5) needs to use hydrolocation during the progression of the needle. The combination of ultrasound and neurostimulation reduced the use of LA compared with neurostimulation alone.[6] A prospective study demonstrated noninferiority between ultrasound-guided femoral catheters placed with an in-plane

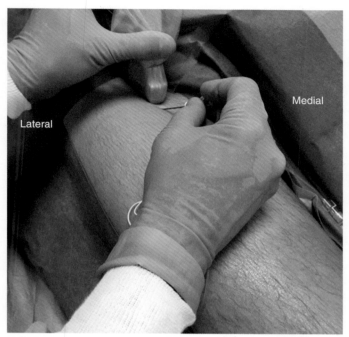

FIG 97.3 High-frequency linear probe and needle position for an in-plane approach of the femoral nerve in a long-axis view.

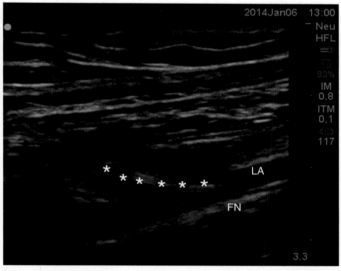

FIG 97.4 High-frequency ultrasound scan showing the catheter inserted in an in-plane approach in a long-axis view and local anesthetic *(LA)*.

approach in a short-axis view of the nerve and neurostimulation in regard to VAS scores and opioid requirement.[27]

Another aspect concerns the extent of the motor and sensory nerve block during CNB. The anatomic description of the usual motor fibers of the quadriceps muscle shows predominance on the dorsal part of the nerve, whereas sensory fibers are more superficial and peripheral.[36] Healthy volunteers in whom femoral catheters were inserted using a short-axis view anteriorly or posteriorly to the nerve were evaluated with voluntary isometric contraction as primary objective.[44] Contraction was significantly reduced in both groups compared with baselines (29% ± 26% and 30% ± 28%, respectively) but without

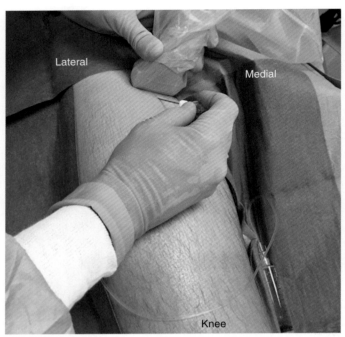

FIG 97.5 High-frequency linear probe and needle position for an out-of plane approach of the femoral nerve.

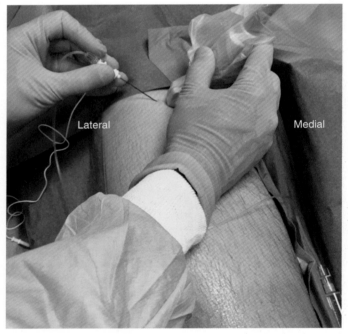

FIG 97.6 High-frequency linear probe and needle for femoral nerve catheter using an in-plane approach. The probe is positioned to obtain a short-axis view.

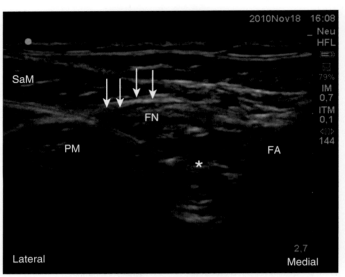

FIG 97.7 High-frequency ultrasound scan showing the tip of the catheter (*) in a transverse view (short axis) located between the femoral nerve (FN) and iliopsoas muscle (PM) within the echoic spread of local anesthetic. *Arrows,* Iliac fascia; *FA,* femoral artery; *SaM,* sartorius muscle.

differences between the anterior and posterior positions after 6 hours of infusion of 0.1% ropivacaine.[44] However, the sensory block was more important on the anterior aspect of the thigh when the catheter was located anteriorly to the femoral nerve.[44]

The motor block might impair active rehabilitation, leading to a risk of falls during mobilization.[41,55,71] A post-hoc analysis[41] of three prospective multicenter studies in hip and knee surgeries found seven falls in six patients in the perineural analgesia groups versus none in the placebo group (three femoral catheters and four posterior lumbar catheters, flow rate 5 to 8 mL/h, time to onset between POD1 and POD4, giving a relative risk of 7% (95% confidence interval [CI], 3% to 15%). In this follow-up analysis, only one case of quadriceps weakness was involved in the falls.[41] A meta-analysis including 1595 patients found a fourfold increase in risk of falls with CNBs.[71] However, the attributable effect of CNBs was low (1.7%), giving a number need to harm of 59.[71] This database did not report the reasons for falls.[71] A multicenter database including more than 190,000 patients found an incidence of falls of 1.6% after orthopedic limb surgery.[55] Multivariate analysis found older age, male sex, comorbidities, general anesthesia (vs neuraxial), and postoperative anemia as predictive factors, whereas nerve blocks (odds ratio [OR] 0.85; 95% CI, 0.71 to 1.03) were not identified as predictive of risk.[45] A follow-up evaluation of 118 patients showed a 24% annual incidence of falls after TKA with an increased risk in the presence of preoperative instability (OR 7.75; 95% CI, 1.72 to 35.71; $P = .008$) and a higher preoperative depression score (OR 1.27; 95% CI, 1.02 to 1.58; $P = .031$).[81] Preoperative muscle weakness increased postoperative dysfunction as well as tourniquet use for surgery.[68] Both of these parameters warrant individual analysis. An outcome study including more than 2000 patients after TKA found a 2.7% incidence of fall with an increased risk in multivariate analysis in the presence of a continuous femoral nerve block (OR 4.4; 95% CI, 1.04 to 18.2; $P = .04$), obesity (OR 2.4; 95% CI, 1.3 to 4.5; $P = .005$), and older age (OR 1.04; 95% CI, 1 to 1.07; $P = .008$).[84] However, no details were available on quality of CNB and the modality of LA infusion.

Individualization of infusion rate and concentration, placement of the catheter tip anterior to the nerve, and preoperative identification of patients at risk of falls or experiencing high levels of preoperative pain would help reduce the risk of fall. Perineural catheters have been widely validated for analgesia and rehabilitation after major knee surgery[17,70] and to reduce the onset of hyperalgesia and inflammation.[7,9,70] Femoral catheters also enabled earlier resumption of ambulation after TKA with a reduction of 53% to obtain ambulation time on the operative day without opiate or pain compared with a single injection of LA followed by placebo during 4 days.[42] On POD1, 43% of patients in the CNB group required temporary interruption of LA infusion for quadriceps weakness compared with 12% in the placebo group.[42] These results were confirmed with a 15-hour reduction in delay to achieve pain relief and ambulation with CNB administered using a patient-controlled perineural mode with 0.2% ropivacaine than a single-injection block of mepivacaine.[45]

Compared with single-injection nerve blocks, CNBs do not improve multidimensional scores assessing the quality of recovery 1 year after surgery.[46,47] However, analgesia is only one of the key elements of recovery after TKA, and these results were extracted from two post-hoc analyses underpowered for this long-term objective.[28,49]

ADDUCTOR CANAL CATHETERS

Clinical Data

In volunteers, a femoral block reduced the strength of leg extension by 83% at 30 minutes and 59% at 60 minutes without impact on hip adduction.[63] In another volunteer study, a subsartorial block using a high volume of LA (0.1% ropivacaine, 30 mL) reduced quadriceps strength by 8%, whereas a femoral block reduced it by 49%.[51] The lesser impairment observed with the subsartorial block suggested a modest effect on the vastus medialis and allowed ambulation 1 hour and 6 hours after injection compared with the femoral block.[51] Some studies compared CNB performed at the subsartorial level after TKA with placebo[37,53] and with a femoral block.[35,52,61] A subsartorial catheter significantly reduced mean opioid consumption by 16 mg, reduced pain scores during mobilization on POD1 and POD2, and provided better muscle recovery on POD2.[37] In this study, all patients received preoperative femoral nerve blockade, and approximately 30% to 35% of patients received intra-articular LA with 10 mg of morphine.[37] Between POD1 and POD2, the mean difference for morphine requirement remained significant (mean reduction −10.6 mg) regardless of whether patients received intra-articular morphine.[37] Compared with placebo, intermittent subsartorial injections of ropivacaine reduced morphine requirement by 30% and VAS scores during knee flexion and improved functional recovery as evaluated by the time up to go (TUG) test.[53] A prospective study compared ultrasound-guided femoral and subsartorial catheters on voluntary isometric contraction of the quadriceps.[52] Patients in the subsartorial group exhibited better isometric quadriceps contraction (mean difference 26%) without any impact on hip adduction but without differences in VAS scores and morphine consumption during the first 24 hours.[52] An adductor canal block was noninferior to femoral block for VAS scores and opioid consumption but was more effective in preservation of quadriceps function.[61] This study was limited by the addition of postoperative epidural analgesia impacting the quality of analgesia.[61] There are no clear data on the use of adductor canal catheters for arthroscopic knee surgery, which is often considered markedly less painful than TKA.

Ultrasound-Guided Subsartorial Catheter

A continuous infusion of 5 mL/h of 0.2% ropivacaine or 0.125% levobupivacaine, with a bolus of 5 mL every 30 minutes, is

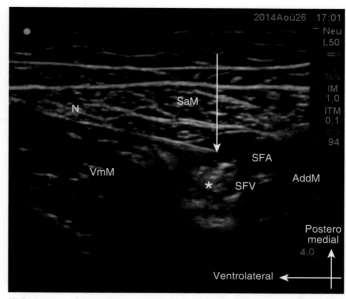

FIG 97.8 Ultrasound view of the subsartorial space after injection. Needle *(N)* was inserted along the fascia of the sartorius muscle *(SaM)*. *AddM,* Adductor magnus muscle; *arrow,* tip of the needle and hypoechoic spread of local anesthetic; **,* location of saphenous nerve and nerve to the vastus medialis muscle; *SFA,* superficial femoral artery; *SFV,* superficial femoral vein; *VmM,* vastus medialis muscle.

commonly used despite the fact that the optimal dose of LA for subsartorial catheters remains to be determined. The needle usually is introduced using a lateromedial approach, and the catheter is inserted with an in-plane technique in the short-axis view (Figs. 97.8 and 97.9). This block also represents an effective analgesic technique in association with intra-articular analgesia or an effective technique to treat severe postoperative pain not relieved by systemic analgesics[50] as well as an effective alternative to femoral block with limited quadriceps impairment. A femoral block using a 6-hour continuous 5 mL/h infusion of 0.1% ropivacaine or 6 hourly bolus doses reduced quadriceps strength similarly by 84% and 83%.[18] Another study confirmed this result where a continuous administration of 4 mL/h of 0.05% or 0.1% levobupivacaine through a femoral catheter reduced quadriceps strength similarly by 30%.[26] A case report described a transient quadriceps motor block after an adductor canal block performed with 20 mL of 0.5% ropivacaine.[19] Another report described an extension to the sciatic nerve in the popliteal fossa after a distal trans-sartorial approach.[32] In the latter case report, the tip of the catheter was close to the inferior hiatus of the adductor canal, and opacification revealed contrast diffusion around divisions of the sciatic nerve.[32] Despite these two reports, such blocks remain a rare event, but they raise the problem of interfascial anatomic variations or the methodologic problems of the level of injection or catheter placement.

SCIATIC CATHETERS

The sciatic nerve is involved in the innervation of the anterior and posterior capsule to the bone surfaces (in particular the tibia) and posterior skin. Several approaches have been described

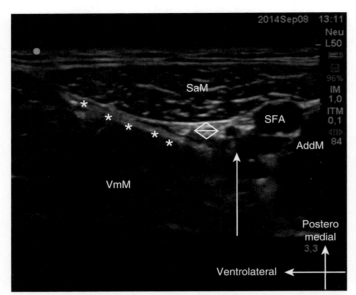

FIG 97.9 Ultrasound view of the subsartorial space after injection. *AddM,* Adductor magnus muscle; *arrow,* tip of the catheter around the saphenous nerve and nerve to the vastus medialis muscle *(white lozenge)* within the hypoechoic halo of local anesthetic; *asterisk,* catheter inserted from a lateral to medial direction and using an in-plane approach; *SaM,* sartorius muscle; *SFA,* superficial femoral artery; *SFV,* superficial femoral vein; *VmM,* vastus medialis muscle.

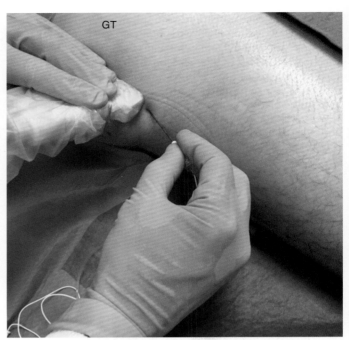

FIG 97.10 Needle and probe position for an in-plane approach in long-axis view of the sciatic nerve in the subgluteal region.

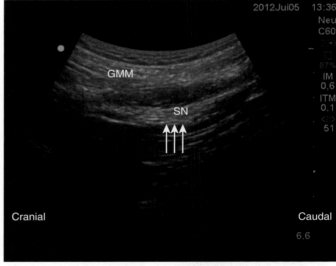

FIG 97.11 Long-axis view of the sciatic nerve *(SN)* at the anterior face of the gluteus maximus muscle *(GMM)* with a 2- to 5-MHz curved array at the subgluteal level. *Arrows,* Tip of the catheter; *,* local anesthetic spread.

including parasacral plexus block, anterior sciatic block, posterior infragluteal block (Figs. 97.10 to 97.13), or selective tibial nerve block more distally.[80] Distal catheters have not been evaluated for major knee surgery. A qualitative analysis comprising three studies favored sciatic catheters for TKA based on VAS scores at rest for the first 24 hours and morphine consumption during the first 24 hours.[24] No benefits were identified for scores during mobilization or in rehabilitation scores.[1] Sciatic catheters were associated with femoral catheters and were inserted using neurostimulation. However, this analysis noted a reduction in the incidence of pain in the posterior part of the knee.[1]

After the publication of this meta-analysis, three other prospective studies were published.[16,79,87] The first compared a femoral catheter alone or associated with a single-injection parasacral block or a continuous parasacral block.[87] No significant differences occurred, but patients in the parasacral catheter group needed less morphine up to POD2 compared with the femoral catheter group, with no differences between the single-injection parasacral nerve and continuous sciatic blocks.[87] The second study assessed a continuous sciatic infragluteal catheter placed with neurostimulation associated with a continuous posterior lumbar plexus block versus placebo with morphine consumption as the primary outcome.[5] The combined continuous lumbar-sciatic nerve block reduced morphine consumption by 75% and VAS scores on knee flexion during the first 48 hours.[16] Ambulation was also achieved faster without falls despite the posterior lumbar block.[16] Finally, the third placebo-controlled study compared an ultrasound-guided sciatic catheter placed through an anterior approach with a single-injection

sciatic nerve block, both associated with a femoral catheter over 48 hours.[79] Results favored the sciatic catheter group for the primary outcome with a 50% decrease in morphine consumption until POD2.[79] The VAS scores were also reduced in the continuous sciatic group over the same period with no difference in maximum knee flexion or the duration of hospitalization.[79] The in-plane (see Figs. 97.10 and 97.11) and out-of-plane (see Figs. 97.12 and 97.13) approaches produce similar results, but the long-axis technique is more difficult and takes more time to perform.

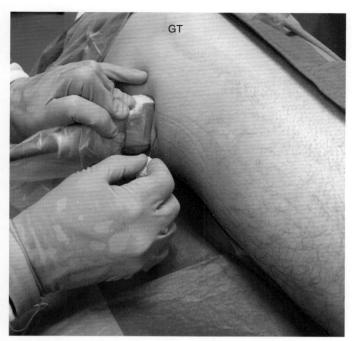

FIG 97.12 Probe and needle position for an out-of-plane approach of the sciatic nerve by a subgluteal block with patient in lateral decubitus. The transducer is usually a 2- to 5-MHz curve-linear probe, but in a thin patient a high-frequency linear 6- to 15-MHz probe can be used. *GT,* Greater trochanter.

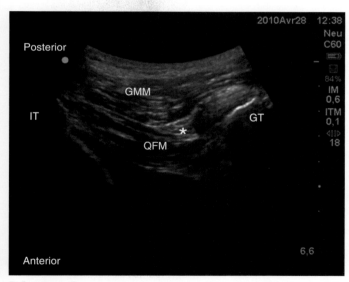

FIG 97.13 Transverse view (short axis) showing the sciatic nerve *(SN)* between the gluteus maximus muscle *(GMM)* posteriorly and quadratus femoris muscle *(QFM)* anteriorly. *GT,* Greater trochanter; *IT,* ischial tuberosity.

INFECTION AND PERINEURAL CATHETERS FOR KNEE SURGERY

The infectious risk associated with perineural catheters is difficult to establish but remains very low—approximately 0.1% if aseptic measures are observed—despite a frequency of colonization ranging from 6% to 57%.[11,54,58,65,89] The femoral localization did not increase the risk in multivariate analysis,[5,15] and femoral catheters appeared to be less often colonized than interscalene catheters (OR 1.18; 95% CI, 1.1 to 1.3; $P = .024$) in a prospective study including more than 700 catheters.[5] There are no data for septic complications after subsartorial catheters, but no infections have been attributed directly to the catheter in prospective studies.[35,37,51-53,61] Diabetes was a recognized risk factor for colonization in a prospective study (OR 2.32; 95% CI, 1.43 to 9.58; $P = .004$)[5] and in a retrospective analysis (OR 2.42; 95% CI, 1.05 to 5.57; $P = .039$).[11] Other risk factors have been identified such as the duration of catheter use,[5,15] prior antibiotic therapy for sepsis,[5] and the absence of antibiotic prophylaxis,[15] the last factor being bypassed by the perioperative prophylaxis used for major knee surgeries. The in-plane approach during ultrasound-guided insertion allows the realization of a subcutaneous tunnel, which is an effective technique to reduce colonization.[22] The identification of patients at risk, strict observance of aseptic guidelines during catheter insertion, and reduction of manipulation of catheters all help reduce the risk of colonization and infection. By comparison, the incidence of colonization of suction drains after TKA reached 25% on POD2.[89]

OBTURATOR NERVE BLOCK

No study has evaluated continuous obturator nerve blockade for knee surgery.[58,65] The obturator nerve block remains controversial for analgesia and rehabilitation. Spread to the knee articular branch from the posterior part of the obturator nerve is likely during the subsartorial adductor canal block, but the unpredictability of its sensory distribution and the difficulty to test its motor component specifically make it difficult to draw conclusions.

CONCLUSION

CNBs are an effective strategy during major knee surgery to reduce pain and inflammation and allow rehabilitation. Ultrasound-guided subsartorial catheters are a promising alternative to conventional femoral catheters, but better prospective evaluation regarding the optimal placement of the catheter and the optimal dose of LA is needed. A meta-analysis documented superiority of subsartorial catheters compared with placebo in regard to VAS scores and opioid consumption, but a limitation in interpreting these results was the variety of perioperative anesthetic strategies used (periarticular infiltration, intrathecal analgesia, general anesthesia, multimodal analgesic drugs), which may have an impact on the results.[54] Periarticular infiltration analgesia is increasingly used, and the subsartorial catheter is a potential associated strategy because 26% of patients after TKA can present with severe postoperative pain.[34,50] Sciatic nerve catheters can be used to optimize posterior knee pain or after revised TKA. The literature on femoral nerve blocks regarding pain relief and rehabilitation is more robust, but caution is needed with ambulation. Complications of CNBs are low and likely depend on compliance with guidelines and the use of ultrasound.

KEY REFERENCES

1. Abdallah FW, Brull R: Is sciatic nerve block advantageous when combined with femoral nerve block for postoperative analgesia following

total knee arthroplasty? A systematic review. *Reg Anesth Pain Med* 36:493–498, 2011.

6. Aveline C, et al: Postoperative efficacies of femoral nerve catheters sited using ultrasound combined with neurostimulation compared with neurostimulation alone for total knee arthroplasty. *Eur J Anaesthesiol* 27:978–984, 2010.

28. Franco CD, et al: Innervation of the anterior capsule of the human knee: implications for radiofrequency ablation. *Reg Anesth Pain Med* 40:363–368, 2015.

31. Fuzier R, et al: Analgesic drug consumption increases after knee arthroplasty: a pharmacoepidemiological study investigating postoperative pain. *Pain* 155:1339–1345, 2014.

34. Grevstad U, et al: Effect of canal block on pain in patients with severe pain after total knee arthroplasty: a randomized study in individual patient analysis. *Br J Anaesth* 112:912–919, 2014.

42. Ilfeld BM, et al: Ambulatory continuous femoral nerve blocks decrease time to discharge readiness after tricompartment total knee arthroplasty: a randomized, triple-masked, placebo-controlled study. *Anesthesiology* 108:703–713, 2008.

46. Ilfeld BM, et al: Health-related quality of life after tricompartment knee arthroplasty with and without an extended-duration continuous femoral nerve block: a prospective, 1-year follow-up of a randomized, triple-masked, placebo-controlled study. *Anesth Analg* 108:1320–1325, 2009.

55. Johnson RL, et al: Falls and major orthopaedic surgery with peripheral nerve blockade: a systematic review and meta-analysis. *Br J Anaesth* 110:518–528, 2013.

57. Kapoor R, et al: The saphenous nerve and its relationship to the nerve to the vastus medialis in and around the adductor canal: an anatomical study. *Acta Anaesthesiol Scand* 56:365–367, 2012.

60. Karmakar MK, et al: Ultrasound-guided lumbar plexus block using a transverse scan through the lumbar intertransverse space: a prospective case series. *Reg Anesth Pain Med* 40:75–81, 2015.

68. Martin F, et al: Antiinflammatory effect of peripheral nerve blocks after knee surgery: clinical and biologic evaluation. *Anesthesiology* 10:484–490, 2008.

70. Méleine M, et al: Sciatic nerve block fails in preventing the development of late stress-induced hyperalgesia when high-dose fentanyl is administered perioperatively in rats. *Reg Anesth Pain Med* 37:448–454, 2012.

71. Memtsoudis SG, et al: Inpatient falls after total knee arthroplasty: the role of anesthesia type and peripheral nerve blocks. *Anesthesiology* 120:551–563, 2014.

82. Walker KJ, et al: Ultrasound guidance for peripheral nerve blockade. *Cochrane Database Syst Rev* (4):CD006459, 2009.

91. Xu J, et al: Peripheral nerve blocks for postoperative pain after major knee surgery. *Cochrane Database Syst Rev* (12):CD01093, 2014.

The references for this chapter can also be found on www.expertconsult.com.

Local Anesthetic Infiltration

John P. Begly, Jonathan M. Vigdorchik

PERIARTICULAR INJECTION

Total knee arthroplasty (TKA) is among the most frequently and most successful procedures performed by orthopedic surgeons today.[22] Despite excellent outcomes, recovery from TKA remains a significant challenge for patients. Postoperative pain may be severe, and can negatively impact the course of rehabilitation.[17,18] Multiple pain management strategies have been used to effectively control postoperative pain, such as parenteral narcotics and peripheral nerve blockade.[18] However, these methods are associated with potentially dangerous side effects, and may provide insufficient postoperative pain control.[1,12,15]

Recently, periarticular injection (PAI) has gained popularity as an additional tool in the multimodal approach to the management of joint arthroplasty pain. PAI has been shown to result in reduced surgical pain and opioid consumption,[16,29,31] and provides pain control comparable to that of epidural anesthesia but without the associated complications of this modality.[2]

The use of PAI allows for decreased dependency on alternative methods of pain control, such as epidural anesthesia, peripheral nerve blockade, and parenteral narcotics, which carry unique risks. Forst et al. reported on significant adverse events associated with the use of continuous femoral nerve blockade, including muscle weakness, nerve damage, and local infection.[18] Heavy postoperative opioid use is associated with respiratory depression, hypotension, motor weakness, and urinary retention, and Dillon et al. have reported that these side effects negatively impact patient recovery.[15] Indeed, Oderda et al. determined that opioid use was associated with longer hospital stays and higher hospitalization costs in surgical patients.[27]

Multiple studies have demonstrated that the use of PAI results in lower opioid use in postoperative arthroplasty patients.[2,16,24,30,31] In a randomized controlled trial, Busch et al. found that patients who received intraoperative PAI used less patient-controlled analgesia at 6, 12, and 24 hours postoperatively, and also reported lower pain scores in the postoperative unit.[10] Mullaji et al. examined the efficacy of PAI by performing periarticular injections in only one operative knee in 40 patients who underwent bilateral TKA. The patients reported improved pain scores and demonstrated superior range of flexion and quadriceps function on the infiltrated side.[24]

Comparing PAI to epidural anesthesia, Thorsell et al. found pain scores to be equivalent between the groups but that patients in the PAI mobilized quicker and reported improved satisfaction.[29] Chaumeron et al. reported similar benefits of PAI, including improved ambulation and quadriceps function compared to femoral nerve blockade.[11] These advantages are significant in shortening inpatient stay and associated perioperative risk and hospital costs.[16] Labrara et al. reported that rapid rehab after knee arthroplasty resulted in decreased length of hospital stay.[23] Shorter inpatient postoperative periods have been associated with decreased risk of respiratory complications and deep venous thrombosis.[20] In a systematic review of multimodal wound infiltration analgesia in TKA, Banerjee et al. reported that PAI resulted in increased mobilization, decreased risk of perioperative infection and complications, and a shortened time to discharge.[7] The addition of liposomal bupivacaine (Exparel) to periarticular regional analgesia has been demonstrated to result in rapid rehabilitation, even in TKA procedures performed in an outpatient setting,[8] although some authors failed to find any advantage.[5]

In a retrospective review, Perlas et al. noted further improvements in early ambulation and a higher incidence of home discharge in patients who received an adductor canal block in addition to PAI, compared to PAI alone or to a continuous femoral nerve block.[28]

FORMULATIONS

PAI typically involves the infiltration of a "pain cocktail" into the local tissues. The effects of this cocktail are dependent on several factors: type of analgesic, percentage of medication, additives or adjuncts, and density of nerve fibers or vascularity of the area to be injected. The composition of this formulation varies according to institution, and multiple effective preparations have been described* (Table 98.1). At the authors' institution, the following formulation is used for unilateral TKA (Fig. 98.1):

- 2.5 mg/mL bupivacaine, 40 mL total
- 5 mg preservative-free morphine (Duramorph), 1 mg/mL, 5 mL total
- 30 mg ketorolac, 30 mg/mL, 1 mL total

In some formulations, epinephrine is included to aid in maintaining anesthetic levels in tissues and to help control bleeding. Consideration must be given to patients' comorbidities. In the setting of significant renal disease and/or allergy, ketorolac is typically held. In patients older than 75 years, or who have a history of peptic ulcer disease, diabetes, or a creatinine clearance of 30 to 50 mg/minute, 15 mg (0.5 mL) of ketorolac is used. The total volume of the formulation is approximately 46 mL.

Recently, the use of liposomal bupivacaine (Exparel, Pacira Pharmaceuticals, Parsippany, NJ) has gained popularity.

*References 2, 9, 10, 13, 14, 15, 18, 20, 23, and 27.

TABLE 98.1	A Selection of Periarticular Infiltration Formulations Described in Peer-Reviewed Literature. The Formulations Described Previously Apply to Unilateral Total Knee Arthroplasty
Publication	**Periarticular Injection Formulation**

Kerr and Kohan[21]	• Total of 150-175 mL
	  • Ropivacaine HCl 2 mg/mL
	  • Ketorolac 30 mg/mL
	  • Epinephrine 10 μg/mL
	  • Normal saline, dilute to total mL

Andersen et al.[2]	• Total of 150 mL
	  • Ropivacaine 2-150 mg/mL
	  • Epinephrine 10 μg/mL

Essving et al.[16]	• Total volume not defined
	  • 400 mg Ropivacaine
	  • 30 mg Ketorolac 30 mg/mL
	  • Epinephrine 0.5 mg

Mullaji et al.[24]	• Total volume not defined
	  • Bupivacaine 2 mg/kg body weight
	  • Fentanyl 100 μg
	  • Methylprednisolone acetate 40 mg
	  • Cefuroxime 750 mg
	  • Normal saline 25 mL

Thorsell et al.[29]	• Total volume of 156 mL
	  • Ropivacaine 2 mg/mL—150 mL
	  • Epinephrine 0.1 mg/mL—5 mL
	  • Ketorolac 30 mg/mL—1 mL

Dalury et al.[14]	• Total of 100 mL
	  • Ropivacaine 5 mg/mL—49.25 mL
	  • Epinephrine 1 mg/mL—0.5 mL
	  • Ketorolac 30 mg/mL—1 mL
	  • Clonidine 0.1 mg/mL—0.8 mL
	  • Normal saline—48.45 mL

Dillon et al.[15]	• Total volume not defined
	  • Ropivacaine HCl 2 mg/mL
	  • Ketorolac 30 mg/mL—1 mL
	  • Dexamethasone—4 mg
	  • Epinephrine—1 mg

Chaumeron et al.[11]	• Total volume 109 mL
	  • Ropivacaine HCl 10 mg/mL—7.5 mL
	  • Ketorolac 30 mg/mL—1 mL
	  • Epinephrine—0.5 mL
	  • Ropivacaine HCl 0.2 mg/mL—100 mL

Guild III et al.[19]	• Total of 60 mL in single syringe
	  • Exparel 266 mg—20 mL
	  • Bupivacaine 2.5 mg/mL—20 mL
	  • Epinephrine 1:200,000
	  • Normal Saline—20 mL

Authors' Home Institution Policy	• Total of 46 mL
	  • Marcaine 2.5 mg/mL—40 mL
	  • Duramorph 1 mg/mL—5 mL
	  • Ketorolac 30 mg/mL—1 mL
	• Exparel injection. 60 mL into 20-mL syringes × 3
	  • 266 mg Exparel—20 mL
	  • Normal saline—40 mL

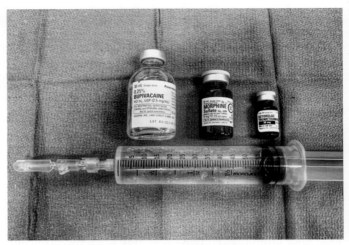

FIG 98.1 Formulation used for periarticular injection at the authors' home institution.

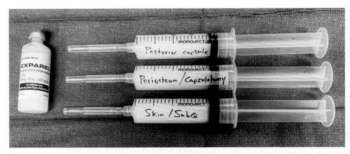

FIG 98.2 Periarticular injection divided into three 20-mL syringes with 21-gauge needles.

days, providing effective longer-term pain control.[8] An osmotic diuresis of Exparel from the lysosomes can be prevented by adding bupivacaine to another cocktail at a dosage of 50% or less of the Exparel dose. Also, lidocaine or ropivacaine should not be used within 20 minutes of Exparel to prevent replacement of the bupivacaine in the lysosome. Per our institutional policy, Exparel is administered separately from the pain cocktail. In unilateral arthroplasty, the maximum dose of Exparel is 266 mg (1 vial, 20 mL). This is combined with 40 mL of normal saline for a total of 60 mL, which is divided into three 20-mL syringes with 18- or 21-gauge needles (Fig. 98.2). Exparel can be expanded up to a total volume of 300 mL with 0.9% normal saline to accommodate larger surgical sites without impacting efficacy. The suspension is injected into the capsule, periosteum and fascia, and subcutaneous tissues. Exparel is viscous and does not diffuse like regular bupivacaine (Fig. 98.3). The goal of injection is to distribute the liposomes across the surgical site and in each layer of the tissue, and thus requires repeated injections.

PREOPERATIVE CONSIDERATIONS

All procedures in orthopedic surgery require effective planning and communication, and periarticular injections are no exception to this rule. Preoperatively, surgeons should discuss the method of pain control with the anesthesiologist, nursing, and the perioperative staff. The type and amount of each medication should be understood by all members of the surgical team.

Exparel is bupivacaine encapsulated by DepoFoam, a multivesicular liposomal product-delivery technology that encapsulates drugs without altering their molecular structure and releases them over a desired period of time. The bupivacaine is released from the vesicles into the soft tissues of the knee over several

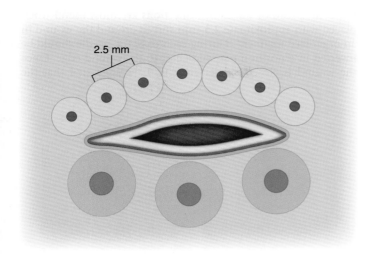

FIG 98.3 Diffusion of Exparel *(purple dots)* compared to that of Marcaine *(teal dots)*. Exparel does not diffuse as much within infiltrated tissues, and therefore additional separate needle sticks are necessary to fully infiltrate a given area of tissue.

Necessary equipment including syringes and needles should be available prior to the start of the procedure. Intraoperative efficiency will be optimized with the preparation and communication of the surgical team.

PERIARTICULAR INJECTION TECHNIQUE

Correct technique is essential in ensuring maximal benefit from periarticular injection during TKA. The use of the small-gauge needle (18-25 gauge) is recommended. Each pass of the needle needs to be to an appropriate and safe depth for the particular tissue under injection. Once this depth is reached, the surgeon should aspirate to ensure that intravascular injection does not occur. Injection of the medication should be performed slowly and continuously as the needle is withdrawn from the tissue (Fig. 98.4).

Ideally, injections should be 2.5 mm apart, leaving approximately 1 to 2 mL in each location (Fig. 98.5). The goal of each injection should be to maximize the amount of fluid within the soft tissues. Pain control from PAI is dependent on adequate tissue infiltration. Each injection should involve a small volume, as injecting too much fluid in a single pass will lead to extravasation.[13]

The rationale behind PAI is based on an understanding of the neuroanatomy of the human knee joint. The density of nerve endings is not homogeneous throughout the joint; rather, pain receptors tend to be localized to specific areas within the knee. In their comprehensive review of PAI, Guild III et al. outline the areas of highest innervation, including the suprapatellar pouch and quad tendon, medial retinaculum, patellar tendon, fat pad, medial collateral ligament and medial meniscal capsular attachments, posterior cruciate ligament tibial attachment, anterior cruciate ligament femoral attachment, lateral collateral ligament and lateral meniscal capsular attachments, and the lateral retinaculum.[19] Throughout the knee joint, the periosteum is also highly innervated. Multiple studies have demonstrated that intra-articular injections provide inferior pain control to that provided by PAI.[2,4]

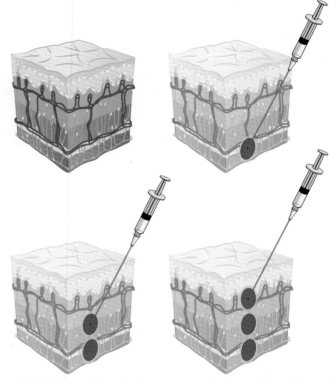

FIG 98.4 Illustration of the correct technique of needle withdrawal from tissue, beginning with the top left and proceeding to the bottom right. *Purple circles* represent injected analgesia.

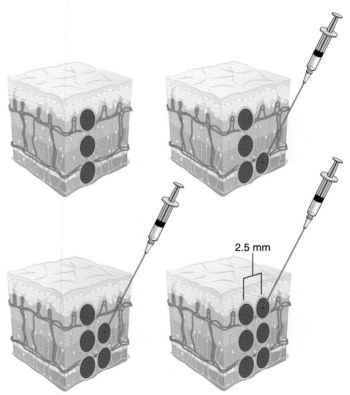

FIG 98.5 Recommended interval distance between individual injections.

The first injections should be placed after the femoral, tibial, and patellar cuts have been performed and before the final components have been inserted. The knee is placed into flexion and laminar spreaders are applied to the lateral and medial joint to provide visualization of the posteromedial and posterolateral structures, respectively (Fig. 98.6). Injection into the posterior capsule must be performed with particular care. Although variation exists, the popliteal artery on average is present approximately 2 cm from the posterior capsule when the knee is positioned in flexion. In more than 95% of patients, the artery is located just lateral to the midline of the joint (Fig. 98.7).[26] A maximal depth of 3 mm is recommended for posterior capsule injection.

The anterior cruciate ligament (ACL) femoral origin and the posterior cruciate ligament (PCL) tibial attachments are highly innervated structures and PAI of these structures may enhance pain control.[19] When using a cruciate-retaining prosthesis design, injection into the PCL should be performed.

Following posterior capsule infiltration, the injection is administered into the lateral femoral and tibial periosteum. The surgeon must be aware of the location of the peroneal nerve while performing lateral injections. As the tissue is infiltrated, a wheal should visibly form. The injection is then administered into the medial femoral and tibial periosteum. Again, watch for the formation of a wheal and confirmation of tissue infiltration (Fig. 98.8).

Once the knee is balanced and the final components are cemented into place, the second syringe may be used for capsular injections. Highly innervated structures to target include sites along the arthrotomy, the proximal extensor mechanism, the patellar periosteum, the retinaculum, the anterior capsule, and the fat pad (Fig. 98.9).

The final syringe is reserved for subcutaneous tissue and skin injections. Often, a significantly lower volume of fluid is necessary for injections into these layers (Figs. 98.10 and 98.11). Surgeons should aim for maximal tissue infiltration and uniform spread of injections. Injections are most useful when placed with approximate 2.5-mm spread around the wound in an organized manner.[21] During each pass, the needle should be inserted in a position perpendicular to the wound edge. Once the wound is closed, Andersen et al. have suggested that the

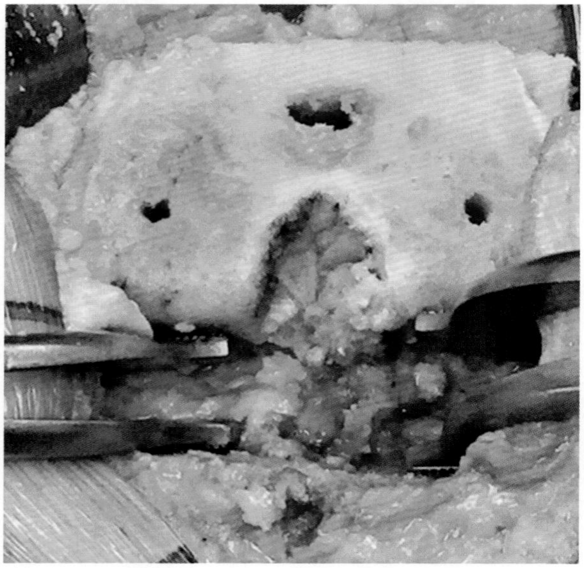

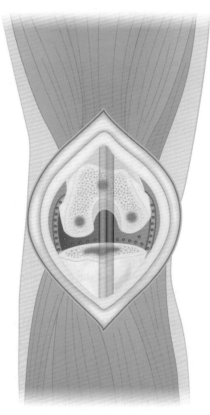

FIG 98.7 Artist rendition of posterior capsule target injection sites *(red dots)*. Note the close proximity of injection sites and posterior neuromuscular structures.

FIG 98.6 Laminar spreaders placed in the knee joint, providing visualization of the posteromedial and posterolateral capsules.

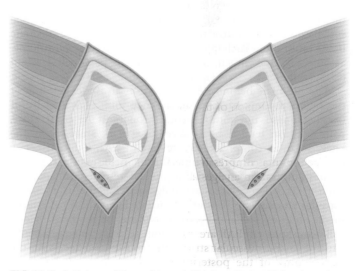

FIG 98.8 Artist rendition of target tibial periosteal injection sites *(red dots)*.

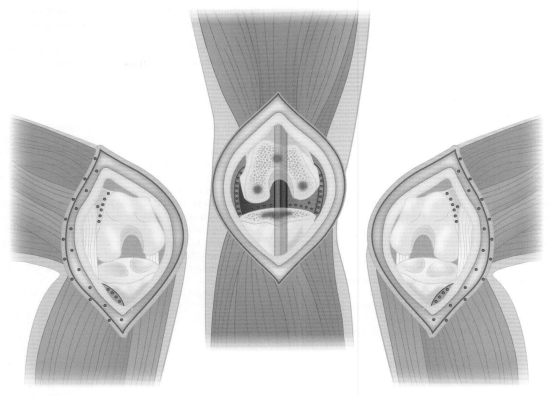

FIG 98.9 Illustration depicting target sites *(red dots)* for periarticular injection of the knee.

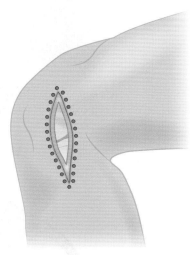

FIG 98.10 Illustration of the locations of superficial layer injection sites.

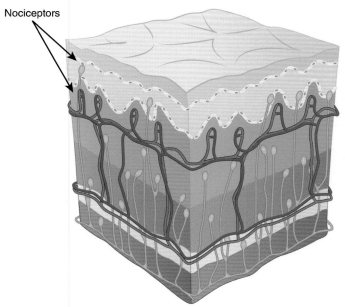

Nociceptors

FIG 98.11 Illustration of layers of the skin with distribution of nerve endings.

application of a compressive bandage may improve the efficacy of local infiltration analgesia.[3]

COMPLICATIONS

Complications of PAI are rare but do exist. These include damage to neurovascular structures, including the neurovascular anatomy of the posterior knee and the peroneal nerve laterally. Additionally, when used incorrectly, the pain medications themselves carry potentially serious systemic risks, such as allergy, cardiotoxicity, renal dysfunction, seizures, gastrointestinal ulceration, and bleeding. However, with knowledge of the patients' baseline medical condition and care in formulation of the injection, PAI may be administered in a safe and effective manner. Exparel has been found to be safe in volumes much higher than those typically used in PAI.[25]

KEY REFERENCES

1. Albert TJ, Cohn JC, Rothman JS, et al: Patient controlled analgesia in a postoperative total joint arthroplasty population. *J Arthroplasty* 6(Suppl):S23–S28, 1991.

2. Andersen KV, Bak M, Christensen BV, et al: A randomized, controlled trial comparing local infiltration analgesia with epidural infusion for total knee arthroplasty. *Acta Orthop* 81(5):606–610, 2010.

4. Andersen LO, Husted H, Otte KS, et al: High-volume infiltration analgesia in total knee arthroplasty: a randomized, double-blind, placebo-controlled trial. *Acta Anaesthesiol Scand* 52(10):1331–1335, 2008.

5. Bagsby DT, Ireland PH, Meneghini RM: Liposomal bupivacaine versus traditional periarticular injection for pain control after total knee arthroplasty. *J Arthroplasty* 29(8):1687–1690, 2014.

7. Berger RA, Kusuma SK, Sanders SA, et al: The feasibility and perioperative complications of outpatient knee arthroplasty. *Clin Orthop Relat Res* 467(6):1443–1449, 2009.

9. Brown NM, Cipriano CA, Moric M, et al: Dilute betadine lavage before closure for the prevention of acute postoperative deep periprosthetic joint infection. *J Arthroplasty* 27(1):27–30, 2012.

12. Cuvillon P, Ripart J, Lalourcey L, et al: The continuous femoral nerve block catheter for postoperative analgesia: bacterial colonization, infectious rate, and adverse effects. *Anesth Analg* 93(4):1045–1049, 2001.

13. Dalury DF: Injection technique to enhance outcomes after periarticular injections for TKR pain control. JBJS Essential Surgical Techniques [In Press].

15. Dillion JP, Brennan L, Mitchel D: Local infiltration analgesia in hip and knee arthroplasty: an emerging technique. *Acta Orthop Belg* 78:158–163, 2012.

18. Forst J, Wolff S, Thamm P, et al: Pain therapy following joint replacement: a randomized study of patient-controlled analgesia versus conventional pain therapy. *Arch Orthop Trauma Surg* 119:267–270, 1999.

20. Husted H, Otte KS, Kristensen BB, et al: Low risk of thromboembolic complications after fast-track hip and knee arthroplasty. *Acta Orthop* 81:599–605, 2010.

23. Labraca NS, Castro-Sanchez AM, Mataran-Penarrocha GA, et al: Benefits of starting rehabilitation within 24 hours of primary total knee arthroplasty: randomized clinical trial. *Clin Rehabil* 25:557–566, 2011.

28. Perlas A, Kirkham KR, Billing R, et al: The impact of analgesic modality on early ambulation following total knee arthroplasty. *Reg Anesth Pain Med* 38(4):334–339, 2013.

29. Thorsell M, Holst P, Hyldahl HC, et al: Pain control after total knee arthroplasty: a prospective study comparing local infiltration anaesthesia and epidural anaesthesia. *Orthopaedics* 33:75–80, 2010.

30. Toftdahl K, Mikolajsen L, Haraldsted V, et al: Comparision of peri- and intraarticular analgesia with FB after total knee arthroplasty: a randomized clinical trial. *Acta Orthop* 78:172–179, 2007.

The references for this chapter can also be found on www.expertconsult.com.

Epidural Analgesia

Rishi Vashishta, Lisa V. Doan

Epidural anesthesia may be used as an adjunct to general anesthesia or as the primary anesthetic for surgical procedures such as those involving the lower extremities. The use of epidural catheters also allows for the use of continuous postoperative analgesia, with numerous studies confirming its superiority over parenteral opioids.[9] Some studies also suggest that postoperative morbidity may be reduced when neuraxial anesthesia is used alone or as an adjunct to general anesthesia, with lower incidences of venous thrombosis, pulmonary emboli, cardiac complications in high-risk patients, and respiratory complications. With regard to postoperative analgesia following hip or knee arthroplasty, epidural analgesia has been shown to be equivalent to peripheral nerve blockade[5] and vastly superior in the immediate postoperative period when compared to systemic opioids.[3]

INDICATIONS AND CONTRAINDICATIONS

Indications for epidural anesthesia are largely based on the type of procedure and the requirement for analgesia, usually in the form of patient-controlled epidural analgesia (PCEA) infusions for postoperative pain control. For procedures on the lower extremities, epidural anesthesia may be used as the sole anesthetic or combined with a general anesthetic or a spinal anesthetic (combined spinal epidural, or CSE).

Absolute contraindications to epidural anesthesia include patient refusal, infection at the injection site, coagulopathy or other bleeding diathesis, and elevated intracranial pressure. The presence of preexisting neurologic diseases or demyelinating lesions should be considered a relative contraindication, given the difficulty of distinguishing the effects of complications from the block from preexisting deficits or disease exacerbation. Although not contraindicated, patients with severe mitral stenosis, aortic stenosis, and hypertrophic obstructive cardiomyopathy are intolerant of acute decreases in systemic vascular resistance, and neuraxial anesthesia should thus be performed cautiously in such cases.

ANATOMY

The epidural space is the space between the bony spinal canal and the dura mater. Deep to the dura is the subarachnoid space, which contains the cerebrospinal fluid (CSF) that surrounds the spinal cord. In adults, the spinal cord terminates at the L1 level, with the cauda equina extending below. Therefore, lumbar epidural injections carry a low risk of injuring the spinal cord. Insertion of an epidural needle involves threading a needle between the vertebrae, through the ligamentum flavum, and into the epidural space. Great care must be taken to avoid puncturing the dura. In general, insertion of the epidural catheter corresponds to the dermatome level of the incision. For lower extremity operations such as total knee arthroplasty, this would correspond to the L2 to L4 levels.

MECHANISM OF ACTION

The precise mechanism of epidural anesthesia remains speculative, although the primary site of blockade is believed to be the nerve roots originating from the spinal cord. Local anesthetic injected into the epidural space bathes the nerve roots to produce anesthetic effects. Blockade of neural transmission in the posterior nerve root fibers interrupts the afferent transmission of painful stimuli. Blockade of the anterior nerve root fibers prevents efferent motor and autonomic outflow. The varying effects of local anesthetics on different types of nerve fibers according to their size and characteristics usually leads to a differential blockade, whereby a sympathetic blockade (temperature sensitivity, vascular tone) forms two segments more cephalad than a sensory block (pain, light touch), which forms several segments more cephalad than the motor block.

POSTOPERATIVE ANALGESIA

Epidural anesthesia may be performed by injection of a local anesthetic solution into the epidural space as a "single shot" or more commonly as a continuous infusion through a catheter that is threaded 3 to 5 cm into the epidural space. For postoperative epidural analgesia, a continuous infusion of a combined local anesthetic and opioid solution is usually administered via PCEA. The combination of a local anesthetic and an opioid in PCEA infusions has been shown to provide analgesia superior to that of an intravenous patient-controlled analgesia (PCA) with opioids alone.[12] Although epidural infusion of either agent alone may be used for postoperative analgesia, the local anesthetic-opioid combination provides superior analgesia with a purported synergistic effect. The use of local anesthetic as a sole analgesic in epidural infusions is less common because of the increased possibility of motor block and hypotension. The use of opioids alone in an epidural infusion or as a single neuraxial dose (epidural or intrathecal) is also effective in providing analgesia, without causing motor blockade or hypotension, and is further discussed in Chapter 100.

The choice of a local anesthetic and an opioid in a combined epidural infusion is variable in clinical practice. In general, the most common local anesthetics used are bupivacaine and ropivacaine since they have a preferential sensory blockade with minimal impairment of motor function. The side-effect profiles of the chosen local anesthetic may also be a consideration, with ropivacaine having fewer cardiotoxic effects than bupivacaine. The choice of opioid is also variable, although many clinicians prefer a lipophilic opioid (fentanyl or sufentanil) since it allows for rapid titration of analgesia and has a lower incidence of adverse effects, including pruritus and respiratory depression.

The concentrations of local anesthetic and opioid in the infused solution are significantly lower than those used for intraoperative epidural anesthesia. Although the optimal dosages of each agent required to provide superior analgesia while minimizing medication-related side effects remains unknown and is multifactorial, common combinations include 0.06% to 0.125% bupivacaine with 2 to 5 µg/mL fentanyl. A continuous infusion rate of 4 to 8 mL/hour is typically used with a PCEA bolus dose of 4 mL and a lockout time of 15 minutes. The low concentration of local anesthetic in particular allows for adequate pain control without producing significant motor deficits.

There are a number of studies comparing epidural infusions to other regional anesthetic techniques used for lower extremity surgery, such as peripheral nerve blocks and intra-articular injections. When compared to continuous femoral nerve blockade (FNB) following total knee arthroplasty, patients with PCEA infusions received fewer systemic opioids, but experienced a higher incidence of nausea and vomiting.[1] Additional considerations when comparing postoperative epidural analgesia to peripheral nerve catheters include the option to discharge a patient home with a catheter in place and the postoperative thromboprophylaxis regimen to be started. In comparing postoperative epidural analgesia to a periarticular injection (PAI) following total knee arthroplasty, patients receiving PAI were shown to have fewer systemic opioid-related side effects, such as nausea and pruritus, but only experienced superior analgesia in the first 24 hours postoperatively.[10] Finally, when using a multimodal approach of PCEA and FNB compared to PAI alone, patients were found to have similar pain scores at rest and discharge timelines; however, the group receiving both PCEA and FNB analgesia experienced significantly less pain on ambulation.[8]

SIDE EFFECTS AND COMPLICATIONS

The most common side effects of postoperative epidural anesthesia are typically a result of adverse or exaggerated physiologic responses to the appropriately placed anesthetic agent. The incidence of persistent or disabling neurologic complications is rare with the use of neuraxial anesthesia and is minimized by an appreciation of the factors that may contribute to injury.

Hypotension may occur from the local anesthetic used in the analgesic regimen, which causes a sympathectomy that decreases systemic vascular resistance. This situation is estimated to occur in approximately 6% of patients receiving postoperative epidural analgesia. If appropriate, hydration may be considered. In addition, the overall dose of local anesthetic administered can be decreased by reducing the infusion rate, decreasing the local anesthetic concentration, or using only an opioid in the epidural solution.[2]

Lower extremity motor blockade may also occur because of the local anesthetic in the postoperative epidural analgesic regimen, with a reported incidence of 3%.[12] This may delay ambulation postoperatively. Fall precautions should be used. Lowering the concentration of local anesthetic or using only an opioid in the epidural infusion may be considered. If a patient continues to experience persistent or worsening deficits after decreasing or stopping the epidural infusion, he or she should be promptly evaluated to rule out epidural hematoma, epidural abscess, or intrathecal migration of the catheter.

Urinary retention associated with neuraxial anesthesia is likely related to the use of opioids in the infusion. Although the exact incidence of urinary retention is difficult to determine since many patients undergoing major surgery are often routinely catheterized postoperatively, the incidence is estimated at 10% and 25%.[4] Management of urinary retention involves placement of a catheter.

Pruritus is one of the most common side effects of epidural or intrathecal administration of opioids, with an incidence of approximately 16%. Although the cause of neuraxial opioid-induced pruritus is uncertain, it is thought to be related to central activation of an "itch center" in the medulla. The most effective treatment for opioid-induced pruritus remains opioid receptor antagonists such as intravenous naloxone.[7]

Nausea and vomiting with epidural analgesia is a side effect of the opioids in the analgesic regimen. The overall data suggests that the incidence of postoperative vomiting is similar for epidural analgesia and systemic opioids, with a higher frequency in women. A variety of medications may be used to treat the nausea and vomiting including naloxone, droperidol, metoclopramide, dexamethasone, ondansetron, and transdermal scopolamine.[4]

Finally, the presence of opioids in the epidural infusion at higher doses may also result in respiratory depression. Treatment is effective with naloxone administered in 0.1- to 0.4-mg increments. Since the clinical duration of action of naloxone is significantly shorter than most opioids, multiple doses or a continuous infusion may be required in addition to close monitoring.

Other rare complications of epidural anesthesia, and often the most feared ones, are largely related to needle insertion and catheter placement and removal. These include postdural puncture headache following a "wet tap" (1 in about 100), bleeding or epidural hematoma (1 in about 168,000), infection or epidural abscess formation (1 in about 145,000), catheter misplacement in the subarachnoid space resulting in total spinal anesthesia (<1 in 1000), and persistent neurologic injury (<1 in 7000).[11] Suspicion of epidural hematoma or abscess requires prompt imaging and neurosurgical consultation.

EPIDURAL ANESTHESIA AND THROMBOPROPHYLAXIS

The American Society of Regional Anesthesia and Pain Medicine (ASRA) has published recommendations regarding neuraxial anesthesia in conjunction with perioperative anticoagulation.[6] When any anticoagulant is administered perioperatively in a patient receiving neuraxial anesthesia, close neurologic monitoring of the lower extremities should be mandated to detect early signs of epidural hematoma formation. The use of certain thromboprophylaxis regimens may limit or preclude the use of epidural analgesia.

KEY REFERENCE

12. Wu CL, Cohen SR, Richman JM, et al: Efficacy of postoperative patient-controlled and continuous infusion epidural analgesia versus intravenous patient-controlled analgesia with opioids: a meta-analysis. *Anesthesiology* 103:1079–1088, 2005.

The references for this chapter can also be found on www.expertconsult.com.

Neuraxial Opioids

Rishi Vashishta, Lisa V. Doan

Neuraxial anesthesia is the use of spinal and epidural techniques to provide analgesia and anesthesia in a wide variety of procedures. Analgesia and anesthesia may be achieved by a single injection, intermittent bolus, or continuous infusion of medication. This chapter discusses the use of opioids in neuraxial analgesia.

MECHANISM OF ACTION

Opioids act primarily at opioid receptors located throughout the body including the brain, spinal cord, and non-neural tissues such as the gastrointestinal tract. Opioid receptors are G-protein coupled receptors and are subdivided into four main classes: mu, kappa, delta, and nociceptin. Analgesia from neuraxial opioid administration is primarily mediated by mu opioid receptors in the dorsal horn of the spinal cord; however, other mechanisms may also be responsible depending on the method of opioid delivery, including cephalad spread to the brain and systemic absorption via diffusion into the vasculature.

INTRATHECAL AND EPIDURAL OPIOIDS

The onset and duration of neuraxial opioid action are dependent on lipid solubility, which in turn affects the degree of cephalad spread. Highly lipid-soluble (lipophilic) opioids such as fentanyl and sufentanil produce a rapid onset of analgesia with minimal cephalad spread and a relatively short duration of action. In contrast, morphine and hydromorphone are poorly lipid soluble (hydrophilic), resulting in a slower onset of analgesia, prolonged duration of action, and increased cephalad spread. With greater cephalad spread, these agents have an increased risk of delayed respiratory depression when compared to fentanyl and sufentanil. Intrathecal opioids are administered in direct proximity of the spinal cord and undergo minimal metabolism within the cerebrospinal fluid (CSF). Thus a much smaller dose of opioid is given intrathecally than when used via the epidural route. While a single dose of an intrathecal opioid may be used for postoperative analgesia, neuraxial opioids are most often used in a continuous infusion through an epidural catheter.

Following epidural administration, variable quantities of opioid will diffuse across the dura into the subarachnoid space to bind the opioid receptors in the dorsal horn of the spinal cord. In addition to diffusing into the CSF, there is also absorption of opioids though the epidural venous plexus into the systemic circulation, allowing them to reach the brain to modulate pain perception and response. In both cases, lipid solubility is again the most important factor affecting the rate of diffusion. As with intrathecal administration of hydrophilic morphine or hydromorphone, the slower absorption and prolonged duration of action results in an increased risk of delayed respiratory depression.

POSTOPERATIVE ANALGESIA

Neuraxial opioids for postoperative analgesia may be administered as a single dose or through continuous epidural infusion. The administration of a single dose of intrathecal or epidural opioid may be effective as a sole analgesic drug. The choice of opioid is primarily dependent on the clinical situation. For example, a single neuraxial dose of a lipophilic opioid (fentanyl or sufentanil) may be advantageous for ambulatory procedures, where a rapid onset of analgesia with a moderate duration of action and minimal risk of respiratory depression is desired. In contrast, a single neuraxial dose of a hydrophilic opioid (morphine or hydromorphone) may be useful for patients who will continue to be monitored on an inpatient basis and require a longer duration of analgesia.

The most common use of neuraxial opioids in postoperative analgesia, however, is in conjunction with a local anesthetic when administered in an epidural infusion. When compared to a local anesthetic or opioid alone, the combination provides analgesia superior to that of intravenous patient-controlled analgesia (PCA) with opioids alone.[5] Although the choice of opioid is variable, many clinicians prefer a lipophilic opioid (fentanyl or sufentanil) since it allows for rapid titration of analgesia. The optimal dosages of local anesthetic and opioid that provide the greatest amount of analgesia while minimizing medication-related side effects remain unknown and largely depends on multiple variables, including the type of surgical procedure, location of the epidural catheter, and the patients themselves.

Opioids may also be used alone for postoperative epidural infusion, with the advantages of not causing a motor block and avoiding hypotension from sympathetic blockade. The particular opioid to be used is variable, although generally the overall advantage of administering a continuous epidural infusion of lipophilic opioids (fentanyl or sufentanil) alone is marginal in comparison to intravenous opioids.[4] Continuous infusion of a hydrophilic opioid (morphine or hydromorphone) allows for a primarily spinal site of analgesic action (Table 100.1).

SIDE EFFECTS

Adverse effects from neuraxial opioids are primarily because of the cephalad spread of the opioid in the CSF or via systemic

TABLE 100.1	Dosing of Neuraxial Opioids[a]		
Drug	Intrathecal or Subarachnoid Single Dose	Epidural Single Dose	Epidural Continuous Infusion
Fentanyl	5-25 µg	50-100 µg	25-100 µg/hr
Sufentanil	2-10 µg	10-50 µg	10-20 µg/hr
Alfentanil	—	0.5-1 mg	0.2 mg/hr
Morphine	0.1-0.3 mg	1-5 mg	0.1-1 mg/hr
Hydromorphone	—	0.5-1 mg	0.1-0.2 mg/hr
Extended-release morphine[b]	Not recommended	5-15 mg	Not recommended

[a]Doses are based on the use of a neuraxial opioid alone. No continuous intrathecal or subarachnoid infusions are provided. Lower doses may be effective when administered to older patients or when injected in the cervical or thoracic region. Units vary across agents for single dose (mg vs. pg) and continuous infusion (mg/hr vs. pg/hr).
[b]See package insert for details on dosage and administration.
From Fukuda K: Opioid analgesics. In Miller RD, ed: Miller's anesthesia, ed 8, Philadelphia, 2015, Saunders, pp 864–914.

absorption from the epidural space. The classic side effects associated with neuraxial opioids are pruritus, nausea and vomiting, urinary retention, and respiratory depression.

Pruritus is the most common adverse effect associated with neuraxial opioids, with an incidence of 16%.[2] Although the exact mechanism of neuraxial opioid-induced pruritus remains unclear, it is postulated that the presence of an "itch center" in the central nervous system, medullary dorsal horn activation, and antagonism of inhibitory neurotransmitters all play a role. The treatment of pruritus may be challenging and includes opioid receptor antagonists such as intravenous naloxone.

The incidence of nausea and vomiting associated with neuraxial opioids is reported between 20% and 50%, and is more common in females and with intrathecal morphine.[4] The precise mechanism also remains unclear, however it is thought to be because of the cephalad migration of the opioid to the chemoreceptor trigger zone. Treatment with anti-emetics is recommended.

Urinary retention associated with neuraxial opioids is primarily mediated by opioid receptors in the sacral spinal cord, which inhibit sacral parasympathetic outflow and lead to detrusor relaxation. While the exact incidence of urinary retention is difficult to determine since many patients undergoing major surgery are routinely catheterized postoperatively, it is estimated to be between 10% and 25%.[1] The conventional management of urinary retention involves placement of a Foley catheter, however, a low-dose opioid antagonist (naloxone) may also be used since urinary retention is not dependent on the dose of opioid administered.

Respiratory depression is the most serious adverse effect caused by neuraxial opioids. Factors increasing the risk of respiratory depression include high opioid dose, elderly patients, concomitant use of sedative medications, lack of opioid tolerance, and the presence of comorbidities such as sleep apnea and pulmonary disease. Early respiratory depression typically occurs with the use of lipophilic opioids such as fentanyl and sufentanil, and is usually seen within 2 hours of administration. Delayed respiratory depression may develop between 6 and 12 hours following neuraxial administration of hydrophilic opioids such as morphine. This is because of the cephalad migration of the opioid within the neuraxis, where it reaches opioid receptors in the respiratory center of the central nervous system. The American Society of Anesthesiologists has published a practice guideline regarding respiratory depression associated with neuraxial opioid administration. These guidelines recommend identifying patients at increased risk for respiratory depression through a focused history and physical examination, using home sleep devices in patients with sleep apnea, carefully monitoring ventilation and oxygen saturation in patients receiving neuraxial opioids, and management with supplemental oxygen, noninvasive positive pressure ventilation, and opioid antagonists such as naloxone, if needed. The guidelines also recommend using the lowest efficacious dose and the preferential use of lipophilic opioids such as fentanyl and sufentanil if possible.[3]

KEY REFERENCE

3. Practice guidelines for the prevention, detection, and management of respiratory depression associated with neuraxial opioid administration: An updated report by the American Society of Anesthesiologists Task Force on Neuraxial Opioids and the American Society of Regional Anesthesia and Pain Medicine. *Anesthesiol* 124:535–552, 2016.

The references for this chapter can also be found on www.expertconsult.com.

Systemic Opioids and Postoperative Nausea and Vomiting

Lisa V. Doan, Rishi Vashishta

SYSTEMIC OPIOIDS

Opioids are commonly used for the treatment of acute postoperative pain. Their use is limited by side effects such as respiratory depression, sedation, constipation, nausea, and vomiting; thus they should be used in the setting of a multimodal analgesic plan. Opioids may be administered via several routes. Parenteral or oral routes are used most commonly in the postoperative period.

Mechanism of Action

The opioid receptor family includes mu-, delta-, and kappa-opioid receptors and the nociceptin receptor. The actions of each type of opioid receptor are listed in Table 101.1. Most opioids used clinically act on the mu-opioid receptor.[3]

Opioid receptors are G-protein–coupled receptors that act on G_i/G_o proteins to inhibit the conversion of adenosine triphosphate to cyclic adenosine monophosphate. Voltage-gated calcium channels are inhibited, and inwardly rectifying potassium channels are activated. This results in decreased neuronal excitability. Mitogen-activated protein kinase cascades are also activated, ultimately leading to changes in gene expression.[1] Particular opioids may also act on nonopioid receptors, such as the N-methyl-D-aspartate receptor and the serotonin receptor.[3]

The analgesic properties of opioids occur primarily through effects in the central nervous system. Opioids act to inhibit ascending transmission of pain signals from the spinal cord and activate descending modulatory circuits from the midbrain periaqueductal gray to the rostral ventromedial medulla and on to the spinal cord. Opioids act presynaptically and postsynaptically in the spinal cord. They may also act in the periphery.[3]

Side Effects

Opioids have several side effects, including respiratory depression, cognitive impairment, nausea and vomiting, constipation, and pruritus (Table 101.2). Long-term use can cause physical dependence, immune suppression, and endocrine changes.

Respiratory depression occurs in a dose-dependent manner. Patients at risk for respiratory depression include opioid-naïve patients, patients at the extremes of age, patients taking other central nervous system depressants such as benzodiazepines, obese patients, and patients with underlying respiratory dysfunction including obstructive sleep apnea. Treatment for opioid-induced respiratory depression includes respiratory support and the use of naloxone, an opioid antagonist.

Cognitive impairment including sedation may occur. Minimizing other central nervous system depressants, lowering the dose, or switching to an alternative opioid may be considered.

Nausea and vomiting are a result of stimulation of the chemoreceptor trigger zone in the medulla. Antiemetics may be prescribed. If nausea and vomiting persist, rotation to a different opioid should be considered.

Constipation is a commonly encountered side effect. It occurs via opioid receptors in the gastrointestinal tract and through spinal and supraspinal mechanisms.[3] Patients should generally be placed on a bowel regimen including a stool softener such as docusate and a laxative such as senna. Osmotic agents may be added as step therapy. Refractory opioid-induced constipation may be treated with the peripheral opioid antagonist methylnaltrexone or oral naloxone.

Pruritus occurs more commonly with the intravenous (IV) than the oral route. It may be independent of histamine release. Opioid rotation may be considered. Low doses of naloxone or nalbuphine, a mu-receptor antagonist and kappa-receptor agonist, may also be considered for management of pruritus.

Specific Opioids

Opioids can be classified in various ways, including chemical structure and action on opioid receptors. Opioids can be divided into agonists, mixed agonist-antagonists, and antagonists. Mixed agonist-antagonists are generally not used in the postoperative period because of a ceiling effect for analgesia. Commonly used mu-opioid agonists are discussed, focusing on parenteral and oral forms.

Morphine is the prototypical mu-opioid agonist. It comes in a variety forms, including parenteral and oral formulations. The oral form is also available as a solution. Morphine is metabolized by the liver to morphine-3-glucuronide, which has no analgesic properties, and morphine-6-glucuronide, an agonist at the mu-opioid receptor. These metabolites are excreted by the kidney. In patients with renal dysfunction, morphine-6-glucuronide may accumulate and lead to adverse events including respiratory depression. Thus morphine should be avoided in renal impairment. IV morphine has an onset of 5 to 10 minutes and a duration of approximately 4 hours.

Hydromorphone is more potent than morphine. It is available in a variety of forms including parenteral and oral formulations. IV hydromorphone has an onset of approximately 5 minutes and a duration of approximately 3 to 4 hours.[3]

IV fentanyl is approximately 100 times as potent as IV morphine. It has a rapid onset and short duration of action.

TABLE 101.1 Pharmacologic Actions of Opioids and Opioid Receptors in Animal Models

	Receptor	Agonists	Antagonists
Supraspinal	μ,δ,κ	Analgesic	No effect
Spinal	μ,δ,κ	Analgesic	No effect
Respiratory function	μ	Decrease	No effect
Gastrointestinal tract	μ,κ	Decrease transit	No effect
Psychotomimesis	κ	Increase	No effect
Feeding	μ,δ,κ	Increase feeding	Decrease feeding
Sedation	μ,κ	Increase	No effect
Diuresis	κ	Increase	—

From Fukuda K: Opioid analgesics. In Miller RD, editor: *Miller's anesthesia*, ed 8, Philadelphia, 2015, Elsevier, pp 864–914.

TABLE 101.2 Adverse Effects of Opioids

Common	Occasional	Rare
Nausea	Hallucinations	Respiratory depression
Vomiting	Mood changes	Delirium
Constipation	Anxiety	Seizures
Sedation	Pruritus	Hyperalgesia
Drowsiness	Myoclonus	Allodynia
Cognitive impairment	Rigidity	Biliary spasm
Miosis	Dry mouth	Noncardiogenic
Cough suppression	Gastric stasis	pulmonary edema
Urinary retention	Bronchoconstriction	Tolerance
		Addiction

From Schug SA: Opioids: clinical use. In McMahon SB, Koltzenburg M, Tracey I, et al, eds: *Wall and Melzack's textbook of pain*, ed 6, Philadelphia, 2013, Elsevier, pp 429–443.

The onset is within a few minutes. The analgesic effects last approximately 1 hour. Fentanyl also comes in transdermal and transmucosal forms, which are typically not indicated in the acute postoperative period.

Oxycodone and hydrocodone are used in oral formulations. They are also available as solutions. They are often used as combination products with acetaminophen.

Codeine is metabolized in the liver via several pathways. O-demethylation via cytochrome P4502D6 produces morphine, the analgesic metabolite of codeine. Poor metabolizers will have no analgesic effects from codeine. Ultrarapid metabolizers will have increased risk of adverse effects from codeine.[9] Codeine is commonly used in an oral preparation in combination with acetaminophen.

Tramadol is a mu-opioid agonist and a norepinephrine and serotonin reuptake inhibitor; these monoaminergic actions work on the descending inhibitory pain pathway. It is considered a weak opioid. It is used as an oral formulation, sometimes in combination with acetaminophen. Because of the possible risk of seizure, caution should be used in patients with a seizure history and those taking serotonin reuptake inhibitors and monoamine oxidase inhibitors.

Patient-Controlled Analgesia

IV patient-controlled analgesia (PCA) is often used in the immediate postoperative period. PCA is based on a feedback loop in which medication is administered when the patient

TABLE 101.3 Common Initial Settings for Opioids Frequently Used for Intravenous Postoperative Nausea and Vomiting

Opioid	Bolus Dose	Lockout Interval (min)
Morphine	1 mg	5-10
Hydromorphone	0.1 mg	5-10
Fentanyl	10-20 μg	5-10

experiences pain. PCA circumvents the wide swings that may occur with intermittent parenteral injections in which patients may have periods of pain followed by periods at risk for respiratory depression or sedation. It is fairly simple to titrate on the bolus dose or lockout interval for analgesic effect and avoidance of side effects.[8] PCA has been shown to provide greater pain control and patient satisfaction compared to intermittent parenteral injections.[7]

The use of continuous basal infusions is generally not recommended in opioid-naïve patients in the postoperative period. Basal infusions have been shown to increase the incidence of respiratory depression.[5]

Table 101.3 provides common initial settings for opioids frequently used for IV PCA.

Transition to Oral Opioids

The transition from IV to oral opioids occurs when patients tolerate oral intake and when pain has been stabilized on parenteral opioids. Short-acting oral opioids can typically be used. Dosing should be coordinated so that patients can benefit from physical therapy sessions. Extended-release opioid preparations may occasionally be needed in some patients.

POSTOPERATIVE NAUSEA AND VOMITING

Postoperative nausea and vomiting (PONV) occurs in approximately 30% of patients.[2] The main causes of PONV after surgery are the use of inhalational anesthetics and opioids (Fig. 101.1).[6]

Pathophysiology of Postoperative Nausea and Vomiting

The nucleus of the solitary tract in the hindbrain and nuclei in the reticular formation are important in the pathophysiology of PONV. Several pathways project to the nucleus of the solitary tract to activate vomiting. Drugs or toxins in the gastrointestinal tract cause enteroendocrine cells to release mediators that stimulate vagal afferent fibers. Vestibular input arises from motion input in the inner ear. The chemoreceptor trigger zone is located in the area postrema. This organ is located directly adjacent to the nucleus of the solitary tract and has a reduced blood-brain barrier to detect circulating drugs or toxins that can trigger vomiting. Forebrain areas are also involved in vomiting.[6]

Risk Factors for Postoperative Nausea and Vomiting

Risk factors for PONV include female gender, history of PONV or motion sickness, nonsmoking status, the use of opioids and certain anesthetic medications, and certain types of surgery.[4] Of note, orthopedic surgeries are typically not considered emetogenic surgeries. Risk assessment scores have been developed for the prediction of PONV; the simplified risk score is presented in Fig. 101.2.

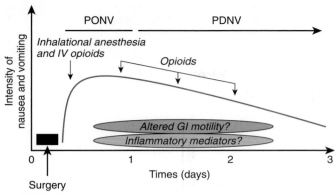

FIG 101.1 Model of the phases and stimuli that contribute to postoperative and postdischarge nausea and vomiting (PONV and PDNV). Both inhalation anesthesia and intravenous opioids (eg, fentanyl) can contribute to PONV, which is defined by most authors as nausea and vomiting experienced in the post-anesthesia care unit (PACU) or as inpatient stay in the hospital. PDNV appears to be the result of opioid analgesic usage. Although not well understood, surgery-related effects on gastrointestinal motility (eg, postoperative ileus) and GI inflammation might also contribute to nausea and vomiting. Patients can develop tolerance to opioid-induced nausea and vomiting. This model is dependent on the type of surgery and may have shorter or longer periods of PONV and PDNV. (From Horn CC, Wallisch WJ, Homanics GE, et al: Pathophysiological and neurochemical mechanisms of postoperative nause and vomiting. *Eur J Pharmacol* 722:55-66, 2014.)

Risk factors	Points
Female gender	1
Nonsmoker	1
History of PONV	1
Postoperative opioids	1
Risk score =	0...4

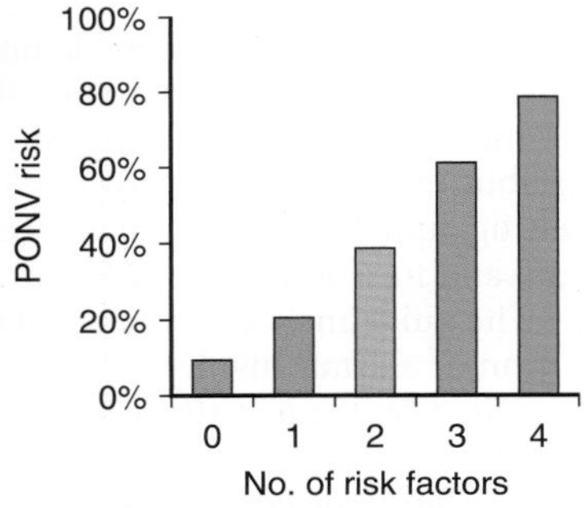

FIG 101.2 The simplified risk score for adults. PONV, Postoperative nausea and vomiting. (From Apfel CC, Laara E, Koivuranta M, et al: A simplified risk score for predicting postoperative nausea and vomiting: conclusion from cross-validation between two centers, (From Apfel CC: Postoperative nausea and vomiting. In Miller RD, editor: *Miller's anesthesia,* ed 8, Philadelphia, 2015, Elsevier, pp 2947–2973.)

Strategies to Reduce Risk

Several strategies may be used in the perioperative period to reduce the risk of developing PONV. These include the consideration of regional anesthesia techniques rather than general anesthesia, the avoidance of inhalational anesthetics and nitrous oxide, and the use of multimodal analgesia to minimize postoperative opioid use.[4]

Prophylaxis and Treatment of Postoperative Nausea and Vomiting

Guidelines have been published for the management of PONV, including those from the Society of Ambulatory Anesthesia. Using the simplified risk score for PONV, patients with a score of 0 to 1 are considered low risk, 2 to 3 medium risk, and 4 high risk. In patients at moderate risk for PONV, it is recommended to administer 1 to 2 antiemetics prophylactically. In patients at high risk for PONV, prophylactic therapy with 2 or more antiemetics is recommended.[4]

Serotonin antagonists include ondansetron, granisetron, and palonosetron. Ondansetron is considered the "gold standard" for antiemetics. Palonosetron is a second-generation serotonin antagonist with a long half-life of 40 hours that is more effective than ondansetron for preventing PONV. Ondansetron and granisetron are usually dosed at the end of surgery, whereas palonosetron is usually given at the beginning of surgery. All serotonin antagonists except palonosetron can affect the QT interval.[4]

Aprepitant is a neurokinin antagonist that has been found to be more efficacious than ondansetron for preventing emesis after surgery. Its use is currently limited because of cost.[4]

The corticosteroid dexamethasone is an effective antiemetic. It may also improve postoperative pain and fatigue. The use of a single dose of dexamethasone likely does not affect the incidence of wound infection. It may increase blood glucose levels and should be used with caution in diabetics.[4]

Dopamine antagonists include metoclopramide and droperidol. Metoclopramide's side effects include dyskinesia or extrapyramidal symptoms. Droperidol is as effective as ondansetron for PONV prophylaxis. However, it carries a US Food and Drug Administration (FDA) black box warning for QT prolongation.[4]

Transdermal scopolamine, an anticholinergic, can be used for PONV prophylaxis. It can be placed the evening before or a few hours before surgery. Side effects include visual disturbances, dry mouth, and dizziness.[4]

If patients continue to experience PONV despite the use of prophylactic therapy, an agent with a different mechanism of action should be tried.

The references for this chapter can also be found on www.expertconsult.com.

Multimodal Pharmacologic Analgesia

Tomas J. Kucera, Sorosch Didehvar, Christopher Gharibo

Total knee arthroplasty (TKA) is one of the most common and successful inpatient operations performed in the United States.[18,41,43] There were 719,000 TKAs performed in the United States in the year 2010.[11] Long-term quality of life, measured by quality-adjusted life years, has been demonstrated to be improved by TKA.[51] The immediate postoperative period may be accompanied by intense pain that may hinder rehabilitation and return to an optimized functional capacity. Pain limited rehabilitation and daily physical function can lead to deconditioning, deconditioning-related pain, frozen knees, secondary orthopedic and neuropathic pain, deep venous thrombosis, pulmonary embolism, cardiac complications, and other adverse events related to immobility. Historically, although opioids have been the analgesics of choice for postoperative pain control, they are associated with side effects and complications that range from nausea, vomiting, and respiratory depression to risks of misuse, abuse, and diversion. Postoperative opioid monotherapy is associated with high-dose oral opioid discharges, which further emphasizes the need for a multimodal plan of care.

Since the publication of its last addition in 2012, the Center for Medicare and Medicaid Services (CMS) has implemented mandatory reporting of hospital quality data through Hospital Consumer Assessment of Healthcare Providers and Systems (HCAHPS).[28] The survey consists of 21 questions on patients' perception of communication with doctors, nurses, cleanliness of the hospital environment, and also two questions that pertain to pain management.[28] Through the CMS Value-Based Purchasing program, a portion of inpatient reimbursement is withheld from each hospital and given to the top performing hospitals.[28] There are two specific questions on pain that ask patients how often, during their hospital stay, their pain was well controlled and how often the staff did everything they could to help alleviate pain. Only a response of "always" is counted toward a hospital's ranking.

> *"During this hospital stay, how often was your pain well controlled?"*
>
> *"During this hospital stay, how often did the hospital staff do everything they could to help you with your pain?"*

Effective pain management is an important factor in achieving a fast, efficient, and safe discharge. The average length of stay (LOS) from a primary TKA went from 7.9 days in 1991 to 3.5 days in 2010 and the trend is continuing for shorter LOS with some centers performing TKA with same day discharge.[34] Shorter LOS is affected by many factors such as regular staff, continuity, managing expectations, early mobilizations, and a multimodal opioid-sparing analgesia.[34]

Multimodal perioperative pain protocols have been advocated for many different types of surgeries such as cardiac, bariatric, hernia repair, and many others including TKA. What exactly is multimodal analgesia?

Kehlet et al. is one of the first groups to describe "multimodal" or "balanced analgesia" in 1993 as the use of different analgesics with different pharmacodynamic mechanisms that result in additive or synergistic analgesia, thereby allowing reduction of the adverse effects seen with higher doses of a single analgesic such as opioids.[39]

This chapter provides a review of different enteral and parenteral medications that can be used in combination to provide a multimodal approach to pain management for TKA.

ACUTE PAIN MEDICINE SERVICE

The institution of a comprehensive acute pain service (APS) that is entrusted with the responsibility of managing postoperative pain control has been demonstrated to improve patient self-reported pain scores.* The most recent practice guidelines of the American Society of Anesthesiologists (ASA) for the establishment of acute pain management in the perioperative setting, updated in 2012, make recommendations on the structure and function of an APS team.[3]

The guidelines recommend that teaching and ongoing education of all staff involved in the care of the surgical patient be provided by the anesthesiologist involved with APS and other associated healthcare professionals.[18] It is also recommended that a standardized approach to optimal pain management be instituted using regular evaluation and treatment of pain, and that the anesthesiologist responsible for perioperative analgesia be available at all times.[3] The ASA guidelines recommend a standardized institutional policy and procedure for perioperative acute pain management.[3]

Using an APS service in perioperative pain management allows patient expectations to be addressed early, allows education of both patients and staff, and allows policies and guidelines to be created to achieve reproducible care across multiple providers.† In the era of HCAHPS scores, value-based purchasing, and quality initiatives, it will become increasingly important to provide quality, evidence-based pain control, with reproducible results in the most cost-effective manner.

---

*References 3, 16, 27, 54, 56, and 64.
†References 16, 27, 54, 56, 64, and 70.

ACETAMINOPHEN

Acetaminophen is a centrally acting analgesic and antipyretic agent. Its mechanism of action is not completely understood. The main mechanism proposed is the inhibition of the cyclooxygenase (COX) system, and recent findings suggest that it is highly selective for cyclooxygenase-2 (COX-2).[29] It is also believed that acetaminophen may involve inhibition of the nitric oxide pathway mediated by neurotransmitter receptors including N-methyl-D-aspartate (NMDA) and substance P.[8]

One randomized controlled trial by Sinatra et al. in major orthopedic surgery demonstrated that intravenous acetaminophen and its prodrug propacetamol both provided significant pain relief, as measured by reduced morphine rescue consumption, of up to 30% compared with the placebo.[61] The rates of adverse events in the acetaminophen and placebo groups were similar. In a further expanded analysis after total hip arthroplasty (THA) and TKA, the same authors reported significantly longer times to morphine rescue dose requirement in the intravenous acetaminophen group compared with placebo after THA and TKA (3.9 and 2.1 hours vs. 0.8 hours in the placebo group, respectively).[62]

A Cochrane review, published in 2013, compared oral acetaminophen plus ibuprofen in acute postoperative patients and found that the combinations provided better analgesia in than either drug alone (at the same dose), with a smaller chance of needing additional analgesia over approximately 8 hours, and with a smaller chance of experiencing an adverse event.[20]

Acetaminophen has potential for severe liver injury and has led to cases of acute liver failure resulting in liver transplant and death.[19] Patients should be advised not to exceed the acetaminophen maximum total daily dose of 4 g/day.[19] Furthermore, it is important to educate patients to abstain from alcohol consumption while taking acetaminophen and it should be avoided in patients with conditions that involve liver damage like hepatitis or chronic alcohol abuse with liver damage.

Although rare, serious skin reactions like Stevens-Johnson Syndrome (SJS) and toxic epidermal necrolysis (TEN) have been linked to acetaminophen use.[19]

NONSTEROIDAL ANTI-INFLAMMATORY DRUGS

Nonsteroidal anti-inflammatory drugs (NSAIDs) have anti-inflammatory, antipyretic, and analgesic effects. NSAIDs exert their mechanism of action both peripherally and centrally. They exert their effects by inhibiting COX production of prostaglandins in the peripheral tissues via the COX system. Prostaglandins are important mediators of pain peripherally. Recent research has demonstrated that NSAIDs also have a significant effect in central inhibition of COX-2 in modulating nociception.[9]

There are many commercially available NSAIDs that inhibit both COX-1 and COX-2 enzymes in varying degrees of selectivity. COX-2 selective inhibitors are specific for COX-2 isozymes and have minimal gastrointestinal side effects as a result of less prostaglandin inhibition in the gastric mucosa.[38] Currently, celecoxib is the only COX-2 selective inhibitor on the market in the United States.[38] Previously commercially available COX-2–selective blockers such as rofecoxib have been withdrawn because of long-term cardiovascular risks.[38] Another COX-2 selective medication is etoricoxib, used predominantly in Europe; it is not approved for use in the United States.[38]

Cardiovascular risks associated with use of NSAIDs have been an increasing concern as more is learned about their effect on patients who use them. In a nationwide cohort study published in *Circulation* in 2011, researchers found that even short-term treatment with most NSAIDs was associated with increased risk of death and recurrent myocardial infarction (MI) in patients with prior MI.[57] The researchers recommended that neither short- nor long-term treatment with NSAIDs is advised in this population.

NSAIDs are strong analgesics that have been shown to be nearly as effective as opioids in postoperative orthopedic patients.[23,32,46,65] In one trial, patients with moderate to severe pain after ambulatory orthopedic surgery experienced comparable analgesia with single doses of hydrocodone and acetaminophen combination as compared with celecoxib. Over a 5-day period, oral doses of celecoxib 200 mg taken 3 times a day demonstrated superior analgesia and tolerability compared with hydrocodone 10 mg and acetaminophen 1000 mg taken 3 times a day.[23]

Perioperative celecoxib doses have been shown to decrease pain and narcotic requirements after TKA[38] and in a systematic review of randomized trials, preoperative celecoxib compared to placebo was found to significantly reduce postoperative pain in most studies.[65]

NSAIDs should not be given to patients with a history of renal insufficiency or gastrointestinal ulcers or bleeding, or in patients with a history of MI and serious cardiovascular risk factors.[57]

KETAMINE

Ketamine is a noncompetitive antagonist of NMDA receptor in the central nervous system (CNS). This mechanism appears to account for most of its anesthetic and analgesic effects.[15] Other proposed ketamine mechanisms of action include a complex interaction with opioid receptors with a smaller affinity for these receptors than for the NMDA receptor.[12]

Numerous studies demonstrate the advantages of using ketamine in multimodal pain management and show that small intraoperative infusion doses of ketamine result in reduced postoperative opioid requirements and reduced postoperative pain scores in surgical patients.[‡]

In one study, researchers found that low-dose ketamine improved postoperative analgesia with a significant decrease of morphine consumption when its administration was continued for 48 hours postoperatively, along with a lower incidence of nausea.[73]

In an interesting study from Switzerland, researchers demonstrated that intranasal ketamine (S-ketamine) spray combined with intranasal midazolam (for prevention of hallucinations and delirium caused by ketamine) was similar in effectiveness, satisfaction, number of demands and deliveries to standard intravenous patient-controlled analgesia (PCA) with morphine in postoperative spine surgery patients.[53]

Adam et al. studied patients undergoing TKA that were assigned to receive a continuous femoral nerve block with ropivacaine starting before the surgery with either an intraoperative ketamine infusion and postoperative ketamine infusion up to 48 hours postoperatively or an equivalent saline infusion

---

‡References 1, 6, 37, 53, 58, 66, and 73.

intraoperatively and 48 hours postoperatively.[1] Additional postoperative analgesia was provided by PCA intravenous morphine. The ketamine group required significantly less morphine than the control group and the ketamine group reached 90 degrees of active knee flexion more rapidly than those in the control group with similar outcomes at 6 weeks and 3 months in each group.[1]

GABAPENTINOIDS

Gabapentinoids (gabapentin and pregabalin) were originally developed as anticonvulsants, but have since been shown to have analgesic effects.[4] They exert their effects by binding to the alpha-2 delta subunit of the presynaptic voltage gated–calcium channels and inhibiting calcium release, thereby preventing the release of excitatory neurotransmitters involved in the dorsal horn.[4,30]

The effectiveness of gabapentinoids in chronic pain conditions such diabetic neuropathy, postherpetic neuralgia, and neuropathic pain is well established.[48]

Perioperative gabapentinoids have been shown to reduce early postoperative pain,[45,68] provide good dynamic and static analgesia, and reduce opioid use by 30% to 60%.[14,50,59,60] Although debated, there is evidence that gabapentinoids may have an effect on reducing the incidence of chronic postsurgical pain.[10,13]

Clarke et al. evaluated different regimens of gabapentin patients undergoing TKA.[14] The investigators found that while self-reported pain scores were similar, patients treated with gabapentin used significantly less PCA morphine up to 2 days postoperatively, and had less opioid-related side effects, but showed more gabapentin-related side effects like dizziness and sedation.[3,56]

In another clinical trial examining the effects of pregabalin on the development of chronic pain, patients undergoing TKA were given either pregabalin (preoperatively and for 14 days postoperatively) or placebo.[10] The study participants had less epidural and oral narcotic use in the pregabalin group.[10] The pregabalin patients also had greater knee flexion at 30 days postoperatively and significantly less neuropathic pain at 3 and 6 months postoperatively.[10]

The most common side effects of gabapentinoids are increased sedation, dizziness, and visual disturbances.[72] Postoperative dizziness in particular is a well-known complication and caution should be exercised, especially in older adults. Other potential adverse effects of gabapentinoids are headache, edema, cognitive disturbances, and ataxia, which are well known from chronic pain studies.[35,72] Gabapentinoids may also exert a positive effect on the mood (mood stabilizing) and have been used off label for alcohol withdrawl.[26]

OPIOIDS

Primary ascending pain fibers (A, δ, and C fibers) from peripheral sites reach the dorsal horn of the spinal cord to innervate the neurons in laminae I and II.[52] Neurons of the dorsal horn give rise to ascending spinothalamic tracts.[52] There are three opioid receptors (mu, kappa, and delta) in the body, which are located in the brain, spinal cord, and digestive tract, respectively.[52] The opioid receptors at the spinal level are located at the presynaptic ends of the neurons and at the interneural-level layers IV to VII in the dorsal horn. Each receptor serves specific functions, with the mu receptor being predominantly responsible for pain relief provided by opioid medications.[52]

Opioids elicit their effects by binding to opioid receptors at different CNS levels. As a result of binding at the receptor in subcortical sites, secondary changes lead to changes in the electrophysiologic properties of these neurons and modulation of the ascending pain information.

Because of their high effectiveness and relative low cost, opioids have been the first-line treatment for acute postsurgical pain for many years.[2] Their usefulness is further enhanced by the different ways of administration (oral, intravenous, sublingual, rectal, epidural, intrathecal).[2,7,49]

However, because of their numerous side effects and high addiction potential, the aim of modern techniques for postsurgical analgesia has been to reduce opioid consumption, reduce associated side effects, and improve patient satisfaction.[7,47,49]

The most promising approach in treating postsurgical pain remains a comprehensive multimodal perioperative approach involving different medication groups like gabapentinoids, NSAIDs, and regional nerve block techniques concomitantly.[40,42,47,55]

Common side effects of opioids include sedation, dizziness, nausea, vomiting, constipation, physical dependence, tolerance, and respiratory depression.[7]

INTERVENTIONAL TECHNIQUES

Regional Blockade

The use of epidural and spinal anesthesia (neuraxial) with or without the use of peripheral nerve blocks (PNBs) has become commonplace in hospitals that provide TKA.[25,63,71] While the recent evidence has not shown that regional or neuraxial techniques improve overall mortality or cardiovascular events, they have shown that pain control is superior to nonregional techniques.[25,31,44,63,71] The use of spinal anesthesia has also been shown to be more cost-effective than general anesthesia in the case of TKA.[24,31]

Periarticular Infiltration

Intraoperative infiltration of the knee joint by the surgeon has been used as an adjuvant modality for pain control in TKA.[25,63] There are studies and published protocols using intra- and periarticular clonidine, ketorolac, ropivacaine, and liposomal bupivacaine.[25,63] It should be noted that all of these injections are "off-label" uses, meaning that these medications are not U.S. Food and Drug Administration (FDA) indicated for periarticular infiltration.[25,63] Since the last edition, long-acting bupivacaine liposome injectable suspension (Exparel) was approved by the FDA in 2011 for infiltrating in bunionectomy and hemorrhoidectomy.[36] It has been used increasingly off label in TKA because of its advertised 72-hour pain relief. In September of 2014, the FDA issued a warning letter stating that it was not approved for periarticular use and that Exparel's 72-hour pain relief claims are unsubstantiated.[21] There is currently no data available on the injection of liposomal bupivacaine into major joints.

The addition of dexamethasone and/or epinephrine to local anesthetic (bupivacaine, lidocaine, ropivacaine) has been shown to prolong the duration of peripheral nerve and periarticular joint injections.[5] There is some concern with intra-articular corticosteroid injections because there is some data showing that all corticosteroids are chondrotoxic and also neurotoxic.[67]

PROTOCOL

Preoperative

- Celecoxib 400 mg or ibuprofen 800 mg by mouth day of surgery
- Pregabalin 100 to 150 mg or gabapentin 900 to 1200 mg single dose by mouth day of surgery
- Oxycodone controlled release 10 mg or oxymorphone extended release 5 mg by mouth
- Acetaminophen 1 g by mouth

Intraoperative

- Regional blockade
- Neuraxial (epidural or spinal-epidural) anesthesia
- Peripheral nerve block with catheter or periarticular infiltration by surgeon

Postoperative

- Celecoxib 200 mg twice daily by mouth (14 days) or ibuprofen 800 mg by mouth three times daily
- Ketorolac 30 mg IM/IV (patients aged <65 years), 15 mg (patients aged >65 years), every 6 hours (not to exceed 120 mg/day)
- Pregabalin 50 mg by mouth twice daily or gabapentin 100 to 300 mg by mouth three times daily (14 days)
- Oxycodone 5 to 10 mg by mouth every 6 hours, as needed (5-10 days) for moderate to severe pain or tramadol 50 mg by mouth every 6 hours for mild pain as needed
- Oral acetaminophen or IV acetaminophen if patient is NPO
- Continue regional block infusion (neuraxial or peripheral)

CONCLUSION

Multimodal analgesia has evolved since it was first suggested in the early 1990s as surgical and anesthetic techniques have improved. TKA has evolved from a surgery that involved a weeklong stay to, in some centers, a same-day surgery. Standardized protocols and strategies of perioperative pain management such as dedicated APS teams have improved function, shortened LOS, improved patients' pain satisfaction, and may be beneficial in patient outcomes. The goal of multimodal analgesia is to provide an optimal pain control regimen that allows the patient to rehabilitate while limiting the adverse side effects of each medication.

The references for this chapter can also be found on www.expertconsult.com.

103

Chronic Pain After Total Knee Arthroplasty

Patrick J. Milord, Hersh Patel, Christopher Gharibo

Fundamental changes in pain processing may occur postoperatively in patients to give rise to the chronic pain state. Chronic pain may be described as pain "beyond the expected temporal boundary of tissue injury and normal healing,"[2] although some have traditionally considered this as pain lasting for greater than 3 months in duration.

Total knee arthroplasty (TKA) poses a particular challenge to clinicians; although early ambulation is paramount to successful long-term rehabilitation and recovery,[25] persistent pain may severely debilitate the patient and contribute to a functional state worse off than their respective preoperative condition. The pain may be intrinsic to the knee itself or may originate from an external source; thus a wide differential of probable diagnoses exists. Therefore it is important that a thorough pain management pathway be established and adhered to, so that the chronic pain is prevented and post-TKA milestones are met in a timely fashion.

Osteoarthritis (OA) is one of the primary reasons to pursue TKA. A painful condition in and of itself, this diagnosis is characterized by gradual degeneration and narrowing of the joint space, along with cartilaginous destruction leading to decreased mobility and function. An estimated 25% to 39% of adults aged 45 to 64 years old experience knee OA symptomatology.[32] Surgery is often reserved for severe cases after conservative measures have proven ineffective (Fig. 103.1).[12]

Total knee arthroscopy is one of the most common orthopedic procedures; between 1991 and 2010 the number of annual TKA procedures in Medicare patients increased 162% from 93,230 to 243,802.[11] Unfortunately, TKA surgery is not always curative, and the knee pain may persist long afterwards. Chronic pain after TKA has a prevalence of approximately 20% to 40%; thus a significant number of patients will likely remain impaired by chronic pain from 3 to 24 months after TKA surgery.[4,6,16,28,29,36] Despite this staggering value, most patients maintain a different perception and generally express the expectation of significant recovery and majority function within 12 weeks.[14] Thus the surgeon must identify those at increased risk for worsened pain, manage expectations appropriately, and mitigate symptoms and sources of pain should they arise.

This chapter will comprehensively address chronic pain after TKA, including etiology and risk factors for development, pathophysiology, diagnostic testing modalities, and treatment options. Specific types of equipment failures and surgical techniques are beyond the scope of this chapter.

ETIOLOGY AND RISK FACTORS

Chronic pain is a multifaceted entity, often with a combination of chemical, neurologic, and psychological components

incorporated into it. In response to local tissue trauma, the milieu of some nerve fibers changes such that subsequent stimuli at the site elicits an enhanced sensory response[38] (hyperalgesia). Nearby nerves may also be affected, such that adjacent dermatomes are activated in addition (secondary hyperalgesia), thereby yielding greater pain along a wider distribution. However, this phenomenon does not occur routinely because most people experience a painful foci as a discrete and time-dependent event. Although for a subset of others, it appears that certain preoperative characteristics may indeed "prime" individuals to develop persistent chronic pain. A systematic review and meta-analysis of 32 studies with approximately 30,000 patients at least 3 months post-TKA aimed to identify key preoperative patient variables associated with persistent pain[24]; it was revealed that (1) other pain sites, (2) catastrophizing, (3) depression/anxiety (mental health state), and (4) preoperative pain score[29] were among the most significant chronic pain predictor variables (Fig. 103.2).

The presence of other pain sites and greater preoperative pain scores[29] may relate to central sensitization, a generalized process by which nociception is effectively recalibrated with a hair-trigger, thereby leading to an exaggerated pain response. The collective data suggest that OA patients specifically possess a lower pain threshold; for example, an experiment demonstrated that OA subjects reported both an enhanced degree and duration of pain in response to intramuscular (IM) hypertonic saline injection.[3] Thus it is postulated that there may be a central component responsible for the chronic pain state rather than local tissue and joint destructive processes.[26]

Catastrophizing is of particular significance because, unlike the other predictive variables, its impact on pain does not disappear over time and it continues to exert an effect many months to years later. In essence, it magnifies and perpetuates pain as a vicious and circuitous cycle to the beholder. Major depression confers a 1.3-fold greater risk of experiencing worse persistent pain after total knee replacement (TKR) versus nondepressed patients[32]; this clearly demonstrates the importance of overcoming psychosocial and emotional barriers in treating the distress of persistent chronic pain.

PATHOPHYSIOLOGY

Typical patterns of pain exist after TKA, which may direct the clinician to the specific reason for failure[32] (Table 103.1).

Pain with movement is considered because of sensitization of both peripheral Aδ and C fibers,[7,19] whereas pain at rest has been associated more to central sensitization.[31] With chronic joint inflammation being the primary intermediary, repeated local injury results in several cascades, which all eventually lead to the activation of terminal protein kinases to yield enhanced depolarizations to subsequent stimuli.[38] Known as "wind-up," the complex interactions necessary for this hypersensitivity are (1) repetitive stimuli inputs, (2) reduced activation of local inhibitory interneurons, and (3) activation of nonneuronal cells, thereby activating proexcitatory factors.

ASSESSMENT AND DIAGNOSTIC TESTING MODALITIES

For Researchers

A limited number of studies have been established to evaluate postsurgical chronic pain, especially with knee arthroplasties. With no objective measurement of pain, researchers rely on

surveys with studied efficacy for the assessment of chronic pain. Various works by both clinicians and researchers have shown that a thorough valuation of chronic pain requires a multifaceted approach.[8,17,23] The Initiative on Methods, Measurement, and Pain Assessment in Clinical Trials (IMMPACT) set forth guidelines on developing surveys and described the following core outcome measures for clinical trials of chronic pain treatment efficacy and effectiveness: intensity, physical functioning, emotional functioning, and patient global impression of change.[15]

Wylde et al. performed a systematic review of 8486 articles (of which 1164 met inclusion criteria) in 2013 to identify the measures currently used to assess chronic postsurgical pain after knee replacements (Table 103.2). The five most common multi-item tools used in these total knee replacement surgeries included the American Knee Society Score, Western Ontario and McMaster Universities (WOMAC) Osteoarthritis Index, Hospital for Special Surgery (HSS) Knee Score, Short Form 36 (SF-36), and Oxford Knee Score (OKS). According to Wylde

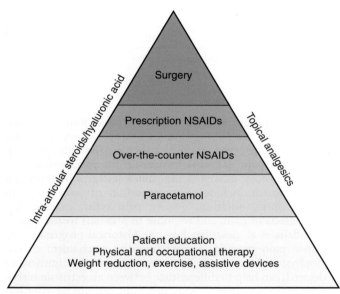

FIG 103.1 Treatment pyramid for osteoarthritis of the knee.

TABLE 103.1 Type of Pain

Night and Rest Pain	Infection
	Joint effusion or referred neurogenic
Pain on descending stairs	Flexion gap instability
Pain on chair raising	Femur malrotation
Anterior knee pain	Patella maltracking
	Overuse tendinitis and neurinoma
Posterior knee pain	Posterior soft tissue tightness
	Popliteus tendinitis
Pain on full extension	Anterior soft tissue impingement
	Posterior tightness
Pain on full flexion	Post impingement (offset/osteophytes)
	Patella impingement or tightness
Starting pain	Loose components
	Tibia and/or femur forceps pain
Weight-bearing pain	Unspecific
	Mainly mechanical cause

	n	Fisher's Z	Lower limit	Upper limit	P-value	I^2	Fisher's Z and 95% CI
Age*	8	−0.047	−0.083	−0.011	0.011	54	
Anxiety*	1	0.172	0.045	0.299	0.008	0	
Catastrophizing*	2	0.316	0.165	0.467	<0.001	0	
Comorbidities	5	0.083	−0.002	0.167	0.055	66	
Depression*	2	0.217	0.113	0.321	<0.001	0	
Education	3	−0.136	−0.314	0.043	0.136	85	
Function*	5	−0.124	−0.240	−0.008	0.036	82	
Gender*	11	0.056	0.011	0.101	0.015	68	
Other pain sites*	1	0.362	0.030	0.693	0.032	0	
Patella resurfacing	3	0.049	−0.089	0.186	0.487	0	
Preoperative pain*	11	0.155	0.043	0.266	0.007	80	
Social support*	2	−0.064	−0.116	−0.012	0.015	0	
Weight*	12	0.057	0.015	0.099	0.008	56	
							−1.0 −0.5 0 0.5 1.0

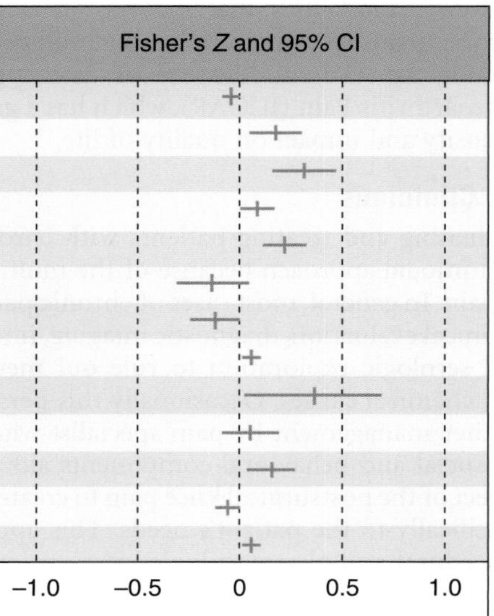

FIG 103.2 Forest plot showing the effect size (Fisher's Z) for predictor variables that were analyzed using univariate models. *p < .05; *CI*, Confidence interval.

TABLE 103.2   Multi-Item Tools Used in More Than Five Studies*

Name of Multi-item Tool	No. of Studies That Used Tool (%)	No. of Items in Tool	No. of Items in Tool Assessing Pain
American Knee Society Score	675 (58)	10	1
WOMAC	267 (23)	24	5
Hospital for Special Surgery Knee Score	184 (16)	7	2
Short Form 36	165 (14)	36	2
Oxford Knee Score	101 (9)	12	5
Short Form 12	54 (5)	12	1
Knee Injury and Osteoarthritis Outcome Score	26 (2)	42	9
EQ-5D	25 (2)	5	1
Feller Patellar Score	20 (2)	4	1
Knee Outcome Survey activities of daily living scale	14 (1)	17	1
Lequesne Index	11 (<1)	12	5
Tegner and Lysholm Score	9 (<1)	8	1
Total Knee Function Questionnaire	9 (<1)	55	1
Nottingham Health Profile	7 (<1)	45	8
Self-Administered Patient Satisfaction Scale	6 (<1)	4	1
Stern and Insall Patellar Score	6 (<1)	1	1
Bristol Knee Score	6 (<1)	9	1
15D	6 (<1)	15	1

*WOMAC, Western Ontario and McMaster Universities Osteoarthritis Index; EQ-5D, EuroQol 5-domain instrument; 15D, 15-dimensional instrument.

et al. none of the tools evaluated pain quality, pain medication use, or participant ratings of global improvement, but the OKS and WOMAC provided the most comprehensive assessment of chronic pain. The AKSS, although the most commonly used survey, provided a single question on pain and had limited utility in pain-related postoperative outcomes.[35]

The WOMAC pain scale considers the pain experienced during five different activities: walking, using stairs, sitting or lying, standing upright, and in bed. The questionnaire uses a 5-point Likert scale ranging from none to unbearable (0 to 4) and the score is converted into a 0 to 100 scale where 0 indicates extreme pain and 100 indicates no pain.[5] The OKS is a twelve question survey that also uses a 5-point Likert Scale to evaluate the functionality and pain associated specifically after treatments performed on the knee.[13]

Newer modalities that incorporate a global approach to chronic pain outcomes are being developed and tested. These include the 11-item Measure of Intermittent and Constant Osteoarthritis Pain (ICOAP), which has a greater focus on pain intensity and impact on quality of life.[18]

For Clinicians

Evaluating and treating patients with chronic pain requires a multimodal approach because of the multidimensional nature of pain. In general, most cases of chronic pain after TKA require a clinical evaluation, diagnostic imaging, microbiologic analysis, and serologic exploration to rule out mechanical, biological, and chemical causes. Occasionally this persistent pain requires further management by pain specialist who focus on the psychosocial and behavioral components along with the physical aspect of the postsurgical knee pain to create treatments tailored specifically to the patient's needs. This approach incorporates procedural and pharmacologic interventions with the goals of relieving pain, increasing physical activity, and managing stress, while minimizing potential for addiction and substance abuse.

The standard medical history and physical exam provides the clinician with a basis for the overall well-being of the patient.

It also offers insight into any comorbid conditions that could be exacerbating the pain symptoms postoperatively, including diabetes mellitus, rheumatoid arthritis, and fibromyalgia. However, the pain specialist focuses on the psychosocial and behavioral history, as well as the pain assessment. A thorough pain assessment includes documentation of pain location, intensity, onset, duration, quality, pain relief, exacerbating factors, effects of pain, and response to previous treatments.

Mandalia et al. describes how the historical progression of the knee pain provides insight into the mechanism of the pathophysiology involved. Time of onset, whether immediate or delayed, can help to differentiate between an extrinsic versus intrinsic source. Extrinsic sources would include referred hip pain, nerve entrapment in the spine, or vascular causes, which present as pain that is unchanged after surgical intervention. In contrast, intrinsic sources of pain gradually develop over time after the surgery. Instability, misalignment, soft tissue impingement, and acute infection are processes with more acute presentations than loosening of components, wear of polyethylene, late ligamentous instability, or fracture. Pain occurring at rest is more indicative of infection or neuropathic pain, hypersensitivity to touch suggests cutaneous neuroma or neuropathic pain, sharp and stabbing points towards mechanical pain, and radiating pain is likely referred pain from hip or spine.[27]

A thorough physical exam also guides the therapeutic approach by narrowing the differential. The general assessment of the knee joint should elucidate any gross deformities, atrophies, discolorations, erythema, swelling, pallor, or cyanosis. Gait, range of motion, tenderness to palpation, and joint temperature may also reveal significant pathologies during the exam. Referred pain in the peripheral nervous system, especially from the hip and spine, should be assessed by evaluating muscle strength, sensation, and stretch reflexes.

With no diagnostic test available for chronic pain, various assessment tools are used to objectify and trend knee pain. Hooten et al. describe some of the modalities used in clinical practice (Tables 103.3 and 103.4).

TABLE 103.3 Clinical Tools—Subjective Indicators of Pain: Simple Assessment Scales versus Comprehensive Assessment Scales

Simple		Comprehensive	
"Faces" Pain Scale (FPS)	Ideal for young children	Body outline markings	Assesses location, intensity, and pattern; reports meds, pain relief, patient beliefs, and interference in quality of life
Numeric Rating Scales (NRS)	Very commonly used; controversial metric of pain as "5th vital sign"	Brief pain inventory	Valid, reliable, easy to use, relevant to primary care setting
Visual Analog Scale (VAS)	Continuous line, fixed endpoints; assumes pain intensity correlates to measured distance	Chronic Pain Grade Scale (CPGS)	Measured parameters: intensity and pain-related disability, as experienced over time
Verbal Descriptive Scales (VDS)	Ideal for older adults and mildly cognitively impaired		Ideal for primary care/outpatient setting, as recall period is 3-6 months

TABLE 103.4 Multimodal, Multidisciplinary Therapeutic Options Matrix

Physical	Psychological	Pharmacological	Salvage Interventions
Physical rehabilitation home exercise weight loss	Meditation hypnotherapy	Nonsteroidals (NSAIDs)	Revision surgery
Massage acupuncture	Support group therapy	Neuropathics (gabapentinoids)	Intrathecal pump
TENS cryotherapy	Pain counseling	Antidepressants, anticonvulsants	Spinal cord stimulator
Minimally invasive procedures (intraarticular)	Psychotherapy (CBT, ECT)	Opioids	

Because psychological factors, such as depression, are risk factors for developing chronic pain after TKR, other assessments that should be used include the Patient Health Questionnaire-9 (PHQ-9) for depression, generalized anxiety disorder (GAD) 7 for anxiety, and CAGE for alcohol abuse.

PREVENTION

Various factors can play an integral role in the prevention of persistent pain after a TKA. Early identification and management of preoperative risk factors, such as mood disorders and catastrophizing, may largely influence the timeline of postoperative recovery experienced by the patient.[22,33] However, studies have yet to show efficacy for pharmaceutical management of these risk factors preoperatively; research will require an emphasis on the risk-benefit ratio of the side effects of preoperative medications and chronic pain as an outcome of surgery.[34] Early preoperative management of the pain itself may help to prevent the chronic state as a result of the close follow-up necessary in its management, as well as the improvement in quality of life for the patient.[10] Furthermore, the synergistic effect of a multimodal approach to chronic pain reduces the individual doses of each drug and consequently the risk of adverse effects.[30] Studies have shown that high pregabalin may diminish the process of hyperalgesia, a major pathway to chronic pain, while producing heavy side effects. Therapies such as perioperative ketamine infusions may decrease perioperative opioid requirements.[1,9] The efficacy of local anesthetics and nonsteroidal anti-inflammatory drugs (NSAIDs) in reducing inflammatory states and opioid consumption has also been shown in various studies related to chronic postsurgical pain.[20,37]

TREATMENT

Although orthopedic revision remains a viable option for many of the intrinsic causes of chronic pain after TKA, many surgeons opt for pharmacologic treatments, especially for neuropathic pain. The multidisciplinary approach includes physical rehabilitation supplemented by analgesics, which include narcotics, NSAIDs, and gabapentinoids, as well as creams and transcutaneous electrical nerve stimulation (TENS) therapy. When the source of pain becomes ambiguous or unresolved for both the physician and patient, a more holistic, long-term pain management regimen is established using a biopsychosocial approach by a pain specialist that may include interventional pain management including spinal cord stimulation.

SELECTED REFERENCES

2. American Society of Anesthesiologists: Practice guidelines for chronic pain management: an updated report by the American Society of Anesthesiologists Task Force on Chronic Pain Management and the American Society of Regional Anesthesia and Pain Medicine. *Anesthesiology* 112:810–833, 2010.

4. Baker PN, van der Meulen JH, Lewsey J, et al: The role of pain and function in determining patient satisfaction after total knee replacement. Data from the national joint registry for England and Wales. *J Bone Joint Surg* 89:893–900, 2007.

5. Bellamy N, Buchanan WW, Goldsmith CH, et al: Validation study of WOMAC: a health status instrument for measuring clinically important patient relevant outcomes to antirheumatic drug therapy in patients with osteoarthritis of the hip or knee. *J Rheumatol* 15:1833–1840, 1988.

12. Creamer P, Hochberg MC: Treatment pyramid for osteoarthritis of the knee. *Lancet* 350(9076):503–508, 1997.

15. Dworkin RH, Turk DC, Farrar JT, et al: Core outcome measures for chronic pain clinical trials: IMMPACT recommendations. *Pain* 113:9–19, 2005.

21. Hooten WM, Timming R, Belgrade M, et al: Institute for Clinical Systems Improvement. Assessment and management of chronic pain. Updated November 2013.

24. Lewis GN, Rice DA, McNair PJ, et al: Predictors of persistent pain after total knee arthroplasty: a systematic review and meta-analysis. *Br J Anaesth* 114(4):551–561, 2015. doi: 10.1093/bja/aeu441.

27. Mandalia V, Eyres K, Schranz P, et al: Evaluation of patients with a painful total knee replacement. *J Bone Joint Surg Br* 90(3):265–271, 2008.

28. Nashi N, Hong CC, Krishna L: Residual knee pain and functional outcome following total knee arthroplasty in osteoarthritic patients. *Knee Surg Sports Traumatol Arthrosc* 23:1841–1847, 2015.

29. Puolakka PA, Rorarius MG, Roviola M, et al: Persistent pain following knee arthroplasty. *Eur J Anaesthesiol* 27(5):455–460, 2010. doi: 10.1097/EJA.0b013e328335b31c.

30. Reuben SS, Buvanendran A: Preventing the development of chronic pain after orthopaedic surgery with preventive multimodal analgesic techniques. *J Bone Joint Surg Am* 89(6):1343–1358, 2007.

31. Schaible HG, Ebersberger A, Von Banchet GS: Mechanisms of pain in arthritis. *Ann N Y Acad Sci* 966:343–354, 2002.

35. Wylde V, Bruce J, Beswick A, et al: Gooberman-hill R: Assessment of chronic postsurgical pain after knee replacement: a systematic review. *Arthritis Care Res (Hoboken)* 65(11):1795–1803, 2013.

36. Wylde V, Hewlett S, Learmonth ID, et al: Persistent pain after joint replacement: prevalence, sensory qualities, and postoperative determinants. *Pain* 152:566–572, 2011.

The references for this chapter can also be found on www.expertconsult.com

Ambulatory Procedures

104

Knee Arthroscopy

Lisa Mouzi Wofford

AMBULATORY SURGERY

With advances in surgical techniques and innovations in the safety and quality of anesthesia care, the number of outpatient cases in the United States has steadily risen to surpass the number of nonambulatory cases performed annually. Costs are lower for ambulatory facilities, scheduling is more predictable, and operating room turn-around times tend to be shorter. Procedures suitable for ambulatory surgery are those associated with short surgical time, low rates of postoperative complications, and postoperative care that can be easily managed by the patient at home. Identifying appropriate patients who can benefit from the efficiency of ambulatory care is also important to minimize the risk of morbidity and mortality.

Mathis et al. sought to guide patient selection for outpatient surgery by identifying patient risk factors contributing to surgical morbidity and mortality. Information was collected from 244,397 outpatient surgeries performed at more than 250 medical centers across the United States from 2005 to 2010. Within this study population, 232 cases (0.1%) experienced a perioperative adverse event. Seven independent predictors of perioperative morbidity or mortality were identified: overweight by body mass index (BMI), obese by BMI, chronic obstructive pulmonary disease, history of transient ischemic attack/stroke, hypertension, previous cardiac surgical intervention, and prolonged operative time. Early postoperative pneumonia, unplanned postoperative intubation, and wound disruption were the most common morbidities identified.[31]

Another recent study evaluating the risk factors for unanticipated hospital admission following ambulatory surgery concluded that length of surgery more than 1 hour, high American Society of Anesthesiologists (ASA) physical status classification (ASA ≥ 3), advanced age (>80 years), and increased BMI were all predictors. The most common reasons identified for admission were surgical (40%), anesthetic (20%), and medical (19%). Plastic; orthopedic; dental; and ear, nose, and throat (ENT) surgery were associated with a reduced risk when compared with general surgery. Because no specific comorbid illness was associated with increased morbidity, the authors suggest that these findings support continued use of the ASA classification for perioperative risk assessment.[39] Ambulatory surgery is no longer restricted to ASA class I and II patients. Procedures on class III and IV patients can be safely performed as long as their comorbid conditions are medically optimized and stable (Table 104.1).

Obese patients are a distinct class of patients and most studies associate obesity with increased risk for perioperative complications. A systematic review assessing perioperative outcome in adult obese patients undergoing ambulatory surgery found that the super obese (BMI > 50 kg/m^2) do present an increased risk for perioperative complications, whereas patients with lower BMIs can safely undergo outpatient surgery as long as comorbidities are optimized before surgery.[23] Because most obese patients have sleep disordered breathing such as obstructive sleep apnea (OSA) or obesity hypoventilation syndrome, it is prudent to consider the presence of these conditions when determining the appropriateness of their care in an ambulatory facility. The ASA recently published updated guidelines on the perioperative management of patients with OSA. Those guidelines state that procedures typically performed on an outpatient basis in non-OSA patients may also be safely performed on an outpatient basis in patients with OSA when local or regional anesthesia is administered. These patients should not be discharged home or to an unmonitored setting until they are no longer at risk for apnea or respiratory depression.[2,11] This may require a longer stay in the recovery room compared to non-OSA patients undergoing the same procedure. Patients with OSA who are at significantly increased risk of perioperative complications are generally not good candidates for outpatient surgery and accommodations should be made in advance for prolonged observation.

The ability to discharge a patient from the recovery room in a time-effective manner is important and also needs to be a consideration preoperatively. Drowsiness, nausea and vomiting, and pain are the most common causes for delays in patient discharge. Especially in the outpatient setting, it is imperative to use carefully considered pain management strategies including multimodal analgesia and regional anesthesia to maximize pain control and minimize opioid use, which subsequently diminishes the incidence of postoperative nausea, vomiting, and oversedation. The ASA has recently updated their guidelines on postanesthesia care to address these issues.[3] To determine eligibility for discharge, the modified Aldrete score and the Home Readiness scale are most often used and a score of 9 to 10 is recommended (Tables 104.2 and 104.3).

The two most frequently performed outpatient surgical procedures on the knee are knee arthroscopy and ligament reconstruction. The advent of arthroscopy has revolutionized diagnosis and treatment of the knee, and although the typical patients undergoing knee arthroscopy and ligament reconstruction are young, healthy, and athletic, many patients undergoing these procedures are older adults with multiple medical comorbidities. The following discussion will review the current recommendations regarding the anesthetic management of knee arthroscopy and knee ligament reconstruction.

TABLE 104.1   American Society of Anesthesiologists Physical Status Classification System

American Society of Anesthesiologists Classification	Definition	Examples, Including but Not Limited to
ASA I	A normal healthy patient	Healthy, nonsmoking, no or minimal alcohol use
ASA II	A patient with mild systemic disease	Mild diseases only, without substantive functional limitations. Examples include (but are not limited to): current smoker, social alcohol drinker, pregnancy, obesity, well-controlled DM/HTN, mild lung disease
ASA III	A patient with severe systemic disease	Substantive functional limitations: One or more moderate to severe diseases. Examples include (but are not limited to): poorly controlled DM or HTN, COPD, morbid obesity, active hepatitis, alcohol dependence or abuse, implanted pacemaker, moderate reduction of ejection fraction, ESRD undergoing regularly scheduled dialysis, premature infant PCA < 60 weeks, history of (>3 months) MI, CVA, TIA, CAD/stents
ASA IV	A patient with severe systemic disease that is a constant threat to life	Examples include (but not limited to): recent (<3 months) MI, CVA, TIA, or CAD/stents, ongoing cardiac ischemia or severe valve dysfunction, severe reduction of ejection fraction, sepsis, DIC, ARD, or ESRD not undergoing regularly scheduled dialysis
ASA V	A moribund patient who is not expected to survive without the operation	Examples include (but are not limited to): ruptured abdominal/thoracic aneurysm, massive trauma, intracranial bleed with mass effect, ischemic bowel in the face of significant cardiac pathology or multiple organ/system dysfunction
ASA VI	A declared brain-dead patient whose organs are being removed for donor purposes	

The addition of "E" denotes Emergency surgery: (an emergency is defined as existing when delay in treatment of the patient would lead to a significant increase in the threat to life or body part).

ARD, Acute respiratory distress; *ASA,* American Society of Anesthesiologists; *CAD,* coronary artery disease; *COPD,* chronic obstructive pulmonary disease; *CVA,* cerebrovascular accident; *DIC,* disseminated intravascular coagulation; *DM,* diabetes mellitus; *ESRD;* end-stage renal disease; *HTN,* hypertension; *MI,* myocardial infarction; *PCA,* postconceptual age; *TIA,* transient ischemic attack.

http://www.asahq.org/resources/clinical-information/asa-physical-status-classification-system.

TABLE 104.2   Modified Aldrete Scoring System for Determining PACU Discharge

Discharge Criteria	Score
Activity: Able to Move Voluntarily or on Command	
Four extremities	2
Two extremities	1
Zero extremities	0
Respiration	
Able to deep breathe and cough freely	2
Dyspnea, shallow, or limited breathing	1
Apneic	0
Circulation	
Blood pressure ±20 mm of preanesthetic level	2
Blood pressure ±20-50 mm of preanesthetic level	1
Blood pressure ±50 mm of preanesthetic level	0
Consciousness	
Fully awake	2
Arousable on calling	1
Not responding	0
Oxygen Saturation	
Able to maintain O_2 > 92% on room air	2
Needs O_2 inhalation to maintain O_2 saturation >90%	1
O_2 saturation <90% even with O_2 supplementations	0

Patients who have a score of 9 or greater and have an appropriate escort are ready to be discharged.
From Aldrete JA: The post-anesthesia recovery score revisited. *J Clin Anesth* 7(1):89–91, 1995.

KNEE ARTHROSCOPY

Knee arthroscopy is one of the most commonly performed orthopedic procedures in the United States. General and neuraxial anesthesia are most often used. However, alternative techniques including peripheral nerve blocks and local anesthesia infiltration intra-articularly and periarticularly are also options. Important aspects that influence the choice of anesthesia are patient and surgeon satisfaction, patient safety, and costs. Because this procedure is typically performed on an outpatient basis, the choice of anesthetic must also result in early patient ambulation, adequate pain relief, and minimal nausea and vomiting leading to timely recovery and discharge (Table 104.4).

General Anesthesia

General anesthesia for knee arthroscopy is easy to perform, yields excellent operating conditions, and is usually the default anesthetic in case of failure of other techniques. Many patients prefer general anesthesia because they would rather be completely unaware during their operation, and many surgeons favor an unconscious patient. However, general anesthesia is not without drawbacks including, but not limited to, postoperative nausea and vomiting, prolonged postoperative drowsiness, and increased postoperative pain. Many studies have compared patient satisfaction scores, operating room times and costs, pain management, and recovery times of general anesthesia with other anesthesia techniques for knee arthroscopy.

Dahl et al. compared general with neuraxial anesthesia for cases of outpatient diagnostic knee arthroscopy and general meniscectomy. The time between the patient's entry to the OR and surgical incision was much shorter in the general anesthesia group; however, emergence from general anesthesia significantly lengthened the time from the end of the operation to arrival in the recovery room, partially negating initial time savings.

TABLE 104.3   PACU Score for Determining Home Readiness

Discharge Criteria	Score
Vital Signs	
Vital Signs Must Be Stable and Consistent With Age and Preoperative Baseline	
Blood pressure and pulse within 20% of preoperative baseline	2
Blood pressure and pulse 20%-40% of preoperative baseline	1
Blood pressure and pulse >40% of preoperative baseline	0
Activity Level	
Patient Must Be Able to Ambulate at Preoperative Level	
Steady gait to dizziness, or meets preoperative level	2
Requires assistance	1
Unable to ambulate	0
Nausea and Vomiting	
Patient Should Have Minimal Nausea and Vomiting Before Discharge	
Minimal: successfully treated with or without medication	2
Moderate: successfully treated with parenteral medication	1
Severe: continues after repeated treatment	0
Pain	
Patient Should Have Minimal or No Pain Before Discharge	
The level of pain that the patient has should be acceptable to the patient.	
The location, type, and intensity of the pain should be consistent with anticipated postoperative discomfort.	
Pain acceptable	2
Pain not acceptable	1
Surgical Bleeding	
Postsurgical Bleeding Should Be Consistent With Expected Blood Loss for the Procedure	
Minimal: does not require dressing change	2
Moderate: up to two dressing changes required	1
Severe: more than three dressing changes required	0

Patients with a score of 9 or greater are fit for discharge.
From Marshall S, Chung F: Assessment of 'home readiness': discharge criteria and postdischarge complications. *Curr Opin Anaesthesiol* 10:445–450, 1997.

TABLE 104.4   Advantages and Disadvantages of Various Anesthesia Modalities for Arthroscopic Knee Surgery

	Advantages	Disadvantages
General anesthesia	• Easy to perform • Excellent operating conditions	• Postoperative nausea/vomiting, pain, sedation • Increased costs
Neuraxial anesthesia	• Easy to perform • Rapid onset • Postoperative pain control	• Cannot be titrated • Delayed discharge from prolonged motor weakness
Regional anesthesia	• Postoperative pain control • Reduced postoperative nausea/vomiting	• Slower onset of anesthesia
Local anesthesia	• Reduced cost • Reduced complication rate • Fast recovery	• Intraoperative pain • Limitations on extent of surgery

Although the level of postoperative pain was generally low, the general anesthesia group did have higher postoperative pain scores and did require more opioid medication during recovery.[4]

When compared with peripheral nerve blocks, general anesthesia is associated with higher postoperative pain scores and opioid use, more nausea and vomiting, and longer time to reach home readiness criteria.[14]

A study comparing general with local anesthesia in 400 patients undergoing knee arthroscopy found that surgeons experienced less technical difficulties during surgery on patients in the general anesthesia group. No intraoperative pain was experienced in the patients under general anesthesia, in contrast with the patients in the local anesthesia group.[18] Thus, general anesthesia was associated with a high level of patient and surgeon acceptance when compared with local anesthesia infiltration.

Cost analyses of outpatient knee arthroscopy have shown that general anesthesia is associated with costs that are up to $600 more per procedure when compared to other anesthetic techniques. This is a result of additional charges related to pharmaceuticals, anesthesia equipment, and lengthier recovery room times.[9,25,38]

The data indicate that alternative techniques like neuraxial, regional, and local anesthetic infiltration are preferable to general anesthesia for many reasons including, but not limited to, better postoperative pain management, decreased use of resources, and overall cost containment. Whenever general anesthesia is used, however, a balanced analgesic technique including the administration of acetaminophen, nonsteroidal antiinflammatory drugs (NSAIDs), and intra-articular morphine with local anesthetic is recommended to enhance patient recovery.

Neuraxial Anesthesia

Spinal and epidural anesthesia are useful for abdominal and lower extremity surgeries. Spinal anesthesia is simple to perform, the onset is rapid and reliable, and it offers the benefit of postoperative pain relief. Epidurals have similar advantages with the additional benefit of an indwelling catheter to allow adjustment of anesthesia density and duration intraoperatively and the prolonged treatment of pain postoperatively. Neuraxial anesthesia does have its disadvantages, however. Spinal anesthesia is a single-injection technique and is limited because it cannot be titrated if its analgesia is not dense enough or its duration is insufficient. Larger doses may be required for adequate anesthesia but are associated with prolonged sensory and motor block and subsequent prolonged recovery. Urinary retention associated with neuraxial anesthesia can also delay discharge. Local anesthetics such as lidocaine, with a short duration of action to facilitate discharge, have a higher incidence of transient neurologic symptoms, which can be quite uncomfortable and unsettling to patients. Additionally, some patients are uncomfortable with the idea of an injection into the spine.

Mulroy et al. compared discharge times, side effects, operating room efficiency, and patient satisfaction levels of spinal, epidural, and general anesthesia for outpatient knee arthroscopy. The anesthesia in all three groups was satisfactory for incision. Patients who had spinals had a higher incidence of side effects in this study, including pruritus and headache, and time in the recovery room was longest in the spinal group, by about 50 minutes. Operating room turnover was no different in the groups. Despite these differences, patient satisfaction was equally high in all three groups.[32]

It is important to keep in mind that a variety of local anesthetics in varying concentrations exist for intrathecal administration. The right selection of local anesthetic can make spinal anesthesia better suited for brief procedures. Although these patients may require longer recovery room stays, they tend to have lower pain scores and require less opioid postoperatively.[4]

Regional Anesthesia

Peripheral nerve blocks have been successfully used for arthroscopic surgery. They allow surgery to be performed on conscious, cooperative patients. Potential advantages include improved postoperative pain management, less postoperative nausea and vomiting, less urinary retention, earlier ambulation, and hastened recovery. Despite these benefits, peripheral nerve blocks as the sole anesthetic are not as commonly used as other anesthetic modalities because of the perception that they take longer to perform, have a slower onset of anesthesia, and have variable success rates.

The femoral and adductor canal block are the most commonly performed peripheral nerve blocks for analgesia in knee arthroscopy. The obturator nerve also provides sensation to the knee and should be blocked for complete anesthesia, but even with a high-volume femoral block, this nerve is usually spared. The psoas compartment block produces reliable blockade of the entire lumbar plexus and has been used as the sole anesthetic for outpatient knee arthroscopy. In a study by Jankowski et al., the psoas compartment block was shown to provide satisfactory operating conditions that were comparable to spinal and general anesthesia. Patients who received this block had no pain at 120 minutes postoperatively and required significantly less analgesics. Patient satisfaction was highest in patients who received a regional technique.[21] A study by Hadzic compared patients who received general anesthesia to those who received a combination of psoas compartment block with sciatic nerve block for outpatient knee arthroscopy. The peripheral nerve blocks were performed in the operating room as was the induction of general anesthesia. The total operating room time did not differ significantly between the two groups, which indicates that the additional time that is required to place the peripheral nerve block at the beginning of the case offsets the emergence and extubation time required in general anesthesia. Patients also had less pain and nausea postoperatively and were able to meet home readiness criteria much sooner than patients who had general anesthesia.[14] The individual nerves (femoral, sciatic, lateral femoral cutaneous, and obturator) that supply the knee can be blocked in lieu of a psoas compartment block with similar positive results.[24]

If general or spinal anesthesia is selected as the primary anesthetic for outpatient knee arthroscopy, a femoral nerve or adductor canal block can be performed for postoperative analgesia. An adductor canal block is preferable for ambulatory procedures because it preserves quadriceps strength and the ability to ambulate better than the femoral nerve block.[19] As part of a multimodal analgesic regimen, an ultrasound-guided block at the adductor canal performed preoperatively has been shown to significantly reduce resting pain scores and opioid consumption in the recovery room and 24 hours postoperatively.[15] Adductor canal blocks are also effective as a rescue block to treat pain after surgery. Espelund et al. demonstrated a significant analgesic benefit in patients with moderate to severe pain. Pain during 45-degree active flexion of the knee, at rest, and during a 5-m walk was considerably reduced and all patients could be mobilized to walk 90 minutes after the block.[8]

Local Anesthesia

Local anesthesia for knee arthroscopy is a well-documented practice and has several advantages over other techniques including low costs and complication rates, faster recovery, and the ability of the patient to be awake and participate in the procedure. However, local anesthesia is not without its downsides. Depending on the extent of the arthroscopic surgery, pain control with local anesthesia can be insufficient, which can make a comprehensive surgical examination technically impossible and may require conversion to general anesthesia.

When local anesthesia is used as the sole anesthetic for knee arthroscopy, it is injected at the portal sites and into the joint capsule. Surgery is initiated 30 minutes after administration to allow the local anesthetic to exert its effects. This would ideally be done in the preoperative area to avoid wasted intraoperative time.

A randomized prospective study by Jacobson et al.[18] from 2000 compared local anesthesia with general and spinal anesthesia for primary elective outpatient knee arthroscopy. Approximately 33% of the subjects underwent purely diagnostic arthroscopy, whereas the other 67% had intra-articular procedures, including recessing plicas, shaving synovia and chondral defects, and partial meniscus resection. The surgeons assessed the technical difficulties to be more intense on patients in the local anesthesia group, the most common reasons being a narrow joint capsule, excess synovitis, and extensive surgery. Intraoperative pain was higher in the local anesthesia group over the spinal and general anesthesia groups. Overall, however, 90% of patients in the local anesthesia group were satisfied with their procedure.

Multimodal pain therapy is recommended for intraoperative and postoperative pain management. The synergistic effects of different groups of analgesics allow lower dosing with less associated side effects to achieve improved pain relief. The combination of local anesthetic with morphine and ketorolac injected intra-articularly has been shown to further decrease pain scores, especially with movement, and analgesic consumption postoperatively when compared to local anesthesia alone.[33]

Local anesthesia is viewed favorably by many because of the cost savings associated with this form of anesthesia. Decreased anesthesia-related fees along with shorter recovery room times are associated with hundreds of dollars in cost savings per patient.[25]

Local anesthesia infiltration is a safe, efficacious, and cost-effective form of anesthesia that can be routinely used for outpatient knee arthroscopy. Patients who want to view the procedure and participate in their surgical management and those without extensive intra-articular pathology, such as hypertrophic synovitis, are the best candidates for local anesthesia.

Summary

Various types of anesthesia have been successfully used for knee arthroscopy procedures in the outpatient setting. All of these techniques provide satisfactory anesthesia for outpatient knee arthroscopy, but the ultimate decision needs to be individualized based on surgeon technique and preference, patient comorbidities and expectations, and institutional practice. The ideal technique should result in high patient satisfaction, yield optimal surgical conditions, enhance operating room efficiency, and result in rapid recovery and discharge. There is no one-size-fits-all anesthetic for outpatient knee arthroscopy and the anesthesia should be tailored appropriately to accommodate each patient's needs.

LIGAMENT RECONSTRUCTION

Anterior cruciate ligament (ACL) injuries are a common problem with an estimated incidence of tears being 100,000 per year in the United States.[34] Because ACL reconstructions comprise a substantial portion of many orthopedic practices, it is important for orthopedic surgeons to understand the anesthetic and analgesic options available to patients. These procedures are increasingly performed on an outpatient basis and can be associated with severe pain unless appropriate measures are taken. There are multiple analgesic modalities available to the surgeon and anesthesiologist to help reduce postoperative pain, nausea and vomiting, and facilitate discharge from the recovery room; however there is no consensus in the current literature about the most appropriate technique. Successful techniques used for postoperative pain management include intra-articular injection, femoral nerve blocks, and adductor canal blocks.

Local Anesthesia Infiltration

Local anesthesia infiltration of the incision and the intra-articular space can be a quick and inexpensive way to provide postoperative analgesia in the patient undergoing ACL repair. Tetzlaff et al. compared intra-articular placebo with bupivacaine and morphine to assess postoperative pain scores and opioid consumption after ACL reconstruction. The group that received 0.25% bupivacaine with 1 mg morphine intra-articularly had significantly lower pain scores upon arrival to the postanesthesia care unit (PACU) and lower fentanyl and hydrocodone use postoperatively.[37] Studies of continuous intra-articular infusions show similar results. Hoenecke et al. randomized patients who underwent ACL reconstruction to receive normal saline or bupivacaine for 48 hours through a catheter at the donor site of the patellar tendon. Both groups received a single intra-articular bolus injection of 35 mL of 0.25% bupivacaine with 5 mg of morphine at the conclusion of surgery. There was a statistically significant decrease in pain scores and narcotic consumption by patients receiving the local anesthetic infusion over the 48-hour period.[16] Morphine is the most commonly used opioid for intra-articular injection. A meta-analysis of the studies in the literature has shown that intra-articular morphine can produce analgesia for up to 24 hours after the injection. The ideal dose has not yet been determined because some studies suggest a dose-dependent effect and others do not.[13]

When continuous patellar wound and intra-articular wound infusion were compared with continuous femoral nerve block in patients who underwent ACL reconstruction, the results showed that patients in the femoral group had significantly lower pain scores at rest and at movement 24 hours after surgery. Additionally, the consumption of morphine and ketorolac was less in the femoral group postoperatively.[5] Somewhat conflicting with these results is a study by Woods et al. that showed no difference in postoperative pain ratings in the two study groups, however significantly more patients in the intra-articular

injection group received intramuscular hydromorphone than the femoral group.[40]

Thus, according to the literature, local anesthesia infiltration appears to be superior to placebo at controlling postoperative pain after ACL reconstruction, but femoral nerve block may provide an even better level of analgesia.

Femoral Nerve Block

Femoral nerve blocks for the postoperative pain management of ACL repair are commonly used because they are quick and easy to perform, inexpensive, and provide a dense sensory block to the anterior aspect of the knee, as well as to the bone in the distal femur and the proximal tibia where tunnels are drilled during the procedure.

Iskander et al. compared femoral nerve block using 20 mL of 1% ropivacaine with intra-articular infiltration using 20 mL of 1% ropivacaine in a prospective randomized study. Pain scores were significantly lower in the femoral group than in the intra-articular group in the recovery room and during rehabilitation. Analgesic duration was longer and morphine consumption postoperatively was almost three times lower in the femoral nerve block group. Because less opioid was administered in the femoral group, there was also a decrease in opioid-related side effects such as nausea and sedation in this group.[17]

Similar results were found in other studies. In patients undergoing ACL reconstruction under spinal anesthesia, those who received a femoral nerve block had better pain control in the first 12 hours after surgery.[12] Souza et al. demonstrated that patients undergoing ACL reconstruction or total knee replacement had less pain, a lower morphine consumption, and less nausea with a femoral nerve block for postoperative pain control compared to those without a femoral nerve block.[6]

There are differing results in some reports, however. A systematic review of 13 studies assessing the efficacy of femoral nerve blocks in controlling pain after ACL reconstruction concluded that there was little added benefit to using these blocks for ACL reconstruction when a multimodal approach to pain was used.[29] A drawback of this review, weakening its assertion, is that it was not a meta-analysis of the literature because the heterogeneity in the studies evaluated was too high.

Overall, the femoral nerve block does provide reliable analgesia for ACL reconstruction, but it is not without drawbacks. As with any peripheral nerve block, infection and bleeding is always a risk. Quadriceps strength has been shown to decrease by a mean of 49% after femoral nerve block,[19] which can put patients at increased risk of falling postoperatively.

Adductor Canal Block

Although the femoral nerve block has been shown to provide effective analgesia, the associated diminished quadriceps strength leading to delayed mobilization and increased risk of falling has led to the investigation of alternative peripheral block techniques that have more sensory and less motor effects. The adductor canal lies in the middle third of the thigh in the anterior-medial compartment. The canal contains the femoral artery and vein, the saphenous nerve, and the nerve to the vastus medialis.[35] Injection of local anesthetic in the adductor canal results in an almost exclusively sensory block of the anterior knee and medial aspect of the leg and although more studies have evaluated its efficacy in controlling pain after major knee surgery such as total knee arthroplasty (TKA), adductor canal blocks are being used for ACL reconstruction as well.[22,35]

Lundblad et al. studied the analgesic effect of the saphenous block specifically after ACL repair and demonstrated improved pain relief when compared to a sham block.[27] Interestingly, these results were not reproduced in a study by Espelund et al.[7] They did not find any additional analgesic benefit of the adductor canal block in patients undergoing ACL repair, but this may have been a result of inadequate sample size and low overall pain scores that did not allow detection of the effect of the block.[7,36]

Adductor canal blocks have been directly compared with femoral nerve blocks for postoperative analgesia in cases of TKA. In patients with severe movement-related pain following TKA, the quadriceps maximum voluntary isometric contraction increased to 193% of the baseline value (postoperative but before block performance) in patients receiving a postoperative adductor canal block and decreased to 16% in patients receiving a postoperative femoral nerve block. Pain scores were similar between groups. According to this study, the adductor canal block provides a clinically relevant increase in quadriceps muscle strength for patients in severe pain after TKA.[10] Multiple studies have shown similar pain scores and amounts of opioid consumption with a trend toward earlier discharge in patients with an adductor canal block for postoperative pain relief when compared to a femoral nerve block.[20,26,28]

Summary

The goals for patients undergoing outpatient ligament reconstruction include adequate pain control, minimal opioid-related side effects, early ambulation, and timely discharge from the recovery room. A multimodal approach to analgesia that includes local anesthesia infiltration, opioids, NSAIDs, and peripheral nerve blocks is ideal. Based on the current literature, adductor canal blocks are becoming the more favorable peripheral nerve block for postoperative analgesia because they provide reliable analgesia and preserve quadriceps strength to facilitate discharge from the recovery room.

KEY REFERENCES

2. American Society of Anesthesiologists Task Force on Perioperative Management of Patients with Obstructive Sleep Apnea: Practice guidelines for the perioperative management of patients with obstructive sleep apnea: an updated report by the American Society of Anesthesiologists Task Force on Perioperative Management of patients with obstructive sleep apnea. *Anesthesiology* 120(2):268–286, 2014.

4. Dahl V, Gierloff C, Omland E, et al: Spinal, epidural or propofol anaesthesia for outpatient knee arthroscopy? *Acta Anaesthesiol Scand* 41:1341–1345, 1997.

5. Dauri M, Fabbi E, Mariani P, et al: Continuous femoral nerve block provides superior analgesia compared with continuous intra-articular and wound infusion after anterior cruciate ligament reconstruction. *Reg Anesth Pain Med* 34(2):95–99, 2009.

9. Forssblad M, Jacobson E, Weidenhielm L: Knee arthroscopy with different anesthesia methods: a comparison of efficacy and cost. *Knee Surg Sports Traumatol Arthrosc* 12(5):344–349, 2004.

11. Gross JB, Bachenberg KL, Benumof JL, et al: Practice guidelines for the perioperative management of patients with obstructive sleep apnea: a report by the American Society of Anesthesiologists Task Force on Perioperative Management of patients with obstructive sleep apnea. *Anesthesiology* 104(5):1081–1093, 2006.

13. Gupta A, Bodin L, Holmström B, et al: A systematic review of the peripheral analgesic effects of intraarticular morphine. *Anesth Analg* 93(3):761–770, 2001.

14. Hadzic A, Karaca P, Hobeika P, et al: Peripheral nerve blocks result in superior recovery profile compared with general anesthesia in outpatient knee arthroscopy. *Anesth Analg* 100:976–981, 2005.

16. Hoenecke HR, Jr, Pulido PA, Morris BA, et al: The efficacy of continuous bupivacaine infiltration following anterior cruciate ligament reconstruction. *Arthroscopy* 18(8):854–858, 2002.

18. Jacobson E, Forssblad M, Rosenberg J, et al: Can local anesthesia be recommended for routine use in elective knee arthroscopy? A comparison between local, spinal, and general anesthesia. *Arthroscopy* 16(2):183–190, 2000.

23. Joshi GP, Ahmad S, Riad W, et al: Selection of obese patients undergoing ambulatory surgery: a systematic review of the literature. *Anesth Analg* 117(5):1082–1091, 2013.

31. Mathis MR, Naughton NN, Shanks AM, et al: Patient selection for day case-eligible surgery: identifying those at high risk for major complications. *Anesthesiology* 119(6):1310–1321, 2013.

34. Prodromos CC, Han Y, Rogowski J, et al: A meta-analysis of the incidence of anterior cruciate ligament tears as a function of gender, sport, and a knee injury-reduction regimen. *Arthroscopy* 23:1320–1325, 2007.

37. Tetzlaff JE, Dilger JA, Abate J, et al: Preoperative intra-articular morphine and bupivacaine for pain control after outpatient arthroscopic anterior cruciate ligament reconstruction. *Reg Anesth Pain Med* 24(3):220–224, 1999.

38. Triessmann HW: Knee arthroscopy: a cost analysis of general and local anesthesia. *Arthroscopy* 12(1):60–63, 1996.

39. Whippey A, Kostandoff G, Paul J, et al: Predictors of unanticipated admission following ambulatory surgery: a retrospective case-control study. *Can J Anaesth* 60:675–683, 2013.

The references for this chapter can also be found on www.expertconsult.com.

PART V

Thromboprophylaxis

105

Thromboprophylaxis and Neuraxial Anesthesia

Yeseniya Aronova, Milad Nazemzadeh

Venous thromboembolism is a major cause of death after trauma to the lower extremities or surgery. This risk is highest in patients undergoing major surgery, particularly hip and knee replacement.[14] Without prophylaxis, venous thrombosis develops in 40% to 60% of orthopedic patients, and 1% to 28% show clinical or laboratory evidence of pulmonary embolism. Fatal pulmonary embolism occurs in 0.1% to 8% of patients (Box 105.1).[4,14]

Improvements in morbidity and mortality have been demonstrated with neuraxial techniques for orthopedic procedures. Specifically, several old studies showed a decrease in the incidence of deep venous thrombosis (DVT) and pulmonary embolism (PE) in patients undergoing knee surgery with epidural anesthesia and not receiving currently recommended pharmacologic prophylaxis.[12,13] Proposed mechanisms for this effect include (1) rheologic changes resulting in hyperkinetic lower extremity blood flow, which reduces venous stasis and prevents thrombus formation; (2) beneficial circulatory effects from epinephrine added to local anesthetic solutions; (3) altered coagulation and fibrinolytic responses to surgery under central neural blockade, resulting in a decreased tendency for blood to clot and better fibrinolytic function; (4) absence of positive-pressure ventilation and its concomitant effects on circulation; and (5) direct local anesthetic effects such as decreased platelet aggregation. It is unclear now how much of this effect persists, given that all patients receive pharmacologic and/or mechanical prophylaxis.

Despite the reduced incidence of DVTs after central neuraxial blockade, additional pharmacologic prophylaxis is needed. Guidelines for antithrombotic therapy, including selection of pharmacologic agent, degree of anticoagulation desired, and duration of therapy, continue to evolve.[4] For patients undergoing hip or knee arthroplasty, administration of low-molecular-weight heparin (LMWH), warfarin, or fondaparinux is recommended.[14] In low-risk patients, however, a multimodal approach including preoperative thromboembolic risk stratification, regional anesthesia, postoperative rapid mobilization, pneumatic compression devices, and aspirin can jointly provide safe and effective thromboprophylaxis for elective primary joint replacement.[18]

Patients receiving perioperative anticoagulants and antiplatelet medications often are not considered candidates for spinal or epidural anesthesia and analgesia because of the risk of neurologic compromise from expanding spinal or epidural hematoma. The actual incidence of hemorrhagic complications associated with neuraxial blockade is unknown; however, the incidence cited in the literature is estimated to be less than 1 in 150,000 epidural and less than 1 in 220,000 spinal anesthetics.[2,15] The frequency of spinal or epidural hematoma is increased in patients who receive perioperative anticoagulation.[2,11,17] Other risk factors include technical difficulties, increased age, nonsteroidal anti-inflammatory drug (NSAID) use during anticoagulation, length of therapy, and history of gastrointestinal (GI) bleed.[2,8]

Spinal hematoma was considered a rare complication of neuraxial blockade until the introduction of LMWH as a thromboprophylactic agent in the 1990s. The calculated incidence (approximately 1 in 3000 epidural anesthetics), along with the catastrophic nature of spinal bleeding (only 30% of patients had good neurologic recovery), warranted an alternate approach to analgesic management following total hip and knee replacement.[6] There is evidence that patients undergoing major orthopedic surgery benefit from thromboprophylaxis, continuous peripheral nerve blocks, or a combination of both.[3] Furthermore, there is no evidence to support a belief that the combination of thromboprophylaxis and continuous peripheral nerve blocks increases the risk of major bleeding compared to either of these treatment modalities alone.[3]

It is reassuring that there are few reports of serious complications following intentional neurovascular sheath cannulation for surgical, radiologic, or cardiac indications. For example, during interventional cardiac procedures, large-bore catheters are placed within brachial or femoral vessels, and heparin, LMWH, antiplatelet medications, and/or thrombolytics are subsequently administered. Despite significant vessel trauma and coagulation deficiencies, neurologic complications are rare, although patients occasionally require a blood transfusion. In addition, all cases of major bleeding (significant decrease in hemoglobin and/or blood pressure) with non-neuraxial techniques occurred after psoas compartment or lumbar sympathetic blockade and involved heparin, LMWH, warfarin, or thienopyridine derivatives. These cases suggest that significant blood loss, rather than neural deficits, may be the most serious complication of non-neuraxial regional techniques in the anticoagulated patient.

Currently there are no prospective data on the use of central neuraxial anesthesia in the presence of anticoagulants. Most of the recommendations and guidelines are based on expert opinions from large case series, case reports, and the pharmacokinetics and pharmacodynamics of the anticoagulants used today. These guidelines specifically include (1) the minimum time interval between the last dose of an anticoagulant and the

---

TABLE 105.1 Summary of Guidelines on Anticoagulants and Neuraxial Blocks

I. Antiplatelet Medications

1. Aspirin, NSAIDs, COX-2 (cyclooxygenase-2) Inhibitors
   Surgery: may continue
   Pain clinic: ASA preferably stopped 2 to 3 days in thoracic/cervical epidurals
2. Thienopyridine derivatives
   a. Clopidogrel (Plavix): discontinue for 7 days
   b. Ticlopidine (Ticlid): discontinue for 14 days
   Do not perform a neuraxial block in patients on more than one antiplatelet drug
   If a neuraxial or deep plexus block has to be performed in patients whose clopidogrel was discontinued <7 days, then a P2Y12 assay should be performed.
3. GPIIB/IIIA: Time to normal platelet aggregation
   a. Abciximab (ReoPro) = 48 hr
   b. Eptifibatide (Integrilin) = 8 hr
   c. Tirofiban (Aggrastat) = 8 hr

II. Warfarin

Check INR; discontinue 4 to 5 days
INR < 1.4 before neuraxial block or epidural catheter removal

III. Heparin

1. Subcutaneous heparin (5000 U SC q 12 hr)
   Subcutaneous heparin is not a contraindication against a neuraxial block
   Neuraxial block should preferably be performed before SC heparin is given
   Risk of decreased platelet count with SC heparin therapy >5 days
2. Intravenous heparin
   Neuraxial block: 2 to 4 hr after the last intravenous heparin dose
   Wait ≥1 hr after neuraxial block before giving intravenous heparin

IV. Low-Molecular-Weight Heparin

No concomitant antiplatelet medication, heparin or dextran
Time interval between placement/removal of catheter after last dose
   a. Enoxaparin (Lovenox) 0.5 mg/kg BID (prophylactic dose): 12 hr
   b. 24-hr interval:
   Enoxaparin (Lovenox), 1 mg/kg BID (therapeutic dose)
   Enoxaparin (Lovenox), 1.5 mg/kg QD
   Dalteparin (Fragmin), 120 U/kg BID, 200 U/kg QD
   Tinzaparin (Innohep), 175 U/kg QD
   LMWH Postop: LMWH should not be started until 24 hr postsurgery
   LMWH should not be given until ≥2 hr after epidural catheter removals

V. Specific Xa Inhibitor: Fondaparinux (Arixtra)

ASRA: If neuraxial procedure has to be performed, recommend single needle, atraumatic placement, avoid indwelling catheter
EXPERT Study:[31] Epidural placement or catheter removal: 36 hr after Fondaparinux (half-lives); subsequent dose 12 hr after catheter removal

VI. Fibrinolytic/Thrombolytic Drugs (Streptokinase, Alteplase [tPA])

Recommended interval: 10 days (ASRA: no definite recommendation)
No data on safety interval for performance of neuraxial procedure

ASRA, American Society of Regional Anesthesia; *BID,* twice daily; *NSAID,* nonsteroidal anti-inflammatory drug; *SC,* subcutaneous.

BOX 105.1 Categories of Risk for Venous Thromboembolism in Surgical Patients

Low Risk

Minor surgery in patients <40 years of age with no additional risk factors present[a]

- Risk of calf DVT: 2%
- Risk of proximal DVT: 0.4%
- Risk of clinical PE: 0.2%
- Risk of fatal PE: <0.01%

Moderate Risk

Minor surgery in patients with additional risk factor present[a] *or* surgery in patients 40 to 60 years old with no additional risk factors

- Risk of calf DVT: 10% to 20%
- Risk of proximal DVT: 2% to 4%
- Risk of clinical PE: 1% to 2%
- Risk of fatal PE: 0.1% to 0.4%

High Risk

Surgery in patients ≥60 years old or surgery in patients 40 to 60 years old with additional risk factors[a]

- Risk of calf DVT: 20% to 40%
- Risk of proximal DVT: 4% to 8%
- Risk of clinical PE: 2% to 4%
- Risk of fatal PE: 0.4% to 1.0%

Highest Risk

Surgery in patients ≥40 years old with multiple risk factors,[a]
   Hip or knee arthroplasty, hip fracture surgery, major trauma, or spinal cord injury

- Risk of calf DVT: 40% to 80%
- Risk of proximal DVT: 10% to 20%
- Risk of clinical PE: 4% to 10%
- Risk of fatal PE: 0.2% to 5%

[a]Additional risk factors include one or more of the following: advanced age, cancer, prior venous thromboembolism, obesity, heart failure, paralysis, or molecular hypercoagulable state (eg, protein C deficiency, factor V Leiden).
DVT, Deep venous thrombosis; *PE,* pulmonary embolism.
Data from Geerts WH, Pineo GF, Heit JA, et al: Prevention of venous thromboembolism: the Seventh ACCP Conference on Antithrombotic and Thrombolytic Therapy. *Chest* 126:338S–340S, 2004.

---

insertion of the neuraxial needle/catheter or catheter removal, (2) the minimum time interval between the insertion of the neuraxial needle/catheter or catheter removal and the next dose of anticoagulant, and (3) the minimum values of coagulation studies needed for the performance of neuraxial techniques.[16] A summary of guidelines on anticoagulants and neuraxial blockade is shown in Table 105.1.[1] This is based on the most recent American Society of Regional Anesthesia (ASRA) guidelines. However, in the near future, a collaboration between the European Society of Anaesthesiology (ESA) and the ASRA on regional anesthesia and antithrombotic agents is expected.[2,5,7,9]

The references for this chapter can also be found on www.expertconsult.com.

Plastic Surgery

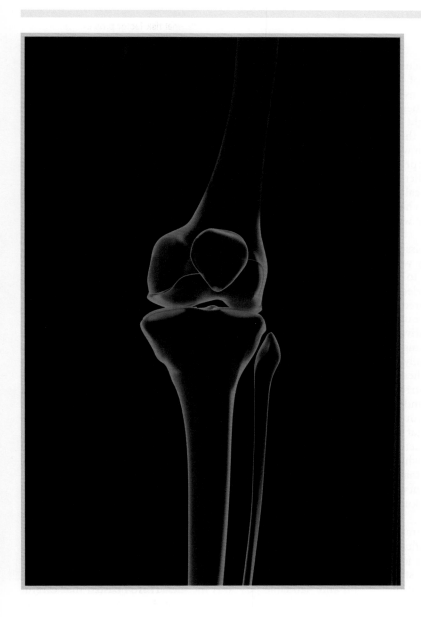

106

Soft Tissue Healing

Susan Craig Scott, Robert S. Reiffel, Kelly L. Scott, Alyssa Reiffel Golas

A patient who is to undergo total knee arthroplasty is focused on relief of pain and increased mobility, major quality of life issues that the operation reliably provides. Considerations of soft tissue healing are not ordinarily present in the patient's mind at the time of initial evaluation. That there might be difficulty with soft tissue healing may well be the furthest thing from a patient's thoughts. It is not unusual for a physician who introduces the subject of wound healing to be met with surprise, disbelief, or even suspicion. Only those who have had difficulty with soft tissue healing in the past are even aware that healing might be an issue. Unfortunately, patients who are likely to have difficulty with soft tissue healing are not limited to those with difficulty in the past.

Responsibility for assessing the condition of the soft tissues and systemic and local factors that might cause difficulty with healing lies with the treating physician. In the past 40 to 50 years, the modern era of total knee replacement, our knowledge of these wound-compromising factors has allowed us to predict with some degree of accuracy those who might have trouble and to assess what we might do preoperatively, intraoperatively, and postoperatively to maximize healing. Our understanding of the normal healing process has also expanded dramatically as molecular biology has contributed the ability to synthesize healing factors.[108] This chapter is a summary of our current knowledge and approach to soft tissue healing. A basic understanding of the biochemical and cellular processes of wound healing helps us appreciate the complexity of a process that we sometimes take for granted. In addition, in exploring factors that influence wound healing, we can better realize at which points interruption of normal healing might occur. Finally, steps that might be taken before and after surgery to influence the wound-healing process favorably become clear if we know where normal healing might go wrong.

Uncomplicated wound healing is a precisely orchestrated series of events. A troublesome wound can cause significant disability and prolonged recovery and result in prosthesis loss, amputation, and in extreme circumstances, death. In the last 20 years, there has been an explosion of research and information about the biochemical aspects of healing, chemoattractants, cytokines and their enumerated growth factors, and recombinant DNA technology, all of which hold promise for furthering our understanding of soft tissue healing.[107] Technology has contributed the ability to identify with a remarkable degree of accuracy the exact three-dimensional size of a wound allowing us to better assess what is needed for repair.[17,21] Although this exciting research has not yet led to acceleration of the normal healing of a wound in a healthy patient, it shows great promise in treating difficult wounds, as this chapter will outline. The normal healing phases will be described and factors that might enhance these phases in a wound that is healing poorly will be identified.

HISTORY

As long as there have been medical writings, attention has been directed to wound healing and attempts to enhance and accelerate it. The use of plant extracts, even bread mold, in healing is at least 2000 years old by written record.[13,68] Two famed papers, the Edwin Smith Surgical Papyrus and the Ebers Papyrus, describe certain of the earliest known wound manipulations—splinting and honey—to influence outcome.[11,26,90] Imhotep, the Egyptian polymath who lived and worked around 2630 BC is credited with composing the Smith Papyrus, which is the earliest known writing dealing with trauma and is named for Edwin Smith, an American antiquities dealer who purchased it in 1862. Composed at some time between 3000 and 2500 BC, the Papyrus is unique for its minimal references to magic and mystical remedies, and its emphasis on sound principles of diagnosis and treatment.[90] Hippocrates, the fourth century Greek physician, is remembered for his insistence on cleanliness and irrigation of wounds with only clean water or wine.[33] In addition, his prescient emphasis on documentation and accurate recording of events is a primary characteristic of good medical practice to this day. Hippocrates's scholarship was followed 300 years later by the Roman Celsus and about 100 years after that by Galen, whose work on wounded gladiators of Asia Minor led to his understanding of the venous and arterial systems, wound care, dressings, and meticulous follow-up. Descartes wrote the first Western physiology text, and Ambroise Paré deserves credit for one of the most significant contributions to our current approach today, the emphasis on gentle handling of tissues and on the harmful effects of trauma on tissue.[33,93] Pare's insight, very much alive today in our emphasis on avoidance of crushing clamps and prolonged vigorous retraction, is all the more remarkable because it was introduced into a medical world in which wounds were treated with boiling oil and "laudable pus" was the ideal. Paré insisted that careful tissue handling was the first step to uncomplicated tissue healing, a point we emphasize as well.

The late 19th and early 20th centuries saw rapid progress in our understanding of the causes of healing difficulties. Joseph Lister's acceptance of Pasteur's germ theory of infection and his application of its conclusions, controversial at the time, bore fruit in his description of aseptic technique and the use of carbolic acid as a topical disinfectant in hospitals in which infection was rampant.[13] His practical application of this sound principle, coupled with the discovery of antibiotics, put in place the last essential component of normal wound healing, control of infection, as the second half of the 20th century began.[37] The life-saving introduction of sulfanilamide came in the late 1930s; the discovery of penicillin soon after resulted in the awarding of the Nobel Prize in Physiology or Medicine in 1945 to Ernst B. Chain, Sir Alexander Fleming, and Sir Howard Florey.

The latter part of the 20th century saw dramatic technologic advances as well as advances in molecular biology, biochemistry, and immunology.[108] At the same time, surgical techniques and scholarship produced replacements for knees, hips, wrists, and elbows and functional replacements for kidneys, lungs, and hearts. It seems that there is no limit to what the confluence of ingenuity, adequate resources, and need might produce. Our challenge remains to follow where these advances lead without losing sight of the basic precepts that have brought us here.

PHASES OF WOUND HEALING

Surgical wound healing may be separated functionally and chronologically into three phases. Although these phases overlap, the events that predominate in each phase are different and together produce the strong, substantial, protective, resilient endpoint that we called a healed wound.[12]

The initial phase of inflammation, the phase which initiates life-saving hemostasis, begins with the formation of a platelet plug occluding a site of blood loss. This platelet plug then starts the cascade of events to follow. At the same time, vasoconstriction occurs, lasting roughly 10 minutes followed in rapid succession by vasodilation; it is vasodilation that allows the influx of cellular elements responsible for cleaning debris from the wound in preparation for the structural events that result in wound closure. The influx of platelets is rapidly followed by the arrival of polymorphonuclear leukocytes, lymphocytes, and macrophages. Vascular permeability moderated by histamine increases dramatically at the wound site. These cellular events result in the release of multiple factors—cytokines, platelet-derived factors, complement, and possibly even prostaglandins—enhancing the local cellular response in preparation for healing.

The elements of these first healing phases result in hemostasis, protection against infection, clearing of cellular debris, char, and necrotic tissue in preparation for the series of structural events that close the soft tissue in a healed wound.

Phase 2, the fibroblastic proliferative phase, uses the cellular elements and chemotactants that have rapidly accumulated in the wound during phase 1 to prepare the wound for the migration of fibroblasts, which are the primary synthesizers of collagen, the substance responsible for the healed wound's strength and durability. This second phase of healing begins within 48 hours after wounding. Fibroblasts climb along the fibrin matrix that has been deposited during the inflammatory phase of platelet aggregation. Interference with this crucially important matrix can be a cause of wound-healing delay.[130] As fibroblasts migrate in and become the predominant cell type in the healing wound around day 5, they produce ground substance, a gel-like combination of hyaluronic acid and chondroitin 4-sulfate, the glycosaminoglycans. This substrate will act as a matrix for the collagen fibrils synthesized most rapidly during the first few days of wound healing. This first collagen synthesized, tropocollagen, is converted to collagen fibrils, which assume structural and biochemical integrity on which wound strength is based; it is in the first 3 or so weeks after injury that we see the most rapid rise in wound strength gains.[74,107] As collagen homeostasis

is reached at approximately 3 weeks, collagen synthesis and degradation rates approach one another. This stage leads to the last and most prolonged phase of wound healing, the phase of remodeling or collagen maturation.

In the phase of collagen maturation, collagen-producing fibroblasts are markedly diminished; the collagen fibrils which have been deposited become measurably more organized and structured in response to a variety of factors, including local mechanical demands. The water content of the wound, along with the measurable ground substance, diminishes; the wound may feel more firm, dense, and indurated. Type III collagen, initially present in large amounts, is reduced and replaced by type I collagen as tissue strength–providing elements much more closely approach the elements that give strength to normal skin. Stronger collagen cross-links create mechanical resistance to disruption in the now-maturing wound. This process continues for many months, even years, after the initiating event.[94,95]

CELLULAR ELEMENTS OF HEALING

Specific cellular elements in wound healing are responsible for stimulation of fibroblasts, ingrowth of new and essential blood vessels, and clearing of debris in preparation for healing. Some medical illnesses, certain medications, and a number of environmental factors can challenge the ability of these cellular elements to perform their essential functions.

T lymphocytes produce a sustained response to injury in the wound. They generate local influences on the vascular endothelial lining in preparation for regrowth of new vessels. In addition, they produce a fibroblast-activating factor, which encourages and regulates fibroblastic activity in the healing wound. T-cell depletion at the time that a wound occurs can significantly deter strength gains in the healing wound.[8,96]

Macrophages migrate into the healing wound and are activated as they participate in the initial inflammatory phase. These cells remain in the wound much longer than other responders and release cytokines responsible for angiogenesis and for stimulating fibroblast proliferation.[71] Some studies have noted significant loss of the essential early functions of fibroplasia and debris clearance if there is interference with the availability, migration, or accumulation of macrophages.[132]

FACTORS AFFECTING SOFT TISSUE HEALING

With a clear understanding of the normal unfolding of events from the time of wounding to the production of a strong, stable, healed wound, a variety of factors that have bearing on tissue healing can be examined for their influence before, during, and after surgery. These factors are consistently present and may be manifested to the benefit or deterrence of tissue healing.

In the practical reality of the daily care of a surgical patient, environmental and physical factors, patient-related factors, and nutrition-related factors, as well as factors related to underlying medical illnesses, can all affect the progress of wound healing. A thorough understanding of the role these factors play helps the physician avoid healing difficulties, encourages patient participation in recovery, and mitigates the effects when healing does not progress as expected.

Scarring and Tissue Perfusion

Adequate levels of PO_2 in the healing wound are essential.[47] The oxygen delivery system whereby inspired oxygen traverses the pulmonary vessels, binds to hemoglobin, and is subsequently released in response to tissue demands is subject to breakdown at several points.[66] Local scarring, irradiated tissue, diabetes with vascular compromise, peripheral vascular disease, and chronic exposure to cigarette smoke can all interfere with the ability of small vessels to provide sufficient oxygen to the healing wound. Even local swelling or increased tissue pressure such as t created by an expanding hematoma might reduce perfusion and result in ischemic injury.[124] Preparation for surgery requires the surgeon to identify and remedy these factors as much as possible. At the molecular level, collagen synthesis by fibroblasts will not occur if tissue oxygenation is not adequate.

The mechanism whereby ischemia causes destructive effects on living tissue, whether the ischemia is the result of poor perfusion, radiation injury, or even small-vessel disease, is believed to be the production of oxygen free radicals, which are atoms or groups of atoms with unpaired electrons. These free radicals, a factor in aging skin and its loss of elasticity, are cytotoxic to both cell membranes and their internal components.[78,135] In addition, free radicals disrupt enzymes and other proteins and cause collagen to degrade prematurely.[127] In fact, white blood cells contribute to tissue ischemia in two ways: they are stiffer and less deformable than red cells and become trapped at the entry to small capillaries, obstructing blood flow. In addition, they are the producers of oxygen free radicals and exist in higher numbers in patients with underlying comorbidities. Minimizing free radical production by ensuring adequate tissue oxygenation is one way of minimizing or even reversing these detrimental effects. Additionally, when blockage occurs, it is possible to augment the body's own fibrinolytic system with agents such as streptokinase.[51]

When local factors dramatically reduce wound perfusion and create severe local ischemia, the only solution is an equally dramatic increase in local tissue oxygenation or local blood supply. The use of a hyperbaric chamber to increase the partial pressure of oxygen in the circulation subjects the patient and wound to an atmosphere of 100% oxygen at twice the normal atmospheric pressure at sea level,[137] creating an elevated PO_2 level in local arterioles, forcing increased amounts of oxygen into compromised tissue (Fig. 106.1). Tissue that is severely ischemic in the postoperative period requires débridement followed by local or distant flap transfer, removing tissue with

circulatory compromise and introducing healthy, well-vascularized tissue to deliver oxygen so that healing may progress.[80]

Smoking

Although cigarette smoking has a deleterious effect on virtually every organ system of the body, the detrimental effects on wound healing can be seen in the postoperative period as progressive wound ischemia and marginal necrosis. Absorbed nicotine and its breakdown product cotinine have an inhibiting effect on capillary circulation and cause necrosis of skin margins to an unpredictable degree. Moreover, in a cigarette smoker, the addition of even a small degree of overzealous traction may cause wound compromise; the effect is additive to the peripheral circulatory effect of inhaled cigarette smoke. In addition, carbon monoxide contained in cigarette smoke forms carboxyhemoglobin, a form of hemoglobin that shifts the oxygen dissociation curve to the left, making oxygen release to ischemic tissue more difficult.[32,42,67,110] This twofold effect of cigarette smoking on tissue oxygenation puts the smoker at risk for wound-healing difficulties. Although there is no consensus among physicians regarding the length of a preoperative period of discontinuation of smoking to ensure uncompromised healing and hard evidence for predictable duration is lacking, we insist on at least 3 weeks' abstention from smoking and require such abstention until skin sutures are removed in the postoperative period.[77] This prohibition applies to exposure to second-hand smoke as well; it is essential to inquire about such exposure at the preoperative interview. In our practice, smokers are required to sign an additional consent form (Fig. 106.2). Smokers can be offered a number of options preoperatively to aid in cessation and some do take advantage of this.

Diabetes Mellitus

The fact that a diabetic patient is prone to a variety of secondary vascular, neurologic, renal, and cardiac difficulties as a result of this chronic illness is well known to surgeons. However, the concept of small-vessel occlusive disease as the primary reason for the wound-healing difficulties sometimes experienced by diabetic patients has not been borne out in multiple studies of ischemia in the diabetic wound; other factors seem to play a larger role.[70]

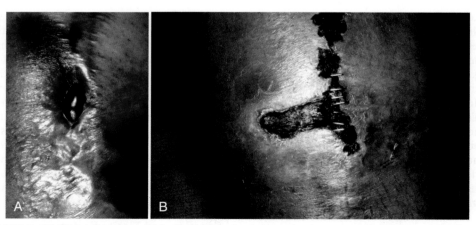

FIG 106.1 (A) Circulation present but compromised. Hyperbaric oxygen (O_2) therapy is indicated. (B) Eschar indicates full-thickness tissue loss, with no circulation. Hyperbaric O_2 therapy is contraindicated.

CONSENT FOR SURGICAL PROCEDURES FOR SMOKERS

Patient _____   Age _____

Dr. _____ and her staff have advised me that I must not smoke or use nicotine substitutes for a **minimum** of three weeks before surgery and after my surgery.

It has been explained to me that the risks of surgery are much greater for smokers, and even if I am refraining from the use of nicotine for three weeks before and after surgery, I may still experience the effects of nicotine in my bloodstream.

There is a greater risk in smokers of bad scarring, hematoma formation, intraoperative bleeding, poor or delayed healing, hair loss, sloughing of the skin (skin loss), infection, increased or prolonged bruising, and hyperpigmentation.

I ACKNOWLEDGE THAT I HAVE READ AND FULLY UNDERSTAND THE ABOVE CONSENT TO OPERATION AND THAT THE RISKS HAVE BEEN FULLY EXPLAINED TO ME, AND I WISH TO PROCEED WITH SURGERY.

Patient signature _____   Date _____

FIG 106.2 Consent form used for patients who smoke cigarettes.

Diabetic patients have increased blood viscosity secondary to a stiffer, less deformable red blood cell, making it more difficult for red cells to pass through the tiny capillaries supplying oxygen to local tissue.[125] The high serum glucose level in a poorly controlled diabetic patient shifts the hemoglobin dissociation curve and inhibits oxygen delivery to the tissue from capillaries, thereby causing lower tissue PO_2 and impaired healing.[24]

Finally, the tibial and peroneal arteries in a diabetic patient seem to be particularly prone to atherosclerotic peripheral vascular disease.[87] Preventive measures regarding these vulnerable patients include preoperative vascular examination of the lower extremities with palpation of the peripheral pulses and further evaluation if abnormalities are noted, meticulous control of the serum glucose level in the perioperative period, and avoidance of extremity edema and the local compounding of a diabetic's rheologic changes.

Other Factors

Anemia. The evidence regarding anemia as a contributing factor in the failure of wounds to heal is inconclusive. Hemoglobinopathies and extreme drops in the hematocrit level, both of which can compromise delivery of oxygen, have not been proved to compromise soft tissue healing.[7,46,55]

Radiation Exposure. Ionizing radiation causes injury not just to the target tissue but also to the tissue that surrounds the target. Radiation was at one time used to aid in wound healing, treat scar formation, and for keloid control in particular; there are patients today who have had such exposure (Fig. 106.3). The damage caused by ionizing radiation is progressive, permanent, and irreversible. Radiation causes an obliterative endarteritis that results in local tissue ischemia and permanent difficulty with wound healing, normal wound contracture, and the formation of healthy granulation tissue. There is some evidence that collateral damage to the proliferation of local fibroblasts adds to these healing difficulties in irradiated tissue.[40,41,117]

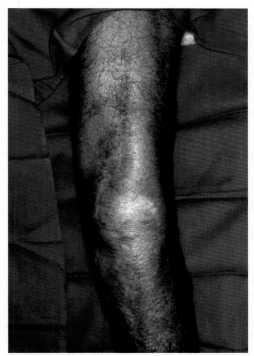

FIG 106.3 Radiation therapy in childhood caused profound scarring. Tissue must be replaced by well-vascularized coverage.

Steroids. It becomes obvious from a discussion of the phases of wound healing that corticosteroids, which inhibit fibrin synthesis, macrophage migration, wound contracture, and the events that lead to the formation and ingrowth of new blood vessels are responsible for the poor progression in wound healing seen in patients receiving corticosteroid therapy. Early and late effects, including failure to gain strength as well as loss of accumulated tensile strength in the healing wound, can both be attributed to steroid intake.

The effect of steroids on wound healing can be minimized by the administration of vitamin A topically or orally. Collagen deposition, increase in wound strength, and functional macrophage support are documented effects of oral vitamin A in a steroid-dependent patient.[28,48,49]

Aspirin and Nonsteroidal Medications. Many prospective total knee replacement patients take nonsteroidal anti-inflammatory drugs (NSAIDs) for pain relief, and a large number of adults take one or more aspirin tablets daily as a cardioprotective regimen. There is evidence that collagen synthesis is inhibited by normal therapeutic dosages of these medications, even in the normal population, and discontinuation of these medications in the perioperative and postoperative periods is recommended, in part because of this effect.

Chemotherapy. Medications used to fight cancer inhibit wound healing. Although there is a great deal of variation in the mechanism of action of this group of drugs, they are all designed to target some aspect of rapidly dividing cells. Molecular biology currently seeks to fight tumors with targeted T cells; this goal is elusive at present, and currently no chemotherapeutic agents are selective enough to protect healing tissue while continuing antineoplastic activity elsewhere.[89,116] It is recommended, when possible, that the perioperative period provide a break in the administration of chemotherapeutic agents.[136] Harmful effects seem to be most evident in the early phases of wound healing; a 2-week postoperative delay in administration can mitigate these harmful effects.[30,31]

Age. It is unclear whether advancing age alone inhibits wound healing. There is ample anecdotal evidence that although very young patients heal with scars that remain hyperemic and indurated for prolonged periods, older patients seem much less prone to this type of healing, a fact that is to their advantage when incisions are placed in cosmetically obvious areas such as the face.[4,25,35,65,134] There is certainly no evidence that the final results of wound healing in terms of ultimate closure and tensile strength are inhibited or influenced by age. In fact, a study from the American College of Surgeons National Surgical Quality Improvement Program using wound dehiscence as the indicator for poor wound healing found no association between dehiscence and advanced age in a review of 25,967 patients. In two groups of patients ages 61 to 70 and ages 70 and older, there was no increased likelihood of the occurrence of this specific measure of impaired healing when compared with younger age groups.[58] Factors that did have a role in poor healing included steroid and tobacco use, and increasing body mass index (BMI).

Nutrition. Nutritional factors play a role in wound healing; a serum protein level below 2 g/dL is indicative of severe nutritional deficiency and can result in a prolonged inflammatory phase and impaired fibroplasia.[100,104,131] Nutritional factors seem to be most important in the first phases of wound healing, when the local inflammatory response and early fibroplasia are most active. However, only when profound malnutrition is present are the phases of wound healing impaired; in the preoperative phase, malnutrition is suspected with a serum albumin less than 3.5 mg/dL, or a transferrin less than 200 mg/dL.[3,59] Although it is most unusual to encounter this problem in today's surgical

environment, many older patients are at least mildly deficient in one or more vitamins essential to healing; obtaining a nutritional consultation plus supplementing these patients prior to surgery when indicated is an excellent part of any preoperative plan.

Vitamin Supplements. An essential element of wound healing, vitamin C (ascorbic acid) is required for the maintenance of tissue integrity in a normal healthy patient.[99] Even a completely healed wound will lose strength over time if vitamin C intake is not adequate. Ascorbic acid is an absolute requirement for the normal synthesis of collagen; if deficient, stable structural elements, including the vessel wall, skin integrity, and the type III collagen of healing tissue, are affected. A truly vitamin C–deficient wound can be separated with only the smallest amount of manual pressure, and hemorrhage from weakened capillaries is common. There may be an added benefit to vitamin C intake in the surgical patient; increased susceptibility to wound infection is seen in the vitamin C deficient patient.[3,9,86a] As much as 2 g per day of vitamin C may be required in the deficient patient, although the recommended dietary allowance is a mere 60 mg per day.[52a] Rarely seen today, vitamin C deficiency is easily remedied when recognized.[15]

Vitamin A, cited above for its role in the steroid dependent patient, may be beneficial for wound healing even if existing levels are adequate, and it is used in doses up to 25,000 IU/day in severely injured patients.[58]

Vitamin E, along with its partner antioxidant vitamin C, has a complex role in skin metabolism and healing. It plays a role in the mobility of polymorphonuclear inflammatory cells in the traumatized patient and can reduce free radicals in wounds.[59,75] Vitamin E has achieved almost mythic properties in popular culture for preserving healthy tissue, particularly for minimizing scar overhealing and keloid formation. The best evidence for vitamin E's beneficial effect indicates that it is a membrane-stabilizing antioxidant that counters the damaging cumulative effect of preoperative irradiation on wounds. In large doses, vitamin E has an inhibitory effect on wound healing that can be reversed by vitamin A.[130]

Although the evidence is conflicting, some studies have demonstrated that vitamin E supplementation lowers the risk for atherosclerotic coronary artery disease, making this vitamin an extremely popular supplement.[113] It should, however, be discontinued before surgery because of its inhibiting effect on platelet adhesion.[52,126] In addition, there is evidence that supplementing a normal diet with vitamin E can cause impaired collagen synthesis and impaired wound healing.[27]

Certainly a careful history of vitamin supplement intake is warranted today; our understanding of the effects of some supplements, both vitamin and herbal, is incomplete.

Micronutrients. Zinc is a trace element present in all human tissue and is required in almost every enzyme reaction. Administration of exogenous zinc increases the rate of wound healing only when there is a zinc deficiency; the surgeon may encounter deficiencies of this trace element in patients with chronic alcoholism, cirrhosis, and gastrointestinal absorption problems, such as short bowel syndrome. Zinc is required in such minute amounts for normal healing that only an extensive loss of absorptive surface will produce a deficiency; in such cases, zinc administration can rapidly and markedly accelerate healing when provided as a supplement.[69,103]

Delay in the early phases of wound healing has been demonstrated in animal studies of zinc deficiency. Compromise in the cellular and humeral immune systems occurs as well.[105,106]

Iron deficiency is not unusual in the postoperative period, particularly if there has been extensive blood loss or diminished oral intake. Its role in the formation of healthy collagen production is less often appreciated than its role in the anemia caused by its deficiency, but it is critically important in oxygen transport and wound healing. Fortunately, iron deficiency is usually obvious in the preoperative evaluation.

Mechanical Stress of Healing. All healing tissue responds to mechanical stress. Expanded tissue gains strength, and its collagen is more precisely oriented to resist disruption than nonexpanded tissue. More specifically, forces on a healing wound, depending on their magnitude and direction, will affect the orientation, amount, and strength of collagen fibers that create healing. The benefit of controlled passive motion on the postoperative wound is not simply a rapid and early gain in range of motion. When hemostasis at the time of wound closure is satisfactory, when swelling is controlled, and when the application of stress across the wound is gradual, the potential for hematoma formation and wound necrosis is minimized. Mechanical stress provides a short-term benefit in diminished adhesion formation, and a long-term benefit of anatomic remodeling and increased wound strength.[36,133]

Skin Closure

The purpose of skin closure is to provide sufficient support over an adequate time period so that wound healing and strength gain occur until support afforded by sutures is no longer needed. Primary suturing of a wound provides skin closure as a temporary barrier to contamination from the skin surface, replicating one function of the skin as an organ system. To this end, an evaluation of closure techniques and materials is in order.

A variety of options exist to effect skin closure—staples, skin sutures, skin tape, skin glue—all of which will coapt the skin margins appropriately. In addition to contributing to wound healing, sutures also have a number of less desirable effects. By penetrating local intact skin to a variable degree, sutures introduce an additional source of local contamination. When tied tightly, sutures can impede local blood supply and, if left in place for a long period, cosmetically unsatisfactory cutaneous marks ("railroad tracks") can be the result (Fig. 106.4).

Suturing of a wound can be accomplished with material that is braided or monofilament and permanent or nonpermanent. Closure can also be achieved with skin staples, which are usually stainless steel and smooth-surfaced. Skin tape made of a variety of materials—plastic, fabric, paper—is bonded to an adhesive and applied to dry skin, where appropriate.

Several important facts are known regarding the materials that we use for skin closure. First, there is excellent evidence that stapled wounds provide superior resistance to infection when compared with sutured wounds. Particularly at lower levels of bacterial contamination, skin staples have a lower infection rate than even the least reactive nonabsorbable suture, monofilament nylon.[54,128]

Second, skin tapes used to close a wound that is dry (but not when continuous oozing loosens the tape) seem to provide the greatest resistance to infection, especially from surface contamination, when compared with other closure techniques.[18] Perfect skin edge to edge coaptation is essential for uneventful wound

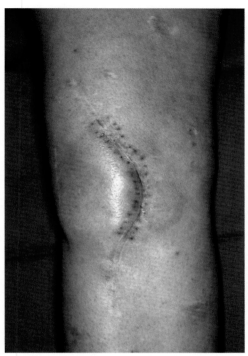

FIG 106.4 Cutaneous sutures in place for 3 weeks epithelialize along suture tracks. Permanent scarring results.

healing. Although manual suturing is perhaps best suited to compensate for the inequalities in skin thickness that result in surface overlap or override, if the deep tissues are accurately approximated, skin staples appear to be an excellent choice for skin closure in total knee arthroplasty. Concern regarding compressive ischemia between the legs of the skin staples is unfounded.

HEALING THE INCISION

The largest organ in the body, the skin is responsible for protecting the underlying tissues from inhospitable elements, potentially invading foreign organisms, trauma, and other undesirable effects. Because infection of an underlying joint space or implant is such a significant problem, maintaining healthy overlying skin and subcutaneous tissues throughout the surgical period is of critical importance, especially because there is no additional muscle layer over the knee to give added protection (Fig. 106.5). Various factors before, during, and after surgery can contribute to the success or failure of that effort.

The patient, as a whole, needs to be in optimal condition to maximize the potential for uncomplicated wound healing. Because circulation is essential to healing, an assessment of the large vessel circulation (popliteal and pedal pulses) must be made to minimize the risk of unknown ischemic problems. Venous inadequacy may also impair circulation and needs to be assessed and managed, if necessary. Small vessel disease as a consequence of diabetes can also exist, and the patient's diabetes must therefore be optimally managed throughout the period. Other external factors such as cigarette smoking, hypotension, or hypothermia with resulting vasoconstriction can reduce nutrient flow to the skin and result in poor healing. Even with adequate blood flow, issues such as anemia and malnutrition or

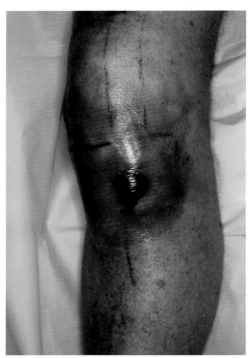

FIG 106.5 Partial-thickness skin circulatory compromise is indicated by skin blistering.

obesity can make the skin less resilient and therefore less able to meet the demands required to achieve rapid, uncomplicated, and complete wound closure.[1,64]

Preoperative Preparation

The operative site must be examined several days prior to the procedure to ensure the skin is clean and intact. Abrasions and similar injuries can contaminate the wound and must be treated appropriately so they are completely healed prior to surgery. Topical dressing with bacitracin or similar antibacterial ointment and an occlusive dressing may be used for minor abrasions. Paper tape or low-allergy bandages cause fewer skin reactions than standard tape. Simple dry, cracked skin may just be kept moist with an over-the-counter emollient, remembering that a cream that comes in a jar is thicker and therefore more effective than a lotion that comes in a bottle. Hair removal should be done immediately prior to surgery with clippers or depilatory cream, not a razor, because the latter can nick the skin and lead to microbiological contamination, especially if performed a day in advance.[1,61,79,123]

Much has been studied regarding the optimal type of preoperative skin preparation.[86] When addressing this issue, several items must be considered. If the surgery is on a body cavity or organ, the potential contaminating microorganisms can come from the skin or the body part itself. However, in orthopedic surgery, one can generally concentrate on the type of organisms that populate the skin. Therefore, the surgical skin preparation should be one that targets them more favorably.

Bacterial contamination at the time of surgery is absolutely inevitable in every operation. It is impossible to achieve absolute sterility, no matter what type of preparation is performed. One key to limiting infection is reducing the bacterial inoculum to a size that the tissue can handle. For ordinary tissue, this has

been calculated to be 10^5 for staphylococcus aureus.[45,62,114] Factors that can lessen the resistance of the native tissues, such as diabetes, cigarette smoking, and obesity, have been mentioned previously. Others such as tissue trauma and suture material will be discussed later.

The skin is colonized by mostly gram-positive bacteria, which live on the surface and extend down hair follicles. Therefore, the skin preparation should be one that removes both the skin oils and dead outer skin cells while targeting the type of bacteria resident. In addition, the time it takes to achieve bacterial death, the longevity of action, and the potential for allergies and skin irritation are important.[29]

Painting a topical solution on the skin surface does not remove the skin oils or dead cells.[129] Therefore, a surgical scrub is preferred. Chlorhexidine gluconate 4% with alcohol has a broad spectrum of activity against both gram-positive and gram-negative bacteria. It has a long duration of activity of at least 6 hours, and its effectiveness is not reduced by blood or other organic matter. It should be noted that Hibiclens (Molnycke Health Care, Göteborg, Sweden) scrub has 4% isopropyl alcohol, which adds to its effectiveness. The fact that it is a surgical scrub allows it to remove the surface oils and dead skin cells before surgery. Its effectiveness is both time-dependent and cumulative, so a scrub for 3 minutes (as per the manufacturer) the night before surgery and again the morning of surgery adds to its effectiveness for maximum benefit. ChloraPrep (CareFusion Corporation, San Diego, California) has chlorhexidine gluconate and 70% isopropyl alcohol, which increases the immediate antibacterial effectiveness. It is a paint, not a scrub, and should be applied to the surgical area in the operating room and allowed to dry completely both to allow for complete effectiveness and prevention of surgical fires because of its alcohol content.[1,10,22,120,121]

Iodophor-containing preparations (Betadine, Purdue Products L.P., Stamford, Connecticut, and others), while popular, may not be the most efficacious in terms of specificity and duration.[138] They must be allowed to dry on the skin, they may be inhibited by blood or other organic matter, and their duration of activity is shorter than chlorhexidine. A newer, water-insoluble iodophor-in alcohol solution, 3M DuraPrep Surgical (3M, St. Paul, Minnesota) has been shown to be at least as effective and longer in duration than the standard two-step iodophor scrub-then-paint regimen.[20,53,97]

Chloroxylenol 3.0% (Technicare, Care-Tech Laboratories Inc., Saint Louis, Missouri) is also a scrub that has the advantage of killing 99.9% of a broad range of bacteria, including MRSA, in 30 seconds, while having a long duration of activity. It is not drying and has no alcohol, so it is not toxic to mucous membranes and corneas.[2]

Although older studies were able to document a decreased bacterial skin count when comparing chlorhexidine-alcohol with povidone iodine, only recently have studies documented a decrease in actual surgical site infection with the former.[20,73,92] Some have included oral and intranasal decontamination preoperatively as well.[57] Although some studies were not able to document a difference, not all of them have specified chlorhexidine and alcohol. Indeed, some of the generic preparations do not have alcohol in them, and because the alcohol is a definite contributor to the overall effectiveness of the product, some generic formulations without it may be less effective.

Another important step in reducing the degree of bacterial contamination of the wound is the use of prophylactic antibiotics, for which timing is important. Administration within 1 hour before the incision is made, and maintaining tissue levels with supplementary doses during longer surgery, is more effective than commencing therapy after the surgery has begun. There is no evidence that administering antibiotics more than 1 hour before surgery is more or less effective. However, the choice of antibiotic is significant. Cefazolin is more effective than vancomycin alone. If the latter must be used for reasons of allergy, a second agent should be administered with it.[1,44,119]

Intraoperative Factors

Inflammation is used by the body as a mechanism to removed damaged tissue. It commences shortly after an injury occurs and continues until the perceived damaged tissue is removed. The process itself can also be damaging and therefore can continue for days, weeks, or even months after an injury. Like a construction crew demolishing and reconstructing a building site, the rebuilding crew does not start working until the demolition crew is finished. Similarly, the body will not start the proliferative phase of wound healing until the inflammatory phase has completed. Therefore, it is essential to minimize the amount of trauma inflicted upon the tissues if one is to maximize the success in achieving rapid primary wound healing.

During the surgical procedure, from beginning to end, there are numerous events that can affect the skin and subcutaneous tissues in a negative manner and render the wound more susceptible to poor healing and possible infection.[81] In healthy individuals with surgery on well-vascularized areas, these issues may be of little importance. However, in the knee area of a patient with local or systemic comorbid conditions, they may rise to a level of significance.

Planning the skin incision is important, especially if there are preexisting scars. When incisions are placed parallel and close to one another, ischemia of the tissue between them can result. In addition, excess traction on a surgical wound can severely damage the skin and surrounding tissue. Retractors, clamps, and the use of electrocautery at the edge of the skin can be damaging. Incision length is not as important as tissue viability. Putting excess intraoperative traction on an incision that is too short to give adequate exposure can prove detrimental. A longer incision that heals primarily is preferable to a shorter one that develops wound healing issues.

Although it is rare for a surgeon to make the skin incision with a cautery, the use of that instrument for deeper dissection is common. It should be remembered that the cautery does not cut only the tissues upon which it is used; it damages the tissue on either side of the wound. This can easily lead to seroma, poor healing, or wound infection. Although this damage is not visible on the surface, it is there underneath. Palpation of the temperature of tissue that has been extensively cauterized can reveal the surprising thermal damage that instrument can cause. Therefore, it should be used at the lowest effective setting, understanding that the goal of minimizing intraoperative bleeding may inadvertently lead to more postoperative wound healing problems. Furthermore, as a method of hemostasis, the current from the unipolar cautery spreads peripherally beyond the tissue being treated, spreading damage. By contrast, damage from a bipolar cautery is mostly limited to the tissue between the forceps tips, minimizing collateral damage.

A newer device, the PEAK Plasma Blade (Medtronic Minneapolis, Minnesota) uses radiofrequency energy to cut and/or coagulate tissue with less collateral damage than standard electrocautery, resulting in less scar tissue and faster healing.[72]

Because skin perfusion is used by the body as a method of regulating body temperature, hypothermia during surgery can diminish skin perfusion and increase the rate of wound infection. Therefore, maintenance of normothermia during surgery is essential.[16,63,76,85] Various factors that may have received little attention can affect this process in either a harmful or beneficial manner. The use of alcohol-based skin preparations can cool the extremity and contribute to hypothermia. The use of underbody type warmers, using the natural tendency of heat to rise, may be more effective than warmers placed on top of the patient. It should be noted, however, that forced-air warming, especially without a suitable air filter in the heating unit, can contaminate the surgical field and lead to an increase in surgical site infections.[82] Therefore, conductive-fabric or mattress-warming from underneath may be preferable. In addition, warming the patient even before surgery has proven beneficial. By contrast, laminar airflow has not generally been shown to decrease the rate of wound infection.[34]

The use of a tourniquet has been shown not to influence the penetration of antibiotics into the knee during surgery, remembering that the antibiotics are to be administrated 1 hour before surgery, allowing time for tissue penetration.[122] By reducing blood loss and therefore anemia, the tourniquet can maintain tissue perfusion during and after surgery. In addition, maintenance of normal glucose levels during surgery and routine use of supplemental oxygen can both maintain better tissue perfusion and decrease surgical site infections.[1]

Another factor that can influence the rate of surgical site infections is the choice of suture material. Because of its inflammatory properties, a single silk suture in a surgical wound can reduce the size of inoculum necessary to produce an infection by a factor of 10, from 100,000 bacteria per gram of tissue to only 10,000 per gram of tissue in an otherwise healthy individual. Wounds closed with braided sutures are also more prone to infection than those closed with monofilament sutures because bacteria within the braids are protected from the activity of phagocytic cells. However, the newer antibiotic-impregnated sutures have shown to reduce the rate of wound infections.[1]

If the quality and thickness of the overlying skin is tenuous, the implantation of acellular dermal matrix from either humans (Alloderm or Allomax) or pigs (Strattice or Xenmatrix) (LifeCell Corporation, Bridgewater, New Jersey, and Davol, a Bard Company, Warwick, Rhode Island, respectively) can augment the tissue thickness and resiliency. It must be remembered, however, that those products must be in direct contact with healthy, well-vascularized overlying tissue to become vascularized themselves. Otherwise, they will necrose.

When a wound is closed, the tissue on either side of the incision must be treated in such a manner as to maximize the likelihood of rapid cell growth and healing. In that regard, factors that can slow down the rate of collagen synthesis and epidermal cell proliferation must be avoided. Excessive use of electrocautery has been mentioned previously. Because suture material encircles live tissue, tight sutures can compress tissue in such a manner as to make it ischemic. Tissues generally swell during the first 24 to 48 hours after surgery, so that sutures that do not appear tight at the end of the procedure may become too tight in the initial postoperative period.

In addition, the outermost layer of the epidermis is composed of dead epidermal cells, which have dried and compacted and lost their nuclei during their 4- to 6-week migration from the living deeper epidermis to the surface. If the wound is closed in such a manner as to fold the outer epidermis inward, there is no chance of proper adherence between the two sides because they are just dead cells. Therefore, it is imperative that the wound be everted, either with vertical mattress sutures, continuous intradermal sutures (actually placed at the dermoepidermal junction), or staples placed in such a manner as to evert the edges properly. This allows better contact between the underlying dermis and the deeper living epidermis, and therefore more rapid healing.

It is also to be remembered that tissues generally swell for the first 24 to 48 hours so that circumferential dressings or splints must be applied properly and inspected frequently to prevent their obstruction of venous or lymphatic flow. Similarly, tape should not be applied in a completely circumferential manner so as to avoid its becoming too constrictive as the extremity swells. Not only can such constriction cause venous or lymphatic obstruction distally, but it can also lead to shearing and blistering of the underlying skin. The use of thigh-high elastic stockings has generally been abandoned because of their propensity to fold at the knee level and cause such an obstruction. If significant peripheral edema is noted, such as from right-sided heart failure, adherence to proper salt intake, leg elevation, and cardiac medication is essential.

Postoperative Factors

Most operating rooms adhere to a strict level of compliance with sterilization procedures and surveillance of the effectiveness of those procedures using biological indicators. However, a rigorous program of monitoring and tracking is essential to ensure that quality. In addition, after surgery, there are a number of opportunities for the patient to come in contact with contaminated surfaces. Therefore, the stretchers, beds, controls, gowns, light strings, and all other devices and equipment that come in contact with the patient, including the hands of health care personnel, must be evaluated on a regular basis to minimize the risk of cross-contamination both before and after surgery.[109,118] In addition, close attention must be given to management of oxygen, hemoglobin and glucose levels, body temperature, and care of indwelling Foley catheters.[19]

Once the wound is closed, it is advantageous to achieve epidermal growth across the incision line as rapidly as possible to minimize the risk of bacterial entry. As noted previously, that endpoint is the culmination of a two-step process. First, the obligatory inflammatory phase must be completed before the desirable proliferative phase of healing will commence. In that regard, measures to limit the amount of trauma to the skin and deeper tissues have already been discussed. However, the type of dressing can have an ongoing influence on that process. Dry environments impede the successful completion of the inflammatory stage and should therefore be avoided.

Similarly, dry environments can slow the rate of epithelialization by half, further interfering with the desired outcome of a closed wound.[56,83] In addition, if the epidermal layer desiccates and dries, the underlying dermis then becomes exposed to air, which it cannot tolerate, so it dies and the damage extends more deeply. Therefore, maintaining a properly moist environment is essential. A wound closed with staples may be dressed with a layer of petrolatum-based ointment such as bacitracin or gauze impregnated with petrolatum such as Xeroform (Covidien, Medtronic Operational Headquarters, 710 Medtronic Parkway, Minneapolis, Minnesota) or Vaseline Gauze (Unilever PLC/Unilever NV) or similar material with dry gauze on top.

For wounds closed with an intradermal suture, either removable or dissolving, the use of a polyurethane film such as Tegaderm (3M) or Bioclusive (Johnson & Johnson, New Brunswick, New Jersey) maintains the proper degree of moisture in a relatively sterile and waterproof environment and can be left in place until epithelialization is complete. The use of Mastisol (Eloquest Healthcare, Ferndale Pharma Group Inc., Ferndale, Michigan) on the skin prior to placement of the film dressing helps maintain adherence longer. Covering the film dressing with a dry gauze which is held in place with picture-frame tape around the edges or a circumferential elastic dressing on an extremity can prevent the film from peeling off prematurely. It is common to see dried blood collect under the film dressing. As long as it stays dry and no fluid leaks out the edge of the film dressing, the dried blood can be safely ignored. It will come off when the film is removed. If fluid does leak out, the entire film must be removed and the wound treated with daily washings, ointment, and gauze, as noted previously, or a wound infection will result.

If a topical ointment is used, proper selection is important. For routine wounds, simple bacitracin is sufficient. If contamination by gram-negative bacteria is of concern, the use of Neosporin (Johnson & Johnson) may prove beneficial. Mupirocin 2% ointment (Bactroban, GlaxoSmithKline, Research Triangle Park, North Carolina) is an excellent alternative. Not only is it effective even against MRSA, but it is rarely allergenic and is a good alternative for those who manifest a topical allergic response to other ointments. Postoperatively, the wound should never be left either wet or exposed to air and allowed to dry out. On a regular basis, it should be gently washed with soap and water to remove the old ointment and any dead skin cells then patted dry. Leaving it open to air leads to desiccation and cell death. Leaving it wet leads to maceration and infection. A new layer of ointment or impregnated gauze is applied until the wound has epithelialized across the incision line, which may take 1 to 2 weeks. It remains susceptible to microbial penetration until that epidermal cell layer has reformed across the incision.

Silver-containing cream, such as Silvadene (Pfizer, New York, New York) is frequently used in burns because of its effective antibacterial properties. However, it also slows down the rate of cell growth, so its duration of use should be limited, if possible, and discontinued when the concern about infection has diminished.[6]

INFLUENCE OF GROWTH FACTORS

A complete discussion of the topical treatment of healing wounds must include a discussion of cytokines, or polypeptides, whose function is to facilitate the cellular, biochemical, and mechanical stages of normal wound healing and regulate many of these processes.[84] Among these cytokines are growth factors that have been explored as topical applications to the open wound to aid in healing. The nomenclature of growth factors is confusing; some are named for the cell from which they are derived, some for the cell that is their target, or in some cases, even for the function for which they are responsible. Growth factors are large polypeptides that function to facilitate the various stages of wound healing. Certain growth factors encourage angiogenesis, others are responsible for cell mitosis, and still others influence the cellular elements in surrounding soft tissue to mobilize in response to injury.

The literature over the last 15 years contains many studies using growth factors to aid in wound healing; the evidence for their use to benefit normal wound healing in terms of speed of healing, strength gain, or ultimate satisfactory cosmesis is conflicting.[14,60,98] Some clinical trials have supported evidence for more rapid shrinkage of an opened wound to which growth factors are applied, whereas other evidence has indicated that the ultimate outcome regarding time to closure and strength gain is unaffected. Considering these agents as an early step in influencing more rapid wound closure is useful because evidence exists to support their importance in aiding the closure of difficult wounds. There is some evidence that growth factors can influence events in disorders of healing skin, such as keloid and hypertrophic scar formation.[50,101,139] That this information will ultimately lead to topical agents that accelerate wound healing, in addition to agents that are useful adjuncts to the basic surgical principles of adequate débridement and edema control in local wound care, is hoped for but not yet ensured.

It is clear that nutrient circulation to healing cells is vital if one is to achieve rapid primary healing and minimize complications. The heart pumps blood to the peripheral tissues. In the ambulatory patient, the activity of the large calf muscles, by constricting the deep veins with their incorporated valves, serves to pump the venous blood upwards. If the patient is immobilized, that pumping action is negated. Therefore, leg elevation and the use of intermittent-compression devices is essential, not only to reduce the risk of deep-vein thrombosis but also to improve nutrient circulation to tissue.

Once a wound shows characteristics of poor healing, one must try to decide the exact factor or factors that have compromised the area. The pattern of skin involvement may provide clues as to the cause. If there is discoloration of the skin of only one side of the incision, a circulatory problem of that particular flap is present. If there is redness, swelling, or discoloration of both sides of the incision, a more general problem is probably present, such as a hematoma and/or an infection. Steroid use, either topically, systemically, or a recent depot injection, can slow down the rate of white blood cell and macrophage activity, thereby lessening the ability to fight infection and produce growth factors necessary for healing. Fibroblast collagen synthesis is impeded, and the wound does not heal properly.

One of the most common and treatable problems to develop is a hematoma beneath the skin flaps.[38] Collections of blood are toxic to the overlying dermis, causing necrosis from below. In the first 2 weeks or so, the blood clot remains a gelatinous mass that will not come out through a drain or an aspiration needle. During that early postoperative interval, if a significant hematoma is recognized, it must be manually drained and irrigated.[91] If this is not done, topical treatment will not be sufficient to halt and reverse the process. Usually, by about 2 weeks, the hematoma has begun to liquefy, causing a soft spot that can be aspirated successfully on one or more occasions. This continues to be an important factor in removing the underlying offending material while treating the surface effects.

A closer look at the wound itself will provide clues as to the cause and extent of the problem. A wound that is bluish but still retains some capillary refill indicates that the epidermis has been compromised, but the underlying dermis, which contains the capillaries and small arterioles, still has some viability. If the color is brown, gray, or black and hard, then the necrosis is full thickness. It is important to assess, as closely as possible, the depth of loss because the functions of the different skin and soft tissue layers that are missing, and therefore need substitution or replacement, differ.

The purpose of the epidermis is to keep the underlying organism clean and moist in a dry, hostile environment. Bacteria and other pathogens are to be kept out. Flexibility is to be allowed. Epidermal cells start off as a living layer at the dermo-epidermal junction, where they grow and start a 6-week migration up to the surface. By the time the journey is complete, they have formed a flat, dry, dead, flexible layer. The epidermal cells extend into the dermis along the adnexal structures such as hair follicles, which extend down into the dermis, and often into the subcutaneous fat. If the epidermal layer has been lost but the dermis is preserved, assuming no further loss of tissue occurs, a new epidermal layer will regenerate. A functional layer will usually develop within about 2 weeks, although it can take 6 weeks for a mature layer to form, able to withstand the usual traumas of daily life.

If the epidermis is lost, a substitute for its function must be provided until it regenerates: a moist environment, simulating the isotonic properties of normal tissue, and preventing bacterial colonization. Various different types of agents are available for this. In choosing which one to use, one must consider effectiveness, ease of use, cost, and any ancillary requirements, such as treatment or prevention of infection. Some of the options for topical wound care have been discussed previously.

Another alternative to treatment of superficial skin loss involves the use of an aloe vera–based agent called Carrasyn Hydrogel (Medline Industries Inc., Mundelein, Illinois), which has been shown not only to increase the rate of skin cell growth, but also to decrease the rate of bacterial growth. It has been compared with silver sulfadiazene, which is highly effective in preventing bacterial growth, but also slows down skin cell growth, as well as salicylic acid cream, which increases skin cell growth but does not fight bacteria.[102] Carrasyn requires two or three dressing changes per day but is highly effective.[115]

A number of hydro gel products are available on the market. Some are thicker and easier to handle. However, none have been shown to increase the rate of skin cell growth, or decrease the rate of bacterial growth, when compared to other modalities.[43]

If the wound is draining, the use of an absorptive layer can remove exudate, limiting maceration and removing potentially toxic enzymes. Calcium or sodium alginate dressings are placed on the wound after cleaning with saline, and covered with a dry gauze.[23] They are changed daily, or less frequently, depending on the amount of drainage.

Hydro fiber dressings, such as Aquacel (ConvaTec, North Carolina) or an equivalent also absorb many times their weight in exudate. They have the advantage of ease of use because they do not fragment upon removal. Aquacel AG is silver impregnated and highly effective against even antibiotic-resistant bacteria. They are used until the infection resolves, then changed to the form without the silver.[4]

If tissue necrosis should develop, it must be dealt with promptly and effectively because dead tissue has no ability to fight infection.[88] The problem that usually arises is deciding what is going to live and what is going to die. Radical early débridement may unnecessarily sacrifice tissue that otherwise would have survived. Wet-to-dry dressings do adhere to necrotic tissue and mechanically remove them. However, in the process, they also damage fragile healthy tissues and are frequently painful. Concentrated solutions of povidone-iodine or hydrogen peroxide are also toxic to fragile cells and should also be avoided. They may be used for cleaning crusted material, but should then be wiped away with saline.

The urgency of the situation depends on the size of the affected area and whether or not exposure of any underlying implant has occurred or is suspected. If the depth of involvement is only into the skin and subcutaneous tissue and the deeper layers are intact, then chemical débridement with collagenase Santyl (Smith & Nephew Inc., Andover, Massachusetts) mixed with topical antibiotic can be effective in removing the necrotic tissue and allowing healing by secondary intention. It should be noted that the enzyme in collagenase may be deactivated by metal ions such as silver and iodine, so the choice of antibacterial ointment with which it is mixed or the type of absorptive dressing on top must be made carefully.

If the defect is larger and deeper, then immediate surgical débridement and secondary closure is essential. However, if the local tissues are not adequate to accomplish this, the temporary use of a negative-pressure or vacuum-type dressing is warranted. It has the advantages of removing draining fluid and increasing vascularity while maintaining a near-sterile environment to protect the underlying tissues and prosthesis until wound closure can be accomplished. It needs a formal dressing change with sterile gloves and instruments usually every 2 to 3 days. It can be performed either as an inpatient or as an outpatient process.

Alternatively, if the site is not infected and the hardware is not exposed, a product called Integra (Integra LifeSciences, Plainsboro, New Jersey) may be used. According to the manufacturer, "It is comprised of a Collagen-GAG matrix made of a three-dimensional porous matrix of cross-linked bovine tendon collagen and glycosaminoglycan. It provides a scaffold for cellular invasion and capillary growth. The scaffold is eventually remodeled as the patient's cells rebuild the damaged site." On top of the matrix layer is a protective silicone layer that maintains the proper level of moisture and protects the underlying matrix. Before application, the site must be thoroughly débrided down to clean, healthy tissue because the Integra must adhere to that layer to become incorporated, much the same way a skin graft does. The Integra is affixed down with either staples or sutures and the area immobilized until incorporation is complete and the silicone layer loosens, typically in 14 to 28 days, at which time a thin epidermal autograft is applied.[39]

The process of healing is not complete when the sutures are removed. In fact, collagen synthesis continues for weeks or months after the incision is closed. Many techniques have been attempted to modify the process and limit the formation of hypertrophic scars. Scar hypertrophy is much like a rope—the greater the lengthwise tension on the rope, the thicker the rope needs to be to resist such tension. Similarly, the body senses lengthwise tension on a scar, especially one that is stretched during movement of a joint and, in response, makes that scar thicker to resist the pull. If the incision can be planned to lie parallel to relaxed-skin tension lines, it is less likely to hypertrophy. If it is designed in a zigzag manner, it can open and fold like an accordion and also is less likely to thicken. However, absent those two possibilities, the use of either paper tape lengthwise on top of the incision, starting at the time of suture removal and continuing 24/7 for a period of 2 to 3 months, or more if necessary, has been shown to diminish the likelihood of scar hypertrophy. This is especially useful around joints.[5,111]

Alternatively, a newer technique of placing a slow-dissolving suture directly from the dermis at one apex of the incision to the other apex and buried under a standard two-layer closure has also been shown to minimize the likelihood of scar hypertrophy without the need for overlying paper tape.[112]

In the end, achieving the desired outcome in the surgical treatment of a patient is the result of the identification and proper management of as many variables and risk factors as possible. In the age of evidence-based medicine, nothing can be taken for granted. Close attention to the minutest details, while seemingly burdensome, may mean the difference between a successful result and a disaster.

KEY REFERENCES

1. Alexander JW, Solomkin JS, Edwards MJ: Updated recommendations for control of surgical site infections. *Ann Surg* 253(6): 1082–1093, 2011.
10. Bebko SP, Green DM, Awad SS: Effect of a preoperative decontamination protocol on surgical site infections in patients undergoing elective orthopedic surgery with hardware implantation. *JAMA Surg* 150(5):390–395, 2015.
17. Chang J, Small KH, Choi M: Three dimensional surface imaging in plastic surgery. *Plast Reconstr Surg* 135(5):1295–1304, 2015.
19. Daines BK, Dennis DA, Amann S: Infection prevention in total knee arthroplasty. *J Am Acad Orthop Surg* 23(6):356–364, 2015.
20. Darouiche RO, Wall MJ Jr, Itani KM, et al: Chlorhexidine-alcohol versus povidone-iodine for surgical-site antisepsis. *N Engl J Med* 362:18–26, 2010.
34. Gastmeier P, Breier AC, Brandt C: Influence of laminar airflow on prosthetic joint infections: a systematic review. *J Hosp Infect* 81(2):73–78, 2012.
39. Gottlieb M, Furman J: Successful management and surgical closure of chronic and pathological wounds using Integra. *J Burns Surg Wound Care* 3(2):4, 2004.
44. Hawn MT, Richman JS, Vick C, et al: Timing of surgical antibiotic prophylaxis and the risk of surgical site infection. *JAMA Surg* 148(7):649–657, 2013.
53. Jarral OA, McCormack DJ, Ibrahim S, et al: Should surgeons scrub with chlorhexidine or iodine prior to surgery? *Interact Cardiovasc Thorac Surg* 12(6):1017–1021, 2011.
56. Junker JPE, Kamel RA, Caterson EJ, et al: Clinical impact upon wound healing and inflammation in moist, wet, and dry environments. *Adv Wound Care (New Rochelle)* 2(7):348–356, 2013.
57. Kalmeijer MD, Coertjens H, van Nieuwland-Bollen PM, et al: Surgical site infections in orthopedic surgery: the effect of mupirocin in nasal ointment in a double-blind, randomized, placebo-controlled study. *Clin Infect Dis* 35(4):353–358, 2002.
62. Krizek TJ, Robson MC: Evolution of quantitative bacteriology in wound management. *Am J Surg* 130:579–584, 1975.
64. Lamplot JD, Luther G, Mawdsley EL, et al: Modified protocol decreases surgical site infections after total knee arthroplasty. *J Knee Surg* 28(5):395–403, 2015.

72. Loh SA, Carlson GA, Chang EI, et al: Comparative healing of surgical incisions created by the PEAK PlasmaBlade, conventional electrosurgery, and a scalpel. *Plast Reconstr Surg* 124(6):1849–1859, 2009.

76. Mahoney CB, Odom J: Maintaining intraoperative normothermia: a meta analysis of outcomes with costs. *AANA J* 67:155–163, 1999.

82. McGovern PD, Albrecht M, Belani KG, et al: Forced-air warming and ultra-clean ventilation do not mix: an investigation of theatre ventilation, patient warming and joint replacement infection in orthopaedics. *J Bone Joint Surg Br* 93(11):1537–1544, 2011.

83. McGrath MH: How topical dressings salvage "questionable" flaps: experimental study. *Plast Reconstr Surg* 67:653–659, 1981.

The references for this chapter can also be found on www.expertconsult.com.

107

The Problem Wound: Coverage Options

Sarah Sasor, Kevin R. Knox, Kelly L. Scott, Susan Craig Scott

INTRODUCTION

Wound complications, including poor healing, skin necrosis and superficial skin infection, occur in up to 20% of patients after total knee arthroplasty (TKA).[35,37] Prompt attention is required to reduce the risk of deep infection and prosthesis exposure.[47]

Goals of soft tissue reconstruction are to achieve a healed wound bed, optimize long-term functional status, provide an acceptable aesthetic appearance, and minimize donor site morbidity.[19]

The focus of this chapter is to discuss preoperative optimization of the difficult wound bed and to review surgical treatment options for soft tissue complications after TKA.

PREOPERATIVE SOFT TISSUE MANIPULATION

Some local conditions, such as previous incisions (Fig. 107.1), a history of radiation in the region, or tobacco use, place a patient at high risk for wound healing difficulties after TKA. Appropriate preoperative planning allows patients the best chance for primary healing. In the problematic wound bed, surgical options include a "sham" incision, tissue expansion, and simultaneous flap coverage at the time of TKA.

Sham Incision

Sham incisions are indicated when the likelihood of primary healing is reasonable but some question remains regarding the health and vascularity of local soft tissue. The procedure is useful in stimulating increased local blood supply; it avoids placing an underlying prosthesis at risk, as it simulates every aspect of the TKA procedure up to but not including the arthrotomy and prosthesis insertion. Approximately 7 to 10 days before the arthroplasty procedure, the intended incision is made through the skin and subcutaneous tissue; flap elevation proceeds proximally, distally, medially, and laterally as though for joint replacement, although the joint is not entered. The incision is then closed. The sham incision acts as a kind of delay: it disrupts the blood supply that traverses the incision and increases demand from the periphery. The mechanism behind the delay phenomenon includes opening of choke vessels between adjacent perforators, hypertrophy and reorganization of existing vessels along the axis of the delayed tissue, vascular ingrowth, and conditioning of tissue in response to tissue ischemia.[8] One week is sufficient time for the delay phenomenon to occur; longer times provide no advantage in the number or size of improved vasculature.[12,39,41]

The usefulness of this approach is that it provides information regarding the health and vascularity of local tissue without violating the knee joint or risking infection of the prosthesis. Primary healing of this incision is a good indication that wound healing will proceed without difficulty after TKA.

The disadvantage is the potential for tissue loss in the wound created by the sham incision. Although this is preferable to tissue loss after TKA, the surgeon is now faced with addressing a nonhealing wound in a patient who has yet to undergo joint replacement.

Soft Tissue Expansion

Scarring from previous surgeries or trauma often leads to thin, fibrotic, contracted skin that is adherent to underlying structures. The concept of tissue expansion (Fig. 107.2) was first introduced in the 1950s[35] and is another option for soft tissue coverage in difficult wound beds. Expansion is based on the principles of biologic and mechanical creep and stress relaxation. When skin is stretched beyond its physiologic limit, a series of events is induced that results in increased mitotic activity and collagen synthesis. Existing collagen fibers elongate and realign parallel to one another. The effect is increased skin surface area when an expanding internal force is applied over time.[52] In addition, the vascularity of the expanded skin is superior to the increased vascularity that results from delay, and the microvascular enhancement of the expanded skin can be of benefit in heavily scarred areas.[22,36]

A tissue expander is inserted into a subcutaneous pocket adjacent to the planned incision at least 8 weeks prior to TKA. The separate access port should be placed proximally to avoid dependent leakage after injections. The expander and access port are completely subcutaneous. Weekly or biweekly injections are carried out with a 23-gauge needle or smaller until adequate expansion is achieved.

The expander is removed at the time of TKA. At closure, the expander pocket is drained separately with a large-bore drain.

Tissue expanders are available in a wide variety of shapes and sizes. Rectangular, crescentic and round expanders are available and provide 38%, 32% and 25% gains in surface area, respectively.[49]

Tissue expansion is a very labor-intensive approach to soft tissue manipulation. There is some discomfort involved in the weekly or biweekly injections, and the manpower requirement in a busy office setting cannot always be met. There is recent evidence that a system of remotely activated carbon dioxide release into an implanted tissue expander may not only reduce expansion time but, when used in a patient-controlled format,

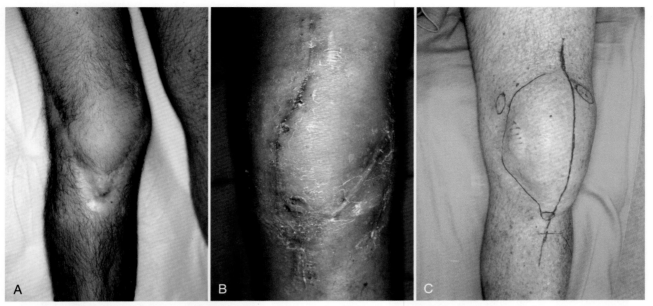

FIG 107.1 (A-C) Patients who have undergone multiple previous surgical procedures through a variety of incisions may be at risk for healing compromise after total knee arthroplasty.

also lead to greater patient satisfaction and less expansion related pain.[1]

Flaps

Every effort should be made to thoroughly evaluate the soft tissues prior to TKA and anticipate which patients will have healing difficulties. Patients who have extensive local soft tissue damage, a large zone of injury, or those who present for revision TKA are at high risk for wound complications. Local soft tissue options are often unavailable. In these patients, flap coverage prior to joint replacement should be considered. Flap surgery should precede TKA by weeks to months to allow sufficient time for healing, although simultaneous TKA and flap transfer may be done successfully in experienced hands. This accomplishes the goal of joint replacement and soft tissue coverage and avoids delays in rehabilitation and mobilization. Specific flap options are discussed later in this chapter.

THE PROBLEM WOUND

Even with appropriate patient selection and preoperative optimization, wound healing complications are common after TKA.[25,37] Soft tissue reconstruction of the knee is challenging because of its unique anatomic and functional requirements. Thin, pliable, tough skin is needed for stable, long-term coverage. Reconstructive options include skin grafting, local flaps, free flaps, or a combination of these modalities.

Skin Grafting

Full thickness tissue loss often results in soft tissue defects that are too large to close primarily. In cases where the joint capsule is completely intact, soft tissue bulk is adequate, and there is no threat of prosthesis exposure, skin grafting may be appropriate.

Skin grafting requires a recipient bed that is well vascularized, hemostatic, and free of infection (Fig. 107.3). Grafts survive by serum imbibition for the first 48 hours. Inosculation initiates vascular ingrowth, and graft circulation sufficient for survival occurs by day 5 to 6.[3,5,6] Shear forces must be minimized to allow for proper revascularization. This can be accomplished by applying a compressive/bolster dressing or a negative pressure wound therapy device.

After 5 to 7 days, the skin graft dressing may be removed and dependence of the limb gradually initiated. Topical ointment should be applied to the graft until it is completely healed. Long term, grafts often require supplemental moisture since they are devoid of sebaceous glands, which are located in the deep or subdermis and are not harvested with the graft.

Skin graft donor sites heal by secondary intention. Multiple options exist for donor site dressings. Evidence suggests that moist occlusive dressings may provide better pain control for patients.[48] Once the donor site has epithelialized, long-term effects such as pruritis, sensitivity, pigment changes, and even scar hypertrophy may occur (Fig. 107.4). While self-limited, these conditions may be addressed with antipruritics, antihistamines, lubricants, or topical silicone sheeting.

Local Flaps

When soft tissue loss is extensive or associated with incomplete joint capsular closure, when the knee joint is exposed, or when exposure of the prosthesis occurs, robust, well-vascularized coverage is mandatory. Local rotation flaps composed of skin and muscle, muscle alone, skin and fascia, or fascia alone are reconstructive options. The location of tissue loss and precise coverage requirements determine the appropriate choice of flap. Local flaps are raised on a vascular pedicle that is rotated or as an island of tissue that is transposed into position as required.

MUSCLE AND MYOCUTANEOUS FLAPS

Gastrocnemius Flap

The gastrocnemius muscle flap is the local workhorse for coverage of defects about the knee. It may be raised with a skin paddle or as a muscle-only flap with an overlying skin graft applied. The gastrocnemius has two heads, medial and lateral, each with

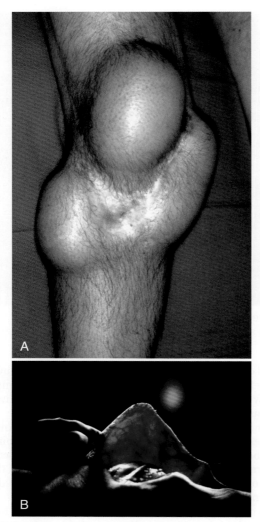

FIG 107.2 (A and B) Tissue expansion can improve the local blood supply in patients with potential healing compromise.

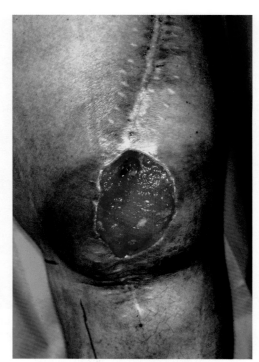

FIG 107.3 A healthy bed with excellent vascularity will support a split-thickness skin graft.

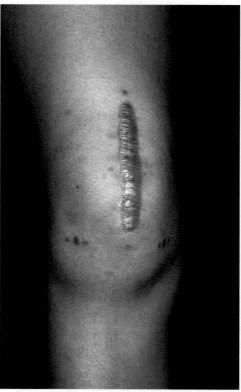

FIG 107.4 Scar hypertrophy such as pictured here will respond to the application of topical silicone sheeting.

a single, dominant blood supply from the medial and lateral sural vessels, respectively.[31] The heads are clearly separated by a fibrous band known as the *median raphe*; the raphe can be split to allow for unilateral muscle harvest or independent muscle use. Each sural artery has a 2 to 5 cm course before it penetrates the deep surface of the muscle, arborizes, and divides within.[30,34,43,46] The medial head is usually the longer of the two heads, extending more distal than the lateral head. The arc of rotation of the medial gastrocnemius muscle flap allows coverage of the proximal third of the tibia, the medial knee joint, the tibial tubercle, and the patella (Fig. 107.5). When taken as an extended flap with overlying skin, coverage can be achieved from the middle third of the tibia to the suprapatellar region. An additional 2 cm in length may be obtained by taking down the origin at the posterior surface of the medial femoral condyle or by scoring the deep muscle fascia.[11]

The lateral head of the gastrocnemius can be used to cover defects of the lateral knee joint and the fibula. It may also be taken with overlying skin when perforators are carefully identified. Proximal dissection and transposition must be done with great care, as the peroneal nerve is in a vulnerable, subcutaneous

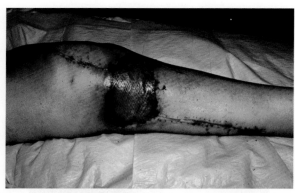

FIG 107.5 The gastrocnemius muscle flap provides reliable soft tissue coverage when needed.

position at the head the fibula. The arc of rotation is limited by the fibular head.[9]

The major drawback to the use of a gastrocnemius myocutaneous flap is the cosmetic deformity created at the donor and recipient sites. Some patients have a thick adipose layer overlying the muscle that, when transposed, appears bulky in comparison to the thin skin of the anterior knee. Patients should be counseled on this risk preoperatively. Using a muscle-only flap, when possible, may minimize this problem.

Other Muscle Flaps

Other local options for knee reconstruction include the distally based anterolateral thigh (ALT),[53] vastus lateralis,[40,45] sartorius,[21,28] and gracilis muscle flaps.[23,32] The reverse-ALT and vastus lateralis flaps rely on retrograde flow through the lateral circumflex femoral system. Sartorius and gracilis muscles receive contributions from the superficial femoral artery (SFA) and/or popliteal artery distally. Sartorius and gracilis muscle flaps may require a two-stage procedure with a vascular delay to ensure adequate blood supply from minor pedicles.[21,32]

Fascial and Fasciocutaneous Flaps

The use of a fasciocutaneous flap for lower extremity reconstruction was first described in 1981 by Pontén.[38] Understanding of these flaps along with their clinical applications continues to evolve.[7,14-16] Fasciocutaneous flaps provide thin, durable coverage when a skin graft or random pattern skin flap is insufficient (eg, for exposed tendon, joint, or prosthesis). They are less bulky than muscle flaps and leave no functional deficit at the donor site. Elevation of fasciocutaneous flaps is relatively simple and fast. Vascular pedicles are variable and must be meticulously defined and preserved; this caution prevents them from being adapted universally as the most satisfactory local coverage option. Several local fasciocutaneous flaps are available for reconstruction of knee defects, including the posterior calf flap, saphenous flap, and lateral genicular artery flap.

Posterior Calf Flap

The posterior calf flap can be raised as a fascia-only or fasciocutaneous flap. It is supplied by the descending cutaneous branch of the popliteal artery, also called the *median sural artery*,[7] which is superficial to and not the same as the medial sural artery. Where the median sural artery is present, the flap extends from the popliteal crease to the junction of the middle and distal third of the posterior leg. Harvest requires careful preoperative planning since the median sural artery is often small or absent-the flap is unusable in approximately one-third of patients.[17]

This flap is useful for thin coverage about the knee. It has several advantages over the gastrocnemius muscle flap in that it provides better coverage of large suprapatellar defects as well as better cosmesis of both donor and recipient sites. It can be harvested with branches of the lateral sural cutaneous nerve to provide protective sensation, and it can easily be re-elevated for future orthopedic procedures.[42]

Saphenous Flap

The saphenous fasciocutaneous flap is based on the saphenous artery, a branch of the descending genicular artery from the SFA, which supplies the skin on the medial aspect of the thigh and superior leg.[13] The saphenous artery is reliably present, originating deep to the sartorius muscle and becoming superficial distal and medial to its insertion. This course makes the artery vulnerable to injury during TKA. The artery and its cutaneous perforators must be dissected with meticulous care before flap incision because adequate anterior perforators are present in only about 45% of dissections.[17] Its arc of rotation limits its use to defects in the proximal third of the knee and distal femur—two areas where wound healing difficulties rarely occur.

Lateral Genicular Artery Flap

The lateral genicular artery fasciocutaneous flap receives its blood supply from a cutaneous perforator of the superior lateral genicular artery, which in turn originates directly from the popliteal artery. The skin island is designed on the lateral aspect of the distal thigh. Its arc of rotation allows the flap to reach the distal third of the thigh and the superolateral aspect of the patella as well as the popliteal fossa. In addition, it is well positioned to provide a vascilarized bone graft from the lateral femoral condyle.[33] Advantages of this flap include excellent contour of the recipient site, a one-stage procedure, and the ability to close the donor site primarily in most cases.[18]

Free Flap Coverage

When local soft tissue is damaged or other attempts at coverage have failed, free tissue transfer is the preferred method of reconstruction. Free flaps may also be required in defects that are too large or complex for local options.

The ideal free flap for knee reconstruction has a predictable blood supply with few anatomic variants and a vascular pedicle of about 12 cm in length to reach the SFA in the adductor canal. Several donor sites exist that meet these requirements; the shape and volume of the defect as well as the experience of the surgeon dictate flap choice.[20,24] Preoperative angiography is not always necessary but should be performed in patients with an abnormal distal pulse, an abnormal ankle-brachial index,[27] or in patients who have had significant trauma to the extremity. Computed angiography is the procedure of choice when preoperative angiography is indicated. Vessels as small as 1 mm can be well visualized.[10]

Latissimus Dorsi Flap

The latissimus dorsi muscle flap is the most common free flap used for soft tissue knee reconstruction (Fig. 107.6).[26,37] It is broad and flat, has a long and predictable thoracodorsal pedicle, and has an abundant vascular network within the muscle,

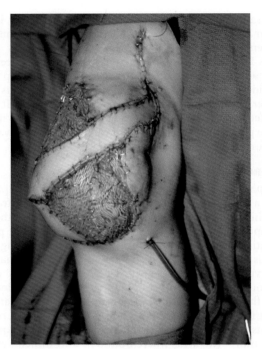

FIG 107.6 Free myocutaneous flap coverage is the ideal solution when local coverage is not available.

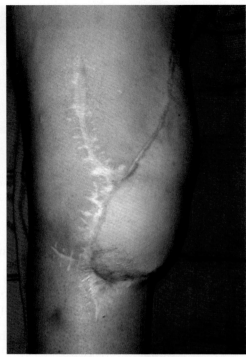

FIG 107.7 The transverse rectus abdominis flap provides thin suitable coverage in selected patients.

making it preferable in irradiated or infected wound bed. These features make the latissimus dorsi a versatile and reliable flap.

The main disadvantage to the latissimus dorsi flap is that harvesting and insetting frequently require a change in body position.

Other Free Flaps

Other free flap options include the ALT,[44] gracilis muscle,[51] rectus abdominis musculocutaneous,[4] and the radial forearm fascial flap.[29] All offer the advantage of supine patient positioning for the duration of the case.

The ALT flap is located in a nearby operative field and can be taken as a fasciocutaneous flap. The donor site can sometimes be closed primarily.[44] The gracilis requires extended local fascial harvest for its skin paddle to reliably survive.[51] The rectus abdominis muscle, although a satisfactory donor in slender patients (Fig. 107.7), can be extremely bulky when combined with skin and subcutaneous tissue. The radial forearm flap, a thin pliable septocutaneous flap, is acceptable for defects with minimal dead space. The donor site is unsightly and often requires skin grafting.

Other Considerations

Numerous recipient vessels are available in the knee region: the profunda femoris, SFA, and descending branch of the lateral femoral circumflex arteries proximal to the knee; the popliteal, genicular, and sural arteries around the knee; and the anterior tibial, posterior tibial, and peroneal arteries distal to the knee. Choice of recipient vessel is based on its proximity to the defect, vessel availability, vessel size match, and concomitant injuries. Complication rates are equivalent.[26]

Approximately 20% of free flaps to the knee require acute reexploration for arterial or venous thrombosis.[26] This take-back rate is quite high when compared with other lower extremity-free flap recipient sites, such as the distal tibia and the foot, which have take-back rates of 6.5% to 7.8%.[2,50] Quite possibly this high rate is related to the fact that the pedicle frequently must cross the knee joint posteriorly to reach the donor artery. In spite of this unusually high take-back rate, free flap reconstruction about the knee has a better than 97% survival rate, a rate similar to free flaps elsewhere in the lower extremity.[4,26]

CONCLUSION

The management of soft tissue defects after TKA is challenging. Every attempt should be made to identify and optimize at-risk patients prior to joint replacement. Options for soft tissue management span the reconstructive ladder. The goals of reconstruction are to provide stable soft tissue coverage and achieve full function of the joint.

KEY REFERENCES

24. Kumar AR, Grewal NS, Chung TL, et al: Lessons from operation Iraqi freedom: successful subacute reconstruction of complex lower extremity battle injuries. *Plast Reconstr Surg* 123(1):218–229, 2009.

26. Louer CR, Garcia RM, Earle SA, et al: Free flap reconstruction of the knee: an outcome study of 34 cases. *Ann Plast Surg* 74(1):57–63, 2015.

34. Moscona RA, Fodor L, Har-Shai Y: The segmental gastrocnemius muscle flap: anatomical study and clinical applicatons. *Plast Reconstr Surg* 118(5):1178–1182, 2006.

The references for this chapter can also be found on www.expertconsult.com.

Fractures About the Knee

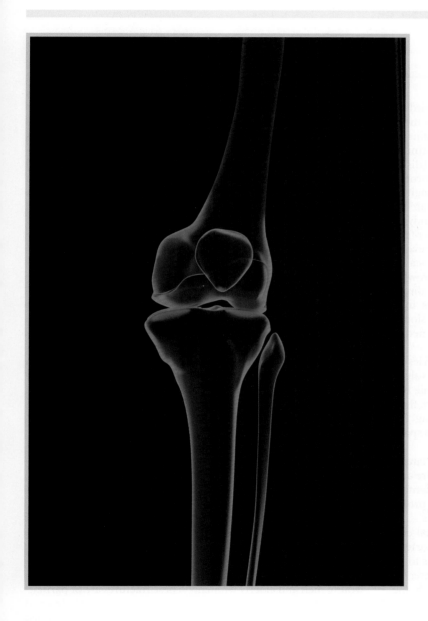

108

Distal Femur Fractures

Ryan Stancil, George J. Haidukewych, Adam A. Sassoon

ANATOMY

General Anatomy

The distal femur extends for approximately the distal third of the femur, or generally the width of the epicondylar axis measured proximally from the end of the femur.[41,46,108] It begins as the canal gradually widens and the cortices thin and continues distally to the joint line. The supracondylar region (distal metaphysis) flares medially greater than laterally in the coronal plane and broadens laterally greater than medially in the sagittal plane. The anterior and distal trochlear groove allows patellar articulation with the distal end of the femur. The intercondylar notch is posteriorly based and houses the cruciate ligaments.

An axial cut through the distal articular surface reveals a trapezoidal shape with the greatest dimension located posteriorly in a lateral-to-medial direction and the narrowest dimension located medially in an anterior-to-posterior direction. The medial side slopes approximately 25 degrees in a posteromedial-to-anterolateral direction. The lateral side slopes approximately 15 degrees in a posterolateral-to-anteromedial direction (Fig. 108.1).[86]

The shaft lies in the anterior two-thirds of the condyles in the sagittal plane and slightly lateral, with a 9-degree valgus orientation in the coronal plane.[46,86,95,135] The joint capsule has greater space anteriorly than posteriorly and extends more than 2 cm proximal to the superior pole of the patella along the anterior aspect of the distal femur. Posteriorly, the joint space extends only to the condyle-shaft junction.

The articular surface involves the entire medial and lateral condyles and is thickest along the distal articular curvature and within the trochlear groove, the regions with the highest contact pressure. Anteriorly, the articular cartilage extends more proximally on the lateral condyle than on the medial condyle.

The critical nervous and arterial anatomy of the distal end of the femur includes the sciatic nerve and the femoral artery. The femoral artery proceeds distally beneath the sartorius to lie between the adductors and the vastus medialis before entering the adductor canal. It then courses posteriorly through the adductor hiatus and into the popliteal fossa, where it changes name and becomes the popliteal artery until its trifurcation. The sciatic nerve lies posterior in the thigh between the long head of the biceps femoris and the semimembranosus. It then divides into the tibial and common peroneal branches before it emerges from the popliteal fossa.

Radiographic Anatomy

The anteroposterior (AP) radiograph demonstrates the 9-degree valgus angle created between the femoral shaft and the distal joint line. It also shows the greater medial condyle flare but does not reveal the trapezoidal shape as seen on an axial computed tomography (CT) image. The lateral radiograph demonstrates an anterior curvilinear sclerotic line representing the trochlear groove and a convergent posterior sclerotic line representing the intercondylar notch (Blumensaat line), both of which end as they meet distally (Fig. 108.2). In addition, a true lateral radiograph of the knee allows identification of the medial femoral condyle as it articulates with the concave medial tibial plateau and the lateral femoral condyle as it articulates with the convex lateral tibial plateau (see Fig. 108.2). Flexion of the knee during the AP radiograph allows visualization of the intercondylar notch.

Surface Anatomy

Palpation of the distal femur demonstrates a medial prominence, the adductor tubercle, which allows for muscle and ligament attachment. A lesser lateral prominence slightly more proximal represents the lateral tubercle. With the knee in the extended position, the inferior pole of the patella corresponds to the level of the tibiofemoral joint line. Approximately two to three fingerbreadths proximal to the superior pole of the patella is the proximal extension of the suprapatellar pouch. Four fingerbreadths proximal to the adductor tubercle is the level where the femoral artery traverses from the anterior half of the femur to the posterior half.

INCIDENCE AND ETIOLOGY

The incidence of supracondylar femoral fractures has a bimodal distribution—young adult patients with higher-energy injuries and elderly patients with lower-energy injuries.[5,41]

The supracondylar femoral fracture is typically the result of an external force, but the amount of force required to cause the fracture can vary significantly and is dependent on bone quality. In a 2000 report on 2165 distal femoral fractures, the distribution of such fractures was found to be bimodal, occurring in young men and elderly women.[76] These fractures are of particular significance in older adults, as their effects on morbidity and overall mortality are comparable to more heavily studied femoral neck fractures.[117] Several studies have shown the following: 18% mortality at 1 year,[113] 18% able ambulate unaided, 23% strictly housebound, and 48.8% mortality at 5 years.[57] Lower-energy injuries are generally the result of ground-level falls or torsional injuries in patients with osteopenic or osteoporotic bone. Periprosthetic fractures are usually low-energy injuries that are encountered most commonly in older sdults as a result of disuse osteopenia, osteoporosis, and/or stress

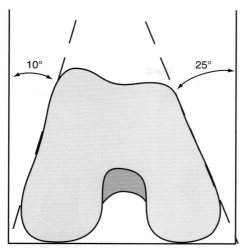

FIG 108.1 Diagram depicting the trapezoidal shape of the distal end of the femur. The 10-degree slope is shown laterally, and the 25-degree slope is shown medially.

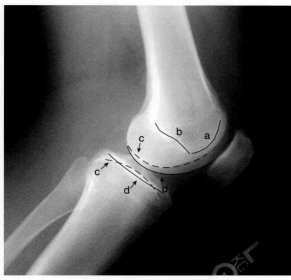

FIG 108.2 Lateral radiograph of the knee showing the trochlear groove (a), the intercondylar notch (Blumensaat line) (b), the lateral distal femoral condylar articular surface with matching lateral tibial convex surface (c), and the medial femoral condylar articular surface with matching medial tibial concave surface (d).

shielding around a prosthetic device or other metallic implant when a stress riser is created in the transition area between the prosthesis and routine bone. Examples include the area distal to a hip stem, proximal to a short supracondylar nail and proximal to a total knee prosthesis. These fracture types are increasing in incidence, as the prevalence of patients with orthopedic prostheses has significantly increased with an aging population.[71]

Paraplegics and quadriplegics have weakened bone and, because of the resultant osteopenia and frequent contractures, are at increased risk for distal femoral fracture through falls from a wheelchair or transfer of the patient. The amount of energy required to cause a supracondylar or distal femoral fracture in young patients with no existing bone pathology is

usually significant, and this fracture is often seen in conjunction with other associated fractures.[6,12,14,24,127] Knee ligament injuries and intra-articular pathology have been reported in approximately 20% to 70% of ipsilateral femoral fractures via post injury examination or magnetic resonance (MR) imaging.[12,24,29,127] Motor vehicle accidents, falls from heights, pedestrian versus auto accidents, and other heavy industrial accidents are common mechanisms of injury.[76]

CLASSIFICATION

A number of classification systems have been proposed for fractures of the distal femur. In 1967, Neer et al. described a classification system that divided fractures into three main categories: minimal displacement, condylar displacement from the shaft, and supracondylar or shaft comminution.[88] Seinsheimer later published a more detailed system.[108] The Swiss Arbeitsgemeinschaft für Osteosynthesefragen/Association for the Study of Internal Fixation (AO/ASIF) group has since developed a comprehensive fracture classification scheme that has become accepted in the trauma community: type A, extraarticular; type B, unicondylar; and type C, bicondylar (Fig. 108.3). This classification is further subdivided by the degree of comminution.[87] The Orthopaedic Trauma Association (OTA) has developed a similar detailed and well-accepted classification system that encompasses the entire axial skeleton.[36]

DIAGNOSIS

History and Physical Examination

As with any traumatized patient, a complete history and detailed physical examination should be conducted. The preinjury level of function and additional medical conditions should be recorded because such knowledge will aid in determining whether conservative or operative treatment should be performed. The mechanism of injury must also be ascertained to help determine the severity of the injury and other associated injuries. The physical examination should include a detailed evaluation of the entire limb and other extremities to rule out ipsilateral and associated fractures.[14] The skin must be circumferentially inspected for open wounds, and a detailed neurologic and vascular examination of the entire extremity should be documented. Higher-energy injuries can result in laceration or rupture of the quadriceps tendon, the femoral artery as it exits the adductor hiatus, the popliteal artery, and knee ligaments.[6,12,29,127] The knee joint itself should be evaluated for an effusion, because an effusion often represents a radiographically unnoticed intercondylar split, an associated tibial plateau or patellar fracture, and/or cruciate ligament rupture.

In higher-energy fractures, the ankle-brachial index should be documented even if palpable pulses are present. A ratio less than 0.9 has been shown to correlate with a high incidence of arterial injury, whereas ratios greater than 0.9 show that vascular intervention was not required. If abnormal, angiography and vascular surgery consultation should be performed.[64,80]

Radiographic Examination

As with any fracture, orthogonal views (AP and lateral) are indicated (Fig. 108.4A). Both knee and femur radiographs are necessary to fully evaluate the fracture and the entire femoral shaft. A traction radiograph may be helpful to better delineate all fracture fragments. Knee views will better diagnose

33-Femur Distal

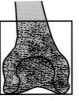

Location

Essence: The fractures of the distal segment are divided into 3 types:
A, extra-articular; B, partial articular; C, complete articular

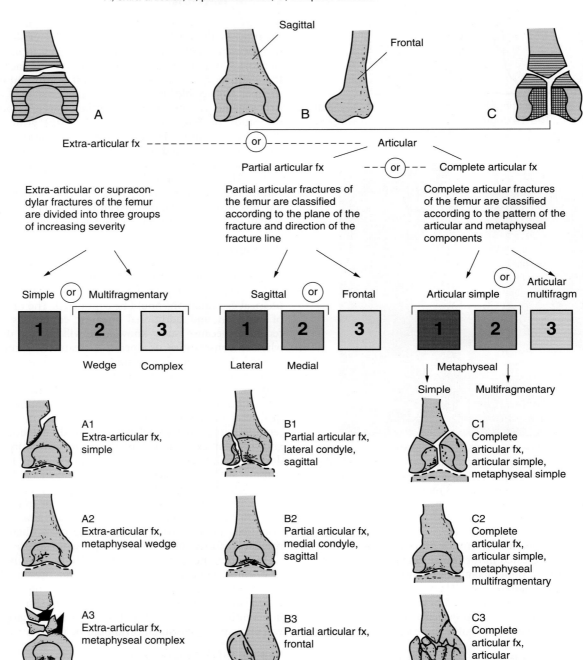

FIG 108.3 AO/ASIF classification. (From Müller ME, Nazarian S, Koch P, et al: The comprehensive classification of fractures of long bones, 1995, Bern, Switzerland, M.E. Müller Foundation.)

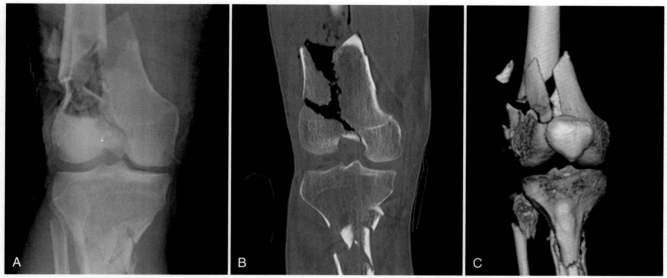

FIG 108.4 Multiple imaging modalities of a polytrauma patient with ipsilateral distal femur and tibial plateau fractures: (A) AP x-ray, (B) coronal cut of CT scan, (C) three-dimensional reformatting from CT scan.

intra-articular extension or comminution and associated patellar or tibial plateau fractures. Femoral shaft radiographs will reveal the proximal extent of the fracture, segmental fracture patterns, or possibly ipsilateral femoral neck fractures. If femoral neck involvement is at all suspected, dedicated hip radiographs must be obtained, because intraoperative discovery of this associated fracture can lead to different instrumentation and patient positioning.[134] Coronal plane condylar fractures (the so-called Hoffa fragment) seen in the lateral view must not be missed because the presence of such coronal splits will influence the selection of fixation devices.[6,51,131] Nork et al. demonstrated an association of 38.1% between coronal plane fractures and supracondylar-intracondylar distal femur fractures in a series of 202 fractures. Coronal plane fractures were 2.8 times more likely in open fractures; 76% of these fractures were unicondylar, of which 85% affected the lateral condyle.[89] CT is indicated for comminuted fractures or if absolute certainty of all fracture lines cannot be gained from plain radiographs. Once all fracture planes are determined, more optimal fixation can be applied. The authors obtain CT scans as standard practice when planning definitive internal fixation (see Fig. 108.4B). In the previously mentioned series, 10 coronal plane fractures were first discovered intraoperatively. None of these patients had a preoperative CT.[89] Additionally, three-dimensional reformatting from CT scans is an emerging technology that produces striking pictures and has practical use in surgical planning (see Fig. 108.4C).

MANAGEMENT

Conservative Versus Operative Management

Nonoperative management should be reserved for patients who are too debilitated and/or bedridden, or who have prohibitive medical comorbid conditions. Other indications for conservative treatment may include nondisplaced, incomplete, and/or avulsion fractures. These situations are extremely rare.

The overwhelming majority of distal femoral fractures should be treated surgically. Operative stabilization allows increased mobility and early knee range of motion. The goals of surgical treatment are to reduce the joint anatomically, restore condyle-shaft alignment, and provide fracture stability to permit uneventful fracture healing and regain early knee range of motion.

Surgical Approaches

Lateral. The lateral approach, the most commonly used approach for supracondylar and distal femoral fractures, is an extension of the lateral approach to the femoral shaft. The patient is positioned supine, and the incision begins along the midlateral aspect of the thigh and extends distally to the lateral femoral epicondyle. If joint visualization is necessary, the incision is extended distally and curved anteriorly toward the midportion of the patellar tendon. The iliotibial band is then incised in line with the skin incision. Distally, the joint capsule is incised as distal as necessary, and medial subluxation of the patella allows intercondylar inspection. Proximally, the fascia of the vastus lateralis is incised and the muscle is dissected in a distal-to-proximal direction from the lateral intermuscular septum and posterior fascia, with ligation of any perforating arteries encountered. The muscle is then retracted anteriorly to expose the distal femoral shaft. The periosteum should be carefully preserved, and no medial dissection should be performed to avoid devascularization of fracture fragments.

Alternative Exposures

Medial. The medial approach is less commonly used because essentially all anatomically designed plates have been created for the lateral aspect of the distal femur. If necessary, however, the medial approach also offers adequate distal femur exposure. The incision is made along the medial aspect of the distal femur, just anterior to the sartorius, while avoiding the saphenous vein. The fascia is incised in line with the skin incision to expose the vastus medialis. The vastus medialis fascia is then incised at the medial intermuscular septum. As with the lateral approach, the muscle is dissected in a distal-to-proximal direction off the fascia (medial intermuscular septum), and any perforating arteries encountered are ligated. The muscle is retracted anteriorly to expose the medial aspect of the distal femur. The femoral artery remains posterior and proximal to the dissection. A long medial plate can safely avoid the femoral artery if placed on anteromedial aspect of the femur, up to 8 cm from the lesser trochanter.[62] This approach may be useful for isolated medial condylar fractures or for corrective distal femur osteotomies.

Anterior. The anterior approach requires a midline incision and a parapatellar arthrotomy. It allows excellent joint exposure but also requires separation of the vastus intermedius, as the approach is extended proximally from the knee joint. A variation of the anterior approach described as the "swash-buckler" also allows for excellent joint exposure and is basically a lateral approach with an anteriorly placed incision.[115] It allows intraoperative flexibility, should the need arise, to switch from a retrograde intramedullary nail to a lateral plate to gain better fixation without having to make a second incision. Other variations of the aforementioned standard approaches have also been described.[81,90]

IMPLANTS: DESIGN AND FUNCTION

Numerous implants have been described and designed for supracondylar and distal femoral fractures. Implant types include retrograde nails, various fixed-angled devices, screws (cortical, cancellous, or fixed angle), and standard compression and buttress plates. Specific examples include long retrograde nails; the AO angled blade plate; the dynamic condylar screw; the condylar buttress plate; and, more recently, locked plates.* The choice of implant is dependent on the location of the fracture, the fracture pattern, existing hardware, bone quality, and surgeon preference.

Intramedullary nails are available as retrograde nails that typically provide multiple distal locking options. If sufficient distal bone is available, retrograde nailing is an excellent fixation option, especially for extra-articular fractures. Careful attention to distal fragment alignment is critical during reaming and nailing. Multiple distal interlock options are available to enhance fixation, including several preassembled locking mechanisms that can statically lock up to four interlock screws.

Plates initially consisted of a condylar buttress-type plate and standard compression plates. The AO angled blade plate and condylar compression screw were the early forms of "fixed"-angle devices; the condylar compression screw allowed an additional degree of freedom and therefore easier insertion. Although the 95-degree angled blade plate does not anatomically match the medial distal femoral angle (99 degrees), the design allows for slight overbending of the plate to create compression of the opposite medial cortex. As the blade is inserted parallel to the joint line, the femoral shaft is reduced to the plate, which causes the "preloaded" plate to compress the opposite cortex. The 95-degree condylar compression screw, however, is extremely rigid and therefore can create a slight varus deformity if inserted improperly. Fixation of unicondylar fractures in the coronal plane (Hoffa fragment) can be achieved

with direct large diameter headless compression screws placed anterior to posterior. Posterior to anterior placed screws or a posteriorly placed buttress plate are also viable fixation options that come at the expense of additional soft tissue dissection and potential neuropraxia.[4,9,119,131]

Additional fixed-angle devices have become available in the form of anatomically designed plates with locking screw technology that can be inserted through a traditional open approach or percutaneously.[34,68] The locking plate design also creates a 95-degree angle between the distal screws and the plate. Proper insertion is achieved with the distal screws parallel to the joint line; this is followed by reduction of the femoral shaft to the plate.[37,102] The advantage of locked plates over the traditional angled blade plate is seen with intercondylar split fractures. Insertion of an angled blade generates significantly more force than is generated by insertion of a threaded locked screw and can therefore displace a nondisplaced or previously reduced and compressed intercondylar split. In addition, rotational freedom during insertion is present with locked plates, as with the condylar screw, and the advantage of a fixed-angle device is gained. Newer anatomically designed locking plates may also allow for variable-angle locked screws that are inserted at the surgeon's preferred angle and then locked to the plate once fully seated.[133] One recent study showed 1 nonunion at 6 months among 31 distal femur fractures treated with dynamic locked plating.[15]

In cases of extreme osteopenia, osteoporosis, tumor, or other conditions with poor bone quality, a second medial implant has been described to add to construct stability.[44,56,77,78,101] The addition of bone cement has been advocated in similar situations to achieve increased screw purchase.[10,118] With the advent of modern locking plate technology, the need for adjunctive medial fixation or cement augmentation has essentially been eliminated.

Primary total knee arthroplasty has also been described for use in elderly patients. Several papers have reported primary total knee arthroplasty for fixation of simple distal femur fractures in patients with preexisting osteoarthritis.[20,99] Although more often used for periprosthetic distal femur fractures, distal femoral replacement has been described as a primary or salvage option for patients with massive bony destruction and severe osteopenia.[11,33,122]

TREATMENT

Initially, as with all fractures, splinting and immobilization were favored over internal fixation. In the 1940s and 1950s, internal fixation was reported, but without overwhelming success.[1,121,132]

As technology advanced and techniques improved, success rates with internal fixation began to increase. The Swiss AO group in 1958 defined the goals of open reduction and internal fixation as follows: (1) anatomic reduction, (2) preservation of the blood supply, (3) stable internal fixation, and (4) early mobilization.[85] Schatzker and Wenzl began documenting improved results with the AO principles and showed open reduction and internal fixation to be superior to conservative management.[103-105,130] Other authors soon reported similar findings.† Today, although slightly modified, the AO principles are still being used, and the results of surgical treatment remain superior to those of nonoperative management for displaced fractures.

---

*References 42, 48, 54, 85, 100, 102, 107, 110, 112, and 138.

†References 19, 45, 81, 90, 111, 112, and 116.

Conservative Treatment

Conservative management of distal femoral and supracondylar fractures has fallen out of favor as surgical techniques, implant designs, and rehabilitation protocols have continued to progress and yield outcomes superior to those of nonoperative treatment.[‡] Certain situations, however, still require nonoperative management; it is therefore necessary to remain familiar with conservative treatment options.

For patients with low-energy, extra-articular, nondisplaced fractures who refuse or cannot medically tolerate a surgical procedure, cast bracing or casting is recommended. Non–weight bearing must be enforced until adequate healing is achieved to avoid creating a deformity or unstable fracture. Knee joint stiffness typically becomes problematic with longer than 6 weeks of immobilization.[39] Special attention must be paid to the skin condition during casting or bracing. Paraplegics and quadriplegics also present a treatment challenge because skin breakdown can occur without warning, leading to additional setbacks and the potential for limb compromise.

Operative Management

The goals of operative stabilization should be to achieve adequate fracture reduction with minimal soft tissue stripping that ultimately allows for preservation of functional knee range of motion and early postoperative ambulation. For extra-articular fractures, anatomic reduction is less important than anatomic alignment. Intra-articular fractures, however, should undergo anatomic reduction to decrease the chance of later arthritis. The more distal the fracture and the greater the mechanism of injury, the higher the likelihood of an unrecognized intra-articular split. Depending on the fracture location, an intramedullary device or a locked plate is typically used to achieve fracture stability. The ideal implant would be inserted with minimal dissection and would allow immediate knee range of motion and early weight bearing.

High-energy injuries involving the distal femur are frequently comminuted and have significant intra-articular involvement (Fig. 108.5A-D). If the fracture is an open fracture, adequate initial débridement must be performed, followed by thorough irrigation and temporary or definitive stabilization. Temporary stabilization is especially appropriate in patients with multiple fractures, requiring several surgical procedures and/or polytrauma patients awaiting hemodynamic, respiratory, or neurologic stabilization.[8] If temporary stabilization is chosen, a spanning external fixator can be used, with the pins for the fixator placed away from the region of future definitive fixation. Two pins are typically inserted anteriorly or laterally into the femur, and two pins into the proximal end of the tibia, with the frame then spanning the knee joint. If the soft tissues appear stable and appropriate studies and implants are available, definitive fixation may be performed at the time of initial débridement. When significant intra-articular comminution warrants a CT scan, a staged approach must be adopted if the CT scan is not available prior to the initial open fracture débridement. The distal femur has better soft tissue coverage than the tibia, so plate application can be safely performed acutely unless significant soft tissue loss and/or excessive gross contamination are present. If tissue transfer is required for bone or plate coverage, or for both, initial spanning external fixation

is more appropriate. Intravenous antibiotic coverage based on the type and degree of soft tissue wounds is necessary, as in all long-bone open fractures. Acute bone grafting of open fractures is not recommended because of the increased risk of infection, although the literature mostly pertains to open tibia rather than open femur fractures.

Operative Treatment: General Principles

Regardless of whether a plate or nail is chosen to stabilize an intra-articular distal femoral fracture, adherence to the following principles is essential:
1. Achieving anatomic reduction with lag screw fixation of the articular surface
2. Maximizing distal fragment fixation
3. Obtaining correct coronal (5- to 7-degree valgus) and sagittal plane alignment
4. Obtaining correct leg length
5. Obtaining correct leg rotation
6. Achieving stable, balanced proximal fragment fixation
7. Preserving fracture fragment viability by avoiding periosteal stripping and medial dissection

Intramedullary Devices. Once the morphology of the fracture has been clearly defined, the surgeon can decide on the most appropriate implant. The authors find retrograde nailing useful for extra-articular fractures with a distal fragment of sufficient length to allow stable distal fixation. Occasionally, a fracture with extensive femoral shaft extension and simple or nondisplaced intra-articular involvement can be managed effectively with lag screws and a retrograde nail. If a retrograde intramedullary nail is selected, an anterior incision is made over the patellar tendon and a lateral mini-arthrotomy is performed on the lateral border of the tendon. The entry point in the trochlear groove must be accurately placed to avoid injury to the anterior cruciate ligament and patella. Ideally, the entry point should cheat a few millimeters medial to center on the AP view and at the intersection of Blumensaat line and the sclerotic line representing the femoral notch on the lateral view.[17] If the nail is inserted in the center and is not directed slightly lateral, to remain in line with the anatomic femoral axis, a varus deformity will result when the nail enters the isthmus of the femoral canal. Because there is no canal fill in the metaphyseal flare of the distal femur, it is easy to create an angular deformity during nail insertion. Vigilance is required to avoid malalignment. It is important to understand that the nail will not reduce the fracture in this situation. A flexion or extension deformity can also be created if reduction in the sagittal plane is not obtained and maintained before reaming and insertion of the nail. Early treatment of supracondylar femoral fractures with a retrograde intramedullary device was reported by Zickel et al. in 1977.[138] Difficulty was noted in achieving stability in patients with intra-articular comminution. A subsequent report by Zickel et al. showed improved results with the intramedullary nail, but half the patients with intra-articular fractures did not regain more than 90 degrees of knee motion.[139]

Antegrade nailing of supracondylar femoral fractures has also been reported as a successful procedure.[72] Its effectiveness is limited with intercondylar fractures, unless adjunctive fixation is used.[72,120] Adequate distal fragment length is necessary to achieve stable distal fixation, which is rare. Tornetta and Tiburzi achieved a 100% union rate with antegrade nailing of supracondylar femoral fractures but reported a 50% incidence of

[‡]References 19, 45, 81, 88, 90, 103-105, 111, 112, 116, and 130.

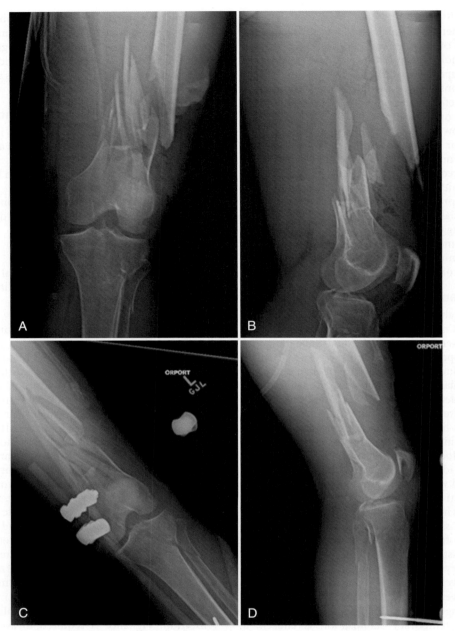

FIG 108.5 Preoperative AP (A) and lateral (B) radiographs demonstrating open distal femur fracture in polytrauma patient. Patient initially treated with irrigation and débridement of open fracture wounds and spanning external fixation, as shown in postoperative AP (C) and lateral (D) radiographs.

valgus malunion in patients in whom nailing was performed in the lateral position.[120] Dominquez et al. also noted successful results with antegrade nailing of distal femoral fractures and had 1 nonunion in a series of 20 fractures.[25]

Retrograde nailing continues to be more popular than antegrade nailing because it is easier to control the distal fragment. Lucas et al. reported union of all 25 fractures in their series with use of the retrograde nail, although 4 fractures did require bone grafting.[73] Danziger et al. also demonstrated successful treatment, with healing of all but 1 of 16 fractures in their series.[22] Kim et al. reported 84% good or excellent outcomes in a series of 31 distal femoral fractures treated with retrograde nailing. Poor results and complications were related

to a high degree of comminution and the most distal fracture line coming within 5 cm of the intracondylar notch.[63] Iannacone et al., however, reported 4 nonunions, 5 delayed unions, and 4 stress nail fatigue fractures in 41 patients.[53] During their series, the nail was changed from an 11-mm nail with 6.4-mm locking screws to 12- and 13-mm nails with 5.0-mm locking screws. All device failures were noted with the 11-mm nail. In a series of fractures in elderly patients that involved the supracondylar region, Janzing et al. reported 89% good or excellent results with use of the retrograde nail.[55] These investigators did, however, comment on poor fixation distally with locking screws in osteoporotic bone. Recently, Hierholzer et al. reported a cohort study that showed no statistically significant difference in time to osseous healing, rate of nonunion, and postoperative complication in a series of 115 distal femur fractures treated with either a retrograde nail (*n* = 59) or minimally invasive locked plating (*n* = 56).[49]

Other materials or implants can be used as adjuncts to the retrograde nail in osteoporotic bone or heavily comminuted fractures. Kim et al. used either cement augmentation or shape memory alloy as augmentation in a series of 13 retrograde nails in osteoporotic patients with satisfactory clinical outcomes.[61] Garnavos et al. reported 100% union in a series of 17 type C distal femoral fractures treated with a retrograde nail and independent condylar compression bolts placed prior to nail insertion.[38] As the intramedullary canal widens in the distal femoral metaphysis, surgeons may have difficulty preventing varus, valgus, or recurvatum deformity of a distal femur fracture when using a retrograde nail. Seyhan et al. reported 100% union in a series of patients treated with a nail and blocking screws used as an adjunctive reduction aid.[109]

Mechanical testing to evaluate various fixation constructs has been reported. Firoozbaksh et al. tested retrograde nailing versus dynamic condylar screw (DCS) plate fixation in a synthetic bone model.[35]

The DCS plate was found to be stiffer in lateral bending and torsion, but no significant difference was found with respect to bending stiffness in varus and flexion. Because the most common clinical forms of failure occurred in varus and flexion, both devices were deemed biomechanically adequate fixation for these fractures.[35] Koval et al. compared a short retrograde nail, an antegrade nail, and a DCS plate in a cadaveric model.[67] They demonstrated that the antegrade nail was the least stable and recommended use of the DCS plate when maximum stiffness is desired. In a comparison of a locked intramedullary nail versus a 95-degree angled plate, David et al. also concluded that the plate provided greater stiffness.[23]

Ito et al. similarly compared the 95-degree angled plate with both the Green-Seligson-Henry (GSH) and the AO supracondylar nail and concluded that the nails were inferior in torsion and varus loading.[54] With respect to specific nail comparison, Voor et al. compared fatigue testing on 5- and 12-hole supracondylar nails and found better fatigue strength in 5-hole nails because of fewer stress risers and therefore recommended their use.[125] More recently, biomechanical comparisons of modern retrograde nails have even been reported.[52] Using both an osteoporotic synthetic bone model and human cadaveric femora, Muckley et al. investigated three intramedullary nails differing in their distal interlock mechanism plus one angular stable plate under torsional and axial loading. The four-screw (two oblique and two lateral to medial with medial nuts) construct was found to have the highest torsional strength and stiffness, the highest axial stiffness, and the highest number of axial cycles to failure in both synthetic and human bone models.[84] The authors routinely use long retrograde nails when treating these fractures. Long nails allow the fit in the femoral diaphysis to assist with proximal fixation and alignment and avoid the need for interlocking screws in the femoral diaphysis; instead, locking screws are inserted more proximally in the femur than short retrograde nails. The authors currently have no indication for short retrograde nails.

Plates. Plate insertion requires knowledge of femoral condylar anatomy in the coronal, sagittal, and axial planes. Although most distal femoral or supracondylar plates are anatomically designed,

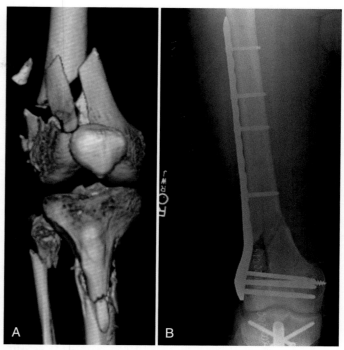

FIG 108.6 (A) Preoperative three-dimensional reconstruction of comminuted distal femur fracture and (B) postoperative radiograph after treatment with lateral locked plate.

they still require correct placement to achieve anatomically aligned reduction. The need for double plating and intramedullary plating for medially comminuted fractures has essentially been eliminated with the advent of locked plating.[73,129,140] The locked plate has replaced the traditional condylar plate and, to a large extent, the condylar screw and blade plate (Fig. 108.6A and B).§ Locked plating has shown equivalent clinical outcomes compared to the traditional condylar screw, with lower risk of early implant loosening.[58] Four locked screws distally have been shown to be equivalent in fixation to the standard blade of a 95-degree blade plate.[66] The locked plates can be inserted percutaneously, thus allowing easier insertion and enhanced stability, especially in comminuted fractures of the medial and lateral columns.[129] The locked plate must be correctly placed on the distal end of the femur to allow precise placement of the locked screws, because the angle of screw insertion is not variable and the screws will lock into the plate only at the predetermined angle. Once correct plate location is achieved in the AP and lateral views, the appropriate femoral length and alignment must be restored before proximal plate fixation.[59,136] As with intramedullary nailing, flexion or extension deformities can occur and are often difficult to assess intraoperatively if an external locking handle of the plate partially obstructs a fluoroscopic image.[70] Provisional fixation of the plate both distally and proximally is encouraged to avoid extensive revision of screw or plate placement, should adjustments be necessary. If the plate is fixed distally first, a small amount of anterior or posterior plate angulation will translate into an increasing amount of plate–shaft mismatch as one progresses proximally. Therefore, a flexion or extension deformity will result as one reduces the plate to the shaft. To

§References 69, 70, 73, 97, 107, and 114.

avoid extensive intraoperative revision, a single initial locked screw can be inserted distally without seating the head to allow rotational freedom of the plate. Once appropriate length is restored through gentle manual traction or the use of a femoral distractor, the plate can be fixed proximally to the shaft. The distal screw is then seated and locked to achieve rotational control. If adjustments are required, distal screw revision is simplified because only a single screw needs to be removed. The surgeon must be extremely vigilant to avoid plate malposition or fracture malalignment, typically valgus of the distal fragment.

Plate fixation of the distal femur with a condylar screw, angled blade plate, or lateral condylar buttress plate is a well-established procedure described in detail elsewhere.[||] Fixation of intra-articular distal femoral fractures with a DCS plate has been compared with nonoperative treatment in elderly patients and has been shown to result in fewer malunions, fewer nonunions, and a decrease in complications such as respiratory infection, deep vein thrombosis, and pressure sores.[16] In a series of 116 type C distal femur fractures treated by a single surgeon with a mean follow-up period of 11 years, patients treated with dynamic condylar screw fixation had a significantly higher rate of good to excellent results compared to condylar buttress and condylar blade plates (96% to 84% to 71%, respectively). Dynamic condylar screw fixation also showed significantly lower rates of pseudarthrosis, varus deformity, and knee stiffness.[94] Other forms of plate fixation have also provided satisfactory results.[¶] Wenzl documented the first series of supracondylar femoral fractures stabilized with the angled blade plate and reported 73.5% good to excellent results.[130] Blade plate fixation has recently been shown to have equivalent International Knee Score and final anatomic axis values compared to condylar screw plates, intramedullary nails, and locked condylar plates.[124] Indirect reduction, pioneered by Mast et al.,[77] has changed fracture fixation techniques and continues to evolve. The lateral condylar buttress plate and angled blade plate combined with indirect reduction techniques have provided 84% to 87% good to excellent results in treating supracondylar femoral fracture with intra-articular comminution.[13,92] It has been shown that malunion and nonunion are often the result of bone loss, severe osteoporosis, and/or medial column comminution.[2,27] Because of medial comminution, osteoporosis, and/or bone loss, double plating, intramedullary plating, bone grafting, and the use of bone cement are some of the techniques described to add additional medial stability and avoid varus collapse or fixation failure.[#]

The locked plated construct, even in osteoporotic bone, has been shown to provide enhanced stability while requiring less additional fixation and bone grafting (Fig. 108.7A-F).[**] Locked plating has evolved as an extension of indirect reduction techniques, and results initially appeared to be better than those of traditional techniques.[††] Weight and Collinge reported on 22 patients with unstable distal femoral fractures (AO/OTA types A2, A3, C2, and C3) stabilized with percutaneous locked plating and documented a 100% union rate.[129] All fractures healed without the need for bone grafting, and no hardware failures were noted. Average knee range of motion was 5 to 114 degrees.

[||]References 1, 13, 79, 92, 100, 110, 121, and 130.
[¶]References 1, 13, 65, 79, 92, and 130.
[#]References 10, 27, 44, 56, 77, 78, 101, 118, and 126.
[**]References 7, 30, 18, 26, 32, 40, 65, 75, 114, 129, and 140.
[††]References 31, 69, 70, 93, 107, and 129.

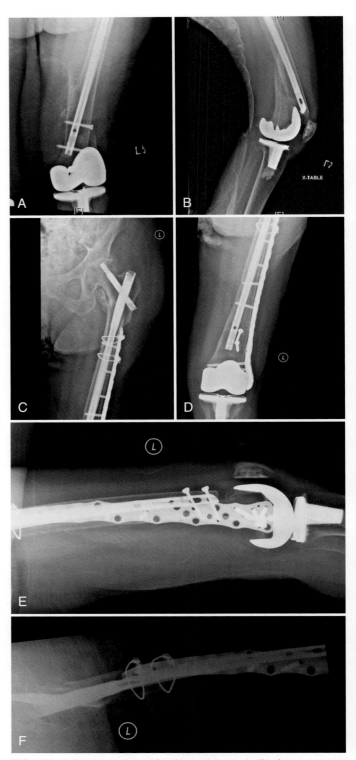

FIG 108.7 Preoperative AP (A) and lateral (B) femur x-rays demonstrating an interprosthetic distal femur fracture in osteoporotic bone. Six-month postoperative radiographs (C-F) after being treated with lag screw fixation and a distal femoral neutralization locking plate demonstrating fracture union with a persistent anterior cortical defect that occurred at the time of injury. The patient is pain free and ambulating with a walker at her most recent follow-up.

Kregor et al. documented similar results in 103 distal femoral fractures stabilized with percutaneous locked plating.[70] They reported a 93% union rate after the initial procedure and average knee motion of 1 to 109 degrees. Only 1 of 68 closed fractures required later bone grafting, whereas 6 of 35 open fractures needed later bone grafting (because of bone loss) to eventually achieve union in all fractures. Of importance was the fact that no fracture sustained loss of distal fixation. Pascarella et al. reported an 87% union rate at a mean time of 16.3 weeks in 77 distal femur fractures.[93] Schutz et al. reported early healing in 37 of 40 patients treated with locked percutaneous plating of the distal femur.[107] Ehlinger et al. recently reported similar positive results of 87% early bony union within 12 weeks postoperatively in 76 patients.[31] Both of these studies, however, reported an overall 20% incidence of a 5-degree deformity in either the frontal or sagittal plane.

These impressive early results have been tempered by recent evidence that locked plating still carries a moderate risk of complication. Although locked plating provides documented advantages, it must be used properly to avoid the increased risk of nonunion because of its increased construct stiffness that can vary widely between different plate systems.[14,106] For instance, Lujan et al. showed that the more flexible titanium plates showed 76% and 71% more callus formation at 6 and 12 weeks postoperatively compared to stainless steel plates.[74] More recent data have shown a higher nonunion rate than earlier studies, from 0% to 32% found in one recent systemic review.[47] Hoffmann et al. reported worse clinical outcomes than in prior studies. This group reported an 18% nonunion rate in 111 distal femur fractures with an improved nonunion rate in fractures treated with submuscular plating (10%) compared to open reduction (32%).[50]

Several studies published since the introduction of locked plating of distal femurs have sought to identify the risk factors for treatment failure. A biomechanical study using osteoporotic cadaveric femurs and 13-hole distal femur locking plates tested the construct stiffness in four groups (all locked, all unlocked, proximal unlocked, and distal unlocked). Only a distal unlocked screw placed nearest the fracture gap had a significant effect on torsional and failure stiffness and therefore dictated working length stiffness.[21] Radiographic posterior cortical continuity at the time of fixation in comminuted fractures treated with locked plating has been shown to be predictive of avoiding the need for secondary bone grafting.[7] Imaging studies support this finding, as locked plating can produce asymmetrical callus formation, with 64% more medially compared to anteriorly and posteriorly.[74] In a series of 335 distal femur fractures with 64 fractures (19%) requiring reoperation to reach union, Ricci et al. looked at both patient and technical factors that increased the rate of nonunion. They identified that smoking, diabetes, increased body mass index, and open fracture unsurprisingly increased nonunion risk. Shorter plate length, however, was a technical factor that increased nonunion risk and was the one variable over which the surgeon had control.[96] Another series of 285 distal femur fractures showed similar results, with the exception of stainless steel plates over titanium being an additional prognostic risk factor of nonunion.[98]

COMPLICATIONS

Complications of nonoperative treatment include skin breakdown from casting, stiffness from prolonged immobilization, malunion, and nonunion. Skin breakdown often occurs in patients who are bedridden and may not be surgical candidates. Stiffness remains the most common complication following intra-articular distal femur fractures.[95] Patello-femoral arthrofibrosis and patella baja are especially problematic with open fractures. Knee stiffness is seen more frequently in nonoperatively treated patients than in operatively stabilized patients because early motion will occur through the fracture site and therefore lengthier immobilization is required. Malunion is also more common with closed treatment because achieving fracture stability is more difficult without internal fixation (Fig. 108.8A and B).[16] Although nonunion can also occur, some bedridden

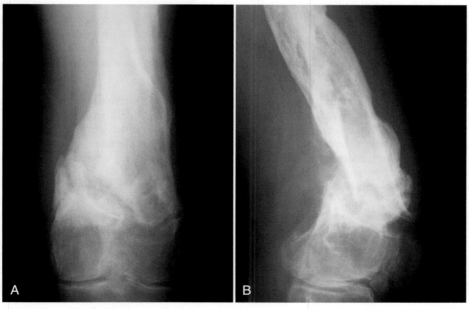

FIG 108.8 (A and B) Radiographs showing malunion of a supracondylar femoral fracture treated 12 years earlier by skeletal traction.

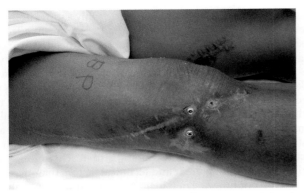

FIG 108.9 Clinical photograph revealing exposed hardware with active drainage from wounds.

patients fare better with nonunion than with a postoperative infection or wound complication. Other complications with conservative care include deep venous thrombosis, respiratory infection, and pressure sores.

Infection remains the most significant complication of operative treatment (Fig. 108.9). Although the infection rate was previously reported to be as high as 20%, advances in surgical technique, patient selection, and perioperative antibiotic therapy have continued to decrease infection rates to below 7%.[‡‡] Factors that contribute to increased risk for infection include open fractures, high-energy trauma, lengthy and extensive surgical dissection, and inadequate surgical stabilization.[46] Infection must always be investigated in distal femoral nonunions, even in presumed aseptic nonunions.[60] Mast and associates pioneered the technique of indirect reduction and biologic, balanced, stable internal fixation.[77] Bolhofner et al. and Ostrum and Geel applied these concepts and reported much improved results when compared with older techniques described in the literature.[13,92] More recent techniques involving percutaneous locked plating have decreased infection rates from 0% to 3%.[70,129]

Open fracture management continues to improve. The tenets of open fracture care include immediate tetanus prophylaxis and appropriate antibiotic administration followed by initial immediate surgical wound irrigation and débridement. Controversy continues regarding the number of débridement sessions required and the optimal timing of wound closure. These issues must be individualized by the surgeon and should take into account the mechanism of injury, the quality of local tissue at the time of initial surgery, and the presence or absence of any gross contamination. Once the tissues are judged to be healthy and clean, definitive wound closure should be performed. The sooner the traumatized region can resume its previous biologic environment, the sooner the healing process can occur. Ostermann et al. demonstrated decreased infection rates in open fractures when antibiotic polymethylmethacrylate beads were inserted into the fracture zone, but no prospective, randomized study has evaluated the routine use of beads in open distal femoral fractures.[91] The authors use beads routinely in high-energy open fractures with bone loss. These beads not only provide high local concentrations of antibiotics but also make subsequent bone grafting easier by reducing dead space.

Nonunion, a possible complication of any fracture, initially occurred in 10% to 19% of patients in early reports of open

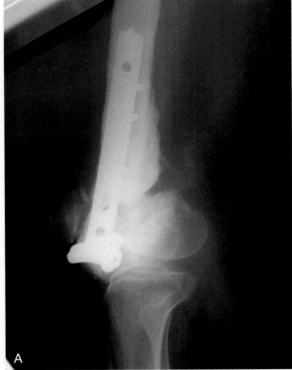

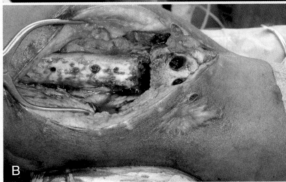

FIG 108.10 (A) Radiograph of fracture nonunion and hardware migration and (B) intraoperative photograph demonstrating fracture nonunion and enlarged screw holes secondary to loosening and bone absorption.

reduction and internal fixation of supracondylar femoral fractures (Fig. 108.10A and B).[83,88,111,137] The current literature describes a significant improvement in the nonunion rate of operatively stabilized supracondylar femoral fractures, which is now reported to be between 0% and 5%.[§§] Several studies have documented successful treatment of distal femoral nonunion with union rates of 95% to 100%.[3,28,43,128] Haidukewych et al. reported on distal femoral nonunion in 22 patients and achieved union in 21 with repeat open reduction and internal fixation and bone grafting. Achieving stable fixation of the distal fragment was critical to successful union. Autogenous bone grafting was used in the vast majority of cases. Wang and Weng documented a 100% union rate in 13 distal femoral nonunions treated with cortical strut allografting, autogenous bone

‡‡References 13, 19, 70, 88, 91, 92, 100, 111, 123, and 129.

§§References 41, 69, 70, 88, 105, 129, 130, and 137.

grafting, and internal fixation with angled blade plates and intramedullary nails.[128] Amorosa et al. documented a series of 71 distal femoral nonunions treated with a 95 degree angled blade plate. The rate of healing with 1 surgery was 91.2% (52 of 57) in aseptic nonunions and 47.6% (10 of 21) in infected nonunions.[3] Fortunately, once bony union is achieved, patients have a reasonable expectation of similar functional outcomes to those patients that achieved bony union on time.[82] As mentioned previously, distal femoral replacement is also a last ditch salvage option in patients with distal femoral nonunions and severe osteopenia.[122]

Malunion, another complication, was initially seen most commonly in fractures with significant medial comminution treated with conventional nonlocking plates. Traditional plating techniques have been associated with malunion greater than 5 degrees in the frontal plane in as many as 26% of patients.[136] Newer plating techniques with anatomically designed locked plates have also resulted in higher than expected rates of malunion greater than 5 degrees in the frontal plane, with reported malunion rates as low as 4.5% to 6% and as high as 20% in some studies.[31,69,107] Percutaneous techniques require vigilance to avoid plate malposition and fracture malalignment. As our experience with and understanding of the newer implants advances, percutaneous locked plating outcomes should continue to improve.

SUMMARY AND FUTURE DIRECTIONS

Internal fixation techniques for distal femoral fractures continue to evolve. More biologically friendly plating techniques using locked screw technology for improved mechanical performance, percutaneous plate insertion, and screw targeting for preservation of fracture vascularity have improved union rates and essentially eliminated varus collapse and decreased the need for bone grafting despite recent reports of more frequent nonunions than initially thought. Newer-generation locking plates offer polyaxial and far cortical locking screws in conjunction with fixed locking screws.[15] Such "hybrid plate" technology will offer even greater versatility in achieving maximal distal fragment fixation while potentially reducing construct stiffness for highly comminuted fractures. The role of orthobiologic agents remains undefined.

KEY REFERENCES

7. Barei DP, Beingessner DM: Open distal femur fractures treated with lateral locked implants: union, secondary bone grafting, and predictive parameters. *Orthopedics* 35:e843, 2012.

14. Bottlang M, Doornink J, Lujan TJ, et al: Effects of construct stiffness on healing of fractures stabilized with locking plates. *J Bone Joint Surg Am* 92:12, 2010.

15. Bottlang M, Fitzpatrick DC, Sheerin D, et al: Dynamic fixation of distal femur fractures using far cortical locking screws: a prospective observational study. *J Orthop Trauma* 28:181, 2014.

47. Henderson CE, Kuhl LL, Fitzpatrick DC, et al: Locking plates for distal femur fractures: is there a problem with fracture healing? *J Orthop Trauma* 25(Suppl 1):S8, 2011.

49. Hierholzer C, von Ruden C, Potzel T, et al: Outcome analysis of retrograde nailing and less invasive stabilization system in distal femoral fractures: a retrospective analysis. *Indian J Orthop* 45:243, 2011.

57. Kammerlander C, Riedmuller P, Gosch M, et al: Functional outcome and mortality in geriatric distal femoral fractures. *Injury* 43:1096, 2012.

59. Karunakar MA, Kellam JF, Zehnter MK, et al: Avoiding malunion with 95-degree fixed-angle distal femoral implants. *J Orthop Trauma* 18:443, 2004.

63. Kim JW, Oh CW, Kyung HS, et al: Factors affecting the results of distal femoral fractures treated by retrograde intramedullary nailing. *Zhongguo Xiu Fu Chong Jian Wai Ke Za Zhi* 23:1311, 2009.

70. Kregor PJ, Stannard JA, Zlowodski M, et al: Treatment of distal femur fractures using the less invasive stabilization system: surgical experience and early clinical results in 103 fractures. *J Orthop Trauma* 18:509, 2004.

74. Lujan TJ, Henderson OE, Madey SM, et al: Locked plating of distal femur fractures leads to inconsistent and symmetric callus formation. *J Orthop Trauma* 24:156, 2010.

82. Monroy A, Urruela A, Singh P, et al: Distal femur nonunion patients can expect good outcomes. *J Knee Surg* 27:83, 2014.

84. Muckley T, Wahnery D, Hoffmeier KL, et al: Internal fixation of type-C distal femoral fractures in osteoporotic bone: surgical technique. *J Bone Joint Surg Am* 93(Suppl 1):40, 2011.

89. Nork SE, Segina DN, Aflatoon K, et al: The association between supracondylar-intracondylar distal femoral fractures and coronal plane fractures. *J Bone Joint Surg Am* 87:564, 2005.

96. Ricci WM, Streubel PN, Morshed S, et al: Risk factors for failure of locked plate fixation of distal femur fractures: an analysis of 335 cases. *J Orthop Trauma* 28:83, 2014.

98. Rodriguez EK, Boulton C, Weaver MJ, et al: Predictive factors of distal femoral fracture nonunion after lateral locked plating: a retrospective multicenter case-control study of 283 fractures. *Injury* 45:554, 2014.

99. Rosen AL, Strauss E: Primary total knee arthroplasty for complex distal femur fractures in elderly patients. *Clin Orthop Relat Res* 425:101, 2004.

129. Weight M, Collinge C: Early results of the less invasive stabilization system for mechanically unstable fractures of the distal femur (AO/OTA types A2, A3, C2, and C3). *J Orthop Trauma* 18:503, 2004.

The references for this chapter can also be found on www.expertconsult.com.

109

Tibial Plateau Fractures

Adam A. Sassoon, Nathan Summers, Joshua R. Langford

Tibial plateau fractures account for 1% to 2% of all fractures but represent 8% of fractures occurring in older adults.[32] Fractures range in severity from simple to extremely complex depending on the extent of articular comminution and status of the soft tissue envelope. Classification systems have been helpful in stratifying these injuries into distinct patterns, which have guided algorithmic approaches to treatment. Furthermore, classification systems have allowed outcome studies to temper postoperative expectations related to specific fracture patterns. Key principles in the treatment of these injuries include a mandatory respect for the soft tissue envelope, restoration of a congruent articular surface, and stable fixation to promote early initiation of knee movement. Minimally invasive percutaneous osteosynthesis, a more recent advance, has promoted the accomplishment of these three objectives and is highlighted in this chapter. Technical pearls, potential pitfalls, and clinical outcomes of minimally invasive percutaneous osteosynthesis techniques are also reviewed. Additionally, the management of posttraumatic arthritis, which can often follow successful treatment of these injuries, is discussed with emphasis on specific demands this injury may place on eventual joint reconstructive efforts.

SURGICAL ANATOMY

The proximal surface of the tibia is divided between the medial and lateral plateaus, which is separated by the intercondylar tibial eminence (or spine). The lateral plateau is convex in the sagittal plane and flat to convex in the coronal plane. The medial plateau is larger than the lateral side and gently concave in both the coronal and the sagittal planes. The articular cartilage on the lateral side is slightly thicker, and in combination with its convex surface, the tibia has an approximately 3 degrees varus alignment across the joint surface, relative to the long axis of the tibia, in the frontal plane. This varus alignment correlates with the lateral distal femoral angle of 9 degrees valgus in the frontal plane. Such knowledge is extremely important during placement of screws from the lateral to the medial side of the proximal end of the tibia because the surgeon, if not cognizant of this anatomy, can easily place a subchondral lateral screw through the articular cartilage of the lower medial side.

Between the plateaus lies a nonarticular area that contains the anterior and posterior tibial spines. The anterior spine is more medial and lies just posterior to the insertion of the anterior cruciate ligament (ACL). This area is often comminuted in high-energy injuries involving the tibial plateau, and although nonarticular, it is important to restore the general width of the intercondylar eminence to appropriately restore the anatomic width of the proximal end of the tibia as a whole. In a normal knee, load is predominantly borne on the medial side. Consequently, the trabecular bone on the medial tibial condyle is stronger and more sclerotic than bone on the lateral side, perhaps explaining why lateral-sided fractures are far more common except in higher energy injuries.

The medial and lateral menisci are both semilunar, triangular-shaped fibrocartilage structures that rest between the femoral condyles and tibial plateaus. They serve an important function in load sharing by protecting the articular cartilage from up to 60% of the load encountered by the knee.[40] The lateral meniscus is larger than the medial meniscus and covers a larger percentage of the lateral plateau. The intermeniscal ligament anteriorly connects the anterior horns of the two menisci. The menisci are attached peripherally by the coronary ligaments to the rim of their respective tibial plateaus. The anterior attachment of the lateral meniscus is slightly posterior to that of the medial meniscus. The medial meniscus also supports deep attachments of the medial collateral ligament (MCL) as it overlies it. It is important to recognize the normal anatomy of these structures because they are often damaged and require repair in the management of tibial plateau fractures.

Important neurovascular structures to recognize include structures in the popliteal fossa: the tibial nerve, artery, and vein. These structures run on the lateral side of midline through the fossa, so care should be taken with any anterior to posterior directed fixation. The common peroneal nerve runs just distal to the fibular head as it moves around to the anterior compartment. High-energy tibial plateau fractures, typically Schatzker types IV through VI, are often associated with knee dislocations, so care should be taken in the neurovascular examination with a low threshold for vascular studies in these patients.[39]

MECHANISM OF INJURY

The predominant pattern producing tibial plateau fractures is a varus or valgus stress, with concomitant axial loading. This combination may be seen with low-energy injuries such as falls from a standing height or with high-energy injuries such as motor vehicle accidents. Isolated valgus or varus loading tends to cause an isolated lateral or medial injury, respectively. The more an axial load predominates, the more likely a patient is to sustain a bicondylar injury. The lateral plateau is involved in 55% to 70% of cases, with medial plateau or bicondylar involvement occurring in 10% to 30% of cases.[32] Simple central depression–type injuries are often the result of low-energy injuries in older patients with osteoporotic bone, and, conversely, bicondylar fractures with axial loading and shearing injuries tend to be seen in high-energy injuries in younger patients.

CLASSIFICATION

Comprehensive anatomic classifications such as the Arbeitsgemeinschaft für Osteosynthesefragen/Association for the Study of Internal Fixation (AO/ASIF) classification and the Orthopaedic Trauma Association (OTA) classification may be useful for research purposes (Fig. 109.1). These classification systems may be cumbersome and difficult for surgeons to use in clinical communication. The most commonly used classification system

in clinical practice is the Schatzker classification system (Fig. 109.2).[36] In the Schatzker classification system, a type I injury is a "pure" split fracture of the lateral tibial plateau. It is typically seen in young patients with strong cancellous bone, and, by definition, there is no associated articular depression. With significant displacement, it is frequently associated with a peripheral tear of the lateral meniscus. Type II fractures are combined split depression fractures of the lateral tibial plateau. Similar to a type I injury, this injury is most commonly caused by a lateral bending force combined with axial loading. Type III fractures, the most common fracture pattern in Schatzker's series (accounting for 36% of injuries), are pure depression

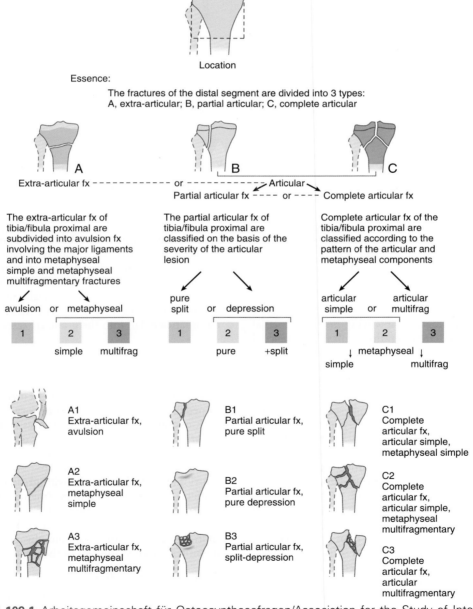

FIG 109.1 Arbeitsgemeinschaft für Osteosynthesefragen/Association for the Study of Internal Fixation (AO/ASIF) classification of tibial plateau fractures. *fx,* Fractures. (From Müller ME, et al: *The comprehensive classification of fractures of long bones,* Bern, Switzerland, 1995, ME Müller Foundation.)

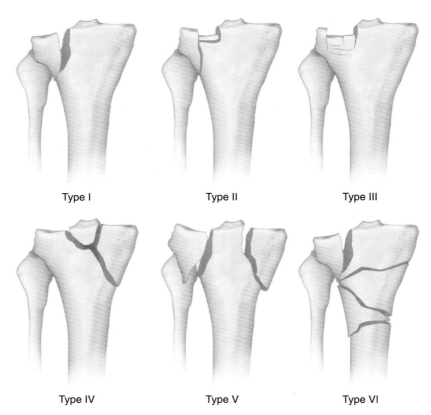

Type I   Type II   Type III

Type IV   Type V   Type VI

FIG 109.2 Schatzker classification of tibial plateau fractures.

fractures of the lateral plateau and are primarily seen in older osteoporotic individuals sustaining lower energy injuries. A type IV fracture is a fracture of the medial tibial plateau. Because the medial plateau is stronger than the lateral side, these fractures are typically secondary to higher energy injuries and have commonly associated ligamentous and soft tissue damage. Type V injuries are bicondylar fractures involving both the medial and the lateral plateaus and are often the result of a pure axial load applied while the knee is in full extension, such as may be seen in a driver pressing on the brake before impact during a motor vehicle accident. Type VI injuries are the highest energy injuries; they involve both the medial and the lateral plateaus and are associated with metaphyseal-diaphyseal dissociation. The AO/OTA and Schatzker classification systems have been associated with high intraobserver (kappa = 0.57 and 0.53, respectively) and interobserver variability (kappa = 0.41 and 0.43, respectively), but this is greatly improved if the fracture descriptors are simply divided into unicondylar versus bicondylar and pure split versus split depression.[5]

Experienced surgeons know that it is the status of the soft tissues and classification of the soft tissue envelope injury that are as important, if not more important, than the underlying osseous injury. The Tscherne classification of soft tissue damage in closed fractures is an excellent means whereby surgeons can evaluate associated soft tissue injuries.[29] A grade 0 injury results from indirect trauma and is associated with negligible soft tissue damage. A grade I injury typically results from low or moderate energy and is identified by superficial abrasions or overlying contusions. In grade II injuries, significant muscle contusion and possible deep contaminated abrasions may be

seen. Grade II injuries may be the result of a bumper strike and are often associated with marked fracture comminution. The highest grade in this classification system is grade III soft tissue injury, which is frequently associated with extensive crushing of soft tissues and subcutaneous degloving. There may be concomitant arterial injury. Patients with compartment syndrome automatically fall into the grade III category.

CLINICAL EVALUATION

History

The type of knee injury that has occurred can usually be determined from a thorough patient history. Differentiating between high-energy and low-energy injuries is important because the occurrence of a high-energy injury often alerts an experienced surgeon to look for other associated osseous injuries that may manifest in predictable patterns. Additionally, high-energy injuries are often associated with greater soft tissue injury and confer a higher risk of compartment syndrome. Patients with polytrauma may be unable to give any history at all because of a closed head injury, intubation, or other distracting injuries. A thorough tertiary survey should always be performed to avoid missing associated injuries in these patients.

Physical Examination

In a patient with polytrauma, primary advanced trauma life support survey protocols and examination to stabilize the patient should be undertaken. During the secondary survey, the entire skeleton should be examined as indicated; if a tibial plateau fracture is present, it is mandatory that the entire affected limb be examined fully. Careful circumferential inspection to rule out open fractures is mandatory, and visual inspection can reveal abrasions, contusions, or early fracture blisters that must be considered because they may markedly alter the recommended surgical management. Palpation may also reveal an effusion or hemarthrosis.

Although examination of the ligaments and menisci is of paramount importance, it is typically too painful for the patient in the acute setting and needs to be performed under anesthesia. Similarly, without the concomitant use of fluoroscopy, it is difficult to determine whether fracture or ligamentous insufficiency has led to perceived instability on physical examination. One cannot overemphasize the importance of a complete neurologic and vascular examination. Knee dislocations leading to vascular or neurologic injury in association with tibial plateau fractures have been reported to reduce spontaneously and may be missed without careful examination, especially in Schatzker types IV through VI.[39] If pulses are not equal on palpation, arteriography may be performed.[33] Use of the ankle-brachial index to compare blood pressure in the arm and ankle can help evaluate the vascular status of the limb further and should be routinely performed in patients with Schatzker types IV through VI fractures in which suspicion of knee dislocation is high. Neurologic injury, most commonly in the form of peroneal nerve palsy, is common.[36] Arduous motor and sensory evaluation of the lower part of the leg must be undertaken carefully and repeated regularly.

Careful evaluation for compartment syndrome should be performed in all patients with tibial plateau fractures. The index of suspicion should be high for Schatzker types IV, V, and VI, but compartment syndrome can also occur in simple fracture patterns associated with high-energy injury. Patients who are at risk for compartment syndrome should be monitored carefully for at least the first 24 to 48 hours after injury and for a similar period after each closed reduction or surgical intervention. If any question about compartment syndrome exists as a result of clinical evaluation, compartment pressures should be measured, and fasciotomies should be performed as indicated. In conjunction with higher Schatzker grades, other radiographic indicators have also been associated with the development of compartment syndrome including tibial widening and displacement of the femur on the tibia.[43]

Imaging

Radiographs should be obtained after all acute knee injuries. The standard knee trauma series should include anteroposterior, lateral, and patellar tangential views. Oblique radiographs can be extremely helpful in diagnosing minimally displaced fractures of the proximal end of the tibia. Alignment, the presence of bony injury, and the details of the soft tissue all should be examined on radiographs. Stress radiographs may occasionally be helpful to define the severity and stability of tibial plateau fractures and associated collateral ligament injuries better. However, stress radiographs have limited benefit because they have not been shown to increase diagnostic accuracy over examination under anesthesia or arthroscopy (or both).

Computed tomography (CT) is perhaps the most valuable test in the evaluation of traumatic knee injuries because it helps rule out the possibility of occult plateau fractures that are missed on plain radiographs. Moreover, it helps define the nature of complex intra-articular fractures. A study by Molenaars and colleagues[28] evaluating CT scans from 127 tibial plateau fractures

demonstrated four recurrent major fracture features: a lateral split fragment, seen in 75%; a posteromedial fragment, seen in 43%; a tibial tubercle fragment, seen in 16%; and a zone of comminution that included the tibial spine and frequently extended to the lateral condyle, seen in 28%.[28] Understanding these patterns aids in the surgical planning of tibial plateau fractures. However, CT is an adjuvant test that should be performed with, and not in place of, plain radiography.

Soft tissue structures such as the menisci and collateral ligaments are poorly visualized on a CT scan. Magnetic resonance imaging (MRI) is superior for determining the status of such structures. The use of MRI for the evaluation of acute knee injuries continues to improve and evolve. The sensitivity and specificity of MRI for meniscal and cruciate ligament injury are greater than 90% when correlated with arthroscopic or intraoperative findings.[11] MRI should not be used indiscriminately in place of a careful clinical evaluation, routine plain films, and CT scanning. The benefit of MRI in tibial plateau fractures lies largely in the exclusion of significant meniscal tears or ligamentous injuries in patients who would otherwise be treated nonoperatively or in a percutaneous fashion such that these injuries would then perhaps be missed. Studies in which MRI was performed on tibial plateau fractures have shown associated soft tissue injuries in greater than 45% of patients.[22] Increasing data have suggested the value of routine MRI in the preoperative evaluation of high-energy tibial plateau fractures, given a reported rate of 71% of these injuries being associated with an injury of at least a single major ligamentous structure and 53% being associated with a disruption of two ligamentous structures.[39]

Angiography

Angiography is indicated when the vascularity of the lower part of the leg is in question. Asymmetrical distal pulses or an ankle-brachial index less than 0.9 should prompt angiographic examination.[26] If a leg is obviously ischemic, although angiography may be helpful in localizing the injured area, it must not delay vascular exploration and subsequent revascularization to the point that viability of the limb would potentially be compromised. In such circumstances, "on the table" angiography performed by the vascular team in the operating room while spanning external fixation is being performed may help expedite the overall care of the patient. Prolonged ischemia, combined with muscular injury from the trauma, may cause a reperfusion compartment syndrome after perfusion is restored. Therefore, prophylactic fasciotomies are commonly performed after revascularization.

TREATMENT

Initial Management

In all tibial plateau fractures, the status of the soft tissues is of paramount importance in determining the timing of internal fixation. Complications arise from the underlying inflammatory cascade that leads to venous congestion, hypoxia, and subsequent necrosis creating the least ideal operative environment.[13,35] Patients with higher energy injuries and significant soft tissue damage should typically undergo temporizing knee-spanning external fixation until the soft tissues have recovered to a state in which a surgical incision can safely be made. Surgical incisions made through acutely traumatized tissue portend a high rate of wound dehiscence, wound infection, and

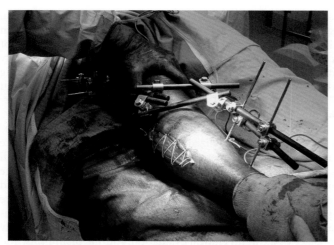

FIG 109.3 Clinical postoperative photograph taken in the operating room after a patient with a tibial plateau fracture and compartment syndrome underwent fasciotomies and spanning external fixation.

subsequent soft tissue complications. In higher energy injuries, it is common for the soft tissue envelope to take several weeks to become amenable to surgical intervention. Sometimes an experienced physician may estimate that the soft tissue envelope will not become amenable to surgical incision for more than 3 to 4 weeks. In such situations, methods other than formal internal fixation will probably need to be used. Delayed definitive internal fixation with the use of temporizing spanning external fixation (Fig. 109.3) has markedly decreased the rate of complications in this difficult patient population. Lower energy injuries, such as injuries seen after a simple fall that results in a depression fracture in an osteoporotic patient, may often be fixed relatively acutely because the associated soft tissue injury is minor. The surgeon's judgment is paramount when evaluating the character of osseous and soft tissue injuries. In general, the return of skin wrinkles and the absence of blisters indicates that the inflammatory cascade is subsiding.

Open fractures of the tibial plateau require emergency irrigation and débridement and initiation of antibiotics. Spanning external fixation is very useful in this setting. Extensions of incisions to expose and débride the fracture or fasciotomy incisions should be undertaken with consideration for the location of future incisions that will probably be needed for the reconstruction as well as future arthroplasty. General principles of open fracture management apply, and definitive internal fixation, when indicated, should be undertaken only after the soft tissue envelope permits and the wounds are deemed to be clean. Grossly contaminated wounds may require multiple débridements to achieve this end. When using temporizing external fixators, pins should be placed well away from the area of planned future incisions to avoid potential bacterial contamination and infection. We typically do not perform the definitive fixation until the soft tissues have recovered.

Nonoperative Management

Although no clear-cut guidelines have been established across all patient ages and activity levels regarding what is acceptable to treat nonoperatively, some general rules can be applied. An articular step-off of less than 3 mm or condylar widening of less than 5 mm tends to have an acceptably low rate of adverse long-term effects if treated nonoperatively. However, function deteriorates with varus tilt, whereas mild valgus tilt up to 5 degrees is generally well tolerated.[18] Nonoperative management would be poorly advised if a tibial plateau fracture were associated with varus or valgus instability in a fully extended knee joint. Age alone is not an absolute contraindication to surgical management because older patients do well functionally with proper treatment.[20] However, surgeons must use their judgment about the expectations, functional demands, medical comorbid conditions, and surgical risks of the specific patient being treated when making a decision regarding the most appropriate intervention. The goal of nonoperative treatment is still to allow early range of motion to include full extension and 120 degrees of flexion. Permanent knee stiffness develops if fractures treated nonoperatively are immobilized for longer than 6 weeks.[12] Nonoperative management can include a period of traction or casting or both, focusing on quadriceps activation and edema control, followed by early range of motion in a cast brace or functional brace. Cast brace treatment of minimally displaced unicondylar fractures tends to yield good results, but outcomes are far less predictable with bicondylar fractures.[8] In general, nonoperative treatment is typically reserved for stable, well-aligned, minimally displaced fractures or fractures in patients with prohibitive medical comorbidity.

Operative Management

General Principles. The keys to successful operative treatment of tibial plateau fracture are respecting the soft tissues, anatomic restoration of the articular surface, and stable fixation to allow for early knee motion. Incision selection should be deliberate and based on the fracture pattern, a detailed description of which is outlined here. Consideration should also be given to the potential need for eventual arthroplasty when selecting an incision location but not at the expense of the primary aforementioned objectives of treatment. Submeniscal arthrotomies are routinely performed for articular visualization and to ensure that the meniscus is not trapped in the fracture site. This practice is supported in that intraoperative fluoroscopy has not been deemed reliable in detecting articular step-offs smaller than 5 mm[15] and by a 30% coincidence of meniscal injuries in the setting of plateau fractures.[38] Furthermore, a transition away from bulky, large fragment plates (screws ≥4.5 mm), which may irritate the surrounding soft tissue envelope, to small fragment constructs is underway, with data indicating equivalent mechanical performance.[42]

Schatzker Type I Injuries. A displaced wedge or split fracture of the lateral plateau is unstable and, in most cases, is an absolute indication for open reduction and internal fixation. In general, reduction may be achieved by applying a varus force manually or by using a laterally based femoral distractor, or reduction may be performed with the use of a large King-Tong clamp or pelvic-type reduction forceps placed percutaneously through small stab incisions (Fig. 109.4). Clamps that are curved may be beneficial in protecting the soft tissues around the anterior face of the tibia from becoming crushed during compression of the fracture. If compression of the fracture site appears to be difficult in that the fracture seems to require significant force to close down completely, the lateral meniscus may be incarcerated in this fracture fragment, and arthroscopic or open removal of the meniscus from the fracture site must be undertaken. It is

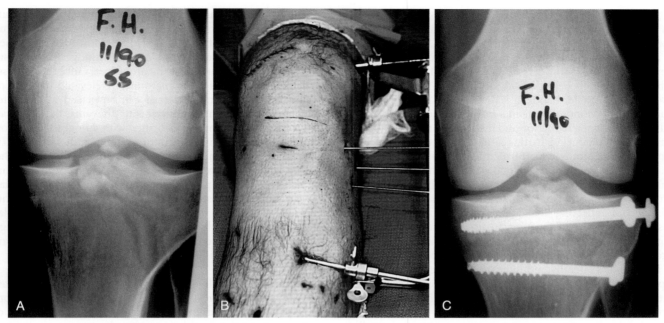

FIG 109.4 Schatzker type I tibial plateau fracture in a 30-year-old man who fell from a ladder. (A) Preoperative anteroposterior radiograph. (B) Intraoperative photograph showing a femoral distractor being used to obtain indirect reduction, with guide wires for the cannulated screws in place. (C) Postoperative anteroposterior radiograph showing anatomic reduction of the tibial plateau.

possible to place so much force on the reduction forceps that the meniscus will simply be crushed within the trabecular bone and the fracture will appear reduced under fluoroscopy. If the split does not close down easily, a mini-open, arthroscopic, or formal open reduction is indicated. Fixation is typically accomplished with two or three large cannulated screws inserted percutaneously. As with all fractures, the screws should be placed perpendicular to the major fracture lines to achieve compression of the fracture without displacing it when the screws are tightened.[23,25] In general, two to three solitary lag screws are adequate for fixation,[24] although an antiglide plate or a buttress plate may be necessary in patients with poor bone quality, especially in the face of a vertically oriented condylar fracture. A gentle varus-valgus stress under real-time fluoroscopy can help determine whether screw fixation alone is adequate. If instability is noted and the screws toggle, buttress plate fixation is indicated. In general, a lag screw–only approach suffices in younger patients with excellent bone quality, whereas supplementing with a buttress plate in patients with poor bone quality is common.

Schatzker Type II Injuries. Schatzker type II injuries are more difficult to treat than type I injuries because of the associated joint depression and, at times, more severe instability than seen with a simple split fracture of the lateral condyle (Fig. 109.5). Minimally invasive techniques such as arthroscopically assisted fixation are rarely indicated but sometimes may be feasible when the lateral cortical disruption is nondisplaced or minimally displaced and the peripheral rim of cortical bone laterally is functionally competent. In this situation, arthroscopically assisted reduction of the joint surface can be performed. The arthroscope is placed in the joint, and a hole is drilled in the medial face of the tibia through a stab incision in a location that

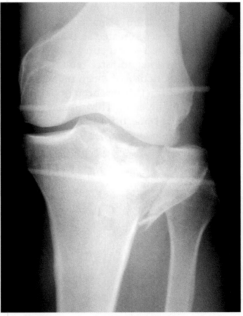

FIG 109.5 Anteroposterior radiograph of a patient with a Schatzker type II tibial plateau fracture.

allows curved or straight bone tamps to reach the area of the depressed lateral plateau. An ACL drill guide may be helpful to position the drill precisely. Bone graft or a bone graft substitute can then be impacted or injected through the tunnel from the medial aspect of the tibia to beneath the area of reduced subchondral bone. The arthroscope can assist in determining when appropriate reduction has been achieved. Over-reduction by 0.5

to 1 mm may be beneficial because subsidence occurs in most cases despite the best efforts of the surgeon. Injectable bioresorbable cement may help alleviate this problem, but long-term data are not yet available. After articular reduction has been achieved, multiple 3.5-mm screws may be placed just under the subchondral bone to help prevent settling and fracture of the lateral condyle. Smaller diameter screws can be placed in close proximity to subchondral bone in a rafting fashion. More commonly, however, open reduction and internal fixation is required for most type II injuries. In this situation, a straight, lateral, parapatellar arthrotomy is performed to allow improved visualization of the joint line. The lateral aspect of the joint may be visualized through a submeniscal approach or by splitting the intermeniscal and anterior coronary ligaments of the lateral meniscus and reflecting the lateral meniscus posteriorly to expose the lateral side of the joint. In almost all cases, a plate is required, and the distal aspect of the lateral parapatellar arthrotomy at the lateral aspect of the tibial tubercle can typically be extended laterally and inferiorly to dissect the anterior compartment muscles extraperiosteally from the proximal end of the tibia and allow placement of a traditional or percutaneous plate.

For simpler fracture patterns requiring a plate, a laterally based submeniscal approach may be adequate (Fig. 109.6). It is important to not strip all the musculature from the lateral condylar fragment, but rather to strip only what is required to allow placement of the plate. The fracture itself acts as access to the subchondral and posterior regions of the lateral plateau in that reduction and grafting can be performed through a fracture line that has been booked open. A femoral distractor and lamina spreader are often helpful for visualizing the joint space and allowing enough space to be created so that the depressed joint line can be elevated without competing with the lateral femoral condyle. Flexion of the knee to force femoral rollback posteriorly also assists with reduction of the joint, especially anteriorly and centrally. After the fracture has been booked open, the joint line is reduced with an impactor. The impactor is used to scrape metaphyseal cancellous bone from beneath the articular fragments so that the articular fragments are reduced indirectly with this metaphyseal cancellous bone. Placing the impactor

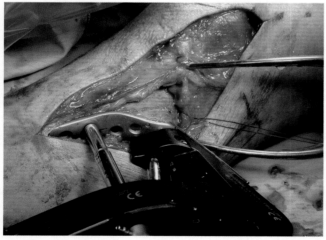

FIG 109.6 Intraoperative clinical photograph of a lateral submeniscal exposure with placement of a lateral submuscular plate.

directly on subchondral bone, although tempting, can often lead to complete cracking of incompletely cracked articular cartilage as a result of overzealous force. Additionally, this metaphyseal cancellous bone makes excellent autograft for the subchondral grafting portion of the procedure. Once the depressed articular surface has been anatomically elevated under direct vision, additional graft material can be placed in the defect, which typically remains inferior to the area that has been reduced. Grafting can be performed with autograft but is commonly performed with allograft or a bone graft substitute (see later discussion). The split condyle is then reduced and held with a large reduction clamp. Fixation of the condyles should be achieved with a periarticular buttress plate. Locked plates have advantages in osteoporotic bone but are reserved for more unstable bicondylar injuries that require more coronal plane stability. The use of locked plates should be selective owing to the added cost and no proven difference in outcomes compared with nonlocked plating of simple fractures.[1]

Schatzker Type III Injuries. Type III fractures of the lateral plateau are pure depression fractures usually found in osteoporotic patients after sustaining a valgus stress; however, they can occur as a result of athletic trauma in younger individuals. Valgus instability of more than 5 to 8 degrees in a patient without significant preexisting arthritis is typically an indication for surgical intervention.

Treatment of this injury is usually performed with arthroscopic or fluoroscopic assistance in a percutaneous fashion (Figs. 109.7 to 109.11). The arthroscope is placed in the joint as previously described for type II injuries. A cortical window is made distally on the medial or lateral face of the metadiaphysis to allow percutaneous bone tamps to be placed through a tunnel to reduce the depressed fracture fragments under arthroscopic visualization. The location of this window can best be determined by the location of the depression needing to be accessed, which is best determined with a CT scan. Very anterior depressions are usually best managed through a medial corticotomy, whereas posterolateral depressions are often best managed from the distal aspect of the lateral tibial metaphysis. An ACL drill guide can be used to place the tunnel more accurately. After the tunnel is completely packed with graft, screws are placed across the joint just under subchondral bone to prevent collapse of the elevated joint surface. If there is any question of reduction, a small vertical osteotomy of the anterior tibial cortex may be performed just lateral to the tibial tubercle in an open fashion. This osteotomy combined with a submeniscal arthrotomy can turn a type III injury into a type II injury.

Schatzker Type IV Injuries. Nonoperative management of type IV injuries has been associated with a high incidence of varus malunion and is indicated only for nondisplaced stable injuries.[9,10] It is crucial to remember that these fractures are often associated with disruption of the lateral collateral ligament complex and should often be thought of as fracture-dislocation variants of knee dislocations. Therefore, neurovascular examination is of the utmost importance (see earlier discussion). The magnitude of the soft tissue injuries associated with medial plateau fractures portends the higher complication rates and the poorer prognosis, more so than the osseous injury itself.

A more recent cohort study has indicated that compared with type II injuries, isolated type IV injuries are more

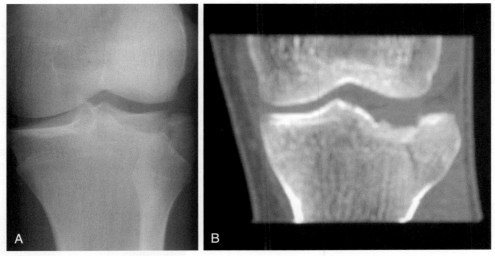

FIG 109.7 (A and B) Preoperative two-dimensional coronal reconstruction of a Schatzker type III tibial plateau fracture amenable to percutaneous treatment.

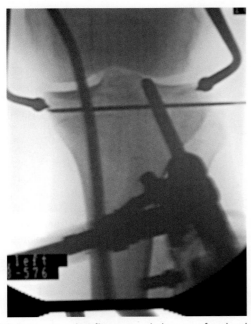

FIG 109.8 Intraoperative fluoroscopic image of reduction of the cortical rim and placement of the arthroscope.

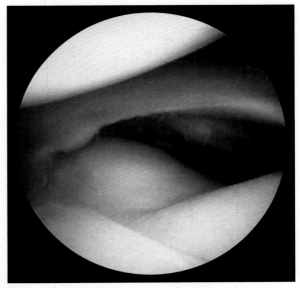

FIG 109.9 Intra-articular view through the arthroscope of the articular depression present before reduction of the articular surface.

commonly associated with low-energy injuries, less initial articular depression, and better functional outcomes.[14] However, because these fractures are typically displaced and comminuted to some degree, open reduction and internal fixation is generally the preferred method of treatment. Additionally, the importance of delaying definitive open reduction and internal fixation in the face of a high-energy fracture should be noted. Temporizing spanning external fixation until the soft tissue envelope has recovered adequately is recommended to minimize complications.

In general, definitive surgery is carried out through a medial parapatellar arthrotomy; after adequate reduction, fixation is achieved with a plate and screws. The plate is typically placed medially, and exposure of an isolated medial condylar fracture requires elevation of the pes anserinus and the superficial MCL in an extraperiosteal fashion. Some authors have advocated placing the plate superficial to this complex; fixation can occasionally be performed in such a manner if the condylar split is near the location of the incision and the entire exposure can be accomplished by booking open the fracture. Placing the plate outside the superficial MCL complex helps preserve the vascularity to the area of the fracture but also, in theory, may lead to increased wound healing complications because the flap that is created is subcutaneous in nature (Figs. 109.12 and 109.13). It may also lead to an increased rate of symptomatic hardware, requiring later removal.

In the rare situation of an isolated posteromedial fracture fragment, a posteromedial incision may be adequate for reduction and fixation. The complexity of the posteromedial fragment as determined by CT scan best establishes whether a single medially based plate would be adequate. A posteromedial fragment that is separate and displaced from the medial condyle proper may require a second posteromedial incision and placement of a posteromedial buttress plate to prevent displacement and subsidence of the posteromedial fragment, which can lead to posterior subluxation of the medial femoral condyle, subsequent instability, and poor results.[23] Biomechanical data indicate that both 10-mm and 20-mm posteromedial fragments were displaced with simulated non–weight-bearing, range-of-motion exercises, indicating the importance of fixation of these seemingly stable fragments.[6]

Schatzker Type V and VI Injuries. Types V and VI fractures are bicondylar tibial plateau fractures, with type VI injury being distinguished by metadiaphyseal dissociation and, often, shaft extension (Figs. 109.14 and 109.15). These injuries should always be considered high-energy injuries, and immediate definitive internal fixation is generally contraindicated. Temporizing spanning external fixation as well as fasciotomies when indicated for compartment syndrome is typically the mainstay of initial treatment (see Fig. 109.3). Occasionally, these bicondylar fractures can be fracture-dislocation variants. In this case, the ability to maintain a reduced joint in spanning external fixation can be very challenging (Fig. 109.16). If there is any question, a simple percutaneous 6.5-mm cannulated screw can be used to temporarily hold the condyles together while in the

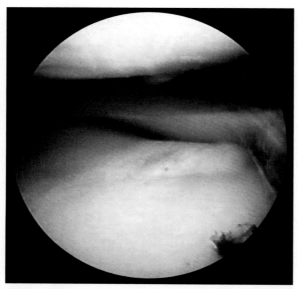

FIG 109.10 Intra-articular view through the arthroscope of the articular surface after reduction.

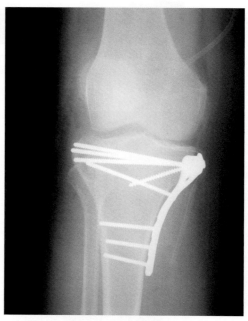

FIG 109.12 Anteroposterior radiograph after open reduction and internal fixation of a Schatzker type IV tibial plateau fracture with a medial buttress plate.

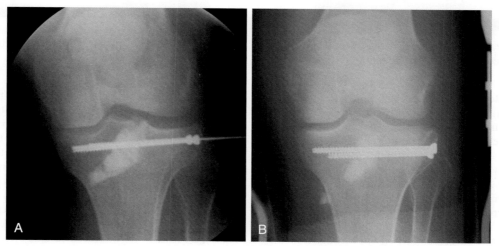

FIG 109.11 (A) Intraoperative anteroposterior radiograph of reduction achieved through a metaphyseal tunnel that was back-filled with calcium sulfate cement. (B) Anteroposterior radiograph of the same patient 6 weeks after surgery showing resorption of calcium sulfate cement.

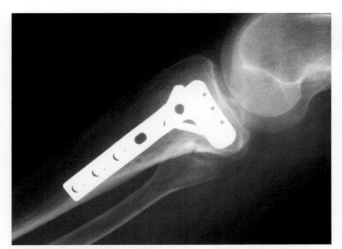

FIG 109.13 Lateral radiograph after open reduction and internal fixation of a Schatzker type IV tibial plateau fracture with a medial buttress plate.

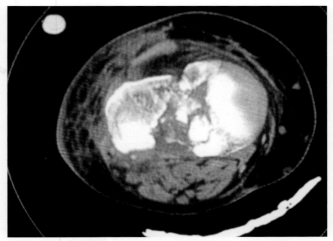

FIG 109.15 Axial computed tomography scan of a Schatzker type VI tibial plateau fracture showing a split of the condyles and comminution in the region of the tibial spines.

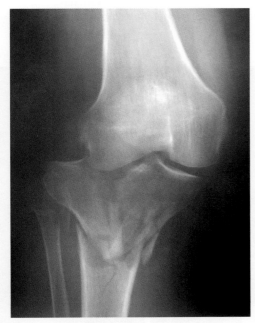

FIG 109.14 Anteroposterior radiograph of a Schatzker type VI tibial plateau fracture.

spanning fixator (Fig. 109.17). This temporary screw is removed when definitive fixation is carried out.

Definitive internal fixation should be carried out only when the soft tissue envelope has recovered to the point at which such fixation is safe and reasonable. This is typically 7 to 10 days after injury but can be up to 3 weeks after injury in more severe injuries. It is prudent to wait until skin wrinkles return and all blistered areas have been epithelialized.

The use of a single anterior incision for definitive fixation has largely been abandoned because of the inherent wound complications from raising large lateral and medial flaps. At the present time, the workhorse for severe bicondylar fractures is a two-incision technique popularized by Barei and colleagues.[3] This technique allows for less total soft tissue dissection and

precise placement of plates through approaches that are familiar to the surgeon for treatment of type II and type IV injuries.

Traditionally, plating both condyles had been required for most of these bicondylar injuries. However, if the medial condylar component is large and relatively simple, a laterally based locked plate may be adequate for maintenance of medial reduction (Fig. 109.18). Early data have been encouraging; however, long-term data on the ability of laterally based locked plates to maintain reduction of the medial side are still unavailable.[22] More recent biomechanical data have also shown that smaller 3.5-mm locking constructs are able to withstand similar loads as their 4.5-mm counterparts along with the advantage of a more low-profile design.[17,42] Locked screws in a plate prevent screw toggle and can prevent varus collapse of coronally unstable fractures without the need for adjuvant medial plating. This concept depends on a medial condylar fragment of sufficient size to be able to be controlled with laterally inserted screws. The biologic advantage of avoiding double plating and the inevitable soft tissue dissection necessary for double plating is intuitive. Gentle varus-valgus stress testing under real-time fluoroscopy can assist the surgeon in deciding whether a lateral locking plate is sufficient fixation.

If double plating through a traditional midline approach is to be performed, it is recommended that the medial plate be placed superficial to the superficial MCL and pes anserinus to prevent what has become known as the "dead bone sandwich," which results from stripping of both the lateral and the medial aspects of the tibial metaphysis (Figs. 109.19 and 109.20).

In general, the use of CT scans to evaluate the complexity of the medial condylar component can help determine whether a lateral locked plate will suffice or whether a medial plate will be necessary. Typically, the more complexity (or higher degree of comminution) observed in the medial fracture, the more likely that a medial plate will be needed. For the posteromedial fragment, a posteromedial approach and plating are necessary for adequate stability. As noted previously, even "seemingly stable" posteromedial fragments may require a separate approach and plate to prevent displacement during postoperative knee flexion.[6] In general, if the medial split is sagittal and the fragment is large, a lateral locked plate will suffice. Another approach

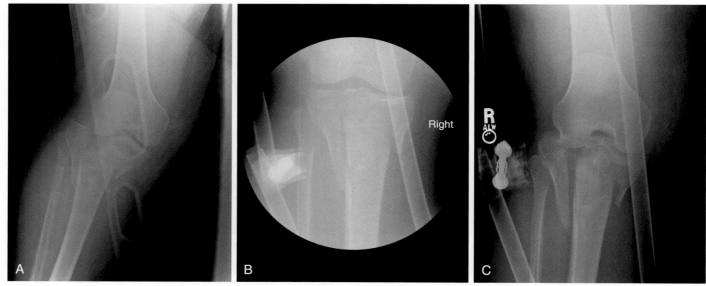

FIG 109.16 (A) Schatzker type VI tibial plateau fracture, which is also a fracture-dislocation variant. (B) The knee was reduced after external fixator application, (C) but on follow-up examination was found to be dislocated within the frame secondary to metaphyseal widening, which the fixator is unable to adequately control.

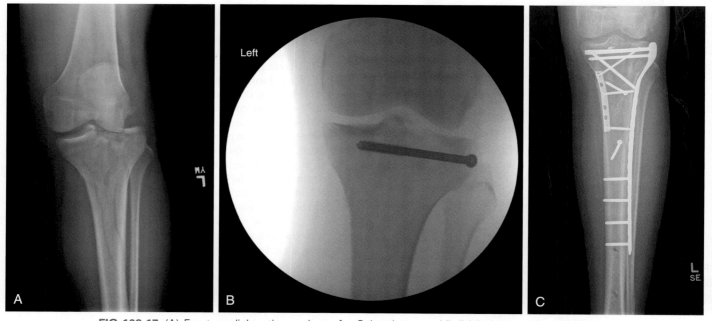

FIG 109.17 (A) Fracture-dislocation variant of a Schatzker type VI tibial plateau injury. (B) Initial treatment consisted of a spanning fixator with placement of a single 6.5-mm cannulated screw to help maintain the knee in a reduced position by preventing gradual widening of the tibial metaphysis. (C) The screw was then reduced when staged definitive fixation was performed, as dictated by soft tissue "readiness."

to these more "simple" type VI fractures that are minimally comminuted, with sagittally directed fracture lines, involves the use of multiple rafting screws and the placement of an intramedullary nail to stabilize the metadiaphyseal dissociation (Fig. 109.21). In cases in which the medial plateau split is coronal or the fragment is highly comminuted, a two-incision, two-plate strategy is preferred.

In patients whose soft tissue envelope is not amenable to formal open reduction and internal fixation within 14 to 21 days or in patients with a markedly comminuted metaphysis and minimal involvement of the articular surfaces, hybrid or fine wire external fixation may be the best option (Fig. 109.22). Multiple percutaneous screws can be placed to lag large fragments at the joint and fine wires, or half-pins can be placed

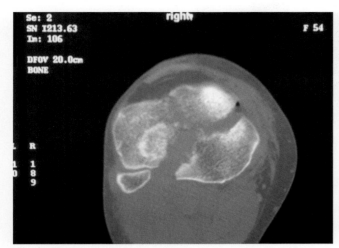

FIG 109.18 Axial CT scan showing a large posteromedial fracture fragment in a Schatzker type VI tibial plateau fracture.

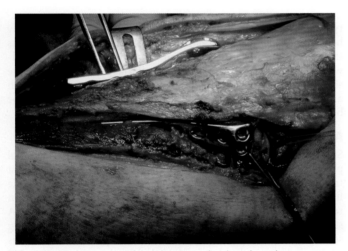

FIG 109.19 Intraoperative photograph showing the exposure for double plating through a midline incision. The medial plate should be placed superficial to the superficial medial collateral ligament.

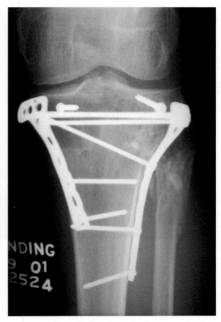

FIG 109.20 Anteroposterior radiograph showing double plating in the same patient shown in Fig. 109.19.

postoperative Western Ontario and McMaster Universities Osteoarthritis Index score was 70, the mean 36-Item Short Form Health Survey (SF-36) physical score was 40, and the mean SF-36 mental score was 47. There were no differences between patients treated with plating or Taylor Spacial Frame. All patients in this study achieved union; however, of the 54 patients treated with operative fixation, 5 (9%) patients had a displacement of greater than 4 mm, including 3 patients (5%) with an articular displacement of greater than 4 mm with a metadiaphyseal angulation of 75 degrees.

Open Fractures. Open fractures of the tibial plateau require emergency irrigation and débridement following immediate administration of intravenous antibiotics and tetanus vaccination when needed. Spanning external fixation is very useful after débridement. Extensions of incisions to expose and débride the fracture or fasciotomy incisions (or both) should be undertaken with consideration for the location of future incisions that will likely be needed for the reconstruction. General principles of open fracture management apply, and definitive internal fixation, when indicated, should be undertaken only when the soft tissue envelope permits and the wounds are deemed to be clean. Grossly contaminated wounds may require multiple débridements to achieve this end. When using temporizing external fixators, pins should be placed well away from the area of planned future incisions to avoid potential bacterial contamination and infection. Definitive fixation should be delayed until the soft tissues have recovered. Additionally, ring fixators, usually combined with joint-holding lag screws, can be used for definitive fixation in these instances and are an excellent choice when the soft tissue envelope is severely compromised.

Bone Grafting and Orthobiologic Agents

Injectable resorbable cement has become popular especially for the percutaneous injection of contained defects in periarticular areas. In 2004, Watson[41] reported a series of eight comminuted

proximally to achieve adequate proximal fixation. Wires and half-pins should be placed at least 15 mm distal to the joint line to prevent penetration of the synovial capsular reflections leading to intra-articular hardware and possible septic arthritis.[7] Olive wires can be helpful for achieving and maintaining reduction. Additionally, external fixation can be used definitively for patients with extensive metadiaphyseal comminution, especially patients with associated significant soft tissue injury (Fig. 109.23).

An additional fragment that requires recognition and fixation is the tibial tubercle fragment. Retrospective data indicate that the incidence of tibial tubercle fractures in the setting of bicondylar tibial plateau fractures is approximately 20%.[27] Fixation of this fragment is imperative to allow for extensor mechanism continuity and early range of motion. Fixation is most commonly accomplished with screws alone or a plate and screws.

Outcomes after treatment of bicondylar tibial plateau fractures with either locked plating or a circular external fixator with 1-year follow-up have been reported.[2] The mean

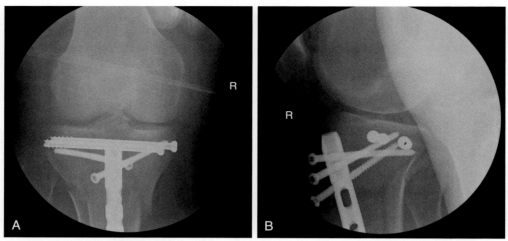

FIG 109.21 Intraoperative anteroposterior (A) and lateral (B) fluoroscopy views demonstrating fixation of a type VI tibial plateau fracture with a tibial nail in conjunction with rafting screws.

tibial plateau or tibial pilon fractures treated with calcium sulfate injectable cement. Although one fracture with a large defect required additional grafting, the other seven fractures healed. At 3 months, greater than 90% of the graft was resorbed radiographically. The same technique has been used for distal radius fractures to assist with stability by percutaneous grafting after closed reduction or external fixation.

Russell and colleagues and others have reported similar findings in prospective randomized trials, even showing calcium phosphate cement to be superior to autograft impaction for subchondral support in tibial plateau fractures.[31] Such agents avoid donor site morbidity associated with autografts and risk of disease transmission associated with allografts. However, simple defects can be managed effectively with allograft croutons.

More recently, structural bone allograft has been gaining favor in the support of bone defects associated with tibial plateau fractures. Berkes and colleagues[4] retrospectively studied the use of Plexur, a composite of nondemineralized bone and resorbable polymers, and fibular strut allografts in the treatment of Schatzker type II fractures and noted no subsidence greater than 2 mm in 77 cases. Sassoon and associates[33] demonstrated success with the use of fibular allograft strut grafting in the treatment of 11 cases of posterolateral depression. The rationale cited for this technique was that traditional locking plates do not often adequately support the posterolateral portion of the tibial plateau. At final follow-up, the mean depression of the posterolateral joint surface was noted to be 0.8 mm. Only one patient demonstrated greater than 3 mm of progressive joint depression.

COMPLICATIONS

Infection

Deep infections in tibial plateau fractures often result from surgical procedures performed through tenuous soft tissue envelopes, with subsequent poor wound healing and bacterial colonization. Superficial wound infections that occur early should be aggressively treated with antibiotics, and surgeons should have a low threshold for surgical débridement. Deep infections may also require irrigation and débridement with arthrotomy and irrigation of the knee joint. Stable implants are typically retained if the fracture has not yet united, and it may be beneficial, when an organism has been isolated, to suppress the infection with antibiotics until union has occurred. Hardware can subsequently be removed as indicated. Loose hardware should be removed. Consultation and co-management with an infectious disease specialist and plastic surgeon may be beneficial.

Arthrofibrosis

Stiffness is one of the most common complications after tibial plateau fractures, especially in more severe injuries. The best treatment is prevention, which can be achieved through stable fixation and early range of motion. Early range of motion requires that the surgeon obtain fixation as stable as possible. A study indicated that the incidence of arthrofibrosis requiring secondary treatment after fixation of tibial plateau fractures is 14.5%.[16] This study also indicated that time in an external fixator before definitive fixation was directly related to the risk of developing arthrofibrosis.[16] Additionally, it demonstrated that the use of a continuous passive motion machine after plateau fixation conferred a protective effect and decreased the incidence of arthrofibrosis.[16] Closed manipulation under anesthesia for posttraumatic arthrofibrosis of the knee has been found to be successful and a low risk for fracture displacement in a series of 22 patients, improving the mean range of motion arc from 59 degrees to 110 degrees at final follow-up.[34] This study failed to find a difference in patients who received manipulation within 90 days of definitive fixation and patients who received manipulation after this 90-day window. This time-independent efficacy has not been universally observed.[16]

Posttraumatic Arthrosis

The articular cartilage and meniscal damage that occur at the time of tibial plateau fracture predispose the joint to arthrosis, often regardless of the adequacy of the reduction. Honkonen[19] reported that 44% of patients had arthrosis at a mean of 7.6 years after injury. In patients who underwent total meniscectomy on the affected plateau, this percentage increased to 74%. However, it is difficult to determine whether it was the meniscectomy or perhaps the increased magnitude of the injury causing the meniscal pathology that led to this change.

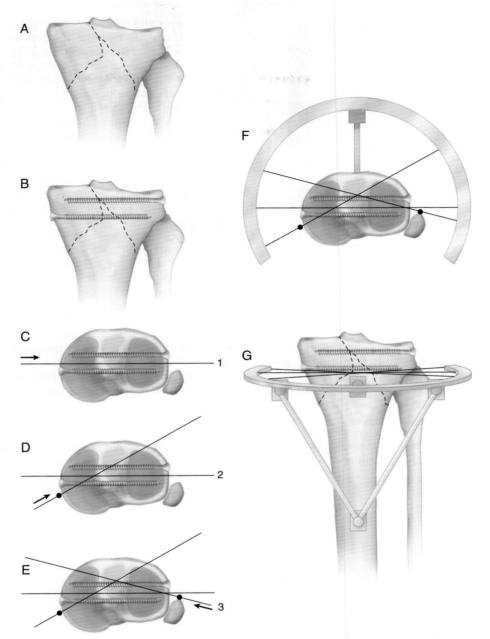

FIG 109.22 Technique for reduction and fixation of a Schatzker type V tibial plateau fracture with cannulated screws and a hybrid external fixator. (A) Reduction is obtained via open or closed methods and held with a reduction clamp. (B) Cannulated screws are placed to hold the articular reduction. (C) A smooth guide wire for the external fixator is placed in the coronal plane, at least 14 mm distal to the joint line. (D) The second wire, with a bead or olive, is passed posteromedially to anterolaterally. (E) A third wire, also beaded, is passed posterolaterally to anteromedially. (F) The wires are appropriately tensioned and fixed to the ring. An optional half-pin can be placed from the anterior to the posterior aspect and attached to the ring for increased stability. (G) Half-pins are inserted into the tibial shaft, and the distal pins are connected to the ring with the appropriate clamps and bars.

The best prognosis was seen in patients with normal or slight valgus limb alignment and an intact meniscus on the affected side. However, many studies have found little correlation between radiographic arthrosis and clinical symptoms.[25,30] Corrective osteotomy, total knee arthroplasty, unicompartmental

arthroplasty, and arthrodesis are potentially viable options for management of symptomatic posttraumatic arthritis that is refractory to conservative management. Decision making is based on the underlying pathology, patient age, and activity. It is important to counsel patients in whom this treatment avenue

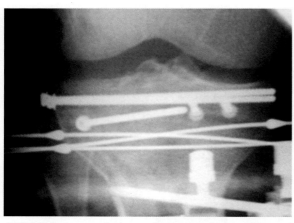

FIG 109.23 Anteroposterior radiograph of a patient with a Schatzker type VI tibial plateau fracture. Extensive metaphyseal comminution and a simple articular fracture are seen. A fine wire fixator and lag screw fixation at the subchondral region were used in this patient because of significant soft tissue injury.

is required because total knee arthroplasties after posttraumatic arthrosis have a higher rate of revision, infection, stiffness, poor wound healing, and other postoperative complications.[21,37] A full discussion of reconstructive options in the setting of post-traumatic arthrosis is beyond the scope of this chapter.

Nonunion

Nonunion of tibial plateau fractures is relatively rare given their metaphyseal location. Nonunion is typically associated with open fractures or higher energy injuries with significant soft tissue damage and typically occurs at the metadiaphyseal junction of bicondylar fractures. In patients who appear to be acutely at risk for nonunion secondary to significant bone loss or a poor soft tissue envelope, bone grafting can be performed at the time of the index definitive procedure, if feasible. However, if healing appears to be delayed in the postoperative course, early bone grafting should be performed. If nonunion has led to fixation failure, revision of this fixation is typically indicated. In some cases, arthroplasty may be a better option. In all cases of nonunion, it is of paramount importance that an infection be ruled out because it can often derail further attempts to treat the nonunion and could be catastrophic if left undiagnosed before an arthroplasty.

CONCLUSION

Tibial plateau fractures are severe injuries that continue to pose a significant challenge to even the most highly trained orthopedic traumatologists. To the frustration of many surgeons, the injuries sustained by the cartilage may cause the development of arthrosis, even when a seemingly perfect postoperative radiograph is obtained. Minimally invasive treatment modalities and locked plating technologies have continued to evolve, and these advances as well as the development of improved bone graft substitutes and structural bone grafting techniques that minimize articular loss of reduction may translate into improvements in outcome. Recognition of the importance of the soft tissue envelope in higher energy injuries and understanding the use of temporizing external fixation before definitive internal fixation have markedly reduced the complication rate in the management of these injuries.

The references for this chapter can also be found on www.expertconsult.com.

110

Fractures of the Patella

Frank A. Liporace, Joshua R. Langford, Richard S. Yoon, George J. Haidukewych

INTRODUCTION

Patella fractures constitute approximately 1% of all bony injuries with traffic accidents and falls being the most common causes.[17] Fractures have also been associated with excessive extensor mechanism contraction, total knee arthroplasty, post-anterior cruciate ligament (ACL) reconstruction, postsurgical stabilization, chronic disease (eg, gout), and severe squatting with weightlifting. Because of its subcutaneous location and the significant joint reactive forces to which it is subjected, the patella is prone to injury.[2,58,76,85,115] Posttraumatic complications include knee stiffness, extensor mechanism weakness, and symptomatic arthritis. A growing body of literature has helped us better understand the extensor mechanism and allowed us to apply various fixation strategies for reliable results.[80] However, despite these advances, outcomes are less than ideal.[61,80] Even so, the goals of treatment remain constant: reconstitution of the extensor mechanism and restoration of articular congruity.

ANATOMY

The patella lies deep to the fascia lata and tendinous rectus femoris, making it the largest sesamoid bone in the body.[98] Its distal-most aspect is termed the *apex* while its proximal end is known as the *basis*.[98] There are seven facets separated by a major and minor vertical ridge with two transverse ridges traversing the major vertical ridge (Fig. 110.1).[98]

The patella's ossification center most commonly presents between 3 and 5 years of age. As this center enlarges, it may be associated with multiple accessory ossification centers, most commonly superolateral bipartite patella.[90] These accessory ossification centers usually have a nonossified cartilaginous connection to the central ossification center.

The Wiberg classification and the Baumgartl modification have been used to classify the patella. Type I has equal medial and lateral facets and progressive types have smaller medial facets finally leading to no medial facet, also known as the Jaegerhut patella.[8,126] Proximally the undersurface of the patella is covered with the thickest articular cartilage in the body while the distal 25% is devoid of articular cartilage.[30]

The four muscles of the extensor mechanism (rectus femoris, vastus medialis, vastus lateralis, and vastus intermedius), the fascia lata, patella tendon, and the retinaculum of the knee all attach to the patella (Fig. 110.2). The rectus femoris is most superficial and central with its fibers running approximately 7 to 10 degrees medial relative to the femur. The vastus medialis has two portions: the longus, with a proximal attachment to the patella, and the obliquus, with a distal attachment to the patella).

These portions attach to the patella at angles of approximately 15 and 50 degrees, respectively. The vastus lateralis attaches proximally on the patella at an angle of approximately 30 degrees. Laterally it fuses with the iliotibial band and the lateral retinaculum. The vastus intermedius is the deepest portion of the quadriceps and attaches directly superior into the patella. The retinaculum of the knee is composed of the overlying fascia lata anteriorly, which blends with the vastus medialis and lateralis and with the capsule. The patella tendon is the terminal soft tissue extension of the extensor mechanism that inserts into the tibial tubercle. It is approximately 5 cm long and is formed by central fibers of the rectus femoris, fascial expansions of the iliotibial band, and patella retinaculum.[17,66,98] Thickenings of the capsule connect the patella to the femoral epicondyles and aid in appropriate tracking with the medial patellofemoral ligament contributing 53% to the lateral stability of the patella.[29]

The blood supply of the patella is composed of the peripatellar plexus, which is derived from six separate arteries (Fig. 110.3). The supreme geniculate artery is derived from the superficial femoral artery at the adductor canal. The four geniculate arteries (superolateral, superomedial, inferolateral, and inferomedial arteries) are derived from the popliteal artery. Finally, the recurrent anterior tibial artery is derived from a branch of the anterior tibial artery at the interosseous membrane.[7,103] The net functional blood supply of the patella is from distal to proximal (Fig. 110.4).[111]

BIOMECHANICS

From full flexion to 45 degrees, the load is shared between the patella and the tendinous portion of the extensor mechanism. At less than 45 degrees of flexion, the only component of the extensor mechanism in contact with the distal femur is the patella. The patella causes an increase in the moment arm of the extensor mechanism by displacing it anteriorly from the knee's center of rotation (Fig. 110.5). This increases the force of the extensor mechanism by up to 50%. The terminal 15 degrees of extension require twice the torque required to extend the knee from full flexion to 15 degrees.[57,66] Thus, the patella functions as a pulley. With total patellectomy, numerous studies have documented up to a 50% decrease in isokinetic strength testing of the extensor mechanism.[95,117,123]

Because of the small area of contact at the patellofemoral articulation, the undersurface of the patella is subjected to some of the highest joint reactive forces in the body, up to 7.6 times body weight, even though the overall tibiofemoral forces are greater.[45,99]

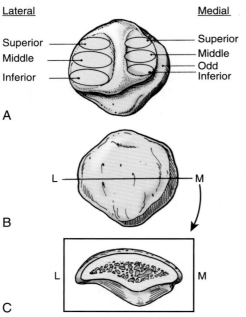

Lateral   Medial

A

B

C

FIG 110.1 (A) The seven patellar facets. (B) The anterior surface. (C) Cross-section of a Wiberg II patella. (From Scuderi G: *The patella,* New York, 1995, Springer-Verlag.)

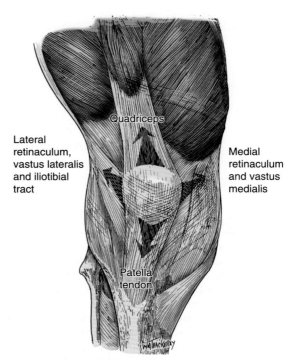

FIG 110.2 The patella is anchored and stabilized to the knee by four structures in a cruciform fashion: the patellar tendon inferiorly, the quadriceps tendon superiorly, and the retinaculum medially and laterally.

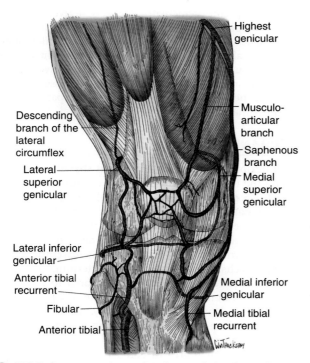

FIG 110.3 Anastomosis at the front of the knee formed by genicular branches from the popliteal artery and descending branches, which connect the femoral artery proximally with the popliteal and anterior tibial arteries distally.

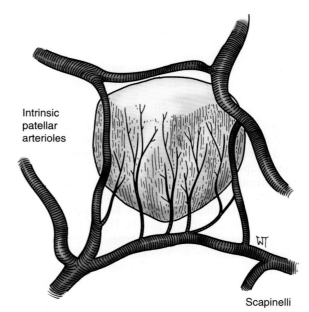

FIG 110.4 Vascular circle around the patella, which, according to Scapinelli,[103] supplies the patella by nutrient arteries that enter predominantly at the inferior pole. The genicular arteries and their branches lie in the most superficial layer of the deep fascia.

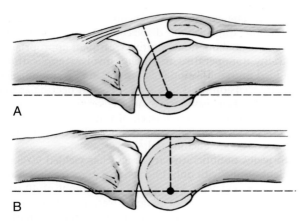

FIG 110.5 In (A), the patella increases the effective moment arm. In (B), after patellectomy, the moment arm is decreased, thereby diminishing extensor force. (From Sanders R: Patella fractures and extensor mechanism injuries. In Browner B [ed]: *Skeletal trauma,* Philadelphia, 1992, WB Saunders.)

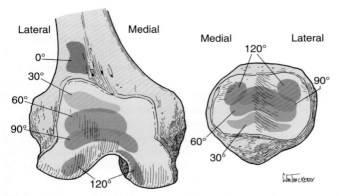

FIG 110.6 Patellofemoral contact zones. (From Aglietti P, Insall JN, Walker PS, et al: A new patella prosthesis. *Clin Orthop Relat Res* 107:175, 1975.)

At any point within the knee's range of motion, a maximum of 13% to 38% of contact of the patella occurs with the femur.[75] Throughout flexion, the area of patellofemoral contact changes. At 20 degrees of flexion, the patella centers within the trochlea groove. As greater angles of flexion are achieved, the area of contact moves proximally on the patella's undersurface and distally on the trochlea (Fig. 110.6).[39]

DIAGNOSIS

History and Physical

Usually the patient will describe a fall or direct blow to the anterior knee that represents direct forces. Indirect forces may be represented by a severe eccentric contraction resulting in a transverse patella fracture. This may occur in the flexed knee with severe quadriceps contraction that literally results in the patella and the retinaculum being torn transversely. Historically, classification systems involved stratifying injury patterns according to their mechanism.[15,17,70] Frequently, injuries are present that represent a combination of direct and indirect forces.

The patient often presents with pain, a large effusion, inability to walk, and inability to straight leg raise or extend the bent knee. It is important to examine for other associated injuries that may be present in high-energy trauma. Also, the quality of the surrounding soft tissues is important when evaluating and treating any patient with an orthopedic injury. If a suspicion of a traumatic arthrotomy or open patella fracture exists, diagnostic injection may help in making the diagnosis. Also, sterile local anesthetic injection following needle aspiration of hematoma may allow for more accurate physical examination. A persistent inability to actively extend the knee implies a concomitant injury to the medial and lateral quadriceps expansions.[17,108]

Diagnostic Studies

Plain radiographs may be useful in determining the type and degree of patella injury. In subtle extensor mechanism injuries, computed tomography (CT) or magnetic resonance imaging (MRI) may prove helpful. The standard plain radiographic series for evaluating the patella include an anteroposterior (AP) view, lateral view, and tangential view of the patellofemoral joint. Using large cassettes (14 × 17 inches) can help evaluate concomitant ipsilateral knee injuries.

The AP view should evaluate the position of the patella relative to the femoral sulcus and the relation of the distal pole of the patella to the distal femoral condyles. At times, the presence of an accessory ossification center (eg, bipartite patella) may be confused for a fracture. Frequently, a bipartite patella is bilateral and at the superolateral aspect of the patella. Usually, a bipartite patella is asymptomatic and does not affect extensor mechanism function. Contralateral radiographs may be useful in confirming this diagnosis.[78] It is rare to have a unilateral bipartite patella. This often represents an old marginal patella fracture.[32] Some recent reports in the literature have documented cases of painful bipartite patella after injury. These have been treated either nonoperatively, with excision, or with lateral release.[23,51,82,91]

Lateral radiographs help define displacement and articular step-off in patella fractures and help in identifying avulsion fractures of the tibial tubercle. These views should be acquired with 30 degrees of knee flexion to allow calculation of the patella's height relative to the long bones of the knee. The Insall-Salvati ratio—the length of the patella tendon compared to the length of the patella—can be calculated. (The distal pole should be at a level tangential to the Blumensaat line—distal physeal scar.) An Insall-Salvati ratio of approximately 1.0 is normal, greater than 1.2 indicates patella alta, and less than 0.8 indicates patella baja.[49,54,100] Some authors have criticized this method since there can be variability of patella shape, which would impact classification of the patella height.[41,54] Alternatively, the Blackburne-Peel index (ratio of the distance from the tibial plateau to the inferior articular surface of the patella to the length of the patella articular surface) can be calculated. Normally, this is approximately 0.8 with a value of greater than 1.0 indicating patella alta.[12,13,107]

The tangential view (Merchant view) is taken with the patient supine and passive positioning of the limb at 45 degrees of flexion.[81] This view may help define vertical fractures, osteochondral fractures, or marginal fractures (Fig. 110.7).

CT has been used to identify stress fractures, especially in patients with osteopenia and hemarthrosis.[5] CT scans have been shown to have a 71% detection rate of these fractures as opposed to a 30% detection rate with bone scans in the setting of negative plain radiographs.[5] With patella pathology, bone scans *with*

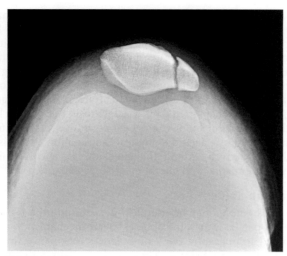

FIG 110.7 Merchant view clearly demonstrates a displaced longitudinal fracture.

indium-labeled leukocytes or gallium scanning may be helpful in evaluating patella osteomyelitis, tumors, and ischemia, however, with the advances in imaging modalities, this scan has largely fallen out of favor[1,35,37,55] CT scans may also be employed to evaluate cases of nonunion, malunion, and patellofemoral alignment disorders.

MRI has been used in evaluation of quadriceps tendon injury, patella tendon injury, and post-patella dislocation. With tendon rupture, the normal low-intensity signal of the tendon will be interrupted with the tendon edges obscured.[128] Even after relocation of a dislocated patella, a set of concomitant injuries is often present (contusion of the lateral femoral condyle, tear of the medial retinaculum, and a joint effusion).[122] In such cases, the use of MRI to diagnose concomitant osteomyelitis and tumors can be extremely helpful.

CLASSIFICATION

No specific classification system has been effective in determining outcomes based on degree of displacement, fracture pattern, or proposed mechanism of injury. Therefore, long-term results have been most commonly associated with the type of treatment.* Reasons for selecting operative treatment have included fractures with a fracture gap greater than 3 mm, articular incongruity greater than 2 mm, and extensor mechanism dysfunction.[15,17,78,108]

Evaluation of the fracture according to its pattern (transverse, vertical, stellate, apical, marginal, osteochondral), the patient's functional capacity, and the surrounding soft tissue envelope provide the surgeon with the most helpful information when determining appropriate treatment (Fig. 110.8).

NONOPERATIVE TREATMENT

Nonoperative treatment is traditionally chosen when there is a lack of significant displacement or articular incongruity and the extensor mechanism is confluent after careful physical examination. The extensor mechanism forces are also perpendicular to the direction of displacement in vertical patella fractures, thus making nonoperative treatment appropriate.

Typically, nonoperative treatment involves application of well-padded immobilization (cast, splint, knee immobilizer) in nearly full extension for 4 to 6 weeks. Weight bearing as tolerated is permitted and isometric quadriceps exercises and straight leg raises are begun within 1 week of injury.[17,19,42] When consolidation is evident on follow-up radiographs, active range-of-motion exercises are encouraged.

Historically, nonoperative treatment has yielded 90% good to excellent results with only 1% having a poor result.[17] A more modern series reviewing nonoperative treatment of 40 patella fractures found that 80% of patients were pain free and 90% had a full knee range of motion at an average follow-up of 30.5 months.[19] The importance of timely, controlled physical therapy is imperative to avoid arthrofibrosis and patella infera.[73] One case report describes patella infera following nonoperative treatment; this case required a tibial tubercle osteotomy that yielded only partial correction and resulted in symptomatic recurrence.[83]

OPERATIVE TREATMENT

Operative intervention has been indicated in patella fractures that are open, with a fracture gap greater than 3 mm, articular incongruity greater than 2 mm, or extensor mechanism dysfunction.[15,17,78,108,119] The goals are to provide adequate reduction with stable fixation while preserving a viable soft tissue envelope to allow early rehabilitation and uneventful healing.

Surgical intervention involves internal fixation, external fixation, or patellectomy (partial or complete). The patient is placed supine with a small bolster under the ipsilateral buttock to allow the patella to face directly anteriorly. A nonsterile tourniquet is applied to the proximal aspect of the ipsilateral thigh. Esmarch exsanguination and tourniquet inflation is conducted just prior to incision unless a grossly contaminated open injury is present. Prior to inflation, the quadriceps mechanism must be pulled distally either manually or with knee flexion.

If the surrounding soft tissue allows, a midline vertical incision extending from well above the proximal pole of the patella to the tibial tubercle will provide adequate exposure while not limiting reoperation in the area. Full-thickness subcutaneous flaps can be made to the mid-axis, both medially and laterally, to expose and assess the entire extensor retinaculum.

Alternatively, a transverse incision can be used in cases of transverse fractures to allow limited soft tissue stripping and provide a cosmetic result.[70,84] Prior to choosing this approach, careful consideration must be made of the potential for subsequent procedures.

In young patients with severely comminuted fractures, good bone quality, and an intact soft tissue envelope, an extensile exposure through a tibial tubercle osteotomy has also been described. After a midline longitudinal incision through skin and subcutaneous tissue, a lateral parapatellar incision is made. The tibial tubercle is predrilled and tapped for eventual large fragment screw fixation. Then it is osteotomized 1.5 cm deep to a healthy bed of dense cancellous bone.[11] Six patients with an average of 31-months of follow-up had four good, one fair, and one poor result with this technique. Clinical union of the osteotomy occurred at an average of 8 weeks with clinical union of the patella at an average of 11 weeks.[11]

*References 15, 17, 18, 70, 79, 89, 93, 110, and 130.

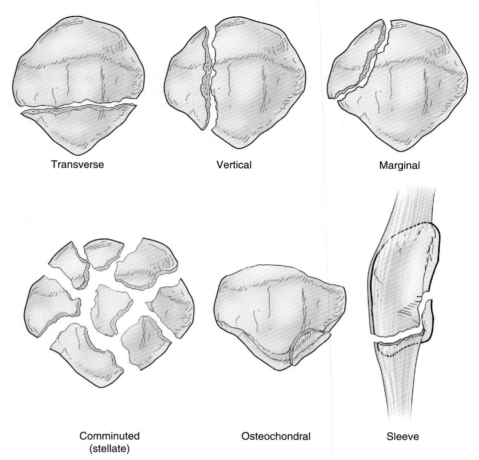

Transverse   Vertical   Marginal

Comminuted   Osteochondral   Sleeve
(stellate)

FIG 110.8 Classification of patellar fractures based on fracture configuration. (Redrawn from Cramer K, Moed B: Patellar fractures: contemporary approach to treatment. *J Am Acad Orthop Surg* 5:323, 1997.)

After the surgical approach, the following steps should be followed. In the case of open fractures, all foreign material and nonviable tissue should be débrided and followed by copious lavage. Careful assessment of the entire extensor mechanism is necessary to avoid neglecting tendinous or retinacular injuries. Evaluation of the distal femoral condyles should also be conducted. Bone fragments that lack soft tissue attachments and are too comminuted for fixation should be removed. Prior to fixation, articular reduction should be attained, including reduction of impacted fragments. Provisional reduction with Kirschner wires, large pointed bone reduction forceps, and patella forceps should be attained prior to definitive fixation. Throughout the procedure, reduction should be assessed via palpation through a retinacular defect, surgical arthrotomy, and orthogonal fluoroscopy, both to the patella and the knee joint itself.

Internal Fixation

Original wiring techniques used circumferential cerclage wires, or wires passed through drill holes were used and were followed by 4 to 6 weeks of cast immobilization. These techniques did not incorporate tension band principles. Results were often suboptimal because of the inability to start early motion, lack of articular compression, and lack of stable fixation.[14,17,106]

In the 1950s the tension band concept was popularized by the Arbeitsgemeinschaft fürOsteosynthesefragen/Orthopaedic Trauma Association (AO/OTA) group. Two 18-gauge stainless steel wires are used. One is placed through the quadriceps and patella tendons in a figure-of-eight configuration anterior to the patella, while the other is placed in a cerclage fashion around the patella.[84] Weber showed that these techniques improved results and were stable enough to allow early range of motion.[125] Modifications to this technique have evolved. The addition of two parallel longitudinal Kirschner wires placed through the patella can prevent toggling of fragments (Figs. 110.9 and 110.10). The Kirschner wires may be placed retrograde through the transverse component of the main proximal and distal fragments and then advanced antegrade once reduction has been attained. The proximal end of the Kirschner wires are bent into a "hook" that is impacted over the tension band wire into the proximal pole of the patella. To be effective, the figure-of-eight tension band wire must be free of slack and come in contact with the posterior aspect of the Kirschner wires and the bone both proximally and distally (Fig. 110.11).

More recently, horizontal wiring versus standard vertical wiring in tension banding was evaluated biomechanically. With this method, the K-wires are inserted in standard fashion, but the figure eight created by the wire around the K-wires lies horizontally versus its classical vertical position. In biomechanical testing, permanent fracture displacement was 67% lower with a horizontal orientation than with the standard vertical orientation.[52]

Lotke et al. described a modified technique for transverse patella fractures called longitudinal anterior band plus cerclage wiring (LABC). Two vertical holes separated by a 1-cm bone bridge are drilled longitudinally with a Beath-Steinmann pin through the reduced patella. A single wire is threaded on the pins and drawn through the patella. The midportion of the wire is folded over the anterior surface of the patella while one end of the wire is passed through this loop and tied. If necessary, a supplementary cerclage wire can be added (Figs. 110.12 and 110.13).[70] In the original series of 16 patients, 13 were asymptomatic while 3 noted some discomfort with stairs or prolonged

activity. All patients had greater than 90 degrees of motion within 6 weeks of the procedure.[70]

When comparing four wiring techniques, circumferential wiring, tension band cerclage, cerclage over Kirschner wires, and LABC, the latter two showed the most stable fixation with displacements of less than 1 mm when subjected to a 90-degree arc of knee motion.[21] This enforces the importance of the tension band principle combined with transosseous fixation.

Braided cable has been proposed as an alternative to the monofilament wire loop.[105] A retrospective review of 51 patella fractures treated with tension band wiring and early motion had a 22% rate of displacement greater than 2 mm in the early postoperative period when monofilament wire was used.[113] It is speculated that the braided cable acts as a wire rope, allowing it conform better to bone surfaces and not kink. Also, its ends are secured with a crimp sleeve that cannot unravel like a twisted monofilament wire knot. In a biomechanical comparison of transverse patella fractures treated by a modified tension loop with either monofilament or braided wire of equal diameter (1.0 mm), the specimens fixed with braided wire had approximately one-third the displacement of those fixed with monofilament wire after cyclical loading.[105]

In an effort to avoid the reported 30% to 50% need for removal of hardware in these fractures,[47,48,88] alternative fixation with suture has been investigated. A biomechanical study compared tension band and LABC fixation of transverse patella fractures with either 1.25-mm (18-gauge) stainless steel wire or braided polyester suture (No. 5 Ethibond). Through a 90-degree arc of knee motion, no significant difference in failure or fracture gapping was appreciated after 1000 cycles.[94] In a similar dynamic model that involved 2000 cycles per specimen, similar results were acquired when using a modified tension band technique.[77] Tensile testing of each material showed that polyester was 75% as strong, but this did not impact dynamic testing.[77]

Clinically, suture fixation has been shown to be adequate. A clinical review of seven patients treated with a modified tension band of No. 5 Ti-cron suture had 100% union with good

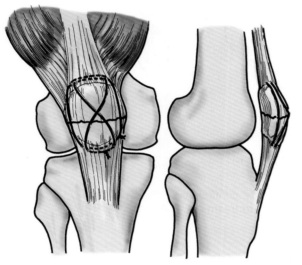

FIG 110.9 Tension cerclage of patellar fractures.

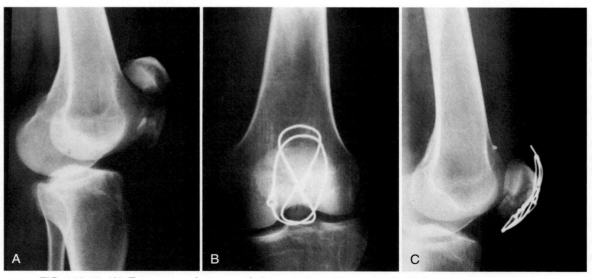

FIG 110.10 (A) Transverse fracture of the patella with some distal fragment comminution. (B and C) Treatment by tension band cerclage with two wires; after 1 month, the fracture showed good healing, with a little step on the articular surface.

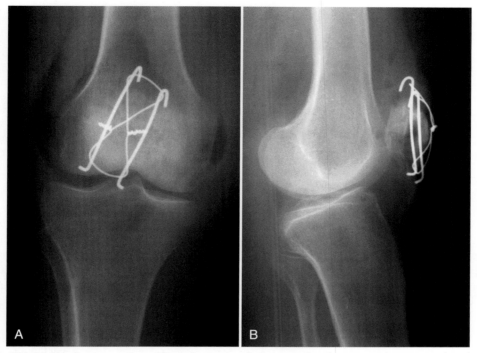

FIG 110.11 (A) Postoperative AP radiograph of the patella demonstrating a tension band construct. (B) Postoperative lateral radiograph of the patella demonstrating a tension band construct.

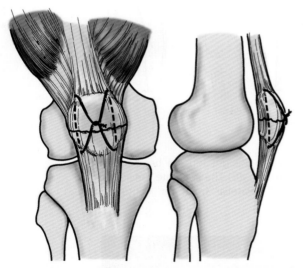

FIG 110.12 Internal fixation of a transverse fracture of the patella according to the method of Lotke and Ecker.

restoration of knee function.[26] In a pediatric case report, No. 1 PDS absorbable suture was used and the patient was allowed range of motion in 2 weeks with uneventful healing and full, asymptomatic function by 1 year.[116] The authors attributed the accelerated healing without displacement after such early range of motion to the fact that pediatric patients have accelerated healing potential compared to adults.[116] A recent biomechanical study using braided suture with a special knot configuration has also shown that knot configuration helps decrease displacement with cyclical loading.[46]

A randomized clinical trial compared the modified tension band technique in 18 patients using biodegradable implants (polyglycolide [PGA] or poly-L-lactide [PLLA] plugs with polyester ligament) to 20 patients using stainless steel fixation.[27] All fractures healed within a mean time of 8 weeks. At an average 2-year follow-up, 72% of patients treated with biodegradable implants had a good result compared to 75% in the metallic group. There were no clinical or radiographic differences between the groups.[25,27]

An alternative to the modified tension band technique replaces the two Kirschner wires with cannulated screws.[10] Screws alone may be used in vertical fracture patterns, in fractures with a simple transverse component in patients with good bone quality, or to fix multiple fragments to create two main fragments that can be addressed with any of the techniques mentioned in this chapter. Cannulated screws may be inserted antegrade or retrograde with the wire tension band loop inserted through the screws. It is important to have the distal aspect of the screw recessed deep to the bony margin. If the screw is prominent, fretting of the wire at the wire-screw interface can result in fixation failure. Also, if one end of the wire is against the screw head and the other end is around the distal aspect of the screw, not against bone, additional compression of fragments cannot be achieved and the tension band is ineffective through range of motion (Figs. 110.14 and 110.15). In a biomechanical study comparing screws with the tension band to screws alone or with a modified tension band with Kirschner wires, the screws with tension band failed at significantly higher loads than the other two techniques. Although screws alone were more stable than the modified tension band with Kirschner wires, this was not statistically significant.[25] A clinical study evaluating 10 patients (3 smokers and 7 with severe osteopenia) with patella fractures treated with cannulated screws and wire

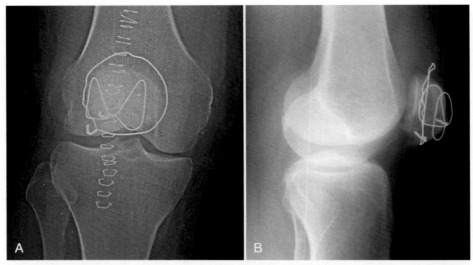

FIG 110.13 (A) Postoperative AP radiograph of the patella demonstrating longitudinal anterior band plus cerclage wiring (LABC). (B) Postoperative lateral radiograph of the patella demonstrating LABC.

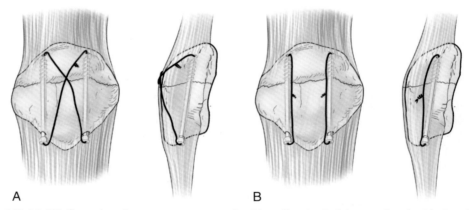

FIG 110.14 (A) Cannulated screws augmented with a figure-of-eight tension band anteriorly. Note that the threads of the screw do not cross the fracture site. (B) The separate tension bands are applied vertically. (Redrawn from Cramer K, Moed B: Patellar fractures: contemporary approach to treatment. *J Am Acad Orthop Surg* 5:323, 1997.)

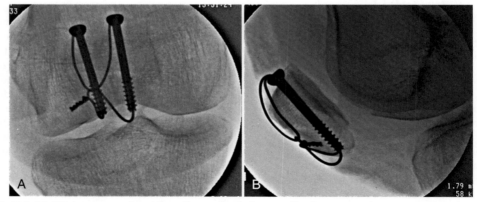

FIG 110.15 (A) Intraoperative AP radiograph of the patella demonstrating a cannulated screw tension band (CSTB) construct. (B) Intraoperative lateral radiograph of the patella demonstrating a CSTB construct.

tension band had 100% clinical union at a mean of 8 weeks and radiographic union at a mean of 13 weeks. Seventy percent had excellent and good results at an average 24-month follow-up.[10]

Arthroscopic assisted reduction and fixation with cannulated screws has also been described.[71,118] With an infrapatellar arthroscope inserted, percutaneous reduction with pointed reduction clamps can be achieved and provisionally maintained with the guide wires for cannulated screws. Screws are inserted over the guide wires, which are subsequently replaced with a wire loop as previously described.[71,118] Tandogan et al. used this technique on five patients, including two with severe osteopenia. All patients had uneventful healing and 80% had full knee range of motion at 28-month follow-up.[118] Makino et al. evaluated five patients treated with this technique at a mean 24-month follow-up. All had uneventful healing and full return of range of motion and preinjury activity level.[71]

Although techniques have continued to evolve, return of completely normal knee function from displaced patella fractures remains elusive. In a recent study, at a mean of 6.5 years follow-up, 20% of patients had an extensor lag of more than 5 degrees. Compared to the normal knee, Biodex testing of these patients revealed a mean isometric extension deficit of 25.5%, an extension power deficit of 31% at an angular velocity of 90 deg/second, and an extension power deficit of 28.9% at an angular velocity of 180 deg/second on the side of the patella fracture.[62]

Future directions for internal fixation will likely focus on materials that are less prone to failure. One such device uses nitinol compression staples for transverse fractures. Under cadaveric testing, this method showed much less displacement than standard tension band techniques and was highly resistant to implant failure.[104] Another device is indicated specifically for comminuted patellar fractures.[68] Liu et al. describe a ring and hook construct that sizes the ring to match the circumference of the anterior patella and is fixed to the bone with hooks.[68] Their initial series included 75 patients with only one failure and no complications. However, with only 1 year of follow-up, the longevity and pragmatic use of this construct remains to be seen.[68]

Domby et al. introduced the idea of using a compressive bolt and nut device that acts as a standalone fixation device that tensions without the need for a traditional tension band construct. In a cadaveric comparison study, however, it did not outperform a standard tension band and cannulated screw construct with both constructs performing well, even at the end of dynamic cyclical testing.[31] While promising in the lab, these products have yet to reach the clinical mainstream.

Another promising technique is the use of mini fragment locking plate fixation for fractures that have comminution or in revision of failed patella fixation. In this situation, the mini fragment locking plate is precontoured and may be placed inferiorly, medially, or laterally (Fig. 110.16). These plates may be used in conjunction with lag screws, thus neutralizing compression as in other fractures.

External Fixation

The use of external fixator techniques with patella fractures has been described in cases of a compromised soft tissue envelope and open injuries with contamination.[6,59,60,65,129] In such severe circumstances, standard internal fixation may result in septic arthritis, failure of fixation, or further soft tissue compromise.

A four-hook external fixation compression clamp has been designed. In its first clinical trial on five patients with open patella fractures (Grades II and III), reduction was percutaneously obtained and the compression clamp applied percutaneously. Union occurred at an average of 13 weeks. At an average follow-up of 25.6 months, 4 of 5 patients returned to their previous activity and had mild to no pain with an average range of motion of 0 to 120 degrees. One patient had recurrent septic arthritis with moderate pain and a range of motion of 10 to 45 degrees.[59] Although promising, very little clinical use or progress has been made.

Alternatively, limited open reduction with external fixator application has also been used.[65] One series of 27 cases evaluating open reduction with subsequent application of two external compressive clamps over wires yielded 24 of 27 patients with excellent and good results. These 24 patients returned to full

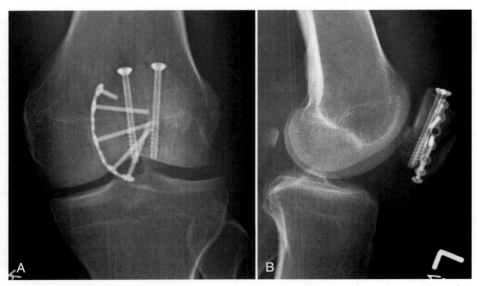

FIG 110.16 (A) Postoperative AP radiograph of the patella demonstrating the addition of a mini fragment locking plate medially to augment fixation. (B) Postoperative lateral radiograph of the patella demonstrating the addition of a mini fragment locking plate medially to augment fixation.

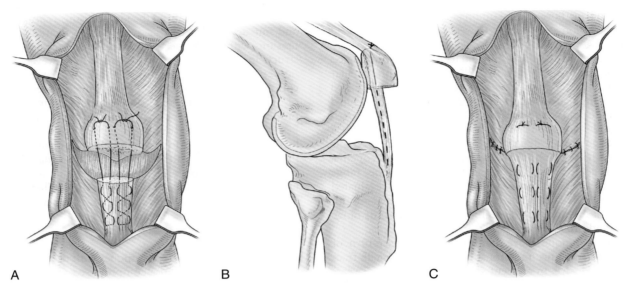

FIG 110.17 Technique of partial patellectomy. Note the placement of the patellar tendon at the articular surface of the remaining patella. A and B, AP and lateral views of the partial patellectomy and tendon advancement via transosseous tunnels prior to retinacular repair. C, Final reconstruction with tendon advancement and retinacular repair. (Redrawn from Cramer K, Moed B: Patellar fractures: contemporary approach to treatment. *J Am Acad Orthop Surg* 5:323, 1997.)

activity and knee range of motion comparable to the contralateral, uninjured extremity.[65]

Reduction with Ilizarov external fixation techniques has been combined with limited percutaneous screw fixation.[6] With this technique, percutaneous olive wires are inserted across the fracture with one olive on either side. Compression across the fracture is then achieved with a tension bow. When the reduction is deemed acceptable, guide wires for percutaneous screws are inserted parallel to the olive wires and screws are then placed. When stable screw fixation is achieved, the olive wires may be removed. A description of the technique and presentation of four cases has been published. Although the authors cite uneventful healing, no specific evaluation of functional outcome was discussed.[6] Another series examined using solely circular external fixation in comminuted patella fractures in conjunction with arthroscopic evaluation. While their series involved only five patients, the mean Lysholm score at follow-up was 94.[127]

Partial Patellectomy

In cases with polar fractures in which the fracture fragments are not of adequate size to support internal fixation, partial patellectomy and extensor mechanism advancement is indicated after stable fixation of any large fragments is completed.[†] Once excision of irreparable fragments is finished, a bony trough should be made in the remaining patella. Then two locking stitches with nonabsorbable braided suture (ie, No. 5 Ethibond) should be placed in the tendon, resulting in one suture tail medially, one laterally, and two centrally. Three holes can then be drilled longitudinally through the patella, one centrally and one on each side. The two central suture tails should be placed through the central hole and the medial and lateral suture tails

passed through their corresponding holes. Finally, the appropriate sutures should be tied to each other at the far end of the patella. A medial and lateral retinacular repair is then achieved (Fig. 110.17). A reinforcing wire or cable may be placed around the patella and through the tibial tubercle. This has been shown to improve the overall strength of the repair.[96]

With partial patellectomy, outcomes comparable to internal fixation, with up to 88% good to excellent results, have been reported[15-17,93,101] Saltzman et al. evaluated 40 patients with partial patellectomy with a mean follow-up of 8 years. Seventy-eight percent had good to excellent results with a mean range of motion of 94% and mean quadriceps strength of 85%.[101] Most reports cite results with distal pole excision and tendon advancement.[15,16,93,101]

No specific correlation has been shown between the size of the retained fragment and the functional outcome.[101] Pandey et al. suggested that retaining any amount of patellar fragment potentially contributes to a biomechanical advantage over total patellectomy.[93] This argument was strengthened by an article looking at distal pole preservation using a basket plate. The group treated with basket plate fixation had less pain, increased level of activity, and better range of motion than the control partial patellectomy group.[56] Another study confirmed these results with a series of 120 patients comparing partial patellectomy (n = 49) to basket plate fixation (n = 71). Using validated outcome tools, they found statistically significant improvement in patellofemoral function with distal pole preservation.[74]

Total Patellectomy

Total patellectomy should be reserved as a salvage procedure when comminution is so severe that it is technically impossible to retain any congruous fragments of patella at the articulation with the trochlea. Functionally, the soft tissue contribution of the extensor mechanism is lengthened with total patellectomy. Therefore, some imbrication is indicated in an attempt to avoid future extensor lag.[102] Soft tissue repair should proceed with

---

†References 4, 30, 48, 84, 93, 101, and 120.

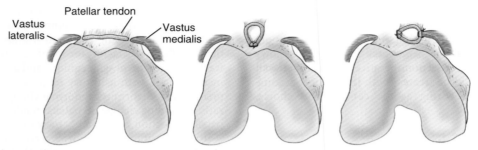

FIG 110.18 Compere technique for patellectomy (see text). Ossification will occur within the tube.

multiple nonabsorbable tendon-grabbing stitches once all bone fragments have been removed. It is imperative that intraoperative flexion of 90 degrees be obtained. If inadequate soft tissue is present, or primary repair or augmentation is needed, an inverted V-plasty "turndown" should be performed.[112] Mobilization may begin within 3 to 6 weeks postoperatively if the repair allows. Up to 2 years may be required before maximal rehabilitation is achieved.[63]

When adequate soft tissue is available, the remaining extensor mechanism can be "tubularized," as described by Compere et al. (Fig. 110.18). At times, ossification will develop within the tube, forming a pseudo-patella to help restore some of the extensor mechanism's mechanics.[28]

While pain relief is common, overall results regarding function and strength following total patellectomy are poor when compared to other treatment options. Sutton et al. reported a 49% reduction in extensor mechanism strength in patients who underwent total as opposed to partial patellectomy.[117] Severe quadriceps atrophy, difficulty with stair climbing, and pain with activity have all been reported.[34] Levack et al. postulated that good results were attainable if patients maintained 70% quadriceps function of the contralateral limb. However, 27 of 34 patients in that series maintained less than 70% of quadriceps strength and did not have a good result.[63] At 7.5 years follow-up, Einola et al. had only 21% of 28 patients with good results and maintenance of 75% quadriceps power.[34]

COMPLICATIONS

Despite advances in fixation strategies and technologies, outcomes following operative fixation of patella fractures remain less than desired.[61] Common complications include functional impairment, which includes limited range of motion, muscle weakness, and anterior knee pain. While nonunion and infection rates remain low, reoperation rates because of symptomatic hardware and persistent pain are exceedingly high.[33,44,97]

Loss of Knee Motion

This may be the most common complication with loss of terminal knee flexion.[30] Usually this does not affect daily function. If severe, manipulation under anesthesia, arthroscopic lysis of adhesions, or quadricepsplasty may be considered. To date, widely accepted standard protocols do not exist for specific interventions.

Although some authors have not reported long-term effects of immobilization up to 6 weeks,[15,17] early motion is generally instituted to promote cartilage healing and potentially decrease short-term stiffness.

Infection

Postsurgical infection for patella fractures ranges from 3% to 10%.[15,47,113] Because of the limited soft tissue envelope around the patella, careful surgical handling is imperative. In cases of concomitant soft tissue injury, avoiding the zone of injury should be attempted. Additionally, adequate débridement of all necrotic and nonviable tissue as well as foreign material should be conducted with open injuries. If suspected deep infection exists, appropriate antibiotics and thorough débridment should be conducted. If healing has not occurred, implants should remain in place with plans for a staged removal after union if infection risk persists.

Loss of Reduction

Loss of reduction after operative fixation has ranged from 0% to 20%.[15,47,113] This may be related to technical errors, unrecognized injury, or patient noncompliance.[63,113] If displacement is minimal, a period of immobilization may be indicated to allow the remaining reduction to heal. If there is severe displacement or discontinuity of the extensor mechanism, revision surgery is indicated.

Osteoarthrosis

Long-term follow-up indicates that rates of osteoarthrosis in a knee that has sustained a patella fracture is greater than in the contralateral, uninjured extremity.[47,114] Severe articular damage at the time of injury may result in osteoarthritis, even with anatomic reduction. Exuberant callous during healing may also contribute to degenerative joint disease.[102] Finally, inadequate restoration of the articular surface may result in osteoarthritis after surgery for patella fracture.

Hardware Irritation

Two separate studies indicate that subcutaneous hardware may become symptomatic in 15% of cases.[47,113] When necessary, it should be removed on an elective basis after full healing has occurred.

Delayed Union and Nonunion

With modern fixation, this complication is extremely rare. Frequently it is an asymptomatic fibrous nonunion with an intact extensor mechanism that does not necessitate further treatment. Bostrom reported 3% incidence of asymptomatic pseudarthrosis regardless of operative or nonoperative treatment.[17] Carpenter et al. had a 1% incidence of nonunion.[24] If a delayed union is present, a period of immobilization will often allow healing to progress. If this fails, revision fixation with bone grafting should be considered. Weber and Cech reported a 100% healing rate with revision surgery.[124] In a recent meta-analysis, Nathan et al. compiled the results of five studies that met inclusion criteria.[86] The authors emphasized the importance of assessing the patient's functional status because low-demand patients can be treated nonoperatively. More functional patients, however, should be treated, with the authors recommending tension band wiring as the construct of choice, according to their review.[86]

PATELLA FRACTURES IN TOTAL KNEE ARTHROPLASTY

Although overall a rare complication of total knee arthroplasty, patella fractures may be the most frequently occurring periprosthetic knee fractures.[67] The range of this complication is 0.33% to 6.3%.[22,40] Operative treatment of these injuries are often fraught with high complication rates and severe functional loss, and is discouraged unless there is frank extensor mechanism disruption or component loosening.

Many risk factors have been associated with patella fractures in total knee arthroplasty.[3] These include patient factors (osteoporosis, rheumatoid arthritis, male sex, overactivity, excessive knee motion); implant factors (central peg, cementless implants, posterior cruciate ligament [PCL]-substituting prosthesis, inset design, osteolysis); and technical factors (excessive resection,

inadequate resection, anterior patella perforation, revision surgery, cement usage, malalignment, patella blood supply disruption).[53,64] In a recent case-control study, Seo et al. determined that significant risk factors for spontaneous periprosthetic patella fracture largely involved technique and alignment. Other than an increased risk with a history of previous surgeries, increasing preoperative deformity, abnormal changes to the Insall-Salvati ratio (including changes to patellar tendon length), and excessive patellar resection, significantly increased risk for fracture.[109]

Insall classified these injuries according to the configuration of the fracture (horizontal, vertical, and comminuted) and traumatic or fatigue fractures. He recommended traumatic, displaced injuries be treated operatively and nondisplaced fatigue fractures with adequate component stability be treated nonoperatively.[50]

Goldberg classified patella fractures according to concomitant extensor mechanism injury. Type I are marginal fractures without component involvement or extensor injury. Type II injuries have disruption of the extensor mechanism or implant-bone interface. Type III involve the inferior pole with type III-A having patellar tendon disruption and type III-B having a competent patella tendon. Type IV fractures have concomitant patellofemoral dislocation (Fig. 110.19).[38]

Treatment is based on competence of the extensor mechanism and stability of the prosthetic component. In Goldberg

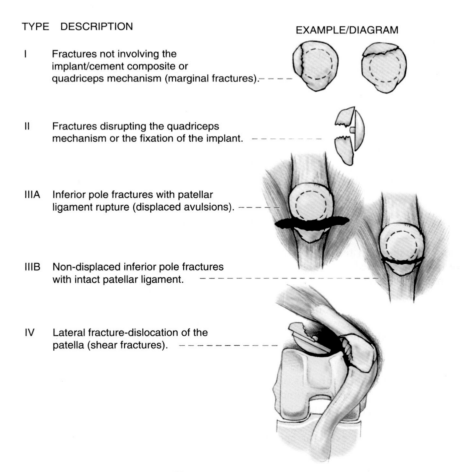

TYPE	DESCRIPTION	EXAMPLE/DIAGRAM
I	Fractures not involving the implant/cement composite or quadriceps mechanism (marginal fractures).	
II	Fractures disrupting the quadriceps mechanism or the fixation of the implant.	
IIIA	Inferior pole fractures with patellar ligament rupture (displaced avulsions).	
IIIB	Non-displaced inferior pole fractures with intact patellar ligament.	
IV	Lateral fracture-dislocation of the patella (shear fractures).	

FIG 110.19 Goldberg classification[38] of patellar fractures after total knee arthroplasty. (From Kolessar D, Rand J: Extensor mechanism problems following total knee arthroplasty. In Morrey B [ed]: *Reconstructive surgery of the joints*, ed 2, New York, 1996, Churchill Livingstone.)

type I fractures, nonoperative treatment is appropriate. With extensor mechanism incompetence (type II and type III-A), surgical repair must be undertaken. Fractures with excessive displacement or extreme component loosening also require operative intervention.[20,38,40] If standard fixation techniques are technically impossible, suture anchor fixation, cerclage fixation, or partial patellectomy with delayed postoperative range of motion may be necessary.[9,36,69,72,121] For type III fractures with severe bone loss, advanced techniques using allograft and/or trabecular metal may be required to restore the extensor mechanism.[3,43,87]

A retrospective study reviewed 85 periprosthetic patella fractures with a mean follow-up of 3.6 years. Thirty-seven of 38 fractures without extensor mechanism dysfunction or component loosening were successfully treated nonoperatively. Eleven of 12 fractures with extensor mechanism disruption were treated operatively. Six had postoperative complications, five of which required reoperation. Of the 28 fractures with a loose patella component, 20 were operatively treated and 9 had complications. This data highlights that periprosthetic patella fractures that require operative intervention in the setting of a total knee arthroplasty have a high complication rate.[92]

SUMMARY

Patella fractures are fairly common injuries. Current classification schemes according to fracture pattern and mechanism of injury do not correlate with functional outcomes. It is relatively clear that maintenance of the patella when possible is superior to total patellectomy. Results of treatment seem to be based on maintenance and adequacy of reduction and fixation. Currently modified tension band techniques with or without screw fixation appear to provide the best results. Biomechanically, cannulated screws and braided wire have added to the stability of repairs, but have not been proven to clinically improve results.

Treatment may be dictated by its subcutaneous location and potential for anterior soft tissue injury. With an intact soft tissue envelope, treatment must be based on surgeon experience and comfort with techniques to obtain the previously discussed treatment goals. Postoperative protocols for initiation of range of motion and strengthening are personalized to patient needs and stability of fixation.

The references for this chapter can also be found on www.expertconsult.com.

111

Treatment of Periprosthetic Fractures Around a Total Knee Arthroplasty

George J. Haidukewych, Steven Lyons, Thomas Bernasek

Periprosthetic fractures remain common complications after total knee arthroplasty. The number of knee arthroplasties performed worldwide continues to increase, and with the growing older population, the number of periprosthetic fractures will also continue to increase. Decision making regarding the management of these fractures is divided according to whether the fracture has occurred in the femur or the tibia or whether the arthroplasty is loose or well fixed. Fractures of the distal end of the femur above a well-fixed arthroplasty are typically treated with some form of internal fixation. The use of fixed-angled, locked, percutaneously inserted plates has revolutionized the treatment of these fractures. Early clinical and biomechanical data are encouraging. Recently, modern retrograde nails that offer multiple plane, angle stable locking screws have demonstrated excellent results. For loose implants, revision is typically considered. Bony defects, areas of osteolysis, osteopenia, and short periarticular fragments all pose challenges to a successful revision arthroplasty in this setting. In older patients, distal femoral replacement tumor prostheses are often required to reconstruct massive bony defects. Attention to specific technical details is necessary for a successful result, and surgeons undertaking such reconstructions should be experienced in arthroplasty and fracture management techniques.

The number of primary knee arthroplasties performed annually in the United States continues to increase. It is estimated that 0.3% to 2.5% of patients will sustain a periprosthetic fracture as a complication of total knee arthroplasty.[1,11,31] Patient-specific risk factors, such as rheumatoid arthritis, osteolysis, osteopenic bone, and frequent falls, common in the older population, and technique-specific risk factors, such as anterior femoral cortical notching, have all been implicated as potential causes of periprosthetic fractures. The economic impact and disability associated with these fractures is substantial; therefore having an effective strategy to manage these challenging injuries is important. Fractures typically occur in the supracondylar area of the femur above a well-fixed total knee arthroplasty (Fig. 111.1).[2,18,24] Fractures of the tibia are much less common and are frequently associated with implant loosening and varus malalignment.[12,17] Decision making regarding the treatment of periprosthetic fractures around a total knee arthroplasty is divided, as noted earlier. In general, patients with fractures around loose implants are considered candidates for revision total knee arthroplasty, whereas fractures around well-fixed implants are candidates for open reduction and internal fixation. Various methods of internal fixation have been described for the treatment of these injuries.[5,33] There has been recent enthusiasm for minimally invasive osteosynthesis of these injuries with the use of locked plates. Revision arthroplasty in this setting can be very demanding, with a unique set of technical challenges. The purpose of this chapter is to review the decision making, contemporary techniques, and potential complications of the management of periprosthetic fractures of the femur and tibia around a total knee arthroplasty. Periprosthetic fractures of the patella are discussed in Chapter 67.

PATIENT EVALUATION

Patients with fractures around asymptomatic, well-fixed implants do not usually require an infection workup. However, in patients with a loose implant or history of prefracture knee pain, routine preoperative evaluation of these patients should include a complete blood count with manual differential, sedimentation rate, C-reactive protein serology, and knee aspiration to exclude occult infection. Medical optimization for these frequently frail older patients is recommended.

High-quality radiographs are necessary to evaluate the fixation status of the arthroplasty and the amount and quality of remaining periarticular bone stock. Computed tomography (CT) scanning can be helpful if more information is needed about remaining bone stock. The history and physical examination should focus on prefracture knee symptoms, such as pain, instability, and stiffness. If available, the operative notes from the original arthroplasty should be obtained. This is especially important if isolated component revision is contemplated. Older implant designs may not offer varying degrees of constraint, augmentation, polyethylene insert sizes, and other factors, and thus compatibility issues may necessitate complete arthroplasty revision. Previous incisions and the status of the soft tissues should be circumferentially evaluated. The neurovascular status of the limb should be carefully documented.

OPEN REDUCTION AND INTERNAL FIXATION

Supracondylar Periprosthetic Fractures

The typical clinical situation that the orthopedic surgeon will encounter is a supracondylar femoral fracture above a well-fixed, well-functioning total knee arthroplasty in an older patient (Figs. 111.2 and 111.3).[1,11] Minimally displaced stable fractures and those impacted in good alignment may be candidates for nonoperative treatment. However, in our experience, these situations are rare. Long-leg casting with or without incorporation

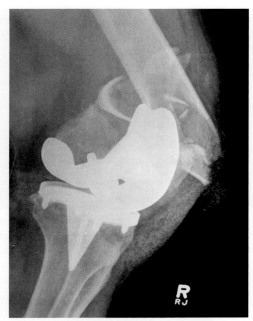

FIG 111.1 Displaced comminuted periprosthetic distal femoral fracture.

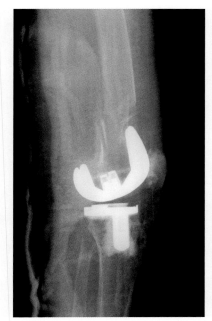

FIG 111.3 Lateral view of the patient in Fig. 86.2. Note the fracture at the level of the anterior femoral flange, the most common fracture location.

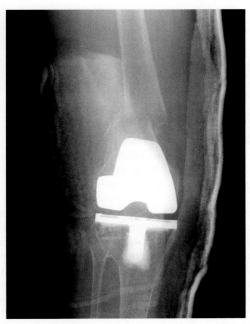

FIG 111.2 Anteroposterior view of a typical distal femoral periprosthetic fracture above a well-fixed total knee arthroplasty.

of a hip guide brace to control leg rotation is recommended. Close radiographic follow-up is indicated, with early surgical intervention if fracture instability is noted. Prolonged attempts at managing unstable fractures with casting may result in further erosion of the distal bone stock and potentially compromise the success of any future reconstruction.

The principles of treatment of these injuries include obtaining bony union, maintaining correct limb alignment, length, and rotation, and avoiding complications. Surgical challenges to achieving these goals include the often short, osteopenic

distal bony fragments, fracture comminution, areas of osteolysis, and parts of the femoral component that can make obtaining stable distal fixation difficult, such as lugs, boxes, and stems. Such fractures usually require an internal fixation device that provides coronal plane stability to avoid the deformity, typically varus collapse, that can occur during the healing process. In the past, such devices as the 95-degree angled blade plate and dynamic condylar screw have been used, with mixed results.*

Because of the extremely distal nature of these fractures, the blade of the blade plate or the lag screw of the dynamic condylar screw must often be inserted more proximally to avoid portions of the femoral component, and thus distal fixation is often suboptimal. The traditional condylar buttress plate offers more freedom of angulation of distal screws but provides no coronal plane stability. Unacceptable rates of varus collapse have been reported when this device was used for unstable fractures.[10]

Retrograde intramedullary nailing has been used successfully in many series to manage these fractures and offers the advantage of soft tissue–friendly, minimally invasive stability for complex periprosthetic fractures.[1,5,11,18-20] Challenges to successful union with intramedullary techniques include the marginal distal fixation provided by locking screws for the typically comminuted, osteopenic distal bony fragments (Figs. 111.4 and 111.5). In addition, intramedullary nailing may be challenging because the femoral housing may preclude in-line access to the intramedullary canal. Careful attention to the starting point is required to avoid hyperextension deformity of the distal femur (Fig. 111.6). Furthermore, biomechanical evidence has suggested that, in the presence of medial comminution, retrograde intramedullary nails may be mechanically more stable than laterally placed locking plates.[4] Modern retrograde nails offer multiplane, fixed-angle distal locking screw options

---

*References 1-3, 5, 8, 18, 31, and 33.

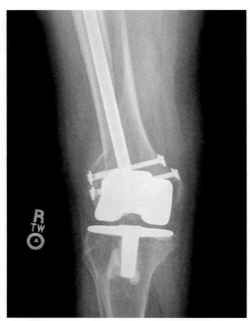

FIG 111.4 Loss of fixation after retrograde nailing because of inadequate distal fixation.

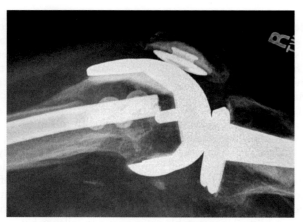

FIG 111.5 Lateral view of the patient in Fig. 86.4.

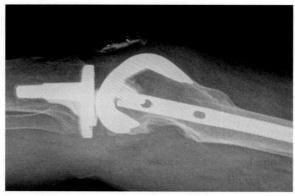

FIG 111.6 Lateral view of a distal femoral periprosthetic fracture. Note the hyperextension deformity because of the femoral trochlea of the femoral component precluding in line access to the femoral canal.

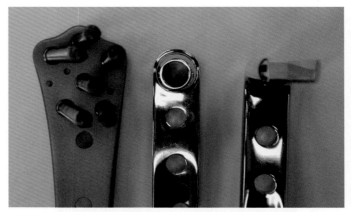

FIG 111.7 En face view of a locked plate, dynamic condylar screw, and blade plate. The versatility and superior ability to obtain distal fixation with the locked plate are obvious.

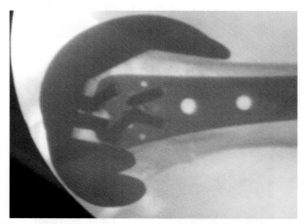

FIG 111.8 Internal fixation with the LISS device (Synthes, West Chester, Pennsylvania). Note the positioning of the screws around distal obstacles, such as femoral lugs.

that can provide excellent fixation even in very short distal segments. Occasionally, antegrade femoral nailing can be used for periprosthetic distal femoral fractures as well, provided that a sufficiently long distal fragment is present. In our experience, such fractures are extremely rare. The main challenge with antegrade techniques is obtaining appropriate alignment and stable distal fixation. In addition, with antegrade techniques, an area of high-stress concentration is created between the distal end of the nail and the femoral component.

Locking plate technology has gained popularity for the management of complex periarticular fractures about the knee.[†] Threads on the screw heads are threaded into corresponding threads in the plate holes, thereby forming a fixed-angle construct and providing coronal plane stability.[15] These devices have been used with excellent results for the management of complex periarticular injuries and have an excellent track record for providing reliable distal fixation. In addition, such devices allow multiple locked screws to be placed around and between portions of the femoral component to improve distal fixation (Figs. 111.7 to 111.9).[38] Kregor et al.[24,25] have reported a series

---

[†]References 7, 16, 21, 23-26, 28, 30, 34, and 35.

of 38 periprosthetic fractures treated with the Less Invasive Stabilization System (LISS) device (Synthes, West Chester, Pennsylvania). There were only two failures (5%). One patient required revision knee arthroplasty and one required bone grafting to achieve solid union. Ultimately, 37 of 38 fractures (97%) healed. Medical and orthopedic complications were uncommon. Leaving metaphyseal comminution undisturbed, thereby preserving vascularity to the fragments, is critical to predictable healing with this technique.

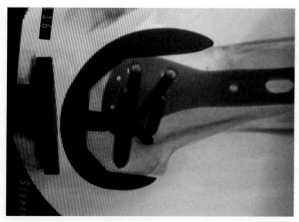

FIG 111.9 Internal fixation with the PolyAx device (DePuy, Warsaw, Indiana), which allows angled polyaxial screws and fixed-angle locking screws as well.

In addition to providing excellent mechanical stability, several locked plating designs also offer the added theoretical biologic advantage of allowing percutaneous insertion.[23] This type of insertion minimizes the need for additional large incisions around the knee and potentially minimizes the soft tissue complications and stiffness associated with the traditional exposures used for open reduction and internal fixation.[16] When percutaneous techniques are used, vigilance is required to avoid malalignment, typically valgus deformity and hyperextension of the distal fragment. Many commercially available locked plating designs offer the surgeon the option of open or percutaneous insertion. When possible, we perform the internal fixation percutaneously to take advantage of the mechanical stability provided by these devices, as well as the advantages that percutaneous insertion allows.[12]

Percutaneous Technique of Distal End of the Femur Using Locked Plating Designs

The patient is positioned supine on a radiolucent table, and intravenous antibiotics are administered. Excellent muscle relaxation and fluoroscopic images are essential. Preparing both legs in the operative field can make it easier to obtain a lateral view of the fractured extremity by lifting the normal extremity out of the C-arm beam (Fig. 111.10). A lateral incision is made at the flare of the lateral condyle. A plate of appropriate length is then inserted in a submuscular extraperiosteal fashion under fluoroscopic control. The plate is positioned as distally as possible on the distal fragment and provisionally held with a guide pin. It is critical to place this guide pin parallel to the knee joint to ensure excellent alignment. Limb length and rotation are

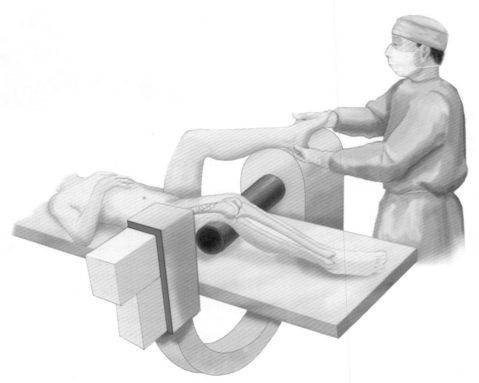

FIG 111.10 Patient positioning with the fluoroscope from the opposite side and inclusion of both lower extremities in the surgical draping. Such positioning allows simple lifting of the well leg to obtain a true lateral view. (Courtesy Mayo Foundation for Medical Education and Research, Rochester, Minnesota.)

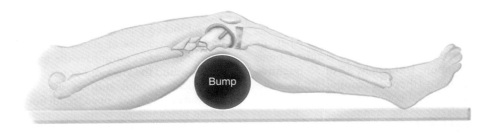

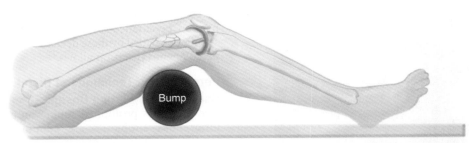

FIG 111.11 Use of a bump to assist in avoiding hyperextension of the distal fragment. A more proximal bump location allows the distal fragment to flex into the appropriate position. Often, multiple attempts with bumps of various sizes and positions are necessary to determine which will reduce the fracture best.

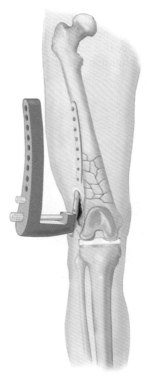

FIG 111.12 Percutaneous, submuscular, extraperiosteal insertion of a locked plate. (Courtesy Mayo Foundation for Medical Education and Research, Rochester, Minnesota.)

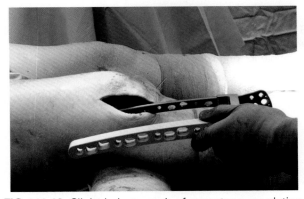

FIG 111.13 Clinical photograph of percutaneous plating.

then adjusted, and a second guide pin is placed proximally into the femoral shaft. Leaving metaphyseal comminution undisturbed by bridging this area is critical to the success of this technique. A combination of gentle manual traction and placement of a small bump under the fracture site can assist with closed reduction, the most difficult portion of the procedure. There is a strong tendency for the distal fragment to tip into hyperextension because of pull of the gastrocnemius muscles (Figs. 111.11 to 111.16). With first-generation locking plates, it is critical to have the plate positioned accurately and have all aspects of the reduction complete before placing any locking screws. These screws will not pull the plate down to bone, nor will they allow fine adjustments in alignment after they are inserted. Newer locking plate designs offer so-called hybrid fixation that allows the surgeon a choice of locked, traditional unlocked, or polyaxial angled locked screws. Distal fixation should be optimized by placing as many distal screws as possible. Typically, screws can pass just posterior to the anterior flange of the femoral component or just above the box of a posterior-stabilized housing. We attempt to use all distal screws and at least four proximal screws.

Fracture stability is assessed by intraoperatively testing flexion and varus-valgus stability under live fluoroscopy. The wound is closed in a routine layered fashion over a suction drain. In general, a hinged knee brace is used postoperatively

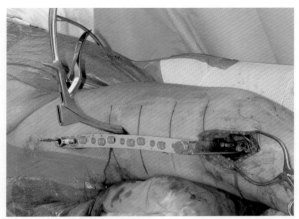

FIG 111.14 Use of percutaneous clamps for reduction and an aiming arm to target percutaneous screws.

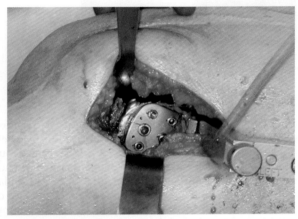

FIG 111.15 Clinical photograph demonstrating the minimally invasive nature of the internal fixation.

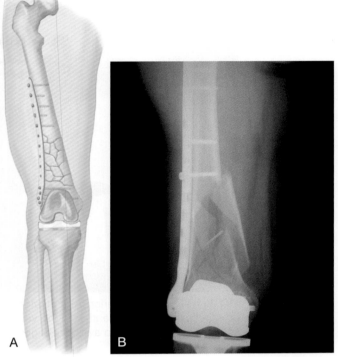

FIG 111.16 (A and B) Bridge plating, leaving the metaphyseal comminution undisturbed and thereby preserving its vascularity. (Courtesy Mayo Foundation for Medical Education and Research, Rochester, Minnesota.)

and knee motion is started when the wound is dry. Toe touch weight bearing is maintained until healing is evident, typically at 10 to 12 weeks post procedure (Fig. 111.17).

Periprosthetic Tibial Fractures

Periprosthetic fractures of the proximal tibia are rare, and no specific incidence has been reported. They typically occur around loose tibial components and are frequently associated with varus malalignment. Felix et al.[13] have reported on 102 periprosthetic tibial fractures below a total knee arthroplasty. Of these, 83 fractures occurred postoperatively and 19 occurred intraoperatively. The authors of this study developed a treatment-based classification system in which fractures were classified into three types based on the fixation status of the implant and four types based on the location of the fracture. Type A fractures occurred around implants that were radiographically well fixed, type B occurred in those that were radiographically loose, and type C fractures occurred intraoperatively. Type I fractures occurred at the tibial plateau, type II were located adjacent to the prosthetic stem, type III occurred distal to the prosthetic stem, and type IV involved the tibial tubercle. Type I fractures were the most common, accounting for 61 fractures. Type II fractures were the second most common, accounting for 22 fractures. Only 17 fractures occurred distal

to the prosthetic stem. Most proximal fractures were associated with a loose prosthesis, and these were managed successfully with revision surgery, typically involving stems to bypass the deficient bone. Fractures around a stable implant were managed successfully by the standard principles for tibial fracture management. No large series has evaluated the outcomes of open reduction and internal fixation of periprosthetic fractures of the tibia below a total knee arthroplasty. Therefore treatment of fractures of the tibia below a total knee arthroplasty is dictated by the location and stability of the fracture and the fixation status of the implant.[1,8,11,17,31] For example, closed reduction and casting may be very successful for spiral, "boot top"–type distal tibial fractures; however, a comminuted midshaft, same-level tibiofibular fracture would probably be difficult to manage nonoperatively.

Fractures of the tibia distal to the arthroplasty can often be managed by closed reduction and casting if appropriate alignment can be obtained. The tibial component obviously precludes the use of routine locked intramedullary nails, and therefore plating may be the best choice for unstable fractures with a healthy soft tissue envelope. Contemporary locked plate technology allows long, fixed-angle plates to be applied percutaneously, thus minimizing soft tissue dissection and the potential disastrous risk of wound infection. In addition, excellent proximal fixation can be obtained with multiple locked screws placed around stems or keels of the tibial component.[7]

Fractures of the proximal end of the tibia in contact with the tibial component are typically associated with loosening of the tibial component and are usually managed with revision arthroplasty in which the deficient proximal bone is bypassed

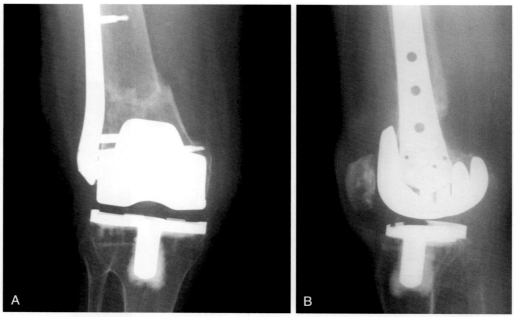

FIG 111.17 Anteroposterior (A) and lateral (B) views at follow-up after locked plating of a periprosthetic fracture. Note the slight valgus malalignment. Careful vigilance and fluoroscopic scrutiny are necessary to avoid malalignment when using percutaneous techniques.

with an intramedullary stem.[1,11,13] The use of metal augmentation or structural bone grafting may be required if insufficient host bone support for the tibial component is available.

The use of external fixation is discouraged because of concern for pin site sepsis and potential contamination of the total knee arthroplasty. When external fixation is unavoidable, meticulous pin site care and extreme vigilance are recommended to minimize pin site infections. Because of this concern, we reserve the use of external fixation as a last resort when treating these injuries.

ROLE OF REVISION ARTHROPLASTY

The need to revise a total knee arthroplasty secondary to a periprosthetic fracture has become less common in our practices with the advent of improved internal fixation devices, such as locked plates. Revision arthroplasty is typically reserved for fractures around a loose prosthesis, fractures with inadequate bone stock to allow for stable internal fixation, or recalcitrant supracondylar nonunion that requires resection and implantation of a so-called tumor prosthesis. Surgeons who treat periprosthetic fractures around a total knee arthroplasty must have the expertise and technical support to be able to perform long-stemmed, revision total knee arthroplasty because one is often unable to determine which reconstructive option is necessary until the fracture has been exposed in the operating room. Bony defects secondary to comminution, multiple previous procedures, presence of broken hardware, and presence of deformity may all present technical challenges to a successful outcome.

Supracondylar Fractures

Revision total knee arthroplasty with intramedullary femoral stems that engage the diaphysis and simultaneously stabilize the fracture can be effective. Cemented stems may be used, but care must be taken to prevent extrusion of cement into the fracture site. Allograft struts with cerclage wiring can be used to reinforce the stability provided by a long-stemmed prosthesis. However, it is unusual to have distal femoral bone stock that is inadequate for internal fixation yet adequate for formal revision. The ideal indication for long-stemmed revision total knee arthroplasty would be the presence of adequate bone stock in the face of a supracondylar fracture with a grossly loose femoral component.[1,11] Most of the clinical data evaluating the outcomes of a simultaneous revision arthroplasty with intramedullary stem fixation of a supracondylar fracture have been gathered from the treatment of distal femoral nonunion in this situation. Kress et al.[27] have reported a small series of nonunions about the knee treated successfully with revision and uncemented femoral stems with bone grafting. Union was achieved in 6 months.

Distal femoral replacement tumor prostheses have been used for salvage of failed internal fixation of supracondylar periprosthetic femoral fractures. The long-term results of the kinematic rotating hinge prosthesis for oncologic resections about the knee have been good, with a 10-year survivorship of approximately 90%.[36] As their success becomes more predictable, the indications for such megaprostheses are expanding. Older patients with refractory periprosthetic supracondylar nonunion or those with acute fractures and bone stock inadequate for internal fixation are reasonable candidates for megaprostheses. Davila et al.[9] have reported a small series of supracondylar distal femoral nonunions treated with a megaprosthesis in older patients. They indicated that a cemented megaprosthesis in this patient population permits early ambulation and return to activities of daily living. Freedman et al.[14] have performed distal femoral replacement in five older patients with acute fractures and reported four good results and one poor result secondary to infection. The four patients with good results regained ambulation in less than 1 month and had an average arc of motion of 99 degrees. All patients had some degree of extension lag.

For a younger, active patient, an allograft prosthetic composite may be a better alternative. Distal femoral reconstruction with an allograft prosthetic composite to provide a biologic interface can help to restore bone stock and potentially make future revision easier.[11,16] Kraay et al.[22] have reported a series of allograft prosthetic reconstructions for the treatment of supracondylar fractures in patients with total knee arthroplasties. At a minimum 2-year follow-up, the mean Knee Society score was 71 and the mean arc of motion was 96 degrees. All femoral components were well fixed at follow-up. The results of this study indicate that large segmental distal femoral allograft prosthetic composites can be a reasonable treatment method in this setting. In our experience, when revision is required because of fracture and distal bone loss, a tumor prosthesis is usually required.

Periprosthetic Fractures of the Tibia

Periprosthetic fractures of the tibia associated with total knee arthroplasty are extremely uncommon. Tibial fractures associated with loose components are best treated with revision arthroplasty, frequently with the use of a long stem to bypass the fracture.[1,11,13] Often, these fractures are associated with extensive osteolysis and may therefore require structural or morselized bone grafting, the use of metal wedges, metaphyseal filling sleeves, trabecular metal cones, or in the most severe cases a proximal tibial megaprosthesis or allograft prosthetic composite. Maximizing host bone support is critical for a good result. The largest series of periprosthetic tibial fractures around loose prostheses was reported by Rand and Coventry.[32] In their series, all 15 knees had varus axial malalignment when compared with those of a control group. Similar studies have confirmed that varus malalignment may be a potential risk factor for periprosthetic tibial fractures.[29,37] Specific technical considerations include careful soft tissue dissection and retraction to minimize soft tissue trauma to the already compromised skin flaps. It is important that surgeons undertaking these reconstructions be experienced in revision arthroplasty and fracture management techniques to achieve a successful outcome.

CONCLUSIONS

Periprosthetic fractures around total knee arthroplasty remain difficult injuries to treat. With the ever-growing older population, the incidence of these fractures will increase. Decision making regarding open reduction and internal fixation or revision arthroplasty is based on the fixation status of the implant, remaining bone quality, physiologic age of the patient, and location and stability of the fracture. Advances in locked plate technology and modern retrograde nailing show promise for improved fixation of such complex fractures, with minimal additional soft tissue trauma. More data are needed to define fully the role of this exciting technology, along with traditional techniques of internal fixation of these fractures. Revision arthroplasty frequently requires modular distal femoral replacement, metal or allograft augmentation of bone deficiency, and long stems to bypass deficient bone. These reconstructions are demanding and fraught with complications. Attention to specific technical details is essential for a successful result.

KEY REFERENCES

3. Bolhofner BR, Carmen B, Clifford P: The results of open reduction and internal fixation of distal femur fractures using a biologic (indirect) reduction technique. *J Orthop Trauma* 10:372–377, 1996.
10. Davison BL: Varus collapse of comminuted distal femur fractures after ORIF with a lateral condylar buttress plate. *Am J Orthop* 32:27–30, 2003.
13. Felix N, Stuart M, Hanssen A: Periprosthetic fractures of the tibia associated with total knee arthroplasty. *Clin Orthop* 345:113–124, 1997.
14. Freedman DL, Hak DJ, Johnson EE, et al: Total knee arthroplasty including a modular distal femoral component in elderly patients with acute fracture or nonunion. *J Orthop Trauma* 9:231–237, 1995.
16. Haidukewych GJ: Innovations in locking plate technology for orthopedic trauma. *J Am Acad Orthop Surg* 12:205–212, 2004.
20. Henry SL, Busconi B, Gold S, et al: Management of supracondylar femur fractures proximal to total knee prostheses with the GSH supracondylar intramedullary nail. *Orthop Trans* 19:153, 1995.
21. Koval KJ, Hoehl JJ, Kummer FJ, et al: Distal femoral fixation: a biomechanical comparison of the standard condylar buttress plate, a locked buttress plate, and the 95-degree blade plate. *J Orthop Trauma* 11:521–524, 1997.
25. Kregor PJ, Hughes JL, Cole PA: Fixation of distal femoral fractures above total knee arthroplasty utilizing the Less Invasive Stabilization System (LISS). *Injury* 32:SC64–SC75, 2001.

The references for this chapter can also be found on www.expertconsult.com.

Pediatric Knee

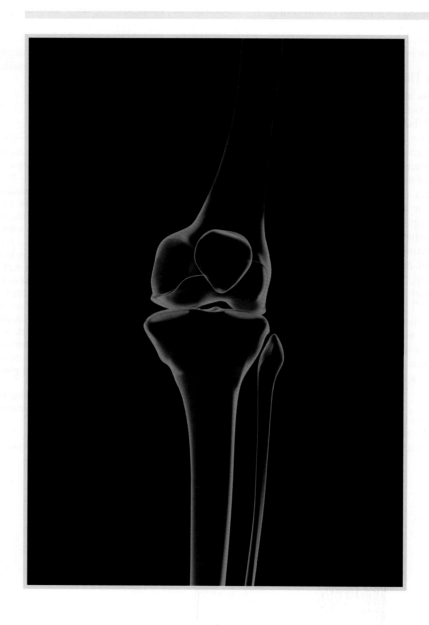

112

Normal Knee Embryology and Development

James G. Jarvis, Hans K. Uhthoff

The term *embryology* infers the study of embryos. However, nowadays embryology generally refers to the entire period of prenatal development and includes the study of embryos and fetuses. Although prenatal development is more rapid than postnatal development and results in striking changes, the developmental mechanisms of the two periods are the same. "Embryology provides a mechanism to help to understand the causes of variations in human structure. It illuminates gross anatomy and explains how both normal relations and abnormalities develop."[23]

OVERVIEW OF EMBRYOLOGY

Prenatal development consists of four sequential stages:
1. *Gametogenesis.* Gametogenesis is the process of formation and development of specialized generative cells called gametes, which unite at fertilization to form a single cell called a zygote.
2. *Early embryonic period (weeks 1 and 2).* The early embryonic phase encompasses the 2-week period from fertilization to implantation of the embryo, during which the zygote repeatedly divides. During week 2 the amniotic cavity and trilaminar embryonic disk are formed. The early embryo usually is aborted if a lethal or serious genetic defect is present, although at this time the early embryo is less susceptible to teratogens than during the remainder of the embryonic period.
3. *Embryo (weeks 3 to 8).* Week 3 is the first week of organogenesis. The trilaminar embryonic disk develops, somites begin to form, and the neuroplate closes to form a neural tube (Fig. 112.1).[41] At week 4 the limb buds become recognizable, and the somites differentiate into three segments. The dermatome becomes skin, the myotome becomes muscle, and the sclerotome becomes cartilage and bone. Serious defects in limb development may originate at this time (Fig. 112.2).[40] By week 8 the basic organ systems are complete.
4. *Fetus (week 8 to term).* The first half of the fetal period is characterized by rapid growth and changes in body proportions. The lower limbs become proportionate, and most bones start to ossify. During the second half of gestation, growth continues, and body proportions become more infant-like (see Fig. 112.2).

TIMING AND STAGING OF DEVELOPMENT

Gestational age based on the date of the mother's last menstrual period overestimates the actual gestational age by more than 2 weeks. To estimate age more accurately, embryos are staged according to the method of Streeter.[43] This system, a derivative of the Carnegie embryonic staging system, divides the embryonic period into 23 stages based on clearly defined details of either external form or the development of structures.[29,30] The maturity of older embryos and fetuses is based on measurement of the crown-rump length.[31]

NORMAL SEQUENTIAL EMBRYOLOGIC DEVELOPMENT OF THE KNEE*

Week 6

Fig. 112.3 shows an embryo at 6 weeks old, Streeter stage 17. The cartilaginous anlagen of femur and tibia are separated by cells of uniform density, the future femorotibial joint. Early evidence of cavitation, a sign of beginning joint formation, in the otherwise homogeneous, uniform interzone is easily recognizable.

Week 7

Fig. 112.4 shows an embryo at 7 weeks old, Streeter stage 19. Already at this stage, the lateral femoral condyle and medial femoral condyle are well formed. The lateral collateral ligament spans from the femur to the fibular head, and the medial collateral ligament connects the femur to the tibia.

Week 8

Fig. 112.5 shows an embryo at 8 weeks old. Not only is the posterior cruciate ligament seen but also the multiple sites of beginning cavitation. Persistence of some of these intra-articular strands may lead to the development of plicae.

Week 10

Fig. 112.6 shows a fetus at 10 weeks old. Between the medial femoral condyle and tibia, the medial meniscus (MM) can be seen. A small plica connects the midpart of the MM with the medial femoral condyle.

Fig. 112.7 also shows a fetus at 10 weeks old. Not only the femur, tibia, and fibular head but also the anterior cruciate ligament are seen in the figure. At this stage, no vascular channels are present in the epiphyses.

---

*NOTE: All specimens are from spontaneous abortions because no therapeutic abortions are permitted in our Catholic institution.

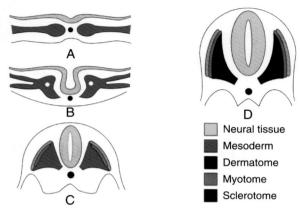

Neural tissue
Mesoderm
Dermatome
Myotome
Sclerotome

FIG 112.1 Trilaminar Disk (A) The neural tube closes. The mesoderm differentiates into dermatome (B) myotome (C), and sclerotome (D). (From Staheli L: Growth. In Staheli L (ed): *Practice of pediatric orthopedics*, Philadelphia, 2001, Lippincott Williams & Wilkins.)

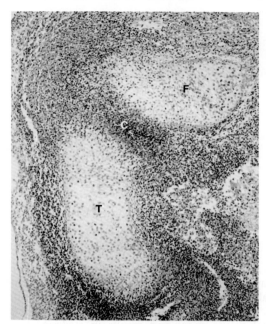

FIG 112.3 Embryo 117N, 6 weeks old, Streeter stage 17, sagittal section (see the text). *C,* Cavitation; *F,* femur; *T,* tibia (Goldner, ×100).

	Age (wks)	Size (mm)	Shape	Form	Bones	Muscles	Nerves
Embryo			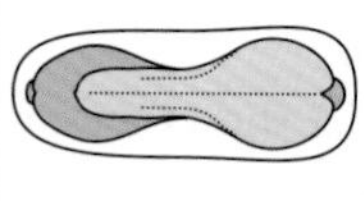	Trilaminar notochord			Neural plate
			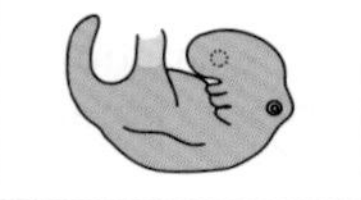	Limb buds	Sclerotomes	Somites	Neural tube
			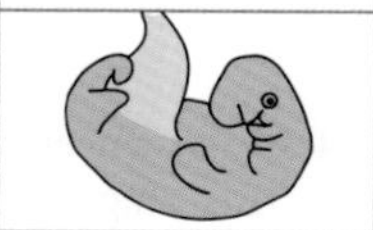	Hand plate	Mesenchyme condenses	Premuscle	
		12	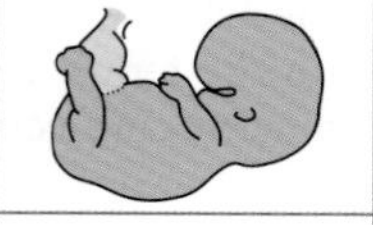	Digits	Chondrification	Fusion myotomes	
		17	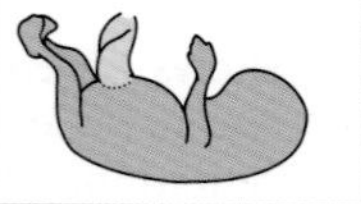	Limbs rotate	Early ossification	Differentiation	
		23	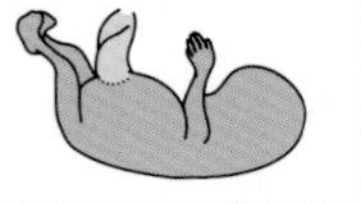	Fingers separate		Definite muscles	Cord equals vertebral length
Fetus	12	156	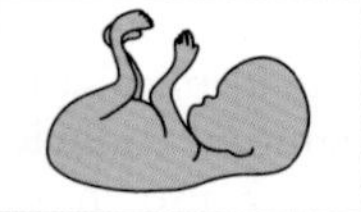	Sex determined	Ossification spreading		
	16	112	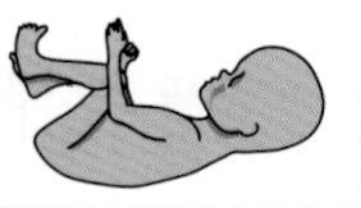	Face human	Joint cavities	Spontaneous activity	
	20 40	160–350	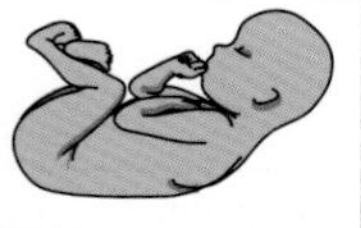	Body more proportional			Myelin sheath forms; cord ends L3

FIG 112.2 Prenatal Development This chart summarizes musculoskeletal development during embryonic and fetal life. (From Staheli L: Growth. In Staheli L (ed): *Practice of pediatric orthopedics*, Philadelphia, PA, 2001, Lippincott Williams & Wilkins.)

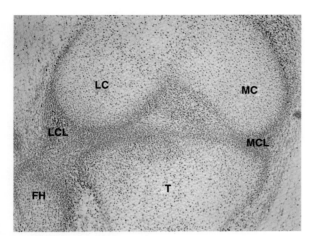

FIG 112.4 Embryo 123N, 7 weeks old, Streeter stage 19, frontal section (see the text). *FH,* Fibular head; *LC,* lateral femoral condyle; *LCL,* lateral collateral ligament; *MC,* medial femoral condyle; *MCL,* medial collateral ligament; *T,* tibia (Azan, ×100).

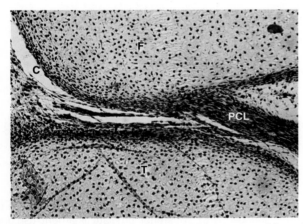

FIG 112.5 Embryo 50N, 8 weeks old, Streeter stage 23, sagittal section (see the text). *C,* Area of cavitation; *F,* femur; *PCL,* posterior cruciate ligament; *T,* tibia (Azan, ×100).

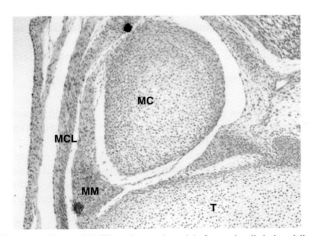

FIG 112.6 Fetus HHF2, 10 weeks old, frontal, slightly oblique section going through the posterior part of the medial compartment (see the text). *MC,* Medial femoral condyle; *MCL,* medial collateral ligament; *MM,* medial meniscus; *T,* tibia (Azan, ×100).

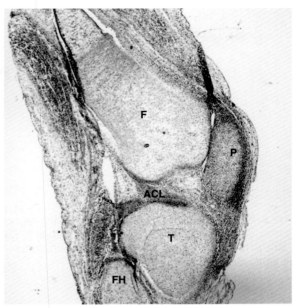

FIG 112.7 Fetus HKSAG3, 10 weeks old, sagittal section (see the text). *ACL,* Anterior cruciate ligament; *F,* femur; *FH,* fibular head; *T,* tibia; *P,* patella (Goldner, ×20).

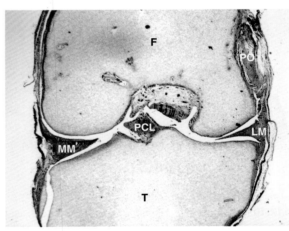

FIG 112.8 Fetus HK24F, 12.5 weeks old, frontal section (see the text). *F,* Femur; *LM,* lateral meniscus; *MM,* medial meniscus; *PCL,* posterior cruciate ligament; *PO,* popliteus muscle; *T,* tibia (Goldner, ×20).

Week 12.5

Fig. 112.8 shows a fetus at 12.5 weeks old. A dense layer of cells covers the articular surfaces of the femur and tibia. Lateral to the lateral femoral condyle, the popliteus muscle is seen. Both menisci are well formed. Vessels are present at their periphery. Vascular channels are present in the femoral epiphysis. The posterior cruciate ligament inserts into the tibia.

Week 15.5

Fig. 112.9 shows a fetus at 15.5 weeks old. The much longer lateral facet of the patella helps to distinguish it from the medial facet. The lateral retinaculum is much denser than the medial retinaculum.

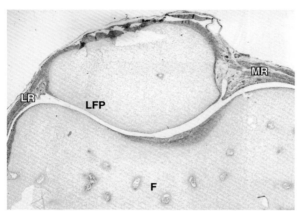

FIG 112.9 Fetus 130N, HKFr, 15.5 weeks old, frontal section going through the patellofemoral joint (see the text). *F*, Femur; *LFP*, lateral facet of the patella; *LR*, lateral retinaculum; *MR*, medial retinaculum (Azan, ×20).

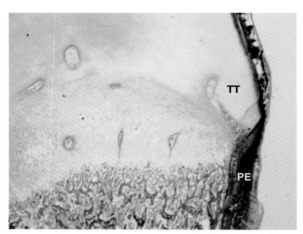

FIG 112.11 Fetus 73N, 18 weeks old, sagittal section (see the text). *PE*, Periosteum; *TT*, tibial tuberosity (Goldner, ×20).

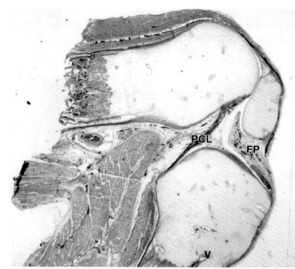

FIG 112.10 Fetus 147N, HKSag, 16.5 weeks old, sagittal section (see the text). *FP*, Infrapatellar fat pad; *PCL*, posterior cruciate ligament; *V*, blood vessels (Goldner, ×5).

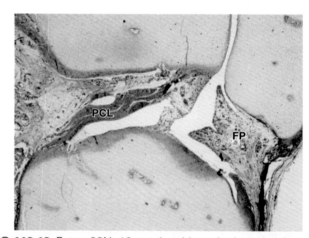

FIG 112.12 Fetus 28N, 19 weeks old, sagittal section (see the text). *FP*, Fat pad; *PCL*, posterior cruciate ligament (Goldner, ×20).

Week 19

Fig. 112.12 shows a fetus at 19 weeks old. Intra-articular tissues at the level of the intercondylar notch are visible in the figure. The fat pad is well developed. The posterior cruciate ligament is extra-articular.

Week 20

Fig. 112.13 shows a fetus at 20 weeks old. Although vessels are seen at the periphery of the MM, no vascular structures can be identified at its inner border.

Fig. 112.14 also shows a fetus at 20 weeks old. The enchondral ossification of the tibia has almost reached its final destination between the metaphysis and epiphysis. Ossification of the TT occurs late and is a postnatal event.[28,37] Strong collagenous tissue binds this apophysis to the PE of the tibia.

Week 16.5

Fig. 112.10 shows a fetus at 16.5 weeks old. The ossification processes that started in the diaphyses of the femur and tibia are progressing toward the metaphyses. At this stage, blood vessels still cross the growth plate. The suprapatellar bursa extends under the quadriceps muscle. The posterior cruciate ligament originates in the intercondylar fossa and infrapatellar fat pad.

Week 18

Fig. 112.11 shows a fetus at 18 weeks old. The formation of the tibial tuberosity (TT) that had started at 14 weeks has continued to separate this apophysis from the tibial epiphysis as a result of an advancing ingrowth of vessels. A thick periosteum (PE) spans from the tuberosity to the tibial metaphysis.

Week 40 (Full Term)

Fig. 112.15 shows the knee of a full-term specimen. Rich vascularity is present at the base of the meniscus. The MM is attached to the medial collateral ligament (not separate).

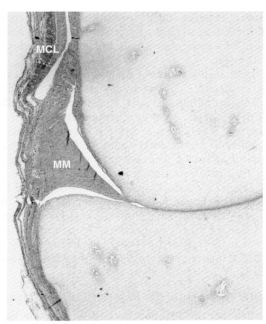

FIG 112.13 Fetus 132N, HKF, 20 weeks old, frontal section of the medial compartment (see the text). *MCL*, Medial collateral ligament; *MM*, medial meniscus (Azan, ×20).

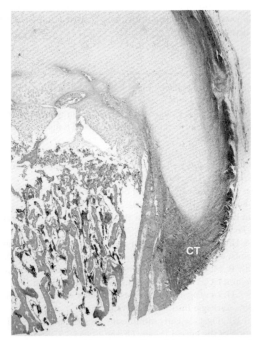

FIG 112.14 Fetus 116N, 20 weeks old, sagittal section at the level of the TT (see the text). *CT*, Collagenous tissue (Azan, ×20).

EMBRYOLOGIC DEVELOPMENT OF VARIANTS AND SPECIFIC ABNORMALITIES

Discoid Lateral Meniscus

Discoid lateral meniscus initially was believed to be a failure of the embryologic degeneration of the center of the meniscus[39]; however, this subsequently was shown not to be the case.[14] It is

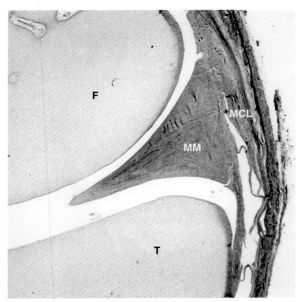

FIG 112.15 Fetus A10917, term, frontal section showing the MM (see the text). *F*, Femur; *MCL*, medial collateral ligament; *MM*, medial meniscus; *T*, tibia (Goldner, ×20).

now known that the lateral meniscus is semilunar in shape from its earliest development.[10,15,18,35,46] Although some discoid menisci (Wrisberg type 1) may be caused by abnormal meniscal attachments, because discoid menisci have been reported in very young children, the condition is likely the result of early development.[1,25]

Morphometric analyses have revealed that in the developing meniscus, the proportion of the area of meniscus to that of plateau is consistently higher in the lateral, compared with the medial, side.[9] Similarly the layered structure of fibers developed earlier in the lateral meniscus than in the medial. The differential development of the lateral and medial sides of the meniscus may be involved in the early development of discoid meniscus.

Congenital Dislocation of the Knee

First described in the early 1800s,[4,34] congenital dislocation of the knee now can be diagnosed in the prenatal period using ultrasound.[6] Although congenital dislocation is seen frequently in association with other hereditary conditions (e.g., Larsen syndrome), it is not believed to be genetic.[5,13,16,19] Uhthoff and Ogata[47] have reported congenital dislocation in a fetus of 19.5 weeks' gestation (Fig. 112.16).

Fig. 112.16 shows a fetus at 19.5 weeks old. This fetus presented with a bilateral (congenital) dislocation of the knee accompanied by rotation. Not only is the knee in hyperextension, but also the tibia is displaced anteriorly; it rides on the anterior surface of the femur. The joint cavity barely reaches under the patella. An unusually strong component of fibrous tissue is noted in the quadriceps muscle.

Multiple causative theories involving intrauterine events have been proposed, including abnormal fetal position of hyperextension,[38] congenital absence of the cruciate ligaments,[16] fibrosis of quadriceps,[22] and intrauterine ischemia causing compartment syndrome–like fibrosis.[7] It has not always been possible to separate cause and effect, but these findings are most likely to be secondary adaptive changes.[47]

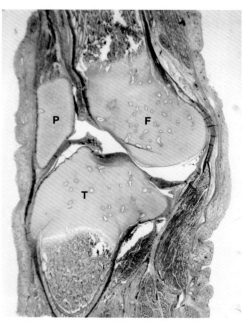

FIG 112.16 Fetus 71N, 19.5 weeks old, sagittal section (see the text). *F,* Femur; *P,* patella; *T,* tibia (Azan, ×5).

Bipartite Patella

Bipartite patella is a phenomenon of secondary ossification and probably a postnatal event.

Synovial Plica

The embryonic knee is partitioned into suprapatellar, medial, and lateral compartments by synovial septa.[21] Synovial plicae are regarded as remnants of the divisions between these compartments that were present in the knee during embryologic development.[32] Although more typically seen in adults than children, residual synovial plicae have been noted in the fetus between 11 and 20 weeks of gestation (see Fig. 112.6).[27]

The suprapatellar plica can be explained as a septum between the suprapatellar bursa and patellofemoral cavitation. The infrapatellar plica may be considered a septum of the medial and lateral femorotibial cavitations. The mediopatellar plica is not a remnant of a septum of a distinct compartment present during the developmental stage but probably constitutes a remnant of mesenchymal tissue caused by developmental circumstances.[27]

Patellofemoral Instability and Congenital Dislocation of the Patella

Recurrent dislocation of the patella usually is caused by lateral malalignment of the quadriceps mechanism. Associated contributing factors, including ligamentous laxity, lateral soft tissue

contractures, external tibial torsion, shallow intercondylar notch of the femur, trochlear dysplasia, patella alta, and vastus medialis insufficiency, play a role but mainly develop in the postnatal period.

In congenital dislocation of the patella, the patella is dislocated at birth and there is usually deformity of the knee. Although the condition has been reported within families,[24] it also is seen in association with other conditions, most notably arthrogryposis and Down syndrome.[17] Stanisavljevic et al.[42] have suggested that dislocation occurs during the first trimester as a result of failure of medial rotation of the myotome that contains the quadriceps mechanism.

Both patellar retinacula can be recognized in the fetus by 9.5 weeks. The lateral retinaculum is dense and fibrous, whereas the medial retinaculum is loosely arranged. The patella is not completely centered in the femoral groove and tends to ride more laterally. These two features may predispose to lateral tracking or dislocation of the patella or both (see Fig. 112.9).[8]

Congenital Absence of the Anterior Cruciate Ligament

The exact timing of the appearance of the cruciate ligaments differs among authors.[20,33] Although typically described in association with congenital dislocation of the knee, congenital absence of the anterior cruciate ligament also has been reported as an isolated finding.[11] Associations with other abnormalities include congenital short femur,[2,12] congenital absence of the meniscus,[44] congenital ring menisci,[3,26] and thrombocytopenic absent radius syndrome.[36,45]

KEY REFERENCES

3. Basmajian JV: A ring-shaped medial semi-lunar cartilage. *J Bone Joint Surg Br* 34:638–639, 1952.
5. Curtis BH, Fisher RL: Congenital hyperextension with anterior subluxation of the knee. Surgical treatment and long-term observations. *J Bone Joint Surg Am* 51:255–269, 1969.
8. Finnegan M, Uhthoff H: The development of the knee. In Uhthoff HK, editor: *The embryology of the human locomotor system*, New York, NY, 1990, Springer-Verlag, pp 129–140.
10. Gardner E, O'Rahilly R: The early development of the knee joint in staged human embryos. *J Anat* 102:289–299, 1968.
13. Johnson E, Audell R, Oppenheim WL: Congenital dislocation of the knee. *J Pediatr Orthop* 7:194–200, 1987.
27. Ogata S, Uhthoff HK: The development of synovial plicae in human knee joints: an embryologic study. *Arthroscopy* 6:315–321, 1990.
30. O'Rahilly R, Muller F: *Developmental stages in human embryos*, Washington, DC, 1987, Carnegie Institute of Washington.
43. Streeter GH: *Developmental horizons in human embryos*, Washington, DC, 1951, Carnegie Institution of Washington.
47. Uhthoff HK, Ogata S: Early intrauterine presence of congenital dislocation of the knee. *J Pediatr Orthop* 14:254–257, 1994.

The references for this chapter can also be found on www.expertconsult.com.

113

Congenital Deformities of the Knee

Charles E. Johnston II

Congenital deformities of the knee include hyperextension and flexion deformities at birth whose severity at first glance may appear to be incompatible with functional ambulation. Except for patellar dislocation, which may not be apparent at birth, these deformities differ from acquired or developmental angular, torsional, or internal derangement problems in that they are usually obvious in the newborn. Once the diagnosis is made and the prognosis defined, rational early treatment can significantly improve the outlook for functional ambulation. This chapter describes and reviews treatment options for these relatively rare but dramatic congenital knee abnormalities.

CONGENITAL DISLOCATION OF THE KNEE

Few orthopedic birth abnormalities are as dramatic and obvious as congenital dislocation of the knee (CDK; Fig. 113.1A). Inexperienced observers may describe the extremity as having the knee on backward because of the unstable excessive hyperextension combined with an element of angular deformity. CDK is rare, being only about 1% as common as congenital hip dislocation.[28] Even if the milder form of congenital hyperextension deformity is included as CDK, the incidence is still less than 0.1%.[8] It can be diagnosed prenatally by ultrasound.[15]

Clinically, the hyperextension deformity is unmistakable, with the femoral condyles often being prominent on the posterior distal thigh. The foot may present at the baby's face or shoulders, and this marked hyperflexion of the hip (see Fig. 113.1B), reflecting the positioning in utero,[48] raises the suspicion of concomitant congenital hip instability. Radiographically, the relationship between the distal femur and proximal tibia should be determined on a true lateral radiograph of the knee, defining that relationship as hyperextended, subluxated, or dislocated (Fig. 113.2). Next, the degree of passive flexion of the knee is important to determine prognosis; a knee that will flex and reduce with gentle stretching of the quadriceps can be immediately classified as grade 1 congenital hyperextension.[10,39] On the other hand, any flexion of the knee may be impossible, and the tibia, which is anteriorly translated in the resting position, may subluxate laterally on the femur when more vigorous flexion is attempted, indicating a grade 3 irreducible dislocation (Fig. 113.3). The latter is always associated with significant quadriceps fibrosis and shortening, which may be the cause of the deformity.[43] An intermediate degree of contracture, a grade 2 subluxation, may be noted when the knee will not flex beyond neutral extension, but the femoral and tibial epiphyses are in contact and do not subluxate readily when flexion is attempted.

Equally important at the initial evaluation is the search for associated anomalies and syndromes. Ipsilateral hip dysplasia and clubfoot are present 70% and 50% of the time, respectively,[5,29] with other anomalies of the upper extremity, face, gastrointestinal (GI), and genitourinary (GU) systems not uncommon. *Bilateral* CDK is almost always syndromic, most commonly associated with laxity syndromes such as Larsen, Beals, or Ehlers-Danlos syndrome. Neurologic conditions, such as arthrogryposis or spinal dysraphism, may have bilateral CDK, or may have one extended (dislocated) knee and one with a flexion deformity. *Unilateral* CDK is most often a teratologic, stiff dislocation related to abnormal fetal position (see Fig. 113.1B). In the teratologic or neurologic types, quadriceps fibrosis and atrophy develop when the knee cannot move and the muscle shortens in the extended position. Hypoplasia of the patella and contracture of the iliotibial band probably result from the same lack of joint and muscle movement.

Ligamentous laxity, with elongation, insufficiency, or absence of the cruciate ligaments, has long been known as a complicating feature of CDK,[4,10,32,50] although it has been downplayed in importance in some reports.[5,55] Cruciate absence is actually typical of bilateral, syndromic cases (see Fig. 113.3D), and should be addressed as part of the comprehensive surgical management (see the following section). Conversely, nonsyndromic CDK (with or without ipsilateral hip or foot deformity) is often unilateral, and once reduced, the knee is relatively stable (anterior cruciate ligament [ACL] present), and thus can been termed *stiff CDK* as opposed to the lax syndromic variety.

Other pathologic findings in grade 3 CDK include anterior subluxation of the posterolateral and posteromedial periarticular tissues, including hamstring tendons and the iliotibial (IT) band, because of the chronic hyperextension and anterior translation of the tibia on the femur (Fig. 113.4).[5,10,29,64] The suprapatellar pouch may be atrophic or obliterated, with adhesions between the hypoplastic patella and the femur and IT band. These intra-articular abnormalities will need to be addressed surgically in the irreducible CDK.

Treatment

Nonoperative Management. Nonoperative treatment should begin as soon as possible in infancy. After determining the radiographic position (see Fig. 113.2A), initial flexibility of the quadriceps contracture is assessed by applying gentle traction to the tibia and attempting flexion of the knee.[34] The tibia, if anteriorly located, engages the distal femur and translates posteriorly with traction and, as the knee is flexed, a stable articulation can be palpated. In simple hyperextension cases, this may be readily achievable and usually maintained with an anterior plaster slab or a long-leg cast. The latter is actually

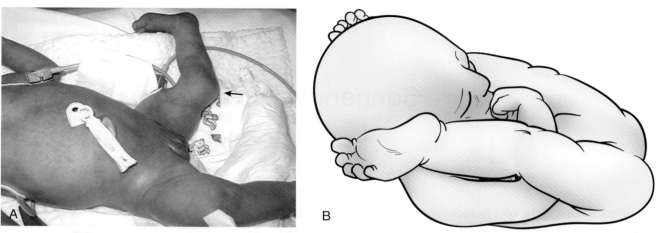

FIG 113.1 (A) Left CDK in a newborn. The femoral condyles in the popliteal fossa are prominent *(arrow)*. (B) Typical intrauterine position associated with CDK, hyperflexion of hips with hyperextended knees. (Redrawn from Niebauer JJ, King D: Congenital dislocation of the knee. *J Bone Joint Surg Am* 42:207, 1960.)

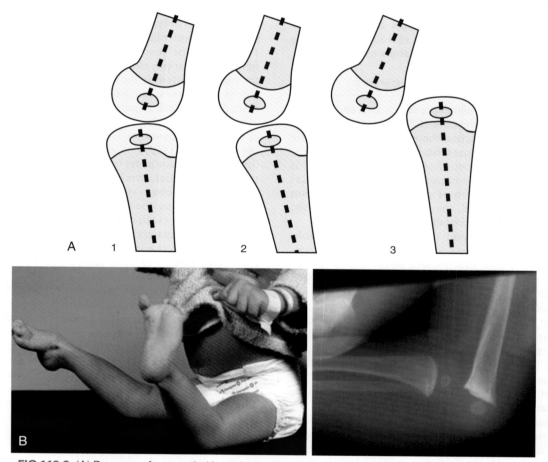

FIG 113.2 (A) Degrees of congenital knee instability: *1*, hyperextension; *2*, subluxation; *3*, dislocation. (B) Clinical and radiographic views of a grade 3 dislocation.

more difficult to apply in the infant and maintain reduction. Obviously, forceful manipulation is contraindicated because of risk of pressure damage to cartilaginous epiphyses or fracture-separation of the proximal tibial physis (Fig. 113.5).[59] Serial manipulations and splinting in increasing flexion proceed until

the knee will flex more than 90 degrees, at which time a removable plastic splint can be used to maintain reduction while allowing some active motion. Alternatively, if the patient also has an ipsilateral CDK, knee flexion can be maintained in a Pavlik harness while the hip is simultaneously addressed.

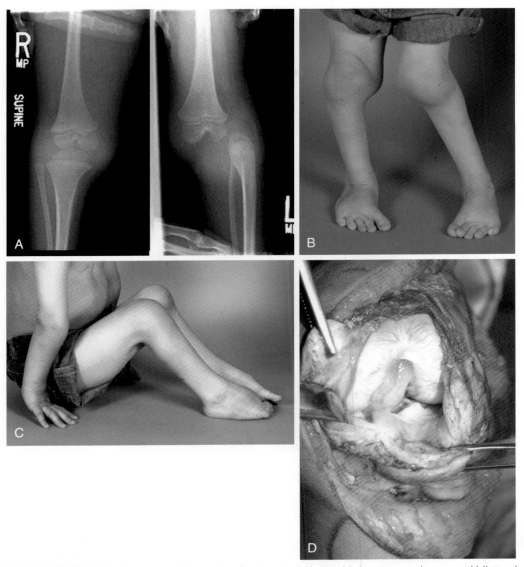

FIG 113.3 (A) Anteroposterior radiographs of a 3-year-old boy with Larsen syndrome and bilateral CDK. (B) Clinical appearance, grade 3 dislocation on the left. (C) The right knee reduces with flexion, grade 1 (see Fig. 113.14). (D) The ACL is congenitally absent.

In knees with more severe quadriceps contracture preventing effective gradual flexion, femoral nerve block or botulinum toxin can been effective. Botox injection of the quadriceps has the added advantage of longer-term paralysis of the quadriceps, allowing gradual stretching to occur with daily physical therapy even when initial flexibility seemed unfavorable for nonoperative reduction (Fig. 113.6). Recent experience has confirmed that a trial of nonoperative management, with or without adjunctive neuromuscular blockade, is appropriate initial treatment in infants up to 12 months of age.

Surgical Management. Surgical treatment is indicated for cases not responding to nonoperative means, and has been advocated for infants as early as 6 months of age.[4,5] Although earlier reduction of the knee may provide greater potential for remodeling of articular surfaces, patients as old as 4 years have had successful initial reduction, and patients as old as 16 years have had late gross instability with reducible but recurrent dislocation

addressed. Considering the current use of femoral shortening to achieve reduction (see the following section), the earliest age for surgery should be when the surgeon thinks that the femur is robust enough to accept meaningful internal fixation to stabilize a shortening osteotomy.

Reduction and flexion with femoral shortening. Classic surgical treatment of CDK has invariably used extensive V-Y quadriceps tendon lengthening (Fig. 113.7; see Fig. 113.4) to gain flexion, and hence reduction, of the joint. Outcomes of such lengthenings are poorly documented in many series, because simple documentation of reduction and reporting the passive range of motion is the extent of the recorded information. Because many patients have other anomalies and comorbidities affecting outcome, the functional results of the knees themselves have rarely been reported. Extensive lengthening invariably leads to weakness and an extensor lag, and the extensive dissection required to obtain such length produces additional fibrosis, limiting flexion. Finally, wound healing over the anterior knee

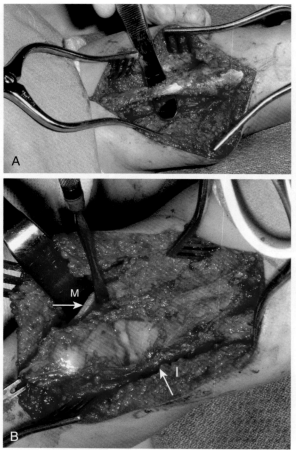

FIG 113.4 (A) Contracted quadriceps tendon prior to V-Y lengthening (not recommended during open reduction). The hip is to the right. (B) Medial hamstrings *(M)* and IT band *(I)* are subluxated anterior to the distal femur (note physis). The patella has been reflected distally with the quadriceps tendon.

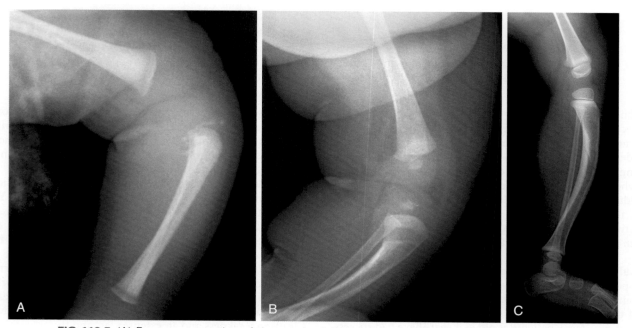

FIG 113.5 (A) Fracture-separation of the proximal tibial epiphysis in a 2-week-old infant initially with a hyperextended knee. (B) Healed fracture at age 4 months. The limb was splinted in the degree of flexion obtained in (A). (C) Residual antecurvatum deformity with otherwise normal growth of the tibia, age 3 years.

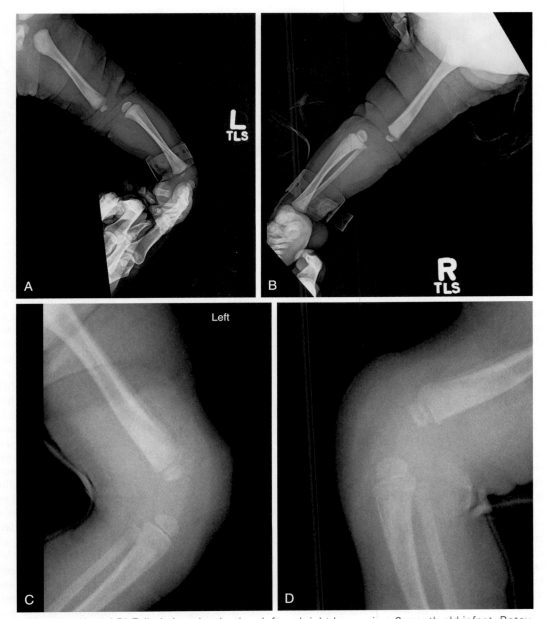

FIG 113.6 (A and B) Failed closed reduction, left and right knees, in a 2-month-old infant. Botox injections to the quadriceps bilaterally, twice at 1-month intervals with daily manipulations, were carried out. (C and D) Full flexion-reduction was achieved 2 months later.

surface is compromised because of tension produced by the flexion stretching the contracted anterior skin (see Fig. 113.7C).

In addition to the quadricepsplasty, arthrotomy must be performed to mobilize the anteriorly subluxated medial and lateral periarticular structures and allow them to relocate to their normal anatomic position as the knee is flexed (see Fig. 113.4B). However, once the knee is reduced in flexion, the redundant posterior capsule resulting from that maneuver has rarely been addressed (by capsulorrhaphy), thus inviting a redislocation into the same incompetent posterior space. The rationale of this oversight can be easily appreciated if one considers that a late open reduction of a congenital hip dislocation would never be completed without performing a capsulorrhaphy to obliterate a potential space into which the femoral

head could redislocate. Thus, if the ACL is also congenitally absent in a CDK that is reduced without capsulorrhaphy, it is hardly surprising that chronic hyperlaxity-instability of the knee at a minimum, and frank redislocation at the other extreme, would be the common outcome of knees treated by such an approach, especially with flexion limited by the scarred fibrotic quadriceps muscle.

As a result, we have abandoned V-Y quadricepsplasty as the primary treatment in favor of femoral shortening to minimize quadriceps dissection and weakening (Fig. 113.8). Acute femoral shortening decompresses the anterior skin and allows knee flexion without surgical lengthening of the muscle. The operative procedure begins with a lateral parapatellar arthrotomy incision that is extended proximally along the lateral femur to

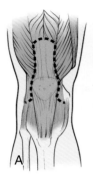 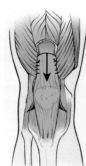 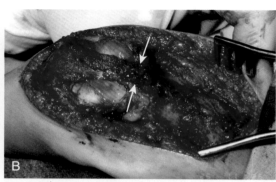 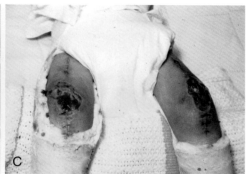

FIG 113.7 (A) Classic V-Y quadricepsplasty. (B) The resulting repair of the quadriceps tendon *(arrows)* is tenuous at best because of the extensive lengthening required to gain knee reduction (same patient as in Fig. 113.4). (C) Wound dehiscence-slough as a result of skin necrosis from knee flexion. ([A] From Curtis B, Fisher R: Congenital hyperextension with anterior subluxation of the knee; surgical treatment and long-term observations. *J Bone Joint Surg Am* 41:255, 1969.)

allow division and mobilization of the distal contracted lateral tissues (IT band, released from its distal insertion, and vastus lateralis from intermuscular septum) and provide subperiosteal access to the supracondylar region for the bone shortening (Fig. 113.9). The quadriceps tendon, patella, and patellar tendon are mobilized (skeletonized) as a continuous longitudinal structure via a medial arthrotomy to allow sharp dissection and elevation of medial periarticular structures (pes tendons), which are subluxated anteriorly. The intercondylar notch is inspected for the presence or absence of the anterior cruciate ligament. Once the femur is acutely shortened and plated—usually approximately 2.0 to 2.5 cm is removed—the knee will usually reduce with flexion, and the only repair necessary is to stabilize the patellar mechanism in the intercondylar groove, generally by medial imbrication and advancement of the vastus medialis obliquus (see Fig. 113.9E and F). The lateral release is repaired only to the extent of covering the internal fixation.

Capsulorrhaphy is performed at the posterolateral corner of the lateral femoral condyle by bluntly dissecting the capsule, with the knee flexed, from the more superficial tissues with an elevator. The dissection is simplified once the IT band and vastus lateralis have been released and mobilized. The lateral side of the posterior capsule is imbricated proximal to the distal following excision of 1 to 1.5 cm of redundant patulous capsule (Fig. 113.10). Shortening of the hamstrings[4,5,29] may be done in conjunction with the capsulorrhaphy (and ACL reconstruction, if necessary; see the following section), but should not be considered a replacement for it.

The posteromedial capsulorrhaphy is performed through a separate 3- to 4-cm incision behind the medial femoral condyle (Fig. 113.11). This incision can be located by placing a blunt instrument from inside the arthrotomy to the posteromedial corner and cutting down on the instrument tenting the skin. The redundant capsule is dissected free of superficial tissues with the knee flexed, a segment excised, and the imbrication performed (see Fig. 113.11B-D). Following the medial-lateral capsulorrhaphies, the knee should lack 45 degrees or more from full extension; the patient will eventually stretch this iatrogenic flexion contracture in 4 to 6 months.

At this point, the knee must be assessed for ligamentous instability, especially using the anterior drawer test with the knee flexed, prior to tying the capsulorrhaphy sutures. If anterior drawer is unacceptable with the knee extended and

capsulorrhaphy sutures tensioned (but not tied), the ligament should be reconstructed, if not during this procedure, as a staged procedure later. If ACL competence is satisfactory, the wounds are closed and the knee casted in 45 to 60 degrees of flexion for 8 weeks, followed by gradual active range of motion exercises, with full extension limited by a brace for the first 4 months.

The long-term outcomes of seven patients (nine knees) who underwent surgical correction of CDK, have been determined by functional outcome assessment (Lysholm knee questionnaire, Pediatric Outcomes Data Collection Instrument [PODCI]) and three-dimensional kinematic and kinetic gait evaluation.[49] The patients were evaluated as a group and compared based on surgical approach (femoral shortening vs. V-Y quadricepsplasty) at an average of 12-year follow-up. A fairly normal total arc of knee motion (112 degrees) was found, with only one patient from each group demonstrating an extensor lag. Although not statistically significant, the femoral shortening group did demonstrate a better range of motion and Lysholm knee scores when compared with the V-Y quadricepsplasty group. Gait analysis of these patients demonstrated that they walked with more flexion during stance and achieved less peak knee flexion during swing as compared with normal controls (Fig. 113.12). Comparison of the gait between the patients with femoral shortening and V-Y quadricepsplasty showed minor differences in the sagittal plane of the knee, which were consistent with increased stiffness in the quadriceps muscle in the V-Y quadricepsplasty group (Fig. 113.13). Because of the small number of patients, caution must be used in drawing definitive conclusions, but overall it does appear that patients treated surgically for CDK maintain functionality fairly well, with femoral shortening providing improved knee motion and self-reported knee function as compared with V-Y quadricepsplasty.

Anterior cruciate ligament reconstruction. ACL reconstruction in a young child is controversial, but in an unpublished review of 22 knees (14 patients) treated at our institution, with up to 15-year follow-up, the 9 knees that underwent reduction by V-Y quadricepsplasty and no ligament reconstruction were uniformly unstable, had poor quadriceps strength, and required full-time bracing or assistive devices (crutches, wheelchair) for community ambulation. Of these nine unsatisfactory knees, eight were in patients with laxity syndromes (predominantly

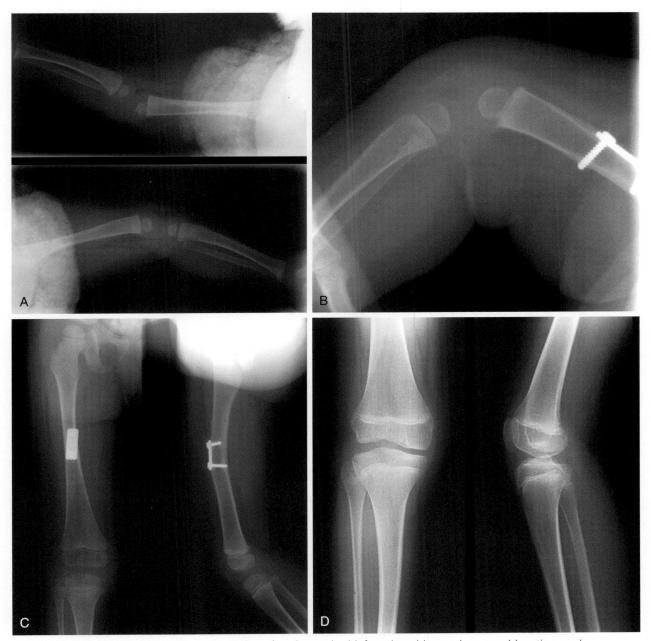

FIG 113.8 (A) Lateral radiographs of a 6-month-old female with persistent subluxation and inadequate flexion. (B) Four months following limited open reduction (no quadriceps tendon lengthening) with femoral shortening. (C) Three years postoperatively. (D) Twelve years postoperatively. Range of motion is 5 to 70 degrees of flexion, with normal quadriceps strength. Note the hypoplastic patella. She is completely asymptomatic other than the limited flexion.

Larsen). The instability was dramatic in that unbraced knees dislocated in the extended position (Fig. 113.14) and, even with bracing, were still unstable, although they were usually capable of weight bearing. As a result of this review, an attempt to reconstruct the ACL-deficient knee in the laxity syndrome group seemed justified in an attempt to improve the uniformly unacceptable results of the earlier cases.

Historically there has been reluctance to attempt intra-articular ACL reconstruction in children, because of fear of physeal injury producing deformity and growth arrest from transphyseal procedures. These concerns are gradually relenting

because clinical and experimental studies have shown that this risk may be overplayed. Options include transphyseal and physeal-sparing techniques. Although drilling an anchoring hole across any physis potentially risks injury, the practice of placing smooth pins across physes for periarticular and physeal trauma is well accepted, especially if the fixation is temporary. Logically, a smooth, centrally placed hole across a physis that is filled with a nonosseous (e.g., tendon) material is no more likely to produce growth disturbance than temporary pin fixation because it is an interposition material. Animal[23,61] and clinical studies[52] using hamstrings, IT band, or patellar tendon as

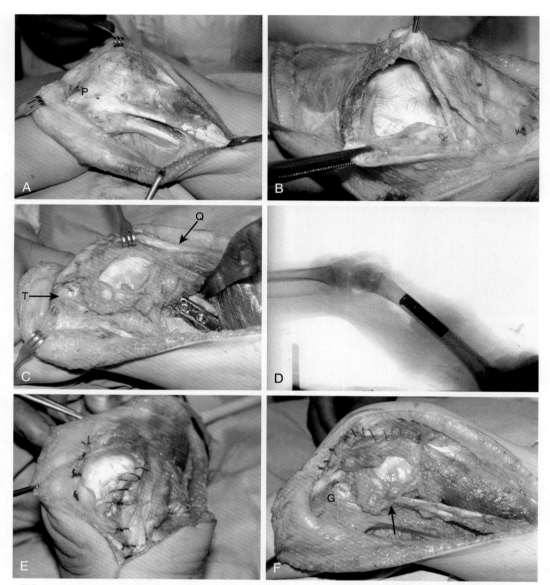

FIG 113.9 (A) Lateral knee, distal femoral exposure. The tibia is dislocated posterolaterally (same patient as in Fig. 113.3, left knee). The IT band and biceps are seen prior to release of the former from its insertion. Anteriorly, the patellar tendon is marked. (B) Medial arthrotomy. The vastus medialis and medial retinaculum are being separated from the quadriceps tendon (inferior clamp). (C) The femur has been shortened and plated. The tibia *(T)* now reduces under direct vision. The quadriceps mechanism *(Q)* is in continuity. (D) Intraoperative radiograph confirming reduction. (E) Anterior view of advancement-imbrication of vastus medialis to hold patella centralized (medial to right). (F) Lateral view of the imbrication. No attempt has been made to close the lateral arthrotomy. The vastus lateralis covers the plate. Posterolateral capsulorrhaphy has been performed deep to the IT band, which has been reattached to the posterolateral condyle *(arrow)*. Reattachment to the Gerdy tubercle *(G)* is impossible and contraindicated.

transphyseal ligament reconstructions have achieved knee stability without limb length or angular deformity.

The pes anserine tendons are conveniently used for ACL reconstruction by physis-sparing or physis-crossing techniques.[2,40,52,54] In the former, the tendon(s) are left attached at their insertion, detached proximally in the posteromedial thigh, pulled distally and rerouted superficially over the anterior tibial surface, passed under the transverse meniscal ligament to penetrate the knee joint, and passed through the intercondylar notch and over the top of the lateral femoral condyle to be anchored to bone and lateral intermuscular septum (Fig. 113.15A). To place such an ACL substitution closer to anatomic position, the tendon(s) may be passed through a transphyseal drill hole exiting the tibial articular surface at the normal ACL insertion point (see Fig. 113.15B). This method is currently our treatment of choice, regardless of patient age. A 6-mm drill hole

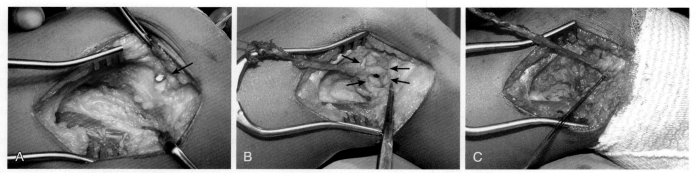

FIG 113.10 (A) Exposure of posterolateral capsule (hip to left). A Freer elevator *(arrow)* has been inserted through the anterior arthrotomy to localize the site of capsular incision. (B) Excision of posterolateral capsule (*arrows* indicating capsule edges) with semitendinosus graft inserted through capsular window. (C) Completed posterolateral capsulorrhaphy.

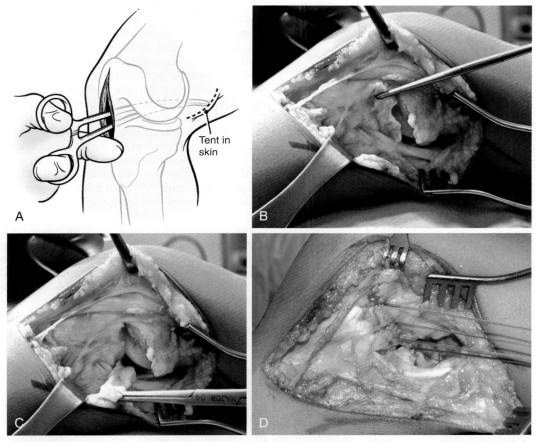

FIG 113.11 (A) Skin incision for the posteromedial capsulorrhaphy. (B) Exposure of posteromedial joint with posteriomedial arthrotomy. (C) Excision of redundant capsule (in clamp). (D) Completed capsulorrhaphy.

has proven technically adequate and noninjurious, with the tendons again anchored over the top of the lateral femoral condyle after traversing the notch. In either technique, care in drilling or passing tendons near the tibial tubercle is most important, because this part of the physis seems most vulnerable. For the same reason, use of the patellar tendon as a ligament substitution is not recommended because of the dissection near this portion of the physis. Several small series[2,40,54] have reported restoration of stability, as documented by KT-1000

instrumentation, improvement in Lachman test, and return to previous levels of sport, without physeal injury in immature patients followed up to 5 years.

An alternative ACL reconstruction involves the use of the IT band in a combined intra-articular and extra-articular technique (see Figs. 113.9 and 113.15C). This method, a modification of the procedure described by McIntosh and Darby, has been popularized by Kocher et al.[35] The technique involves rerouting a central slip of IT band, which is left attached distally to the Gerdy tubercle, in an over-the-top position. The tendon is sutured to the lateral femoral condyle to secure its position and routed through the intracondylar notch. The tendon can then exit the knee in the over-the-front position under the transverse meniscal ligament or it can be routed through a more

anatomically positioned drill hole through the tibial articular surface, as described earlier. Good results were reported with this technique in their series of 44 skeletally immature patients, with a 95% graft survival at an average follow-up of 5.3 years. If this technique is used in a child with CDK, it may be helpful to use the anterior third instead of the middle third of the IT band for the reconstruction. This minor modification would allow the most anterior aspect of the IT band to be detached, eliminating this deforming structure of the knee dislocation.

We have previously used the IT band transfer rerouted through the intercondylar notch, as described by Insall and associates.[27,58,65] It is readily detached from the Gerdy tubercle during the approach described for the open reduction of the knee (see Figs. 113.9 and 113.15D), and mobilized proximally to be passed antegrade over the top of the lateral femoral condyle and through the notch prior to completing the capsulorrhaphy. The tubed tendon is anchored in the proximal tibia through a drill hole within the epiphysis (see Fig. 113.15E), and is tensioned prior to wound closure with the tibia in maximum posterior drawer and the suture tied over a button on the anterior tibial skin or over a suture staple in the tibial metaphysis. The drill hole should be placed with radiographic control to minimize the possibility of oblique transphyseal placement; the tunnel must include the ossification center to provide tendon-to-bone anchorage. Alternative transphyseal placement through a more vertical, centrally placed tunnel can be attempted if enough tendon length is available. The postoperative care is the same as for the knee reduction procedure.

The advantage of the Insall technique, as opposed to other ACL substitution procedures in which the IT band is rerouted as a passive restraint,[44,47] is that it is an active transfer in which only the insertion of the tendon is rerouted. The structure being transferred is also a deforming force maintaining the CDK in the first place, so its rerouting should be beneficial. In any case, it will be dissected and mobilized as part of the open reduction-shortening procedure. The disadvantage of the antegrade transfer is poor maintenance of adequate anchorage of the insertion in a diminutive, mostly cartilaginous tibial epiphysis. This has been noted visually in two cases of revision performed for recurrent anterior instability, in which the IT band insertion was severely attenuated 2 to 3 years after the initial transfer. Also, this transfer

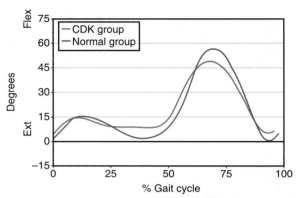

FIG 113.12 Gait Plot for the Sagittal Plane of the Knee for the Normal Controls and CDK Group. *CDK,* Congenital dislocation of the knee.

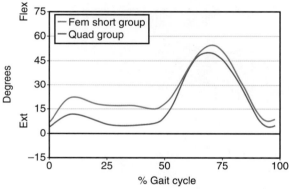

FIG 113.13 Gait Plot for the Sagittal Plane of the Knee for the Quadricepsplasty and Femoral Shortening Groups.

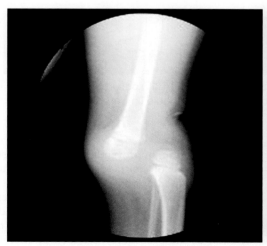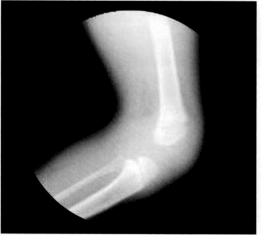

FIG 113.14 Right Knee of Patient in Fig. 113.3 Showing Dislocation in Extension and Reduction in Flexion.

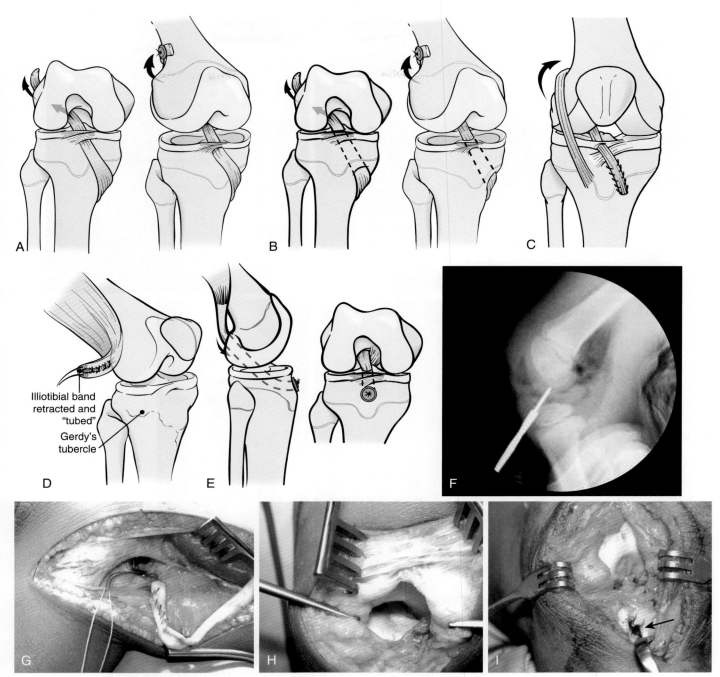

Illiotibial band retracted and "tubed"

Gerdy's tubercle

FIG 113.15 (A) Complete physeal-sparing ACL reconstruction using pes tendon(s). No drill holes cross any physes. (B) Transtibial physis reconstruction using pes tendon(s). (C) McIntosh ACL reconstruction using IT band. (D and E) Insall-type reconstruction using IT band, rerouted antegrade over the top of the femoral condyle, anchored within the proximal tibial epiphysis (physeal-sparing). (F) Intraoperative placement of epiphyseal tunnel for IT band transfer. A guide wire is placed entirely within the epiphysis, followed by cannulated drill. (G) Tubed IT band tendon ready for rerouting over the top of the lateral femoral condyle. (H) Congenital absence of ACL. (I) Transferred IT band has been anchored in epiphyseal hole *(arrow)* created in (E).

retains the possibility of physeal injury at the proximal tibia, a feared complication that has restrained the use of transphyseal ACL substitutions, except in adolescents nearing skeletal maturity. Three knees in two children younger than 5 years have undergone this reconstruction simultaneously with the index

open reduction procedure, with one physeal arrest (Fig. 113.16). This complication occurred in the first of bilateral reconstructions in a boy with Larsen syndrome, operated at age 18 months. He underwent the identical procedure on the second knee at age 3, with no physeal injury apparent at 9-year follow-up. The first

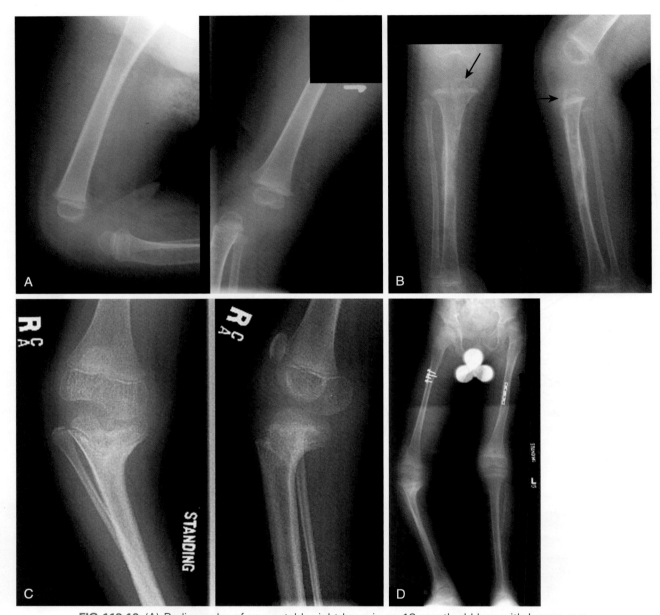

FIG 113.16 (A) Radiographs of an unstable right knee in an 18-month-old boy with Larsen syndrome after closed reduction of CDK. (B) Five months after ACL reconstruction using IT band (tunnel visible in epiphysis). A tibial diaphyseal bone graft had been harvested previously for a cervical fusion. (C and D) At age 12, a flexion-varus deformity has developed, subsequently corrected by osteotomy. No deformity is seen in the left knee, which had an identical procedure performed at age 3.

side eventually developed a varus-flexion deformity, corrected uneventfully by a simple open wedge proximal tibia osteotomy at age 12. Both knees are painless and stable, with 0- to 120-degree range of motion and normal quadriceps strength. The third knee in the series, in a second child with fibular hemimelia, is stable and painless, and the patient actively runs and plays using a Syme amputation prosthesis on the operated side. Although other investigators[47] have reported satisfactory stability without physeal injury using this technique in older children (age 12 years), the combined problems of gradual stretching out of the insertion and possibility of physeal injury has led us to favor transphyseal hamstring reconstruction

Summary

This imposing birth deformity should no longer present as a disabling or unreconstructable problem as a result of joint instability and quadriceps insufficiency. Early treatment (newborn) often succeeds in gaining closed reduction[55] and, with the use of adjunctive nerve block or Botox, even grade 3 dislocations can be successfully reduced nonoperatively. Late reduction in syndromic knees (after walking age) using femoral shortening and capsulorrhaphy and early ACL reconstruction, simultaneous with the open reduction or staged, can still provide a stable and functional outcome if the treatment approach described here is effectively applied. Although transphyseal ACL reconstruction will remain controversial, especially in children younger than 5 years undergoing CDK reduction, some form of ACL reconstruction is indicated to provide a functional knee to a patient with perhaps other syndromic orthopedic disabilities as well. The stability provided by the early ACL reconstruction is invaluable to the function of such syndromic patients and, should a physeal growth disturbance occur, it can always be reconstructed later by appropriate osteotomy and/or lengthening.

CONGENITAL DISLOCATION OF THE PATELLA

Patellofemoral instability is a common and well-known problem familiar to all orthopedists, and describes a continuum of deformities, which in the severest form is a congenital dislocation of the patella. This should be defined as a laterally displaced, hypoplastic patella, present at birth, diagnosed by age 10, associated with a flexion contracture of the knee and a valgus and external rotation deformity of the leg, and basically irreducible (fixed dislocation) by closed means.[16,62] The continuum or grades of congenital patellar dislocation and dysplasia are also described as recurrent, habitual, or obligatory dislocations,[14] in which the patella is sometimes reducible in extension but unstable in flexion, resuming its laterally displaced position as the knee is flexed (Fig. 113.17), because of a variety of soft tissue contractures and/or deficient lateral femoral condyle. Regardless, an attempt to discuss all grades and types of patellofemoral instability, such as those associated with adolescence, including developmental, rotational (miserable malalignment), and possibly traumatic causes, is beyond the scope of this chapter, which will limit the discussion to the irreducible or obligatory congenital lesion just described.

Clinical Features

Goldthwait[20] first described the surgical treatment of a permanent dislocation of the patella in 1899, and Conn[9] described the release of the contracted lateral soft tissues and advancement of the vastus medialis in 1925. However, the true cause and pathoanatomy for the dislocated patella was probably not described until Stanisavljevic et al.,[62] in 1976, described the failure of the internal rotation of the quadriceps myotome in the fetus. They noted that the laterally placed thigh structures normally rotate internally in the first trimester of fetal development and that when this fails to occur, the patella remains laterally displaced on the lateral femoral condyle and the entire quadriceps mechanism remains rotated anterolaterally. The actual diagnosis of this situation may be delayed because of the inability to palpate the true position of the patella in the newborn or young child and inability to document its position radiographically until later. Normal ossification of the patella occurs at around age 3 but is often delayed further when the patella is hypoplastic, as in congenital dislocation.

Diagnosis of the condition may not occur until the child presents for a disability of the leg, including delayed weight bearing.[17,41] There may be a valgus and flexion deformity with external tibial torsion, with seeming lateral instability during weight bearing and an empty intercondylar space at the anterior distal femur when the knee is flexed. The patella may not be palpable, as noted, because of its hypoplasia and fixation to the lateral femoral condyle; therefore, it is mistaken for the latter structure. Quadriceps insufficiency, denoted by an extension lag (and thus the flexion contracture deformity), may be the most obvious physical finding, suggesting the diagnosis in the infant. On the other hand, in patients with less quadriceps insufficiency and a mobile patella reducible in extension, the lateral dislocation of the patella with flexion will confirm the diagnosis (see Fig. 113.17). It may be possible to demonstrate an inability to extend the knee against resistance from a flexed position, when the patella is dislocated, whereas strength-tested in extension, when the patella is more normally positioned, is almost normal. Depending on the degree of quadriceps dysfunction, the child may do relatively well in the first decade, only to begin falling or have increasing disability as increasing body size overstresses the quadriceps mechanism. This scenario is often seen in patients with syndromic associations underlying their patellar dislocation, such as children with Down, Rubinstein-Taybi, or

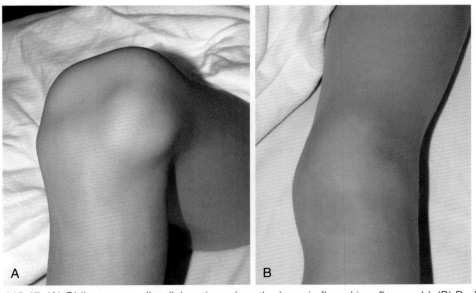

FIG 113.17 (A) Obligatory patellar dislocation when the knee is flexed in a 5-year-old. (B) Reduction in extension.

nail-patella syndrome. It may be necessary to resort to ultrasonography, computed tomography (CT), magnetic resonance imaging (MRI) or, rarely, open exploration, to make the diagnosis in some cases.[17,36]

Treatment

Treatment for congenital dislocation of the patella is surgical, because this dislocation is by definition irreducible or unstable. The goal is to realign the quadriceps mechanism and place the patella in the intercondylar groove, balancing the muscle insertions so that the reduction is stable. The groove, congenitally hypoplastic because of anterior flattening of the lateral femoral condyle, should deepen as normal patellar tracking ensues.[14] The classic procedure involves the concepts of Judet[31] and Stanisavljevic et al.[62] in dissecting the vastus lateralis from the lateral intermuscular septum from origin to insertion and subperiosteally rotating the entire quadriceps muscle mass medially. Thus, the skin incision basically extends from the greater trochanter to the lateral parapatellar area and distally to just beyond the tibial tubercle if infrapatellar realignment is necessary (Fig. 113.18). Distally, in the thigh, the lateral retinaculum and muscle insertions are abnormally contracted and must be divided to free the patella from these tethering structures (see Fig. 113.18C), which actually produce the flexion deformity by being displaced posterior to the axis of knee motion. Transversely dividing the iliotibial band corrects the external tibial rotation, genu valgum, and knee flexion

deformity. Lengthening the quadriceps tendon by Z- or V-Y plasty has been advocated, if necessary, to remedy the obligatory dislocation caused by quadriceps contracture.[14] Femoral shortening (see previous section) may be a better solution if the quadriceps is that severely contracted. The biceps may also require division to completely reduce the tibial subluxation-valgus.[38] Once the patella and quadriceps can be centralized, a medial imbrication is necessary to maintain the reduction. A medial arthrotomy is performed to mobilize the vastus medialis insertion, which is advanced distally and laterally to maintain centralization of the patella (see Fig. 113.9E and F). There is no need to close or otherwise repair the large lateral retinacular defect, although some have described excising the fascia lata and using it as a graft to cover the defect and close the joint.

The final step is to realign the patellar tendon insertion if it remains too lateral. The classic Goldthwait transfer of the lateral half of the patellar tendon, split longitudinally from the medial half, sharply dissected from its insertion, and passed medially under the intact medial portion to be reattached to bone-periosteum for distal medial advancement, is generally used in immature patients for this purpose.[20] Others prefer complete release and reinsertion of the entire patellar tendon,[14,38] although the risk of tibial tubercle physeal injury[22] or excessive patellofemoral joint compression[42] may be increased by this method. Prior to closure, the knee is ranged to ascertain whether the suprapatellar or infrapatellar imbrications are too tight, preventing passive flexion to at least 45 degrees. Alternatively, if

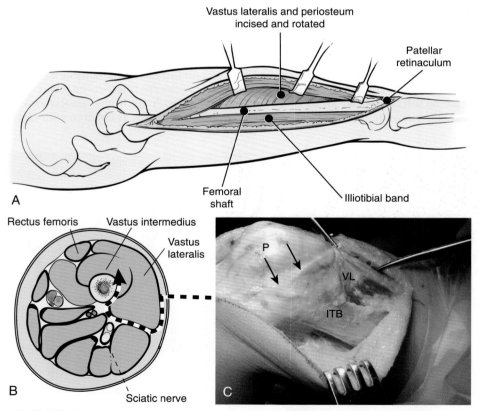

FIG 113.18 (A) Incision and mobilization of vastus lateralis, intermedius, and rectus for Judet-Stanisvljevic quadricepsplasty. (B) Dissection posterior to vastus lateralis with subperiosteal mobilization of vasti lateralis and intermedius. (C) Abnormal lateral insertions of vastus lateralis *(VL)* and IT band into patellar retinaculum *(P)*. *ITB,* Iliotibial band.

the patella continues to dislocate laterally, additional proximal lateral release (see the following text) and/or a revision of the medial imbrication is indicated. In the most severe cases, a semitendinosus transfer[3,14] may be added as an additional checkrein to continued lateral subluxation. Normally, 6 to 8 weeks of cast immobilization in slight flexion is required to achieve stability following the medial imbrication and Goldthwait and Dewar procedures, followed by vigorous rehabilitation.

Often, the extensive quadriceps dissection and mobilization into the proximal thigh described earlier are unnecessary. Although it may seem logical to perform this dissection to address the pathoanatomy completely, the dissection can often be limited to the distal third of the thigh, avoiding filleting the thigh from trochanter to knee to rotate the entire quadriceps. A competent and adequately tensioned medial imbrication is stable, even if there appears to be some persistent lateralization of the proximal thigh musculature. If intraoperative stability through 45 to 60 degrees of flexion is documented, additional dissection of the intermuscular septum proximally is unnecessary. Furthermore, early range-of-motion exercises can be started after 2 to 3 weeks for wound healing if the medial imbrication is competent and the patella stable. Similar experiences have been reported.[17]

Results and Comments

Unfortunately, the results of quadriceps realignment are not that well documented, with many classic procedures and recent advancements in technique being reported in individual case reports or small case series with little outcome data. A 10% incidence of recurrent dislocation has been reported[16,21,30] at an average 5-year follow-up, and extension lag is generally improved, although not always in the more severe arthrogrypotic or skeletal dysplasia patients.[38] Other complications include medial dislocation, presumably from overzealous vastus medialis advancement, and peroneal nerve palsy. In patients with Down syndrome, in whom patellar instability occurs in 5% to 8% of affected persons, and includes fixed persistent dislocation and frank obligatory instability, the indication for patellar stabilization has been questioned because of the frequent absence of symptoms or functional deficit.[13,63] Operative treatment for patients with poor function secondary to instability has been reported successful in up to 86% of patients[42] and in patients followed up to 15 years, although most series have been small, with short follow-up. Readers can draw their own conclusions concerning the effectiveness of patellar stabilization in this group of patients with notorious laxity and consequent risk of recurrence.

Because the main indication for patellar stabilization surgery is the local functional deficit caused by the impaired quadriceps function and the flexion-valgus-external rotation deformity, any outcome that improves the extension lag, instability in gait, and overall function with a range of knee motion compatible with normal activities (generally 0 to 90 degrees of motion) should be considered worthwhile, even if a repeat operation is necessary later to deal with recurrence. Ultimately, it is assumed that chronic patellar dislocation, fixed or recurrent-obligatory, will degenerate into significant painful arthritis, at which time other reconstructive procedures, including patellectomy or total arthroplasty, may not be attractive because of long-standing quadriceps and periarticular soft tissue laxity or insufficiency. Thus, there is always an indication for surgical reduction of congenital patellar dislocation with any functional impairment

except in cases such as Down syndrome, where symptoms and long-term disability are generally infrequent.

FLEXION DEFORMITY OF THE KNEE

A knee flexion contracture (KFC) of up to 45 degrees is a normal finding in the neonate, with further flexion to 160 degrees, the normal intrauterine position of the knee at term, also possible. As long as the quadriceps function is normal and there are no other neurologic or dysmorphic features, this congenital contracture gradually resolves in the first few months of life. By age 6 months, a significant amount of fixed knee flexion (45 degrees or more), with or without limitation of further flexion, will probably have been noted if there is a local or syndromic condition affecting the extremity. In general, such a knee deformity would be a manifestation of one of the underlying conditions in Box 113.1, which would probably have been recognized because of other orthopedic deformities or syndromic features.

Establishing the associated diagnosis underlying the knee flexion deformity has important prognostic and therapeutic value. In conditions in which femoral-tibial extension is blocked by intrinsic bony deformity (eg, skeletal dysplasias), early soft tissue releases are probably of little value to increase extension, and thus correction by osteotomy or growth manipulation will be considered and probably delayed until technical considerations and ambulatory status indicate treatment. On the other hand, in soft tissue contracture syndromes, early aggressive treatment may be important to prevent development of secondary joint deformity precluding full extension and irreversible quadriceps dysfunction, which will impede ambulatory capability. Finally, treatment of the knee in the limb reduction anomalies (eg, femoral deficiency, tibial hemimelia) is dictated by overall function, knee stability, and limb length considerations, and whether the involvement is unilateral or bilateral. This section will focus on soft tissue webbing syndromes, in which early reconstructive knee surgery may be of benefit; the skeletal dysplasias and limb reduction anomalies, requiring a combination of angular and growth manipulations of the entire extremity, will not be discussed further here.

BOX 113.1   Conditions Associated With Congenital Knee Flexion Deformity

Localized Dysplasia Affecting the Extremity Only
Congenital femoral deficiency
Tibial hemimelia type 1a, 1b
Congenital quadriceps/patellar tendon dysplasia
Congenital dislocation (fixed) of the patella

Syndromes With Soft Tissue Contracture
Arthrogryposis
Popliteal pterygium syndrome
Escobar (multiple pterygium) syndrome
Beals syndrome (congenital contractural arachnodactyly)
Paralytic (sacral agenesis, myelodysplasia)

Skeletal Dysplasia With Bony Flexion Deformity
Diastrophic dysplasia
Metatropic dysplasia
Miscellaneous skeletal dysplasias

Correcting a congenital KFC, or any significant KFC, is often a frustrating and complication-riddled proposition. The decision to proceed must involve an overall evaluation of the prognosis for functional ambulation, appreciating the extent of involvement of the ipsilateral hip and foot as well as any neurodevelopmental implications for function. A KFC exceeding 30 degrees alters gait adversely because of overstressing of the quadriceps.[56] It is often problematic to determine the pretreatment status of the quadriceps when a significant KFC is present. Furthermore, significant hip flexion deformity or severe equinus may have to be corrected simultaneously, or else these uncorrected deformities will induce recurrent knee flexion to maintain overall sagittal alignment for upright posture. The absolute prerequisite for KFC treatment is the identification of a functional quadriceps, without which any extension obtained through treatment will be certainly lost as the unopposed forces producing the original contracture persist.

PTERYGIUM SYNDROMES

These congenital syndromic deformities produce soft tissue webbing on the flexion side of various joints. The popliteal pterygium syndrome (PPS, also known as faciogenitopopliteal syndrome) includes, in addition to the popliteal web restricting extension, cleft lip and palate, intraoral webbing sometimes requiring surgical release to open the mouth, intercrural webs distorting the external genitalia, and finger and toe syndactylies with nail abnormalities (Fig. 113.19). Patients have normal intelligence and development. In multiple pterygium (Escobar) syndrome, webs occur across every flexion area, with particular involvement of the neck (85%) and popliteal (60%) areas, and with less common involvement of the axilla, antecubital area, and fingers. Severe kyphoscoliosis and short stature (adult height, 135 cm [53 inches]) are typical of Escobar patients, who may also show little abnormality at birth but then the webs develop with growth. In arthrogryposis and Beals syndrome (Fig. 113.20), multiple joints are typically involved, with stiffness, lack of active motion, and absence of flexion creases noted, especially in classic arthrogryposis. In sacral agenesis and myelodysplasia, lack of motion is also obvious, related to the neurologic deficit of spinal cord origin.

Pathoanatomy

The hallmark of popliteal pterygia is the extension of a fibrous band from the ischium to the calcaneus, with a subcutaneous cord (the calcaneoischiadicus muscle) and the sciatic nerve, or one of its divisions (usually tibial), intimately adherent within the web (Fig. 113.21). There is often a longitudinal skin marking of a lighter color outlining the path of the subcutaneous cord. The cord is covered by a tent of muscle or fascia that fills the web and connects to the medial and lateral intramuscular septae of the thigh and leg. Abnormal muscle bellies and aberrant nerve paths piercing the pterygium fascia should be expected in any surgical dissection.

The obstacles to correction of a pterygium contracture include the following: (1) the calcaneoischial cord, which is generally not flexible and intuitively invites excision, usually with a Z-plasty of the skin; (2) the shortness of the sciatic or tibial nerve division accompanying the cord,[24,51] which cannot be stretched acutely; and (3) intra-articular incongruity, secondary to flattening of the femoral condyles caused by persistence of growth in flexion. The latter is an important argument

for early surgical correction before the joint deformity per se prevents full extension because of misshapen articular surfaces. Recurrence of the contracture is extremely frequent because of reconstitution of the calcaneoischial cord and popliteal scar formation, and secondarily by ankle equinus from the calcaneal insertion; the knee must flex to accommodate the persistent or recurrent equinus. The role of a weak quadriceps is obvious, although in practice the actual strength is difficult, if not impossible, to test or document—the pretreatment strength of the muscle cannot be determined in an infant or toddler with a rigid flexion deformity that prevents extension. About all that can be determined is whether the muscle contracts when the leg is stimulated.

In arthrogryposis and similar conditions, the obstacles to correction are mainly the periarticular fibrosis and underlying muscle paralysis. These joints are congenitally rigid, because of lack of intrauterine movement—for example, as evidenced by absence of flexion creases. Periarticular tissue and joint capsules are contracted as a result. Early attempts to mobilize these joints with physical therapy are usually unrewarding because of lack of active movement, but should always be attempted. At some point, in the 12- to 24-month-old patient, a decision must be made about prognosis for ambulation based on active movements of the lower extremities and, in particular, the presence of quadriceps function. In cases of total absence of quadriceps function, the decision to accept the flexed knee position and consequent nonambulatory status, and thus forego knee flexion deformity treatment, is completely justified.

The prognosis for obtaining and maintaining correction of congenital KFC of these causes, and thus useful ambulation, is guarded, at best, because of the often insurmountable problem of recurrence. Treatment must anticipate that recurrence to some degree is inevitable and that functional gains are elusive because of numerous possible complications, including nerve stretching and neuropathic pain, joint damage from extensive dissection producing avascular necrosis of epiphysis and physis, incongruity and cartilage necrosis (Fig. 113.22), and inadequate muscle strength to allow nonsupported knee extension.

Treatment

Acute Correction: Pterygium and Arthrogryposis. Correction by surgical release of popliteal structures, combined with femoral and possibly tibial shortening, is first-line treatment for deformities of moderate severity, up to perhaps 60 degrees. The popliteal release may be best accomplished with the patient prone, although if hip mobility is adequate to allow full internal and external rotation, the patient can be positioned supine, allowing access to anterior and posterior structures simultaneously. Anterior exposure is needed to inspect the intercondylar notch and patellofemoral joint following posterior release, because there is often a soft tissue pulvinar in the notch blocking full extension, which must be excised. In arthrogrypotic patients, the patellofemoral joint is often scarred or obliterated and the quadriceps mechanism must be freed from the femur and a suprapatellar pouch created (Fig. 113.23).

Regardless of the patient position, the skin over the ischiocalcaneal band must be incised longitudinally with multiple Z-plasties and the actual cord exposed circumferentially from ischial tuberosity to calcaneal tuberosity. The exposure of the cord will encounter the sciatic nerve and its tibial, peroneal, and sural components, which should be completely dissected,

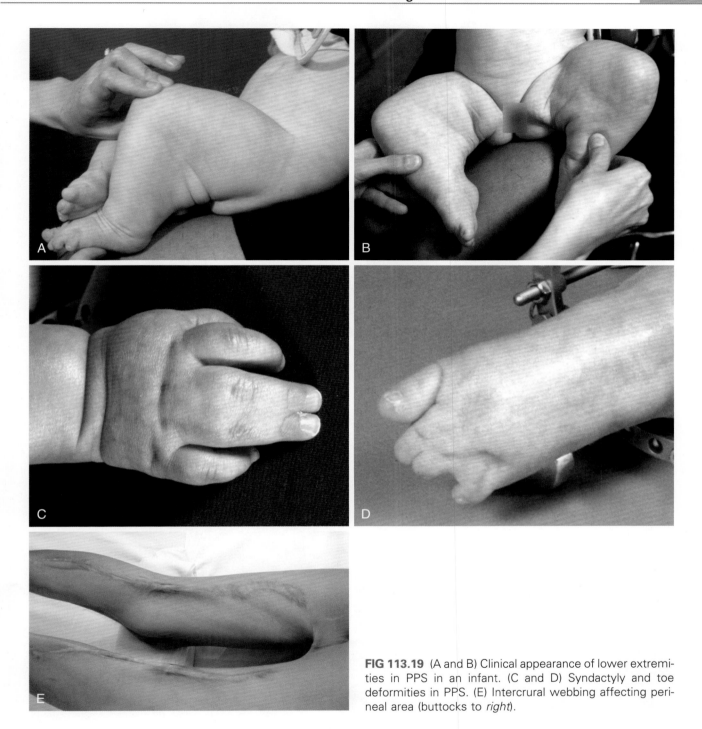

FIG 113.19 (A and B) Clinical appearance of lower extremities in PPS in an infant. (C and D) Syndactyly and toe deformities in PPS. (E) Intercrural webbing affecting perineal area (buttocks to *right*).

mobilized, and protected (see Fig. 113.21). The ischiocalcaneal structure is excised. The arcade of fascia enveloping the band can then be safely followed to the medial and lateral intermuscular septae and divided transversely, just like a fasciotomy of the leg. This fascial division is best accomplished close to the joint, near the axis of rotation, but can also be accomplished at points proximal and distal to the knee. Deeper structures in the popliteal fossa can then be dissected and released sharply, obviously protecting the vascular structures deep midline, which are in the normal anatomic location (see Fig. 113.21C). Beginning laterally, the biceps and iliotibial band are released

(Henry approach); posterior capsulotomy of the knee is the ultimate goal of the dissection. Medially, the hamstring tendons are released, leading to complete posteromedial capsulotomy. However, in spite of what appears to be a comprehensive, thorough posterior knee release, the limiting factor—the sciatic nerve or its tibial component—usually prevents adequate extension, and bowstrings in the popliteal area so severely that skin closure over the nerve may be an issue (see Fig. 113.21D).

The femur should be shortened,[51,57] as much as 3 to 4 cm if necessary, to achieve as much extension as possible (see Figs.

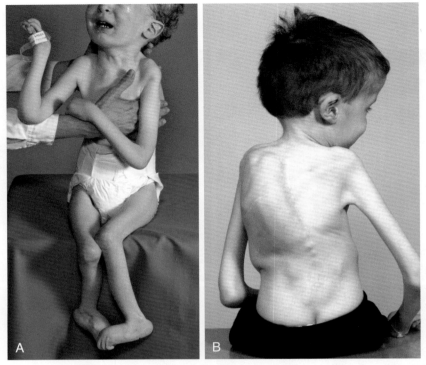

FIG 113.20 (A) Congenital contractural arachnodactyly (Beals syndrome)—elbow and knee flexion contractures in a 1-year-old. (B) Spinal deformity in Beals syndrome.

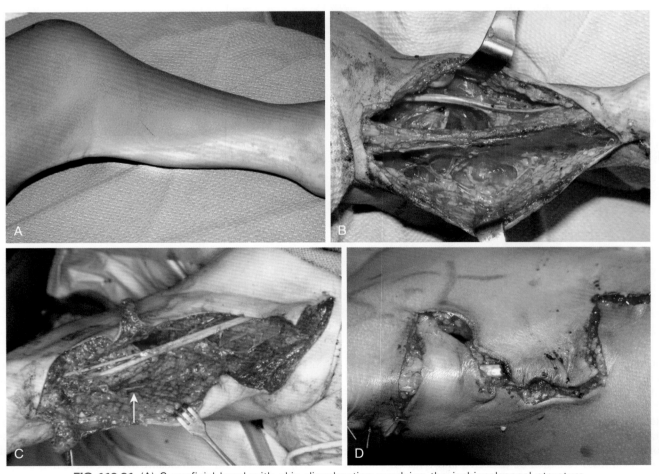

FIG 113.21 (A) Superficial band with skin discoloration overlying the ischiocalcaneal structure (foot to *right*). (B) Ischiocalcaneal muscle and band, with the sciatic nerve isolated. (C) All popliteal soft tissue structures have been released except the major nerve divisions and the vascular bundle *(arrow).* (D) Following wound closure, the sciatic nerve is bowstrung directly under the skin.

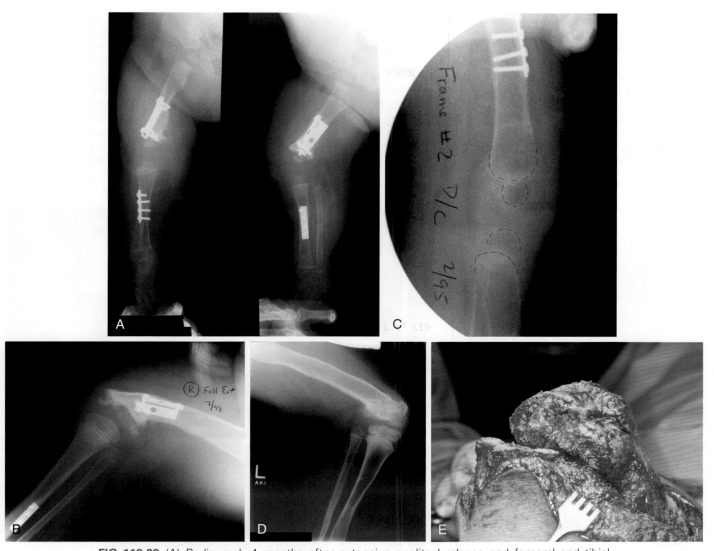

FIG 113.22 (A) Radiograph 4 months after extensive popliteal release and femoral and tibial shortening were performed on the right lower extremity of the patient in Fig. 113.16. (B) Avascular necrosis of the distal femoral epiphysis and physis resulted. (C) Left knee radiograph, showing full extension, of the same patient after second attempt at distraction arthrodiastasis correction with Ilizarov method (see also Fig. 113.25). Soft tissue release and femoral shortening followed the second frame correction. (D) The result was recurrent deformity with severe degenerative changes 2 years later. (E) Intraoperative view of destroyed distal femur in (D). The articular surface is covered with pannus and cartilage cannot be identified. Knee fusion with rotationplasty was performed.

113.22A and 113.23E and F). This effectively decompresses the tissue around the knee, much like femoral shortening applied to the reduction of a late-diagnosed congenital dislocation of the hip,[6] allowing extension without undue tension on the nerves. This can be accomplished in the distal diaphysis by plating the femur laterally or posteriorly; the latter is theoretically preferable because the plate will be on the tension side of the osteotomy when the knee is extended with some force. An overly aggressive popliteal soft tissue release combined with a distal femoral shortening can result in avascular injury to the distal femoral physis (see Fig. 113.22B). The tibia can also be shortened to benefit the ankle equinus and decompress the popliteal structures further. Hyperextension osteotomy of the

distal femur has been used to correct KFC[12] but, in a young child, provides only temporary improvement because of remodeling by the distal physeal growth.

As suggested earlier, anterior arthrotomy must be considered for removal of fibrofatty soft tissue, which often fills the intercondylar notch and prevents the final 10 to 15 degrees of extension (see Fig. 113.23D). The patellofemoral joint may need to be inspected to assess whether full passive extension is possible. Finally, plication of the patellar tendon should be considered following the femoral shortening to remove excessive redundance, which will compromise eventual quadriceps strength. In children younger than 2 years, this may not be necessary, but one will never be criticized for this final step in attempting to balance and augment the extension function in this deformity, in which such function is often lacking.

Once maximum extension has been achieved, the incisions are closed and a spica cast is applied to control the proximal thigh, because a long-leg cast has inadequate purchase on the thigh following femoral shortening. As soon as the osteotomies are healed the patient is vigorously mobilized, concentrating on active extension and unencumbered weight bearing. Bracing in full extension can be used if quadriceps weakness appears to be allowing excessive flexion. Long-term night bracing in full extension is often recommended, but its efficacy is unknown.

As noted, the tendency for recurrence is overwhelming, so attempts to delay it by long-term bracing are appropriate.

In spite of vigorous treatment of KFC in arthrogryposis, over half of patients lose ambulatory ability because of ineffective correction or recurrence, and thus do not remain community ambulators.[46,60] A recent report[26] of functional outcomes following knee release in patients with arthrogryposis found only 31% of patients to be independent ambulators, with the remainder being wheelchair-bound for community mobility at a mean follow-up of 12 years after surgical release. Despite the observation of increased recurrence rate of flexion contracture

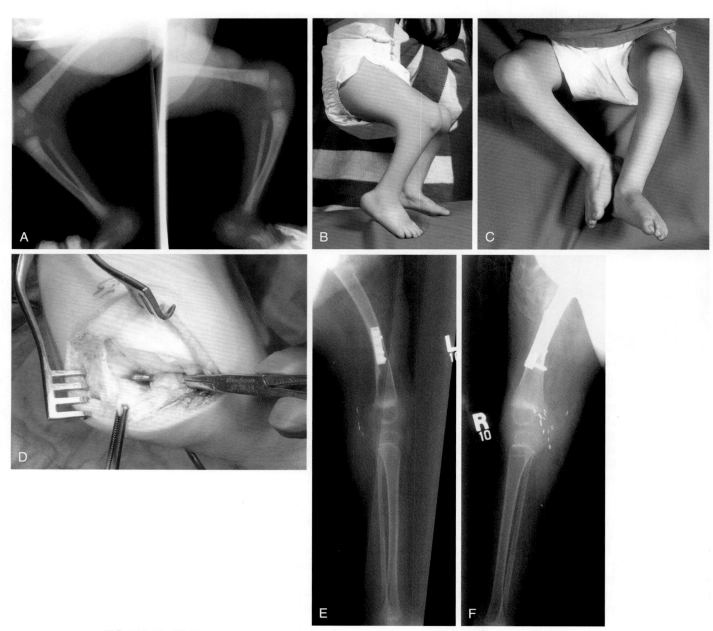

FIG 113.23 (A) Knee radiographs of an infant boy with multiple pterygia (Escobar syndrome). (B and C) Clinical appearance of lower extremities. (D) Anterior arthrotomy to excise fibrofatty soft tissue obstructing the intercondylar notch, blocking full extension. (E and F) Radiographs at age 3½ years after staged popliteal releases, femoral shortening, and anterior arthrotomy, with latissimus dorsi free flaps for soft tissue closure of the popliteal fossae.

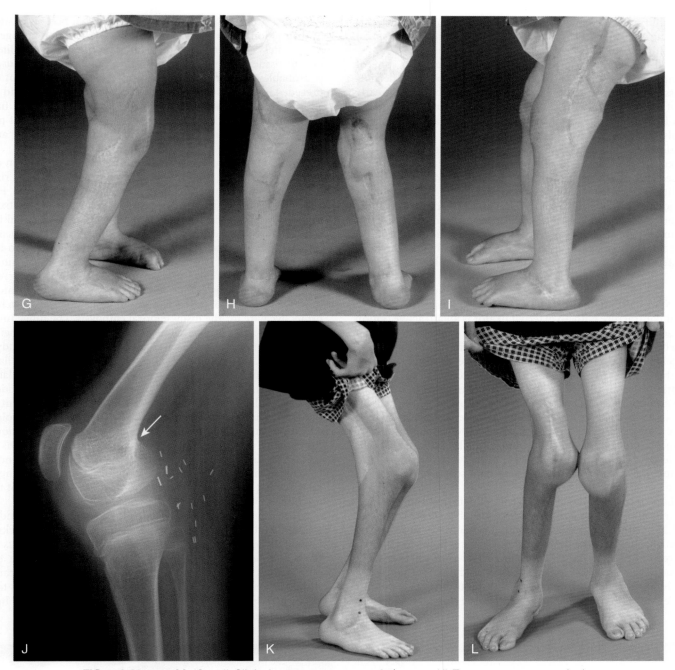

FIG 113.23, cont'd (G to I) Clinical appearance at age 3½ years. (J) Ten years postoperatively, a significant flexion deformity has recurred on the right. Premature growth arrest at the posterior physis is suspected *(arrow)*. Joint incongruity is also apparent. (K and L) Clinical appearance at age 14.

with extended follow-up, improved functional mobility scores, functional independence scores, and self-reported sports and physical functioning scores with increased knee extension were documented. This study reinforces the difficultly in treating KFC in arthrogryposis. Although short- and intermediate-term function may be improved with aggressive surgical management, long-term ambulatory ability invariably declines with the inevitable recurrence. For PPS patients, many will remain community ambulators with repetitive surgery, depending on initial severity,[51,53] provided that the knees do not succumb to painful

degenerative arthritis (see Fig. 113.22). Knee disarticulation may be appropriate in the latter situation.

Microvascular free tissue transfer has been used in place of Z-plasty in an attempt to decompress the popliteal scarring further, which contributes to recurrence. Limited experience with latissimus dorsi free transfer (see Fig. 113.23) has shown that KFC recurrence can be delayed, but cannot be prevented simply by supplying noninvolved healthy tissue to cover the popliteal space. Because of the possible untoward effects of bilateral free latissimus flaps on development of spinal deformity, this method may be appropriate only for patients nearing skeletal maturity, in whom the risk of progressive spinal deformity is minimal.

Full passive extension is almost never achieved in spite of comprehensive surgery, usually because of incomplete decompression of neurovascular structures, but also because of early joint incongruity. A form of gradual extension improvement can be attempted postoperatively with serial casts in progressively more extension or with the use of an extension-desubluxation hinge cast (Quengel hinges; Fig. 113.24). The latter allow casting in flexion, with progressive extension produced once early wound healing has occurred, retaining the ability to translate the tibia anteriorly during correction to avoid knee subluxation. Care is required to avoid decubiti at the anterior distal thigh, where careful padding and judicious cast trimming are crucial to prevent skin complications as progressive extension is achieved. A spica cast is recommended to avoid posterior proximal thigh skin pressure caused by the Quengel technique when a long-leg–only cast is placed.

Gradual Correction: Ilizarov Technique. Gradual correction of joint contracture with an external fixator is an attractive option for severe congenital KFCs. The amount of corrective force that can be applied to the bony skeleton is not limited by skin tolerance and, because the skeletal elements are controlled directly by the external fixation, joint subluxation can be avoided. The sciatic nerve and its branches, the structures directly limiting the amount of acute correction, tolerate slow stretching. Circular and monolateral devices using a hinge distractor method have been reported.[7,45] Improvement in extension and total arc range of motion, changed to a more functional range, can be achieved. The problem, as with acute correction, remains maintenance of correction whether or not soft tissue release has been performed simultaneously.[11,18,25]

Loss of correction with recurrence of deformity and stiffness are common in our limited experience (Fig. 113.25; see Fig. 113.22). Although gradual correction remains attractive, it still does not eliminate the problem of recurrences following Ilizarov correction of pterygia. The question arises as to whether a soft tissue release prior to frame correction is advisable. The reasoning might be that the distraction arthrodiastasis actually induces increased fibrous tissue as the surgically treated popliteal

structures are lengthened, in the same way that bone is created by distraction forces after osteotomy. Such distraction histogenesis invites recurrence by the stimulation of new popliteal fibrous tissue, becoming apparent after frame removal. Thus, it is probable that Ilizarov correction of pterygia should not be preceded by soft tissue release; instead, the deformity should be addressed by external fixation–arthrodiastasis alone. At first sign of recurrence (loss of extension), following healing of pin tracts, it can be subjected to formal soft tissue release and femoral shortening, as described for acute correction.

The frame is constructed with double points of fixation on the femur and tibia, usually with an arch proximally and a ring distally on the femur, and two rings for the tibia (see Fig. 113.25A). The foot should be included in a static frame, fixed to the tibia in neutral position, whenever there is potential for significant equinus during correction, which in practice means essentially every case of KFC. An extra point of fixation to the distal femoral ring is a transverse wire through the femoral epiphysis to protect this physis from separation during correction,[11] although this is not mandatory; monolateral fixators have successfully corrected KFCs,[45] obviously without such a protective wire for the distal femoral epiphysis. The hinge must be placed as a distraction hinge, with the axis of rotation being just distal to the anterior distal edge of the distal femoral condyle (see Fig. 113.25D). This is intended to prevent articular cartilage pressure damage, but this is probably the least controllable complication of the procedure. The rate of angular correction can be calculated using the triangulation formula or concentric radii,[25] but in practice is generally tailored to the patient's tolerance and the appearance of any neuropraxic complications. Empirically, 4 mm/day distraction on the motor rod seems to correct the deformity efficiently. Distal neuropathy, as evidenced by hyperesthesia or dysesthesia of the foot, warrants a temporary slowing or pause from correction and consideration of the use of gabapentin (Neurontin) if it does not resolve.

Once full extension is achieved, it is generally recommended to maintain the frame locked in full extension for 4 to 6 weeks.[45] Rapid flexion and extension through an arc of 30 degrees or more can be attempted during this period to mobilize the periarticular tissues once full extension is reached. The frame should be removed and the knee casted for an additional 4 to 6 weeks to help maintain correction and allow pin tracts to heal

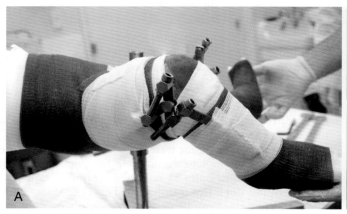
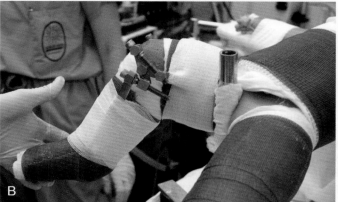

FIG 113.24 (A and B) Extension-desubluxation hinge cast applied immediately following acute correction surgery. The proximal threaded screw extends the knee and the distal one translates the tibia anteriorly to prevent posterior subluxation.

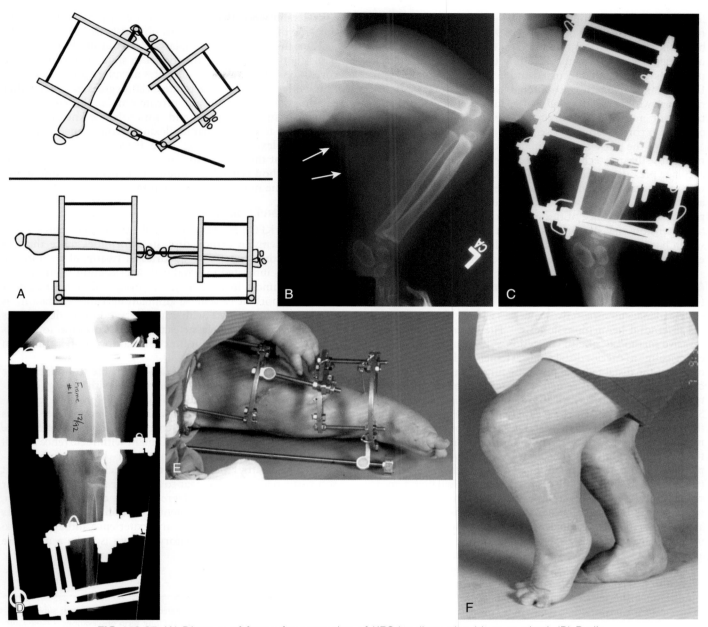

FIG 113.25 (A) Diagram of frame for correction of KFC by distraction hinge method. (B) Radiograph of left lower extremity (patient in Fig. 113.19) prior to frame application. The soft tissue edge of the pterygium can be seen *(arrows)*. (C) Radiograph of initial position in frame. (D) Full extension achieved. Note position of the knee hinge at the anterior edge of the distal femur to accomplish joint distraction with extension. (E) Clinical appearance with knee extended. Failure to incorporate the foot allowed uncontrolled equinus, contributing to recurrence. (F) Recurrent deformity 1 year later. This extremity was treated a second time (see Fig. 113.22C), with a similar outcome.

in preparation for possible additional surgery, such as ischiocalcaneal cord excision and femoral shortening, to decompress the correction. Such surgery should be considered as soon as recurrence or loss of extension becomes apparent. Although long-leg bracing is commonly recommended once the final cast is removed, this is mechanically ineffective in young children because of the limited control of the thigh, especially if the femur has been shortened. A nighttime extension orthosis may be the most practical for post-treatment splinting.

Results of Ilizarov correction of KFCs are far more encouraging than for acute correction, except for PPS patients, for whom recurrence is almost expected. The results indicate that 60% to 85% of knees gain significant correction and maintain it at up to 5-year follow-up. Brunner et al.[7] have corrected 11 of 13 knees from 39 degrees flexion to 17 degrees at follow-up, without frame-related complications. Herzenberg et al.[25] have achieved good to excellent results in 9 of 14 knees, starting from an average 60-degree contracture, corrected to 16 degrees at follow-up without complications. Damsin and Ghanem[11] have reported 13 corrections of more than 90-degree contracture—by far the most severe contractures ever reported—to an average of 10 degrees at follow-up, excluding two cases with multiple pterygia syndrome that recurred and needed further treatment. Damsin and Ghanem encountered three fractures and one nerve palsy in their series, and 5 of 13 knees remained stiff after treatment, more a reflection of the severity of the joint pathology than a complication per se.

Perhaps the most discouraging aspect of severe KFC correction by the Ilizarov technique is the potential joint damage from cartilage pressure necrosis (see Fig. 113.22). There is no agreed method to avoid this complication, other than to proceed slowly and to ensure that the joint is distracted during the extension period. The recurrence of flexion deformity after correction to full extension may also be related to an inadequate quadriceps, which has not been addressed by patellar tendon plication, for example, in any series of Ilizarov corrections to date.

Anterior Femoral Guided Growth (Hemiepiphysiodesis). Mild (10- to 25-degree) flexion deformities are amenable to nonoperative management, soft tissue releases with casting, or anterior distal femoral hemiepiphysiodesis.[37] The latter is a minimally invasive method to obtain correction via a hemiepiphysiodesis effect using an anterior distal femoral tethering device. It requires only that the distal femoral physis be functional and have sufficient growth potential remain to obtain adequate correction, typically more than 2 years of growth remaining. Kramer and Stevens[37] have reported their experience with this technique, first using traditional epiphyseal staples and more recently using nonlocking eight-plates.[33] They found promising results using the eight-plates for fixed knee flexion deformities, with 17 of 18 patients having significant improvement of their deformities (total mean correction, 15 degrees). They calculated a mean correction of 1.4 degrees/month, with few complications (one wound breakdown, one knee effusion, one rebound deformity after plate removal). Comparing these results with their results using epiphyseal staples, they believe that the eight-plates offer a more reliable and faster correction of the flexion deformity.

Despite these promising early results, long-term data are needed to determine whether rebound deformity will be problematic once the hardware is removed. Additionally, we have found anterior femoral hardware to be prominent, with potential for soft tissue problems when used in very young or small children, who are typically the population with less severe deformity in whom this technique may be most successful. This technique is worth considering when an extensive surgical release or osteotomy is being considered for a less severe deformity, or with younger children with more severe deformities if significant growth potential is remaining and anterior femoral soft tissue coverage is deemed sufficient.

Amputation, Arthrodesis, and Rotationplasty. Failure to achieve a functional knee position, especially if accompanied by pain not amenable to bracing or medication, after perhaps two attempts to correct a severe KFC, is an indication for knee fusion or disarticulation. Any discussion of treatment of severe KFC must include a realization that especially if the failure is primarily unilateral, these are appropriate and useful alternatives. Because most congenital KFC cases are bilateral, these salvage procedures are usually considered when one knee is considerably worse than the other. The decision to proceed with this type of salvage surgery must obviously be individualized.

Knee fusion with rotationplasty[1,19] should also be considered if the foot and ankle are functional in spite of the failed knee correction. The procedure simulates an internal knee amputation, with the limb being rotated 180 degrees externally after excising the distal femur and proximal tibia. This converts the ankle to a functional knee and, with a below-knee prosthesis fitted to the foot, ankle plantar flexion becomes knee extension, with dorsiflexion becoming knee flexion. The rotated foot should be at the level of the contralateral knee, so use of this salvage method generally is limited to patients with one sound limb and one requiring knee ablation.

Summary and Comments

Congenital KFC presents some of the most challenging treatment problems in orthopedics. In deformities more than 45 degrees, with a functional quadriceps, treatment to improve extension is indicated to avoid gait deterioration from quadriceps mechanical insufficiency. In young children, treatment may be important to achieve ambulation if the contracture is severe, and in patients with multiple syndromic deformities (arthrogryposis is the classic example), the decision to treat is difficult if the prognosis for functional ambulation is uncertain or poor.

Milder deformities are generally amenable to nonoperative management (bracing), soft tissue releases with casting (including extension-desubluxation hinges), or possibly growth-modulating hemiepiphysiodesis. In the more severe cases described in this chapter, extensive surgical approaches are indicated but unfortunately are fraught with recurrence as well as complications. Gradual correction by arthrodiastasis-extension (Ilizarov) methods are more effective, with or without soft tissue release, and appear to be the treatment of choice for deformities greater than 60 degrees. Frame correction, however, is no panacea, because the potential for complications is just as great as with acute correction, and experience and attention to correction details are mandatory if there is to be a moderate chance of lasting success.

KEY REFERENCES

10. Curtis B, Fisher R: Congenital hyperextension with anterior subluxation of the knee; surgical treatment and long-term observations. *J Bone Joint Surg Am* 41:255, 1969.
17. Ghanem I, Wattincourt L, Seringe R: Congenital dislocation of the patella. Part I: pathologic anatomy. Part II: orthopedic management. *J Pediatr Orthop* 20:812, 2000.
25. Herzenberg JE, Davis JR, Paley D, et al: Mechanical distraction for treatment of severe flexion contractures. *Clin Orthop* 301:80, 1994.
26. Ho CA, Karol LA: The utility of knee releases in arthrogryposis. *J Pediatr Orthop* 28:307, 2008.
33. Klatt J, Stevens PM: Guided growth for fixed knee flexion deformity. *J Pediatr Orthop* 28:626, 2008.
35. Kocher MS, Garg S, Micheli LJ: Physeal sparing reconstruction of the anterior cruciate ligament in skeletally immature prepubescent children and adolescents. *J Bone Joint Surg Am* 87:2371, 2005.
52. Paletta GA, Jr: Special considerations. Anterior cruciate ligament reconstruction in the skeletally immature. *Orthop Clin N Am* 34:65, 2003.

The references for this chapter can also be found on www.expertconsult.com.

114

Meniscal Disorders

Matthew Beran, Dennis E. Kramer, Mininder S. Kocher, Kevin Klingele

MENISCAL TEARS

Meniscal tears are being seen with increasing frequency in the pediatric population.[12] Potential causes of this include a rise in organized sports participation in younger children, an improved awareness of the diagnosis among common practitioners, and wider availability and improved quality of magnetic resonance imaging (MRI).[40]

Anatomy and Classification

Pediatric meniscal tears are believed to have a greater healing potential compared with adult tears.[13] This may be in part the result of the vascularity of the developing meniscus. The meniscus is completely vascular at birth, but its vascularity gradually diminishes over time, resembling the adult meniscus by age 10.[25] The peripheral 25% to 30% of the adult meniscus has a direct vascular supply from the perimeniscal capillary plexus and so is termed the *red-red zone*. This area is thought to have the greatest potential for healing. The remainder of the meniscus obtains its nutrition through synovial diffusion, with the middle third termed the *red-white zone* and the central third termed the *white-white zone* to emphasize a diminishing vascular supply.

Other factors may also contribute to the healing potential of pediatric and adolescent meniscal tears. Pediatric meniscal tears usually occur following a specific injury to a previously normal meniscus. Simple nondegenerative tear patterns are most common and include longitudinal and bucket handle tears in the red-red zone.[17] In a study of 378 meniscal tears in young athletes with stable knees, the medial meniscus was involved 70% of the time, with the most common tear pattern found to be a vertical longitudinal tear (78%) through the posterior horn (75%).[72] Degenerative tear patterns, such as parrot beak, horizontal cleavage, and complex tears, are more often seen in the adult population and have lower healing potential. These patterns are also more suggestive of underlying discoid morphology if isolated and in younger patients.

In addition, many pediatric meniscal injuries occur in the setting of anterior cruciate ligament (ACL) tears.[69] The highest healing rates for meniscal repair have traditionally been seen in the setting of concomitant ACL reconstruction. Samora et al. found a prevalence of meniscal injury of 69.3% in association with acute ACL tears in skeletally immature patients. Tears were most common in the posterior horn of the lateral meniscus through the vascular zone and were usually in a repairable configuration.[64]

In contrast, a more recent cross-sectional study delineating the pattern of meniscus tears in children and adolescents found that meniscus tears in this population may be more complex and often less repairable than previously reported in the literature.[66] The factors found to be associated with greater meniscal tear complexity were male gender and greater body mass index.

Diagnosis

Isolated meniscal tears in children younger than 10 years generally occur in the setting of a discoid meniscus. Nondiscoid tears most commonly occur in the adolescent age group following a twisting injury during sports activities and often with associated ligamentous injury. Children usually present with knee pain and swelling. Mechanical symptoms, such as locking or catching, suggest meniscal tear instability. A locked knee (unable to be fully extended or flexed) is highly suggestive of a displaced bucket handle meniscal tear. In these cases, displaced meniscal tissue occupies the intercondylar notch area to block motion. A hemarthrosis is a strong indicator of potential meniscal pathology. In one report, meniscal tears were identified in approximately 45% of children ages 7 to 18 years who presented with an acute knee hemarthrosis.[69] In this series the medial meniscus was more commonly torn (70% to 88%) and a concurrent ACL tear was noted in 36% of the adolescents.

On physical examination, a knee effusion is often accompanied by joint line tenderness. Range of motion should be carefully assessed to identify mechanical blocks to motion. Provocative physical examination maneuvers on children may be difficult, limited by pain and apprehension. The traditional McMurray test for meniscal pathology requires 90 degrees of knee flexion, which may be uncomfortable for children following a knee injury. The test has been modified for children: the knee is flexed to 30 to 40 degrees and a rotational varus or valgus stress is placed on the knee.[12,14] Joint line pain following this maneuver is indicative of meniscal pathology. When performed by an experienced examiner, the physical examination can be reliably used to diagnose both medial (62% sensitivity; 80% specificity) and lateral (50% sensitivity; 89% specificity) meniscal tears in children.[37] Other potential diagnoses must be considered in this population, including patellar dislocation, osteochondritis dissecans (OCD), osteochondral injury, and plica syndrome. The ipsilateral hip should be assessed because knee pain may be indicative of hip pathology (eg, slipped capital femoral epiphysis) in this age group.

A meticulous ligamentous examination of the knee is necessary for children with suspected meniscal tears. Concurrent injuries, such as ACL tears, are common.[69] The Lachman test is reliable in the pediatric population for the diagnosis of ACL insufficiency, but the test findings must be compared with those of the contralateral knee because normal tibial translation is increased in younger patients.[19] In addition, unstable, displaced meniscal tears may prevent anterior translation, thereby producing a false-negative Lachman exam. Knee radiographs are standard following knee injuries in children. A complete radiographic series in children includes an anteroposterior (AP), lateral, intercondylar notch (tunnel), and Merchant (sunrise) views. Tunnel views are helpful to identify OCD lesions located posteriorly on the femoral condyles, whereas sunrise views can show patellar subluxation or osteochondral loose bodies indicative of patellar dislocation.

MRI, when used appropriately, can aid in the diagnosis of meniscal pathology. In the proper clinical setting, MRI findings can support a presumptive diagnosis of meniscal tear in children. However, overuse of MRI in young patients has its drawbacks. A high rate of false-positive MRI findings has been noted in the pediatric population.[48] The increased vascularity of the pediatric meniscus causes intrameniscal signal change, which can be misinterpreted as a meniscal tear (Fig. 114.1). MRI has lower sensitivity and specificity when used to evaluate meniscal pathology in children compared with adults and in younger children compared with older children.[69] MRI sensitivity (61.7%) and specificity (90.2%) for the diagnosis of meniscal tears in children younger than 12 years has been reported and compared unfavorably with children aged 12 to 16 years old (sensitivity 78.2%; specificity 95.5%).[37] Advances in MRI have improved these percentages in the adolescent age group.[46] A study evaluating the use of a 3-Tesla MRI for the diagnosis of intra-articular knee pathologies in a pediatric and adolescent patient population showed a sensitivity and specificity of 81.0% and 90.9%, respectively, for medial meniscus tears and 68.8% and 93%, respectively, for lateral meniscus tears.[65]

A retrospective review found the overall diagnostic accuracy of presurgical clinical evaluation (95.3%) and MRI (92.7%) in the assessment of traumatic intra-articular knee disorders in children and adolescents to be quite high.[22] The most common diagnoses missed on either clinical exam or MRI, but found at arthroscopy, were discoid meniscus (26.7%) and lateral meniscus tears (18.8%).

Treatment

The majority of meniscal tears in pediatric patients require some form of surgical treatment, with the goal being meniscal repair and preservation whenever possible. Asymptomatic meniscal tears noted incidentally on MRI can be observed over time for healing. Likewise, small symptomatic meniscal tears noted on physical exam or MRI scan may be initially treated with a trial of conservative management but persistent symptoms warrant surgical intervention. However, large tears should be addressed surgically in a prompt fashion because higher healing rates have been reported when the tear is repaired within 3 months of injury.[73] Meniscal tears identified during arthroscopy should be assessed for stability because small (<10 mm), stable (manually displaceable <3 mm), or partial-thickness tears may heal spontaneously.[76] Meniscal trephination and synovial rasping are commonly used techniques to stimulate bleeding near the tear site.

Arthroscopic management is standard, with meniscal repair favored over partial or total meniscectomy. The menisci reduce contact stress in the knee, thereby protecting the articular cartilage. Removal of part or all of the meniscus significantly increases contact forces in the knee[44,67] and may accelerate degenerative changes,[49] which may have profound consequences in the long term for young, active patients. Total meniscectomy increases contact stresses by 235%,[9] whereas removal of a small bucket handle medial meniscus tear increases stress by 65% and débridement of 75% of the posterior horn of the medial meniscus increases contact forces equivalent to a total meniscectomy.[20] Long-term results are poor following meniscectomy in young patients. One group, reporting 5-year follow-up after partial or total meniscectomy in 20 children, showed that 75% were symptomatic and 80% showed radiographic signs of early osteoarthritis.[47] A review noted that 50% of patients who underwent total meniscectomy had radiographic changes, symptoms, and functional loss consistent with osteoarthritis at 10- to 20-year follow-up.[45] Unfortunately, no studies to date have demonstrated a long-term reduction in the incidence of early osteoarthritis following meniscal repair in this young, active population.

Most pediatric meniscal tears are amenable to repair. Longitudinal peripheral tears in the red-red zone are the most common tear type (50% to 90%) and are ideal tears to repair.[20] Other repairable tear types include bucket handle tears, meniscal root tears, and most tears that extend into the red-red or red-white zones. Many meniscal repairs in children are done in

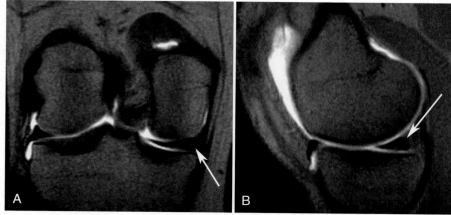

FIG 114.1 Coronal (A) and sagittal (B) T1-weighted MRI images of the knee showing intrameniscal signal abnormality (*white arrow*) consistent with the high vascularity of the meniscus in the skeletally immature child. This can easily be mistaken for a meniscal tear.

the setting of ACL reconstruction, which increases the potential for success.[43] Given the increased healing potential in children, paired with the poor results following meniscectomy, most surgeons are aggressive in meniscal preservation attempts. Even tears extending into the white-white zone, such as cleavage-type tears, can be partially débrided back to the red-white zone, removing the unstable portion followed by repair of the remaining rim. Complex degenerative, adult-type meniscal tear patterns, such as horizontal cleavage tears and radial tears, are less commonly seen in the pediatric population and may reflect a genetic or structural weakness of meniscal tissue.[40] These tears are generally treated with partial meniscectomy, with an attempt to preserve as much meniscal tissue as possible.

Arthroscopic techniques for meniscal repair can be divided into three groups—inside-out, outside-in, and all-inside repair. For all techniques, the tear is first identified and probed to evaluate the size, location, pattern, and stability. Repairable tears are then reduced, and the tear site is prepared through rasping of the nearby synovium and meniscal tissue to create a bleeding surface for repair. Inside-out arthroscopic techniques have traditionally been the gold standard method of repair for most midbody and posterior horn tears. This technique relies on the use of double-armed absorbable or nonabsorbable sutures linking long flexible needles. The flexible needles are placed through curved cannulas and across the meniscal tear in a horizontal or vertical mattress fashion. The sutures are spaced approximately 3 to 5 mm apart and must be retrieved through and tied down to the capsule through a separate medial or lateral incision, thereby protecting the posterior neurovascular structures as well as the saphenous nerve medially and peroneal nerve laterally (Fig. 114.2).[24] Outside-in repair is a similar technique used mostly for anterior horn tears that relies on sutures fed through spinal needles percutaneously placed across the tear site. After passing through the tear, the sutures are retrieved and tied down to the capsule anteriorly through a small separate incision.

Recently, arthroscopic all-inside meniscal repair techniques have gained in popularity. These techniques rely on newer generation implants that are suture-based, flexible, and low profile, providing secure fixation across the tear site while minimizing risk of adjacent chondral injury (Fig. 114.3). These implants rely on capsular penetration for deployment during repair of tears. There is still considerable concern in younger children with smaller knees in using adult-sized implants, given the closer proximity of the posterior neurovascular bundle and the risk of overpenetration of the capsule. In these cases a standard inside-out repair with protection of the posterior neurovascular structures through an accessory incision is safest. All-inside techniques may also be used in combination with inside-out sutures, forming a so-called hybrid construct, particularly in the repair of large bucket hangle tears.[11] Regardless of the technique used, preparation of the repair site, anatomic

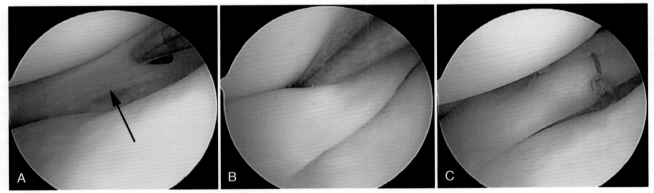

FIG 114.2 Reduction and Repair of a Bucket Handle Meniscal Tear Using an Inside-Out Technique (A) Bucket handle meniscal tear is identified *(black arrow)*. (B) Meniscal fragment is reduced with probe, and tear is identified. (C) Meniscal repair using inside-out technique with horizontal mattress suture.

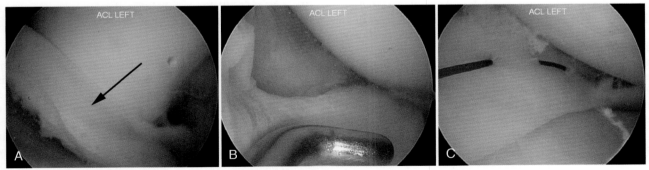

FIG 114.3 All-Inside Meniscal Repair (A) Meniscal tear is identified *(black arrow)*. (B) Tear is assessed for stability with a probe. Note the displacement of the meniscus. (C) All-inside meniscal repair with two sutures.

reduction of the meniscal tissue, and protected postoperative mobilization are key principles of any repair. Newer "enhancements," such as fibrin clot and protein rich plasma, may help to improve healing rates but are not yet standardized.

Postoperative protocols vary following meniscal repair. In most cases a combination of limited weight bearing, bracing, and restricted motion is used for a period of 4 to 6 weeks. Physical therapy is prescribed with the goal of obtaining full knee range of motion and strength. Return to sports occurs at 4 to 6 months. Patients are clinically assessed for meniscal healing, and the routine use of postoperative MRI is not recommended unless warranted by patient symptoms.

Outcome

Prior studies have published promising results on meniscal repair in children as part of a larger cohort of adult patients.[16,71] Despite the perception that the pediatric meniscus has greater healing potential, there is a paucity of data on success rates of meniscal repairs in this population. In the first published report, 26 patients, mean age 15.3 years (range: 11 to 17 years), underwent 29 meniscal repairs (12 medial and 17 lateral), with 15 of the patients (58%) undergoing simultaneous ACL reconstruction.[50] All repairs were performed arthroscopically, 25 with an inside-out technique and 4 with an all-inside technique. At mean 5-year follow-up, no meniscal symptoms were noted, all meniscal repairs were believed to have healed, and 27 of 29 patients returned to preinjury level sports. Another series reported results on 71 children and adolescents, mean age 16 years (range: 9 to 19 years), following repair of complex meniscal tears extending into the central avascular region.[53] At a mean 51-month follow-up, 75% of tears were deemed clinically healed. Notably, a higher rate of healing (87%) was found in patients undergoing simultaneous ACL reconstruction.[53]

A retrospective case series of 45 isolated meniscal repairs in children, mean age 16 years (range: 10 to 18 years), reported clinical success in 80% of simple tears, 68% of displaced bucket handle tears, and 13% of complex tears at a mean follow-up of 5.8 years.[42] Of these, 17 repairs (38%) failed at a mean time of 17 months (range: 3 to 61 months) and required reoperation. Failure was associated with a rim width greater than 3 mm from the meniscosynovial junction, suggesting a tear location outside the red-red zone. The same group later reported improved meniscal repair results in the setting of ACL reconstruction. In 96 children, mean age 16 years (range: 13 to 18 years), clinical success was 84% for simple tears, 59% for displaced bucket handle tears, and 57% for complex tears.[43] Another group included adolescents in a larger adult series and reported an 82% healing rate (based on second-look arthroscopic evaluation) for bucket handle meniscal repairs done in the setting of ACL reconstruction.[17]

The most recent study published to date on meniscal repair isolated to children and adolescents was a retrospective review on 29 meniscal repairs, patient mean age 15 years (range: 4 to 17 years).[41] Eleven patients underwent simultaneous ACL reconstruction. There were 26 longitudinal or bucket handle tears. The method of fixation was all-inside in 25 cases and outside-in in 4 cases. In 10 of the cases the tear extended into the white-white zone. At a mean follow-up of 2.3 years, 24 out of 29 meniscal tears had healed clinically. Four patients had reruptured their menisci at an average of 15 months after surgery, following a new injury.

Complications of meniscal repair in children are rare but can include neurovascular injury, arthrofibrosis, complex regional pain syndrome, and chondral injury from a protruding implant. In the studies noted, only two cases of arthrofibrosis and one painful neuroma of the infrapatellar branch of the saphenous nerve following inside-out repair were reported.[50] Although success rates following meniscal repair in the adolescent population are encouraging, long-term data are lacking and it remains to be seen whether meniscal preservation through repair will translate into lower rates of early osteoarthritis for these young active patients.

DISCOID MENISCUS

Since its first description in a cadaveric specimen by Young in 1889,[81] discoid lateral meniscus has become a well-documented meniscal abnormality seen in children. Although often synonymous with so-called snapping knee syndrome, discoid lateral menisci may manifest in a variety of ways. The true incidence of discoid lateral meniscus is unknown because many children may remain asymptomatic and few present with a true snapping knee. Nonetheless, the incidence is thought to be 3% to 5% in the general population, slightly higher in Asian populations.[15,30,31,38] Discoid morphology almost exclusively occurs within the lateral meniscus, but medial discoid menisci also have been reported.[13] In addition, the incidence of bilateral abnormality has been reported to be 20%.[5,10,59,68]

Cause

Debate exists over the exact cause of a discoid lateral meniscus but is likely multifactorial. Although initially thought to represent an arrest in embryologic development with failure of central resorption of the meniscus,[68] this theory has been disputed because the normal meniscus has been shown to not be discoid-shaped at any point during development.[13,33] Thus discoid menisci likely represent a congenital anomaly. Further theories have claimed that increased mobility with subsequent repetitive microtrauma leads to the thickened discoid morphology,[51] though hypermobility alone does not explain the formation of the commonly seen stable discoid meniscus with intact peripheral attachments.[77] Most authors now consider discoid meniscus as an anatomic variant with a propensity for tearing because of mechanical stresses and hypermobility because of a thicker, less vascular structure that often lacks peripheral attachments.[13,38,51] Studies have reported a different ultrastructure of discoid menisci, including a decreased number of collagen fibers and a disorganization and discontinuity of the collagen network.[8,56] Reports of familial transmission and occurrence among identical twins support the congenital theory.[30]

Classification

The most widely documented classification system is that of Watanabe et al.[75] who have described three types of discoid lateral menisci based on arthroscopic appearance (Fig. 114.4). Discoid menisci with intact peripheral attachments are complete (type I), covering the entire tibial plateau, or incomplete (type II). Type III discoid lateral menisci, the so-called Wrisberg ligament type, are complete or incomplete in morphology and lack posterior capsular attachments, with the exception of the posterior meniscofemoral ligament (ligament of Wrisberg). This type of discoid meniscus is thought to produce the classic snapping knee syndrome.[15]

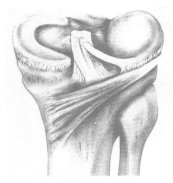 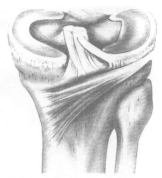 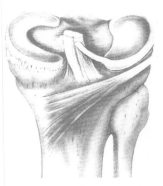

Type I   Type II   Type III

FIG 114.4 Watanabe Classification of Discoid Lateral Meniscus Type I is a complete variant, type II is a partial variant, and type III is a Wrisberg variant.

TABLE 114.1 Jordan Classification of Discoid Lateral Meniscus			
Classification	**Correlation**	**Tear**	**Symptoms**
Stable	Complete, incomplete	Yes, no	Yes, no
Unstable with discoid shape	Wrisberg type	Yes, no	Yes, no
Unstable with normal shape	Wrisberg variant	Yes, no	Yes, no

More recent reports have described variability, not only in the morphology of the lateral menisci but also in the attachments at the peripheral rim.* As a result, newer classification systems have been proposed. Jordan et al.[30,31] have suggested a system based on peripheral stability, type of discoid meniscus (complete or incomplete), presence of associated meniscal tear, and presence or lack of clinical symptoms (Table 114.1).

The true incidence of the Wrisberg-type, or unstable, discoid meniscus is difficult to assess. Previous series have documented between 0% and 33% of symptomatic discoid menisci as unstable.[24,25,28,49,59] With variability in the morphology and the subjective nature of assessing hypermobility, reporting stability is problematic. In a review of 128 cases of discoid menisci, Klingele et al.[36] reported a 28% prevalence of peripheral rim instability, with 47% detached along the anterior horn, 11% at the middle third, and almost 39% at the posterior third peripheral attachment. Good et al.[23] have reported a 77% prevalence of meniscal instability, documenting a 53% prevalence of anterior horn detachment or hypermobility, defined as the ability to evert the meniscus or translate the anterior horn to the posterior half of the tibial plateau. Such studies suggest that the classification of discoid menisci should be based on shape (complete or incomplete), stability (stable or unstable), and presence or absence of a meniscal tear. The assumption that an unstable discoid meniscus, or what many describe as a Wrisberg type, is present at birth may not hold true. With varying locations of instability identified, discoid menisci may begin as

stable and become unstable, or hypermobile, because of the repetitive stress placed on a thicker, histologically abnormal meniscus.

Diagnosis

The clinical presentation of a discoid lateral meniscus varies. Symptoms often are related to the type of discoid present, peripheral stability of the meniscus, and presence or absence of an associated tear.† Stable discoid menisci without associated tears often remain asymptomatic, identified only as incidental findings during MRI or arthroscopy. Unstable discoid menisci more commonly occur in younger children and in those with complete discoid menisci.[36] Peripheral rim detachment or hypermobility may produce the so-called snapping knee syndrome. In such cases a painless and palpable audible or visible snap is produced with knee range of motion, especially near terminal extension. This snap is thought to be secondary to reduction of the subluxed unstable meniscus as the joint space widens with knee extension. Limitation of knee extension by 10 degrees or more has been shown to correlate with unstable and complete discoid menisci.

In children with stable discoid lateral menisci, symptoms often present when an associated tear is present. In contrast to acute meniscal tears, such symptoms may present insidiously without previous trauma. Signs and symptoms of a meniscal tear may exist, including pain, swelling, catching, locking, and limited motion. On physical examination, there may be joint line tenderness, popping, limited motion, effusion, terminal motion pain, and positive provocative test results (eg, McMurray maneuvers, Apley test). Degenerative horizontal cleavage tears are the most common type of tear seen, reported in the largest series to occur in 58% to 98% of symptomatic discoid menisci.[5,10,59]

It is important to keep in mind the potential for bilateral involvement, particularly in children who present at a young age or with a complete or Wrisberg type discoid meniscus, because these patients have been shown to be at increased odds of symptomatic discoid meniscus in the contralateral knee, even several years later.[58] Patients under 12 years of age at initial treatment were 4.6 times more likely to require surgery on both

---

*References 8, 9, 23, 36, 52, and 79.

†References 6, 15, 18, 30, 52, 62, 77, and 79.

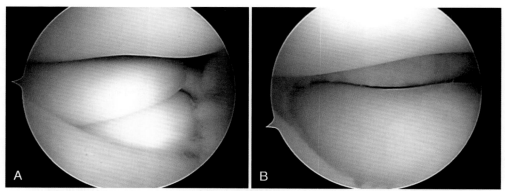

FIG 114.5 Saucerization of a Partial Discoid Lateral Meniscus (A) Presaucerization. (B) Postsaucerization.

knees, whereas those with an unstable discoid meniscus were 8.4 times more likely to have current or future bilateral symptoms.

Imaging Studies

Radiographic evaluation is often helpful to aid in diagnosis. Standard plain radiographs of both knees should be obtained, including AP, lateral, Merchant, and tunnel views. Characteristic findings on plain radiographs are often subtle but include a widened lateral joint line, calcification of the lateral meniscus, squaring of the lateral condyle with concomitant cupping of the lateral tibial plateau, mild hypoplasia of the tibial spine, and an elevated fibular head. Ha et al. have described hypoplasia of the lateral femoral condyle as seen on a tunnel view radiograph, terming this the condylar cutoff sign.[26] This is seen as a decreased prominence on the lateral femoral condyle adjacent to the intercondylar notch.

On MRI, discoid meniscus is seen as three or more successive sagittal slices with continuity between the anterior and posterior meniscal horns or a transverse meniscal diameter of greater than 15 mm or greater than 20% of the tibial width on transverse images. In addition, MRI can detect the presence of an associated meniscal tear. MRI has a high positive predictive value for discoid meniscus.[37] That is, when MRI is positive, discoid meniscus is almost always present. However, MRI has been shown to have a low sensitivity for identifying a discoid meniscus. That is, discoid meniscus still may be present despite negative MRI. When there is strong clinical suspicion for discoid meniscus despite negative MRI, the diagnosis still should be considered, and diagnostic arthroscopy may be necessary. Complete discoid menisci are detected more easily than partial discoid menisci. Normal morphology with detachment or hypermobility can be difficult to detect on MRI. Techniques to improve the detection of discoid meniscus include newer meniscal sequences, finer cuts, and increased MRI and pediatric imaging experience. Ahn et al.[4] have proposed a classification of discoid menisci based on MRI visualization of peripheral attachments.

There is growing interest in the use of ultrasound in orthopedics. Ultrasound has been used in the evaluation of discoid menisci and offers the advantage of a dynamic assessment of the meniscus to correlate extrusion with knee snapping during provocative maneuvers.[32] Although easily available and low cost, the use of ultrasound remains highly operator dependent.

Treatment

If the diagnosis of a symptomatic, discoid lateral meniscus is confirmed, surgical intervention is indicated. For stable, complete, or incomplete discoid menisci, partial meniscectomy, or so-called saucerization, is the technique of choice. If instability with peripheral detachment also exists, meniscal repair should also be performed. Traditionally, complete meniscectomy via open or arthroscopic means was suggested for such lesions. However, the long-term results of complete or near-total meniscectomy in children are poor, with early degenerative changes.[‡] Although there remains the rare case in which salvage of a discoid meniscus is impossible, improved arthroscopic techniques and instrumentation have made meniscal preservation through saucerization and repair the ideal treatment.

Arthroscopic saucerization should débride the discoid meniscus to a peripheral rim of 6 to 8 mm (Figs. 114.5 and 114.6).[§] Often, an indentation on the meniscus from the overlying lateral femoral condyle guides the depth of resection needed. If a meniscal tear is present, typically of the horizontal cleavage type, incorporation of its débridement into saucerization is most commonly performed. If the tear extends into the peripheral vascular zone, repair should be attempted. Arthroscopic saucerization can be challenging to an inexperienced surgeon because visualization and performance within the lateral joint space can be limited by the thickened meniscus and small size of the knee in pediatric patients. Saucerization is best begun with the knee in flexion by the aid of a straight biter or scissor punch. Smaller baskets are available and are more appropriate for pediatric knees. A meniscal or cartilage knife can aid in contouring the abnormal meniscus, especially the anterior horn. The knee can be placed in the figure-of-four position for further work. A combination of small arthroscopic shavers and biters further facilitates saucerization. With horizontal cleavage tears, often the smaller of the meniscal flaps is débrided, leaving an intact peripheral rim to the remaining tissue. Resection to widths more than 8 mm is thought to increase the risk of recurrent tear.

A careful and methodical assessment of peripheral rim stability and attachment must be carried out after saucerization.[23,36]

‡References 1, 16, 27, 39, 47, 49, 60, 61, 63, and 78.
§References 21, 28, 29, 39, 54, 57, and 70.

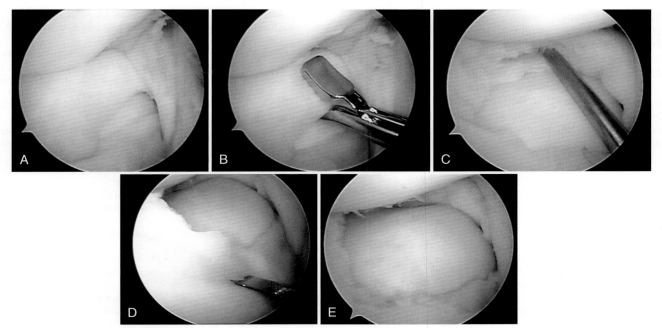

FIG 114.6 Saucerization of a Complete Discoid Lateral Meniscus (A) Presaucerization. (B) Excision of the central portion in the flexed knee position. (C) Probe within the horizontal cleavage tear. (D) Arthroscopic knife excision of the excess anterior horn. (E) Postsaucerization.

The frequency of peripheral rim instability mandates a systematic probing of the remnant meniscus at all peripheral attachments. In contrast to the posteriorly unstable Wrisberg type, anterior or middle horn detachment may also be seen. If peripheral instability is identified, meniscal repair is indicated. We prefer to perform meniscal repair using numerous inside-out sutures, zone-specific cannulas, and an open posterolateral incision to retrieve and tie the sutures, thereby protecting the peroneal nerve. All-inside devices may be inappropriate for discoid lateral meniscus repair, given the extreme meniscal instability and the size of the implants. For anterior horn instability, an outside-in technique is used, with a spinal needle used to pass sutures across the meniscocapsular junction (see Fig. 114.6).

Postoperatively, protected motion and weight bearing followed by progressive mobilization and rehabilitation are necessary. Younger children may be unable to ambulate effectively with crutches or comply with motion and weight-bearing restrictions.

The results of arthroscopic saucerization with or without repair have not been established. The studies showing short-term results report good outcomes.[52,62,77] Ahn et al.[3] have reported on 28 knees that underwent saucerization and peripheral rim repair. At minimum 2-year follow-up, all patients were able to return to full activity, with improved Lysholm and Hospital for Special Surgery (HSS) knee scores. Ogut et al., in a retrospective study of 10 knees treated with saucerization for complete discoid menisci, showed excellent results in 9 of 10 knees, with no degenerative changes identified on radiographs at 4.5-year follow-up.[55] In a consecutive series of 27 knees treated with saucerization and repair, peripheral instability was identified in more than 75% of knees and excellent clinical results were reported in 21 patients at 3-year follow-up.[23]

Studies reporting longer follow-up do suggest progressive degenerative changes of the lateral compartment. Despite showing good or excellent results in 85% of cases at 5-year follow-up, Atay et al. demonstrated radiographic flattening of the lateral femoral condyle in a significant percentage of patients.[7] Most recently, Ahn et al. reported outcomes following either saucerization, saucerization and repair, or subtotal meniscectomy in 48 knees at a mean follow-up of 10.1 years.[2] Although 94% of cases showed excellent or good clinical results, progressive degenerative changes appeared in 40% of patients. The subtotal meniscectomy group (88%) had significantly increased degenerative changes compared with the saucerization alone group (23%) or the saucerization with repair group (39%). Meniscal allograft transplantation may be an option for those patients with meniscal deficiency following total meniscectomy for a discoid lateral meniscus, with encouraging short- and intermediate-term clinical results.[34,80]

The biomechanics of the knee are certainly altered in the presence of and following treatment of a discoid meniscus. In a retrospective study of 158 patients older than 40 years who ultimately required treatment for a discoid lateral meniscus, those with a torn discoid meniscus had a higher prevalence of varus knee deformity and a higher prevalence of osteoarthritis.[35] Wang et al. demonstrated that the axial alignment of the lower limb changed to increasing valgus inclination rather acutely following saucerization of a discoid lateral meniscus.[74] Further long-term studies are needed to determine whether this change in alignment following treatment is protective to the knee or concentrates excessive stress on the lateral femoral condyle leading to degenerative changes or the development of lateral femoral condyle osteochrondritis dissecans (OCD) lesions, which have also been described in the setting of a discoid meniscus.

With further understanding of discoid menisci and the potential for developing peripheral rim instability, treatment of a stable asymptomatic discoid remains debatable. Classic teaching has been to treat asymptomatic discoids or those found incidentally without surgical intervention.

Unstable discoid menisci, which may be harder to salvage, more commonly present in younger patients with complete discoid morphology. Saucerization prior to symptoms and/or peripheral rim detachment may prevent future instability or the development of degenerative cleavage meniscal tears.

KEY REFERENCES

5. Aichroth PM, Patel DV, Marx CL: Congenital discoid lateral meniscus in children. A follow-up study and evolution of management. *J Bone Joint Surg Br* 73:932–936, 1991.
13. Clark CR, Ogden JA: Development of the menisci of the human knee joint. Morphological changes and their potential role in childhood meniscal injury. *J Bone Joint Surg Am* 65:538–547, 1983.
15. Dickhaut SC, DeLee JC: The discoid lateral-meniscus syndrome. *J Bone Joint Surg Am* 64:1068–1073, 1982.
29. Ikeuchi H: Arthroscopic treatment of the discoid lateral meniscus. Technique and long-term results. *Clin Orthop* 67:19–28, 1982.
30. Jordan MR: Lateral meniscal variants: evaluation and treatment. *J Am Acad Orthop Surg* 4:191–200, 1996.
33. Kaplan EB: Discoid lateral meniscus of the knee join: nature, mechanism, and operative treatment. *J Bone Joint Surg Am* 39-A:77–87, 1957.
36. Klingele KE, Kocher MS, Hresko MT, et al: Discoid lateral meniscus: prevalence of peripheral rim instability. *J Pediatr Orthop* 24:79–82, 2004.
40. Kramer DE, Micheli LJ: Meniscal tears and discoid meniscus in children: diagnosis and treatment. *J Am Acad Orthop Surg* 17:698–707, 2009.
47. Manzione M, Pizzutillo PD, Peoples AB, et al: Meniscectomy in children: a long-term follow-up study. *Am J Sports Med* 11:111–115, 1983.
49. Medlar RC, Mandiberg JJ, Lyne ED: Meniscectomies in children. Report of long-term results (mean, 8.3 years) of 26 children. *Am J Sports Med* 8:87–92, 1980.
50. Mintzer CM, Richmond JC, Taylor J: Meniscal repair in the young athlete. *Am J Sports Med* 26:630–633, 1998.
60. Raber DA, Friederich NF, Hefti F: Discoid lateral meniscus in children. Long-term follow-up after total meniscectomy. *J Bone Joint Surg Am* 80:1579–1586, 1998.
68. Smillie IS: The congenital discoid meniscus. *J Bone Joint Surg Am Br* 30B:671–682, 1948.
73. Vandermeer RD, Cunningham FK: Arthroscopic treatment of the discoid lateral meniscus: results of long-term follow-up. *Arthroscopy* 5:101–109, 1989.
79. Wroble RR, Henderson RC, Campion ER, et al: Meniscectomy in children and adolescents. A long-term follow-up study. *Clin Orthop* 279:180–189, 1992.

The references for this chapter can also be found on www.expertconsult.com.

115

Osteochondritis Dissecans

Benton E. Heyworth, Theodore J. Ganley

INTRODUCTION

Osteochondritis dissecans (OCD) was recently defined by Research in OsteoChondritis of the Knee (ROCK), an international study group[23] of high-volume OCD surgeon-investigators, as "a focal, idiopathic alteration of subchondral bone with risk for instability and disruption of adjacent articular cartilage that may result in premature osteoarthritis."[24] OCD is a relatively uncommon cause of knee pain and dysfunction in the child and adolescent, with the incidence recently established among patients 6 to 19 years old as 9.5/100,000 per year, with rates of 15.4 per 100,000 among males and 3.3 per 100,000 among females. Although the cause of OCD is unknown in most cases, repetitive microtrauma and athletic overuse patterns have been most commonly implicated.[13,17,33,59,75] Traditionally subclassified into "juvenile" and "adult" forms, modern understanding of treatment of knee OCD has classically relied on assessing the status of the distal femoral physis, with more than 50% of cases in patients with open physes demonstrating healing within 6 to 18 months after initiation of nonoperative treatment.[15,34,38,64,71] Standard of care treatment of OCD in patients with closed physes is operative intervention, given relatively low rates of healing with nonoperative modalities.[4,15] Close monitoring of all patients with OCD is essential, given that the natural history of untreated OCD is lesion progression towards instability and separation of the involved osteochondral fragment, leading to osteochondral defects, localized osteoarthritis, and possibly diffuse joint degeneration.[48,70]

HISTORY AND CAUSES OF OSTEOCHONDRITIS DISSECANS

Several factors have been implicated in the origin of OCD: inflammation, genetics, ischemia, accessory centers of ossification, and repetitive trauma. In 1887 König suggested an inflammatory origin, using the name "osteochondritis dissecans."[43] However, further study did not support inflammation as a primary cause of OCD. Ribbing ascribed OCD to an ossification abnormality of the distal femoral epiphysis in 1955,[62] a theory more comprehensively articulated by Laor et al., who conceptualize OCD more as a disturbance in the secondary ossification process of epiphyseal growth.[46] Based on their anatomic and histologic findings, Green and Banks[34] proposed that ischemia was implicated in OCD, although some additional studies have failed to find avascular necrosis of the OCD fragment.[16,41,61,63] There are conflicting studies regarding the presence of an ischemic watershed at the commonly affected areas of the femoral condyles.[16,41,61,63,68] Some investigators have

suggested a genetic predisposition to OCD, a theory which has generated renewed interest with more modern genetic studies.[8,55,60,79] In 1933 Fairbank suggested that OCD might be because of a "violent rotation inwards of the tibia, driving the tibial spine against the inner condyle."[26] Although anterior tibial spine impingement may not be the cause of lesions in the most common location of the posterolateral aspect of the medial femoral condyle, the frequent occurrence of OCD in patients who are involved in sports with repetitive impact supports a repetitive trauma etiology.[27] Trends in youth sports, such as loss of free play, early sport specialization, multiple leagues in a single sport, and intensive training, may be contributing factors. In summary, although subsets of OCD populations may demonstrate features of genetic, traumatic, ischemic, developmental, or metabolic pathophysiologic pathways, most cases are likely to have a multifactorial etiology and the continued study of the causes of OCD will be an important research initiative in the coming decades towards the treatment and prevention of OCD.

DIAGNOSIS

Clinical Presentation

The presenting complaints of most children and adolescents with OCD are vague and nonspecific, with variably localized aching and activity-related knee pain as the most common complaints.

Physical examination findings are often subtle. Children and adolescents with stable OCD lesions may walk with a slight antalgic gait. With careful palpation through varying amounts of knee flexion, a point of maximum tenderness can sometimes be located over the anterior aspect of the knee, medially or laterally, depending on the condyle. With stable lesions, knee effusion, crepitus, and extreme pain are rarely observed through a normal range of motion. Wilson sign, in which the knee is flexed to 90 degrees, then the tibia internally rotated as the knee is extended from 90 degrees toward full extension, eliciting pain at approximately 30 degrees, may be helpful but often is not present.[18,77] Mechanical symptoms are more pronounced in the less common circumstance of unstable lesion. An antalgic gait and knee effusion, possibly associated with crepitus during range of motion assessments, may be detected. In the case of both stable and unstable presentations, both knees should be examined, given the high rate of bilateral lesions, even when symptoms are not reported on the contralateral side.[19]

Imaging Studies

Imaging protocols have received close attention in the literature because of the varied success of nonoperative treatment. The goals of imaging are to characterize the lesion, determine the prognosis of nonoperative management, and monitor healing of the lesion (Fig. 115.1A to C).

Imaging workup begins with plain radiographs: anteroposterior (AP) (Fig. 115.2A), lateral, tunnel/notch, and Merchant/sunrise/skyline views. The tunnel view is particularly valuable because typical OCD lesions may affect the lateral portion of the medial femoral condyle (see Fig. 115.2B) or the posterior aspect of both the medial and lateral condyles. Because patellar and trochlear OCD lesions may be difficult to appreciate in the standard AP and lateral views, the Merchant or sunrise/skyline view should also be included. In older children the status of the physis (open, closing, or closed) should be assessed because this has major implications in the prognosis for healing. Plain radiographs usually characterize and localize the lesion and rule out other bony pathology of the knee region. In children 10 years old and younger the distal femoral epiphyseal ossification center may exhibit irregularities that simulate the appearance of an OCD. Contralateral radiographs may be helpful in differentiating these developmental variants from true OCD pathology (Table 115.1),[81] and given the minimal radiation and cost and availability of x-rays, screening radiographs of the other knee, which can detect treatable bilateral OCD before it progresses to more advanced stages, may become standard of care for OCD patients.[19]

Although computed tomography and technetium bone scans have been used to characterize OCD lesions and obtain information about the biologic capacity of an OCD lesion to heal, these modalities have not been widely used and may pose unnecessary risks related to radiation exposure in children.[14,48,58]

Magnetic resonance imaging (MRI) is the gold standard for accurately quantifying the size of the lesion and the status of the involved cartilage and subchondral bone. The extent of adjacent bony edema, the presence of a subchondral cyst and a fluid-like signal zone beneath the fragment (Fig. 115.3A to C), and the presence of other loose bodies are important findings on the initial MRI (Table 115.2). Evidence suggests that a high signal line on T2-weighted images, representing healing vascular granulation tissue or articular fluid beneath the subchondral bone, is a predictor of instability. A breach in the subchondral bone plate or cartilage, as seen on T1-weighted MRI, may help to predict treatment failure, particularly when seen in conjunction with a high signal line on T2-weighted images.[57] Because investigations of the relationship between gadolinium enhancement and healing have been inconclusive, noncontrast MRI remains the gold standard modality over intravenous contrast studies.[11,44,74]

TABLE 115.1 Features That May Differentiate Developmental Ossification Variation and Juvenile Osteochondritis Dissecans

Ossification Variation	Juvenile Osteochondritis Dissecans
Demographics	
Girls <10 years of age, boys <13 years of age	Girls or boys >8 years of age
MRI Features	
No adjacent bone marrow edema	Adjacent bone marrow edema
Posterior third location ± extension to middle third; not anterior third	Usually middle third location
No intracondylar extension	—
Spiculation, puzzle pieces, accessory ossification centers	—
>10% residual cartilage	Rare with >30% residual cartilage
Deeper lesion (lesional angle <105 degrees)	Flatter lesion (lesional angle >105 degrees)
—	Disruption of secondary physis
—	Widened overlying unossified epiphyseal cartilage

From Zbojniewicz AM, Laor T: Imaging of osteochondritis dissecans. *Clin Sports Med* 33(2):221–250, 2014.

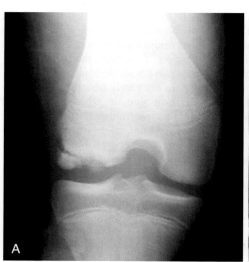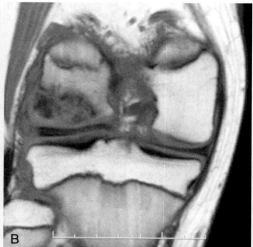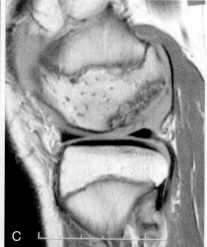

FIG 115.1 (A) AP x-ray of a large OCD of the lateral femoral condyle in an adolescent patient. (B) AP and (C) lateral T1-weighted images of a large OCD lesion in the posterolateral aspect of the lateral femoral condyle.

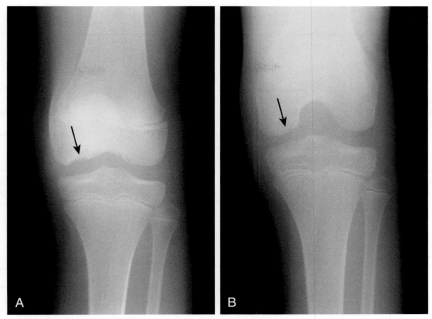

FIG 115.2 (A) AP and (B) tunnel plain radiographs demonstrating OCD *(arrows)* of the lateral aspect of the medial femoral condyle.

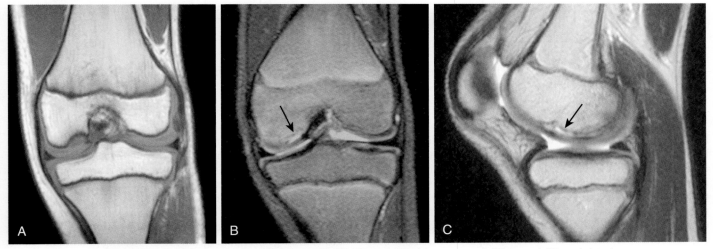

FIG 115.3 (A) AP T1-weighted image, (B) AP T2-weighted image, and (C) lateral T1-weighted image show classic location of an OCD lesion at the lateral aspect of the medial femoral condyle with fluid shown beneath the lesion *(arrows)*.

TABLE 115.2 Magnetic Resonance Imaging Classification of Juvenile Osteochondritis Dissecans

Stage	Magnetic Resonance Imaging Finding
I	Small change of signal without clear margins of fragment
II	Osteochondral fragment with clear margins, but without fluid between fragment and underlying bone
III	Fluid visible partially between fragment and underlying bone
IV	Fluid completely surrounding the fragment, but the fragment is still in situ
V	Fragment completely detached and displaced (loose body)

Data from Hefti F, Berguiristain J, Krauspe R, et al: Osteochondritis dissecans: a multicenter study of the European Pediatric Orthopedic Society. *J Pediatr Orthop B* 8(4):231–245, 1999.

NONOPERATIVE MANAGEMENT

Nonoperative management is the preferred initial treatment for skeletally immature children with stable knee OCD lesions (Fig. 115.4).[71] Although there are continued controversy and a limited body of literature-based evidence to support any one nonoperative treatment protocol,[29] the common denominator in all programs is activity modification in the form of cessation of impact activities, such as running, jumping, cutting, and pivoting sports. Because the primary goal of treatment is regeneration of affected subchondral bone, knee bracing is favored by many to provide immobilization or to help to unload the bone to allow for healing. Although casting remains a viable option for immobilization, many view this as more of a histori-cal treatment approach, given that hinged knee braces can be

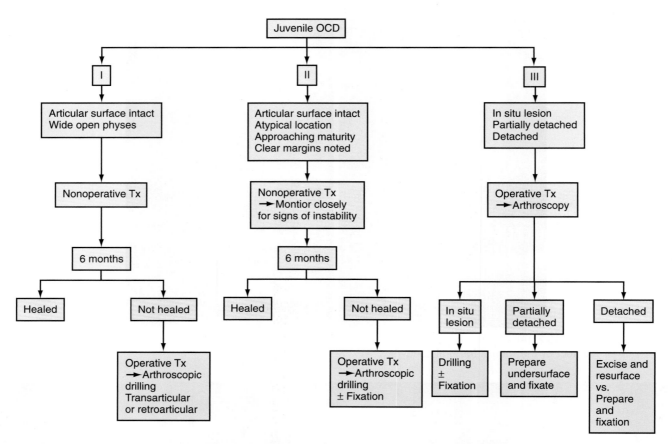

FIG 115.4 Algorithm for the treatment of osteochondritis dissecans in the pediatric patient. *OCD,* Osteochondritis dissecans.

locked and achieve a similar degree of immobilization but can be removed for bathing and possibly physical therapy. However, data have shown that casts are efficacious for healing and do not adversely affect long-term range of motion or strength in this population.[72] An alternative to locked hinged bracing is unloader bracing, and commercially available pediatric versions of the adult-type unloader braces, originally designed to unload an osteoarthritic medial or lateral compartment, have the benefit of allowing normal walking and range of motion. Non-weight bearing or partial weight bearing with crutches represents another alternative or compliment to bracing, although compliance with prolonged weight-bearing protection in the typical preadolescent or adolescent OCD population may be a challenge and has not been well studied.

Although patients with open physes have a better prognosis for healing than those closed physes, not all lesions in skeletally immature knees heal, and a patient or family's willingness to pursue these forms of treatment for many months may be limited, when operative options, despite carrying more significant risks, are theorized to speed the rate of healing. However, for amenable patients, repeat nonoperative treatment can be considered if radiographs show failure to heal, recurrence, or worsening of the radiographic appearance of the lesion or symptom recurrence. The duration that such nonoperative modalities should be pursued before recommending surgical alternatives is one of the most controversial topics in knee OCD management, although significant healing should generally not

be expected before 3 months, with most studies involving a protocol of a minimum of 6 months avoidance of impact activities before lesions are declared "unhealed." If any healing is seen within 3 months of nonoperative treatment, as seen on repeat radiographs or MRI, often families can be encouraged that continued healing may be likely, and analysis of risk factors for failed healing can be used to prognosticate on long-term healing without surgery. A nomogram for the healing potential of stable lesions in children was proposed by Wall et al., who found that after 6 months of nonoperative treatment, 16 (34%) of 47 stable lesions did not progress to healing. Large lesion size on MRI was the strongest prognostic variable for poor healing, with mechanical symptoms at presentation (giving way, swelling, clicking, locking) also representing a significant predictive sign of failure to heal with nonoperative measures.[76] A similar study by Krause et al. demonstrated that older patient age, larger OCD width, and presence of larger subchondral "cystlike lesions" were the strongest predictors for failed healing.[45]

OPERATIVE MANAGEMENT

Surgical treatment is the typical treatment for patients with unstable lesions, in patients with closed or closing physes, and in those whose stable lesions have not resolved after a reasonable period of nonoperative management.[4,13,25,36,39] The broad goals of operative treatment are to promote healing of subchondral bone, maintain joint congruity, rigidly fix unstable fragments,

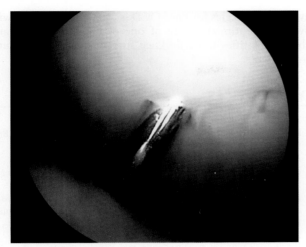

FIG 115.5 Drilling OCD lesion with smooth K-wire.

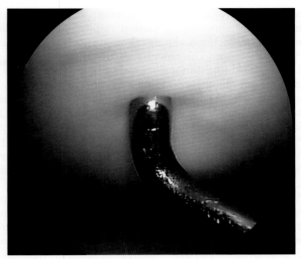

FIG 115.6 Probe demonstrates softening of a femoral condyle OCD lesion.

or perform advanced cartilage resurfacing procedures to replace osteochondral defects that arise in the setting of failed stabilization or detached lesions that are not considered salvagable.[32,64]

Arthroscopic drilling of the OCD lesion, which creates channels between the affected subchondral bone and adjacent healthy bone to promote revascularization and bony healing, is indicated for stable lesions with an intact articular surface (Fig. 115.5). The most common and best studied technique is referred to as "transarticular drilling," in which a small Kirschner wire (K-wire) (eg, 0.045 inch) is advanced multiple times in perpendicular, retrograde fashion through the articular cartilage under arthroscopic visualization (Fig. 115.6), across the subchondral bone of the lesion and into the deeper, unaffected bone.[6,42] "Retroarticular drilling" involves anterograde multiple passes of a similarly sized or slightly larger K-wire (eg, 0.062 inch) through the healthy condylar bone into the affected subchondral bone under fluoroscopic visualization, taking care to avoid advancement through the articular cartilage of the lesion.[1,12,22] Although the transarticular approach does not rely on fluoroscopy and may allow for optimized localization of the lesion and the drilling passes, the retroarticular approach has the theoretical advantage of preserving the chondral surface from injury. However, both techniques are currently widely used for treatment of stable lesions, with similarly favorable healing rates, which was likely to occur between 4 and 6 months postoperatively, and medium-term improvement in knee-specific functional outcome measures.[37] Younger age has been shown to be a predictor of a more favorable Lysholm score,[42] whereas factors associated with inadequate healing after drilling may include those in atypical locations, multiple lesions, and patients with underlying medical conditions.[28]

Treatment of unstable OCD lesions also involves drilling but must also include stabilization of the lesion with fixation in the form of rigid metal screws or bioabsorbable tacks or screws.[2] In the setting of a grossly unstable lesion that can be easily hinged open arthroscopically, additional steps to curretage the fibrous tissue and necrotic, sclerotic, or unstable bone found interposed between the subchondral bony portion of the fragment and underlying healthy portion is warranted. To optimize the healing environment at the bony interface of the fragment and parent bone, impaction of autologous, morcelized cancellous bone graft, following harvest from the femoral condyle or proximal tibial metaphyses of the affected knee or ipsilateral iliac crest, may be warranted if extensive curettage is performed or preoperative MRI demonstrates large or multiple cystlike lesions deep to the affected subchondral bone. All curettage, bone grafting, and fixation techniques may be performed arthroscopically or in open fashion, typically with a peripatellar arthrotomy on the side of the affected condyle, with both techniques and various implant options showing good rates of healing seen at a mean of approximately 6 months postoperatively in most series.* In cases of failed healing following fixation or presentation with an unsalvageable fragment, cartilage resurfacing techniques are used to attempt to optimize the local biology in the area of the lesion and the congruity of the articular surface. Although OCD fragment excision and simple débridement of the crater has been proposed as an initial treatment option,[3] progression of osteoarthritic "Fairbank" radiographic changes suggest a poor prognosis for lesions larger than 2 cm.[5] Marrow stimulation techniques with small drills or K-wires, sometimes referred to as "nanofracture," or awls/picks, commonly known as "microfracture," are designed to recruit pluripotential cells from the adjacent marrow that preferentially differentiate into fibrocartilage.[65] However, these techniques should also be reserved for smaller lesions, given that fibrocartilage does not respond to shear stress as effectively as native hyaline cartilage, and deterioration over time of the resurfaced region has been reported.[52]

Transfer of cylindrical autologous osteochondral plugs, also known as "mosaicplasty" or Osteochondral Autograft Transfer System (OATS) procedures (Arthrex, Naples, Fla), which are obtained from non–weight-bearing regions of the same knee (eg, the edge of the intercondylar notch or trochlear ridge), remains a viable option for osteochondral defects associated with OCD.[9,10,31,47] Good results have been reported in recent studies, both in patients with open growth plates and in those who have reached skeletal maturity.[58,80] A recent prospective, randomized study of 47 patients compared outcomes of patients treated with microfracture versus those treated with autologous

---

*References 4, 20, 21, 51, 66, 67, 69, and 78.

osteochondral plugs. Both microfracture and osteochondral autografts gave encouraging clinical results; however, lesions treated with osteochondral plugs showed superior outcomes at 4.2-year follow-up.[35] The potential disadvantage of osteochondral grafts, including donor site morbidity, are balanced by the advantages of biologic internal fixation.[40] Osteochondral allograft transfer for lesions large enough to require multiple mosaicplasty plugs has also been described for knee OCD,[30] with two studies suggesting successful incorporation in 90% to 100% of cases and mean International Knee Documentation Committee (IKDC) scores of 75, although 35% underwent secondary procedures, including revision allografting in 4 of 26 OCD patients at a median of 2.7 years, in one series.[49,56]

Autologous chondrocyte implantation (ACI) has been used in younger patients without coronal plane knee malalignment for resurfacing of large, isolated femoral defects. Three different series have reported good to excellent results between 4 and 6 years postoperatively in the majority of adolescents treated with ACI for knee OCD.[50,53,54] For deeper lesions with subchondral bone loss greater than 7 mm, good results also have been shown when a bilayer collagen membrane ("sandwich" technique) is used, which involves packing morselized cancellous bone graft into the osseous defect, covering the graft with a collagen membrane, then implanting cells in this and a second, overlying membrane.[7,73]

SUMMARY

Our understanding of the debilitating effects of knee OCD, when not diagnosed or appropriately treated early in the natural history of the condition, on the function and quality of life of both children and young adults, is improving. Because stable lesions with an intact articular surface can most often be treated successfully without long-term sequelae, early detection is critical, with MRI representing the gold standard for comprehensive diagnosis and staging of the lesion. Despite the challenges of imposing strict activity restrictions and forms of bracing or weight-bearing protection on an otherwise healthy and often active patient population who may be minimally symptomatic, nonoperative measures allow for healing of stable lesions in a substantial portion of patients with open physes. For stable lesions in patients with closed physes or those with closed physes do not show signs of healing despite these nonoperative modalities, arthroscopic drilling should be considered to prevent progression to an unstable lesion. Unstable lesions should undergo drilling and fixation, with a variety of implants and technique variations demonstrating successful healing. Because excision of large unsalvageable lesions generally yields poor long-term results, chondral resurfacing techniques should be used to decrease the risk of subsequent arthrosis. Future higher-level research into the best diagnostic, therapeutic, and prevention strategies for knee OCD is critical and may provide answers for optimizing care of one of the most challenging pathologic entities faced by knee surgeons caring for young, active patients.

KEY REFERENCES

2. Adachi N, Motoyama M, Deie M, et al: Histological evaluation of internally-fixed osteochondral lesions of the knee. *J Bone Joint Surg Br* 91(6):823–829, 2009.
5. Anderson AF, Pagnani MJ: Osteochondritis dissecans of the femoral condyles. Long-term results of excision of the fragment. *Am J Sports Med* 25(6):830–834, 1997.
9. Bentley G, Biant LC, Carrington RW, et al: A prospective, randomised comparison of autologous chondrocyte implantation versus mosaicplasty for osteochondral defects in the knee. *J Bone Joint Surg Br* 85(2):223–230, 2003.
12. Boughanem J, Riaz R, Patel RM, et al: Functional and radiographic outcomes of juvenile osteochondritis dissecans of the knee treated with extra-articular retrograde drilling. *Am J Sports Med* 39(10):2212–2217, 2011.
18. Conrad JM, Stanitski CL: Osteochondritis dissecans: Wilson's sign revisited. *Am J Sports Med* 31(5):777–778, 2003.
22. Donaldson LD, Wojtys EM: Extraarticular drilling for stable osteochondritis dissecans in the skeletally immature knee. *J Pediatr Orthop* 28(8):831–835, 2008.
27. Flynn JM, Kocher MS, Ganley TJ: Osteochondritis dissecans of the knee. *J Pediatr Orthop* 24(4):434–443, 2004.
35. Gudas R, Simonaityte R, Cekanauskas E, et al: A prospective, randomized clinical study of osteochondral autologous transplantation versus microfracture for the treatment of osteochondritis dissecans in the knee joint in children. *J Pediatr Orthop* 29(7):741–748, 2009.
38. Hefti F, Beguiristain J, Krauspe R, et al: Osteochondritis dissecans: a multicenter study of the European Pediatric Orthopedic Society. *J Pediatr Orthop B* 8(4):231–245, 1999.
42. Kocher MS, Micheli LJ, Yaniv M, et al: Functional and radiographic outcome of juvenile osteochondritis dissecans of the knee treated with transarticular arthroscopic drilling. *Am J Sports Med* 29(5):562–566, 2001.
45. Krause M, Hapfelmeier A, Moller M, et al: Healing predictors of stable juvenile osteochondritis dissecans knee lesions after 6 and 12 months of nonoperative treatment. *Am J Sports Med* 41(10):2384–2391, 2013.
51. Makino A, Muscolo DL, Puigdevall M, et al: Arthroscopic fixation of osteochondritis dissecans of the knee: clinical, magnetic resonance imaging, and arthroscopic follow-up. *Am J Sports Med* 33(10):1499–1504, 2005.
53. Micheli LJ, Moseley JB, Anderson AF, et al: Articular cartilage defects of the distal femur in children and adolescents: treatment with autologous chondrocyte implantation. *J Pediatr Orthop* 26(4):455–460, 2006.
76. Wall EJ, Vourazeris J, Myer GD, et al: The healing potential of stable juvenile osteochondritis dissecans knee lesions. *J Bone Joint Surg Am* 90(12):2655–2664, 2008.

The references for this chapter can also be found on www.expertconsult.com.

116

Reconstruction of the Anterior Cruciate Ligament in Pediatric Patients

Allen F. Anderson, Christian N. Anderson

An intrasubstance tear of the anterior cruciate ligament (ACL) is uncommon in pediatric patients, although it is a common injury in adults. Typically, knee trauma in a child or adolescent results in a bone or physeal injury.[49] However, the reported incidence of debilitating ACL injury in children has risen because of their increased participation in competitive sports and improved ACL diagnostic techniques.

A torn ACL in a skeletally immature patient is a treatment dilemma for the physician. In such cases, two basic treatment options are available: nonoperative and operative. Each option has its own set of challenges and possible long-term consequences for the child. The nonoperative approach can lead to instability, meniscal tears, and cumulative degenerative changes,* whereas operative treatment can result in iatrogenic leg length discrepancy or angular deformity.†

No consensus has been reached on the best method of treatment for a torn ACL in children and adolescents, primarily because of the paucity of basic science research on physeal growth and its response to injury. Although several retrospective studies on ACL tears in children have been conducted, the methods of the studies and the quality of the data have been inadequate.‡

Consequently, the treatment of ACL tears remains controversial in the pediatric population. Despite the lack of consensus, by using the current pediatric literature on the natural history of ACL tears, average growth and development patterns, and the response of the physis to injury, a reasonable treatment plan can be developed that is based on the consequences of iatrogenic growth disturbance. This chapter presents an evaluative approach to ACL reconstruction and describes three surgical techniques that may be used in the pediatric population.

NATURAL HISTORY OF ANTERIOR CRUCIATE LIGAMENT INJURY

The natural history of ACL tears in pediatric patients is not fully understood. However, evaluating the results of nonoperative treatment of ACL tears leads to some understanding of it. Physicians often favor nonoperative treatment for ACL injury because of the risks involved in operating on a skeletally immature patient. Nonoperative treatment may include activity

modification, bracing, and rehabilitation. However, studies have shown that these nonoperative approaches have poor efficacy,§ predominantly because pediatric patients are noncompliant, especially with modification of sports activity, and patients may be injured during free play. Noncompliance often leads to recurrent and sports-related instability and damage to the menisci.

Weak evidence in the older literature suggests that the efficacy of nonoperative treatment is related to the severity of the ACL tear. Kannus and Jarvinen[26] treated 32 patients nonoperatively with grade II (partial) and grade III (complete) ACL tears. At 8-year (on average) follow-up, 25 patients in this series with grade II tears had good to excellent outcomes. Seven patients with complete grade III tears had poor outcomes that included chronic instability and posttraumatic arthritis. These outcomes led the authors to reject nonoperative treatment of grade III ACL tears in pediatric patients. Angel and Hall also reported poor outcomes, including pain and limited activity, with nonoperative treatment of 27 pediatric patients with grade III ACL tears.[6] Most children younger than 14 years of age (92%) had functional knee disability at follow-up evaluation. Graf et al. found new meniscal tears after 15 months of nonoperative treatment in 87.5% of pediatric patients.[17] In a study of 38 adolescent patients, McCarroll et al. reported that 97% of patients experienced episodes of instability and 71% had symptomatic meniscal tears.[35] Mizuta et al. found degenerative changes in 61% (11/18) of patients within 51 treatment months[39] and concluded that these outcomes were unacceptable.

Several studies with a higher level of evidence have evaluated the consequences associated with delay in ACL reconstruction. In a study of 39 pediatric patients with an average age of 13.6 years, Millet et al.[38] (level of evidence [LOE]: 3) compared the concurrent injuries in a cohort of patients who had acute reconstructions (less than 6 weeks) with another cohort who had chronic reconstructions (more than 6 weeks). A highly significant relationship was found between the time of surgery and medial meniscus tears. Thirty-six percent of patients in the chronic cohort sustained medial meniscus tears compared with only 11% in the acute cohort. Lawrence et al.,[30] in a (LOE: 3) cohort study of 70 patients, found with logistic regression analysis that time to surgical reconstruction greater than 12 weeks (odds ratio: 4.1) and a single episode of knee instability (odds ratio: 11.4) were independently associated with medial

---

*References 1-3, 6, 17, 30, 31, 35, 38, and 39.
†References 5, 28, 29, 36, 46, and 52.
‡References 2, 5-7, 9, 10, 12, 17, 31, 35, 37, 45, and 54.

§References 3, 6, 13, 16, 17, 19, 22, 26, 35, 38, 39, 43, and 48.

meniscal tears. Time to surgery was also independently associated with medial and lateral compartment chondral injuries (odds ratio: 5.6 and 11.3, respectively).

Anderson and Anderson,[3] in a (LOE: 3) study of 135 patients found that delay in reconstruction increased the risks of secondary meniscal and chondral injury. Sixty-two patients were treated with ACL reconstruction within 6 weeks, 37 had surgery between 6 and 12 weeks, and 36 were treated after 12 weeks. Increased time to surgery had a bivariate association with lateral and medial meniscal tears ($P = .16$ and $.007$, respectively). Independent risk factors for incidence of lateral meniscal tears were younger age ($P = .028$) and return to sports activity before surgery ($P = .007$). Patients with one episode of recurrent instability had threefold higher odds of a higher grade of lateral meniscal tears. Compared with acute reconstruction, subacute and chronic reconstruction patients had 1.45 and 2.82 times higher odds, respectively, of lateral meniscal tears severity ($P = .012$). Another correlate of severity of lateral meniscal tears was any episode of recurrent instability (odds ratio: 3.15). Independent risk factors for the incidence of medial meniscal tears were older age ($P = .01$) and any recurrent instability episode ($P = .01$). The odds ratio for increased severity of medial meniscal tears include any recurrent instability episodes (odds ratio: 5.6), playing sports before reconstruction (odds ratio: 15.2), and time to surgery greater than 3 months (odds ratio: 4.3). Seventeen patients had 23 chondral injuries in this cohort. The risk factors for increased incidence and grade of chondral injuries included time to surgery ($P = .005$) and any recurrent instability episodes ($P = .001$).

Newman et al.[43] performed a (LOE: 3) study of 66 patients who were younger than 14 years to 165 patients who were 14 to 19 years old to determine the prevalence and severity of concurrent meniscal and chondral injuries. A multivariable logistic regression analysis was used to identify factors related to the presence of concomitant injuries. They found a significant relationship between time to surgery and the development of an irreparable meniscal injury ($P \le .05$) in both younger and older patients. Time to surgery correlated with severity of chondral injuries in the young cohort ($P = .03$) but not the older cohorts ($P = .88$). In the younger cohort, only a delay in surgery greater than 3 months (odds ratio: 4.8; $P = .003$) was significantly predictive of the presence of an injury that required an additional operative procedure. In the older patients, return to activity before surgery (odds ratio: 3.8; $P = .003$) and obesity (odds ratio: 2.5; $P = .038$) were significantly predictive of an injury that required additional operative procedures. They concluded that a delay in surgery correlated with increased severity of injury among both older and younger patients. A delay in surgery greater than 3 months was the strongest predictor of the development of concomitant injuries in the younger cohorts.

Other studies have evaluated additional injuries when ACL reconstruction was delayed for at least 6 months after the initial injury. Henry et al.[22] in a retrospective study of 56 patients (LOE: 2) compared concurrent injuries with surgery delayed by a mean of 30 months with those who had surgery delayed by 13.5 months. They found a statistically higher rate of medial meniscal tears (41% vs. 16%) and lower subjective International Knee Documentation Committee (IKDC) scores (83.4 vs. 94.6) in those with surgery delayed by 30 months. Dumont et al.[13] (LOE: 3) evaluated the incidence of meniscal and chondral injuries in patients undergoing early (<150 days; $n = 241$)

compared with delayed ACL reconstruction (>150 days; $n = 129$). Medial meniscal tears were significantly more common in the delayed treatment group (37.8% vs 53.5%; odds ratio: 1.8; $P = .014$) but the incidence of lateral meniscal tears were similar between groups. They also found that patients with meniscal tears were more likely to have chondral injuries in the same compartment. Guenther et al.[19] conducted a retrospective review (LOE: 4) of 112 adolescents with a mean age of 15 years. A comparison of magnetic resonance imaging (MRI) findings after the initial injury (mean: 79 days) with surgical findings at the time of reconstruction (mean: 342 days) showed patients who waited significantly longer for surgery (445 vs 290 days) had new or worsened medial meniscal tears. In addition, bucket-handle meniscal tears increased steadily in frequency for more than a year after ACL injury.

In contrast to the findings of these studies, a few studies have found that delayed reconstruction is a reasonable option. Woods[54] (LOE: 4) compared a group of 13 adolescents with a mean age of 13.8 years at the time of injury who had surgery delayed for a mean of 70 weeks with a group of 116 adolescents with a mean age of 15 years. The skeletally mature group had a mean time interval from the injury to surgery of 14.1 (0.3 to 355) weeks. The rate of meniscal injuries was 20% higher and the number of irreparable medial meniscal tears was greater when surgery was delayed by 6 months. The rate of additional knee surgeries was 62% when surgery was delayed by more than 6 months and 27% when surgery was performed within 6 months. Despite these differences, the authors concluded that there was no significant difference with respect to meniscal and chondral injuries between the groups, although they admitted that one of the limitations was the lack of statistical power because of the small sample sizes.

Another study of Moksnes et al.[40] compared 20 children 12 years old or younger treated nonoperatively with six children who had delayed reconstruction. Of the nonoperative group, 65% returned to their preinjury activity level and 50% were classified as copers at follow-up. Only 9.5% of the non-copers had secondary meniscal injuries. Based on the large number of copers in the nonoperative group and relatively low number of meniscal injuries, a treatment algorithm based on function and patient satisfaction was suggested that may identify patients who could participate in sports activities until skeletally immaturity, when ACL reconstruction would be considered.

In a follow-up (LOE: 4) study of this algorithm,[41] the same authors evaluated 40 children with 3.0T MRI at the time of injury and 3.8 years later. Patients in this cohort had a 19.5% chance of developing a meniscal tear not related to initial injury. Ultimately, 32% had ACL reconstruction because of recurrent instability, meniscal injury, and significant reduction of activity level. The authors recommended further follow-up to evaluate the long-term knee health in these children.

A recent meta-analysis and a systematic review evaluated the literature to determine the harms associated with nonoperative treatment or delay in surgical reconstruction. Vavken and Murray[52] systematically reviewed the current evidence for nonoperative and surgical treatment of ACL tears in skeletally immature patients. They identified 47 studies that met the inclusion criteria. Nonoperative treatment was found to result in poor clinical outcomes and a higher incidence of secondary defects, including meniscal and chondral injuries. They concluded that surgical stabilization should be considered the preferred treatment and nonoperative treatment should only be considered as a last resort.

Ramski et al.,[48] in a meta-analysis, systematically analyzed aggregated data from the literature to determine if superiority of treatment outcomes exists for nonoperative or early operative treatment for ACL tears in pediatric patients. They found six studies (217 patients) that compared operative to nonoperative treatment and five studies (353 patients) that compared early with delayed ACL reconstruction. Three studies reported that posttreatment instability occurred in 13.6% of patients after operative treatment and 75% of patients after nonoperative treatment ($P \leq .01$). Two studies found that symptomatic medial meniscal tears were 12 times more likely after nonoperative treatment ($P = .02$). Two additional studies reported return to activity; none of the patients in the nonoperative group returned to previous activity level of play compared with 85.7% of patients who were treated operatively ($P \leq .01$). The authors concluded that multiple trends favor early surgical stabilization over nonoperative or delayed treatment in pediatric ACL tears.

Although operative treatment has serious risks, these risks can be mitigated by careful evaluation of skeletal and sexual maturity of the patient and by selection of the appropriate surgical technique based on these presurgical evaluations.

SKELETAL MATURITY

Although chronologic age is a good indicator of mean skeletal maturity in large populations, an individual child can vary widely from the mean. The skeletal age of the pediatric patient is a key factor in determining appropriate treatment for an ACL tear. By estimating the skeletal age of the patient, the physician can gauge the potential risks and consequences of iatrogenic injury to the physis. As a rule, the younger the skeletal age (ie, the more growth remains in the distal femur and proximal tibial physes), the greater the consequences should growth disturbances occur.

Skeletal age is determined with radiographs. The most common method of determining skeletal age is to compare an anteroposterior radiograph of the patient's left hand and wrist with the age-specific radiograph in the Greulich and Pyle atlas.[18]

Although skeletal age is essential to determining the relative risk of ACL reconstruction, the physiologic age of the patient is also important and should be considered when planning treatment. Physiologic age can be determined using the Tanner staging of sexual maturation.[51] Tanner stages can determine whether the child is prepubescent (stages I and II), pubescent (stage III), or postpubescent (stages IV and V) through the presence or absence of secondary sexual characteristics (ie, pubic axillary hair, development of breasts and genitalia) (Table 116.1).

Preliminary staging should be assigned before surgery by asking the patient about the onset of menarche or the growth of axillary hair. To spare the child the trauma of genital examination, a thorough examination should be completed after the child is under anesthesia, but before surgery, for precise determination of the Tanner stage.

GROWTH AND DEVELOPMENT

The most rapidly growing physes in the body are located on the distal femur and proximal tibia. The distal femoral physis

TABLE 116.1 Tanner Stages of Sexual Characteristics Development

Tanner Stage	Boys	Girls
I (Prepubescent)	No pubic hair	No pubic hair
	Testes <4 mL or <2.5 cm	No breast development
II	Minimal pubic hair at base of penis	Minimal pubic hair on labia
	Testes 4 mL or 2.5-3.2 cm	Breast buds
III (Pubescent)	Testes 12 mL or 3.6 cm	Pubic hair on mons pubis
	Pubic hair over pubis	Elevation of breast; enlargement of areolae
	Voice changes	—
	Muscle mass increases	Axillary hair
		Acne
IV	Adult pubic hair	Adult pubic hair
	Testes 4.1-4.5 cm	Areolae enlargement
	Axillary hair	—
	Acne	—
V (Postpubescent)	No growth	No growth
	Adult testes	Adult breast shape
	Adult facial hair	Adult pubic hair
	Adult physique	—

contributes approximately 40% of the overall lower extremity length, and the proximal tibial physis contributes approximately 27%.[4] The distal femur grows at the annual rate of 1.3 cm but slows in the last 2 years of growth to an annual rate of 0.65 cm.[47] In boys, the mean peak height velocity occurs at age 13.5 years, with a range from 13 to 15 years of age. Peak height velocity in boys usually occurs at Tanner stage IV. However, approximately 20% of boys do not reach peak height velocity before Tanner stage V. Girls reach peak height velocity earlier than boys. The mean age for girls is age 11.5 years, with a range from 11 to 13 years of age. Onset of menarche typically occurs 1 year after peak height velocity is reached.

The severity of iatrogenic growth disturbance can be predicted by the skeletal maturity of the patient at the time that injury occurred. A 3-cm discrepancy in leg length—nearly three times normal variance—is estimated to occur from complete closure of the proximal tibial physis in an average 12-year-old boy, complete closure of the distal femoral physes in a 13-year-old boy, or complete closure of the femoral and tibial physes in a 14-year-old boy.

Although leg length discrepancy is an undesirable result of surgery, angular deformity is the more serious surgical complication. A valgus/flexion deformity of the distal femur can be caused by an over-the-top femoral groove if the perichondral ring of LaCroix is damaged, and recurvatum of the knee can occur if the anterior tibial physis is damaged. Wester et al. estimated that partial tibial physeal arrest in a 14-year-old boy with 2 cm of growth remaining in the distal femur could result in a 14-degree valgus deformity with a lateral femoral epiphysiodesis or 11-degree recurvatum with a partial tibial physeal arrest.[53]

Each of the studies reviewed in the following section illustrates the potential consequences of iatrogenic injury to the physis during surgical treatment. Patients at greatest risk are prepubescent (Tanner stages I and II), followed by pubescent patients (Tanner stage III). Patients at least risk are those nearing and those who have reached sexual maturity (Tanner stages IV and V).

BASIC RESEARCH ON PHYSEAL INJURY

Although there is a dearth of basic research on physeal injury in pediatric patients, several animal studies have evaluated the consequences of drill hole damage to the physis and of insertion of a soft tissue graft through a transphyseal hole. In 1988 Mäkelä et al. studied the effects of 2.0- and 3.2-mm transphyseal femoral drill holes in rabbits.[33] The cross-sectional area of the physis destroyed was 3% for the 2-mm drill hole and 7% for the 3.2-mm drill hole. Results showed that 7% cross-sectional destruction of the physis resulted in permanent disruption of growth.

Guzzanti et al. evaluated the effects of placing a soft tissue graft across the physis in immature rabbits.[20] ACL reconstruction was performed with the semitendinosus tendon using 2-mm transphyseal femoral and tibial holes. Drill hole damage to the femoral physis was seen in 11% of the transverse diameter and 3% of the cross-sectional diameter. The extent of damage to the tibial physis was 12% of the transverse diameter and 4% of the cross-sectional area. A valgus deformity developed in approximately 9% (2/21) of tibiae, and one incident of tibial growth disruption was noted. Based on these data, the authors recommended extreme caution when transphyseal reconstruction is considered in pediatric patients.

Transphyseal ACL reconstruction in a rabbit model using four tunnel diameters ranging from 1.95 to 3.97 mm was conducted by Houle et al.[23] Larger drill hole size was associated with increased and substantial deformity, and physeal arrest occurred despite the soft tissue graft. This study suggests that no more than 1% of the physis should be disrupted in children during an ACL reconstruction. In a rabbit model, Babb et al. evaluated the potential for growth arrest in three groups.[8] Group 1 was the control group; tunnels were drilled in the femur and tibia and were left open. In group 2 the tunnels were filled with a soft tissue autograft, and in group 3 the autograft was seeded with mesenchymal stem cells. Angular deformity and growth arrest were prevented only in group 3.

In contrast to these three studies, which found that soft tissue provided no protection, the following two studies demonstrated that a soft tissue graft across the physis prevents growth disturbance. In rabbit femurs, drill holes of 1.7, 2.5, and 3.4 mm were evaluated, in which one hole was left empty and the contralateral one was filled with an autograft of soft tissue.[25] Growth was retarded when 7% to 9% of the distal femoral physis was destroyed, but not when 4% to 5% of the cross-sectional area of the physis was destroyed. Bone cylinders were observed around the soft tissue grafts, but solid bone bridging did not occur. Prevention of bony bridge development or growth disturbance was also found in a canine model subsequent to a soft tissue graft placement in transphyseal drill holes.[50]

Other researchers have evaluated the effects of graft tension. Edwards studied the effect of tensioning a graft across open physes in a canine model at 80 N.[14] This technique resulted in the development of valgus femoral and varus tibial deformities without radiographic or histologic evidence of physeal bar formation. Chudik et al. also tensioned autografts at 80 N using transepiphyseal, transphyseal, and over-the-top femoral positions.[11] They found growth disturbances with each technique. However, the transepiphyseal technique was more anatomic

and caused less growth disturbance. These results are predicted by the Hueter-Volkmann principle (ie, when compressive force is applied perpendicular to the physes, longitudinal growth is inhibited). This suggests that even physeal-sparing procedures pose a risk for ACL reconstruction in pediatric patients.

CAUSES OF IATROGENIC GROWTH DISTURBANCE

Decisions about the surgical technique used in ACL reconstruction of a skeletally immature knee should be made after the potential for growth disturbance is weighed. Basic research, although incomplete and not entirely generalizable to humans, provides some evidence to assess the risk factors. Studies by Guzzanti et al.[20] and by Houle et al.[23] found that the risk for arrested growth is greater in the proximal tibial physis than in the femoral physis.

The risk of growth disturbance is generally associated with the extent of damage to the cross-sectional area of the physis. It is not completely understood, in animal models or in children, which drill hole size and orientation can be used without risk of disturbing growth. In animal models, the threshold for drill size growth disturbance appears to be between 1% and 7% of the cross-sectional area of the physis.[20,23,25, 33] Damage to the cross-sectional area of the physis can be diminished by making drill holes perpendicular rather than oblique to the surface of the physis. Although study results are not uniform, soft tissue grafts placed across the physis are probably protective against bone bridging and arrested growth. The physes are sensitive to compression forces,[14] so excessive ACL graft tension should be avoided.

Rare complications, such as angular deformity and significant leg length discrepancies have been reported in children who underwent ACL reconstruction.[28,29,31,52] Kocher et al. found 15 cases of growth disturbance in a survey of 140 physicians.[28] Lipscomb and Anderson[31] had one case of valgus deformity following ACL reconstruction in skeletally immature patients.

SURGICAL OPTIONS

Although there is a growing body of evidence indicating that nonoperative treatment is associated with meniscal and chondral injuries and sports-related disability, the decision to perform surgery depends on the risk and efficacy of the alternative, surgical reconstruction. Most authors have not reported growth disturbance after physeal-sparing ACL reconstruction in pediatric patients; however, Frosch et al.[16] in a meta-analysis of 55 studies including 935 patients who had either a physeal-sparing, partial physeal-sparing, or transphyseal reconstruction found that the risk of leg-length discrepancy or angular deformity after surgical treatment was 1.8%. In the systematic review of 31 studies ($n = 479$ patients), Vavken and Murray[52] found three patients developed angular defects and two had leg-length discrepancies. They also analyzed the literature to determine if surgical treatment was the best option for pediatric ACL tears. Nine studies with evidence level 2 or 3 compared surgical treatment to nonsurgical treatment ($n = 6$), immediate with delayed reconstruction ($n = 2$), and surgical treatment with mature versus immature patient ($n = 1$). These studies unanimously reported significantly better clinical scores and knee laxity after surgical reconstruction compared with nonoperative treatment. They also found no difference in the risk of growth disturbance.

Some operative approaches in pediatric patients, such as primary repair[12,15] and extra-articular replacements,[17,35] have also resulted in poor outcomes. It is possible to minimize the risk of physeal injury using a modified physeal-sparing intraarticular replacement.[32,42] Parker and coworkers reconstructed an ACL by passing hamstring tendons through a groove in the anterior aspect of the tibia and over the top of the lateral femoral condyle.[45] In 44 Tanner stage I or II patients, Kocher et al. used a combined intra-articular/extra-articular ACL reconstruction technique.[27,37] This technique places the iliotibial band around the lateral femoral condyle extra-articularly and passes it through the intercondylar notch. It is then sutured to the periosteum of the proximal tibia. In 42 of the 44 patients a mean IKDC subjective score of 96.7 was reported. Mean growth from surgery to follow-up was 21 cm. Lachman examinations were normal in 23 patients, nearly normal in 18, and abnormal in one patient. Pivot-shift test results were normal in 31 patients. Functional outcomes were excellent, and growth disturbance was minimal. Two patients had graft failure and subsequent reconstruction. Transphyseal tibial holes and over-the-top femoral positions with autografts[9,12] and allografts[5] have also been used.

In Tanner stage I patients, Guzzanti et al. suggested reconstructing the ACL using single-stranded semitendinosus and gracilis tendon grafts with a transepiphyseal tibial hole and an over-the-top femoral position.[21] No growth disturbances have been reported with over-the-top procedures, but lack of isometry can be an issue with this technique. The femoral over-the-top position has resulted in a mean graft elongation of 10 mm as the knee approaches full extension.[44] Avoid rasping with the over-the-top femoral position because this may damage the perichondral ring of LaCroix.

Controversy continues over ACL replacement procedures that use intra-articular transphyseal graft placement, because of deficiencies in basic science and clinical literature. Clinical studies that demonstrate the safety of transphyseal replacements have included postmenarchal girls and postpubescent boys with physes near closure.[5,7,34,35] Intra-articular replacements were performed by Pressman et al. in a series of 18 patients, 7 with open physes and 11 with closed or nearly closed physes.[46] Other surgeons have also performed intra-articular ACL replacements, but patients in these cohorts had only 2.3 to 4.5 cm of postoperative growth. In other case series, average patient age was greater than 14 years at the time of surgery, so the risks of angular deformity and leg length discrepancy were low compared with those in younger children.

Children in Tanner I and II stages are at greatest risk for growth disturbance as a consequence of ACL surgery. Few patients in the early Tanner stages have participated in studies of transphyseal procedures; therefore the safety of these procedures in preadolescent patients is not documented in the clinical literature. Furthermore, basic research has not proven the safety of drilling across the physis or of placing a soft tissue graft across the physis.

In an effort to minimize physeal trauma in Tanner stage II and III patients, Guzzanti et al. used a semitendinosus graft passed through 6-mm or smaller transphyseal femoral holes and transepiphyseal tibial holes.[21]

Anderson performed transepiphyseal replacement in a series of 12 patients (Tanner stage I, $n = 3$; Tanner stage II, $n = 4$; Tanner stage III, $n = 5$), using a modified adult ACL reconstruction procedure that did not transgress the physes of the tibia or the femur.[2] At the 4-year follow-up, mean growth from surgery was 16.5 cm. No clinically significant differences were noted in lower leg lengths, as determined by long leg radiographs. The mean IKDC Subjective Knee Form score was 96.5. The ligament laxity testing performed using a KT-1000 arthrometer showed a mean side-to-side difference at 1.5 mm at 134 N. According to the criteria of the Objective 2001 IKDC Knee Form,[24] the rating was normal for seven patients and nearly normal for the remaining five. At 4 years post surgery, one patient, who rated 100 on the IKDC Subjective Score at follow-up year 2, ruptured his ACL graft during a sporting event.

This technique or the all-epiphyseal technique shown in this chapter was subsequently performed on an additional 64 patients (76 total, Tanner stages I and II, $n = 53$; Tanner stage III, $n = 23$). Four of the 76 patients have ruptured their ACL grafts. One was in a motorcycle accident 8 weeks post surgery, sustaining a grade III injury to the ACL graft, as well as an injury to the medial collateral ligament. In another patient the graft failed, and no history of trauma was reported. The other complications included four patients who had a break in the EndoButton continuous loop after surgery. These patients had an excellent recovery after removal of the washer without residual pathologic laxity.

ANTERIOR CRUCIATE LIGAMENT RECONSTRUCTION RECOMMENDATIONS

Determining the best technique for ACL reconstruction in skeletally immature patients is not always easy or straightforward. The surgical literature is the most important factor in determining the best treatment. Unfortunately, the literature does not provide evidence to guide recommendations. Increased scientific rigor provided by multicenter research is necessary to clarify the contradictions in the literature and to help in determining the best method of treatment for pediatric patients with ACL injuries. Until a higher level of evidence is available, our bias is to modify the surgical procedure based on the patient's physiologic and skeletal age; this approach identifies the consequences should a growth disturbance occur.

For patients at highest risk—those in Tanner stages I and II (prepubescent males younger than 12 and females younger than 11 years)—a transepiphyseal or all-epiphyseal ACL reconstruction procedure is recommended because it does not transgress the tibial or femoral physis, thus minimizing the risk of physeal injury, but follows the accepted principles of adult ACL reconstruction. Some surgeons concerned about the technical difficulty of these procedures prefer the physeal-sparing procedure described by Kocher et al., which uses an iliotibial graft.[27] The functional results of this procedure are also good, although the iliotibial band is a weaker graft and is not isometrically placed on the tibia or the femur.

Intermediate-risk patients in early Tanner stage III (pubescent boys 13 to 16 years old and girls 12 to 14 years old) may be treated with the same procedures.

For lower-risk patients in later Tanner stage III or IV, the recommended procedure is a transphyseal replacement using quadruple hamstring grafts fixed with a proximal EndoButton and a distal screw and post. The recommended procedure for Tanner stage V patients (ie, boys older than 16 years and girls older than 14 years) is a standard adult ACL replacement procedure.

SURGICAL TECHNIQUES AND POSTOPERATIVE REHABILITATION PROCEDURES

ALL-EPIPHYSEAL RECONSTRUCTION

Setup

The patient is positioned supine on the operating table. The operative leg is placed in an arthroscopic leg holder one hand-breadth above the patella. The leg holder is then raised to elevate the operative knee above the contralateral extremity. Raising the leg holder facilitates visualization in the lateral plane while using fluoroscopy. The C-arm is placed on the side of the table opposite the injured knee, with the monitor at the head of the table on the same side as the operative extremity. Before the leg is prepared and draped, the tibial and femoral physes should be visualized in both anteroposterior (AP) and lateral planes. The C-arm is then rotated 30 degrees to visualize the extension of the tibial physis into the tibial tubercle on the lateral view of the tibia.

Graft Harvesting and Preparation

The hamstrings are harvested through a 3 to 4 cm oblique incision made at the level of the pes anserinus. The semitendinosus and gracilis tendons are isolated from the undersurface of the sartorius with a 90-degree hemostat and dissected free of any adhesions proximally. Then a standard tendon stripper is used to detach the tendons at the musculotendinous junction. The tendons are then sharply removed from their distal insertion. Next, the tendons are doubled, and a no. 2 FiberWire suture (Arthrex, Naples, Florida) is placed in the ends using a locking whipstitch. The doubled tendons are then placed on the back table under 4.5 kg of tension using the Graft Master device (Acufex-Smith Nephew, Andover, Massachusetts).

Diagnostic Arthroscopy and Notch Preparation

The arthroscope is introduced into the anterolateral portal, and a probe is inserted through the anteromedial portal. An intra-articular examination is then performed in a standard manner, and tears of the menisci can be repaired at this time. The ACL stump is then removed from the intercondylar notch so its anatomic footprint on the femur can be visualized.

Femoral and Tibial Tunnel Placement

The OrthoPediatrics (Warsaw, Indiana) all-epiphyseal ACL set has all the necessary instrumentation to perform each step. For femoral tunnel drilling, the arthroscope is placed in the anteromedial portal and the ACL drill guide in the anterolateral portal. The tip of the guide is placed in the center of the ACL footprint on the femur (Fig. 116.1). A minimal notchplasty may be required to visualize the footprint adequately. The handle of the guide is elevated 30 degrees anteriorly so the drill hole does not damage the lateral collateral ligament or popliteus tendon attachment. At this point, the C-arm is used in the AP plane to place the drill guide and guide wire distal to the femoral physis. After adequate distance between the femoral physis and guide wire is confirmed, the wire can be advanced across the femoral epiphysis (Fig. 116.2A and B). Using the arthroscope, the guide wire is then visualized entering into the center of the anatomic footprint of the ACL on the femur. The appropriately sized reamer is then placed over the guide wire to confirm the femoral tunnel will be distal to and not encroach upon the physis. The

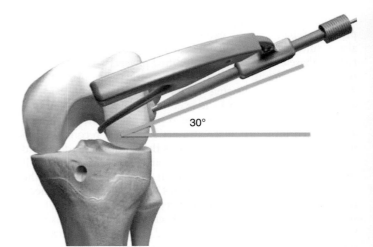

FIG 116.1 The Femoral Guide The handle of the guide should be elevated approximately 30 degrees to avoid damaging the lateral collateral ligament and popliteus tendon during reaming. (Copyright 2013 OrthoPediatrics Corp., with permission.)

femoral guide wire is left in place, and the arthroscope is switched back to the anterolateral portal for tibial guide wire placement. To visualize the tibial physis extending into the tibial tubercle, the C-arm is rotated approximately 30 degrees from the lateral plane. The tip of the tibial drill guide is introduced into the anteromedial portal and positioned anterior to the free edge of the lateral meniscus in the footprint of the ACL (Fig. 116.3). The guide wire is positioned on the anteromedial tibial epiphysis between the physis and joint surface and advanced using real-time fluoroscopic imaging through the epiphysis into the tibial footprint (Fig. 116.4).

Before proceeding, the diameter of the quadruple hamstring graft is measured using tendon sizers; these grafts typically range from 6 to 8 mm in diameter. We recommend selecting a reamer size that result in a tight fit for the graft in the tunnels. The tunnels are then reamed using live fluoroscopy. After reaming, the anterior intra-articular aspect of the femoral tunnel is chamfered using a rasp.

Graft Fixation

The first step in graft fixation on the femoral side is to insert the ShieldLoc sleeve into the femoral hole. The ShieldLoc sleeve (OrthoPediatrics, Warsaw, IN) is designed to protect the physis from radial pressure caused by the insertion of the interference screw. First, the counter bore reamer is inserted into the femoral hole until it bottoms out on the lateral femoral cortex (Fig. 116.5). During this step, the counter bore is inserted to a depth of 8 mm and increases the diameter of the femoral hole by 2 mm. The small amount of bone removal occurs rapidly. The iliotibial band should be retracted and soft tissue immediately around the hole is removed to allow for clear placement of the ShieldLoc sleeve. The appropriately sized ShieldLoc sleeve is then screwed on to the insertion device (Fig. 116.6A) and gently tapped it into the femoral tunnel (see Fig. 116.6B). The fluted fins on the outside of the ShieldLoc sleeve prevent the device from backing out of the femoral tunnel while removing the insertion device. After the ShieldLoc has been inserted, the Graft Passer from the Disposable Kit is placed through the femoral tunnel and retrieved through the tibial tunnel with an arthroscopic grasper. One of the free ends of both the

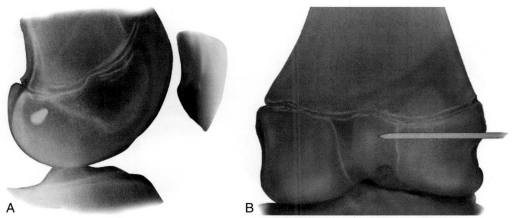

FIG 116.2 Anteroposterior (A) and lateral (B) fluoroscopic images demonstrating the position of the guide wire in the femoral epiphysis. (From Anderson AF, Anderson CN: Anterior cruciate ligament reconstruction in skeletally immature patients. In Prodromos C, Brown C, Fu FH, et al (eds): *The anterior cruciate ligament: reconstruction and basic science.* Philadelphia, PA, 2008, Saunders, p 464, with permission.)

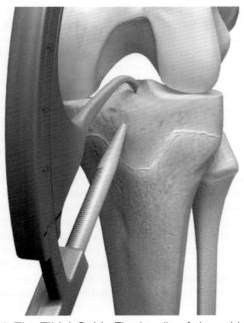

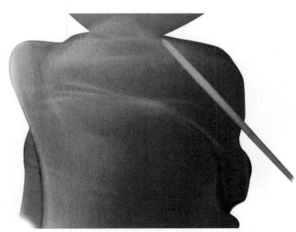

FIG 116.4 Lateral fluoroscopic image demonstrating the position of the tibial guide wire. (From Anderson AF, Anderson CN: Anterior cruciate ligament reconstruction in skeletally immature patients. In Prodromos C, Brown C, Fu FH, et al (eds): *The anterior cruciate ligament: reconstruction and basic science.* Philadelphia, PA, 2008, Saunders, p 464, with permission.)

FIG 116.3 The Tibial Guide The handle of the guide is positioned medial to the tibial tubercle to allow the guide wire to be advanced through the anteromedial epiphysis. (Copyright 2013 OrthoPediatrics Corp., with permission.)

semitendinosus and gracilis tendons are placed through the Graft Passer loop on the femoral side (Fig. 116.7). The tibial end of the Graft Passer is pulled, bringing the graft through the femoral tunnel into the tibial tunnel. Approximately 1 to 2 cm of the graft is pulled outside of the anterior tibial cortex to allow installation of the ArmorLink implant. The ArmorLink provides suspensory fixation on the tibial side. A hemostat is used to pass the ArmorLink around the tendons (Fig. 116.8A). The free ends of the graft coming out of the femoral tunnel are pulled to seat the ArmorLink on the tibial cortex (see Fig. 116.8B). The ArmorLink may be positioned in any orientation. Observe the ShieldLoc sleeve when pulling the free strands of the graft to make sure the ShieldLoc does not catch on the sutures in the

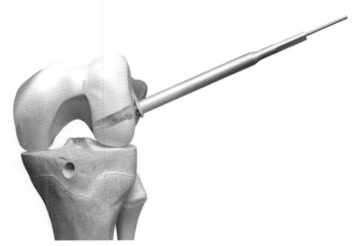

FIG 116.5 The counter bore reamer. (Copyright 2013 Ortho-Pediatrics Corp., with permission.)

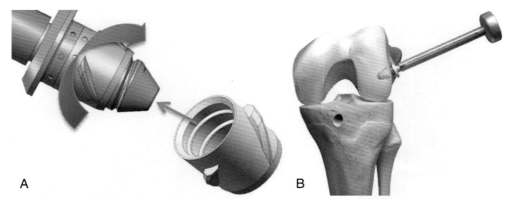

FIG 116.6 The ShieldLoc sleeve is screwed on the insertion device (A) and tapped into the femoral tunnel (B). (Copyright 2013 OrthoPediatrics Corp., with permission.)

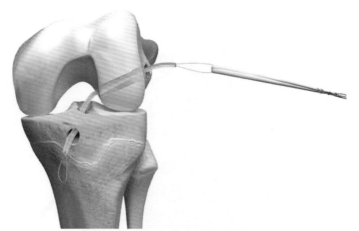

FIG 116.7 The Graft Passer loop is used to shuttle the graft through the femoral tunnel into the tibial tunnel. (Copyright 2013 OrthoPediatrics Corp., with permission.)

free ends of the graft and become displaced. If the ShieldLoc sleeve moves when pulling the tendons through, it can be stabilized with a hemostat to prevent displacement. With the knee in approximately 20 to 30 degrees of flexion, tension is applied to the graft using a graft tensioner and the corresponding screw is inserted into the ShieldLoc sleeve (Fig. 116.9). The graft is evaluated for intercondylar notch impingement, and the free ends of the semitendinosus and gracilis are trimmed after satisfactory stability is confirmed (Figs. 116.10A and B). The wounds are closed in a standard fashion.

POSTOPERATIVE ALL-EPIPHYSEAL REHABILITATION

Rehabilitation following the transepiphyseal ACL reconstruction procedure has three phases. Phase I begins when the patient awakens from surgery. Encourage the patient to perform straight-leg raises and to contract the quadriceps muscle. Use cryotherapy for 5 to 10 minutes each hour. The day after surgery, the patient performs range-of-motion exercises and hamstring stretches from a prone position. Patients without meniscal repairs may ambulate with crutches and partial bearing weight for 4 weeks. For patients who required meniscal repair, only toe

touch weight bearing is allowed for first 6 weeks. The 1-week post-surgical goal is to have a range of motion from 0 degrees of extension to 90 degrees of flexion.

Rehabilitation phase II is the strengthening phase and may last for 2 to 11 weeks. During this phase, patients perform active range-of-motion exercises and patellar mobilization and undergo electrical muscle stimulation. Patients should work at a comfortable pace. At post-surgical week 2, the patient is fitted with a functional knee brace and is encouraged to bear weight. Exercises should be introduced in order of increasing difficulty, including hamstring stretches, quadriceps muscle stretches and strengthening, proprioception exercises, and functional strengthening. Finally, strengthening exercises are performed in the pool. The goal is for the operative knee to have the same range of motion as the normal knee by postsurgical week 6.

The goal of the final rehabilitation phase is regaining full functional ability of the knee. This phase lasts from 12 to 20 weeks. Rehabilitation activities during this phase include functional strengthening exercises, straight-line jogging, plyometric exercises, sport cord exercises for jogging, lateral movement, and foot agility exercises. Between post-surgical weeks 16 and 20, patients may resume functional activities (ie, full-speed running) while wearing the brace. At post-surgical week 32, patients may fully engage in all activities, including competitive sports.

Physeal-Sparing Anterior Cruciate Ligament Reconstruction With the Iliotibial Band

This iliotibial band technique was previously described by Kocher et al.,[27] who modified it from the McIntosh and Darby intra- and extra-articular ACL reconstruction.[37] Kocher had good functional results despite the fact that this is not an anatomic ACL replacement. One cautionary note: this technique causes a defect in the iliotibial band over the vastus lateralis muscle that should be closed to prevent a cosmetic problem caused by herniation of the muscle.

The procedure begins with the patient in a supine position with a tourniquet on the proximal thigh. Make a 6- to 10-cm-long incision from the lateral joint line along the superior border of the iliotibial band. Expose the band and make incisions along its superior and inferior margins from Gerdy's tubercle to 15 to 20 cm proximal to the joint line, depending on the size of the patient. Detach the iliotibial band proximally and dissect it free from the lateral capsule; tabularize it with a

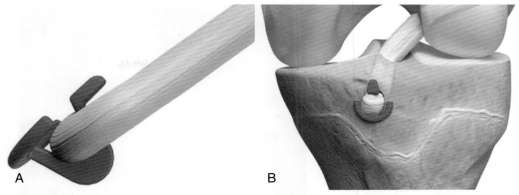

FIG 116.8 The ArmorLink device is passed around the loops formed from doubling over the hamstring tendons (A) and seated on the anteromedial tibia by pulling the free ends of the tendons proximally (B). (Copyright 2013 OrthoPediatrics Corp., with permission.)

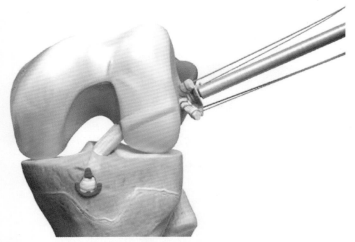

FIG 116.9 The interference screw is then inserted into the ShieldLoc with the knee in 20 to 30 degrees of flexion. (Copyright 2013 OrthoPediatrics Corp., with permission.)

whipstitch using a no. 2 Ethibond suture. Using the arthroscope through the anteromedial and anterolateral portals, resect remnants of the torn ACL and fat pad and perform a small notchplasty. Remove soft tissue from the over-the-top position of the lateral femoral condyle, taking care to avoid injury to the perichondral ring. Make a second incision parallel to the medial border of the patellar tendon, extending 4 cm distally from the joint line, and carry the dissection down to the periosteum. Use a Keith needle to identify the physis. Place a curved clamp under the intermeniscal ligament, and make a groove in the proximal tibial epiphysis using a small curved rasp; be careful not to damage the anterior tibial physis. Pull the iliotibial band graft into the knee using a full-length clamp or a tendon passer. Pass it through the anteromedial portal, over the top of the lateral femoral condyle, and out the lateral capsule. Then pass the clamp under the intermeniscal ligament, grasp the graft again, and pull it into the medial incision. The graft can now be seated into the groove in the tibial epiphyses. After placing it under tension, suture it to the lateral femoral condyle at the insertion of the lateral intermuscular septum with the knee placed in 90 degrees of flexion and 15 degrees of external rotation (Fig. 116.11). Incise the periosteum distal to the physis, and make a

trough into the metaphysis. Next, with the knee placed in 20 degrees of flexion, place the graft under tension and suture it to the periosteum. Close the defect over the vastus lateralis muscle that was created when the iliotibial band was harvested. Leave the lateral patellar reticulum open to avoid excessive pressure on the lateral facet of the patella. Close the wounds using standard technique, and place the knee in a hinged knee brace.

Postoperative Rehabilitation

Keep the knee in the hinged knee brace for the first 6 postoperative weeks. For the first 2 postoperative weeks, a continuous passive motion (CPM) machine is used with the range of motion set at 0 to 90 degrees. The patient should be maintained on partial weight bearing for 6 weeks. Rehabilitation otherwise should proceed in the same manner as that for the transepiphyseal ACL reconstruction.

TRANSPHYSEAL ANTERIOR CRUCIATE LIGAMENT RECONSTRUCTION

Place the lower limb in an arthroscopic leg holder at 60 degrees flexion. Make an oblique incision 4 cm long over the semitendinosus and gracilis tendons and dissect the tendons free. Transect the tendons at the musculotendinous junction using a standard tendon stripper, and detach them at the distal end. Place a no. 2 FiberWire suture in each end of the tendons, using an interlocking whipstitch. Measure the diameter of the quadruple hamstring grafts with tendon sizers; they typically range in size from 6 to 8 mm. Double the tendons, and place them under 4.5 kg (10 lb) of tension on the back table with the Graft Master device (Acufex-Smith Nephew). Next, insert the arthroscope into the anterolateral portal, and insert a probe through the anteromedial portal. Perform a systematic intra-articular examination using standard methods. Remove any debris found in the intercondylar notch, and perform a minimal notchplasty to visualize the anatomic footprint of the ACL on the femur. Note that the femoral physis is in close proximity, and be careful to avoid enlarging the posterior arch of the intercondylar notch. At this point in the procedure, repair any significant tears in the meniscus.

Insert the point of the tibial drill guide through the anteromedial portal. With the guide set at a 55-degree angle, orient it so that the guide pin enters the anteromedial aspect of the tibia

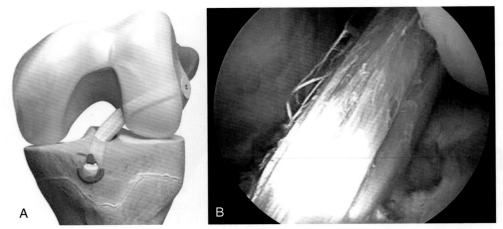

FIG 116.10 The final construct (A). Arthroscopic view of the graft after fixation (B). (Copyright 2013 OrthoPediatrics Corp., with permission.)

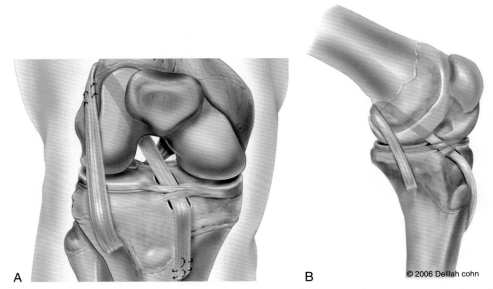

© 2006 Delilah cohn

FIG 116.11 Anteroposterior (A) and oblique (B) views of the over-the-top reconstruction after the graft has been passed over the lateral femoral condyle, through the knee, under the intermeniscal ligament, and into the groove in the proximal tibia. (With permission from Delilah Cohn.)

at a 65- to 70-degree angle in the coronal plane. Ensure that the pin enters the joint at the level of the free edge of the lateral meniscus and in the posterior footprint of the ACL on the tibia. Ream the tibial hole over the guide wire with a standard cannulated drill bit. Ensure that the fit of the graft is tight within the tibial tunnel by using the smallest drill bit possible to ream the tibial hole. After drilling is complete, remove debris using a shaver.

Before inserting the femoral guide wire, flex the knee to at least 90 degrees. Use a flexible reamer (Stryker Corp., Kalamazoo, Michigan) to advance a 2.7-mm passing pin through the guide and lateral femoral condyle, penetrating the lateral femoral cortex. It should be possible to palpate the pin under the skin just distal to the tourniquet. Using a flexible acorn reamer matched to the diameter of the graft, create the femoral tunnel. Drill a 30- to 35-mm hole in the femur at the anatomic site of the ACL attachment. The depth of the femoral hole

should be 10 mm greater than the desired graft insertion in the lateral femoral condyle to allow for rotation of the EndoButton. Drill the 4.5-mm EndoButton reamer over the guide wire and out the lateral femoral cortex. Chamfer the hole to minimize fraying of the graft. Measure the length of the femoral tunnel using the EndoButton depth gauge from the anterolateral femoral cortex to the opening of the intercondylar notch. Use the EndoButton continuous loop that leaves 20 to 25 mm of graft within the femoral tunnel. Pass the no. 5 Ethibond suture in the EndoButton to facilitate its passage through both the tibia and the femur. Then, use the no. 2 Ethibond suture in the other EndoButton hole to rotate the EndoButton after it exits the anterolateral femoral cortex. Pass the hamstring grafts through the EndoButton continuous loop, thus creating a quadruple graft. Thread both suture strands through the eye of the 2.7-mm flexible passing pin. Insert the pin up through the tibial and femoral holes, piercing the quadriceps and the skin proximal to

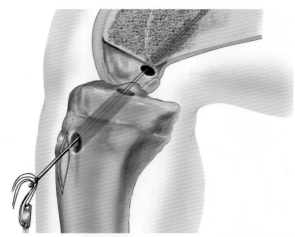

FIG 116.12 The passing pin is placed through the tibial and femoral tunnels and pulled proximally to pass the sutures. (With permission from Delilah Cohn.)

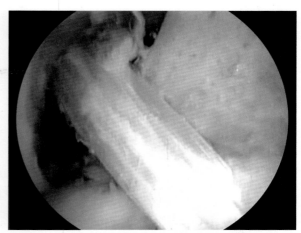

FIG 116.14 Arthroscopic view of the graft.

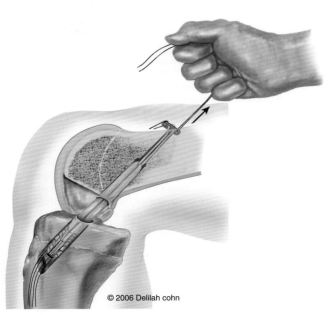

FIG 116.13 The graft is pulled into the femoral socked by pulling the no. 5 suture. The EndoButton is flipped by pulling the no. 2 suture. (With permission from Delilah Cohn.)

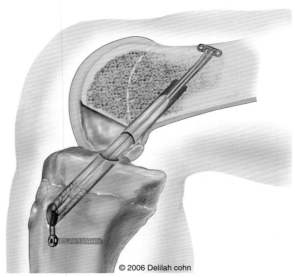

FIG 116.15 The graft is pulled distally to lock the EndoButton on the femoral cortex, and the hamstring graft is tied distally over a tibial screw and post. (With permission from Delilah Cohn.)

the knee (Fig. 116.12). Pass the suture by pulling the pin out of the femur. Pull the no. 5 suture first, and advance both the EndoButton and the graft into the femoral hole (Fig. 116.13). To lock the EndoButton on the outside of the femoral cortex, pull the graft distally. It should feel securely fixed in place. Use C-arm visualization to confirm proper EndoButton position.

At this point, remove both sutures from the EndoButton. Pre-tension the graft by cycling the knee through the ranges of motion several times. Next, place the graft under tension and extend the knee. Using the arthroscope, ensure that the graft is not being impinged by the intercondylar notch (Fig. 116.14). It may be necessary to remove a small portion of the anterior outlet of the intercondylar notch. Place a tibial screw and post medial to the tibial tubercle apophysis and distal to the proximal

tibial physis. With the knee in 20 degrees of flexion, secure the quadruple hamstring graft distally by tying the no. 5 FiberWire sutures over the tibial screw and post (Fig. 116.15). A graft that extends through the tibial drill hole should also be secured to the periosteum of the anterior tibia with several no. 1 Ethibond sutures using a figure-of-eight pattern. After closing the subcutaneous tissue and the skin with standard methods, apply a hinged brace.

Fig. 116.15 shows a more vertical graft position when the transtibial hole is used to create the femoral hole compared with the transepiphyseal technique. Postoperative radiographs show the drill holes and fixation in a male with a chronologic age of 12 years 9 months and a bone age of 14 years (Fig. 116.16).

Postoperative Rehabilitation

The postoperative rehabilitation protocol for the transepiphyseal ACL reconstruction should be used following this surgery.

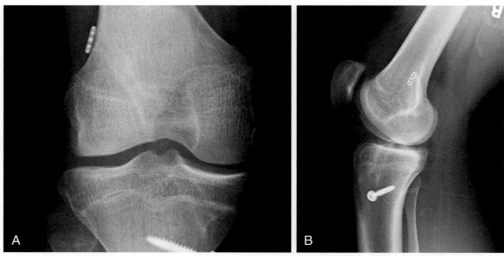

FIG 116.16 Anteroposterior (A) and lateral (B) radiographs of the knee 2 years after transphyseal ACL reconstruction in a patient with a bone age of 14 years at the time of surgery.

CONCLUSION

Ideally, operative treatment of ACL injuries in skeletally immature patients could be postponed until physeal closure. However, most of the evidence indicates that nonoperative treatment may actually result in substantial risks to the knee. In contrast, current methods of ACL reconstruction are highly effective in preventing additional injuries and sports-related disability. Consequently, the treatment of choice for pediatric ACL tears is early reconstruction (within 3 months).

KEY REFERENCES

2. Anderson AF: Transepiphyseal replacement of the anterior cruciate ligament in skeletally immature patients a preliminary report. *J Bone Joint Surg* 85A:1255–1263, 2003.

3. Anderson AF, Anderson CN: Correlation of meniscal and articular cartilage injuries in children and adolescents: timing ACL reconstruction. *Am J Sports Med* 43(2):275–281, 2015.

30. Lawrence JTR, Argawal N, Ganley TJ: Degeneration of the knee joint in skeletally immature patients with a diagnosis of an anterior cruciate ligament tear: is there harm in delay of treatment? *Am J Sports Med* 39(12):2582–2587, 2011.

43. Newman JT, Carry PM, Terhune B, et al: Factors predictive of concomitant injuries among children and adolescents undergoing anterior cruciate ligament surgery. *Am J Sports Med* 43(2):282–288, 2015.

48. Ramski DE, Kanj WW, Franklin CC, et al: Anterior cruciate ligament tears in children and adolescents: a meta-analysis of nonoperative versus operative treatment. *Am J Sports Med* 42(11):2769–2776, 2014.

52. Vavken P, Murray M: Treating anterior cruciate ligament tears in skeletally immature patients. *Arthroscopy* 27(5):704–716, 2011.

The references for this chapter can also be found on www.expertconsult.com.

117

Tibial Spine Fractures

Dennis E. Kramer, Yi-Meng Yen, Mininder S. Kocher

INTRODUCTION

Tibial spine (eminence) fractures occur in skeletally immature children and represent chondroepiphyseal avulsions of the anterior cruciate ligament (ACL) insertion on the anteromedial tibial spine.[21] These injuries usually occur in individuals between the ages of 8 and 14 with no predilection for gender. This is still a relatively rare injury accounting for about 2% of knee injuries or 3 per 100,000 children per year.[30] Originally believed to be the pediatric equivalent of the adult midsubstance ACL tear, it is now well known that isolated midsubstance ACL tears can also occur in skeletally immature children.[22] In a tibial spine fracture, excessive tensile force on the ACL in skeletally immature children leads to failure through the cancellous bone beneath as the ACL attachment site is broad and stronger than the underlying bone.[59] Recent authors have described a purely cartilaginous variant of tibial spine fractures that has been seen in patients younger than 9 years old.[8] Subtle anatomic differences may predispose children to a tibial spine avulsion or midsubstance ACL tear. Kocher et al.[22] compared 25 skeletally immature patients with midsubstance ACL tears to 25 similarly aged patients with tibial spine avulsions and noted a significantly narrower notch-width index in patients who had midsubstance ACL tears.

Fractures of the tibial spine are avulsion fractures of the ACL insertion, and in addition to disrupting ACL continuity may, depending on the size of the fracture, involve the articular surface of the tibia.[41,59] Noyes et al. has shown that as the subchondral bone fails, a elongation or stretch of the ACL occurs.[41] This has led many authors to equate this injury to a midsubstance ACL rupture in adults.*

Historically, treatment has evolved from closed treatment of all fractures to operative treatment of certain types. Garcia and Neer[17] reported 42 fractures of the tibial spine in patients ranging in age from 7 to 60 years with successful closed management in half their patients. Meyers and McKeever[37] recommended arthrotomy and open reduction for all displaced fractures, followed by cast immobilization with the knee in 20 degrees of flexion. Gronkvist et al.[14] reported late instability in 16 of 32 children with tibial spine fractures, and recommended surgery for all displaced tibial spine fractures, particularly in children older than 10 years of age because of increased demand on the ACL–tibial spine complex. In a comparison of displaced tibial spine fractures, McLennan[35] reported on 10 patients treated with closed reduction or with arthroscopic reduction with or without internal fixation. After a second-look arthroscopy at 6 years, those treated with closed reduction had more knee laxity than those treated arthroscopically.

Modern treatment is based on fracture type. Fractures that are nondisplaced or minimally displaced but reducible with knee extension can be treated with immobilization. Hinged and displaced fractures that do not reduce require open or arthroscopic reduction with internal fixation. A variety of treatment options have been reported with the goal of treatment to obtain a stable, pain-free knee. The prognosis for closed treatment of nondisplaced tibial spine fractures and for operative treatment of displaced fractures is good. Most series report healing with an excellent functional outcome despite some residual knee laxity.† Potential complications include nonunion, malunion, arthrofibrosis, residual knee laxity, and growth disturbance.‡

MECHANISM OF INJURY

Classically, pediatric tibial spine fractures occurred from bicycling accidents, although they are also seen with pedestrian–motor vehicle accidents or sports injuries.[37] With increased participation in youth sports at earlier ages and higher competitive levels, fractures resulting from sporting activities are being seen with increased frequency. The differential injury patterns of an ACL tear versus a tibial eminence fracture in the skeletally immature knee may be because of loading conditions, biomechanical properties, and anatomical differences.[22,41,57,59] The most common mechanism of tibial eminence fracture is forced valgus and external rotation of the tibia, although tibial spine avulsion fractures can also occur from hyperflexion, hyperextension, or tibial internal rotation. Slower loading rates, relative weakness of the incompletely ossified intercondylar eminence compared to the ligament midsubstance, greater elasticity of the ACL, and a wider intercondylar notch are believed to preferentially result in tibial spine avulsion fracture.[22,41,57,59] Although far less common, tibial spine fracture can occur in adults and frequently involve lesions of the meniscus, capsule, or collateral ligaments because they are associated with higher energy mechanisms.[45]

PHYSICAL EXAMINATION

Evaluation should consist of a thorough history and physical examination. Tibial spine fractures often present with a painful

---

*References 4, 5, 14, 16, 57, and 58.

†References 3, 4, 5, 19, 23, 25, 32, 35, 40, 52, 57, and 58.
‡References 3, 4, 5, 13, 19, 23, 25, 32, 35, 40, and 54.

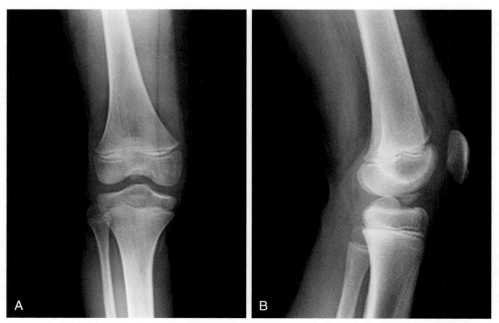

FIG 117.1 (A) Anteroposterior radiograph of displaced tibial spine fracture. (B) Lateral radiograph of displaced tibial spine fracture.

swollen knee, limitation of knee motion, and difficulty with weight bearing. On exam, a large hemarthrosis is typically seen and knees are usually held flexed because of hamstring spasm and may lack full extension if the fragment is elevated. Lachman's test can reveal anterior laxity similar to an ACL tear. Gentle varus valgus stress testing should be performed to detect insufficiency of the medial collateral ligament (MCL) or ateral collateral ligament (LCL). The contralateral knee should be assessed for physiologic laxity. A complete neurological and vascular examination should be performed. Pain may make thorough examination of the knee difficult. Patients with a late malunion of a displaced tibial spine fracture may lack full extension because of a bony block and may have increased knee laxity as demonstrated by a positive Lachman and pivot-shift.

IMAGING

Standard roentgenograms and anteroposterior, lateral, and notch radiographic views are usually diagnostic. The fracture is best seen on the lateral and notch views (Fig. 117.1). Radiographs should be carefully scrutinized because the avulsed fragment may be mostly nonossified cartilage with only a small, thin ossified portion visible on the lateral view. If necessary, computed tomography (CT) scanning allows refined definition of the fracture anatomy and may be necessary to best evaluate the size of the fragment and the amount of displacement. It is important to keep in mind that these are not "articular" fractures but rather functional fractures that contribute to ACL stability. Therefore, the most important aspect of assessing the reduction is to ensure that the ACL insertion on the tibia is reduced.

Magnetic resonance imaging (MRI) is not typically necessary to make the diagnosis of tibial eminence fractures in children. MRI may be helpful, however, to confirm the diagnosis in cases with a very thin ossified portion of the avulsed fragment and to evaluate associated collateral ligament, chondral, meniscal, or physeal pathology. If distal pulses are abnormal or

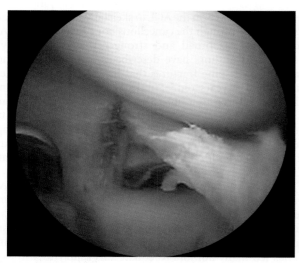

FIG 117.2 Meniscal tear in conjunction with a tibial spine fracture.

a knee dislocation is suspected, an arteriogram should be obtained.

ASSOCIATED INJURIES

Intercondylar eminence fractures may include or be associated with any combination of bone, chondral, meniscal, or ligamentous injuries. In a series of 80 skeletally immature patients who underwent surgical fixation of tibial eminence fractures, Kocher et al. found no associated chondral injuries and associated meniscal tear in only 3.8% (3/80) of patients (Fig. 117.2).[21] Other more recent studies have reported higher rates of meniscal pathology especially in type 2 and 3 injuries.[18] Mitchell et al. found no injuries in type 1 fractures, whereas type 2 fractures had 29% meniscal entrapment, 33% meniscal tears, 7% chondral injuries, and type 3 fractures had 48% meniscal entrapment, 12% meniscal tears, and 8% chondral injuries.[38] Associated collateral ligament injury or proximal ACL avulsion in conjunction with a tibial spine fracture have also been reported.[18,56]

CLASSIFICATION

The classification system of Meyers and McKeever based on the degree of displacement is widely used to classify fractures and to guide treatment (Fig. 117.3).[36,37] Zaricznyj later modified this classification to include a fourth type, comminuted fractures of the tibial spine.[60]

1. Type 1: minimal displacement of the tibial spine fragment from the rest of the proximal tibial epiphysis
2. Type 2: displacement of the anterior third to half of the avulsed fragment, which is lifted upward but remains hinged on its posterior border which is in contact with the proximal tibial epiphysis
3. Type 3: complete separation of the avulsed fragment from the proximal tibial epiphysis, usually associated with upward displacement and rotation

The interobserver reliability between type 1 fractures and type 2 and 3 fractures is good; however, differentiation between type 2 and 3 fractures may be difficult.[22]

SURGICAL AND APPLIED ANATOMY

Between the condyles, the intercondylar eminence or spine is the insertion point for portions of the menisci and the ACL and posterior cruciate ligament (PCL). The tibial eminence is triangular and refers to the portion of the proximal tibia where there are two ridges of bone and cartilage. In the immature skeleton, the proximal surface of the eminence is covered entirely with cartilage. The ACL attaches distally to the anteromedial portion of the tibial intercondylar eminence (Fig. 117.4). The PCL inserts on the posterior aspect of the proximal tibia, distal to the joint line. Both menisci insert into the tibia in the region

between the lateral and medial eminences, but there is no direct connection between the ACL and the menisci. In 12 patients with displaced tibial spine fractures that could not be treated by closed reduction, Lowe et al.[28] reported that the anterior horn of the lateral meniscus and the ACL were attached simultaneously and pulling in different directions.

Meniscal or intermeniscal ligament entrapment under the displaced tibial eminence fragment can be common and may be a rationale for considering arthroscopic or open reduction in displaced tibial spine fractures (Fig. 117.5).[6,7,21] Meniscal entrapment can prevent the anatomic reduction of the tibial spine fragment, which may result in increased anterior laxity or a block to extension and knee pain after the fracture has healed.[16,35,42] Mah et al. found medial meniscal entrapment preventing reduction in 8 of 10 children with type 3 fractures undergoing arthroscopic management.[31] In a consecutive series of 80 patients who underwent surgical fixation of tibial eminence fractures that could not be treated by closed reduction, Kocher et al. found entrapment of the anterior horn medial meniscus ($n = 36$), intermeniscal ligament ($n = 6$), or anterior horn lateral meniscus ($n = 1$) in 26% of type 2 fractures and 65% of type 3 fractures.[21] The entrapped meniscus can typically be extracted with an arthroscopic probe and retracted with a retaining suture (Fig. 117.6).

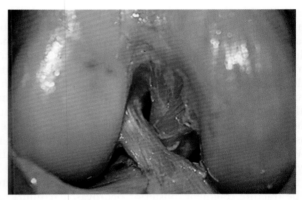

FIG 117.4 ACL insertion onto the anteromedial portion of the tibial eminence.

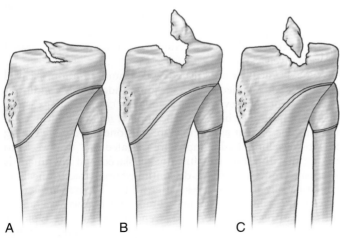

FIG 117.3 Meyers and McKeever Classification System of Tibial Spine Fractures in Children. (A) Type 1: minimal displacement. (B) Type 2: displaced and hinged posteriorly. (C) Type 3: complete displacement.

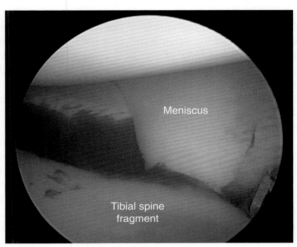

FIG 117.5 Anterior horn of the medial meniscus entrapped under tibial spine fragment.

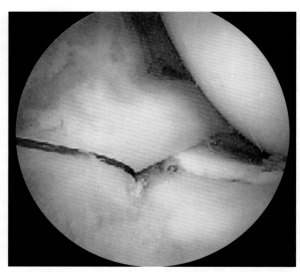

FIG 117.6 Use of a retention suture to retract the anterior horn of the medial meniscus.

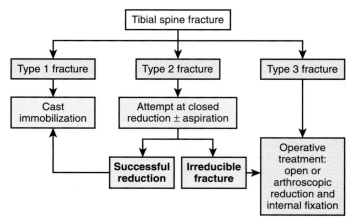

FIG 117.7 Treatment recommendations.

CURRENT TREATMENT OPTIONS

Current treatment options include cast immobilization,[25,39] closed reduction with immobilization,[42,58] open reduction with immobilization,[39] open reduction with internal fixation,[40,58] and arthroscopic reduction with immobilization.[34] Arthroscopic reduction is also available with a variety of fixation methods including suture fixation,[19,25,26,31,51] wire fixation,[3] screw fixation,[5,25,34] anchor fixation,[55] suture-button fixation,[2,15] suture bridge fixation (using anchors),[46] and bioabsorbable nail fixation.[49] All have been used with success, but the most common methods of fixation reported are suture or screw. Although some biomechanical studies have shown a slight increase in construct strength for suture repair,[48] clinical studies have not shown a clear advantage to either technique.[10] Suture fixation may be favored in small or comminuted fractures because it has the advantage of eliminating the risks of further comminution of the fracture fragment, posterior neurovascular injury, and the need for hardware removal.[1,26,49,51]

The goal of treatment of a tibial spine avulsion is anatomic reduction, but there is controversy regarding whether the tibial spine should be over-reduced. Theoretically, over-reduction may lead to excessive tightening of the ACL and limitation of knee motion.[29] On the other hand, it is likely that permanent intrasubstance stretching of the ACL occurs before the fracture,[41] and therefore over-reduction could be performed to account for this. Although further clinical or in vitro research is required, long-term evaluation of well-reduced tibial eminence fractures shows subtle increases in anteroposterior knee laxity without functional deficit.[4,23,52,57]

Closed treatment is typically used for type 1 fractures and for type 2 or 3 fractures that can be successfully reduced by closed reduction. Aspiration of the hematoma is performed first and closed reduction is achieved by placement of the knee in full extension or 20 to 30 degrees of flexion. If the fracture fragment extends into the medial or lateral tibial plateaus, full extension may aid reduction through pressure applied by medial or lateral femoral condyle congruence, whereas fractures confined completely within the intercondylar notch may not reduce. Portions of the ACL are tight in all knee positions;

therefore, there may not be any one position that exists without traction being applied by the ACL, which may prevent anatomic reduction. Radiographs are used to assess the adequacy of reduction.

Closed reduction can be successful for some type 2 fractures, but is frequently not successful for type 3 fractures. In their series, Kocher et al. reported closed reduction in approximately 50% of type 2 fractures (26/49) with unsuccessful closed reduction in all 57 of the type 3 fractures.[21] Arthroscopic or open reduction with internal fixation of type 2 and 3 tibial eminence fractures that do not reduce has been advocated because of the potential for clinical instability and loss of extension associated with closed reduction and immobilization, the ability to evaluate and treat injuries, and the opportunity for early mobilization.[6,7,23,31] For displaced type 2 and 3 fractures, Wiley and Baxter found a correlation between fracture displacement with measured knee laxity despite good patient function.[57]

AUTHOR'S PREFERRED TREATMENT

The author's algorithm for treatment of tibial spine fractures is shown in Fig. 117.7. It should be emphasized that displacement may be difficult to determine on radiographs. If uncertain, a CT scan can be obtained to accurately measure displacement. In addition, proximal displacement of the anterior-most portion of the tibial spine may not be clinically relevant. If most of the ACL insertion on the tibia is reduced, the fracture can be treated conservatively.

Type 1 fractures are treated with immobilization. A local anesthetic can be injected into the joint under sterile conditions if the patient is in severe pain. A long-leg cast, cylinder cast, or locked hinged knee brace may be applied in 0 to 20 degrees of flexion. The patient and family are cautioned to elevate the leg to avoid swelling. Radiographs are repeated in 1 to 2 weeks to ensure that the fragment has not displaced and alignment is adequate. Immobilization is discontinued upon fracture healing, which usually occurs 6 weeks after injury. The patient is then placed into a hinged ACL knee brace and physical therapy is initiated to regain motion and strength. Patients are typically allowed to return to sports at 3 months after injury if they demonstrate fracture healing and adequate motion and strength. A sports ACL brace is recommended for the first 6 to 12 months post-injury. Type 2 fractures are initially treated with an attempt at closed reduction. The hematoma is aspirated and local anesthetic is injected into the knee under sterile conditions. Reduction is attempted at full extension and at 20 to 30 degrees of flexion. Radiographs are taken to assess reduction. If anatomic reduction is obtained, an immobilization is applied in the position of reduction and the protocol for type 1 fractures is followed. If the fracture does not reduce adequately or if the fracture displaces later, operative treatment is performed.

Type 3 fractures may be treated with attempted closed reduction; however this is usually unsuccessful and operative treatment is typically performed. The author's preferred operative treatment is arthroscopic reduction and internal fixation. Open reduction through a medial parapatellar incision can also be performed per surgeon preference and experience or if arthroscopic visualization is difficult.

ARTHROSCOPIC REDUCTION AND INTERNAL FIXATION WITH EPIPHYSEAL CANNULATED SCREWS

A standard arthroscopic operating room setup is used. The patient is placed supine and general anesthesia is typically used. A standard arthroscope can be used in most patients, whereas a small (2.7-mm) arthroscope is used in smaller knees. An arthroscopic fluid pump is used at 35 torr to prevent excess bleeding and a tourniquet is routinely used. A high anterolateral viewing portal is made at the inferolateral border of the patella, and a lower anteromedial working portal is placed at the joint line, just medial to the patellar tendon. Accessory superomedial

and superolateral portals are necessary for screw insertion. The hematoma is evacuated prior to insertion of the arthroscope.

A thorough arthroscopic examination of the entire knee joint is conducted to evaluate for concomitant injuries. Frequently, we excise some portion of the anterior fat pad and ligamentum mucosum with an arthroscopic shaver for complete visualization of the intercondylar eminence fragment. An entrapped meniscus or intermeniscal ligament can be extracted with an arthroscopic probe and retracted with a retention suture inserted from outside-in (see Fig. 117.6). The base of the tibial eminence fragment is elevated (Fig. 117.8A) and the entire fracture bed débrided with an arthroscopic shaver and hand curette (see Fig. 117.8B). The arthroscope can be passed under the tibial spine fragment and into the fracture bed to confirm that débridement is complete. It is often preferred to leave the hinged portion of fracture intact to facilitate reduction. A small amount of excess subchondral cancellous bone can be removed from the base of the fracture site to help with over-reduction of the fragment to better tension the ACL. The tibial spine fragment is often thin and the surgeon should avoid removing any bone from the tibial spine fragment itself.

Screw fixation is most applicable to larger (>1 cm^2) tibial spine fracture fragments. Anatomic reduction is obtained using a probe, blunt obturator, or Kirschner wire with the knee in 30 to 90 degrees of flexion (see Fig. 117.8C). The tibial spine fragment is often hinged laterally and this hinge can be used as a key to reduction. The reduction is then assessed by visualizing the medial and lateral borders of the fragment in relation to the medial and lateral tibial plateau. Over-reduction by 1 to 2 mm

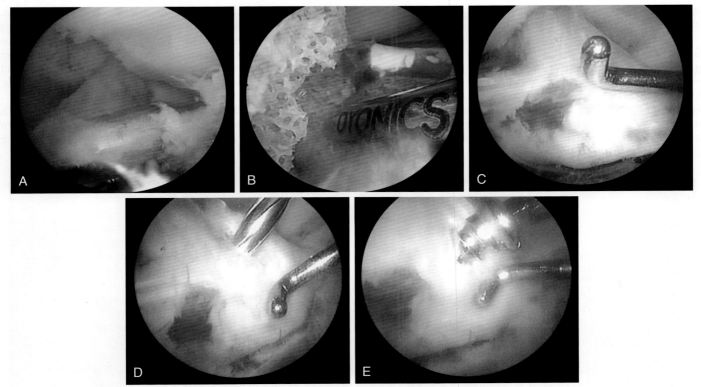

FIG 117.8 Arthroscopic Reduction and Insertion of Cannulated Screw Internal Fixation for a Displaced Tibial Spine Fracture. (A) Tibial spine fragment. (B) Elevation and débridement of the fracture bed. (C) Reduction of tibial spine fragment. (D) Drilling with a cannulated screw system. (E) Insertion of 3.5-mm screw.

is preferable to account for any stretch in the native ACL. Cannulated guide wires are placed just off the superomedial and superolateral borders of the patella through the accessory portals. Fluoroscopic assistance is used to confirm anatomic reduction, guide correct wire orientation, and to ensure avoidance of the proximal tibial physis. Once the tibial spine fragment is stabilized with a guide pin or pins, the angle of the knee must be maintained to avoid wire bending. A cannulated drill is used over the guide wires and one or two screws are inserted based on the size of the tibial eminence fragment (see Fig. 117.8D). Partially threaded 3.5-mm diameter screws (see Fig. 117.8E) are most commonly used depending on fragment size. It is recommended to use a tap prior to placing the screw to prevent the tibial spine from fragmenting. The knee is evaluated through a full range of motion to ensure rigid fixation without fracture displacement and to ensure that there is no impingement of the screw head in extension.

Postoperatively, patients are placed in a hinged knee brace and maintained at touchdown weight bearing for 6 weeks postoperatively. Motion is restricted to 0 to 30 degrees for the first 2 weeks and then slowly increased toward full range of motion at 6 weeks postoperatively. The brace is locked in extension for sleeping. Radiographs are obtained to evaluate maintenance of reduction and fracture healing at 2 and 6 weeks (Fig. 117.9). Cast immobilization in 20 to 30 degrees of flexion for 4 weeks postoperatively may be necessary in younger children who are unable to comply with protected weight bearing and brace immobilization. Physical therapy is used to achieve motion, strength, and sport-specific training. Patients are typically allowed to return to sports at 12 to 16 weeks postoperatively depending on knee function and strength. Screws are not routinely removed. Functional ACL bracing is used for 6 to 12 months postoperatively and may be continued if there is residual knee laxity.

ARTHROSCOPIC REDUCTION AND SUTURE FIXATION

Arthroscopic setup and examination is similar to the technique described for epiphyseal screw fixation. Accessory superomedial and superolateral portals typically are not used. A small incision is made just medial and distal to the tibial tubercle as would be performed for an ACL reconstruction. After the fracture is débrided and slightly over-reduced, a tibial ACL guide system with the tibial guide set at 50 to 60 degrees is used to place two guide wires through the base of the fracture bed in the tibia. It is important here to maintain at least a 1-cm tibial bone bridge between the guide wires at the proximal medial tibia. Drilling the more lateral tunnel is difficult and should be done first. Using two separate guide wires for drilling the tunnels ensures the bone bridge is adequate on the tibia. It is not necessary for the guide wires to pass through the tibial spine fracture fragment itself. The smooth guide wires may traverse the proximal tibial physis, but no cases of growth arrest after suture fixation have been reported.[12]

The guide wires are exchanged for looped suture passers and two sutures are passed through the suture passers and the base of the ACL using a suture passing instrument (Fig. 117.10). With the arthroscope in the anterolateral portal, a curved suture passer (typically used in shoulder arthroscopy) is placed through the anteromedial portal and used to pass a suture sequentially through the medial suture retriever, around the base of the ACL at its insertion on the tibial spine fragment, and through the lateral suture retriever. It is easiest to retrieve the suture from an accessory trans-patellar tendon portal to keep the anterolateral portal free for viewing. The process is then repeated with a second suture. The first suture passes through a more posterior portion of the ACL base and the second suture passes through the anterior aspect of the ACL base. It is not necessary for the sutures to pass through the actual bone of the tibial spine fragment. The sutures are retrieved through the tibial tubercle incision by pulling the looped suture passers simultaneously. It is important at this step to make sure that there is no entrapped meniscal tissue anteriorly. With the knee at 30 degrees of flexion, each suture is pulled taut and tied to itself over the bone bridge of the proximal medial tibia. The tibial incision here should be large enough to expose each tunnel and ensure that the suture knots are tied down to bone without intervening soft tissue and that there is at least a 1-cm bone bridge between the tunnels. The postoperative protocol is the same (Fig. 117.11).

Absorbable and nonabsorbable sutures may be used with this technique. No differences in clinical outcome have been shown with different suture material, but a recent cadaveric

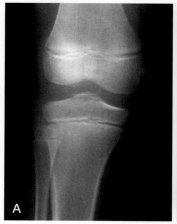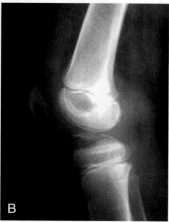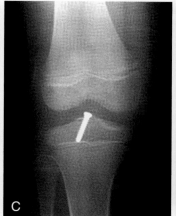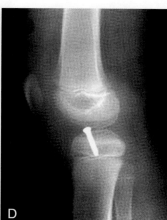

FIG 117.9 Type 3 Tibial Spine Fracture Treated With Arthroscopic Reduction and Screw Fixation. (A) Preoperative anteroposterior radiograph. (B) Preoperative lateral radiograph. (C) Postoperative anteroposterior radiograph. (D) Postoperative lateral radiograph.

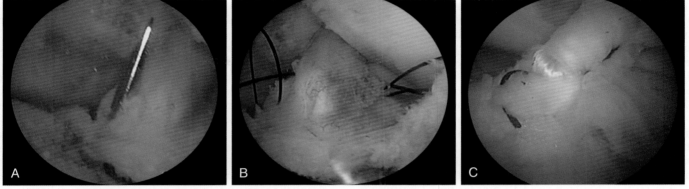

FIG 117.10 Treatment of a Type 2 Tibial Spine Fracture With Arthroscopic Reduction and Suture Fixation. (A) Drilling of a guide wire with an ACL guide system. (B) Hewson suture passers on each side of the ACL and passage of absorbable sutures through the ACL. (C) Final appearance after suture fixation.

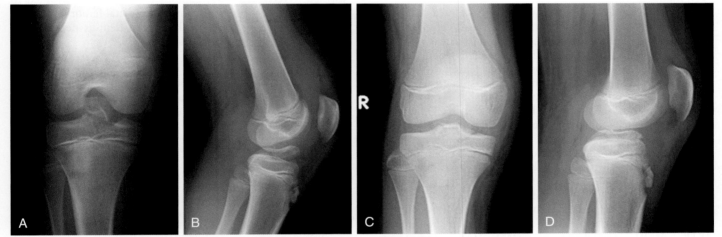

FIG 117.11 Type 2 Tibial Spine Fracture Treated With Arthroscopic Reduction and Suture Fixation. (A) Preoperative anteroposterior radiograph. (B) Preoperative lateral radiograph. (C) Postoperative anteroposterior radiograph. (D) Postoperative lateral radiograph.

study compared polydioxanone suture (PDS) II (Ethicon, Somerville, NJ), Vicryl (Ethicon, Somerville, NJ), and Fiber-Wire (Arthrex, Naples, FL) and found that FiberWire yielded a superior ultimate failure load, Vicryl presented comparable results under cyclic conditions, and PDS II was inferior.[47]

PEARLS AND PITFALLS

When managing tibial eminence fractures with closed reduction, follow-up radiographs should be obtained at 1 and 2 weeks post-injury to verify maintenance of reduction. Late displacement and malunion can occur, particularly for type 2 fractures. The injection of local anesthetic under sterile conditions can be helpful to minimize pain and allow for full knee extension in attempts at closed reduction.

During arthroscopic reduction and fixation of tibial spine fractures, visualization can be difficult unless the large hematoma is evacuated prior to introduction of the arthroscope and bleeding from the fracture is controlled. Adequate inflow and outflow is essential for proper visualization, and we routinely use an arthroscopic pump and a tourniquet to achieve this. Careful attention should be paid to prepare the fracture bed to

provide optimal conditions for bony healing. A slight over-reduction of the fracture is preferable.

Epiphyseal cannulated screw fixation of small or comminuted tibial eminence fragments can fail because of inadequate bony purchase or further comminution. For these cases, suture fixation is preferred. If epiphyseal cannulated screw fixation is used, fluoroscopy is necessary to ensure that the screw does not traverse the proximal tibial physis, which may result in a proximal tibial physeal growth arrest.[11]

Early mobilization is useful to avoid arthrofibrosis, which can occur with prolonged immobilization.[43,53] Recent studies have reported improved outcomes (more rapid return to activity and lower incidence of arthrofibrosis) in patients treated with earlier (within 4 weeks) postoperative range of motion.[44] However, in younger children, compliance with protected weight bearing and brace use can be problematic, and casting can be considered in these cases.

PROGNOSIS AND COMPLICATIONS

The overall prognosis for tibial eminence fractures is good to excellent if satisfactory reduction is achieved. However, the level of evidence supporting various treatments is low. A recent systemic review concluded that there was insufficient evidence to support open versus arthroscopic approaches, or screw versus suture fixation.[12] Many studies have reported asymptomatic residual knee laxity following open or closed management of all tibial eminence fracture types.[§] Baxter and Wiley found excellent functional results without symptomatic instability in 17 pediatric knees with displaced tibial spine fractures, despite a positive Lachman examination in 51% of patients and increased measured mean knee laxity up to 3.5 mm.[4,57] Willis et al. reported excellent clinical stability in all 50 children treated with closed or open reduction despite a positive Lachman exam in 64% of patients and instrumented (KT-1000) knee laxity of 3.5 mm for type 2 fractures and 4.5 mm for type 3 fractures.[58] Similarly, Janarv et al. and Kocher et al. found excellent functional results despite persistent laxity in up to 80% of patients, even with an anatomic reduction.[16,23] No major clinical outcome differences have been seen in studies comparing arthroscopic to open management.[9,56]

Clinical outcomes, especially with regard to knee laxity, are better in patients with type 1 and type 2 fractures compared to type 3 or type 4 injuries. Increased laxity has been reported in type 3 or 4 injuries and those with associated ligament tears.[**] This is likely because of intrasubstance stretching of the ACL, which occurs at injury. At the time of tibial spine fixation, the ACL often appears hemorrhagic within its sheath, but grossly intact and in continuity with the bony bed of tibia. However, a complete ACL tear following previous tibial spine fracture is rare.

Clinical results in adults treated with surgical repair of tibial spine fractures are also good. Koukoulias et al. recently reported on 12 patients with a mean age 30 years (range, 18 to 45) treated with arthroscopic suture fixation for tibial spine avulsions.[24] At a mean of 50 months postoperatively, mean Lysholm score was 98, mean International Knee Documentation Committee (IKDC) was 94.7, and all knees were stable.[24] Other studies have reported slightly lower functional outcomes in older patients.[33]

Poor results may occur after eminence fractures that are associated with unrecognized injuries to the collateral ligaments or physeal fracture.[8] In addition, hardware across the proximal tibial physis may result in a growth disturbance with a recurvatum deformity.[11] Malunion of type 2 and 3 fractures may cause bony impingement of the knee during full extension.[32] This can be corrected by excision of the malunited fragment[50] and anatomic reinsertion of the ACL, or ACL reconstruction can be considered when deemed necessary.

The incidence of nonunion following tibial spine fractures is low, but is more commonly reported following children treated by immobilization versus internal fixation.[12,14] Nonunion of type 2 and 3 tibial spine fractures can usually be managed by arthroscopic or open reduction with internal fixation with or without bone graft.[20,27,54] Débridement of the fracture bed and the fracture fragment to bleeding bone is essential to optimize bony healing and bone grafting may be required in some cases. Excision of the fragment and ACL reconstruction can be considered in adults and older adolescents.

Arthrofibrosis, particularly loss of extension, can occur after tibial spine fracture, even after anatomic reduction.[13] This is believed to result from the local increase in blood supply during healing, which leads to spine enlargement, which can cause a mechanical block to extension. A recent report noted that delayed surgery (more than 7 days from injury) and prolonged operative time (>120 minutes) were significant risk factors for arthrofibrosis.[56] Early range of motion and mobilization are essential to prevent loss of motion. Dynamic splinting and aggressive physical therapy may be used during the first 3 months post-fracture if stiffness is present. If stiffness persists after three months, a manipulation under anesthesia in conjunction with an arthroscopic lysis of adhesions can be performed. Overly vigorous manipulation should be avoided to prevent injury to the proximal tibial or distal femoral physis. A notchplasty can be performed if the patient is near skeletal maturity to help regain extension.

KEY REFERENCES

9. Edmonds EW, et al: Results of displaced pediatric tibial spine fractures: a comparison between open, arthroscopic, and closed management. *J Pediatr Orthop* 2014.

10. Eggers AK, Becker C, Weimann A, et al: Biomechanical evaluation of different fixation methods for tibial eminence fractures. *Am J Sports Med* 35(3):404–410, 2007.

12. Gans I, Baldwin KD, Ganley TJ: Treatment and management outcomes of tibial eminence fractures in pediatric patients: a systematic review. *Am J Sports Med* 42(7):1743–1750, 2014.

16. Janarv PM, Westblad P, Johansson C, et al: Long-term follow-up of anterior tibial spine fractures in children. *J Pediatr Orthop* 15(1):63–68, 1995.

21. Kocher MS, Micheli LJ, Gerbino P, et al: Tibial eminence fractures in children: prevalence of meniscal entrapment. *Am J Sports Med* 31(3):404–407, 2003.

22. Kocher MS, Mandiga R, Klingele K, et al: Anterior cruciate ligament injury versus tibial spine fracture in the skeletally immature knee: a comparison of skeletal maturation and notch width index. *J Pediatr Orthop* 24(2):185–188, 2004.

23. Kocher MS, Foreman ES, Micheli LJ: Laxity and functional outcome after arthroscopic reduction and internal fixation of displaced tibial spine fractures in children. *Arthroscopy* 19(10):1085–1090, 2003.

24. Koukoulias NE, Germanou E, Lola D, et al: Clinical outcome of arthroscopic suture fixation for tibial eminence fractures in adults. *Arthroscopy* 28(10):1472–1480, 2012.

38. Mitchell JJ, et al: Incidence of meniscal injury and chondral pathology in anterior tibial spine fractures of children. *J Pediatr Orthop* 35(2):130–135, 2015.

53. Vander Have KL, et al: Arthrofibrosis after surgical fixation of tibial eminence fractures in children and adolescents. *Am J Sports Med* 38(2):298–301, 2010.

The references for this chapter can also be found on www.expertconsult.com.

118

Physeal Fractures About the Knee

Corinna C. Franklin, David L. Skaggs, Jennifer Weiss

BACKGROUND

Physeal fractures about the knee include distal femoral physeal fractures, proximal tibial physeal fractures, tibial tubercle fractures, tibial eminence fractures, and patellar sleeve fractures. Diagnosis and treatment of these fractures and their complications can be challenging. Even physeal fractures that are not displaced can lead to complications of physeal arrest, making proper treatment and long-term follow-up essential.

DISTAL FEMUR

Distal femoral physeal fractures are most common in older children and tend to occur from high-energy trauma.[36] Most commonly, these fractures are Salter-Harris II fractures.[25] The most common mechanisms of injury are motor vehicle accidents and falls.[25] Most commonly, a valgus force leads to medial physeal separation extending into an oblique fracture through the lateral metaphysis.[10] Less commonly, a hyperextension injury is responsible, with risk of neurovascular injury.[10] The distal femoral physis is at risk for fracture in this scenario because the anterior cruciate ligament (ACL), posterior cruciate ligament (PCL), lateral collateral ligament (LCL), and medial collateral ligament (MCL) do not span or protect it. This fracture is four times more common in boys than in girls.[25]

Imaging should begin with anteroposterior (AP), lateral, and oblique radiographs. Stress radiographs may provide a definitive diagnosis but risk further physeal damage and can cause significant pain; therefore these are no longer recommended.[40] If nonstress radiographs are inconclusive, magnetic resonance imaging (MRI) is less painful for the patient and can provide more information.[3]

Suspicion for popliteal vascular injury should be high, with the incidence of popliteal artery injury reported at 3%.[15] Angiography is the gold standard for evaluation of arterial injury in the setting of a fracture about the knee.[15] Prompt recognition and intervention for vascular injury in this scenario decreases the risk of catastrophic complications such as loss of limb. Other complications can include compartment syndrome, peroneal nerve palsy, ligamentous laxity, and loss of range of motion.[40]

A recent systematic review found that 52% of distal femoral physeal fractures had a growth disturbance, with Salter Harris type IV fractures having the highest rate and Salter Harris I fractures having the lowest rate. Even fractures without displacement resulted in growth disturbance in 31% of cases, although it was much more likely in displaced fractures.[2]

At least 20% of distal femoral physeal fractures lead to angular deformity and growth arrest requiring reconstructive surgery.[25] Factors that predict outcome include type of fracture, initial fracture displacement, and exactness of reduction.[25] Growth disturbances are usually evident within 6 months to 1 year, but follow-up may be considered until skeletal maturity.[37]

Anatomic reduction of extra-articular distal femoral physeal fractures (Salter-Harris types I and II) can usually be done via closed reduction. To address the flexion deformity, the knee may be flexed to relax the gastrocnemius muscle. Once the knee is flexed, assessment of coronal plane alignment can be challenging. Closed reduction attempts should be gentle and repeated attempts minimized because these may exacerbate trauma to the physis. The reduction maneuver should consist of 90% traction and 10% manipulation to minimize iatrogenic damage to the physis. Open reduction may be necessary because periosteum may be interposed.

At times, interposed periosteum may be removed through a relatively small incision with a skin hook. If the Thurston-Holland fragment is large enough, lag screws may be placed for relatively rigid fixation (Figs. 118.1 to 118.4). Thomson and associates demonstrated that 43% of fractures reduced without fixation displaced during cast treatment, whereas no fractures treated with internal fixation displaced.[38] Smooth pins can be placed percutaneously to maintain reduction with little risk to the physis.[8,13] Once the fracture reduction is maintained, the knee can be extended again to assess coronal plane alignment.

Anatomic reduction of intra-articular distal femoral physeal fractures (Salter-Harris types III and IV) frequently requires open reduction. Visualization of the articular surface is encouraged if there is any doubt about the reduction. When a large metaphyseal fragment permits, cannulated screws can be used for secure fixation in extra-articular and intra-articular physeal fractures of the distal femur. Titanium screws should be considered because they can facilitate future MRI scanning. MRI may be of interest because these patients can have concomitant intra-articular injury to the ligaments or meniscus. MRI can also be useful in evaluating for physeal bar formation.

Postoperative care of these fractures should include a long-leg cast or brace applied with the knee in 0 to 30 degrees of flexion. In patients with short, thick thighs, a waist band may be considered. Non–weight bearing is recommended for 3 weeks. When pins are used, the pins are removed at 4 weeks after surgery because pin tract infection can lead to a septic knee. Immobilization should be continued until 6 weeks postoperatively. Screw removal is not mandatory, and no studies

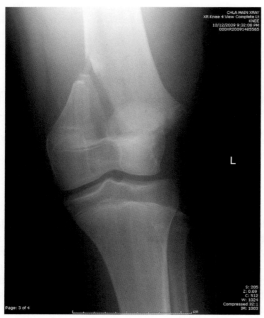

FIG 118.1 AP radiograph of distal femoral physeal fracture. (Image property of Children's Orthopedic Center.)

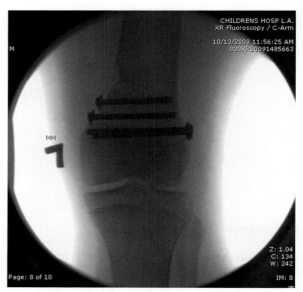

FIG 118.3 AP radiograph post closed reduction internal fixation distal femur physeal fracture. (Image property of Children's Orthopedic Center.)

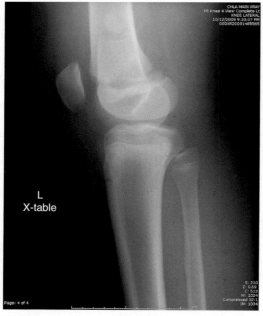

FIG 118.2 Lateral radiograph of distal femoral physeal fracture. (Image property of Children's Orthopedic Center.)

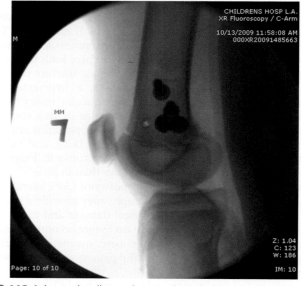

FIG 118.4 Lateral radiograph post closed reduction internal fixation distal femoral physeal. (Image property of Children's Orthopedic Center.)

have compared outcomes in patients with retained versus removed hardware in this location.

Figs. 118.1 to 118.4 illustrate a distal femoral Salter-Harris III fracture treated with closed reduction and internal fixation.

PROXIMAL TIBIA

Physeal fractures of the proximal tibia are extremely rare. The stabilizing anatomy of the hamstrings, MCL, and LCL protects this region, and high energy is required to disturb the area. Peak incidence of proximal tibia physeal fractures occurs between the ages of 10 and 12 years. Extension is the predominant mechanism of injury for these fractures.[28] Salter-Harris type I and II fractures predominate in this age group, and Salter-Harris type III and IV fractures tend to occur at a later age (14 years).[28,32] Proximal tibial triplane fractures have also been described, but are rare.[35]

When injury to the proximal tibia is suspected, imaging consists of anteroposterior and lateral radiographs of the knee.

Stress views should be avoided because they may cause further physeal damage. If radiographs are inconclusive, MRI can be used to further investigate for physeal injury.[3]

As in fractures of the distal femur and in knee dislocations when there is posterior placement of the tibia, suspicion of injury to the popliteal artery should be high. Angiography is the standard of care in diagnosing popliteal injury, and vascular consultation should be obtained promptly.[15] Shelton and Canale reported popliteal artery injuries resulting in vascular insufficiency in 2 of 39 patients.[34]

Anatomic reduction of proximal tibial fractures is necessary to protect the articular surface and the physis. Direct visualization may augment radiographic evaluation of the articular surface and is recommended if there is any doubt about articular congruity. Arthroscopic assistance to assess the reduction is well reported in the adult literature and can be considered for adolescents.[7] If a large metaphyseal fragment is present, cannulated screws can be used as fixation. If the physis must be crossed, smooth pins should be used. Because they may need to enter the knee joint itself, early removal of these pins is recommended to prevent infection. Fig. 118.5 shows operative fixation of a proximal tibial physeal fracture with Kirschner wires (K-wires).

Complications of proximal tibial physeal fractures include popliteal artery injury (associated with posterior displacement of the tibial shaft), compartment syndrome, peroneal nerve palsy, growth disturbance, and traumatic arthritis.[34] Because of the high energy required to cause this fracture, and the risk of compartment syndrome, inpatient admission for observation should be considered for even minimally displaced proximal tibial physeal fractures. Initially, regaining range of motion can be challenging. Vigilant follow-up to evaluate for growth plate injury in the form of angular deformity or leg length discrepancy should continue for at least 1 year after surgery. Standing radiographs from hip to ankle should be reviewed at 6 months and 1 year postoperatively.

Cozen Fractures

A particular phenomenon described by Jackson and Cozen in 1971 is now often referred to as a "Cozen fracture," and describes a pediatric proximal tibial fracture that results in genu valgum.[19] This deformity may progress for up to 2 years following the initial fracture and may occur despite acceptable initial alignment of the fracture.[1,19,43] In most cases, this deformity will correct or resolve adequately with nonoperative management or observation, and corrective osteotomy is usually not indicated.[1,19,43] Treatment consists of a long-leg cast with a varus mold.

Tibial Tubercle Fractures

Tibial tubercle fractures occur when the tibial tubercle physis is closing at the age of 11 or 12. These fractures occur much more frequently in boys than in girls.[5] They are classified according to the Watson-Jones classification, which was modified by Ogden and Tross in 1980 to include "A" and "B" subsets.[29] A type I fracture is a small fragment of the tuberosity, which is avulsed and displaced upward. Type IA is an incomplete separation of the fragment from the metaphysis, and type IB is a complete separation. In a type II fracture, the entire lip of the tibial tuberosity is displaced upward. A type IIA fracture has no comminution, and a type IIB fracture has comminution. A type III fracture is one in which the entire tuberosity is fractured at its base, and the fracture line extends superiorly into the proximal tibial intra-articular surface. A type IIIA fracture has a single displaced fragment, and a type IIIB fracture includes comminuted displaced fragments. This classification system was further expanded by Ryu and Debenham.[33] They added a type IV fracture, which is an avulsion fracture of the proximal tibial

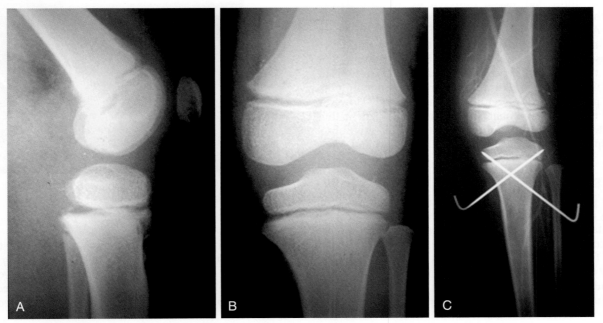

FIG 118.5 (A and B) Proximal tibial physeal fracture that is minimally displaced. (C) Fixation of this fracture with percutaneous pins.

epiphysis that extends into the posterior cortex of the tibia.[18] This type of flexion avulsion fracture of the proximal tibia is seen most commonly in the prepubescent patient age 13 or older.[28] Jumping with eccentric contraction of the quadriceps mechanism is the most common mechanism of injury.

Physical examination reveals point tenderness at the tibial tubercle, and the bony fragment can be palpated frequently. The extensor mechanism may not be intact, and the patient may not be able to initiate or maintain a straight-leg raise. A clinical pearl: any time an injured patient cannot actively bring their knee into full extension, consider the possibility of an injury somewhere along the extensor mechanism (quadriceps tendon, patella, patellar sleeve, patellar tendon, or tibial tubercle). The injury is most evident on the lateral radiograph. A recent study by Pandya et al. suggested that radiographs alone may underestimate the severity of injury, particularly with regard to intra-articular involvement. The authors suggest that advanced imaging with computed tomography (CT) or MRI should be performed with plans for arthroscopy or arthrotomy in the case of intra-articular extension.[30]

Operative indications for tibial tubercle fracture include displacement or intra-articular extension into the proximal tibia.[29] Because these fractures usually occur when the tibial tubercle physis is beginning to close, treatment involves screw fixation across the fracture and physis without concern for growth disturbance in those approaching the end of growth. Type IV tibial tubercle fractures that extend to the posterior aspect of the tibia must also be fixed by securing the tibial tubercle. Although these fractures may appear similar to proximal tibial physeal fractures, they are on a continuum with tibial tubercle fractures (particularly in terms of mechanism and energy of injury) and should be treated as such.

Complications. Compartment syndrome can occur in displaced tibial tubercle fractures as the result of damage to the recurrent branch of the anterior tibial artery. Because this physis is beginning to close, genu recurvatum is actually a rare complication.[29] Genu recurvatum may occur, however, in the rare patient younger than the age of 11 or 12 who sustains a tibial tubercle fracture. Avulsion of the tibialis anterior muscle has been reported in concert with a type III tibial tubercle fracture.[20]

The case pictured in Figs. 118.6 to 118.12 illustrates a type IV tibial tubercle fracture that was treated incorrectly. The proximal tibial physeal fracture was secured with smooth pins, and this portion of the fracture did in fact heal. However, the tibial tubercle component did not heal. The patient thus went on to sustain a tibial tubercle fracture. This was subsequently appropriately treated with open reduction and screw fixation.

Patellar Sleeve Fractures

Although proximal patellar sleeve fracture has been reported, they are a rarity because almost all patellar sleeve fractures are of the distal pole of the patella.[4,6,26] Patellar sleeve fractures are the most common type of patellar fracture in children.[13] Because the distal fragment of bone can be small, it is easy to overlook this entity on radiographs. MRI is helpful when physical examination and radiographs are inconclusive; ultrasound may also be a useful diagnostic tool.[14] Fig. 118.12 shows that the distal fragment may be very subtle, and that the fracture can be easy to overlook. Suspicion of this injury should be great after a mechanism of eccentric contraction of the quadriceps is noted.

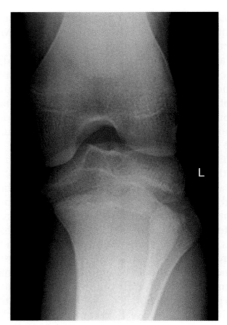

FIG 118.6 AP radiograph of type IV tibial tubercle fracture. (Image property of Children's Orthopedic Center.)

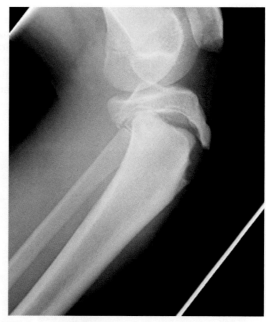

FIG 118.7 Lateral radiograph of type IV tibial tubercle fracture. (Image property of Children's Orthopedic Center.)

Physical examination is characterized by an inability to actively extend the knee. Point tenderness will be present over the distal or proximal pole of the patella, and a defect may even be palpable (Fig. 118.13). In the rare, truly nondisplaced patellar sleeve fractures, cylinder casting is the treatment of choice. When the fracture is displaced, treatment consists of open reduction with internal fixation in the form of tension band fixation.[12] If reduction and fixation are not achieved in a timely

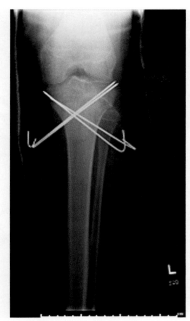

FIG 118.8 AP radiograph post smooth pin fixation of type IV tibial tubercle fracture. (Image property of Children's Orthopedic Center.)

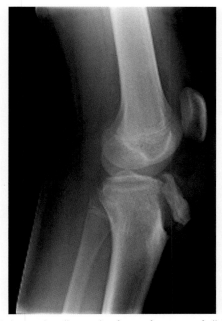

FIG 118.10 Lateral radiograph after refracture of tibial tubercle following incorrect treatment with smooth pins. (Image property of Children's Orthopedic Center.)

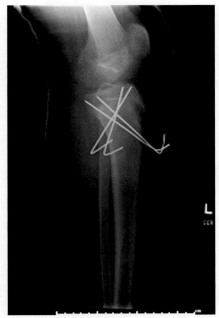

FIG 118.9 Lateral radiograph post smooth pin fixation of type IV tibial tubercle fracture. (Image property of Children's Orthopedic Center.)

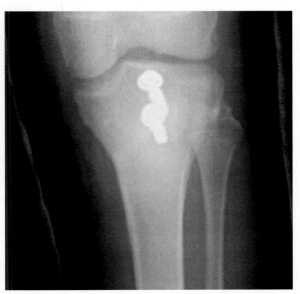

FIG 118.11 AP radiograph of correct treatment of tibial tubercle fracture with screw fixation. (Image property of Children's Orthopedic Center.)

fashion, there is risk of patellar elongation and disruption of patellofemoral joint mechanics.

Fig. 118.14 shows the intraoperative appearance of the patellar sleeve fragment. Note the large size of the distal fragment, which was difficult to appreciate on the radiograph. Fig. 118.15 shows the postoperative appearance of a healing patellar sleeve fracture after open reduction and internal fixation.

Tibial Eminence Fractures

Several mechanisms of injury for a tibial eminence fracture have been proposed, including hyperextension coupled with lateral loading, and knee flexion with an internally rotated tibia.[23] Patients with a narrow intercondylar notch may be more susceptible to ACL tears, whereas those who sustain a tibial eminence fracture are believed to have a slightly wider notch

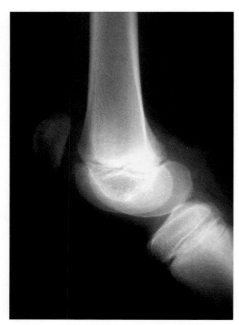

FIG **118.12** Lateral radiograph of correct treatment of tibial tubercle fracture with screw fixation. (Image property of Children's Orthopedic Center.)

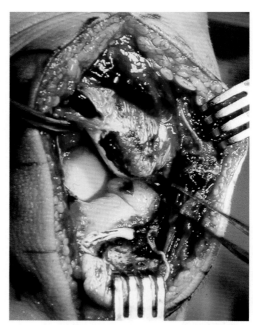

FIG **118.14** Intraoperative photograph demonstrating patellar sleeve fracture. (Photograph property of Children's Orthopedic Center.)

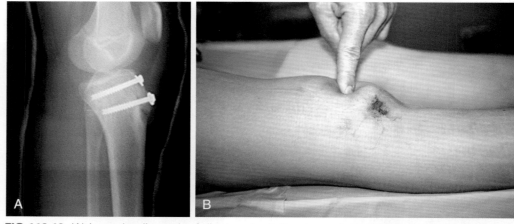

FIG **118.13** (A) Lateral radiograph of displaced patellar sleeve fracture. (B) Physical examination of patellar sleeve fracture demonstrating palpable defect at fracture site. (Images property of Children's Orthopedic Center.)

index.[22] The peak age for tibial eminence fracture is 10 years.[28] Tibial eminence fractures are associated with other injuries almost 40% of the time; these injuries include meniscal, capsular, and collateral ligament injuries, as well as osteochondral fractures.[23] MRI imaging is often useful in the workup of these fractures.

Tibial eminence fractures are classified by the Myers and McKeever system.[27] Type I fractures are nondisplaced. Type II fractures are displaced, with elevation of the anterior portion of the spine and hinging of the posterior aspect of the spine (Figs. 118.16 and 118.17). Type III fractures are displaced and detached.

Nondisplaced fractures are treated with a long-leg cast with the leg in extension. Type II, or hinged, fractures may be reduced with knee extension to 30 degrees or full extension. The intermeniscal ligament may prevent reduction, in which case open or arthroscopic reduction with fixation is indicated. Type III, or detached and displaced, fractures require reduction and fixation.

Concomitant meniscal tears can occur with tibial spine fractures. Unstable torn menisci and the intermeniscal ligament can become trapped under a displaced tibial spine fracture. A benefit of arthroscopic treatment of these fractures is the ability to evaluate the menisci and treat tears at the same time.

Arthroscopically assisted reduction and fixation is an excellent alternative to open reduction and internal fixation for these fractures. Different techniques have been described for fixation, including suture fixation, metallic screw fixation, K-wire fixation, and absorbable implant fixation.[11,17,24] A physeal-sparing arthroscopically assisted technique has been reported with

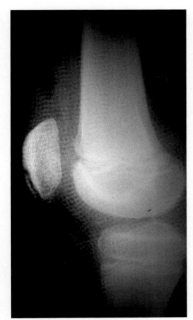

FIG 118.15 Postoperative radiograph after fixation of patellar sleeve fracture demonstrating healing. (Image property of Children's Orthopedic Center.)

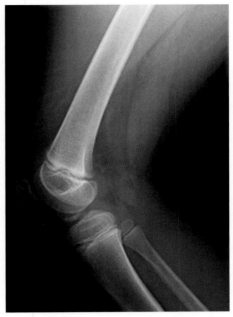

FIG 118.17 Lateral radiograph of displaced tibial spine fracture. (Image property of Children's Orthopedic Center.)

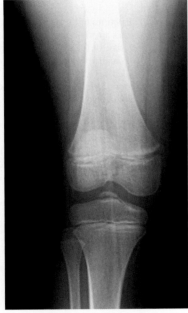

FIG 118.16 AP radiograph of displaced tibial spine fracture. (Image property of Children's Orthopedic Center.)

good results.[16] In 2003, Kocher et al. reported on six patients who underwent this surgery. Five of their six patients had an abnormal Lachman examination, and two of the six had an abnormal pivot-shift examination. Functional outcomes, which were evaluated by Lysholm scores, were excellent.[21] Because laxity may result from interstitial damage to the ACL, these authors recommend slight countersinking of the fragment to combat this laxity.

Edmonds et al. compared displaced tibial eminence fractures treated with open fixation, arthroscopic fixation, or closed fixation. They found that surgical treatment resulted in better reduction but more risk for arthrofibrosis, whereas closed treatment had less risk for arthrofibrosis but higher risk for laxity or impingement requiring later surgery. The authors recommend surgical management for fractures with greater than 5 mm of fracture displacement, and did not find a significant long-term difference between open and arthroscopic management.[9]

Wiley and colleagues reported objective loss of extension in 100% of patients treated operatively and nonoperatively for tibial spine fractures. Subjective stiffness was noted in 65% of patients.[41] Vander Have et al. reported on a series of patients with arthrofibrosis after surgical management of tibial eminence fractures, and found that most of these required reoperation to regain knee motion.[39] Patel et al. implemented mobilization within 4 weeks of treatment of tibial eminence fractures, and found that this resulted in earlier return to full activity as well as decreased arthrofibrosis.[31]

Figs. 118.18 and 118.19 depict fractures after arthroscopically aided reduction and fixation.

FOCAL PERIPHYSEAL EDEMA

Several recent studies have noted an abnormality in closing physes called focal periphyseal edema, or FOPE. This phenomenon presents as vague, activity-related knee pain; MRI imaging demonstrates a starburst pattern of edema centered on a thinning physis in the knee (distal femur, proximal tibia or fibula) and extending into the epiphysis and metaphysis. Although not a fracture, it may be an explanatory cause of knee pain in adolescents and should be considered when other injuries are not found. FOPE may be treated conservatively, with nonsteroidal antiinflammatory drugs (NSAIDs), physical therapy, and/or bracing.[42]

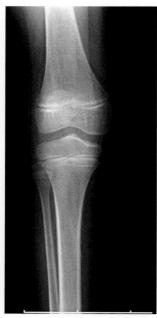

FIG 118.18 AP radiograph after surgical fixation of displaced tibial spine fracture. (Image property of Children's Orthopedic Center.)

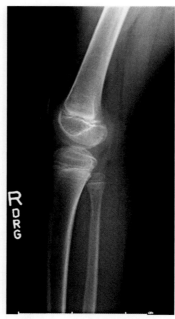

FIG 118.19 AP radiograph after surgical fixation of displaced tibial spine fracture. (Image property of Children's Orthopedic Center.)

KEY REFERENCES

3. Berquist TH: Osseous and myotendinous injuries about the knee. *Radiol Clin North Am* 45(6):955–968, 2007. doi: 10.1016/j.rcl.2007.08.004.
5. Bolesta MJ, Fitch RD: Tibial tubercle avulsions. *J Pediatr Orthop* 6:186–192, 1986.
10. Edwards PH Jr, Grana WA: Physeal fractures about the knee. *J Am Acad Orthop Surg* 3(2):63–69, 2013. <http://www.ncbi.nlm.nih.gov/pubmed/10790654>.
12. Gao GX, Mahadev A, Lee EH: Sleeve fracture of the patella in children. *J Orthop Surg (Hong Kong)* 16(1):43–46, 2008. doi: 10.1177/036354659101900521.
15. Harrell DJ, Spain DA, Bergamini TM, et al: Blunt popliteal artery trauma: a challenging injury. *Am Surg* 63:228–231, 1997.
21. Kocher MS, Foreman ES, Micheli LJ: Laxity and functional outcome after arthroscopic reduction and internal fixation of displaced tibial spine fractures in children. *Arthroscopy* 19:1085–1090, 2003.
23. Lafrance RM, Giordano B, Goldblatt J, et al: Pediatric tibial eminence fractures: evaluation and management. *J Am Acad Orthop Surg* 18(7):395–405, 2010.
25. Lombardo SJ, Harvey JP: Fractures of the distal femoral epiphyses. Factors influencing prognosis: a review of thirty-four cases. *J Bone Joint Surg Am* 59:742–751, 1977. doi: 10.1016/S0022-3468(78)80081-5.
27. Meyers MH, McKeever F: Fracture of the intercondylar eminence of the tibia. *J Bone Joint Surg Am* 52:1677–1684, 1970.
28. Mubarak SJ, Kim JR, Edmonds EW, et al: Classification of proximal tibial fractures in children. *J Child Orthop* 3(3):191–197, 2009. doi: 10.1007/s11832-009-0167-8.
29. Ogden JA, Tross RB, Murphy MJ: Fractures of the tibial tuberosity in adolescents. *J Bone Joint Surg Am* 62(2):205–215, 1980.
34. Shelton WR, Canale ST: Fractures of the tibia through the proximal tibial epiphyseal cartilage. *J Bone Joint Surg Am* 61(2):167–173, 1979.
36. Skak SV, Jensen TT, Poulsen TD, et al: Epidemiology of knee injuries in children. *Acta Orthop Scand* 58(1):78–81, 1987.
38. Thomson JD, Stricker SJ, Williams MM: Fractures of the distal femoral epiphyseal plate. *J Pediatr Orthop* 15:474–478, 1995.
41. Wiley JJ, Baxter MP: Tibial spine fractures in children. *Clin Orthop* 255:54–60, 1990.

The references for this chapter can also be found on www.expertconsult.com.

119

Patellar Instability

Richard Y. Hinton, Richard G. Levine, James C. Dreese

Patellofemoral instability is a common cause of knee complaints in the pediatric and adolescent population. Conditions may vary from developmental dysplasias to traumatic injuries in high-demand scholastic athletes. As discrepant as these scenarios may seem, they have in common a relative imbalance of the normal envelope of patella stabilization.[37] The medial patellofemoral ligament (MPFL) is the primary soft tissue structure in this envelope, and there is growing interest in the structure, function, and surgical restoration of this ligament. However, when caring for younger patients, this enthusiasm must be coupled with a full understanding of growth and development about the knee and the myriad of variables that may play a role in the underlying condition. This chapter focuses on patellofemoral instability in young, athletically active patients. We review age-specific anatomy, discuss underlying risk factors, overview current operative and nonoperative treatment concepts, and detail our preferred technique for MPFL reconstruction.

EMBRYOLOGY

The appendicular skeleton appears very early in embryologic development. By the fourth week of gestation, the limb buds are easily identifiable, with maturation of the lower extremities trailing the upper extremities by several days. The leg buds begin to bend anteriorly at the developing knee during the fifth week. By week 7 the distal end of the femur and the patella have undergone chondrification, and the patellofemoral articulation is recognizable in its adult form. The lower limbs initially extend from the torso with the soles of the feet facing medially, toward one another. By the eighth week of gestation, the lower limbs complete a 90-degree internal rotation, which brings them into their adult orientation.[40,104,125,141] Failure of rotation leaves the extensor mechanism in a contracted, lateral position relative to the distal end of the femur and is thought to play a role in congenital patellofemoral dislocation.[55,56,145]

Initial formation or malformation of the patellofemoral joint appears to be genetically driven without dependence on function.[40,77] Kim et al.[78] have reported that, although absolute size measurements increase with age, the relative osteochondral morphology of the patellofemoral joint is constant from early childhood to adulthood. Abnormalities, such as a trochlear dysplasia, patellar hypoplasia, and patella alta, often coexist within a constellation of dysplastic changes. This suggests common temporal development. Progressive extensor mechanism dysfunction can occur with abnormal motion and stress across a dysplastic patellofemoral articulation. In cases of congenital, developmental, and obligatory dislocation, early surgical restoration toward a more normal extensor mechanism may lead to partial normalization of patellofemoral architecture.[52,56,82]

ANATOMY AND BIOMECHANICS

The osteochondral architecture of the patellofemoral joint plays a significant role in stability. Patella alta, trochlear dysplasia, increased tibial tuberosity–trochlear groove (TT-TG) distance, and patellar hypoplasia all have been suggested as risk factors for initial and recurrent patellar instability.[41,49,68,77] The patella lies within the trochlea of the femur, bounded by the medial and lateral femoral condyles. Cartilaginous at birth, the patella begins ossification from multiple centers during early childhood. Apparent lack of patellofemoral congruity and excessive shallowness of the femoral sulcus in the child's knee are in large part an illusion (Fig. 119.1).Nietosvaara et al.[111] have shown that, although the osseous patellofemoral sulcus angle is inversely proportional to age, ultrasound measurements of the cartilaginous sulcus are almost constant throughout growth. Gradual thinning of the articular cartilage from the outer areas of the sulcus and retropatellar facets leads to apparent deepening of the sulcus with age.[117]

Patella alta is one of the best substantiated radiographic risk factors for patellar instability.* With the knee in full extension, the patella rests lateral and superior to the trochlea. Engagement occurs between 10 and 30 degrees of flexion. This is dependent on relative patellar tendon length, and, in individuals with patella alta, engagement will occur later in flexion. This can lead to instability in early knee flexion. FF or the normal adolescent and young adult population, the Insall ratio has been measured as 0.98 ± 0.13 for males and 1.08 ± 0.15 for females.[87,128] In a study of 104 patellar dislocators, Runow[128] found that the average Insall ratio was greater than 1.0 in all patients and that a ratio greater than 1.3 was significantly correlated with recurrent and bilateral dislocation. Generating standard Insall ratio measurements is limited by the cartilaginous nature of the patella and the tibial tubercle in the younger patient.[156] Alternative methods aim to minimize these effects. The Caton-Deschamps index is a simple method defined by the ratio of the articular facet length of the patella and the distance from the lower edge of the facet to the corner of the superior tibia.[18] The Blackburne-Peel[16] modification is similar and uses the relationship between posterior facet length and the distance to the tibial articular surface. Koshino and Sugimoto's method[81] is

---

*References 10, 49, 68, 93, 101, and 128.

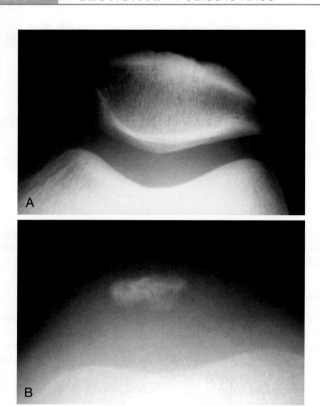

FIG 119.1 Sunrise view of the patellofemoral joint in an adult man (A) and an 8-year-old boy (B). (From Hinton RY, Sharma KM: Acute and recurrent patellar instability in the young athlete. *Orthop Clin North Am* 34:285–396, 2003.)

more complex, using relationships of the midpatella to the midepiphyseal lines of the tibia and femur (Fig. 119.2). Aparicio et al.[8] found the Caton method to be most reproducible. Caton indices greater than 1.2 suggest consideration of distal realignment, and values greater than 1.4 point to consideration of distalization coupled with realignment.[26,36,45] Although not as routinely available as lateral radiographs, magnetic resonance imaging (MRI) and ultrasound can also be used to compensate for the variability of osseous landmarks in generating patella height in the skeletally immature.[15,75,152]

Trochlear dysplasia includes abnormalities in trochlear shape, orientation, and increases in TT-TG distance. It is associated not only with patella maltracking and instability but also with joint incongruity and increased joint contact forces.[129] A normal sulcus angle for young individuals has been reported to be less than 138 ± 3 degrees.[126,157] Trochlear dysplasia has been classified into subtypes A to D[32,79,86] (Fig. 119.3). As can be seen, the condition is not a simple flattening of the lateral condyle but a combined hyperplasia of the lateral trochlear facet with hypoplasia of the medial trochlear facet. This results in a flattening and medial shift of the groove.[129] Mild trochlear dysplasia corresponds to a sulcus angle of 143 degrees, moderate dysplasia to an angle of 149 degrees, and severe dysplasia to an angle of 171 degrees.[31] Runow[128] found the average sulcus angle in a large group of young patients with documented patellar dislocation to be increased to 146 ± 6 degrees. A similar increase to 147 degrees has been reported by Aglietti et al.[2] in symptomatic patellar subluxers. Although MPFL reconstruction can be

effective in the face of moderate trochlear dysplasia, studies have found high-grade trochlear dysplasia to be associated with increased rates of MPFL reconstruction failure.[69,110,116] In these cases, consideration may be given to combining reconstruction with distal realignment or trochleoplasty.

The Q angle is subtended by a line drawn from the anterior superior iliac spine to the center of the patella or the trochlear groove and a second line drawn from the center of the tibial tubercle. An increased Q angle suggests a greater lateralizing vector on the patella. An increased Q angle is often discussed as a risk factor for instability, but it has not been uniformly associated with patellar instability in many large studies.[10,23,43,88] Unfortunately, no agreed-upon standards are available for Q angle measurement with regard to the most appropriate degree of knee flexion, weight-bearing status, and quadriceps activity. Axial MRI or computer tomography (CT) scans can currently be used to generate more reproducible measurements of relative tibial tubercle "lateralization" by providing anterior TT-TG distances[134] and tibial tubercle–lateral condylar (TT-LC) angles.[106] Normalized TT-TG distance (Fig. 119.4) has been identified in the adult population at approximately 13 mm, with values greater than 15 mm considered abnormal. Values greater 20 mm are viewed as a significant risk factor for patella dislocation, recurrent instability, and rationale for distal realignment at time of surgery.[36] However, TT-TG distance is an absolute value and is dependent on the overall size of the knee. Several investigators have addressed this by reporting TT-TG distance as a ratio with overall knee size, as measured in various fashions.[11,67,153] The concept of TT-TG distance can also be converted to an angular measurement that is knee size independent.[67,106]

A few studies[11,34,121] have begun reporting on pediatric/adolescent-specific TT-TG distance data and have found high intra- and inter-rater reliability using MRI. Values increase with age and height but tend to plateau, taking on near adult values by the early teen years. Importantly, as with adults, increased TT-TG values are associated with increased risk of patella instability. Dickens et al.[34] found a group of 495 normal children (average age: 11 years 11 months) to have a median TT-TG of 8.5 ± 0.3 mm and a similar age group of patella instability patients to have a value of 12.2 ± 1.1 mm. Pennock et al.[121] showed similar findings in a group of 45 instability patients (average age: 15.4 years) whose TT-TG mean was 16.3 mm versus an age-matched control with a mean value of 11.7 mm. Although increased TT-TG is associated with patellofemoral instability, what absolute values are the upper limit that warrant distal realignment in the young population is uncertain. This will require longer-term study on surgical outcomes.[121]

Another consideration for distal realignment is that the tibial tubercle undergoes gradual ossification during childhood. Genu recurvatum is a potential complication with tubercle osteotomies. It is generally suggested that such procedures are put off until skeletal maturity; however, the appropriate age cutoff is not well described. Older case series[63,90] report such complications in patients younger than but not older than 14 years. Tibial tubercle fractures are routinely fixed with open reduction and internal fixation in young males above this age, and significant growth disturbances are rare.[1,70,118] Pandya et al.[119] have reported recurvatum deformities after tubercle avulsion fracture and fixation in two young males aged 12.8 and 13.2 years. Tubercle osteotomy for distal realignment may be considered as the adolescent is "approaching" skeletal

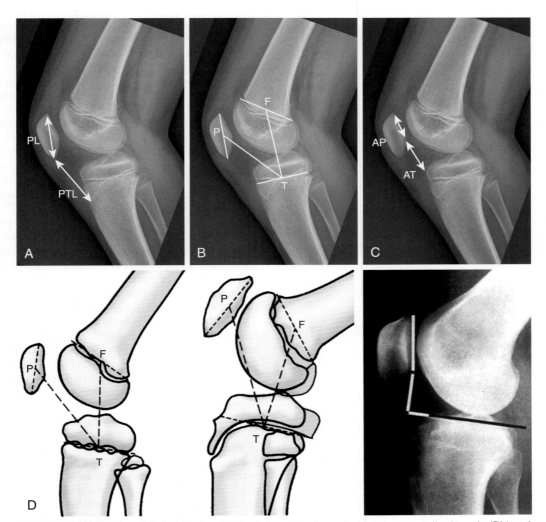

FIG 119.2 (A) The Insall-Salvati index (IS) is defined by the ratio between patellar length *(PL)* and patella-tibia length *(PTL)*. IS = PTL/PL. (B) The Koshino index (KI) is defined by the ratio between patella-tibia distance (PT) and femur-tibia distance (FT). KI = PT/FT. (C) The Caton-Deschamps index (CDI) is defined by the ratio between the articular facet length of the patella *(AP)* and the distance between the articular facet of the patella and the anterior corner of the superior tibial epiphysis *(AT)*. CDI = AT/AP. In young children the anterior superior margin of the tibia was defined as being the most anterior point of the proximal tibial epiphysis. (From Thevenin-Lemoine C, Ferrand M, Courvoisier A, et al: Is the Caton-Deschamps index a valuable ratio to investigate patellar height in children? *J Bone Joint Surg Am* 93:e35, 2011) (D) A new method of measuring patellar height. (From Blackburne JS, Peel TE: A new method of measuring patellar height. *J Bone Joint Surg Br* 59:241–242, 1977.)

maturity, but an exact age is uncertain and is dependent upon gender, skeletal age, and growth remaining.

The multilayer soft tissue envelope about the patellofemoral joint has been described as having three layers on the medial side.[33,142,144,157] The second layer includes the MPFL, parapatellar retinaculum, and superficial medial collateral ligament (MCL) (Fig. 119.5). Several studies[20,33,54,64,114] undertaken to compare the roles of the MPFL, medial patellar retinaculum, patellotibial ligament, patellomeniscal ligament, and lateral retinaculum have found that the MPFL provides between 70% and 80% of soft tissue restraint to lateral patellar displacement in early knee flexion. The MPFL is relatively isometric between full extension and to approximately 40 degrees of flexion, at which

point the structure is nonisometric over the remainder of full flexion.[132,142,147,150,155]

The MPFL is an hourglass-shaped, sail-like ligamentous structure that runs transversely from the posterior part of the medial epicondyle, approximately 1 cm distal to the adductor tubercle, to the superomedial part of the patella. Although present as a distinct structure in 90% of specimens, this ligament can vary greatly in size and strength.[20,33,64] The ligament appears to have two functional bundles. The straight inferior bundle is the main static stabilizing portion and the superior oblique bundle, which is intimately associated with the underside of the vastus medialis obliquus (VMO), serves a more dynamic role.[76,132,135] The femoral origin is intimately associated

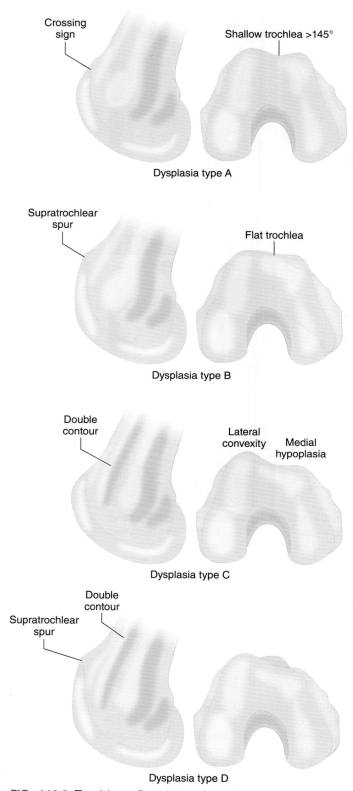

FIG 119.3 Trochlear Dysplasia Classification of trochlear dysplasia. Type A: crossing sign, with trochlear morphology preserved (fairly shallow trochlea [>145°]). Type B: crossing sign, supratrochlear spur, and flat or convex trochlea. Type C: crossing sign, with double contour. Type D: crossing sign, supratrochlear spur, double contour, asymmetry of trochlear facets, and vertical link between medial and lateral facet (cliff pattern). (From Dejour D, Le Coultre B: Osteotomies in patello-femoral instabilities. *Sports Med Arthrosc* 15:40, 2007.)

with insertions of the adductor tendon and superficial MCL (Fig. 119.6). The MPFL originates in the saddle area distal to the adductor tubercle, just superior to the MCL origin and posterior to both.[114,123,142] Radiographically, on a true lateral view, the center of femoral origin is 1 mm anterior to an extension line from the posterior cortex, 2.5 mm distal to the origin of the medial femoral condyle, and proximal to the level of the posterior point of the Blumensaat line (Fig. 119.7).[108,136] Replicating this femoral insertion is paramount in biomechanically and clinically successful MPFL reconstruction. The ligament courses from its femoral origin to attach to the superior medial border of the patella and the undersurface of the VMO.

There is growing consensus that the femoral origin of the MPFL is just distal to the femoral physis.[44,66,108,132] On a lateral x-ray the attachment may actually appear proximal to the growth plate.[76,108,132] However, the femoral physis is cup-shaped at its periphery. Although the attachment appears superior to the more central physeal plate, it is below the physis at its medial peripheral zone of attachment (Fig. 119.8). This must be taken into consideration when drilling tunnels or using various fixation devices for the femoral side of MPFL reconstructions. These must be angled downward away from the curving physis, not in line with the ligament peripheral femoral attachment and inadvertently into the physeal plate more centrally. As will be discussed in later text, erring slightly distal with the femoral insertion of an MPFL reconstruction has fewer potential adverse consequences for the biomechanics of the graft than a graft placed too proximal.

Imaging and surgical exploration reports have found the MPFL to be routinely injured at the time of patellar dislocation in young acute patella dislocators.[†] Injury may be complete or partial, isolated to the patella or femoral insertion, combined with intersubstance injury, and involve soft tissue or bony avulsion. Several studies have found a significantly higher percentage of MPFL injury at the patella insertion in younger patients rather than the femoral avulsion more commonly seen in adults.[47,60,122,137] Sillanpää et al.[140] have classified these patella insertion injuries as ligamentous, avulsion from the medial nonarticular margin, and bony avulsion with articular cartilage fragment requiring internal fixation.

Muscle contraction may affect patellofemoral stability by "seating" the articulation as a result of increased joint reaction forces or by generating dynamic displacement forces.[144] Relative vectors of the individual quadriceps muscular components are determined by their level of attachment, angle of pull, and cross-sectional area. The VMO is a dynamic stabilizer to lateral dislocation. It is intimately associated with the MPFL. The VMO can be injured, along with the MPFL, in patella-side injuries in the young population.[137] A focus of rehabilitation after injury or surgery is optimizing quadriceps function. Although often discussed, independent function, disuse, or rehabilitation of the VMO separate from the remaining quadriceps is questionable.[7,83,124] In addition to maximizing quadriceps activity; there is a growing interest in the concepts of core strengthening, hip function, and core sporting postures in the treatment of patellofemoral instability. This is very similar to evolving anterior cruciate ligament (ACL) injury and prevention protocols.

---

†References 47, 94, 122, 131, 133, and 137.

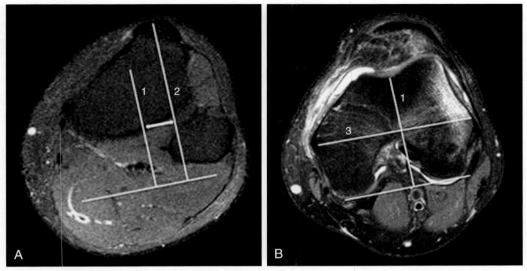

FIG 119.4 **Measurement of TT-TG Distance** (A) The first line *(1)* was drawn through the deepest point of the trochlear groove, perpendicular to the posterior condyle tangent. The second line *(2)* was drawn in parallel to the trochlear line through the most anterior portion of the tibial tubercle. The distance between these two lines represented the TT-TG distance. (B) The third line *(3)* measured the total width of the distal femur from the medial to the lateral epicondyle, parallel to the posterior condyle tangent. (From Balcarek P, Jung K, Frosch KH, Sturmer KM: Value of the tibial tuberosity-trochlear groove distance in patellar instability in the young athlete. *Am J Sports Med* 39:1756–1761, 2011.)

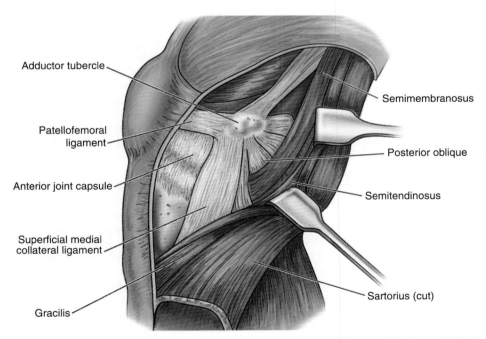

FIG 119.5 Diagram of layer II medial-side knee structures. (From Clarke HD, Scott WN, Insall JN, et al: Anatomy. In Insall JN, Scott WN [eds]: *Surgery of the knee*, Philadelphia, PA, 2001, WB Saunders, p 52.)

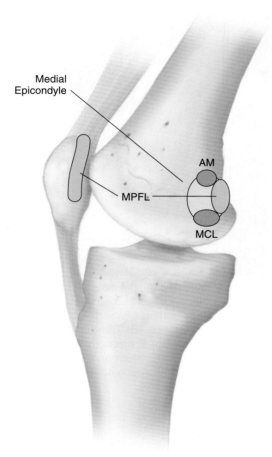

FIG 119.6 Schematic diagram shows the medial femoral epicondyle and its attachments for the AM, the MPFL, and the MCL. *AM,* Adductor magnus tendon; *MCL,* medial collateral ligament; *MPFL,* medial patellofemoral ligament. (From Smirk C, Morris H: The anatomy and reconstruction of the medial patellofemoral ligament. *Knee* 10:221–227, 2003.)

RISK FACTORS

As with other musculoskeletal injuries, risk factors for patellofemoral instability are best viewed within the triad of *host* (patient characteristics), *agent* (energy exchange), and *environmental* (physical and social) risk factors.[68,98] We have found it useful to classify young patients with patellofemoral instability into two large, somewhat overlapping groups (TONES and LAACS) based on "relative" risk factors, natural history, and patient characteristics (Table 119.1). In general, TONES patients have a relatively structurally normal knee subjected to macrotraumatic overstress, and LAACS patients have more significant underlying biomechanical risks factors.

Host factors that may play an important role in patellar instability include age, gender, previous history of patellar instability, generalized ligamentous laxity, and patellofemoral dysplasia. Patellar dislocation rates are highest during the second decade of life[10,49,128] probably because of higher athletic activity during this period and an underlying musculoskeletal predisposition in this age group. During a period of rapid growth, early adolescents are in the seemingly dichotomous situation of simultaneous musculotendinous tightness and relative ligamentous laxity. This is particularly apparent with the

TABLE 119.1	Classification of Patellofemoral Instability in Young Patients: TONES and LAACS
T	Traumatic, sports-related injury mechanisms
O	Older at initial dislocation, Osteochondral fractures more common
N	Normal patellofemoral architecture, Normal ligamentous function
E	Equal gender distribution
S	Single occurrence, Single-leg involvement
L	Laxity, generalized, Lower age at onset
A	Atraumatic in nature
A	Abnormal patellofemoral architecture, Abnormal ligamentous laxity
C	Chronic in nature, Contralateral involvement
S	Sex dependent, with greater number of females

strap-like, two-joint musculotendinous units crossing the knee. Tightness in the iliotibial band, abductors, and lateral hamstrings may lead to increased valgus vector on the patella, which may be poorly balanced by underdeveloped quadriceps musculature coupled with immature core sporting postures and abilities. Age is also a significant risk factor for recurrence, with earlier initial dislocation being a positive predictor of higher recurrence rates.[‡] Generalized ligamentous laxity is correlated with earlier onset, more frequent recurrence, and dislocations that occur with lesser trauma.[128] Patellofemoral markers that have been linked most reliably to increased dislocation and recurrence risk are patella alta, increased sulcus angle, and lateral dominance of the retropatellar surface. These dysplastic changes often occur as a constellation and are more often seen in younger, LAACS-type patients (see Table 119.1). However, subtle abnormalities in these measurements, particularly some mild trochlear dysplasia,[122] are often also noted among TONES-type patients (see Table 119.1). Another key host characteristic of recurrent dislocation is a history of previous dislocation.[49]

Trauma, in varying degrees, is almost always associated with patellar dislocation. A large population-based study conducted by Atkin et al.[10] points to the "agent" of high sports participation as the major risk factor for first-time, acute patellofemoral dislocators. The most common mechanism of patellar dislocation—noncontact external rotation of the lower part of the leg on a planted foot, resulting in valgus overload of the extensor mechanism—is common in sports participation. In their group of TONES-type patients, the investigators[10] reported no predictive role for gender, family history, increased Q angle, or excessive hip rotation. Patella alta was the one traditional factor associated with higher risk in this patient group. In TONES patients, patellar dislocation is a more traumatic event, with higher rates of MRI-documented disruption of the MPFL, VMO, and medial retinaculum. Fithian et al.[49] suggested that increased soft tissue trauma is a sign of macrotrauma to normal structures and that given adequate chance to heal, a lower risk of recurrence will be seen than in cases in which the patella dislocates with less trauma. Osteochondral fracture rates are significantly higher in TONES patients as a result of the greater

---

‡References 21, 49, 50, 101, 102, and 128.

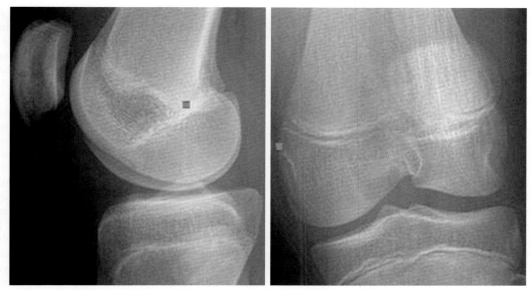

FIG 119.7 Cross-reference of the physis on the lateral view onto an anteroposterior view shows that the same point *(dot)* that is projected on or proximal to the physis on the lateral view is distal to the physis on the anteroposterior view. (From Nelitz M, Dreyhaupt J, Reichel H, et al: Anatomic reconstruction of the medial patellofemoral ligament in children and adolescents with open growth plates: surgical technique and clinical outcome. *Am J Sports Med* 41:58–63, 2013.)

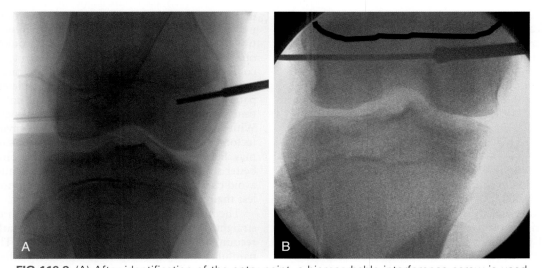

FIG 119.8 (A) After identification of the entry point, a bioresorbable interference screw is used to secure the graft within the medial condyle distal to the physis. (B) Anteroposterior view of the knee showing the guide wire and acorn drill entering distal to the physis. The distal femoral physis is outlined by a *bold black line*. (A, From Nelitz M, Dreyhaupt J, Reichel H, et al: Anatomic reconstruction of the medial patellofemoral ligament in children and adolescents with open growth plates: surgical technique and clinical outcome. *Am J Sports Med* 41:58–63, 2013.)

stress required to dislocate the patellofemoral joint in patients with more normal soft tissue function and bony anatomy. It is interesting to note that fractures tend to be avulsion-type or intra-articular osteochondral in nature, but the two rarely occur concurrently.[140,157] An initial avulsion may serve to decompress the patellofemoral joint, thus decreasing stress between the retropatellar surface and the lateral femoral condyle.

Sports, dance, and other high-demand activities are often the primary cause of injury in initial dislocators. Using the

NHSS-RIO database, Mitchell et al.[105] found the overall rate of patella instability to be 1.95 per 100,000 athletic exposures for scholastic athletes. The highest rates were seen in the high-demand sports of girls' gymnastics, boys' football, and boys' wrestling with rates of 6.19, 4.10, and 3.45 episodes, respectively, per 100,000 athletic exposures. Although girls had an overall lower rate of patella dislocation (thought to be because of higher participation in lower demand sports), the injury rate was higher for girls than boys (1.47 vs. 0.88 in gender-comparable sports like soccer and lacrosse). Young athletes nowadays are playing sports in an environment of relatively more game-versus-practice time, consistently higher competitive levels, and early specialization in single sports. These factors combine to increase injury exposure and risk.

CLASSIFICATION

A myriad of classification systems for patellofemoral instability and maltracking have been devised. In his classic treatise on patellofemoral instability, Runow[128] grouped initial dislocators into four groups (Table 119.2). Group I had only minimal patella alta (Insall ratio of 1.0 to 1.3), minimal trochlear dysplasia, and no generalized hyper laxity. Seventy-six percent of these patients experienced significant trauma causing the dislocation; they had an average age at initial onset of 19 and a low rate of recurrence, and osteochondral fractures occurred in 63%. Group II had generalized hyperlaxity and an Insall ratio of 1.0 to 1.3, and group III had normal soft tissue function but an Insall ratio greater than 1.3. Group IV demonstrated both hyperlaxity and severe patella alta. Among group IV patients the age at onset was 13, the recurrence rate was 74%, bilateral involvement occurred in 68%, significant trauma played a role in only 28%, and osteochondral fractures occurred in only 17% (see Table 119.2). In a comprehensive population study, Fithian et al.[49] classified acute dislocators into those with and without a history of previous dislocation. Those with a history of previous dislocation were more likely female and had a higher risk of future dislocation, a positive family history for patellar instability, higher rates of dysplastic hip disease, and increases in patella alta, patellar tilt, and patellar subluxation. As discussed earlier, we have found that grouping patients generally into the TONES and LAACS classifications is useful in assessing risk factors, discussing the natural history, and guiding treatment options (see Table 119.1).

NATURAL HISTORY

Population-based studies have estimated the per capita risk for first-time dislocation in children and adolescents to be between 29 and 43 per 100,000.[10,49,111] The natural history of this fairly common major knee malady is not benign. A significant number of patients experience recurrent instability and/or patellofemoral pain related to maltracking or osteochondral injury. For nonoperative patients, reported redislocation rates vary widely from 15% to 45%, and 30% to 50% may be expected to suffer anterior knee pain.[12,68] Fithian et al.[49] in their group of first-time

dislocators, reported recurrent instability in 49% of patients with a previous history of preceding instability symptoms. Runow[128] reported a redislocation rate of only 13% in his group I patients without laxity or patellofemoral dysplasia. However, the rate jumped to 74% in group IV patients with both generalized hypermobility and patellofemoral dysplasia. In their study of 100 young acute dislocators, Mäenpää et al.[91] found a redislocation rate of 44%, patellofemoral pain in 19%, and no complaints after nonoperative treatment in only 37% of patients. In a randomized study of nonoperative and operative treatment, Nikku et al. reported recurrent instability rates of 20% in their nonoperative group and 18% in their operative group and overall better function in their nonoperative patients.[113] In a large group of male Army conscripts with an average age of 20 years who underwent surgery for acute or recurrent patellar dislocation, Mäenpää et al.[91] found that only 19% had excellent results. Only 35% were able to finish their military service normally after surgical intervention.

Systematic reviews, reviews, and meta-analyses on first-time dislocators speak to the lack of a definitive treatment algorithm for treating young patients with acute patellar dislocation.[148,154] Many studies are retrospective in nature, are short term in follow-up, use various surgical interventions, suffer from subject/treatment selection bias, and lack defined outcomes variables. To date, nonoperative care is generally recommended for first-time dislocators unless there is concurrent osteochondral injury, early recurrent dislocation, substantial disruption of the MPFL-VMO-adductor mechanism, other knee injury necessitating surgical care, or failure to progress with nonoperative care. We follow similar guidelines but would also offer early operative intervention to LAACS-type patients (often requiring combined procedures) who have had contralateral instability requiring surgery and to high-demand athletes, TONES-type patients whose competitive schedules will not tolerate downtime or future dislocation (MPFL reconstruction or repair). With better understanding of host and environmental risk factors for recurrence and surgical failure, surgical selection may become more appropriately focused. This may lead to better surgery for the large group of young patients looking to avoid currently high rates of recurrence after nonoperative and less than perfect surgical care to date.[154]

The history of an acute patellar dislocation is not always as straightforward as it may seem. The young athlete is able to recount a major injury but rarely the details. The athlete has a painful, swollen, guarded knee but rarely a fixed dislocation. Although injuries can occur as the result of a direct fall onto the patella, most occur through the noncontact mechanisms

TABLE 119.2	**Classification of Patellar Instability**								
Instability Grade	Joint Laxity	Insall Index >1.3	Percent of Total Group	Age at Onset, Yr	Frequent Dislocations (Fraction)	Bilateral Dislocations (Fraction)	Moderate Trauma (Fraction)	Fracture(s) (Fraction)	Instability Score
0	—	—	—	—	—	—	—	—	—
I	—	—	16	19	0.13	0.13	0.76	0.63	2.1
II	+	—	35	15	0.26	0.19	0.69	0.38	2.7
III	—	+	19	15	0.60	0.35	0.55	0.33	3.6
IV	+	+	30	13	0.74	0.68	0.26	0.17	5.0
Total/average			100	15	0.46	0.37	0.55	0.33	3.6

From Runow A: The dislocating patella: etiology and prognosis in relation to generalized joint laxity and anatomy of the patellar articulation. *Acta Orthop Scand Suppl* 201:1–53, 1983.

previously described. Children and younger adolescents can have a hard time differentiating this plant-twist mechanism from that leading to a noncontact ACL injury. Both result in a sense of traumatic giving way, pain, hemarthrosis, and significant impairment. Both diagnoses must be considered and carefully ruled out in an acutely injured knee. Patients with recurrent acute dislocation usually relate a history and a feeling of "sameness" to the current dislocation episode. Symptomatic osteochondral fractures may result in complaints of mechanical locking and persistent effusion. Complaints associated with chronic subluxation are often vague. The child often complains of generalized anterior knee pain or burning and a sense of the knee giving way with quick stops, jumping, or change of direction. A history of multiple physician consultations and sporadic efforts at rehabilitation is often reported.

In getting one's "clinical hands" around a patient with patellofemoral instability, the following questions are important to answer. (1) What is the personality of the injury? Is this a mechanically normal knee subjected to macrotrauma, or did the dislocation occur with minimal trauma in a patient with significant underlying mechanical risk factors? (2) Is this problem an aggravation or a disability, as gauged by lost play/practice time or the presence of chronic quadriceps atrophy? (3) Has truly adequate nonoperative care been provided, and what was the response? (4) Are signs or symptoms of concurrent knee injury present, such as osteochondral fractures, other extensor mechanism overuse syndromes, or missed ligamentous injuries? (5) Is the instability truly first-time, acute recurrent, or chronic? (6) Is the patella grossly unstable during clinical examination or daily activities? (7) What are the age, activity level, and athletic participation/potential of the patient?

PHYSICAL EXAMINATION

Fortunately, the patellofemoral articulation is very accessible for physical examination. Efforts should be made to specifically correlate underlying anatomic structures with superficial palpation. For example, zone-specific injury to the MPFL may be inferred from specific tenderness at its patella or femoral origins. In the acute setting, arthrocentesis is both diagnostic and therapeutic. Hemarthrosis and fatty globules can be documented. Instillation of a local anesthetic and decompression of the joint may improve the quality of the examination. Pain is decreased, and early range-of-motion and quadriceps activities are improved. A standard ligamentous examination of the knee should be performed to rule out concurrent injury. A sense of the overall tissue trauma should be established. Large palpable rents in the VMO, adductors, or MPFL and a grossly dislocatable patella are relative indicators for surgical intervention in a TONES-type patient.

The young patient with patella instability should receive a holistic review of potential risk factors. Overall alignment of the lower extremities should be determined in a weight-bearing position. This examination includes an assessment of generalized joint laxity, knee valgus, femoral/tibial rotation, and foot posture. Walking, jogging, jumping, and other sport-specific activity should be evaluated if symptoms allow. Total lower extremity flexibility/strength and core strength should be assessed. Particular emphasis is placed on the following: hip abductor/adductor strength balance, iliotibial band and hip flexor tightness, quadriceps atrophy, and painful arcs of resisted knee motion. The patient should be assessed for excessive guarding about the knee, hypersensitivity to light touch, and other signs of saphenous nerve irritation or early reflex sympathetic dystrophy.

More specific evaluation of the patellofemoral joint can then be carried out. Evaluation includes assessing the Q angle in full extension and at 20 degrees of flexion. Patellar apprehension testing is then performed by attempting to displace the patella laterally over the lateral femoral condyle while observing the patient for signs of apprehension or discomfort. This is done in both a static and dynamic fashion. Medial and lateral patellar translation and endpoint compliance are assessed. The patella normally can be displaced both medially and laterally between 25% and 50% of the width of the patella. Patellar tilt should be evaluated. Lateral retinacular tightness may prevent the lateral facet from being tilted above the horizontal. Patellar tracking is evaluated through a full range of motion with and without patellofemoral compression. Late engagement, J sign, patella alta or baja, lateralization, and painful arcs of motion are documented.

IMAGING

With regard to patellofemoral instability, diagnostic imaging serves two broad functions. It provides information on traumatic injury, and it assesses underlying anatomy that may predispose to maltracking and instability. Unfortunately, most imaging studies are static and do not reflect the dynamic nature of the patellofemoral joint.

Radiographs should begin with standard anteroposterior, bent-knee weight bearing, true lateral views at 20 to 30 degrees, and sunrise views at 20 degrees. A true lateral radiograph can be helpful in assessing patellar tilt, trochlea depth, dysplastic changes, and patella alta.[79,93] Some time should be devoted to assessment of patella alta because it is one of the radiographic risk factors that is most correlated with symptomatic instability.[§] Many different methods and standard ratios are used.[8,16,22,81,152] For children and younger adolescents, we recommend the method of Caton-Deschamps,[22] Blackburn and Peel,[16] or Koshino-Sugimoto.[81] For a skeletally mature patient the modified or standard Insall-Salvati method is appropriate.[71] Lateral x-rays are examined for trochlear dysplasia.[25,32,79] Sunrise view at 20 degrees is used to assess patella tilt and subluxation. The Merchant view[103] is taken at 45 degrees of knee flexion and yields information on the patellofemoral relationship in a more seated position. The congruence angle defines the relationship of the patella apex to the bisected femoral trochlea, and the sulcus angle defines the depth of the trochlear groove. Normal and dysplastic values have been noted earlier in the text.

MRI is routinely obtained on all acute dislocators to evaluate TT-TG distance[11,34,121] to define the zone of MPFL injury.[**] These areas are discussed in the anatomy section of this chapter. MRI is also used to identify osteochondral injuries. Plain radiographs miss a high percentage of osteochondral fractures that occur at the time of patellofemoral dislocation. Dainer et al.[30] found that 40% of arthroscopically documented lesions were missed on initial films. In a group of adolescent dislocators, Stanitski[146] found that only 34% of arthroscopically diagnosed osteochondral injuries were apparent on standard radiographs.

---

§References 10, 41, 84, 101, 128, and 152.
**References 47, 94, 122, 131, 137, and 144.

Correlation of MRI with arthroscopic findings, though not perfect, is significantly better than plain films. Medial patellar avulsion fractures and osteochondral fractures from the retropatellar surface or lateral condyle are common. Discussion of current techniques for patellofemoral imaging, including specific sequences, magnetic resonance arthrography, and dynamic MRI, are available.[11,34,99,121,159]

TREATMENT

A number of factors must be considered in deciding on treatment of patellofemoral instability in a young patient, including the chronicity of the instability, the presence of predisposing mechanical risk factors, the degree of instability, the existence of concurrent injury, the age and activity level of the athlete, progression with nonoperative care, and the desires of the athlete and family. Most patients with patellofemoral instability should be treated initially with a comprehensive, well-monitored nonoperative program. However, the indications for initial surgical intervention and earlier reconstruction are evolving.

Nonoperative Care

Nonoperative treatment remains the most common treatment for first-time patellar instability. Clinical studies provide little support for surgical intervention over nonoperative care for first-time instability events.[9,25,100,139,143]

Most dislocations will spontaneously reduce on the field with terminal knee extension. If this does not happen, reduction should be done in a controlled setting. Intra-articular lidocaine injection, full passive extension, and gentle pressure are usually adequate for successful relocation. As discussed earlier, arthrocentesis is preformed for diagnostic and therapeutic benefit. There is no consensus regarding immobilization in the treatment of primary patellar instability.[73] Recommendations range widely from immediate brace-free mobilization to brace immobilization in extension for 6 weeks. Immobilization in extension may allow the medial structures a better opportunity to heal but predisposes to stiffness, weakness, and loss of limb control. A study of primary patellar dislocations found that those treated with casting in extension for 6 weeks had the lowest risk of recurrent dislocation but also suffered most frequently from stiffness.[92] Quad sets, straight-leg raises, and single-plane motion are begun early and are progressed as tolerated. Early guarded motion and exercise are beneficial. It is unlikely that single-plane controlled motion will stress the healing MPFL or cause recurrent instability. It is repetition of the valgus, plant-twist injury mechanism or mechanically similar activities that must be avoided in the healing period.

As strength and symptoms allow, patients progress out of their brace in the protected environment of physical therapy to single-plane walking, running, cutting, and finally sport-specific activity. Early modalities and exercise are aimed at decreasing pain and effusion while triggering quadriceps activity. It is much easier to maintain quadriceps function than to retrieve it after a period of complete immobilization and inactivity. Early motion also helps to maintain articular cartilage health.

Rehabilitation involves optimizing the environment for quadriceps activity, restoring extensor mechanism balance, and improving overall core strength and sports posture/basic skills. Retropatellar irritation is a potential source of problems during extensor mechanism rehabilitation. Pain leads to significant quadriceps inhibition and may indicate increasing articular cartilage damage. Exercises should be done in a pain-free range and incorporate closed-chain exercises. Patellar taping as described by Gilleard et al.[57] has been shown to decrease pain, allow increased quadriceps activity, and improve weight acceptance in functional activities during the early rehabilitation period. The exact mechanism of the beneficial effects is unclear. Possibilities include changes in patellofemoral compressive forces, proprioceptive feedback to improve recruitment of quadriceps activity, and subtle improvements in dynamic patellar tracking.

Despite traditional focus on VMO activity, the quadriceps function in a complex, coordinated fashion.[7,83,124] EMG studies suggest that a balanced relationship exists between the VMO and VL in maintaining position of the patella. Numerous studies have shown that EMG activity of the VMO and VL in the normal population is nearly balanced during a wide variety of activities.[27,29] Studies have shown that physical therapy can positively alter delayed-onset firing of the VMO relative to the VL in individuals with patellofemoral syndromes.[28] Quadriceps activity should be incorporated into functional patterns as soon as possible. Examples include working lateral pelvic tilts (hip abduction) or hip adduction (ball squeezes) with concurrent quadriceps. Control of the thigh and pelvic muscles is critical to minimizing increases in the dynamic Q angle and the valgus force on the patellofemoral joint.[100] Acute lateral patellar dislocations most commonly occur when the femur internally rotates on a fixed externally rotated tibia. In a recent study, subjects with patellofemoral pain syndrome exhibited delayed gluteus medius activation relative to control subjects.[19] In addition, gluteal muscle strength has also been shown to be decreased in female patellofemoral pain subjects, with hip abduction and external rotation strength decreased 26% to 36% versus age- and activity-matched controls.[72] Closed-chain gluteal rehabilitation aids in externally rotating the femur and as a result decreasing the Q angle during the gait cycle.[35] Selective stretching is required to achieve a balanced extensor mechanism. Stretching of the upper and lower iliotibial band, hamstrings, gastrocnemius, and hip flexors is important. Relative internal rotation of the lower extremity increases the lateralizing vector on the patella. Excessive or prolonged midfoot pronation may be a contributor, and semirigid orthotic devices are helpful in selected patients. Dynamic hip anteversion may also be improved by proximal strengthening. Core strengthening of the abdominals, hips, and low back is an essential part of the rehabilitation and prevention program.

Operative Care

Surgical interventions for patellofemoral instability are numerous. The phrase "over 100 procedures" has become synonymous with any discussion of surgery to address patellofemoral instability. Despite the recent trend towards "anatomic" restoration of the MPFL, there is not yet full consensus with regard to repair versus reconstruction, surgical approaches, graft options, fixation techniques, origin and insertion points, and dynamic versus static constructs. Soon, the "over 100 procedures" may apply to MPFL surgeries alone. Surgical algorithms must include decision points on proximal, distal, or combined reconstructive procedures. As surgical techniques and outcomes improve, the indications for operative intervention of acute patella dislocation may expand. They currently include: (1) concurrent osteochondral injury that necessitates operative intervention, (2) other concurrent injury requiring surgery, (3) grossly palpable disruption of the MPFL-VMO-adductor mechanism, (4) early repeat dislocation, and (5) failure to progress with rehabilitation. We would include a discussion of early nonoperative care for the first-time dislocator in the following circumstances: (1) history of contralateral instability requiring surgical intervention and (2) high level athlete who has some underlying anatomic risk factors and whose schedule poorly tolerates a repeat dislocation.[4]

Surgical Decision Making. In general, surgery addressing the MPFL is appropriate when the primary deficiency is of medial soft tissue restraints. If significant functional malalignment exists, a distal realignment is required. In a combined deficiency, MPFL repair or reconstruction may be used in combination with distal realignment. Age-dependent data for TT-TG and patella alta in young normal and patella dislocators have been reported.[††] However, critical values that should trigger distal realignment, distalization, or trochlearplasty in young patients are uncertain. MPFL reconstruction alone appears to be successful in the face of mild-to-moderate trochlear dysplasia and has been reported to actually decrease moderate preexisting patella alta.[41] However, "significant" trochlear dysplasia and patella alta are predictors of failure of isolated MPFL reconstruction.[120,138] Extrapolating from the adult literature, markers for a distal procedure might include TT-TG >15 to 20 mm, Caton index of 1.2, and distalization for Caton indices more than 1.4.[26,36,80] Consideration for distal or combined procedure may also be appropriate when there is a constellation of dysplastic changes with lesser individual values. Feller et al.[46] have also suggested the presence of significant J tracking necessitating a distal realignment procedure.

Gade III and IV articular cartilage lesions are associated with poor functional outcomes in the adolescent population.[110] Oblique osteotomies can provide not only realignment but also off-loading for lateral and distal lesion patellofemoral and cartilage restorative procedures. Tubercle osteotomy techniques for the adolescent are similar to those in the adult and have been fully discussed elsewhere.[36,79] Conceptually, these techniques may provide more medialization for realignment and more anteriorization for off-loading. For significant patella alta, tubercle osteotomies can also be distalized. In younger patients, distal realignment must be accomplished with soft tissue procedures, which avoid physeal injury of the tubercle. The safe age for tibial tubercle osteotomy is not well defined. However, a bone age of 14 to 15 years for boys and 13 to 14 years for girls should avoid iatrogenic recurvatum.[63,90]

The two most common soft tissue distal realignment procedures are the Galeazzi semitendinosus tenodesis[51] and the Roux-Goldthwait[24] hemipatella tendon transfer. Numerous modifications of each technique can be found. Historically, both procedures have often been combined with proximal procedures of lateral release, medial retinaculum repair, and VMO imbrications. Good to excellent results in a skeletally immature population have been achieved in 62% to 82% of cases.[85] However, more recent reviews suggest that recurrent subluxation and subjective knee complaints may be higher than initially reported.[59] Both procedures secondarily address patella alta, as well as medialization. Other soft tissue realignments include the Nietosvaara technique[112] a modification of the

Galeazzi procedure that reconstructs the MPFL and the patellotibial ligaments. Luhmann et al.[89] and Garin et al.[53] have described a distal medial, hemipatella tendon transfer that may mimic MPFL function more than the Roux-Goldthwait (Fig. 119.9). Andrish[6] has described a soft tissue, patellar tendon imbrications to address patella alta in the skeletally immature who are not candidates for tubercle osteotomy. In skeletally immature patients with a significant patella alta, reconstruction of the MPFL may be augmented by using a limb of the hamstring graft to reconstruct the patellotibial ligament, in addition to the MPFL.[6,112] As noted previously, Fabricant et al.[41] have reported patella alta to improve with MPFL reconstruction.

In the young child, correction of lateral vector related to increased knee valgus may be achieved through guided growth. Indications include at least a 10-degree valgus deformity in a child with adequate corrective growth remaining. Correction of 0.7 degrees per month from the femur and 0.3 degrees per month from the tibia has been reported. This approach is not indicated before the age of 8 because spontaneous correction can occur. Devices can be removed after correction and reapplied if necessary.[17,42,61,65,130]

Indications for trochlearplasty have included Dejour changes C or greater, grade B with gross patella instability at 30 degrees of flexion or greater, and "severe" trochlear dysplasia.[107,129] Reconstruction of the MPFL coupled with trochleoplasty may be considered in young patients with severe trochlear dysplasia. Various techniques have been described including reshaping the trochlear groove via deepening, osteochondral flapping into a deepened trochlear groove, or raising the lateral condyle. The authors have not used this technique but refer the reader to a 2-year follow-up on combined MPFL and trochlearplasty.[107]

Medial patellofemoral ligament surgery: general concepts. The injured MPFL may be addressed by repair, repair with augmentation, or reconstruction. Outcomes appear to be better with reconstruction than repair, but complications other than recurrence may also be higher. Although the trend is toward reconstruction, we feel that repair still has some viable indications: (1) as the proximal part of a combined procedure in which there is adequate MPFL tissue as judged on MRI and at time of operation; (2) in an acute injury in which there is an isolated zone of injury at the patella or femoral insertions as judged by MRI and operative investigation, coupled with minimal underlying patellofemoral dysplasia; and (3) when clinical history and examination under anesthesia are suggestive of only mild instability. Acute repairs may be performed with suture to periosteum, suture anchors or fixation of avulsion fractures, as indicated. Ahmad and et al.[4] emphasized the importance of concurrently assessing the femoral attachment of the VMO, which may be ruptured. Specific repair techniques and the necessary anatomic dissection have been described by previous authors.[3,54,144] Several arthroscopic soft tissue balancing techniques for lateral patellar instability have been reported. These are essentially medial advancements coupled with an arthroscopic lateral release.[18,62,95] They offer the advantages of being minimally invasive and not burning any treatment bridges for young patients. Ahmad and Lee[3] described making an incision in the medial retinaculum, which is then repaired in a pants-over-vest fashion. The distance that sutures are passed from the edge of the incision will determine the degree of imbrication. Halbrecht[62] reported the use of suturing to bunch and tighten the medial retinaculum without incising it. These authors combined medial reefing with arthroscopic lateral

---

††References 11, 34, 41, 110, 121, and 152.

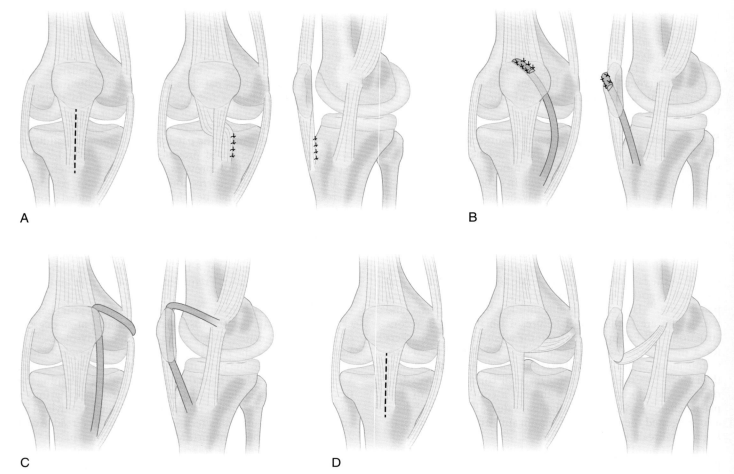

FIG 119.9 Distal Realignment Procedures (A) Roux-Goldthwait. (B) Galeazzi procedure. (C) Nietosvaara technique. (D) Hemipatella tendon transfer. (From Weeks KD III, Fabricant PD, Ladenhauf HN, Green DW: Surgical options for patellar stabilization in the skeletally immature patient. *Sports Med Arthrosc* 20:194–202, 2012.)

release. The procedures may be best performed in patients with more subtle instability, good soft tissue quality, and relatively normal patellofemoral bony architecture. These procedures may also be used as an adjunct to distal realignment.

If necessary, a repair may be reinforced with local tissues, such as a turndown of part of the adductor tendon or quad tendon. In addition, advancement and repair of the native MPFL is always a part of our reconstructive procedure when using a free hamstring graft.

When reconstructing the MPFL, there are a variety of options for graft material, placement, fixation, and tensioning. Graft options include free and distally attached hamstring autografts, a slip of adductor tendon, quadriceps tendon, iliotibial band, and allograft materials. The MPFL may be reconstructed alone or in combination with the medial patellotibial ligament. Fixation on the patellar side can be achieved with the use of suture anchors, suture, or bone tunnels. On the femoral side, suture anchors or punch lock devices, tunnel with interference screw fixation, direct suturing, post with a washer, and sling fabrication from the MCL, adductor tendon, or intramuscular septum have been described (Fig. 119.10). In a skeletally immature patient, hardware and graft tunnels must be kept out of the femoral growth plate and excessive dissection about the

peripheral growth plate must be avoided. The undulating anatomy of the distal femoral physis was discussed earlier. Live-time x-ray should be available for all MPFL cases.

A single best technique has not emerged, but there is a growing body of biomechanical information laying the groundwork for basic concepts of successful surgery and improved outcomes. Paramount among these are adequately re-creating the normal femoral and patella insertion sites of the ligament, followed by appropriate graft tensioning and mimicking native MPFL biomechanics with the graft.[‡‡] Fixation on the femoral side may be fixed or dynamic (through a soft tissue sling). We think that femoral and particularly patella fixation should minimize bone loss and best replicate the superficial blending attachment of the native ligament. Several authors[39,132,142] have investigated the isometricity of various origin and insertion positions for MPFL reconstruction. Inappropriate graft placement can result in increased patellofemoral contact pressures and poor graft tension though knee range of motion. Best results are obtained by using the anatomic femoral and patellar attachments. Proximal displacement of the femoral insertion

---

[‡‡]References 76, 132, 147, 149, 150, and 155.

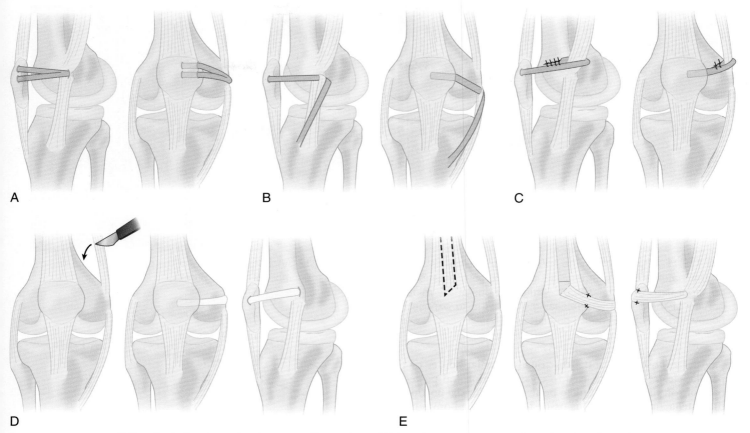

FIG 119.10 Proximal Realignment Procedures (A) Free hamstring autograft (authors' preferred method). (B) MCL pulley. (C) Adductor sling. (D) Adductor tendon graft. (E) Hemiquadriceps tendon transfer. (From Weeks KD III, Fabricant PD, Ladenhauf HN, Green DW: Surgical options for patellar stabilization in the skeletally immature patient. *Sports Med Arthrosc* 20:194–202, 2012.)

results in increased distance between insertion sites as the knee moves into greater flexion, which can lead to loss of knee flexion or disruption of the graft. Anterior malposition coupled with a shorter than anatomic MPFL graft substitute appears to result in significantly increased medial patellar tilt and retropatellar pressure.[39] Distal displacement of the femoral insertion results in lesser changes in graft length and tension during the first 40 degrees of knee flexion.

If using a bone tunnel and interference screw fixation on the femoral side, it must be recognized that the graft will rest in the anterior part of the tunnel, not the center. Selecting the center of the femoral insertion site combines radiographic evaluation on an intraoperative true lateral of the knee. This is combined with a clinical check of isometricity of the graft through 0 to 40 degrees of flexion. The patella attachment should be broadly applied to the medial patella centered at the junction of the superior one-third/inferior two-thirds of the patella, reflecting its two-bundle nature.

Another important factor is graft tensioning. The MPFL graft is to serve as a tether, not a shortened restrictor of normal patellofemoral tracking. In the normal knee, the native MPFL sees significant strain only when a valgus force is applied. The graft should be tensioned with low force. There is no consensus on knee flexion angle at which to tension the graft. Full

extension, 30 flexion, and 45 degrees of flexion have all been suggested.[132] We tension at 20 to 30 degrees flexion. At this angle the patella is initially engaged in the trochlear groove, and this is a knee flexion angle at which the knee functions in many sporting activities. The graft must be assessed for appropriate translation, endpoint quality, and normal full motion of the knee. Before final fixation we check relative isometricity from 0 to 40 degrees for both limbs of our graft. This is done initially with sutures from the patella side anchors and then via preliminary fixation of each limb of the graft before final suturing. Our technique for MPFL reconstruction in the young patient uses a free hamstring autograph and is similar to the technique reported by Nelitz and Williams.[109]

Preferred MPFL reconstruction technique. For MPFL reconstruction, we currently use one incision midway between the medial border of the patella and the medial epicondyle. Access to the medial border of the patella is best achieved with the knee in extension, whereas knee flexion allows optimal access to the MPFL femoral insertion site. Dissection is performed to create anterior and posterior subcutaneous flaps to access these areas. A second incision is made for hamstring graft harvest, which can be performed using any standard technique. Our preferred graft is the semitendinosus, although a robust gracilis tendon may be adequate.

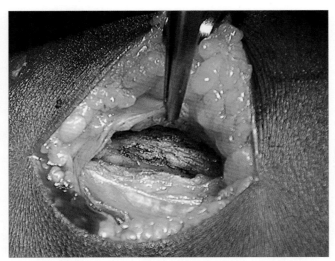

FIG 119.11 After exposing the soft tissue on the medial border of the patella, electrocautery is used to create anterior and posterior flaps of soft tissue by cutting to bone at the midaxial portion of the patella and releasing this tissue to expose the bony surface of the medial patella.

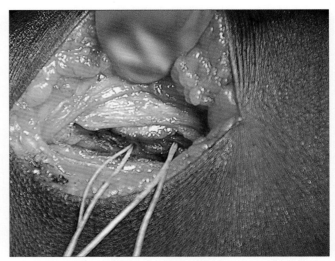

FIG 119.12 Anchors are placed in the proximal to mid one-third of the medial border of the patella.

After exposing the soft tissue on the medial border of the patella, electrocautery is used to create anterior and posterior flaps of soft tissue by cutting to bone at the midaxial portion of the patella and releasing this tissue to expose the bony surface of the medial patella (Fig. 119.11). Exposure should be done to allow for anchor placement in the middle to proximal portion of the patella. We currently use two 1.7-mm all-suture anchors (Fig. 119.12). After placement of the anchors, it is important to ensure that the sutures slide smoothly through the anchor for later graft fixation to bone. The knee is then flexed to allow access to the femoral insertion site for the graft.

The optimal location for graft fixation is posterior and distal to the adductor tubercle. A 0.62-mm K-wire is placed under direct visualization and checked using fluoroscopy. On a true lateral view, the center of the femoral origin is 1 mm anterior to an extension line from the posterior cortex, 2.5 mm distal to the origin of the medial femoral condyle, and proximal to the level of the posterior point of the Blumenstaat line (see Fig. 119.7). The sutures from the previously placed patella anchors are then wrapped around the K-wire, and the knee is brought through a range of motion to assess isometry. The sutures should be slightly looser in flexion than extension to avoid placing a graft that will exhibit increased pressures on the patellofemoral articulation once the patella engages the trochlea in flexion. After the optimal femoral insertion site has been located, the K-wire is replaced with a 5.5-mm suture anchor. This should be angled away from the undulation of the femoral physis in the skeletally immature patient. The hamstring graft is then folded in half, and the U portion of the graft secured to the patella using the previously place anchors. Several locked suture passes are placed in the graft from each anchor, leaving a gap between the suture entry site equal to the distance between the two suture anchors (Fig. 119.13). The opposite suture from each anchor is then used to slide the graft to bone.

After the graft is secured to the medial border of the patella, the same sutures are used to create a soft tissue tunnel by passing the sutures through the previously created anterior and

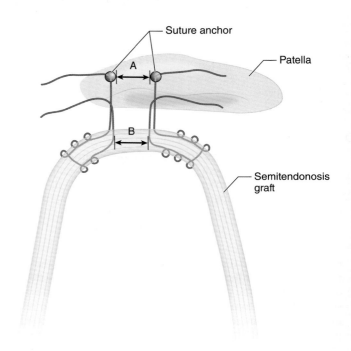

FIG 119.13 Distance between suture anchors A and B should be equal to the distance between the entry site of sutures in the graft. Graft is doubled and secured to patella using suture anchors.

posterior soft tissue flaps in a vest over pants fashion (Fig. 119.14). Each limb of the graft is then individually tensioned and secured to the femoral insertion site. With the knee flexed 60 degrees, a limb of the graft is held over the femoral anchor site to approximate the location of suture entry. Two locking suture passes are then placed in the graft, and the graft is temporarily held at the femoral insertion site by pulling tension on the opposite limb of suture through the anchor. The knee is then brought through a range of motion to assess the graft tension before committing to the femoral fixation. The graft should be slightly tighter in extension than flexion. Excess

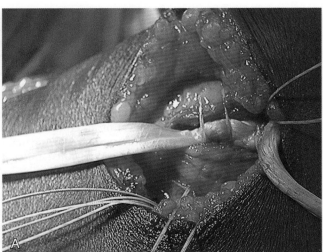
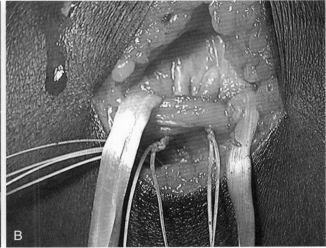

FIG 119.14 After the graft is secured to the medial border of the patella (A) the same sutures are then used to create a soft tissue tunnel by passing the sutures through the previously created anterior and posterior soft tissue flaps in a vest-over-pants fashion (B).

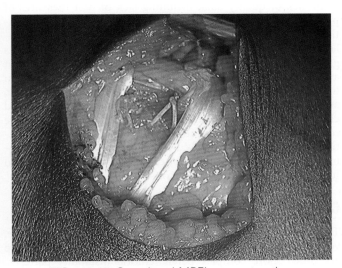

FIG 119.15 Completed MPFL reconstruction.

tension in flexion will lead to increased patellofemoral pressure and potentially pain and long-term arthrosis.

The goal of our reconstruction is to allow the patella to enter the trochlear groove in a centered position and then allow the bony anatomy of the patellofemoral articulation to allow for stability in higher degrees of flexion. If graft tension is satisfactory, then two more locking passes are placed and the graft is secured to the femur. The femoral fixation is then reinforced by removing the excess graft leaving a 1-cm stump of graft posterior to the femoral insertion site and securing this to the adjacent soft tissue with the sutures from the anchor. The process is then repeated using the other limb of the graft. This allows each limb of the graft to be individually tensioned (Fig. 119.15).

OTHER MEDIAL PATELLOFEMORAL LIGAMENT RECONSTRUCTION OPTIONS

The use of a pedicle quadriceps allograft is gaining popularity.[48,109,115,127] Advantages include a native attachment of the graft to the patella (avoiding hardware or potential fracture from tunnels or hardware) and the possibility that a superficial medal quad tendon graft may more closely approximate the geometry and biomechanical function of the native MPFL. Numerous techniques have been reported[48,109,115,127] with favorable outcomes. With all techniques, close care must be given to the harvest of the quad tendon toward the patella attachment to avoid graft compromise of the quad tendon graft as it turns laterally off the superior medial patella toward the femoral insertion site (Fig. 119.16). Transfer of a slip of adductor magnus tendon from the femoral attachment side offers potential benefits similar to those of the quadriceps tendon. To avoid hardware near the femoral physis, several different sling fixation techniques are available. Graft can be looped around or through a sling in the insertion of the adductor tendon or MCL. In addition, some have suggested that this more dynamic insertion may have biomechanical benefits. There is also some interest in the dynamic nature of the MPFL, particularly the superior bundle with its close association with the VMO.

SURGICAL COMPLICATIONS

Surgical complications after MPFL reconstruction are not rare, being reported between 15% and 25% of cases.[13,87,120,151] Complications may be related to technical mistakes, inappropriate patient selection, or more general surgical complications. Complications can be reduced with a thorough understanding of patellofemoral anatomy and adhering to basic concepts, such as anatomic restoration, limiting bone loss, avoiding stress risers, not relying on soft tissue procedures with significant underlying bony misalignment, or not artificially constricting normal motion. Complications may include recurrent lateral instability, iatrogenic medial side instability (which is more frequent with lateral release and underlying trochlear dysplasia), graft malposition and loss of motion or insufficient graft function, patella fracture, femoral bony tunnel enlargement, increased patellofemoral compression, and hardware irritation. Tubercle osteotomies can be associated with proximal tibial or tubercle shingle fracture, hardware irritation, and recurvatum

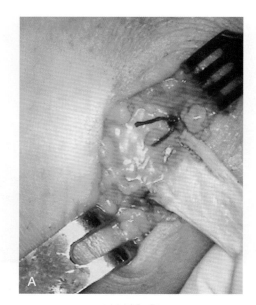

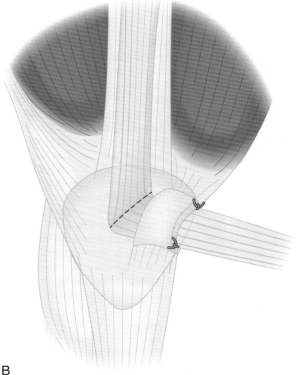

B

FIG 119.16 (A) The QT strip is fixed with two sutures at the medial patella border. (B) Schematic drawing showing the final location of the QT strip. (From Fink C, Veselko M, Herbort M, Hoser C: MPFL reconstruction using a quadriceps tendon graft: part 2: operative technique and short term clinical results. *Knee* 21:1175–1179, 2014.)

if performed too early in skeletal maturity. Nonantomic distal soft tissue realignments may overconstrain the knee, gradually loosening with time. Knee stiffness and significant loss of quadriceps function can also be seen if appropriate rehabilitation, and quad activation are not begun in the early postoperative period. In a comprehensive review of complications and

failures associated with MPFL reconstruction, Shah et al.[138] reported an overall complication rate of 26% after MPFL reconstruction. In this review, there were a total of 164 complications in a group of 629 MPFL reconstructions. Most common (32%) was recurrent lateral apprehension or instability. The most serious complication was patella fracture, of which there were four, all in patients who had undergone MPFL reconstruction with patella side fixation with patella bone tunnels. A surprisingly high 22 patients (13% of all complications) sustained a postoperative loss of knee motion requiring manipulation under anesthesia. Painful hardware was noted in 19 patients.

OUTCOMES AND RETURN TO ACTIVITY

There is a paucity of data reporting on the return to sporting activity after MPFL reconstruction.[96,97] Return to play at the same level has been reported to vary between 40% and 65%, not the 100% that most patients expect. Time for return to play has been reported to be between 4 months and 2 years.[96,97,109] Although children and adolescents appear to have higher recurrent instability rates, they also have higher return-to-sports and functional levels than older adults. The current literature suffers from lack of quality data, including lack of best measures of preoperative and postoperative activity levels, lack of preoperative risk factor documentation, and mixing of instability populations. It is our impression that return-to-play time varies greatly among different patients. TONES-type patients without articular damage and a history of athletic participation return to full activities quicker than do LAACS-type patients. However, articular cartilage damage is a risk factor for delayed return and chronic patellofemoral pain. We also think that comprehensive return-to-play testing including video and core sports functional analysis should be used in MPFL patients. Close, long-term objective follow-up can often reveal an extended time to full recovery, similar to ACL reconstruction patients.

COMPLEX PATELLOFEMORAL INSTABILITY

This chapter has focused on patellofemoral instability in active, young patients. Certainly, within the pediatric population there are much more complex patellofemoral instability patterns. Although a full discussion is beyond the scope of this chapter, Weeks et al.[158] have offered a useful classification system.

Syndromic: Dislocation associated with genetic syndromes and connective tissue disorders.

Congenital: Persistent or fixed lateral dislocation of the patella detected at or near birth. It is manifested as knee flexion contracture with the patella tethered lateral to the femoral condyles. The probable cause is failure of normal embryologic rotation of the quadriceps myotome during lower extremity development.

Fixed lateral: Remains laterally dislocated, irreducible.

Obligatory: Dislocation with spontaneous reduction that occurs with every flexion-extension cycle. It is associated with significant patellofemoral dysplasia and tightness of the extensor mechanism.

Ghanem et al.[55,56] pointed out that true congenital, in utero fixed dislocation of the patella is rare. It may occur as a result of arthrogryposis, skeletal dysplasia, and other related abnormalities. However, it should be differentiated from syndromic dislocation, in which the extensor mechanism is located normally at birth but progressively dysfunctional later in childhood.

The probable cause of congenital dislocation is failure of normal medial rotation of the quadriceps myotome during in utero development.[55,145] In contrast, the patellar dislocation often associated with Down syndrome, as well as nail-patella syndrome, acquired quadriceps fibrosis, and various neuromuscular conditions, is related to abnormal biomechanical forces on an initially normally located patella. Although congenital dislocation is usually associated with more severe deformity, developmental dislocation can progress to a similar phenotypic manifestation of fixed lateral patellar dislocation, severe quadriceps contracture, and functional disability. It appears that early, comprehensive surgical realignment affords the best chance to normalize lower extremity function.[38,56,58,74] Such realignment involves aggressive mobilization of the entire patella/quadriceps mechanism, division of the lateral soft tissues, imbrication of the medial soft tissues, and possible transfer of the insertion of the patellar ligament.

Obligatory dislocators present with spontaneous dislocation and reduction of the patella with every flexion-extension cycle of the knee. This condition does not significantly delay the age or ability of early ambulation. Consequently, it is usually diagnosed later, at 5 to 10 years of age. It is relatively painless and is not voluntary in nature. In contrast, recurrent dislocation is typically episodic, is often a result of minor trauma, is painful, and can lead to swelling. Some degree of extensor mechanism contracture is usually seen in obligatory dislocators. Several authors describe the underlying pathology as quadriceps muscle contracture.[5,14] In contrast to the more common recurrent dislocation, treatment of habitual dislocation would routinely require quadriceps lengthening and lateral release.

SUMMARY

Patella instability is a common pediatric/adolescent knee problem. Traditionally, patella dislocation has been treated with varying periods of protection, sporadic rehabilitation, and anticipated return to full sports activity. The reality is that many young athletes may suffer with continued instability, pain, and extensor mechanism dysfunction. There is growing interest in the structure, biomechanics, and surgical restoration of the MPFL. When caring for younger patients, there must be a full understanding of growth and development about the knee and the myriad of risks factors that may play a role in the underlying condition. Normative age-specific data for patellofemoral dislocators and the normal population are being developed and will increasingly help to drive treatment decisions. Successful MPFL reconstruction is dependent upon exacting technique and comprehensive rehabilitation. Isolated MPFL procedures appear appropriate even with moderate underlying patellofemoral dysplasia and patella alta; however, more significant underlying dysplasia necessitates distal or combined realignment procedures. As surgical techniques improve and better postoperative outcomes are documented, the indications for surgery may expand. Return-to-sports expectation and predictors are complex and are similar to those seen in ACL reconstruction in the high-risk skeletally immature population. Development of comprehensive prevention and return to play programs are required for best outcomes.

KEY REFERENCES

11. Balcarek P, Jung K, Frosch KH, et al: Value of the tibial tuberosity-trochlear groove distance in patellar instability in the young athlete. *Am J Sports Med* 39:1756–1761, 2011.

34. Dickens AJ, Morrell NT, Doering A, et al: Tibial tubercle-trochlear groove distance: defining normal in a pediatric population. *J Bone Joint Surg Am* 96:318–324, 2014.

44. Farrow LD, Alentado VJ, Abdulnabi Z, et al: The relationship of the medial patellofemoral ligament attachment to the distal femoral physis. *Am J Sports Med* 42:2214–2218, 2014.

47. Felus J, Kowalczyk B: Age-related differences in medial patellofemoral ligament injury patterns in traumatic patellar dislocation: case series of 50 surgically treated children and adolescents. *Am J Sports Med* 40:2357–2364, 2012.

65. Hennrikus W, Pylawka T: Patellofemoral instability in skeletally immature athletes. *J Bone Joint Surg Am* 95:176–183, 2013.

66. Hensler D, Sillanpaa PJ, Schoettle PB: Medial patellofemoral ligament: anatomy, injury and treatment in the adolescent knee. *Curr Opin Pediatr* 26:70–78, 2014.

107. Nelitz M, Dreyhaupt J, Lippacher S: Combined trochleoplasty and medial patellofemoral ligament reconstruction for recurrent patellar dislocations in severe trochlear dysplasia: a minimum 2-year follow-up study. *Am J Sports Med* 41:1005–1012, 2013.

108. Nelitz M, Dreyhaupt J, Reichel H, et al: Anatomic reconstruction of the medial patellofemoral ligament in children and adolescents with open growth plates: surgical technique and clinical outcome. *Am J Sports Med* 41:58–63, 2013.

109. Nelitz M, Williams SR: Anatomic reconstruction of the medial patellofemoral ligament in children and adolescents using a pedicled quadriceps tendon graft. *Arthrosc Tech* 3:e303–e308, 2014.

110. Nelitz M, Williams RS, Lippacher S, et al: Analysis of failure and clinical outcome after unsuccessful medial patellofemoral ligament reconstruction in young patients. *Int Orthop* 38:2265–2272, 2014.

120. Parikh SN, Nathan ST, Wall EJ, et al: Complications of medial patellofemoral ligament reconstruction in young patients. *Am J Sports Med* 41:1030–1038, 2013.

121. Pennock AT, Alam M, Bastrom T: Variation in tibial tubercle-trochlear groove measurement as a function of age, sex, size, and patellar instability. *Am J Sports Med* 42:389–393, 2014.

132. Sanchis-Alfonso V: Guidelines for medial patellofemoral ligament reconstruction in chronic lateral patellar instability. *J Am Acad Orthop Surg* 22:175–182, 2014.

137. Seeley M, Bowman KF, Walsh C, et al: Magnetic resonance imaging of acute patellar dislocation in children: patterns of injury and risk factors for recurrence. *J Pediatr Orthop* 32:145–155, 2012.

The references for this chapter can also be found on www.expertconsult.com.

Joint Replacement and Its Alternatives

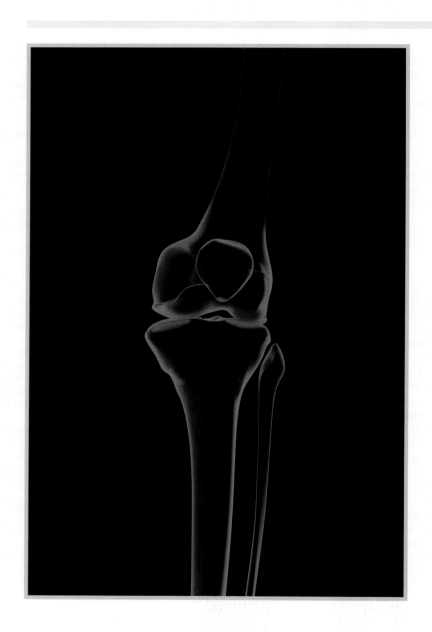

120

Nonoperative Treatment of Knee Arthritis

Zan A. Naseer, Louis Okafor, Anne Kuwabara, Harpal S. Khanuja

Osteoarthritis affects an estimated 26.9 million adults in the United States and is the most common joint disease in adults throughout the world.[194] The prevalence of osteoarthritis is 14% in adults aged 25 years or older and 34% in those 65 or older. Symptomatic osteoarthritis of the knee is present in 16% of adults aged 45 years or older, affecting approximately 19% of women and 14% of men in this age group.[162] An estimated 37% of US adults aged 60 or older have radiographic evidence of knee osteoarthritis, with 12% having symptomatic knee osteoarthritis.[372]

Nonoperative treatment of knee arthritis is aimed at alleviating symptoms. As our understanding of the disease process grows, interventions will likely be directed to earlier stages with the goals of repair and prevention. This chapter reviews the nonoperative treatments currently available for knee osteoarthritis.

Many treatment options are available for osteoarthritis of the knee, and the choice depends on the severity of symptoms. Although a radiographic diagnosis of osteoarthritis is relatively straightforward, similar findings are commonly seen in asymptomatic individuals. Therefore, radiographic changes alone do not warrant treatment. It is important to exclude other sources of knee pain such as hip and spinal abnormalities. The questions of whether the patient has osteoarthritis and whether the disease accounts for the patient's symptoms should be carefully considered before deciding on a course of therapy.

The differential diagnosis for joint pain covers the spectrum of rheumatologic, orthopedic, neurologic, and vascular diseases. It includes soft tissue disorders ranging from muscle and ligament strains to pes anserine bursitis or meniscal problems. Inflammatory arthropathies can mimic osteoarthritis and include crystal arthropathy (which has a predilection for the knees and other large joints) rheumatoid arthritis, and systemic lupus erythematosus. Spontaneous osteonecrosis of the knee typically presents in women older than 55 years. Secondary or idiopathic osteonecrosis may present in younger patients, especially those with certain risk factors (eg, corticosteroid or alcohol use). Other causes of knee pain include neurologic conditions (radiculopathy, peripheral neuropathy, spinal stenosis), vascular conditions (claudication, insufficiency), malignancy, and infection.

Knowledge of the natural history of osteoarthritis influences the aggressiveness of treatment. Although end-stage disease can be extremely painful and debilitating, osteoarthritis, in general, is not relentlessly progressive. In a recent longitudinal, population-based study of the progression of knee osteoarthritis, Murphy et al.[247] estimated that each year 6% of the population develop only knee symptoms, defined as pain, aching, and stiffness, and approximately 2% develop symptomatic knee osteoarthritis, defined as radiographic osteoarthritis and symptoms in the same knee. Although the incidence of radiographic and symptomatic knee osteoarthritis rises with increasing age, with the highest rates among those older than 75 years, only the incidence of radiographic osteoarthritis was found to be statistically different between age groups. This shows that, as patients age, radiographic changes associated with knee osteoarthritis may increase, but symptoms are not rapidly progressive. In a survey of 682 older adults, the prevalence and severity of symptoms of osteoarthritis about the knee remained constant through the seventh, eighth, and ninth decades of life.[102] In another study documenting radiographic progression in patients older than 54 years, the percentage of patients with the most severe changes did not increase with age.[193] However, in a recent cross-sectional study by Matsumoto et al.,[220] radiographic analysis of the knee suggested that aging is significantly associated with structural changes in the knee such as lateral curvature of the femoral diaphysis, decreasing condylar shaft angle, and widening condylar plateau angle. These changes may contribute to the initiation of knee osteoarthritis as patients age. In a study that followed symptomatic osteoarthritic defects over 2 years using magnetic resonance imaging, 81% of the defects increased, 15% remained unchanged, and 4% regressed.[67] Age and the area of bone affected were predictors of progression. Osteoarthritis is a chronic disease with a waxing and waning course. With proper management, many patients can maintain reasonable comfort and function.

The source of pain in osteoarthritis is not completely understood. Cartilage itself is avascular and aneural. Proposed causes of pain include muscle strain caused by overuse, microfractures in the subchondral trabeculae, irritation of periosteal nerve endings, ligamentous stress caused by bone deformity or effusion, and venous congestion caused by remodeling of subchondral bone.[212,233] Different mechanisms likely play a role in different patients. The variety of potential mechanisms underscores the need to define the sources and mediators of pain more thoroughly so that the most effective treatments can be selected.

Synovitis is a prime candidate for pain generation in osteoarthritis. Synovium is richly innervated.[174] Patients with early-stage osteoarthritis may show little evidence of synovial inflammation. However, in patients with more advanced disease, synovial inflammation is common and may be a major source of pain. Animal studies have suggested that the early, transient synovial inflammation observed in rats injected with monosodium iodoacetate (which causes chondrocyte death) may be the primary cause of initial pain in these animals, whereas later, more persistent pain has been correlated with changes in joint histology.[34,307] Recent studies show that increased concentrations of proinflammatory cytokines such as tumor necrosis factor (TNF)-α and interleukin (IL)-6 are correlated with higher pain scores, and that a diverse group of cytokines play a role in the pathogenesis of synovitis in osteoarthritic knees.[206,261] These cytokines, individually and in combination with different cell modulators, are responsible for tissue damage and repair. For example, TNF-α has been shown to be associated with pain generation, whereas IL-6 is correlated with joint function.[261] Inflammation in osteoarthritis may be induced by cartilage fragments[85] or proteoglycans[32] released by damaged cartilage. Synovitis leads to the release of inflammatory mediators, sensitizing nociceptive cells and damaging cartilage directly. If synovial inflammation is the predominant source of pain, corticosteroids and anti-inflammatory medications are rational therapies. However, inflammation in osteoarthritis is much less intense than in rheumatoid arthritis. In an arthroscopic study of patients with mild or moderate radiographic osteoarthritis of the knee, almost 50% of those examined had no appreciable synovitis. No relationships between severity, size, or location of lesion and synovitis were noted.[250]

Pain (P) fibers have been found in multiple locations in the knee. Immunohistochemistry stains identify substance-P fibers in structures that include the periosteum, subchondral bone, fat pad, and capsule.[91,367] Evidence also indicates there may be a decreased threshold to noxious stimuli in limbs affected by osteoarthritis.[260]

Our understanding of the pathophysiology of osteoarthritis is limited, and treatment options will improve as our knowledge grows. A clinical practice guideline for the nonarthroplasty treatment of osteoarthritis of the knee was published in 2013 by the American Academy of Orthopaedic Surgeons (AAOS).[3] This guideline was based on an extensive systematic review of the published literature. The Osteoarthritis Research Society International (OARSI) has published similar guidelines.[186,359]

PATIENT EDUCATION

The goals of patient education are to reduce anxiety and make patients aware of treatment and activity modifications so they can participate in their care proactively. Patient education and self-management programs have proven beneficial in reducing the pain[59] associated with knee arthritis. Regular contact with patients pertaining to their arthritis may be beneficial. A large randomized controlled trial (RCT) showed that telephone contact leads to improvements in pain and functional status and is cost-effective.[186,359]

A meta-analysis of studies contrasting patient education with ibuprofen therapy concluded that there is a significant reduction of pain, but not disability, with education.[329] There was some evidence for a synergistic effect of both interventions.

Education allows for a better understanding of activity modification. For example, activities that lead to excessive loading of the knee should be avoided when possible.[203] Loading activities are better performed in short periods; rest periods of 30 minutes between activities may help reduce pain and allow greater overall productivity. Several shorter periods of standing are preferable to a single prolonged period.

Education is important not only to manage symptoms, but also to engage patients in their disease and overall health. The provider caring for knee arthritis is in a unique position to discuss the implications of weight loss, smoking cessation, and general health. Surgical risk factor modification should be encouraged early in the encounter with these patients, so if nonoperative management fails there is time to optimize surgical outcomes.

PHYSICAL THERAPY, WEIGHT LOSS, AND OTHER MODALITIES

Physical Therapy

The proven benefits of physical therapy (PT) coupled with the absence of adverse effects argues for a prominent role of this modality in the treatment of early stages of osteoarthritis. The advantageous risk-benefit ratio is further amplified in older adults, a population at greater risk of adverse effects from pharmacologic or surgical intervention. It is important to note, however, that PT in cases of advanced osteoarthritis may not be justified and can delay further intervention. Fehring et al.[89] reported that PT may actually increase disease activity, rather than reduce pain in patients with advanced osteoarthritis. Therefore, PT may not be suitable for all patients; rather, risks and benefits should be assessed individually according to osteoarthritis severity. The rehabilitation goals in treating patients with osteoarthritis of the knee are to increase and maintain current function and to prevent further joint deterioration. PT uses multiple modalities to achieve these goals, including braces, orthoses, exercises, educational plans, and physical modalities (eg, temperature, electrical stimulation, ultrasound). In general, a PT program involves the use of heat, cold, or other modalities followed by an exercise program. This section provides a brief description of these modalities and reviews the literature regarding their efficacy and indications.

Exercise. Exercise programs have been devised with diverse goals, including increasing strength, endurance, and range of motion (ROM) in patients with knee arthritis. Much of the published and ongoing research is directed at the quadriceps mechanism.* Different types of exercise include passive exercises, in which the joint, and thus muscles, are moved by the therapist or a continuous passive motion machine without active input by the patient. Active or active-assisted exercises are performed by active contraction of muscles with assistance by the therapist. Resistive exercises are accomplished by active contraction of muscles by the patient against mechanical or manual resistance. Isometric, isotonic, and isokinetic contractions may all be used. Stretching exercises to increase joint motion and flexibility are frequently part of the regimen.

Range of motion and stretching exercises. ROM and stretching exercises are conservative management strategies that should be considered for all patients with osteoarthritis. Beneficial effects include maintenance of function, reduction of edema, stimulation of flexion-extension reflexes, and preparation of the limb for active exercise. Stretching exercises can restore or maintain ROM.[265,349] Care should be taken with inflamed joints, because passive ROM exercise has been shown to increase joint inflammation. In a study by Weng et al.,[360] 132

---

*References 73, 83, 84, 90, 94, 95, 96, 146, 156, 185, 214, 215, 234, 235, 243, 255, 283, 324, 333, and 339.

patients with bilateral knee osteoarthritis underwent an 8-week stretching exercise program. Patients were randomly divided into groups and performed isokinetic muscular strengthening exercises, bilateral knee static stretching, or proprioceptive neuromuscular facilitation stretching. At the end of the 8-week period, patients in all groups had statistically significant reductions in knee pain scores.

Strengthening exercises. In knee arthritis, loss of strength and function occurs rapidly. A muscle can atrophy up to 30% in 1 week. A muscle at complete rest will lose strength at a rate of 3% per day.[94,96,243] Despite a wealth of published literature, consensus regarding optimum amount, type, and frequency of exercise for strengthening the quadriceps is lacking. In a recent single-blind RCT, patients were assigned to a 12-week strengthening program for the hip or leg.[209] Both programs consisted of strengthening and flexibility exercises, which were performed on 3 to 5 days per week. Participation in the program led to statistically significant improvement in knee pain, function, and overall quality of life in patients with knee osteoarthritis. In one case study,[214] isometric strengthening of the quadriceps muscles led to improvements in quadriceps torque, clinical status, and pain after walking. This program consisted of exercises performed three times weekly for 6 weeks with the knee flexed to 60 degrees. Other studies have demonstrated improvement in function of quadriceps-trained individuals, but most of these studies failed to compare the results with those of patients who rested. Three RCTs[83,90,156] in patients with knee osteoarthritis who underwent quadriceps strengthening with isometric, isotonic, or resistive exercises showed significant improvements in quadriceps strength, knee pain, and function compared with controls. A recent systematic review and meta-analysis of eight RCTs focused on the efficacy of strengthening or aerobic exercise on pain relief in people with knee osteoarthritis.[330] Trials comparing the effects of exercise intervention with those of nonintervention or psychoeducational intervention were collected. The investigators concluded that muscle strengthening exercises, with or without weight-bearing and aerobic exercises, are effective for pain relief, with the greatest relief in patients who participated in non–weight-bearing strengthening exercises.

Although beneficial, strengthening exercises must be used with caution. Increased force across the joint with strengthening exercises may increase inflammation and pain. Isometric contraction is less likely to increase joint pain and inflammation. Dynamic (repetitive) exercises are appropriate using isotonic or isokinetic muscle contraction after pain is controlled. Isokinetic exercises can be used for patients with ligamentous stability and no internal derangement. Deep knee bends, however, may increase intra-articular pressure and should be avoided.[45] The AAOS clinical practice guidelines strongly recommend weight-bearing and non–weight-bearing exercises for the treatment of knee osteoarthritis and suggest that strength training can significantly improve physical function.[3]

Aerobic conditioning. In addition to weakness, patients with osteoarthritis often experience decreased cardiovascular endurance.[146] Aerobic exercise can increase the overall vitality, activity, and feeling of well-being in these patients. Suitable endurance exercises include cycling, swimming, and low-impact aerobics. The effects of high-impact loading activities such as jogging are uncertain in regard to osteoarthritis progression. Several studies have reported no significant association between recreational running and joint health.[44,184,267,334] However, a recent systematic review identified long-distance running at the elite level to be a significant risk factor for osteoarthritis progression.[75] Nevertheless, it remains difficult to isolate the effects of running on joint health because of numerous confounding variables. For example, it is known that habitual running can influence important risk factors associated with osteoarthritis such as body mass index, muscle strength, and joint injury. Joint injury secondary to running has been shown to be associated with an increased risk of osteoarthritis development.[334] A clear recommendation for or against running cannot be made. Increased aerobic fitness not only improves patients' overall health but specifically improves their arthritic symptoms. In 102 patients with knee osteoarthritis participating in an 8-week supervised fitness walking program, Kovar et al.[185] found improvements in 6-minute walking distance and reductions in pain and the use of medications in the exercise group compared with controls. In the recently published Intensive Diet and Exercise for Arthritis (IDEA) RCT, 454 overweight or obese adults (aged ≥55 years with body mass index values between 27 and 41) with pain and radiographic knee osteoarthritis were assigned to 18-month diet and exercise programs. Participants were randomized to one of three groups: diet-induced weight loss only, diet-induced weight loss plus exercise, or exercise-only (control). Knee joint compressive forces and plasma IL-6 levels were used as primary outcome measures for osteoarthritis progression. Among overweight and obese adults with knee osteoarthritis, participants in the diet and diet plus exercise groups had more weight loss and significant reductions in IL-6 levels and joint forces compared with patients in the exercise-only group.[230]

Roddy et al.[301] published a systematic review of 13 RCTs. They reported a significant treatment effect for aerobic conditioning and quadriceps strengthening in patients with osteoarthritis of the knee.

Weight Loss

Weight reduction should be encouraged in overweight patients. A 1-pound weight loss represents a 3- to 4-pound decrease in load across the knee joint. Studies have shown that weight loss in middle-aged and older women significantly reduces the incidence of symptomatic osteoarthritis in the knee.[29,228,229,287] OARSI guidelines published in 2014 suggest that achieving a loss of 5% of total body weight within a 20-week period is most effective for treatment of knee osteoarthritis.[263]

Therapy regimens are generally prescribed in a programmatic fashion rather than in isolation. The Arthritis, Diet, and Activity Promotion Trial (ADAPT) estimated the relative contribution of various modalities.[228] In this trial, 316 overweight patients with knee osteoarthritis were randomized into four groups: healthy lifestyle (education), diet only, exercise only, and diet plus exercise. At the end of the 18-month trial, the diet-plus-exercise group showed improvement in self-reported function, 6-minute walking distance, stair climb time, and knee pain. The exercise-only group showed improvement in walking distance. The diet-only group performed no better than the education group. Whether the benefits persist over the long term is unknown.[345]

Other Modalities

Yoga. Yoga has become increasingly popular. The practice of yoga in complementary medicine originates from traditional Indian philosophy and focuses on promoting healing by establishing a connection between the mind and body through exercise. Yoga consists of meditation, breathing exercises, and manipulation of poses, which theoretically alleviate the symptoms of osteoarthritis by stretching and strengthening the muscles around joints. A pilot study by Cheung et al.[51] assessed the feasibility and efficacy of a yoga program in older women (mean age, 72 years) with knee arthritis. Participants were randomly assigned to an 8-week yoga program or a wait-list control group. Participants in the treatment group exhibited significantly greater improvement in their Western Ontario and McMaster Universities Osteoarthritis Index (WOMAC) pain and stiffness scores and maintained a study retention rate of 95%. The authors concluded that a weekly yoga program is feasible and may provide a therapeutic benefit as a complementary approach to knee arthritis management. A more recent study by Moonaz et al. also suggested that a yoga routine consisting of two weekly classes and one at-home session per week for 8 weeks significantly improved pain, flexibility, general health, vitality, and mental health in sedentary individuals with osteoarthritis.[238] Furthermore, the AAOS clinical practice guidelines strongly recommend that patients with knee osteoarthritis participate in low-impact exercises and physical activity such as yoga.[3]

Biomechanical Treatment. The modalities described in this section are used in an attempt to change the biomechanical forces across the joint to decrease loading of the diseased areas.

Taping. Cushnaghan et al.[63] found that taping the patella medially reduced knee pain in patients with patellofemoral arthritis. In their randomized, single-blind, crossover trial with 14 subjects, medial taping was superior to lateral or neutral taping for pain, other symptoms, and patient preference. Cho et al.[52] investigated the short-term effects of Kinesio taping on various types of pain, active ROM, and proprioception in patients with knee osteoarthritis. Kinesio taping with proper tension to the quadriceps has been shown to attenuate pain and improve active ROM and proprioception in osteoarthritis patients. Although taping is not recommended as a sole therapy for knee osteoarthritis, studies have shown the usefulness of taping in providing immediate and short-term pain relief and improving knee function while the tape is worn.[6,62,136,356]

Knee bracing and orthotics. The usefulness of bracing for the treatment of knee osteoarthritis has been controversial.[105,176,306,324] Most clinical and biomechanical studies have shown little or no benefit from these devices. A recent Cochrane database systematic review of 13 RCTs focusing on the benefits and risks of braces and foot/ankle orthoses in the treatment of patients with osteoarthritis of the knee found little evidence supporting the utility of bracing for pain, stiffness, and function in the treatment of patients with medial compartment knee osteoarthritis.[77]

There are two goals of knee bracing: achieving mechanical stability and changing the biomechanical forces across the joint. In fitting a patient for a brace, it is important to define the abnormal motion and alignment that the brace should control.

A Swedish knee cage or a hinged knee brace may provide support by limiting extension and may help decrease pain.[306] There are a number of three-point pressure braces to control medial or lateral instability.[324] In some patients, these devices can be effective. Kirkley et al.[176] found that valgus-producing functional knee braces were much more effective for the treatment of medial compartment osteoarthritis of the knee than a simple neoprene sleeve. Furthermore, quality-of-life (WOMAC)

scores of both braced groups exceeded those of a control group receiving standard medical treatment in a prospective, parallel group RCT. The use of unloader braces has also been shown to provide short-term pain relief and improved function[11,36,366]; however, a study of patient compliance found that only 28% of patients regularly wore their unloader braces (twice per week, 1 hour at a time) and reported lack of symptom relief, brace discomfort, poor fit, and skin irritation as reasons for discontinuing brace wear.[327] Subsequently, most patients opt for total knee replacement on the symptomatic knee.[366] Because of a lack of appropriate studies and limited data, the AAOS clinical practice guidelines are inconclusive regarding the use of a valgus directing force brace for medial compartment unloading.[3]

Assistive devices: cane or walker. The cane can successfully unload the knee joint and provide symptomatic relief.[237,320] Assistive devices to unload the knee joint are most effectively used on the opposite side; a single crutch or cane will reduce the joint load by approximately 50%. A quadruped cane can be used instead of a straight cane when balance is a problem. A study in which 64 patients were assigned to no cane use or cane use every day for 2 months showed that cane use can improve knee pain and function in patients with osteoarthritis.[161] Although patient energy expenditure increases within the first month while the patient adapts to cane use, this returns to baseline levels within the second month.

Hydrotherapy. The buoyancy of water is useful to minimize stress on the knee joint by effectively neutralizing the force of gravity. This is especially useful when ROM and strengthening exercises are prescribed for obese patients. The external application of water for therapeutic purposes can provide heat or cold. Many physiologic effects have been reported in patients treated with warm-water hydrotherapy. These include a rise in body temperature, increased sweating, superficial vasodilation, increased peripheral circulation, decreased blood pressure after immersion, sedative effect on nerve endings, and muscle relaxation. The water temperature should be between 34°C and 37°C.[240] Contraindications to hydrotherapy include skin infections or lesions, open wounds, and cardiovascular disorders.

Water-based exercises have been shown to be an effective alternative for the management of osteoarthritis of the knee.[100,109,317] A systematic review of 26 RCTs focusing on the effectiveness of aquatic exercise in the management of musculoskeletal conditions found that aquatic exercise had moderate beneficial effects on pain, physical function, and quality of life in adults with osteoarthritis. These benefits appear to be similar to those achieved via land-based exercise.[20] The AAOS clinical practice guidelines include hydrotherapy as a subset of low-impact aerobic exercises that are strongly recommended for patients with symptomatic knee osteoarthritis.[3]

Electrical and Related Energy Treatments

Heat modalities. Therapeutic heat can be applied superficially or to a deep location, usually at temperatures of 41°C to 45°C. Superficial heat can elevate soft tissue temperatures by 3°C at a depth of 1 cm, thus penetrating the knee joint.[152] Some studies have demonstrated that the threshold for pain can be raised in humans and animals by applying superficial or deep heat.[199] The effect is produced by muscle relaxation and analgesia of free nerve endings (peripheral nerves and gamma fibers of muscle spindles).[200] Local heat may also relieve pain by acting on sensory afferents and closing the "pain gate" or increasing local blood flow and thus washing out pain-inducing metabolites and inflammatory mediators produced in osteoarthritis. All heat treatment modalities should be used as adjuncts or precursors to other treatment regimens such as exercise, mobilization, or stretching. They should be used cautiously because heat may increase inflammation and joint damage. Use of heat therapy in patients with inadequate thermal sensation is contraindicated.

The five general methods that produce superficial heat are diathermy (shortwave) microwaves, ultrasound, radiation (infrared), conduction (heating pad, water bottle), and convection (sauna, steam room).[69,79,259,288] Moist heat produces a greater temperature elevation than dry heat and may be preferable for clinical applications.[152] For all of these modalities, care must be taken to avoid burns, especially with uneven application. A towel-wrapped hot water bottle, gel-filled hot pack, or thermostatically controlled electric heating pad provides a simple method for superficial heat application.

Diathermy. Deep heat affects the viscoelastic properties of collagen.[346] Diathermy can use shortwave (11.062-m wavelength, 27.12-MHz frequency) radiation delivered via two electrodes or an induction cable for approximately 20 minutes.[288] This treatment leads to an increase in skin temperature, blood flow, and pain threshold. The effects are maintained for 15 to 30 minutes after cessation of treatment.

Diathermy has produced clinical benefit when used in combination with exercise but should not be used indiscriminately.[288] Shortwave diathermy can exacerbate knee arthritis because of the heat-induced proliferation of collagenous tissue, leading to the development of adhesions and thus a decreased ROM. Microwave electromagnetic radiation (12.2 cm at 2456-, 915-, and 433.9-MHz frequencies) is used less frequently, probably because of safety concerns.[69] However, local microwave diathermy has also been shown to have significant short-term benefits. Rabini et al.[294] showed that diathermy (three times a week for 4 weeks) significantly improved knee pain and function in patients with moderate knee osteoarthritis, with benefits lasting at least 12 months after treatment.

Ultrasound. Ultrasound is a well-established deep-heating modality that can penetrate more deeply than shortwave or microwave diathermy.[189,333] Several early studies showed the efficacy of ultrasound in relieving osteoarthritic pain.[79,199,332] Its effects are attributed to thermal and mechanical mechanisms. Ultrasound is absorbed by and creates heat in structures with high protein content. The physiologic effects of local tissue heating, as described earlier, include an increase in pain threshold, reduction of muscle spasms, and promotion of the healing process. The nonthermal or mechanical effects include microstreaming, or small fluid movements around cells that alter cell membrane permeability, promote collagen synthesis, and alter electrical activity in painful nerve afferents.

Ultrasound therapy requires the use of a coupling agent (water or mineral oil) to prevent attenuation of the sound waves in air. Energy exposures of 0.5 to 4.0 W/cm² for 5 to 10 minutes are commonly used. The therapist must keep the ultrasound applicator in constant motion to decrease excessive focal heating.

A pilot study focusing on low-intensity therapeutic ultrasound (LITUS) showed benefits in regard to osteoarthritis relief. This form of ultrasound is novel in that it can be applied for a longer duration without causing pain or thermal damage. This research was conducted using a battery-powered, wearable LITUS device. A retrospective analysis showed a statistically significant 52% reduction in pain, which is similar to pain reductions in patients using ultrasound therapy for chronic muscle and shoulder pain.[189] Ultrasound may be a useful adjunct to other modes of treatment but should not be a mainstay of therapy.

Interferential Therapy. Interferential therapy uses two medium-frequency (approximately 4 KHz) alternating currents applied to the skin through suction cups or adhesive padding. The resultant current has a low frequency that is the difference between the two original frequencies applied. This current is typically applied to the knee for approximately 15 minutes and is experienced by the patient as a prickling sensation. Various pain-relieving mechanisms that block unmyelinated nociceptive fibers and activate A-delta and C-fibers, releasing enkephalins and endorphins, or that activate the opioid system, have been proposed.[288] The AAOS clinical practice guidelines are inconclusive regarding the use of interferential therapy or other electrotherapeutic modalities for the treatment of knee osteoarthritis.[3]

Transcutaneous Electrical Nerve Stimulation. Transcutaneous electrical nerve stimulation (TENS) delivers short-pulse-width (50- to 250-μs), low-frequency waves (2- to 150-Hz) that are used specifically for pain relief.[157] As with interferometry, a prickling sensation is produced. Carbon-rubber electrodes with a coupling gel on the skin or with self-adhesive electrodes are used to deliver pulses for 30 to 60 minutes once or twice daily. The finding that large-diameter, cutaneous nerve fibers are preferentially stimulated by TENS is thought to account for its efficacy. These fibers inhibit the transmission of painful stimuli to the spinal cord. A recent systematic review and meta-analysis of 18 RCTs by Chen et al.[49] found that TENS significantly decreased pain compared with controls, but there was no statistical difference in WOMAC scores. However, Cherian et al.[50] showed that the use of TENS for 3 months led to significant reduction in pain as determined by visual analog scale (VAS) scores, as well as improved knee function and quality of life. The AAOS clinical practice guidelines are inconclusive regarding TENS because of few published studies and conflicting data.[3]

Acupuncture. Interest in traditional Chinese medicine in general, and acupuncture specifically, has been increasing. Information from the National Health Interview Survey[21] showed that approximately 3 million patients receive acupuncture treatments in the United States annually, many of them for musculoskeletal ailments. The technique has been applied to many conditions, including postoperative pain, arthritis, obesity, and nicotine addiction.

Although interest in acupuncture is strong, scientific evidence of its efficacy is lacking. Studies involving acupuncture frequently have major methodologic deficiencies such as lack of placebo control and lack of blinding. Most studies also report small sample sizes.

Ezzo et al.[86] systematically reviewed acupuncture studies specific to osteoarthritis of the knee. In the seven studies identified, there was limited evidence that acupuncture is more effective in improving pain and function than standard treatment. They found that several studies reported significant improvements in pain scores, an effect that lasted more than 1 month after cessation of treatment. This improvement was not seen in two of three studies in which sham acupuncture was used. In a recent RCT of 282 patients aged 50 years or older, Hinman et al.[144] found that neither laser nor needle acupuncture conferred benefit over sham acupuncture for pain or function.

An AAOS working group performed a meta-analysis of nine RCTs on the effectiveness of acupuncture for the treatment of osteoarthritis.[3] They found that the treatment effect on pain and function was much smaller in studies in which patients were blinded and the blinding was confirmed. Furthermore, the most recent AAOS clinical practice guidelines strongly recommend against use of acupuncture, citing studies that show no statistical significance in pain relief in patients with knee osteoarthritis.[3]

Cryotherapy. Cold can be used to decrease pain. Joints are cooled by the application of ice packs or commercial gel hydropacks.[259] The pack should be applied for 15 to 20 minutes and should be separated from the skin by a towel to prevent freezing of the skin. Decreasing skin and muscle temperature may reduce muscle spasms by reducing muscle spindle activity and raising the pain threshold. Cryotherapy may also provide functional improvements with an increase in passive ROM and a decrease in joint stiffness.[197] Cold therapy is contraindicated in patients with Raynaud's disease and should be used cautiously in patients with cold hypersensitivity and peripheral vascular disease.

PHARMACOLOGIC MEASURES

Analgesics

Acetaminophen. Acetaminophen is one of the most commonly used over-the-counter medications for knee osteoarthritis[249] and is the only non-narcotic analgesic available in the United States. Alternately classified as a peripheral or central analgesic, its mode of action is poorly understood. Acetaminophen readily penetrates the central nervous system, and its analgesic action may be mediated through the diffuse noxious inhibitory control pathway.[335]

The efficacy of acetaminophen is debated. A 2006 Cochrane review of 15 RCTs concluded that nonsteroidal anti-inflammatory drugs (NSAIDs) were superior to acetaminophen but that acetaminophen was superior to placebo.[337] In contrast, the AAOS downgraded its recommendation on acetaminophen from moderate in 2008 to inconclusive in 2013.[4] Their systematic review identified only one study that tested it against placebo,[231] finding no statistical difference compared with placebo when using a maximum of 4000 mg of acetaminophen per day. Dosage should be lower in patients with renal or hepatic impairment.[278,309] Machado et al.[211] recently reviewed 13 RCTs to determine the efficacy and safety of acetaminophen in the treatment of hip and knee osteoarthritis. They determined that acetaminophen provides significant, but not clinically important, pain relief in the short term in patients with knee osteoarthritis. Furthermore, they found that patients who chronically take this medication are four times as likely to have abnormal liver function tests. Ultimately, they concluded that acetaminophen is ineffective at providing clinically important pain relief in patients with knee osteoarthritis, and its use should therefore be reconsidered.

Previously, acetaminophen had been viewed as a safe, short-term medication to treat knee osteoarthritis. A 2010 systematic review and a 2012 safety review raised concerns about liver toxicity and suggested that this medication should be used more conservatively in dosing and duration.[60,148] Additionally, a population-based cohort study of 958,397 people from the United Kingdom reported a relative risk of 3.6 for upper gastrointestinal (GI) complications from acetaminophen at doses higher than 2 g/day.[116] The relative risks of these complications were 2.4 and 4.9 for low-to-medium and high doses of NSAIDs, respectively. Other studies have shown that patients taking higher doses of acetaminophen are at increased risk for GI events, including hospitalizations, ulcers, and dyspepsia, compared with those taking lower doses.[295] In patients with early renal failure, acetaminophen has been associated with further decline.[101] This drug has also been associated with an increase in hypertension in both men and women.[103,104] Because of inconclusive data and minimal evidence of pain relief compared with placebo, we no longer recommend acetaminophen as a first-line treatment for symptomatic knee osteoarthritis. It may be indicated if patients are seeking conservative management and cannot tolerate NSAIDs because of GI effects.

Opioids. For patients who have failed nonpharmacologic and conservative pharmacologic therapies and are not candidates for arthroplasty, tramadol and opioids may offer pain relief.

Opioids were found to have a small to moderate benefit compared with placebo in a 2009 Cochrane review, but these benefits were outweighed by large increases in the risk of adverse events.[256] Therefore, it was recommended that they not be used, even if osteoarthritic pain is severe. However, the American College of Rheumatology recommends the use of opioid analgesics and conditionally recommends the use of duloxetine.[145] The American Pain Society and the American Academy of Pain Medicine have recommended the use of opioid analgesics for chronic noncancer pain.[54] These recommendations provide structured guidance on opioid treatment options, dosing information, indications and contraindications for opioid therapy, and management of opioid-related adverse effects. Referral of patients who have failed nonoperative approaches and are not candidates for surgery to physicians familiar with opioid management can be considered.

Tramadol, a synthetic opioid with a dual mechanism of action, has been of interest for the treatment of osteoarthritis because it does not produce the GI bleeding or renal injury associated with NSAIDs. It activates opiate receptors and descending inhibitory pain systems and inhibits the reuptake of serotonin and norepinephrine.[125,202] When tramadol is taken as an immediate-release oral formulation, the pain relief usually occurs within 1 hour.[169] However, similar to opioids, its benefits appear to be small in relation to pain reduction, with a number of adverse events that cause patients to stop taking the medication.[92] Although various medications are available to reduce pain related to knee osteoarthritis, their safety profiles should be considered when initiating treatment, and they should not be viewed as sustainable, long-term treatment. Two high-strength and three moderate-strength studies with 8- to 13-week follow-up periods compared tramadol with placebo. Ten of 14 outcomes were statistically better in the treatment group. A novel once-daily, long-acting formulation of tramadol, called tramadol contramid, has also been suggested to provide sustained analgesia with a favorable safety profile. Fishman et al.[97] reported significantly better pain control, as measured by the WOMAC pain scale, using tramadol contramid doses of 200 mg and 300 mg compared with a lower dose of 100 mg. Beaulieu et al.[24] found similar treatment effects of long-acting tramadol compared with diclofenac measured by WOMAC pain, stiffness, and function subscales. The researchers suggest that sustained-released tramadol is effective in relieving pain and may have fewer adverse effects than NSAIDs. Given the risks and potential for dependence, however, we rarely prescribe opioids and tramadol in our practice. The AAOS clinical practice guidelines are inconclusive about the use of opioids for the treatment of knee osteoarthritis.[3]

Nonsteroidal Anti-Inflammatory Drugs

The AAOS strongly recommends NSAIDs for symptomatic osteoarthritis on the basis of a review of 19 studies with 202 favorable outcomes comparing selective, nonselective, or topical analgesics with placebo.[4]

NSAIDs bind to the cyclooxygenase (COX) enzyme, blocking the conversion of arachidonic acid to prostaglandins. This is most likely the main mechanism for their anti-inflammatory and analgesic effects.[22] The COX-1 isoform of the enzyme is expressed in many normal tissues. Prostaglandins produced by COX-1 play a role in normal tissue hemostasis such as mucosal defense and repair in the GI system, as well as renal perfusion.[216,311] COX-1 is also found in platelets and plays a role in platelet aggregation.[155,216] The COX-2 isoform, although found in normal tissue, is also an inducible enzyme and appears in areas of inflammation and injury.[165]

Traditional NSAIDs were nonselective in that they bound to and inhibited the COX-1 and COX-2 isoforms. Isolated COX-2 inhibitors, commonly called coxibs, were developed to avoid the adverse effects associated with nonspecific COX inhibition.

Nonselective Nonsteroidal Anti-Inflammatory Drugs.
Inhibition of prostaglandin synthesis has detrimental effects. Prostacyclin (PGI_2) and prostaglandin E2 (PGE_2) are vasodilators that are important in maintaining renal perfusion during hypovolemia. Prostaglandin inhibition leads to sodium retention in the kidneys, which may worsen congestive heart failure. A number of medical conditions depend on renal prostaglandins to maintain renal profusion, including congestive heart failure, cirrhosis, certain forms of hypertension, and dehydration. In patients with such conditions, exposure to NSAIDs leads to a decline in renal function, even if creatinine clearance was normal before treatment.[58,248] This decline is usually reversible; however, NSAIDs may increase the overall risk of chronic renal failure.[278] Acute interstitial nephritis has also been noted with most NSAIDs but is seen most commonly with fenoprofen.[39,213] Sulindac[361,362] and nabumatone[12] are purported to be less likely to cause deterioration in renal function.[41] Oral NSAIDs should not be used in patients with chronic kidney disease stage IV or V (estimated glomerular filtration rate, <30 mL/min). In patients with chronic kidney disease stage III (estimated glomerular filtration rate, 30–59 mL/min), the decision should be made on an individual basis.[145]

Although NSAIDs are a short-term treatment option, their adverse effects make them a poor long-term treatment. A comparative effectiveness review in 2011 indicated that NSAIDs are associated with increased risk of serious GI, cardiovascular, and renal injury compared with placebo.[55] It has been estimated that 15% to 35% of all peptic ulcer complications are attributable to these drugs.[131,132,134,140,190]

NSAID plus aspirin use is responsible for approximately 15 deaths per 100,000 users, with approximately one-third of

deaths likely attributable to low-dose aspirin use.[188] Upper GI symptoms caused by NSAIDs include dyspepsia, ulceration, hemorrhage, and GI perforation.[113,118,322] There is an estimated three- to fivefold higher relative risk of GI bleeding from the use of NSAIDs.[139] Risk factors for developing a bleeding complication with the use of these medications include a history of peptic ulcer disease, concomitant use of corticosteroids or anticoagulants, and poor general health.[111,117,316,319] Toxicity from NSAIDs is additive, so the use of more than one NSAID at a time is contraindicated.[43,232] The concomitant use of NSAIDs in patients who are also taking systemic corticosteroids should be avoided, if possible, because the risk of bleeding complications and death is significantly elevated.

In patients aged 75 years or older, topical NSAIDS can be considered a safe and well-tolerated treatment, although they are associated with a higher risk of adverse dermatologic effects.[92] If the patient has a history of a symptomatic or complicated upper GI ulcer but has not experienced upper GI bleeding in the past year and is not at high risk of cardiac disease, a COX-2 selective inhibitor can be considered.[326]

If the patient is taking low-dose aspirin (≤325 mg/day) for cardioprotection, a non-selective NSAID other than ibuprofen should be used in combination with a proton-pump inhibitor[191] because of a recognized pharmacodynamic interaction between ibuprofen and low-dose aspirin that decreases aspirin's effectiveness.[239] Diclofenac and celecoxib have not demonstrated this effect.[239]

Selective Cyclooxygenase-2 Inhibition.
COX-2 inhibitors are associated with a lower risk of adverse GI events and complications.[68,80,311] Two large, prospective, randomized outcome studies were performed for celecoxib and rofecoxib.[31,318] Celecoxib was compared with diclofenac and ibuprofen, and rofecoxib was compared with naproxen. The risk of symptomatic ulcers or ulcer complications was lower with the selective COX-2 inhibitors. A 2011 comparative effectiveness review also found that celecoxib was associated with a lower risk of ulcer complications compared with nonselective NSAIDs but was associated with a moderately higher risk of cardiovascular complications, highlighting the need to use the lowest required dose of NSAIDs to achieve pain relief and to avoiding prolonged use.[92]

The selectivity of COX-2 inhibitors, although beneficial to the GI mucosa, may lead to problems with thrombosis, as well as salt and fluid imbalance.[368] The incidence of acute myocardial infarction was significantly higher for patients taking rofecoxib than for those taking naproxen in this study, and the former medication has been removed from the market. Recent evidence suggests that coxibs increase the risk of ischemic cardiovascular disease, heart failure, hypertension, and cardiac arrhythmia in patients with high-risk cardiac profiles.[164,173,338] Two large chemoprevention trials for adenomatous polyps, one with celecoxib and one with rofecoxib, were discontinued after demonstrating increased cardiovascular risk.[227,341] Although coxib use is associated with cardiovascular risk, several studies have shown that the risk appears to be dose-dependent, with moderate, low-dose use in healthy patients conferring no substantial risk.[7,46,338] It is recommended that coxibs be avoided when possible in patients with elevated risk of cardiovascular disease. Patients should be started on a nonselective NSAID. For patients with GI issues, coxibs can be used, but for the shortest possible duration and at the lowest effective dose. In patients with substantial cardiovascular risks, naproxen with GI protection can be used. There are insufficient data to recommend one agent over another.

The exact mechanism for increased cardiac risk associated with COX-2 inhibition has not been elucidated. In addition to vasoconstriction, other factors may exist. COX-2 enzyme expression is found in endothelial cells in response to injury.[165] It is also found in atheromatous plaques and may play a role in decreasing vascular inflammation.[314] There is no COX-2 expression on platelets, and unlike their nonselective counterparts, they do not block formation of thromboxane, which plays an important role in platelet aggregation and vasoconstriction. Fitzgerald[98] reported that rofecoxib and celecoxib suppress the formation of PGI_2, which may be the primary mechanism by which coxibs elevate blood pressure and accelerate atherogenesis, predisposing patients to an exaggerated thrombotic response. This may explain the apparent increased cardiovascular risk of coxibs over traditional NSAIDs. However, a recent trial of anti-inflammatory drugs in patients with Alzheimer disease indicated that naproxen, 220 mg, was associated with an increased cardiovascular risk that was higher than that associated with celecoxib, 200 mg, in older patients.[2] In a report of population-based National Health Insurance data from Taiwan, four NSAIDs were examined.[153] There were no differences in the risk of serious long-term events in those treated with etodolac, ibuprofen, naproxen, nambutone, or celecoxib for a 180-day period. In this study, a previous history of cardiovascular disease was the greatest predictor of risk.

Hypertensive effects of coxibs seem equal to those of nonselective NSAIDs. It appears that the COX-2 enzyme is responsible for prostaglandin production, which is important for fluid balance. Blocking its production affects fluid retention, which can result in hypertension.[165] The COX-2 enzyme is also responsible for the production of PGI_2, which is a vasodilator.[99] A number of products of the COX-1 enzyme have vasoconstrictive effects. Therefore, the selective inhibition of COX-2 favors vasoconstriction, which plays a role in hypertension and heart disease.

Possible Chondroprotective Action of Nonsteroidal Anti-Inflammatory Drugs.

The traditional view that osteoarthritis is an inevitably progressive disease resulting from wear and tear of the cartilage has been replaced by an understanding of the biochemical and biomechanical factors that contribute to the disease and its progression. Because cartilage is continuously undergoing degradation and renewal, an ideal medication would promote anabolic activity of cartilage and inhibit its degradation. The evidence for these beneficial activities of NSAIDs is mixed.[143]

A chondroprotective effect of NSAIDs has been postulated.[74] Proposed mechanisms include improved biomechanics as a result of decreasing arthralgia and inhibiting cartilage catabolism. Cartilage matrix proteoglycans are degraded by enzymes such as metalloproteases and serine proteases. Some NSAIDs are effective inhibitors of these enzymes.[37,119,201] Release of oxygen free radicals and other inflammatory mediators may also be suppressed by NSAIDs.[142,274,276] Other NSAIDs may actually stimulate glycosaminoglycan production, as indicated by increased sulfate incorporation.

The net effect of NSAIDs on cartilage remains to be determined and may vary among NSAIDs.[266] The effects of COX-2 inhibitors on articular cartilage have not been extensively studied. The effects of celecoxib and diclofenac on human chondrocyte metabolism were compared in an in vitro model.[82] Celecoxib increased the synthesis of hyaluronan and proteoglycans in explanted cells, whereas diclofenac had no such effect.

Other studies[217,218] have also demonstrated a potential chondroprotective effect of COX-2 inhibitors in vitro. Human articular cartilage cells exposed to celecoxib in culture have demonstrated increased proteoglycan synthesis and decreased proteoglycan release.[217]

Recommendations. If nonpharmacologic measures fail, nonselective NSAIDs may be tried as a first-line measure, with an understanding of the potential GI complications associated with their use. A low dose (≤1200 mg/day) of ibuprofen often provides effective pain relief. If ibuprofen is not effective at an analgesic dose, anti-inflammatory doses of ibuprofen or other nonselective NSAIDs may be tried. As a first-line pharmacologic treatment, the AAOS clinical practice guidelines recommend NSAIDs.[3]

In patients with GI risk, acetaminophen or COX-2 inhibitors may be used.[3,373] All NSAIDs should be used cautiously in older adults and in patients with hypertension or history of cardiac or renal disease. Scheiman and Fendrick[312] have provided an algorithm to help determine the appropriate NSAID on the basis of GI and cardiovascular risk (Table 120.1).

Once relief is achieved with NSAIDs, periodic withdrawal of therapy with substitution of a simple analgesic is prudent, especially in older adults. NSAIDs should be avoided in high-risk patients such as those with a history of ulcer disease, GI bleeding, congestive heart failure, or renal insufficiency and those taking concurrent oral corticosteroids. Nonacetylated salicylates, salsalate, choline magnesium trisalicylate, or renal-sparing NSAIDs such as sulindac may have a role in the treatment of these patients.

Other Medications

Injectable Corticosteroids. Injectable corticosteroids were introduced by Hollander et al.[151] in the 1950s. Despite their long

---

TABLE 120.1   Clinician's Guide to Anti-Inflammatory Therapy

Cardiovascular Risk	NSAID GASTROINTESTINAL RISK	
	None or Low	**Risk Present**
None (without aspirin)	Nonselective NSAID (cost consideration)	COX-2 selective or nonselective inhibitor; NSAID + PPI; COX-2 selective inhibitor + PPI for those with prior GI bleeding
Cardiovascular risk (with aspirin)	Naproxen; addition of PPI if GI risk of aspirin-NSAID combination warrants gastroprotection	PPI irrespective of NSAID; naproxen if cardiovascular risk outweighs GI risk; COX-2 selective inhibitor + PPI for those with previous GI bleeding

COX, Cyclooxygenase; GI, gastrointestinal; NSAID, non-steroidal anti-inflammatory drug; PPI, proton pump inhibitor. (Adapted from Scheiman JM, Fendrick AM: Summing the risk of NSAID therapy. Lancet 369:1580–1581, 2007.)

history and widespread use, there is little research to guide the physician about the optimal corticosteroid preparation, appropriate frequency of dosage, and length of treatment. In addition, there are few well-controlled studies documenting their efficacy. Concern also persists about the possible deleterious effects of these medications on cartilage. The 2013 AAOS clinical practice guidelines are inconclusive for the use of intra-articular corticosteroids.

Corticosteroids inhibit phospholipase A2 expression, which blocks the COX and lipoxygenase pathways.[87] This is likely their main mechanism of action, although they also affect ribonucleic acid protein synthesis and cellular metabolism.[23]

Various injectable corticosteroids are available. Their duration of action appears to be related to the solubility of the compound.[23] Hydrocortisone acetate is absorbed rapidly from the knee (half-life, 1-2 hours) and provides only a few days of relief; triamcinolone hexacetonide is the longest acting, with a half-life of several weeks.[70]

Systemic absorption of these compounds from the joint can occur. Suppression of the hypothalamic-pituitary axis is possible if multiple joints are injected or if injections are given at close intervals.[264] Decreased serum cortisol levels have been noted from even a single intra-articular injection.[195] Suppression of the hypothalamic-pituitary axis does not persist for more than 2 days, and adrenocorticosteroid secretion returns to normal in 3 to 6 days.[179] Systemic absorption is rarely a clinical problem.

Hollander[149] reported on 231 patients who received corticosteroid injections over a period of 20 years in 1953. Of those patients, 87% reported complete pain relief. Since that time, a systematic review[141] found only six level-I trials in five reports (279 total knees)[72,110,114,159,296] comparing intra-articular corticosteroid injections with placebo. A 2015 Cochrane review identified 27 trials (1767 total knees) comparing intra-articular corticosteroid against sham injection and no treatment.[163] The results of these reviews demonstrated a short-term benefit of intra-articular corticosteroid injections versus placebo. At 1 week, all studies reported an approximate one-third decrease in pain as measured by the VAS, which was statistically significant. Functional improvement was also noted in the corticosteroid group. Between 2 and 3 weeks, there was inconsistent evidence for pain reduction. At 4 to 24 weeks, no statistically significant difference in pain or functional status was noted in any of the analyzed studies. Both reviews concluded that intra-articular corticosteroid injections were associated with clinically important improvement in pain 1 week after injection but with little evidence for longer-term benefit. Triamcinolone was used in most trials, and methylprednisolone and betamethasone were also used. Data were inconclusive with regard to the efficacy of one form of corticosteroid over any other.

Recognized complications from corticosteroid injections include intra-articular infection and inflammatory flair.[129,130] Intra-articular infection is extremely rare, even when rigorous aseptic technique is not used. The incidence is estimated at 0.005% to 0.01%.[313] Postinjection flair is far more common, with an incidence of 2% to 5%. Inflammation occurs within hours of injection. It is a neutrophil-dependent inflammatory response, most likely caused by the corticosteroid crystals themselves.[225] It is almost always self-limiting and resolves within 1 to 3 days.

Dark-skinned individuals may have local discoloration of the skin from subcutaneous injection, which may be permanent.[253] This cosmetic discoloration is not serious but can lead to dissatisfaction on the part of the patient and therefore should be a part of informed consent. Temporary disturbances may include an elevated blood sugar level, arterial hypertension, and facial flushing.[160,269] Diabetic patients should be cautioned about potential elevations in glucose levels to heighten their vigilance after injection.

There are also concerns about increased risk of periprosthetic infection in patients receiving intra-articular corticosteroid injections before total knee arthroplasty.[268] However, a meta-analysis of eight studies found that preoperative steroid injections have no significant effect on rates of deep or superficial infections after subsequent total joint arthroplasty.[47] Another meta-analysis and review of 12 studies with 2068 participants found no evidence of a link between injection and deep joint infection.[226]

Effects on cartilage. The evidence for the effects of injected corticosteroids on cartilage metabolism is mixed. Corticosteroids are potent inhibitors of anabolic and catabolic processes in cartilage. Weekly injections into rabbit joints have produced histologic and macroscopic evidence of cartilage degeneration and depressed synthesis of collagen and proteoglycan.[25,242] Weight-bearing joints were more strongly affected. Conversely, injection of corticosteroid provided significant protection from cartilage breakdown in secondary arthritis in rabbits.[37a] Similar protective effects have been noted in primates and dogs.[126,273,275,365] An in vitro study of human chondrocytes demonstrated that dexamethasone administration decreases proteoglycan concentration.[328] Whether inhibition of anabolic or catabolic functions predominates in humans is unknown.

Anecdotal reports linking intra-articular corticosteroid therapy with accelerated joint destruction have not been substantiated by clinical experience or historical data. Even in those uncontrolled studies, this was a rare occurrence.[129,172,370] Historical data covering more than 330,000 injections have put the incidence of this complication at less than 1%, which is well within the realm of coincidence.[17] Nevertheless, given the possibility of a deleterious effect on the joint, many physicians are reluctant to inject a joint more frequently than every 4 to 6 weeks. Our current practice is, at most, every 3 months.

Theoretically, pain masking may lead to overuse and subsequent accelerated breakdown. Therefore, some recommend a period of joint rest after corticosteroid injection.[150,223,252] In patients with rheumatoid arthritis, those who had a period of rest after triamcinolone hexacetonide injection experienced a longer period of relief than ambulatory patients. In an animal study, articular cartilage damage produced by corticosteroids in meniscectomized rabbits seemed to be potentiated by exercise.[242]

In summary, intra-articular corticosteroid therapy is appropriate as a "stopgap" measure for acute pain in osteoarthritis. It should be considered a long-term treatment only for patients in whom other regimens have failed and surgical treatment is not indicated. It appears prudent for patients to rest for a time immediately after injection.

Chondroprotective Agents

Attention has focused on the development of agents or interventions that could actually slow or reverse the progression of disease. Such agents are called chondroprotective agents, or disease-modifying osteoarthritis drugs. Although no agreed-upon definition exits, Ghosh and Brooks[123] proposed that a chondroprotective agent should enhance chondrocyte and hyaluronan synthesis, inhibit cartilage degradation, and reduce joint pain and inflammation. With these guidelines in mind, we will examine the scientific evidence for several agents.

Hyaluronic Acid. Hyaluronic acid (HA), also referred to as hyaluronate or hyaluronan, is a key constituent of cartilage ground substance and synovial fluid. It is composed of continuously repeating sequences of glucuronic acid and N-acetylglucosamine. Type-B synovial cells synthesize and secrete HA into the joint space. It has several important roles in the viscous and elastic properties of synovial fluid. The precise mechanism of action remains elusive. HA is believed to provide joint lubrication and shock absorbancy,[277] promote chondrocyte proliferation and differentiation,[171] stabilize proteoglycan structure,[154,325] and down-regulate the expression of proinflammatory cytokines such as IL-8 and TNF-α.[355]

Early osteoarthritis is characterized by loss and degradation of HA from cartilage and synthesis of lower-molecular-weight HA by synoviocytes.[358] As a pharmacologic agent, HA has been shown to have anti-inflammatory, antinociceptive, and cartilage anabolic effects.[120,121] Thus, the purpose of HA injection in patients with mild to moderate osteoarthritis is not only to act as an analgesic but also to increase the viscosity of synovial fluid and promote endogenous HA production.[15]

Intra-articular HA has been used in veterinary practice for at least 30 years. Beneficial effects have been noted in several species, including horses and dogs.[14,38,115,305] Experience in human subjects began in 1974, when Peyron and Balazs[280] reported a beneficial effect of intra-articular HA in a double-blind, placebo-controlled study of 28 patients. Since that time, many clinical studies, including some prospective RCTs, have lent credence to the assertion that injected HA has a beneficial effect in osteoarthritis. Despite this lengthy and sustained clinical and laboratory interest in HA as a possible treatment for osteoarthritis, its use and efficacy remain controversial.[64,65,66,121,177] The 2013 AAOS guidelines[4] for nonoperative treatment of osteoarthritis of the knee strongly recommend against the use of intra-articular HA, citing lack of efficacy, not potential harm.

In a pilot study of 40 patients treated with 20 mg of HA interarticularly once weekly for 5 weeks, Frizziero et al.[112] found that 30% of patients had morphologic improvement in cartilage and synovial membranes compared with baseline. Improvements included reconstitution of the superficial amorphous layer, improvements in chondrocyte density and vitality, and reduction in synovial inflammation. However, 60% of patients showed no improvement, 7% worsened, and the study included no placebo control group. In a recent prospective study by Watik et al.,[357] 75 patients with painful grade-1, -2, or -3 knee osteoarthritis (based on the American College of Rheumatology radiological criteria[170]) were treated with three weekly injections of intra-articular sodium hyaluronate. The efficacy parameters included a VAS and Lequesne index. It was determined that at 3 and 6 months after injection, there were statistically significant improvements in VAS and Lequesne index scores.

Interpretation of clinical efficacy studies of HA injection is confounded by different study designs, injection regimens, and outcome evaluation criteria, as well as failure to control for concurrent NSAID use. Furthermore, it is well recognized that the placebo effect becomes more pronounced as the therapy becomes more invasive. Given that more than 75 RCTs have investigated the effects of HA and hylan derivatives in the treatment of knee osteoarthritis, meta-analysis becomes an important tool to determine the efficacy of HA. Presently, there are several published meta-analyses that review the literature.[13,26,207,236,354] Each meta-analysis reviewed similar papers, and many of the same trials were used in each analysis. All levels of osteoarthritis severity were included in patients between 55 and 75 years of age. A validated outcome measure was used such as the VAS, WOMAC, Lequesne, or numeric rating scale. Observation periods varied but typically did not exceed 1 year. Most studies included in the meta-analyses used lower-molecular-weight HA but all FDA-approved HA products were included.

Lo et al.[207] performed the first meta-analysis evaluating the efficacy of HA. They observed a small improvement in pain compared with placebo; the effect size was comparable to that observed with NSAID administration. Wang et al.[354] performed a similar analysis and came to the same conclusions as Lo et al. They also noted that studies with lower methodologic quality reported higher estimates of HA efficacy. In the analysis by Arrich et al.,[13] significant improvement in rest pain and exercise pain were noted between 10 and 30 weeks after treatment but the authors suggested that the findings were inconclusive because of excessive heterogeneity in the data. Modawal et al.[236] determined the causes of heterogeneity among the data in their meta-analysis using random-effect regression models. Study quality, pain, and form of HA used were the three causes, with study quality being predominant. When the lowest-quality studies were eliminated, heterogeneity improved, allowing the authors to conclude that HA is moderately effective in relieving rest pain between 5 and 12 weeks compared with placebo. Bellamy et al.[26] performed a large meta-analysis and obtained similar results to the previous meta-analyses, with improvements in rest pain and weight-bearing pain, particularly between 5 and 13 weeks. Notably, no meta-analysis was able to differentiate between lower- and higher-molecular-weight HA preparations. In a recent systematic review of 14 overlapping meta-analyses comparing treatment of knee osteoarthritis with intra-articular HA versus oral NSAIDS, intra-articular corticosteroids, intra-articular platelet-rich plasma (PRP), and placebo, Campbell et al.[40] identified areas of similarity and discordance. They concluded that intra-articular HA is a viable option for knee osteoarthritis, providing significant reductions in knee pain and gains in function, with effects lasting up to 26 months. They also showed that the positive effects of HA are optimal between 5 and 13 weeks but were less robust than effects induced by intra-articular PRP injections.[40]

Intra-articular HA is generally well tolerated, but problems occasionally arise. The risk of infection is small and, although not specifically reported, may be assumed to be of the same magnitude as that reported for corticosteroid injection. A local inflammatory reaction is a more frequent occurrence.[1,258] One study reported local inflammation in 11% of injections and 27% of patients; occurrence was unpredictable and symptoms lasted up to 3 weeks.[285] Three of the five meta-analyses discussed adverse effects. Wang et al.[354] noted three major adverse effects among the 1002 injected knees—an episode of severe knee swelling, a vasculitis, and a hypersensitivity reaction. The relative risk of minor adverse events was 1.19 and included transient mild increases in local pain or swelling.

Despite positive clinical and laboratory evidence, the question of the efficacy of injected hyaluronates remains. No evidence exists to support the use of one commercially available preparation over another, nor are the optimal dosage, injection regimen, or patient selection criteria known at this time.

Glucosamine. Glucosamine has been shown in culture studies dating back to the 1950s to enhance secretion of mucopolysaccharides in cartilage-derived fibroblasts. As early as 1994, McCarty[224] advocated for research into the use of glucosamine as a treatment for arthritis, citing animal and human studies that demonstrated a beneficial effect on the prevention and treatment of arthritis. Support for the use of glucosamine increased in the popular media and scientific circles, culminating in the blinded, randomized, placebo-controlled Glucosamine-Chondroitin Arthritis Intervention Trial (GAIT) of 2006.[57] OARSI has issued and revised expert consensus guidelines for the management of hip and knee osteoarthritis by systematic review and meta-analysis of studies conducted mainly in European countries and the United States. In their most recent guidelines for the nonsurgical treatment of knee osteoarthritis, OARSI made an inconclusive recommendation for the use of glucosamine for symptom relief, citing two systematic reviews that found inconclusive data and no statistically significant benefit for pain relief.[221] The AAOS strongly recommends against the use of glucosamine because of no statistically significant improvement in pain or function compared with placebo. Data from 21 prospective studies were considered in this recommendation.[4]

Rationale for glucosamine. Glucosamine is a simple amino sugar that serves as a substrate for the synthesis of glycosaminoglycans (GAGs) and HA. Glucosamine is synthesized directly by the chondrocyte, but when supplemented, it can be used directly to synthesize larger macromolecules. Most preparations are derived from chitin in crustacean shells. In in vitro and animal models, a wide variety of effects have been documented. These can be broadly classified as substrate, transcriptional, antireactive, and antiarthritic effects.

As far back as 1956, Roden[302] noted an increased production of GAGs and collagen when glucosamine sulfate was added to cartilage-derived fibroblast cell cultures. Other studies have confirmed this effect.[351,352] Karzel and Domenjoz[167] later demonstrated that glucosamine sulfate was efficiently incorporated into mucopolysaccharides.

In addition to functioning as a simple substrate, glucosamine has been shown in other studies to affect gene transcription within the chondrocyte. Jimenez and Dodge[158] demonstrated a twofold increase in perlecan and aggrecan messenger ribonucleic acid (mRNA) levels and a moderate increase in stromelysin mRNA in chondrocyte cultures incubated with 50 µM of glucosamine. They also found a dose-dependent downregulation of metalloproteinase I and II (enzymes important in the degradation of cartilage) mRNA in the same model. A more recent study demonstrated the differences in chondroprotective effects of glucosamine in combination with other agents.[342] Animal knee joints injected with glucosamine hydrochloride in combination with chondroitin sulfate and other herbal extracts were associated with significantly lower levels of immune modulators responsible for arthritis and cartilage degeneration compared with placebo.

Glucosamine may be effective in upregulating cartilage metabolism in arthritic or stressed cartilage. Lippiello[204] found an increase in glycosaminoglycan synthesis in arthritic cartilage explants under various types of stress when exposed to glucosamine compared with young or nonstressed explants. Investigating a biologic marker of type-II cartilage degradation, Christgau et al.[56] determined that patients with higher rates of cartilage turnover (higher levels of cross-linked telopeptide type II collagen in the urine) benefited the most from glucosamine supplementation.

Glucosamine increases the synovial production of HA, which has itself been shown to have anti-inflammatory effects, induce anabolic activity in chondrocytes, decrease joint pain, and increase mobility in vivo and in clinical studies.[224] Animal studies have demonstrated an anti-reactive effect of glucosamine, finding that glucosamine prevents an inflammatory response to certain irritants known to cause inflammation in rats but has no inhibitory effects on inflammation caused by inflammatory mediators such as bradykinin, serotonin, or histamine.[315] Importantly, glucosamine did not show any inhibition of the COX system, thus lending some credibility to the claim of GI tolerability. In fact, glucosamine may stimulate the production of protective mucopolysaccharides in the gastric mucosa and therefore may be useful in ulcer therapy.[241]

An antiarthritic effect of glucosamine has been demonstrated in animal models for inflammatory arthritis, mechanical arthritis, immunoreactive arthritis, and generalized inflammation. Efficacy in these models was lower than with indomethacin but toxicity was significantly lower, so the overall therapeutic margin was much more favorable.[315] Therefore, glucosamine may have a place in the therapy for inflammatory arthritis, in addition to osteoarthritis.[315]

Human studies of glucosamine. Glucosamine sulfate has been heavily studied in patients with arthritis over the past 30 years. Studies have been performed in many countries, including Italy,[61] Germany,[30,78,81,246] Spain,[208] Portugal,[331] China,[286] and the Philippines[284] in patients with arthritis of the hand, spine, shoulders, hips, and knees. The results were consistent; all showed a beneficial effect of glucosamine. Improvement in pain occurred slowly over a period of several weeks. Subjects continued to improve while taking the study drug, although patients taking the placebo did not. Patients maintained improvement for weeks to months after the drug was discontinued. Response to treatment was high, ranging from 56% to more than 90%.[61,284] Equally important, no study reported major adverse effects. Early clinical uncontrolled trials performed in Germany beginning in 1969 used an injectable form at a dosage of 400 mg/day. Injections were intra-articular, intramuscular, or intravenous. All studies reported diminution of pain, some improvement of mobility, and no major adverse effects.[344] In a recent randomized, double-blind, placebo-controlled trial by Tsuji et al.,[340] patients received 100 mg of N-acetyl glucosamine daily for 24 weeks. The primary outcome was based on VAS score, and secondary outcomes were based on the Japanese Knee Osteoarthritis Measure score and physical activity and performance. At the end of the 24-week period, it was determined that glucosamine administration of 12 weeks or longer had a significantly positive effect on self-reported knee function and household physical activity. In another double-blind, multicenter RCT, the efficacy of glucosamine hydrochloride in combination with chondroitin sulfate was compared with that of celecoxib in patients with grade-2 or -3 knee osteoarthritis.[147] A total of 606 patients were randomized to receive treatment for 6 months, at which time both groups reported a 50% decrease in pain (as determined by the WOMAC score), and both groups had a reduction of more than 50% in joint swelling.

Interest in glucosamine accelerated in Europe with the synthesis of an easily absorbable oral preparation. Since the early 1980s, numerous controlled studies, including a number of double-blind studies,[†] have been conducted. Of these, at least five were double-blind, single-joint, placebo-controlled studies using a validated outcome tool.[245,254,270,297,298]

Criticism of the older research on glucosamine has centered on the small numbers of patients studied, short time periods, and relative lack of studies independent of corporate sponsorship. Methodologic concerns, specifically the failure of most studies to control for NSAID use, have also been raised.[178] Meta-analyses have generally supported the use of glucosamine. Towheed et al.[336] evaluated 16 RCTs, 12 comparing glucosamine with placebo and four comparing it with an NSAID. They concluded that glucosamine is safe and effective. McAlindon et al.[222] reviewed six studies of glucosamine involving 911 patients. Combined results showed a moderate treatment effect of glucosamine. Of the six meta-analyses published on the subject, five supported a mild treatment effect,[198,222,282,300,337] and one reported no difference compared with placebo.[28]

Interest in glucosamine has been tempered since the publication of the GAIT study.[57] In this large, multicenter, randomized, placebo-controlled trial, 1583 patients with osteoarthritis of the knee were randomized to glucosamine, 1500 mg/day; chondroitin, 1200 mg/day; glucosamine and chondroitin in combination; celecoxib, 200 mg/day; or placebo. Acetaminophen, up to 4000 mg/day, was used as a rescue medication. Glucosamine and chondroitin were associated with a decrease in pain levels from baseline but not significantly greater than placebo and not as much as celecoxib, which was significantly better than placebo. However, in patients with moderate to severe pain, the response to combined glucosamine-chondroitin therapy was significantly greater than placebo (79% versus 54%; $p > .002$). Two-year follow-up results from the GAIT study show that no treatment achieved a clinically important difference in WOMAC pain or function scores compared with the placebo. Glucosamine and celecoxib, however, showed beneficial but not significant effects. Adverse reactions were similar among treatment groups.[310]

Chondroitin. Several other amino sugars, or GAGs, are commercially available for the treatment of osteoarthritis. These include chondroitin sulfate, glycosaminoglycan-peptide association complex (Rumalon), glycosaminoglycan polysulfuric acid (GAGPS; Arteparon), and sodium pentosan polysulfate (Cartrophen). Although these compounds have some laboratory and clinical support, they have not gained the popularity, nor have they been as well studied as glucosamine and HA.

Chondroitin sulfate (galactosaminoglycuronoglycan sulfate) is a mucopolysaccharide, which together with keratan sulfate and a protein core, forms aggrecan. Aggrecan, in turn, associates with hyaluronan to form a hygroscopic macromolecule largely responsible for the physical elasticity of cartilage. During aging, the ratio of keratan sulfate to chondroitin sulfate in aggrecan increases, reflecting a relative loss of chondroitin. Also, chondroitin sulfate from diseased cartilage is shorter in length than normal.[35]

As a pharmaceutical, chondroitin exhibits anti-inflammatory properties similar to those of other GAGs and GAG precursors.[16] It is well tolerated in humans and has few adverse effects and reasonable bioavailability.[304] Also, like other GAG precursors, stimulatory effects on cartilage have been reported.[168] Chondroitin

sulfate has also been shown to neutralize catabolic processes such as IL-1 production and metalloproteinase activation in human osteoarthritis chondrocyte tissue culture.[219,342,371,374]

Several RCTs demonstrating a beneficial effect of chondroitin sulfate have been published. In a double-blind, placebo-controlled RCT with 2-year follow-up of 605 participants with chronic knee osteoarthritis, Fransen et al.[108] showed that chondroitin plus glucosamine led to significant reduction in joint space narrowing. Another RCT by Wildi et al.[364] concluded that supplementation with chondroitin sulfate alone led to significant reductions in cartilage volume loss in knee osteoarthritis starting at 6 months of treatment. Studying 120 patients with knee osteoarthritis, Uebelhart et al.[343] found the group given chondroitin sulfate had better functional outcomes and less joint space narrowing on standard radiographs at 1 year compared with controls. Verbruggen et al.[347] also reported on two studies in which patients with erosive arthritis of the hand experienced less progression and fewer new lesions when given chondroitin compared with a control group.

Glucosamine-Chondroitin Synergy. When considering the definition of a chondroprotective agent, according to Ghosh and Brooks,[123] it is clear that neither glucosamine alone nor chondroitin alone satisfies all criteria. Because they act through different mechanisms, it is reasonable to suppose that they could have a synergistic effect (Table 120.2). Lippiello et al.[205] published a dramatic study of a rabbit instability model of knee osteoarthritis. They compared glucosamine alone, chondroitin alone, and both in combination. Although chondroprotective effects of glucosamine and chondroitin alone were noted, the combination almost completely prevented the onset of osteoarthritis (Figs. 120.1 to 120.3). In a recent double-blind RCT, Hochberg et al.[147] demonstrated that chondroitin, in combination with glucosamine, had comparable efficacy to celecoxib in reducing pain, stiffness, functional limitation, and joint swelling/effusion after 6 months in patients with painful

TABLE 120.2	**Postulated Synergistic Mechanism Between Glucosamine and Chondroitin Sulfate**	
Chondroprotective Agent	**Characteristics**
Glucosamine	Stimulates chondrocyte and synoviocyte metabolism
Chondroitin sulfate	Inhibits degradative enzymes; prevents fibrin thrombi in periarticular tissues

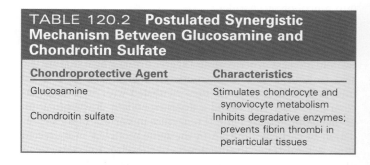

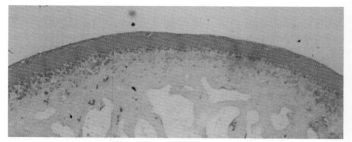

FIG 120.1 Cross-section of normal rabbit femoral condyle. Cartilage is of normal thickness and shows normal glycosaminoglycan staining (safranin O).

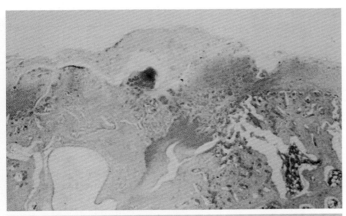

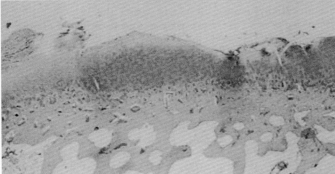

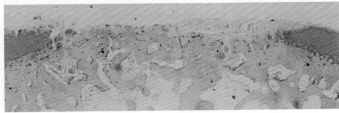

FIG 120.2 Cross-section of an experimental animal treated with placebo. Extensive loss of glycosaminoglycan and cartilage destruction can be noted (safranin O).

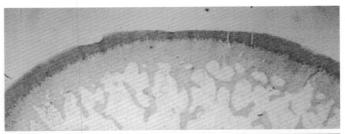

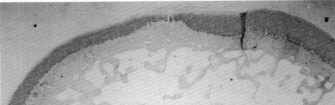

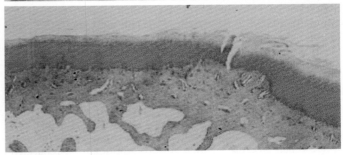

FIG 120.3 Experimental animal treated with a glucosamine-chondroitin combination. Cartilage shows near-perfect preservation (safranin O).

knee osteoarthritis. These data, however, contrast the GAIT study's 2-year follow-up data. These discrepancies illustrate the need for further research. In their most recent treatment guidelines for the nonoperative management of knee osteoarthritis, the AAOS and OARSI recommended against the use of glucosamine and chondroitin supplementation.[3]

"Nutraceuticals." In the United States, "nutraceuticals" are considered nutritional supplements and are therefore not regulated by the Food and Drug Administration. The nutritional supplement industry is regulated by the Dietary Supplement Health Education Act, which simply requires that the percentages of active ingredients match claims on the label. There is no requirement for safety, efficacy, or bioavailability of the product. Reports have cast doubt that even the percentages claimed on labels are accurate. Until the Food and Drug Administration begins to regulate these agents, it will be incumbent on the physician to investigate the purity and efficacy of individual formulations before recommending them to patients.

Agents primarily directed at inhibiting enzymatic or inflammatory cartilage destruction are being investigated. These include bovine superoxide dismutase (Orgotein), IL-1 receptor antagonists, S-adenosyl methionine,[‡] and sodium pentosan polysulfate (Cartrophen). Although some encouraging data have been reported,[§] these compounds should be considered investigational at this time.

Future Medications

COX-inhibiting nitric oxide donors (CINODs) are a recently developed group of analgesic and anti-inflammatory medications. It is theorized that the addition of the nitric oxide will counteract some of the known complications seen with COX inhibitors, specifically elevated blood pressure and GI upset.[353] The release of nitric oxide causes vasodilation of blood vessels, which decreases systemic blood pressure and decreases platelet aggregation. The first drug in this class is AZD3582, or nitronaproxen, a combination of nitric oxide and naproxen.

In a pharmacologic study using a murine model of peritonitis,[5] a naproxen based CINOD, NCX 429, elicited significant anti-inflammatory activity beyond the simple COX inhibition or pure nitric oxide release. An in vivo experiment has also demonstrated that NCX 429 inhibited inflammatory cell influx after cytokine administration.[5]

White et al.[363] compared the effects of naproxen alone versus naproxcinod on blood pressure. The treatment protocols for the four comparison groups were as follows: (1) 750 mg

---

[‡]References 19, 127, 137, 183, 192, 210, 244, 271, 281, and 350.
[§]References 18, 42, 106, 107, 122, 124, 182, 251, 272, 303, 308, 323, and 348.

nitronaproxen twice daily; (2) 375 mg naproxcinod twice daily; (3) 500 mg naproxen twice daily; and (4) placebo twice daily. The authors found that neither dose of nitronaproxen resulted in increased blood pressure compared with the naproxen group. Patients who had a diagnosis of hypertension before beginning the study and who were treated with naproxen alone had blood pressure that was 6.5 mmHg higher than those hypertensive patients in the 500-mg nitronaproxen treatment arm.

In a phase-2, randomized, double-blind study, Karlsson et al.[166] found the most efficacious dose of nitronaproxen was 750 mg twice daily. They included patients treated with 25 mg daily of the COX-II inhibitor, rofecoxib. They found no significant differences in WOMAC pain scores for those treated with nitronaproxen, 750 mg twice daily; nitronaproxen, 1125 mg twice daily; or rofecoxib, 25 mg daily. However, patients on these regimens had better pain relief than those taking a once-daily dose of nitronaproxen, 750 mg, or placebo. The authors also reported a decreased mean systolic blood pressure in the cohort treated with naproxcinod and an increase in the mean systolic blood pressure of patients treated with rofecoxib.

Although these early results are promising, long-term studies of the CINODs must be conducted to identify possible adverse effects that have not yet been discovered.

Stem Cells. Mesenchymal stem cells (MSCs) are multipotent cells that can be isolated from human tissues. MSCs have been tested in animal models and have potential applications in tissue repair because of their immunomodulatory, reparative, and anti-inflammatory properties.[27] In a rabbit model of osteoarthritis, animals receiving intra-articular injections of scaffold-free MSCs obtained from bone marrow had less cartilage degeneration, osteophyte formation, and subchondral sclerosis compared with controls.[321] Although the exact mechanism is unknown, MSCs can induce proliferation and differentiation of resident progenitor cells and have an innate differentiation potential to become chondrocytes to regenerate articular cartilage.[133] In a pilot study, 12 patients with refractory knee pain caused by osteoarthritis received intra-articular injections of autologous expanded bone marrow MSCs. Eleven of the patients exhibited rapid and progressive improvement in function by 1 year, a highly significant decrease in poor cartilage areas, and improvement in cartilage quality.[262] A systematic review of the use of MSCs for the treatment of cartilage lesions included 72 preclinical studies and 18 clinical trials.[93] In regard to the clinical trials focusing on cartilage degeneration, there were no randomized trials, five comparative studies, six case series, and seven case reports. Of further note, two studies involved the use of adipose-derived MSCs, five the use of bone marrow concentration, and eleven the use of bone marrow–derived MSCs. Although multiple studies showed positive effects of MSCs for the treatment of osteoarthritis or other cartilage defects, the authors acknowledged that these results are preliminary because of weak methodology, small sample sizes, and short-term follow-up.[93] Safety concerns have also arisen surrounding the use of MSCs because of their neoplastic potential caused by their proliferative capacity and risk of infection given their immunomodulatory effects.[92] A systematic review to evaluate the safety of MSCs did not identify any major safety issues but rather identified less severe complications such as transient fever.[187] Stem cell therapy appears to be a promising treatment to halt disease progression and regenerate articular cartilage. However, studies of higher quality are needed to determine the safety, efficacy, and optimal source and preparation of cells for the treatment of knee osteoarthritis.

Growth Hormone. Only one study has reported on the use of intra-articular recombinant human growth hormone (GH). The study quantified the additive effects of GH administered with HA. After intra-articular collagenase injection, 30 mature rabbits were assigned to three groups (normal saline control, HA, or HA plus GH). After 9 weeks of observation, lameness was significantly less severe and shorter in duration in the HA plus GH group compared with the groups that received normal saline or HA alone, suggesting that co-injection of intra-articular HA and recombinant human GH is more effective than HA injections alone in an osteoarthritis model.[175]

Platelet-Rich Plasma. In recent years, the use of PRP has expanded beyond the treatment of tendon and ligament injuries to the treatment of cartilage disease such as knee osteoarthritis. PRP is derived from centrifuging whole blood to obtain an increased platelet concentration.[71] There are various formulations and preparations of PRP with different constituents, depending on the preparation.

PRP has been shown to have healing and anti-inflammatory properties. In terms of healing properties, an in vitro study demonstrated that PRP had a proliferative effect on autologous chondrocytes and MSCs.[135] When Petrera et al.[279] compared chondrocyte supplementation with fetal bovine serum or platelet-poor plasma, PRP provided the most significant enhancement of in vitro formation of cartilage and increased overall GAG content. In a randomized study of dogs with documented symptomatic arthritis in a single joint, animals that received a single injection of PRP had 55% improvement in comfort as measured by lameness scores and function and a 12% increase in weight placed on the affected limb at 12 weeks compared with a control group that received a saline injection.[88,92]

In regard to PRP's anti-inflammatory properties, PRP has reduced several effects of IL-1β, which is involved in the catabolism of articular cartilage in knee osteoarthritis.[9] A prospective study of 115 knees receiving three consecutive PRP injections reported statistically significant improvements in all clinical scores at 12 months with maximal improvement at 6 months.[180] Compared with HA, PRP has better results in younger patients or patients with early osteoarthritis and similar efficacy in older patients with advanced disease.[181] In early knee osteoarthritis, a single dose of PRP is as effective as two doses.[128] Different PRP formulations induced distinct effects on human articular chondrocytes in vitro, emphasizing that differences in technique and PRP composition may produce different outcomes in the treatment of knee osteoarthritis and present difficulties in comparing the results of various studies.[92] However, PRP has shown promise as a useful treatment for mild knee osteoarthritis compared with HA. Additional studies are needed before conclusions regarding efficacy can be confirmed, especially in regard to optimal PRP composition.

OTHER TREATMENTS

Botulinum Toxin

Newer injection therapies have been implemented for the treatment of knee osteoarthritis. Recent studies demonstrate the therapeutic utility of botulinum toxin injection.[92] Botulinum toxin type-A (BoNT-A) has been shown to have an anti-inflammatory effect in an arthritic knee rat model.[369] Yoo et al.[369] investigated joint inflammation using histopathologic and immunofluorescent techniques. A BoNT-A injection group was compared with a saline injection control group. Subsequent histologic analysis 1 to 2 weeks after BoNT-A injection showed significant reductions in joint inflammation and destruction. The expression of IL-1β immune-reactive cells, normally involved in the catabolism of articular cartilage, was significantly attenuated in the injected areas.[369] A pilot study by Boon et al.[33] investigated the safety and efficacy of BoNT-A in 60 patients with moderate to severe knee osteoarthritis. Patients were randomized into three groups: single injection of corticosteroid; low-dose intra-articular injection of BoNT-A; or high-dose intra-articular injection of BoNT-A. The primary outcome was pain on a VAS at 8 weeks. Only the low-dose BoNT-A group experienced a statistically significant reduction in pain. WOMAC scores for pain, stiffness, and function were significantly improved for all groups without any serious adverse events noted.[33] Use of botulinum toxin type-B (BoNT-B) has also shown efficacy in the treatment of chronic degenerative knee arthritis pain.[8] One study suggested the involvement of BoNT-B in the inhibition of cell mediators involved in pain generation, thereby reducing the effects of local inflammation at the injected site.[8] These studies support the role of botulinum toxin injection as a treatment option for symptomatic knee arthritis and have elucidated the need for further randomized, double-blind studies.

Holistic/Complementary Medicine

Treatments for knee osteoarthritis are derived from a multidisciplinary approach. The US Agency for Healthcare Research and Quality has called for the development of new therapies and has reported no clear benefit from the use of any one approach.[299] The chronic and debilitating nature of knee osteoarthritis has forced patients to seek alternative and complementary medicine routes.[257]

Prolotherapy

Prolotherapy, commonly known as *proliferative therapy*, has been used by practitioners for more than 70 years.[292] Prolotherapy involves injection of hypertonic dextrose, an irritant solution, into the painful joint space and around the ligament and tendon insertions.[289] This causes a local inflammatory response with an up-regulation of chemical mediators.[292]Although the exact mechanism of chemical up-regulation is not understood at this time, it is thought that chemical mediators induce a therapeutic response leading to stronger connective tissues, improved biomechanics, and soft tissue recovery.[290] The earliest report of this therapy in allopathic literature referred to the method as *sclerotherapy* because of the therapeutic nature of the scar-forming properties of the early injectants.[292] Although this form of therapy has been used for several years, only recently has a study demonstrated its efficacy. A single-arm uncontrolled study with 1-year follow-up by Rabago et al.[291] concluded that dextrose injection may mitigate the pain and stiffness experienced by patients with knee osteoarthritis, resulting in significant and sustained improvement in knee function. In this study, 36 patients with moderate to severe knee osteoarthritis received an average of four injections over 17 weeks. Fifteen percent dextrose extra-articular injections along with 25% dextrose intra-articular injections were given at weeks 1, 5, and 9, and at weeks 13 and 17 as needed. The WOMAC was used as a primary outcome measure and showed significant improvement within 4 weeks of the first injection with progressive improvement during the 1-year follow-up period.[293] This intervention may provide symptomatic relief but further investigation is needed.

Moxibustion

Moxibustion is a traditional East Asian intervention that has been widely used to treat the symptoms of osteoarthritis, stroke, and hot flashes in Korea, China, Japan, and Vietnam.[53] It is a form of thermal stimulation achieved by burning herbs, primarily *Artemisia vulgaris,* at specific acupuncture sites on the skin.[48] A multicenter RCT in South Korea compared the outcomes of 212 patients with knee osteoarthritis, half of whom were allocated to moxibustion and half to usual care.[196] Moxibustion therapy on the affected knee was offered at six standard acupuncture points. WOMAC scores improved significantly at 13 weeks; however, adverse events related to treatment were common. These included first- and second-degree burns, pruritus, and fatigue.[196] A recent systematic review[53] on the use of moxibustion reported on its use in clinical practice for the treatment of rheumatologic and inflammatory disease states, but there has been no conclusive evidence of its effectiveness in the treatment of knee osteoarthritis. There have been few full-scale RCTs of moxibustion, which makes the recommendation for moxibustion weak.[53]

AMERICAN ACADEMY OF ORTHOPAEDIC SURGEONS GUIDELINES SUMMARY

In their clinical practice guidelines, the AAOS has provided a list of recommendations, including conservative and pharmacological alternatives, for the management of knee osteoarthritis. The recommendations were established using evidence-based medicine and are not meant to be the sole guide in the overall management of individual patients. Rather, management is multifactorial. Recommendations are labeled as strong, moderate, or inconclusive.[4]

The AAOS strongly recommends that patients with symptomatic osteoarthritis of the knee engage in physical activity, including low-impact aerobic exercises, muscular strengthening, and self-management programs such as the Arthritis Self-Management Program. Furthermore, it is strongly recommended that NSAIDS or tramadol be used to treat symptoms. Weight loss for patients with a body mass index value of 25 or greater carries a moderate recommendation.

In contrast, the AAOS is unable to recommend for or against the use of acetaminophen and opioids. Recommendations for other forms of therapy, including injections of intra-articular corticosteroids, PRP, and GH, are also inconclusive because of the lack of efficacy demonstrated in recent studies.[4]

KEY REFERENCES

3. American Academy of Orthopaedic Surgeons: *Treatment of osteoarthritis of the knee: Evidence-based guideline,* ed 2, 2013, pp 1–1200.

26. Bellamy N, Campbell J, Robinson V, et al: Viscosupplementation for the treatment of osteoarthritis of the knee. *Cochrane Database Syst Rev* (2):CD005321, 2006.

67. Davies-Tuck ML, Wluka AE, Wang Y, et al: The natural history of cartilage defects in people with knee osteoarthritis. *Osteoarthritis Cartilage* 16(3):337–342, 2008.

141. Hepper CT, Halvorson JJ, Duncan ST, et al: The efficacy and duration of intra-articular corticosteroid injection for knee osteoarthritis: a systematic review of level I studies. *J Am Acad Orthop Surg* 17(10):638–646, 2009.

153. Huang WF, Hsiao FY, Wen YW, et al: Cardiovascular events associated with the use of four nonselective NSAIDs (etodolac, nabumetone, ibuprofen, or naproxen) versus a cyclooxygenase-2 inhibitor (celecoxib): a population-based analysis in Taiwanese adults. *Clin Ther* 28(11):1827–1836, 2006.

194. Lawrence RC, Felson DT, Helmick CG, et al: Estimates of the prevalence of arthritis and other rheumatic conditions in the United States: Part II. *Arthritis Rheum* 58(1):26–35, 2008.

275. Pelletier JP, Martel-Pelletier J: The pathophysiology of osteoarthritis and the implication of the use of hyaluronan and hylan as therapeutic agents in viscosupplementation. *J Rheumatol Suppl* 39:19–24, 1993.

322. Smalley WE, Ray WA, Daugherty JR, et al: Nonsteroidal anti-inflammatory drugs and the incidence of hospitalizations for peptic ulcer disease in elderly persons. *Am J Epidemiol* 141(6):539–545, 1995.

329. Superio-Cabuslay E, Ward MM, Lorig KR: Patient education interventions in osteoarthritis and rheumatoid arthritis: a meta-analytic comparison with nonsteroidal antiinflammatory drug treatment. *Arthritis Care Res* 9(4):292–301, 1996.

354. Wang CT, Lin J, Chang CJ, et al: Therapeutic effects of hyaluronic acid on osteoarthritis of the knee. A meta-analysis of randomized controlled trials. *J Bone Joint Surg Am* 86-A(3):538–545, 2004.

373. Zhang W, Moskowitz RW, Nuki G, et al: OARSI recommendations for the management of hip and knee osteoarthritis, Part II: OARSI evidence-based, expert consensus guidelines. *Osteoarthritis Cartilage* 16(2):137–162, 2008.

The references for this chapter can also be found on www.expertconsult.com.

121

Osteotomies About the Knee

Andrew Feldman, Guillem Gonzalez-Lomas, Stephanie J. Swensen, Daniel J. Kaplan

In the setting of lower extremity malalignment, increased forces across a compartment have been associated with accelerated cartilage degeneration and increased symptoms in that compartment. In these cases, realignment osteotomies provide the ability to unload the compartment—potentially delaying arthroplasty and preserving the native joint. Although technically challenging, osteotomies about the knee represent an important treatment option in young, active patients because, in contrast to arthroplasty, they facilitate a return to high-level activities. Additionally, osteotomies may alleviate the biomechanical stresses on cartilage-sparing procedures, meniscal repairs or transplantation, and ligamentous reconstructions, augmenting their success rates. As older demographic groups increase their activity levels and intensity, indications for osteotomy have expanded. Modifications in surgical techniques, instrumentation, and fixation devices have facilitated more reproducible and reliable outcomes.

The most common types of osteotomies are the high tibial osteotomy (HTO) for varus deformity, distal femoral osteotomy (DFO) for valgus deformity, and tibial tubercle osteotomy (TTO) for patellofemoral malalignment. The choice of osteotomy is highly individualized and based on careful preoperative measurements. This chapter reviews the indications, preoperative decision making, surgical techniques, and clinical outcomes of these challenging procedures.

HIGH TIBIAL OSTEOTOMY FOR VARUS KNEE

Indications

HTOs were used in the early 1900s for correction of valgus or varus deformities of the knee caused by rickets or poliomyelitis. In 1958, Jackson[44] published results of proximal tibial osteotomies for treatment of osteoarthritis. Original osteotomies consisted of a dome transection distal to the tibial tubercle, realignment of the shaft to "make the knee straight," and subsequent casting. Several reports followed, with modifications of the original technique touting a success rate of 85%.[45] Coventry reported his results in a 1965 publication but was pessimistic about long-term outcomes. Koshino introduced the use of a blade plate for maintaining correction and allowing early motion, and Hernigou and Debeyre recognized the importance of maintaining the sagittal slope while the coronal plane was being corrected. The modern HTO is a direct descendant of the Coventry osteotomy. In adults, it is used primarily in the setting of a varus knee with medial compartment arthritis and symptoms of medial sided knee pain. Indications have expanded to include use of HTO in joint preservation surgery, to unload a cartilage restoration site (i.e., microfracture, autologous

chondrocyte implantation [ACI], osteochondral autograft or allograft), and to modify the sagittal slope in cruciate ligament insufficiency. Patients generally have better outcomes when osteotomy is performed before medial compartment arthritis has become severe and subchondral bone has been exposed.[42,67] HTO is contraindicated in the following settings: significant symptomatic chondral injury to the patellofemoral or lateral compartments, tricompartmental arthritis, inflammatory arthritis, age older than 60 years, and motion limitations (arc of motion <120 degrees and flexion contracture >5 degrees) (Table 121.1).

There are other situations that require special attention. Patients who present with anterior knee pain are unlikely to improve after a coronal plane correction and may actually do worse. Patients should also be carefully screened for their potential to endure the requisite postoperative rehabilitation. The recovery from an HTO is long and arduous, typically requiring a period of protected weight bearing followed by extensive lower limb muscular re-education and training. Preoperatively, patient expectations should be managed judiciously. Patients must understand that recovery to a pain-free state of full activity takes an average of 6 months.

Globally, indications for HTO have been found to differ by region. In the United States, patients older than age 60 are typically offered total knee arthroplasty (TKA) or unicompartmental knee arthroplasty (UKA) over an HTO. Outside the United States, HTO is still routinely performed in older, fit patients, who are aware that they may obtain only partial symptom relief.[2]

The ideal patient is nonsmoking, is younger than 60 years old, and has an active lifestyle precluding arthroplasty. Obesity has been variously described as a contraindication in an older patient (because of the increased stresses that the osteotomy site must support) and a relative indication (in the setting of a younger patient in whom arthroplasty is indicated). A large-scale population-based study looking at 2671 patients who had undergone an HTO before conversion to a TKA found that certain factors lowered HTO survival rates, including older age, female sex, concurrent ligament injuries, and prior meniscectomy.[48] In that study, the mean survival at 10 years was found to be 67%.

History and Physical Examination

A thorough history should distinguish between patients with a prior traumatic knee injury and patients with an insidious onset of medial compartment arthritis. Previous trauma may denote other concomitant injuries, including chronic ligamentous laxity. Current patient activity level, expectations, and overall health should be noted. Patients with varus knees can be identified by observing them standing and walking, although observation alone is notoriously unreliable, especially in cases of large body habitus.

Any patient who is suspected to have a varus knee (or any patient who is a potential candidate for an osteotomy) should undergo a three-joint standing mechanical axis radiograph to evaluate the coronal alignment objectively. Examination of gait is also critical because the varus knee not only overloads the medial compartment but also creates an increased knee adduction moment. Over time, this stresses the lateral ligamentous structures in tension. Noyes and Simon[66] classified the relationship of varus malalignment with lateral ligament

laxity into primary varus, double varus, and triple varus knee syndromes (Fig. 121.1). Over time, primary mechanical axis varus may lead to lateral ligament insufficiency (double varus.) Chronically stressed knees may further develop varus recurvatum, becoming "triple varus knees." Most double varus and triple varus knees represent the sequelae of previous anterior cruciate ligament (ACL) injuries with resultant ACL insufficiency. These knees often have increased external knee extension moments and knee hyperextension during the stance phase.[64,65] In double varus and triple varus knees, management of the ligament insufficiencies should be performed in addition to HTO to optimize outcomes.

Imaging

A complete radiographic evaluation includes the following: a full-length, three-joint (bilateral hip to ankle on the same cassette) weight-bearing view in full extension with the feet in a neutral position; a 45-degree flexion posteroanterior view to assess for posterior femorotibial compartment narrowing; a lateral view to measure patellar height and observe the patellofemoral joint (PFJ); and a skyline view for further patellofemoral compartment evaluation (Table 121.2). Preoperative patellar height indices (Insall-Salvati index, modified Insall-Salvati index, Caton-Deschamps index, Blackburne-Peel index) should be calculated because both opening and closing wedge HTOs have had patella baja reported as a sequela (Fig.

TABLE 121.1 **Indications and Contraindications for High Tibial Osteotomies**	
Indications	**Contraindications**
Joint preservation surgery	Age >60 years
Unload a cartilage restoration	Tricompartmental arthritis
Modify sagittal slope in cruciate ligament insufficiency	Significant symptomatic chondral injury to patellofemoral or lateral compartments
	Inflammatory arthritis
	Motion limitations

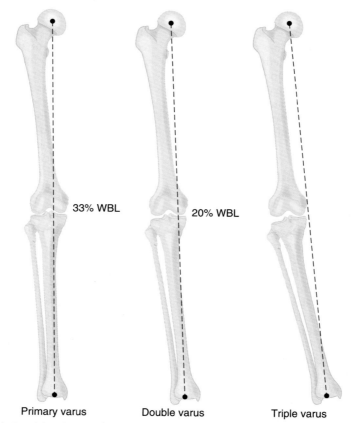

33% WBL   20% WBL

Primary varus   Double varus   Triple varus

FIG 121.1 The relationship of varus malalignment with lateral ligament laxity has been classified into primary varus, double varus, and triple varus knee syndromes. Over time, primary mechanical axis varus may lead to lateral ligament insufficiency (double varus.) Chronically stressed knees may further develop varus recurvatum, becoming "triple varus knees."

TABLE 121.2 Radiographs Evaluate a Patient for High Tibial Osteotomy

Radiographs	Evaluate
Full-length, three-joint weight-bearing view	Alignment
45° flexion PA view	Posterior femorotibial compartment narrowing
Lateral view	Patellar height and patellofemoral joint
Skyline view	Patellofemoral compartment

PA, Posteroanterior.

121.2).[28,69,75] If a patient has a preexisting patella baja, HTO should be approached with caution.

A lateral radiograph also helps to establish the posterior tibial slope baseline. The tibia is triangular in cross section. Because of this, a medial opening wedge osteotomy is in actuality cutting from anteromedial to posterolateral. Therefore, the tibial slope increases as the osteotomy site is opened. The concept is similar, but in reverse, for a lateral closing wedge osteotomy. In this case, the cut is in an anterolateral-to-posteromedial direction, decreasing the tibial slope.

Tibial slope changes have a direct effect in a knee with cruciate ligament deficiencies. An increased tibial slope accentuates

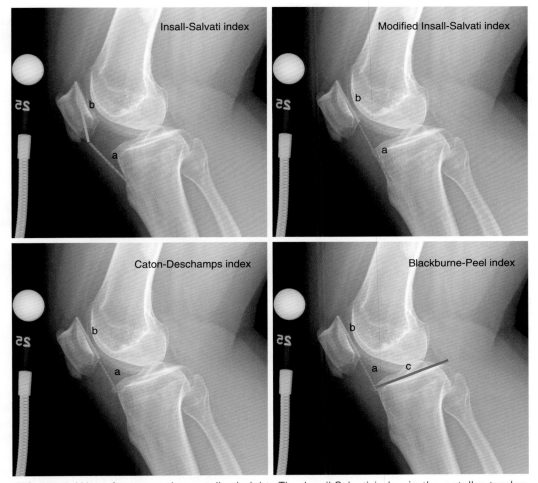

FIG 121.2 Ways for measuring patellar height. The Insall-Salvati index is the patellar tendon length *(a)*/the patellar length *(b)*. This is the length of the posterior surface of the tendon from the lower pole of the patella to its insertion on the tibia divided by the greatest pole-to-pole length. The modified Insall-Salvati index uses slightly different measurements. It measures the distance from the inferior margin of the patellar articular surface (as opposed to the lower pole of the patella itself) to the patellar tendon insertion *(a)*. This is divided by the length of the patellar articular surface *(b)*. The Caton-Deschamps index measures the ratio of the distance between the upper tibia and inferior patella *(a)* divided by the length of the articular surface of the patella *(b)*. The Blackburne-Peel index uses a horizontally drawn line at the level of the tibial plateau *(c)*. Perpendicular to this line, a vertical line is drawn *(a)* at the patella between the horizontal line and the inferior aspect of the patellar articular surface. A second measurement *(b)* is made along the patellar articular surface.

PCL insufficiency, whereas a decreased tibial slope increases instability in an ACL-deficient knee. However, these tibial slope changes can be used to the surgeon's advantage because the converse is also true. Increasing the tibial slope may be desirable to enhance stability in an ACL-deficient knee, whereas decreasing the slope can help stabilize a PCL-deficient knee.

Magnetic resonance imaging (MRI) can evaluate soft tissue pathology such as ligament injuries, meniscus tears, osteochondral defects, or subchondral bone edema. The authors recommend it as part of their standard preoperative workup.

Preoperative Decision Making

Medial Opening Wedge High Tibial Osteotomy Versus Lateral Closing Wedge High Tibial Osteotomy.

The preoperative mechanical axis deviation and the degree of medial compartment arthrosis determine the amount of correction needed. Either a medial opening wedge osteotomy or a lateral closing wedge osteotomy can be performed at the discretion of the surgeon.

Coventry[16,17] helped popularize the lateral closing wedge osteotomy in the 1960s. Closing wedge HTOs allow for immediate weight bearing, have lower rates of malunion and nonunion, and theoretically carry lower risks of increasing the posterior sagittal slope and creating patella baja. Disadvantages include a narrow window for modification once the bone wedge is removed, bone loss, a more involved exposure that violates the anterior compartment of the leg, a possible concomitant fibular osteotomy, and risks associated with peroneal nerve exposure (Table 121.3).

In the last 2 decades in the United States, medial opening wedge HTOs have become more popular, largely as a result of innovations in lower profile plates and fixation techniques, broader bone grafting options, and the ease of the exposure and approach. Medial opening wedge osteotomies avoid exposing the lateral aspect of the leg, decreasing the risks associated with peroneal nerve exposure, anterior compartment dissection, and fibular osteotomies. They facilitate correction and allow for fine-tuning in both the coronal and the sagittal planes, although the osteotomy cut must still be carefully planned. The exposure is direct. Disadvantages include an association with inadvertently increasing the sagittal tibial slope and a historically higher rate of nonunion. Nevertheless, a meta-analysis found equivalent union rates in closing and opening wedge HTOs (Table 121.4).[82]

Degree of Correction Planning. The degree of correction depends on the desired location of the mechanical axis line through the knee. The method described by Dugdale and colleagues[23] applies to both medial opening and lateral closing wedge osteotomies. For most cases of genu varum resulting from arthritis, the desired reference point on the tibial plateau is set at 62.5% of its width as measured from the medial cortex (Fig. 121.3). The idea is to have the mechanical axis pass lateral to the center of the knee to help unload the medial compartment. In cases of mild degenerative changes within the lateral compartment, massive corrections, or subtle corrections with a concomitant cartilage transplant, the reference point can be moved to the midline of the knee to avoid overloading the lateral side.

From the reference point, line A is drawn to the center of the femoral head. Line B is drawn to the center of the ankle. The

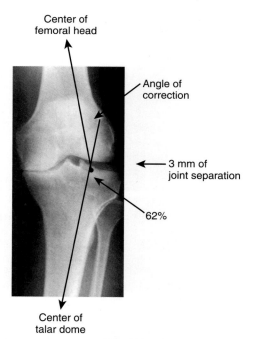

FIG 121.3 Method of calculating the correction angle for a high tibial osteotomy using a radiograph. The lines from the centers of the femoral head and tibiotalar joint converge at the 62% coordinate to form the desired angle of correction.

TABLE 121.3 **Advantages, Disadvantages, and Complications of Lateral Closing Wedge Osteotomy**

Advantages	Disadvantages	Complications
Immediate weight bearing	Narrow window for modifications once bone wedge removed	Peroneal nerve injury
Lower malunion/nonunion rates	Bone loss	Fibular osteotomy
Lower risk of increasing posterior sagittal slope and patella baja	More involved exposure violating anterior compartment	Nonunion
	Possible concomitant fibular osteotomy	Medial tibial cortex fracture
	Risk associated with peroneal nerve exposure	Anterior compartment syndrome

TABLE 121.4 **Advantages, Disadvantages, and Complications of Medial Opening Wedge Osteotomies**

Advantages	Disadvantages	Complications
Avoid exposing lateral aspect of leg	Increasing sagittal tibial slope	Lateral tibial plateau fractures
Facilitate correction and allow for fine-tuning	Higher nonunion rate	MCL injuries
Direct exposure		Hardware irritation
		Loss of correction/nonunion

MCL, Medial collateral ligament.

angle of the intersection of these two lines is the angle of correction, called the alpha angle. In most knees, the correction angle is proportional to the amount of osteotomy distraction at the level of the medial cortex in a 1-degree to 1-mm correlation.

Lateral closing wedge osteotomies have their correction angle calculated using the same technique. The first osteotomy line is drawn on the tibia, perpendicular to its axis and approximately 2 cm below the joint line. The second osteotomy line is drawn using the 1-degree to 1-mm equivalence at the lateral cortex below the initial osteotomy. The two lines border the wedge that will be removed. The sagittal slope must be assessed throughout to avoid significant slope perturbations.

Surgical Techniques

Medial Opening Wedge. A 5-cm longitudinal skin incision is made midway between the tibial tubercle and the medial border of the tibia, beginning 1 cm below the medial joint line. The incision is carried down to the pes anserinus. A full-thickness, inverted, "trapdoor," L-shaped flap can be elevated or the pes tendons can be retracted distally after dividing the sartorial fascia. The proximal medial tibia is then exposed subperiosteally. The distal superficial medial collateral ligament fibers must be elevated off the medial tibia. If the distal superficial medial collateral ligament attachment is left intact, medial compartment pressures may increase as the ligament is tensioned across the joint during distraction of the osteotomy.[1]

Meticulous subperiosteal dissection is required, particularly posteriorly, with protection of the posterior neurovascular structures. The patellar tendon is then identified just proximal to its attachment on the tubercle, and a retractor is placed in the anterior interval to protect the tendon from the saw blade. When the proximal-medial tibia is fully exposed, a guide wire is inserted from the anteromedial border of the tibia, starting just proximal to the tibial tubercle and aiming toward the tip of the fibular head.

A second guide wire can be placed posteriorly to determine the angle of the cut in the sagittal plane. This angle can exert an effect on the tibial sagittal slope. The more superior the posterior guide wire is placed, the flatter the cut will be, resulting in a reduction in posterior tibial slope. The more inferior the wire is placed, the greater the increase in posterior slope. Some osteotomy systems have a saw guide that can be introduced over the guide wires at this point.

The osteotomy begins with a small oscillating saw to cut the anteromedial cortex. Osteotomes are advanced to a point within 1 cm of the lateral tibial cortex. The tip of the osteotome should lie where the vertical distance to the lateral plateau is 1.25 times the horizontal distance to the lateral tibial cortex (Fig. 121.4). This minimizes risk of fracture propagation into the lateral plateau. The tibia is then gently stressed in valgus to ensure that the osteotomy opens up slightly (Fig. 121.5). Calibrated wedges are sequentially introduced to open the osteotomy the desired amount (Fig. 121.6). The new mechanical axis can be confirmed by placing an alignment rod or a Bovie cord from the center of the hip to the center of the ankle and seeing where it crosses the knee.

Fixation. Overall, plate fixation seems to outperform external fixation.[84,96] Plates with spacer wedges have a lower failure rate than plates without.[84] Comparing modified Puddu plates (Arthrex, Naples, FL) with TomoFix plates (Synthes, West

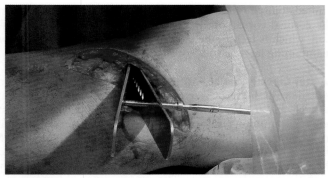

FIG 121.4 An adjustable osteotome is placed into the osteotomy, which will be gapped open slowly to allow for plastic deformation. This can be adjusted depending on the degree of correction desired.

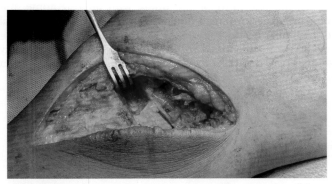

FIG 121.5 View of the open wedge created in the tibia.

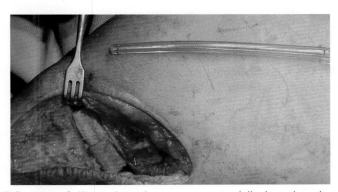

FIG 121.6 Calibrated wedges are sequentially introduced to open the osteotomy the desired amount and maintain the open wedge.

Chester, PA), Stoffel and coworkers[86] found that both plates provided adequate initial stability. However, if a lateral cortex fracture did occur, only the TomoFix plates maintained stability without requiring additional lateral fixation.

More recently, a nonabsorbable polyetheretherketone (PEEK) implant wedge placed flush with the medial cortex and secured by PEEK screws (iBalance; Arthrex) has been introduced (Fig. 121.7). Purported advantages of the implant include less hardware prominence and the option to perform concomitant ligamentous reconstructions through the plate.[21] Additionally, the device is inserted using a system that provides nearly circumferential protection to the soft tissues and neurovascular structures around the knee. Potential disadvantages include a limited ability to modify the sagittal slope independently from the coronal correction; the circumferential protector application, which is technically onerous; and insufficient rigidity for maintaining larger corrections (>12 degrees).[34]

Lateral Closing Wedge. An inverted anterolateral "L" incision is made with the vertical arm along the lateral edge of the tibial tubercle and the horizontal arm 1 cm distal to the lateral joint line. The common peroneal nerve is dissected 2 to 2.5 cm distal to the proximal fibular styloid, crossing the fibular neck, and protected. The incision is carried down to the periosteum, and the anterior compartment muscle is elevated subperiosteally from the anterolateral tibia. The anterior interval between the patellar tendon and the anterior tibia is protected with a retractor. Lateral closing wedge HTOs require management of the proximal tibiofibular joint. Options include disrupting the tibiofibular joint (usually with an osteotomy), resecting the medial one-third of the fibula with an osteotome and rongeur, or performing a fibular shaft osteotomy 10 cm distal to the fibular head.

The joint is identified with two needles, and the osteotomy guide is placed parallel to the needles and approximately 2 cm

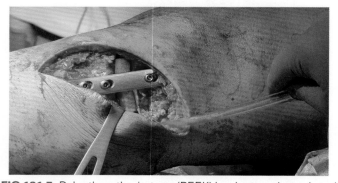

FIG 121.7 Polyetheretherketone (PEEK) implant wedges placed flush with the medial cortex and secured by PEEK screws.

below the joint line. Two smooth pins are then placed through the osteotomy guide to secure it to the bone. The plate can be provisionally applied over the pins to ensure that it will be parallel to the tibia's posterior slope. With the posterior neurovascular structures and the patellar tendon protected with retractors, the osteotomy is first made with a saw and then with osteotomes. The tip of the osteotome should end 2 cm distal to the joint line and 1 cm from the medial tibial cortex. A 5-mm drill hole can be placed in this location to relax stresses on the cortex.[47] Using the osteotomy guide, the desired amount of bone is resected. The plate is then reapplied over the smooth pins, and the pins are replaced with screws. The osteotomy is slowly closed using a clamp around the plate and through a distal 3.2-mm cortical hole in the tibia in line with the plate. Once the osteotomy is compressed, the remaining screws can be inserted and tightened (Fig. 121.8).

Dome Osteotomy. When the desired angle of correction exceeds 20 degrees, a dome osteotomy may be indicated. The osteotomy is typically performed as an inverted U–shaped bone cut proximal to the level of the tibial tubercle. This maintains the patellar height and allows for anterior translation of the tubercle (by shifting the distal tibia anteriorly). This may be beneficial in cases of concomitant patellofemoral disease. Dome osteotomies typically require resection of a portion of the fibular shaft.

A jig is placed, and anterior-to-posterior drill holes are created proximal to the tibial tubercle in a half-barrel configuration. The amount of angular correction is predetermined on the jig and denoted by Steinmann pins left in the proximal and distal fragments. The jig is removed, the posterior cortex is carefully violated with osteotomes, and the desired correction is performed including anteriorization of the distal fragment (with the tibial tubercle). Fixation is normally achieved with an external fixator. Disadvantages of dome HTOs include increased operative time and complexity, pin-site infections and patient discomfort while the external fixator is in place, and need for frequent follow-up visits. In adults, the procedure is generally reserved for massive corrections.

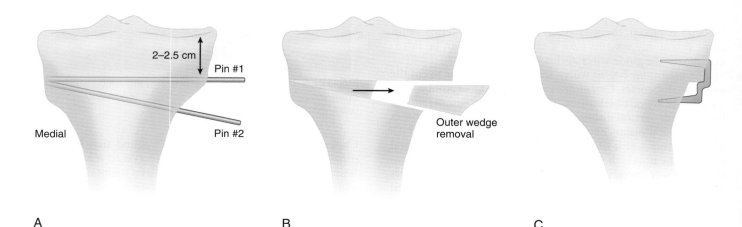

A   B   C

FIG 121.8 (A) The first guide wire is inserted parallel to the tibial articular surface approximately 2.0 to 2.5 cm below the joint line. The second guide wire, inserted at a point distally based on the preoperative calculation of actual tibial wedge height, is advanced obliquely to intersect at the medial tibial cortex with the first guide wire. (B) The outer 50% to 75% of the wedge is initially removed to allow completion of the inner portion of the wedge. (C) The tibia is stabilized by the insertion of two stepped staples bridging the osteotomy site.

Sagittal Deformity. The preservation of a normal sagittal slope (0 to 18 degrees) during an HTO is critical for isolated cases of coronal deformity. However, if desired (e.g., in cases of cruciate ligament insufficiency), the sagittal slope can be modified to augment stability. Medial opening wedge HTOs allow for some slope manipulation once the cut has been made. Although the tendency is for the slope to increase in these osteotomies, if the cut is made slightly posterosuperior to anteroinferior, and the spacer is placed posteriorly, the slope can be reduced. A closing wedge osteotomy also reduces the tibial slope. A reduced, flatter slope limits anterior translation in cases of ACL insufficiency. Conversely, an anteriorly placed spacer in an opening wedge HTO increases the posterior slope further. This may be desirable in cases of PCL insufficiency to mitigate posterior tibial translation.[75]

Outcomes

Opening Wedge Versus Closing Wedge. Overall, outcomes for opening wedge and closing wedge osteotomies for varus deformities are equivalent and are good to excellent. Closing wedge osteotomies have been found to have a survival of 95% at 5 years and 60% at 15 years. Birmingham and colleagues looked at 126 patients prospectively and demonstrated improved clinical outcomes and preservation of neutral alignment. In a trial of opening wedge versus closing wedge osteotomies, Brouwer and associates found both to be similar in terms of knee outcome scores, pain symptoms, and walking ability. A meta-analysis of nine comparative clinical trials concluded that opening wedge HTOs led to increased posterior slope, increased mean correction angle, and decreased patellar height.

Functional outcomes including pain scores and complications did not differ between the two techniques. A long-term follow-up comparative study of 412 Dutch patients concluded that opening wedge HTOs had a better 10-year survival than closing wedge HTOs (90% vs 75%) but a higher rate of complications including removal of hardware (71% in opening wedge, 48% in closing wedge). The rate of peroneal nerve sensory deficits in the closing wedge group was 4%. The rate of persistent pain at the iliac crest in the opening wedge group was 9.8%.[24,25] A 6-year follow-up randomized trial from the same group found a higher rate of conversion to TKA for the closing wedge group (22% vs 8% in the opening wedge group).[24] There were no differences in functional outcomes in patients who did not require conversion to a TKA.

Several studies have documented undercorrection of deformities with both techniques.[8,62] However, other studies have found good and equivalent correction accuracy.[33] A radiographic comparison study by Nerhus and associates[62] found that opening wedge HTOs increased sagittal slope by 1 degree even with careful preoperative planning, and closing wedge HTOs decreased it by 2.5 degrees. In their study, leg length was increased by a mean of 3.1 mm in opening wedge HTOs and decreased by a mean of 5.7 mm in closing wedge HTOs.

High Tibial Osteotomy Versus Unicompartmental Knee Arthroplasty. Several studies have confirmed that outcomes for UKA and HTOs are comparable. Broughton's 1986 retrospective study found 76% good results with UKA versus only 43% good results with lateral closing wedge HTO; however, newer studies have shown no difference in outcomes. Dettoni found similar clinical and radiographic outcomes between opening wedge HTO and UKA. Brouwer's meta-analysis determined there were no significant differences in outcomes between the two procedures. The 10-year survival does not differ between UKA and HTO.

A significant difference between the two procedures is that UKA requires patients to modify their activity postoperatively. This may make UKA better indicated for older patients. Furthermore, recovery from an HTO does have to take into account the requisite bone healing. HTOs are typically more painful in the immediate postoperative weeks. A meta-analysis by Spahn found similar 9- to 12-year survival for UKA and HTO (HTO 84.4% vs UKA 86.9%). Smith and colleagues[83] looked at cost-effectiveness of UKA versus TKA versus HTO and concluded that HTO provided better age-stratified cost-effectiveness in patients younger than age 60, whereas UKA was better in patients older than 60.

High Tibial Osteotomy and Subsequent Total Knee Arthroplasty. Any HTO changes fundamental anatomic relationships in the knee region, potentially complicating an ensuing TKA. Lateral closing wedge osteotomies have been implicated in problems including everting the patella, ligament balancing, and retained hardware necessitating removal. The risk of patella baja and changes in the sagittal slope may need to be addressed at the time of arthroplasty. van Raaij and associates[90] found longer surgical time, additional combined procedures, and greater postoperative knee stiffness in patients undergoing TKA after HTO. However, at midterm and long-term follow-up, there were no differences in outcomes between primary TKAs or post-HTO TKAs. Erak and colleagues found that 36 TKAs done after a prior opening wedge HTO had worse knee scores and more pain compared with 1315 primary TKAs.[28a] Han and coworkers[38] performed a systematic review of TKAs performed after opening wedge versus closing wedge HTOs and found that ultimately there were no differences in outcomes. However, the closing wedge group resulted in more intraoperative technical complexity during the TKA including a greater incidence of quadriceps snip, lateral tissue release, and TTO.[38]

Complications

Complication rates for HTOs between 7% and 55% have been reported. Asik and colleagues found that 9% of opening wedge HTOs required additional procedures. As with any procedure, there is a learning curve, and evidence points to reduced complication rates with accrued experience.[89] Amendola and associates[3] found that complication rate decreased from 15% to 8% over the course of several years.

For opening wedge HTOs, complications have included lateral tibial plateau fractures, medial collateral ligament injuries, hardware failure, hardware irritation (up to 40%), loss of correction, and nonunion.[3] Complications in closing wedge HTOs include peroneal nerve injury, fibular osteotomy nonunion, medial tibial cortex fracture, and anterior compartment syndrome.

In a large series of HTOs, Floerkmeier and colleagues concluded that positive predictors of postoperative Oxford Knee Score included male sex, no preoperative opioid use, and no operative complications. Age, body mass index, and smoking did not appear to have a negative effect on the score.

High Tibial Osteotomies and Concurrent Cartilage Procedures

Unloading cartilage has a favorable effect on healing. In the setting of a chondral restoration procedure, a concomitant

HTO may improve outcomes. In a series by Bauer and colleagues,[5] 18 patients with an HTO performed in conjunction with matrix-induced ACI had clinical improvement at 5 years, although MRI showed poor infill. Wong and colleagues[94] reported good clinical outcomes with HTO and mesenchymal stem cell intra-articular injections.

A systematic review assessed HTO with and without articular cartilage procedures or meniscus allograft transplantation and concluded that HTO combined with cartilage procedures led to excellent short-term and midterm survival and strong clinical outcomes, with deterioration after 10 years.[40] Bode and coworkers[6] published a series of 43 patients with HTO and ACI that showed improved cartilage survival and a decreased rate of revision in patients with mild varus of less than 5 degrees. Evidence for neutralizing the mechanical axis in the setting of a cartilage procedure continues to mount.

High Tibial Osteotomy and Anterior Cruciate Ligament Reconstruction

In cases of chronic ACL deficiency and knee varus, a combined procedure may yield satisfactory results. A systematic review by Li and associates[54] showed that in patients with a mean varus of 7.1 degrees and concomitant ACL deficiency, an HTO led to subjective improvements in knee scores. However, they also reported an overall high complication rate with a deep venous thrombosis rate of 7.7%. Trojani and colleagues[88] reported pain relief in 70% and return to sport in 80% of patients (mean age 43) after the combined ACL reconstruction/HTO procedure.

DISTAL FEMORAL OSTEOTOMY FOR VALGUS KNEE

Indications

Restoration of the mechanical axis is essential for the prevention of cartilage degradation and progression of arthritis in painful, valgus knees.[57,72] Although Coventry[18] and other authors[81] described proximal medial closing wedge tibial osteotomies for genu valgum deformity, they also suggested that DFOs were preferable if the valgus deformity exceeded 12 to 15 degrees or if the joint line obliquity was expected to exceed 10 degrees after the tibial osteotomy.

Using an HTO for severe valgus deformity can result in joint line obliquity and instability.[59,71,76] Conversely, DFO has the ability to address a complex valgus deformity by creating a transcondylar line perpendicular to the mechanical axis, minimizing medial-sided ligamentous laxity.[18] Similar to HTO for varus deformities, appropriate patient selection is critical for achieving optimal outcomes after DFO. Candidates for DFO include younger, active patients with valgus deformity and resultant isolated lateral compartment osteoarthritis. Patients younger than 60 years old are typically considered candidates; however, age must be considered within the context of other patient factors, such as activity level and overall health.[72]

Commonly accepted contraindications for DFO include inflammatory disease, ligamentous instability, extreme valgus deformity, severe tricompartmental osteoarthritis, osteonecrosis of the lateral femoral condyle, and bone loss. DFO is generally contraindicated in patients with rheumatoid arthritis or other inflammatory conditions because of associated ligamentous pathology and propensity for development of global knee arthritis. Valgus deformity greater than 20 degrees is a

TABLE 121.5   Indications and Contraindications for Distal Femoral Osteotomies

Indications	Contraindications
Valgus deformity	Inflammatory disease
Younger active patient	Ligamentous instability
Isolated lateral compartment syndrome	Extreme valgus deformity
	Severe tricompartmental osteoarthritis
	Osteonecrosis of lateral femoral condyle
	Bone loss
	Valgus deformity >20°

contraindication to DFO because of likely associated ligamentous instability (Table 121.5). This point was made emphatically by Puddu and colleagues,[72] who argued that severe valgus deformity associated with tibial subluxation of greater than 1 cm should be an absolute contraindication to osteotomy.

Whether obesity should be a contraindication remains unclear. Studies have demonstrated an association between obesity, defined as 1.32 times the normal weight or body mass index greater than 30 kg/m^2, and poorer outcomes after osteotomies about the knee.[7,18] However, some authors have argued that osteotomy provides a superior treatment option in obese patients compared with arthroplasty.[72] In all cases, weight loss should be encouraged, and general health must be optimized before considering DFO.

Whether or not to perform a DFO in the presence of concomitant patellofemoral compartment osteoarthritis is also controversial. Patellofemoral osteoarthritis has historically been considered a contraindication to DFO.[79,85] However, more recent studies suggest that a DFO decreases the Q angle and medializes the anterior tibial tubercle, reducing the lateral traction force on the patella and unloading the lateral patellofemoral compartment.[92,95] A study by Zarrouk and colleagues[95] examining DFO in patients with associated patellofemoral osteoarthritis found no difference in functional results compared with patients with isolated lateral unicompartmental osteoarthritis.

Physical Examination. A thorough physical examination is necessary for appropriate patient selection and preoperative planning. The examination should begin with inspection of the lower extremities, focusing on overall clinical alignment on both sagittal and coronal planes. Rotational malalignment may also be appreciated on examination. Palpation of the knee may reveal lateral joint line tenderness in the case of isolated lateral compartment arthritis. Patellofemoral arthritis and crepitus may also be detected with direct palpation. Range of motion (ROM) is an essential component of the preoperative examination. Although few studies have examined ROM and DFO, a study by Bonasia and coworkers[7] demonstrated that a preoperative ROM of less than 120 degrees of flexion is a negative prognostic factor in HTO.

A focused ligamentous examination is essential to determine knee stability. Varus and valgus stress testing at 0 and 30 degrees of flexion should be performed to assess fixed deformity. Meniscal injury is an important cause of progressive cartilage deterioration and deformity, and meniscal testing must be included in the examination. Gait analysis is useful to evaluate dynamic valgus deformity. A complete physical examination is important to rule out other causes of knee pain, such as spinal etiologies or referred pain from the hip.

Imaging

Complete radiographic evaluation allows for detailed characterization of the patient's deformity and is necessary for corrective osteotomy planning (Fig. 121.9). Initial assessment begins with standard anteroposterior, lateral, and sunrise views. Additionally, the posteroanterior weight-bearing 45 degrees flexion view (Rosenberg view) is useful to identify multicompartmental osteoarthritis.[74] Systematic reviews have found the Rosenberg view to have a higher sensitivity for detecting medial or lateral tibiofemoral compartment arthritis than standing anteroposterior views.[26] This view also has a strong predictive value for joint deformity associated with cruciate deficiency, as evidenced by chondral damage in the posterior tibial plateau.[72,74] The tibial slope can be evaluated on the standing lateral view of the knee. Finally, standing full-length weight-bearing lower extremity alignment films are used to measure the anatomic and mechanical axes.

Advanced imaging modalities are also useful for detecting associated knee pathology and alignment. MRI allows for adequate visualization of soft tissue structures including ligaments, menisci, and cartilage. MRI has the ability to identify early stages of osteoarthritis by demonstrating stress response of the subchondral bone.[71] Computed tomography (CT) can help to further characterize rotational malalignment; however, CT is associated with increased radiation exposure and is not always necessary.

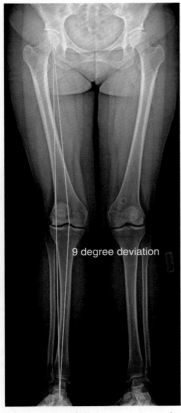

9 degree deviation

FIG 121.9 Weight-bearing full lower extremity x-ray demonstrating valgus deformity. This patient has 9 degrees of deviation from the mechanical axis.

Preoperative Decision Making

Preoperative planning is critical to determine the appropriate osteotomy and degree of correction for each individual patient. Options reported in the literature for valgus deformity include medial closing wedge DFO, lateral opening wedge DFO, dome osteotomy, and tibial lateral opening wedge osteotomy for tibial deformities.

Lateral opening wedge osteotomy is currently the preferred technique in the literature. The theoretical advantages of a lateral opening wedge technique include a single bone cut, better control over the degree of correction, avoidance of vascular structures, maintenance of axial and rotational stability with an intact medial hinge, and more anatomic correction of the typical pathoanatomy of excessive distal femoral valgus.[10,11] Potential disadvantages include irritation of lateral knee structures by hardware or surgical trauma and possibility of delayed union or nonunion.[10]

A medial closing wedge osteotomy has been suggested as a more favorable technique for patients with comorbidities predisposing to nonunion, such as smoking and obesity.[41,46,89] A distal femoral dome osteotomy offers the advantages of minimal surgical dissection, simultaneous correction of multiplanar deformity, high union rate, and avoidance of leg length discrepancy.[35,56] This technique may be preferable for patients with complex valgus deformities or existent leg length inequality.

Planning Degree of Correction

The degree of correction is based on measurements obtained from lower extremity alignment films. The mechanical axis of the lower extremity is measured from a straight line drawn from the center of the femoral head to the center of the talus and indicates the weight-bearing line of the knee. Sagittal plane deformity is assessed on the lateral radiograph, and tibial slope is measured. The osteotomy is planned according to the method originally described by Dugdale and colleagues.[23] The weight-bearing line is placed at a selected position 48% to 50% across the width of the tibial plateau as measured from the medial cortex. A line is then drawn from the center of the femoral head to weight-bearing position selected on the tibial plateau. Another line is drawn from the center of the talus to the same selected point on the tibial plateau. The correction angle is the angle formed by the intersection of these two lines. The wedge size for the osteotomy is determined by measuring the width of the femur at the proposed osteotomy site (Fig. 121.10).

The overall goal of correction differs between osteotomies for valgus and varus deformities. Although studies have demonstrated superior results with overcorrection of the deformity for valgus tibial osteotomies,[7] overcorrection has traditionally been discouraged for DFO, with a goal of producing a 0- to 2-degree difference between the mechanical and anatomic axes.[72] However, a biomechanical study by Quirno and coworkers[73] has challenged the concept of neutral correction for valgus deformity as a goal. The cadaveric study demonstrated progressive unloading of the lateral femoral compartment with increasing osteotomy angles, suggesting that overcorrecting the osteotomy by 5 degrees may restore near-normal contact pressures in the lateral compartment.

Surgical Technique

Lateral Opening Wedge Osteotomy. The patient is placed supine on the operating table with a small bump under the ipsilateral

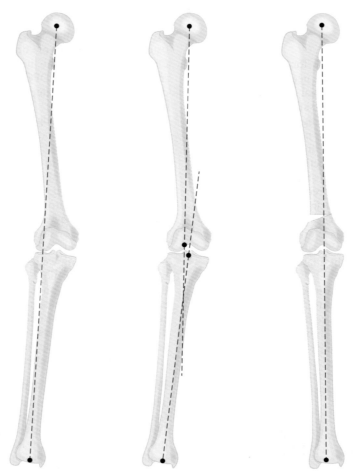

FIG 121.10 Assessment and planning of the amount of correction. The weight-bearing line is placed at a selected position 48% to 50% across the width of the tibial plateau as measured from the medial cortex. A line is then drawn from the center of the femoral head to weight-bearing position selected on the tibial plateau. Another line is drawn from the center of the talus to the same selected point on the tibial plateau. The correction angle is the angle formed by the intersection of these two lines. The wedge size for the osteotomy is determined by measuring the width of the femur at the proposed osteotomy site.

hip to maintain neutral alignment of the limb. A 10- to 15-cm longitudinal incision is made over the lateral aspect of the distal femur, starting approximately two fingerbreadths distal to the lateral epicondyle and extending proximally in line with the femur. The iliotibial band is incised in line with the incision, and the vastus lateralis is dissected off of the lateral intermuscular septum and retracted anteriorly. A retractor is placed posteriorly to protect the neurovascular structures. The femoral shaft and metaphysis is visualized, and the joint capsule typically remains intact. The knee is then flexed to 30 degrees to relax the posterior structures.

Two guide wires are passed through the distal femur under direct fluoroscopic guidance (Fig. 121.11). The first guide wire is passed parallel to the joint line through the epiphysis, and the second wire is inserted approximately three fingerbreadths above the lateral epicondyle and trochlear groove, angled obliquely at a 20-degree angle from proximal to distal toward the medial epicondyle. The cutting guide is placed perpendicular to the femur, and a 1-cm cut into the lateral cortex is made with an oscillating saw (Fig. 121.12).

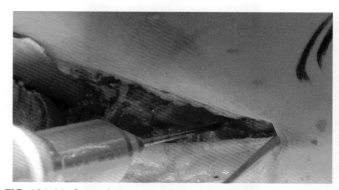

FIG 121.11 One of the two guide wires passed through the distal femur under direct fluoroscopic guidance can be seen being inserted here. The first guide wire is passed parallel to the joint line through the epiphysis, and the second wire is inserted approximately three fingerbreadths above the lateral epicondyle and trochlear groove, angled obliquely at a 20-degree angle from proximal to distal toward the medial epicondyle.

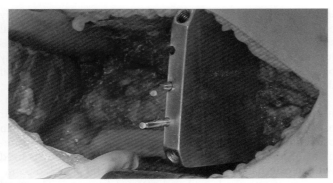

FIG 121.12 The cutting guide is then placed perpendicular to the femur, and a 1-cm cut into the lateral cortex is made with an oscillating saw.

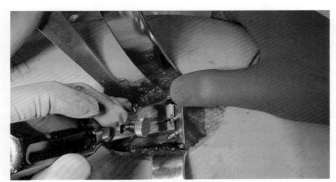

FIG 121.13 The osteotomy is completed with an osteotome, leaving a 1-cm medial hinge. The osteotomy site is distracted with gentle varus stress, and fluoroscopy is used to evaluate the mechanical axis.

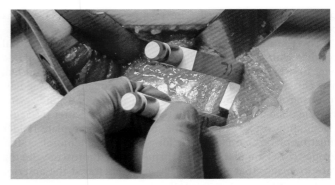

FIG 121.14 Tines of the wedge osteotome are placed within the osteotomy and slowly advanced. Marking on the tines can be used as a rough estimate of the angle of correction.

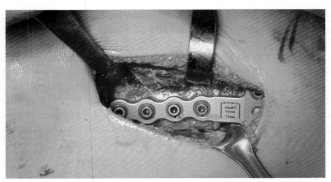

FIG 121.15 The plate is placed carefully on the bone so that the anterior tine does not impinge the patellofemoral joint at the lateral trochlea.

The osteotomy is completed with an osteotome, leaving a 1-cm medial hinge. The osteotomy site is distracted with gentle varus stress, and fluoroscopy is used to evaluate the mechanical axis (Fig. 121.13). The osteotomy should be opened equally, anteriorly and posteriorly. A plate or external fixator is used to achieve fixation at the osteotomy site at the desired level of distraction.[10,72,89]

Numerous different plates and instrumentation have been developed for lateral opening wedge DFO (Fig. 121.14). The mechanical advantage of lateral plates compared with medial-sided plates is that they act as a tension band. In a severely valgus knee, the mechanical axis is shifted laterally, resulting in the medial side of the knee becoming the tension side (Fig. 121.15). However, after the osteotomy, the mechanical axis is shifted medially, and the lateral femoral cortex becomes the tension side. This is due to the body weight acting as an extrinsic varus component.[72] The most commonly used implants available at the present time include the 95-degree blade plate, Puddu plates (Arthrex), VS plates (Biomet, Warsaw, IN), and TomoFix plates (Synthes, West Chester, PA). External fixation methods have also been employed to stabilize the osteotomy.[78]

Several types of graft materials are used to fill the gap formed by the osteotomy. The "gold standard" graft is iliac crest bone graft; however, it is associated with significant donor site morbidity, pain, and infection risk. Therefore, other graft options with osteoinductive, osteoconductive, or osteogenic properties have been increasingly used. Such grafts include allograft bone grafts and injectable synthetic bone substitutes (hydroxyapatite, beta-tricalcium phosphate, bone cement).[76] More recent studies have also suggested the use of platelet-rich plasma and growth factors for osteotomy graft sites.[49]

Medial Closing Wedge Osteotomy. The distal femoral medial closing wedge osteotomy was historically the most commonly performed osteotomy for genu valgum deformity. McDermott and colleagues[59] first described the technique using a 90-degree AO blade plate. In this approach, a straight 10- to 15-cm midline incision is made to expose the medial aspect of the distal femur. The approach has the benefit of allowing for easy conversion to TKA.

A medial skin flap is developed, and the vastus medialis is elevated from the medial septum and retracted anteriorly, exposing the medial femoral condyle. Contrary to a lateral opening wedge osteotomy, a small arthrotomy is made just proximal to the adductor tubercle to locate the joint line and intercondylar notch. Subperiosteal dissection of the medial femoral cortex assists in protecting the femoral vessels in the adductor canal. The knee is then flexed to 90 degrees, and a guide wire is placed across the joint, parallel to the articular surface of the femur.

Another guide wire is inserted approximately 2 cm proximal to the first pin in an anteromedial-to-posterolateral direction. This pin facilitates entry of the blade plate chisel. A third guide wire is inserted proximal and parallel to the second guide wire at the upper margin of the anterior aspect of the femoral condyle articular surface. The position of the guide pins is confirmed with fluoroscopy.

Three holes are drilled into the medial cortex of the femoral condyle with a 4.5-mm drill just proximal to the second guide wire to prevent cortical comminution as the chisel is inserted. The chisel is then placed through the holes in an anteromedial-to-posterolateral direction, parallel to the second guide wire. For the plate to be in line with the femoral shaft after insertion (facilitating osteosynthesis), the long arm of the plate holder must be placed parallel to the long axis of the femoral shaft.[93] Proper chisel angulation is confirmed with fluoroscopy, taking care to ensure that the chisel has not penetrated the anterior femoral cortex or intercondylar notch.

Converging pins placed medial to lateral are used to perform the osteotomy. Methylene blue (or another marking device) is used on the medial cortex to demarcate the levels of osteotomy. The distal osteotomy line is drawn along the line of the third guide wire, and the proximal osteotomy line is drawn 5 to 8 mm proximal to the first line medially and intersects with the first line laterally. An oscillating saw is used to perform the medial osteotomy. The 5- to 8-mm wedge of bone is removed, and the lateral cortex is perforated with three drill holes using a 4.5-mm drill bit. A varus stress is applied to the lower extremity to close the osteotomy site, and the 90-degree blade plate is applied along the medial femoral cortex. If the 90-degree blade plate is placed appropriately parallel to the transcondylar axis, the tibiofemoral angle will be 0 degrees (Figs. 121.16 and 121.17).[59,93]

Dome Osteotomy. The dome osteotomy is a less commonly employed technique that has the theoretical benefits of minimal surgical dissection and early rehabilitation. The technique was initially described for tibial osteotomy but has subsequently been modified by several authors for application in femoral deformities.[35,37,56]

Various techniques have been described, including percutaneous and open approaches, but all involve a semicircular osteotomy created with drill holes and completed with an osteotome. Correct alignment based on preoperative measurements is assessed with fluoroscopy, and the osteotomy is fixed with an external fixator,[56] lateral distal femoral plate,[35] or combination of retrograde nail and external fixation.[37] The distal femoral dome osteotomy has been reported for use in 20 degrees of correction and achieves stability with direct bone contact between the circular fragments, supporting earlier weight bearing and more efficient consolidation (Fig. 121.18).[56]

Tibial Osteotomies for Valgus Deformity. Before performing an osteotomy for genu valgum, it is important to determine the location of the deformity. Although femoral deformities are the most common causes of valgus malalignment, tibial-sided deformities may occasionally be the culprit, such as after a remote lateral tibial plateau fracture. When this is suspected, measurement of the center of rotation of angulation becomes critical.[14,58] The center of rotation of angulation is the angle formed from the intersection of the proximal and distal anatomic or mechanical axes of an extremity.

Both tibial medial closing wedge and tibial lateral opening wedge osteotomies have been described for use in correction of valgus deformity. As demonstrated by studies performed by Coventry,[18] Chambat and colleagues,[13] and Marti and colleagues,[58] tibial medial closing wedge osteotomy is a successful procedure when the joint surface tilt is less than 10 degrees.[72] Correction of greater than 10 degrees results in progressive lateral subluxation of the tibia.[81] Tibial osteotomies have the benefit of unloading the joint in both extension and flexion, whereas DFO is capable only of correcting in extension.[13] The indications for this procedure are less common than the indications for DFO, and most patients with indications for tibial-based procedures have posttraumatic deformity.[58]

The tibial medial closing wedge osteotomy is performed with the same medial proximal tibial approach that is used for the medial tibial opening wedge osteotomy. A pin is inserted from

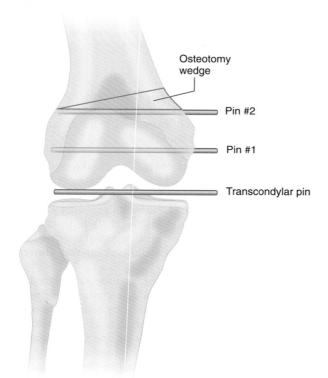

FIG 121.16 Diagram depicting placement of the transcondylar pin, the location of pin no. 1 for entry of the blade plate, and the location of pin no. 2 used for the inferior portion of the osteotomy wedge. A truly parallel position of the transcondylar pin and blade plate entry is essential to obtain a neutral mechanical axis.

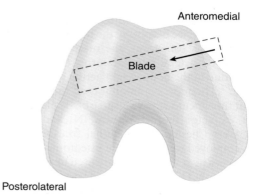

FIG 121.17 The blade plate should be inserted obliquely in an anteromedial-to-posterolateral direction to avoid penetration of the intercondylar notch or the anterior femoral articular surface.

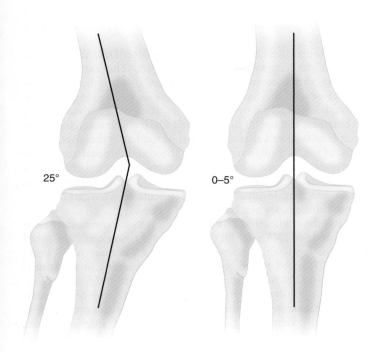

25°   0–5°

FIG 121.18 Dome osteotomy demonstrating the anatomic axis angle is corrected at a value of 0 to 5 degrees sliding the proximal fragment through the semicircular osteotomy.

medial to lateral and from distal to proximal. The osteotomy is performed with an oscillating saw and completed with an osteotome. Care is taken to leave approximately 5 mm of intact lateral tibial cortex. A varus stress is applied, and restoration of the mechanical axis is assessed with fluoroscopy. The osteotomy is then fixed with a plate or staples.

Collins and associates[14] have described the technique for tibial lateral opening wedge osteotomy as a viable surgical option for patients with genu valgum and tibial deformity. An anterolateral longitudinal incision is made lateral to the tibial tuberosity, and anterior compartment muscles are elevated off the tibia and retracted posteriorly. The capsule of the proximal tibiofibular joint is incised anteriorly, and the posterior soft tissues are elevated off the tibia. Care is taken to protect the neurovascular structures. The osteotomy is performed with the use of a guide pin positioned 1.5 to 2.0 cm below the level of the articular surface and 1 to 1.5 cm from the medial cortex. A microsagittal saw is used to begin the osteotomy, and it is completed with an osteotome. The saw blade must be positioned parallel to the tibial slope to prevent changes in the sagittal kinematics of the knee. The osteotomy site is distracted and fixed with a plate. Bone graft is often used.

Clinical Outcomes

Numerous more recent studies have demonstrated good to excellent functional outcomes and survival for lateral distal femoral opening wedge osteotomy to correct valgus deformity of the knee. Puddu and colleagues[72] presented excellent results with the use of their Puddu plate, which has subsequently been used in other studies. Dewilde and coworkers[21] performed DFOs secured with the Puddu plate and used calcium phosphate cement to fill the osteotomy gap. These authors demonstrated

a significant improvement in average knee scores and 82% survival rate at 7 years of follow-up.[21] Thein and associates[87] similarly demonstrated significant improvement in functional and satisfaction scores with lateral opening wedge DFO and iliac crest bone graft. Additionally, they found no worsening of arthritic changes on subsequent radiographs, full incorporation of bone graft, and no hardware failure with a median follow-up of 6.5 years. Ekeland and colleagues[27] reported their good functional results with lateral opening wedge DFO with Puddu plates and iliac crest bone graft. Their findings were consistent with prior studies with an osteotomy survival rate of 88% at 5 years and 74% at 10 years.[27]

Favorable results have also been demonstrated with other types of implants for lateral opening wedge DFO. The TomoFix plate has frequently been used for proximal tibial osteotomies and is considered to be more stable, allowing earlier weight bearing.[76,86] Jacobi and coworkers[46] reported 14 patients who underwent lateral opening wedge DFO. They found delayed osteotomy healing and significant hardware irritation as a result of the iliotibial band rubbing on the plate. The outcomes improved to 86% satisfactory once the plate was removed and the osteotomy healed.[46] Saithna and colleagues[77] used both Puddu plates and TomoFix plates, with bone graft used if wedge opening was greater than 12 mm. These authors also noted significant improvement in pain scores, with a 5-year survival rate of 79%. Although not statistically significant, four patients in the study required revision fixation, and three of these patients had their original fixation with Puddu plates.[77] Overall, reoperation rate was common for hardware prominence, nonunion, loss of correction, infection, and persistent symptoms including pain and stiffness.

There is a greater body of literature examining the outcomes of medial closing wedge osteotomies. Most studies report on outcomes using the 90-degree blade plate, but good functional results have been demonstrated with the use of a malleable semitubular plate[85] and angle-stable locking plate.[30] Wang and Hsu[92] reported 83% satisfactory results and 87% 10-year survival using the McDermott technique with a 90-degree dynamic compression plate. Improvement in patellar tracking was also noted in seven of eight knees with associated patellofemoral arthritis.[92]

Backstein and associates[4] performed one of the longest term outcome studies of distal femoral medial closing wedge osteotomies in the literature and found results similar to Wang and Hsu at 10-year follow-up. However, the authors noted a precipitous decrease in survival after 10 years with a reported 45% survival rate at 15 years.[4] Kosashvili and colleagues[51] also noted satisfactory outcomes within the first 10 years after medial closing wedge DFO and conversion to TKA is expected to be required in approximately half of all patients at a mean of 15.6 years.

Complications. The complications of DFO are frequently divided into intraoperative and postoperative complications.[76] Intraoperative complications include fracture, hinge disruption, and neurovascular injury. Fractures may propagate proximally, through the far cortex, or may become intra-articular if the guide pin is placed too close to the articular surface. Disruption of the medial hinge during lateral wedge opening may result in displacement of the osteotomy, requiring a contralateral screw or staple.[72,76] Neurologic injury is most common after tibial-sided osteotomy but may occur during distal femur closing wedge osteotomy owing to the proximity of neurovascular structures supplying the vastus medialis muscle.[91] The etiology of neurologic injury is most commonly traction or compression and less commonly secondary to laceration or pin penetration. The risk of neurologic injury may be mitigated with careful retractor placement including protection of neurovascular structures during the approach.

Postoperative complications may further be divided into minor and major complications. Minor complications include superficial infection, pin-site infection with use of external fixators, hardware prominence and irritation, and arthrofibrosis. Hardware irritation is more significant for lateral opening wedge DFO.

Major postoperative complications are less common and include thromboembolic events, deep infection, compartment syndrome, nonunion, malunion, loss of correction, and overcorrection. The rate of deep venous thrombosis has been reported to be comparable to the rate in TKA.[76] The risk of compartment syndrome is small and is greater in tibial-sided osteotomies.[52] Nonunion is more common for opening wedge DFO. The use of bone autograft may also result in postoperative pain and donor site morbidity (Table 121.6).

Distal Femoral Osteotomy and Concurrent Cartilage Preservation Procedures

Combining DFO and cartilage preservation procedures is appealing in young patients because it both corrects the malalignment—the source of uneven load distribution and resultant cartilage damage—and addresses the cartilage deficiencies. The most commonly performed concomitant procedures are meniscal transplantation and articular cartilage repair, both of which have reported successful functional outcomes.[11,22,39] Of the various cartilage procedures, the most frequently used are microfracture, ACI, and osteochondral autograft or allograft. Although these procedures have an overall high rate of reoperation, they have been demonstrated to significantly delay the need for TKA in most patients. Cameron and colleagues[11] compared a group of patients with isolated symptomatic lateral compartment arthritis who underwent DFO alone with patients who underwent DFO and joint preservation procedures and found the conversion rate to TKA at 5 years to be 26% in the isolated DFO group and 8% in the DFO and joint preservation group.

Total Knee Arthroplasty After Distal Femoral Osteotomy

Although successful outcomes have been reported with DFO procedures in recent decades, many patients eventually require TKA. Numerous studies have reported on the results of TKA after HTO; however, there is a paucity of data regarding TKA after DFO.

Postoperative changes in alignment after DFO may present several challenges for subsequent TKA. The extra-articular femoral varus deformity that is produced through the osteotomy may result in the femoral anatomic axis intersecting with the lateral femoral condyle instead of the intercondylar notch. Therefore, the use of an intramedullary alignment guide may result in relative varus angulation of the femoral component.[61] Also, resection of more bone of the distal femoral condyle is necessary to create a neutral mechanical axis in patients with a postoperative femoral varus extra-articular deformity. This resection may result in lateral ligamentous laxity, which may pose difficulties when balancing the knee.[60]

For the studies that do exist, satisfactory outcomes have been reported for TKA after DFO. Nelson and coworkers[61] evaluated nine patients who underwent TKA at an average of 14 years after DFO and found significant improvement in functional scores and arc of motion (average of 81.8 to 105.9 postoperatively). A constrained prosthesis was required in 5 of 11 knees. Despite these results, the authors noted that the procedure is technically demanding and associated with inferior results compared with primary procedures.[61] Kosashvili and associates[50] noted similar improvement in functional results in their cohort of 22 patients and concluded that standard components provide satisfactory stability in TKA, and history of DFO does not dictate the need for constrained components.

TIBIAL TUBERCLE OSTEOTOMY FOR PATELLOFEMORAL JOINT ARTHRITIS

Indications

Patellofemoral arthritis is an extremely common[63] and often crippling condition that has confounded practitioners for years. Although often refractory to treatment, new understanding of the complexities and mechanics of the regional anatomy has expanded treatment options. TTO (or tibial tubercle transfer), with or without chondral resurfacing, has been incorporated into the armamentarium for treatment of patellofemoral arthrosis and joint overload.

Anatomy and Biomechanics

The PFJ is biomechanically complex. Comprehensive understanding of its anatomy, mechanics, and static and dynamic restraints will help triage the best surgical candidates (Fig. 121.19). Bony stability is provided by the congruency between the patella and trochlea. Soft tissue restraints include an envelope surrounding the patella with the medial structures (medial patellofemoral ligament, medial patellar retinaculum) being stronger than the lateral ones.[12]

During normal knee flexion and extension, large amounts of contact and sheer stresses are placed across the PFJ. Joint reactive forces increase more with knee flexion (Fig. 121.20).[43] Activities such as squatting and stair climbing can increase forces across the compartment to multiple times body weight. With repetitive high stresses, wear patterns on the trochlea, patellar facets, or both can develop. Risk factors for accelerated wear include hypermobility, tilting (lateral overload), patellar height (alta vs baja), and increased Q angle (Fig. 121.21). Abnormal limb alignment including excessive femoral

TABLE 121.6	Possible Complications of Distal Femoral Osteotomies	
	POSTOPERATIVE	
Intraoperative	**Minor**	**Major**
Fracture		
Hinge disruption	Superficial infection	Thromboembolism
Neurovascular injury	Pin site infection	Deep infection
	Hardware prominence/ irritation	Compartment syndrome
	Arthrofibrosis	Nonunion/malunion
		Loss of correction/ overcorrection

anteversion and varus or valgus malalignment can overload the PFJ further (Table 121.7).Wear patterns tend to concentrate[32] more laterally than medially, suggesting lateral overload as an overriding factor in facet arthritis.

The primary indications for TTO in the setting of PFJ arthritis are persistent pain, swelling, and mechanical symptoms despite conservative treatment. The specific type of procedure used depends on a multitude of factors. TTO should be considered if the patella is excessively lateral to the tuberosity as a result of extensor mechanism malalignment (e.g., tibial tuberosity–trochlear groove [TT-TG] distance >20 mm) or excessively high (Caton-Deschamp index >1.2) in patients with large focal defects of the patella or trochlea.[80] The TT-TG distance is the space between the tibial tubercle (TT) and trochlear groove of the femur (TG). It is calculated by drawing a line tangent to the posterior epicondyle and then drawing a line perpendicular to it, through the deepest point of the trochlea, and a third line parallel to the second through the most anterior portion of the tibial tuberosity. Large TT-TG distances are associated with patellar instability.[12] The Caton-Deschamp index is a ratio of the distance between the lowest articular point on the patella to the top of the tibial plateau, divided by the length of the articular surface of the patella. Caton-Deschamp index greater than 1.2 is considered patella alta. Patients with normal proximal and medial patellar cartilage surfaces may be considered for an isolated anteromedialization (AMZ) of the tibial tubercle (or Fulkerson osteotomy).

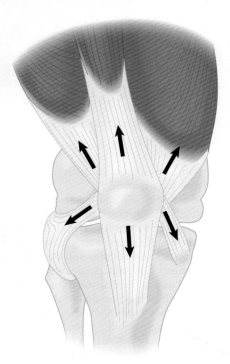

FIG 121.19 The multiple forces being pulled on the patella including the various quadriceps muscles and surrounding ligaments.

TABLE 121.7 Factors That Increase the Amount of Wear on Patellar Cartilage
Variously shaped bones
Hypermobility
Tilting (lateral overload)
Patellar height (alta vs baja)
Increased Q angle
Femoral version rotation
Varus or valgus alignment
Core strength
Pelvic obliquity
Quadriceps dynamics

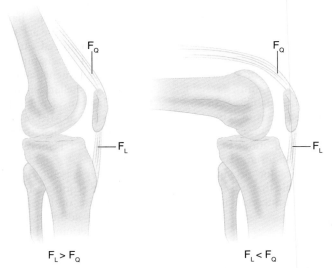

$$F_L > F_Q \qquad F_L < F_Q$$

FIG 121.20 It can be seen how the ratio of force on the patella engaged in flexion to patella (not engaged) in extension changes drastically. While in flexion, there is considerably more stress.

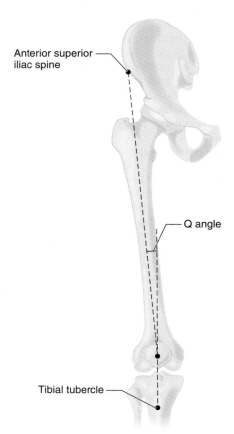

FIG 121.21 The Q angle is calculated as the angle formed by a line drawn from the anterior superior iliac spine to the central patella and a second line drawn from the central patella to the tibial tubercle. An increased Q angle is a risk factor for patellar subluxation because this indicates increased lateral pull on the patella. The normal angle is 14 degrees for men and 17 degrees for women.

The indications for AMZ in patients with TT-TG distances of 15 to 20 mm are less clear. In the treatment of lateral patellar or trochlear chondral disease or lateral facet overload syndrome, AMZ may play a role in cases of borderline tuberosity positions (TT-TG distance = 15 mm), in which case the goal remains to normalize and not overmedialize.[80]

Straight anteriorization is indicated to unload large distal patellar chondral lesions, bipolar kissing lesions, or arthritis in the setting of a normal TT-TG distance (<15 mm). Straight anteriorization is not indicated for patellar instability.[80] In any AMZ, overmedialization should be stringently avoided because it would overload the medial patella and trochlea. However, AMZ is not a panacea, and patients with indications for AMZ must be selected judiciously. A study by Pidoriano and colleagues[70] showed poor results in surgeries for proximal or medial chondrosis of the patella. It is possible that novel chondral resurfacing procedures may improve outcomes in these patients.

History and Physical Examination

A trial of conservative treatment should be exhausted before considering surgical options. A history of swelling, catching, or locking may suggest a chondral lesion. The onset, nature, and

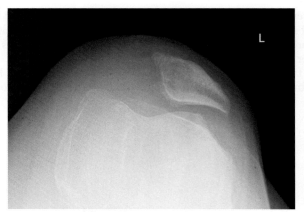

FIG 121.22 Merchant view demonstrating a laterally set patella.

location of the pain are essential in differentiating a degenerative condition from pure instability.

Patellofemoral syndrome and secondary evaluation of degenerative arthritis is not limited to the joint itself. An overall assessment of the lower extremity is vital. This includes core strength, hip rotation, quadriceps strength, symmetry, and foot alignment. A complete knee examination should be performed to rule out other sources of pain. A concentrated examination of the patella should include evaluation of patellar height, patellar tilt, retinacular tightness, Q angle (14 degrees for men and 17 degrees for women on average), the J sign, crepitus, and palpation for effusions. Instability should be assessed by the apprehension test. It is very important to differentiate between pure instability, instability combined with chondral lesions, and pure osteoarthritis. The potential treatment options differ with each diagnosis.

Imaging

Routine and advanced imaging studies are necessary to gain a better understanding of the location and extent of chondral damage. Patellar tilt, patellar height, degenerative patterns, and subluxation all can be assessed with basic x-rays. Radiographic views should include weight-bearing anteroposterior, flexed, standard lateral, and Merchant (Fig. 121.22) or Lauren views.[15]

Multiple techniques have been derived to measure patellar height. Among these are the Insall-Salvati index (the length of the patella compared with the patellar tendon), Labelle-Laurin index, Caton-Deschamps index, and Blackburne-Peel index. These measurements all can be derived by standard x-rays or MRI or CT. Patellar height is particularly important if distalization is being considered. Patellar tilt is evaluated by the Merchant view on x-ray or MRI or CT. This measurement is important if lateral release or lengthening is being considered to alleviate lateral overload. Femoral anteversion is best evaluated with CT scan.

If surgery is being considered, imaging studies such as MRI and CT are required. These advanced studies provide a better understanding of the particular wear patterns and the extent of damage. In addition, evaluation of the three-dimensional anatomy ascertained by these studies is critical in determining the exact nature of the surgical intervention. The individual's unique interactions between the tibial tubercle, patella, trochlea, and femoral anteversion can be assessed, and this information can be used to form a patient-specific surgical approach.

The TT-TG distance described by Dejour and colleagues[20] is defined as the distance between the trochlear groove and the tibial tubercle (Fig. 121.23) and is critical to operative planning. This distance can be obtained by either CT scan or MRI. A TT-TG distance greater than 15 mm on CT—MRI has been shown to slightly overestimate the TT-TG distance by 2 to 3 mm—is consistent with instability. Trochlear depth is also an important factor that needs to be determined preoperatively. This can be measured with the crossing sign—a term used to determine the floor of the trochlea crossing the lateral lip of the trochlea.

Preoperative Planning and Patient Selection

A patient must be prepared for an extensive rehabilitation period and the possibility of further procedures in the future. After all x-rays and advanced imaging studies have been obtained, assessing the exact wear pattern or location of chondral defects is imperative. This assessment allows the surgeon to determine and customize the TTO to best fit the lesion or location of the degenerative joint disease, providing the proper amount of medial or anterior movement of the osteotomy.

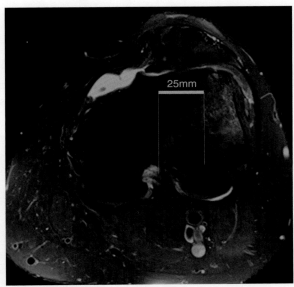

FIG 121.23 Magnetic resonance imaging–derived tibial tubercle–trochlear groove measurement. This measurement is ascertained by superimposing two cuts, one clearly demonstrating the groove and one of the tubercle, and measuring the distance between the two. A value greater than 15 mm is concerning for patellar subluxation.

AMZ, or straight anteriorization, may be contraindicated with wear patterns that are localized either proximally or medially, potentially overloading the contact stress in these regions (Fig. 121.24). Additionally, patellar height, tilt, and instability patterns, if present, need to evaluated for proper preoperative planning. With the popularization of chondral-sparing technologies, the indications for TTO have expanded. However, incorporation of these techniques with TTO requires additional planning. Autologus Chondrocyte Implantation (Vericel, Ann Arbor, MI), BioCartilage (Arthrex), and shelf allograts (Biomet) must be obtained and available during the index TTO.

Diagnostic arthroscopy and possible scraping procedures are often used as an adjunct to TTO to evaluate the exact size and location of the wear patterns or lesions. Evaluation and location of normal cartilage may define the amount and angle of necessary mechanical realignment and thus influence clinical outcomes.[70]

Surgical Techniques for Patellofemoral Osteotomy

Anteromedialization. Popularized by Fulkerson in 1983,[31] AMZ is the workhorse for TTO and addresses both degenerative conditions and instability patterns. An arthroscopic examination is often done to confirm the subtleties of the wear pattern, which might influence the bony cut. Lateral release, if indicated, should be performed at this time. This oblique osteotomy is performed through a midline incision based over the tibial tubercle. The incision is lengthened proximally if additional chondral procedures are indicated necessitating patellar eversion. Guided systems are available for more precise osteotomy and tissue protection (Fig. 121.25). Skin flaps are raised, and the patellar tendon is freed. Capsulotomies of the patellar tendon are performed medially and laterally and continued distally.

Subperiosteal dissection of the anterior lateral musculature is performed, and retractors are gently placed to protect the lateral neurovascular structures (anterior tibial artery and deep peroneal nerve). Full medial and lateral visualization of the patellar tendon is essential before proceeding with the osteotomy. The shingle is now marked and prepared.

The slope of the cut is determined by the amount of anteriorization indicated. The greater the slope, the more the contact stress is relieved. A 45-degree or 60-degree slope cut is standard depending on the amount of unloading desired. With constant anteriorization of 15 mm, a 60-degree slope creates approximately 9 mm of medialization, whereas a 45-degree slope provides 15 mm of medialization. Less medialization can also be achieved with less anteriorization.[80]

A 5- to 6-cm, slightly oblique cut tapering anteriorly or distally is made from proximal to distal, slightly longer

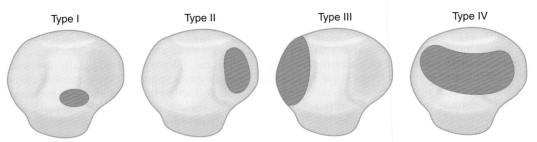

Type I   Type II   Type III   Type IV

FIG 121.24 Quadrants of the patella. It is important to consider localized patellar wear patterns that are localized either proximally or medially, potentially overloading the contact stress in these regions.

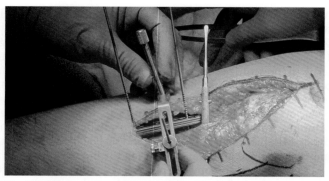

FIG 121.25 Anteromedialization guide placed over the tibia, determining the extent of the medial-to-lateral cutting. The stylus can be placed to determine where the saw blade will emerge.

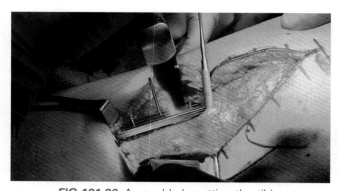

FIG 121.26 A saw blade cutting the tibia.

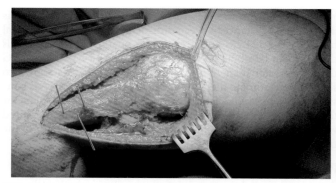

FIG 121.27 Once the osteotomy is placed, two bicortical pins and one cross pin are inserted to keep the osteotomy in place.

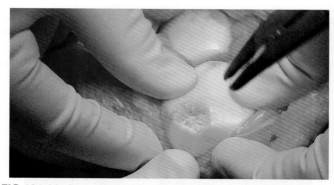

FIG 121.28 A patellar articular surface localized cartilage lesion.

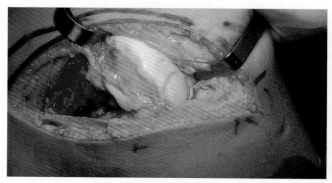

FIG 121.29 An osteochondral allograft being used to fill a defect on the lateral femoral condyle.

if distalization of the patella is indicated. Cutting guides and alignment tools (e.g., Arthrex, Depuy) should be used to assist the surgeon in making the precise osteotomy, while protecting soft tissue and avoiding fracture. A large saw is used from antero-medial to posterolateral to begin the cut (Fig. 121.26), but it is completed with large osteotomes for safety. The osteotomy is completed with proximal transverse cuts, and the shingle is gently toggled. Typically, only 1 to 1.5 cm of movement is needed to correct the abnormal TT-TG distance. Care is taken to avoid fracture to the most distal part of the shingle, and gentle medi-alization and anteriorization of the tuberosity is performed. Temporary fixation (Fig. 121.27) is then achieved, while the alignment, ROM, and tracking are evaluated. Once the surgeon is satisfied with x-ray confirmation, the osteotomy is perma-nently fixed with two lag 4.5-mm compression screws, counter-sinking each screw. The wound is closed in a standard fashion, and the fascia may be left open to avoid potential compartment issues if the surgeon chooses.[31] Straight anteriorization tech-niques such as the Maquet have been obviated by AMZ modifi-cation and extreme slope precluding the need for bone graft. This can minimize the potential complications associated with the Maquet osteotomy, such as nonunion or delayed union, kneeling pain, skin necrosis, and graft site pain. These proce-dures have fallen out of favor because of the deterioration of pain relief over time and relatively high complication rate.[53]

Associated Chondral-Sparing Procedures

Younger patients with associated chondral lesions are ideal candidates for AMZ with concomitant cartilage-sparing proce-dures (Fig. 121.28). As we have gained insight into the benefits

of these treatments, the surgical indications have expanded for TTO. Unloading the patella and trochlea can be achieved with a combined approach. The osteotomy can be performed with a variety of potential off-the-shelf and cell-based technologies, including ACI, DeNovo, and BioCartilage associated microfrac-ture as well as chondral allograft (Fig. 121.29) and autograft techniques. Newer shelf allografts for trochlear defects are becoming more popular for their abilities to custom fit the graft.

Microfracture of the patella does not seem to have the same positive results as with the femoral condyle and should not be used in and of itself as a primary chondral-sparing procedure. Adjuncts such as BioCartilage or Autologous Matrix-Induced Chondrogenesis (AMIC) may in the future prove to enhance results by promoting tissue fill, although long-term studies are still pending. DeNovo (juvenile allograft chondrocyte) (Fig.

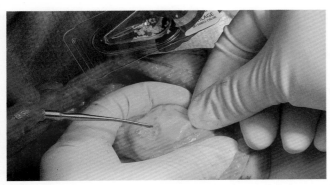

FIG 121.30 DeNovo (juvenile allograft chondrocyte) being used to fill the lesion.

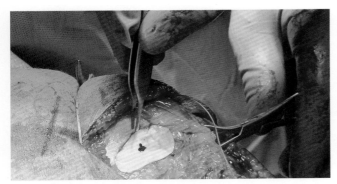

FIG 121.31 The membrane is soaked in autologous chondrocyte and stitched using 6-0 suture. The seal should be watertight.

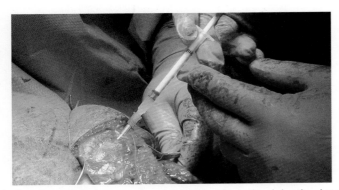

FIG 121.32 Autologous chondrocyte implantation injection into the potential space created by the sewn membrane.

121.30) is an off-the-shelf one-stage technique that has shown promising results when combined with AMZ[9]; however, long-term studies are still pending. ACI (Figs. 121.31 and 121.32), although an expensive two-procedure technique, currently holds the most promise when combined with AMZ for long-term relief of symptoms, with studies showing up to 11 years of relief.[36]

Complications

The results of these techniques are far from predictable, and even with the most meticulous surgical procedure, chronic postoperative pain can exist. Patients must be prepared for the long and arduous rehabilitation process and subsequent mechanical education that is associated with an optimal outcome. Nonunion of the osteotomy has been reported in 5.9% of cases.[55] Proximal tibia fracture has also been reported. Wound infections and skin necrosis from overzealous anteriorization is common. Compartment syndrome, a more serious complication, has also been reported, and early recognition of this syndrome is of paramount importance.

Outcomes

Outcome trends associated with positive results seem to be related to a combined approach that includes AMZ with chondral-sparing procedures. As mentioned earlier, the study by Pidoriano and colleagues[70] showed good results with AMZ for distal and lateral lesions and worse results with proximal and medial degeneration. Fulkerson[19] had success for up to 12 years with TTO, especially in the younger patient population with osteoarthritis (OA). However, the study by Farr[29] showed vast improvement in success rate when combining AMZ with ACI. Results seem to be better in younger patients with focal rather than global pathology. Pain relief may take 3 years in some instances.

CONCLUSION

Properly selected patients who have failed conservative treatments may be candidates for TTO, often combined with biologic procedures. This synergistic approach can improve the eventual outcome and has created new indications for reconstructive degenerative patellofemoral surgery. Meticulous preoperative planning and determination of the proper amount of correction can lead to predictable positive results in younger patients with focal lesions, minimizing complications frequently associated with older techniques.

KEY REFERENCES

2. Amendola A, Bonasia DE: Results of high tibial osteotomy: review of the literature. *Int Orthop* 34:155–160, 2010.
10. Bugbee WD: Distal femoral varus osteotomy for correction of valgus deformity. In Shetty A, Kim S-J, Nakamura N, et al, editors: *Tech Cartil Repair Surg*, 2014, pp 35–47.
12. Caton JH, Dejour D: Tibial tubercle osteotomy in patello-femoral instability and in patellar height abnormality. *Int Orthop* 34:305–309, 2010.
18. Coventry M: Proximal tibial varus osteotomy for osteoarthritis of the lateral compartment of the knee. *J Bone Joint Surg Am* 69:32–38, 1987.
19. Buuck DA, Fulkerson JP: Anteromedialization of the tibial tubercle: a 4- to 12-year follow-up. *Oper Tech Sports Med* 8:131–137, 2000.
21. Dewilde TR, et al: Opening wedge distal femoral varus osteotomy using the Puddu plate and calcium phosphate bone cement. *Knee Surg Sports Traumatol Arthrosc* 21:249–254, 2013.
29. Farr J: Autologous chondrocyte implantation improves patellofemoral cartilage treatment outcomes. *Clin Orthop Relat Res* 463:187–194, 2007.
32. Fulkerson JP, Buuck DA: Patellar tilt/compression and the excessive lateral pressure syndrome (ELPS). In Merrit J, editor: *Disord Patellofemoral Jt*, ed 4, Philadelphia, 2004, Lippincott Williams & Wilkins.
72. Puddu G, et al: Which osteotomy for a valgus knee? *Int Orthop* 34:239–247, 2010.
74. Rosenberg T, et al: The forty-five-degree posteroanterior flexion weight-bearing radiograph of the knee. *J Bone Joint Surg Am* 70:1479–1483, 2013.

75. Rossi R, et al: The role of high tibial osteotomy in the varus knee. *J Am Acad Orthop Surg* 19:590–599, 2011.

80. Sherman SL, et al: Tibial tuberosity osteotomy: indications, techniques, and outcomes. *Am J Sports Med* 42:2006–2017, 2013.

82. Smith TO, et al: Opening- or closing-wedged high tibial osteotomy: a meta-analysis of clinical and radiological outcomes. *Knee* 18:361–368, 2011.

84. Spahn G, et al: Biomechanical investigation of different internal fixations in medial opening-wedge high tibial osteotomy. *Clin Biomech (Bristol, Avon)* 21:272–278, 2006.

89. Uquillas C, et al: Osteotomies about the knee: AAOS exhibit selection. *J Bone Joint Surg Am* 96:e199, 2014.

The references for this chapter can also be found on www.expertconsult.com.

122

Osteotomy for the Arthritic Knee: A European Perspective

Simone Cerciello, Sébastien Lustig, Elvire Servien, Philippe Neyret

OSTEOTOMY: GENERAL CONCEPTS AND INDICATIONS

Before the introduction of unicompartmental* and total knee arthroplasty (TKA) into clinical medicine,[32,39,101] an osteotomy of the knee was the treatment of choice for gonarthrosis.[24,29,57,81] It has a long past dating back to the 19th century.[125] Today however, an osteotomy is considered technically difficult for many surgeons and demanding for the patient. Nevertheless, osteotomies remain an important treatment option for arthritis of the knee in our daily practice because they offer several advantages over prostheses, such as proprioceptivity, bone stock preservation, return to a high level of activity including sports,[2] and lower costs. In addition, they can be associated with specific treatments for cartilage damage such as abrasion, microfractures, and autologous chondrocyte transplantation or meniscal allograft with encouraging results.[16,42,110] Finally, they can delay the need for total knee prosthesis in young and active patients. The indications for osteotomy should be defined and numerous variables have to be taken into account: the type of arthritis, clinical and radiologic criteria, and the level of expectations of the patient.

Why an Osteotomy?

The surgical management of gonarthrosis includes three types of interventions: osteotomies, unicompartmental arthroplasty (UKA), and TKA. Considering the improvement of the outcome of total[32,39,101] and unicompartmental[20,64,91] knee arthroplasties reported in recent years, the legitimate question arises of the necessity of osteotomies. The final choice of intervention will largely depend on the patient's history, functional complaints, motivations, clinical examinations, and radiologic findings.

Anatomic and Clinical Findings. Anatomic findings have to be considered: the stage of osteoarthritis (OA), the analysis of the deformity and its reducibility, ligamentous status (frontal and sagittal laxity), and the range of motion. Clinical findings are of course essential too: weight, age, level of activity, autonomy, general conditions (diabetes, rheumatoid arthritis, use of anticoagulants), and surgical history. The decision to perform a certain type of intervention is also sometimes influenced by geographic factors (an osteotomy is more frequently performed in regions close to the poles, and a prosthesis is more common in regions away from the poles), cultural factors (osteotomy is more frequent in Asia and in Muslim countries, prosthetic surgery more frequently in English-speaking countries), and economic factors (UKA is not recognized and taught as a treatment option in certain countries because of the cost of other procedures).

Patient Expectancy and Information. Satisfaction after an intervention is a function of the difference between the patient's expectations (functional expected result) and the obtained functional result. This relationship emphasizes that vital information must be given to the patient and adapted to the patient's level and expectations. If the patient does not understand their situation, their satisfaction can be adversely affected.

The concept of the functional envelope by Dye applied on gonarthrosis (Fig. 122.1).[33] The x-axis represents the frequency of the applied forces or load whereas the y-axis represents the intensity of the applied forces/load. The surface under the curve defines the functional envelope of the knee. The upper limit thus defines the threshold above which a clinical reaction may be observed (discomfort, pain, swelling, stress fracture). The definition of the functional envelope remains a theoretical concept with a large variation between individuals and over time. It remains difficult to determine the individual upper and lower thresholds. Nevertheless, the profile of the functional envelope will be modified by medication, surgery, and rehabilitation. Each type of intervention modifies the functional envelope in a specific way: for instance, the change in the aspect of the curve will be different for a TKA versus an osteotomy.

Remember that patients can modify their activity (or their body weight) to re-enter the functional envelope, and the aim of surgery is to enlarge this envelope. If a zone of the envelope will be reduced, it has to be clearly explained to the patient. If the patient applies excessive forces, above the threshold, the risk for failure is increased.

Functional result of an osteotomy
- Pain free (95%), forgotten knee (80%), stability (90%), unlimited walking distance, normal stair climbing and descent, no limp, no use of crutches, no swelling.
- All sports (impact and contact) are possible but are not recommended. A recent study reported 92.3% of patients

---

*References 20, 25, 64, 91, 103, and 116.

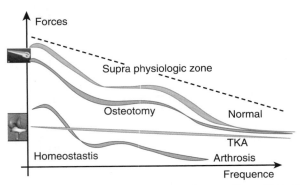

FIG 122.1 Functional envelope according to Dye. *TKA,* Total knee arthroplasty.

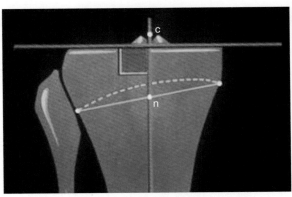

FIG 122.2 Epiphyseal axis defined by Levigne: line connecting the middle of the tibial joint line and the middle of the line connecting the tibial epiphysis. This axis forms a constant angle of 90 ± 2 degrees to the lateral tibial plateau.

returned to preoperative sports activities after surgery; however a reduction in the duration of these activities and a shift away from high-impact sports to lower-impact sports was reported.[36]

- Full extension, flexion to 145 degrees
- Activity limits: weight bearing is not allowed until 2 months after surgery; 5 days' hospitalization, return to home, functional autonomy and driving (75 days); it takes 4 to 6 months to adapt to the modified biomechanics and degree of valgus.
- Revision TKA is easy.
- Survival rate is 70% at 10 years,[48] with a revision rate for progression of OA from 14%[38] to 31% (mainly to TKA)[52] and the infection rate is less than 0.5%.

Radiologic Workup. The radiologic workup is the same for all types of osteotomies and in our daily practice, is not different from the workup for unicompartmental and total knee prosthesis. The workup includes the following:

- Unipodal weight bearing: type of arthrosis, localization, presence of osteophytes, cysts, foreign bodies, obliquity of the joint line, and so on.
- Unipodal stance profile at 30 degrees of flexion: presence of a cupule, patella height, tibial slope, anterior tibial translation, malunion with flexion deformity. This view is the most important view for antirecurvatum osteotomies.
- Sky-line view of the patella in 30 degrees of flexion: to exam the patellofemoral joint.
- Bipedal stance at 45 degrees of flexion view (schuss view). This view is excellent for evaluating femorotibial joint space width narrowing, which is frequently underestimated on the previously mentioned views.
- Bipedal stance full leg film: allows measurement of the different angle and axes.

The mechanical femoral axis is represented by a line connecting the center of the femoral head and the middle of the tibial spine. The mechanical tibial axis connects the middle of the tibial spine and the middle of the ankle joint. The mechanical femorotibial axis represents the overall deformity of the lower limb. This view will define the origin of the deformity (at the level of the femur or tibia) and will thus indicate the level at which to perform the osteotomy, the importance of the overall deformity, and the amount of correction necessary.

- Stress X-rays in varus and valgus will illustrate articular laxity and reducibility of the deformity.

- Measurement of the constitutional varus: (epiphyseal axis defined by Levigne[68]): line connecting the middle of the tibial joint line and the middle of the line connecting the tibial epiphysis. This axis forms a constant angle of 90 ± 2 degrees to the lateral tibial plateau (Fig. 122.2). The constitutional deformity of the tibia is defined as the angle between the epiphyseal axis and the tibial mechanical axis (Fig. 122.3). Sometimes it is difficult to determine the middle of the tibial joint line and to perform the measurement. Therefore we prefer to determine the level of the original tibial plateau by the line tangent to the normal contralateral tibial plateau. Subsequently the mechanical tibial axis is drawn. The angle between these axes is the angle alpha. The constitutional varus is defined by the complementary angle 90-alpha (Fig. 122.4).

Additional radiologic investigations: a computed tomography (CT) scan will determine the presence of rotational problems. Certain patients with a frontal valgus or varus deformity have developed a unilateral arthritis at the side of the convexity of the malunion. This lateralization of the degenerative process can be explained by the rotational problem. An internal medial rotation will cause a lateral femorotibial arthrosis, whereas an external rotation of the femur will cause a medial femorotibial arthrosis.

Ideal Indication. The indication is often a compromise and a choice made by the patient and the surgeon. For teaching purposes, we would like to remind you that it is not always possible to have ideal indications. Sometimes one or more criteria will make the indications limited or disputable.

Physical examination. The following are ideal physical indications for osteotomy: pain localized on the femorotibial joint line, normal range of motion, ligamentous status (but anterior cruciate ligament [ACL] or posterior cruciate ligament [PCL] insufficiency is not a contraindication), nonreducible deformity, no inflammatory arthritis, less than 70 years old, no obesity.

Radiologic findings. The following are ideal radiologic indications for osteotomy: Partial or complete joints space width narrowing in one compartment, no contralateral femorotibial joints space width narrowing or patella femoral joints space width narrowing, extra-articular deformity more than 5 degrees.

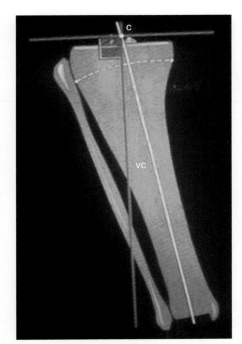

FIG 122.3 The constitutional deformity of the tibia is defined as the angle between the epiphyseal axis and the tibial mechanical axis.

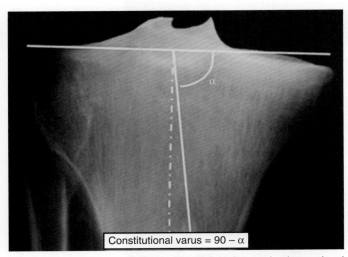

Constitutional varus = 90 − α

FIG 122.4 The level of the native tibial plateau is determined by the line tangent to the normal contralateral tibial plateau. Subsequently the mechanical tibial axes are drawn. The angle between both axes is the angle alpha. The constitutional varus is defined by the complementary angle 90 − α.

Disputable indications. The following are disputable indications for osteotomy: Patellofemoral arthritis, flexion less than 100 degrees or fixed flexum deformity, extra-articular deformity, age greater than 70 years, obese female.

Patient Expectations. The patient's preoperative level of activity and the expected postoperative level of activity will influence the indications for osteotomy. We are more likely to treat even an older patient with a high level of activity, including sports, by an osteotomy.

What Type of Osteotomy?
Type of Arthritis

Medial gonarthrosis. The following elements support the performance of an osteotomy:

- The origin of the medial gonarthrosis is most likely on the tibial site and usually in the proximal metaphyseal region. The result of a high tibial osteotomy (HTO) is better for varus deformity mainly because of bowing than a deformity that is essentially a result of wear.[17,71]
- The clinical outcome of an osteotomy in medial gonarthrosis is reported to be good, reliable, and durable with a survivorship of approximately 70% at 10 years.[8]
- An osteotomy restores the morphology with a horizontal joint line.
- Technically, the objective of this procedure is to obtain a hypercorrection between 3 and 6 degrees of valgus, as measured on the mechanical femorotibial angle between 183 degrees and 186 degrees.[1,14,46,51,56]

Opening wedge osteotomy. There are many advantages of an opening wedge osteotomy in comparison with a closing wedge osteotomy: a more accurate correction is possible, there is no peroneal nerve injury (palsy), and it can be combined with an ACL reconstruction through the same incision.[100] The disadvantages include the need for a graft (bone graft, ceramic, etc.), the consolidation may be longer (8 to 10 weeks), there is tensioning of the extensor system and to a lesser degree the medial collateral ligament and medial tendinous structures, and the leg length is increased (average 5.5 ± 4.4 mm).[75] Our tendency is to prefer an opening wedge HTO in the young patient with pre-OA or limited OA.

Closing wedge osteotomy. The advantages of the closing wedge osteotomy are a shorter consolidation (7 to 8 weeks) and a natural tendency to decrease the tibial slope angle. The disadvantages are the risk for damaging the peroneal nerve, more variability in the obtained correction, and a decrease in leg length (average 2.7 ± 4.0 mm).[75] We prefer a closing wedge HTO in the somewhat older patient with advanced OA. In cases of evolved OA secondary to chronic anterior laxity, this is the technique of choice.

Lateral gonarthrosis. This type of OA with valgus deformity is of mixed origin on the femur and the tibia, and in our experience the clinical outcome is less reproducible. Similar to other authors, we aim for a normocorrection between 0 and 2 degrees of varus.

Opening wedge distal femoral osteotomy. Because the origin of the valgus knee is situated in the distal femur, an osteotomy of the distal femur seems logical. Nevertheless, we must understand that a correction by osteotomy is only obtained in the frontal plane, in extension (Fig. 122.5). The anatomy and alignment are not changed in flexion and thus a valgus knee will persist in flexion after a distal femoral osteotomy. Therefore, the indication for a distal femoral osteotomy is a valgus knee in extension (Fig. 122.6). Currently we believe that the classification of the valgus knee according to the origin of the deformations is not yet well understood and that the deformities at a level of the diaphysis are not yet included. A distal femoral osteotomy requires a rigid fixation and is associated with more blood loss and a high risk of arthrofibrosis.

We generally perform a distal femoral osteotomy in younger patients with a valgus of distal femoral origin. The patients should be well motivated.

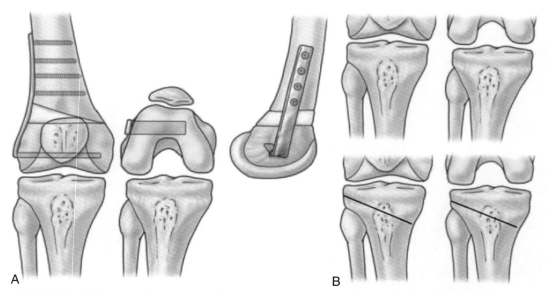

FIG 122.5 (A) A correction by femoral osteotomy is only obtained in the frontal plane, in extension. (B) HTO for varisation (medial closing wedge HTO) on the contrary will have an effect both in extension and in flexion. (Courtesy Dr. Chambat).

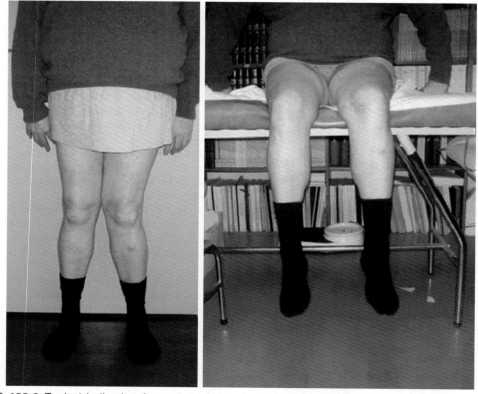

FIG 122.6 Typical indication for a distal femoral osteotomy: valgus knee in extension and no valgus in flexion.

High tibial osteotomy for varisation (medial closing wedge high tibial osteotomy). In contrast, this type of osteotomy will have an effect in extension as well as in flexion. (It is the only osteotomy with an action in flexion.) It is indicated and justified in valgus knees of mixed origin. However, it is accompanied by a risk for an important obliquity in the joint line. This obliquity, if greater than 10 degrees, can lead to excessive stress on the patellofemoral joint, especially on the medial side. We propose a medial closing wedge HTO for the patient around 60 years of age with a high level of activity including sport, with a valgus knee of mixed origin or of tibial origin that is inferior that is less than 8 degrees.

Clinical Criteria. The age of the patient must be taken into account: in a young patient with limited or early medial OA, we prefer an opening wedge HTO. The patient's weight can also influence the decision: morbid obesity has a negative influence because of loss of correction in the osteotomy and difficulties during the non-weight-bearing period. Arthritis secondary to ACL rupture can influence the choice of the technique because a wear pattern located more posterior on the tibial plateau (owing to the ACL rupture) decreases the tibial slope and limits the anterior tibial translation. Therefore a closing wedge HTO seems to be more appropriate.

Radiologic Criteria. The origin of the deformation is important:

- If an extra-articular constitutional or malunion deformation is involved, the osteotomy is considered corrective because it will correct the bony deformity.
- If intra-articular wear is involved, the osteotomy is considered palliative because the wear deformation is compensated by creating a bony deformity.

HIGH VALGUS TIBIAL OSTEOTOMY

In cases of medial OA in association with a genu varum morphotype, an HTO remains an important surgical option. The long-term clinical outcome at 10 years continues to be favorable in more than 70% of the patients if the frontal angular malalignment has been corrected to 3 to 6 degrees of valgus. The main reasons for failure are as follows:

1. Hypocorrection with the presence of a residual varus deformity
2. Overcorrection with progressive lateral gonarthrosis
3. Development of patellofemoral arthritis

Despite the progression in cartilage degeneration over time, this type of intervention remains indicated, especially in the middle-aged patient.

Two surgical techniques are available. On the one hand we have the opening wedge medial HTO, which should be associated with the use of a bone graft. On the other hand we have the lateral closing wedge HTO associated with a fibular neck osteotomy. The clinical outcome is more predictable in patients who are not obese. Therefore we generally provide information on hygiene (and smoking cessation) and calorie intake preoperatively. If we are confronted with a young and sports-minded patient, the osteotomy still remains the option of choice before an arthroplasty.

Radiologic Workup

The height of the opening wedge to obtain a valgus correction of 3 to 6 degrees is calculated as a function of the width of the tibia at the level of the osteotomy and the angular correction needed.

Lateral Closing Wedge High Tibial Osteotomy

Installation. The patient is in a supine position. A tourniquet is generally used. The patient is draped using an extremity sheet and the image intensifier is installed. A slightly oblique, almost horizontal, anterolateral skin incision is used. The incision starts 1 cm above the anterior tibial tuberosity and goes lateral 1 cm below the fibular head. The insertion of the tibialis anterior is released as a Z-plasty. Subsequently the tibialis anterior

muscle and the long toe extensor muscle are released from the tibial metaphysis using a large periosteal elevator.

Osteotomy of the Neck of the Fibula. The neck of the fibula is identified and presented. A periosteal elevator is slid around the neck, always staying in contact with the bone. This protects the peroneal nerve. Four holes are drilled in the neck using a 3.2-mm drill. Using the osteotome, the four holes are interconnected and the segment is removed using a large grasper. The fibular shaft should be mobile. Care is taken to ensure that the peroneal nerve is not entrapped in the osteotomy.

Peroneal nerve protection
- Distally release enough the tibialis anterior muscle.
- Distally, the fibular neck is identified and presented. A periosteal elevator is slid laterally around the neck always staying in contact with the bone. This protects the peroneal nerve.
- Four drill holes are made in the neck.
- First the two distal drill holes are interconnected with the osteotome.
- Subsequently the proximal drill holes
- The bone segment can be removed using a large grasper.

Closing Wedge Osteotomy of the Tibia. Specific instruments are available to perform, in a reproducible way, the HTO and its fixation. The osteotomy is performed proximal to the tibial tubercle in an oblique direction. Imaging intensifier control of the pin position is not necessary if the following rules are respected:

- Laterally, the osteotomy should start distally from the peroneotibial joint and should cross the tibial tubercle proximally. In this direction the tibial plateau is not in danger.
- The patellar tendon should be protected during the procedure and should not be damaged.
- Always check with an image intensifier to ensure that the appropriate alignment correction was obtained during the operation.

We now use a new fixation device with locked-in screws (Lepine) for the fixation. This blade plate–screw system is specifically designed to minimize subcutaneous irritation. Different blade and screw lengths are available to adapt to the different widths of the tibia. A small guide pin is introduced at the level of the joint line and an alignment guide is subsequently introduced over this guide pin. The alignment guide will automatically give the position and direction of a second guide pin parallel with the joint line and 1 cm distal to it. We then introduce the blade reamer over the second guide pin. The length of the blade should be 1 cm shorter than the total width of the tibia. The box preparation guide is introduced over the guide pin and impacted. Four drill holes are made 6 mm in diameter. The HTO blade is introduced and impacted into the box (Fig. 122.7). The distal cut of the closing wedge osteotomy is performed. Many surgeons use a guide pin for the distal cut of the osteotomy. We do not feel this is necessary. The posterior surface of the tibia is protected by a large periosteal elevator; the patellar tendon is retracted anteriorly. An oscillating saw is used to perform the distal cut. An angled cutting guide (6–8–10 degrees) is introduced in the distal cut of the osteotomy. The proximal cut is performed using this angle. The cutting guide should be introduced and impacted on the medial cortex. An oscillating saw is used. The bone wedge is removed (Fig. 122.8). The medial cortex is weakened with a 3.2-mm drill. Distal to the osteotomy, a provisional unicortical screw is positioned. This screw will be used as a support for the reduction clamp. The wedge is closed with the reduction clamp (Fig. 122.9A). Using a long metal bar positioned on the center of the femur head and in the middle of the ankle joint, the mechanical femorotibial axis is evaluated

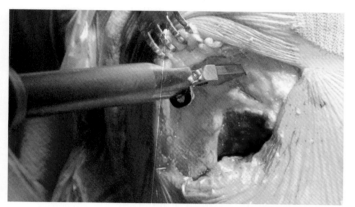

FIG 122.7 Introduction and impaction of the blade.

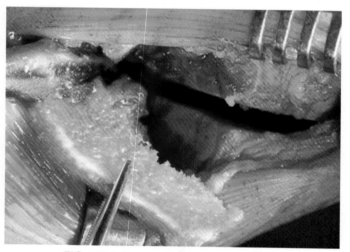

FIG 122.8 Removal of the bone wedge.

(see Fig. 122.9B). The metal bar should pass just lateral to the lateral tibial spine. The osteotomy is fixed with two bicortical long screws, which are introduced through the blade into the distal tibia (Fig. 122.10). The muscle insertions are closed over a drain. The skin is closed with separate sutures.

Other Fixation Devices and Guiding Jigs Are Available. The following devices and jigs are also available:
- The "swan-neck" blade plate[30,71]
- Classical blade plates[62,90]
- Staples[12,26,45,128,132]

A recent study showed the biomechanical superiority of plate fixation for proximal tibial osteotomy.[43] There is no advantage in using staples as a means of fixation because the plates and blade plates currently available are more stable and do not carry additional risks of complications.

Medial Opening Wedge High Tibial Osteotomy

Installation and Skin Incision. The patient is in a supine position. A tourniquet is applied. An extremity sheet is used for the knee and a small square field is applied on the ipsilateral iliac crest. A small cushion is positioned underneath the buttocks to obtain a better exposure of the iliac crest. An 8-cm-long horizontal anteromedial skin incision is made starting anteriorly just proximal to the tibial tubercle. The pes anserinus tendons are retracted. The superficial medial collateral ligament is incised at the level of the osteotomy (Fig. 122.11). The posterior surface of the tibia is exposed using a large periosteal elevator. During the osteotomy, this periosteal elevator is left in place. Anteriorly, the patellar tendon is retracted using a Farabeuf retractor.

Osteotomy of the Tibia. The osteotomy is performed proximally to the tibial tubercle and through the superficial medial collateral ligament, which has previously been incised. The plane of the osteotomy is horizontal (slightly different from the closing wedge medial HTO, which is more oblique). First two Kirschner 20/10 guide pins are introduced from the medial side. Laterally, these guide pins should be just superior to the head of the fibula. An image intensifier is used to evaluate the correct position of the guide pins. The direction can be adjusted if

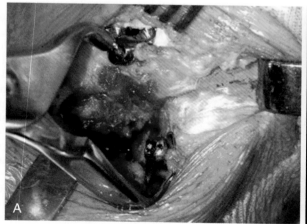
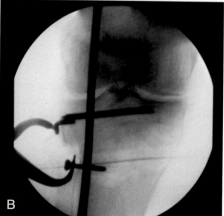

FIG 122.9 (A) Closing of the wedge with the reduction clamp. (B) Using a long metal bar positioned from the center of the femur head to the middle of the ankle joint, the mechanical femorotibial axis is evaluated. The metal bar should pass just laterally to the lateral tibial spine.

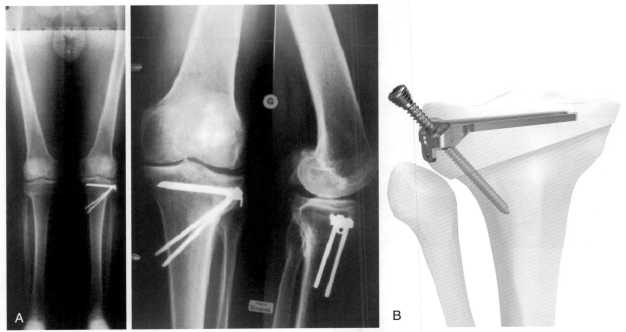

FIG 122.10 (A) Closing wedge high osteotomy of the tibia with 5 years FU, and (B) new fixation device with locked-in screws (Lepine).

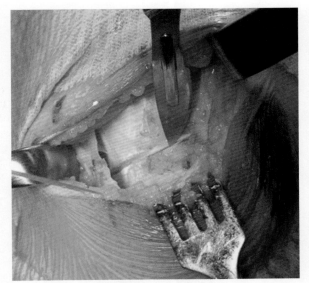

FIG 122.11 Incision of the superficial medial collateral ligament at the level of the osteotomy.

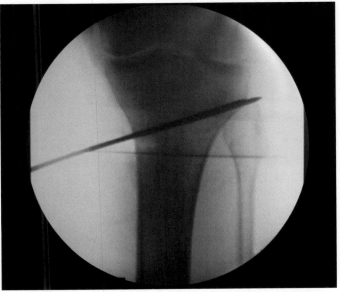

FIG 122.12 Control of the correct position of the guide pins with imaging identifier. The pins should be introduced medially and be just superior to the head of the fibula laterally.

necessary (Fig. 122.12). Using an oscillating saw, the tibial cut is performed underneath these guide pins, but always staying in contact with them (Fig. 122.13). First, the center of the tibia is cut, followed by the anterior and posterior cortex. The cuts are completed using an osteotome, especially on the anterior cortex where the patella tendon is in danger. It is necessary to have an intact lateral hinge for this type of osteotomy. This is ensured with a number of drill holes. Subsequently a Lambotte osteotome (thickness of 2 mm corresponding to approximately 2 degrees of angular correction) is introduced into the osteotomy.

A second osteotome is introduced below the first. To gently open the osteotomy, several more osteotomes are introduced between the first two (Fig. 122.14). If an insufficient opening of the osteotomy is obtained, the bony bridges anteriorly and posteriorly should be carefully fragilized using an additional osteotome. In general, the opening is more important anteriorly than posteriorly. Three complications can be encountered during this type of osteotomy:

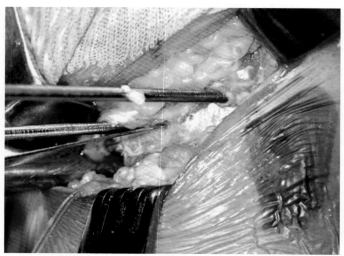

FIG 122.13 The tibial cut is performed underneath two guide pins introduced medially.

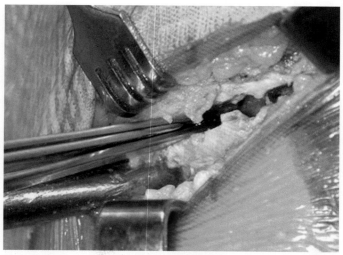

FIG 122.14 Progressive and controlled opening up of the osteotomy with several osteotomes introduced between the first two.

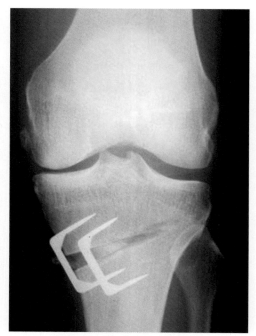

FIG 122.15 Fixation with staples.

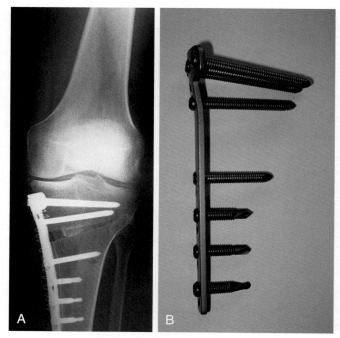

A   B

FIG 122.16 Tomofix plate.

- A fracture of the lateral hinge is frequently observed in important corrections beyond 10 to 15 degrees.[123] This results in a surgical undercorrection of the deformity and delayed osteotomy gap filling by the host.[109]
- A fracture of the lateral tibial plateau is observed if the lateral hinge has been insufficiently fragilized or if one forcefully tries to open the osteotomy with a valgus maneuver or if the osteotomes are impacted too deep. Usually plate and screw fixation suffice to overcome this complication.
- Variations in tibial slope. Increased tibial slope was frequently encountered in cases of anteromedial approach and fixation with a conventional Puddu plate.[99] Lustig et al. have demonstrated greater increase in medial compartment slope than in the lateral one.[73] This complication, which may worsen an anterior laxity, is less frequent with new plates.[98]

The obtained angle of correction is evaluated using a long metal bar centered on the hip and ankle. The angular correction is evaluated at the level of the joint line. If necessary an additional osteotome is introduced or removed.

Osteosynthesis. To avoid loss of correction in the postoperative period, the fixation should be strong and stable. Previously, we ensured the fixation with two to three Blount or Orthomed staples (Fig. 122.15). Over the past few years we have been using a Tomofix locking plate (Fig. 122.16). The Arbeitsgemeinschaft für Osteosynthesefragen (AO) group developed the Tomofix, a plate-fixator based on the internal fixator principle that allows secure fixation of locking head screws in the plate. Plates are adapted to the anatomy of the lateral femur and of the medial or lateral tibia. Lobenhoffer[69,70] and Staubli[114] reported good results of opening wedge osteotomy without graft stabilized with this medial plate. Other types of fixation are also possible (Surfix Plate, Chambat Plate (Fig. 122.17). The opening wedge may be left empty or can be filled with a tricortical bone graft harvested from the ipsilateral anterior iliac crest (Fig. 122.18). In the first instance, its filling by host bone is reduced in heavy smokers, whereas it is not positively influenced by early full

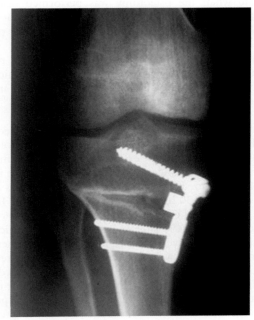

FIG 122.17 Fixation with Puddu-Chambat plate.

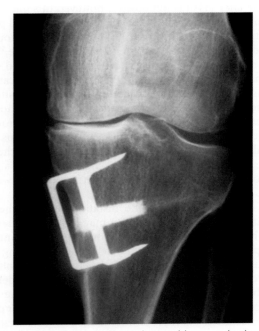

FIG 122.18 Orthomed staples and bone substitute.

weight bearing.[109] Bone substitutes are also available and can be used instead of the bone graft. These grafts are impacted, taking care not to overcorrect. The superficial medial collateral ligament is approximated over the staples.

Postoperative Guidelines

The postoperative guidelines are identical for the closing wedge and the opening wedge HTO.
- No weight bearing for 2 months has been our general indication. However, recent reports show better clinical results after an opening wedge HTO with an angular locking plate and without a bone graft if early partial weight bearing is allowed.[109]
- Walking is permitted only with the protection of two crutches.
- Thrombosis prophylaxis is used for 1 month.
- Bracing in extension is used for 2 months.
- Flexion is limited to 120 degrees the first 15 days. After that date, flexion can be progressively augmented.
- The drain is removed between day 2 and day 4.
- Hospital stay is between 4 and 5 days.
- Skin sutures are removed around day 12.
- Driving a car is not allowed for 10 weeks (except with an automatic gearbox).
- Physical work is not allowed for 3 to 4 months.
- Strenuous sports are allowed after 6 months.

The patient is invited for a clinical visit 2 months after the intervention. Radiographs should be taken. If bony healing is observed, weight bearing can be started. If delayed union is suspected, weight bearing is allowed and the patient is invited to come back in 1 month.

Results

The results of HTO have been studied and reported extensively since the 1960s. Insall[55] and Healy[44] reviewed the experience of the 1960s through the 1990s. They drew several conclusions from these reviews:
1. After an HTO, pain recurs in most knees, and most knees eventually require TKA.[85]
2. Younger patients with moderate varus deformities have the best results; obesity, undercorrection, and overcorrection[25,85] are adverse factors.
3. The overall preoperative state of the knee is the most important determinant of an eventual good result.[49]
4. Preoperative arthroscopic assessment of the knee is not useful.[58]
5. Previous medial meniscectomy[96] and anterior cruciate deficiency are not contraindications, but previous lateral meniscectomy may be.
6. The addition of tibial tubercle elevation to the osteotomy in the case of associated patellofemoral arthritis is unnecessary, and it increases the complication rate.[51,94]

Some complementary information has been added in recently published results. Reported recent outcomes are quite variable, but suggest that HTO provides satisfactory and durable results if the procedure is accurately performed in selected patients. In addition, both clinical outcomes and survival are similar between closing and opening osteotomies.[13,107] The negative influence of the passage of time on the results of HTO has been confirmed repeatedly. Many HTO series reveal satisfactory results at 5 to 7 years follow-up (FU), but the rate of satisfactory clinical results diminishes significantly thereafter

TABLE 122.1   Survival Success Series of High Tibial Osteotomy

Author	Year	n	10-Year Survival Rate (%)
Cass[21]	1988	86	69
Ritter[102]	1988	78	58
Rudan[105]	1991	128	80
Coventry[27]	1993	87	66
Naudie[92]	1999	85	80
Billings[15]	2000	64	53
Majima[76]	2000	48	61
Hernigou[47]	2001	245	85
Aglietti[3]	2003	102	78
Sprenger[113]	2003	66	74
Van Raij[123]	2008	100	75
Babis[9]	2008	54	76
Akizuki[6]	2008	132	97.6
Schalleberger[107]	2011	71	92
Hui[52]	2011	394	79
Howells[50]	2014	164	79

(Table 122.1). A recent meta-analysis reviewing 19 previous HTO publications reported good or excellent results in 75.3% of patients at 60-month FU and in 60.3% at 100-month FU,[124] but we would like to emphasize that the results are influenced by the quality of the selection criteria. The importance of precise postoperative alignment has been stressed in many reports.[†] There is no general agreement, however, about the optimal postoperative femorotibial alignment. If one tries to define a consensual ideal postoperative hip-knee angle, the obtained value approximates 3 to 6 degrees valgus, although Yasuda et al.[129,130] recommend a larger overcorrection, of up to 10 degrees valgus. On the contrary, undercorrection of less than 5 degrees was strongly related to a high failure rate.[130] The importance of the preoperative grade of OA on the long-term result of HTO has also been confirmed.[‡] A preoperative Alback grade I or grade II is predictive of a good long-term result. HTO for medial OA is a successful procedure for selected patients. The ideal patient would typically be younger than 65 years, have less than 12-degree angular deformity, unicompartmental disease, ligamentous stability, and a preoperative range-of-motion arc of at least 90 degrees.[14] The axial correction should be accurate, and stable internal fixation with an early range of motion is advisable. Despite the remarkable results of knee arthroplasty, a place should remain for this surgical procedure aimed at maintaining the natural knee.

Complications

Infection. Deep infection is rare after HTO. Compiling the complications of 10 clinical series, for a total of 804 osteotomies, Insall found 5 deep and 55 superficial infections; 37 occurred when an external fixator was used. Maquet et al.[79] in a series of 700 osteotomies, noted a 2.8% rate of skin necrosis and a 7.7% infection rate. Lortat-Jacob[72] reported six cases of early reintervention for infection after HTO. In four cases, the

internal fixation was left in place, with a good end result. One patient with gas gangrene required amputation, and another died from septic shock. Lemaire,[66] in a series of 201 dome osteotomies, reported three infections: one was treated successfully by general antibiotics, and two were treated by curettage and antibiotic-impregnated polymethylmethacrylate beads left temporarily in the wound. The infection rate after HTO justifies routine antibiotic prophylaxis.

Nonunion. Delayed union or nonunion of the osteotomy is rare. The reported rate of nonunion ranges from 0% to 3%.[21,54,119,120] Jackson and Waugh[57] reported a threefold increase in the nonunion rate when the osteotomy was performed below the tuberosity rather than above it. Insall[55] believed that a thin proximal fragment was a risk factor for nonunion, perhaps because of avascular necrosis.

Treatment of nonunion after osteotomy usually requires bone grafting and compression fixation in cases in which rigid fixation was not used initially.[44] This fixation may be internal. For some authors an external fixator may be used.[19,26,103]

Peroneal Nerve Dysfunction. Fibular osteotomy or resection of the fibular head can induce a common peroneal nerve palsy[28] or an isolated weakness of the extensor hallucis longus muscle.[60] Kirgis and Albrecht define two high-risk regions for an isolated injury of the motor branches to the extensor hallucis longus, the first one about 30 mm and the second one 68 to 153 mm distal to the fibular head.[60] Maquet[77] recorded a 3.1% rate of motor deficit and a 4.1% rate of sensory deficit, of which 1.2% and 1.5% were definitive. Idusuyi and Morrey[53] documented 32 postoperative peroneal nerve palsies in a retrospective review of 10,361 consecutive total knee arthroplasties performed at the Mayo Clinic. They showed that epidural anesthesia for postoperative control of pain was significantly associated with peroneal nerve palsy. The anesthesia should not produce prolonged sensory and motor blockade.

Compartment Syndrome. The exact incidence of compartment syndrome after HTO is unknown[41]; however, in some series it has been reported to be less than 1%.[67] Some technical precautions can help decrease this risk. The fascial incision should not be closed tightly.[65] A suction drain should be left in place.[41,65,78,126] The tourniquet should be released before closure, and careful hemostasis should be performed. Epidural anesthesia can mask the signs of an impending ischemia. If epidural anesthesia is used, the amount of local anesthetic that is given should be sufficient to make the patient comfortable without producing prolonged sensory and motor blockade, and the status of the leg should be observed even more closely. If in doubt, the tissue pressure should be monitored, and high pressure is a strong indication that fasciotomy should be performed.

Patella Baja. By changing the distance between the tibial tuberosity and the joint line, HTO may have an influence on patellar height. In an opening wedge osteotomy the joint line is shifted proximally resulting in a patella baja. In closing wedge osteotomies the joint line is distalized. It should result in an increased patellar height[35,40]; however, clinical evidence of patella baja is more common.[10,59,108] This may be the consequence of postoperative immobilization and scarring or patellar tendon slackness because of the reduction of metaphyseal thickness.

[†]References 1, 14, 27, 46, 51, 56, 58, 71, 92, 93, 95, 97, 104, 105, 112, 113, 121, 129, and 130.
[‡]References 14, 46, 56, 71, 95, 104, and 105.

Future Improvements

Several points may improve results in the near future:

- Inclusion of the femoral rotation component in preoperative planning for the desired angle of correction.
- Computer-assisted surgery to achieve and evaluate the obtained mechanical femorotibial axis is currently under investigation.
- Better accuracy in reaching this target (thanks to computer-assisted surgery).
- A gait analysis probably should become part of the preoperative assessment for all patients undergoing HTO to adapt the amount of overcorrection according to the importance of the adduction moment.
- Association of HTOs with stem cell treatment and growth factors.[61]

HIGH TIBIAL VARUS OSTEOTOMY

The high tibial varus osteotomy is indicated in the young and active patient with lateral arthritis of the knee and a moderate valgus knee. This surgical procedure results in a durable and satisfying clinical outcome up to 8 to 12 years if the lower limb has been corrected to neutral.[120] This procedure addresses both the valgus in extension as well as in flexion. Because it frequently results in an obliquity of the joint line, it is usually proposed in cases of mild to moderate mechanical angle deformation (<10 to 12 degrees).[83] It has also been proposed in ligament-deficient knees such as in grade 3 chronic PCL injuries with associated genu varus alignment to avoid ligament reconstruction.[7] This surgery should be conceived as an alternative to a knee prosthesis (TKA or UKA). The surgical technique consists of a closing wedge osteotomy on the medial side of the tibia. The exception is a lateral opening wedge osteotomy done to correct an initial hypercorrection of a closing wedge HTO (Fig. 122.19).

Radiological Workup

The amount of correction needed to obtain a mechanical femorotibial axis of approximately 180 degrees is calculated as a function of the width of the metaphyseal area of the tibia. The evaluation of the valgus deformity remains more difficult than the evaluation of a varus deformity.

Medial Closing Wedge High Tibial Osteotomy

Positioning of the Patient. The patient is placed in a supine position and a tourniquet is used. The lower limb is covered with an extremity sheet. The image intensifier should be available. The surgical approach is identical to the surgical approach for an opening wedge HTO. The anteromedial, slightly oblique, almost horizontal skin incision starts 1 cm proximal to the tibial tubercle and continues medially over a distance of 8 cm. The hamstring tendons are identified and retracted. The superficial medial collateral ligament is incised horizontally at the level of the osteotomy. The proximal fibers of the superficial medial collateral ligament are elevated proximal and distal to the incision over a distance of a couple of millimeters (a function of the height of the wedge that will be resected). A periosteal elevator is introduced posterior to the metaphyseal area of the tibia, always staying in contact with the bone. The periosteal elevator is kept in place once the lateral side of the posterior tibia is reached. It will protect the posterior structures during the osteotomy. A Farabeuf retractor is introduced underneath the patellar tendon to retract and protect it during the osteotomy.

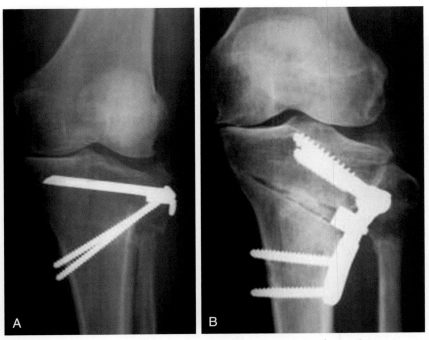

FIG 122.19 Exceptionally, a lateral opening wedge osteotomy is performed to correct an excessive hypercorrection of a closing wedge HTO. (A) 14bisa preoperative X-ray. (B) 14bisb postoperative X-ray.

Tibial Osteotomy. The tibial osteotomy is performed just proximal to the level of the tibial tubercle. It is almost horizontal in the coronal plane, slightly oblique, and up-sloped from medial to lateral. Two Kirschner wires (K-wires) serve as guide pins for the proximal cut of the osteotomy. The pins are introduced medially and will emerge laterally just proximal to the fibulo-tibial joint. After the introduction of two guide pins, their correct position is verified using an image intensifier. The proximal cut of the osteotomy is done with an oscillating saw on the two guide pins. First the middle part of the tibia is done, followed by the anterior and posterior cortex; the lateral cortex should not be transected. The lateral cortex will serve as a hinge during the procedure. Subsequently, the distal cut is performed. In the sagittal plane, it should be parallel to the proximal cut, and in the frontal plane, it should converge on the lateral side. The distance between the cuts at the level of the medial cortex is defined during the surgical planning. The wedge is removed using a large grasper. The lateral hinge is now gently perforated with a drill to fragilize it. The osteotomy will progressively be closed by introducing an osteotome into the osteotomy and gently further fragilizing the lateral hinge. An intraoperative evaluation of the correction is mandatory. A long metal bar is placed in projection from the center of the femoral head to the center of the ankle joint. At the level of the knee, this bar should pass through the center of the knee. An overcorrection should be avoided. Therefore the height of the resected wedge should not be excessive. A frequent error of overcorrection is that the surgeon did not include the thickness of the saw blade in the resection width. The osteotomy is fixed using two to three Blount or Orthomed staples on the medial side (Fig. 122.20). Use of other fixation devices such as plate and screw fixation is of course possible, but we prefer to use less space-filling types of fixation in this area of the knee. The pes anserinus is closed over the staples. A drain is positioned in proximity of the osteotomy and the skin is closed using interrupted sutures.

Lateral Opening Wedge High Tibial Osteotomy

Positioning of the Patient. Patients are positioned supine on a radiolucent operating table with a lateral thigh support; a tourniquet is used. The image intensifier should be available. A 6- to 8-cm longitudinal or slightly oblique incision is performed between the tibial tubercle and fibular head. The incision extends from the joint line distally to a point approximately 1 cm distal to the level of the tibial tuberosity. After blunt dissection of the subcutaneous tissue, the fascia is incised along the tibial edge leaving approximately 1 cm of fascia attached to the tibial crest for closure. The tibialis anterior and the long toe extensor muscle are released from the tibial metaphysis using a large periosteal elevator. This maneuver is usually more extensive than a valgus-producing osteotomy to facilitate mobilization of the peroneal nerve. The fibular head may be released by incising the capsule of the proximal tibiofibular joint or performing an osteotomy of the fibular head. The patellar tendon is carefully released to avoid any damage at the time of the osteotomy.

Fibular Osteotomy. Fibular osteotomy is our preferred option in the absence of malunion. Two options are available: distal and proximal osteotomies. A distal diaphyseal osteotomy is performed approximately 10 cm below the tip of the fibula. However, at this level, risk of denervating the extensor hallucis longus muscle exists.[111] A proximal osteotomy is associated with a risk of peroneal nerve damage, both during surgery and postoperatively as a consequence of nerve stretching. For this reason, the nerve should be identified at the lateral aspect of the fibular neck and mobilized from surrounding soft tissues. A periosteal elevator is placed around the lateral cortex of the fibular neck. Although it is crucial to protect the nerve, its lateral retraction should be avoided because it may stretch the nerve. Two holes are made with a 3.2-mm drill bit in the neck to mark the osteotomy site. The osteotomy is then

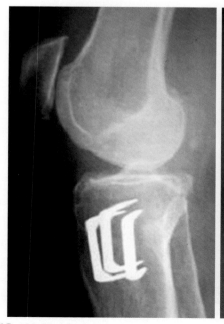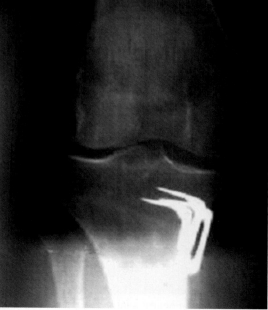

FIG 122.20 Medial closing wedge HTO using two to three Blount or Orthomed staples on the medial side.

completed with an osteotome with the periosteal elevator still in place.

Tibial Osteotomy. Once the posterolateral aspect of the tibial metaphysis has been released from soft tissues, an elevator is placed around the posterior aspect of the tibial. The elevator must be positioned in contact with the bone to avoid neurovascular injury. Anteriorly, a retractor is placed behind the patellar tendon just proximal to the tibial tuberosity to avoid any damage. The osteotomy begins just above the level of the tibial tuberosity and extends proximally and medially to a point approximately 1 cm below the medial joint line. Generally, the osteotomy is performed more horizontally than a medial opening-wedge osteotomy. Two K-wires wires are positioned under fluoroscopic control to mark the desired path. The osteotomy is carried out with an oscillating saw just below the two K-wires, starting with the middle portion of the tibia and proceeding to the anterior and posterior cortices. The medial cortical hinge must be preserved; thus before opening the osteotomy, it should be weakened by perforating it with a 3.2-mm drill bit and the anterior and posterior cortices should be completely cut. The desired opening is gradually achieved using several osteotomes. The first one is placed in the osteotomy site just below the K-wires and advanced to the opposite cortex. The second is placed directly below it, whereas the third is advanced between the first two osteotomes, opening the osteotomy site. To avoid the medial hinge fracture, the third osteotome should not be advanced as far as the first two osteotomes. However, it is mandatory to reach the medial cortex with the first two osteotomes before opening the osteotomy. This can be confirmed by the sound change when the osteotome hits the opposite cortex or with fluoroscopic control. The desired correction is achieved with additional osteotomes and maintained with a lamina spreader. In case of large corrections, a staple can be placed between Gerdy's tubercle and the tibial tubercle to provide additional stability. At this time the alignment is confirmed, with direct visual check of the overall limb alignment, and under fluoroscopy with a radio-opaque bar that is centered over the middle of the femoral head and the ankle. Fluoroscopy also confirms the integrity of the medial hinge.

Fixation. Fixation must be relatively rigid to avoid any loss of correction postoperatively. Several fixation devices are available including staples, standard plates, and a variety of precontoured plates. We prefer to use staples because they require minimal bone bridge proximal to the osteotomy and can often be more easily placed than plates. In addition, standard plates require extensive dissection of the anterior soft tissues and a larger incision or additional incisions for percutaneous screw placement. Finally, precontoured plates often do not fit well with the local anatomy because many of these patients have somewhat abnormal proximal tibial anatomy owing to prior osteotomies. If staples are used, the first is placed obliquely between the tibial tuberosity and Gerdy's tubercle and the second is placed more lateral in a more vertical position. We use an iliac crest corticocancellous bone graft or bone substitutes (calcium triphosphate) in all cases, even those with relatively small correction.

Postoperative Guidelines

The patient should receive information on the postoperative guidelines prior to the surgery.

These postoperative guidelines are identical to those for valgisation osteotomies.

Results

Collins reported the outcomes of his series of 24 lateral opening wedge tibial osteotomies at an average FU of 52 months.[23] After changing the mechanical axis from 2.4 ± 2.4 degrees valgus to 0 ± 2.6 degrees varus, the Lower Extremity Functional Scale (LEFS) and Knee Injury and Osteoarthritis Outcome Score (KOOS) values improved from 48 ± 15.9 to 61.8 ± 15.6 and from 51.3 ± to 67 ± 17.6, respectively.

Complications

The following complications can occur:
- Errors of correction: hypocorrection is more frequent than hypercorrection.
- Nonunion and fixation failures are rare.
- Delayed union can be observed in cases of imperfect fit between the osteotomy cuts.
- The osteosynthesis material can cause pain or discomfort. Removal of it is in many cases sufficient.
- The clinical outcome of a medial closing wedge HTO can decline after approximately 7 to 20 years (Fig. 122.21). In those cases, a TKA can be performed without any major difficulties.

Future Improvements

Future improvement will involve the following:
- Exact calculation of the correction should improve results.
- Better reproducibility of the desired correction: computer-assisted surgery and navigation could result in a more precise evaluation of the mechanical femorotibial axis.
- Improvement in the fixation of the osteotomy allowing earlier weight bearing.
- Application of specific growth factors to improve early consolidation.

DISTAL FEMORAL OSTEOTOMY FOR THE TREATMENT OF A VALGUS DEFORMITY

Opening Wedge Osteotomy

The overall aim of this osteotomy is to correct the mechanical axis of the lower limb to a normal varus (0 to 3 degrees of varus). In general it is better to slightly overcorrect than to undercorrect. During the preoperative planning, one can determine the desired angle of correction and the opening that will be needed to obtain this correction. The radiographs not only help determine the proper indications but also measure the correction needed. The major drawback of femoral osteotomies is that they correct the deformity in extension but they do not have any influence on the alignment in flexion.

Positioning and Approach. With the knee in 90 degrees of flexion, a lateral skin incision starts 15 cm proximal to the joint line and ends at a level of Gerdy's tubercle (Fig. 122.22). The fascia lata is incised slightly anteriorly in the direction of its fibers and the lateral vastus muscle is elevated. The perforating arteries of the vastus lateralis are carefully coagulated or ligated. The vastus lateralis is elevated from the lateral border of the femoral diaphysis using a periosteal elevator. The patella tendon is identified and a limited lateral arthrotomy is performed to

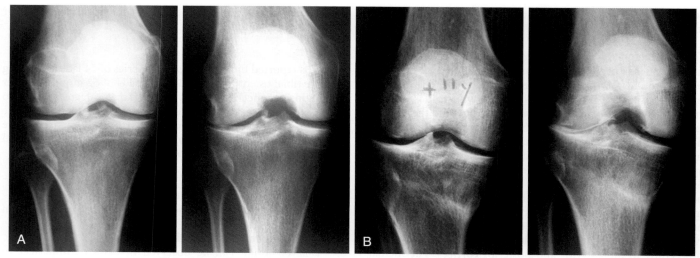

FIG 122.21 Same case. (A) Preoperative X-rays. (B) 11 years follow-up.

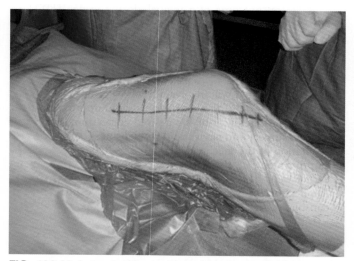

FIG 122.22 Lateral skin incision for distal opening wedge femoral osteotomy: it starts 1 cm proximal to the joint line and ends at the level of Gerdy's tubercle.

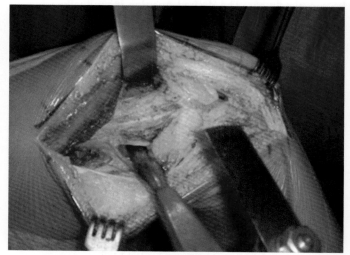

FIG 122.23 Exposure of the lateral distal part of the femoral diaphysis with elevation of the vastus lateralis. With the knee at 90 degrees of flexion, the posterior side of the metaphyseal region is exposed. A landmark is made with the oscillating saw; it will serve as a guide to determine the rotation.

expose the orientation of the trochlea and the condyles. Two guide pins are inserted into the joint: one at the femorotibial joint line, another in the patella femoral joint. The guide pins help guide the blade plate and reduce the radiation owing to image amplification. Next, the zone of the osteotomy is prepared. The osteotomy is horizontal, just proximal to the lateral part of the trochlea. With the knee in extension, the suprapatellar approach is elevated and with the knee at 90 degrees of flexion, the posterior side of the metaphyseal region is elevated. With the oscillating saw, a landmark is made on the lateral side of the femur perpendicular to the horizontal osteotomy. This serves as a guide to determine the rotation (Fig. 122.23).

Introduction of the Blade. The blade should be introduced into the epiphyseal region 30 mm proximal to the joint line (Fig. 122.24). The blade plate is 5.6 mm in thickness, 16 mm in width, and the distance between the screw holes is 16 mm. The

guide for the blade plate should be introduced ventrally and proximally to the femoral insertion of the lateral collateral ligament. The angle of insertion depends on the level of the deformation. If the deformation is located at a diaphyseal level, the blade should be introduced oblique to the joint line. To introduce the blade parallel to the joint line, the angle should be 85 degrees since the blade plate angle is 95 degrees (complementary angle is 180 less 95). To obtain a varisation of 10 degrees (angle of correction) the angle should be set at 75 degrees (85 less 10). If the deformation is situated at the metaphyseal level, the blade should be introduced parallel to the joint line. This is the most common situation. When introducing the blade parallel to the joint line, a correction to a normal anatomic femoral valgus of 5 degrees is automatically obtained by introducing a 95-degree angle blade plate. In others words,

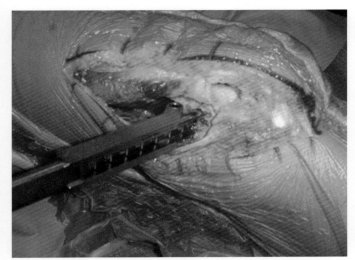

FIG 122.24 Introduction of the blade into the epiphyseal region.

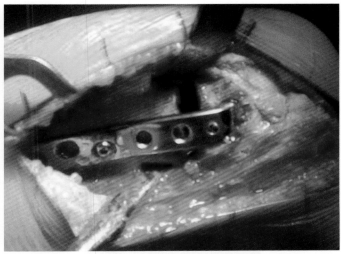

FIG 122.26 Impaction of the blade plate and progressive opening of the osteotomy.

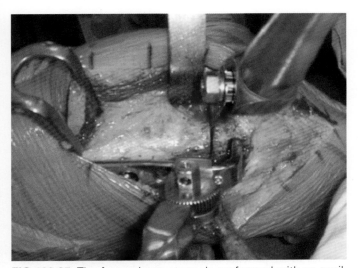

FIG 122.25 The femoral osteotomy is performed with an oscillating saw. Introduction of the blade plate.

if the femur is normal, no correction is obtained when the blade plate is introduced parallel to the joint line. If we are confronted with a combined deformation or mixed with a metaphyseal component (lateral condyle hypoplasia or diaphyseal malunion), the angle of introduction should be even smaller and the blade plate should be introduced in a smaller angle. The preoperative planning is essential to evaluate the correction needed.

Intraoperative Control. The position of the blade can be checked using the image intensifier. The angle of correction can be measured on a printout by drawing a line tangent to the medial and lateral condyle and another line tangent to the blade.

The Osteotomy. The femoral osteotomy is performed with an oscillating saw. The medial cortex should not be cut. Once the blade plate is introduced, the medial cortex is fragilized using a drill bit (Fig. 122.25). Two or more osteotomes are then introduced into the osteotomy. It is, however, the impaction of the

blade plate that will progressively open up the osteotomy once in contact with the diaphysis (Fig. 122.26). A screw is temporarily placed in the distal oval screw hole. The blade plate is now impacted. The screw is in the proximal zone of the hole. A screw is introduced in another screw hole and the former is removed. The impaction of the blade plate is continued and the osteotomy will progressively open up until the blade plate is in full contact with the lateral side of the femoral diaphysis. Progressive impaction allows opening of the osteotomy. Provisional fixation with one screw helps to control the correction and gives additional stability. By playing with the impaction and the positioning of the screws, one can increase or decrease the opening. If the blade plate is impacted with the screw left in place, the correction is halted. Conversely, if an additional screw is again placed in the distal part of the screw hole and the former screw is taken out, the correction can be increased. Final fixation of the blade plate is achieved by four cortical screws of 4.5-mm diameter (Fig. 122.27). Cortical and cancellous iliac crest bone grafts are used to fill the opening wedge osteotomy. The soft tissues and skins are closed over a drain, which is introduced underneath the fascia lata.

Lateral Closing Wedge High Tibial Osteotomy

Positioning and Approach. The technique was initially described by McDermott et al.[86] The osteotomy is performed just proximal to the adductor tubercle and the anterior margin of the femoral articular surface through an anteromedial skin incision that begins from the joint line and extends proximally for 15 cm. The vastus medialis is reflected laterally from the medial intermuscular septum, and care is taken to protect the neurovascular bundle medially in the adductor canal by performing the dissection subperiosteally. A medial arthrotomy of the knee is often used. A medially based wedge of bone is removed from the proximal femur using guide wires placed parallel to the articular surface. Biplanar fluoroscopy is used. Typically the osteotomy is fixed with a 90-degree dynamic compression blade plate.[82]

Fixation. Fixation with staples is not recommended. Recently, Wang and Hsu[127] described a technique using blade-plate

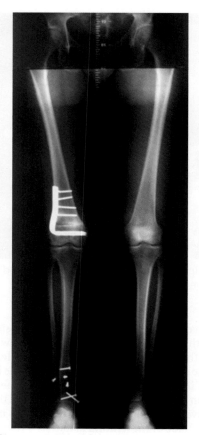

FIG 122.27 Six month FU of lateral opening wedge osteotomy with blade plate.

fixation with a derotational screw. Also, van Heerwaarden et al.[122] have described a technique using a TomoFix plate fixator. McDermott et al.[86] state that a flexion contracture of as much as 20 degrees can be corrected by adding extension to the osteotomy. The final correction achieved by the medial distal femoral closing wedge osteotomy should bring the mechanical axis to 50% of the tibial plateau.

Postoperative Guidelines

Continuous passive motion is allowed immediately postoperatively. The flexion should be limited to 120 degrees for the first 15 days postoperatively. Non–weight-bearing is continued for 2 months and an extension brace is applied. Complications are observed somewhat more frequently than after a tibial osteotomy; in particular, postoperative blood loss can be important, and stiffness of the knee and delayed union are more frequent. Possible complications should be avoided using a strict surgical technique and a specific postoperative rehabilitation protocol.

Results

As with HTO, variable success with distal femoral osteotomy has been reported (Table 122.2). Patient selection factors, good surgical technique, appropriate postoperative alignment, and the passage of time all affect the final clinical outcome. The ideal candidate should be younger than 65 years and have good bone stock and isolated OA of the lateral compartment (at an Ahlback stage I or II), minimal ligamentous laxity, a range of motion arc

TABLE 122.2 Survival Success Series of Distal Femoral Osteotomy

Author	Year	n	Follow-Up	Survival Rate (%)
Mc Dermott[87]	1988	24	4	92
Miniaci[88]	1989	35	5.4	86
Terry[118]	1992	35	5.4	60
Edgerton[34]	1993	24	8.3	71
Finkelstein[37]	1996	21	11	64
Cameron[18]	1997	49	7	87
Mathews[84]	1998	21	3	57
Marin Morales[80]	2000	17	6.5	75
Aglietti[4]	2000	18	9	77
Backstein[11]	2007	40	10	82
Sternheim[115]	2011	45	10	89.9
Dewilde[31]	2013	19	7	82
Saitnha[106]	2014	21	5	79
Madelaine[74]	2014	29	80.2	87.6

of more than 90 degrees, and flexion contracture of less than 20 degrees.

Cognet[22] reported the results of 75 closing wedge supracondylar osteotomies fixed with a guided blade plate, with an average FU of 8.7 years (range 5 to 14 years). The mechanical axis at FU was 0.1 degrees varus. Of all the patients, 77% were satisfied or very satisfied. In one study with 5 to 11 years FU,[34] the success rate was 77% if the alignment was corrected to neutral or varus, as opposed to 60% success in patients left in some degree of valgus. For us, the postoperative alignment goal is a tibiofemoral angle of approximately 0 degrees (neutral alignment) for a supracondylar osteotomy.

Only a few series report the outcomes of opening wedge osteotomies. Dewilde et al., using the Puddu plate, reported a survival rate of 82% at 7 years.[31] Zarrouk et al., using a Strelizia-type blade plate, had 91% survivorship at 8 years.[131] Saithna reported the outcomes of his technique (with a Puddu plate) in a series of 21 patients at an average FU of 4.5 years.[106] After achieving a mechanical axis of 37% (from medial to lateral) the cumulative survival rate was 79%. Madelaine et al., in a series of 29 opening wedge osteotomies, reported improvement in Knee Society Score (KSS) functional values from 50.4 to 68.5 at 80.2 months.[74]

Complications

Supracondylar femoral osteotomy is technically demanding and is not performed frequently. It has a high rate of complications. Cameron et al.,[18] reporting on 49 consecutive patients treated by supracondylar varus closing wedge osteotomy stabilized with a blade plate, had six cases of delayed union, one case of loss of fixation, and one case of rotational deformity. Teinturier,[117] in a series of 131 lateral supracondylar osteotomies, reported four infections, one nonunion, and five deep vein thromboses. Mironneau[89] analyzed the results of 28 supracondylar osteotomies all fixed with a blade plate. The morbidity was high, with three fixation losses, one fracture, one nonunion, and one arthrofibrosis. The reported complication rate varies. As stated by Aglietti,[5] avoiding entering into the knee joint should reduce the incidence of stiffness. A rigid internal fixation is mandatory, given the high rate of loss of fixation and nonunion when staples are used.

DOUBLE OSTEOTOMY

There are two different indications for double osteotomy.

The first indication is when a unipolar osteotomy (on the femur or on the tibia) will result in an oblique joint line to address a major angular deformity (> to 10 degrees) in the frontal plane (in valgus or varus [Fig. 122.28]). This obliquity creates shear forces cross the knee joint, which could lead to early failure. Additionally, in case of a unipolar correction by an opening wedge osteotomy, the stability of the osteotomy is compromised. In a closing wedge unipolar osteotomy, the proximal and distal ends will not adapt sufficiently and this can cause problems for future TKA. A distal femoral osteotomy combined with a proximal tibial osteotomy can correct the axis of the lower limb and maintain an acceptable obliquity of the joint line (Fig. 122.29).

The second indication is for the treatment of OA secondary to a malunion of the femur. In these cases, the aim of the procedure is to address the frontal or torsional malunion on the femur by a normocorrection and to address the arthritis with a tibial osteotomy. It is of major importance to know that the femoral malunion situated close to the knee joint is more severe than the others. A femoral osteotomy can only correct a deformation in extension and not in flexion. Double osteotomy has certain difficulties and complications:

1. The risks for a delayed union or malunion are increased compared to a normal osteotomy.
2. Calculation of the correction remains difficult and complicated. In a femoral malunion, one could perform the interventions separately starting with the femoral derotation and perform the tibial osteotomy at a different time. If computer-assisted navigation is available, correction in the frontal and horizontal planes can be combined in the same intervention.

Nevertheless, indication for a double osteotomy remains rare.

The Principles

Varus Knee. In the case of a varus knee with a mechanical axis less than 165 degrees, the combination of a lateral closing wedge distal femur osteotomy with a lateral closing wedge HTO or medial opening wedge HTO is indicated. The advantage of an opening wedge HTO is the preservation of the length of the lower limb. In that case, the skin incision is laterally placed on the femur, crosses the midline at the level of the tibial tubercle, and continues medially on the tibia. An isolated lateral femoral incision can be combined with an isolated medial tibial incision. Commonly, however, in case of a closing wedge HTO, a laterally based long skin incision is used.

Valgus Knee. In case of a valgus knee with a mechanical axis more than 190 degrees, a combination of an opening wedge lateral distal femoral osteotomy with a closing wedge medial HTO is indicated. This combination results in an acceptable orientation of the joint line and the risk for apraxia of the peroneal nerve remains low.

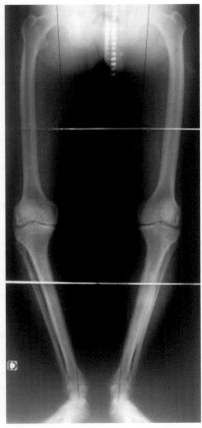

FIG 122.28 Double osteotomy for major angular deformity in varus.

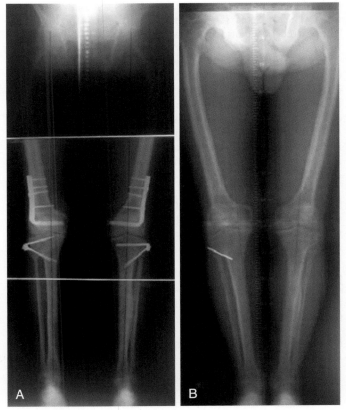

FIG 122.29 A distal femoral osteotomy combined with a proximal tibial osteotomy is able to correct the axis of the lower limb and maintain an acceptable obliquity of the joint line.

Malunion With Torsional Problem. In case of OA secondary to a femoral malunion with a torsional problem more than 15 degrees and a frontal deviation superior to 10 degrees, we advise including a derotation osteotomy on the femur.

Surgical Technique

On the Femur. The approach has been described in detail in the section on femoral osteotomy for varisation.

Lateral opening wedge osteotomy for valgus knee. (See section on femoral osteotomy for varisation.)

Lateral closing wedge osteotomy for the varus knee. The area for the osteotomy is prepared. Two additional Kirschner guide pins are introduced in the femur as guide pins for the future osteotomy. One pin is introduced parallel to the joint line approximately 50 mm proximal to the joint line. The second pin is introduced proximally to the first on the lateral cortex but converging with the first medially. This represents the angle and the wedge that will be resected. The quadriceps muscle is retracted at a level proximal to the trochlea with the knee in extension; the posterior side of the knee is cleared. A superficial mark on the lateral cortex of the femur with the oscillating saw can serve as a landmark for determining the rotation. The blade plate has to be introduced in the epiphyseal area approximately 30 mm proximal to the joint line. The blade is 5.6 mm thick, 16 mm in width, and the distance between the holes is 16 mm. Its entry point is ventral and proximal to the lateral collateral ligament, the entry angle has been determined by the specific instruments and the specific reamer is used. For a calculated valgus correction of 8 degrees, the guide instrument is set at 93 degrees (85 + 8 degrees; this is the complementary angle to the desired anatomic angle of 95 degrees, plus the angle of correction). The blade is subsequently introduced into the femur. The correct angulations are again checked using the image intensifier.

Derotation osteotomy in case of femoral malrotation. The area of the osteotomy is prepared in the same manner. Two superficial saw marks are made on the lateral cortex indicating the desired angle of the derotation. Thus an isolated derotation osteotomy can be performed as well as a derotation osteotomy in combination with an opening wedge or a closing wedge femoral osteotomy. The derotation osteotomy should not interfere with the patella tracking or create a step on the anterior cortex.

On the Tibia. For these surgical techniques, please see the section on tibial osteotomy. The bone graft obtained in case of a closing wedge femoral osteotomy is used to fill the opening wedge tibial osteotomy.

CONCLUSIONS

In conclusion, osteotomy is still a treatment of choice for OA. Our main indications are presented here.

Medial Femorotibial Arthrosis

- Opening wedge HTO:
  - Young patient
  - Early OA: stage 1 and 2
  - Extended indication: combination ACL reconstruction and osteotomy
  - In the exceptional case of a constitutional varus knee without OA (constitutional varus more than 8 degrees, if

bilateral or with more than four finger widths of space between the condyles). In this rare case, the aim is to leave some residual varus (2 to 3 degrees).
- Closing wedge HTO:
  - Older patient but still active
  - Stage 3 and 4
  - Associated patella infera
  - Chronic anterior laxity with posterior wear on the tibial plateau
- Femoral osteotomy and double osteotomy are exceptional: these techniques are indicated in arthritis secondary to malunion, vitamin D deficiency, and so on.

Lateral Femorotibial Arthrosis

- Tibial osteotomy:
  - We prefer a medial closing wedge osteotomy.
  - To correct abnormalities of mixed origin (femoral and tibial) only if the obliquity of the joint line will not be superior to 10 degrees after osteotomy and in a valgus knee less than 8 degrees.
  - Lateral opening wedge HTO with a reosteotomy of the fibula is only indicated secondary to an excessive closing wedge HTO with an overcorrection.
- Femoral osteotomy:
  - Valgus knee of femoral origin
  - If valgus with a fixed flexion deformity or a hyperextension of more than 20 degrees: this pathology can be addressed more appropriately with a femoral osteotomy than with a tibial osteotomy. However, the morbidity of the femoral osteotomy is more important and has to be integrated into the indications flowchart to prevent complications.
- In case of a large deformation: Double osteotomy combining a lateral distal femoral opening wedge osteotomy and a medial closing wedge HTO.

Some pictures of this text have already been published in "My Knee Practice"

Elsevier, Paris, 2007.

KEY REFERENCES

6. Akizuki S, Shibakawa A, Takizawa T, et al: The long-term outcome of high tibial osteotomy: a ten- to 20-year follow up. *J Bone Joint Surg Br* 90:592–596, 2008.

7. Arthur A, LaPrade RF, Agel J: Proximal tibial opening wedge osteotomy as the initial treatment for chronic posterolateral corner deficiency in the varus knee: a prospective clinical study. *Am J Sports Med* 35(11):1844–1850, 2007.

35. El-Azab H, Glabgly P, Paul J, et al: Patellar height and posterior tibial slope after open- and closed-wedge high tibial osteotomy: a radiological study on 100 patients. *Am J Sports Med* 38(2):323–329, 2010.

36. Faschingbauer M, Nelitz M, Urlaub S, et al: Return to work and sporting activities after high tibial osteotomy. *Int Orthop* 39(8):1527–1534, 2015.

52. Hui C, Salmon LJ, Kok A, et al: Long-term survival of high tibial osteotomy for medial compartment osteoarthritis of the knee. *Am J Sports Med* 39(1):64–70, 2011. doi: 10.1177/0363546510377445.

61. Koh YG, Kwon OR, Kim YS, et al: Comparative outcomes of open-wedge high tibial osteotomy with platelet-rich plasma alone or in combination with mesenchymal stem cell treatment: a prospective study. *Arthroscopy* 30(11):1453–1460, 2014. doi: 10.1016/j.arthro.2014.05.036.

73. Lustig S, Scholes CJ, Costa AJ, et al: Different changes in slope between the medial and lateral tibial plateau after open-wedge high tibial

osteotomy. *Knee Surg Sports Traumatol Arthrosc* 21(1):32–38, 2013. doi: 10.1007/s00167-012-2229-6.

74. Madelaine A, Lording T, Villa V, et al: The effect of lateral opening wedge distal femoral osteotomy on leg length. *Knee Surg Sports Traumatol Arthrosc* 24(3):847–854, 2014.

99. Ozel O, Yucel B, Mutlu S, et al: Changes in posterior tibial slope angle in patients undergoing open-wedge high tibial osteotomy for varus gonarthrosis. *Knee Surg Sports Traumatol Arthrosc* 2015. [Epub ahead of print].

107. Schallberger A, Jacobi M, Wahl P, et al: High tibial valgus osteotomy in unicompartmental medial osteoarthritis of the knee: a retrospective follow-up study over 13–21 years. *Knee Surg Sports Traumatol Arthrosc* 19(1):122–127, 2011. doi: 10.1007/s00167-010-1256-4.

109. Schröter S, Freude T, Kopp MM, et al: Smoking and unstable hinge fractures cause delayed gap filling irrespective of early weight bearing after open wedge osteotomy. *Arthroscopy* 31(2):254–265, 2015. doi: 10.1016/j.arthro.

110. Schuster P, Schulz M, Mayer P, et al: Open-wedge high tibial osteotomy and combined abrasion/microfracture in severe medial osteoarthritis and varus malalignment: 5-year results and arthroscopic findings after 2 years. *Arthroscopy* pii:S0749–S8063(15)00104-8, 2015. doi: 10.1016/j.arthro.2015.02.010.

123. van Raaij TM, Brouwer RW, de Vlieger R, et al: Opposite cortical fracture in high tibial osteotomy: lateral closing compared to the medial opening-wedge technique. *Acta Orthop* 79(4):508–514, 2008.

124. Virolainen P, Aro HT: High tibial osteotomy for the treatment of osteoarthritis of the knee: a review of the literature and a meta-analysis of follow-up studies. *Arch Orthop Trauma Surg* 124:258–261, 2004. doi: 10.1007/s00402-003-0545-5.

131. Zarrouk A, Bouzidi R, Karray B, et al: Distal femoral varus osteotomy outcome: is associated femoropatellar osteoarthritis consequential? *Orthop Traumatol Surg Res* 96:632–636, 2010.

The references for this chapter can also be found on www.expertconsult.com.

123

Scoring Systems and Their Validation for the Arthritic Knee

Adam C. Brekke, Philip C. Noble, David Rodriguez-Quintana, Brian S. Parsley, Kenneth B. Mathis

BACKGROUND AND RATIONALE

Total knee replacement (TKR) has proven to be a highly effective surgical intervention for improving the health-related quality of life of patients suffering from knee arthritis. Published data shows that approximately 700,000 knee replacements are performed in the United States annually, at a total cost of over $11 billion.[59,86] Moreover, it is projected that the demand for TKR in the United States will approach 3.5 million cases per year by 2030, an increase of 673% over current usage.[81] At current rates, 52% of males and 51% of females with symptomatic knee osteoarthritis will receive a primary TKR in their lifetime.[131]

Although the arrival of the baby boomer generation and longer life expectancy are contributing to the increased demand for total knee arthroplasty (TKA), the obesity epidemic and the resulting prevalence of osteoarthritis are driving younger patients (ie, <65) to seek primary and revision knee replacement at astounding rates.[43] In fact, Kurtz et al. previously projected that, if current trends continue, younger patients will constitute most (>50%) of the demand for primary knee replacement and revision knee surgery by 2016, and this was noted early in this decade, with more than 50% of the demand for revision knee surgery.[80]

Postoperatively, patients have reported reduced pain, restored range of motion (ROM), high satisfaction, and the ability to return to a more active lifestyle.[18,56,60,100,101] Moreover, detailed economic analysis has confirmed the favorable cost-effectiveness of the procedure.[86] Recent data show that for a male age 60 to 64 who undergoes knee replacement surgery, improvement in the 36-Item Short Form Survey (SF-36) functional score is consistent with a 20- to 21-percentage point higher probability of being employed, $4300 to $4700 increase in annual household income, and six fewer missed work days for those who are employed, and a decline in probability of receiving Social Security Income (SSI) payments for disability.[26]

Although there are marked benefits from the procedure, recent focus on quantifying these improvements has shifted toward a more subjective evaluation of the outcomes, based upon the patient's own assessment of their outcome and the extent to which their expectations have been fulfilled after undergoing the procedure. It has been shown that 10% to 20% of patients are not satisfied with the outcome of TKR, primarily because of unmet preoperative expectations and the presence of persistent knee symptoms.[15] This level of dissatisfaction has been reported most recently in younger, more active TKA patients who expect and require a higher postsurgical level of activity.[108] As a consequence, there has been increasing emphasis on the role of surgeons in addressing the preoperative expectations of patients regarding the outcome of joint replacement in an effort to reduce the incidence of dissatisfaction following surgery.

As increasing numbers of patients elect to have their knees replaced, the need for revision surgery will also increase. Among those who undergo a primary TKR, the risk of subsequent revision is 14.9% for males and 17.4% for females, further increasing the future costs of joint replacement surgery.[131] As a result, measures to control the risk of complications and the resulting financial burden must become top priorities in the formulation of health care policy.[81,134] Today, the effectiveness of TKRs and other costly surgical interventions are subject to increased scrutiny. In this environment, it is of paramount concern to patients, health care providers, device manufacturers, and the community that the health-related benefit and cost-effectiveness of TKR be demonstrated in an objective and scientifically valid manner.[113]

Quantification of the success of these procedures can be achieved in a number of ways, principally driven by the definition of a "successful" versus an "unsuccessful" procedure.[102] The simplest measure of the clinical success of knee arthroplasty is crude survivorship, defined as retention of the artificial joint in situ, regardless of the function of the patient or the degree of relief from knee symptoms (pain, swelling, and stiffness). More recently, researchers have highlighted the importance of adding patient perspectives of their outcome to provide a complete assessment of treatment impact and expectations.[7,29,138] However, to establish any insight into surgical outcomes, especially as they relate to subjective evaluations, more comprehensive assessment methods are required and have recently been included in the literature.[133] The outcomes movement, a collection of efforts by investigators to address this concern, has spurred the development of several assessment systems that measure patient health status.[16]

Certainly, one can gather patient information and present the attributes of successful surgeries as a series of case reports. However, conclusions drawn from this approach generally lack broad applicability and do not allow valid comparisons of outcome with variations in patients and treatments. In attempting to provide an objective evaluation of the patient's condition before and after surgery, measurement tools have been developed that allow the outcome of surgical treatment to be quantified on an individual basis.[15] Most often, these tools consist of questionnaires, surveys, or interviews that the patient and/or surgeon can complete during clinic visits or research studies, along with some data derived from the clinical exam.

Traditional methods of evaluating different treatments have relied on objective endpoints with little relevance to how the patient was affected by the treatment itself.[16] The methods also neglected patient expectations and preoperative activity level and placed most of their weight on pain control and arc of motion achieved after surgery or rates of postoperative complications, including revision. Wright posited that a fundamental task for clinicians when evaluating patients or interpreting the results of clinical trials is to decide if a particular outcome assessment relates to an important improvement in patient health. In this sense, contemporary outcome instruments measure the effect of treatment on those treated, and the quality of their lives after receiving the treatment.[48,56] But because TKR is generally an elective procedure, patient goals and expectations need to be clearly determined if the outcome is to be accurately appraised.[135]

Although there is no universally accepted instrument for evaluating the outcome of patients after TKR, it is generally agreed that a quantifiable rating (usually a scoring system, ie, 0 to 100 points) provides the most concise, clear measure, especially for comparing large groups of patients and treatments. Scoring systems are generally categorized as overall generic health measures (ie, global health) or specific health measures (ie, disease-specific), and each system may contain one or more domains that address a particular facet of health (ie, functional capabilities, pain, mental health, etc.). Recently, new outcome instruments have been developed with their own specific focus.[33,34,112] With pain, range of motion, distance walked, ability to climb stairs, ability to rise from a sitting position, and presence of a flexion contracture weighting heavily on these scores, new scores have been introduced that accommodate variations between the lifestyles and expectations of individual patients.[97,120,121] The procedures adopted for determining each instrument's composition and the methodologies for scoring and reporting the results are still the source of much debate and will likely continue to be long into the future. The variations between these rating systems makes it difficult for them to achieve their purpose—to compare patient outcomes and to assess the merits of treatments across studies.[75] Despite methodological differences, scoring systems that have been subjected to formal validation and the rigors of standard psychometric testing and item response theory (IRT), have broad applicability and are generally accepted across the orthopedic community.

SCORING SYSTEM STRUCTURE

Numerous factors affect the response of individual patients to a specific orthopedic treatment, many of which are based on subjective perceptions. As a result, investigators have had difficulty in reaching a consensus as to how the outcome of treatments should be measured. Given the existence of a multitude of measurement instruments and the assortment of methodologies for patient evaluation, it can be difficult to compare different measures of patient outcome directly or to draw appropriate or practical conclusions from data collected by different instruments.[34,75] In the case of TKR, the ability to compare outcomes across different studies is imperative for the following stakeholders:

- patients and physicians considering different treatment options,
- surgeons attempting to predict postoperative outcome based on the patient's clinical characteristics,

- surgeons counseling patients to establish reasonable expectations,
- surgeons assessing whether a patient's preoperative expectations will be met by knee replacement surgery,
- patents wondering if they will be able to participate in their favorite high-demand activities after knee replacement surgery, and
- implant manufacturers developing new technologies or surgical techniques.

As early as 1975, Kettelkamp and Thompson recognized the potential for discord and postulated that a uniform rating system should fulfill the following requirements[71]:

- It should be based on important measurable characteristics of the knee.
- It should avoid arbitrary assignment of point values.
- Points assigned to a knee condition according to the rating system should be related to clinical results.
- The rating system should be simple and should be based on clinical variables that can be easily quantified.

Regardless of the type of instrument used, the responses elicited will be influenced by the patient themselves (ie, their personality, educational and cultural background, health history, etc.) as well as the design and content of the instrument itself.[58] Therefore, an understanding of the structure and scoring methodology adopted by an outcome assessment instrument is critical for the interpretation of its results.

Item Development

In practice, relief of symptoms, restoration of function, and promotion of satisfaction and a feeling of well-being are among the most important outcomes of TKA and are universally recognized as central concerns of patients and physicians alike.[41] Consequently, any instrument that attempts to measure the outcome of treatment of the arthritic knee must assess these multidimensional facets of each patient's experience.[126] Patient outcome measures, especially self-assessed measures, are all subject to the patients' attitudes, abilities, expectations, and motivations to undergo surgery.[126] Whether the assessment instrument is designed to evaluate the patient's general health or only the physiologic function of the knee in isolation, optimally designed instruments clearly define these health dimensions and measure, with full coverage, the underlying trait or condition of interest.[20]

Designers of outcome instruments start by first identifying the intended scope of their instrument and what it intends to measure. Those interested in the overall impact of an arthritic knee or a knee replacement on a patient's health consider different outcome variables than those interested in the knee in isolation from the patient's other health issues. In general, instrument scoring systems contain items assessing pain, function, ROM, and satisfaction, among other components.[18,19,34] Certain outcome instruments assess each of these components of patient health in different ways. For example, assessments interested in patient function may include any one or more of the following traits: the ability to walk, the dependence on supports or walking aids, the presence of a limp, the ability to sit for an extended period, the ability to rise from a chair, the ability to ascend or descend stairs, and the ability to run.[34]

The components of a patient's health are interdependent, and all contribute to a patient's overall outcome. For example, physical activity is likely associated with the patient's

- capabilities (eg, ROM, stability),
- knee symptoms (eg, pain, stiffness, comorbidities),

- attitude (eg, personal importance of each activity, expectations and willingness to tolerate pain), and
- contextual factors (eg, age, occupational status).

However, there is no exclusive causal relationship between these variables. In other words, symptoms could limit physical activity, or abstaining from activity may exacerbate persistence of symptoms. Furthermore, the true relationship between these components and a patient's satisfaction or overall assessment is variable. Certain patients may have very different, even dynamic expectations of their knee function and may change their personal definition of a satisfactory outcome. All of the interrelated health factors contribute to a patient's priorities, their internal processes of assessment of the need for surgery, and the value of the level of restored function and symptom relief that the procedure provides.[70] Therefore, the items in an assessment instrument must distinguish among these contributing factors in striving to characterize patient outcome.[41,95,126,135]

Designers of assessment instruments must establish clear definitions and parameters for each variable they will use to measure outcome. This step is critical, yet it is subject to much debate. For example, instruments commonly contain items asking patients about any persisting pain ("Have you had any sudden, severe pain—shooting, stabbing, or spasms—from the affected joint?"),[29] but only a few consider whether the patient's perceptions of symptoms are mitigated through their use of analgesics.[28] Knee assessment instruments often focus on function as an outcome as well, but some inquire about the patient's capabilities or limitations in performing a specific activity ("What degree of difficulty do you have bending to the floor?"),[9,10] whereas others ask about the extent or frequency of a patient's participation in the activity ("How often do you participate in squatting?").[14,103,139] Because patient-based assessment instruments are subject to interpretation and context, accurate wording of items is important to account for subtle differences in meaning and inference.[111]

It is also important that the items in an outcome instrument reflect the clinical outcome of all patients who fall within its intended scope, inclusive of variations in age, diagnosis, and treatment. As the demand for TKRs expands, especially among young or active patients, and because the technologies and techniques used are in constant development, a growing spectrum of patients will be reporting a myriad of conditions and outcomes.[80,81,134] Broad applicability allows differentiation to be made, even at the extremes of the distribution of patients, such as those who are very young or very old, very active or very sedentary, or very healthy or burdened with complications or comorbidities.[28,57,76,83] This means that investigations that quantify outcomes in terms of the ability to perform physical activities should include items that distinguish among those who are limited and those who are relatively active.[65,103,132] An example of this approach is the University of California Los Angeles (UCLA) activity-level rating, introduced by Zahiri et al. in 1998, which distinguishes between patient activity levels as follows[139]:

Regularly participate in impact sports
Sometimes participate in impact sports
Regularly participate in very active events
Sometimes participate in mild activities
Mostly inactive: restricted to minimal activities of daily living
Wholly inactive: dependent on others, cannot leave residence

From an array of patients with a broad spectrum of conditions, instruments aim to identify, accurately and distinctly, those who will benefit from a treatment and those who would be better served using an alternative approach.[18,28,79,111]

It is difficult for one item to completely measure a patient's true condition or trait in isolation from the patient's other related conditions. Most outcome instruments are based on questionnaires with multiple items that assess manifestations of the same symptom (eg, pain), which are not completely independent, and therefore have a significant statistical association with each other.[41] This characteristic of patient conditions is referred to statistically as *covariance*. Thus, when attempting to measure covariant traits, there is a high risk of sampling the same underlying trait repeatedly through questionnaire items that are not entirely independent.[111] This redundancy, whether overt or subtle, can distort the measurement of the patient's true condition and lead to spurious conclusions, such as overrepresentation of an underlying dimension of outcome. All of these considerations speak to the importance of ensuring that the individual items measure only the condition of interest, without simultaneously measuring additional unrelated traits.[111,126]

Scoring Methodology

Outcome measures quantify or summarize the patients' responses in the form of a numerical score or classification. Although most instruments adopt a systematic approach to scoring a patient's response, many features of their scoring systems were established arbitrarily and can vary widely from one another.[34] There are two factors contributing to variations in scoring methodology: (1) the response formats and (2) the scoring allocation or classification system.

For most outcome instruments, test items have nominal, partial-credit, graded, or other polytomous (more than two response categories) response formats for assessing multidimensional abilities.[126] Current instruments contain items whose responses are scaled in many different ways, sometimes with too many response categories, other times with too few.[20] When asking a question such as, "Do you have swelling in your knee?" some instruments offer responses in a Likert-scale format, with ordinal responses, corresponding to increments in symptom frequency or severity (eg, "never/rarely/sometimes/often/always").[116,117] Other measurement systems use a dichotomous ("yes/no") response format for the same question. Items with too few response categories may not differentiate between patients with clinical differences, whereas those with too many response categories may introduce unnecessary error because of variations in each patient's definition of the gradations corresponding to the ordinal scale. Both of these issues can confound data and mask a patient's true condition.[136] Moreover, most Likert-scale data is condensed into fewer categories in subsequent analysis as clinicians view subjective assessment of symptoms in dichotomous (ie, present/absent) or possibly trichotomous terms (eg, absent/mild/intense). This raises the question: "Is there value in the use of multiple level options if responses are subsequently analyzed and discussed in a condensed format without weighting the frequency or severity within each category?"

The appropriateness of alternative response formats can be assessed through statistical testing. For example, Bach et al. used interobserver correlation analysis to conclude that assessment of pain is most reliably attained using a simple four-point scale ("no pain/mild or occasional pain/moderate pain restricting activity/severe pain disturbing rest") as in the Bristol Score or the Hospital for Special Surgery Score as opposed to a more complex six-point or seven-point scale.* Because the responses to each item contribute to a patient's score, the item's response format can have a significant impact in distinguishing patients' outcomes.

Despite the proliferation of many different outcome scores in the literature, there has been a movement toward the standardization of scoring systems. This has arisen because the scores allocated by different systems have proven difficult to compare, causing uncertainty of how outcome scores truly relate to patients' clinical outcomes. If a scoring system uses a scale from 0 to 100 points, as many do, those points are allocated, or awarded, based on responses to items throughout the instrument. However, the way in which these points are allocated varies widely between instruments.[34] In a review of 34 different rating systems that are used to evaluate patients after TKR, Drake et al. reported that the total points awarded for a perfect outcome ranged from 10 to 110, with scoring based on summation of points, deductions from a baseline score, or a combination thereof.[34] The contribution, or weight, of certain components to the total score was notably diverse. For example, the contribution of pain symptoms to the total score ranged from 7% to 69%, whereas the ROM of the joint was assigned between 4% and 30% of the total score. Diverse weightings for patients' ability to perform functional tasks were also reported, with items such as the ability to climb stairs making up 4% to 50% of the total outcome score.[34] With the advent of instruments focused on patient satisfaction and expectations, investigators can potentially determine the primary subjective factors affecting patients' postoperative satisfaction and their motivations for undergoing surgery. As investigators elucidate these and other factors affecting outcome, guidelines will be developed to allow more consistent and appropriate weighting of each component to outcome scores.

In addition to component weighting, understanding a system's point value allocation to specific responses is critical. For example, two different systems may assign a maximum of 50 of the scale's 100 total points to responses quantifying pain; however, on one scale, 40 points may be assigned if patients experience pain "once a month," whereas the second scale may assign 50 points to the same response. Moreover, the point scores necessary to achieve a particular categorical designation (ie, 90 to 100 points is "Excellent," 80 to 90 points is "Good," etc.) are somewhat arbitrary and inconsistent across studies.[18] Component point values could be the same in different scoring systems, but interpretation of the responses can vary.[34] In one system, an "excellent" or "acceptable" outcome may correspond to a score of at least 90 out of 100, whereas it may correspond to at least 80 out of 100 in another.[1,34] Therefore, it is important to consider the scoring system's weighting, allocation, and categorization methodology when interpreting a patient's score.

Because patient outcome is multidimensional, consideration of the outcome total score, in and of itself, does not necessarily shed light on the patient's true condition. By analyzing a patient's raw total outcome score (eg, 70 out of 100), an investigator has no insight into which conditions are primarily affecting the patient's outcome. With this limitation, a raw total outcome score cannot readily describe or relate to a clinically relevant outcome. Jones et al. affirm that a simple summative

score may dilute the important effects of confounding conditions (eg, other symptomatic joints, psychiatric disorder), thereby masking the true effect of other conditions on functional recovery.[70] Therefore, several investigators have emphasized the need for component subscores in addition to, or as opposed to, a sum raw total score.† A separation of health outcome components, sometimes called a dual rating system, can eliminate the falsely inflated or deflated scores associated with co-variables in assessment systems that aggregate different parameters into a global score.[65,75] Components of health, such as function, pain, and mental health, can be separated so that their component scores can be considered independently and as an aggregate composite score. Based on trends and comparisons of component scores, one can identify patient conditions that benefit most from treatment or even those that tend to predict success. With a distinct component scoring system, characterization of scores to clinically relevant outcomes is more feasible and appropriate.

STATISTICAL REQUIREMENTS

Psychometric Principles

Outcome instruments are most useful as a means of comparing large sets of data (sets of patient subgroups, surgical techniques, component designs, rehabilitation protocols, etc.), so they must adhere to statistical principles that ensure broad applicability and comparison across groups. McDowell stated that a well-constructed and acceptable rating system uses "statistically correct procedures to refine an instrument whose content is based on clinical wisdom and common sense."[95] The conventional method of statistical testing, generally referred to as classical test theory (CTT), states that valid methods of outcome assessment must adhere to three psychometric properties: validity, reliability, and responsiveness.‡

The *validity* of an instrument is its ability to accurately measure the health of a patient or the effectiveness of a treatment regimen. In other words, a valid instrument is one that measures what was intended, yielding results corresponding to the true state of the trait being measured.[41,95]

Many of the established assessment instruments consist of questionnaires designed to measure traits such as symptoms or pain, which are grouped together to form scales. Scaling systems allow subjective reports of health to be quantified and analyzed. Three general forms of validity—content validity, criterion validity, and construct validity—are tested in assessing whether a scale is truly valid.[41,95] These forms of validity are defined as follows:

1. Content validity: Refers to the comprehensiveness of a measurement instrument in covering the scope of the trait it is intended to measure and nothing more. The content validity of different instruments is undermined by three main forms of distortion of the trait being measured. These sources of error are commonly termed the floor effect, the ceiling effect, and the skew of the true frequency distribution.[41,95]

   a. Floor and ceiling effects: Patients who score the best possible score on a questionnaire, for example, cannot demonstrate improvement on a subsequent application of the same questionnaire, even if they have improved clinically. This is referred to as the *ceiling effect* and describes a measurement instrument that awards the maximum score too easily for a significant proportion of its target population. Conversely, the *floor effect* refers to measurement instruments that award the minimum score too easily for a significant proportion of its target population.

b. Skew of frequency distribution: The skew of the distribution of the outcome scores quantifies the deviation of scores from a normal distribution.[37] Outcome measures may over-rate or under-rate the underlying trait of subjects, thereby distorting the relevant component of the health status of the respondents.

2. Criterion validity: This is present when the outcome measure is correlated with a directly observable phenomenon that is generally accepted as a surrogate for the condition being measured, or when the outcome measure provides a classification of subjects generally in agreement with standard accepted measures of the same trait.[41,95]

3. Construct validity: To be valid, an outcome instrument must actually quantify the trait that it intends to measure, and not something else. Thus, a valid knee function instrument ranks patients with clearly different degrees of impairment in the expected order, and awards similar scores to patients who appear to have the same or similar degrees of impairment on clinical examination.[41,95] Although this concept may seem self-evident, it becomes particularly important in developing new instruments when there is no pre-existing rating system that is accepted as the "gold standard."

When assessing patient outcomes after treatment of knee arthritis, there is no universally accepted instrument. Therefore, constructs are sometimes validated through comparison against other questionnaires or against surgeons' conceptual definitions of patient health. This circuitous logic is problematic and should be considered when examining construct validity.[37]

The *reliability*, or reproducibility, of a measurement instrument is the extent to which it yields similar results when administered at different times, to different patients, or by different observers when the measured trait remains constant. According to CTT, every assessment instrument has an inherent error because of its design, wording, response formats, and other contextual factors that influence individuals' responses.[58,95] Consequently, as individuals complete outcome instruments, the responses elicited, and any scores derived from them, are a combined function of the patient's true responses and this inherent measurement error. The proportion of variation of the observed scores that is attributable to the true outcome is defined as the reliability of an instrument.[95] In practice, the reliability of an outcome instrument can be measured through its test-retest reproducibility, which is most frequently estimated using an indicator of internal consistency called *Cronbach's alpha*. Cronbach's alpha represents the average of all intercorrelations among test items of an instrument. It is used when the instrument's items have more than two response options (eg, 5-point Likert scale), and it indicates the degree to which a set of items measures an underlying latent trait.[95]

Reliability and validity are not altogether independent. Reliability is a necessary but insufficient property of valid instruments; an unreliable measurement cannot be valid, and a valid instrument must be reliable.[41,95] When a measurement is reliable, any change noted in a patient's scores can be attributed confidently to a true change in the clinical status of the patient.

Because the most direct measure of patient health outcomes after TKR often includes subjective measurements (ie, pain, function, satisfaction), a measurement tool that minimizes sources of variability and bias while maintaining reliability can instill confidence in those depending on its measurements.[136]

Responsiveness is a crucial component of outcome measures to distinguish those patients who benefit from a procedure from those who do not. A more responsive test is more sensitive to subtle changes in the patient's health status.[79] Thus, highly responsive scales allow clinical trials to be performed using fewer patients.[137] Several methods of determining responsiveness have been introduced. Generally, the change in mean raw scores of a given sample of patients divided by the standard deviation of the sample will yield a measure of responsiveness of an instrument, which is commonly called the *standard effect size*.[95] Alternatively, the change in raw score may be normalized with respect to its standard error (*t*-test approach) or to the standard deviation of the changes in scores of all respondents (standardized response mean).[95] Although no clear consensus exists as to how responsiveness should be demonstrated, it is generally agreed that a responsive instrument will be sensitive enough to detect changes in health or physical functioning that are revealed by existing established measures of the same or similar traits. Accordingly, the responsiveness of new knee function scales can be assessed by comparing the distribution of scores derived from the new instrument against those determined with a basket of conventional instruments (eg, Knee Injury and Osteoarthritis Outcome Score [KOOS], Oxford, SF-36).[41,95]

For an outcome measure to be effective, it must accurately and reliably quantify a set of data that is often comprised of subjective as well as objective measurements describing the health of a variety of patients, spanning a broad range of conditions and perspectives. To date, there have been a number of established methods proposed to assess patients' quality of life and the cost-effectiveness of alternative procedures, yet few have been proven to be valid and reliable.[5,34] When an outcome measure has been demonstrated to be valid and reliable, its responsiveness may be an additional factor in its selection to measure the outcome variables of interest.[95]

Item Response Theory

The multidimensional character of patient perspectives impacts the score of the instrument by introducing error and variability in responses. CTT, including psychometric testing, although valuable and essential, has its limitations. To determine validity and responsiveness, CTT uses estimates based on correlational data, most often maximizing Cronbach's alpha. Analyses of response data using CTT may reflect only a small part of the underlying condition and may depend on the size and nature of the sample of patients and set of items present in the instrument.[111] CTT assumes that systematic differences between responses of patients are due only to variation in the patients' underlying conditions of interest; other sources of variations are ignored and assumed to be constant or random by nature.[126] CTT is also limited by the fact that the patients' abilities and item difficulties cannot be estimated separately. Also, CTT yields only a single reliability estimate and corresponding standard error of measurement, despite the fact that precision of measurement is known to vary by the patients' ability levels.[59] In other words, CTT methods do not capture the notion that different types of patients (eg, male vs. female or active vs.

sedentary) exhibit different response patterns, which could affect the estimate of instrument reliability.

The recent development of a modern statistical analysis method, called IRT, stems from recognition of these limitations. IRT addresses the need for deeper insight into patient response processes and into the interaction among the items of an assessment instrument and the abilities of the respondent.[126] Using specified mathematical models, IRT can describe the association between a respondent's underlying condition and the probability of a particular item response.[58,126] These IRT models are designed to cope with natural experimental error, noise, and other confounding variables that are unavoidable under less rigorous standardization of assessment, such as self-administered surveys.[126] Application of IRT to outcome instruments has begun to enhance investigators' ability to evaluate, modify, compare, and score existing instruments to reveal more useful health outcome information. Investigators have even used IRT methods to create and validate outcome instruments. One such instrument was administered by Parsley and colleagues to TKR patients who received two different prosthesis designs. Patients receiving a posterior cruciate ligament (PCL)-sacrificing design reported less ability to perform specific functional activities than those receiving PCL-retaining designs.[25] These results were unexpected because, in the same patient groups, conventional instruments developed using CTT testing regimens showed no difference in clinical outcome of the two prosthesis designs.[25] This demonstrates that instruments developed using IRT may facilitate the identification of clinically significant factors that would have otherwise gone unnoticed. Going forward, IRT can also be used to develop briefer, more flexible, more efficient, and more precise instruments than could be constructed using classical approaches.[20,58,76]

Although the content of the questions in an outcome measure is certainly important, IRT models are explicitly directed at the rating scale.[20] IRT models (eg, Rasch and Generalized Partial Credit Models) describe how difficult an activity is and the degree to which the patient's response varies as his or her condition changes. Using sets of patient response data, the models are also used to measure the level of agreement between the observed and model-predicted probabilities of selecting each response option. IRT models can calculate a differential item function that identifies inefficient, inaccurate, or inappropriate items whose responses differ systematically across groups of respondents.[76] For example, in an IRT analysis of common assessment items, the responses to the item, "need help with grooming," differ significantly between males and females. The responses for "difficulty getting in and out of bed" are shown to differ significantly between patient age groups.[76] These items, although appearing to have face validity, may be inappropriate for a standard instrument applied to a diverse set of total knee patients. After an instrument has been tested using IRT models, its items should measure a single concept, fit the chosen IRT model, and should not function differently across groups.[76]

Compared to CTT estimates, IRT models may better depict patients' actual response patterns, and IRT estimates more accurately reflect patients' true conditions.[20,57] Thus, use of IRT for large sets of patient responses should lead to an outcome assessment that is more sensitive to true cross-sectional differences and more responsive to change in health over time.[20,57] The models use measurement units with interval measurement properties that remove the bias at the extreme ends of a patient condition. Therefore, they can be used to discriminate among patients who are very active or very disabled.[20,57] This capability to discriminate between levels of an underlying trait enhances the usefulness of IRT models in relating the results to clinically relevant outcomes, especially within single diagnostic groups.[20]

Compared to more conventional statistical analyses, IRT is more difficult to perform and understand, although it results in discriminative, informative, nonredundant items adhering to psychometric principles. Therefore, IRT could best be used in conjunction with CTT.[111] For future development of outcome measures using IRT, it is essential that collaborative efforts be successful between statisticians and clinical investigators, leading to a consensus regarding acceptable standards for use and reporting of outcome data.[57]

CLASSIFICATIONS OF OUTCOME MEASURES

Generic Outcome Measures

Some investigators have assessed the outcome of knee arthroplasty using generic health questionnaires on the basis that the value of medical treatment should be reflected in improvement in patients' health-related quality of life. Generic measures assess overall health as well as the impact of side effects and comorbidities.[72] These instruments typically ask questions in the spheres of physical health, physiologic function, mental health, and social function, and so can measure different aspects of health across different patients being treated with different interventions for different symptoms.

One of the most widely accepted and most often used instruments for measurement of generic health outcomes is the SF-36 developed in 1988 by Ware at the Health Institute at New England Medical Center.[128,129] The SF-36 measures three major health attributes and eight health concepts[113]:

1. Functional status
   a. Physical functioning
   b. Social functioning
   c. Role limitations attributed to physical problems
   d. Emotional problems
2. Well-being
   a. Mental health
   b. Energy/fatigue
   c. Pain
3. Overall evaluation of health
   a. General health perception

The SF-36 questionnaire has been validated and proven reliable[77,78] and the resulting score has been shown to be an effective measure of the effect of interventions, including TKA, on overall patient health and quality of life.[12,113] The responsiveness of the SF-36 and the minimal clinically important difference (MCID) of scores generated by this instrument have been reported in the literature.[40,72] However, the SF-36 may not be practical for application with large populations of subjects because of its length. This has led to the development of a shorter version, the 12-Item Short Form Health Survey (SF-12) consisting of the 12 items from the functional status and well-being sections of the SF-36 that were found to be most predictive of the original outcome score.[130] The SF-12 has been validated and demonstrates exceptional test-retest reliability, and is therefore an appropriate alternative to the lengthier and less responsive SF-36.[37,130] One comparison study even demonstrated that, according to statistical testing, the SF-12 had the best overall ranking compared to other frequently used generic health instruments, and was thus recommended for use in a cross-sectional discriminative application.[36] Recently, Clement et al. reported the MCID for outcome scores derived from the physical, pain relief, and functional components on the SF-12.[24]

Because of their generic nature, the SF-36 and SF-12 have not demonstrated high sensitivity or responsiveness to subtle changes among subjects with varying severity of knee problems or levels of recovery.[12,73] Therefore, many investigators support the inclusion of a generic and a specific outcome measure for comprehensive assessment of patient outcomes in studies.

Specific Outcome Measures

Although a number of outcome measures have been established for use in the general population, these instruments have not been designed to detect subtle, clinically important changes in a patient with arthritis of the knee. Many investigators emphasize the need for more specific health instruments to objectively measure the effect of specific treatments on the function of individual systems or body functions, as in the case of TKA for treatment of degenerative joint disease affecting the knee. These instruments can still measure different aspects of health, but the intended subject is limited to those with symptomatic or replaced knees. Specific outcome measures can be further qualified as global knee rating systems, disease-specific, patient-specific, functional outcome measures, etc.

Global Rating Systems

A global knee rating system has been operationally defined as an outcome instrument that includes, at a minimum, assessments of pain, function, and ROM, and summarizes these outcomes as a single score on a global scale.[18,19,34] In a review of the literature from 1972 to 1992, Drake et al. recognized 34 different global knee rating systems.[34] In this review, and in others, the most commonly used outcome measure was the Hospital for Special Surgery (HSS) Knee Scoring System.[18,19,28,34,66] Introduced in 1976 by Insall et al., the HSS knee score generates a maximum of 100 points derived from six categories:

1. Pain (30 points)
2. Function (22 points)
3. ROM (22 points)
4. Muscle strength (10 points)
5. Flexion deformity (10 points)
6. Instability (10 points)
7. Deductions, if applicable
   a. Dependence on walking aids
   b. Extension lag
   c. Varus/valgus deformity

Patient outcomes can be classified as Excellent for scores better than 85, Good for scores of 70 to 84, Fair for 60 to 69, and Poor for any scores less than 60.[28,66] This scaling system is heavily weighted toward pain, ROM, and function. The global assessment of function, particularly, is notable because its measure of walking and stair-climbing ability may be confounded by comorbidities or factors other than the function of the knee. Additionally, the assessment of pain makes no attempt to investigate the patient's use or dependence on analgesics.[28] Although the HSS scoring system has been widely used and has been validated, its limitations and demonstrations of poor reliability have caused it to fall out of favor as an outcome measure following knee replacement surgery.[28,34]

In 1989, Insall et al. published the Knee Society (KS) Clinical Rating System, which recognized some of the limitations of the HSS score and implemented a scoring method that has been widely adopted and supported.[§] The KS Score segregates the knee score from the functional score, both of which consist of distinct 100-point scales and should be based on findings in the last 4 weeks prior to completion. The KS knee score is clinician administered, whereas a clinician or the patient may complete the pain and function subscales. Separate scores enable surgeons to assess the patient's knee conditions independent of any functional deterioration as a result of comorbidities.

The KS "Objective" knee score measures:
1. Pain (50 points)
2. ROM (25 points)
3. Stability (25 points)
4. Deductions, if applicable
   a. Flexion contracture
   b. Extension lag
   c. Malalignment

The KS function score measures:
1. Walking (50 points)
2. Stair climbing (50 points)
3. Deductions for reliance on walking aids

Again, any use or dependence on analgesics for patient pain management is not taken into account. The KS Clinical Rating System avoids the arbitrary classification of composite scores into categorical ratings, such as Excellent, Good, etc.[28,34,65] Psychometric testing has shown that the KS Objective Score has poor reliability with acceptable responsiveness, whereas the KS Function Score has good reliability with questionable responsiveness.[5,28,79,84] This has led to the use of both measurement tools, a practice that has been widely accepted in clinical use and is supported by some validation trials.[5,28,84]

Critics of the KS Rating System cite the fact that the original Knee Society Score (KSS) was developed for a significantly older and less active population compared to those seeking knee replacement surgery today. Given that the KS functional score only measures stair climbing and walking in its functional evaluation, outcomes for patients expecting a much higher activity level may not be well represented by this rating system in today's patient population. Younger and more active patients undergoing TKA today demand a more thorough evaluation of their results, including the possibility of remaining active in specific recreational activities far beyond walking and stair climbing.[104] Also, given the increased incidence and need for revision knee surgery, reliable outcome scores for evaluation of revision surgery are needed in today's literature.[50]

Given the weaknesses of the original KS score, and the need for contemporary outcome measures to better account for preoperative patient expectations, satisfaction, and physical activities of the younger, more diverse population of TKA patients, a New KSS has been developed and formally validated.[104,120] This New KSS is based on information from two domains: surgeon-generated objective measures and subjective patient-derived measures. The surgeon-generated component is based on the objective component of the original Knee Society scoring system, which grades the technical outcome of the procedures on the basis of pain, ROM, alignment, and stability. The subjective measures are determined by the individual patient and include knee function, satisfaction, and fulfillment of expectations. This subjective score represents a departure from the original KSS in that the new score calls upon

---

§References 5, 28, 36, 65, 75, and 79.

the patient to assess the extent to which the function of the knee allows the patient to perform his or her preferred activities. By evaluating patient expectations, satisfaction, and surveying preoperative ability to participate in a broad range of activities, the New KSS is more representative of both the younger and the traditional TKR patient.

The New KSS consists of four sections:

1. Objective Knee Score (seven items; 100 points)
   a. Anteroposterior (AP) alignment (25 points)
   b. Stability/instability (25 points)
      i. Medial/lateral (15 points)
      ii. Anterior/posterior (10 points)
   c. ROM (25 points)
   d. Symptoms (25 points)
   e. Deductions (malalignment/flexion contracture/extensor lag)
2. Satisfaction Score (five items; 40 points)
   a. Pain level while sitting (8 points)
   b. Pain level while lying in bed (8 points)
   c. Knee function while getting out of bed (8 points)
   d. Knee function while performing light household duties (8 points)
   e. Knee function while performing leisure recreational activities (8 points)
3. Expectation Score (three items; 15 points)
   a. Pain relief (5 points)
   b. Ability to carry out activities of daily living (5 points)
   c. Ability to perform leisure, recreational, or sport activities (5 points)
4. Functional Activity Score (19 items; 100 points)
   a. Walking and standing (five items; 30 points)
   b. Standard activities (six items; 30 points)
   c. Advanced activities (five items; 25 points)
   d. Discretionary activities (three items; 15 points)

The functional activity score in this New KSS takes into account the discrepancies in perception of outcome that exist between surgeons and patients.[51,102] It includes more detailed patient-specific activities that can include sports and recreational activities if the patient is active enough preoperatively. The MCID estimates for the KSS and 2011-KS have not been identified for patients undergoing TKR. Also, during validation studies of the Dutch translation of the New KSS, it was found to be a reliable, valid, and responsive questionnaire without showing preoperative floor effects or ceiling effects at 6 months after TKR.[32,127] Validation in French and Japanese versions are also recently available.[31,54]

Historically, given their length and answering time, translation of valid outcome scores like the New KSS into the clinical setting has led to decreased response rates and decreased usefulness for everyday follow-up of knee replacement patients. To address these issues, and to provide the benefits of the New KSS, a short form of the New KSS was developed and validated by Scuderi et al.[121] During validation, the short form proved to be a more responsive instrument, and was capable of discriminating clinically different groups of patients before and after TKA with virtually the same estimated effect size as the original functional activities subscale of the new Knee Society Knee Score.

The New Knee Society Knee Score Short Form consists of the following three domains of the long form:

1. Symptoms: three items
2. Satisfaction: one item
   a. Satisfaction while performing light household activities

3. Functional score: maximum total 100
   a. How long can you walk: 20
   b. Walking on an uneven surface: 15
   c. Climbing or descending stairs: 15
   d. Getting up from low couch or chair without arms: 15
   e. Running: 20
   f. Discretionary activity: 15

Although the short form of the New KSS is a valid alternative in the clinical setting to monitor patient outcomes and is expected to improve the rate of patient completion, authors of both scores recommend the use of the long form for research studies and for more sensitive measurement of the outcomes of individual patients.[121]

Disease-Specific Rating Systems

Disease-specific outcome scales, sometimes referred to as condition-specific scales, focus on complaints that can be attributed to a specific diagnosis or patient population. Disease-specific scales tend to have a narrower focus and stronger responsiveness compared to generic health status measures.[12,137]

The most popular disease-specific outcome measure for hip or knee osteoarthritis is the Western Ontario and McMaster Universities Osteoarthritis Index (WOMAC), which measures the course of the disease and symptoms as well as the effectiveness of any treatment.** The WOMAC was also recently introduced and validated for evaluation of older adult patients with femoral neck fractures.[17]

The WOMAC was originally introduced and validated in 1988 by Bellamy et al. and consists of three subscales containing a total of 24 Likert-scaled items:

1. Pain (five items)
2. Stiffness (two items)
3. Physical function (17 items)

Reports conclude that the WOMAC demonstrates validity, strong reliability, and specific responsiveness, especially in assessment of pain and function.[12,14,37,79,137] Online versions of the WOMAC may be administered without compromising its validity, which facilitates its inclusion in database registries.[42,94] The WOMAC, and its subscales, have undergone extensive validity, reliability, and responsiveness testing†† and are even used as a tool for validating other instruments.[47,84] The MCID for outcome scores derived from the WOMAC instrument is reported to be 15 points.[40]

One instrument that was compared to the WOMAC for its validation testing is the Oxford 12-Item Knee Score (Oxford-12) developed by Dawson et al. in 1998.[29,37] The Oxford-12 assesses the health outcomes of TKR patients on the basis of responses to 12 items that query pain, physical function, and limitations associated with the knee, each scored on a five-point scale.[28,29] The scoring system produces a single score instead of distinct subscores, and has demonstrated validity, including acceptable floor and ceiling effects, and reliability.[28,37] In fact, after statistical testing in a comparative study, the Oxford-12 was the highest ranked among the disease-specific instruments investigated in the study and was recommended for cross-sectional discriminative applications.[37] A recent study has shown that using a specific prediction model, results from the KSS and the Oxford Knee Score can be compared.[89] In general,

---

**References 9, 10, 12, 14, 37, 56, 84, and 137.
††References 10, 12, 28, 37, 47, 79, and 137.

the Oxford-12 is considered to be a simple and reliable tool for assessment of outcome. One of the strengths of the Oxford-12 is that it has proven responsive to clinically important changes over time, which facilitates comparisons between different patient groups and different treatment regimens, including TKR.[28,37,55,68] The MCID of the Oxford knee score has recently been reported as 5.0 points.[24]

A recent trend toward using the Oxford-12 as a predictor of patient satisfaction and as a measure of achievement of patient expectations has been published, but further studies correlating the Oxford-12 score with the New KSS, which includes functional, satisfaction, and expectation subscores, have yet to be made.[24,131]

Functional Rating Systems

Once pain relief has been attained by patients undergoing knee replacement, restoration of normal function often becomes the primary goal and a key indicator of the perceived success of the procedure. Because TKR is being performed more frequently in younger and more active patients, the functional outcome of the procedure has assumed greater importance since the initial introduction of the procedure. Functional rating systems can measure many components of outcome with a focus, not only on capabilities and limitations, but also on the extent to which patients can participate in activities related to daily living, sports, and recreation. Functional rating systems tend to be very responsive and several have been proven valid and reliable.[14,28,34]

The KOOS was developed in 1998 by Roos et al. as an extension of the WOMAC with adaptations from some of the same subscales as the WOMAC.[116] The KOOS was originally intended to measure the condition of younger, more active patients who suffer from early-stage osteoarthritis or knee symptoms. It has since emerged as an appropriate outcome measure for arthroplasty patients as joint replacement is becoming a viable treatment option for some relatively young, active patients with expectations of returning to demanding physical activities.[14,39,107,116,117]

The KOOS is a 42-item, self-administered, self-explanatory questionnaire that queries patients concerning the following:
1. Pain (nine items)
2. Symptoms (seven items)
3. Function during activities of daily living (17 items)
4. Sport and recreation function (five items)
5. Quality of life (four items)

Each item is measured using a five-point Likert scale, and each subscale is reported separately.[116,117] The KOOS, like the WOMAC, has been demonstrated to be a valid, reliable, and responsive assessment instrument, especially for patients with expectations of physical activity or for those investigating physical function as a primary outcome.[109,117]

To assess the physical demands of activities performed by patients before and after joint replacement, Zahiri et al. created the UCLA rating score.[139] The UCLA score groups patients into one of 10 descriptive levels according to the frequency and type of activities that they regularly perform, ranging from "wholly inactive and dependent on others" to "regular participation in impact sports." These data can be useful in determining a patient's functional capabilities as well as the types of demands placed on the implanted component.[14,139]

More recently, another instrument, the Lower-Extremity Activity Scale (LEAS), has been introduced by Saleh et al. in an attempt to ascertain the change in actual daily physical activity that occurs prior to and following lower-limb arthroplasty.[118] The LEAS is a self-administered, self-assessed, 18-item survey that differentiates between those who (1) are housebound with limited walking ability, (2) walk more ordinarily about the house, (3) walk about the community, and (4) work and exercise a substantial amount. There is a fine gradation between activity level classifications, especially at higher activity levels, without any perceived overlap. The LEAS has been subjected to psychometric testing, including comparisons to the WOMAC, and has exhibited acceptable validity, reliability, responsiveness, and is readily seen in today's knee replacement literature.[22,38,118]

Performance-Based Rating Systems

Although other specific outcome measures can be very useful, they may be intended for measuring a narrow range of patients or treatments, which limits their applicability.[52] Rather than rely on global health scores that indirectly measure function or self-administered self-assessments of physical activity, some investigators endorse the use of performance-based measures, especially as a supplement to generic or global health ratings.[11,47,52]

Common performance-based systems include the 6-minute walk and the 30-second stair climb, established by Guyatt in 1985 and Bolton in 1994, respectively.[11,52,53] Both of these tests involve submaximal exercises that objectively assess capability even for those impaired by joint symptoms or those recovering from joint replacement surgery. The 6-minute walk assessment tests how many times a patient can walk back and forth down a level, 30-m-long surface in 6 minutes.[52,53,79] The 30-second stair climb task records the number of times a patient can walk up and down a 12-step flight of stairs in 30 seconds.[11,79] When performing these tasks, the patients are instructed to proceed at a pace within their capacity and are usually supervised by an instructor. Another performance-based test is the Timed Up and Go (TUG) test, which records the time required for a patient to rise from a chair, take a few steps, return, and sit back down in the chair.[49,110]

Each of these instruments measures capability objectively, without bias, and can track a patient's progress over time, but they do not consider any comorbidities that may inhibit function. Although the reproducibility of these tests is acceptable, low correlation with conventional measures, such as the WOMAC or SF-36, has limited their validity.[11,47,53,110] However, given the direct measure of functional capability, some urge that performance-based measures should be administered along with conventional instruments.[80]

Patient-Specific Rating Systems

In general, the fundamental task of outcome instruments, especially those that are patient-based, is to determine if a particular outcome relates to an important improvement in the patient's health.[145] Because many instruments do not clearly specify or determine individual patient goals, the effectiveness and benefits of the treatment are not assessed with reference to improvements valued by the individual rather than an "average" patient or physician. Patient-specific health assessments focus on evaluating individual patient concerns and provide a forum to discuss patient expectations and subsequent satisfaction with the treatment.[135]

The McMaster Toronto Arthritis Patient Function Preference Questionnaire (MACTAR) is one of the most often used patient-specific rating systems.[14,135,137] Originally designed in 1987 by Tugwell et al. for patients with rheumatoid arthritis, the

MACTAR is an individualized functional priority approach for assessing improvement in physical disability.[125] It allows patients to identify and rank their five most important complaints preoperatively, and then rate the changes in the complaints postoperatively. Predictably, the MACTAR has been shown to be highly responsive, although the quantification of patient improvements may be considered inflated because the MACTAR only measures the five most important complaints or expectations.[137] Regardless, the MACTAR has met testing requirements for validity and reliability.[8,124,133,135]

Introduced in 2012 by Noble and colleagues, the Total Knee Function Questionnaire (TKFQ) is a self-administered instrument that identifies those physical activities that are important to TKR patients, the frequency of patient participation in each activity, and the prevalence of symptoms during their participation.[103,132] The TKFQ is designed as an inventory of 33 different activities spanning the least demanding (walking and standing) to the most demanding (running, downhill skiing), which were selected on the basis of initial studies using a larger battery of possible activities. The TKFQ consists of 55 Likert-scaled multiple choice questions regarding the following:

1. Symptoms and activities
   a. Activities of daily living (17 items)
   b. Movement and lifestyle activities (eight items)
   c. Recreational activities, exercises, and advanced activities (eight items)
2. Walking and running (five items)
3. Satisfaction (one item)
4. Activity level and expectations (three items)
5. Pain and other symptoms (four items)
6. Patient information (nine items)

Unlike previous questionnaires, the TKFQ is designed on the assumption that no patient will perform all of the activities listed, and so the activities selected will differ from patient to patient on the basis of their individual lifestyles and activity levels. Consequently, outcome scores are generated for each specific activity, and in aggregate for all of the activities performed by each individual patient. This approach overcomes the limitations of many of the earlier outcome instruments because the outcome score is based on the activities that are actually performed by patients rather than activities selected by the authors of the questionnaire. This makes it possible to assess each patient's function in performing activities that are personally important, as well as those that are not, by definition, essential to the lowest level of physical function (ie, recreational, sporting, and exercise activities). In addition, the inclusion of items that explicitly inquire into satisfaction and expectations can lend insight into the patient's own consideration of the TKR's impact on his or her overall quality of life.[70] The TKFQ has been validated, but its responsiveness, which could be expected to be acceptable, has not been reported.[25,101,103,132]

Patients' expectations are becoming important predictors and indicators of outcome. The Hospital for Special Surgery Knee Replacement Expectations Survey (KRES) was developed to ascertain the importance of symptoms to patients and their concerns about treatments.[91] The KRES explicitly inquiries into expectations that are strongly related to patients' assessments of outcome. The KRES consists of 17 items that relate to the patient's expectations of how their treatment will impact their

1. pain (one item),
2. psychological well-being (one item), and
3. physical function (15 items).

The response format for each item asks patients whether they have that expectation and, if so, how important it is to them. Through familiarity with patients' expectations, physicians can provide more focused care, more guided patient education, and perspectives for shared decision making. The KRES has been tested and has been shown to demonstrate acceptable validity and reliability.[91]

PATIENT FACTORS AFFECTING OUTCOME

An evidence-based understanding of the relationship between patient attributes and the outcomes of different treatments is critical to rational decision making in health care. However, in the realm of treatment of the arthritic knee, no single universal set of factors can be expected to predict the outcome of any intervention in terms that are applicable to all patients. Nonetheless, studies using knee scoring systems have identified several traits that could be factors in patient outcomes. When patients present for treatment with these or other factors that portend a certain outcome, physicians should counsel patients accordingly.

Pain Relief

Pain relief has been, and continues to be, a primary patient expectation of treatments for their arthritic knees.[56] Patients' postoperative satisfaction is dependent, in part, on the effectiveness of TKR in relieving their pain.[56,101] Previous reports and a recent randomized controlled trial have demonstrated that contemporary knee replacements succeed in relieving patients' pain postoperatively,[30,56,60,115] although complete relief is not necessarily experienced immediately.[70] Using contemporary outcome instruments to determine any causal relationships between the severity of preoperative pain and a specific outcome is difficult, however, because the assessment of pain is very subjective and depends on several patient factors as well as assessment instrument design factors. However, as one might expect, a higher level of preoperative pain has been shown to correlate with more severe postoperative pain.[56,105] Although some conflicting data exist, according to outcome scores, patients with greater preoperative pain have reported similar increments of pain relief as patients with less preoperative pain, thus patients with greater preoperative pain do not experience the same postoperative relief as those with less preoperative pain.[70,83,92,122]

Range of Motion

Because knee function is critical for participation in many functional activities, some degree of the normal ROM of the joint is a minimum expectation of all patients postoperatively. Mechanically, at least 65 degrees of knee flexion is required for ambulatory function, and about 105 degrees is necessary to rise from a low chair.[70] In a review, Ritter et al. showed that postoperative ROM of approximately 130 degrees correlated with the best pain and functional results. They also concluded that outcomes are compromised for patients with limited motion, accentuated hyperextension, or flexion contracture, according to KSSs.[114] In a therapeutic study, Argenson et al. reported that patients with postoperative knee flexion around 130 degrees experienced restored function, satisfaction, and pain relief such that most were able to return to their previous level of sporting activity.[2] Studies have shown that patients' preoperative ROM is a reliable predictor of postoperative ROM, although patients with poor or restricted preoperative ROM are shown to gain more knee joint motion after TKR than patients with mid- to high-range knee motion.[70] Surgeons should, therefore, be able to educate their patients about the importance of ROM and how it may affect their success in achieving their functional goals postoperatively.[85]

Age

It may be expected that as people age, the prevalence of comorbidities and musculoskeletal pathology will increase, leading to more frequent knee symptoms and reduced functional abilities. It has been noted, however, that people continue to participate in physical activities as they age, although the nature of the activities varies with age.[103] Reports indicate that TKR is effective in restoring some function to patients who are older than 65 years compared to nonsurgical treatment.[49,123] Noble et al. qualified that notion by demonstrating that patients' postoperative physical activity, especially high-demand activity, is not fully restored compared with nonoperated age- and gender-matched controls, and that the limitation is not attributable to the effects of normal aging.[103] In addition, Franklin et al. reported that total knee patients older than 80 years may regain less knee function after TKA than those who are younger.[43] In addition, it is well recognized that the outcome of surgery is more often compromised in older patients as a result of postoperative complications.[89,96]

Nonetheless, increased age is certainly not a contraindication for TKR. Older adult patients have reported pain relief, implant survivability, and satisfaction that parallels or exceeds that of younger patients.[9,56,60] In fact, one review reports a greater risk of moderate to severe postoperative pain in primary and revision patients younger than 60 years than in those who are older.[122] As the prevalence of knee arthritis and the concurrent demand for TKR is increasing, especially among a younger, more active cohort, surgeons should consider the aspects of outcome that tend to be impacted by age when referring, treating, and counseling patients.[67]

Gender

It is recognized that men and women vary in terms of knee anatomy, as typified by differences in lower-extremity alignment and distal femoral anatomy.[87] Additional differences have been reported in patterns of patient recall of the preoperative status of their knees after surgery, and their motivation for seeking a TKR. This is to be expected as more women of 55 to 85 years of age live alone, potentially limiting their ability to rely on others for assistance with daily activities. All of these apparent gender differences may theoretically impact self-assessed outcome.[56,83] Despite these potential confounders, outcome instruments have been used to demonstrate that women report moderate to severe postoperative pain as well as preoperative pain, swelling, use of analgesics, and functional limitations with greater propensity than males, although the prevalence of concomitant musculoskeletal problems is equal.[††] Using validated, reliable instruments, men typically report higher knee scores than women, pre- and postoperatively. However, women have been shown to experience about the same improvement in knee scores after TKA, although the differences between

genders vary with the measurement instrument. Thus, women report greater improvements in WOMAC scores when compared to men, equal improvements in SF-12 scores, and less improvement than men in KSS function and KSS total scores.[87,106] Although women may undergo TKA for treatment of more severe symptoms than men, and may experience more pain, stiffness, and swelling postoperatively, TKR seems equally effective in improving the health status of male and female patients, independent of gender.

Obesity

Currently, opinions are mixed regarding the effect of obesity on long-term patient outcomes after knee replacement. Some surgeons are hesitant to recommend TKR for patients who are morbidly obese, citing concerns about high rates of mechanical failure of the prosthesis and increased risks of intra- and postoperative complications (eg, infection).[56,70] Others posit that, when controlled for comorbidities, obesity is not correlated with long-term complications and may show comparable outcomes compared to non-obese patients.[4,6,56,70] However, there is agreement among investigators that knee replacement in morbidly obese patients is associated with relatively poor functional gains postoperatively, although the personal significance of these gains has not been evaluated in quantitative terms.[43,56] Although increased body mass index (BMI) is linked to decreased function and possible increase in perioperative complications, it is not a strong predictor of postoperative pain or survivorship of the prosthesis.[56] In summary, although obesity is certainly of clinical concern because of its impact on patient health, it still does not appear to have a significant adverse effect on the outcome of knee replacement, and may not be a contraindication for this procedure.

Mental Health

Future research is still needed to refine assessment instruments to clarify the relationship between coexisting mental or emotional conditions and outcomes after total joint replacement. With recent reports linking preoperative anxiety and depression with worse patient-reported outcomes, many surgeons regard psychiatric disease as a relative contraindication for surgical intervention.[35,61] For patients with lesser levels of psychological dysfunction that do not preclude them from surgery (eg, clinically defined trait anxiety, mild depression, limited coping skills, etc.), the mental health component of the SF-36 can be used to relate mental health status to the outcome of knee replacement.[3,60] A low mental health score does not conclusively indicate clinical depression but is a general measure that may be affected by an acute event or chronic condition. It is difficult to identify a causal relationship between mental health and outcome after knee replacement; it is not known if poor mental health can determine a certain outcome or if an outcome partially influences a patient's mental condition after this procedure.[56] Nonetheless, it is generally accepted that preoperative mental health can have an impact on a patient's perception of pain, satisfaction, and functional status postoperatively, negatively affecting patient-reported outcome.[23] Lower preoperative mental health scores have been shown to be an independent predictor of patient dissatisfaction with total joint replacement.[23,46] In several studies, lower preoperative mental or emotional health scores are associated with smaller improvements in physical function postoperatively.[3,35,43,60,83] Assessment of mental health status can, perhaps, enable clinicians to modify

---

††References 22, 56, 64, 83, 87, 106, and 122.

the way they manage patients to reduce any psychological distress and to establish common expectations that will help optimize the patient's outcome after knee replacement.

Comorbidities and Diagnosis

Current scoring systems, especially questionnaires, are imperfect, and their results can be confounded by factors other than the condition of interest that affect the calculated outcome score.[70] Common sources of error are the presence of comorbid and preoperative conditions, which can lead to erroneous assessments of patient outcomes.[36] Of course, some comorbidities may preclude surgery as a possible treatment altogether, but even those patients who are candidates for TKR often have coexisting medical conditions (some reports indicate more than 80% of patients).[3] Comorbidities can significantly complicate the surgical procedure and the patient's postoperative medical management, and may also limit the patient's ability to attend or participate in rehabilitative treatment sessions.[3,60] Hence, Dunbar et al. demonstrated that patient comorbidities, as stratified by a modified Charnley classification, were significant determinants of the outcome score generated by all questionnaires tested, regardless of the specificity of the questions concerning the treated knee.[36]

Conflicting results from assessment instruments highlight the complexity of the relationship between comorbidities and outcome. Patients presenting with two or more comorbid conditions generally achieve lower global rating scores compared to those without comorbidities.[19] The Charlson comorbidity index has been developed to weight the effect of comorbidities in predicting the risk of patient mortality.[21] In a recent prospective review, Elmallah et al. correlated a higher preoperative Charleston Comorbidity Index with improved patient reported outcomes for up to 5 years following knee replacement surgery.[38] Other authors have shown that the presence of comorbid conditions is associated with more severe short-term postoperative pain and lower postoperative function at 1 and 2 years.[70,83] In contrast, Ayers et al. found that patients' comorbidities did not relate to impaired 12-month physical function when adjusted for preoperative baseline function.[3] As long as the patient's coexisting medical conditions do not preclude him or her from undergoing surgery, it appears that TKR is still a reasonably effective treatment for advanced osteoarthritis.

The correlation between physical traits and an outcome score is indicative of an average health status of individuals who typically have some form of underlying disabling condition. Logically, this relationship, and hence the validity of the outcome instrument, will vary between individuals with different diseases (eg, osteo- and rheumatoid arthritis). Consequently, clinicians should be wary of comparing the outcome scores of patients with different diagnoses. Studies using instruments to assess the outcome of unicompartmental, bicompartmental, and TKR patients have shown that average postoperative outcome scores are lower for patients with rheumatoid arthritis compared to those with osteoarthritis.[18,19] Therefore, surgeons may need to counsel their patients that their clinical outcome may be compromised somewhat because of their diagnosis or coexisting conditions.[3,60,83]

Physical Activity

As the demand for TKR continues to increase among younger patients, the operation, prosthesis, and the outcome assessment need to accommodate the patient's ability to perform physical activities as an important element of a successful procedure. The recent introduction of the New KSS and its consideration of patient-specific physical activities have increased the value placed on a patient's activity level and subjective perception of outcomes. Physical activity depends on a complex network of factors, including the patient's knee function, motivation, and environment. Outcome scores suggest that patients' exercise and physical activity levels shortly after TKR may contribute to long-term functional gains.[44] Adherence to a more active rehabilitation program that consists of more daily exercise repetitions is correlated with greater 6-month postoperative functional improvement compared to less physical activity.[44]

Other reports indicate that many patients place significance on certain physical activities and regularly participate in exercises and even demanding sports despite experiencing symptoms. In these individuals, postoperative physical activity is associated with satisfaction, improved function, fulfillment of expectations, and excellent clinical outcomes.[93,98,103,132] The impact of TKR on postoperative physical function appears to be linked to the patient's baseline preoperative functional status; patients with severe preoperative functional impairment had worse 3-year outcomes compared with patients whose preoperative function was better.[82] Although certain surgical techniques or prosthesis designs may limit postoperative capability, thereby limiting patients' functional activities, most design features and treatment options (ie, total vs. unicompartmental knee replacement) tend to result in improved postoperative physical function in comparison with preoperative levels.[27,69] Especially given the trend for younger, more active patients presenting for knee replacement, physicians can customize their recommendations for physical activity based on findings from functional components of scoring systems.

Expectations

Preoperative expectations critically influence patients' subjective assessment of the success of any treatment affecting musculoskeletal function. Patient expectations are important, in part, because they are linked to requests for elective surgery and have a significant influence over patient satisfaction with the procedure.[74,91,119] Expectations have even been suggested to contribute more than clinical baseline variables in predicting pain and functional outcomes after TKR.[39] Newly introduced outcome instruments like the New KSS and the KSS short form have improved how patient expectations are now measured following knee replacement surgery. Mancuso et al. established that patients' multiple expectations in the areas of symptom relief, physical function, and psychosocial function can vary by diagnosis.[91] Noble et al. concluded that before most patients undergo knee replacement surgery, they expect that the procedure will relieve pain, stiffness, and swelling and restore knee function. The postoperative correlation analysis revealed that the satisfaction of those patients was primarily determined by whether or not the treatment met their expectations as opposed to their absolute level of functioning.[101] These findings reiterate the importance of establishing realistic expectations through individual preoperative counseling, shared surgeon-patient decision making, and preoperative patient educational classes in maximizing the satisfaction of each patient with TKR.[90]

KEY REFERENCES

3. Ayers DC, Franklin PD, Ploutz-Snyder R, et al: Total knee replacement outcome and coexisting physical and emotional illness. *Clin Orthop* 440:157–161, 2005.

14. Bourne RB: Measuring tools for functional outcomes in total knee arthroplasty. *Clin Orthop* 466(11):2634–2638, 2008.

29. Dawson J, Fitzpatrick R, Murray D, et al: Questionnaire on the perceptions of patients about total knee replacement. *J Bone Joint Surg Br* 80(1):63–69, 1998.

34. Drake BG, Callahan CM, Dittus RS, et al: Global rating systems used in assessing knee arthroplasty outcomes. *J Arthroplasty* 9(4):409–417, 1994.

36. Dunbar MJ, Robertsson O, Ryd L: What's all that noise? The effect of co-morbidity on health outcome questionnaire results after knee arthroplasty. *Acta Orthop Scand* 75(2):119–126, 2004.

37. Dunbar MJ, Robertsson O, Ryd L, et al: Appropriate questionnaires for knee arthroplasty. Results of a survey of 3600 patients from the Swedish Knee Arthroplasty Registry. *J Bone Joint Surg Br* 83(3):339–344, 2001.

42. Franklin PD, Lewallen D, Bozic K, et al: Implementation of patient-reported outcome measures in US total joint replacement registries: rational, status and plans. *J Bone Joint Surg Am* 96(Suppl 1):104–109, 2014.

47. Gandhi R, Tsvetkov D, Davey JR, et al: Relationship between self-reported and performance-based tests in a hip and knee joint replacement population. *Clin Rheumatol* 28(3):253–257, 2009.

60. Heck DA, Robinson RL, Partridge CM, et al: Patient outcomes after knee replacement. *Clin Orthop* 356:93–110, 1998.

78. Kosinski M, Keller SD, Ware JE Jr, et al: The SF-36 Health Survey as a generic outcome measure in clinical trials of patients with osteoarthritis and rheumatoid arthritis: relative validity of scales in relation to clinical measures of arthritis severity. *Med Care* 37(5 Suppl):MS23–MS39, 1999.

84. Lingard EA, Katz JN, Wright RJ, et al: Validity and responsiveness of the Knee Society Clinical Rating System in comparison with the SF-36 and WOMAC. *J Bone Joint Surg* 83-A(12):1856–1864, 2001.

91. Mancuso CA, Sculco TP, Wickiewicz TL, et al: Patients' expectations of knee surgery. *J Bone Joint Surg* 83-A(7):1005–1012, 2001.

101. Noble PC, Conditt MA, Cook KF, et al: The John Insall award: patient expectations affect satisfaction with total knee arthroplasty. *Clin Orthop* 452:35–43, 2006.

102. Noble PC, Fuller-Lafreniere S, Meftah M, et al: Challenges in outcome measurement: discrepancies between patient and provider definitions of success. *Clin Orthop* 471(11):3437–3445, 2013.

103. Noble PC, Gordon MJ, Weiss JM, et al: Does total knee replacement restore normal knee function? *Clin Orthop* 431:157–165, 2005.

104. Noble PC, Scuderi GR, Brekke AC, et al: Development of a new knee society scoring system. *Clin Orthop* 470(1):20–32, 2012.

116. Roos EM, Roos HP, Lohmander LS, et al: Knee Injury and Osteoarthritis Outcome Score (KOOS)—development of a self-administered outcome measure. *J Orthop Sports Phys Ther* 28(2):88–96, 1998.

121. Scuderi GR, Sikorskii A, Bourne RB, et al: The Knee Society short form reduces respondent burden in the assessment of patient-reported outcomes. *Clin Orthop* 474(1):134–142, 2015.

129. Ware JE Jr, Gandek B: Overview of the SF-36 Health Survey and the International Quality of Life Assessment (IQOLA) project. *J Clin Epidemiol* 51(11):903–912, 1998.

132. Weiss JM, Noble PC, Conditt MA, et al: What functional activities are important to patients with knee replacements? *Clin Orthop* 404:172–188, 2002.

The references for this chapter can also be found on www.expertconsult.com.

124

Historic Development, Classification, and Characteristics of Knee Prostheses

John N. Insall,[†] *Henry D. Clarke*

The era of modern total knee replacement (TKR) is rapidly approaching 50 years old and the evolution in prosthesis design is not merely of historic interest. Surgeons with some years of experience will have noticed that fashion tends to repeat itself. For example, in the early years (1970 to 1974), a range of prostheses (unicondylar, bicondylar, and hinged) were used, depending on the preoperative condition and deformity. Many of these devices and concepts fell out of favor, and for a while, except in select centers, tricondylar resurfacing prostheses were in vogue for almost all procedures. Over the past 15 years, we have witnessed renewed interest in a graduated approach to knee replacement, with increased use of unicondylar and bicondylar prostheses for the femorotibial and patellofemoral compartments. Growth in the use of these devices has been in large part the result of the increased emphasis on less invasive surgical techniques and more rapid postoperative recovery, as well as changing attitudes about how patient outcomes are evaluated. In addition to the resurrection of partial knee replacements, we have seen increased use and acceptance of constrained condylar and hinged knee prostheses over the past decade for a variety of difficult cases. As the problems encountered in revision TKR have become more challenging because of osteolysis and bone loss, these devices have assumed an important place in our surgical armamentarium. Yet another example of a trend that is reemerging is the concept of uncemented fixation in TKR. After more than a decade of limited application of this form of fixation, new materials that mimic the structure of natural cancellous bone, and the near universal adoption of this mode of fixation in total hip replacement (at least in North America), have prompted renewed interest.

The resurrection of the concepts and devices noted, which have been investigated in one form or another, is often fueled by promises from the device manufacturers for design improvements that will theoretically eliminate the less desirable outcomes seen with previous generations of implants (and surgeons). Whether these developments will provide significant advantages at this time still remains to be proven. The proliferation of newer materials, such as ceramics and cross-linked polyethylene, as well as prosthesis design changes to maximize flexion, minimize potential backside wear, optimize kinematics, better accommodate gender and racial anatomic variation, and allow prosthesis insertion through minimally invasive approaches, has led to more unanswered questions in the field of TKR.

While many new developments present opportunities for improvement in patient outcomes, there is also increased risk with the use of new devices. It is concerning that many of these concepts have been embraced in widespread clinical use prior to the publication of scientific results to support these changes. At this important time in the field of TKR, when the original pioneers are being succeeded by a new generation of joint replacement surgeons, it is important to emphasize that change should only be embraced once three criteria have been met:

1. A problem that needs a solution should exist.
2. The solution should be based on solid basic science research.
3. The introduction of new devices and techniques should be performed in a graduated manner with scrutiny of clinical outcomes.

To help guide this pursuit of continuing improvement in TKR, we believe that it is useful to look at what has not worked in the past. Finally, it is important to note that although the manufacturers of current systems are acknowledged, only the names of earlier devices are used. In some cases, early prostheses were manufactured by more than one company and, in other cases, the original manufacturers have vanished or merged, which makes accurate acknowledgment difficult at times and often meaningless in the context of this review.

EARLY PROSTHETIC MODELS

Interposition and Resurfacing Prostheses

The concept of improving knee joint function by modifying the articular surfaces has received attention since the 19th century. In 1860, Verneuil[281] suggested the interposition of soft tissues to reconstruct the articular surface of a joint. Subsequently, pig bladder, nylon, fascia lata, prepatellar bursa, and cellophane were some of the materials used for this purpose. The results were disappointing. In 1860, Ferguson[78] resected the entire knee joint, which resulted in mobility of the newly created subchondral surfaces (Fig. 124.1). When more bone was removed, the patients enjoyed good motion but lacked the necessary stability, whereas with less bone resection, spontaneous fusion often resulted. These early attempts were usually performed on knees damaged by tuberculosis or other infectious processes. The results of this procedure were sufficiently poor to discourage anything more than occasional attempts in severe cases.

Encouraged by the relative success of hip cup arthroplasty, Campbell[46] reported the successful use of a metallic interposition femoral mold in 1940. A similar type of arthroplasty was developed and used at Massachusetts General Hospital. The results, published by Speed and Trout[267] in 1949 and by Miller and Friedman[198] in 1952, were not very good, and this type of knee arthroplasty never achieved wide recognition.

†Deceased.

In 1958, MacIntosh[180] described a different type of hemiarthroplasty that he had used in treating painful varus or valgus deformities of the knee. An acrylic tibial plateau prosthesis was inserted into the affected side to correct deformity, restore stability, and relieve pain. Later versions of this prosthesis[181] were made of metal (Fig. 124.2), and the somewhat similar McKeever prosthesis[70,194,242] showed considerably more success and was extensively used, particularly in patients with rheumatoid arthritis. Gunston[38,107] carried MacIntosh's ideas a step further and, instead of using a simple metal disk interposed within the joint, substituted metallic runners embedded in the femoral condyles that articulated against polyethylene troughs attached to the tibial plateau. To make a four-part system of this type feasible, it was necessary to find a means of fixing the components rigidly to the bone. The solution was provided by acrylic cement.

Although the Gunston polycentric prosthesis[38,107] was the first cemented surface arthroplasty of the knee joint, the work of Freeman et al.[84,91] has had an even greater influence on the direction of prosthetic design and surgical technique. The design objectives for a prosthesis (Fig. 124.3) were outlined in 1973 by Freeman et al.[91] The most important of these objectives are the following and remain mostly valid today:

1. A salvage procedure should be readily available.
2. The chances of loosening should be minimized by avoiding unnecessary constraint, reducing friction within the device, and by spreading the loads at the prosthesis-bone interface as widely as possible.
3. The rate of production of wear debris should be minimized, and the debris produced should be as innocuous as possible.
4. The probability of infection should be minimized.
5. A standard insertion procedure should be available.
6. The prosthesis should give motion from 5 degrees of hyperextension to at least 90 degrees of flexion and any hyperextension limiting arrangement should be progressive and not sudden in action.
7. Some freedom of rotation should be resisted.
8. Excessive movements in any direction should be resisted by the soft tissues, particularly the collateral ligaments.

Other early examples of resurfacing prostheses (Figs. 124.4 and 124.5) were the Geometric,[57,58,278] Duocondylar,[222,261] UCI (University of California at Irvine),[292] and Marmor.[186-190]

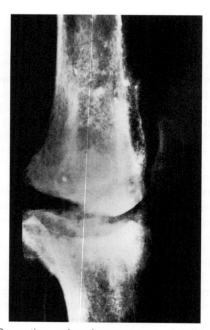

FIG 124.1 Resection arthroplasty creates a mobile but usually unstable joint.

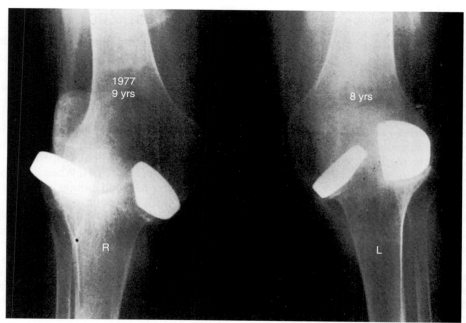

FIG 124.2 Use of the MacIntosh hemiarthroplasty in patients with rheumatoid arthritis often restored alignment and stability for a few years. However, as in this bilateral case, late dislocation and sinkage were common. *L*, Left; *R*, right.

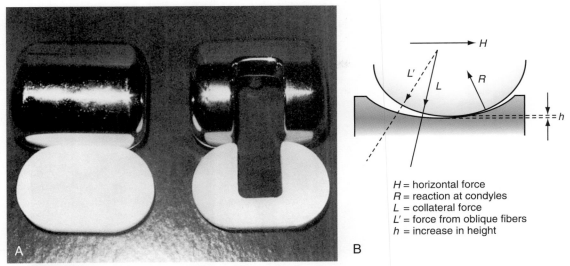

H = horizontal force
R = reaction at condyles
L = collateral force
L' = force from oblique fibers
h = increase in height

FIG 124.3 (A) The original Freeman-Swanson prosthesis used two one-piece components. (B) Stability was obtained by the roller-in-trough concept; dislocation could occur only if one component ran uphill on the other. Distraction was resisted by capsular and collateral ligament tension.

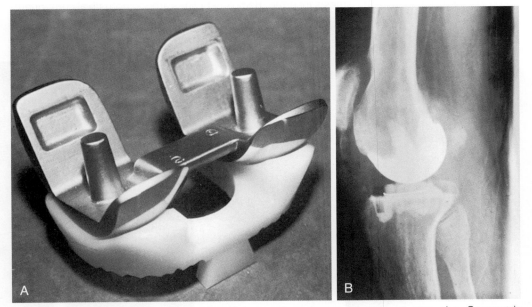

FIG 124.4 (A and B) An early and widely used surface replacement was the Geometric prosthesis.

Constrained Prostheses

A second line of development in knee arthroplasty occurred parallel to the concepts of interposition and, later, surface replacement. In 1951, Walldius[288] developed the hinged prosthesis that bears his name. The device was initially made of acrylic and later of metal.

Shortly thereafter, Shiers[254] described a similar device with even simpler mechanical characteristics (Fig. 124.6). A hinged prosthesis has considerable appeal. Technically, it is easy to use because the intramedullary stems make the prosthesis largely self-aligning and all the ligaments and other soft tissue constraints can be sacrificed because the prosthesis is self-stabilizing. The extent of damage to the knee is therefore of no consequence, and even the most extreme deformities can be corrected by dividing the soft tissues and resecting sufficient bone. Of course, the early hinged designs were uncemented, although later developments such as the GUEPAR (Fig. 124.7) were designed from the outset to be used with methylmethacrylate cement. Because of inherent limitations with a simple hinge, including limited range of motion (ROM) and transmission of stress to the prosthesis-cement interface, the early hinged prostheses were supplanted by rotating hinge devices that constrain the prosthesis in the coronal and sagittal planes, but allow

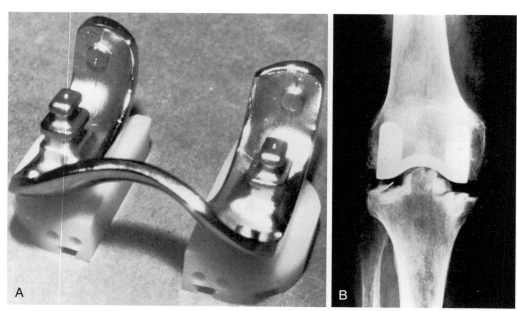

FIG 124.5 (A) The Duocondylar prosthesis was anatomic in concept and retained both cruciate ligaments when present, but did not resurface the patellofemoral joint. Sinkage and loosening of the tibial components were an eventual problem with this design. (B) Anteroposterior radiograph with the Duocondylar prosthesis inserted. Radiolucent lines around both tibial components are visible.

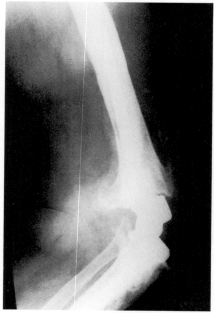

FIG 124.6 The Shiers Prosthesis Was a Simple Uniaxial Metallic Hinge.

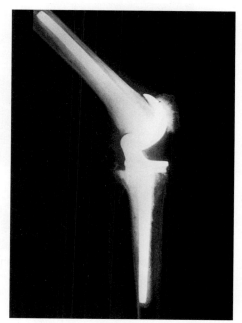

FIG 124.7 The GUEPAR hinge was similar to the Shiers uniaxial metallic hinge, but with the axis placed more posteriorly and femoral resurfacing for the patellar articulation.

rotation in the axial plane. Early designs included the Spherocentric (Fig. 124.8) prosthesis. In addition to linked, hinged devices, unlinked but constrained devices were also introduced in some centers. These devices were well suited to the significant deformities and bone loss encountered during the early years of TKA that exceeded the indications for the basic resurfacing

systems available at the time, but where the maximal constraint of hinged devices was not required. The primary characteristic of these devices was a cam-and-post mechanism, similar to that found in a posterior-stabilized (PS) prosthesis, but thicker and taller, that provides resistance not only to posterior translation but also to varus and valgus stress. Historical devices included

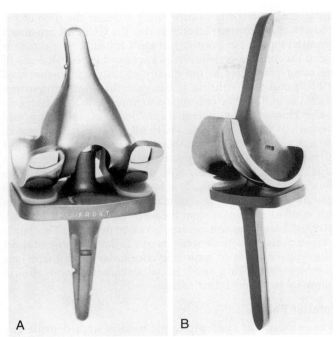

FIG 124.8 Spherocentric Prosthesis (A) Standard version. (B) Long-stemmed variant with a patellar flange. (Courtesy Dr. H. Kauffer and Dr. L.S. Matthews.)

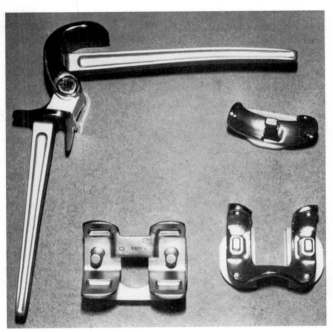

FIG 124.10 The graduated system concept selected the prosthesis according to the degree and extent of damage. The prostheses shown here in a clockwise direction are the unicondylar, Duocondylar, Geometric, and GUEPAR prostheses.

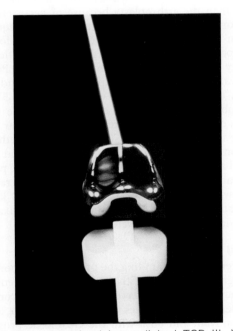

FIG 124.9 The constrained but unlinked TCP III. Varus and valgus constraints were provided by the rectangular central peg on the tibial component.

the Total Condylar Prosthesis III (TCP III; Fig. 124.9)[63] and the Constrained Condylar Knee (CCK).[159]

EVOLUTION OF PROSTHETIC DESIGN

The prostheses discussed up to this point are now more or less obsolete. Although the early results were encouraging, further follow-up demonstrated various problems. The literature

relevant to TKR includes many articles that report the clinical results of designs no longer in common use.*

These published reports on early models are somewhat difficult to compare because different rating methods were used. A review conducted at the Hospital for Special Surgery (HSS) between 1971 and 1973 is probably representative. This review[129] compared four different models (Fig. 124.10): the unicondylar (Fig. 124.11), Duocondylar, Geometric, and GUEPAR. The results were expressed by using the HSS 100-point knee rating scale.

Postoperative knees were classified into four groups according to their scores on the HSS scale:

Excellent: 85+. These knees approached the normal and were obviously much improved in the opinion of the patient and the examiner.

Good: 70 to 84. These knees showed obvious improvement after arthroplasty, but the result was not as good as in the excellent group.

Fair: 60 to 69. This group mostly consisted of knees in which the result of arthroplasty was deficient in some way (eg, pain, moderate instability, unsatisfactory motion), but also included some in which the rating of the arthroplasty was downgraded by the patient's general condition (eg, multiple joint involvement).

Failure: Less than 60. These knees were evidently unsatisfactory and below the rating achieved by knee fusion, which scored a 60 on the HSS knee rating scale.

*References 4, 9, 10, 12-14, 16, 25, 36, 38, 45, 48, 49, 53, 59, 63, 65, 74-76, 81, 83, 85, 89, 90, 92, 95, 98, 104, 108, 117, 122, 123, 125, 126, 129, 132, 134-138, 140, 144, 159, 165, 167, 172-174, 183, 184, 191, 192, 203, 205, 215, 217, 223, 226, 228, 229, 231, 237, 252, 253, 255, 256, 258-260, 263, 273, 277, 280, 293, 294, 301, and 308.

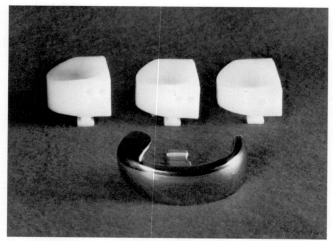

FIG 124.11 The unicondylar prosthesis was designed to resurface only the affected femorotibial compartment. The shape and curvature of the component were similar to that of the duocondylar design.

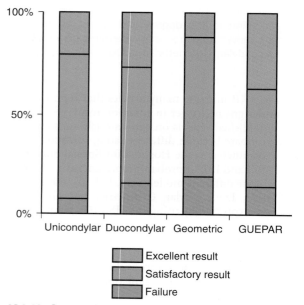

FIG 124.12 Graph Showing the Comparative Results of Four Early Prosthetic Models.

improvement in the HSS knee rating scale. At the time of the study, the conclusion reached was that the GUEPAR prosthesis appeared superior in a number of ways. It had been selected for use in the most severely involved knees and yet equaled any of the other prostheses in the quality of results in rheumatoid arthritis and osteoarthritis. It also gave the lowest proportion of failures and was the only model to improve ROM postoperatively. However, the potential problems of loosening and mechanical failure with the GUEPAR prosthesis were noted. More than 100 GUEPAR prostheses were used at the HSS almost 40 years ago, and these expected problems materialized to a large extent. Approximately 80% of the prostheses were loose clinically and radiographically at long-term follow-up, although they are not necessarily symptomatic (Fig. 124.13A). There were also numerous cases of stem breakage (see Fig. 124.13B) and, as noted later, infection became a major problem. This study therefore reached some erroneous conclusions because of short follow-up—a point of great relevance today when many new prostheses are being used in patients with scant clinical follow-up to support their merits.

Patellar Pain

None of the four early prosthetic models studied made any provision for patellofemoral function. Patellectomy did not seem to offer a solution to the problem of patellofemoral arthritis (Fig. 124.14). In the early study, 38 patellectomies were performed in the group as a whole, 3 of which were done at a later date than the arthroplasty because of persistent patellar pain. Importantly, pain after patellectomy was as frequent as in patients in whom patellectomy had not been performed. In addition, patients who underwent patellectomy suffered from inadequacy of the extensor mechanism. In the GUEPAR group of 45 knees, pain on patellar compression was found in 22 on follow-up, and patellar erosion was observed in 5 patients. Patellar subluxation frequently occurred with the GUEPAR prosthesis, despite wide lateral release of the patellar retinaculum at the time of arthroplasty (Fig. 124.15). Nonetheless, the subluxation was often not apparent to the patient and was considered an incidental finding. Subluxation of the patella did not necessarily correlate with complaints of postoperative pain. However, with the Geometric prosthesis, 29 of 50 knees had pain on patellofemoral compression. Patellar subluxation was found in nine knees and all were painful.

Loosening

A radiolucent line surrounding the prosthetic components was seen with great frequency. With the condylar replacements, the radiolucency was usually observed around the tibial component. It was present in 70% of knees with the unicondylar, 50% with the Duocondylar, and 80% with the Geometric prosthesis. A radiolucent line was observed around the femoral component in 45% of the patients with a GUEPAR prosthesis. The radiolucent line was slightly more frequent in patients with osteoarthritis than in those with rheumatoid arthritis and it was observed in all knees with osteoarthritis in which the Geometric prosthesis was used. Radiolucent lines are by no means always symptomatic, but when complete, progressive, and associated with pain on weight bearing, they generally indicate failure of fixation. Subsequent experience has shown that the incidence of partial radiolucencies for these early prostheses did not correlate with the eventual amount of component loosening at 10- to 12-year follow-up (Fig. 124.16).

Considering the entire group of 178 arthroplasties studied in the four different models (23 unicondylar, 60 Duocondylar, 50 Geometric, and 45 GUEPAR), the results were considered excellent in 47 (26%), good in 66 (37%), fair in 37 (21%), and poor in 28 (16%; Fig. 124.12). There was no statistically significant difference among the results obtained with each of the four prostheses studied. However, because it is easier to improve a bad knee than a relatively good one, the percentage of improvement was much greater with the GUEPAR than with the unicondylar (120% vs. 45%).

Three specific problems were identified from this study: patellar pain, component loosening, and surgical technique. However, because the GUEPAR hinge was inserted into the worst knees originally, it gave the greatest percentage of

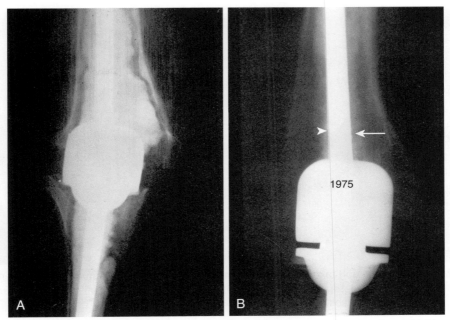

FIG 124.13 (A) Radiograph of a grossly loose GUEPAR prosthesis 5 years after initial insertion. (B) Stem breakage occurred with the GUEPAR prosthesis, usually at the site shown here *(arrows)* in the radiograph, 5 cm proximal to the joint.

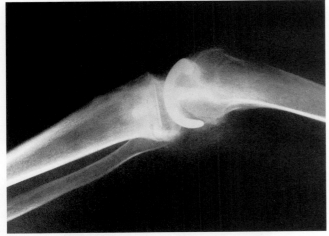

FIG 124.14 Patellectomy is not a satisfactory solution to patellofemoral pain. Patellectomy was performed in conjunction with the implantation of a unicondylar prosthesis.

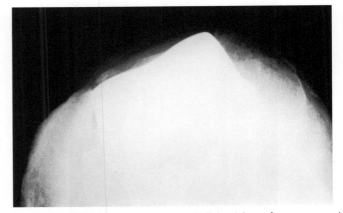

FIG 124.15 Patellar subluxation and dislocation often occurred with the GUEPAR prosthesis. It was not always symptomatic.

On the basis of early analysis of these data, it was clear that tibial loosening represented a failure in prosthetic design. The flat cancellous surface of the upper part of the tibia is not a suitable bed for a flat prosthetic component because of poor resistance to shear stress. Moreover, this bone is not of sufficient strength to resist subsidence of the tibial component, even if excavations are made to accommodate fixation fins or lugs on the bottom of the tibial prosthesis (Figs. 124.17 and 124.18). It was concluded that some form of cortical fixation would be essential for a successful TKR series.

Prosthesis Selection and Surgical Technique

Early in the experience with knee arthroplasty, as previously noted, the concept of a graduated system, in which selection of

a prosthesis depended on the severity of damage found in the arthritic knee, was quite popular (see Fig. 124.10). For example, knees with cartilage erosion restricted to one femorotibial compartment were replaced with a unicondylar prosthesis, whereas a hinged prosthesis was used in the most severely damaged and deformed knees. The bicondylar prosthesis occupied an intermediate position with respect to the severity of arthritis. Although the use of a hinged prosthesis is not technically demanding, the early condylar designs were difficult to insert and align, and there was very little margin for error. Obviously, the advantage of even the most sophisticated prosthetic design is lost if surgical placement is incorrect. Another inherent drawback in a graduated system of prostheses is that a model may be used for degrees of deformity exceeding the limits for which the prosthesis was intended. This error can itself be a cause of failure (eg, dislocation; Fig. 124.19). The

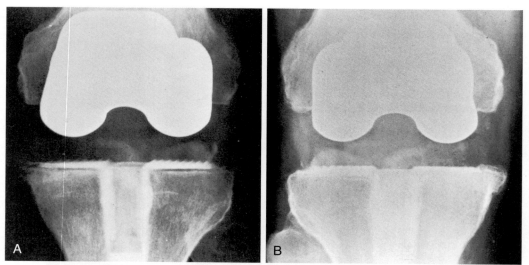

FIG 124.16 (A) Radiograph taken 1 year after implantation shows a pronounced radiolucent line beneath the medial and lateral tibial plateaus. (B) Radiograph of the same knee taken at 5 years shows a barely visible radiolucency.

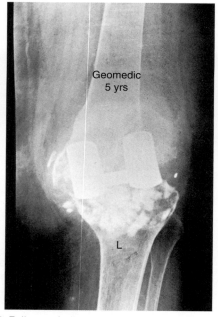

Geomedic
5 yrs

L

FIG 124.17 Failure of tibial fixation was a frequent problem with many early prosthetic designs. The problem was primarily attributable to collapse of the cancellous bone of the upper part of the tibia along with sinkage of the component. *L,* Left.

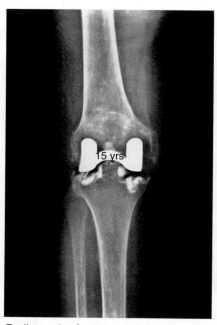

15 yrs

FIG 124.18 Radiograph of a 15-year follow-up of a duocondylar prosthesis that had two separate tibial components. There is the appearance of osteopenia around the femoral component runners. The knee continued to function well.

merits of graduated knee systems still remain a source of debate. Indeed, after a relative hiatus from use in the 1990s, unicondylar and bicondylar replacements achieved renewed support for use in patients with less extensive knee arthritis since the beginning of the 2000s.

Infection

Although deep periprosthetic infection was not a frequent cause of failure for the condylar designs, it has subsequently proved to be a major problem with the GUEPAR prosthesis. With further follow-up, 15 of 108 prostheses (14%) became infected

(4 became infected early and 8 later). There have been reports of similar occurrences in the literature.[10]

At the HSS, dissatisfaction with the early prostheses led to the design of the Total Condylar and Duopatellar prostheses, which were based on different concepts of how to manage the posterior collateral ligament (PCL).[219,232,241] During the 1980s, prosthetic characteristics diverged further and were generally linked to whether the prosthesis was designed to substitute for or preserve the PCL. However, during the 1990s, there was a convergence of prosthetic designs, particularly in the United States.

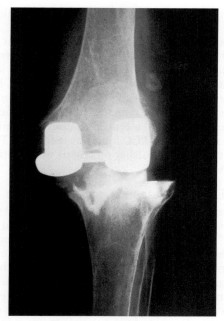

FIG 124.19 This Geometric prosthesis translocated and dislocated. This was the condition of the knee before the prosthesis was inserted and represents an error in prosthesis selection.

TYPES OF PROSTHESES

Most simply, a prosthesis can be a surface replacement or a constrained design. These two categories may be further subdivided. Surface replacements comprise unicondylar and bicondylar designs. Unicondylar prostheses are discussed elsewhere in this text.[†]

Bicondylar prostheses can be cruciate-retaining, cruciate-sacrificing, or cruciate-substituting prostheses. Constrained prostheses can be hinged or unlinked. Most hinged devices are now designed to allow rotation in the axial plane and eliminate motion in the coronal plane. Although in original designs the load was transmitted solely through a metal axle that linked the femoral and tibial components, many contemporary designs allow for condylar load bearing between the femur and tibia, as found in surface replacement designs or, at a minimum, load sharing between the axle and femorotibial articulation. The primary characteristic of unlinked designs, such as the Zimmer-Biomet Legacy Constrained Condylar Knee (LCCK), or Stryker Triathlon Total Stabilizer, is a robust cam-and-post mechanism. This mechanism provides resistance not only to posterior translation but also to varus and valgus stress and rotation. Although these devices offer less constraint in the coronal plane than a rotating hinged prosthesis, they are more constrained in the axial plane. Concerns with the high degree of rotational constraint in these fixed-bearing, unlinked, constrained devices, has led to the development of mobile-bearing, unlinked, constrained prostheses, such as the DePuy PFC Sigma TC3. However, to date, there is little information about which type of constrained device will demonstrate superior survivorship in the long term.

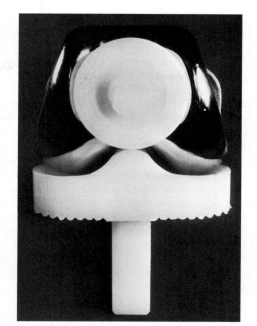

FIG 124.20 The Total Condylar Prosthesis.

Early Surface Replacement Designs

In the following sections, we discuss early surface replacement designs.[284] Supplemental information about the individual innovators and the tremendous advances in TKR during the early years of the modern era can be found in the three historical reviews by Robinson,[232] Ranawat,[219] and Scott[241] that should be compulsory reading for all students of knee arthroplasty. Much of the early debate about prosthesis design and the techniques used to implant the components, including how to address the cruciate ligaments, arose from conceptual differences among the pioneers about whether it was better to design a knee prosthesis from an anatomic (PCL-retaining) or functional (PCL-sacrificing or PCL-substituting) perspective. The current generation of prostheses has converged in many ways, with most designs incorporating characteristics from each category that seem to have optimized long-term outcomes—for example, side-specific femoral components with optimized trochlear geometries from the anatomic approach and the moderately conforming coronal and sagittal geometry that was more closely associated with the functional approach.

Total Condylar Prosthesis

Although originally coined as the name of a specific prosthesis, the term TCP has been used generically to describe a whole range of surface replacement prostheses that share general characteristics with the original (Fig. 124.20).[‡]

The TCP, designed in 1973, was a true total replacement of the knee in that the patellofemoral joint was replaced as well as the femorotibial compartment. Designed from a functional perspective, the inherent geometry of the prosthesis was intended to substitute for the anatomic function of the cruciate ligaments, native articular geometry, and menisci. The salient features of the design are discussed in the following sections.[232]

[†]References 15, 47, 111, 155, 156, 164, 166, 185, 189, 200, 201, 246, and 249.

[‡]References 3, 7, 72, 79, 97, 115, 120, 121, 126, 127, 130, 131, 133, 143, 153, 170, 220, 238, 247, 282, and 283.

Femoral Component. Made of cobalt chromium alloy, the femoral component contained a symmetrically grooved anterior flange that separated posteriorly into two symmetrical condyles, each of decreasing radius posteriorly, with a symmetrical convex curvature in the coronal plane.

Tibial Component. The tibial component was made of high-density polyethylene in one piece with two separate biconcave tibial plateaus that articulated precisely with the femoral condyles in extension, thus permitting no rotation in this position. In flexion, the fit ceased to be exact and rotation and gliding motions were possible. The symmetrical tibial plateaus were separated by an intercondylar eminence designed to prevent translocation or sideways sliding movements. The peripheral margin of the articular concavities was of an even height anteriorly and posteriorly. The undersurface of the component had a central fixation peg 35 mm in length and 12.5 mm in width. The anterior margin of the peg was vertical but the posterior margin was oblique, thereby conforming to the posterior cortex of the tibia.

Patellar Component. Made of high-density polyethylene, the patellar component was dome-shaped on its articular surface, closely conforming to the curvature of the femoral flange. A dome was selected because this shape did not require rotary alignment as an anatomic prosthesis would. The bony surface of the prosthesis had a central, rectangular fixation peg.

Duopatellar Prosthesis

The TCP was designed as a cruciate-sacrificing prosthesis. In contrast, the Duopatellar prosthesis,[76] a sibling prosthesis designed from an anatomic perspective at the HSS as a replacement for the Duocondylar model, was intended to preserve existing cruciate ligaments, particularly the PCL.[219,232,241] The general shape of the tibial runners was anatomic in the sagittal plane. Coronally, the condyles were flat with a median curvature.

The anterior connecting bar of the Duocondylar prosthesis was extended into a femoral flange. The initial version of the Duopatellar model had two separate tibial plateaus identical to the Duocondylar design: flat in the sagittal plane, but with a median curvature coronally to prevent translocation. The deep surface was dovetailed for cement fixation. Later, the two components were joined, and a central fixation peg similar to that of the TCP was added. A PCL cutout was provided. The patellar component of the Duopatellar prosthesis was identical to that of the TCP.

Cruciate Excision, Retention, and Substitution

The TCP and Duopatellar prostheses were designed to sacrifice the ACL and the PCL, or to sacrifice the ACL and retain the PCL.[6,8,64,86,90] Subsequent modifications to the TCP incorporated a cam on the femoral component and a central post on the tibial polyethylene (Fig. 124.21). This cam-and-post mechanism was designed to act as a functional substitute for the PCL and produce femoral rollback during flexion. With the development of this so-called PS prosthesis, it was apparent that excision of both cruciates alone was not optimal. However, the relative merits of PCL retention versus PCL substitution have been debated vigorously within the orthopedic community for many years.[29,60,210,272,302] The development of total knee prostheses has historically occurred along two distinct evolutionary paths based on these different principles.[232] Potential advantages of PCL substitution include easier correction of deformity, more reproducible kinematics, and improved ROM; disadvantages include the potential for increased risk of loosening and reduced proprioception.[210] Although advocates of both concepts still argue the merits of each principle, excellent results can be obtained with a prosthesis of either general design.[61,231] However, it has become clear that if the PCL is retained, the function of

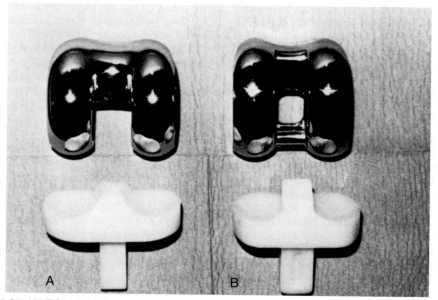

FIG 124.21 (A) TCP. (B) PS condylar knee, a newer derivative providing posterior cruciate substitution by means of a central cam mechanism. (From Insall JN, Lachiewicz PF, Burstein AH: The posterior stabilized condylar prosthesis: a modification of the total condylar design: two- to four-year clinical experience. *J Bone Joint Surg Am* 64:1317–1323, 1982.)

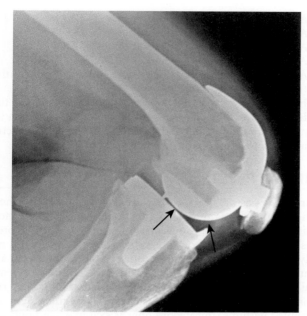

FIG 124.22 Sagittal radiograph of a nonfunctional PCL. There has been roll-forward rather than rollback with knee flexion *(arrows)*. The anterior margin of the femoral component abuts the anterior margin of the tibial component, as it does in a total condylar–type design.

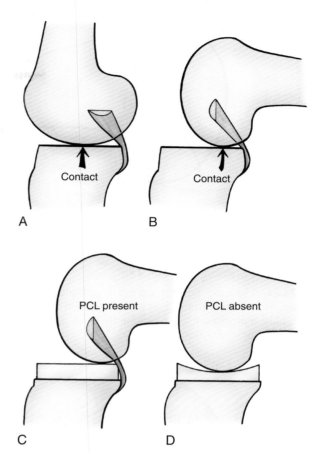

FIG 124.23 Effect of PCL Retention on Prosthetic Design (A and B) Because of the rollback enforced by the PCL, the prosthetic tibial surface must be flat to allow this movement. The femoral tibial contact point *(black arrow)* moves posteriorly during knee extension (A) to knee flexion (B). (C and D) When the PCL is absent, a dished tibial plateau is used.

the ligament must be optimized through a balancing technique. Difficulties with balancing the PCL, as well as late PCL rupture leading to flexion instability and paradoxical anterior translation of the femur seen on fluoroscopic analysis, have led to the development of the *deep-dish* or anterior-stabilized (AS) polyethylene inserts that are offered as part of many knee prosthesis systems (Fig. 124.22).[211,272,291] These inserts have moderately conforming articular surfaces in the coronal and sagittal planes, together with an anterior lip that limits paradoxical anterior translation of the femur on the tibia. This is one example of how prosthesis design has converged in the past 2 decades, thus making it more difficult to trace the origins of any particular design. The anatomic function of the cruciate ligaments, relative advantages and disadvantages of cruciate ligament excision, retention, and substitution will be briefly reviewed here, but are discussed in more detail in the separate chapters elsewhere in this book that discuss the specific prostheses.

ANATOMIC FUNCTIONS OF THE CRUCIATE LIGAMENTS

One function of the cruciate ligaments, in addition to providing static anterior and posterior stability, is to impose certain movements on the joint surfaces relative to one another. The anterior cruciate ligament (ACL) is often absent in arthritic knees and until recently was not believed to be of much consequence in TKR. The importance of the ACL may have been underestimated inasmuch as unconstrained prostheses have increased sagittal plane laxity and fail more often when the ACL is absent.[297] Although the PCL is often attenuated in arthritic knees, it is usually present. It has been considered the collateral ligament for the medial compartment of the knee.[69] The PCL causes the femoral condyles to glide and roll back on the tibial

plateau as the knee is flexed.[142] In a normal knee, the shape of the plateau does not restrain this motion and the laxity of the meniscal attachments allows the menisci to move posteriorly with the femur. This femoral rollback is crucial in prosthetic design. If the cruciates are excised, a more conforming tibial polyethylene component can be used to provide some degree of anterior and posterior stability. However, without the function of the PCL, femoral rollback will not occur, which theoretically limits the ultimate flexion that can be obtained. If the PCL is retained, the tibial surface must be flat or even sloped posteriorly (Fig. 124.23). If a more conforming component is used in these circumstances, posterior impingement will occur (Fig. 124.24). Substitution of the PCL with a cam-and-post mechanism not only re-creates femoral rollback, but also allows a conforming articulation to be used without risk of posterior impingement (Fig. 124.25). These considerations were reflected in the design of early prostheses including the Total Condylar, Duopatellar, PS, and various PCL-retaining (cruciate-retaining [CR]) prostheses, and remain important today in the subsequent derivatives of these designs.

Further confusion regarding the best management of the cruciate ligaments has occurred more recently as a result of the re-introduction of prostheses that are designed to work in

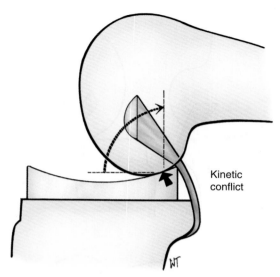

FIG 124.24 Kinematic conflict occurs if concepts are mismatched. In this case, the PCL is preserved with the use of a dished tibial component. Impingement *(thick black arrow)* occurs posteriorly with flexion.

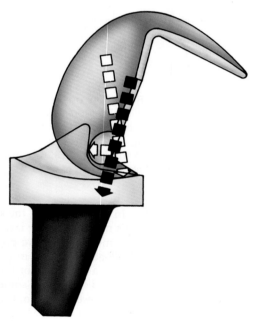

FIG 124.25 The cam mechanism of a posterior-stabilized knee simulates the function of the posterior cruciate ligament and causes rollback of the femur on the tibia with flexion. The resulting vector of forces passes distally through the fixation peg. (From Insall JN, Lachiewicz PF, Burstein AH: The posterior stabilized condylar prosthesis: a modification of the total condylar design: two- to four-year clinical experience. *J Bone Joint Surg Am* 64:1317–1323, 1982.)

conjunction with both native cruciate ligaments, (bicruciate-retaining prosthesis) or substitute for both cruciate ligaments (bicruciate-substituting prosthesis). Therefore, currently five philosophies exist about how to create the best knee kinematics after TKR:

1. ACL sacrifice with PCL retention (CR TKR)
2. ACL sacrifice with PCL substitution (PS TKR)
3. ACL sacrifice with PCL substitution (AS TKR)
4. ACL and PCL retention (bicruciate-retaining TKR)
5. ACL and PCL sacrifice with ACL and PCL substitution (bicruciate substituting TKA)

In some knee prosthesis systems, devices are offered that address each of these surgeon preferences. Our bias is to the posterior stabilized school of thought, but this remains an active area of debate despite more than 30 years of evidence.

CURRENT PROSTHESIS DESIGN

During the past 20 years, early clear distinctions in prosthesis design between anatomic and functional concepts have, to a large degree, vanished, and at this point, many aspects of prosthesis design are common to a variety of prostheses. This not only includes articular surface geometry, but also fixation and bearing options. To the extent possible, the types of currently available implants are discussed under broad headings in terms of similarities and differences. Specific implants and systems are presented within each category only as examples; certainly, the intent is not to present a comprehensive list of all current total knee prostheses marketed in the United States and elsewhere.

Fixed-Bearing, Surface Replacement Prostheses
Traditional Cruciate-Retaining and Posterior-Stabilized Prostheses. The early knee prostheses described in the preceding sections have given rise to derivatives (Fig. 124.26). The TCP led to a series of PS prostheses initially developed by Insall and Burstein, including the IB PS prosthesis, and modular IB II (IB II PS) prostheses (Figs. 124.27 to 124.29).[§] These devices evolved into the Zimmer NexGen LPS and LPS Flex prostheses (Figs. 124.30 and 124.31) and more recently the Zimmer-Biomet Persona PS (Fig. 124.32). Although the basic elements of the original prostheses that have proven successful, such as the moderate sagittal and coronal plane conformity (Fig. 124.33), have endured, modifications have been made over time. These changes include more size options to better fit a wider variety of the ethnic and gender variations that are now appreciated; side-specific femoral and tibial components; a greater number of polyethylene insert thicknesses to allow easier soft tissue balancing; extension of the posterior condylar geometry to improve contact areas in high flexion; and improvements to the tibial polyethylene locking mechanism. In addition to this extended family of PS knees, the Press-Fit Condylar (PFC) PS and its successor, the PFC Sigma PS prosthesis (Fig. 124.34), were developed from the same TCP foundation as were the Optetrak PS and Advance PS prostheses; the PCL-preserving Duopatellar prosthesis evolved into the Kinematic I and II and PFC CR prostheses (Fig. 124.35).[232,305]

During the consolidation of the PFC CR and PS variants under the PFC Sigma brand more than a decade ago, the coronal plane geometry of the CR and PS implants was made identical.[241] This highlights the trend that has occurred over the past 15 years where, to some degree, prosthesis design has converged with several seemingly important elements becoming common not only to CR and PS variants in the same implant system from

---

[§]References 1, 2, 80, 105, 110, 128, 232, 244, 245, 269-271, and 299.

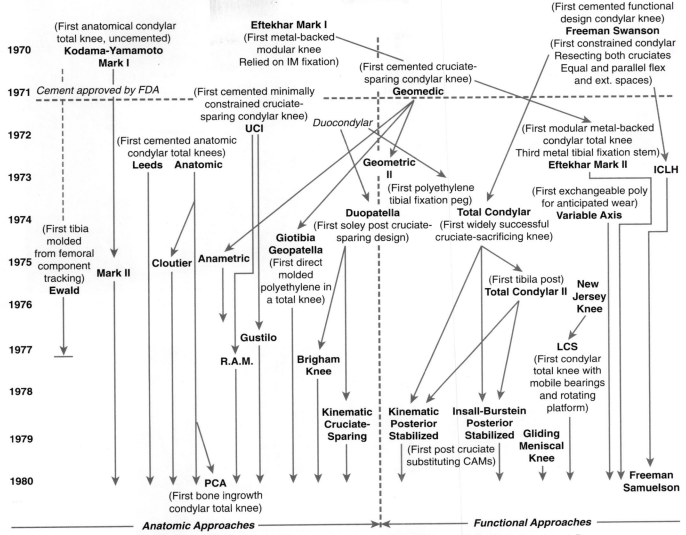

FIG 124.26 The evolution of the condylar total knee from 1970 to 1980. *FDA,* Food and Drug Administration; *IM,* intramedullary; *LCS,* low-contact stress; *PCA,* porous coated anatomic. (Adapted from Robinson RP: The early innovators of today's resurfacing condylar knees. *J Arthroplasty* 20[Suppl 1]:2–26, 2005.)

one manufacturer, but also across manufacturers. These desirable features of fixed-bearing, surface replacement prostheses include the following:

1. Multiple sizing options to match a broader range of native anatomy.
2. Side-specific femoral components with anatomically oriented trochlear grooves designed to accommodate native and resurfaced patellae.
3. Front-loading, modular, metal-backed tibial components for ease of potential revision and optimization of soft tissue balancing; moderately conforming round-on-round femorotibial geometry in the coronal plane to minimize edge loading and polyethylene wear.
4. Femoral components with the so-called J curve, multiradius sagittal plane geometry that is moderately to highly conforming during the early arc of flexion to optimize contact areas under weight-bearing conditions, but where the radius

of curvature decreases toward the posterior condyles, which facilitates rollback and ROM.[221]

Examples of CR and PS knee prostheses that currently incorporate most or all of these concepts include the Zimmer-Biomet Persona, DePuy Attune, Smith & Nephew Legion, and Zimmer-Biomet Vanguard systems. Other systems, such as the Stryker Triathlon, Smith & Nephew Journey Bi-Cruciate Stabilized, and Microport Evolution Medial Pivot Knee, incorporate alternative unique elements that theoretically change the function of the devices. The features of this latter group of devices, which are considered guided motion prostheses, are described here.

Guided Motion Prostheses. Although traditional PS knees may be considered guided motion prostheses to some degree, the kinematics of traditional surface replacement prostheses are less rigidly dictated by the design than in the prostheses introduced predominantly during the past 10 years, which are usually

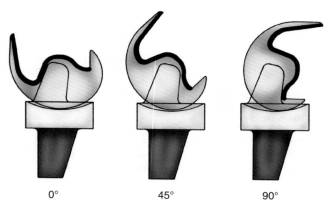

0°   45°   90°

FIG 124.27 The TCP II was a precursor of the posterior-stabilized knee that provided a passive stop against posterior displacement in flexion as well as a hyperextension stop in extension. (From Insall JN, Tria AJ, Scott WN: The total condylar knee prosthesis: the first five years. *Clin Orthop* 145:68–77, 1979.)

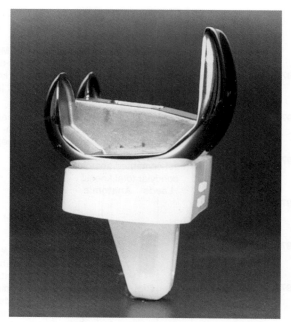

FIG 124.28 The Original Insall-Burstein Posterior-Stabilized Prosthesis.

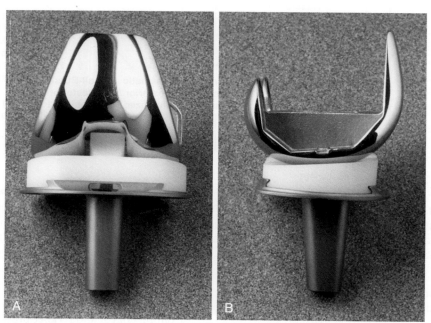

FIG 124.29 The Modular Insall-Burstein II Posterior-Stabilized Prosthesis (A) Front view. (B) Side view.

considered to be guided motion devices. Each of these devices has similar elements that attempt to compel the components to move in a more specific way. Two common features include a femoral component with a single sagittal axis of rotation to at least 90 to 100 degrees of flexion, rather than the J curve noted earlier, and articular surfaces that are molded and shaped to encourage rotation and rollback of the lateral condyle on the tibia while the medial femoral condyle remains relatively static. As noted in the previous section, most current traditional fixed-bearing surface replacement prostheses have a femoral component with posterior condylar geometry that incorporates a

number of different axes of rotation. This effectively creates a decreasing sagittal radius of curvature of the posterior condyles, which facilitates rollback in flexion. However, although the J curve theoretically facilitates rollback and improves flexion, the decreasing radius of curvature reduces the contact area of the articulating surfaces as the knee flexes, which may lead to increased polyethylene stresses.[221] However, in most surface replacement designs, the effects of this J curve do not occur during the initial 30 to 40 degrees of flexion; therefore, the increased joint forces generated during the weight-bearing portion of the gait cycle are accommodated by articular surfaces

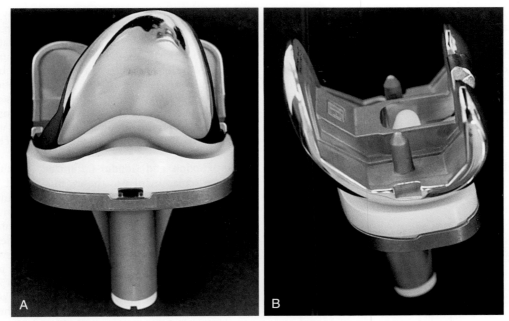

FIG 124.30 The Legacy Posterior-Stabilized Prosthesis (A) Front view. (B) Oblique view. (Zimmer, Warsaw, Indiana.)

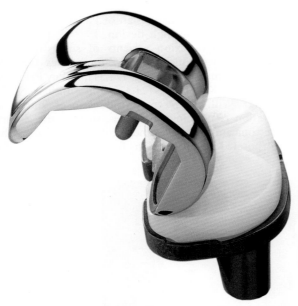

FIG 124.31 The LPS Flex prosthesis was optimized for use in patients with good preoperative motion to allow safer flexion. (Courtesy Zimmer, Warsaw, Indiana.)

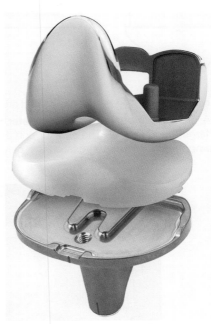

FIG 124.32 The Persona PS prosthesis (Zimmer-Biomet, Warsaw, Indiana) is a fifth-generation PS replacement descended from the original TCP. Contemporary features include geometry designed to accommodate high flexion, 21 femoral size options to better fit the gender and ethnic diversity now appreciated, and asymmetric right and left tibial baseplates designed to optimize tibial coverage and component rotation. (Courtesy Zimmer-Biomet, Warsaw, Indiana.)

with moderate to high combined coronal and sagittal plane conformity, which reduces this potential for wear; indeed, topside polyethylene wear has not been a significant clinical problem for most types of modern resurfacing prostheses. Another criticism of J curve prostheses is that the decreasing radius of curvature results in decreasing tension on the collateral ligaments as the knee flexes. This reduction in soft tissue tension has been implicated in the phenomenon described as mid-flexion instability, in which some patients experience pain and instability with activities performed with the knee in moderate flexion, such as stair climbing or rising from a chair.[289]

This is a controversial subject; however, in a minority of modern fixed-bearing surface replacement prostheses, it has led to the incorporation of a fixed single sagittal radius of curvature through an extended arc of motion exceeding 90 to 100 degrees. The Stryker Triathlon prosthesis (Fig. 124.36) and the Scorpio knee that preceded it, along with the Wright Medical Technologies Advance Medial Pivot Knee, are designs that incorporate this concept of a single sagittal axis of rotation. However, at higher degrees of flexion, these devices actually incorporate a gradual reduction of the sagittal radius of curvature to allow better rollback. Other theoretical advantages of a prosthesis with a constant sagittal radius of curvature and a more posterior flexion-extension axis that lengthens the extensor moment arm are improved quadriceps function and reduced anterior knee pain.[182]

The second design element that is common to these guided motion devices is that the articular surfaces are designed with a unique geometry that attempts to replicate the kinematics of

the normal knee. This is accomplished by encouraging the medial femoral condyle to rotate but remain relatively static in the sagittal plan while the lateral condyle rotates, rolls back, and slides posteriorly on the tibial articular surface as the knee flexes. Although potential advantages have been attributed to the single sagittal axis of rotation and motion guided by the articular geometry, it is also possible that kinematic conflict can occur between the motion driven by the prosthesis design and the motion that the surrounding soft tissues will accommodate; this can create problems unique to the devices.[178]

High-Flexion and Gender-Optimized Prostheses. Traditional surface replacement prostheses, in CR and PS variants, have been associated with excellent clinical outcomes. However, despite successful pain relief and improvements in functional outcomes, the increased desire among patients to pursue activities associated with greater degrees of knee flexion, especially in certain Asian populations, has driven the development of knee prostheses designed to accommodate better and even facilitate higher degrees of flexion, exceeding 140 to 150 degrees. Design elements that have been used in many of these included enhanced posterior condylar geometry of the femoral component to improve contact areas in high flexion, thereby reducing the risk of polyethylene wear; modifications to the anterior aspect of the tibial polyethylene insert to reduce the potential for extensor mechanism impingement in high flexion; and optimization of the cam-post design of PS variants to reduce the risk of dislocation in high flexion.[11,151,193,221] Examples of these optimized high-flexion variants of successful surface replacement prostheses include the Zimmer Nex Gen Flex-Fixed CR and PS implants (see Fig. 124.31), DePuy PFC Sigma CR150 High Flex Knee (Fig. 124.37), and Smith & Nephew Genesis II-HF. With the recent introduction of fourth- and fifth-generation resurfacing prostheses, such as the Zimmer-Biomet Persona and DePuy Attune, most of these features have been incorporated into the designs from the beginning of the

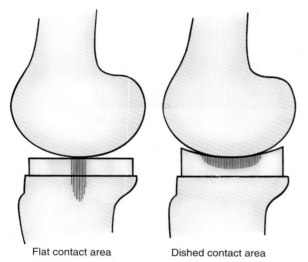

Flat contact area　　Dished contact area

FIG 124.33 A dished component permits greater conformity, and hence a larger contact area. The smaller contact area with a flat tibial component increases stress on the polyethylene.

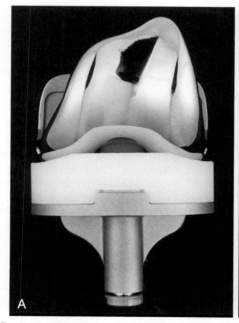
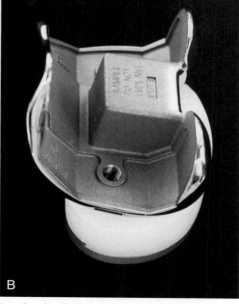

A　　B

FIG 124.34 The Press-Fit Condylar Sigma Prosthesis (DePuy, Warsaw, Indiana) (A) Front view. (B) Oblique view.

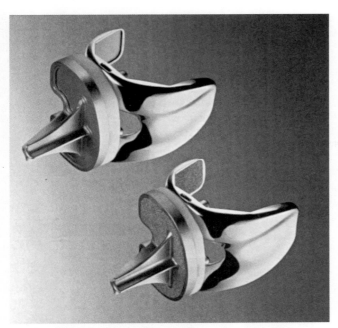

FIG 124.35 Press-fit Condylar Prosthesis.

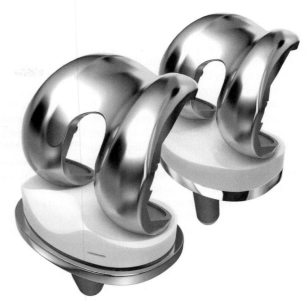

FIG 124.37 PFC Sigma CR150 High Flex Knee, mobile-bearing *(front)* and fixed-bearing *(rear)* variants. (Courtesy DePuy, Warsaw, Indiana.)

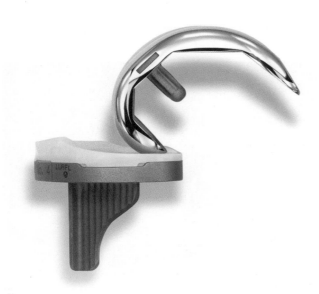

FIG 124.36 The Triathlon CR prosthesis. This device has a single sagittal radius of curvature from 10 to 110 degrees that is centered about the transepicondylar axis. This differs from the so-called J curve common to many surface replacement total condylar-type femoral components. (Courtesy Stryker, Mahwah, New Jersey.)

development process rather than as specific high-flexion variants. This has, from a practical perspective, eliminated the distinctions between high-flexion and standard protheses, with all new systems essentially representing devices that are optimized for the high-flexion environment.

To date, studies of high-flexion TKR prostheses have provided little data to support the theoretical advantages attributed to the optimized designs. In a meta-analysis on this topic, Ghandi et al.[94] noted that high-flexion designs are associated with improved ROM compared with traditional implants, but offer no clinical benefits. Similarly, Meneghini et al.[196] were unable to demonstrate any functional benefit from flexion of more than 125 degrees after TKR. Studies of individual prostheses are also inconclusive. Kim et al.[152] reported on a prospective randomized study of 50 patients who underwent simultaneous bilateral TKR with a standard fixed-bearing Zimmer NexGen LPS knee prosthesis on one side and a high-flexion, fixed-bearing NexGen LPS-Flex knee prosthesis on the opposite side. The Knee Society and HSS scores were not significantly different for either knee preoperatively or postoperatively. Moreover, there were no statistically significant differences in ROM at any time point preoperatively or postoperatively; at final follow-up, the standard prosthesis had a mean ROM of 135.8 degrees (range, 105 to 150 degrees) versus a mean of 135.8 degrees for the high-flexion prosthesis. The same authors have also reported their results from an identical prospective randomized study of 54 bilateral TKR patients comparing the Zimmer Nex Gen CR prosthesis on one side with the CR version of the NexGen Flex prosthesis on the other side.[151] Similar to their results demonstrated with the PS prostheses, no statistically significant differences in knee scores or ROM were identified between the two groups at any time, preoperatively or postoperatively.

Similar results using the same implant system have been reported from a second center in South Korea. In a trial of patients who had been randomized to receive the Zimmer fixed-bearing Nex Gen CR or the Nex Gen CR Flex-Fixed prosthesis, Seon et al.[250] did not identify any statistical differences in postoperative ROM between the two groups. Similar results have been reported from Western patients with the same Zimmer NexGen prostheses. Nutton et al.[207] compared patients who had been randomized to receive a standard or high-flexion version of the Zimmer NexGen LPS fixed-bearing design. No significant differences in outcomes or knee flexion were noted between the two groups of patients. Published information on other high-flexion prostheses is also limited. McCalden et al.[193] reported on a prospective randomized trial comparing the Smith & Nephew Genesis II PS fixed-bearing prosthesis with the high-flexion version of the same implant. At short-term follow-up, no differences in outcome scores or ROM were demonstrated; at 2 years postoperatively the mean ROM for the standard prosthesis was 123 versus 124 degrees for the high-flexion variant. Therefore, there is no clear evidence that these fixed-bearing, high-flexion devices help obtain improved ROM or are associated with better clinical results at the 2- to 3-year range. However, it is still possible that the theoretical improvements in contact area at high flexion may result in lower long-term wear and reduced rates of aseptic loosening and osteolysis at 10 years and beyond.

In addition to surface replacement designs that were optimized for the high-flexion environment, increased acknowledgment of the anthropomorphic variation that exists among different genders, races, and ethnic groups has also led to the introduction of optimized components that better accommodated these differences.**

These changes chiefly involved modifications to the mediolateral to anteroposterior (AP) ratio of the femoral components that made the component narrower for any given AP dimension, as well as modifications to the orientation and thickness of the trochlear groove and anterior flange.[30,103,197] Examples of these modified prostheses included the Zimmer Gender Solutions Nex Gen High Flex CR and LPS prostheses, and Zimmer Gender Solutions Natural and Smith & Nephew Legion Narrow femoral components. Early results examining the use of gender-optimized devices have been controversial. Although radiographic and anatomic studies have demonstrated the gender bias of standard implants toward white male anatomy, little data exist to date to support the contention that this bias has adversely affected clinical outcomes in white females or patients of other races.[52,113,179] In addition to modifications made to existing surface replacement prostheses to make them more compatible with the greater diversity of femoral sizes and shapes that is now better appreciated, new knee implant systems have been introduced during the past decade that have attempted to embrace these concepts of expanded sizing options from the initial product launch. In a similar manner to the evolution that has occurred with the concepts of high flexion and subsequent incorporation into all systems as they are introduced, the distinctions between standard and gender-optimized designs have, from a practical point, been eliminated as most now provide a wide variety of sizes. Examples of these systems include the Smith & Nephew Journey Bi-Cruciate Stabilized Knee, Stryker Triathlon, Zimmer-Biomet Persona, and DePuy Attune knee prostheses.

Cementless Fixation. Concerns about the long-term durability of cement fixation prompted the development of a variety of knee prostheses designed for cementless use during the 1980s. Because of theoretical concern about the increased stress transferred to the prosthesis-bone interface in PS designs that could potentially limit successful bone ingrowth, these uncemented devices were all designed to retain the PCL. The first design, developed by David Hungerford, was the Porous Coated Anatomic (PCA) knee prosthesis (Fig. 124.38).††

** References 30, 103, 113, 158, 176, and 279.
†† References 22, 50, 56, 62, 82, 118, 119, 154, 202, 233, 235, and 266.

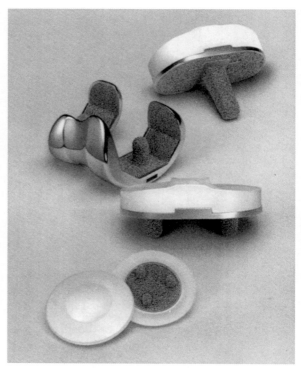

FIG 124.38 Porous Coated Anatomic Prosthesis.

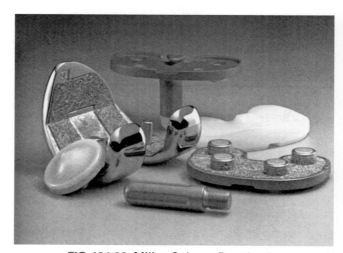

FIG 124.39 Miller-Galante Prosthesis.

Other examples included the PCA II, Miller-Galante (Fig. 124.39),[157,161,234] Miller-Galante II, Tricon M,[168,206] Genesis (Fig. 124.40), and Ortholoc prostheses.[298] The Freeman-Swanson prosthesis[90,92] was modified into the Freeman-Samuelson prosthesis[87,88,236] (Fig. 124.41), which still used serrated polyethylene pegs for cementless fixation but offered a metal baseplate with intramedullary rods for the tibia and an intramedullary rod on the femoral component.

Unfortunately, the initial enthusiasm in some circles for these devices was not supported by the long-term results. Aseptic loosening and failure to achieve initial fixation, as well as confounding problems caused by the flat-on-flat geometries used in most of these designs, led to higher failure rates than noted with comparable cemented prostheses during the first

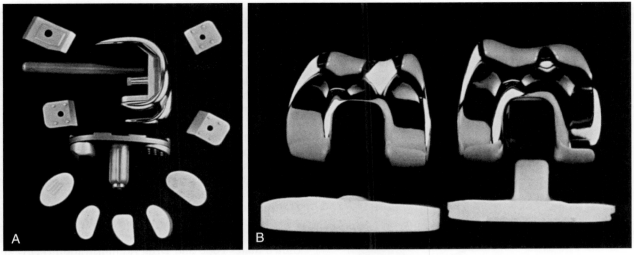

FIG 124.40 (A and B) Genesis prosthesis.

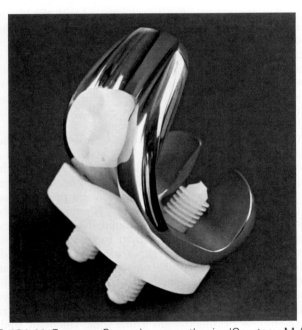

FIG 124.41 Freeman-Samuelson prosthesis. (Courtesy M.A.R. Freeman.)

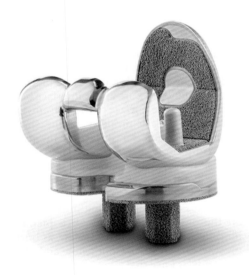

FIG 124.42 Persona PS prosthesis with porous metal in-growth surfaces. (Courtesy Zimmer-Biomet, Warsaw, Indiana.)

decade.[66,227] Consequently, these first-generation uncemented devices did not achieve widespread acceptance. More recently, the development of new bone ingrowth materials, especially those based on porous tantalum and titanium, have prompted renewed interest in this area (Fig. 124.42). Many current CR and PS knee systems now offer uncemented fixation options for the femur, tibia, and patella that can be used in conjunction with cemented components. Thus, the early division between cemented PS knees and uncemented CR knees is no longer pertinent. Individual surgeons may choose fully cemented, fully uncemented, or hybrid components used in conjunction with CR, cruciate-sacrificing, and cruciate-substituting articular options. At this time, long-term results of this next generation of uncemented and hybrid implants are not yet available.

Mobile-Bearing, Surface Replacement Prostheses. Conventional fixed-bearing knee prostheses have proven clinically successful, with favorable results at 10 to 15 years.[54,146,183] However, with only a few exceptions, these results were obtained in older, less active patient populations.[61,67] Concern exists regarding the long-term durability of current prostheses in younger, more demanding patients, especially regarding problems related to polyethylene wear and osteolysis. Polyethylene wear may be reduced by radical improvements in the inherent qualities of the material itself—for example, through cross linking, or incorporation of antioxidants such as vitamin E, and by decreasing the contact stress at the articular surfaces. Reduction in contact stress could be accomplished by increasing the conformity of the femoral component and polyethylene insert. However, because of the inherent trade-off between conformity and freedom of motion that exists in fixed-bearing prostheses, significant improvements in contact stress are not feasible

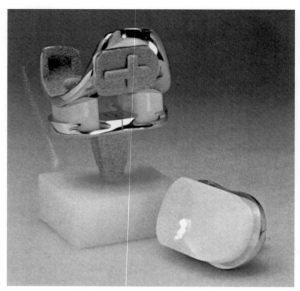

FIG 124.43 Low-Contact Stress Prosthesis.

without potentially restricting ROM. Mobile-bearing prostheses represent a theoretically appealing solution to this problem.[124] A mobile bearing eliminates the relationship between articular conformity and freedom of rotation that exists in fixed-bearing prostheses because rotation occurs at the interface between the tibial baseplate and the undersurface of the polyethylene insert, and articular conformity is a property of the shape of the femoral component and superior surface of the polyethylene insert. Articular conformity can be maximized in a mobile-bearing prosthesis, thereby reducing contact stress and wear on the superior surface of the polyethylene while freedom of rotation is theoretically maintained.

The many nuances of mobile-bearing prosthesis design are reviewed more thoroughly in a subsequent chapter. Briefly, the concepts behind these prostheses are not new, as borne out by the Oxford prostheses.[‡‡] In 1976, Goodfellow and O'Connor[100] introduced a bicondylar knee that attempted to solve the potential problem of polyethylene wear by providing a meniscal bearing—that is, a polyethylene tibial component that is fully congruent with the femoral component but free to move on a metallic tibial base tray. This concept hoped to provide the best possible wear characteristics with complete lack of constraint. The designers of the Oxford knee now recommend that this prosthesis be used only as a unicompartmental prosthesis when the ACL and PCL are present and can be preserved. An absent ACL is considered a contraindication to the use of the Oxford knee. Buechel et al.[39-41] developed the meniscal-bearing concept into a series of prostheses known as the DePuy Low-Contact Stress (LCS) knee prostheses[23] (Fig. 124.43). These devices possessed a femoral component similar to the TCP that was designed to be mated with a bicondylar meniscal-bearing tibial component or, alternatively, a rotating platform for use when cruciate excision was performed. A metal-backed patellar component with a swiveling polyethylene surface of anatomic design was also offered with this system. Unlike the Oxford knee, the LCS model has a femoral component of decreasing

radius posteriorly. Congruency is reduced when the knee is flexed so the contact area decreases in flexion, thereby losing a potential advantage of the original design.

A puzzle created by meniscal designs, particularly the Oxford model, was in deciding the position of the actual joint axis. Flexion takes place between the femur and superior surface of the polyethylene bearing, whereas AP sliding and rotation occur at the inferior surface (a position 8 to 10 mm distal to the true joint line). Whether this curious anomaly has clinical significance has not been studied extensively.

In Europe, a large number of other mobile-bearing knees have been in clinical use for over a decade. In distinction, in the United States, the LCS prosthesis was the only available mobile-bearing knee until the merger of DePuy and Johnson & Johnson. This merger allowed the development of mobile-bearing variants of the PFC Sigma CR and PS prostheses (see Fig. 124.37). Excluding these notable exceptions, the complexity of gaining United States Food and Drug Administration (FDA) approval for new devices restricted widespread introduction of other mobile-bearing prostheses. Subsequently, Zimmer also introduced a mobile-bearing version of the Nex Gen LPS into the US market. Important differences compared with the LCS and Sigma mobile-bearing prostheses are a more anterior pivot, a rotational stop that limits rotation to 20 degrees internally and externally, and a smaller contact area between the post of the metal base plate and the cutout of the polyethylene insert that allows rotation at the undersurface. Long-term follow-up will show whether these design features provide better long-term wear characteristics than contemporary fixed-bearing designs or the LCS-based mobile-bearing designs.

Although mobile-bearing prostheses have appealing theoretical advantages versus fixed-bearing knee designs, they are also associated with unique complications that result from their increased complexity. The movement that occurs on the proximal and distal surfaces of the polyethylene bearing introduces the potential for wear at both surfaces.[93] It remains unresolved whether the larger wear surfaces in mobile-bearing knees result in more total volumetric wear than in fixed-bearing knees. There are concerns that the wear particles that are generated in mobile-bearing knees are smaller than those generated in fixed-bearing devices, and these smaller particles may be more likely to result in osteolysis than larger particles. However, in vivo analysis has failed to show a consistent result.[106] Another criticism of mobile-bearing designs is that some kinematic studies of in vivo prostheses have shown that little rotation is actually occurring at the undersurface of the polyethylene, effectively resulting in a fixed-bearing implant. In one recent study, almost 50% of the prostheses demonstrated axial rotation of 3 degrees or less with deep flexion.[290] Finally, dislocation of the bearings has also been reported.[23] Interestingly, in clinical practice, the potential advantages and disadvantages of mobile-bearing devices have not translated into convincingly better or worse outcomes versus those in fixed-bearing knees.[96,160,212,306] Prosthesis survivorship and clinical outcomes for the LCS prosthesis into the second decade and beyond are similar to the results noted with the best fixed-bearing CR and PS designs.[§§] At this time, although the LCS prosthesis has proven successful in the clinical setting, after 3 decades of experience with mobile-bearing knees, they remain a niche product in North America.

‡‡References 19, 32, 34, 99-102, 276, and 300.

§§References 39, 44, 54, 116, 146, and 183.

Constrained Prostheses

Constrained Unlinked Prostheses. Constrained but unlinked prostheses are primarily intended for use in cases in which the medial and lateral soft tissue restraints about the knee have been compromised.[5,16,88,159] The original TCP III[51,63,114,145,150] evolved into the CCK prostheses, which in turn became the Zimmer LCCK prosthesis (Fig. 124.44). Improvements to the LCCK included the incorporation of the same features found on the third-generation PS prostheses, such as side-specific femoral components with anatomically oriented trochlear grooves; front-loading, modular, tibial polyethylene inserts; and an optimized cam-and-post mechanism. In addition, a full range of femoral and tibial augments and offset stem extensions added greater usefulness for the complex primary and revision cases. Constrained unlinked prostheses provide posterior stability and medial-lateral stability by means of an enlarged post that articulates closely with a femoral cam (Fig. 124.45). In distinction to the post and cam of a PS prostheses, the augmented mechanisms in constrained prostheses also limit rotation. The theoretical advantages of constrained prostheses include improved stability, but this comes with the risk of increased polyethylene wear and greater risk of loosening because of

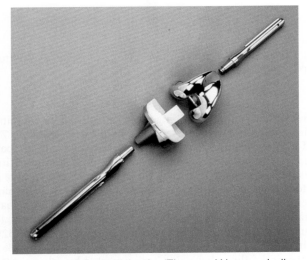

FIG 124.44 LCCK prosthesis. (Zimmer, Warsaw, Indiana.)

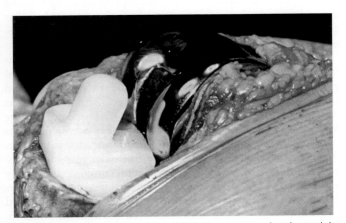

FIG 124.45 Articulation of the TCP III, a constrained condylar knee. A rectangular tibial post fits within a central femoral box or cavity, thereby providing varus and valgus stability as well as posterior restraint.

increased stress transmission to the prosthesis-cement-bone interface.

In its TCP III form, Donaldson et al.[63] found no loosening in 15 primary cases monitored for more than 2 years; all stems were cemented. The CCK was initially used primarily for revision cases, but based on this good experience with the TCP III in primary knees, these constrained devices have proven successful in managing difficult primary knees with predominantly valgus deformities in low-demand patients.[5,68,159] Avoidance of extensive release procedures and possible peroneal nerve complications has hastened recovery and lessened morbidity.

Although the clinical success of these devices has been demonstrated in difficult cases, potential risks remain. Therefore, in general, increased articular constraint is only used when the native soft tissues cannot be adequately balanced to provide medial and lateral stability. Importantly, the LCCK metal components can be used with a constrained polyethylene tibial insert or a standard PS polyethylene insert. Thus, during a difficult knee arthroplasty, if the LCCK metal components are inserted, an intraoperative decision can be made concerning the degree of constraint needed.

It has been our practice to use stem extensions when using a constrained articulation in the primary and revision settings, but good results with constrained implants without stem extensions used in the primary setting with good bone stock have also been reported at short-term to intermediate-term follow-up. In a study of 55 valgus knees that were managed without strict soft tissue balancing and a constrained unlinked prosthesis without stems, there were no cases of loosening or failures at a mean of 44.5 months.[5] Although stems potentially improve prosthesis fixation and help transfer stress from the prosthesis-cement-bone interfaces that may reduce long-term loosening rates, they increase the operative time, potentially increase fat embolization because of violation of the canal, are more difficult to remove at the time of revision, and add cost to the implant. At this time, long-term data are not available to answer the question of whether stems are necessary when a constrained prosthesis is used in a primary setting with good bone stock. However, in the revision setting, in which the bony surfaces of the femur and tibia have been compromised, we recommend that shorter cemented stems or longer uncemented, diaphyseal-engaging stems are used.

Numerous additional designs of constrained unlinked prostheses are now available. Many provide the full range of modular stems and augments along with PS and constrained articulations that allow easy intraoperative management of bony and soft tissue problems in the complex primary and revision settings. These include the Zimmer LCCK, DePuy PFC Sigma TC3, Smith & Nephew Legion Revision, Biomet Vanguard SSK Revision, and Stryker Triathlon TS systems. One unique feature of the DePuy PFC Sigma TC3 system is the availability of a mobile-bearing tibial (MBT) insert (revision tray) Fig. 124.46, which provides medial-lateral stability through the interaction of the cam and post, but also allows rotational freedom through the undersurface of the tibial bearing. Potential advantages include a reduction in polyethylene post wear and reduced transmission of stresses to the prosthesis-cement-bone interface. However, bearing dislocation is a potential disadvantage. At this time, no long-term data are available that clarify whether this mobile-bearing constrained articulation is associated with superior clinical results than the more traditional fixed-bearing constrained prostheses.

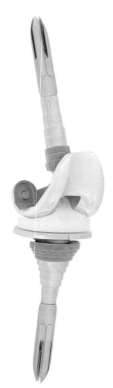

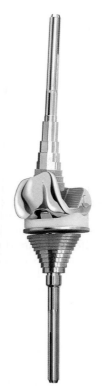

FIG 124.46 PFC Sigma TC3 prosthesis with the MBT mobile-bearing revision tray. (Courtesy DePuy, Warsaw, Indiana.)

FIG 124.47 S-ROM Noiles rotating hinge prosthesis. (Courtesy DePuy, Warsaw, Indiana.)

Constrained Rotating Hinge Prostheses. Early results with hinged devices, as previously noted, were not encouraging, with high rates of infection, loosening, and prosthesis failure. However, in parts of Europe, especially Germany, the use of hinged devices remained popular, even in primary TKR. Bohm and Holy[28] have reported excellent 20-year results with the Blauth prosthesis, a relatively simple early hinge prosthesis. With worst-case survivorship exceeding 85% at 20 years, the results are comparable to the rates noted with surface replacement prostheses from the same era. Newer designs of hinged prostheses were developed to reduce the risk of loosening and improve the kinematics through the incorporation of rotating bearings that eliminated the rotational constraint of the earlier prostheses. Good results from Germany in primary knee replacement have also been reported with these more modern hinges.[214]

In North America, hinged devices were relegated to use in the worst cases of bone loss or ligamentous incompetence, often in the setting of oncologic reconstruction or multiple revised joints. Rand et al.[225] reported the results on 50 Kinematic Rotating-Hinge TKRs performed at the Mayo Clinic. The indications were ligamentous instability, loss of bone, or both. The follow-up was 50 months (range, 29 to 79 months). There were 14 excellent, 12 good, 5 fair, and 5 poor results. Progression of radiolucent lines was observed in 13 knees, and 5 knees probably had radiographic loosening. The rate of sepsis was 16%, patellar instability developed in 22%, and breakage of the implant occurred in 6%. In these patients, 74% of the operations were revisions—a first revision in 17, a second revision in 16, a third revision in 3, and a fourth revision in 1. The authors combined the incidence of complications reported for several

series with a total of 1099 hinged implants. In these combined series, loosening was reported in 27% of knees, sepsis in 7%, and wound-healing problems in 5.5%. Based on this comparison, it was concluded that the Kinematic Rotating-Hinge prosthesis, although possessing theoretical advantages, gave no better results than the older nonrotating hinges. In a more recent report from the Mayo Clinic involving 69 Kinematic Rotating-Hinge knees at a mean of 75 months follow-up, the results were similar, with an overall complication rate of 32%, an infection rate of 14.5%, and component breakage in 10%.[268] Mechanical failures have also been reported by others.[129,148,225] Other centers in North America with experience using rotating hinge devices in the revision setting have also reported similar concerns with the same device, as well as other similar prostheses, such as the Finn Rotating hinged prosthesis.[216,295]

Regardless of these concerns, use of a hinged device remains the best option in some cases. Contemporary rotating hinged prostheses include the DePuy S-ROM Noiles (Fig. 124.47) and Limb Preservation System Rotating Hinges, Zimmer Nex Gen Rotating Hinge Knee (RHK), Biomet Orthopedic Salvage System (OSS), and Stryker Global Modular Replacement System (GMRS). Many of these systems incorporate design features that have theoretical advantages over the older hinged devices. For example, the geometry of the femoral component in many systems is now more similar to contemporary surface replacement prostheses; in particular, the trochlear has been optimized to accommodate native and resurfaced patellae. In addition, some newer designs allow for condylar load bearing between the femur and tibia, as found in surface replacement designs or, at a minimum, load sharing between the axle and femorotibial articulation. In distinction, many older hinge designs bore most of the load through the axle, which contributed to bushing wear and axle failure. It is likely that with improvements, these devices will be associated with better outcomes than previously noted but, unfortunately, the underlying limitations inherent in the multiply failed joint that these devices are used to address and infection will dictate the overall complication rates. Nonetheless, early reports have suggested that superior outcomes will be achieved.[17,139]

GENERAL PROSTHETIC FEATURES

Interchangeability of Sizes

The natural variation that occurs between individual knee joints means that prosthetic components based on average dimensions do not always fit the femur and tibia of a particular joint equally well. Interchangeability of sizes, such that the femoral, tibial, and patellar components can be selected independently of each other according to the fit on their respective bones, becomes an attractive feature. Although it has long been possible to match patellar components with various femoral sizes, similar adaptability between the femoral and tibial components is a newer feature and one that is available to varying degrees in different systems. In some systems, a wide range of femoral and tibial sizes may be mated together, whereas in others, each femur may only be combined with a limited number of tibial sizes, such as one size smaller or one size larger than the natural match. As with other aspects of knee arthroplasty, some compromises are involved, chiefly in regard to the degree of articular congruity or the inventory of parts that must be carried. Flatter tibial articular geometry improves options for interchangeability, but a curved femur on a flat tibia results in a smaller contact area that potentially increases wear. The contact patch can be enlarged by also flattening the femoral surfaces (Fig. 124.48). However, malalignment or any situation that leads to asymmetrical loading, even those occurring during the normal gait cycle, shifts the loading area to the periphery. This type of "edge" loading has been shown experimentally[20,284,286] to produce the greatest stress at the prosthesis-bone interface, perhaps offsetting any benefits obtained from more complete tibial coverage. To some degree, this compromise in congruity can be offset by increased inventory so that an increased variety of polyethylene inserts can be manufactured to allow increased interchangeability.

Articular Geometry

Conforming joint surfaces should have the best wear resistance, particularly when the polyethylene is relatively thick.[20] However, conforming articulations, as noted, are not fully interchangeable, may conflict with PCL kinematics, and can theoretically cause greater fixation stress.

Thatcher et al.,[274] discussing inherent laxity in knee prostheses, have stated that laxity is a function of joint conformity. They believe that the implanted prosthesis should compensate for soft tissue structures that are deficient or removed. They think that the optimal laxity profile has not yet been determined but suggest that the articular geometry should possess partial conformity, and comment on the classic inherent design compromise. The greater the conformity, the larger the contact area and the less intrinsic stress and wear. However, conforming prostheses will create greater fixation stress, which may lead to loosening.

Wear is an increasing problem in TKR. Several factors have been implicated, including the quality of the polyethylene, the manufacturing process, the thickness of the tibial components, and articular geometry.[265] It is also true that in the best of circumstances, polyethylene is not an ideal bearing material,[304] but attempts to improve its performance have historically not been successful.[303] Many cases of severe wear and delamination of tibial components have been reported,[71,149] mainly involving thinner polyethylene components. Manufacturing processes

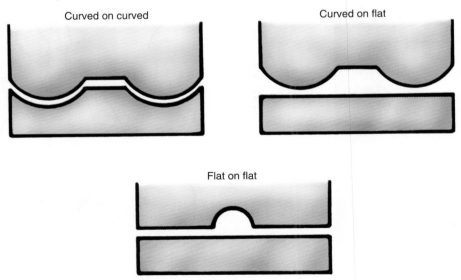

FIG 124.48 The more conforming the articulation, the larger the contact area and the less stress on the polyethylene. In the frontal plane, curved-on-curved geometries are the best. Curved-on-flat geometry is the worst. Flat-on-flat surfaces can provide a good area of contact but are sensitive to edge loading whenever the prosthesis is loaded unevenly, such as in leaning or pivoting movements.

(including heat-pressing[27] the polyethylene to give a smoother surface and gamma sterilization in air leading to free radical formation) have been identified as detrimental factors in the development of polyethylene wear. In addition to these manufacturing issues, prosthesis design factors have certainly contributed to this problem, considering that other prostheses manufactured using similar polyethylene treatments have not shown the same degree of damage. In particular, flat articular designs susceptible to edge loading and increased polyethylene stresses during condylar liftoff appear to be particularly susceptible. Finally, surgical technique is also important, with malalignment and instability potentially contributing to early failures. However, in general, more conforming round-on-round articular surfaces in the coronal plane, which help reduce polyethylene stresses, particularly if condylar liftoff occurs, have become popular in a variety of CR and PS prostheses. As noted in the discussion on guided motion prostheses, considerable debate remains regarding whether a single axis or multiple axes of rotation in the sagittal plane is the optimal design. The J curve that results from the multiple axis of rotation theoretically optimizes flexion but results in decreasing contact areas as the knee flexes.

Design and Fixation of the Tibial Component

An important difference between prostheses is the method of tibial fixation.[175] The TCP and IB PS and Kinematic prostheses used a central peg. The PFC had a central tri-fin post. These prostheses are primarily designed for cement fixation. Long-term studies with a variety of cemented designs have shown tibial component loosening to be rare (Fig. 124.49).[54,146,183]

Others that can be inserted with or without cement have two to four short studs, augmented in some cases by screws.

There is good evidence from early experience with knee arthroplasty that separate tibial components are susceptible to fixation failure. Neither an anterior bar nor the use of fixation studs is helpful. Extensive work has been performed to identify optimal design features.[21,285-287] Walker et al.[285] tested a variety of tibial components by applying compressive load with AP force, rotational torque, or varus-valgus moment (Fig. 124.50). The relative compressive and distractive reflections were measured between the component and the bone. The fewest deflections occurred with one-piece metal components. Whether a central peg or two lateral studs were used did not seem to make much difference. Thick plastic components behaved much like metal-backed ones, except when a cruciate cutout was made.

Railton et al.[218] found metal backing of the polyethylene without a central stem to be of little value in enhancing fixation. They did not address the question of optimal stem length or the use of cement. Yamamoto et al.,[307] discussing the results of the Kodama-Yamamoto Mark II prosthesis, which has an all-polyethylene tibial component with four small studs and is inserted without cement, have expressed the opinion that a stem is unnecessary. They reported a 4.4% incidence of femoral loosening accompanied by tibial sinkage in some patients, but cases with only tibial sinkage were not observed.

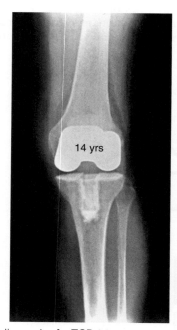

FIG 124.49 Radiograph of a TCP 14 years postoperatively. Note the thin cement mantle clearly showing ridges in the cement caused by the design of the tibial polyethylene. There is no evidence of cracking or fragmentation of the cement. This type of appearance was seen frequently in the more than 10-year follow-up of this prosthesis and indicates that a thick cement mantle is unnecessary.

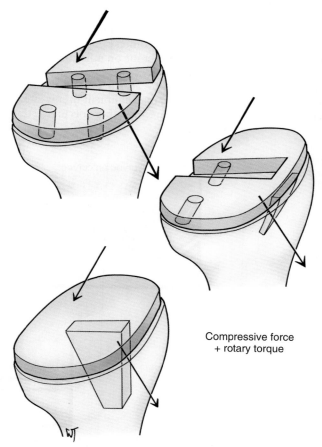

Compressive force + rotary torque

FIG 124.50 The same compressive force and rotatory torque *(arrows)* applied to different tibial component designs produce different deflections at the bone-cement interface. (Courtesy Dr. Peter Walker.)

Lewis et al.[175] tested the fixation of six tibial component configurations by finite element analysis. They concluded that metal-backed, single-post designs provide the lowest system stress overall when cement is used.

Clinical data on implants using metal tray and small stud fixation are mostly applicable to cementless fixation. Computer simulations of bone remodeling around porous-coated implants[208] have demonstrated stress concentrations around small tibial pegs. This resulted in denser bone, with a decrease in density in more peripheral locations. This finding agrees with the clinical observation that bone in-growth occurs most predictably around fixation pegs. Walker et al.,[286] in a comparative study of uncemented tibial component designs, found that central stemmed and bladed designs perform better than short pegs placed near the periphery.

Support of the plastic by means of a metal tray or endoskeleton is certainly desirable when the bone of the upper part of the tibia is deficient (eg, in severe erosive arthritis or revision operations), but when the bone is of good quality, metal backing may not offer an advantage. One-piece plastic components with a central peg have a low rate of loosening, but in 30% to 40% of cases, a partial radiolucency develops. For the most part, these radiolucencies appear within the first year, are nonprogressive, and are of dubious clinical significance. The addition of a metal tray reduces the incidence of radiolucency and also seems to reduce the incidence of late tibial loosening (Fig. 124.51).

Modular Augments and Stems

Modularity, in the sense under discussion, refers to the ability to add stems, augments, and wedges to standard components so that to a degree, the surgeon can make a custom prosthesis intraoperatively (Fig. 124.52). Most manufacturers, such as the DePuy PFC Sigma TC 3, Biomet Vanguard SSK Revision System, Smith & Nephew Legion Revision System, Stryker Triathlon TS, and Zimmer LCCK, now offer a complete knee prosthesis system that includes all these modular components. Modularity is particularly useful for revision surgery when the bone deficiencies cannot be completely anticipated. It is also of value for primary knee replacement when dealing with bone defects.

Metal augments are screwed or cemented to their components. Screw fixation, although mechanically satisfying, creates the possibility of metallic debris formation by micromotion (fretting). Cement may also not be the ideal bonding material between metal surfaces. At present, one or the other method must be used. Alternatives to metal augmentation include cement alone,[177] cement and screws et al.,[230] and bone grafting.[37,169]

Prosthetic stems of varying lengths intended for use with and without cement are also an important part of modular knee systems. Early use of stems about the knee, especially cemented stems, had a stigma that was related to their use with hinges and other constrained models. Murray et al.,[204] from the Mayo Clinic, have reported 5-year results with the use of cemented stems in conjunction with the Kinematic Stabilizer prosthesis in 40 revision TKRs. The incidence of radiolucent lines was 13% around the femoral stems and 32% around the tibial stems. However, most were incomplete, nonprogressive, and less than 1 mm. Only one femoral component and one tibial component were radiographically loose. Theoretical concerns regarding stress shielding were not noted in these cases. Longer-term follow-up of the same cohort at 10 years, as reported by Whaley et al.,[296] demonstrated continued good results with survival free of revision for any reason in 96% of these cases.

Similar results have also recently been reported from France, with no cases of stem loosening at a mean of 12.5 years postoperatively in a group of younger patients who underwent knee reconstruction with a constrained prosthesis following oncologic resection.[162] Therefore, it appears that in this time frame, exceeding 10 years, cemented stems function adequately without significant complications. However, concerns remain regarding potential bone loss and increased surgical difficulty at revision.

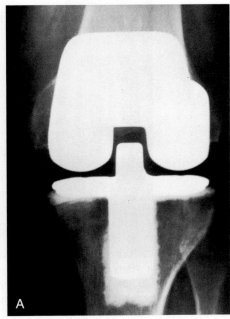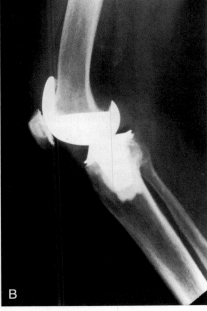

FIG 124.51 (A and B) AP and lateral radiographs of a tibial component with an endoskeleton. Metal backing of this type reduces tibial loosening at long-term follow-up.

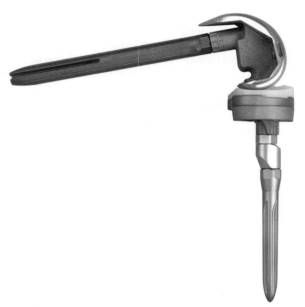

FIG 124.52 Contemporary modular revision knee system (Triathlon TS prosthesis). The components can be customized intraoperatively with a variety of straight or offset cemented or uncemented stems, augments, and PS or constrained tibial polyethylene inserts of varying thicknesses. (Courtesy Stryker, Mahwah, New Jersey.)

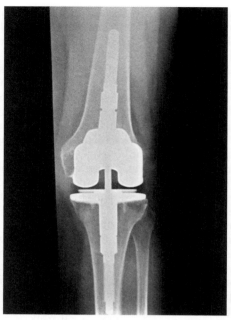

FIG 124.53 Radiograph of a knee prosthesis showing so-called dangle stems. These uncemented stems rest in the intramedullary canal and do not make contact with the cortices. Even so, roentgenographic stereophotogrammetric analysis data have shown that uncemented stems of this type on the tibial side have low rates of migration and inducible displacement.

If the intention is merely to provide additional component support, in the case of deficient bone, stems need not be associated with constraint and do not need to be cemented.[109,199] Freeman advocated use of an uncemented stem of fixed diameter and did not attempt to obtain a press-fit (the so-called dangle stem; Fig. 124.53).[24] Using this technique, the development of radiopaque lines adjacent to the stem occurred in 88% of cases. In another study, similar radiolucent lines were observed about 67% of femoral rods and 69% of tibial rods; however, at a mean follow-up of 42 months, only 3% of the prostheses had failed because of loosening.[109] A sclerotic halo around the tip of the prosthesis has also been noted in some cases (Fig. 124.54).[24] The importance of these findings and the potential for long-term loosening is not fully understood but is concerning. Therefore, to avoid failure when using uncemented stems, longer diaphyseal-engaging stems appear to be better than short metaphyseal stems, especially in patients with more extensive bone loss. At a mean of 5 years, 9 months follow-up, Shannon et al.[251] from the Mayo Clinic reported that 16% of the prostheses inserted with limited cement around the body of the implant and uncemented stems had been revised for aseptic loosening or were considered radiographically loose. In this series, it was noted that stems of varying lengths had been used but the failures were not subdivided by stem length. The higher failure rate noted in this series is different than the more favorable results previously noted from the same institution with cemented stems.[296] Fehring et al.[77] have also reported concerns regarding the use of short metaphyseal uncemented stems with cemented components in revision TKR. In their series of 95 uncemented metaphyseal stems at a minimum of 2-year follow-up, 10% were loose and 19% were considered possibly loose. In contrast, of the 107 cemented metaphyseal stems in the same report, 97% were considered stable, with only 7%

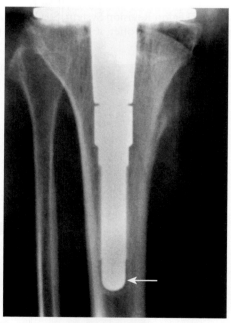

FIG 124.54 Radiograph showing sclerosis at the tip of an uncemented stem *(white arrow)*. The interpretation of this finding, which is fairly constant, is arguable. In part, it is probably caused by bending of the more flexible bone, but it may also be indicative of the stem's role in resisting tilting movements.

possibly loose.[77] One potential advantage of diaphyseal-engaging uncemented press-fit stems compared with shorter metaphyseal stems is that unless there is an unusual anatomic variation, or prior deformity from trauma or osteotomy, diaphyseal-engaging stems help restore anatomic alignment of the extremity. Based on current data, it is the surgeon's choice whether to use cemented or uncemented stems in revision TKR; however, if uncemented stems are used, they should be longer diaphyseal-engaging stems.

Custom Prostheses

Prior to the advent of comprehensive revision systems with modular augments and stems, custom prostheses were occasionally manufactured to help manage particularly challenging anatomic variations, posttraumatic deformities, and most commonly, deformity caused by prior high tibial osteotomy where abnormal metaphyseal/diaphyseal offset was encountered (Fig. 124.55). Modular revision components have greatly reduced the need for custom prostheses in these difficult circumstances, but there is still a role in some especially challenging cases. Advances in computer-aided design and 3D printing have certainly simplified the production of one-off components by traditional orthopedic device manufacturers. In addition, recent advances in 3D printing technology have dramatically reduced the cost of capable 3D printers that has made in-office production of accurate 3D bone models a reality for practicing orthopedic surgeons.[239] These 3D models can now be easily produced using readily available software on inexpensive desktop computers, and printed in a plastic material that can be subsequently worked with standard orthopedic tools. Consequently, these models essentially allow "mock" surgery to be performed in the sawbones lab prior to the operating room. This has been very helpful for improving surgeons' understanding of complex

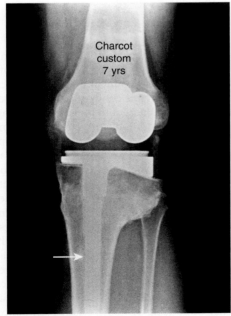

FIG 124.55 Radiograph of a custom prosthesis with a lateral wedge and offset stem *(arrow)*. The prosthesis was designed for a patient with a neuropathic joint who previously underwent high tibial osteotomy. The knee migrated into excessive valgus, leaving a lateral defect and an offset of the tibial diaphysis.

deformities and evaluating treatment options before the time constraints of live surgery are encountered.[239]

Although custom prostheses have traditionally been used to help manage complex deformities, a new application of patient-specific prostheses has been developed over the past 5 years for use in patients undergoing primary knee replacement. Using preoperative computed tomography (CT) scans, patient-specific partial and total knee prostheses can now be designed and produced in 6 weeks or less using just-in-time inventory concepts. These individualized implants match the size and geometry of the patient's native anatomy. The iTotal (ConforMIS, Bedford, Massachusetts) is the first example of this new category of high-volume, patient-specific, total knee prostheses.[240] Rather than using generic and symmetric radii of curvature for the medial and lateral femoral condyles, as are typically used in standard total knee femoral components, the femoral condyles of the iTotal femoral component have individual radii of curvature (J curves) that match the patient's specific native J curves.[240] This is also true for the J curve of the trochlea groove. In addition to re-creating the individual shape of the condyles for each patient, the distal and posterior offsets of the femoral components are patient specific and are accommodated by offset polyethylene inserts for the tibia that are specific for each compartment and each patient (Fig. 124.56). Potential advantages of this anatomic approach, which re-creates the condylar geometry, joint line, and offset, are improved stability, less need for ligament releases, more normal knee kinematics, and significantly larger femorotibial contact areas.[240] Compared to contemporary fixed-bearing devices, the contact area in the iTotal CR prosthesis is 2 to 4 times greater.[240] Although some most aspects of these custom implants are patient specific, other features and concepts used in these individualized implants are based on well-performing features of conventional knee arthroplasty, including the geometry of the trochlear flange, and implantation of the components perpendicular to the mechanical axes of the femur and tibia.[240]

These new individualized, custom implants represent a return to the anatomic philosophy of knee replacement design that proved challenging to implement with prior technology and manufacturing processes. In particular, the increased inventory that results from the numerous modular parts required to allow close intraoperative matching of individual anatomy with conventional, "off-the-shelf" prostheses can be expensive and poses logistical challenges.[240] For example, the Zimmer-Biomet Persona system offers 21 different PS femoral components that come in 2-mm increments in the AP dimension, with standard and narrow widths (Fig. 124.57). These are matched with 18 different, side-specific, asymmetric tibial components that accept polyethylene inserts that are available in 1-mm increments. All these options require an extensive inventory of expensive and bulky parts that must be maintained and stored at individual hospitals.[240] In distinction, patient-specific implants eliminate most of these inventory issues by delivering an individualized prosthesis at the time of surgery using just-in-time manufacturing principles long used elsewhere in industry.

Although patient-specific prostheses have theoretically appealing features, including the individualized anatomic fit and reduced inventory, it remains to be seen whether truly custom devices will provide patient outcomes that are superior to other modern off-the-shelf resurfacing prostheses, and whether they can be produced in a cost-effective, timely manner.

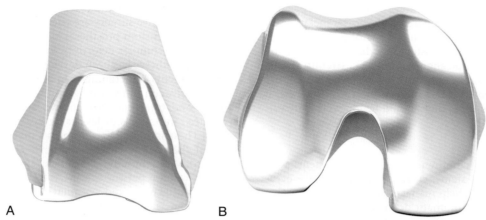

FIG 124.56 The custom, patient-specific iTotal CR prosthesis has asymmetric medial and lateral femoral condyles with patient-specific radii of curvature, and individualized distal (A) and posterior (B) offsets that restore the patient's native anatomy. (Courtesy ConforMIS, Bedford, Massachusetts.)

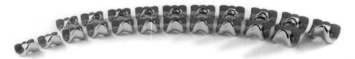

FIG 124.57 The Persona PS prosthesis (Zimmer-Biomet, Warsaw IN) has 21 femoral sizes including 10 standard width components and 11 narrow components.

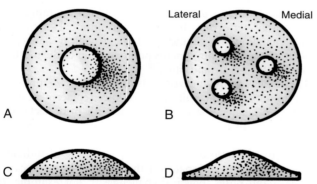

FIG 124.58 Patella Shapes and Methods of Fixation (A and C) Dome patella with a central fixation lug. (B and D) Sombrero patella with three fixation pegs.

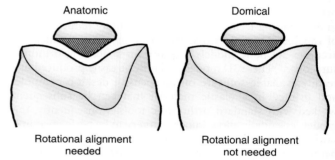

FIG 124.59 Rotational alignment is needed with a patellar replacement of anatomic shape.

Patellar Prostheses

Resurfacing. In rheumatoid arthritis, the patella should always be replaced to remove all articular cartilage from the joint. Some surgeons recommend selective resurfacing of the patella for patients with osteoarthritis.[248,257,262] Others think that the result is more predictable with routine patellar resurfacing.[73,224,243,264] Undoubtedly, patellar resurfacing has its share of iatrogenic complications, such as fracture[275] and soft tissue overgrowth with impingement.[112] Fixation holes in the patella weaken its structure, central holes probably more so than peripheral ones (Fig. 124.58).

Configuration. Traditionally, most patellar components were dome-shaped. This configuration is not ideal because the convex contour might be expected to wear poorly on the basis of engineering experience—in an articulation, the softer material should be concave. A component that is anatomic (eg, PCA and LCS) has a more desirable configuration in this respect but requires careful rotary alignment to prevent binding against the femur (Fig. 124.59). In addition, correct static alignment, even if achieved at surgery, may not predict the functional pull of the quadriceps in active use, and the more desirable wear characteristics can be offset by increased torque on the component caused by malalignment. The LCS patellar design attempts to solve this problem by having an anatomic polyethylene articulation swivel on a metal baseplate. This design has been used for more than 2 decades and has been clinically successful. The tendency of the universal patellar dome to deform has led to the use of oval and sombrero shapes.[35] An oval patella provides greater coverage of the patellar bone and a sombrero shape theoretically has more attractive wear characteristics. Others have advocated inlaying the prosthesis into the central portion of the patellar bone (Fig. 124.60).[171] However, concerns exist regarding the potential for impingement of the unresurfaced peripheral bony rim. Therefore, most surgeons who resurface the patellar chose a cemented all-polyethylene onlay component. Although retrieval analysis has documented deformation of the plastic, clinically significant wear with a dome-shaped

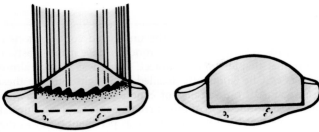

FIG 124.60 In-setting the patella allows greater thickness of polyethylene and the use of metal backing. There is a rim of peripheral exposed bone that can impinge against the femur.

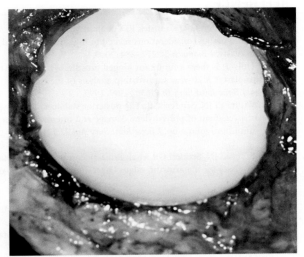

FIG 124.61 Patella showing considerable lateral polyethylene wear. This amount of polyethylene damage is unusual and was caused by lateral subluxation of the patella. Normally, only slighter flattening and deformation of dome-type patellae are noted.

all-polyethylene patellar component is a rare problem in long-term clinical studies (Fig. 124.61).

Metal-Backed Patellar Component. Metal backing of the patellar component was inspired in part by the good experience with tibial component design and in part by the wish to obtain bone ingrowth.[82] It is now apparent that many early metal-backed patellae were designed with inadequate polyethylene thickness. This has resulted in catastrophic failures related to polyethylene dissociation from the baseplate and wear-through (Fig. 124.62).

It has proven difficult to design an onset patellar component with the necessary thickness of polyethylene to avoid wear-through without producing an unacceptably bulky component. This design difficulty caused a widespread return to all-polyethylene patellar components generally used with cement, although press-fit inlaid components have been used without cement.[26] The optimal patellar design remains uncertain.[55,171] A new generation of metal-backed patellae was introduced in the 2000s as a result of the development of new ingrowth materials. Porous trabecular metals offer excellent in-growth potential and allow intrusion of the polyethylene into the metal backing, which not only creates an excellent bond but also allows the thickness of the polyethylene to be optimized. Currently, this

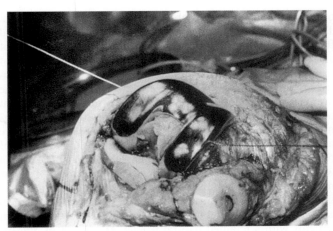

FIG 124.62 Kinematic prosthesis showing central wear-through of a metal-backed patellar component.

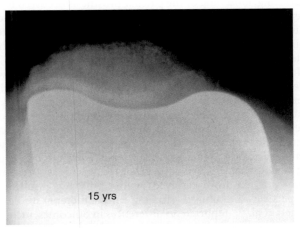

15 yrs

FIG 124.63 Skyline radiograph showing an unresurfaced patella 15 years postoperatively. In this case, the patella has remodeled to fit the femoral groove. The knee is functioning satisfactorily, has good function on stairs, and is pain-free.

new generation of metal-backed patellae represents only a small percentage of the patellar components used, with most comprised of cemented, all-polyethylene domes, ovals, and sombrero-style onlay components.

Prosthetic Patellar Problems. Regardless of how the patella is treated, patellofemoral symptoms on stair climbing and other flexed-knee activities remain a troublesome problem that is not yet fully resolved. Avoidance of a high shoulder profile of the femoral component in the junctional area between the flange and condylar runners in favor of a smooth, uniformly curved trochlear groove reduces patellofemoral strain.[195] Technical factors, such as the orientation of the patellar osteotomy and thickness of the patellar prosthesis composite, are important, as is avoidance of patella infra as a result of proximal alteration of the prosthetic joint line.

Determining Whether the Patella Should Be Resurfaced. Some patellar problems can be avoided if the patellar prosthesis is omitted altogether (Fig. 124.63). Keblish et al.[147] reported on patients who underwent bilateral TKR with patellar resurfacing on one side and retention of the natural patella on the other. The patients expressed no preference between the two sides and there were no differences in stair climbing or the incidence of anterior knee pain. Barrack et al.[18] also reported the results of a prospective randomized study on patellar resurfacing involving 86 patients. They were unable to detect differences in the overall Knee Society, pain, or function score, or in assessment of patellofemoral function. Although the results were not significantly different between the two groups, a clear difference in complications was noted. A significantly higher rate of reoperation was noted in the group in which the natural patella was retained, with a 12% prevalence of subsequent patellar resurfacing in this group. In contrast, there were no reoperations in the resurfaced group. Boyd et al.[33] also reported that in early to midterm follow-up, increased complications occur in patients with a retained natural patella. At a mean of 3 years, the overall complication rate in the group with patellar resurfacing was 4% versus 12% in the unresurfaced group. Among patients with rheumatoid arthritis who underwent patellar resurfacing, loosening of the patellar prosthesis occurred in 1%, whereas a 13% reoperation rate for subsequent resurfacing occurred in the group that initially retained the natural patella. Kajino et al.[141] noted superior pain relief in patients with rheumatoid arthritis after patellar resurfacing.

In a meta-analysis by Parvizi et al.,[213] similar findings were noted, with approximately a 10% risk of reoperation for subsequent patellar resurfacing and a greater risk of anterior knee pain. Another meta-analysis also favored resurfacing but noted exceptions for which not resurfacing the patella could be considered, including in patients younger than 60 years, with minimal arthritic changes of the patella.[31] However, it is important to note that this issue of patellar resurfacing is still controversial and far from resolved, with conflicting results from prospective randomized studies. Two different studies by Burnett et al.[42,42] reported no differences in outcomes, including reoperation rates, at 10-year follow-up.

Our experience suggests slightly better results after patellar resurfacing, particularly when careful surgical technique is used. However, it may be preferable to leave the natural patella intact in certain cases including[31]:

1. The patient is morbidly obese. Stern and Insall[270] have shown that with resurfacing, pain and complications are more frequent in obese patients.
2. The patella is too small or too eroded to accept a prosthesis.
3. The patient is young and active, which theoretically increases the risk of loosening, wear, and fracture.[209]

It is important to note that while these cases are relative contraindications to resurfacing, absence of the patella precludes patellar resurfacing. However, patellectomy is not a contraindication to knee arthroplasty and acceptable results have been reported after total knee arthroplasty in this situation.[163] To allow the option to omit patellar resurfacing, it seems wise to design the femoral component to be compatible with the natural patella. Most current PS and CR resurfacing prostheses are available in side-specific configurations with an extended trochlea, which has a more gradual transition with the distal condyles to accommodate the natural patella as well as the resurfaced patella.

ACKNOWLEDGMENTS

I would like to acknowledge the unequaled contributions of John N. Insall to the success of modern knee arthroplasty. In his original chapter on this subject, which was written almost 30 years ago, he eloquently detailed his insight into prosthesis design gained from decades of experience. His original work remains the foundation of this current chapter and it is interesting to note that his observations are as pertinent today as they were when first published. All students of knee arthroplasty will find pearls of wisdom in these pages. I remain eternally grateful for his mentorship and guidance.

KEY REFERENCES

11. Argenson JN, Scuderi GR, Komistek RD, et al: In vivo kinematic evaluation and design considerations related to high flexion in total knee arthroplasty. *J Biomech* 38:277–284, 2005.

28. Bohm P, Holy T: Is there a future for hinged prostheses in primary total knee arthroplasty? A 20-year survivorship analysis of the Blauth prosthesis. *J Bone Joint Surg Br* 80:302–309, 1998.

54. Colizza WA, Insall JN, Scuderi GR: The posterior stabilized total knee prosthesis: assessment of polyethylene damage and osteolysis after a ten-year-minimum follow-up. *J Bone Joint Surg Am* 77:1713–1720, 1995.

68. Easley ME, Insall JN, Scuderi GR, et al: Primary constrained condylar knee arthroplasty for the arthritic valgus knee. *Clin Orthop* 380:58–64, 2000.

69. Elias SG, Freeman MAR, Gokcay EI: A correlative study of the geometry and anatomy of the distal femur. *Clin Orthop* 260:98–103, 1990.

77. Fehring TK, Odum S, Olekson C, et al: Stem fixation in revision total knee arthroplasty. *Clin Orthop* 416:217–224, 2003.

103. Greene KA: Gender-specific design in total knee arthroplasty. *J Arthroplasty* 22(Suppl):27–31, 2007.

113. Hitt K, Shurman JR, II, Greene K, et al: Anthropometric measurements of the human knee: correlation to the sizing of current knee arthroplasty systems. *J Bone Joint Surg Am* 85:115–122, 2003.

128. Insall JN, Lachiewicz PF, Burstein AH: The posterior stabilized condylar prosthesis: a modification of the total condylar design: two to four-year clinical experience. *J Bone Joint Surg Am* 64:1317–1323, 1982.

129. Insall JN, Ranawat CS, Aglietti P, et al: A comparison of four models of total knee replacement prostheses. *J Bone Joint Surg Am* 58:754–765, 1976.

131. Insall JN, Scott WN, Ranawat CS: The total condylar knee prosthesis: a report of two hundred and twenty cases. *J Bone Joint Surg Am* 61:173–180, 1979.

210. Pagnano MW, Cushner FD, Scott WN: Role of the posterior cruciate ligament in total knee arthroplasty. *J Am Acad Orthop Surg* 6:176–187, 1998.

213. Parvizi J, Rapuri VR, Saleh K, et al: Failure to resurface the patella during total knee arthroplasty may resulting more knee pain and secondary surgery. *Clin Orthop* 438:191–196, 2005.

232. Robinson RP: The early innovators of today's resurfacing condylar knees. *J Arthroplasty* 20(Suppl 1):2–26, 2005.

268. Springer BD, Hanssen AD, Sim FH, et al: The kinematic rotating hinge prosthesis for complex knee arthroplasty. *Clin Orthop* 392:283–291, 2001.

272. Stiehl JB, Komistek RD, Dennis DA, et al: Fluoroscopic analysis of kinematics after posterior-cruciate-retaining knee arthroplasty. *J Bone Joint Surg Br* 77:884–889, 1995.

The references for this chapter can also be found on www.expertconsult.com.

125

Unicompartmental, Bicompartmental, or Tricompartmental Arthritis of the Knee: Algorithm for Surgical Management

Sridhar R. Rachala, Rafael J. Sierra

DEFINITIONS

- Total knee arthroplasty (TKA): Replacement of the tibiofemoral joint with or without patellar resurfacing.
- Partial knee arthroplasty (PKA): Replacement of one of the compartments of the tibiofemoral joint with or without patellar resurfacing or replacement of the patellofemoral (PF) joint only.
- Unicompartmental knee arthroplasty (UKA): One form of PKA; replacement of the medial or lateral compartments.
- Bicompartmental arthroplasty (BCA): Replacement of the medial or lateral compartments and the PF joint simultaneously.

INTRODUCTION

The knee joint is a modified hinge that can be arbitrarily divided into three compartments: medial, lateral, and PF. Arthritis from a surgical standpoint involves loss of articular cartilage with narrowing of joint space. The loss of cartilage can be focal or more diffuse, with a more diffuse pattern seen commonly in degenerative arthritis. When this process is limited to only one compartment, it is defined as unicompartmental arthritis. Bicompartmental arthritis involves either the medial or lateral compartments with involvement of the PF compartment. Tricompartmental arthritis by definition involves all three compartments.

When faced with an articular pathology of the knee that has failed appropriate nonoperative management, the options for surgical management include either joint preservation or joint-sacrificing procedures—the former, in the form of cartilage restoration procedures and/or osteotomies done alone or in combination, and the latter in the form of a partial or total knee replacement or arthrodesis of the knee. The goal of any of these procedures is primarily pain relief and secondarily improved function with restoration of an active lifestyle.

The single most important factor in surgical decision making is the surgeon's philosophy and experience with nonarthroplasty or arthroplasty options. Furthermore, it is aided by numerous other factors, such as the age of the patient, extent and severity of articular pathology, clinical appearance and examination of the knee, and patient expectations with regards to activity, pain, and function. Although in some cases the decision may appear simple, in others all these factors must be taken into account to decide the correct operation for the patient. The development of a fixed algorithm is therefore quite difficult.

Although the joint-preserving surgeries are less predictable,[12,14,25,26] when done with appropriate indications, they may afford long-term solutions with minimal need for activity restrictions. In contrast, joint-sacrificing or replacement procedures are more predictable[5,6,19-21] in terms of pain relief but may need activity restrictions, especially in the young patient.

SURGICAL OPTIONS

Joint Preservation

The components of joint preservation include restoration of cartilage and restoration of alignment and joint stability. Restoring cartilage while leaving the limb malaligned or unstable is a setup for failure.

The ideal patient for a cartilage restoration is the young patient with a focal cartilage defect with a well-aligned, stable limb or one that can be aligned by an osteotomy procedure. It is also ideal for the patient with early arthritis that may require other concomitant procedures, such as meniscal allografts or anterior cruciate ligament (ACL) or posterior cruciate ligament (PCL) reconstruction.

Joint-Sacrificing Procedures

These include either arthroplasty or arthrodesis. With the success of arthroplasty, the role of arthrodesis in the primary treatment of arthritis has become mostly obsolete, except in the patient with a native knee infection in whom this might still be an option.

PKA has gained popularity in the past decades as an alternative to TKA. As a group it has historically been reserved for the relatively older patient with more advanced unicompartmental or bicompartmental arthritis, but with the improvements in surgical design and technique, PKA is currently also an option for the younger patient. The middle-aged patient for example with limited disease who is quite active is also a good candidate for a PKA.[18]

TKA is the gold standard against which all procedures are compared. It traditionally has been described as the most predictable procedure for pain relief for any form of arthritis, either unicompartmental, bicompartmental, or tricompartmental. However, because of the sacrifice of the ACL and occasionally the PCL, it is also the most kinematically different from a normal knee. Its best indication is in the patient with tricompartmental degenerative arthritis or in those knees with an inflammatory component to their arthritis.

FACTORS AFFECTING DECISION MAKING

Severity and Extent of Arthritis

Inflammatory Arthritis. Inflammatory arthritis is a contraindication for osteotomy or PKA.

Compartment(s) Involved. The number of compartments involved and severity of arthritis determine the type of procedure that could potentially be performed. Advanced cartilage loss is associated with poorer results after an osteotomy, and therefore it would be reasonable to recommend a realignment osteotomy in patients with isolated medial or lateral unicompartmental arthroplasty that is not endstage,[24] or in the extremely young patient (<40) with moderate arthritis. Severe unicompartmental arthritis of the tibiofemoral joint in middle-aged or in older patients may benefit from PKA. The presence of tricompartmental arthritis would preclude a limited unicompartmental or bicompartmental replacement. The presence of either medial or lateral compartment arthritis with significant PF arthritis would be a reasonable indication for limited BCA, which replaces either the medial or lateral and the PF joint.

Patellofemoral Joint. One of the most controversial subjects in TKA or PKA is the PF joint. Whether the patella should be resurfaced or not has been a matter of debate for years in patients undergoing TKA[4] and is also a controversy in patients undergoing PKA.

Radiographic evidence of arthritis without clinical symptoms emanating from the PF joint is currently not a contraindication for medial UKA. Furthermore, users of mobile-bearing designs do not believe that anterior knee pain in the presence of radiographic signs of PF arthritis, as long as there are no major grooves in the PF joint or involvement of the lateral patellar facet, is a contraindication to its use.[8,19] The designers report that patient symptoms improve after UKA as the PF joint is unloaded. In addition, long-term follow-up studies have shown low revision rates for progression of PF arthritis. A similar scenario may apply to an osteotomy, especially a varus-producing distal femoral osteotomy as PF joint kinematics are improved.[25]

However, the location of the patellar arthritis is important. Lateral patellar facet arthritis commonly requires replacement. Studies have shown that medial patellar facet arthritis may not be that critical and can be ignored when performing a medial UKA. This is not the case with lateral unicompartmental arthritis; if PF arthritis is present, then the PF joint should be replaced, most commonly in the form of TKA.

Clinical Symptoms and Exam

Some surgeons perform the "single digit test" when assessing a patient for unicompartmental arthroplasty.[3] This is done by asking the patient to point with one finger at the area that generates the most pain. If the patient points to the medial, lateral, or PF joint and has all the other prerequisites on clinical examination for unicompartmental arthroplasty, then the patient could be the best candidate for a PKA. However, the sensitivity and specificity of the "single digit test" has not been determined, but for the surgeon with early experience using PKA it may serve as a good way to screen best candidates for the procedure. In practice, referral patterns about the knee are highly variable and may have very little clinical relevance to the location of the arthritis.

There are two critical exam findings that determine whether a patient is a good candidate for either joint-preserving surgery, PKA, or TKA. In general, the presence of the anterior cruciate ligament and the ability to correct the deformity are important prerequisites[8,10] in patients in whom a PKA is entertained.

Patients who have significant "touch me not" pain with tender points all over the knee may not be good candidates for any type of surgical intervention. The amount of deformity should be noted because patients with significant stiff deformities (varus >15 degrees or fixed flexion contracture >15 degrees) may be best treated with TKA, whereas patients with passively correctable deformities are better candidates for UKA or osteotomy. In our practice, patients who are believed to be candidates for unicompartmental arthroplasty undergo a stress x-ray with the knee flexed to 20 degrees to see whether both the medial or lateral compartments are corrected to predisease state and the joint space in the contralateral compartment is maintained.

Expectations

The patient who wants to return to high-impact activities must be counseled about the possibility of early failure after arthroplasty. In the appropriate candidate, especially if extremely young, an osteotomy should be entertained. However, joint-preserving surgeries are generally less predictable in their pain relief and in return of function when compared with arthroplasty options. There are data to suggest that some patients with UKA have achieved high levels of activity, but recommending that a patient undergo arthroplasty and go back to high-impact sporting activities would be unacceptable for most surgeons.

Age

Although age was once thought to be a critical factor in the decision making, it is currently not considered as much.[5,18] Younger patients, because of their higher activity level and life expectancy, are at higher risk for revision at some point in their life, but if activity-limiting tricompartmental arthritis exists, this should not be ignored. There is long-term data to suggest that TKA is durable in the young patient[5]; however, these patients would likely benefit from less invasive arthroplasty techniques or osteotomy as long as tricompartmental arthroplasty does not exist. The extremely young patient, less than 40, is likely the best candidate for osteotomy. The older patient (>40) is probably a good candidate for some form of arthroplasty, and PKA should be entertained as both temporizing and definitive management in this patient population.

Previous Surgery

Previous upper tibial osteotomy may be a relative contraindication to medial or lateral UKA if the knee has not failed back into its preoperative deformity. It has traditionally been described as an absolute contraindication for a mobile-bearing design used on the medial side.

LONG-TERM CLINICAL RESULTS OF SURGICAL OPTIONS

Osteotomy

An osteotomy helps by mechanically realigning the knee and unloading the affected compartment while relatively

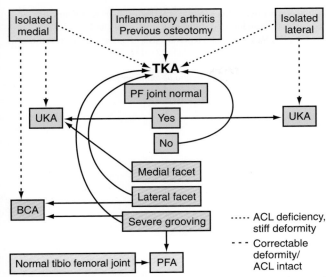

FIG 125.1 Authors' algorithmic approach to the patient with knee arthritis. The use of unicompartmental replacement has proven efficiency and durability in the literature. The use of BCA is in relatively early stages and is currently not recommended by the authors until further long-term studies are available, but it is included in the algorithm for completeness. *ACL,* Anterior cruciate ligament; *BCA,* bi-compartmental arthroplasty; *PF,* patellofemoral; *PFA,* patellofemoral arthroplasty; *TKA,* total knee arthroplasty; *UKA,* unicompartmental knee arthroplasty.

overloading the normal compartment. The review of the literature[23-26] shows that the results of the treatment deteriorate with time. Even in the best-case scenario, the survivorship of the osteotomy is approximately 50% at 20 years.

Unicompartmental Knee Arthroplasty

Unicompartmental arthroplasty has the advantage of being a less invasive surgery, thereby aiding in a fast recovery period.[11,15] In addition, patients have a more natural feel to their knees because the kinematics of the knee are not altered.[17]

Unicompartmental arthroplasty is a surgical option in the middle-aged to older patient with advanced arthritis and symptoms largely confined to one or two compartments. It can be done if the arthritis is confined to the medial compartment and medial patellar facet arthritis or lateral joint without PF arthritis. Using fixed-bearing UKA, Berger et al. reported 96% survival and 92% good or excellent result at a minimum of 10 years.[2] Using Oxford meniscal bearing UKA, Price et al. reported a 15-year survival of 93% in 439 knees, with 91% good or excellent clinical results.[19]

If a patient has isolated lateral compartment arthritis with no PF disease, a lateral unicompartmental arthroplasty may be a reasonable option affording durable results.[1,9,13,16] Even though not as frequently performed, the results are comparable to medial UKA. If PF arthritis coexists with lateral unicompartmental disease, either a TKA or BCA is indicated.

Bicompartmental Arthritis

A combined UKA and PF replacement can be done as a BCA, if there is medial or lateral unicompartmental arthritis with

advanced PF arthritis. A BCA known as the Deuce, has had fair to good reports in the literature and has been subsequently withdrawn from market. Currently, the role of BCA in the management of knee osteoarthritis is questionable, based on the inferior outcomes compared with TKA.[7,22]

Total Knee Arthroplasty

TKA is the gold standard in the treatment of osteoarthritis, and all other forms of surgical treatments are compared with it in terms of efficacy. Long-term follow-up studies of total knee replacement show a 90%[20] good to excellent results and a 15-year survivorship of 92% to 93%[5,6,20,21] with revision for any reason as endpoint.

CONCLUSION

The authors present their algorithm for surgical management in Fig. 125.1. For the extremely young patient with early-stage unicompartmental arthritis, osteotomy may be an option. Joint arthroplasty is the preferred treatment in patients with end-stage arthritis. Whether unicompartmental, bicompartmental, or tricompartmental replacement is performed is highly dependent on surgeon experience and philosophy. The algorithm presents a decision tree approach for the surgeon who is interested in using PKA as an alternative to TKA.

KEY REFERENCES

1. Ashraf T, Newman JH, Evans RL, et al: Lateral unicompartmental knee replacement survivorship and clinical experience over 21 years. *J Bone Joint Surg* 84B:1126–1130, 2002.
2. Berger RA, Meneghini RM, Jacobs JJ, et al: Results of unicompartmental knee arthroplasty at a minimum of 10 years follow-up. *J Bone Joint Surg* 87A:999–1006, 2005.
3. Bert JM: Unicompartmental knee replacement. *Orthop Clin North Am* 36A:513–522, 2005.
4. Burnett RS, Boone JL, Rosenzweig SD, et al: Patellar resurfacing compared with nonresurfacing in total knee arthroplasty. A concise follow-up of a randomized trial. *J Bone Joint Surg* 91A(11):2562–2567, 2009.
6. Dixon MC, Brown RR, Parsch D, et al: Modular fixed-bearing total knee arthroplasty with retention of the posterior cruciate ligament. A study of patients followed for a minimum of fifteen years. *J Bone Joint Surg* 87A(3):598–603, 2005.
12. Magnussen RA, Dunn WR, Carey JL, et al: Treatment of focal articular cartilage defects in the knee: a systematic review. *Clin Orthop* 466(4):952–962, 2008.
16. Ohdera T, Tokunaga J, Kopayashi A: Unicompartmental knee arthroplasty for lateral gonarthrosis: midterm results. *J Arthroplasty* 16:196–200, 2001.
17. Patil S, Colwell CW, Jr, Ezzet KA, et al: Can normal knee kinematics be restored with unicompartmental knee replacement? *J Bone Joint Surg* 87A:332–338, 2005.
18. Pennington DW, Swienckowski JJ, Lutes WB, et al: Unicompartmental knee arthroplasty in patients sixty years of age or younger. *J Bone Joint Surg* 85A:1968–1973, 2003.
19. Price AJ, Waite JC, Svard U: Long term clinical results of the medial Oxford unicompartmental knee arthroplasty. *Clin Orthop* 435:171–180, 2005.
20. Rasquinha VJ, Ranawat CS, Cervieri CL, et al: The press-fit condylar modular total knee system with a posterior cruciate-substituting design. A concise follow-up of a previous report. *J Bone Joint Surg* 88A(5):1006–1010, 2006.

21. Rodricks DJ, Patil S, Pulido P, et al: Press-fit condylar design total knee arthroplasty. Fourteen to seventeen-year follow-up. *J Bone Joint Surg* 89A(1):89–95, 2007.

22. Rolston L, Siewert K: Assessment of knee alignment after bi-compartmental knee arthroplasty. *J Arthroplasty* 24(7):1111–1114, 2009.

23. Stukenborg-Colsman C, Wirth CJ, Lazovic D, et al: High tibial osteotomy versus unicompartmental joint replacement in unicompartmental knee joint osteoarthritis: 7-10-year follow-up prospective randomized study. *Knee* 8:187–194, 2001.

25. Wang JW, Hsu CC: Distal femoral varus osteotomy for osteoarthritis of the knee. *J Bone Joint Surg* 87A(1):127–133, 2005.

The references for this chapter can also be found on www.expertconsult.com.

126

Patellofemoral Arthroplasty

Jess H. Lonner

INTRODUCTION

Isolated patellofemoral (PF) arthritis can be the source of great pain and disability. Often this clinical entity is treated effectively with nonsurgical interventions, such as weight reduction, physical therapy, and judicious use of injectable or oral medications. However, when the pain is refractory to these efforts, surgery may be considered. A number of surgical options have been used for PF arthritis, including arthroscopic débridement and lavage, patellar unloading procedures (such as tibial tubercle elevation or tibial tubercle anteromedialization), patellectomy, cartilage grafting techniques, patellar resurfacing, patellofemoral arthroplasty (PFA), and total knee arthroplasty (TKA). This chapter discusses the role of PFA for isolated PF chondral degeneration. Results may be optimized by limiting the procedure to those patients with arthritis and pain localized to the anterior compartment of the knee and without significant patellar malalignment and by accurately aligning the trochlear prosthesis perpendicular to the anteroposterior axis of the femur to enhance patellar tracking.

Inlay style trochlear designs predispose to a relatively high rate of failures from patellar maltracking, catching, and anterior knee pain, whereas newer and improved onlay style trochlear designs have reduced the incidence of PF dysfunction.* These improved outcomes, as well as an interest in single compartment resurfacing, have led to growing enthusiasm for PFA.

EPIDEMIOLOGY

Chondromalacia patella has been observed in 40% to 60% of patients at autopsy and in 20% to 50% of patients at the time of arthrotomy for other diagnoses.[62] The prevalence of isolated PF arthritis is high, occurring in one study in as many as 11% of men and 24% of women older than 55 years with symptomatic osteoarthritis of the knee.[49] This gender predilection is undoubtedly related to the often subtle patellar malalignment and dysplasia that is common in women. The PF cartilage is also vulnerable to direct traumatic injury, considering its unprotected location in the body.

NONSURGICAL TREATMENT

Nonsurgical management is the mainstay of treatment for isolated PF arthritis; to be certain, it is the minority of patients who ultimately require an operation. A directed therapy program emphasizing short arc quadriceps strengthening, stretching of the lateral retinacular structures, and preservation of motion is frequently successful in mitigating symptoms. There is some evidence to suggest that vastus medialis obliquus dysfunction may be associated with PF pain.[63] This serves to reinforce the importance of a directed strengthening program. When the anterior knee pain associated with PF arthritis is refractory to months of nonoperative interventions, such as weight reduction, physical therapy, and judicious use of injectable or oral medications, surgery may be considered.

SURGICAL ALTERNATIVES

Arthroscopic Surgery

Arthroscopic options for PF chondromalacia and arthritis include lavage or débridement, with or without marrow stimulation. Arthroscopic débridement and lavage may be beneficial in those patients who have recurrent effusions, by decreasing the debris load which may be a source of inflammation. Furthermore, removal of an unstable chondral flap lesion on the patella or trochlear groove can improve the mechanical symptoms. However, these interventions have varied results, and patients should be counseled regarding the likelihood of only partial and temporary symptomatic relief and the persistence of functional limitations. The poor intrinsic healing capabilities of articular cartilage limit the value of arthroscopic treatments for PF arthritis, particularly in the absence of mechanical symptoms.

Various technical modalities are available for débridement of chondromalacia, including mechanical shavers, thermal devices, and lasers. Lasers have shown limited, short-term improvement in symptoms but have extremely worrisome potential complications, including extensive damage of the cartilage and necrosis of subchondral bone. Thermal devices have had more predictable results. In one study comparing thermal versus mechanical débridement, the short-term results of radiofrequency ablation were superior to those using a shaver. However, the long-term effects of thermal energy on articular cartilage have yet to be defined; thus its use should be approached with prudence.

Federico and Reider analyzed a series of 36 patients who underwent arthroscopic chondroplasty for isolated chondromalacia patella without patellar malalignment.[17] Those patients with traumatic chondromalacia had 60% good or excellent results compared with 41% good or excellent results in all others. Lateral retinacular release, after chondral degeneration

*References 7, 29, 38, 39, 41, 42, 43, and 61.

has already occurred, is often ineffective in resolving anterior knee pain.[53] Schonholtz and Ling performed chondroplasty for varying degrees of chondromalacia of the patella to remove loose fibrillation but not to penetrate through subchondral bone or débride intact cartilage.[57] At a mean 40-month follow-up the authors reported good to excellent results in 49% of patients and fair results in 44% of patients. They noted that 78% of patients were satisfied and that the grade of chondromalacia did not correlate with the outcome. Marrow stimulation techniques, such as microfracture, have also fared relatively poorly in treating lesions of the PF articulation. The reparative fibrocartilage tissue, composed primarily of type I collagen, is incapable of withstanding the excessive shear stresses common to the PF articulation.

Tibial Tubercle Unloading Procedures

Anteromedialization of the tibial tubercle is a time-tested and well-established procedure for the treatment of patellar maltracking associated with PF malalignment.[19,20,21] Although anteriorization of the tibial tubercle reduces the PF joint reaction forces by increasing the angle between the patellar tendon and quadriceps tendon and increases the lever arm for extensor mechanism function, medializing the tibial tubercle improves the Q angle and thereby decreases the strong lateral vectors acting upon the patella. Combining these two components can therefore both improve patellar tracking and relieve pain associated with subchondral overload of the lateral patellar facet. The obliquity of the tibial tubercle osteotomy allows for adjustment in the extent of anteriorization, and bone graft is not necessary. The angle can be adjusted to accommodate varying degrees of subluxation and articular cartilage damage. Although Fulkerson has reported excellent to good results in 89% of patients followed up for more than 5 years, no patients achieved excellent results, and satisfaction was only 75% in the presence of substantial chondromalacia (Outerbridge grade III or IV).[20]

Direct anteriorization of the tibial tubercle has also been advocated in patients with PF arthrosis, when there is no patellar subluxation or malalignment.[48] Symptom improvement with the classic Maquet osteotomy has ranged from 30% to 90%.[18,24,48] Biomechanical studies have demonstrated reductions in contact pressures; however, contact areas may shift proximally, paradoxically overloading the proximal portion of the patella in deep flexion.[11] The optimal patient to benefit from a Maquet osteotomy is one with posttraumatic arthritis or chondromalacia involving the inferior half of the patella. Those patients with proximal arthritis or diffuse PF arthritis and those with multiple prior PF surgeries will have compromised outcomes. Its limited indications, unpredictable results, and risk of complications, such as wound necrosis or osteotomy nonunion, restrict the practical application of this procedure.

Cartilage Grafting

Autologous chondrocyte implantation for isolated patellar cartilage lesions has produced satisfactory results in approximately 75% at 2- to 10-year follow-up.[10,51] The proponents advise that residual patellar malalignment is a common reason for failure of this technique and should therefore be addressed prior to or simultaneous with autologous chondrocyte implantation.[51] Autologous osteochondral transplantation has been advocated by its innovator for PF lesions.[22] Although the duration of follow-up is not clear, Hangody reported 79% satisfactory results in those with patellar and/or trochlear mosaicplasties.[22]

Patellectomy

Patellectomy has been shown experimentally to reduce extension power by 25% to 60%, with a concomitant requisite increase in quadriceps force of 15% to 30% to achieve adequate extension torque.[8,28] Tibiofemoral joint reaction forces may increase as much as 250%, explaining the propensity for tibiofemoral arthritis after patellectomy.[15] Variable pain relief, residual quadriceps weakness, and secondary instability, with failures as high as 45%, truly relegate this to being a salvage procedure for the rare patient who does poorly with other more successful interventions[26]. In addition, results of TKA can be compromised after patellectomy.[54] Therefore patellectomy is less desirable than PFA or TKA for the treatment of isolated PF arthrosis.

Total Knee Arthroplasty

TKA is generally effective for older patients with isolated PF arthritis, yielding good and excellent results in 90% to 95% of patients at midterm follow-up, although anterior knee pain has been reported in as many as 7% to 19% of patients.[32,52,55] In one study comparing TKA for isolated PF arthritis with that for tricompartmental arthritis, Knee Society clinical scores, bipedal stair climbing capacity, and ability to rise from a seated position were all significantly better in the former group.[32] Given the predictably good results of TKA, it is preferable to PFA in the older patient with isolated PF arthritis. However, in younger patients with isolated PF arthritis, PFA may be favorable.

Patellofemoral Arthroplasty

PFA may be considered in the treatment algorithm for patients with localized PF arthritis or severe recalcitrant chondromalacia (Fig. 126.1A to F). Early designs resurfaced only the patella, using a metal implant, leaving the trochlea untouched. Although the patella is commonly more degenerated than the trochlea, results have been variable with this technique.[2,47] Recognition that residual anterior knee pain may have been related to trochlear chondromalacia, first-generation PF resurfacing arthroplasties were developed, using a polyethylene patellar component and metallic trochlear component.[9,47]

PATIENT SELECTION FOR PATELLOFEMORAL ARTHROPLASTY

The outcome of PFA can be optimized by limiting its application to patients with isolated PF osteoarthritis, posttraumatic arthritis, or severe chondrosis (Outerbridge grade IV) on either the patellar or trochlear surfaces, after a supervised program of various nonoperative measures. In addition, this option is best reserved for patients with isolated retropatellar and/or peripatellar pain and functional limitations, with considerable discomfort with provocative activities, such as stair or hill ambulation, squatting, or prolonged sitting. The procedure should not be performed in patients with inflammatory arthritis or chondrocalcinosis involving the menisci or tibiofemoral chondral surfaces, nor should it be offered to patients with inappropriate expectations.[†] The presence of medial or lateral joint line pain suggest more diffuse chondral disease and should be considered contraindications to isolated PF resurfacing. Alternative etiologies of anterior knee pain, such as patellar tendonitis, synovitis, patellar instability, sympathetic mediated

---

[†]References 29, 33, 36, 38, 40, and 42.

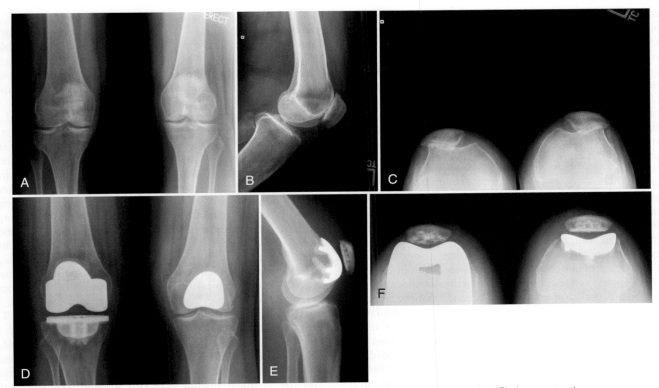

FIG 126.1 Weight-bearing anteroposterior (A), lateral (B), and axial radiographs (C) demonstrating advanced PF arthrosis with sparing of the tibiofemoral compartments. (D to F) Postoperative radiographs after successful PFA (Gender Solutions Patellofemoral Arthroplasty, Zimmer, Warsaw, Indiana).

pain, or pain referred from the back or ipsilateral hip, should be excluded.

Although it can be most effective for treating PF dysplasia,[23] PFA should be avoided in patients with considerable patellar maltracking or malalignment, unless they are corrected. However, this is not to say that moderate patellar tilt, observed on preoperative tangential radiographs or at the time of arthrotomy, or trochlear dysplasia should be considered contraindications for this procedure. In such cases a lateral retinacular recession or release may be necessary at the time of arthroplasty.[36,38,40] Persistent patellar subluxation may cause pain and snapping and potentially polyethylene wear of the prosthesis. Patients with excessive Q angles should undergo tibial tubercle realignment before or during PFA (although some trochlear prosthesis shapes may accommodate a slightly increased Q angle). In addition, the presence of tibiofemoral arthritis should discourage isolated PFA. The presence of even focal grade III tibiofemoral chondromalacia can compromise the outcome after PFA, although these patients will often acknowledge resolution of the most prominent component of pain. Combining PFA with medial or lateral unicompartmental knee arthroplasty or autologous osteochondral grafting are sound considerations in these situations.[6,45]

Although there are intuitive concerns, there are no data available on whether obesity or cruciate ligament insufficiency put the PFA at risk for failure. There are no strict age criteria for PFA provided the other criteria are met. Patients who require narcotics for PF arthritis are not good candidates for PFA because their pain tends to persist and satisfaction is low in this

cohort. Efforts should be taken to wean patients off narcotics before offering PFA.

CLINICAL EVALUATION

Evaluation of the patient under consideration should be thorough to confirm that the pain is indeed localized to the anterior compartment of the knee and that it emanates from the PF chondral surfaces and not soft tissues. This can usually be done by taking a detailed history of the problem and by performing a meticulous physical examination.

The key elements of the history that should be elaborated include whether there was previous trauma to the knee, a history of patellar dislocation, or prior PF "problems." A history of recurrent atraumatic patellar dislocations may suggest considerable malalignment, which may need to be corrected. These patients may have severe trochlear flattening or even convexity, which can be improved with the trochlear component. A clear description of the location of the pain is important—discomfort anywhere but directly retropatellar, or just lateral or medial to the patella will not be relieved with a PFA. PF pain often is exacerbated by such activities as stair climbing and descent, ambulating on hills, standing from a seated position, sitting with the knee flexed, and squatting. Walking on level ground should not be as painful. A description of anterior crepitus is common. After establishing the location and quality of pain, it is important to ascertain whether there were previous interventions, such as physical therapy, weight reduction, medications, injections, or surgery.

With respect to the physical examination, pain on patella inhibition testing, PF crepitus, and retropatellar knee pain with squatting are typical. Any associated medial or lateral tibiofemoral joint line tenderness should raise one's suspicion of more diffuse chondral disease (even in the presence of relatively normal radiographs) and may be a contraindication to isolated PFA. It is also essential to rule out other potential sources of anterior knee pain, such as pes anserinus bursitis, patellar tendonitis, prepatellar bursitis, instability, or pain referred from the ipsilateral hip or back. Careful assessment of patellar tracking and the Q angle also are important. As stated above, even subtle tracking abnormalities and malalignment can predispose to inferior outcomes, particularly with certain designs. Therefore in patients with high Q angles a tibial tubercle realignment procedure (anteromedialization) should be performed prior to or concurrent with PFA. Anterior or posterior cruciate ligament insufficiency is not a contraindication for this procedure; however, cruciate ligament reconstruction may be advisable to reduce the risk of anterior knee pain and instability and to potentially preserve the tibiofemoral articular cartilage.

Weight-bearing radiographs are generally ample imaging studies. Standing anteroposterior and midflexion posteroanterior radiographs are critical to determine the presence of tibiofemoral arthritis. Mild squaring-off of the femoral condyles and even small marginal osteophytes may be accepted, provided the patient is devoid of tibiofemoral pain with functional activities and on physical exam and that there is minimal chondral degeneration during arthroscopy or arthrotomy. Lateral x-rays will occasionally demonstrate PF osteophytes but usually are more useful in identifying whether there is patella alta or baja. Axial radiographs will demonstrate the position of the patella within the trochlear groove and the extent of arthritis, although on occasion there will be relative radiographic PF joint space preservation with minimal or no osteophytes, despite significant cartilage loss (see Fig. 126.1A to F). Newer magnetic resonance imaging (MRI) sequences may be useful for evaluating PF arthrosis, but more importantly it can be used to evaluate the medial and lateral compartments for evidence of chondral wear. If committed to performing a PFA, patients should consent to autologous osteochondral grafting for associated focal condylar defects or unicompartmental knee arthroplasty (as part of a bicompartmental resurfacing) if there is more diffuse degeneration.[6,45] Photographs from prior arthroscopic treatment will provide valuable information regarding the extent of anterior compartment arthritis and the status of the tibiofemoral articular cartilage and menisci.

SURGICAL TECHNIQUE

During arthrotomy, it is essential to avoid cutting normal articular cartilage or the menisci. Before proceeding with PFA, carefully inspect the entire joint to make sure the tibiofemoral compartments are free of disease. As mentioned above, if the weight-bearing condylar surfaces have a focal, full-thickness cartilage defect, consider an autologous osteoarticular graft. If there is more diffuse medial or lateral compartment wear, consider a bicompartmental arthroplasty or a TKA.

In addition to the design features of some contemporary components that have substantially improved patella tracking, instrumentation has been developed that is low profile, accurate, and conducive to less invasive surgical techniques. Early-generation implants required freehand preparation of all of the bony surfaces, which contributed to inaccurate trochlear component alignment. Second-generation implants typically neither offered a means for preparing the distal femur for the intercondylar tail of the implant, nor were they amenable to more contemporary, less invasive surgical techniques, because they tended to be quite bulky. Newer systems have simplified the procedure and improve the anatomic mating of the implant to the articular surfaces of the transition zones.

The trochlear component should be externally rotated perpendicular to the anteroposterior axis of the femur (Whiteside axis) or parallel to the epicondylar axis to enhance patellar tracking.[38,40] Osteophytes bordering the intercondylar notch should be removed. The trochlear component should maximize coverage of the trochlea, without extending beyond the mediolateral femoral margins anteriorly, encroaching on the weight-bearing surfaces of the tibiofemoral articulations, or overhanging into the intercondylar notch. The medial and lateral transitional edges of the prosthesis should be flush with or recessed approximately 1 mm from the adjacent condylar articular cartilage.[40] The proximal edge should be flush with the anterior femoral cortex, and the distal tip should be flush with the articular cartilage and not extend into the intercondylar notch. The patella is resurfaced by the same principles observed in TKA, restoring the original patella thickness and medializing and proximalizing the component. The exposed cut surface of the lateral patella that is not covered by the patellar prosthesis is removed or beveled to avoid the potentially painful articulation on the trochlear prosthesis.[37] This may also enhance patella tracking by releasing tension on the lateral retinaculum.

Assessment of patellar tracking is performed with the trial components in place. Attention is paid to identify patellar tilt, subluxation, or catching of the components. Patellar tilt and mild subluxation usually can be addressed successfully by performing a lateral retinacular recession or release. As stated earlier, more severe extensor mechanism malalignment may require proximal or distal realignment.

POSTOPERATIVE MANAGEMENT

Currently most PFAs can be performed safely on an outpatient basis. Isometrics and active, as well as passive, range-of-motion exercises are started immediately. Continuous passive motion is not routinely used. Full weight bearing is permitted immediately, with support of crutches and a cane until there is adequate recovery of quadriceps strength. In some circumstances, full recovery of quadriceps strength can take 6 months or longer, considering the severe preoperative quadriceps atrophy that is encountered in some patients with PF arthritis. Thromboembolism prophylaxis is used for 4 to 6 weeks. This author uses aspirin for 4 weeks for standard risk patients, and alternatives, such as low-molecular-weight heparin, for high-risk patients. The incidence of venous thromboembolic events after PFA with early mobilization and risk-stratified thromboprophylaxis, but primarily with aspirin, is well less than 1%.[34] Appropriate precautions regarding antibiotic prophylaxis for dental procedures or other interventions should follow standard recommendations of the American Academy of Orthopaedic Surgeons.[23]

DESIGN FEATURES THAT IMPACT PATELLAR TRACKING

With a few exceptions, the clinical results of PFA have improved as the trochlear designs evolved over 30 years.[7,38,39,41] There are a variety of specific design features of the trochlear components

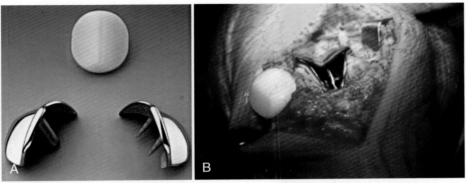

FIG 126.2 (A and B) Richards II and III patellofemoral arthroplasties. (Courtesy Smith Nephew Richards, Memphis, Tennessee).

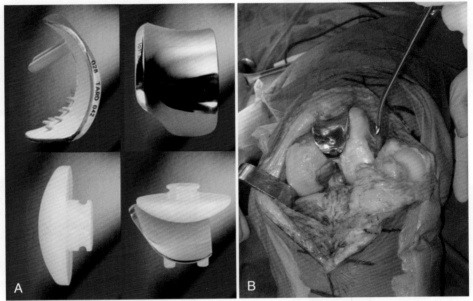

FIG 126.3 (A) Autocentric patellofemoral arthroplasty. (B) Operative appearance of Autocentric PFA 10 years after implantation. Revision to TKA was necessary for progressive tibiofemoral arthrosis. (A, Courtesy Depuy, Warsaw, Indiana.)

that impact patella tracking and the success of the PFA, including the sagittal radius of curvature, proximal extension of the trochlear flange, thickness of the trochlear component, mediolateral width, and constraint of the trochlear groove. In addition, whether they are onlay- or inlay-type designs and asymmetric or symmetric will impact PF performance.‡

The sagittal radius of curvature of some trochlear components, usually inlay-type designs, such as the Lubinus, Richards Mod I and II, and Low Contact Stress (LCS), is obtuse. It is difficult to implant these flush with both the anterior femoral cortex and the medial, lateral, and distal margins of articular cartilage. The trochlear prostheses in those systems are therefore often implanted in a flexed position, leaving them prominent proximally where they can cause patellar snapping, clunking, and maltracking when the patella transitions on to it (Fig. 126.2A). Other trochlear designs have a sagittal radius of curvature far more accommodating of most femora (Fig. 126.2B).

This allows flush implantation on the anterior femoral surface, as well as on the intercondylar surface of the knee, without the need to flex the implant, thereby reducing the risk of patellar catching.

There is also variability in the mediolateral width of the anterior flange of the available implants. Some are very narrow, a feature that is unforgiving of even subtle patellar subluxation, and can result in catching on the medial and lateral edges of the trochlear component (Fig. 126.3A and B). Others are considerably broader (Fig. 126.4A and B), covering nearly the entire anterior surface of the distal femur. This latter feature allows a greater degree of freedom for patellar excursion and tracking; however, if the component is too wide, overhang into the soft tissues can cause painful soft tissue impingement and perhaps limit flexion.

The proximal extension of the trochlear flange on the anterior femur also differs between products (Figs. 126.5 and 126.6). Onlay implants are typically designed to extend considerably more proximal than the articular margin of the trochlear so that the patellar component articulates entirely with the trochlear

‡References 16, 25, 29, 35, 38, 41, 43, and 61.

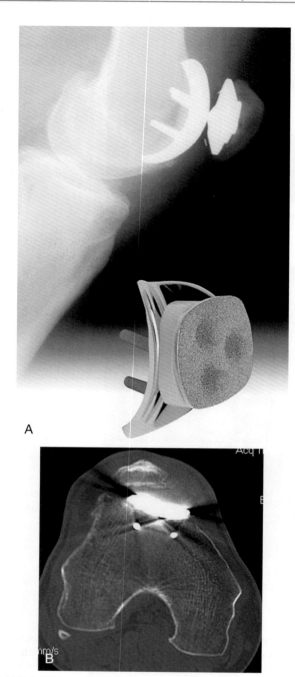

A

B

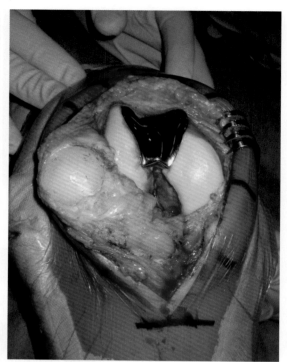

FIG 126.5 Lubinus patellofemoral arthroplasty (Link, Hamburg, Germany).

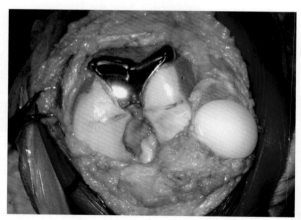

FIG 126.6 Avon patellofemoral arthroplasty (Stryker Orthopaedics, Mahwah, New Jersey).

FIG 126.4 (A) Low Contact Stress patellofemoral joint. (B) Axial CT scan of an inlay-style implant demonstrating internal rotation relative to the anteroposterior axis of the distal femur, resulting in lateral patellar catching and subluxation. This was treated successfully with revision to an onlay-style implant, rotating the trochlear component perpendicular to the anteroposterior axis of the femur. (A, Courtesy Depuy, Warsaw, Indiana.)

component in extension (Fig. 126.7). In contrast, inlay designs, such as the Lubinus and LCS components, and custom designs, such as the Kinamed, do not extend proximal to the articular cartilage margin of the trochlea (Fig. 126.8). The patellar prosthesis in those latter designs therefore articulates with the natural anterior femoral surface in full extension before it

transitions onto the trochlear prosthesis. This predisposes these designs to catching and snapping in the initial 30 degrees of flexion, particularly if the trochlear prosthesis is flexed or offset anteriorly (Fig. 126.9).

As stated earlier, some trochlear designs are an inlay style, whereas others are an onlay-type component. The former design is inset into the trochlea and tends to be more bone conserving; the latter is implanted flush with the anterior surface of the femoral cortex and removes the entire anterior trochlear surface. However, given the variability in distal anterior femoral morphology, inlaid trochlear components often do not accurately mate with the articular geometry of the trochlear region of the femur, resulting in potential offset on any of its edges (Fig. 126.10). This typically results in patella catching on

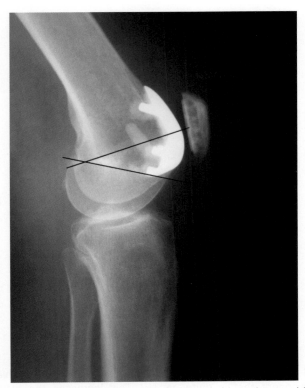

FIG 126.7 Greater proximal extension of this onlay trochlear implant above the physeal scar ensures that the patella articulates with the femoral prosthesis at all times in extension. (From Lonner JH: Patellofemoral arthroplasty: the impact of design on outcomes. *Orthop Clin N Am* 39:347–354, 2008.)

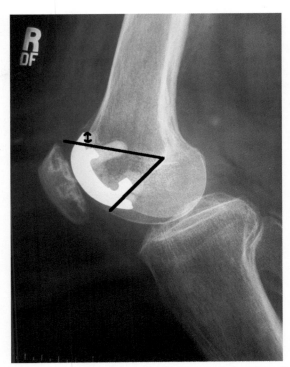

FIG 126.8 Very limited proximal extension above the physeal scar predisposes this typical type of inlay style prosthesis to catching and subluxing as the patella transitions from the native femur onto the prosthesis in the initial 30 degrees of flexion. (From Lonner JH: Patellofemoral arthroplasty: pros, cons, design considerations. *Clin Orthop* 428:158–165, 2004.)

the trochlear component, either proximally as the knee proceeds from extension to flexion, or distally as the knee proceeds from deep flexion to extension. In this regard, the onlay device is more suitable for a larger variation in trochlear geometries. Unlike the inlay designs, it can be applied in patients with trochlear dysplasia without risk of having the component sit proud relative to the surrounding articular cartilage (Fig. 126.11). It is this author's opinion that trying to inset a trochlear component into the bone is analogous to implanting a potato chip onto the anterior aspect of the knee. If the two surfaces are geometrically mated then the outcome will be absolutely perfect. But if there is a mismatch, then there is an increased risk for relative component malalignment and malposition relative to the articular surfaces, which is why patella maltracking is more common with that style of implant.[41] Perhaps the most compelling explanation for the differences in outcomes and incidences of patellar maltracking and instability in inlay compared with onlay devices stems from the native trochlear surface being inherently internally rotated relative to the transepicondylar axis, even in dysplastic knees.[27] This finding explains the propensity to malrotate internally inlay-style trochlear components, which by design are positioned so that their medial and lateral edges are flush with the surrounding articular cartilage surfaces. Like internally rotated femoral components in TKA, internal rotation of the trochlear component in PFA effectively medializes the trochlear groove, increases the Q angle, and puts tension on the lateral retinaculum, all of which predispose to patellar maltracking and instability (see Fig. 126.4B).

CLINICAL RESULTS

Most series have reported good and excellent results in approximately 80% to 90% of cases at short- and mid-term follow-up (Table 126.1). However, clinical results of PFA are affected by trochlear component design features (particularly inlay vs. onlay style designs), as well as patient selection and surgical technique.[7,38,39,41] Outcomes and PF performance have improved, and the need for secondary soft tissue surgery to enhance patellar tracking after PFA has decreased, because of trochlear design improvements that have occurred as we have moved from inlay to onlay trochlear implants. The radius of curvature, width, thickness, tracking angle, and extent of constraint of the trochlear component impact patellar tracking and outcomes. Contemporary onlay designs, positioned perpendicular to the anteroposterior axis of the femur, have substantially reduced the incidence of PF complications, leaving tibiofemoral arthritis as the major source of failure of PFAs.[7,38,39,41]

Blazina et al. reported 81% good results after a follow-up period of less than 2 years in 55 knees using a first-generation inlay PFA with a trochlear implant constrained with a sharp trochlear groove.[9] Thirty subsequent procedures were necessary in their series either to realign the extensor mechanism or to revise malpositioned components. Although the investigators credited technical errors as the reason for most secondary surgeries, component design (ie, trochlear constraint, an obtuse radius of curvature, and narrow implant width) most certainly also contributed to the failures.

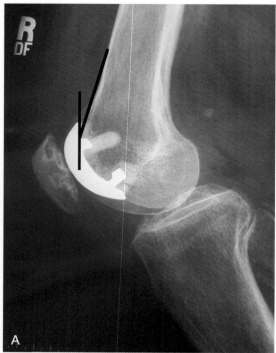

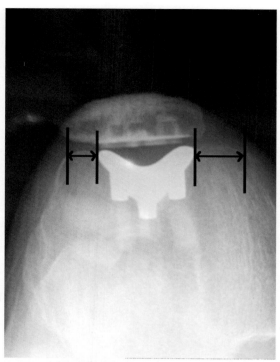

FIG 126.10 Axial radiograph of a "large-" sized inlay trochlear component that is quite narrow. This increases the risk of subluxation with even small degrees of maltracking. There is little room for freedom of excursion. The arrows show the extent of uncapped cartilage anteriorly.

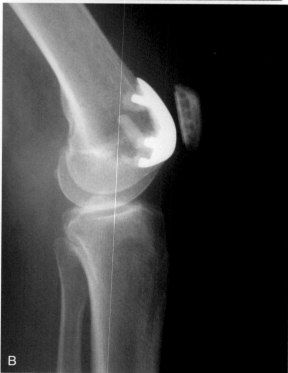

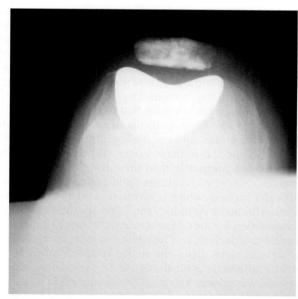

FIG 126.9 (A) Lateral postoperative radiograph after PFA using an inlay prosthesis illustrates one of the potential problems with this design, namely that the trochlear implant must be flexed, leaving it offset from the anterior femoral shaft, and making the patella prone to catching and subluxing. (B) Postoperative radiographs after PFA using an onlay trochlear prosthesis. The postoperative lateral radiograph shows the implant to be flush with the anterior femoral cortex. The radius of curvature is approximately 90 degrees.

FIG 126.11 Broad anterior trochlear coverage provided by this onlay prosthesis accommodates patellar tracking.

TABLE 126.1 **Patellofemoral Arthroplasty Clinical Outcomes**

Series	Implant	No. of PFAs	Age	Diagnosis	Duration of F/U (years)	% of Good/ excellent Results
Blazina[9] (Fig. 8A and B)	Richards types I and II	57	39 (range: 19-81)	NA	2 (range: 8-42 months)	NA
Arciero[3]	Richards type II (14); CFS-Wright (11)	25	62 (range: 33-86)	OA (25); malalignment or instability (14)	5.3 (range: 3-9 years)	85
Cartier[12]	Richards types II and III	72	65 (range: 23-89)	Dysplasia/grade IV chondromalacia (29); PTA (3); chondrocalcinosis (5)	4 (range: 2-12 years)	85
Argenson[4] (Fig. 10)	Autocentric	66	57 (range: 19-82)	Dysplasia or dislocation (22); PTA (20); OA (24)	5.5 (range: 2-10 years)	84
Krajca[31]	Richards types I and II	16	64 (range: 42-84)	Primary OA (10) PTA (2) Recurrent dislocation (1)	5.8 (range: 2-18 years)	88
Tauro[60] (Fig. 9)	Lubinus	62	66 (range: 50-87)	PTA (2); Primary OA (74)	7.5 (range: 5-10 years)	45
deWinter[14]	Richards type II	26	59 (range: 22-90)	Primary OA (17); malalignment (8); PTA (1)	11 (range: 1-20 years)	76
Ackroyd[1] (Fig. 11)	Avon	95	NA	NA	2-5 years	83
Smith[59]	Lubinus	45	72 (range: 42-86)	Primary OA (44); PTA (1)	4 (range: 6 months-7.5 years)	69
Kooijman[30]	Richards type II	45	50 (range: 20-77)	OA (45)	17 (range: 15-21 years)	86
Lonner[38]	Lubinus	30	38 (range: 34-51)	Primary OA (26); PTA (4); [s/p tibial tubercle realignment (10)]	4 (range: 2-6 years)	84
Lonner[38]	Avon trochlea; Nexgen patella	25	44 (range: 28-59)	Primary OA (25); [s/p realignment (2)]	6 months (range: 1 month-1 year)	96
Merchant[50] (Fig. 12)	LCS	15	49 (range: 30-81)	Chronic sublux or recurrent dislocation with secondary DJD (13); chondrosis (2)	3.8 years (range: 2.3-5.5 years)	93
Sisto[58]	Kinematch PFR	25	45 (range: 23-51)	OA (25) [s/p tibial tubercle elevation (6); s/p arthroscopic lateral release and débridement (13)]	73 months (range: 32-119 months)	100
Cartier[13]	Richards types II and III	79	60 (range: 36-81)	Dysplasia and patellar subluxation (70%); primary OA (12%); grade IV chondromalacia (7%); isolated chondrocalcinosis (6%); post patella fracture (5%)	10 years (range: 6-16 years)	77
Argenson[5]	Autocentric	66	57 (range: 21-82)	Dysplasia or dislocation (21); PTA (18); OA (18)	16 years (range: 12-20 years)	NA
Ackroyd[1]	Avon	109	68 (range: 46-86)	OA (106); dislocation (2); PTA (1)	5.2 years (range: 5-8 years)	80
Lonner[16] (Fig. 7)	Gender Solutions	70	51 (range: 36-80)	Primary OA (32); dysplasia/instability (32); PTA (6)	4.9 years (range: 2.3-7.4 years)	NA

DJD, Degenerative joint disease; *F/U,* follow-up; *LCS,* low contact stress; *NA,* not available; *OA,* osteoarthritis; *PFA,* patellofemoral arthroplasty; *PTA,* post-traumatic arthritis.

Cartier et al. had 85% good or excellent results in 72 first-generation inlay PFAs followed for an average of 4 years.[12] There were numerous concomitant surgical procedures performed to enhance patellar tracking, including soft tissue realignment or tibial tubercle transfer. Longer-term follow-up of those patients, at a mean of 10 years (range: 6 to 16 years) after surgery, found that results deteriorated over time, primarily because of the development of tibiofemoral arthritis. That is not surprising, given the average patient age of 60 at the time of the initial PFA in that series. At most recent follow-up, 80% of those who retained their PF prostheses were pain free and 20% had moderate or severe pain, primarily from tibiofemoral arthritis. Stair ambulation was considered normal in 91% of patients. No cases of patellar or trochlear loosening were identified. The authors noted that early failures peaked at 3 years and were related to

inappropriate indications for the surgery and presumably to patellar maltracking problems that could likely be traced to implant design quirks. They identified a later peak in failures in the 9th and 10th years, which corresponded to the development of symptomatic tibiofemoral osteoarthritis. The authors reported a survivorship of 75% at 11 years.[13] Kooijman et al. reported an 86% long-term success rate with the same first-generation PFA, even though early secondary soft tissue surgery was necessary in 18% of patients and revision of the PFA was necessary for catching, imbalance, or malposition in 16%.[30]

In a consecutive series of 30 first-generation inlay trochlear implants and 25 second-generation onlay implants, this author found that results varied depending on which trochlear design was used.[38] The incidence of PF dysfunction, subluxation, catching, and substantial pain was reduced from 17% with the inlay design to less than 4% with the more contemporary onlay product. In another series, 14 of the same first-generation inlay PF implants were revised to a second-generation onlay implant that had a more favorable topography for patellar tracking and that converted an internally rotated trochlear component to one positioned perpendicular to the anteroposterior femoral axis. The etiologies of failure of the primary procedures were component internal rotation, resulting in patellar subluxation, polyethylene wear, or overstuffing. After revision there was statistically significant improvement in knee scores and patellar tracking at a mean 5-year follow-up. Mild femorotibial arthritis (Ahlbach stage I) was predictive of a poorer clinical outcome. At most recent follow-up, there was no evidence of wear, loosening, or subluxation. This study showed that significant improvement can be obtained when revising the failed PFA with a more accommodating implant design, and particularly by repositioning the trochlear component in more optimal rotation, provided there is no tibiofemoral arthritis.[17]

Ackroyd reported on 306 second-generation onlay PFAs and found that patellar tracking was substantially improved compared with first-generation inlay implant. In that series, patellar subluxation occurred in 3% and residual anterior knee pain was noted in 4%. Four percent required revision to TKA, mostly for tibiofemoral arthritis and none for mechanical loosening or wear.[1]

Argenson reported on 66 second-generation PFAs in patients with a mean age of 57 and with a mean follow-up of 16 years.[5] Although most patients had substantial and sustained pain relief, 25% were revised to TKA for tibiofemoral arthritis (at a mean of 7.3 years after PFA) and 14% for aseptic trochlear component loosening, many of which were uncemented (at a mean of 4.5 years after PFA). The authors reported the best results when the procedure was performed for posttraumatic PF arthritis or patellar subluxation and the least favorable in those with primary degenerative arthritis. The development of tibiofemoral arthritis was the most frequent cause of failure; however, at the time of initial PFA, 14% had concomitant tibiofemoral osteotomies for early arthritis, which confounds the results. In those who retained their PFAs at most recent follow-up, there were significant improvements in Knee Society scores. The authors continue to advocate for the procedure as an intermediate stage before TKA in the absence of tibiofemoral arthritis or coronal plane malalignment.[5]

The Australian Orthopaedic Association National Joint Replacement Registry has provided insight into the experience with and outcomes after PFA performed between 1999 and 2008. In that registry, 75.6% of the 977 PFAs performed in Australia were in women, usually in patients under the age of 55 (37.5%) or between the ages of 55 and 64 (29.1%). The tendency for revision after PFA varied between component types, with a substantially higher failure rate within 2 years noted with inlay trochlear components compared with onlay components, presumably because of patellar instability.[7]

In a study of 70 PFAs performed using a contemporary (third generation) onlay design, at a minimum follow-up of 2 years (mean: 4.9 years), the mean range of motion and Knee Society Knee and Function scores improved significantly (*p* < .0001), and less than 4% of patients required revision arthroplasty. There was no radiographic evidence of component loosening or wear and no clinical or radiographic evidence of patellar instability. Despite these improvements, new Knee Society scores indicated that fewer than two-thirds of patients

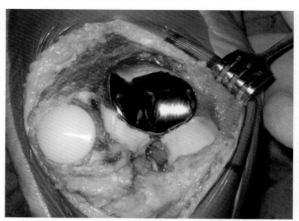

FIG 126.12 Gender Solutions PFJ (Zimmer, Warsaw, Indiana).

were satisfied or had their expectations met. Dissatisfied patients and those whose expectations were not met had significantly lower Mental Health scores according to the Short Form-36, following PFA. Therefore, despite the clinical and radiographic success of onlay style PFAs, patient satisfaction may be lower than expected, which may be partially explained by poor mental health. Surgeons should consider screening patient mental health as a criterion for surgical intervention in the setting of PF arthritis (Fig. 126.12).[29]

COMPLICATIONS

As stated, early inlay designs had a tendency to have a high incidence of patellar snapping and instability, requiring secondary surgery to realign the soft tissues or revise the trochlear prosthesis. These problems were often attributed to trochlear implant design features, as well as soft tissue imbalance or extensor mechanism malalignment, but most likely they were related primarily to internal rotation of the trochlear components. Contemporary onlay designs have substantially reduced the tendency for patellar maltracking or dysfunction because prosthetic trochlear geometries are more accommodating of patellar tracking and because the trochlear components can be positioned perpendicular to the anteroposterior axis of the femur.[16,29,43]

Although anterior knee pain and dysfunction from patellar instability, resulting from soft tissue imbalance or component malalignment, were the major reported etiologies of failure with early PFA designs, these are much less common with some contemporary trochlear designs. A small percentage of patients will have mild anterior knee pain from soft tissue impingement but this occurs with a similar frequency that we see in TKA. Late failures from component subsidence, polyethylene wear, or loosening may eventually develop in the long term, but these problems occur in less than 1% of published cases combined. Trochlear component loosening may be more common in cementless designs.[5,6]

The development of tibiofemoral arthritis is the most common failure mechanism with contemporary designs, even in earlier designs that managed to avoid patellar instability, occurring in approximately 20% of knees at 15 years.[5,13,30] This is more common when the underlying diagnosis is primary osteoarthritis and less common in PF dysplasia or posttraumatic arthritis.[5] In the event that revision to TKA is necessary to treat progressive arthritis, typically the all-polyethylene patellar component can be retained if not worn or loose, and standard total knee components can be used without the need for stems, augments, or bone graft, and without compromising the results.[44,46]

Arthrofibrosis is uncommon after PFA. Although it has been reported with an incidence of 7.6% to 12% in two series, both included a number of patients who had undergone concomitant unicompartmental tibiofemoral arthroplasty but did not mention whether the tendency for arthrofibrosis was increased in those with bicompartmental arthroplasty.[3,4]

Wear of the adjacent articular cartilage from articulation of the patellar prosthesis on the uncapped femoral cartilage is a concern after PFA. It is established that the PF joint reaction forces increase in a normal knee from approximately 3.3 times body weight at 60 degrees of loaded flexion to 7.8 times body weight at 130 degrees of squatting.[56] Beyond 60 degrees, the edges of the patellar components or the cut, exposed lateral osseous patellar surface, may begin to articulate at least in part with the adjacent femoral condyles, as the trochlear components taper distally, and this can predispose to wear of the exposed articular cartilage. Presently there is no ideal bearing surface for the patella that can optimally articulate with both the femoral prosthesis and the surrounding articular cartilage.

As with any arthroplasty procedure, infection and thromboembolic complications are potential complications, and standard prophylactic strategies should be followed.

SUMMARY

PFA can be an effective treatment alternative for PF arthritis resulting from primary osteoarthrosis, dysplasia, or posttraumatic arthritis in patients with normal or correctable patella alignment and tracking.

PFA may provide patients with substantial pain relief of isolated PF arthritis; however, the results can be impacted by the geometric features and positioning of the trochlear component and technical issues. Residual instability may result in early failure, highlighting the importance of excluding those patients with uncorrectable patellar instability or malalignment. Implant malposition, potentially hastened by particular designs, may also contribute to failures from maltracking and mechanical catching of the patella.[36,38,60] At this time optimization of patellar tracking is best done with an onlay-style trochlear component positioned perpendicular to the anteroposterior axis of the femur; inlay style trochlear components have an excessive rate of patellar instability because of internal rotation of the implants and may be best avoided. Sparing of the tibiofemoral compartments, menisci, and cruciate ligaments allows preservation of a more kinematically sound knee joint than TKA.

Although sparse, long-term data suggest that loosening of cemented trochlear and all-polyethylene patellar components is uncommon and that the need for additional surgery for progressive tibiofemoral arthritis may be only approximately 25% at a mean of 15 years after PFA.[30] With emerging designs, the incidence of anterior knee pain after PFA should be comparable to that after total knee replacement surgery, namely approximately 4% to 7%.[32,52] Finally, despite significant improvement in functional outcomes after PFA using contemporary onlay-style trochlear components, patient selection and expectation management remain important determinants of success.

KEY REFERENCES

1. Ackroyd CE, Newman JH, Evans R, et al: The Avon patellofemoral arthroplasty: five-year survivorship and functional results. *J Bone Joint Surg Br* 89B(3):310–315, 2007.
5. Argenson JN, Flecher X, Parratte S, et al: Patellofemoral arthroplasty: an update. *Clin Orthop* 440:50–53, 2005.
13. Cartier P, Sanouiller JL, Khefacha A: Long-term results with the first patellofemoral prosthesis. *Clin Orthop* 436:47–54, 2005.
16. Dy CJ, Franco N, Ma Y, et al: Complications after patello-femoral versus total knee replacement in the treatment of isolated patello-femoral osteoarthritis. A meta-analysis. *Knee Surg Sports Traumatol Arthrosc* 20(11):2174–2190, 2012.
25. Hendrix MR, Ackroyd CE, Lonner JH: Revision patellofemoral arthroplasty: 3-7 year follow-up. *J Arthroplasty* 23:977–983, 2008.
29. Kazarian GS, Tarity TD, Hansen EN, et al: Significant functional improvement at 2 years after isolated patellofemoral arthroplasty with an onlay trochlear implant, but low mental health scores predispose to dissatisfaction. *J Arthroplasty* 31(2):389–394, 2015. doi: 10.1016/j.arth.2015.08.033.
30. Kooijman HJ, Driessen AP, van Horn JR: Long-term results of patellofemoral arthroplasty. *J Bone Joint Surg Br* 85-B(6):836–840, 2003.
33. Leadbetter WB, Seyler TM, Ragland PS, et al: Indications, contraindications, and pitfalls of patellofemoral arthroplasty. *J Bone Joint Surg Am* 88A(Suppl 4):122–137, 2006.
38. Lonner JH: Patellofemoral arthroplasty: pros, cons, design considerations. *Clin Orthop* 428:158–165, 2004.
39. Lonner JH: Patellofemoral arthroplasty. *J Am Acad Orthop Surg* 15:495–506, 2007.
41. Lonner JH: Patellofemoral arthroplasty: the impact of design on outcomes. *Orthop Clin North Am* 39:347–354, 2008.
43. Lonner JH, Bloomfield MR: The clinical outcomes of patellofemoral arthroplasty. *Orthop Clin North Am* 44:271–280, 2013.
44. Lonner JH, Jasko JG, Booth RE: Revision of a failed patellofemoral arthroplasty to a total knee arthroplasty. *J Bone Joint Surg Am* 88A(11):2337–2342, 2006.
45. Lonner JH, Mehta S, Booth RE: Ipsilateral patellofemoral arthroplasty and autogenous osteochondral femoral condylar transplantation. *J Arthroplasty* 22:1130–1136, 2007.
58. Sisto DJ, Sarin VK: Custom patellofemoral arthroplasty of the knee. *J Bone Joint Surg Am* 88A(7):1475–1480, 2006.

The references for this chapter can also be found on www.expertconsult.com.

127

Unicompartmental Knee Arthroplasty: A European Perspective

Matthieu Ollivier, Sebastien Parratte, Jean-Noël Argenson

Isolated unicompartmental knee arthritis remains a challenging problem.[9] Surgical management of unicompartmental knee arthritis includes conservative treatment such as arthroscopic débridement or high tibial osteotomy (HTO) and nonconservative treatment such as unicompartmental arthroplasty or total knee arthroplasty (TKA).[9,21] These procedures, however, have a finite life span in young and active patients, and concerns like functional recovery and the ability to return to sports activities should be considered.[9,21,44,48] During the last decade, enthusiasm for the use of HTO has declined.[44] It has been demonstrated that HTO remains an attractive conservative procedure to avoid a knee prosthesis for patients younger than 50 years with low-grade unicompartmental osteoarthritis (OA) and a varus knee.[21] However, the HTO risk of failure increased dramatically for patients with OA who were rated as Ahlback[1] grade 2 or higher. In these cases, nonconservative treatment should be considered even in young patients.[48] Unicompartmental knee arthroplasty (UKA), which has been performed since the 1970s, in a patient in whom only one compartment of the knee is affected, may provide better physiologic function and quicker recovery than TKA and preserves the bone stock.* Furthermore, patient satisfaction is greater because the knee feels more natural.† UKA has specific modes of failure such as progression of the disease in the remaining compartments or polyethylene wear.‡

In a 2006 survey of the American Association of Hip and Knee Surgeons, UKA was the preferred procedure for 11.4% of the surgeons for a 45-year-old active male and for 29.5% of the surgeons for a 45-year-old active female to manage medial compartment arthritis, assuming a mechanical axis of 7 degrees of varus with an intact anterior cruciate ligament and mild patellofemoral symptoms.[11] Improper patient selection combined with limited instrumentation and suboptimal designs may explain the less-than-satisfactory results originally published for UKA and the subsequent decreased interest, especially in the United States.[11] Interest in UKA has been maintained in Europe since the first experience in the 1970s, and different new designs arrived in the 1980s.§ Since the early 1990s, new implant designs have been introduced with reliable instrumentation, which make the procedure as reliable as TKA.** With proper

patient selection and a more reliable surgical technique, the 10-year results of modern UKA are now available and show survivorship greater than 90% after 10 years of follow-up.[3,45,51,59] The other potential advantage over tricompartmental replacement is the preservation of the bone stock in the remaining compartment and the preservation of the ligaments.[4,9] Thus modern UKA, as a conservative resurfacing arthroplasty of the knee, can preserve the cruciate mechanism, acting as a four-bar linkage guiding the femorotibial movements.[4,9] In vivo kinematics studies performed in patients implanted with a UKA showed a femorotibial pattern similar to those observed in the normal knee.[4,9]

The most important evolution in UKA during the last decade is so-called mini-invasive surgery (MIS).[4,53] Concerning UKA, MIS is defined as the ability to implant the components without an incision in the quadriceps tendon or the vastus medialis or lateralis (depending on the compartment to be replaced) and without everting the patella.[5,44] Minimizing the trauma of the extensor mechanism should allow for an earlier start of walking and active muscle exercises.[4,53] Repicci and Eberle proposed this mini-incision for the implantation of unicompartmental components as a resurfacing procedure using limited instrumentation.[54] With the evolution in instrumentation over the last 5 years, it is possible to perform partial knee arthroplasty with cutting guides fixed only on the replaced compartment, preserving the integrity of the unaffected tibiofemoral compartment.[10] New worldwide interest in UKA is a result of the fast recovery potential and minimal surgical morbidity of MIS and improvement in UKA design allowing greater and safer motion capabilities, especially for active patients who are candidates for a UKA.[9,10]

UNICOMPARTMENTAL KNEE ARTHROPLASTY: THE EUROPEAN EXPERIENCE

After Marmor's initial experience in the United States in 1972, many variations of the Marmor modular knee were introduced in Europe. Marmor published his own experience later, in the mid-1980s, but the concept of resurfacing the tibial and the femoral side of one femorotibial compartment gained great attention in several European countries.[36] The principles of these resurfacing systems were to minimize saw cuts by adapting the femoral component to the condyle and use an inlay polyethylene tibial component cemented in the subchondral tibial bone, while preserving the cortical rim. The St. George Sled, mostly used in Northern Europe, was based on the same

---

*References 9, 3, 13, 15, 27, 51, and 58.
†References 9, 3, 13, 15, 27, 51, and 58.
‡References 9, 3, 13, 15, 27, 51, and 58.
§References 9, 3, 15, 51, 19, 23, 53, and 56.
**References 9, 3, 15, 51, 19, 23, 53, and 56.

concept. The second generation of Marmor-like designs introduced a metal backing of the tibia, to bring modularity to the procedure and to distribute the weight-bearing forces more uniformly on the cut surface of the plateau. Although the initial results seemed satisfactory in terms of a more friendly surgical technique, wear failure of the tibial plateau was attributed mainly to the use of 6-mm-thick polyethylene. It is now recognized that the minimum thickness should be 8 mm for flat-bearing designs.[7] The unicondylar knee prosthesis was used in the United States and Europe as an alternative to the polycentric knee or the duo-condylar design,[10] and resurfacing both tibiofemoral compartments of the knee and preserving the cruciate ligaments represented the first form of the Oxford mobile bearing system by Goodfellow and O'Connor in 1978.[23] The concept was used for unicompartmental arthroplasty and is based on a fully congruent mobile articulating surface, which aims to increase the area of contact and reduce polyethylene wear. Measurement of retrieved bearings has shown a mean linear wear rate of 0.03 mm/year or less (0.001 mm/year) after normal function of the knee is restored.[6]

Cartier, in France, introduced instrumentation specifically dedicated to UKA. Cartier's instrumentation promoted the concept that UKA was not a half-TKA, and that the same type of persistence under correction of the deformity was suitable as opposed to the principle of TKA (Fig. 127.1A).[15,16] These principles were underlined and accurately described by Kennedy and White[29] in their paper describing the postoperative targets in terms of angle restoration after UKA (see Fig. 127.1B). The cutting jig systems brought the same type of instrumentation as the instrumentation used for TKA with posterior and chamfer cuts of the femoral condyle based on intramedullary instruments. The advantage of this type of instrumentation was to provide a reproducible surgical technique, allowing the component to be placed perpendicular to the mechanical axis as previously determined on preoperative radiographs. Most of these designs have been used widely in Europe and the United States since the late 1980s, and long-term follow-up information on the Brigham, Duracon, PFC Uni, and Miller-Galante is now available through the Swedish Registry.[18,41,56] Independent publications have also reported survivorship comparable to that reported for TKA.[††] Most of this experience was realized using cemented components, which are still the standard for UKA in Europe. The first reported use of porous-coated designs was not encouraging, but hydroxyapatite coating has gained some limited acceptance in some European centers.[19]

PATIENT SELECTION

The indications for UKA are painful OA or osteonecrosis limited to one compartment of the knee associated with significant loss of joint space on radiographs.[3,10,47,48] In fact, results after UKA for osteonecrosis limited to one compartment of the knee (ie, idiopathic or posttraumatic osteonecrosis) were comparable to results observed for OA at a mean of 12 years.[47] Any type of inflammatory arthritis, such as rheumatoid arthritis, is recognized as a formal contraindication for UKA because this can be a cause of rapid degeneration of the unreplaced compartments. Mild chondrocalcinosis, which is mostly a radiographic finding, may be accepted as an indication to perform

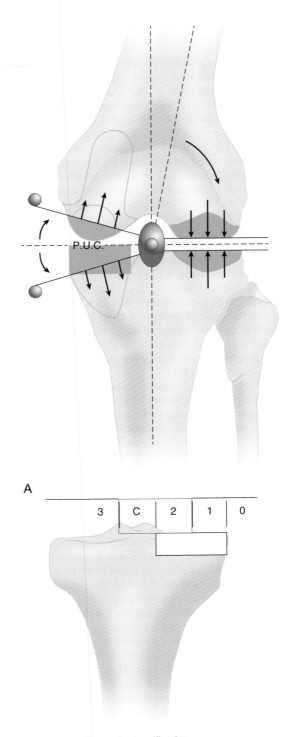

Kennedy classification

B

FIG 127.1 (A) Diagram showing the mechanism of overcorrection leading to progression of osteoarthritis in the unreplaced compartment after UKA. (B) These principles have been emphasized and accurately described by Kennedy and White[29] in their paper describing postoperative targets in terms of angle restoration after UKA.

[††]References 3, 13, 19, 45, 58, and 59.

UKA, in contrast to the productive chondrocalcinosis often associated with cyclic effusion of the knee.

Age and Weight

Age and weight may still represent debatable issues for the indication of UKA because the procedure is often presented as an alternative to osteotomy or TKA. As previously mentioned, and according to the results of previously published series, we consider the HTO as an attractive and efficient conservative procedure for patients younger than 50 years with low-grade unicompartmental OA and a varus knee.[21] However, the HTO risk of failure increased dramatically for patients with OA who were rated as Ahlback grade 2 or higher, which is why in those cases we consider UKA even in younger patients.[48,50] Regarding age and based on the comparative results at 10 years of UKA and TKA, Scott et al. considered that UKA might now assume a role in two groups of patients—middle-aged osteoarthritic patients (especially women undergoing a first arthroplasty) and osteoarthritic octogenarians having their "first and last" arthroplasty.[58] With survivorship studies of modern UKA comparable to TKA after the first decade, the selection process must be reconsidered and patients in their 60s and 70s would seem to have a greater chance of living out their life with a TKA or a UKA, which in any case would be easier to revise.[9,18,35] And thus, we reported very good survivorship in patients younger than 50, despite greater polyethylene wear than for older patients, as we also observed after TKA.[48]

Early reports of UKA considered obesity as a relative contraindication for UKA, but recent studies found no correlation between weight and outcomes and we concur with the idea that wear is more related to activity than to weight.[7] Obesity itself is consequently not a contraindication and has no effect on outcomes.[49]

Clinical Evaluation

The clinical examination of the knee before choosing UKA as a treatment option needs to focus on a range of motion with a minimum range of knee flexion of 100 degrees. A femoral contraction may be improved by only a few degrees after UKA, and this should be recognized preoperatively. The clinical evaluation of the patellofemoral joint is also mandatory to determine any type of anterior knee pain described by the patient during stair climbing and descending or during squatting. The stability of the joint must be evaluated carefully in the sagittal plane for the anterior cruciate ligament (ACL) and in the frontal plane using dedicated tests. The unicompartmental implant fills the gap left by the worn cartilage, bringing the collateral ligament back to normal tension after the procedure. The clinical results of UKA using a mobile meniscal or fixed bearing and the in vivo kinematics have highlighted the importance of a functional ACL for unicondylar knee replacement.[5] The clinical outcome for sedentary patients with a probable secondary distention of the ACL confirmed that correct clinical function of the knee might be achieved in these low-demand patients using fixed bearings, despite ACL deficiency. For these patients, we concur with the findings of Hernigou and Deschamps,[25] who studied the effect of posterior tibial slope on the outcome of UKA and recommended avoiding a posterior slope greater than 7 degrees when the ACL is absent at the time of the implantation.[25] For younger patients, a combined ACL/UKA surgery can be considered with good results in terms of pain and stability, but with more limited range of motion as compared with isolated UKA (Fig. 127.2).

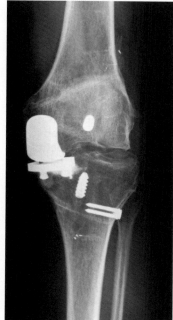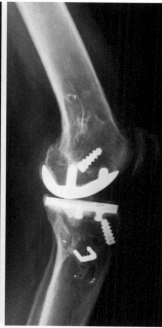

FIG 127.2 For younger patients, a combined ACL-UKA surgery can be considered with good results in terms of pain and stability but with more limited range of motion as compared with isolated UKA, as in this case at 12-year follow-up.

Radiologic Evaluation

Our radiologic analysis systematically includes anteroposterior (AP) and mediolateral (ML) views of the knee, full-length x-rays in bipedal and single leg stance, varus and valgus stress radiographs, and skyline views at 30, 60, and 90 degrees of knee flexion.[22] On full-length x-rays, the angle between the mechanical axis of the femur and the anatomic axis of the femur can be calculated and reproduced during the procedure at the time of the distal femoral cut. Full-length x-rays also evaluate any extra-articular bony deformity that cannot be corrected by the unicompartmental implant and searches for any femoral long hip stem that might require the use of a shorter intramedullary road or the use of an extramedullary rod. Kozinn and Scott first, and various authors thereafter, have suggested that UKA should be limited to preoperative varus or valgus deformity of the lower limb of less than 15 degrees. These authors have also suggested that greater deformities may represent a contraindication for UKA because the correction of such deformities may require collateral ligament release, which should not be performed when doing UKA because that may lead to frontal femorotibial subluxation.[31] It is also important to consider any important (>7 degrees) metaphyseal varus deformity of the proximal tibia, because in these rare cases, combined or staged HTO/UKA surgery can be considered (Fig. 127.3).

Varus and valgus stress X-rays, performed with the patient supine using a dedicated knee stress system, are very important; first, to assess the presence of full-thickness articular cartilage in the uninvolved compartment, and second, to confirm the full correction of the deformity to neutral (Fig. 127.4).[22] If there is absent, insufficient, or overcorrection of the deformity, this view indicates the need for soft tissue management and therefore the use of TKA. The lateral view of the joint confirms the

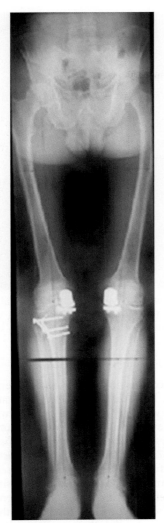

FIG 127.3 Staged opening wedge tibial osteotomy and UKA performed in a 46-year-old man who had a preoperative 8-degree metaphyseal varus deformity and a global varus deformity of 16 degrees. The patient returned to equestrian competition.

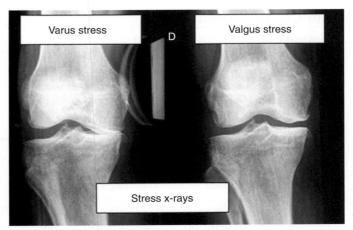

FIG 127.4 Varus and valgus stress x-rays, obtained with the patient supine using a dedicated knee stress system, are important to assess the presence of full-thickness articular cartilage in the uninvolved compartment and to confirm full correction of the deformity to neutral.

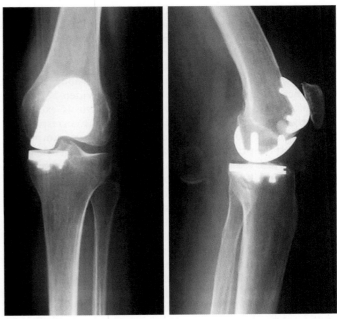

FIG 127.5 In cases of associated wear in the medial and patellofemoral compartments, bicompartmental arthroplasty combining medial UKA and patellofemoral arthroplasty can be considered during the same procedure. Shown here are the results at 2 years after bicompartmental arthroplasty in a 62-year-old woman. She returned to hiking.

absence of anterior tibial translation greater than 10 mm, referencing the posterior edge of the tibial plateau, and shows that tibial erosion is limited to anterior and mid-portions of the tibial plateau. The height of the patella should also be analyzed as a patella baja will limit the exposure during MIS procedures.[10]

The radiographic analysis should ensure that there is no patellofemoral loss of joint space on skyline views at 30, 60, and 90 degrees of flexion. The presence of periarticular osteophytes may not be a contraindication for unicondylar replacement, and these osteophytes can be removed even through a minimally invasive incision. Although the status of the patellofemoral joint is not a criterion of suitability for some authors, the full loss of patellofemoral cartilage is currently, for us, a contraindication to unicondylar replacement. In these cases of associated wear in the medial and in the patellofemoral compartment, bicompartmental arthroplasty combining medial UKA and patellofemoral arthroplasty can be considered during the same procedure (Fig. 127.5).[50] When there is a question regarding the status of

the ACL following the clinical exam, magnetic resonance imaging may be useful in confirming that the ACL is intact.

Laskin analyzed 300 knees undergoing TKA, evaluated the selection criteria presented by Kozinn and Scott, and found that 15% of the knees were eligible for UKA at intraoperative inspection.[31,33] This 15% rate of indication for UKA corresponds to the figures currently reported in Europe, in contrast to the 6% rate of potential candidates for a UKA reported by Ritter et al.[55]

SURGICAL TECHNIQUE

Approach

The procedure can be performed under general or epidural anesthesia on a routine operating table using two leg holders: one at the lateral aspect of the thigh and the second one below the foot. The knee is flexed 90 degrees for the skin incision, the thigh tourniquet is inflated, and the foot rests on the table. The length of the skin incision varies from 8 to 10 cm depending on skin elasticity and patient morphotype. It is important to maintain proper visualization throughout the procedure, which depends in part on the variation in tissue elasticity. Sufficient visualization is important throughout the procedure and this can be achieved by frequent extension-flexion manipulations to preferentially visualize the femoral side or the tibial side. When the proper visualization of the anatomic structure or the component is not obtained by shifting the position of the knee, it might be necessary to extend the size of the incision. One of the classical pitfalls of the procedure is related to the length of the incision, which should not be too small, particularly at the beginning of the learning curve. In fact, insufficient exposure may lead to skin damage as a result of excessive tension, to implant malposition, or to inadequate knee balancing. The upper limit of the incision is the superior pole of the patella extending distally toward the medial for a medial UKA or the lateral for a lateral UKA of the tibial tuberosity, but ending 2 cm distal to the joint line previously located (see Video 127.1). The proximal part of the incision is more essential for the procedure and two-thirds of the incision should be located above the joint line. Once the synovial cavity is opened (see Video 127.2), the part of the fat pad in the way of the condyle is excised to properly visualize the condyle, the ACL, and the corresponding tibial side of the tibial plateau (see Video 127.3). It is important to note that the principles of ligament balancing in TKA cannot be applied to UKA because the collateral ligaments should not be released in UKA. To protect the collateral ligament and safely perform the cuts, a dedicated, curved, thin Homan retractor is placed on the medial or lateral side of the incision.

Before proceeding to the bone cuts, the first step is to bring the knee to 60 degrees of flexion to evaluate the joint by checking the resistance of the ACL with an appropriate hook and evaluating the state of the opposite tibiofemoral joint and the patellofemoral joint (Fig. 127.6). The osteophytes are removed on the medial or lateral side of the femoral condyle, in the intercondylar notch, to avoid late impingement with the ACL on the notch. This point is very important to preserve the ACL and avoid the so-called Marie-Antoinette effect. This effect is famous in Europe and is related to the osteophytes that develop in the intercondylar notch, which have a guillotine effect on the ACL (see Video 127.4). Finally, the osteophytes are also removed from around the patella and the tibial plateau. After removing the peripheral osteophytes, there is a relative lengthening of the medial collateral ligament and capsule, allowing passive correction of the deformity.

Tibial Cut

Once the status of the patella, the ACL, and the opposite compartment have been checked, the next step is the bone cuts. It is important to remember that in UKA the proper tension in the ligaments will be restored by filling the gap left by the worn cartilage with the unicompartmental components, and UKA is therefore a so-called surfacing procedure.

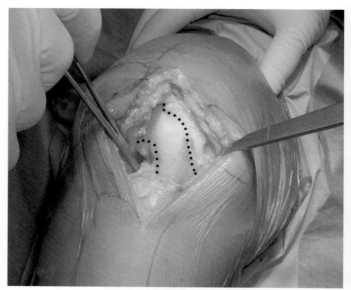

FIG 127.6 Operative view through a minimal incision shows the osteophytes to be removed and the ACL, with the knee at 45 degrees of flexion.

In our practice, the tibial cut is always performed first for UKA and TKA, however because the cuts are independent, surgery can start with the femoral side as well when considering the intramedullary technique for the femur. *N.B.: Various cutting-guide versions based on dependent distal femoral and tibial cut* (Fig. 127.7A) *or full intramedullary instrumentation are available.* The extramedullary technique is based on the correction of the deformity of the leg in extension using an extramedullary rod that references the ankle and the femoral head. This will determine the direction and the level of the femoral distal cut performed first and link that parallel to the tibial cut made with the knee brought into flexion.

The tibial cut is made using an extramedullary rod (see Fig. 127.7B). The guide is placed distally around the ankle with the axis of the guide lying slightly medial to the center of the ankle joint. The proximal part of the guide rests on the anterior tibia pointing toward the axis of the tibial spines; with modern instrumentation it is possible to have the cutting part of the guide resting only on the upper tibia (medial or lateral) to be resected. The diaphyseal part of the guide is parallel to the anterior tibial crest, and the anteroposterior position of the guide is adjusted distally to reproduce the natural upper tibial slope, usually between 5 and 7 degrees of posterior slope (see Video 127.5). The amount of resection is decided after using a 4-mm probe located on the deepest part of the affected plateau, and particular care should be taken to properly define the level of the cut. To do so, it is important to control the level of resection using an "angel-wing" probe to mimic the cut, not only on the anterior part of the plateau, but also on the posterior aspect (see Video 127.6). To complete the tibial cut, the sagittal tibial cut should be made. This can be done using one of the sagittal marks provided by the guide or made as a freehand cut. When the cut is made free hand, the cut should be aligned close to the tibial spine eminence, the anterior starting point decided after checking the alignment of the edge of the femoral condyle on the tibial plateau when the knee is brought from flexion close

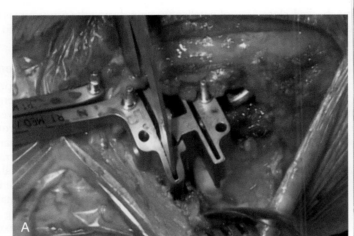

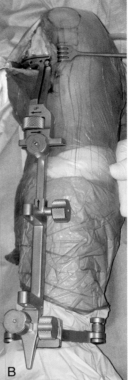

FIG 127.7 (A) Presenting another version of the ancillary based on dependent distal femoral and tibial cutting guides. (B) The tibial cut is made with an extramedullary cutting guide aligned on the tibial crest in the frontal plane and with a 5-degree posterior slope in the sagittal plane. The cutting jig is fixed on the superomedial part of the tibia (for a medial UKA).

to full extension. At this step, once again, particular care should be taken to protect the ACL (see Video 127.6).

Femoral Cut

The entrance hole of the distal femur for the intramedullary technique is centered above the roof of the intercondylar notch and prepared using an osteotome to conserve the cartilage. The drilling of the femoral medullary canal through a short incision often requires bringing the knee to 60 degrees of flexion. In fact, in flexion, the tension from the patella on the intramedullary (IM) guide might induce incorrect alignment. Once the guide has been properly introduced, the distal femoral cut can be made reporting the angle between the anatomic and mechanical axis (previously evaluated on the full weight-bearing view). This angle is usually 4 to 6 degrees. It is critical to carefully protect the skin at the proximal part of the incision while performing this cut to avoid any skin damage (see Video 127.7). The amount of bone resected from the distal femur corresponds exactly, millimeter for millimeter, to the femoral prosthesis. The remainder of the femoral cuts (posterior cut and chamfrains) are completed using the appropriate cutting block. First, the size of the femoral implant should be determined using the cutting block. The size is determined once this femoral finishing guide is positioned on the distal femoral cut and a search is performed for the best compromise between an anatomically centered position on the femoral condyle and a long axis perpendicular to the resected tibial plateau. The top of this finishing guide should be localized 1 to 2 mm above the deepest layer of the

cartilage to avoid a potential notch between the femoral implant and the patella. In others words, ideally, the femoral block should be slightly smaller anteriorly than the original femoral condyle (see Video 127.8). To control the mediolateral position of the femoral cutting guide, which determines the position of the final implant, the use of tibial referencing based on the previously made tibial cut is probably the best landmark. Because the divergence of the medial condyle is different from one knee to another, checking the mediolateral position of the guide on the femoral condyle is also recommended. Once the posterior cut has been made and the cutting guide removed, removal of any posterior osteophytes is necessary using a curved osteotome to increase the range of flexion and avoid any posterior impingement with the polyethylene in high flexion (see Video 127.9).

Tibial Finishing and Trials

The size of the tibial tray should now be determined by managing the best compromise between maximal tibial coverage and overhang, which might induce pain. The anteroposterior size of the tibial plateau sometimes differs from the mediolateral plateau, especially in women, and thus different sizing trials are necessary to find the best compromise. It is important to keep the depth of the tibial cut as conservative as possible to take advantage of the strength of the tibial cortex and the increased area of contact proximally. The knee is brought into maximal flexion and externally rotated. The final preparation of the tibia is completed with the appropriate guide with the underlying keel impacted in the subchondral bone. Using a minimal incision, it is important to carefully locate the posterior margin of the tibial plateau to correctly position the keel in the anteroposterior direction. It is useful to precut the future location of the keel using a reciprocating saw blade or an osteotome (see Video 127.10).

The flexion-extension gaps should be tested with the trial components in place and with the insertion of a trial polyethylene liner. Common causes of impingement are residual bone eminence, incorrect position of the tibial or femoral component, or an oblique tibial cut. Once this has been verified, it is important to look for a 2-mm protective laxity checked close to full extension to avoid any overcorrection of the deformity leading to progression of OA in the unreplaced compartment. It is also important to avoid residual varus deformity, as recently reported, to minimize the risk of polyethylene wear when using flat polyethylene inserts. The ideal correction, as measured on the postoperative full weight-bearing view, will probably consist of a tibiofemoral axis crossing the knee between the tibial spines and the lateral third of the tibial plateau for a medial UKA, as outlined by Kennedy and White in their classification (Fig. 127.8).[29] We cement all components for better fixation because long-term results suggest that loosening is not a common mode of failure with modern cemented, metal-backed components. The tibial component is cemented first with the knee in full flexion and externally rotated for a medial UKA to improve the exposure of the medial compartment. When cementing the components, it is important to avoid leaving any cement at the posterior aspect of the knee, and a 90-degree curved probe is useful for removing any posterior cement when using a minimal incision. Once the femoral implant has been cemented, bringing the knee close to extension helps remove any posterior cement with the polyethylene inserted last (see Video 127.11). Patellar tracking should be checked before closing; the absence of patellar eversion during the procedure is helpful for that step. The tourniquet is released before closure to adequately perform hemostasis (see Video 127.12).

Lateral Unicompartmental Replacement[42]

The skin incision, using a minimal approach of the lateral compartment (Fig. 127.9), must be lateral, especially at the distal portion, because of the frequent divergence of the lateral femoral condyle. When the lateral arthrotomy is performed, visualization of the joint is often easier than on the medial side because of the natural mobility of the lateral tibiofemoral joint. The tibial resection should remain minimal, because the disease is more often on the femoral side. If there is femoral dysplasia, it is often necessary to use a more proximal distal femoral cut.

The alignment of the femoral cutting guide on the tibial cut is crucial because of the natural shape of the lateral femoral condyle. The "screw-home" mechanism[38] is considered a key element in knee stability for standing upright, because this is the rotation between the tibia and femur. At the end of knee extension, between full extension and 20 degrees of knee flexion, external rotation of the tibia occurs and results in tightening of both cruciate ligaments, which locks the knee. At this point, the tibia is in a position of maximal stability with respect to the femur. As a result of this phenomenon, surgeons must remember that a good femoral implant position in flexion may lead to excessive internal rotation in extension and impingement on the tibial spine eminence (Fig. 127.10).

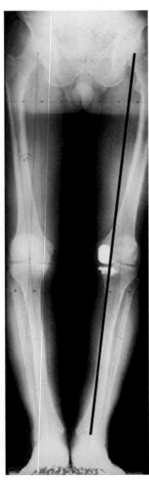

FIG 127.8 Full weight-bearing view of the limbs shows a hip-knee-ankle axis crossing the knee joint just medial to the tibial spines, leaving an undercorrected 3-degree varus deformity after a medial UKA.

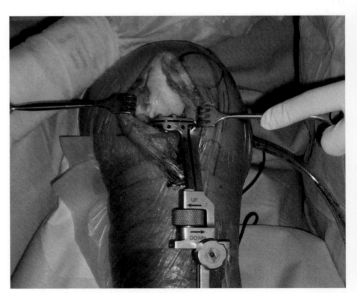

FIG 127.9 Lateral parapatellar approach performed during a lateral UKA implantation.

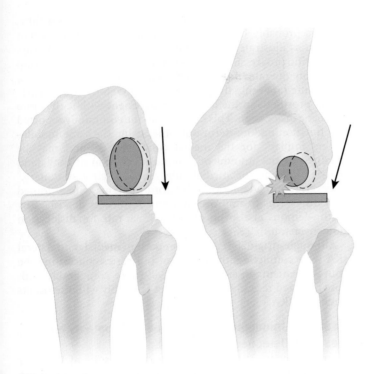

FIG 127.10 As a result of the screw-home mechanism, when positioning the femoral component, it is frequently necessary to mark the correct alignment in extension rather than in flexion to avoid any medial edge loading and impingement between the femoral implant and the tibial spines.

Therefore, the positioning in flexion should exaggerate the lateral rotation and the lateral positioning (almost on the lateral osteophytes to obtain a satisfactory position in extension).

The polyethylene insert for lateral UKA is often thicker than for the medial side in case of femoral dysplasia, even if the principle of undercorrection of the deformity for all cases of lateral UKA remains the basis for successful long-term results.

In our practice, lateral UKA represents 10% of the indications for UKA; our published long-term results confirm results previously published and that lateral OA can be treated successfully by unicondylar replacement.[8] The in vivo kinematic evaluation of patients implanted with lateral UKA found a greater posterior displacement of the femorotibial contact point during flexion as compared with patients implanted with medial UKA.[5]

Postoperative Care

In our practice, one intraarticular drain is left for 36 hours. Immediate weight bearing on two crutches is recommended postoperatively after removal of the femoral nerve block catheter (left 12 hours postoperatively) for a period of 1 or 2 weeks. Manual range-of-motion physiotherapy is performed the day after surgery. Deep venous thrombosis prevention is managed using mechanical devices and low-weight heparin for 3 weeks postoperatively.

RESULTS

Survivorship studies generated from early unicompartmental series show that survivorship rates at 10 years decrease into the 85% range. With better patient selection and reproducible instrumentation, more recent series show 10-year survivorship regularly at 90% or greater.[46,59] Many authors now also support the view that revision of a modern UKA is a relatively common and simple procedure.[18,35] Patients from the Swedish registry are more satisfied after revision of a failed UKA than after a revision of a TKA.[56]

Results of Medial Unicompartmental Knee Arthroplasty for Degenerative Arthritis

Mid- and long-term studies suggest reasonable 10-year survivorship of 95% for UKA performed for medial OA.[8,38,41] Mobile-bearing UKA of a specific design (Oxford; Biomet; Warsaw, IN) has shown a recent increase in use. Murray et al.[39] reported 98% cumulative prosthetic survivorship at 10 years. Price et al.,[52] using the same implant, found 92% survivorship at 15 years. However, the author[52] noted a high frequency (50%) of complete radiolucent lines around their tibial components.

For fixed-bearing metal-backed tibia UKA, we reported[2,10] that the two most common causes of failure were progression of arthritis in the uninvolved compartments (65%) and polyethylene wear (25%). The average time for conversion to TKA or addition of a patellofemoral implant was 13 years (range, 3 months to 21 years). According to Kaplan-Meier analysis, the 20-year survival free of revision for any reason was $74 \pm 7\%$.

In contemporary practice, the discussion has focused on UKA versus TKA results. A recent paper based on 27-year data from the Finnish joint registry provided comparative outcomes between those two strategies.[41] The authors found 4713 patients with UKA for primary OA (mean age, 64 years; mean follow-up, 6 years) who had surgical revision between 1985 and 2011. From this cohort,[41] the Kaplan-Meier survivorship for revision performed for any reason was calculated and compared with the survivorship of 83,511 patients (mean age, 70 years; mean follow-up, 6 years) with TKAs treated for primary OA during the same period. Data were adjusted for age and gender in a comparative analysis. Kaplan-Meier survivorship of UKAs was 89% at 5 years, 81% at 10 years, and 70% at 15 years. The corresponding rates for TKAs were 96%, 93%, and 88%, respectively. UKAs had inferior long-term survivorship compared with cemented TKAs, even after adjusting for the age and gender of the patients (hazard ratio [HR], 2.2; $p < 0.001$).[41] The authors acknowledged that comparing survival directly by using arthroplasty register survival reports might be inadequate because of differences in indications, implant designs, and patient demographics in patients having partial knee replacements (PKRs) and TKAs.[41] Despite these limitations, their conclusions outlined that PKR offers tempting advantages compared with a TKA. However, long-term revision risks are higher with a PKR.[41]

Results of Medial Unicompartmental Knee Arthroplasty in Young Patients

Recently Walker et al.[60] reported that UKA allowed patients younger than 60 years to return to regular physical activities with almost two-thirds of the patients reaching a high activity level (UCLA ≥ 7). In a study[48] evaluating the results of UKA in patients under 50 years of age, our results suggested that (1) UKA for unicompartmental arthritis is reliable in improving function in patients and allowed a return to previous levels of activity, (2) satisfying radiologic results can be achieved in terms of implant fixation and alignment and in restoring lower-limb alignment, and (3) survivorship is acceptable but lower than the previously reported survivorship for older patients. In fact, revisions for polyethylene wear or progression of arthritis in the patellofemoral joint remain important concerns in altering the survivorship of the implant in this group of patients. Our experience[48] shows that knee function can be restored after UKA in patients under 50 years of age and that UKA may be a reliable option for middle-aged patients; however, wear after 10 years remains a problem in this category of patients. In our series, four of the six revisions were related to polyethylene wear. We were unable to identify specific causes such as malalignment or body mass index in this group of patients to account for this wear. In the four cases, a direct exchange of the worn polyethylene insert for a new one was easily performed through a minimally invasive incision.[34] The functional results according to the Knee Society scoring system for these patients were comparable to those obtained for the unrevised patients at last follow-up. In our series there was one case of OA progression that required revision with a standard posterior stabilized TKA. Price et al.[50] reported a multicentric comparison of 512 patients older than 60 and 53 patients younger than 60 years implanted with an Oxford UKA.[50] The results of this comparison suggested that the Oxford medial UKA functions well and is durable in patients younger than 60 years, even if the calculated survivorship in this series was lower for these patients (91% at 10 years in the <60 group vs. 96% in the >60 group).[50]

UKA may be a reliable option for middle-aged patients; however, wear after 10 years remains a problem in this patient category.

Results of Patient-Specific Instrumentation-Unicompartmental Knee Arthroplasty

To increase the likelihood that good alignment will be achieved during surgery, smart tools such as robotics or patient-specific instrumentation (PSI) have been introduced.[20] Very limited scientific data are available concerning PSI UKA: Studies disagree about whether PSI improves alignment in patients undergoing UKA.[12,17,28,30] We designed[43] a randomized controlled trial to verify that UKA performed with PSI would improve implant positioning, patient-reported outcomes, and gait compared with conventional techniques. One year after surgery we found no benefit in any radiologic or functional outcomes (Knee osteoarthritis outcomes score [KOOS], short for [SF]-12) and no difference in gait parameters when PSI was used.[43]

Results of Lateral Unicompartmental Knee Arthroplasty

Unicompartmental femorotibial OA usually affects the medial compartment of the knee, and more rarely the lateral compartment.[57] In addition to osteotomy for correction of a valgus deformity, the surgical treatments for lateral femorotibial OA include TKA or UKA arthroplasty. The results of our study[8] have shown that lateral UKA can provide satisfactory long-term clinical and radiographic results and survivorship at 10, 16, and 22 years is comparable with the survivorship obtained for medial UKA in the literature. Our results at a maximum follow-up of 23 years ranged between the results of the old and recent studies of lateral UKA reported in the literature.[8] Recent studies reported a very low failure rate, whereas the results of older series were more controversial. As previously mentioned,

we observed a significant improvement of the results over time, which is probably linked first to an improvement in patient selection as illustrated by the two cases revised before 3 years for arthritic progression in patients older than 80 years (group of patients operated before 1989). Gunther et al.[24] reported a 21% failure rate using the mobile-bearing Oxford unicompartmental prosthesis in the lateral compartment with a 10% rate of bearing dislocation. This differs from the commonly reported high functioning long-term outcomes using the same mobile-bearing implant for the medial compartment, and may be explained by the amount of femoral translation of the lateral condyle, whereas the medial side remains fairly stationary.[5] However, recent adaptation of Oxford implants with a domed tibial tray seems to improve midterm results, as described by Weston-Simons et al. who report a 1.5% rate for dislocation and conversion to TKA.[61]

Although original reports comparing medial and lateral UKA were conflicting, the results of our series concerning the group of patients operated after 1989 were comparable with those reported recently and compares favorably with the results of medial UKA.

Results of Unicompartmental Knee Arthroplasty for Avascular Osteonecrosis of the Knee

In a retrospective study,[47] we analyzed the results of UKA for osteonecrosis using a modern implant and strict inclusion criteria, first regarding the limitation of the osteonecrosis to one compartment of the knee even for the cases of secondary osteonecrosis, and second regarding the status of the uninvolved compartment of the patellofemoral articulation and of the anterior cruciate ligament. The data suggest that the UKA is reliable in osteonecrosis for alleviating pain and improving function, restoring proper lower-limb mechanical axis, and achieving a durable survivorship at 12 years.[47] Few studies have reported the results of a continuous series of UKA implanted for osteonecrosis.[32,37,40] A review of the literature showed varying outcomes after UKA for spontaneous osteonecrosis of the knee and better outcomes with TKA.[40] Nonetheless, the authors noted an improvement in outcome scores for the most recent series of UKA for osteonecrosis of the knee with strict selection criteria. These studies reported results of UKA only for spontaneous osteonecrosis. The outcomes of UKA reported in our study[47] for osteonecrosis are comparable with the average results of TKA for osteonecrosis with a revision rate of 3% and a mean global knee score of 85 points. The 96.7% survival at 12 years reported in the present study is encouraging, and this favorable outcome may be related to different considerations. Patient selection included osteonecrosis limited to a single femorotibial compartment, a fully correctable deformity on stress radiographs, a healthy patellofemoral joint, and an intact anterior cruciate ligament. Heyse et al.[26] presented similar results for their 28 knees at a mean of 10 years after surgery; the authors described 93.1% survival without implant revision for any cause. Bruni et al.[14] found a 10-year Kaplan-Meier survivorship with revision for any reason as the endpoint of 89%.

These data were consistent with the few other long-term series published in the literature with fixed[37] and mobile-bearing UKA[32] and suggested that UKA is reliable in osteonecrosis for alleviating pain and improving function, restoring the lower-limb mechanical axis, and achieving durable survivorship.

SUMMARY

Unicondylar knee replacement should not be considered as a temporary procedure, and the 10-year survival can be as good as with TKA if patient selection and surgical principles are followed carefully. The advantages of UKA compared with TKA include retention of both cruciate ligaments, preservation of bone stock in the opposite compartment and the patellofemoral joint, and better functional results. For young and active patients, a modern UKA represents a valid alternative to bridge the gap between HTO and TKA with isolated unicompartmental tibiofemoral noninflammatory disease (Ahlback grade 3 or greater). Although component loosening and progression of the arthritis in the remaining compartments has become rare with appropriate patient selection and adequate surgical technique, polyethylene wear, associated with flat metal backed component, remains a problem, particularly in youngest, active, and heavy patients. The last decade, evolutions in terms of surgical technique and instrumentation and in terms of implant designs have made unicompartmental arthroplasty the standard of treatment for patients with severe OA limited to one tibiofemoral compartment.

KEY REFERENCES

2. Argenson J-N, Blanc G, Aubaniac J-M, et al: Modern unicompartmental knee arthroplasty with cement: a concise follow-up, at a mean of twenty years, of a previous report. *J Bone Joint Surg Am* 95:905, 2013.

3. Argenson J-N, Chevrol-Benkeddache Y, Aubaniac J-M: Modern unicompartmental knee arthroplasty with cement: a three to ten-year foll ow-up study. *J Bone Joint Surg Am* 84:2235, 2002.

5. Argenson J-N, Komistek RD, Aubaniac J-M, et al: In vivo determination of knee kinematics for subjects implanted with a unicompartmental arthroplasty. *J Arthroplasty* 17:1049, 2002. doi: 10.1054/arth.2002.34527.

8. Argenson JN, Parratte S, Bertani A, et al: Long-term results with a lateral unicondylar replacement. *Clin Orthop* 466:2686, 2008.

10. Argenson J-N, Parratte S, Flecher X, et al: Unicompartmental knee arthroplasty: technique through a mini-incision. *Clin Orthop* 464:32, 2007.

21. Flecher X, Parratte S, Aubaniac J-M, et al: A 12-28-year follow-up study of closing wedge high tibial osteotomy. *Clin Orthop* 452:91, 2006.

27. Insall J, Walker P: Unicondylar knee replacement. *Clin Orthop* 83:5, 1976.

34. Lunebourg A, Parratte S, Galland A, et al: Is isolated insert exchange a valuable choice for polyethylene wear in metal-backed unicompartment al knee arthroplasty? *Knee Surg Sports Traumatol Arthrosc* 2014. doi: 10.1007/s00167-014-3392-8.

35. Lunebourg A, Parratte S, Ollivier M, et al: Are revisions of unicompartmental knee arthroplasties more like a primary or revision TKA? *J Arthroplasty* 30:1985–1989, 2015. doi: 10.1016/j.arth.2015.05.042.

42. Ollivier M, Abdel MP, Parratte S, et al: Lateral unicondylar knee arthroplasty (UKA): contemporary indications, surgical technique, and results. *Int Orthop* 38:449, 2014.

43. Ollivier M, Parratte S, Lunebourg A, et al: The John Insall Award: no functional benefit after unicompartmental knee arthroplasty performed with patient-specific instrumentation: a randomized trial. *Clin Orthop* 2015. doi: 10.1007/s11999-015-4259-0.

47. Parratte S, Argenson J-N, Dumas J, et al: Unicompartmental knee arthroplasty for avascular osteonecrosis. *Clin Orthop* 464:37, 2007.

48. Parratte S, Argenson JN, Pearce O, et al: Medial unicompartmental knee replacement in the under-50s. *J Bone Joint Surg Br* 91:351, 2009.

51. Price AJ, O'Connor JJ, Murray DW, et al: A history of Oxford unicompartmental knee arthroplasty. *Orthopedics* 30:7, 2007.

57. Scott RD: Lateral unicompartmental replacement: a road less traveled. *Orthopedics* 28:983, 2005.

The references for this chapter can also be found on www.expertconsult.com.

128

Unicomparmental Knee Replacement With ACL Reconstruction

Paolo Adravanti, Giuseppe Calafiore, Aldo Ampollini

Intra-articular knee damage as a result of chronic anterior cruciate ligament (ACL) injury,[8] with meniscal, chondral, and capsular degeneration, commonly occurs in the medial compartment.[9,29] The result is often varus morphometry, with medial cartilage and meniscal wear leading to gradual thinning of the internal articular rim, which can be appreciated on weight-bearing radiography with distension of the lateral capsule.[2] Surgical treatment options include isolated ACL reconstruction, valgus tibial osteotomy with or without ACL reconstruction, and total or partial knee arthroplasty combined with ACL reconstruction. The choice of treatment depends upon patient indications including age and presenting symptoms. The advantages of unicompartmental knee arthroplasty (UKA) over total knee arthroplasty (TKA) include superior joint function, proprioception, and bone conservation, with reported excellent long-term outcomes.[20,27,28]

ACL deficiency or absence is commonly considered a contraindication to UKA because of the high prosthesis failure rate associated with early loosening of the tibial plateau. Goodfellow et al. reported a 22% revision rate within the first 2 years after replacement with a mobile bearing UKA design.[12] The cause of early failure was theorized to be altered knee biomechanics as a result of posterior subluxation of the femur resulting from increased eccentric loading on the tibial plateau.[12] In vivo and cadaveric studies demonstrated that single-bundle ACL reconstruction could restore normal joint biomechanics in knees undergoing UKA.[23,25] More recently, UKA combined with ACL reconstruction was shown to provide a valid alternative for young adults with medial compartment osteoarthritis (OA) and ACL rupture, and is reported to ensure the same joint stability, joint biomechanics, and prosthesis survivorship in the midterm as isolated UKA.[30,32]

ETIOLOGY

ACL rupture alters knee biomechanics, resulting in increased anterior tibial translation,[19] which is partially restrained by the so-called brake stop function of the posterior horn of the medial meniscus.[19] However, tibial translation is further increased due to the greater tibial slope and injury to the posteromedial corner.[4] Damage to the medial cartilage is caused by rupture of the internal meniscus secondary to chronic ACL injury and by anterior subluxation of the medial tibial condyle, particularly of the posterior aspect of the internal tibial plateau, which occurs in internal valgus rotation (pivot shift).[7] In addition, varus morphometry can lead to further severe medial

chondral damage. ACL rupture can also progress secondary to OA when an imbalance on the frontal plane is associated with external femoral and internal tibial rotation, as well as progressive sliding of the tibial spines that conflict with the external condyle. Thereafter, osteophyte formation narrows the intercondylar groove, gradually destroying the ACL. This difference may explain conflicting reports following partial arthroplasty in ACL-deficient knees. Boissonneault et al. reported similar short-term survival rates after partial arthroplasty, with or without ACL reconstruction in patients with ACL deficiency secondary to OA, but not primary ACL injury.[3]

DIAGNOSIS AND PREOPERATIVE EVALUATION

Candidates for combined ACL reconstruction and UKA are young adults with a history of knee joint instability secondary to post-traumatic ACL rupture and secondary OA of the medial compartment. Clinical tests are similar to those performed to assess ACL injury, with careful evaluation of associated peripheral ligament lesions, which although rarely present, are a contraindication to surgery.[30] However, tests may have negative results in a setting of advanced OA where osteophytes and the increased concavity of the tibial plateau stabilize the knee. Because the pivot test is often negative[31] and the Lachman test has a specificity of 33%,[16] clinical and diagnostic findings need to be integrated in the overall assessment.

Anteroposterior (AP) weight-bearing and Rosenberg radiographic studies are optimum for documenting the location and degree of OA, and the presence or absence of osteophytes in the intercondylar groove. Additionally, a lateral weight-bearing radiographic study will reveal evidence of anterior subluxation of the tibial plateau,[4] suggesting ACL rupture (Fig. 128.1).

Axial views of the patella at 45 degrees of knee flexion may demonstrate lateral OA of the femoral patella. Other essential imaging studies include long, bilateral weight-bearing AP radiographs to evaluate the mechanical axis. Also, varus-valgus stress radiographs may be used to assess reducibility of the deformity and to exclude restricted external rotation, which is a sign of lateral femorotibial OA.

In addition to confirming ACL rupture, magnetic resonance imaging (MRI) studies are useful for excluding chondral, external meniscus, femoropatellar injury, chondral edema, and/or tibial stress fractures.[16-22] However, cartilage degeneration may be overestimated with MRI.[15]

Contraindications to UKA combined with ACL reconstruction are the same as those for isolated UKA: irreducible varus

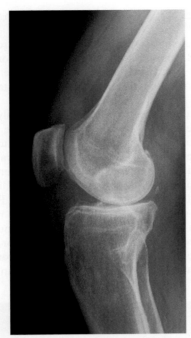

FIG 128.1 Preoperative weight-bearing radiograph reveals subluxation of the medial femoral condyle with posteromedial arthrosis and ACL rupture.

deformity greater than 15 degrees, knee contracture greater than 5 degrees, severe genu recurvatum, advanced lateral femoropatellar OA, and inflammatory arthropathy.

REVIEW OF RELEVANT LITERATURE

Various early studies have reported high short-term failure rates after UKA with different types of prostheses in ACL-deficient patients. Deschamps et al. reported a 25% failure rate in a series of 79 Lotus UKAs (Howmedica Orthopaedics, East Rutherford, NJ) with a follow-up of more than 5 years. In a further retrospective evaluation, it was noted that 13 failures occurred among the patients with an anterior tibial translation greater than 10 mm on preoperative lateral weight-bearing radiograph.[10] The study concluded that the ACL should be carefully evaluated before considering UKA and that lateral weight-bearing radiography is essential during the preoperative assessment. Moreover, Goodfellow et al. reported a 16.2% failure rate in a series of Oxford UKA prostheses in ACL-deficient patients with a follow-up of 3 years.[12] These data were later reconfirmed in a review of the series by the same authors.[13]

Following on the optimal outcomes after partial knee replacement, Pandit et al. and Krishnan et al. published promising results obtained with medial UKA combined with ACL reconstruction performed during a single surgical session.[17,24] More recently, Tinius et al. reported optimal midterm follow-up results following UKA combined with ACL reconstruction.[30] Other studies have demonstrated encouraging short-term results following medial UKA in ACL-deficient patients.[3,5,6,11] However, because follow-up was short in these studies, no conclusions can be drawn regarding intermediate or long-term results.[3]

In a recent review, Mancuso et al. analyzed outcomes following UKA.[21] They reported that the revision rate was significantly lower when anterior cruciate ligament reconstruction (ACLR) was performed. Moreover, the authors reported similar survival rate data of fixed versus mobile bearing in UKA.

It is important to distinguish the post-traumatic ACL rupture versus ACL rupture secondary to OA in which progressive tearing of the ligament is due to the increased friction accompanying cartilage degeneration.[14] Most of authors agree that post-traumatic ACL reconstruction combined with UKA is indicated because the OA is isolated to the posteromedial compartment and the varus deformity can be corrected.[14] In the second case, the OA progresses from the anteromedial to the posteromedial compartment, leading to a varus deformity that cannot be corrected because of flexion/extension contractures as a result of retraction of the superficial medial collateral ligament.[13]

Rotation deformity is commonly identified as the cause of early degeneration of the lateral and the patellofemoral compartments.[18] In such cases, total knee replacement is correctly indicated. However, other authors have reported that UKA is indicated in selected cases, given the better functional results obtained with UKA than with TKA. This evidence comes from studies on patients with ACL deficiency secondary to OA in which the osteoarthritic changes and joint adaptations (osteophyte formation) stabilize the knee joint.[11]

Upon intraoperative knee assessment, the ACL in an arthritic knee can be classified into four categories: normal with synovial damage, longitudinal splits, friable and fragmented, or absent. In a recent study, Boissonneault et al. reviewed 46 UKA cases in which the ACL was classified as friable and fragmented in 33 and absent in 13. The authors found no difference in prosthesis survivorship after 5 years follow-up between UKA with or without an intact ACL. All patients had minimal sagittal instability and lateral arthritis of the non–weight-bearing area.[3] These results complemented those from an earlier study published by the same group in which the authors concluded that a series of ACL-deficient patients with medial OA could have been candidates for UKA, but that further studies were needed to better define which type of patient could benefit from such treatment.[3]

A variety of surgical techniques are available for restoring knee joint stability in UKA without ACL, including reduction of the tibial slope to render it neutral, complete covering of the tibial plateau, and tensioning of the medial collateral ligament.[11] In such cases, removal of osteophytes from the intercondylar groove is indicated if the ACL is present but impinged against the intercondylar notch.[1] If the ACL is absent, osteophytes should be removed with care to maintain a functional degree of joint stability.[26]

SURGICAL TECHNIQUE

The combined procedures are performed in well-defined steps beginning with arthroscopic evaluation to confirm the correct surgical indication: exposure of the posteromedial bone of the tibial plateau will demonstrate OA progression in patients with traumatic rupture of the ACL. Marked osteophytosis with joint space narrowing in the intercondylar groove will be noted in such patients. The intercondylar groove is restored with wide notchplasty. Pandit et al. prefer to perform this combined surgery "open" to restrict infection complications.[24] We prefer to perform the femoral tunnel arthroscopically so that its orientation is more anatomically accurate. The femoral tunnel is positioned through the low anteromedial portal. Before harvesting the graft, the tunnel is predrilled arthroscopically (6 mm in diameter and 20 mm in length); this affords greater accuracy within the ACL anatomic stump and independent positioning of the femoral and tibial tunnels.

We often encounter cartilage defects adjacent to the tibial spine on the lateral tibial plateau, which are a result of altered biomechanics because of chronic ACL injury (Fig. 128.2).

However, these defects are not cause for concern, because restoration of natural rollback will shift the resultant load to the lateral aspect of the knee, thus reducing the risk of late clinical complications.

The second step of the operative procedure involves a standard medial parapatellar approach to the knee in which a snip of the vastus medialis oblique muscle is performed. The incision is extended several centimeters distally on the tibia to allow harvesting of the semitendinosus tendon. The harvested tendon is looped to create a four-stranded graft in which the ends are secured with nonabsorbable suture (Fig. 128.3). The graft length and size are measured using calipers.

The tibial surface is prepared by carefully removing the osteophytes in the intercondylar groove and around the tibial spine. Any remaining osteophytes can cause inaccurate tibial bone cuts or neoligament rupture due to impingement,[1] and the sagittal tibial bone cut is made. Combined UKA and ACL reconstruction is different than isolated UKA because the tibial resection should be made several millimeters medial to the anatomic ACL insertion site to permit correct positioning of the tibial tunnel. Although essential to prevent biomechanical conflict, this approach can create a mismatch between the AP and the mediolateral size of the tibial component. If the mismatch is too great, the sagittal bone cut may be adjusted to reduce external rotation of the UKA component.

In UKA combined with ACL reconstruction, an anatomic tibial slope should be re-created, whereas in UKA in ACL-deficient knees, the slope should be reduced to obtain better joint stability.[11,26]

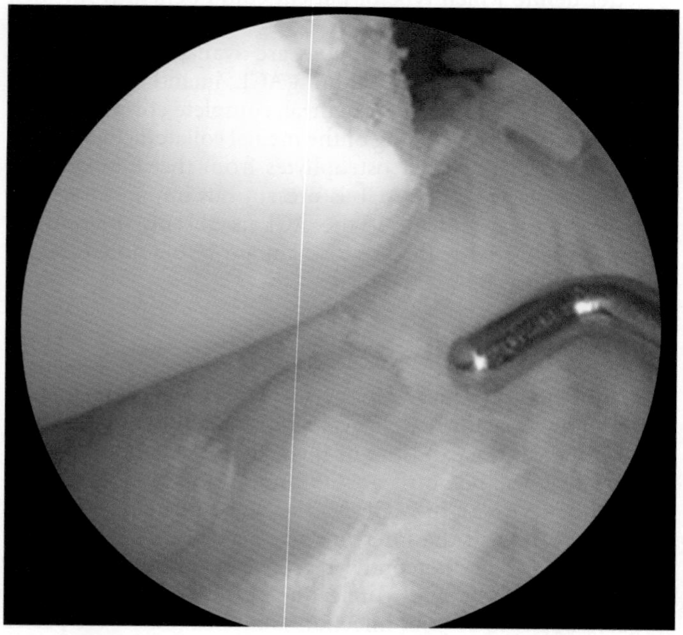

The femoral surface is prepared in a standard manner for UKA. The ACL femoral tunnel is performed accordingly to the diameter and length of the graft, whereas the tibial tunnel is prepared in an open procedure using a standard guide (Fig. 128.4).

The tibial tunnel should be positioned laterally and close to the tibial tuberosity to avoid weakening of the medial tibial plateau and conflict with the prosthesis. Care should be taken to prevent impingement with the external femoral condyle, the posterior cruciate ligament, or the tibial component.[17] This situation underscores the importance of separate drilling of the two tunnels in ACL reconstruction (Fig. 128.5A and B).

The tibial surface is prepared by carefully removing the osteophytes in the intercondylar groove and around the tibial spine, to prevent inaccurate tibial bone cuts or neoligament rupture due to impingement. The sagittal and horizontal tibial bone cuts are made following the preferred technique.

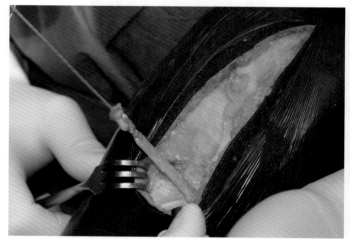

FIG 128.3 Extended incision to allow harvesting of the semitendinosus tendon. The harvested tendon is secured with nonabsorbable suture.

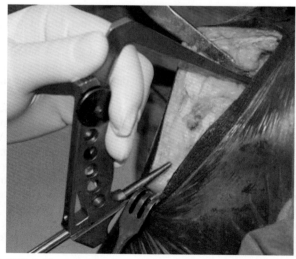

FIG 128.4 The positioning of the tibial guide is vertical and close to the tibial tuberosity.

FIG 128.2 Cartilage defects on the lateral tibial plateau frequently occur following ACL injuries due to trauma.

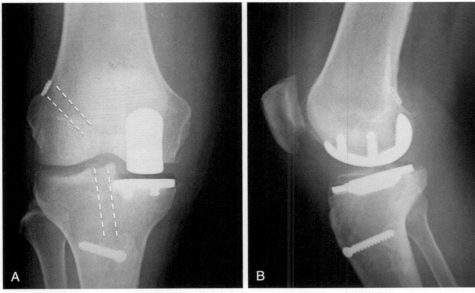

FIG 128.5 (A) AP radiograph shows the complete separation of the tunnels, which allows an anatomic ACL reconstruction. (B) Lateral radiograph showing correct placement of the tunnels and the hardware.

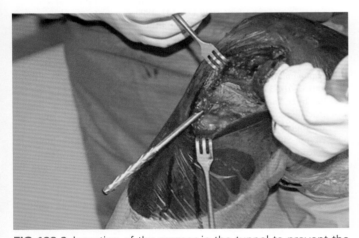

FIG 128.6 Insertion of the reamer in the tunnel to prevent the cement from entering the tunnel.

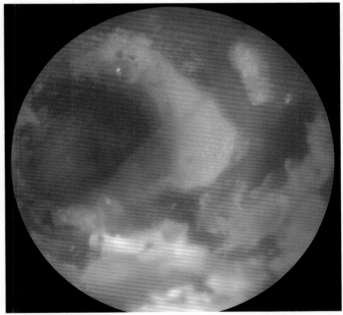

FIG 128.7 Arthroscopic inspection revealing no cement overflow in the prepared tunnels.

After preparing the prosthesis components and the tunnels for the neoligament, the medial meniscus and posteromedial osteophytes are removed. This procedure is easy to perform because the absence of the ACL allows optimum visualization of the posteromedial corner with external rotation of the tibia. One of the final steps is cementing the prosthesis components. We routinely use a fixed bearing design SIGMA HP (DePuy Synthes Inc., Warsaw, IN). A reamer equal in size to the tunnel diameter is inserted into the tunnel to prevent the cement from entering the tunnel and creating problems with the neoligament (Fig. 128.6).

Following polymerization of the bone cement, the tunnel is visually inspected with the arthroscope for cement overflow and cleaned if necessary (Fig. 128.7).

The tendon graft is fixed to the femur with an EndoButton (Smith & Nephew, Memphis, TN) (Fig. 128.8).

The type of tibial fixation is decided intraoperatively depending on bone quality, tunnel orientation, and size. Generally, we prefer not to use absorbable interference screws because they can weaken the biomechanical hold of the tibial plateau. Instead, we usually use nonabsorbable sutures tied around a screw that is used as a post for tibial fixation (Fig. 128.9).

Finally, we suggest selecting the insert thickness following the neoligament placement. In this way, the risk of excessive stabilization of the knee joint, overcorrection, and lateral compartment overloading can be avoided.

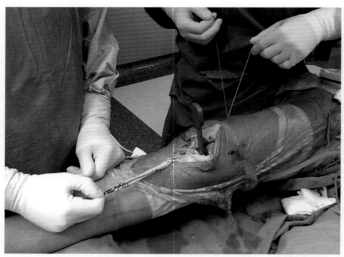

FIG 128.8 Fixation of the tendon graft with the EndoButton. The trial insert is left in situ and helps with the correct choice of the final implant after the ACL reconstruction.

INTRA- AND POSTOPERATIVE TREATMENT

A thigh tourniquet is applied and the surgery is performed under spinal anesthesia. To prevent heavy bleeding, tranexamic acid is administered intravenously in two doses. Intra-articular infiltration of a local anesthetic, adrenaline, and multimodal analgesia are administered during surgery. The treated knee is kept in flexion for 4 hours and drains are removed 24 hours following surgery. Protected ambulation is permitted on the first postoperative day with bracing and crutches under physiotherapist supervision. The patient is generally discharged from the hospital on postoperative day 3. A knee brace is worn for the first 14 days, with instructions for protected weight-bearing using crutches for 25 days postoperatively.

CONCLUSION

In conclusion, in young and active patients with medial OA secondary to ACL rupture, combined ACL reconstruction with

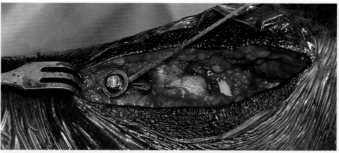

FIG 128.9 Intraoperative image showing the use of the nonabsorbable sutures secured around the screw used as a post to avoid weakening the bone below the implants.

UKA may be indicated. In cases of ACL rupture secondary to progressive OA, total knee replacement is be preferred. Finally, in selected, low-demand patients with early-stage OA, isolated UKA with specific technical adaptations may be indicated.

KEY REFERENCES

7. Dejour D: Laxite chonique anterioeure et arthrhose et pre-arhrose. *8èmes Journ Lyon Chir Genou* 127–131, 1995.
11. Engh GA, Ammeen DJ: Unicondylar arthroplasty in knees with deficient anterior cruciate ligaments. *Clin Orthop Relat Res* 472:73–77, 2014.
21. Mancuso F, Hamilton TW, Kumar V, et al: Clinical outcome after UKA and HTO in ACL deficiency : a systematic review. *Knee Surg Sports Traumatol Arthrosc* 24(1):112–122, 2016. doi: 10.1007/s00167-014-3346-1.
25. Pandit H, Van Duren BH, Gallagher JA, et al: Combined anterior cruciate reconstruction and Oxford unicompartmental knee arthroplasty: in vivo kinematics. *Knee* 15(2):101–106, 2008.
32. Weston-Simons JS, Pandit H, Jenkins C, et al: Outcome of combined unicompartmental knee replacement and combined or sequential anterior cruciate ligament reconstruction: a study of 52 cases with mean follow-up of five years. *J Bone Joint Surg Br* 94(9):1216–1220, 2012.

The references for this chapter can also be found on www.expertconsult.com.

129

Fixed-Bearing Medial Unicompartmental Knee Arthroplasty

Hassan Alosh, Erdan Kayupov, Craig J. Della Valle

INTRODUCTION

Among reconstructive procedures for degenerative joint disease (DJD) of the knee, unicompartmental arthroplasty (UKA) has experienced the greatest growth in recent years. Between 1998 and 2005 the annual increase in rate of UKA was approximately 30% per year, in comparison to approximately 9.5% per year for total knee arthroplasty (TKA), in the United States.[28] The rate and number of UKAs performed have also eclipsed the projected rate of patients expected to undergo revision TKA and is currently between 6% and 8% of all knee arthroplasties performed.[8] Medial compartment UKA was originally developed in the 1960s, with promising initial results. Both the McKeever and MacIntosh design represented the earliest UKA prosthesis, with 70% to 90% pain relief at intermediate follow-up.[14,22] Unfortunately, in subsequent years, flawed designs, improper patient selection, and technical errors led to declined application of this operation. Furthermore, the rapid evolution of TKA design and increasingly favorable results of total knee replacement lead some to all together abandon the concept of UKA. The fixed-bearing UKA was resurrected with increased interest in minimally invasive techniques and bone-preserving procedures in 1990s. Furthermore, recent emphasis on decreasing length of stay and rapid postoperative mobilization have made UKA an increasingly attractive option for the appropriate candidate.

Among the various iterations of UKA design, the two prostheses most commonly compared are fixed- and mobile-bearing designs. Advocates of the mobile-bearing design argue that meniscal bearings reduce surface contact stresses by allowing a greater degree of conformity between articular surfaces.[1] Furthermore, some have suggested that the mobile-bearing knee recreates tibiofemoral kinematics more accurately than fixed-bearing prosthesis, arguing that this is more aligned with the demands placed by younger, active patients undergoing UKA.[16] The Oxford mobile-bearing UKA was introduced in 1978 and initial midterm results demonstrated an impressive 98% survivorship at 10 years.[25] However, subsequent studies have suggested lower survivorship with mobile-bearing UKA, particularly in institutions where the prosthesis is not used frequently.[16] Furthermore, the technical difficulty of achieving a balanced mobile-bearing UKA has been cited frequently, and liner dislocation is a complication unique to this prosthesis that has been attributed to improper soft-tissue balancing or impingement of the bearing against posterior femoral osteophytes.[21,29] Although some theoretical advantages have been ascribed to mobile-bearing UKA, there is sparse clinical data to suggest that it has resulted in improved clinical outcomes or survivorship when compared with a fixed-bearing design.

Fixed-bearing UKA has been used in the earliest UKA prosthesis designs and continues to demonstrate excellent and consistent outcomes in long-term series. The earliest UKA designs consisted of an all-polyethylene tibial component, dating back to Marmor's original prosthesis design. Subsequent investigations have demonstrated higher rates of tibial loosening and failures with all-polyethylene bearings, which has contributed to the rise of modular tibial component designs. Though requiring slightly more tibial resection, modular tibia in fixed-bearing UKA has an excellent record of survivorship and successful clinical outcomes.

INDICATIONS

Among the early reasons for failures of medial UKA was a misunderstanding of the surgical indications and criteria for this procedure. Since then, this operation has emerged as a viable surgical solution for medial compartment osteoarthritis (OA) or osteonecrosis. Despite the progress that has been made in the past several decades, controversies continue to exist regarding appropriate patient selection for medial UKA. Among these issues, the appropriate age for UKA, the degree of residual deformity acceptable, the competency of the anterior cruciate ligament, and perhaps the least elucidated, the status of the patellofemoral joint, have all been debated as the criteria for medial UKA continues to be delineated.

From the standpoint of age, a bimodal distribution of patients has been observed in many series of UKA. As a bone-preserving procedure with more accurate restoration of normal knee kinematics, medial UKA presents an ideal arthroplasty option for a younger, more active population. In a series of 41 patients (45 knees) under the age of 60 who underwent UKA with Miller-Galante system, 93% (39 knees) had excellent outcomes as assessed by Hospital for Special Surgery (HSS) scores and good for three (7%) knees with a mean follow-up of 11 years. Three patients required revision, two for polyethylene wear and one for tibial loosening.[27] A more recent investigation demonstrated excellent results in a series of 75 patients under the age of 55 (mean, 49 years; range, 33 to 55) who had undergone medial UKA with a mean 4 year follow-up (range, 2 to 12 years).[7] Prosthesis used were the Miller-Gallante (7 knees) or

Zimmer UKA (88 knees) (Zimmer, Warsaw, Indiana). At follow-up, Knee Society scores improved from 49 to 95.1. Three patients underwent revision to TKA, two for lateral compartment progression and one for pain. The estimated survivorship was 96.5% at 10 years.

Among older patients with isolated medial compartment disease, UKA is an attractive alternative to TKA because it is a less morbid procedure with lower complication rates than TKA. A multicenter analysis has confirmed the decreased complication burden of UKA. In a review of 2235 TKAs and 605 UKA performed at three institutions, overall risk of complications was 11% with TKA and 4.3% with UKA ($p < .0001$).[9] In comparison to UKA, TKA was associated with increased rates of intensive care unit admission (odd ratio [OR], 7.4; $p = .049$) and had longer hospital stays (mean, 3.3 vs. 2.0 days; $p < .0001$). Although not statistically significant, the study also revealed greater trends towards transfusion, deep infection, and thromboembolic events with TKA. Therefore in the elderly population with less physiologic reserves, UKA presents an attractive alternative to the morbidity of TKA in the appropriate candidate.

The majority of the arthroplasty population considering either UKA or TKA will present with predominantly medial compartment disease typical of varus gonioarthrosis. Within that broad-range patient with medial compartment disease, optimal medial UKA candidacy requires relatively normal knee kinematics. Adequate range of motion, with near full extension and flexion of greater than 110 degrees, has been cited as a prerequisite for UKA given the difficulty in correction flexion contractures with single compartment arthroplasty. With limited access to the posterior capsule and inability to use bony cuts to address residual flexion contracture, UKA presents limited options to correct this deformity in patients presenting with a significant contracture. In a study investigating the relationship between residual flexion contracture following UKA and postoperative (HSS) knee scores, 109 knees were followed for a mean of 4.9 years (range, 3 to 19.9 years).[30] Among these patients, 90 (82.6%) demonstrated good-to-excellent scores using the HSS knee scoring system. Patients who had a residual flexion contracture after surgery demonstrated a significantly reduced improvement in clinical outcomes scores.

Furthermore, minimal fixed varus deformity is tolerated in medial UKA, and attempts to correct a fixed varus deformity with UKA have historically led to failure secondary to overstuffing the medial compartment. Fixed varus deformity results in either excess stress placed on the medial UKA, leading to loosening, or acceleration of lateral compartment disease secondary to excessive force placed on that compartment. Some authors have advocated obtaining stress radiographs with the knee in 15 to 20 degrees of flexion to assess the full extent of correctibility of varus deformity prior to embarking on UKA.[13] However, the utility of a varus stress radiograph prior to UKA has been challenged in recent investigations. In a series of 84 patients (91 knees) undergoing TKA for varus knee arthritis, hip-to-ankle standing films, anteroposterior (AP) standing radiographs, and valgus stress radiographs were reviewed and compared with intraoperative Outerbridge grading of the lateral compartment.[34] Varus stress radiographs were obtained with 20 degrees of knee flexion and a valgus force applied to the knee. On stress radiographs, lateral compartment joint space width and corrected mechanical alignment were evaluated (corrected falling between 3 degrees varus to 3 degrees valgus of neutral

mechanical alignment). The authors determined that lateral compartment joint space did not correlate with intraoperative Outerbridge grading of the lateral compartment. They also found that 93% of knees (55/59) with 10 degrees or less of mechanical varus on full-length films were correctable to within 3 degrees of neutral mechanical alignment. A subsequent study investigated a series of 50 patients undergoing robotically navigated UKA and compared the degree of assessed the degree of varus deformity correctibility on stress radiographs varus the correction achieved intraoperatively.[20] In contrast, this investigation found that preoperative stress radiographs insufficiently assessed the degree of deformity correction because 74% of patients were not correctable to neutral mechanical alignment preoperatively. After osteophyte removal, a significantly greater degree of correction was obtained to a mean corrected alignment of 1.6 ± 2.5 degrees of varus (range, 6 degrees varus to 4 degrees valgus). In conclusion, literature suggests that stress radiographs may not provide a complete assessment of how correctable a varus deformity is when planning for a medial UKA.

An incompetent anterior cruciate ligament (ACL) is a relative, though not absolute, contraindication to fixed-bearing UKA, in contradistinction to mobile-bearing UKA, which risks bearing dislocation in the setting of an incompetent ACL. In general, patients with an intact ACL will meet the other criteria for UKA, including high degrees of preoperative range of motion and minimal deformity. Preoperatively, lateral radiographs can help to identify an anteromedial wear pattern typical of ACL-deficient knees. If a fixed-bearing UKA is to be pursued with an incompetent ACL, it is advisable to reduce the tibial slope to neutral to minimize the shear forces on the implant. A cadaveric study investigated the effects of sectioning the ACL and altering the tibial slope in the setting of a fixed-bearing medial UKA.[33] The investigators found that when the ACL had been sectioned, sagittal motion predictably increased with pivot shift and Lachman testing. When the tibial component was inserted at neutral slope, the sagittal motion of the knee was similar to that of an ACL-competent knee; however, the kinematics of the pivot-shift test remained abnormal.

Obesity has historically been considered a contraindication for medial UKA, and early authors cited concerns for early loosening to justify this position. Some reports have suggested that survivorship is not adversely associated with obesity. In a retrospective series of 212 UKA performed with the HLS UKA prosthesis (Tornier, Grenoble, France), patients with a body mass index (BMI) less than 30 had a survivorship of 94%, versus those with a BMI of greater than 30 had survivorship of 92%, which was not significantly different. There was also no significant difference in Knee Society scores (KSSs). However, this investigation did not address perioperative medical complications. A much larger database review of 15,770 patients who had undergone UKA between 2005 and 2011 strongly implicates obesity as a risk factor for revision[17]; 1823 patients were obese (BMI 30 to 30.9), and 1019 were morbidly obese (BMI >40). Major complications were defined as pulmonary embolism, deep vein thrombosis, postoperative infection, and myocardial infarction. Obese patients had a twofold greater risk of major complications (5.3% vs. 2.3%), and morbidly obese patients had a three-fold increase (7.2% vs. 2.3%). Morbidly obese patients had a 1.8-fold increased rate of revision, and obese patients had 2.2-fold increased revision rate versus nonobese patients. However, the reader should keep in mind that studies of TKA have similarly shown a higher risk of complications and revisions in the obese patient, and hence it is unclear which is a better option for this patient population.

Although medial compartment degenerative disease is the most common indication for medial UKA, osteonecrosis isolated to the medial compartment is also an excellent indication for this operation. Marmor originally reported on a series of 34 knees who underwent UKA for medial compartment DJD with a minimum 2 year follow-up (mean, 5.5 years).[24] He reported four patients with unsatisfactory clinical results of which two were because of progression of osteonecrosis to the lateral compartment. The reasons for persistent pain in the other two patients were not identified. More recently, a series of 84 patients with magnetic resonance imaging (MRI)-confirmed isolated medial compartment osteonecrosis were followed after undergoing UKA with the Depuy Preservation prosthesis (Depuy, Warsaw, Indiana) for a minimum of 3 years (mean, 98 months; range, 63 to 145 months).[10] The authors reported 89% survivorship at 10 years, with 10 patients (12%) undergoing revision. Four revisions were for subsidence of the tibial component, three for aseptic loosening of the tibial component, medial tibial fracture in one, and infection in one patient. Patients who did not undergo revision had a significant improvement in clinical outcomes scores and range of motion. Visual pain scores improved from a mean of 8.6 ± 1.6 (7 to 10) to 1.7 ± 2.5 (0 to 3), and flexion improved from 102 ± 5 degrees to 130 ± 10 degrees. In summary, medial UKA appears to be a viable treatment option for isolated medial compartment osteonecrosis, although one must be cognizant of the possibility for failure secondary to failure of component fixation or the presence of osteonecrosis in the lateral compartment.

Perhaps the most poorly understood criterions for UKA is the status of the patellofemoral joint. Although historical guidelines have suggested the presence of patellofemoral disease as a contraindication to medial UKA, recent findings have prompted revisiting this issue. Some authors have considered the presence of moderate patellofemoral disease to be an absolute contraindication based on their few failures being attributed to progression of disease in this compartment.[1] However, subsequent investigations of fixed-bearing prosthesis in which the appearance of the patellofemoral joint was ignored have demonstrated good results. Biswal and Brighton reported on a series of 128 knees undergoing UKA with the Allegretto prosthesis.[6] Patients with radiographic patellofemoral disease were included unless they complained of patellofemoral symptoms. At an average of 5.7 years (range, 3 to 8 years), there were a total of nine revisions, none of which were for patellofemoral disease. A longer-running series reviewing 203 UKA performed with the St Georg sled (Link, Hamburg, Germany), a fixed-bearing, all-polyethylene tibia prosthesis, also ignored patellofemoral disease if clinically asymptomatic.[32] At a mean 14.8 year (range, 10 to 29 year) follow-up, the authors reported a revision rate of 7.9% (16 knees). Only one of these revisions was for patellofemoral disease. In comparison to fixed-bearing prosthesis, series using the Oxford prosthesis (Biomet, Bridgend, UK) have reported on performing UKA in patients with intraoperative full-thickness defects in the trochlea and patella, with no decrease in Knee Society total scores at 1 year, although they did have worse Knee Society function scores.[2] In addition, the authors reported on a series of 100 Oxford UKAs performed with 2-year follow-up, in which 54% (54 knees) had anterior knee pain.[3] The authors demonstrated no significant difference

in Oxford or American Knee scores at 2 years in comparison with patients without patellofemoral disease or anterior knee pain.

In general, what we observe most commonly intraoperatively is some degenerative changes of the medial facet of the patella and trochlea; however, the lateral side of the patellofemoral joint is usually intact, and this appearance seems to be associated with minimal risk of persistent postoperative pain or arthritis progression. However, the surgeon should be wary of the patient who has disease of the lateral side of the patellofemoral articulation, either on the plain x-rays or upon intraoperative inspection when performing medial UKA, because this combination appears to have a worse prognosis.

In summary, ideal indications for medial UKA include radiographic evidence of noninflammatory arthritis that predominantly affects the medial compartment (Fig. 129.1).

In our practice, age is not heavily considered in the decision-making process because potential advantages exist for both the younger and older patient, so long as the patient does not desire a return to running sports. As has been seen with TKA, suboptimal results can be expected if full-thickness cartilage damage is not obvious on the plain x-rays because patients with less severe disease oftentimes have poorer outcomes. Ideally patients should have a minimal flexion contracture, flexion that typically exceeds 120 degrees and minimal deformity, which is usually associated with an intact ACL. In general, evidence either on the plain x-rays or intraoperatively of lateral compartment disease is not tolerated given the risk of lateral compartment progression. What is less clear is how important degenerative changes of the patellofemoral joint or symptoms of anterior knee pain are to the success of the procedure. In our own practice, we have become much more tolerant of degenerative changes of the patellofemoral joint, particularly if isolated to its medial side.

SURGICAL TECHNIQUE

Medial UKA at our institution is typically performed with neuraxial anesthesia or an adductor canal block. The knee is flexed at 90 degrees for skin incision, which is typically a straight line with its distal end along the medial aspect of the tibial tubercle (TT) and its proximal extent at the proximal pole of the patella (Fig. 129.2).

A common error made, particularly early in the learning curve of this procedure, is insufficient incision length, resulting in excess tension on the edges of the wound and improper exposure, leading to additional errors. Subvastus and midvastus approaches have been described for medial UKA, although we use a standard medial parapatellar approach. When making the arthrotomy, care is taken to avoid damage to the trochlea. Periarticular injections of a local anesthetic plus ketorolac have been shown to be advantageous and are used routinely.[18] As the fascial layer is identified during the exposure, a wheal is developed with the local anesthetic along the path of the fascial incision. The periosteum of the tibia and femur adjacent to the bony cuts is also infiltrated with the anesthetic injection as they are encountered during the exposure.

Excess synovium obstructing the medial compartment is removed along with the anterior horn of the medial meniscus. A minimal medial release of the deep medial collateral ligament (MCL) is performed just distal to the joint line for the purposes of exposure. Over-release of the MCL can lead to overcorrection of varus deformity, which has been recognized as a mode of

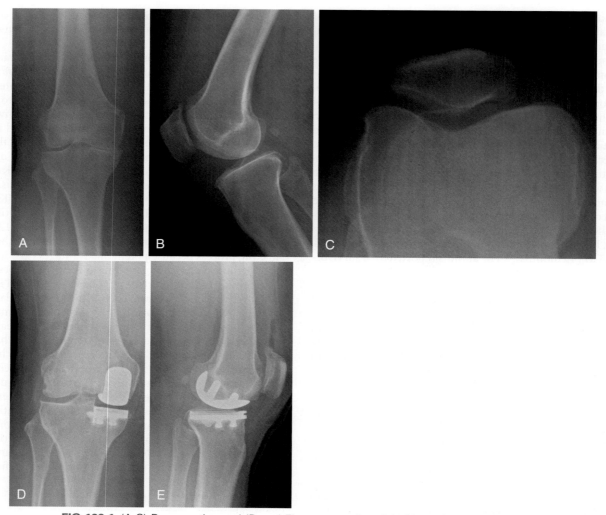

FIG 129.1 (A-C) Preoperative and (D and E) postoperative plain films of a medial UKA.

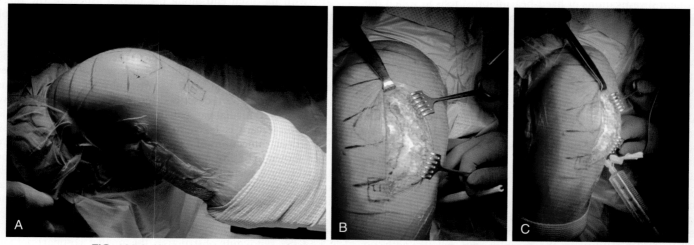

FIG 129.2 (A) Incision relative to patella (P) and tibial tubercle (TT). (B) Medial parapatellar arthrotomy. (C) Injection with periarticular local anesthetic during the exposure.

failure. Partial resection of the infrapatellar fat pad may be required for visualization, although this typically is much less than that required for a TKA. At this point the knee is inspected to ensure competency of the ACL and that the lateral and patellofemoral compartments are acceptable for a medial UKA (Fig. 129.3).

We then proceed with careful removal of femoral and tibial osteophytes, which also facilitates exposure and balancing the UKA. Excision of notch osteophytes helps to avoid later impingement with the ACL. Any osteophytes along the medial side of the patella are also resected at this time (Fig. 129.4).

The knee is then flexed to approximately 60 degrees, and an intramedullary pilot hole is drilled into the femur. The pilot hole is centered over the femoral notch. An intramedullary cutting jig set at 4 degrees of valgus is then used for the distal femoral cut (Fig. 129.5).

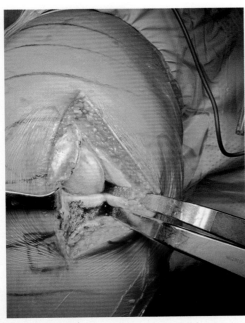

FIG 129.3 Limited medial release with exposure.

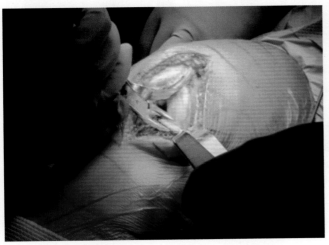

FIG 129.4 Resection of medial osteophytes.

Although extramedullary instrumentation can be used, we prefer intramedullary instrumentation. The advantages of an intramedullary cutting jig include its familiarity to arthroplasty surgeons who perform TKA. In addition, it ensures the angle of the distal femoral cut is made with an easily reproducible fashion relative to the axis of the femur. Finally, the intramedullary rod can be used to help to retract the patella from the surgical field, as demonstrated in Fig. 129.5C. As also noted from the figure, the medial collateral ligament is protected at all times while the distal femoral cut is made. Confirmation of the appropriate thickness of distal femur resection is performed to ensure appropriate balance; in general, the distal femoral resection should equal the thickness of the femoral component it replaces, although in general we will accept slight underresection to account for the distal femoral bone loss, which is often seen in anteromedial arthritis (Fig. 129.6).

The tibial cut is then made using an extramedullary guide. The guide axis should be in line with the center of the ankle joint and parallel in the coronal plane to the tibial crest (Fig. 129.7A). The anteroposterior position of the guide should be positioned to match the patient's native tibial slope. In the scenario of an ACL-deficient knee, it is advisable to cut the tibia with less slope, as previously described. Excessive tibial slope will result in more strain on the ACL with knee flexion. A minimal tibial resection of 2 to 3 mm should be the goal of the tibial cut, so as to allow the prosthesis to sit on stronger subchondral bone. A thin polyethylene liner (8 to 9 mm) has demonstrated good long-term results, and wear is an infrequent mode of failure in UKA in our experience. A reciprocating saw is then used to finish the tibial cut in the sagittal plane in line with the tibial eminence with care to protect the ACL; however, the surgeon should get as close to the ACL as possible to maximize tibial size, which enhances the surface area for fixation of the implant (see Fig. 129.7B and C).

Upon completing the tibial cut, a spacer block corresponding to the composite prosthesis thickness may be used to determine if the flexion and extension gaps are equivalent and if enough tibia has been resected. The extension and flexion spaces should accommodate a spacer that is 2 to 3 mm thicker than the smallest polyethylene liner available, to ensure adequate laxity. If the spacer is tight in both flexion and extension, more tibia needs to be resected. If the spacer is "ok" in extension but tight in flexion, it typically means that the distal femur has been over-resected or that the tibial slope is inadequate. Similarly, if the extension space is tight but the flexion space is adequate, either the distal femur was under-resected or tibial slope is excessive. Alignment of the tibial cut with a drop rod is also checked at this time (Fig. 129.8).

With the knee in extension, the remnant of the posterior horn of the medial meniscus is easily accessible for removal.

The knee is then flexed and attention is then turned to sizing the femoral component. When sizing the femoral component, a balance must be achieved between placing a component that is anatomically located versus one that may potentially impinge on the patella. We aim to have the most anterior extension of the femoral component just below the subchondral line of the distal femur (Fig. 129.9). When in doubt, choose the smaller component to eliminate the risk of the patella impinging on the femoral component. The rotation of the posterior femoral cutting guide should be parallel to the tibial cut.

After making the cuts, posterior osteophytes are easily accessible for removal with a curved osteotome or curette. The tibial

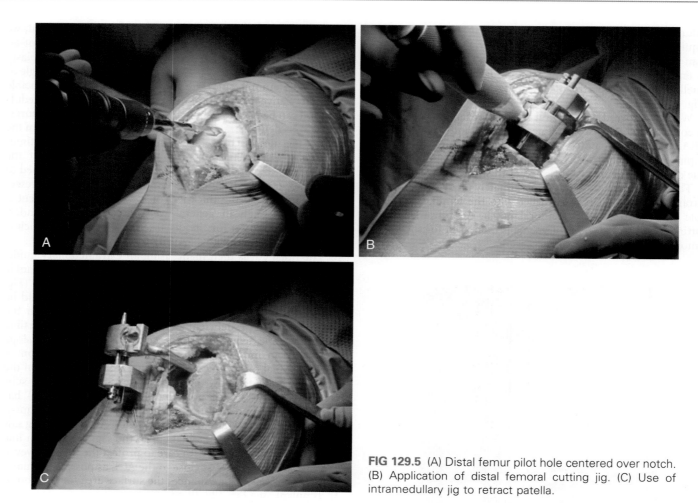

FIG 129.5 (A) Distal femur pilot hole centered over notch. (B) Application of distal femoral cutting jig. (C) Use of intramedullary jig to retract patella.

FIG 129.6 A measured resection of the distal femur. The thickness removed from the distal femur (A) is similar to the thickness of the component to be implanted (B) accounting for the thickness of the saw blade.

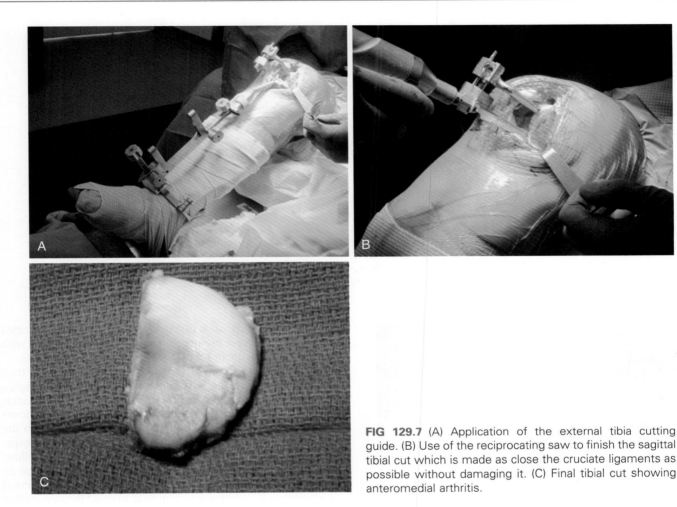

FIG 129.7 (A) Application of the external tibia cutting guide. (B) Use of the reciprocating saw to finish the sagittal tibial cut which is made as close the cruciate ligaments as possible without damaging it. (C) Final tibial cut showing anteromedial arthritis.

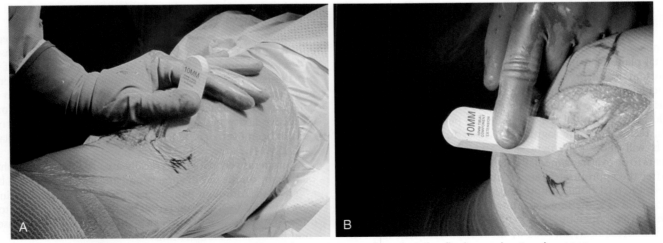

FIG 129.8 (A and B) Use of a calibrated spacer to confirm that the flexion and extension gaps are similar in size and that adequate tibial bone has been resected. In the system we use, an 8-mm polyethylene is the thinnest available, and hence we ensure that the 10-mm spacer block fits in both flexion and extension. If only the 8-mm block fits, additional tibia should be resected.

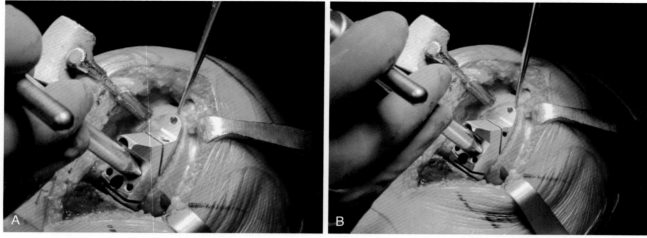

FIG 129.9 (A) This size is too large, overhanging the subchondral bone, risking impingement against the patella. (B) Application of a correctly posterior femoral cutting guide.

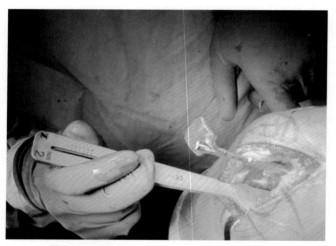

FIG 129.10 Sizing of the tibial component.

component can then be sized using measuring gauge in the sagittal plane or using the excised tibial bone as a guide. It is important to ensure no overhang of the tibial component, particularly in the coronal plane, because this can lead to soft tissue irritation or edge-loading of the component. However, we do strive to fit as large a component as possible, and in some cases, recutting of the sagittal cut closer to the cruciate ligaments will allow placement of a larger component if there appears to be overhang medially but not anteriorly (Fig. 129.10).

After the appropriately sized components have been determined, the trial tibial component is inserted with the knee in flexion; this is sometimes facilitated by placing a valgus stress on the knee to "open up" the medial compartment. The femoral trial is inserted next, followed by the trial polyethylene liner. At this point, the surgeon must ensure that the femoral component tracks centrally on the tibia without overhang medially as this will lead to edge loading of the polyethylene and rapid wear. Furthermore, we aim to have approximately 2 to 3 mm of laxity in both flexion and extension.[1] This helps to guard against overcorrection of the varus deformity, which has been shown to lead to progression of disease in the lateral compartment. We

assess this amount of laxity using 2- and 3-mm calibrated spacers with the knee in extension and flexion, respectively, with all trial components in place (Fig. 129.11).

With satisfactory trial placement, the bony surfaces are then prepared for cementing. After cleansing with pulsatile lavage, a small drill can be used to enhance cement penetration in areas of sclerotic bone. Our preference is to use one unit of cement that is pressurized using an angled tip that is placed into the tibial lug holes. A thin layer of cement is applied to the remaining tibia, with care to compress the cement into the cancellous bone of the proximal tibia using the surgeon's finger and/or an osteotome (Fig. 129.12). The tibial component itself is inserted in a posterior to anterior direction so as to avoid the aggregation of cement behind the tibia (Fig. 129.13). Insertion of the tibial component is mostly easily performed with the knee flexed and with a slight valgus stress applied. The lugs for the femoral component are pressurized with cement from the gun, with additional cement placed on both the component and the remaining cut bony surfaces.

The liner trial is then placed, and the cement is allowed to cure with the knee in extension. A curved probe is often useful to excise residual cement from the posterior aspect of the prosthesis. With removal of the trial liner any excess cement is more easily accessible (see Fig. 129.13). After the cement has cured, a 2-mm spacer is again used to confirm that enough protective laxity has been obtained and the varus deformity has not been overcorrected, and the appropriate liner is placed (Fig. 129.14).

Postoperatively patients typically are ambulated with physical therapy on the day of surgery and are allowed to weight bear as tolerated. Although patients traditionally have had an inpatient stay of 1 to 2 days, in recent years, many have opted to go home the same day of surgery, with no apparent increase in complications or readmissions.

REPORTED OUTCOMES

Early reports of the outcomes of UKA were discouraging, with nearly 30% failure rates. Since then, multiple series have established that long-term outcomes and survivorship of fixed-bearing UKA prosthesis rivals that of TKA. These studies have

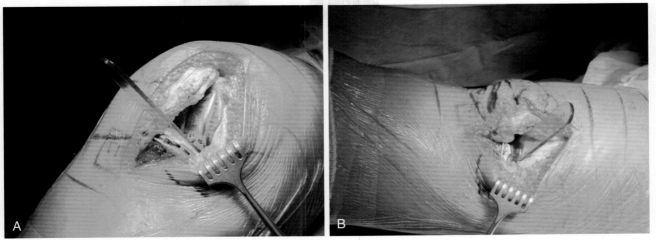

FIG 129.11 (A and B) Use of the 2-mm calibrated spacers in flexion and extension to confirm appropriate laxity with trial components in place.

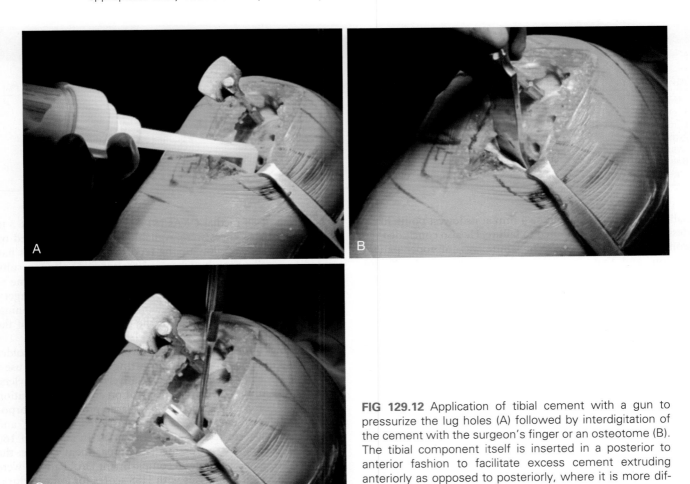

FIG 129.12 Application of tibial cement with a gun to pressurize the lug holes (A) followed by interdigitation of the cement with the surgeon's finger or an osteotome (B). The tibial component itself is inserted in a posterior to anterior fashion to facilitate excess cement extruding anteriorly as opposed to posteriorly, where it is more difficult to remove (C).

helped to transform the perception of UKA from an intermediate procedure until a TKA is required, to a definitive surgical solution in the appropriately selected patient (Table 129.1).

Among the first earliest fixed-bearing designs was the Marmor prosthesis (Richards, UK), which used an all-polyethylene tibial component. The implantation technique was resurfacing based and consisted of implanting the prosthesis onto subchondral bone with minimal bone resection. Marmor reported on a series of 60 knees with a minimum of 10 years follow-up (mean, 11 years, range 10 to 13).[23] He reported 21 failures, with the majority being caused by loosening of the tibial component. The polyethylene tibial component in the

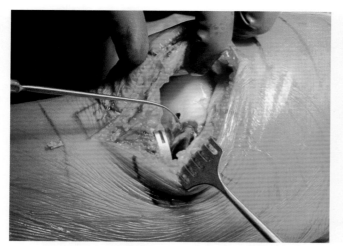

FIG 129.13 Removal of excess cement after removal of the trial liner but prior to placement of the final polyethylene.

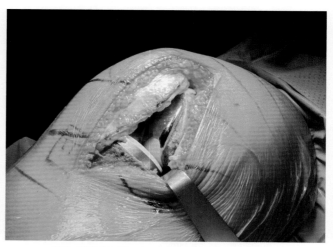

FIG 129.14 Final components in position.

TABLE 129.1   Summary of Fixed Medial Unicompartmental Survivorship and Clinical Outcomes

Author	Publication Year	Implant	# Unicompartmental Arthroplasty at Follow-Up (n)	Mean Follow-Up (Years)	Ten-Year Survivorship (%)
Marmor[23]	1988	Marmor	60	11	65
Scott et al.[31]	1991	Brigham	64	10	85
Cartier et al.[11]	1996	Marmor	60	12	93
Argenson et al.[1]	2002	Miller-Galante	160	5.5	94
Naudie et al.[26]	2004	Miller-Galante	97	10	90
Berger et al.[5]	2005	Miller-Galante	49	12	98
Steele et al.[32]	2006	St Georg Sled	134	14.8	80

smallest Marmor tibia could be 4 mm at its lowest point, likely a design issue that contributed to failure. He also concluded the second most common cause of failure was improper patient selection, and that six patients in the series had adjacent compartment disease that proved too advanced to be indicated for UKA.

The St Georg Sled, another resurfacing-based prosthesis with an all-polyethylene tibia, demonstrated reasonable survivorship at long-term follow-up.[32] Steele et al. reported on a series of 203 UKAs, which had survived a minimum of 10 years (mean, 14.8 years; range, 10 to 29). Survivorship in that series was reported at 85.9% at 20 years. The majority of revisions (16 knees) was progression of arthritis (7 knees), wear of polyethylene (3 knees), and tibial loosening (4 knees).

The next iteration of fixed-bearing prosthesis designs consisted of metal-backed tibias with an inset implantation design. With an inset design, angular cuts are made to prepare the cancellous bone for implanting the prosthesis similar to a TKA. The metal-backed tibia had several advantages, including facilitation of cement removal and allowing titration of the protective laxity required for UKA longevity. The early metal-backed tibial designs did not fare well with regard to longevity, mainly because of prosthesis design issues. The Porous Coated Anatomic Knee (Stryker, Mahwah, NJ) had a constrained prosthesis geometry design coupled with an early generation polyethylene liner. This resulted in a high rate of failure secondary to component loosening and/or excessive wear of the polyethylene liner. Bergenudd reported on a series of 108 knees

consisting of 88 medial UKAs (81%) with a follow-up of 3 to 7 years.[4] Ninety knees were available for follow-up. Based on HSS scores at last follow-up, he reported 61% of patients had good-to-excellent results, whereas 39% had fair or poor results. There was a total of 27 revisions (30%) with average time to revision being 39 months (range, 11 to 80 months) after surgery. Most revisions[13] were because of femoral component loosening. He also reported severe wear of the polyethylene in 14 of the revisions.

Building upon the lessons of previous series with older prosthesis designs, modern fixed-bearing UKA evolved to use a cemented metal-backed tibia, a relatively thick polyethylene liner, and a minimally constrained, flat on concave articulation geometry. For example, the Miller-Galante prosthesis incorporated these elements and has demonstrated longevity and excellent long-term results in several series. In a study of 160 UKAs, 145 (91%) were for medial compartment disease, the balance being done for lateral compartment OA.[1] Patients were followed at annual intervals with HSS scores for a mean duration of 66 months (range, 36 to 112 months). Moderate patellofemoral disease was not considered a contraindication to surgery in that series. Using Kaplan-Meier analysis, the 10-year survival rate was 94%. Two knees were revised for progression of patellofemoral disease, one was for progression lateral compartment disease, and two for polyethylene wear. Subsequent series have confirmed long-term success with this prosthesis design. Naudie et al. reported on 97 medial UKAs performed with the Miller-Galante prosthesis and a mean follow-up of 10 years (range, 3 to 14 years).[26] They reported excellent clinical relief, with 90% survival at 10-years with revision as the end point. Eleven knees were revised: four for lateral compartment disease, three for polyethylene wear, one for MCL injury, and one for retained cement and pain. None were revised for patellofemoral symptoms.

From our center, we reported on 62 UKAs performed in 51 patients, using the Miller-Galante prosthesis with a minimum 10 year follow-up.[5] Patients were deemed appropriate candidates for UKA if they demonstrated unicompartmental OA or osteonecrosis, only mild degeneration of the patellofemoral joint, range of motion of greater than 90 degrees, a flexion contracture of less than 15 degrees, and an age of greater than 50. Fifty-nine (95%) of these patients underwent medial UKA, the remainder involved the lateral compartment. No patients were lost to follow-up, but 13 patients died less than 10 years after their operation for causes unrelated to their arthroplasty. Therefore 38 patients (49 knees) were followed for an average of 12 years (range, 10 to 13 years). Patients were followed with HSS knee scores prospectively on an annual basis. Patients' HSS scores improved from 55 points (range, 30 to 79 points) preoperatively to 92 points (range, 60 to 100 points) at last follow-up. Thirty-nine knees (80%) had an excellent result (85 to 100 points), six (12%) had a good result (70 to 84 points), and four (8%) had a fair result (60 to 69 points). Among the four patients who had a fair result, two underwent conversion to TKA, and the other two had severe cardiopulmonary disease and had limited walking ability. Kaplan-Meier analysis demonstrated 98% survival at 10 years, with revision for any reason or loosening as an endpoint.

Subsequently, this cohort of patients was reassessed to achieve a minimum 15 year follow-up (mean, 19 years; range, 15 to 21 years).[15] Nineteen UKAs in 16 patients were available for this study; 34 patients had died, and one was lost to follow-up. At last follow-up, all but four patients had HSS scores of greater than 75. No patients had evidence of component loosening or osteolysis. Two additional patients were converted to TKA. In all, four patients were converted to TKA: one for patellofemoral and lateral compartment degeneration, one for lateral compartment degeneration, one for polyethylene disengagement and metallosis, and one for pain of unclear cause. Kaplan-Meier analysis with revision or radiographic loosening as an endpoint revealed 93% survivorship at 15 years and 90% survivorship at 20 years.

Fixed-bearing medial UKA has proven to be a successful and durable surgical option for medial compartment OA. The surgical technique and implant design has evolved substantially in the past three decades to provide long-term outcomes and survivorship that is comparable or greater than those for TKA. As a bone-preserving, less invasive procedure with a lower risk of complications, medial UKA is an appealing option for arthroplasty candidates at either end of the age spectrum. Given the remarkable results and renewed attention UKA has received in the arthroplasty community, historical contraindications to medial UKA are being challenged in recent studies. Further investigation is required to delineate the degree of adjacent compartment disease tolerated in the setting of UKA.

The references for this chapter can also be found on www.expertconsult.com.

130

Medial Unicompartmental Knee Arthroplasty Mobile Bearing

Hemant Pandit, David Murray, Christopher A.F. Dodd

This chapter provides an overview of the medial Oxford unicompartmental knee arthroplasty (OUKA) (Fig. 130.1). It covers the historical perspective, indications, surgical principles and surgical technique, complications, and results. A link to a surgical video is also provided.

INTRODUCTION AND HISTORY

Osteoarthritis of the knee is one of the most common causes of painful loss of mobility in middle-aged and older people and is the main indication for knee replacement surgery. Demand for knee arthroplasty is estimated to increase by more than 600% by the year 2030, with nearly 3.5 million patients needing a knee replacement in the United States alone.[12]

Traditionally, two types of knee arthroplasty are offered to patients with symptomatic end-stage knee arthritis—unicompartmental knee arthroplasty (UKA) or total knee arthroplasty (TKA). UKA usage is low and typically used in 5% to 8% of cases undergoing knee replacement, with the remainder undergoing TKA.

Although for many decades it has been recognized that arthritis is often limited to the medial (or lateral) compartment of the knee, the majority of surgical opinions concluded that osteoarthritis of the knee was a disease of the whole joint (like osteoarthritis of the hip) and that common sense required the replacement of all the articular surfaces to provide long-term relief of symptoms. However, the longitudinal studies by Ahlbäck had already suggested that unicompartmental osteoarthritis does not inevitably spread to other parts of the knee.[1] In addition, numerous post-mortem descriptions published in the 1970s and 1980s had revealed the almost universal presence of cartilage lesions in some parts of the joint in middle-aged and older people, implying that their presence is consistent with normal knee function.

In 1974 John Goodfellow and John O'Connor introduced congruous mobile bearings for knee prostheses. The first "Oxford Knee" had a metal femoral component with a spherical articular surface, a metal tibial component that was flat, and a polyethylene mobile bearing, spherically concave above and flat below, interposed between them. The device was fully congruent at both interfaces throughout the range of movement (to minimize polyethylene wear) and fully unconstrained (to allow unrestricted movements and minimize the risk of loosening). These features of the Oxford Knee have remained unchanged to the present day. At first, the implant was used bicompartmentally, as a total joint replacement, with two sets of components inserted, one medially and one laterally. The nonarticular surface of the femoral component of the original design (phase 1) had three inclined facets and was fitted to the femur by

making saw cuts. It became apparent that good results were only achieved if the anterior cruciate ligament (ACL) was intact. Another observation was made: if the ACL was intact, then the arthritis tended to be confined to the anteromedial part of the tibia and the distal part of the medial femoral condyle. In these cases, all ligaments were functionally normal. This disease was called anteromedial osteoarthritis (AMOA).[37] On the basis of these two observations, in 1982 the device began to be used unicompartmentally and the primary indication was AMOA. In 1987 the phase 2 implant was introduced specifically for unicompartmental arthroplasty. The posterior femoral condyle was prepared by a saw cut and its inferior facet was milled by a spherically concave bone-mill rotating around a spigot in a drill hole in the condyle. By shortening the spigot, measured thicknesses of bone could be milled incrementally from the inferior surface of the condyle, allowing the gaps in flexion and extension to be balanced intraoperatively and simultaneously shaping the bone to fit the implant. This accurate system for restoring ligament tension to normal not only decreased the bearing dislocation rate to very low levels but also restored normal knee kinematics.

The long-term results of the phases 1 and 2 Oxford Knee were published by the designers in 1998.[17] An independent surgeon, Dr. Svard in 2001[32] demonstrated for the first time that the long-term survival of UKA can be as good as that achieved by TKA. The phase 1 and 2 prostheses were implanted through an open approach with dislocation of the patella, as in TKA. In 1998 the phase 3 prosthesis was introduced specifically for medial unicompartmental use with a minimally invasive approach. The single size of femoral component (used in all the phase 1 and 2 implants) was replaced by five parametric sizes, the universal tibial plateau was replaced by right- and left-handed tibial components, and the bearings were modified to diminish the likelihood of impingement and rotation. The instruments were miniaturized to facilitate their use through a small parapatellar arthrotomy. The functional results and speed of recovery of phase 3 were found to be better than those of phase 2.[25] In 2004 cementless components based on phase 3 (Fig. 130.2) were first used, although they are still not available for use in the United States because they are not yet US Food and Drug Administration (FDA) approved.

DESIGN RATIONALE

The natural meniscus is an integral part of the tibial articular surface, serving to maximize the contact area without limiting angular and translational movement between the bones. Therefore load is transmitted at an average pressure that the articular cartilage can withstand. Evidence of the importance of this mechanism is provided by the observation that excision (or dysfunction) of a meniscus results in osteoarthritic degeneration of the remaining cartilage surfaces in the affected compartment. During flexion-extension and axial rotation of the native knee, the natural meniscus not only changes its position on the tibial plateau, as the movements of the femoral condyle dictate, but also changes shape to fit the various curvatures of the polyradial femoral condyle. In full extension, the large radius of the inferior surface of the condyle forces the limbs of the meniscus apart in an anteroposterior direction. As the knee flexes and the smaller radius of the posterior condyle is offered, the anteroposterior measurement of the meniscus diminishes appropriately, possibly because divergence of the tibiofemoral contact areas forces the two menisci apart, drawing their anterior and posterior limbs closer together. Changes in the shapes of the menisci are reflected in the differences in anteroposterior movements of the anterior and posterior horns and in the mediolateral movements of the medial and lateral edges of the two menisci observed by Vedi et al.[35]

The mechanical advantages conferred by the natural meniscus can be enjoyed by an artificial knee if it is provided with two joint interfaces instead of one. The design of the articular surfaces of the Oxford Knee has not changed since its first implantation in 1976. The femoral component made of metal has a spherical surface, and the metal tibial component is flat. The polyethylene meniscal bearing has a spherical upper surface and a flat lower surface. The meniscofemoral interface (ball-in-socket) allows the angular movements of flexion-extension, the meniscotibial interface (flat-on-flat) allows translational movements, and axial rotation is allowed by a combination of translation and spinning movement at both interfaces. The unconstrained mobile bearing does not resist the movements demanded by the soft tissues, muscles, and ligaments. Restoration of natural mobility and function may be expected. The surfaces of the prosthesis experience mainly compressive forces, features which should minimize component loosening. A low loosening rate is reflected in a high survival rate.

WHY USE A SPHERICAL AND NOT A POLYRADIAL FEMORAL CONDYLE?

A rigid polyethylene bearing can model only the mobility of the natural meniscus and not its compliance. It cannot change shape and therefore cannot fit more than one of the several radii offered by a polyradial condyle. The only pairs of shapes that can maintain congruity in all relative positions of the components are a sphere in a spherical socket and a flat surface on a flat surface.

Low Wear

Various studies assessing in vivo wear rates after OUKA have demonstrated that the theoretical expectation of a low polyethylene wear rate has been fulfilled in practice.

Twenty-three bearings were retrieved from 18 failed bicompartmental Oxford arthroplasties, 1 to 9 years after implantation.[2] The minimum thickness of each was measured with a dial gauge and compared with the mean thickness of 25 unused bearings. The mean penetration rate was very low; calculated

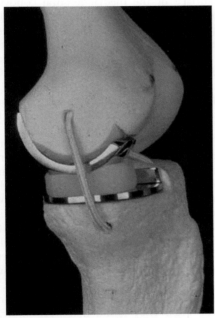

FIG 130.1 Oxford UKA in sawbones.

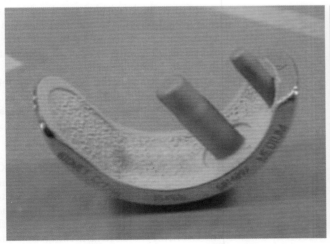
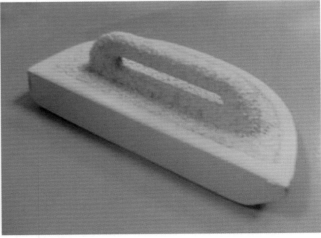

FIG 130.2 Cementless OUKA components.

by two methods, it was either 0.043 or 0.026 mm/year. There was no correlation between the initial minimum thickness of the bearings (range: 3.5 to 10.5 mm) and their rate of wear. Kendrick et al.[6] used the same method to study a further 47 phase 1 and 2 bearings retrieved after OUKA at a mean time to revision of 8.4 years (standard deviation [SD]: 4.1). Twenty had been implanted for more than 10 years (maximum: 17 years). Thirty-one of the 47 bearings showed evidence of impingement, and the mean penetration rate in these was 0.07 mm/year. The rate for the 16 bearings without impingement was 0.01 mm/year. The penetration rate of phase 1 bearings (machined from blocks of Hostalen RCH1000 polyethylene) was approximately double that of phase 2 bearings (individually compression molded from Montel Hifax 1900H powder). However, the impingement rate in phase 1 implants (91%) was also much higher than in phase 2 implants (58%). Kendrick et al. further stratified the impinged bearings into a group showing evidence only of extra-articular impingement damage and those showing articular surface damage from impingement. Those showing intra-articular impingement had a penetration rate 2.5 times that of the group with extra-articular damage alone, whereas the latter had a penetration rate 5 times higher than those (0.01 mm/year) free of impingement damage.

The rate of penetration of the Oxford bearings was also much lower than that reported by Wroblewski[39] for the acetabular component of the fully congruous Charnley hip (0.19 mm/year). This is not surprising because the projected area of contact is larger in the OUKA than in the Charnley hip, and the contact stresses are correspondingly lower. They are also much lower than the mean rate of 0.49 mm/year reported for 81 retrievals of various round-on-flat fixed-bearing designs by Collier et al.[3]

Indications

Anteromedial OA is the most common indication for UKA and is present in approximately half the patients needing knee replacement. The condition can be recognized by a consistent association between the clinical/radiologic signs and the pathologic lesions that cause them.

Principal Physical Signs

1. Knee pain on standing and is severe with walking.
2. With the knee (as near as possible) fully extended, the leg is in varus (5 to 15 degrees), and the deformity cannot be corrected.
3. With the knee flexed 20 degrees or more, the varus can be corrected.
4. With the knee flexed to 90 degrees, the varus corrects spontaneously.

Principal Anatomic Features

At surgery, knees with the above physical signs regularly demonstrate the following anatomic features.

1. Both cruciate ligaments are functionally normal, although the ACL may have suffered some damage and may have longitudinal splits.
2. The cartilage on the medial tibial plateau is eroded, and eburnated bone is exposed, anteriorly and/or centrally. An area of full-thickness cartilage is always preserved at the back of the tibial plateau.
3. The cartilage on the inferior articular surface of the medial femoral condyle is eroded, and eburnated bone is exposed.

The posterior condylar surface retains its full-thickness cartilage.
4. The weight-bearing articular cartilage of the lateral compartment, although often fibrillated, preserves its full thickness. In many cases a full-thickness ulcer can be present on the medial border of the lateral femoral condyle.[7]
5. The medial collateral ligament (MCL) is of normal length.
6. The posterior capsule is shortened, causing flexion deformity.

Correlations

The observed sites of articular surface damage, together with the intact cruciate ligaments and the MCL, explain the symptoms and physical signs.

1. The cruciate ligaments maintain the normal pattern of "rollback" of the femur on the tibia in the sagittal plane and thereby preserve the distinction between the damaged contact areas in extension (the anterior tibial plateau and the inferior surface of the medial femoral condyle) and the intact contact areas in flexion (the posterior tibial plateau and the posterior surface of the femoral condyle).
2. The varus deformity of the extended leg is caused by loss of cartilage and bone from the contact areas in extension.
3. The varus deformity corrects spontaneously at 90 degrees as the articular cartilage is intact in the areas of contact in flexion. Therefore the MCL is drawn out to its normal length every time the patient bends the knee, and structural shortening of the ligament does not occur. Thus an intact ACL ensures an MCL of normal length, as demonstrated by manual correction of the varus when the posterior capsule is relaxed with the knee flexed to 20 degrees or more.

The association of an intact ACL with the focal pattern of cartilage erosions described previously is striking. White et al.[37] described 46 medial tibial plateaus excised sequentially from a series of OA knees treated by OUKA, all of them with an intact ACL and with cartilage erosions exposing bone (Ahlbäck stages 2, 3, and 4). The erosions were all anterior and central. They rarely extended to the posterior quarter of the plateau and never reached the posterior joint margin. Harman et al.[5] examined the tibial plateaus excised from 143 osteoarthritic knees during operations for TKA. They found that wear in ACL-deficient varus knees was located a mean 4 mm more posterior on the medial plateau than wear in ACL-intact knees ($P < .05$). The ACL-deficient knees also exhibited more severe varus deformity. The site and extent of the tibial erosions can be determined reliably from lateral radiographs. Keyes et al.[8] studied the preoperative lateral radiographs of 50 OA knees in which the state of the ACL had been recorded at surgery (25 ACL deficient and 25 ACL intact). Using four blinded observers, they found 95% correlation between preservation of the posterior part of the medial tibial plateau on the radiograph and an intact ACL at surgery and 100% correlation of erosion of the posterior plateau on the radiograph with an absent or badly damaged ACL.

Other Indications

Focal spontaneous osteonecrosis of the knee (SONK): SONK of the medial femoral condyle or, more rarely, of the medial tibial plateau presents anatomic features very similar to those of AMOA (focal loss of bone and cartilage in the medial compartment with the ligaments intact) and therefore is theoretically suitable for OUKA. Preoperative investigation should include magnetic resonance imaging (MRI) in addition to the radiographs. MRI will help to identify cases of SONK prior to subchondral collapse. MRI also helps to understand the extent of pathology and in ruling out multifocal SONK, which is rare but does occur. MRI tends to overestimate the extent of the damage because of the surrounding edema associated with SONK in the acute phase, and this should be ignored in assessing extent of the disease. Unlike AMOA, varus stressed radiographs of knees with AVN lesions usually do not show full-thickness cartilage loss because the tibial cartilage is often preserved. The MRI substantially overestimates the extent of the damage because of the surrounding edema associated with the condition in the acute phase. When assessing the extent of the disease, the edema should be ignored.

Anterior Cruciate Ligament Deficiency

If the ACL is ruptured and there is medial osteoarthritis, the erosions tend to extend to the back of the tibia so the disease is called posteromedial OA. In addition, there is usually cartilage loss on the posterior femur. However, the patho-anatomy is different depending on whether the primary condition was AMOA with secondary ACL rupture or primary ACL rupture with secondary OA.

With primary AMOA the disease begins anteriorly and centrally on the tibia with a varus deformity in extension. As the disease progresses posteriorly and the ACL fails, the varus deformity occurs also in flexion. The MCL shortens and the varus deformity becomes fixed. In addition, the lateral subluxation of the tibia becomes fixed with increasing damage to the lateral side. After these fixed deformities and lateral damage have occurred, the only solution is TKA.

In primary traumatic ACL rupture with secondary medial compartment arthritis, the cartilage defect and bony erosion tend to be central and posterior on the tibial plateau. This is likely to be because of recurrent episodes of giving way in which posterior femoral subluxation in the medial compartment can place a heavy load on the posterior horn of medial meniscus and posterior articular cartilage of the tibia, producing meniscal tears and arthritis. In some cases the rest of the knee joint remains essentially intact with no shortening of the MCL. This is probably because in extension the intact distal femoral cartilage is in contact with the intact anterior tibial cartilage, so the varus deformity is corrected and the MCL is of normal length.

In cases of primary traumatic ACL rupture and secondary OA, which typically occur in younger patients (as compared with the usual cohort of AMOA), we offer combined ACL reconstruction and OUKA, either as a single-stage or a two-stage procedure—ACL reconstruction followed by OUKA implantation.

Previous High Tibial Osteotomy

Thornhill and Scott,[33] using the Brigham implant, referred to some successes in using UKA after failed high tibial osteotomy (HTO) but noted technical problems with ligamentous instability. Vorlat et al.[36] reviewed 38 medial OUKAs, of which six were performed on knees with failed HTO. Two of these had to be revised because of progression of arthritis in the lateral compartment. The failure rate of 33% in the HTO group was compared with a 6.3% failure rate in the group with primary OA. Rees et al.[26] collected data (from three sources) on 631 OUKAs, 18 of which had been performed for failed HTO and the remainder for primary anteromedial OA. The reason for revision of the original HTO was persistent medial pain in every

case, and in all but one there had been undercorrection of the varus deformity. The mean cumulative follow-up times of the two groups were similar (5.6 years and 5.4 years, respectively), and there were no significant differences between their mean ages or gender ratios. The mean time to revision was 2.9 years for the HTO group (five knees) and 4.1 years for the primary OA group (19 knees). The cumulative survival rates at 10 years were 66% and 96%, respectively (log rank comparison $P <$ .0001). The reason for all the OUKA failures in the HTO group was persistent pain and accelerated lateral wear. The failure rate was independent of the type of osteotomy. The explanation for this mode of failure may be biomechanical. OUKA corrects the varus deformity intra-articularly. If the varus has already been corrected (even partially) by an extra-articular osteotomy, valgus alignment may result, with overloading of the lateral compartment.

Valenzuela et al.[34] compared clinical and radiologic outcomes between UKA after HTO ($n = 22$); TKA after HTO ($n = 18$); and primary UKA ($n = 22$). Oxford Knee Score (OKS), American Knee Society Score (AKSS), AKSS-O American Knee Society Score (Objective), AKSS-F American Knee Society Score (Functional), hip-knee-ankle angles, mechanical axis, and patella height were evaluated preoperatively and postoperatively. At a mean of 64 months (range: 19 to 180) postoperatively, the mean OKS were 43.8, 43.3, and 42.5, respectively ($P = .73$), with similar AKSS-O (Objective) and AKSS-F (Functional). The authors' conclusion was that UKA can be safely performed after HTO.

There may be a role for OUKA after failed HTO. However, the indications for this are unclear. We believe that previous tibial osteotomy is a contraindication to OUKA. The revision rate of 34% at a mean follow-up of 5.4 years is much worse than the results reported for TKA after HTO by Meding et al.[16] (one implant failure in 33 knees followed for a mean of 8.7 years after TKA revision of failed tibial osteotomies).

Contraindications

UKA is contraindicated in the inflammatory forms of arthritis because they are diseases of the synovium and therefore cannot be limited to one compartment. Other anatomic contraindications are as follows:

- absent or severely damaged ACL (or posterior cruciate ligament [or PCL] or MCL)
- failure to demonstrate eburnated bone-on-bone contact in the medial compartment
- intra-articular varus not fully correctable
- mediolateral subluxation, not corrected on valgus-stressed films
- flexion deformity greater than 15 degrees
- flexion range less than 100 degrees (under anesthesia)
- thinning or erosion of central cartilage in the lateral compartment
- bone loss (BL) with eburnation and grooving in the lateral part of the patellofemoral joint.

Unnecessary Contraindications

The suggested contraindications for UKA are based on Kozinn and Scott's 1989 publication that stated that patients who weigh more than 82 kg, were younger than 60 years, undertook heavy labor, had exposed bone in the patellofemoral joint (PFJ), or had chondrocalcinosis were not ideal candidates for unicompartmental knee replacement (UKR).[10] We wanted to establish whether these potential contraindications should apply to patients with OUKA. To do this, the outcome of patients with these potential contraindications was compared with that of patients without the contraindications in a prospective series of 1000 OUKAs.[22] The outcome was assessed using the Oxford Knee Score, American Knee Society Score, Tegner activity score, revision rate, and survival. The clinical outcome of patients with each of the potential contraindications was similar to, or better than, those without each contraindication. Overall 678 UKR (68%) were performed in patients who had at least one potential contraindication and only 322 (32%) in patients deemed to be ideal for UKR. The 10-year survival was 97% (95% confidence interval [CI]: 93.4 to 100) for those with potential contraindications and 93.6% (95% CI: 87.2 to 100) in the "ideal" patients. Each of these contraindications, and others, are discussed in detail in this chapter. This difference was also maintained at 15 years. The 15-year survival was 94% (95% CI: 88 to 100) for those with potential contraindications and 90% (95% CI: 78 to 100) in the "ideal" patients.

Surgical Principles

In anteromedial OA the MCL and the cruciate ligaments are intact and have the same mechanical effects as in the normal joint. However, the posterior capsule tends to be shortened, and there is an associated fixed flexion deformity. The effect of this is to close down the medial compartment gap before full extension is reached. For this reason, we assess the gap with the knee flexed at 20 degrees to ensure that the posterior capsule is slack. In all positions of flexion greater than 20 degrees, the medial condyle can be distracted the same distance as in the normal knee because the gap is limited by the normal MCL and cruciates. Therefore distraction in flexion restores normal alignment of the leg. The medial gap appears wider than normal only because cartilage and bone have been lost from the joint surfaces.

In OUKA, medial release should never be undertaken. The MCL is of normal length in anteromedial OA; mobility and stability of the joint, alignment of the leg, and entrapment of the bearing all depend upon its integrity. Balancing the ligaments means adjusting the position of the femoral component relative to the femur (by removing bone) so that the medial distraction gap is the same in flexion and extension. In other words the "flexion gap" and "extension gap" should be equal. As explained previously, the extension gap is measured in 20 degrees flexion because the posterior capsule is slack. The flexion gap is measured at 90 degrees to this, at 110 degrees of knee flexion. The instrumentation is designed to adjust the extension gap without changing the flexion gap. The flexion gap is established first, then the extension gap is adjusted to match it by milling bone from the inferior femoral condyle.

OPERATIVE TECHNIQUE

Preoperative Planning

Preoperative Work-Up. Radiography is the most useful adjunct to physical signs in demonstrating the suitability of a knee for OUKA. Radiographs should demonstrate presence of bone-on-bone arthritis in the affected medial compartment, functionally intact ACL and MCL and presence of full-thickness cartilage in the weight-bearing portion of the lateral compartment. Antero-posterior radiographs, taken in the standard way with the patient weight bearing on the extended leg, can demonstrate loss of articular cartilage medially by showing that the condyles articulate bone on bone (Ahlbäck stage 2 or more). However, in some cases in which there is full-thickness cartilage loss, this method fails to reveal it. A better projection for this purpose is a Rosenberg view with the patient standing with the knee 45 degrees flexed, with the x-ray beam appropriately tilted, to be parallel to the joint surface. A varus-stressed film is more reliable than either of these methods (Fig. 130.3A).

Valgus-stressed radiographs (see Fig. 130.3B) are used to ensure that there is a normal thickness of articular cartilage in the lateral compartment and to demonstrate that the intra-articular varus deformity is correctable (ie, the MCL is not shortened). We have found no other method of investigation to be so satisfactory in confirming these two key requirements for

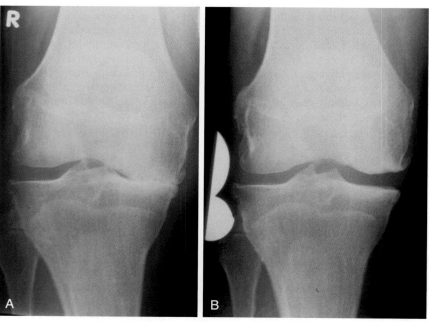

FIG 130.3 Varus-valgus stress radiographs.

successful UKA. When the patient stands on a knee with a varus deformity, body weight tends to distract the lateral joint surfaces. Therefore, to measure the thickness of the lateral compartment cartilage, the lateral condyles must be firmly apposed to one another by applying a valgus force to the otherwise unloaded limb.

Technique. The patient lies supine on the x-ray couch, with a support under the knee to flex it 20 degrees. The x-ray beam is aligned 10 degrees from vertical (to allow for the average posterior inclination of the tibial plateau so it is parallel to the joint surfaces). The surgeon (wearing protective gloves and apron) applies a firm valgus couple of forces through the knee, ensuring that the leg is in neutral rotation. Alternatively, a device can be used by a radiographer to apply stress. The radiographs should be examined to ensure they are of adequate quality. The radiograph should show the joint surfaces end on, and the patella should be approximately central. If the quality is poor, they should be repeated. We have recently developed a stress device that allows the radiographers to carry out the stress views without input from a surgeon. This saves time, the x-rays are reproducible, and there is the added advantage that the surgeon does not get exposed to unnecessary radiation.

In addition to these radiographs, routine work-up as for any major surgery is needed (including cardiopulmonary assessment and routine blood tests).

Instruments and Setup. The trays containing the tibial instruments, templates, and trial components are used with all sizes of femur. The five sizes of femoral component have different spherical radii of curvature. For each femoral size, there is a matching set of meniscal bearings in seven thicknesses, from 3 to 9 mm. There is a separate tray of instruments for each femoral size. The trays contain color-coded instruments and trial components specifically for use with one size of femoral component. They must not be mixed up, so it is safer just to open one size.

In addition to the instruments in the set, it is important to have the thigh support designed for the OUKA and appropriate saw blades. Three saw blades, reciprocating, oscillating, and keel cut, have been designed specifically for the OUKA and can be obtained in a three pack or individually. The reciprocating and oscillating saws have markings to guide the surgeon to the correct depth. The keel cut saw has two parallel blades with some of the teeth bent in. The saw will not only accurately cut the slot but also remove the residual bone between the cuts.

Size of the Femoral Component. The size of the femoral component can be estimated preoperatively from the height and gender of the patient (Table 130.1). During the operation, based in part on the size of the femoral condyle and tibial component, the size may be adjusted. Preoperative x-ray templating is not often used.

A medium-size femoral component is appropriate for most patients. In small women, it is better to use the small size and, in large men, the large size. The extra-large and extra-small sizes are rarely used. If there is doubt between small/medium, or large/medium, it is usually safer to use the medium. Similarly, if there is doubt between extra-small and small, or between extra-large and large, use the small or the large, respectively.

Positioning the Limb. A thigh tourniquet is applied, and the leg is placed on a thigh support with the hip flexed to approximately

TABLE 130.1 Guide to Size of Femoral Component Based on Information About Height and Gender and the Size of the Tibial Component

Height	Femur	Matching Tibia
Women		
<60 inch, <153 cm	Extra-small	A, B
61-65 inch, 155-165 cm	Small	A, B, or C
66-69 inch, 165-175 cm	Medium	C or D
>69 inch, >175 cm	Large	E
Men		
<63 inch, <160 cm	Small	A, B
63-67 inch, 160-175 cm	Medium	C or D
67-73 inch, 170-185 cm	Large	E or F
>73 inch, >183 cm	Extra-large	F

40 degrees and abducted, and the leg hanging freely. When the leg hangs freely, the knee should be flexed to approximately 110 degrees. The knee must be free to be flexed to at least 135 degrees (Fig. 130.4). The thigh support must not intrude into the popliteal fossa, so that risk of damage to the great vessels is minimized.

Incision. A paramedial skin incision is made from the medial pole of the patella to a point just medial to the tibial tubercle—two-thirds above the joint line to one-third below (Fig. 130.5). The medial margin of the patella is identified. The retinacular incision is made along the medial side of the patella and patella tendon. The anterior tibia is exposed. At its upper end, the retinacular incision is extended proximally for 2 to 3 cm into the vastus medialis. Part of the retropatellar fat pad is excised, and the anterior portion of the medial meniscus removed. Self-retaining retractors are inserted into the synovial cavity. The ACL, lateral side, and PFJ can now be inspected. If the ACL appears damaged, check its integrity by pulling on the ligament with a tendon hook (absence of a functioning ACL is a contraindication for OUKA). A full-thickness ulcer on the medial side of the lateral condyle and exposed bone in the PFJ can be ignored.

Excision of Osteophytes. Large osteophytes must be removed from the medial margin of the medial femoral condyle and from both margins and roof of the intercondylar notch (Fig. 130.6). Full clearance of the lateral side and apex of the notch is essential to ensure the ACL does not get damaged and that the fixed flexion deformity corrects. Osteophytes are removed from the anterior tibia because they interfere with seating of the tibial saw guide. In addition, there is usually an anvil-shaped osteophyte anterior to the insertion of the ACL on the tibia. This should be removed.

Tibial Saw Cut

With the knee in 110 degrees flexion, insert the 1-mm-thick femoral sizing spoon (of appropriate size based on the preoperative estimate) and under the center of the medial condyle. Its handle should lie approximately parallel with the long axis of the femur. With all retraction removed, assess the ligament tension by twisting the spoon. It should freely twist approximately 20 degrees in both directions. Usually the 1-mm-thick

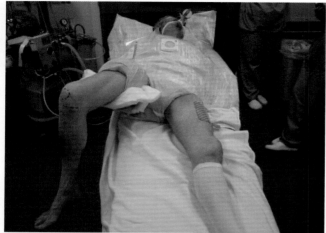

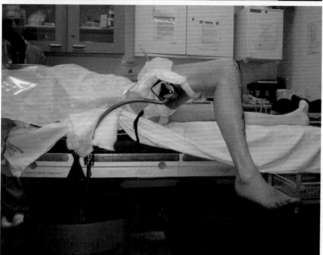

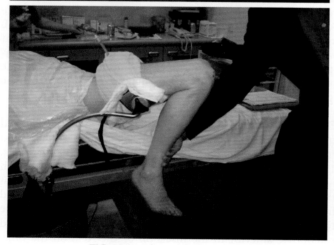

FIG 130.4 Setup for surgery.

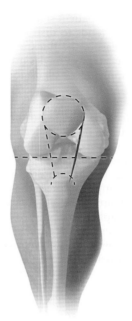

FIG 130.5 Skin incision.

femoral sizing spoon achieves the proper ligament tension; if not, replace it with a thicker sizing spoon until the proper tension is achieved.

Apply the tibial saw guide assembly, with its shaft parallel with long axis of the tibia in both planes (Fig. 130.7). The ankle yoke should be pointing towards the ipsilateral anterosuperior iliac spine (ASIS) in the tibial flexion plane. The tibial saw guide has 7 degrees of posterior slope built in. The femoral sizing

spoon, tibial saw guide, and G-clamp, when used together, will accurately establish the level of bone resection. Select either the 3 or 4 G-clamp and apply to the femoral sizing spoon and to the medial side of the tibial saw guide to ensure access to pin holes in the guide. Although there is an option to adjust the height of the tibial cut using different shims, the zero shim must always be used with the G-clamp. In general, a 3 G-clamp is used for extra-small and small femurs and 4 for the rest, although surgeons starting out with the OUKA should use the 4 G-clamp.

Confirm that the knee is flexed to 110 degrees. Manipulate the upper end of the guide so that its face lies against the exposed bone. Push the guide laterally so its recess accommodates the patellar tendon. Engage the cam on the G-clamp by pulling the lever downwards to lock the three components together. Fix the saw guide in place using one headed pin through the central or lateral hole in the tibial saw guide. Unlock the G-clamp and remove along with the femoral sizing spoon.

Vertical Tibial Cut

Identify the apex of the medial tibial spine with a diathermy (Bovie). Use the reciprocating saw designed for the OUKA (Fig. 130.8). The saw cut should be just medial to the apex of the medial tibial spine. It will pass through the edge of the ACL insertion. Point the blade towards the ASIS, the position of which can be demonstrated by the assistant or align the blade in the tibial flexion plane. The saw must reach the back of the tibial plateau and a little beyond. This is achieved by lining up the appropriate mark on the saw with the anterior tibial cortex. Advance the saw vertically down until it rests on the surface of the saw guide. The saw must remain parallel to the guide. Do not lift the saw handle because this will damage the posterior cortex and increase the risk of tibial plateau fracture.

Horizontal Tibial Cut

Before making the horizontal cut, remove the shim from the tibial resection guide and insert the slotted zero shim. Also

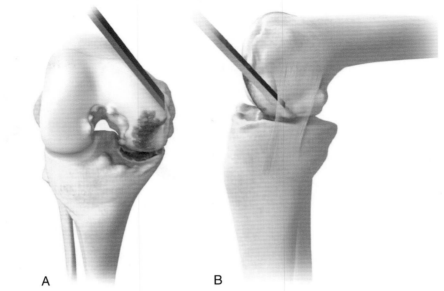

FIG 130.6 Excision of osteophytes (A) from medial margin and (B) from under the MCL.

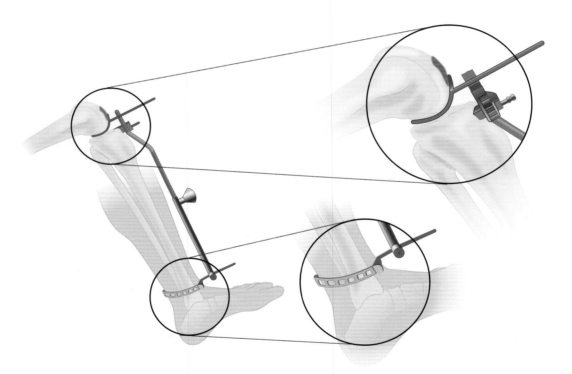

FIG 130.7 Tibial jig assembly.

insert a MCL retractor (sometimes called a Z or curly-whirly retractor). Ensure this retractor lies between the saw and the MCL, protecting the deep fibers of the ligament.

Use the 12-mm-wide oscillating saw blade, designed for the OUKA, with appropriate markings to excise the plateau (Fig. 130.9). Ensure the saw blade is guided along the MCL retractor to cut the medial cortex completely without damaging the MCL. Slightly undermine the vertical cut. When the cut is complete, the plateau usually moves. The tibial "biscuit" should be removed using a Kocher clamp and extending the joint. The excised plateau should show the classical lesion of AMOA:

erosion of cartilage and bone in its mid and anterior parts and preserved cartilage posteriorly. Lay templates of the opposite side on the cut surface of the excised plateau to choose the tibial component with the appropriate width, ignoring medial osteophytes.

Femoral Drill Holes and Alignment

With the knee in approximately 45 degrees flexion, make a hole into the intramedullary (IM) canal of the femur with the 4-mm drill. This should be completed with the 5-mm awl (Fig. 130.10A and B). The hole must be situated 1 cm anterior to the anterior

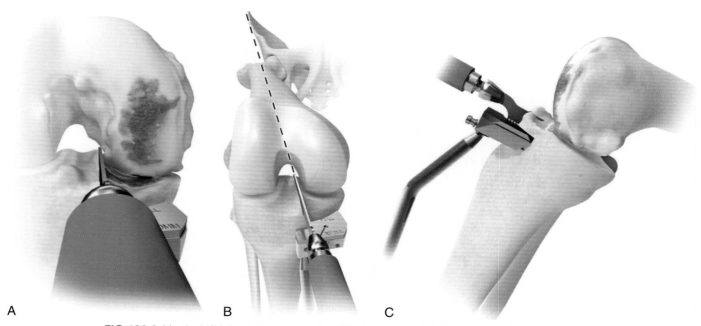

A   B   C

FIG 130.8 Vertical tibial cut demonstrating (A) placement, (B) direction, and (C) technique.

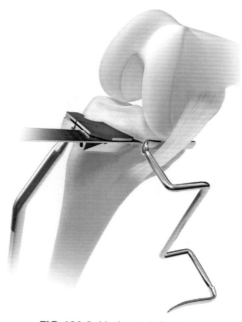

FIG 130.9 Horizontal tibial cut.

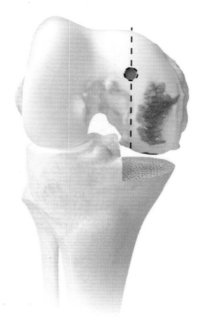

FIG 130.10 IM rod placement.

edge of the intercondylar notch and in line with its medial wall. It should aim for the ipsilateral ASIS. The longer IM rod should then be inserted using the yellow introducer.

Flex the knee to 110 degrees. This must be done with care because the medial border of the patella abuts the IM rod. Using a marker or diathermy, draw a line down the center of the medial femoral condyle. Insert the femoral drill guide for the appropriate size, set to the size of the G-clamp used, either 3 or 4. If the correctly adjusted femoral drill guide cannot be inserted or feels tight, set it to 3. If it still is too tight, remove approximately 1 mm of cartilage off the posterior femur using a chisel. There should be no need to recut the tibial plateau. Insert the

IM link into the IM rod and into the lateral hole of the femoral drill guide (Fig. 130.11). If necessary, tap it gently in with a hammer. The link ensures correct alignment of the guide. It will not necessarily position the guide in the correct medial/lateral position. This needs to be adjusted.

Femoral Saw Cut

Insert the posterior resection guide into the drilled holes, and tap home. Insert a retractor to protect the MCL. Using the oscillating saw blade, excise the posterior facet of the femoral condyle (Fig. 130.12). Remove the guide with the slap hammer, ensuring that it is withdrawn in line with the femoral drill guide

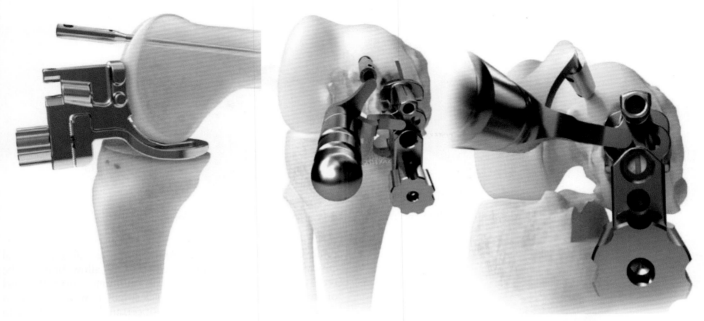

FIG 130.11 IM link showing lateral view, AP view, and magnified AP view to highlight placement of the link in the correct holes.

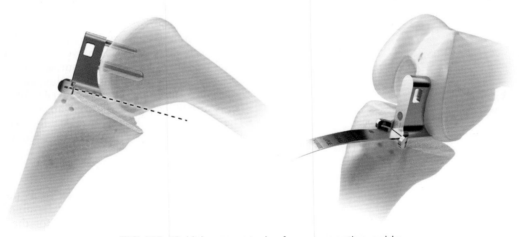

FIG 130.12 Using a posterior femur resection guide.

holes so as to not damage them. (Use of the slap hammer is counterintuitive. The handle should be pushed towards the knee so as to lock the device onto the component while the hammer is used to pull the component off.) Remove the bone fragment. There is now good access to the back of the joint, and any remnants of the medial meniscus should be removed. In the region of the MCL a small cuff of meniscus should be left to protect the MCL from the tibial component. The posterior horn should be completely removed.

First Milling of the Condyle. Insert the 0 spigot, which has the thickest collar, into the large drill hole and tap until the collar abuts the bone. This ensures that the dual reference at the bottom of the hole and on the surface of the condyle are aligned. By extending the knee slightly and retracting the soft tissues, maneuver the spherical cutter (mill) onto the spigot (Fig. 130.13) and into the wound so that the teeth touch the bone. When milling, push firmly in the direction of the spigot axis,

taking care not to tilt the mill because this will damage the hole. Mill until the cutter will no longer advance and the spigot can be seen, in the window, to have reached its end stop. If in doubt, continue to mill; the mill cannot continue beyond the amount permitted by the collar of the selected spigot. Remove the mill and spigot, and trim off the bone protruding from the posterior corners of the condyle that lie outside the periphery of the cutting teeth (Fig. 130.14). These corners should be removed tangentially to the spherically milled surface with a half inch (12 mm) chisel, taking care not to damage the flat posterior surface of the femoral condyle. In addition, any retained posteromedial osteophytes on the femur should be removed.

Measuring the Flexion Gap. Insert the tibial template and apply the single-peg femoral trial component or, if available, the 2-peg without anterior extension, to the milled condyle, tapping it home while holding the femoral impactor angled at 45 degrees to the femoral axis. With the knee in approximately 110 degrees

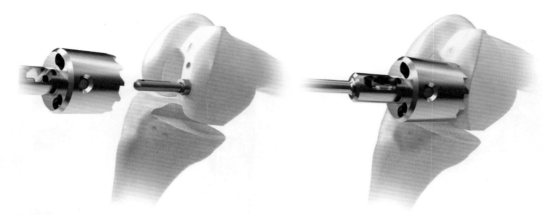

FIG 130.13 Using spherical mill to remove bone and cartilage from the distal femoral condyle.

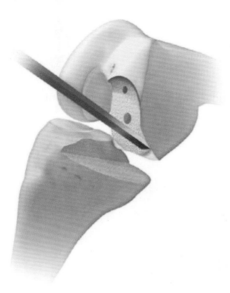

FIG 130.14 Removing the extra bone from the sides of femur after milling.

of flexion, carefully measure the flexion gap with the gap gauges. (In the unlikely event the 3-mm gauge cannot be inserted, replace the tibial cutting guide and redo the tibial cut without the shim.) The gauge thickness is correct when natural tension in the ligaments is achieved. In these circumstances, the gap gauge when held between finger and thumb will easily slide in and out but will not tilt. Confirmation of the correct size is obtained by demonstrating that a 1-mm-thicker gauge is firmly gripped and a 1-mm-thinner gauge is toggling loosely.

Measuring the Extension Gap. Having measured the flexion gap (say 4 mm), remove the gap gauge, fully extend the knee, then flex to approximately 20 degrees flexion. The surgeon should hold the leg and apply a gentle valgus load to take up any slack in the MCL. Use the gap gauges to measure the extension gap (say 1 mm), which is always less than or equal to the flexion gap. Confirm the size of the gap by using a gap gauge 1 mm thicker and 1 mm thinner. If a 1-mm gauge is too tight or cannot be inserted, assume the extension gap is zero. Calculate the amount of bone to remove by subtracting the extension gap from the flexion gap (4 − 1 = 3). It is therefore necessary to

remove a further 3 mm of bone from the inferior femoral condyle. The spigots (numbered 1 to 7) allow bone to be removed in measured quantities (in millimeter) from the level of the first mill cut. The number 3 spigot removes 3 mm, so should be used. If the surgeon is not certain how much bone to remove, it is best to be cautious and remove too little rather than too much bone.

Second Milling

With the appropriate spigot in place (in this case a 3), use the spherical mill to remove the required additional thickness of bone from the condyle. Remove the corners of bone with a chisel tangential to the milled surface. If a collar of bone has appeared around the 6-mm hole, this can be removed with the bone collar remover. Reinsert the trial femoral component, and remeasure the gaps. The flexion gap should not have changed. The extension gap should now equal the flexion gap. Occasionally if the extension gap is still too narrow, a third milling is necessary.

Third Milling

By subtracting the extension gap from the flexion gap, the amount of bone to be removed is determined (say 1 mm). Add this to the size of the spigot used for the second milling to determine the size needed for the third milling. Insert the appropriate spigot, but do not hammer it in. Because the small central collar of bone has been removed, it should not be touching the surface of the bone but is referenced off the bottom of the hole. Repeat milling, and reassess gaps.

Preventing Impingement. Apply the anti-impingement guide to the condyle (Fig. 130.15), and use the anterior mill assembly to remove anterior bone and create clearance for the front of the bearing in full extension. Take great care to ensure the mill does not damage the tibia or patella. The leg needs to be held in approximately 45 degrees of flexion for this milling procedure. Before starting the mill, engage it on the peg and ensure the spring-loaded mechanism moves freely. When milling, push firmly in the direction of the peg axis, taking care not to tilt the mill. Mill until the cutter will not advance further. Leave the anti-impingement guide in place, and use the osteophyte chisel to remove any posterior osteophytes. This should be done medially and laterally, as well as centrally. Remove the guide, and, using the osteophyte chisel, break off any attached osteophytes and sweep them down off the posterior capsule, and

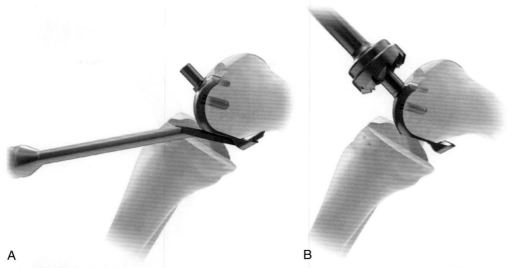

A   B

FIG 130.15 Use of anti-impingement guide demonstrating clearing (A) posterior and (B) anterior sites of potential impingement.

remove them. If possible palpate, with a little finger, the proximal part of the condyle to ensure all posterior osteophytes are removed.

Insert the tibial template, the twin peg femoral trial component, and a trial bearing of appropriate thickness (as determined when measuring flexion and extension gaps). With these components in place, manipulate the knee through a full range of motion to ensure there is no impingement of bone against the bearing in full extension and full flexion. If the bearing impinges in flexion, the knee will open up like a book. If this happens the osteophyte chisel should be used again to ensure all posterior osteophytes are removed.

Final Preparation of the Tibial Plateau. To ensure the correct size, position the tibial template with its posterior margin flush with the posterior tibial cortex. This is facilitated by passing the universal removal hook over the posterior cortex of the tibia. Pull the hook and thus the template forward until it is flush with the posterior cortex. The tibial template should be flush with the medial cortex (ignoring osteophytes) or overhanging slightly. If it overhangs by 2 mm or more, use a smaller size tibial template. The front of the tibial template should also be within 3 mm of the front of the tibia. If it is not, redo the vertical cut so that a larger size can be used. Force the tibial template laterally against the vertical cut and hammer the tibial template nail into place, ideally in the posterior hole. Hold the nail throughout sawing to prevent movement of the template.

Introduce the keel cut saw into the front of the slot, and saw until it has sunk to its shoulder (Fig. 130.16). The saw blade is lifted up and down as it is advanced posteriorly. Confirm the cut is complete by holding the pin and feeling the saw hit the front and back of the keel slot. After the saw cuts are complete, remove the tibial template, and wash the cut surfaces. Insert the trial tibial component and tap with the tibial impactor until fully seated. Ensure that the component is flush with the bone and that the posterior margin of the component is flush with the back of the tibia. If the component does not seat fully, remove it and clean the keel slot out with the appropriate tibial groove cutter. The cementless groove cutter is designed to be

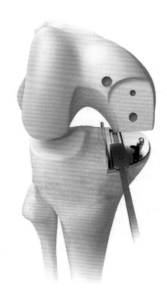

FIG 130.16 Using the keel cut saw.

used through the Microplasty template, whereas the cemented groove cutter should be used without the template. Use only the toffee hammer to avoid the risk of plateau fracture.

Final Trial Reduction. Insert the twin-peg femoral trial component, and ensure it is fully seated by tapping home with the femoral impactor. Insert a trial meniscal bearing of the chosen thickness (Fig. 130.17). With the bearing in place, manipulate the knee through a full range of motion to demonstrate the stability of the joint, the security of the bearing, and the absence of impingement. The thickness of the bearing should be such as to restore the ligaments to their natural tension, so that when the bearing extractor is applied and gently lifted, the front of the bearing lifts 2 to 3 mm. In addition, when a valgus force is applied to the knee, the artificial joint surfaces should distract a millimeter or two. This test should be done with the knee in

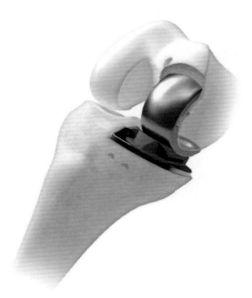

FIG 130.17 Final reduction of trial bearing and trial implants in place.

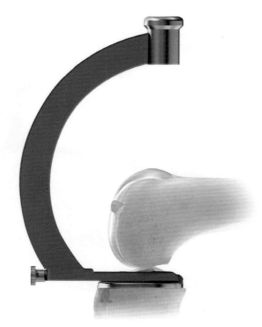

FIG 130.18 Using right angled tibial impactor.

20 degrees of flexion. In full extension, the bearing will be firmly gripped because of the tight posterior capsule. Remove the trial bearing with the bearing extractor.

Cementing the Components. Roughen the femoral and tibial surfaces including the posterior condyles, by making multiple small drill holes with the cement key drill. Clean the bone surface with a pulse-lavage and dry with a swab. When surgeons start using the Oxford prosthesis, we strongly recommend that the components are fixed with two separate mixes of cement.

The tibial component. Place a small amount of cement on the tibial bone surface, and flatten to produce a thin (approximately 1 mm thick) layer covering the whole surface. Insert the component and press down, first posteriorly and then anteriorly, to squeeze out excess cement at the front. Because there is evidence to suggest that early application of cement to implant aids fixation, an alternative approach is to spread a thin layer of cement on the undersurfaces of the tibial component in addition to the layer on the tibia. If this is done, an osteotome should be used to force the cement into the surface of the tibia and sweep the remaining cement off the tibial surface.

Use the right-angled tibial impactor (Fig. 130.18) with a small mallet, applied from posterior to anterior, to complete the insertion. Ensure there is no soft tissue under the component. Remove excess cement with a Woodson cement curette from the margins of the component. Insert the femoral trial component, and pressurize cement by inserting the appropriate thickness feeler gauge. With the feeler gauge inserted, hold the leg in 45 degrees of flexion while the cement sets. Do not fully extend or flex the leg because this may rock the component and compromise the fixation.

After the cement has set, remove the feeler gauge and trial femoral component and look carefully for, and remove, cement that may have extruded. Finally, slide the flat plastic probe along the tibial articular surface, feeling for cement at the edges and posteriorly.

The femoral component. From the second mix, force cement into both femoral drill holes and fill the concave surface of the

femoral component with cement. Apply the loaded component to the condyle and impact with the punch held at 45 degrees to the long axis of the femur. Remove excess cement from the margins with a Woodson cement curette. Pressurize the cement by inserting the appropriate feeler gauge with the knee at 45 degrees of flexion and holding the leg in this position. Do not fully extend or flex the knee because this may rock the components and may loosen them. After the cement has set, remove the feeler gauge. Clear the medial and lateral margins of the femoral component of any extruded cement. The posterior margin cannot be seen directly but can sometimes be seen reflected on the tibial surface and can be palpated with a curved dissector.

Experienced surgeons may wish to cement both tibial and femoral components with one mix. This is acceptable provided they are comfortable that they can do this and leave minimal cement to be removed from the back of the knee. Cement with a long working time should be used. An assistant should apply cement to the components. After the tibial cement has been briefly compressed with the femoral trial and feeler gauge, these should be removed and then excessive cement removed from around the tibia. The femur should then be cemented. Final pressurization is achieved with a feeler gauge inserted with the knee at 45 degrees flexion.

Bearing insertion. Reassess the gap by inserting a gap gauge then trial bearing. Occasionally a smaller size is needed because of gap closure from the cement mantle. Complete the reconstruction by snapping the chosen bearing into place. Close the wound in a routine manner.

Postoperative Management

Intraoperative Local Anesthesia. We have found that a useful technique is a local anesthetic block injected into the damaged tissues in the last stages of the operation. Ropivacaine 300 mg, ketorolac 30 mg, and epinephrine 0.5 mg are made up to a total volume of 100 mL with normal saline. Adrenaline is added to a ratio of 1:200,000. The mixture is put into two 50-mL syringes. Before the components are implanted, the mixture is injected through a 19-gauge spinal needle into any tissue that was damaged during the operation. This is done methodically so that no area is missed, with particular attention being paid to the posterior capsule (3 times 10 mL of the solution are instilled through the posterior capsule and into popliteal space), the periosteum around the implant, and the margins of the incision in the quadriceps muscle. The skin is infiltrated up to 3 cm from the margins of the wound, and 10 mL is reserved until the end of the procedure to inject around the drain site.

In the early postoperative period, good pain control is essential. Regimens of pain management appropriate for TKA may not be suited to the very rapid mobilization that is possible after UKA through a minimally invasive approach. A multimodal approach is best with minimal opiate use. Different regimens are used successfully in different institutions.

Rehabilitation

Range of Motion. Patients recuperate from UKA more rapidly and more predictably than after TKA and do not require formal exercise regimens or outpatient physiotherapy appointments to recover knee movement. Vigorous exercises may even be counterproductive by making the knee more painful and swollen.

Ambulation. Most patients start to walk approximately 2 to 3 hours after the operation. Early walking seems to improve the pain relief. If there is quadriceps weakness, splinting the knee may help.

Early Discharge. With rapid recovery, it is possible to discharge patients from the hospital early. Repicci and Eberle[27] were able to treat 80% of their patients with less than 24 hours in hospital. Increasingly patients having the Oxford UKA are being discharged on the day of surgery. Up to 80% of patients undergoing UKA in some centers are discharged on the same day. These patients undergo a prior rigorous health check-up, have a detailed outpatient consultation (including counseling about advantages of day case surgery), and are provided adequate support (including visits and 24-hour telephone service) after surgery. Patients are prescribed antiinflammatory tablets and oxycodone for break-through pain, and preoperatively femoral/sciatic nerve blocks are avoided. Early outcomes have been shown to be better than or as good as those with conventional discharge without any increase in readmission rates or mortality or morbidity.[4]

Postoperative Radiology

Good postoperative radiographs are necessary as a baseline for comparison with subsequent films and to allow "quality control" of the surgical technique.

For these purposes the standard methods of aligning the x-ray beam are neither sufficiently accurate nor repeatable enough. To assess the positions of the two metal components, the x-ray beam must be centered on one component and aligned with it in two planes. The resulting projection of the other component can then be used to deduce their relative positions. We therefore suggest that fluoroscopically aligned radiographs are taken (screened x-rays). If this is not possible, reasonably good radiographs can be obtained using a digital system. Low-dose images are used to adjust the position. When good alignment is achieved, a standard image is obtained.

In the anteroposterior projection, the patient lies supine on the x-ray table, and the leg and x-ray beam are manipulated under fluoroscopic control until the tibial component appears exactly end-on in silhouette, and the radiograph is then taken (Fig. 130.19). In this projection the alignment of the beam with the flat orthogonal surfaces (horizontal tray and vertical lateral wall and keel) allows great accuracy and reproducibility. In the lateral projection the patient lies supine on the couch with the knee flexed 20 to 30 degrees. The fluoroscope is rotated through 90 degrees, so that the x-ray beam is parallel to the floor and centered on the femoral component (Fig. 130.20). (The tibial implant is not so useful in this projection because it offers no vertical surface and its horizontal surface is obscured by its lateral wall.) Therefore the lateral projection is not as precise or as reproducible as the anteroposterior projection. Radiographs

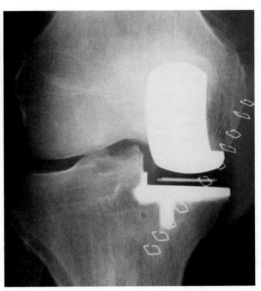

FIG 130.19 Postop. AP radiograph.

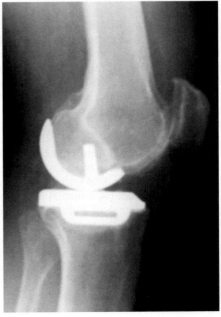

FIG 130.20 Postop. Lateral radiograph.

taken in this way can be repeated at any time interval in the knowledge that (at least in the anteroposterior films) the projections of the tibial component are always the same. Therefore small changes in the relationships of the components to one another and to the bones can be detected. Furthermore, because the x-ray beam is parallel to the tibial plateau, the state of its bone-implant interface is always reliably imaged. Without properly aligned postoperative films for comparison, later radiographs are difficult or impossible to interpret. Subsequent radiographs should be undertaken using the same technique to allow accurate comparison.

Results

The results of Oxford UKA can be gathered from three main sources: the reports of the national registers, observational studies (both comparative and case series), and randomized controlled trials.

National Registers

The National Joint Registry (NJR) for England and Wales was established in 2003 and is currently the largest database of joint replacements in the world. In NJR, like other joint registries, longitudinal data are collected from large numbers of participating institutions before being assembled centrally. The principal aim of any joint registry is to facilitate the identification of poorly performing implants at the earliest possible stage, allowing modification or abandonment of such implants before large numbers are implanted. In addition to patient demographics and surgery details, data on revision operations are collected. A revision operation is defined to have occurred the second time an implant is inserted in a particular joint. Using this information, cumulative revision rates (CRRs) can be calculated.

Although registers are our best source of information on the epidemiology and demography of arthroplasty, they remain imperfect tools to measure outcome. The large number of cases reported and the reliance on operating units to report their cases limit the quantity of data that can be gathered on each patient. In all national registers the primary measure of outcome is the rate of revision surgery; although this has the benefit of being objective and easy to measure, it has several deficiencies. When a revision occurs, the implant is considered to have failed. If it has not been revised, it is considered to have survived and be a success even if it is painful and has poor function. Implant survival is a solid endpoint and has been described as the point at which both the surgeon and the patient agree that revision is preferable to continuing with the prosthesis in situ. As a result of the way data are collected by the registers, revision is considered to occur if a new implant is inserted. The most common revision is therefore removal of a joint replacement and replacement with a new one. The addition of an extra component, such as secondary resurfacing (after TKA), the addition of a lateral or patellofemoral replacement (to a medial UKA with osteoarthritis progression), or exchange of a bearing (for a dislocation or a washout) are therefore also considered to be a revision, whereas replacement of the original bearing after a dislocation is not. Using the same definition, an amputation, a knee fusion, or death resulting from surgery would not be considered a "revision" and so the knee arthroplasty would be considered a success. Therefore it is important to consider a whole series of different endpoints, other than just revision, to assess success or failure of a joint replacement. These could include all adverse events, such as reoperations, complications, mortality, and morbidity, and patients with poor outcome scores and/or dissatisfaction.

COMPARISON OF UNICOMPARTMENTAL KNEE ARTHROPLASTY AND TOTAL KNEE ARTHROPLASTY

All National Registers have found that the revision rate of UKA is approximately 3 times that of TKA. As a result, registers tend to conclude that UKAs have more poor results than TKAs and discourage the use of UKA. This conclusion is probably not justified.

There are many reasons why the revision rate of UKA is higher than that of TKA. Perhaps the most important is that as revising a UKA is usually far more straightforward than revising a TKA, the threshold for revision of UKA is much lower than that of TKA, and therefore the higher revision rate does not necessarily suggest that UKAs have worse outcomes than TKAs.

For different types of implants, there are different thresholds for revision, and these thresholds have a profound effect on the revision rate of the implant. This effect can be so large that comparison of revision rates between implants may lead to misleading conclusions. There is evidence to suggest that the threshold for revision influences the comparison between UKA and TKA. The New Zealand Joint Registry (NZJR), as well as collecting data about revision, also collects Oxford Knee Scores (OKSs) 6 months after the operation. The OKS is subcategorized into poor, fair, good, and excellent. Data from the NZJR demonstrate that UKAs not only have more excellent results but also fewer poor results than TKAs (Fig. 130.21). Therefore the high revision rate of UKAs is not because UKAs have more poor results. The NZJR also compares the 6-month OKS with the subsequent revision rate. The graph in Fig. 130.21 is based on the NZJR data. It demonstrates that, for each outcome score, the revision rate of UKAs is approximately 5 times higher than that of TKAs. The most striking difference in revision rate

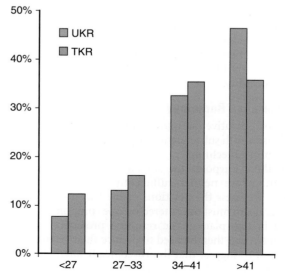

FIG 130.21 NZJR data demonstrating Oxford Knee Scores (OKS) at 6 months for UKA and TKA (OKS [0 to 48]; < 27: poor; 27 to 33: fair; 34 to 41: good; >41: excellent).

occurs in patients who are likely to have a worse score postoperatively than preoperatively (OKS < 20). These patients have a 10% chance of being revised if they have had a TKA and a 60% chance of being revised if they have had a UKA. This is not surprising because the revision of a UKA is usually a simple conversion to a primary TKA and the outcome of this is generally expected to be good. In our hands, except for revision indications of infection or fracture, almost always a primary TKA can be performed usually with a slightly thicker polyethylene. In contrast, a revision of a TKA is often complex, requiring the use of stems, wedges and stabilized implants, and the outcome of this type of revision can be unpredictable.

Matched Comparisons of Unicompartmental Knee Arthroplasty and Total Knee Arthroplasty

When national registers compare different implants, they tend to use raw, unmatched data. Based on raw data, the revision rate of UKA is approximately 3 times higher than that of TKA. Raw data relating the death rate after UKA and TKA are also contained in the registers and shows that the death rate 5 years after a total knee is approximately twice as high as after a partial knee. This difference in death rate is clearly not a simple manifestation of the different types of operation and demonstrates how invalid a comparison using raw data is. The reason for the dramatic difference in the death rate is that UKAs tend to be implanted in younger and more active patients than total knees. An identical explanation must at least in part explain the difference in the revision rate because young and active patients tend to have a higher revision rate. Raw data comparison is therefore misleading. To address this deficiency, Liddle et al.[13] compared adverse events in matched UKA and TKA. Data were obtained not just from the NJR for England and Wales but also the Hospital Episodes Statistics (HES) database and the Office for National Statistics (ONS); 25,334 UKAs were matched against 75,996 TKA patients using a propensity score analysis on 20 variables, including preoperative score, patient demographics, comorbidities, and deprivation indices. Based on the matched cohort, it was found that there were many advantages of UKA compared with TKA. For example, the length of stay was 1.38 (CI: 1.33 to 1.43) days shorter with a UKA. The re-admission rate within the first year (0.65; CI: 0.58 to 0.72), intraoperative complications (0.73; CI: 0.58 to 0.91), and transfusions (0.25; CI: 0.17 to 0.37) were all less. Complications also occurred significantly less frequently; for example, the incidence of thromboembolism was 0.49 (CI: 0.39 to 0.62), infection was 0.5 (CI: 0.38 to 0.66), stroke was 0.37 (CI: 0.16 to 0.86), and myocardial infarct was 0.53 (CI: 0.30 to 0.90).

The mortality following UKA was also significantly lower. For example, during the first 30 days the hazard ratio was 0.23 (CI: 0.11 to 0.50; P < .001) and during the first 90 days it was 0.46 (CI: 0.31 to 0.69; P < .001). The difference in mortality was not just seen in the short term. The survival curves progressively separated for approximately 4 years and thereafter remained parallel until the study stopped at 8 years, suggesting that the effect of surgery on mortality lasted for 4 years. At 8 years the mortality following UKA was 0.87 that of TKA (CI: 0.80 to 0.94; P < .001). Overall there was an appreciable difference in death rate. If 62 patients (95% CI: 43 to 116) were treated with a UKA rather than a TKA, then over the 8-year period one life would be saved. Furthermore, if within the National Health Service the proportion of knee replacements that were UKA increased from approximately 7% to 20% then approximately 160 deaths per year would be saved. In the matched comparison, it was found that the revision rate and reoperation rate were still higher after UKA than TKA. At 8 years the revision rate was 2.12 (CI: 1.99 to 2.26) times higher and the overall reoperation rate was 1.38 (CI: 1.31 to 1.44) times higher with UKA. However, to put the adverse outcomes in perspective, it was concluded that "if 100 patients receiving TKA received UKA instead, the result would be around one less death and three more reoperations in the first 4 years after surgery."

Liddle et al., in a separate matched study,[14] compared the patient-reported outcome measures (PROMS) of UKA and TKA; 3519 UKAs were matched with 10,557 TKAs. The main outcome measure was the OKS. Excellent matching was achieved with the preoperative knee scores (UKA being 21.8 [SD 7.6] and TKA being 21.7 [SD 7.7]). At 6 months following UKA, the OKS was significantly better (P < .0001), with the UKA being 38 and the TKA 36. Although this difference in Oxford Score is relatively small, many more patients achieved an excellent OKS (>41) with UKA rather than TKA (odds ratio: 1.59; CI: 1.47 to 1.73; P < .001). EuroQol five dimensions questionnaire (EQ-5D) (EuroQuol, Rotterdam, The Netherlands) was also collected, and a significantly better overall score was achieved with UKA rather than TKA (P < .001). Furthermore, the four subscales relating to mobility, pain, function, and self-care were significantly better, but in the subscale of anxiety there was no significant difference. The level of patient satisfaction was also assessed and more (odds ratio: 1.3 times; CI: 1.3 [SD 1.2 to 1.4; P < .0001]) patients achieved excellent satisfaction with UKA compared with TKA.

The most important reason for high revision rate with UKA is likely to be because of surgical inexperience. In the national registers, most surgeons are found to be doing very small numbers, whereas, in published series, surgeons tend to do large numbers. The data from the NJR would suggest that approximately half the surgeons doing knee replacement do some UKAs. For those doing UKA, the most common number implanted per year is one and the second most common number is two. The average number is five. When the number of UKAs performed per surgeon per year was compared with the revision rate, it was found, not surprisingly, that the surgeons doing small numbers have a very high revision rates (Fig. 130.22). The surgeons doing one or two UKA per year have a 4% failure rate per year, which would equate to approximately 60% survival at

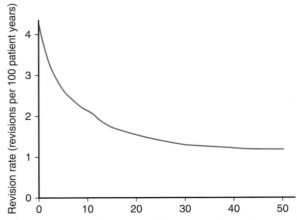

FIG 130.22 Impact of number of cases performed on revision rate.

10 years. The revision rate dramatically decreases with increasing numbers. Surgeons doing approximately 10 UKA per year have a revision rate of 2% per year, whereas surgeons doing approximately 30 per year or more have a revision rate of 1% per year. The data would suggest that surgeons should do at least 10 per year and ideally at least 30 per year.

Over the years we have encouraged surgeons to increase their numbers of UKAs, but these efforts have had little effect. This is not surprising because surgeons cannot easily increase the size of their practice. However, there is an alternative way of increasing the number of UKAs: increasing the proportion of their knee replacements that are unicompartmental; in effect increasing the usage of UKA to TKA in their own practice. To do this, they would have to broaden their indications for UKA. In 1989 Kozinn and Scott defined the ideal indications for UKA and implied that surgeons who extended the indications would have a higher revision rate. Subsequently, Stern et al.[30] and Ritter et al.[28] found that, based on the Kozinn and Scott criteria, approximately 5% of patients would be considered ideal for UKA. It would therefore be expected that the lowest revision rate would be achieved when surgeons did 5% per year and that the revision rate would increase with higher usage. This is far from what actually happens: the revision rate for surgeons with a 5% usage is very high, approximately 3% per year, which equates to a 70% survival at 10 years. As the usage increases, the revision rate dramatically decreases until 20% usage. Thereafter, for the Oxford UKA, with increasing usage there is a slow but steady decrease in the revision rate with the optimal usage being approximately 50%. There are two main reasons why the revision rate decreases with increased usage up to 50%. Firstly with increased usage, surgeons do increased numbers and their results improve. Secondly, their indications change. Surgeons doing small numbers tend only to use UKA when there is early disease and the rest of the knee is pristine. In these circumstances, particularly only with partial-thickness cartilage loss (PTCL), the revision rate is very high.[18] To achieve good results, surgeons not only need to do reasonable numbers but also to use the appropriate indications. The evidence would suggest that, if surgeons have a low usage, they should either stop doing UKAs or change their indications so they are doing at least 20%. For optimal results, surgeons should increase their usage to approximately 50%. If the recommended indications for the OUKA are adhered to, then approximately 50% of a surgeon's knee replacements would be UKAs.

Liddle et al., in their propensity-matched cohorts of UKA and TKA, assessed the effect of usage. Overall, in the unmatched cohort, the revision rate of UKA was 3.2 times higher than TKA but, when the patients were matched, the subhazard ratio for revision became 2.12 (CI: 1.99 to 2.26) that of TKA. However, in the subset of patients in whom the surgeons were considered to have optimal usage rates (40% to 60%), the revision rate of UKA was only 1.4 times higher than TKA. Revision is in some ways a biased outcome measure and reoperation rate is probably a fairer measure with which to compare UKA and TKA. Out to 8 years for UKAs done by surgeons with 40% to 60% usage, there was no significant difference in reoperation rate between matched UKAs and TKAs.

Oxford Unicompartmental Knee Arthroplasty Versus Total Knee Arthroplasty—Nonregistry Studies

Sun et al.[31] randomized 56 patients to either an Oxford UKA or an AGC TKA (both Biomet, Warsaw, Indiana) and reported the results with a mean follow-up of 52 months. The UKA group had a shorter operative time, less blood loss, a lower transfusion requirement and fewer deep vein thromboses (DVTs) than TKA. KSS-Objective and mean range of movement was higher in the UKA group, but neither are described as being statistically significant. Seven patients in the UKA group required revision for tibial loosening (six patients) or subsidence. The authors attribute this to the learning-curve effect because all were performed within the first 2 years of use of the OUKA. There were no revisions in the TKA group.

A case-control study by Lombardi et al.[15] compared early (mean: 31 months) outcomes for TKA and UKA, with particular emphasis on speed of recovery; 103 consecutive UKA patients (115 knees) were matched to the same number of TKA patients (and knees) on the basis of age, gender, BMI, and bilaterality. The number of revisions was similar, as were the number of complications. Stiffness requiring manipulation under anesthetic (MUA) was significantly more common in TKA (7/115 vs. 0/115; $P = .007$). Patients with UKA had a higher mean hemoglobin at discharge (12.1 g/dL vs. 11.3 g/dL; $P < .001$), shorter hospital stays (1.4 days vs. 2.2 days; $P < 0.001$), and a better mean range of movement (77 degrees of flexion vs. 67 degrees; $P < .001$). There was no statistically significant difference in KSS-Functional or KSS-Objective.

In the United States an independent telephone survey done by Washington University compared the level of satisfaction and extent of residual symptoms in a series of 353 mobile UKAs, 104 fixed-bearing UKAs, and 661 TKAs implanted in four centers. Patients were asked about satisfaction with various activities (Fig. 130.23A and B). Overall, the results of mobile UKA were better than fixed UKA or TKA. The fixed-bearing UKA did better than TKA on some questions and worse on others.

Health Economic Studies. Various studies have been conducted comparing cost effectiveness of UKA versus TKA. In 2006 Soohoo et al.[29] analyzed cost effectiveness using a decision

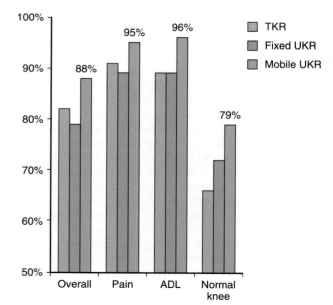

FIG 130.23 Data from an independent telephone survey comparing different types of knee replacements.

model. The study supported UKA as a cost-effective alternative for the treatment of unicompartmental arthritis when the durability and function of a UKA are assumed to be similar to those of a primary TKA. Using nonmatched data from the NJR, Willis-Owen et al.[38] at a 3-year follow up, reported cost savings of £1761 (approximately $2650) per knee treated with UKA compared with TKA. Conversely, Koskinen el al.,[9] using the Finnish Arthroplasty Register, report that in the short term UKA was associated with lower costs, but in the long term, because of the higher revision rate, total knee replacement (TKR) was the more cost effective.

Cohort Studies of Oxford Unicompartmental Knee Arthroplasty. In this section, we first summarize the 20-year and longer results of the Oxford Knee. These results relate primarily to the phase 1 and 2 Oxford Knee because the phase 3 was introduced only in 1998. We then summarize the 10- and 15-year results of the phase 3 Oxford Knee (Tables 130.2 and 130.3). There are numerous short-term studies of the Oxford Knee. We will not discuss these in depth, but we will present the results of a meta-analysis of all published phase 3 studies.

Dr. Ulf Svard is a surgeon who works in Skövde in Sweden. In 1983 he visited Oxford and learned how to use the Oxford Knee. He has been using it since then and following his patients. Initially a group of four surgeons did the operations, but more recently he has done them alone, so the majority of the patients had their surgery done by him. Currently he has implanted Oxford Knees in more than 1100 patients (mean age: 69). At the time of his various reviews, none were lost to follow-up. His 20-year data were first presented in 2006. At that stage, there were 638 OUKA and the 20-year survival was 92% (95% CI: 77 to 100). At 10 years, when 187 patients were reviewed, 90% had good or excellent Hospital for Special Surgery (HSS) scores. These data were subsequently published in 2011, with a 20-year survival of 91%.[24] There had been 29 revisions, 10 for lateral arthrosis, nine for component loosening, five for infection, two bearing dislocations, and three for unexplained pain. The next review was based on the first 1000 implants (125 phase 1, 271 phase 2, and 604 phase 3), and at 20 years the survival rate was 87% (CI: 79 to 95). The survival was also 87% at 22 years. Dr. Svard also reviewed his 125 phase 1 implants. These had been implanted between 1983 and 1988. At the time of review, 80% were dead and the remainder were reviewed with an average follow-up of approximately 25 years. At time of death or last review, 90% had not been revised and had a good or excellent HSS score. This demonstrates that, when used correctly with the correct indications, the Oxford Knee could be considered to be a definitive knee replacement. We are not aware any other implant, either UKA or TKA, that has achieved as good or better results.

At 20 years, approximately 2% of cases had failed from progression of the disease in the lateral compartment. It is generally believed that arthritis will inevitably progress in the lateral compartment after medial unicompartmental replacement. The very low incidence of progression demonstrates that this is not the case and that progression should be considered

---

TABLE 130.2 Survival Rates for Oxford Medial Arthroplasties Phases 1 and 2 at 10, 15, and 20 Years

Implant	Principal Surgeon/Author	Date	No. of Knees	Age (Years)	Time (Years)	Survival (%)	No. of Revisions	Reasons for Revision
Phase 2	Emerson	2010	54	64	20	84	9	—
Phase 1-2	Murray	1998	143	71	10	98	1	Disease progression (2), infection (1), pain (1), loosening (1)
Phase 2	Rajesekhar	2004	135	70	10	94	—	—
Phase 1-2	Kumar	1999	100	71	10	85	7	Patient selection, disease progression (2), fracture (1)
Phase 1-2	Price	2005	52	56	10	91	—	Survival >60 96%, <60 91%
Phase 2	Vorlat	2006	149	66	10	84	24	—
Phase 1-2	Koskinen	2007	1113	64	10	85	—	—
Phase 1-2	Lidgren	2010	749		10	86	—	—
Phase 1-3	Svard	2011	683	70	15	92		Disease progression (10), loosening (9), infection (5), pain (3), bearing dislocation (2)
					20	91	29	

Only the Most Recent Report of a Series is Included.

TABLE 130.3 Reported 10-Year Survival of Oxford Phase 3

Principal Surgeon/Author	Date	No. of Surgeons	No. of Knees (at start)	10-Year Survival (%)	% Of Knee Replacements That Are UKA
Pandit	2011	2	1000	95	>50
Yoshida	2013	1	1279	95	>50
Kristensen	2012	1	794	95	30-50
Jones	2012	56	1000	94	>50
Lim	2012	1	400	94	—
Davidson	2012	—	124	90	20-30
Keys	2013	1	107	97	—
Briant-Evans	2013	35	827	91	20-30
Faour-Martin	2013	1	416	95	—

UKA, Unicompartmental knee arthroplasty.

to be a rare event. Barrington and Emerson also presented 20-year results of the Oxford Knee, and in this study, which was originally started as part of an Investigational Device Exemption (IDE) study in the United States for phase 2, there were 54 knees in 48 patients. At 20 years, the survival was 85%. Nine knees in seven patients had been revised, six for disease progression. As part of the surgical technique, a medial release was undertaken to allow for insertion of a retractor. This may have contributed to the incidence of progression of lateral compartment arthritis.

The 15-year results of the first consecutive 1000 cemented medial Oxford UKA implanted by two designer surgeons were recently reviewed. The mean follow-up was 10 years.[20] At 10 years the mean OKS was 40 (SD: 9), with 79% of the knees having excellent or good outcome. There were 52 implant related reoperations at a mean of 5.5 years (range: 0.2 to 14.7 years). Progression of arthritis in the lateral compartment (2.4%) followed by bearing dislocation (0.7%) and unexplained pain (0.7%) were the most common indications. When implant related reoperations are considered failures, the 15-year survival is 91% (95% CI: 83 to 98). When revisions of the tibial or femoral components are considered failures, 15-year survival is 93% (95% CI: 86 to 99). When revision requiring TKA components are considered failures, the 15-year survival is 99.7% (95% CI: 98 to 100). There were no cases of a revision performed for wear, progression of patellofemoral joint osteoarthritis (PFJOA), or periprosthetic fracture. With 3- or 4-mm bearings ($n = 712$), the 15-year survival was 94.3% (CI: 87.1 to 100), with 5 mm or greater ($n = 86$) 15-year survival was 75.0% (CI: 28.5 to 100). Although the reasons for these differences are not fully understood, it seems sensible to aim for a 3 or 4 bearing. If this is achieved, the 15-year survival is as good as the best TKA.

The 10-year survival rate ranges from 82% to 98%. The series with the second lowest survival rate, by Vorlat et al.,[36] had broad indications and included patients who had undergone previous HTO and also patients with inflammatory arthritis. Similarly, in the series by Kumar et al.,[11] four of the seven revisions were attributed to undiagnosed inflammatory disease. Approximately one-third of the revisions (33%) were for disease progression, 19% were for bearing dislocation, and 14% were for loosening. There were no revisions for wear. In the designer series, which should be indicative of the best results that can be achieved, the survival was 98%.

Functional Outcome

The clinical outcome of the phase 3 OUKA was reported in 2006.[21] The mean objective Knee Society Score improved from 33 to 92, and the mean function score improved from 46 to 80, with 85% considered excellent. The mean flexion deformity decreased from 6 to 2 degrees, and the mean flexion limit increased from 115 to 133 degrees. The Knee Society Score is not a good tool for assessing the outcome of UKA. For example, it does not give credit for flexion beyond 125 degrees. A study by Choy et al. from Korea of 188 knees in 166 patients, with a mean follow-up of 6.5 years, found that the mean flexion limit increased from 135 degrees preoperatively to 150 degrees (140 to 165 degrees) postoperatively; 81% of the patients could squat and 91% could sit cross-legged, both activities that require full flexion in Korea. The very high preoperative range of motion reflects the social practices of that country.

Price et al.[25] compared the rate of recovery (measured by the time taken to achieve straight-leg raising, 70 degrees of flexion,

and independent stair climbing) in 40 OUKAs performed through a short incision medial to the patellar tendon, without dislocation of the patella, using phase 3 instrumentation, with 20 OUKAs implanted through an open approach with dislocation of the patella. Both groups were compared with 40 AGC (Biomet, Swindon, UK) TKAs performed for osteoarthritis during the same time period. The average time (in days) to straight leg raise, manage stair independently, and flex the knee beyond 70 degrees after the short-incision UKA was twice as fast as after open UKA and 3 times as fast as after TKA.

Complications. In the long term the most common cause of failure is progression of arthritis to the lateral compartment, although the incidence is low. In the NJR, there is a much higher incidence of revision for pain or loosening than in the designer series (Table 130.4). This is likely to be, at least in part, because of misinterpretation of tibial radiolucency. Inexperienced surgeons often consider the common stable radiolucency to be a source of pain or indicative of loosening when the evidence suggests it is not. The dislocation rate of 0.1% in the NJR is surprisingly low, perhaps because surgeons do not consider treatment of a dislocation to be a revision. There are no failures because of patellofemoral joint problems.

Infection. The incidence of infection after UKA is approximately half that after TKA. The methods of investigation of suspected infection are the same in OUKA as in TKA except that radionuclide uptake studies are not helpful. After OUKA, activity in the bone beneath the implants persists for several years, and so the presence of a "hot" area on the scan is not necessarily evidence of infection (or loosening). The C-reactive protein or erythrocyte sedimentation rate are the most useful diagnostic tests but may not be positive in the first 2 to 3 weeks. We do not have any experience of using new synovial fluid markers to diagnose suspected prosthetic joint infection.

Treatment

Acute Infection. In the early postoperative period, acute infection is diagnosed and treated in the same way as after TKA. Early open débridement and change of meniscal bearing and intravenous antibiotics can arrest the infection and save the arthroplasty. The use of arthroscopic lavage is not recommended because it is not as reliable as open débridement and exchange of bearing.

TABLE 130.4 **Reasons for Reoperation in the Designer Series and NJR Based on PTIR**		
Indication for Reoperation/Revision	**Designer Series Phase 3, % at Mean 10 Years**	**NJR Data % at 10 Years**
Progression of arthritis in the lateral compartment	2.4	2.6
Bearing dislocation	0.7	0.1
Unexplained pain	0.7	1.9
Infection	0.6	0.5
Aseptic loosening	0.2	3.6
Fracture	0	0.2
Other	0.6	3.5

NJR, National Joint Registry; *PTIR*, Patient Time Incident Rate.

Late Infection. Failure of treatment of an acute infection, or infection of later onset, is diagnosed from the clinical and radiologic signs and bacteriologic studies, as in TKA. The earliest radiologic signs may be thinning of the articular cartilage and juxta-articular erosions of the lateral joint margin (in the retained lateral compartment) of an infected knee after medial OUKA; evidence of chondrolysis by the infecting organism; and chronic synovitis. (Note that acute rheumatoid synovitis can produce a similar appearance.) The eventual appearance of thick (>2 mm), ill-defined progressive radiolucencies beneath the components, quite different from the thin radiolucent lines with radiodense margins that outline most normally functioning OUKA, is diagnostic (Fig. 130.24). Treatment is by removal of the implant and excision of the inflammatory membrane, followed by one- or two-stage revision to TKA. We prefer the two-stage procedure, with removal of the implant and excision of the articular surfaces of the retained compartment at the first stage. An antibiotic-loaded spacer is left in the joint to maintain the gap and allow movement until the infection is eradicated and the second stage can be safely undertaken. We favor a bicompartmental spacer after the first stage because this allows removal of all infected articular cartilage at the first stage. The spacer can be static or an articulating prosthesis depending on surgeon preference. The second-stage TKA may require a stemmed tibial implant (with additional medial augments) if there is substantial tibial BL.

Medial Tibial Plateau Fracture

The 2014 NJR reports 0.30 revisions for periprosthetic fracture per 1000 years (CI: 0.24 to 0.37) in UKA. However, registers underestimate the incidence of fracture because many are fixed rather than revised. In our series of 1000 phase 3 cemented OUKAs, we did not encounter a single fracture.

Fractures occur with all types of UKA; for example, four plateau fractures occurred in 62 UKAs reported by Berger et al., and there are other occasional reports in the literature. We have reported on a series of eight cases of tibial plateau fractures after Oxford UKA[23] (which occurred over a period of 7 years) collected from various institutions in the United Kingdom. The study confirmed that these fractures are rare and tend to occur in inexperienced hands.

Treatment. Management depends on the stage at which the fracture is diagnosed and the degree of varus deformity.

Intraoperative Diagnosis. Several reports suggest that if the fracture is diagnosed during the operation it should be reduced and internally fixed. Thereafter the UKA can be completed in the expectation of a good result. If the medial fragment is comminuted, it is best fixed with a medial buttress plate. The alternative option is to use 6.5-mm cancellous screws inserted through the medial fragment under image intensifier control.

Postoperative Diagnosis. The following algorithm is suggested but may need to be modified according to the circumstances.
Within 3 months of surgery:
A. If the fracture is minimally displaced or undisplaced, use external splinting to maintain alignment while awaiting union.
B. If there is significant displacement, use open reduction and internal fixation with an AO buttress plate or interfragmentary screws (Fig. 130.25).
Later than 3 months after surgery:
A. If the fracture is united and the varus deformity is acceptable, no action is required.
B. If the fracture is united but causing pain, suspect tibial component loosening. If this is confirmed revise to a TKA.
C. If the fracture is not united, revise to a TKA with a stemmed tibial component. This can also require the use of metaphyseal sleeves or cones.

What constitutes "acceptable" varus deformity? In this context, up to 5 degrees of varus is probably acceptable. In UKA, varus malalignment does not have the same sinister implication as it has in TKA; indeed, many practitioners aim always to leave the operated limb in a few degrees of varus.

Dislocation of a Mobile Bearing. In the NJR the incidence is reported as 1.2 revisions for dislocation/subluxation per 1000 years (CI: 1.05 to 1.37) for mobile-bearing UKA. In a meta-analysis of published or presented studies on phase 3 OUKA, it is 0.73% (34 studies, total number of knees 10,125 with 74 dislocations at a mean follow-up of 54 months [range: 24 to 138 months]). In the phase 3 cohort the dislocation rate was 0.5%.

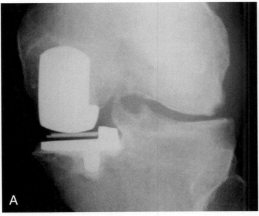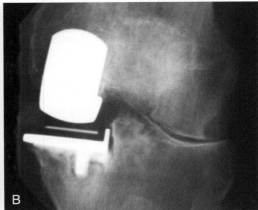

FIG 130.24 Radiograph of an infected knee demonstrating (A) subchondral erosion in the retained lateral compartment (B) pathologic radiolucency.

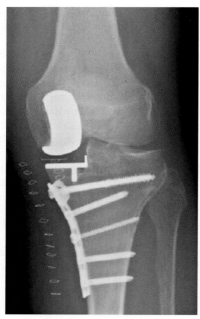

FIG 130.25 Use of a buttress plate for treating a displaced medial tibial plateau fracture after OUKA (components are of a cementless OUKA).

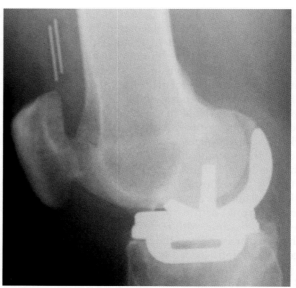

FIG 130.26 Dislocated meniscal bearing in the suprapatellar pouch.

Causes. Primary dislocations are usually caused by a combination of distraction of the joint and displacement of the bearing because of impingement. They are the most common type of dislocation. They occur early and are because of surgical error. The following mistakes all increase the risk of dislocation:

1. Failure to remove osteophytes from the back of the femoral condyle, causing impingement in flexion, stretching of the ligaments, and anterior displacement of the bearing, particularly in patients who achieve high degrees of flexion.
2. Inequality of the 110 degrees and 20 degrees flexion gaps or MCL damage.
3. Retained cement protruding above the tibial plateau surface.
4. Femoral component (and therefore the bearing) sited too far from the lateral wall of the tibial component so that the bearing is free to rotate through 90 degrees. This is unlikely to be a problem with anatomic bearings, which are now routinely used.
5. A bearing that is much too thin relative to gap width may, theoretically, dislocate, and beginners, fearful of dislocation, tend to insert the thickest bearing possible, but this is a mistake. "Overstuffing" the knee should be avoided because it increases the risk of dislocation, pain, and delayed recovery.

Secondary dislocation is the result of loss of entrapment from loosening (and subsidence) of the metal components. Spontaneous elongation of ligaments over time does not seem to occur unless there is impingement, when forced flexion or extension may stretch ligaments. Secondary dislocation is rare. Traumatic dislocation has occasionally been encountered when a normally functioning OUKA has been forced into an extreme posture and the MCL has been momentarily stretched or damaged.

Diagnosis. Dislocation occurs when the knee is unloaded or at the moment when load is reapplied (eg, rising from a chair or getting out of bed). It is usually a dramatic event, and the patient seeks urgent advice, but dislocation can occur relatively silently. Walking may be resumed with the bearing displaced; the weight is borne (painlessly) through the opposed metal components. Radiographs demonstrate the site of the displaced bearing and may suggest its cause (eg, osteophytes, retained cement, displacement of a metal component).

Because the anterior rim of the bearing is higher than its posterior rim, posterior dislocation requires more distraction of the joint than anterior dislocation (5 mm compared with 3 mm). Therefore the displaced bearing is most commonly found in the anterior joint space, often in the suprapatellar pouch (Fig. 130.26). Displacement into the posterior joint space suggests that the bearing has rotated through 90 degrees, from which position it is as easy for it to dislocate backwards as forwards because the entrapment has decreased to 2 mm. Introduction of the anatomic bearing has significantly reduced the incidence of posterior dislocation, as the long lateral side prevents bearing rotation. Occasionally the bearing is found to be tilted into the intercondylar space where it may stabilize in a subluxed position.

Treatment. Manipulation can result in relocation. On a few occasions reduction has occurred, more or less spontaneously, under anesthesia. However, arthrotomy is almost always required to remove the bearing and to determine the cause of its displacement. The bearing can usually be retrieved through a small anterior incision, even if it is in the back of the joint, but an additional posterior arthrotomy has sometimes been needed. We are aware of two cases in which the bearing, which could not be retrieved from the back of the knee, was left and did not cause problems. The femoral component was dislodged on one occasion while retrieving the bearing and was successfully recemented.

Primary Dislocation. When both the metal components are found to be securely fixed to the bones, other causes of dislocation need to be sought.

Any bone or cement that might impinge on the bearing is removed. Retained posterior osteophytes can be removed with the posterior osteophyte chisel. An anatomic bearing, usually one size thicker, is inserted. It is important not to overtighten the ligaments. If there is recurrent dislocation, MCL damage or a serious mismatch between the 110 and 20 degrees flexion gaps, TKA should be performed. Since the introduction of a fixed-bearing tibial plateau to articulate with the OUKA femoral component, some surgeons have converted to this in cases in which instability of the mobile bearing is the only defect in the arthroplasty. However, it should be noted that Australian Orthopaedic Association National Joint Replacement Registry data demonstrate that revisions of failed UKA to another UKA have generally been less successful than revisions from UKA to TKA. Recurrent dislocation is rare and should be treated by conversion to TKA.

Traumatic Dislocation. The few patients in which this has occurred have been successfully managed by either closed reduction of the displaced bearing or open insertion of a new bearing.

Loosening of a Fixed Component

Causes. Over the years, we have gained a good insight into why loosening of cemented components occurs and how it can be prevented. Loosening is one of the most common causes of failure in the national registers. In the NJR the loosening rate is 4.01 (CI: 3.73 to 4.32) per 1000 patient-years. It is much less common in the published series. For example, our series of 1000 cemented OUKAs with up to 15-year follow-up, we have encountered one case each of femoral and tibial loosening. A possible reason for the high rate seen in registers relates to misdiagnosis of physiologic radiolucencies.

Diagnosis. In OUKA, the only reliable radiographic evidence for loosening of a metal component is its displacement. For example, a loose tibial component may tilt or a femoral component may rotate about its peg. As has been discussed elsewhere, stable radiolucencies are very common at the bone-cement interfaces and are not evidence of loosening. Displacement is diagnosed by comparing two radiographs taken with a time interval between them; however, small changes in position can only be detected if the x-ray beam was aligned, on both occasions, in the same relation to one of the components. The required accuracy can only be achieved if both radiographs were taken with the beam aligned by fluoroscopy or by carefully adjusting it while taking multiple low-dose images with a digital system.

Early failures are probably the result of poor initial fixation. Immediate postoperative radiographs and retrieved specimens have often revealed unsatisfactory cementing of the tibial component; in addition, the tibial component is often too small and does not reach the posterior cortex. We have had several reports of sudden displacement of the femoral component in the immediate postoperative period, but usually it occurs a few years later and is associated with clunking, attributable (in retrospect) to poor initial fixation of its posterior facet and lack of cement in the 6-mm hole. Use of the two peg femoral component should decrease the incidence of femoral loosening.

Treatment. In early loosening, if the bone has not been seriously eroded, cementing a new component is a possible option and has been successful on several occasions. However, in late loosening, the bone will already be more extensively damaged and revision to TKA is better undertaken immediately.

Lateral Compartment Arthritis

Our series of 1000 cemented phase 3 OUKAs with up to 15-year follow-up noted that lateral progression requiring revision occurred in 25 cases (2.5% cases) at a mean of 7.0 years (range: 1.9 to 11.4 years). In this series, cases with lateral progression were matched with controls but no factors leading to progression were identified. In Svard's 20-year series the revision rate for lateral compartment OA was 2.3%.

Diagnosis. Pain in the knee, usually but not always on the lateral side, is the main symptom. The first radiographic sign is narrowing of the lateral compartment joint space, and this may long precede the onset of pain. Subchondral sclerosis and disappearance of the joint space ensue. Osteophytes around the margins of the lateral compartment are very common and do not necessarily portend progressive arthritis.

Causes. Some authors have regarded arthritis of the contralateral compartment in UKA as a time-dependent consequence of the gradual, but inevitable, spread of osteoarthritis throughout the joint, perhaps hastened by the presence within the joint cavity of the foreign materials of the prosthesis. If this were true, there would be evidence of progressive arthritis in both the lateral and PFJ. A comparison between 1- and 10-year postoperative radiographs shows that this does not happen. Furthermore, the incidence of revision because of progression is rare (approximately 2.5% at 15 to 20 years), and revision for PFJ progression virtually never occurs. It would seem that in general in AMOA disease progression is arrested by OUKA, suggesting that the underlying disease is a focal mechanical problem. In the few cases when progression does occur, it is likely to relate to some issue with the indications or technique or perhaps an element of inflammatory arthritis or a low-grade infection.

Most authors believe, as we do, that overcorrection of the varus deformity into valgus is the usual cause, and many surgeons recommend aiming to leave the UKA knee in a few degrees of varus to avoid this. Choosing the postoperative tibiofemoral angle is not an option in the OUKA operation because the thickness of the bearing is selected to match the lengths of the ligaments, not to provide an arbitrary alignment of the limb. Therefore an intact MCL is all-important if overcorrection is to be avoided.

To minimize the risk of progression of lateral compartment OA, we recommend valgus stress radiographs to assess the lateral compartment preoperatively, very careful intraoperative preservation of the MCL (particularly its deep fibers), and avoidance of "overstuffing" of the medial compartment with a thicker bearing than the ligaments will easily accommodate.

Treatment. If the symptoms warrant surgical treatment, revision to TKA is indicated. However, experienced surgeons may choose to do a lateral UKA if the medial compartment is satisfactory. We tend to open and extend the old incision and then do a lateral parapatellar approach. In our series of 27 cases with a mean follow-up of 4 years, we have had no failures. Furthermore, we find that patients recover more rapidly (length of stay: 3.3 vs. 4.7 days) and with less morbidity and have better outcomes than after TKA.

PAIN

Pain can be a problem and often leads to unnecessary revision. It is most commonly encountered over the proximal tibia and is anteromedial in distribution. This type of pain is not unusual in the first 6 months and usually settles spontaneously. Review of our patients showed that the incidence has decreased with time and is now 2% at 1-year follow-up. In other series it has been higher, particularly with surgical inexperience. Other sites of pain are much less common. The NZJR reports pain as a cause of revision in 38% of UKA revision. The data from the NJR suggest 23% of UKA revisions are for pain. There are numerous proposed causes and many may be multifactorial. Unexplained pain is the most common presentation, but there is increasing evidence that inappropriate indications or bone overload may be the cause. Impingement, soft tissue irritation, cementing errors (Fig. 130.27), pes anserinus bursitis, or neuroma have all been implicated. Three common reasons are highlighted below along with relevant explanation.

Partial-Thickness Cartilage Loss

It is generally thought that UKA is best used in young patients with early arthritis. We strongly disagree with this and recommend that the Oxford UKA is only offered to patients with bone-on-bone arthritis. Cadaveric studies have shown that asymptomatic PTCL is common. So if a patient has pain and PTCL, the PTCL is not necessarily the cause of pain. In a study[19] comparing the outcome patients with PTCL and matched patients with bone exposed (BE) or BL, it was found those with PTCL had a worse outcome score and greater variability than BE and BL (OKS 36 [SD: 10] vs. 43 [SD: 4] and 43 [SD: 5], respectively). Furthermore 21% of the PTCL group were worse or had no substantial improvement (ΔOKS < 6) after the surgery, whereas all patients in the BE and BL groups reported substantial improvement. In the study, there were four complications, all of which were pain related and all occurred in the PTCL group. Although some patients with PTCL do well with OUKA, a sizeable proportion do not. Until it can be predicted which will do well, it is sensible to avoid doing UKA in patients with PTCL. In the future it may be possible to predict with a bone scan or MRI which patients will do well, but as yet this has not been shown to be possible. Therefore it is important to

be able to distinguish between those with PTCL and those with bone on bone. We do this with a series of radiographs, including standing anteroposterior (AP), varus stress, or Rosenberg. If there is preserved joint space on these views, we would then do an arthroscopy and proceed to OUKA only if exposed bone is seen on both sides of the joint. If there is not bone on bone, we would treat the patients conservatively. The pain either tends to improve or the arthritis worsens in which case a UKA can be performed.

Bone Overload

Both cadaveric studies and finite element analysis (FEA) studies have shown that the tibial strain increases following UKA anteromedially below the tibial component (Fig. 130.28). This may explain why anteromedial pain occurs postoperatively and why the pain settles as remodeling occurs and the strain returns to normal.

The FEA demonstrates a 60% increase in strain with a perfect tibial resection. There is a further increase in strain with a deep vertical cut, a medial vertical cut, and a deep tibial resection. Clearly surgeons should take all measures to avoid these errors. The Microplasty instrumentation was designed to help to address these issues.

Component Overhang. We performed a study to assess the impact of tibial component overhang. We showed that medial overhang of more than 3 mm was associated with pain and poor function that tended to get worse with time. Presumably this was as a result of irritation of medial soft tissues. The tibial component increases in size parametrically by 2 mm, so overhang of 2 mm or more can be avoided by selecting the appropriate component size. Anteromedial femoral component overhang may also cause pain and should be avoided.

Treatment of Unexplained Pain. The temptation for early revision should be avoided. The threshold for revision is necessarily low, and many patients are revised early for unexplained pain in all national registries. In most patients revised for

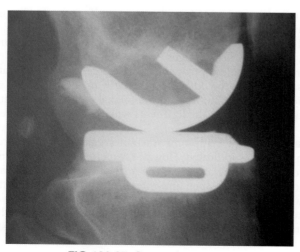

FIG 130.27 Cementing errors.

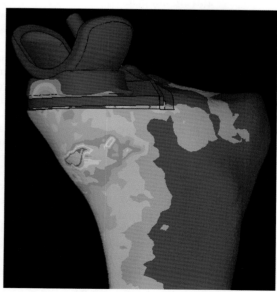

FIG 130.28 Finite element study showing tibial strain after UKA.

unexplained pain, the pain does not improve. In our retrieval study, 75% of patients who were revised to TKA and had no mechanical problems had no improvement in symptoms.

Patients should be treated conservatively because then pain tends to settle spontaneously. Warn the patient before surgery that they are likely to have some pain for 3 to 6 months and that there is a small chance it may take 1 or even 2 years to fully settle. If patients have pain, advise them to decrease their level of activity and use a walking stick. If the pain is focal, it is worth trying a steroid injection. If the pain persists beyond 6 months and the patient is becoming anxious, it is worth requesting a second opinion from a surgeon who is experienced with the OUKA because they will tend to reassure the patient, which is very helpful.

Limited Motion

Knee movements are usually recovered rapidly, particularly because we have used a small incision without dislocation of the patella. Early flexion need not be encouraged because it occurs spontaneously in most patients. However, MUA has been occasionally used if the knee has not recovered 90 degrees flexion at 6 weeks. In these cases, unlike manipulation of a stiff joint after TKA, there are no adhesions in the suprapatellar pouch that need to be ruptured and the knee flexes fully with the application of little force.

Extension improves spontaneously after OUKA and seldom lacks more than 2 to 3 degrees at the end of the first year. If a fixed flexion deformity persists, it is usually because osteophytes in the roof of the notch or on the tibia in front of the ACL insertion have not been removed at the time of surgery.

Implant Fracture

We are not aware of any cases in which the tibial component has fractured. There have been a few cases in which there have been fractures of the femoral component. These have almost all occurred when the femoral component has been used with the fixed-bearing Vanguard M tibia. The fractures tend to occur just posterior to the 6-mm peg and are probably the result of inadequate posterior support.

Fourteen instances of fracture of an OUKA bearing have been reported to date in the literature. We have also been told about a few other fractures. Fracture usually, but not always, occurs with the thinnest (3.5 mm) bearings and is associated with impingement. Treatment is by replacement with a new bearing, usually one size bigger, and addressing the impingement. From a surgical point of view the most significant factor is wear caused by impingement. The surgeon should therefore ensure that impingement does not occur.

Results of Revision Surgery

The national registers have shown that the re-revision rate after a UKA to UKA revision is higher than a UKA to TKA revision. Therefore the general recommendation is that UKA should be revised to TKA. However, there are certain circumstances when a UKA to UKA revision should be considered because the patient recovers quicker, with less morbidity and a better functional outcome. These include replacing a bearing for a dislocation; a lateral or medial UKA for disease progression; and implanting a new component for loosening with minimal BL.

The results of conversion of OUKA to TKA have been reported in a number of studies and are variable. If there is a mechanical cause for the failure, such as disease progression,

component loosening, recurrent dislocation, or damage to deep fibers of the MCL, and there is not substantial BL, the conversion to a primary TKA is straightforward. The tibial resection should be at the level of the top of the medial defect. The remaining defect, which is contained, can be filled with cement or bone graft from resected bone. A 14- or 16-mm tibial bearing is usually needed. The results tend to be as good as those of a primary TKA.

If there is no mechanical cause for the pain then, although the conversion to a primary TKA is straightforward, the results are poor. The typical case is a patient with early arthritis and PTCL who is treated with a UKA. The UKA does not relieve the pain, and the surgeons misinterpret the physiologic radiolucency as indicative of loosening. At revision surgery, although the tibia is secure, it is easily removed when hit hard, so it is recorded as "loosening" in the registry. The conversion to TKA does not relieve the pain, and further re-revision may be done. The message is clear—do not implant an OUKA for partial-thickness disease and do not revise unless there is a definite mechanical problem.

If there is severe BL (eg, following tibial plateau fracture, a two-stage revision for infection, a deep tibial resection, gross ligament instability), then a revision TKA with stems, augments, and increased constraint will be necessary. The results of this type of surgery may be similar to the results of revision TKA.

CONCLUSIONS

OUKA is the only fully congruent, freely mobile design that is approved by the FDA and, when used in correct indications with optimal surgical technique, gives superior functional outcome, is associated with significantly reduced risks, and has equivalent implant survival rates when compared to TKA.

KEY REFERENCES

10. Kozinn SC, Scott R: Unicondylar knee arthroplasty. *J Bone Joint Surg Am* 71(1):145–150, 1989.
13. Liddle AD, Judge A, Pandit H, et al: Adverse outcomes after total and unicompartmental knee replacement in 101,330 matched patients: a study of data from the National Joint Registry for England and Wales. *Lancet* 384(9952):1437–1445, 2014.
14. Liddle AD, Pandit H, Judge A, et al: Patient-reported outcomes after total and unicompartmental knee arthroplasty: a study of 14,076 matched patients from the National Joint Registry for England and Wales. *Bone Joint J* 97-B(6):793–801, 2015.
17. Murray DW, Goodfellow JW, O'Connor JJ: The Oxford medial unicompartmental arthroplasty: a ten-year survival study. *J Bone Joint Surg Br* 80(6):983–989, 1998.
18. Niinimaki TT, Murray DW, Partanen J, et al: Unicompartmental knee arthroplasties implanted for osteoarthritis with partial loss of joint space have high re-operation rates. *Knee* 18(6):432–435, 2011.
19. Pandit H, Gulati A, Jenkins C, et al: Unicompartmental knee replacement for patients with partial thickness cartilage loss in the affected compartment. *Knee* 18(3):168–171, 2011.
20. Pandit H, Hamilton TW, Jenkins C, et al: The clinical outcome of minimally invasive phase 3 Oxford unicompartmental knee arthroplasty: a 15-year follow-up of 1000 UKAs. *Bone Joint J* 97-B(11):1493–1500, 2015.
21. Pandit H, Jenkins C, Barker K, et al: The Oxford medial unicompartmental knee replacement using a minimally-invasive approach. *J Bone Joint Surg Br* 88(1):54–60, 2006.
22. Pandit H, Jenkins C, Gill HS, et al: Unnecessary contraindications for mobile-bearing unicompartmental knee replacement. *J Bone Joint Surg Br* 93(5):622–628, 2011.

23. Pandit H, Murray DW, Dodd CA, et al: Medial tibial plateau fracture and the Oxford unicompartmental knee. *Orthopedics* 30(5 Suppl):28–31, 2007.

24. Price AJ, Svard U: A second decade lifetable survival analysis of the Oxford unicompartmental knee arthroplasty. *Clin Orthop* 469(1):174–179, 2011.

26. Rees JL, Price AJ, Lynskey TG, et al: Medial unicompartmental arthroplasty after failed high tibial osteotomy. *J Bone Joint Surg Br* 83(7):1034–1036, 2001.

28. Ritter MA, Faris PM, Thong AE, et al: Intra-operative findings in varus osteoarthritis of the knee. An analysis of pre-operative alignment in potential candidates for unicompartmental arthroplasty. *J Bone Joint Surg Br* 86(1):43–47, 2004.

37. White SH, Ludkowski PF, Goodfellow JW: Anteromedial osteoarthritis of the knee. *J Bone Joint Surg Br* 73(4):582–586, 1991.

38. Willis-Owen CA, Brust K, Alsop H, et al: Unicondylar knee arthroplasty in the UK National Health Service: an analysis of candidacy, outcome and cost efficacy. *Knee* 16(6):473–478, 2009.

The references for this chapter can also be found on www.expertconsult.com.

131

Bicompartmental Knee Arthroplasty

Michael S. Shin, V. Karthik Jonna, Alfred J. Tria, Jr.*

Partial knee arthroplasty developed in the 1950s with such devices as the McKeever and MacIntosh implants.[8,16,17,19] Unicondylar knee arthroplasty (UKA)[†] and patellofemoral arthroplasty (PFA) prostheses[1,5,6] were used in the late 1970s, and publications showed acceptable results at midterm follow-up. Some surgeons combined UKA and PFA when the pathology presented itself at the time of the surgical procedure. The results were once again acceptable at midterm follow-up and had the advantage of ligament preservation and improved proprioception. However, long-term follow-up showed a high revision rate.[2] As the total knee arthroplasty (TKA) designs improved, there was less interest in partial knee arthroplasty until Repicci and Eberle[21] and Romanowski and Repicci[24] offered a smaller incision for UKA. Limited incisions for knee arthroplasty became more popular, and partial knee arthroplasty became more common.[7,9]

The bicompartmental replacements from the early 1970s had some recognized advantages over TKA, including improved proprioception, easier range of motion, and faster recovery. However, the two separate implants removed a considerable amount of bone, and the operative procedure was complex. Attempts were then made to combine the femoral resurfacing into one single component, and there are presently two designs available. Rolston et al.[22,23] modified a previously existing TKA femoral component and combined this with a UKA-type tibial resurfacing (Journey-Deuce; Smith & Nephew, Memphis, Tennessee). The prosthesis removes less bone and spares all the ligaments of the knee. A similar design is also available that makes cutting blocks based on preoperative computed tomography (CT) imaging of the involved knee. The blocks fit anatomically on the native femur and allow shaping of the surface for the implant (iDuo; Conformis, Burlington, Massachusetts). The tibia is cut with more traditional instrumentation. These newer prosthetic designs borrow technology that has been developed for UKA and TKA. This chapter will review the status of the combined procedures and present the surgical technique for the single-piece femoral component.

HISTORICAL PERSPECTIVE

Partial arthroplasty of the knee started with the work of Marmor[18] in the early 1980s. The UKA that he designed replaced the medial aspect of the knee without interfering with the other two compartments. The early results were acceptable after some problems with the manufacturing were overcome; however, the approach did not become popular among surgeons in the United States because of the increasing interest in TKA. Berger et al.[3,4] and Kozinn and Scott[12] maintained interest in UKA and developed newer designs in the late 1980s that began to show more promise for the technique. Long-term results are now available, which indicate that the prostheses mimic the results of current TKA for the first 10 years after surgery and may even be similar in the second decade.

Repicci's limited surgical approach in the 1990s increased interest in UKA and supported investigations into newer designs and minimally invasive surgical incisions. The instruments have continued to be modified, with some support from the field of navigation. There is even some interest in a robotic application to increase the degree of accuracy and perhaps improve on the long-term results.

PFA also dates back to the early 1980s, when attempts were made to resurface only the patellar side of the articulation in the belief that the patella was the more involved surface. A metallic implant was used, with only moderate success.[11] The implants were modified to include a metal trochlear surface and a polyethylene patella. The early designs did not include many sizes, and the prostheses were not anatomically correct.[1] Krajca-Radcliffe and Coker[13] reported on 30 of 60 knees, with 2- to 18-year follow-up. The results were excellent or good in 84% of the cases. The anatomy was subsequently readdressed, and with modification of the implants the more recent results are much improved but still do not come up to the level of the TKA.[14]

In the late 1980s European surgeons who were performing partial knee arthroplasties looked at the other areas of the knee during surgery and sought to combine partial implants without moving to a total replacement. Argenson et al.[1] operated on 181 knees for primary patellofemoral disease and added a medial replacement in 57%. The early results were encouraging and similar to those of TKA in the first few years; however, there was a 30% revision rate into the second decade.[2] It was concluded that the results may have been compromised by limited early instrumentation and the combination of implants that were not entirely compatible. Cartier and colleagues[5] performed 87 PFAs and included a medial UKA in 36 knees (41%). They reported 86% excellent or good results with 2 to 12 years of follow-up.

Lonner[15] has continued to pursue bicompartmental replacement using two separate implants that are now more anatomically correct. Early results are encouraging, but there is no long-term follow-up.

*The senior author (AJT) is a consultant for Smith & Nephew Orthopaedics, Memphis, Tennessee. Neither of the other authors received any benefits in relation to this article.
†References 3, 4, 10, 12, 18, and 20.

Rolston et al.[22] designed a single-piece femoral component that combined the femoral trochlear groove with the medial femoral condyle replacement. This articulated with a unicondylar type of tibial plateau insert and with an all-polyethylene patellar component. The instruments were designed to accommodate the complex nature of the femoral component; the tibial resection guide was a more traditional extramedullary instrument.

Based on a CT image of the knee, a second technology converts an individualized single-piece femoral component that resurfaces the diseased areas of the knee by using a custom-made shaping instrument that is also designed from the CT information. The tibial tray and patellar resurfacing are completed in a more traditional way with more standard instruments. This approach is very similar to the magnetic resonance imaging (MRI), patient-specific cutting blocks that are now available for TKA; however, the femoral component is manufactured as an individual custom design for each knee.

SURGICAL TECHNIQUE

The surgical techniques for the separate replacement of the patellofemoral joint and medial tibiofemoral joint are presented elsewhere in this textbook and will not be reviewed again here. The two approaches can be combined at the same surgical sitting and are now more compatible with each other because of improvements in the anatomy. However, it does require planning by the operative surgeon and the patience to be sure that both implants are completed with equal precision.

The single-piece femoral components were developed in an attempt to simplify the surgical technique and make the operation similar to a TKA. The procedure can be performed through a limited, minimally invasive surgical approach if the surgeon is comfortable with this option (Fig. 131.1). Otherwise, a standard arthrotomy is acceptable. The tibial resection is performed using an extramedullary guide that is first set for the varus and valgus alignment with reference to the tibial shaft (Fig. 131.2). The depth is set at 2 mm below the deepest point on the medial articular surface. The sagittal alignment, or slope, should be between 5 and 7 degrees and is best if it is set to copy the preexisting tibial slope. Occasionally a tibia will have a slope that is in excess of 10 degrees, especially in a patient of Eastern descent. It is best not to increase the slope above 10 degrees. If this angle is decreased, the flexion gap will be tightened and

some adjustment will need to be made to match the extension gap.

The tibial resection is completed using a power saw for the vertical and horizontal cuts. A pin can be inserted through the cutting guide that protects the remaining tibial surface from any undercutting. After the cut is completed, a spacer is placed into the knee in 90 degrees of flexion and in full extension (Fig. 131.3). The two gaps should be equal at this point. The most common presentation will be a flexion gap that is smaller than the extension gap because of a preexisting flexion contracture. This can be corrected by resecting more bone from the distal femur at the time of the distal resection. If the flexion gap is bigger than the extension gap, the slope of the tibial cut is usually too great and the slope should be decreased by removing bone from the anterior aspect of the tibial cut, using the guide with a change in the slope.

After the gaps have been evaluated, the anteroposterior femoral axis (AP axis) is drawn on the surface of the femur for rotational reference, and an intramedullary hole is made into the femoral canal just above the insertion of the posterior cruciate ligament at the base of the AP axis. The anterior femoral resection is performed with an instrument that is inserted over the intramedullary rod and set parallel to the AP axis (Fig. 131.4). The cut is made flush with the anterior femoral cortex,

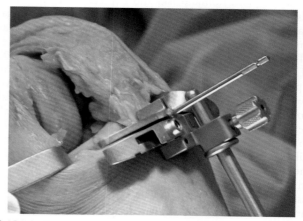

FIG 131.2 The extramedullary tibial guide references the medial tibial plateau surface.

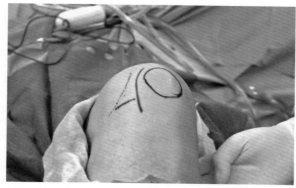

FIG 131.1 A minimally invasive medial incision can be used for this procedure.

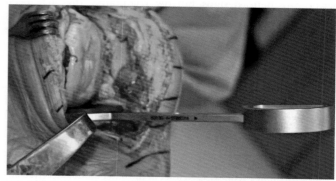

FIG 131.3 The spacer block is placed into the flexion gap and used as a reference for the extension gap.

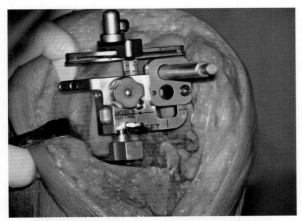

FIG 131.4 The first femoral guide references the posterior medial femoral condyle and sets the depth and rotation for the anterior cut.

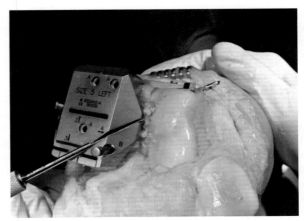

FIG 131.6 The femoral finishing block references the width of the medial femoral condyle and the lateral femoral cortex.

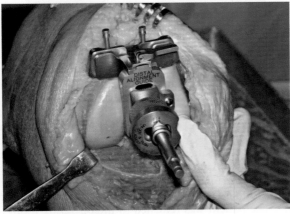

FIG 131.5 The distal femoral cut references the medial femoral condyle for the depth of resection and the lateral femoral cortex for the proper angulation.

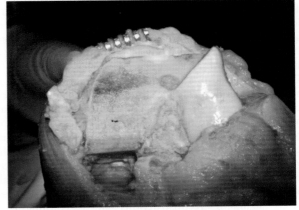

FIG 131.7 Finished cut surfaces of the femur.

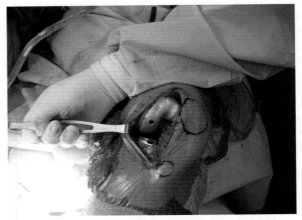

FIG 131.8 The trial components are positioned, and the tracking, balance, and gap laxity are all evaluated.

similar to the cut for a traditional TKA. The distal cut is made with another instrument that locks onto the intramedullary rod (Fig. 131.5). The depth is set on the medial side to equal the flexion gap, and the angle of the distal cut is set with reference to the lateral femoral cortex. This is done so that the final cut will set the prosthesis flush with the lateral cortex and with the cartilaginous surface of the lateral femoral condyle. This cut is critical and is difficult to set to the exact depth.

After the distal femoral resection is completed, the space in flexion and full extension is again checked to ensure that the two are equal. If they are acceptable, the medial femoral condyle is sized by referring to the AP thickness. A finishing block is placed on the distal femoral cut surface and references the medial femoral condyle width and location of the lateral femoral cortex (Fig. 131.6). This is another step that is unique for the bicompartmental surgery and is not typical for TKA.

The final cuts are completed on the femoral side (Fig. 131.7). The tibial tray size is chosen, and the trial components are inserted into the knee (Fig. 131.8). The patellar surface is resected with an oscillating saw or rotary blade and an onlay or inlay patellar component is positioned on the cut surface.

The knee is moved through a complete range of motion to evaluate the patellar tracking and the relationship of the medial femoral condyle to the tibial articular surface implant. The components are removed, the surfaces are lavaged, and all components are cemented in position at the same time.

The wound is closed over drains, and a light dressing is applied so that motion can be instituted on the day of surgery. The patients are all anticoagulated and discharged within the first 2 to 3 days after surgery.

MATERIALS, METHODS, AND RESULTS

There has been only one report of results using the single-piece femoral component with a minimum of 2-year follow-up. Tria et al.[25] studied 40 patients who underwent bicompartmental knee arthroplasty. The patients were chosen for the operation on the basis of the preoperative office interview, physical examination, and x-ray evaluation.

The patients were asked to indicate the location of their pain and its prevalence. If the pain was medial tibiofemoral with associated medial patellofemoral symptoms, the patient was considered a good candidate. The indications were very similar to those used for UKA but allowed more symptoms relating to the patellofemoral joint. Mild lateral tibiofemoral pain was acceptable if the patient was older than 75 years but was not considered ideal. The older patient's symptom presentation was similar to the presentation of a patient who would usually undergo TKA rather than UKA. Global knee pain that was equally distributed in all areas of the knee was a definite contraindication, despite any physical examination and x-ray findings to the contrary.

The physical examination included medial tibiofemoral and patellofemoral tenderness. The clinical deformity did not exceed 10 degrees of varus or flexion contracture. When the varus deformity corrected to neutral with valgus stress, the knee was more ideal for the replacement. However, it was not absolutely necessary for the knee to be corrected. All ligaments were clinically intact. Some degree of anterior laxity related to anterior cruciate ligament deficiency was accepted, but grade 4 instability was not included. Inflammatory arthritis and knees with previous ligament reconstructions or osteotomies were excluded.

The standing AP x-ray showed an anatomic varus deformity that was less than 10 degrees, with minimal translocation of the tibia beneath the femur. Patellofemoral arthritic changes of any extent were acceptable. Mild lateral osteoarthritic changes were considered acceptable. If there were changes in the lateral compartment, there should be no significant symptoms of pain or tenderness on physical examination.

The outpatient follow-up visits were at 2 weeks after surgery and then 6 weeks, 3 months, 6 months, 1 year, and 2 years. X-rays were taken 2 weeks after surgery and then annually, unless otherwise indicated by the clinical presentation.

There were 40 patients (17 men and 23 women). There were two bilateral operations, thus accounting for 42 knees. There were 16 right and 26 left knees. The average age of the patients was 70 years, with a range from 49 to 89 years. The average weight was 185 lb (84 kg), with a range from 114 lb (52 kg) to 262 lb (119 kg). The average body mass index (BMI) was 30 (range: 20 to 42). The average operative time (including surgery and anesthesia) was 114 minutes. The average tourniquet time was 68 minutes. The average cell saver blood return was 110 mL, with a hematocrit of 41%. There were no pulmonary emboli, proximal thigh deep vein thromboses, myocardial infarctions, infections, or mortalities. The average length of stay was 3 days (range: 1 to 6 days). The average preoperative flexion was 122 degrees (range: 115 to 130 degrees). The postoperative flexion

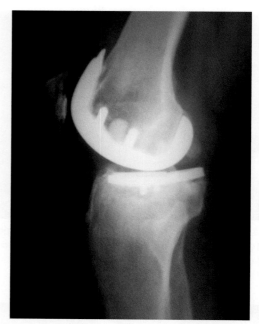

FIG 131.9 Lateral x-ray showing fracture of the tibial tray.

at 2 to 4 weeks after surgery was 102 degrees and increased to 120 degrees at the last recorded office visit. The average preoperative anatomic axis was 3 degrees of varus, and average postoperative axis was 2 degrees of valgus. The Knee Society score improved from 49 to 84, and the function score from 57 to 81.

One patient died after the first year of follow-up. One patient developed a subluxing patella in deep flexion at 6 weeks after the surgery. The components were not malaligned or internally rotated, and there was no disruption of the medial retinacular closure. The patient was returned to the operating room for a lateral release and went on to have a good result.

Five knees have global pain (12%). One has been revised to a standard TKA, with a good result. At the time of the revision, the prosthesis did not appear to have any specific indicating factors for the failure. One patient was lost to follow-up and considered to be a revision. The remaining three patients continued to be followed but are expected to be revised. Persistent anterior knee pain was seen in 10 patients (24%). One tibial tray fractured in the coronal plane at 17 months after surgery, with initial pain that has resolved enough to avoid revision at this time (Fig. 131.9). One tray settled anteriorly at 20 months after surgery, with a reverse in the tibial slope (Fig. 131.10). The patient's pain is presently tolerable without revision.

SUMMARY

The results show a revision rate of 5% (1 knee with global pain and 1 knee lost to follow-up for 2 of 42 knees) in the first 2 years, with another 12% (3 knees with global pain, 1 knee with a tray fracture, and 1 knee with tray collapse [5 of 42 knees]) that might require revision in the near future. None of the cases were technically overcorrected or malaligned. The incidence of anterior knee pain (24%; 10 of 42 knees) is high but has not led to any revisions to date.

The surgical results were studied for malalignment or overcorrection, and there were no contributing factors. The one area

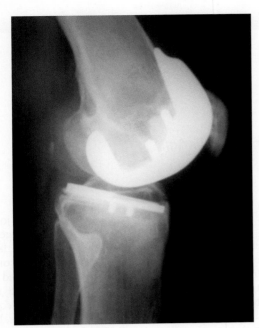

FIG 131.10 Lateral x-ray showing collapse of the tibial tray anteriorly, with reverse slope.

of great difficulty in the surgical procedure was matching the remaining lateral femoral condyle surface to the surface of the femoral implant. One millimeter of separation or offset may lead to some patellofemoral symptoms but would not explain the cases with global knee pain. There are now newer instruments to position the femoral component, and these may make a difference with respect to the lateral interface.

The prosthetic design may need to be revised. The tibial tray fracture occurred in the coronal plane, where the polyethylene slides into the posterior slot for the plastic. This is an area of a stress riser, and the tray may need to be slightly thicker. The tibial tray that collapsed anteriorly might have been more solidly fixed if the pegs were slightly bigger.

The advantages of bicompartmental knee arthroplasty include preservation of the ligaments of the knee, less invasive surgery, and a quicker postoperative recovery. The knee should have more normal proprioception than TKA. Unfortunately, the clinical results have never been better than TKA with two

separate implants or with a single-piece femoral component. It is surgically easier to perform a TKA or UKA than a bicompartmental replacement. However, with the present state of the art, we no longer perform bicompartmental arthroplasty.

KEY REFERENCES

1. Argenson JN, Guillaume JM, Aubaniac JM: Is there a place for patellofemoral arthroplasty? *Clin Orthop* 321:162–167, 1995.
2. Argenson JN, Sebastian P, Aubaniac JM: The outcome of bicompartmental knee arthroplasty at 5- to 23-year follow-up. Presented at the Knee Society Annual Meeting, AAOS, Las Vegas, Nev, February 28, 2009.
3. Berger RA, Meneghini RM, Jacobs JJ, et al: Results of unicompartmental knee arthroplasty at a minimum of ten years of follow-up. *J Bone Joint Surg Am* 87:999–1006, 2005.
6. Cartier P, Sanouiller JL, Khefacha A: Long-term results with the first patellofemoral prosthesis. *Clin Orthop* 436:47–54, 2005.
7. Chen AF, Alan RK, Redziniak DE, et al: Quadriceps sparing total knee arthroplasty: initial experience with two to four year results. *J Bone Joint Surg Br* 88:1448–1453, 2006.
9. Gesell MW, Tria AJ, Jr: MIS unicondylar knee arthroplasty: surgical approach and early results. *Clin Orthop* 428:53–60, 2004.
10. Goodfellow JW, Kershaw CJ, Benson MK, et al: The Oxford knee for unicompartmental osteoarthritis. The first 103 cases. *J Bone Joint Surg Br* 70:692–701, 1988.
11. Insall JN, Tria AJ, Aglietti P: Resurfacing of the patella. *J Bone Joint Surg Am* 62:933–936, 1980.
12. Kozinn SC, Scott R: Unicondylar knee arthroplasty. *J Bone Joint Surg Am* 71:145–150, 1989.
14. Lonner JH: Patellofemoral arthroplasty: the impact of design on outcomes. *Orthop Clin North Am* 39:347–354, 2008.
18. Marmor L: Marmor modular knee in unicompartmental disease. Minimum four-year follow-up. *J Bone Joint Surg Am* 61:347–353, 1979.
20. Price AJ, Webb J, Topf H, et al: Oxford Hip and Knee Group: rapid recovery after Oxford unicompartmental arthroplasty through a short incision. *J Arthroplasty* 16:970–976, 2001.
21. Repicci JA, Eberle RW: Minimally invasive surgical technique for unicondylar knee arthroplasty. *J South Orthop Assoc* 8:20–22, 1999.
22. Rolston L, Bresch J, Engh G, et al: Bicompartmental knee arthroplasty: a bone-sparing, ligament-sparing, and minimally invasive alternative for active patients. *Orthopedics* 30(Suppl):70–73, 2007.
25. Tria AJ, Shin MS, Jonna VK: Bicompartmental arthroplasty of the knee using a single piece femoral component. Presented at the Annual Closed Meeting of the Knee Society, October 9, 2009.

The references for this chapter can also be found on www.expertconsult.com.

132

Bicondylar Knee Replacement

Francesco Benazzo, Stefano M.P. Rossi, Matteo Ghiara, Priyadarshi Amit

Bicompartmental knee arthroplasty (BKA) refers to the association of two different implants in the same knee. It is used to address the degeneration secondary to osteoarthritis (OA) of the compartments involved without sacrificing the healthy portion of the articular surface or the anterior cruciate ligament (ACL)and posterior cruciate ligament (PCL) (Fig. 132.1). BKA can be performed in three combinations:

- Medial unicompartmental prosthesis (Uni) with patellofemoral arthroplasty (PFA) (Fig. 132.2)
- Lateral uni with PFA (Fig. 132.3)
- Medial with lateral uni (Fig. 132.4)

In the 1950s, implants were devised by McKeever, MacIntosh, and Swanson for bicompartmental metallic hemiarthroplasty of the knee to tackle arthritis of both medial and lateral compartments using a metal tibial plateau resurfacing implant.[25,27] They were used with some success. Inadequate pain relief was the main reason for their decline in popularity, and they were then replaced by surface arthroplasty of both the tibial and the femoral surface. Resurfacing the femoral condyle with metal and the tibial condyle with all-polyethylene (metal-plastic) with metal backing on the plastic meniscus (metal-plastic-metal) formed the basis of Marmor modular bicompartmental arthroplasty in the 1970s.[19] Savastano and sledge prostheses were also devised at same time for the same purpose.[9]

The Oxford meniscal bearing prosthesis, developed by Goodfellow and O'Conner, was used separately in medial and lateral compartments.[13] The implant design (metal tibia with flat articular surface and femoral component with spherical articular surface, with fully congruent and unconstrained plastic meniscal bearing) offered the advantage of a congruent surface where a large contact surface with small contact stress lead to less wear and creep. Tension in ligaments and geometry offer stability to the mobile bearings. Additionally, separate condylar components negate the effect of persistent varus or valgus, which would otherwise cause lift-off of a component in one compartment as a result of compression loading on the other. Despite good short-term clinical outcomes, these implants failed principally because of loosening of the tibial component and dislocation of the meniscus in the long-term. Poor patient selection, remote implant design with a thinner polyethylene insert leading to increased wear, and crude instrumentation were the main reasons for initial failure and subsequent revision to total knee arthroplasty (TKA).

Since the introduction of Insall's total condylar design, bicompartmental arthritis of the knee (even in young patients) has been treated with TKA.[16] Good results with TKA have led to decreased interest in BKA. Improved unicondylar implant design has renewed interest in unicompartmental knee arthroplasty (UKA). The use of resurfacing in the patellofemoral joint for isolated patellofemoral arthritis has led to the emergence of patellofemoral resurfacing in BKA. At the present time, because combined arthritis of the medial and patellofemoral compartment is more common than arthritis of the medial and lateral compartment, bicompartmental arthroplasty of the medial compartment with PFA is being performed more frequently than bi-unicondylar arthroplasty. Studies demonstrate, by way of magnetic resonance imaging (MRI) findings, that approximately 30% of patients who undergo TKA can be treated just as well with BKA.[32] The outcome is more favorable nowadays because of improved implant design and patient selection criteria.

Being a bone- and ligament-sparing procedure, surface arthroplasty of the two compartments is considered minimally invasive surgery in the true sense. The skin incision and subcutaneous dissection are not smaller as such, but the procedure does permit the preservation of all the cruciate and collateral ligaments and bone stock.[22] Bone removal is approximately 3.5 to 4 times less than in TKA. Hence, it is an alternative option for isolated bicompartmental arthritis in younger patients with high demands and probability of revision. In addition, ligament preservation means improved proprioception, kinematics more akin to that of a natural knee, greater stability, and improved gait pattern. It is evident that the resurfacing of the medial with patellofemoral compartment eliminates anterior knee pain and slows disease progression in the third compartment. Moreover, BKA can be performed as an additional procedure for progression of arthritis in a second compartment.[21,28]

IMPLANT DESIGN

It has been demonstrated that knee arthritis progresses from the medial compartment to the patellofemoral compartment and then to the lateral compartment. Hence, there are three possible BKA combinations—medial with patellofemoral (most common), lateral with patellofemoral (least common), and medial with lateral.[28] Traditionally, two separate implants are implanted in different compartments, which adds to the modularity of the construct. In 2005, one single component for two diseased compartments was devised to simplify the procedure. This implant is known as monolithic or nonmodular.

Modular

Modular BKA consists of unlinked components in two compartments. A medial or lateral condylar prosthesis is a normal UKA implant (i.e., metal-backed tibial component and femoral component with polyethylene insert). The patellofemoral component consists of an onlay-style trochlear component and a dome-shaped all-polyethylene patellar button. It offers the advantage of two procedures being performed independently in different compartments, with independent orientation and alignment. Modular BKA (medial and patellofemoral) yielded excellent results in a study by Kamath and colleagues[17]; range of motion increased by 10 degrees with most patients achieving more than 120 degrees of flexion, and alignment improved from 6 to 2 degrees varus and 10 to 7 degrees valgus. In addition,

there was no progression of joint space narrowing in the third component; no patellar instability or deep infection; and no progressive radiolucent line, component subsidence, or implant loosening or wear. However, one patient developed tibiofemoral instability and so underwent revision TKA.

Nonmodular or Monolithic

A monoblock off-the-shelf BKA prosthesis (Journey-Deuce; Smith & Nephew, Memphis, TN) was introduced in 2005 mainly for medial and patellofemoral compartment arthritis and used a single-linked femoral component for the medial femoral condyle and trochlear groove. The tibial component is the same as that used in UKA (pegged titanium base plate) with an ultra–high-molecular-weight polyethylene component. The patellofemoral surface functions with either a nonresurfaced patella or a resurfaced patella with an all-polyethylene patellar button as in TKA. This has the theoretical advantage of implanting fewer parts in one surgical, guided procedure. However, the literature shows inconsistent results. Early results suggest that it helps restore normal alignment, achieve normal kinematics, and deliver clinical and functional results very similar to TKA.[10] Various other studies report unfavorable outcomes including inconsistent pain relief and functional results and high revision rate.[20,23,29] For perfect implant positioning and alignment, the lateral edge of the component needs to be flush with the lateral femoral condyle, providing smooth transition between the trochlea and lateral femoral condyle. Morphologic variability of the distal femur as well as the fact that the femoral component is available in only a few different sizes means that the positioning of the component may vary, which may adversely affect sizing and alignment along the mechanical axis. This could explain the adverse outcome of this implant.[1] In addition, compromised implant position in the coronal plane, resulting in transposition of the implant, may also explain the high incidence of anterior knee pain and patellofemoral complications such as

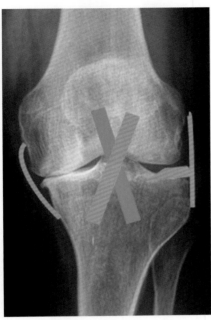

FIG 132.1 Degeneration of medial compartment with healthy ligaments and lateral compartment.

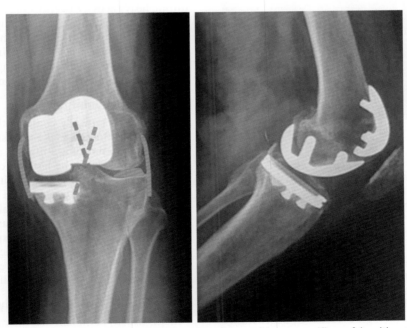

FIG 132.2 Medial uni with patellofemoral arthroplasty without sacrifice of healthy portions of the knee.

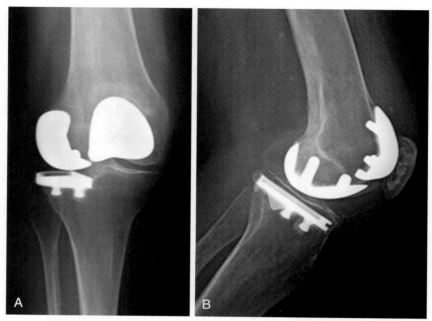

FIG 132.3 (A, B) Lateral uni with patellofemoral arthroplasty.

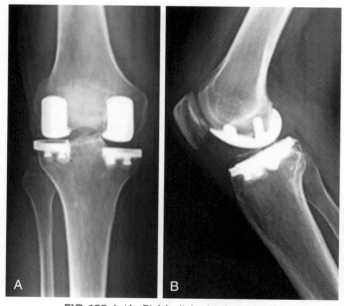

FIG 132.4 (A, B) Medial with lateral uni.

patellar fracture or subluxation.[29] A patient-specific custom monoblock BKA prosthesis has been designed to deal with such implantation problems. However, long-term experience with such implants is awaited.

PATIENT SELECTION

Patients with severe OA, posttraumatic arthritis, or osteonecrosis of the knee joint involving only two compartments with intact cruciate and collateral ligaments are suitable candidates for BKA. There must be no radiologic evidence of degenerative arthritis, painful symptoms, or tenderness on palpation or crepitus in the third compartment.

Pain

In unicompartmental and patellofemoral disorders, pain is usually medial or lateral with associated anterior localization. Although this pain is not immediately well localized and is initially referred to as diffuse by the patient, a further interview and examination can identify the specific location, medial or lateral, with a positive "one finger sign" associated with positive signs and symptoms of the patellofemoral joint. Pain can also sometimes be referred to the whole knee. Although rare, posterior knee pain is also possible, especially when there is an articular effusion with posterior cyst.

The occurrence of pain can vary. It can be experienced during heavy activity, overloading the joint, improving with rest or mild loading, and present at night. The most difficult and painful activities include bending the knee while bearing weight, kneeling, or going up or down stairs. When the patellofemoral compartment is involved, prolonged sitting with the knees flexed is a classic way to cause or increase anterior knee pain.

Stiffness or Instability

These patients typically come to the surgeon complaining of knee pain. Stiffness can be an associated problem (patients usually refer to morning stiffness), and range of motion can be reduced especially at the last few degrees of flexion. Kneeling becomes a problem, as does cycling. Some also complain of flexion contracture, but it must be mild (less than 10 degrees) for this kind of implant to be suitable.

Objective instability with knee laxity is usually not a problem unless the patient has previously experienced an ACL injury. In most of these cases, the development of OA usually reinstates intrinsic stability. Some patients refer to a lateral thrust phenomenon as a sensation of instability

Limitations in Activities of Daily Living

Patients usually complain that their everyday life is limited. Pain and stiffness limit everyday activities such as walking, going up or down stairs, sitting on chairs, cycling, or practicing sports.

PHYSICAL EXAMINATION

The first thing to do in the physical examination is watch the patient while he or she walks into the room. This simple act is insightful because the patient is still behaving naturally at this point. It is then important to observe the patient's unclothed legs and feet to assess the axis of the lower limbs, whether varus, valgus, or neutral. Coronal and rotational alignments are observed as is tibial torsion and limb discrepancy. Extensor mechanism alignment is checked, and the Q angle can be evaluated. The possibility of flat foot should be considered, especially in the case of valgus knee. Walking will reveal any instability in varus, valgus, or lateral thrust during the gait. Rotational deformities are especially evident during gait. Muscle hypotrophy can be noted. Any limp will be evident. Evaluation of the patient while he or she is standing on one leg is also important.

The patient should then be examined in a supine position. First, it is important to exclude any hip problems by examining the range of motion and checking for any pain. The physician should then focus on the knee joint. Effusion and warmth should be checked for. Range of motion should be tested, evaluating flexion limitation or contracture.

All maneuvers to test stability and ligament competence should be carried out. Varus and valgus stress and whether the deformity is correctable or not must be ascertained. Provoked pain can be evaluated, focusing on the compartments involved. In the varus or valgus knee, the medial or lateral compartment is as painful as the opposite compartment, much less painful, or not painful at all. At this moment, asking the patient to pinpoint the painful part of the knee with a finger ("one finger sign") helps to identify a unicompartmental pathology.

The patellofemoral joint should be evaluated. With the patient supine and the limb extended, the Q angle can be measured. In normal individuals, values will generally not exceed 20 degrees. Asking the patient to contract both quadriceps while pushing the patella distally and rasping tests are effective ways to confirm patellofemoral arthritis. Assessing which is the more painful facet of the patella also assists correct indication.

IMAGING

Radiologic criteria for BKA include arthritic degeneration of Outerbridge grade 3 or 4 or Ahlback grade 2 or more in involved compartments and arthritic degeneration of Outerbridge grade 0 or 1 or Ahlback grade less than 2 in the uninvolved compartment.[21,22] In most cases, a simple x-ray examination is sufficient.

- Long-standing weight-bearing x-rays as well as a Schuss/Rosenberg view of the knee should be evaluated in all patients to establish who is a candidate for single or double UKA.
- A lateral view of the knee and an axial view of the patellofemoral joint are needed to correctly evaluate the patellofemoral joint.
- Varus and valgus stress radiographs can also be performed. These can indicate how fixed the deformities are; uncorrectable deformities are considered contraindicated for BKA.[22]

MRI can provide valuable information on the cruciate ligaments, cartilage, and subchondral bone and can reveal the presence and extension of avascular necrosis of condyles. Because MRI can overestimate the extent of the disease, the images should always be carefully correlated with the clinical picture of the patient. Dynamic MRI does not provide any additional significant information. Computed tomography (CT) scan can be useful in posttraumatic cases in which assessment of the overall limb alignment with torsional deformity and tracking of the patella with quadriceps contraction is considered important by the surgeon.

Although arthroscopy before BKA helps decide whether the patient needs a UKA, BKA, or TKA by precisely quantifying the degeneration in each compartment, we do not recommend its routine use. It is wiser to get the patient's consent for BKA while planning for UKA. If there is painful patellofemoral chondromalacia, especially over the lateral facet or lateral trochlea, additional PFA is warranted. Involvement of the medial facet or trochlea alone does not justify PFA.[28]

INDICATIONS AND CONTRAINDICATIONS

The indications and contraindications are listed for the different surgical procedures starting from single uni. The association of two implants does not carry the exact sum of the indications for the single implant (Table 132.1).

Unicompartmental Arthroplasty
Indications

- Unicompartmental disease (medial or lateral) with mild degeneration of one or both of the other compartments
- Deformity of the anatomic axis of the limb caused by narrowing of the joint line as a result of degenerative disease, not deformity of the tibia (Schuss or Rosenberg view of the knee; posteroanterior weight-bearing views taken with the knee in 30 degrees of flexion)
- Positive "one finger" sign—the patient indicates the painful area of the knee with one finger on the medial (or lateral) side
- Varus/valgus deformity less than 10 degrees
- Flexion contracture less than 10 degrees
- Range of motion greater than 90 degrees
- Intact ACL and PCL
- Minimal patellofemoral joint disease
- Age older than 60 years

TABLE 132.1   Resuming Summary Indications

Physical Examination and Imaging	Indication
Varus knee from narrowing of joint space, correctable (any reason)—AVN	UKR
Varus + medial facet	UKR (but limb realignment regained)
Varus + lateral facet	UKR + PFA (TKA remains an option)
Varus+ trochlear incongruence (patellofemoral maltracking), OA	UKR + PFA (TKA remains an option)
Valgus knee due to narrowing of the joint space, correctable (any reason)	UKR
Valgus + lateral/medial facet or trochlear groove incongruence, OA	UKR + PFA (TKA remains an option)
No or minor axial deviation, both compartments involved, central pivot competent	Bilateral UKR Bi-unicompartmental replacement

AVN, Avascular necrosis; *OA,* osteoarthritis; *PFA,* patellofemoral arthroplasty; *TKA,* total knee arthroplasty; *UKR,* unicompartmental knee replacement.

- Weight less than 90 kg
- Low to moderate activity level

Wider Indications

- Age younger than 60 years
- Body mass index greater than 30 (but < 32)
- Presence of degenerative patellofemoral joint without anterior knee pain (and no full-thickness chondral lesions or lateral facet involvement)
- ACL-deficient knee, in low-demand patients; keep the tibial slope less than 5 degrees; no mobile bearing to be used

Contraindications

- Inflammmatory OA
- Fixed flexion deformity greater than 10 degrees
- Fixed valgus/varus deformity greater than 10 degree
- ACL deficiency in young active patients
- Patellar lateral facet OA degeneration
- Severe lateral thrust

Patellofemoral Arthroplasty
Indications

- Primary degenerative OA limited to patellofemoral joint
- Degenerative OA resulting from misalignment/dysplasia with or without instability, with or without previous surgery (unloading procedures)
- Posttraumatic patellofemoral OA

Contraindications

- Associated remarkable tibiofemoral OA
- Systemic joint disease
- Patella baja
- Limited range of motion
- Uncorrected tibiofemoral misalignment

Unicompartmental Prosthesis and Patellofemoral Arthroplasty
Indications

- Unicompartmental disease (medial or lateral) with mild degeneration of one or both of the other compartments, associated with patellofemoral OA with evident clinical symptoms, both subjective and objective (positive signs of patellofemoral pain)
- Arthritis of the patella lateral facet, even with slight or mild symptoms, in association with unicompartmental disease[2,3]
- Deformity of the anatomic axis of the limb as a result of narrowing of the joint line caused by degenerative disease, not deformity of the tibia, with evident patellofemoral incongruency on skyline view owing to patellar misalignment but unrelated to the deviation of the mechanical and anatomic axis of the limb
- Posttraumatic patellofemoral OA associated with overload of one compartment (medial or lateral)
- Varus/valgus deformity less than 10 degrees
- Flexion contracture less than 10 degrees
- Range of motion greater than 90 degrees
- Intact ACL and PCL

Contraindications

- Involvement of all three compartments
- Severe lateral thrust

Bi-Unicompartmental Arthroplasty
Indications

- Medial and lateral degenerative involvement of tibiofemoral compartment
- No ligament imbalance
- No or mild patellofemoral symptoms
- Varus/valgus deformity less than 10 to 15 degrees
- ACL/PCL intact
- No or minimal flexion contracture (<10 degrees)
- Flexion greater than 110 degrees
- Age older than 50 years
- Neuropathy (poliomyelitis) with good quadriceps function (proprioception)

Contraindications

- All deformities requiring extensive releases (including fixed varus and valgus deformity)
- Stability of the construct is solely dependent on the cruciate and collateral ligaments; hence procedure is contraindicated in patients with coronal or sagittal plane instability or previous ligament reconstruction

Two very specific additional surgeries can be considered:

- ACL reconstruction together with UKR (usually medial, more common in male patients) and with UKR and PFA
- Osteotomy and UKR and PFA (when narrowing of the joint space is accompanied by varus deformity of the tibial metaphysis and the patellofemoral joint is affected in any way)

BIOMECHANICS

It has been demonstrated that preserving both the cruciate ligaments, especially the ACL, is essential to maintain normal knee joint kinematics.[21] Results suggest that the PCL alone (without the ACL) cannot reproduce femoral rollback and causes paradoxical anterior translation of the femur over the tibia during deep flexion.[8,26] By preserving both the ACL and the PCL, theoretically, BKA provides for a more physiologic knee and improved knee kinematics, which includes medial pivot rotation, tibial internal rotation, lateral femoral rollback, and posterior femorotibial translation with flexion. Furthermore, intact ligaments provide anteroposterior and mediolateral stability. Restoration of the mechanical axis in arthroplasty is one of the principal ways to achieve a successful clinical outcome. After BKA, undercorrection or overcorrection leads to unequal load distribution over the tibial plateau, leading either to the loosening of the replaced compartment or the progression of arthritis in the uninvolved compartment. Rolston and Siewert[24] reported successful restoration of the mechanical axis after nonmodular BKA in 95% of their 137 bicompartmental knee cases.

Unicondylar with patellofemoral BKA reproduces kinematics more similar to the native knee. This prosthesis gives maximum flexion similar to that in UKA. In addition, it reinstates "normal knee" femoral external rotation and posterior translation of the lateral femoral condyles. With step-up and step-down tasks, there are two phases of motion. One phase, 0 to 30 degrees of flexion, is accompanied by a 10-mm posterior translation of both femoral condyles. The other phase, 30 to 55 degrees of flexion, is accompanied by a 3-mm anterior translation of the medial condyle and a 3-mm posterior translation of the lateral condyle, resulting in 12 degrees of external femoral rotation. In contrast, the bi-unicondylar knee has less maximum flexion, lateral femoral condyle posterior translation, and femoral external rotation. This is probably because replacing the lateral condyle means there could be less posterior translation and hence less rotation. Nonconforming and flat polyethylene inlay may also contribute to less rotation.[31] While evaluating kinematics after monoblock BKA, Park and colleagues[21] observed that femoral external rotation varies according to the angle of flexion and different weight-bearing activities. Posterior tibial slope and mild abnormality in retained ligaments are also influencing factors.

This prosthesis also causes overstuffing of the patellofemoral joint owing to implantation of the rigid trochlea causing posterior shift of the tibiofemoral contact point, which increases extension moment arm. Therefore, less quadriceps strength is required for extension of the knee joint. In addition, greater MCL strain is observed especially during deep flexion.[14]

Gait pattern after monolithic BKA has been reported differently by various authors. Isokinetic strength testing and gait analysis have reported normal gait pattern after monolithic BKA.[30] However, Leffler and coworkers[18] reported slower walking speed with short stance phase and lower cadence for any motor task performed after monolithic BKA, probably as a result of loss in quadriceps strength. Additionally, peak knee extension at midstance is lower, as is, subsequently, the range of motion for the stance phase. These knees also tend to exhibit increased tibial internal rotation and increased varus during the swing phase.

Investigations on kinematics of Bi-unicompartmental arthroplasty have been performed on cadaveric knees, tested under different experimental conditions with KUKA robot, simulating walking, climbing and descending stairs, and lunge (Benazzo et al, personal communication, November 2015). Results are expected in the near future.

SURGICAL TECHNIQUES

Bi-Unicompartmental Arthroplasty

The association of two unicompartmental prostheses in the same knee is a unique operation. As has already been emphasized, a fixed bearing is recommended. Considering the limited number of indications, achieving the perfect balance required by mobile bearing, mainly on the lateral side, would be a challenge even for the most experienced surgeons. The indications have already been presented; however, there are a few additional remarks to be made.

The main purpose of this surgery is to preserve the natural kinematics and proprioception of the knee, conserving the cruciate ligaments, the patellofemoral joint, and the extensor mechanism while barely changing the patellofemoral tracking. However, the key point is the preservation of the natural alignment of the lower limb along with the medial pivoting/lateral shifting mechanism via the substitution of the medial congruent combination of prominent condyle/concave tibia/interposed meniscal bearing and gliding surface, with a fixed-bearing, noncongruent plastic and metal device. Therefore, it is fundamental that the ligaments and extensor mechanism are in good condition and function well before and after surgery.

Planning is also important. Because surgery must result in no major changes to limb alignment, it is important to observe the joint line on long-standing weight-bearing films and in Schuss or Rosenberg view because component position depends on the joint line inclination. Ideally, in the medial uni, the varus

of the medial joint can be (or according to some surgeons, must be—Cartier angle) respected when filling the lost space with plastic and metal. The lateral compartment will consequently be loaded as it was in the native knee. In the double uni, despite the fact that two compartments are involved, one is usually more affected than the other; this side must be treated first, with a filling effect, whereas the other has to be replaced respecting the thickness of the tissue removed. As far as component inclination is concerned, the varus alignment in the medial compartment loses importance because treating both sides means a new joint line is created that respects the overall alignment of the limb.

The main steps of the surgical procedure are as follows:
- Incision and dissection
- Step-by-step core procedure
- Cementing
- Closure
- Postoperative rehabilitation

Incision. The use of a tourniquet depends on the surgeon's preference. There are no major issues concerning patellofemoral tracking in bi-unicompartmental arthroplasty surgery. A midline incision, long enough to expose the medial and lateral aspect of the capsule, is made. The midline incision allows access to both compartments and leaves an "open door" for safe future revision and conversion to a total joint arthroplasty. If the subcutaneous tissue is well represented, it must be detached from the capsule and the patellar tendon; the entire anterior section of the knee must be in full view.

First Uni. The medial compartment is the first to be addressed because it is usually the most involved in varus alignment. It is possible to start from the lateral side in the case of valgus prevalence of the anatomic axis. The technique adopted depends on the design of the component and the surgeon's preference. The measured resection design is usually the most suitable for the double uni because condyle wear is negligible and balanced.

The usual rules of the uni must be followed: removal of osteophytes on the medial side, lateral placement of the femoral component, no removal of osteophytes in the lateral compartment until the components are in final position, and slightly internal rotated tibial plate to accommodate the natural motion of the knee. This rule can be disregarded if the amount of tibial spine bone is to be significantly reduced in the anterior edge. The slope on the medial side must respect the native slope and not exceed 5 degrees. An extra 1 mm of bone should be resected on the tibial side to allow for a little joint looseness, and the trial liner should be 1 mm thinner than the final one. The major risk to be avoided is fracture of the tibial spine from excessive pulling force of the ACL while addressing the opposite compartment. Some surgeons suggest preventive fixation of the spine with an oblique Kirschner wire.

Once the trial implants have been implanted, the capsule is provisionally sutured, and the opposite compartment is then addressed (Fig. 132.5). The slope in the lateral compartment must be the same as the native slope, or just a few degrees more. The combination of flat surfaces with less congruency than the pristine condyle-on-tibia design and insufficient slope can exert pulling forces on the spine. Final balancing adjustments can be made using liners of the appropriate thickness; needle crusting releases of the ligaments can be added if necessary, although it is not the rule.

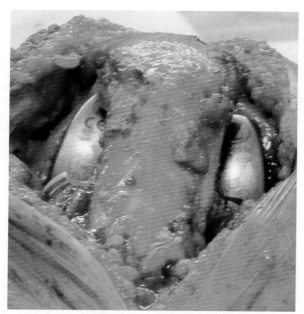

FIG 132.5 Trial implants during Bi-uni arthroplasty.

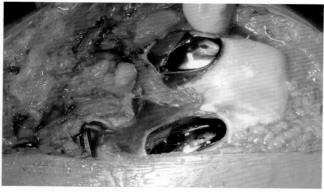

FIG 132.6 Bi-uni implants in place without liners.

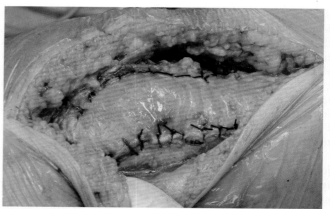

FIG 132.7 Closure of the medial and lateral approaches.

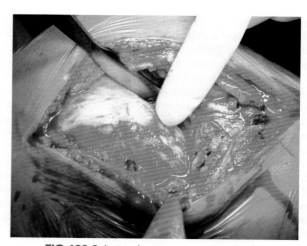

FIG 132.8 Lateral compartment arthritis.

Cementing. The trial components are removed on both sides (Fig. 132.6). Bleeding control with temporary deflation of the tourniquet can be carried out; otherwise, inflation of the tourniquet for cementation can be done at this point. Pulse lavage is mandatory. Infiltrations with cocktails of anesthetic and other substances can be carried out at this point, where all the soft tissues are easily reached.

Cementation is started in the first compartment treated. Using a thinner liner due to the above mentioned risks, a shim can be interposed and the knee secured in forced extension to allow for maximum cement penetration into the bone. The final liners are then inserted as they were in the trials.

Povidone-iodine (Betadine) lavage is carried out before closure. Sutures are placed per the surgeon's judgment (Fig. 132.7). One drain is sufficient. Tranexamic acid can be given via intraarticular injection, the drain kept closed, and the knee is placed in flexion for 2 hours to reduce bleeding.

Postoperative Rehabilitation. Double capsular incision calls for caution in aggressive rehabilitation. This should be the determining factor for the surgeon and physical therapist. Same-day surgery can be carried out in centers well experienced in this rapid line approach. Passive movement not exceeding 60 degrees of flexion can be started the following day. This can be progressively increased each day, reaching 90 degrees on the third day.

Unicompartmental Prosthesis and Patellofemoral Arthroplasty

The combination of a uni, either medial or lateral, and a patellofemoral prosthesis has the potential to address one of the most common problems of the degenerative knee, in which OA, either primary or secondary to trauma, has caused frontal misalignment of the limb, associated with selective degeneration of the patellofemoral joint (Fig. 132.8). By definition, the other compartment is not affected by the disease, and the central pivot is intact. In these situations, knee realignment with a uni is insufficient to also address the patellofemoral joint.

Many studies have demonstrated that only a certain degree of patellofemoral joint generation is acceptable in uni surgery and that realignment of the limb is sufficient to improve the patellofemoral tracking.[2,3] However, other studies report that one of the most common causes of uni failure and patient dissatisfaction is the secondary degeneration of this joint.

The indications for uni and PFA are based on the following:
- Patient symptoms: complaints of medial or lateral pain at the joint space ("finger sign") along with anterior pain when going up or down stairs or sitting.

- Objective clinical evaluation: pain at the joint space and pain on passive motion of the patella (grinding).
- X-rays showing patellofemoral joint involvement: entire surface with osteophytes and narrowing of the space or diseased lateral facet in a varus knee. Dynamic CT scan or MRI can be better at defining patellofemoral tracking; surgical technique and patellofemoral joint implant design can be different in cases of lateral displacement in flexion or under contraction.

Choice of Implants. The patellofemoral prostheses and ancillary instruments (for correct implantation) currently available on the market are "third-generation" designs. Usually, the use of two small implants such as uni and patellofemoral joint in the same knee involves combining two prostheses made by the same company, even though there is no specific design for this particular association. This combination is the responsibility of the surgeon, and as it involves no-contact/gliding surface components, there are no official arguments against combining different brands of implants, provided that correct alignment and patellofemoral tracking are achieved. In theory, the surgeon can choose the uni design he or she is accustomed to (resurfacing or measured resection, fixed or mobile bearing) and the patellofemoral joint design specific to the problem at hand (usually a deeper sulcus of the femoral component to accommodate maltracking). In the case of nickel allergy, zirconium oxide components are the only solution at the present time.

The main steps of the surgical procedure are as follows:
- Incision and dissection
- Step-by-step core procedure
- Cementing
- Closure
- Postoperative rehabilitation

Incision. The use of a tourniquet depends on the individual surgeon. However, we suggest leaving it deflated to avoid any changes in the patellofemoral tracking and inflating it only for cementation. The incision can be medial or lateral, depending on the compartment involved. A midline incision is also an option to consider—it means that you are not forced to use a lateral incision if the procedure is revised to TKA. The incision must be long enough, considering the thickness of the subcutaneous layer of adipose tissue, to expose the entire joint. The patella must be fully displaced laterally or medially, and the entire trochlea must be exposed. To avoid excessive incision of the quadriceps tendon, a mini trivector approach can be used.[4] The synovial tissue of the pouch must be removed if inflamed, and the border between the articular surface and anterior cortical bone, together with the lateral ridge, must be exposed. All adhesions between the vastus intermedius and the bone must be freed to allow free patellofemoral tracking. It is not necessary to completely evert the patella if not required by the instrument used to prepare the articular surface.

Core Procedure. The uni must be implanted first. The two main reasons are that the two uni components will realign the limb, and the patellofemoral tracking will be returned to more physiologic kinematics similar, if not identical, to the native knee and not affected by progressive malalignment. The size of the trochlear component can be chosen after deciding the size of the femoral component, not the other way around. A forced reduction in femoral component dimension can adversely

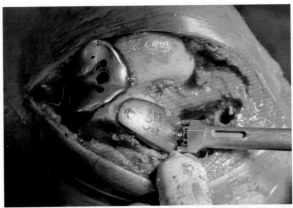

FIG 132.9 A remaining portion of cartilage must separate the two components.

affect the long-term duration of the implant owing to subsidence. There are usually no issues with reducing the size of the trochlear component, provided that the plastic button is dynamically congruent with the metal surface. Moreover, some millimeters of cartilage must remain interposed between the two metal components, which is the demonstration of the good level of depth given to them and of the realization of a smooth gliding surface (Fig. 132.9).

The uni is implanted according to the required surgical technique, the design, and the surgeon's past experience. The patellofemoral joint is addressed second. The position of the trochlear component is important and must be decided according to the preoperative investigations and the intraoperative findings once the trial uni is in place. The ancillary instruments help the surgeon find the correct position, adopting either intramedullary or extramedullary alignment in the femur. However, the surgeon has to take into account that the position must be fine-tuned according to the functional anatomy, and so three different positions must be matched to optimize tracking: rotational alignment, varus/valgus alignment, and flexion/extension position.

Rotational Alignment. In the patellofemoral joint, rotation of the component has nothing to do with flexion space. Therefore, it can be decided on according to the patellar tracking; more external rotation of the component will accommodate lateral tracking of the patella and the opposite in the case of less external rotation. In the case of maltracking, less rotation will help contain the patella, but correct balancing of the medial patello-femoral ligament (MPFL) and lateral patello-femoral ligament (LPFL) is essential to avoid painful tension or patellar dislocation (Fig. 132.10).

Varus/Valgus Alignment. This position affects the engagement of the plastic button with the metal in the first degrees of flexion. Therefore, a more valgus position is indicated for valgus knees and for women with a large pelvis. Surgeons need to be aware that some designs include an augmented Q angle feature.

Flexion/Extension Position. A slightly flexed position generally improves flexion, whereas an extended position prohibits full flexion and increases contact pressure. Position is correlated with the depth of component implantation. The emphasis here

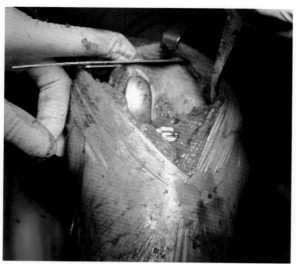

FIG 132.10. Once the trial component of uni has been implanted, native inclination of the trochlea is assessed for decision making on rotational alignment.

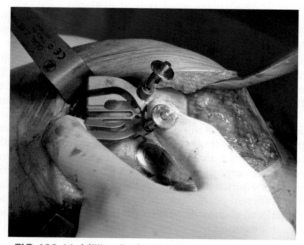

FIG 132.11 Milling jig for the trochlear preparation.

is more on avoiding potential mistakes rather than improving patellofemoral tracking.

Three rules can be followed:

- Distal tip of the implant cannot be proud on or below the roof of the notch.
- Distal triangular area should be congruent to articular cartilage.
- Avoid femoral notching.[12]

Preparation of the trochlear component location is carried out using the power tools provided. It could be a milling guided procedure (Fig. 132.11) with fixed-depth cartilage and bone removal, or a reaming procedure where the surgeon calculates and controls the depth. Whatever the method, the basic principle to respect is that the metal needs to be positioned 1 mm below the remaining cartilage to ensure bump-free smooth gliding of the patella. The size of the remaining cartilage between the two femoral components is not important as long as a smooth gliding motion has been achieved.

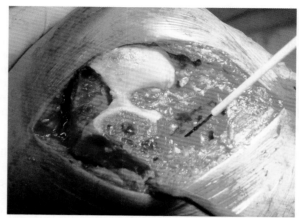

FIG 132.12 Final aspect after bone cuts and milling, before cementing the components.

The final step is the preparation of the patella. There are no data in the literature regarding groups of patients without patellar replacement. Disappointing results warn against this choice. In the authors' experience, a small series of patients had resurfacing done in a second procedure as a result of anterior knee pain. It was unclear if this was due to the design or to suboptimal implantation owing to lack of surgical experience.

The thickness of the patellar bone can be reduced if advisable. The position of the button can be chosen according to the tracking: higher for a low-riding patella and medialized or lateralized according to the position of the femoral component. Excess bone can be trimmed if necessary.

Cementing. The trial components are removed (Fig. 132.12). The tourniquet can be inflated at this point for cementation. Pulse lavage is mandatory. Anesthetics and other medications can be administered at this point, where all the soft tissues are easily reached.

Cementation comes after the surgical steps: uni first, with a thicker liner to increase pressure during the curing of the cement mantle to allow maximum cement penetration, followed by the femoral trochlear component and finally the patella. The knee must be kept at 90 degrees flexion to apply pressure on the patellofemoral joint. The final liner is then inserted according to the trial.

Betadine lavage is carried out before closure. Sutures can be performed per the surgeon's judgment. One drain is sufficient. Tranexamic acid can be given via intraarticular injection, the drain kept closed, and the knee positioned in flexion for 2 hours to reduce bleeding.

Postoperative Rehabilitation. Rehabilitation can be aggressive. Passive flexion can be started on the same day. Active flexion and extension can be started the first day after surgery. Same-day surgery can be done in centers well-experienced in this rapid line approach.

CLINICAL RESULTS

Initial studies documented poor clinical outcomes with high revision rates. With continually developing implants, instrumentation, and techniques, results have improved drastically and are now comparable to results of TKA in selected patients.

Modular

In 2010, Heyse and colleagues[15] reported good midterm and long-term results in nine patients with high satisfaction after independent medial arthroplasty and PFA in an average follow-up period of 11.8 ± 5.4 years (range, 4–17 years). All patients were either satisfied or very satisfied in terms of clinical and functional score (Knee Society score [KSS] and Western Ontario and McMaster Universities Osteoarthritis Index [WOMAC]). Two knees had early manipulation for stiffness. Assessment showed degeneration in the lateral compartment in five patients, radiolucent line beneath the tibial component in two patients and the femoral component in one patient, osteolysis around the tibial screw in one patient, and wear in polyethylene inlays in five patients. However, none of these cases had surgical revision because all patients were satisfied.

In contrast, another midterm to long-term study by Parratte and associates,[22] also published in 2010, reported (for 77 knees) a 17-year survival of only 54%. However, alleviated pain and improved functional scores were achieved. Of knees, 27 were revised for aseptic loosening (20 in patellofemoral and 7 in tibial implant), and 1 was revised for septic loosening. In addition, 15.5% had asymptomatic radiolucency at the tibial bone-cement interface, and a further 7.8% developed asymptomatic arthritic degeneration in the lateral compartment. Correct and stable knee alignment was achieved.

In the same study, Parratte and associates[22] reported more favorable results with bi-unicondylar BKA. The 17-year survival was 78%. Of cases, 16% were revised for aseptic loosening of the tibial implant, and 1% had disease progression in the patellofemoral joint. Asymptomatic degeneration of the patellofemoral joint was observed in 18.2% of patients but did not require revision. Confalonieri and colleagues,[7] in a comparative study of bi-unicondylar BKA with TKA, reported shorter hospital stay and better WOMAC function and stiffness scores in their retrospective matched pair study of 22 patients. However, other parameters, such as surgical time; blood transfusion; and function measures such as KSS, GIUM (specific unicompartmental prosthesis score adopted by the Italian Orthopaedic Unicompartmental Knee Replacement Users Group), and WOMAC pain score, did not differ significantly between the two groups in the 48-month follow-up period.

We performed modular BKA in 30 patients with bicompartmental arthritis (27 medial with patellofemoral and 3 lateral with patellofemoral).[5] In a mean follow-up period of 59 months, the Oxford Knee Score, KSS and HSS scores significantly improved in all patients. Revision surgery was performed on three patients. Two underwent second-stage patellar resurfacing in cases with only trochlea implant, and one was converted to TKA because of loosening of the all-polyethylene tibial component. Apart from these cases, we had no other loosening or component migration complications.

Nonmodular

The literature gives mixed results for monoblock BKA. Engh and coworkers[11] achieved good results with nonmodular BKA in 20 patients. In contrast, Palumbo and associates[20] reported very poor survival and very low satisfaction in their study of 36 monolithic BKA cases. Postoperatively, 81% of patients still experienced pain, and 39% had poor KSS-F and WOMAC score. The tibial bone-cement interface exhibited progressive radiolucency in 61% of patients. Revision rate was high (14% after a mean interval of only 19 months), all for tibial implant

loosening, and one patient had a tibial baseplate fracture. Monoblock prosthesis has become less popular following this study.

COMPLICATIONS

The incidence of complications in BKA in the three possible versions can be high and disappointing. First, the learning curve is not straightforward. As already emphasized, the indications are not simply the sum of those for uni or for PFA, and surgery as well is not the sum of two different procedures. A reasonable number of BKA cases need to be performed on a regular basis. Despite the old design of the components and the crude surgical technique of those times, good long-term results have been reported by the surgeons who prefer this kind of knee surgery.[22]

Improvements in implants and instrumentation have dramatically reduced complications. Nonetheless, aseptic loosening of components (tibial more than lateral, secondary to polyethylene wear) is still the most common reason for revision surgery.[20,22] However, cemented trochlear components are more associated with loosening. Fracture of the tibial tray is sometimes observed (especially in obese patients) mostly secondary to the excessive concentration of load on a specific point over the tibial plateau in the presence of an intact ACL.[20,29] Design needs to be improved to avoid this complication. Persistent pain and progression of arthritis in the uninvolved compartment is also a reason for revision surgery. However, this can be minimized with careful patient selection.[15,20,29] The surgeon can manage disease progression in the uninvolved compartment with an isolated replacement of the compartment rather than resorting to the more invasive TKA. In general, the common complications of prosthetic knee surgery may occur.

Less than 1 mm deep asymptomatic radiolucency is often observed at the bone-cement interface, mostly on the tibial side. Micromotion at the tibial baseplate bone-cement interface owing to greater strain in BKA resulting in micromotion of the fibrocartilaginous tissue could possibly explain radiolucency. However, it is nonprogressive, and its association with symptomatic loosening has not yet been established.[20,22] Patellofemoral complications such as patellar fracture, subluxation, and persistent anterior knee pain are often seen after monolithic BKA and are one of the main causes of prosthesis failure.[29] Another documented intraoperative complication observed during bi-unicondylar BKA is iatrogenic avulsion fracture of the anterior tibial spine resulting from excessive traction on the ACL. This can be managed with intraoperative fixation using screws or nonabsorbable suture. However, it does not have any bearing on the final outcome.[7,22]

BKA is technically demanding surgery and is associated with longer operating time. Nonetheless, the systemic complications associated with TKA are less frequent with BKA because of the minimally invasive nature of the procedure. Theoretically, in cases of failure, it seems easier to revise BKA to TKA. However, this sometimes results in a poorer clinical outcome than primary TKA owing to frequent need of tibial stem and augments or hinged prosthesis. Revision BKA is less complicated than revision TKA because bone stock is preserved.[22]

NEWER TECHNOLOGY

Computer-assisted techniques and robotic technology are used for component positioning in BKA as in TKA.[6,31] This technology requires computer-assisted preoperative planning of implant positioning and bone resection based on three-dimensional CT scans. Tibial and femoral tracking arrays placed with two intracortical pins and articular surface are probed to register the femur and tibia to the preoperative CT scans. Different compartments of both tibia and femur bones are prepared independently using a virtually constrained robotic arm equipped with a high-speed burr followed by implantation. Additionally, real-time dynamic measurement of tibiofemoral motion permits quantitative assessment of soft tissue laxity and accurate soft tissue balancing. Studies report excellent early clinical and radiographic outcomes. Long-term study proving its efficacy is awaited.

CONCLUSION

BKA is a bone-sparing and ligament-preserving surgery. The goal is to preserve bone stock and attain more natural knee kinematics. BKA provides an alternative for treating arthritis limited to two compartments of the knee, especially in young patients who are at higher risk of revision surgery. This procedure strictly requires intact cruciate and collateral ligaments for stability. In carefully selected patients, the short-term and midterm results are equivalent to results of TKA; however, long-term studies are required to confirm its clinical efficacy.

KEY REFERENCES

2. Beard DJ, et al: The influence of the presence and severity of pre-existing patellofemoral degenerative changes on the outcome of the Oxford medial unicompartmental knee replacement. *J Bone Joint Surg Br* 89:1597–1601, 2007.

3. Beard DJ, et al: Pre-operative clinical and radiological assessment of the patellofemoral joint in unicompartmental knee replacement and its influence on outcome. *J Bone Joint Surg Br* 89:1602–1607, 2007.

4. Benazzo F, Rossi SMP: The trivector approach for minimally invasive total knee arthroplasty: a technical note. *J Orthop Traumatol* 13:159–162, 2012.

5. Benazzo F, et al: Partial knee arthroplasty: patellofemoral arthroplasty and combined unicompartmental and patellofemoral arthroplasty implants—general considerations and indications, technique and clinical experience. *Knee* 21(Suppl 1):S43–S46, 2014.

10. Engh G: A bi-compartmental solution: what the Deuce? *Orthopaedics* 30:770–771, 2007.

12. Farr J, Barrett D: Optimizing patellofemoral arthroplasty. *Knee* 15:339–347, 2008.

14. Heyse TJ, et al: Biomechanics of medial unicondylar in combination with patellofemoral knee arthroplasty. *Knee* 21(Suppl 1):S3–S9, 2014.

15. Heyse TJ, et al: UKA in combination with PFR at average 12-year follow up. *Arch Orthop Trauma Surg* 130:1227–1230, 2010.

17. Kamath AF, et al: Minimum two-year outcomes of modular bicompartmental knee arthroplasty. *J Arthroplasty* 29:75–79, 2014.

21. Park BH, et al: Kinematics of monoblock bicompartmental knee arthroplasty during weight-bearing activities. *Knee Surg Sports Traumatol Arthrosc* 23:1756–1762, 2015.

22. Parratte S, et al: Survival of bicompartmental knee arthroplasty at 5 to 23 years. *Clin Orthop Relat Res* 468:64–72, 2010.

23. Rolston L, et al: Bicompartmental knee arthroplasty: a bone-sparing, ligament-sparing, and minimally invasive alternative for young patients. *Orthopaedics* 30(Suppl 8):70–73, 2007.

28. Thienpont E, Price A: Bicompartmental knee arthroplasty of the patellofemoral and medial compartments. *Knee Surg Sports Traumatol Arthrosc* 21:2523–2531, 2013.

29. Tria AJ: Bicompartmental knee arthroplasty: the clinical outcome. *Orthop Clin North Am* 44:281–286, 2013.

32. Yamabe E, et al: Study of surgical indication for knee arthroplasty by cartilage analysis in three compartments using data from Osteoarthritis Initiative (OAI). *BMC Musculoskelet Disord* 14:194, 2013.

The references for this chapter can also be found on www.expertconsult.com.

133

Bicruciate Total Knee Arthroplasty

Stephen Gregorius, Christopher L. Peters

INTRODUCTION

Total knee arthroplasty (TKA) has transformed the treatment of knee arthritis. Initially considered a surgical option for older adults or low-demand patients, TKA is now commonly performed in younger patients with higher expectations and increased functional needs. Although there have been substantial improvements in TKA design over the past several decades, the results of TKA in terms of patient satisfaction remain imperfect. As many as 18% of patients are unsatisfied with their surgical result at 1 year postoperatively.[34] Similarly, activity levels after TKA are less than age-matched controls, with only 16.5% reaching daily walking activity guidelines.[22] Although patient satisfaction and functional results are multifactorial, proprioceptive changes and abnormal kinematics from cruciate ligament resection may be contributing factors to suboptimal patient satisfaction and functional improvement.

Despite the anterior cruciate ligament (ACL) being present in more than 60% of patients undergoing TKA, the majority of implant designs sacrifice one or both cruciate ligaments.[11] Retaining both cruciate ligaments has the theoretical advantage of more natural knee kinematics with improved proprioception and better knee function. Retention of the cruciate ligaments also has the potential to minimize stress transferred to the bone-implant interface and the implant itself. This in turn may minimize the need for added prosthetic constraint, which may enhance implant longevity. General acceptance of bicruciate-retaining TKA designs has been limited because of multiple concerns, including surgical technique challenges, ligament balancing, and difficulty with implant fixation. In addition, there is concern regarding late ACL failure and possible need for added constraint. Nevertheless, a number of bicruciate-retaining TKA designs have shown promising clinical and radiographic results, and some results have hinted at the prospect of improved patient satisfaction.[8,29,31]

HISTORY

Gunston developed the polycentric knee in the 1960s using a nonhinged design with acrylic cement for component fixation (Fig. 133.1).[16] The implant consisted of two semicircular stainless steel runners in the femoral condyles that articulated with two tracks of polyethylene in the tibia plateau while retaining both cruciate ligaments. The geometric knee prosthesis was another bicruciate-retaining design of this era that had a single femoral component (Fig. 133.2).[9,10] This avoided the need for aligning the femoral condyles separately. These designs were the precursors to modern condylar-type TKA implant designs and,

although they preserved both cruciate ligaments, high early failure rates were largely because of crude surgical techniques (lack of instrumentation), poor initial fixation, and lack of condylar femoral implant geometry.[21,32]

Townley designed the anatomic total knee in the early 1970s.[36] This implant was an attempt to maintain normal joint anatomy and function by limiting bone and ligament resection to preserve normal knee kinematics and to create a more normal functioning knee.[36] Cloutier's design consisted of a more modern condylar femoral component and single U-shaped tibial component as an improvement over the technically demanding bicompartmental prostheses (Fig. 133.3).[7] This more contemporary knee allowed for patellofemoral replacement, improved ligament tensioning and deformity correction with asymmetric femoral condyles, and a nearly flat tibial surface.[7] The surgical technique required the use of a knee joint distractor that was attached to Steinmann pins placed transversely through the distal femur and proximal tibia in the coronal plane (Fig. 133.4). The distractor aided in axial alignment and ligament tensioning. Despite clinical success, Cloutier bicruciate TKA (Hermes 2C) was not widely accepted, likely because of the difficulty of the surgical technique.

Other examples of bicruciate retaining TKA included the UCI Knee, Leeds Knee, Ewald Knee, Kodama-Yamamoto Mark I, Duopatella Knee, LCS Bicruciate Knee, Geomedic, and Anametric Knee.[5] In general, bicruciate-retaining TKA lost favor during the period spanning 1990 to present, largely due to perceived difficulty with surgical technique and the widespread clinical success of posterior cruciate-retaining, sacrificing, and substituting designs from multiple manufacturers.

KINEMATICS

The kinematics of the native knee are highly complex and dependent on multiple factors. In the modern era, total knee implant designs have focused largely on excision of one or both cruciate ligaments and less on preservation of these anatomic structures. Sacrificing this tissue complex may result in improved tibial fixation, correction of fixed deformities, ease of technique (largely because of the ability to completely sublux the tibia forward during tibial preparation), removal of posterior cement, avoidance of intercondylar impingement, and the potential for improved motion.[13] Despite these perceived benefits, the cruciate ligaments are fundamental in creating and maintaining normal knee kinematics.[2,4] When both ligaments are retained, patients display more normal function compared with those who have had the cruciate ligaments sacrificed.[15]

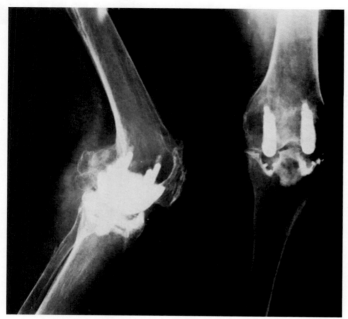

FIG 133.1 Radiograph of Gunston polycentric knee prosthesis.

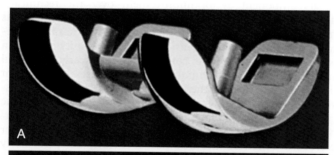

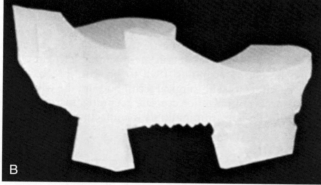

FIG 133.2 Geometric knee prosthesis. The Geomedic knee was a geometric design that had a single femoral component made of Vitallium (A) and a high-density polyethylene tibial plateau (B).

The ACL functions as the primary constraint to anterior translation of the tibia, whereas the remaining ligaments and capsular structures act as secondary constraints.[4] The ACL is described as having two functional fiber bundles consisting of the anteromedial bundle (tight in flexion) and the posterolateral bundle (tight in extension).[26] At 30 and 90 degrees of knee flexion, the ACL provides 86% of the anterior restraining force.[4] In the native knee, while entering terminal extension, the medial

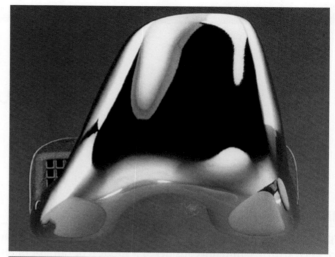

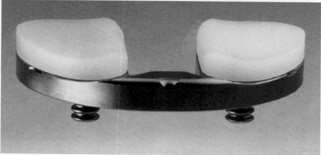

FIG 133.3 Cloutier's knee prosthesis (Hermes 2C).

tibia experiences prolonged anterior glide compared with the lateral tibia, because of the longer articular surface and the aid of the posterior cruciate ligaments (PCLs).[17,19] The anterior glide produces external tibial rotation and is termed the screw-home mechanism.[12,24] As the knee flexes from terminal extension, posterior tibial glide occurs first on the longer medial condyle aided by the ACL, creating relative tibial internal rotation.[19,27]

Multiple studies have proposed that retention of both cruciate ligaments leads to more natural kinematics.[1,15,20,25,35]

Andriacchi et al. performed a gait analysis on patients after total knee replacements with different designs during level walking and stair climbing.[1] The implants used in the study included cruciate-sacrificing, posterior cruciate-preserving, and bicruciate-preserving prostheses. Those with the least constrained, bicruciate-retaining designs were the only subjects with normal motion during ascent and descent of stairs. The authors reasoned that the contact point between the femur and tibia exhibited more posterior translation than the constrained designs, thereby improving the mechanical advantage of the quadriceps.

Stiehl et al. completed an in vivo weight-bearing fluoroscopic analysis of bicruciate-retaining versus posterior cruciate-retaining knee replacements.[35] Individuals performed a deep knee bend, and the anterior to posterior position of the condyles were recorded. The bicruciate-retaining knees had a more anterior contact point in full extension, exhibited posterior femoral roll back in flexion, and had minimal anteroposterior translation. The posterior cruciate-retaining knees maintained a more posterior condylar contact point in extension lateral femoral condyle (LFC −12.1 mm vs. −3.3 mm) and exhibited

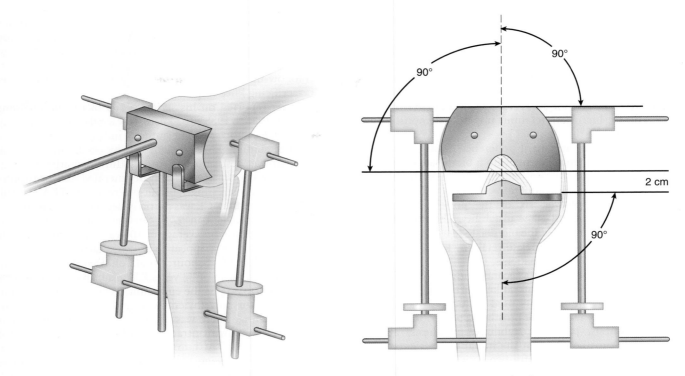

FIG 133.4 Knee joint distractor for Cloutier cruciate-retaining prosthesis.

anterior translation of both condyles in deep flexion. Some subjects in the bicruciate-retaining knee group had a dysfunctional ACL. These knees demonstrated kinematics similar to posterior cruciate-retaining knees. The authors concluded that the posterior cruciate-retaining knees exhibited more abnormal kinematics.

Komistek et al. performed a fluoroscopic kinematic analysis of 30 patients with 15 bicruciate and 15 posterior stabilized knee replacements.[20] The posterior stabilized knees had more kinematic variability, whereas the bicruciate knees on average demonstrated more normal mechanics. Retention of both cruciate ligaments resulted in more consistent anteroposterior contact patterns, more normal axial rotation, and posterior femoral rollback. Three of the 15 bicruciate knees were found to have increased posterior contact points in the stance phase of gait. This was similar to the posterior stabilized knees, likely because of ACL dysfunction.

Moro-oka et al. investigated the kinematics of nine bicruciate-retaining knees and five posterior cruciate-retaining knees by using fluoroscopy and shape matching during different activities.[25] There were statistically significant differences between the two designs, with posterior condylar translation in three settings. At maximum flexion and during stair activity from 30 to 70 degrees flexion, the bicruciate knees had more posterior translation of the lateral femoral condyle. Similarly during the stance and swing phase of gait, the bicruciate knees had more posterior translation of both condyles. The authors concluded that retention of both cruciate ligaments resulted in more normal kinematics during the tested activities.

Retention of the ACL in knee arthroplasty may also have the added value of improved proprioception. In a study by Fuchs et al. the investigators compared a unicondylar prosthesis implanted in both the medial and lateral compartments with retention of both cruciate ligaments to the contralateral

nonreplaced knee in 15 subjects and 11 healthy controls.[14] The individuals performed a single-leg stance on a force place and the change of the projected center of gravity was used to test proprioception. There was no statistically significant difference with sway measurements between the surgical knee versus the contralateral knee or the healthy individual. They concluded that retention of both cruciate ligaments prevents proprioception deficits after knee arthroplasty.

CLINICAL OUTCOMES

Cracchiolo et al. reported on his experience with the first-generation bicruciate-retaining knee arthroplasties.[10] He prospectively compared 119 polycentric and 92 geometric knee replacements, with a mean follow-up of 3.5 years. The polycentric knee had an 11% failure rate with 86% good results, and the geometric knee had a 16% failure rate with 83% good results. The authors stated that the polycentric and geometric prostheses provided excellent relief of pain.[10]

Lewallen et al. investigated 209 polycentric knee replacements with a 10-year follow-up.[21] Patients were considered having successful results if they did not require an assistive device and reported no pain or mild discomfort. At 10 years 42% of those who remained alive had successful results. An additional 24% were successful prior to 10 years but had died or were lost to follow-up. The authors predicted a 66% success rate for the implant at 10 years. Causes of failure included 13% instability, 7% aseptic loosening, 4% patellofemoral pain, and 3% infection.

Townley reviewed the 11-year outcome of 532 anatomic bicruciate-retaining TKAs.[36] The study reported excellent results if the knee motion was greater than 90 degrees, the pain level and activity restriction were mild or none, and the patient did not use a walking aid. The outcomes were 89% good-to-excellent results and 4% poor or failed. The implant failures included 10 with loose tibial trays, 4 with patellar implant dislodgements, 3 with residual ligamentous imbalance, and 2 with patellar dislocations and patellar tendon avulsions.

Buechel and Pappas reported on the 12-year results of a bicruciate-retaining meniscal bearing prosthesis.[3] The 46 knee implants were followed for 12 years. The overall survivorship was 90.9% for the bicruciate-retaining implants, demonstrating good survivorship of this design.

Pritchett published on patient preference in 50 individuals who had staged knee replacements with a bicruciate design on one side and a posterior cruciate-retaining design on the other.[28] Both groups had similar postoperative motion. All bicruciate knees were stable; however, six of the posterior cruciate-retaining knees had sagittal plane instability. The study found that 70% of patients preferred the bicruciate retaining knee and 10% preferred the posterior cruciate-retaining knee. No preference was noted in 20% of the patients.

In 2011 Pritchett performed a second study on 440 patients who also underwent staged bilateral knee arthroplasties using differing designs.[29] The implants used included a bicruciate-retaining prosthesis, medial pivot prosthesis, posterior cruciate-retaining prosthesis, posterior stabilized prosthesis, and a mobile-bearing prosthesis. All of the initial 492 patients were diagnosed with osteoarthritis. Fifty-two patients were excluded because of lack of follow-up or because they had fair or poor results on one or both knees. At 2 years, 89.1% of patients favored the bicruciate-retaining knee over the posterior stabilized knee. The authors proposed that differences in proprioception, sense of stability, and sagittal plane kinematics were factors in the patients' preference.

In a similar group of patients, Pritchett studied noise-related symptoms generated by knee prostheses.[30] He prospectively evaluated 465 patients randomized to have a different implant on each knee. The types of implants tested were medial pivot, bicruciate, posterior cruciate-retaining, posterior stabilized, and mobile-bearing knees. Patients reported the least amount of noise in the bicruciate knees (4%) and the most in the posterior stabilized (33%) and mobile bearing (42%) knees.

In 2015 Pritchett published a report on 489 bicruciate-retaining knees that were implanted from 1989 to 1992.[31] The mean follow-up was 23 years; 51% of patients had died, and 8% were lost to follow-up, leaving 214 knees for evaluation. Survivorship was 89% with revision surgery as the endpoint. The mean postoperative flexion was 117 degrees. The mean Knee Society score was 91. Twenty-two knees were revised, with a mean time to revision of 12 years. The most common reason for revision was polyethylene wear, which occurred in seven knees. All revisions except one (six of seven knees) had the anterior cruciate and PCL intact at the time of revision surgery. The author concluded that bicruciate-retaining implants have good long-term survivorship and function at more than 20-year follow-up.

Migaud et al. reviewed 38 bicruciate-retaining and 30 posterior cruciate-retaining knee replacements at a mean follow-up of 5.5 year.[23] No statistically significant difference in functional scores or range of motion was noted between the two groups. Anterior tibial translation was noted to be higher when a 10-degree increase in posterior tibial slope was present. The authors determined that posterior slope has a higher influence on anterior tibial translation than ACL preservation.

Jenny and Jenny performed a short-term, 2- to 3-year, prospective study comparing 32 bicruciate-retaining with 93 posterior cruciate-retaining knee implants.[18] No statistically significant difference was seen in mean operative time, revision rates, complication rates, functional scores, flexion angle, or radiographic findings. The authors concluded that at short-term follow-up there were no advantages to ACL-sparing over ACL-sacrificing knee implants.

Cloutier reported on his series of 163 bicruciate-retaining knees from 1986 to 1988[8]; 107 knees were available for follow-up at an average of 10 years. The author's indication for placing a bicruciate retaining knee implant was by observing a normal anterior drawer test prior to surgery. Intraoperative findings noted 41% of knees had a partially degenerated ACL or rupture of many fibers. Interestingly, bicruciate-retaining TKA was still performed when the ACL was partially degenerated. The results were good or excellent in 97%. Survival with revision as an endpoint was 95% at an average of 10 years. A macroscopically abnormal ACL did not appear to be a risk factor for failure.

A second report by Sabouret et al. followed the same group of patients for a mean of 22 years.[33] The survival rate was 82% with revision surgery as the endpoint. The reasons for revision included 12% for polyethylene wear and 4% for aseptic component loosening. There was no statistically significant difference between knees, with intraoperative findings of a degenerated ACL versus a normal ACL for revision rate, polyethylene wear, or American Knee Society scores. The authors interpreted these results as demonstrating that at a mean of 22 years the ACL remained functional and provided stability despite some being partially degenerated at the time of surgery.

In 2013 a new US Food and Drug Administration (FDA)-approved bicruciate-retaining TKA design was introduced by Biomet Inc. The Vanguard XP (Biomet Inc, Warsaw, Indiana) was comprised of an anatomically shaped cobalt-chromium femoral component and a U-shaped cobalt-chromium tibial component with two anterior fixation pegs and two posterior fixation rails (Fig. 133.5). Independent medial and lateral bearings made of vitamin E–impregnated, highly cross-linked

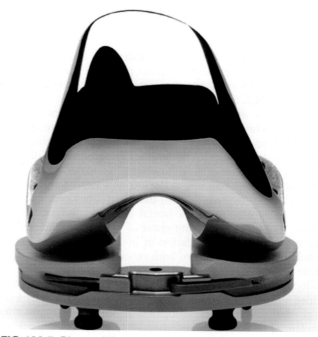

FIG 133.5 Biomet XP knee prosthesis. (Courtesy Biomet.)

polyethylene were made available in 1-mm sizes (9 to 14 mm). In a recently published retrospective study, clinical and radiographic results of 66 bicruciate TKA (Vanguard XP) were compared with 237 posterior cruciate-retaining TKAs (Vanguard). At a minimum 1-year follow-up, the knees in the bicruciate group had a higher frequency of all-cause revision (5% [three of 66] vs. 1.3% [three of 237]; hazard ratio [HR]: 7.44; 95% confidence interval [CI]: 1.24 to 44.80; $P = .028$). Knees in the bicruciate group had a higher frequency of irrigation and débridement with component retention (HR: 0.07; 95% CI: 0.02 to 0.28; $P < .001$). No differences were found between groups for subsequent manipulation (HR: 0.34; 95% CI: 0.08 to 1.42; $P = .137$). The proportion of radiolucent lines was greater in the bicruciate group (HR: 2.93; 95% CI: 1.62 to 5.32; $P < .001$) compared with the posterior cruciate-retaining group. There were no differences between the groups in terms of the Patient-Reported Outcomes Measurement Information System (PROMIS) Physical Function Computerized Adaptive Test scores, PROMIS Global 10 health scores, or knee range-of-motion outcomes. Given this was our initial experience with a new implant design, we continue to clinically and radiographically monitor these patients.[6] Multiple prospective studies are underway to determine if this implant design can improve patient satisfaction after TKA.

TECHNIQUE

Bicruciate TKA can be performed using standard instrumentation similar to a posterior cruciate-retaining knee arthroplasty with some notable changes.

Exposure

The knee is exposed in a standard fashion through a medial parapatellar approach, being careful not to damage the ACL fibers as the capsulotomy, fat pad removal, and meniscal resection are performed. It is infrequently necessary to perform major ligament releases because the ACL seldom remains functional in the setting of severe deformity.

Femoral Preparation

A drill is used to enter the intramedullary canal of the femur, an intramedullary guide is placed, and a distal femoral cutting guide is positioned at the surgeon's preoperatively planned angle of resection. Accurate distal femoral resection (usually 9 mm) is critical to restore the normal joint line. Excessive resection can lead to elevation of the joint line, whereas insufficient resection can lead to increased strain on the ACL; both of which can adversely affect the function of the ACL.

It may also help to protect the ACL by flexing the knee past 90 degrees while performing this resection. After the distal resection is performed, the femur is sized in the standard fashion and rotation is matched parallel to the epicondyle axis and perpendicular to Whiteside's line. A 4-in-1 cutting guide is placed and the anterior, posterior, anterior chamfer, and posterior chamfer cuts are performed. It is recommended that the surgeon switches to a narrow saw blade and, if present, uses the knee system's ACL protector that fits into the cutting guide while performing the posterior and posterior chamfer cuts. If osteophytes are seen within the notch that may cause impingement of the ACL, resection at this time with an osteotome or rongeur is appropriate.

Tibial Preparation

An extramedullary guide is used to set the proximal tibial resection. The guide is positioned parallel to the mechanical axis of the leg. The depth of resection will typically be more than is performed in a standard knee replacement to not raise the joint line. A typical depth of resection may be 4 mm from the medial low point or 11 to 12 mm from the lateral high point of the tibial plateau. An attempt to match the patient's native posterior slope should be made. A common posterior slope angle is 7 degrees. A vertical resection guide is placed to delineate the tibial eminence cut. Additional attention should be spent during this step to determine the medial to lateral position of the tibial implant because the position and rotation of the implant will be determined by the position and rotation of the retained tibial eminence bone island. A trial tibial tray can be used to estimate the end position of the implant with respect to the planned position of the tibial eminence bone island. The vertical cut is made using a reciprocating saw, being careful not to dive with the saw and damage the posterior cortex of the proximal tibia. Next, using a narrow oscillating blade, the horizontal resection is performed. Care is taken during resection of the lateral compartment to protect the patellar tendon. Posterior osteophytes are removed. Single-compartment spacer blocks are trailed to ensure adequate tibial resection and symmetric flexion and extension gaps. The anterior extent of the ACL fibers is noted and a bone cutter is used to resect the anterior tibial bone up to these fibers to allow space for the U-shaped tibial tray. A flat rasp is used to remove rough edges or bone off the tibial eminence bone island, as well as fine-tune the tibial resection. A tibial slope check gauge can be used to ensure the medial and lateral tibia cuts are coplanar.

Trialing

Spacer blocks are used to check the flexion and extension gap sizes. The tibia is next prepped using a tibial template. It is important to place the tibial tray as posteriorly as possible to prevent posterior edge loading. It may be necessary to remove more anterior bone from the tibial eminence bone island to achieve this. The trial tibial and femoral implants are placed. The independent trial bearings are placed. While ranging the knee, it is important to identify any impingement that may occur between the ACL and the femoral implant because this may cause early failure. If the knee does not come to full extension, care must be taken to not force the knee into extension because this may rupture the ACL or fracture the tibial eminence bone island.

Final Implant Placement

The trial implants are removed. Any sclerotic bone should be perforated with 2-mm holes to allow for adequate cement penetration. The bony surfaces are irrigated with a pulse lavage and then dried with a lap sponge. A thin layer of cement is placed on the undersurface of the tibial implant. Cement is then placed on the proximal tibia, preferably using a pressurized nozzle to penetrate and pressurize the cement into the bone. An osteotome can also be used to pressurize the cement into the bone. The tibial implant is placed onto the tibia, manually engaging the posterior structures first to extrude the excess cement anteriorly. A tibial impactor is used in a posterior to anterior fashion to extrude the cement anteriorly. The excess cement is removed and special care is taken to check the posterior aspect of the knee for any remaining cement. In a similar fashion the femur is cleaned with a pulse lavage and dried with a lap sponge. A thin layer of cement is placed on the undersurface of the femoral component. A layer of cement is then placed on the femur, taking time to pressurize the cement with either a pressurized nozzle or manually. The femoral component is placed with a femoral impactor, and the excess cement is removed. It is important to note if the femoral implant is fully seated. If it remains proud, the extension gap will be decreased and tension on the ACL will be dramatically increased. This may possibly lead to ACL failure or tibial eminence fracture. Thus complete seating of the femoral component with the knee in flexion is imperative. The trial bearings are placed, and the knee is ranged once again. The trial bearings are removed, final cement removal is performed, and the final bearings are placed. It is recommended to use two separate batches of cement for placing the tibial and femoral implants, especially early in the learning the curve.

CHALLENGES

Despite the appeal of retaining both cruciate ligaments, there are intraoperative challenges that arise while attempting to achieve this goal. While performing the distal femoral resection, it is possible to injure the ACL with the saw blade, especially during the posterior chamfer resection. To avoid this, a narrow saw blade is recommended, as well as a blocking guide to protect the ACL. The central location of the cruciate ligaments creates challenges for exposure. Anterior subluxation of the tibia is limited because of the intact ACL. This requires in situ resection of the tibia while working around the central tibial eminence, which will often block easy access to the lateral compartment because of the close proximity of the patellar tendon in a medial parapatellar approach. It is important not to undercut the tibial eminence because this can lead to a fracture and failure of the ACL. A narrow saw blade is useful for these reasons during the tibial resection. In addition, the location of tibial eminence guides the rotation and medial to lateral position of the tibial component, requiring the surgeon to be cognizant of this and avoid the pitfall of tibial component overhang and malrotation. With bicruciate ligament retention, it is important to not elevate the joint line. This often requires a larger than typical tibial resection compared with an ACL-sacrificing technique. Under-resection of either the tibia or the distal femur may lead to ACL rupture or tibial eminence fracture. Similarly if the femoral implant does not seat completely, the extension gap will decrease and potentially lead to the same complication.

The central location of the cruciate ligaments also creates design challenges, especially with the tibial component. Independent medial and lateral implants or a U-shaped implant is necessary to preserve the tibial insertion of the ACL. This feature decreases the contact interface between the implant and bone. It also limits the ability to place large fins or keels, requiring instead the use of smaller rails or pegs for component fixation. This may lead to suboptimal tibial component fixation. In U-shaped tibial component designs, the anterior connection between the medial and lateral portion of the tibial implant is also a point of concern, because of the risk of fatigue fracture. However maintaining a single tibial component does decrease the chance of medial to lateral posterior slope mismatch.

CONCLUSION

It would seem reasonable that the retention of both cruciate ligaments is essential to achieve the goal of creating a prosthetic knee that maintains the kinematic subtleties of a native knee. Despite the challenges presented with bicruciate-retaining knee implants, the potential for improved function, higher patient satisfaction, and longer survivability continues to encourage the orthopedic community to pursue this design concept. Multiple studies have shown promising results, suggesting that retaining both cruciate ligaments can lead to more normal knee kinematics, as well as longevity, and patient outcomes similar to ACL-sacrificing knee implants. It remains to be seen whether the notion of bicruciate-retaining knee replacement will succeed in creating a normal-feeling, high-functioning, and long-lasting knee.

KEY REFERENCES

2. Bates NA, Myer GD, Shearn JT, et al: Anterior cruciate ligament biomechanics during robotic and mechanical simulations of physiologic and clinical motion tasks: a systematic review and meta-analysis. *Clin Biomech (Bristol, Avon)* 30(1):1–13, 2015.

6. Christensen JC, Brothers J, Stoddard GJ, et al: Higher frequency of reoperation with a new bicruciate-retaining total knee arthroplasty. *Clin Orthop* 2016. [Epub ahead of print].

11. Cushner FD, La Rosa DF, Vigorita VJ, et al: A quantitative histologic comparison: ACL degeneration in the osteoarthritic knee. *J Arthroplasty* 18(6):687–692, 2003.

12. Freeman MA, Pinskerova V: The movement of the normal tibio-femoral joint. *J Biomech* 38(2):197–208, 2005.

14. Fuchs S, Tibesku CO, Genkinger M, et al: Proprioception with bicondylar sledge prostheses retaining cruciate ligaments. *Clin Orthop* 406:148–154, 2003.

19. Kim HY, Kim KJ, Yang DS, et al: Screw-Home Movement of the tibiofemoral joint during normal gait: three-dimensional analysis. *Clin Orthop Surg* 7(3):303–309, 2015.

20. Komistek RD, Allain J, Anderson DT, et al: In vivo kinematics for subjects with and without an anterior cruciate ligament. *Clin Orthop* 404:315–325, 2002.

25. Moro-oka TA, Muenchinger M, Canciani JP, et al: Comparing in vivo kinematics of anterior cruciate-retaining and posterior cruciate-retaining total knee arthroplasty. *Knee Surg Sports Traumatol Arthrosc* 15(1):93–99, 2007.

31. Pritchett JW: Bicruciate-retaining total knee replacement provides satisfactory function and implant survivorship at 23 years. *Clin Orthop* 473(7):2327–2333, 2015.

33. Sabouret P, Lavoie F, Cloutier JM: Total knee replacement with retention of both cruciate ligaments: a 22-year follow-up study. *Bone Joint J* 95-B(7):917–922, 2013.

35. Stiehl JB, Komistek RD, Cloutier JM, et al: The cruciate ligaments in total knee arthroplasty: a kinematic analysis of 2 total knee arthroplasties. *J Arthroplasty* 15(5):545–550, 2000.

The references for this chapter can also be found on www.expertconsult.com.

134

Bicruciate Total Knee Arthroplasty: An Alternate View

Bertrand W. Parcells, Jared S. Preston, Alfred J. Tria, Jr.

INTRODUCTION

Arthroplasty of the knee changed radically with the introduction of methyl methacrylate in 1969 for hip arthroplasty. Hinges and noncemented devices were quickly replaced by designs that accommodated the ligaments of the knee and could be better fixed to the underlying bone surface. These initial offerings were more sophisticated but experienced early loosening and failure. The designing surgeons learned that the cement could afford fixation but the implant would still require significant bone surface contact. Sacrifice of at least the anterior cruciate ligament (ACL) appeared to be the answer. The ICLH knee resected both of the cruciates and included surface constraint to stabilize the knee.[11] The total condylar knee included similar cruciate resection but changed the surface constraint to allow more motion. The total condylar knee led to the introduction of the posterior stabilized total knee arthroplasty (PS-TKA) designs that resected both of the cruciate ligaments and substituted for the posterior cruciate ligament (PCL) with a tibial post. The cruciate retaining total knee arthroplasty (CR-TKA) designs were able to retain the PCL and still afforded enough surface area for implant cementing. Since the 1980s, the PS- and CR-TKAs controlled the market for replacements, with most further advances representing an evolution in these two themes.[27]

During the same period, however, there were two major groups that continued to investigate the bicruciate retaining (BCR) TKA. Townley developed the anatomic TKA and was able to retain the tibial bone island with bicruciate ligament retention.[34] He presented his results to the Knee Society in 1988 with 11-year follow-up and only 2% loosening. Cloutier was also interested in the design and believed that cruciate ligament retention afforded a degree of proprioception that was extremely desirable, particularly in the younger patient population. He reported 10-year results with 97% excellent or good follow-up.[5]

The BCR TKA never garnered a substantial following despite such findings by two respected surgeons. The notoriety of the earlier failed BCR designs, the greater technical challenges of BCR implantation, and the concern over complications unique to the BCR design, specifically tibial bone island fractures and decreased bone-component contact,[6] likely conspired to prevent widespread use. Furthermore, the PS- and CR-TKAs were developed by famous designers with a strong following around the world. Thus, the BCR supporters continued to work through the 1990s without an updated design coming to market.

Toward the end of the 1990s, some designs for both CR and PS began to emphasize knee kinematics as a means to improve patient satisfaction. These investigations were partially prompted by the studies on UKA designs that indicated preservation of cruciate ligament function produced the most normal kinematics.[8,14,23] More normal motion led to increased range of motion of the knee and, hopefully, a more normal feeling knee joint. New BCR designs are now being released that preserve both of the cruciates and incorporate improved instrumentation.

BENEFITS

The future of total knee arthroplasty aims for a design that infers a more natural feeling knee to improve activity and satisfaction. Currently, most TKA designs demonstrate excellent long-term survival, which is only further improving with the emergence of highly cross-linked polyethylene. Yet patient satisfaction in TKAs without complication remains around 80%.[10,26] The notable limitations that patients cite include the inability to completely kneel, squat, and return to prior athletics, and the inability to restore a "normal" feeling knee. The BCR design may address these areas of dissatisfaction through improvements in kinematics and proprioception.

Kinematics

A balance between articular geometry and soft tissue tension guides the unique motion profiles of the medial and lateral femoral condyles during knee motion.[15,22] The cruciate ligaments play a central role in the soft tissue tensioning.

Increasing attention to the normal ligaments has been central to the progress of TKA design, from the ICLH[11] to modern components. The PCL is believed to be critical to promoting femoral rollback during flexion, and its function is thus preserved either by saving the ligament, in the CR-TKA, or by substituting for its function, in the PS-TKA. Femoral rollback appears to be essential for full range of motion by preventing early impingement of the distal femur.[3] Thus, the main debate among TKA designs in the past decades has been over the approach to preserving PCL function.

Although most current primary TKA designs preserve the collateral ligaments and the PCL function, the ACL is sacrificed without substituting for its function despite evidence that the ACL has a significant effect on normal knee kinematics.[9] An ACL-deficient knee translates the tibia anteriorly during extension and may limit normal femoral rollback during flexion.[9,29] The function of the ACL in knee arthroplasty has been studied in part by comparing UKA, which traditionally requires an intact ACL, with the standard ACL-sacrificing TKA designs.[8,19,23] These studies demonstrate that the UKA designs recreated normal knee kinematics in contrast to the TKA designs. While the two procedures do not offer an isolated view of ACL function, as the UKA preserves not only the ACL but also much of the remaining articular surface, it does suggest that the ACL is important to knee function and that matching knee physiology corresponds to normal knee kinematics.

The BCR designs, similar to the UKA, preserve both cruciate ligaments and may offer improved kinematics by recreating natural soft tissue tension during range of motion. Improved soft tissue tension theoretically decreases the reliance on articular surface design and muscle contraction to guide motion. This in turn restores the normal balance of forces affecting knee motion and improves TKA kinematics.

Proprioception

Studies suggest preservation of the cruciate ligaments not only encourages physiologic movement but also improves proprioception. Proprioception is the information about movement and position of the knee. Afferent nerve receptors located within the ligaments and capsule[13,30] gather information during motion and send signals to both the gamma reflex and somatosensory pathways to adjust muscle contractions. Knee stability relies on complex communication between the soft tissue and the nervous system. Preservation of knee proprioception should lead to a more stable knee, which feels more normal and less like a prosthetic device.

Histologic studies of healthy appearing ACLs have identified proprioceptive receptors, including Pacini, Ruffini, and Golgi organ receptors.[30] Immunohistochemical analysis of the PCL at time of TKA demonstrated the presence of these receptors in degenerative appearing ligaments.[7,18] These findings highlight the functional role of the cruciate ligaments despite ligamentous degeneration in osteoarthritic knees. Clinical studies, in the sports medicine literature, have shown a correlation between ACL injury and loss of knee proprioception. Yet proprioception after TKA is somewhat difficult to evaluate. Preservation of the PCL alone does not seem to demonstrate a significant benefit.[18,32,35] Simmons et al. compared TKA and UKA designs and found no differences in proprioception between the groups.[31] Wada et al. specifically found no change in postoperative proprioception after TKA in patients with lax or absent ACLs, suggesting that the role of the ACL in proprioception may diminish with degeneration.[36]

However, one study comparing a BCR TKA with the contralateral nonoperated knee found no significant loss in proprioception.[12] Furthermore, histologic staining of the PCL in the CR-TKA design demonstrates persistence of the mechanoreceptors seen in knees after undergoing TKA.[37] This finding highlights the potential for these structures to remain functional. The role of the cruciate ligaments in proprioception has been well established in the healthy knee, yet their role after TKA appears controversial despite signs of functional mechanoreceptors.

INDICATIONS

The BCR prosthesis is designed to address multicompartmental arthritis in a select cohort of patients. However, the BCR is not intended to replace all primary TKA designs on the market. The prosthesis uses the normal surrounding structures to guide kinematics and thus requires functional cruciate ligaments for optimal performance. Absent or dysfunctional cruciate ligaments are a contraindication for the BCR knee. Yet identifying

the integrity of cruciate ligaments in a knee with advanced osteoarthritis remains challenging and controversial. Studies evaluating the ACL in osteoarthritic knees have questioned the baseline integrity of the ACL.[1] Further investigation has suggested that most ligaments at the time of TKA demonstrate signs of wear yet remain functionally intact.[16] Studies that evaluated cruciate integrity years after UKA and BCR implantation suggest persistent function despite signs of degeneration.[14,28]

The surgical approach to the BCR design combines many elements of the standard TKA with the ligament preserving UKA. Thus, the relative inclusion and exclusion criteria for the BCR strike a balance between these procedures. Kozinn and Scott were the first to standardize UKA indications based on integrity of soft tissues and degree of contracture.[17,33] The BCR design shares some contraindications because the cruciate preservation limits the extent of bony and soft tissue corrections. A fixed deformity greater than 10 degrees in any plane may be applied as a relative contraindication to the BCR knee. The applicability of other relative contraindications to UKA, such as high activity, younger patients, or heavy laborers, are less applicable to the BCR; thus the BCR should have greater usefulness.

Prosthetic Design and Surgical Technique

A new TKA must consider both the prosthetic design itself and the instruments. The design must be tested both for tolerance to the intraarticular surface forces and for the fixation to the underlying bone. The femoral component will not be particularly unique and in most cases it will be "borrowed" from a pre-existing CR type of design that will have an open intercondylar notch that will accommodate the tibial bone island and cruciate retention (Fig. 134.1). Cruciate retention requires preservation of the bone island on the tibial side (Fig. 134.2). It is possible to design a "U" shaped polyethylene modular insert, but this makes it difficult to have varying thicknesses of the polyethylene on the medial and lateral sides without a

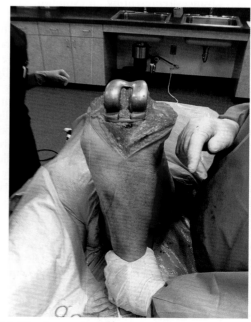

FIG 134.1 The femoral component has an intercondylar notch that accommodates the tibial bone island.

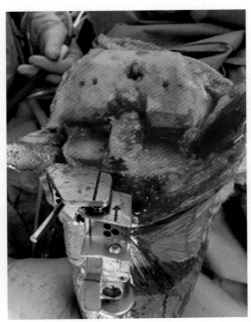

FIG 134.2 The tibial bone island is preserved to maintain the ACL and the PCL.

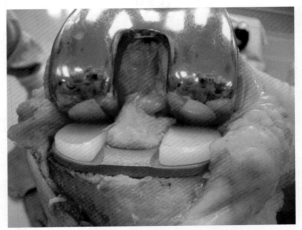

FIG 134.3 Separate tibial polyethylene inserts allow for modification of the thickness on each side.

significant increase in the inventory. It is more advantageous to have a separate polyethylene insert on the medial and lateral side that can be anatomically shaped and varied in thickness (Fig. 134.3). The medial insert should be concave and the lateral more convex to mimic the normal anatomy. Some build up is necessary on the side that abuts the bone island to control coronal plane shifting of the femoral component throughout the range of motion of the knee. The tibial tray is "U" shaped to extend around the bone island and preserve the coplanar surfaces on the medial and lateral sides. The bridge from the medial to the lateral aspect of the tray must be reinforced to prevent stress fracturing (Fig. 134.4). Most tibial trays for the PS TKA incorporate a central keel for stabilization. This will not be possible with the bone island preservation. Many of the CR knee designs use short pegs for fixation on the medial and lateral aspects of the tray, slightly peripheral to the center of the tibia. A combination of pegs and a keel should enhance stability.

The instruments for the knee will have to be modified on the tibial side to allow for the bone island preservation (Fig. 134.5). Undercutting the bone can lead to loss of the island integrity, and this has been reported with one of the new designs.[6] It is critical to make the instruments user friendly yet accurate. It is best to incorporate some form of protection for the island when bone saws are used. If the bone island is compromised during the procedure, it may be possible to transfix it with a screw and a washer, but the fixation must certainly be fully confirmed to avoid postoperative bone island fracture.

Results

Townley reported 2- to 11-year follow-up with only 2% loosening with his BCR knee.[34] Cloutier reported 95% survivorship at 9 to 11 years,[5] but dropped to 82% at 22 years follow-up, including any reason for revision.[28] Overall aseptic loosening was only 4.3%, and 12% of his reported knees were revised because of

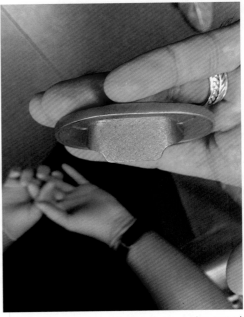

FIG 134.4 The tibial tray has a bridge across the anterior aspect connecting the medial and lateral surfaces, assuring that they are coplanar. The anterior undersurface keel protects the bridge from stress fracture.

polyethylene wear.[28] Buechel reported 90.9% survival rate with a meniscal bearing design.[4] Romagnoli had experience with a type of BCR knee that used a traditional femoral component with two separate unicondylar tibial inserts.[2,21,27] He reported 2- to 11-year follow-ups, with only one failure because of ligament instability and an average range of motion of 116 degrees. Pritchett reported 89% survivorship at a 23-year follow-up. Polyethylene wear, not prosthetic loosening, was his main mode of failure.[25] These reports are equal to many of the reports in the literature for the CR and PS-TKAs; yet the designs did not thrive during that period of time. The CR and PS-TKAs had strong supporters, and the surgical techniques were not difficult for most orthopedic surgeons. The BCR knee designs were less familiar and required more steps and precision. Most of the

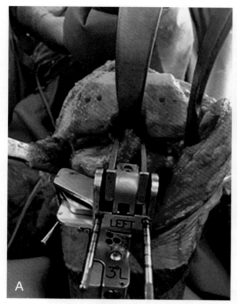 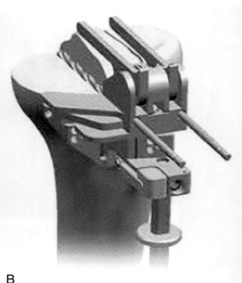 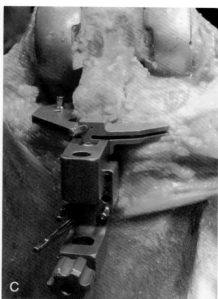

FIG 134.5 (A) The extramedullary tibial cutting guide lines up with the bone island with correct external rotation. (B) The medial tibial resection is completed with a protective pin at the base of the bone island to protect the island from any undercutting. (C) The lateral tibial plateau resection is completed with a saw capturing guide that references the previously completed medial resection to assure a coplanar cut.

results were reported by designing surgeons who were intimately familiar with the prostheses and the instruments.

In the past 5 to 10 years, the evaluations of the results of TKA have become much more complex and include proprioception, kinematics, and patient satisfaction.*

Earlier TKA designs were not subject to such scrutiny. Approximately 15% to 20% of patients are not satisfied with their TKA result and look for something better.[10] There is no doubt that proprioception and kinematics will play a central part in the designing of implants in the future. Preservation of all of the ligaments of the knee improves both kinematics and proprioception.[14,24]

With the renewed interest in the BCR knee, there are now two designs available in the United States. The XP-Preserving Knee (Biomet-Zimmer, Warsaw, Indiana) has had some bone island fractures, but the designers appear to be addressing the issue and improving the early results.[6] The Journey XR Knee (Smith and Nephew Orthopedics, Memphis, Tennessee) is kinematically almost identical to the normal knee. However, it has just been released and does not have any early clinical reports.

CONCLUSIONS

Retention of all of the ligaments of the knee makes good clinical sense. The problems in the past have centered on the difficulty of combining the surface geometry of the implant and the surrounding soft tissue structures in a manner that allows for the most normal motion of the knee with a design that will stand the test of time in vivo. Kinematics and proprioception

should go hand in hand to improve the clinical results, and hopefully, the BCR TKA will be the answer in the future.

CONFLICTS OF INTEREST

Authors BWP and JSP have no conflicts of interest. Author AJT is a royalty bearing surgeon for Smith and Nephew Orthopedics and a consultant for Smith and Nephew Orthopedics, Medtronic, and Pacira.

KEY REFERENCES

2. Banks SA, Fregly BJ, Boniforti F, et al: Comparing in vivo kinematics of unicondylar and bi-unicondylar knee replacements. *Knee Surg Sports Traumatol Arthrosc* 13(7):551–556, 2005.
4. Buechel FF, Pappas MJ: Long-term survivorship analysis of cruciate-sparing versus cruciate-sacrificing knee prostheses using meniscal bearings. *Clin Orthop* 260:162–169, 1990.
5. Cloutier JM, Sabouret P, Deghrar A: Total knee arthroplasty with retention of both cruciate ligaments. A nine to eleven-year follow-up study. *J Bone Joint Surg Am* 81(5):697–702, 1999.
6. Della Valle CJ, Andriacchi TP, Berend KR, et al: Early experience with bi-cruciate retaining TKA. Poster presentation at the Annual Meeting American Academy of Orthopaedic Surgeons, 2015.
9. Dennis DA, Mahfouz MR, Komistek RD, et al: In vivo determination of normal and anterior cruciate ligament-deficient knee kinematics. *J Biomech* 38(2):241–253, 2005.
10. Dunbar MJ, Richardson G, Robertsson O: I can't get no satisfaction after my total knee replacement: rhymes and reasons. *Bone Joint J* 95-B(11 Suppl A):148–152, 2013.
17. Kozinn SC, Scott R: Unicondylar knee arthroplasty. *J Bone Joint Surg Am* 71(1):145–150, 1989.
20. Nam D, Nunley RM, Barrack RL: Patient dissatisfaction following total knee replacement: a growing concern? *Bone Joint J* 96-B(11 Suppl A):96–100, 2014.

*References 2, 10, 12, 14, 20, and 32.

24. Pritchett JW: Patients prefer a bicruciate-retaining or the medial pivot total knee prosthesis. *J Arthroplasty* 26(2):224–228, 2011.

25. Pritchett JW: Bicruciate-retaining total knee replacement provides satisfactory function and implant survivorship at 23 years. *Clin Orthop* 473(7):2327–2333, 2015.

27. Romagnoli S, Verde F, Bibbiani E, et al: Bi-unicompartmental knee prostheses. In Scuderi GR, Tria AJ, editors: *Minimally invasive surgery in orthopedics*, New York, USA, 2010, Springer, pp 327–340.

28. Sabouret P, Lavoie F, Cloutier JM: Total knee replacement with retention of both cruciate ligaments: a 22-year follow-up study. *Bone Joint J* 95-B(7):917–922, 2013.

34. Townley CO: The anatomic total knee resurfacing arthroplasty. *Clin Orthop* 192:82–96, 1985.

37. Zhang K, Mihalko WM: Posterior cruciate mechanoreceptors in osteoarthritic and cruciate-retaining TKA retrievals: a pilot study. *Clin Orthop* 470(7):1855–1859, 2012.

The references for this chapter can also be found on www.expertconsult.com.

135

European Analysis and Results of Partial Knee Replacement

Emmanuel Thienpont

UNICOMPARTMENTAL KNEE ARTHROPLASTY VERSUS TOTAL KNEE ARTHROPLASTY: FUNCTION AND SURVIVAL

Total knee arthroplasty (TKA) achieves excellent outcomes on a range of measures. Patient postoperative satisfaction after TKA is high and is typically reported as being more than 80%,[34] primarily because of achieving a satisfactory level of pain relief.[35] However, patients may experience significant limitations, such as impaired functional activity[64] and persistent postsurgical pain (PPSP).[58,59,67,88] A multicenter survey found that, although 90% of patients reported overall satisfaction with the functioning of their knee, only 66% felt that their knee was "normal," with 33% to 54% reporting residual symptoms and functional problems.[58] There is, therefore, clearly a need for other implant concepts that can improve outcomes, particularly from the patient perspective.

Unicompartmental knee arthroplasty (UKA) is an alternative to TKA for the treatment of isolated bone-on-bone arthritis or osteonecrosis of the medial or lateral femorotibial knee compartments.[15,16] UKA is a less-invasive procedure than TKA, and results in faster rehabilitation, greater preservation of bone stock, reduced blood loss, and a lower risk of infection.[4,26,46,72,74] Moreover, UKA preserves the cruciate ligaments, the contralateral compartment and patellofemoral anatomy, and allows for knee kinematics that match more closely those of the native knee.[2,36,41] The procedure also resurfaces more than replacing the distal and posterior femoral anatomy, thus retaining at least 60% of the natural articular surfaces of the knee. This may result in a more normal gait, as well as reduced perioperative trauma, greater range of motion, and faster rehabilitation.[26,70,73] The result is a joint reconstruction that not only moves in a fashion very similar to the patient's predisease knee but also feels more like a natural knee.[3,81]

Reported survival rates for UKA are nevertheless consistently lower than those for TKA. The Australian Orthopaedic Association National Joint Replacement Registry found 10-year survival rates with TKA and UKA in primary osteoarthritis of 94.4% and 84.9%, respectively,[61] a disparity that is also reflected in the Swedish Knee Arthroplasty Register and National Joint Registry for England and Wales annual reports.[62,63] A systematic review of cumulative data from six national registries and clinical studies found that primary TKA was associated with a mean revision rate of 1.29 revisions per 100 component observed years versus 1.53 revisions per 100 component years for UKA.[47] Furthermore, an analysis of data on 3929 UKAs performed on 3645 patients from the Register of Prosthetic Orthopedic Implants (RPOI) in Italy yielded a 10-year survival rate of 86.6%, with patient age found to significantly influence prosthesis survival.[15] To adjust for any potential confounding in registry data because of comparing patients with different baseline characteristics and indications, Liddle et al. used propensity matching to compare 25,334 UKAs and 75,996 TKAs from the National Joint Registry for England and Wales. They found that UKA had worse implant survival in terms of both revision and revision/reoperation than TKA at 8 years, at hazard ratios of 2.12 and 1.38, respectively.[50] There has been some debate over the usefulness of revision rates in determining the success of UKA, with Goodfellow et al. arguing that the threshold used to revise a painful UKA is lower than that for TKA, and therefore revision per se is not an objective measure.[29] However, this was refuted by an analysis of data from the National Joint Registry of England and Wales, which highlighted that pain is not the most common reason for revision of UKA.[9] Nevertheless, an analysis of the Norwegian Arthroplasty Register by Furnes et al. suggested that UKA is more than 11 times more likely to be revised for pain than TKA, at a relative risk of 11.3 ($p < 0.001$).[28]

Despite the increased revision rates reported for UKA, Liddle et al. found that the average length of stay; rate of complications such as thromboembolism, myocardial infarction, and stroke; and rate of readmission were all higher for TKA than for UKA.[50] In addition, 30-day and 8-year mortality was lower with UKA than with TKA in this study, at hazard ratios of 0.23 and 0.85.[50] Hunt et al., in an analysis of 467,779 primary knee replacements from the same registry, found that UKA was associated with substantially lower 45-day mortality than TKA, at a hazard ratio 0.32 ($p < 0.0005$).[38]

Whether UKA yields better clinical outcomes than TKA, and whether the theoretical advantages of UKA in terms of kinematics have a clinical impact, remains a matter of debate. A study based on data from the National Joint Registry for England and Wales matching 3519 UKA patients with 10,557 TKAs indicated that mean 6-month patient-reported outcome measures (PROMs), including the Oxford Knee Score (OKS) and the EuroQol (EQ-5D) index, were better with UKA than with TKA.[52] UKA patients were also significantly more likely to report excellent results than those who underwent TKA, at an odds ratio of 1.59 ($p < 0.001$) and were less likely to report complications. The researchers therefore suggest that the differences in revision rates between the two procedures may not be because of differences in functional outcomes.[52] These findings contrast with the results of a study by Baker et al., in which a minimum of 6 months of postoperative PROMs data were compared for 23,393 TKAs and 505 UKAs. Once adjustments were made for case-mix differences and preoperative score, there were no significant differences in improvements on both the OKS and the EQ-5D ($p = 0.96$ and $p = 0.37$, respectively).[10]

It is therefore clear that, when deciding whether to offer UKA or TKA to a patient, the higher revision/reoperation rate of UKA should be set against its lower rates of complications, readmission, and mortality, alongside the known benefits in terms of postoperative function. For every 100 patients undergoing UKA instead of TKA, there would be approximately one fewer death but three more reoperations in the first 4 years after surgery with the less-invasive procedure. UKA may therefore still represent a valuable alternative for patients who do not require the more invasive TKA.[37]

Proponents of UKA also state that revision of UKA to TKA (Uni to Total) is a relatively easy procedure that offers advantages over revision of primary TKA.[21] However, approximately 50% of patients undergoing conversion from UKA to TKA have significant bone defects, and stemmed implants and/or augments are required in 33% of cases.[11,19,89] Using data from the New Zealand Joint Registry from 1999 to 2008, Pearse et al. examined 4284 UKAs, of which 236 required revision.[68] Of those, 205 were Uni to Total knee revisions and 31 received a second UKA. In addition, 34,369 primary TKAs were included in the analysis. The rate of revision for Uni to Total was four times higher than for primary TKA, at rates of 1.97 and 0.48 per 100 component years, respectively ($p < 0.05$). Moreover, the rate of revision for patients who had a second UKA was 13 times higher than for a primary TKA. The mean OKS was also significantly worse in the Uni to Total group than in the primary TKA group, at 30.02 versus 37.16 ($p < 0.01$). The researchers conclude that UKA should not be used as a "conservative" procedure to delay TKA, even in the younger patient.[68]

Despite these limitations, UKA can be a viable alternative to TKA, particularly in situations where reduced length of hospital stay, avoidance of complications, a shorter rehabilitation period, and the preservation of bone stock are priorities, such as in the younger or the more elderly patient. Design improvements and the careful selection of patients are likely to yield better outcomes, and it is conceivable that survival rates will approach those seen with the more invasive TKA.

FAILURE ANALYSIS IN UNICOMPARTMENTAL KNEE ARTHROPLASTY

Modes of failure in UKA have been documented in a number of registries.[8,15,48,61] Although the proportion of failures ascribable to each cause varies widely between registries, the most common cause of failure in both the Swedish Knee Arthroplasty Register and the National Joint Registry for England and Wales was aseptic loosening (Table 135.1).[8,48] This finding was supported by Bordini et al. in their analysis of RPOI data, in which all types of aseptic loosening combined accounted for 59.2% of failures.[15] This finding was followed by pain without loosening and infection, which accounted for 15.2% and 11.2% of failures, respectively. Bordini et al. found that the mean time to failure

TABLE 135.1 Modes of Failure in Medial Unicompartmental Knee Arthroplasty

Mode of Failure	Swedish Registry[48] ($n = 1331$)	National Joint Registry[8] ($n = 995$)
Aseptic loosening	400 (30.1)	449 (45.1)
Osteoarthritis progression	60 (4.5)	251 (25.2)
Pain	327 (24.6)	—
Instability	116 (8.7)	27 (2.7)
Infection	73 (5.5)	42 (4.2)
Wear	25 (1.9)	51 (5.1)
Bearing dislocation	35 (2.6)	15 (1.5)
Malalignment	74 (5.6)	21 (2.1)
Fracture	29 (2.2)	23 (2.3)
Tibial subsidence	—	32 (3.2)
Other[a]	192 (14.4)	84 (8.4)

[a]Including patellar problems, arthrofibrosis, stiffness, other and unknown causes. All values n (%).

for UKA ranged from 1 to 6 years, with most common causes of failure clustered around 2 to 3 years.[15] In the Australian Orthopaedic Association National Joint Replacement Registry, the three most common causes of UKA failure were disease progression (43.7%), implant loosening/lysis (20.5%), and pain (13.4%).[61]

Data from the Norwegian Arthroplasty Register suggest that the risk of UKA revision is lower in hospitals that perform more than 40 procedures per year than in those that perform fewer than 10 per year, at a risk ratio adjusted for age, diagnosis, and sex of 0.59 ($p = 0.01$), primarily because of an increase of failure due to dislocation, instability, malalignment, and fracture in low-volume hospitals.[6] The association between hospital volume and failure rates is supported by data from the New Zealand Joint Registry,[60] and an analysis of the National Joint Registry of England and Wales by Baker et al.[7] indicating that the risk of revision decreased as center volume and surgeon volume increased for the most commonly used implant in England and Wales. Baker et al. suggest a minimum number of procedures performed per year of 13, taking into account both surgeon and hospital volume.[7] Because it might be difficult for surgeons to increase the size of their practice, the solution to increase UKA volume is to better select the patients undergoing a TKA and identify UKA candidates instead of replacing the entire joint.[52] Studies have estimated that between 25% and 48% of patients presenting with knee osteoarthritis are candidates for UKA.[76,87]

An essential aspect of UKA, in terms of the restoration of normal knee kinematics and the prevention of the other knee compartment or component wear, is proper component alignment.[17] However, the procedure is technically challenging, and it has been estimated that, with conventional techniques, 40% to 60% of UKA components may be malaligned by greater than 2 degrees from the preoperative plan.[20,42] Malalignment might lead to disease progression of the other compartment, along with aseptic component loosening and pain, and therefore be misclassified as the primary reason for revision in national registries. This might explain the comparatively small numbers of patients listed as having revision because of malalignment (see Table 135.1). Indeed, Bordini et al. did not list malalignment at all as a potential cause of failure.[15]

UKA failures because of component malpositioning are again associated with procedure volume,[5,55] which may be related to the surgeon's learning curve concerning the procedure.[33] As far back as 1986, Weinstein et al. demonstrated that varus-valgus alignment in the frontal plane is directly correlated with the magnitude of the adduction moment during level walking, leading them to suggest that increased precision in component placement should improve long-term outcomes.[86] Their conclusion still holds today, and issues of component alignment have slowed the adoption of UKA,[45] with failure rates remaining persistently high despite improvements in surgical techniques.[6] Technologies to improve alignment accuracy may therefore benefit UKA even more than they have benefited TKA.[71]

The accuracy and consistency of component positioning can be improved with computer navigation over conventional techniques in UKA,[85] with significant reductions in the number of outliers.[20,57] Nevertheless, outliers may still occur in up to 40% of UKA procedures.[40] A further refinement to computer navigation are robotic systems, including image-free, surgeon-controlled handheld robotic sculpting tools. Surgical planning is performed as with any conventional surgical navigation system. However, the surgeon receives continuous, real-time feedback on knee kinematics, range of motion, and implant placement during the procedure to offer component placement accuracy at least comparable to that reported for other robotic-assistive devices,[20,23,54,79] albeit with reduced total surgical times and little, if any, learning curve.[39,77]

A more recent introduction is patient-specific instrumentation (PSI), which may improve the limited precision of standard instrumentation while reducing the perioperative time loss with navigation. Rather than relying on the intraoperative identification of anatomic landmarks by the surgeon, PSI involves manufacturing instruments based on computed tomography (CT) or magnetic resonance imaging (MRI) to match the individual patient's anatomy.

PSI has been shown in some studies to enhance implant alignment,[13,22] which should, theoretically, improve surgical outcomes and reduce the risk of revision. However, other studies have not indicated improvements in implant accuracy with PSI versus the conventional technique.[65] The reasons for these divergent results have not yet been clarified.

Cemented Versus Cementless Unicompartmental Knee Arthroplasty

Most UKA designs rely on cement to achieve bone fixation.[1] However, many UKAs are performed using a minimally invasive technique, making the insertion and extrusion of cement challenging.[1,53] Cementation errors may cause excess wear, ultimately leading to loosening and pain, which are two of the most common reasons for revision in national joint registries.[53,61,66] Cementless UKA has thus been suggested as a way of reducing failures and achieving more reliable fixation, which is especially important in younger patients.[1] Cementless UKA has consequently become increasingly popular in recent years.[32,53]

In joints with loose implants, the bone-implant or bone-cement interface is replaced by a layer of fibrocartilage, seen radiographically as a thick, poorly defined radiolucent area.[56] These radiolucencies are less common following UKA with cementless fixation than in cemented UKA. In an analysis of 63 knees in 62 patients that underwent either cemented or cementless UKA with the Oxford Partial Knee, Pandit et al. found that there were significantly more radiolucencies in the cemented than in the cementless group, at 20 of 30 knees versus 2 of 27 knees ($p < 0.001$). Moreover, there were nine complete radiolucencies in cemented knees, as opposed to none in the cementless group ($p = 0.01$).[66] The radiolucencies did not progress between 1 and 5 years, while radiolucencies associated with inadequate seating of the tibial tray disappeared within the first year. Functional outcomes were comparable between the groups, and it was noted that cementless fixation required a significantly shorter mean operative time compared with cemented fixation, at 86.5 minutes versus 95.7 minutes ($p = 0.049$).[66] These results were confirmed by a recently published radiostereometric analysis. This analysis revealed that although the femoral components migrated significantly during the first postoperative year by a mean of 0.16 mm with cemented fixation and 0.24 mm with cementless fixation, there was no significant migration between 1 and 2 years ($p = 0.92$).[44] Again, there were significantly fewer radiolucencies associated with cementless fixation than with cemented components ($p = 0.02$).[44]

It should be noted, however, that radiolucencies are not always associated with pain or loosening, but rather indicate suboptimal fixation.[43] It is therefore commonly believed that fixation is of higher quality if the fibrocartilage layer is not present.[66] Anteromedial tibial pain can frequently occur in the early postoperative period and usually resolves spontaneously,[66] which may be a result of changes in bone stresses following surgery.[78] Surgeons who are relatively unfamiliar with radiolucencies may attribute this pain to the presence of a radiolucent line, and convert the UKA to a TKA.[66] This is often unnecessary, as a fine, well-defined radiolucent line may be present at the bone-cement interface even in well-functioning cemented UKAs.[24,31,66,84]

Some rare complications have nevertheless been reported for cementless UKA, including early subsidence of the tibial component into a valgus position.[51] The researchers hypothesized that if the femoral component is positioned slightly too far laterally relative to the tibial component, impingement of the mobile bearing on the lateral wall may occur. This would then result in subluxation of the femur in the bearing and subsequent tilting of the bearing relative to the tibial tray, which may cause the tibial component to subside into valgus.[51]

A cadaveric study also indicated that cementless implants may be more susceptible to periprosthetic tibial plateau fracture (PTPF),[75] although this may be because of implantation errors known to dispose toward PTPF, such as a deep posterior cortical cut in the tibia and perforating the posterior cortex perforation during keel preparation.[53] The risk can be minimized by the use of a "keel cut" saw blade, clearing the peg and keel slots, and careful impaction.[53]

Overall, cementless UKA is a promising technology, although more research is required and cemented fixation remains the gold standard.

Fixed Versus Mobile Unicompartmental Knee Arthroplasty

The different design concepts for UKA can be divided into two main categories: fixed bearing (FB) and mobile bearing (MB).[14,25,79,80] While the theoretical advantages of MB prostheses over FB designs have made it increasingly popular in recent years,[18] it does not appear to offer any benefits in terms of rotational and anteroposterior (AP) tibiofemoral translation.[12] The choice of design for UKA therefore remains controversial.[49]

To resolve the issue, several meta-analyses have been conducted. Peersman et al. reviewed 44 comparative and noncomparative studies involving 9463 knees[69] and found that after stratification by age and follow-up time, there appear to be no major differences in survival rates between FB and MB implants. However, the mean time to revision was shorter for MB knees, at 2.5 ± 1.8 years and 6.7 ± 2.5 years, respectively ($p < 0.001$), which applied to all causes of revision ($p < 0.001$), aside from postoperative infection. Time to revision was also significantly shorter with MB implants compared to FB knees in elderly patients, at 4.2 years versus 7.4 years ($p < 0.001$). No other significant differences were found between the implants, although comparisons were hampered by a lack of long-term FB studies in younger patients.[69] The researchers conclude that the findings underscore the importance of patient selection when choosing UKA implants, and that the shorter time to revision supports the view that there is a substantial learning curve with MB UKA, with a high technical standard required to achieve good outcomes.[70] Indeed, Epinette et al. found, in a large multicenter study of 418 failed UKAs, that 19% of revisions were performed within the first postoperative year, and 48.5% were carried out within 5 years.[27]

In another meta-analysis, Cheng et al. examined nine studies involving 915 knees that compared FB and MB UKA. Again, they found no significant differences between the implants in terms of revision rates, clinical outcome scores, range of motion, or radiographic findings, such as limb alignment, implant positioning, and the incidence of radiolucencies.[18] There was, however, a significant difference in the mean time to revision, at 5.0 years for MB knees and 6.3 years for FB implants ($p = 0.016$). Interestingly, early failures in MB patients were linked to bearing dislocations, while later failures in the FB group were more commonly because of polyethylene wear.[18]

Smith et al. identified five studies comparing FB and MB implants for medial and lateral UKA, involving a total of 165 and 159 knees, respectively.[80] There were no significant differences between the implant types in medial UKA in terms of clinical outcome, and no differences in complication rates. Only one study examined lateral UKA procedures and, again, there were no differences in either clinical outcome or complication rates.[80] One study of medial UKA found that there were fewer radiolucent lines with MB than with FB implants ($p = 0.02$). The authors suggested that this might be because of the former more closely approximating normal knee kinematics.[49] Overall, Smith et al. pointed out that the evidence base was small, particularly when assessing lateral UKA, and there were a number of methodological issues, such as inadequate randomization and concealment prior to allocation, limited details on the patient populations, and a lack of assessor and patient blinding prior to group allocation.[80]

In conclusion, any decision between FB and MB designs in UKA is hampered by a lack of robust and well-designed studies, and an evidence base limited to observational studies and small, randomized controlled trials. Nevertheless, it appears that there are no major differences between the two implant types.

The European analysis of results in unicompartmental arthroplasty helps surgeons understand the dilemma. The choice between UKA and TKA according to available literature is still a choice of survivorship over function.[82] Better preoperative analysis of the patient's disease process leading to arthritis progression[83] and better understanding of pain after knee arthroplasty[30] could reduce the number of unnecessary revisions to TKA. Malalignment and aseptic loosening should be addressed by better instrumentation and surgeon education. If the technical failure aspect of UKA can be reduced to the same rate as for TKA patients with isolated bone-on-bone arthritis of one compartment can benefit from the multiple advantages of this type of resurfacing surgery.[50]

KEY REFERENCES

7. Baker P, Jameson S, Critchley R, et al: Center and surgeon volume influence the revision rate following unicondylar knee replacement: an analysis of 23,400 medial cemented unicondylar knee replacements. *J Bone Joint Surg Am* 95:702–709, 2013.

13. Bell SW, Stoddard J, Bennett C, et al: Accuracy and early outcomes in medial unicompartmental knee arthroplasty performed using patient specific instrumentation. *Knee* 21(Suppl 1):S33–S36, 2014.

15. Bordini B, Stea S, Falcioni S, et al: Unicompartmental knee arthroplasty: 11-year experience from 3929 implants in RIPO register. *Knee* 21:1275–1279, 2014.

30. Grosu I, Lavand'homme P, Thienpont E: Pain after knee arthroplasty: an unresolved issue. *Knee Surg Sports Traumatol Arthrosc* 22:1744–1758, 2014.

36. Heyse TJ, El-Zayat BF, De Corte R, et al: UKA closely preserves natural knee kinematics in vitro. *Knee Surg Sports Traumatol Arthrosc* 22:1902–1910, 2014.

38. Hunt LP, Ben-Shlomo Y, Clark EM, et al: 45-day mortality after 467,779 knee replacements for osteoarthritis from the National Joint Registry for England and Wales: an observational study. *Lancet* 384:1429–1436, 2014.

44. Kendrick BJ, Kaptein BL, Valstar ER, et al: Cemented versus cementless Oxford unicompartmental knee arthroplasty using radiostereometric analysis: a randomised controlled trial. *Bone Joint J* 97-B:185–191, 2015.

50. Liddle AD, Judge A, Pandit H, et al: Adverse outcomes after total and unicompartmental knee replacement in 101,330 matched patients: a study of data from the National Joint Registry for England and Wales. *Lancet* 18:1437–1445, 2014.

52. Liddle AD, Pandit H, Judge A, et al: Patient-reported outcomes after total and unicompartmental knee arthroplasty: a study of 14,076 matched patients from the National Joint Registry for England and Wales. *Bone Joint J* 97-B:793–801, 2015.

65. Ollivier M, Parratte S, Lunebourg A, et al: The John Insall Award: no functional benefit after unicompartmental knee arthroplasty performed with patient-specific instrumentation: a randomized trial. *Clin Orthop Relat Res* 474(1):60–68, 2015.

69. Peersman G, Stuyts B, Vandenlangenbergh T, et al: Fixed-versus mobile-bearing UKA: a systematic review and meta-analysis. *Knee Surg Sports Traumatol Arthrosc* 23(11):3296–3305, 2014.

74. Schwab PE, Lavand'homme P, Yombi JC, et al: Lower blood loss after unicompartmental than total knee arthroplasty. *Knee Surg Sports Traumatol Arthrosc* 23(12):2014. doi: 10.1007/s00167-014-3188-x.

83. Thienpont E, Schwab PE, Omoumi P: Wear patterns in anteromedial osteoarthritis of the knee evaluated with CT-arthrography. *Knee* 21(Suppl 1):S15–S19, 2014.

82. Thienpont E, Baldini A: Unicompartmental knee arthroplasty: function versus survivorship, do we have a clue? *Knee* S1:S1–S2, 2014.

The references for this chapter can also be found on www.expertconsult.com.

136

Posterior Cruciate Ligament Retention in Total Knee Arthroplasty

Brian M. Culp, Aaron G. Rosenberg

The debate over whether to preserve the posterior cruciate ligament (PCL) in total knee arthroplasty (TKA), so-called cruciate-retaining (CR), or to substitute for it, so-called posterior stabilized (PS), continues to engage orthopedists. Although multiple differing design philosophies have come and gone over the past several decades, no consensus has been reached as to which knee is preferable. Several factors account for this. First, no clear benefits or drawbacks are apparent for either type of implant to the extent that either is clearly superior. In addition, multiple confounding factors are present in the comparative evaluation of implants (eg, function, patient satisfaction, implant longevity, complication rates), as well as the influence of tradition in the implant choices of most surgeons, which makes comparison difficult. However, it should be noted that of primary importance in understanding the debate over implant choice in knee replacement is the difficulty in "hitting" a moving target.

Analysis of the available data is limited by two issues. First, the implants we now use are frequently different in both big and small (but perhaps no less important) ways from those reported on in most of the long-term follow-up studies. Second, these longer-term studies may reflect a significantly different patient population than that currently presenting for knee replacement. In the early decades of knee arthroplasty surgery, some series reflected as many as half of patients having inflammatory (most commonly rheumatoid) arthritis.[36] Young age, large size, primary or secondary degenerative osteoarthritis, and what were considered high physical activity demands generally were not thought to be ideal indications for TKA. Concerns about implant longevity, as well as a relatively higher complication rate and fear of early failure, led many surgeons to delay arthroplasty of the knee until more advanced disease was present, along with a lower likelihood that the patient would stress the implant construct.

Advances in implant design, surgical technique, and rehabilitative procedures, following careful critical assessment of results, have led to systematic improvement in the quality and consistency of TKA results, such that better pain relief, improved function, and better longevity can be expected for most patients undergoing TKA. These advances have given surgeons the confidence to offer knee replacement to afflicted individuals not previously deemed sufficiently debilitated or aged to warrant the risk. Current indications have subsequently expanded to younger and less severely affected individuals. Thus the surgeon must be aware of the fact that data in the literature may reflect implant and patient types that are not identical to those seen in today's practice.

PS designs have been suggested to offer easier correction of deformity without concern for obtaining appropriate tension on the PCL, a more conforming polyethylene surface that results in decreased polyethylene wear, and more reliable rollback of the femur on the tibia in flexion.[65] Proponents of the PS design note the more widespread clinical usefulness, in that it can be used in knees without a PCL,[37] as well as the potential benefit of avoiding late posterior instability from PCL rupture, which has been reported in osteoarthritic patients[53] and in those with inflammatory arthritis.[44,49]

Proponents of CR[3,4,8,15,29] have suggested that advantages include preservation of an important central stabilizing ligamentous structure, transfer of stress to a functional ligament rather than a mechanical structure with subsequent reduction in wear and fixation stress, more consistent preservation of the joint line,[30] improvement in stair climbing ability,[4] and greater conservation of bone. In addition, problems that appear to be unique to PS designs—patellar clunk and post breakage and wear—are absent from CR designs.[45,48] Lombardi et al. also reported a higher incidence of femoral condyle fractures associated with the box resection in older designs for PS knees.[47] Finally, the concept of simply resurfacing the joint and maintaining as much of the normal structures as possible is a philosophically appealing one, and indeed clinical data support both the quality and the longevity of the cruciate–retaining total knee arthroplasty (CR TKA).

RESULTS OF POSTERIOR CRUCIATE LIGAMENT-RETAINING TOTAL KNEE ARTHROPLASTY

Long-term series of many different CR TKA systems demonstrate excellent longevity and clinical results.* These results reflect 3 decades of evolving implant designs, which have corrected some of the problems noted in previous implant designs and materials and have reflected improvements in surgical technique and understanding of the technical requirements of implanting a knee that retains the PCL. These include improved patellofemoral design characteristics; better understanding of modularity, locking mechanisms, and the adverse effects of backside wear; improved understanding of the relationship

---

*References 8, 12, 17, 25, 33, 35, 45, 54, 55, 60, 62, and 71.

between implant surface kinematics and normal knee function and motion requirements; and improved manufacturing and sterilization of polyethylene. Although earlier studies of older-generation CR systems frequently showed 10-year survivorship of 90%, newer-generation systems have demonstrated improved 10-year survivorship to 96% to 100%.[†]

Aseptic loosening as a mode of failure is relatively rare in both CR and PS TKA, with no clear advantage seen for either type.[22,39,67] However a relative weakness in much of the literature is that it reflects single surgeon series (frequently performed by the implant designer or in an academic setting by individuals who perform high volumes of TKA) and so is less likely to give a balanced view of a particular knee's performance, hence the importance of registry studies and large database reviews. The few of these that are available do show differences in outcome by implant type.

A study of all primary TKAs performed at the Mayo Clinic over a 22-year period noted several trends.[59] Overall survivorship of 84% at 15 years was a significant improvement from the 69% noted in an earlier study from the same institution. Significant risk factors for failure included young age, male gender, noninflammatory arthritis, and the use of metal-backed patellae. Of note with regard to survival of CR versus PS implants, the 10-year survival rate of the CR TKA group was 91% as compared with 76% with posteriorly stabilized designs.

Additional multicenter investigational cohort studies support this finding. Heck et al.[38a] reported a survey of 563 TKAs performed by 43 community surgeons and found that one of the factors related to maximal performance was PCL retention; in addition, the annual reoperation rate was 0.43 per year with CR knees as opposed to 0.51 in the PS design. Both studies indicated that CR implants have better long-term survivorship than PS implants. A recent evaluation of PS versus CR knees of the same design (Smith and Nephew Next Gen II) showed equivalent survival at 10 years.[63]

FUNCTIONAL COMPARISONS

Several studies claim that sensitive functional measures show better performance in deep flexion for the CR knee[24]; however no substantial body of evidence indicates that sacrifice, substitution, or retention leads to consistently "better" knee function.[39,41] Multiple studies have noted no difference between the two in ultimate range of motion or in traditional knee outcome ratings. Studies comparing patients with a CR TKA on one side and a PS on the other have failed to reveal a persistent patient preference for one TKA type over the other.[10,14,67,68]

KINEMATICS

In the normal knee, the PCL serves several functions. It guides rollback of the femoral condyles on the tibial plateau during flexion, thereby allowing the posterior condyles to "clear" the posterior aspect of the tibia in high degrees of flexion and improving the mechanical efficiency of the extensor mechanism.[3] From the standpoint of stability, it prevents posterior subluxation of the tibia on the femur in flexion, while playing a strong secondary role in varus/valgus stability of the knee in flexion.

The history of knee arthroplasty is replete with studies evaluating the kinematic performance of total knee replacement in vivo. Multiple techniques have been used and multiple claims promoted.[‡] Indeed, controversy continues regarding the ability of the surgeon to successfully preserve the PCL in a way that is clinically meaningful. Several authors have claimed that maintaining PCL function following TKA is impossible, and that the kinematic demands of PCL retention require design considerations contrary to maximizing implant longevity.[37]

In the late 1990s Komistek, Dennis, Steihl et al. studied in vivo knee performance in flexion by measuring rollback of the femur on the tibia in PS and CR knees via digital analysis of video fluoroscopy. Their initial studies showed a consistent pattern of anterior translation of the femur on the tibia in flexion in all CR knees studied.[26-28,50,69] This finding was the reverse of the expected rollback of the femur and was termed paradoxical motion (Fig. 136.1A and B). These reports implied that no evidence suggested that the retained PCL was functioning in its expected role. It should be noted that these studies did not describe the surgical technique used or the type of CR knee used. Yet the same group subsequently demonstrated that preservation of the PCL, combined with appropriate implant design, preserves femoral rollback in a study of an unselected group of CR TKAs performed by a single surgeon using a standardized technique with the use of a specific implant design, specific instrumentation, and a specific technique to adjust PCL tension.[13] In this group of 20 patients all but one demonstrated essentially normal patterns of femoral rollback. More recent studies of the same implant design, implanted by three different surgeons using differing techniques,[43] revealed consistent rollback in all patients, thus indicating that these findings are not surgeon dependent but rather are influenced by component design and technique. Results strongly implied that routine PCL preservation could be accomplished with functionally appropriate tensioning.

Additionally, Banks et al.[7] used three-dimensional kinematic assessment with fluoroscopy in a group of total knee replacements with intact PCLs that had essentially normal axial rotation and condylar translation; those with a post-and-cam substitution and no PCL had the smallest in vivo range of rotation and translation. This was seen again in a recent study by Hamai et al. who used compared radiographic imaging matching techniques to assess anterior-posterior stability in midflexion. This comparison showed higher maintenance of anterior-posterior stability of CR knees compared to PS knees.[38]

Of course, the articular surfaces must be designed to be compatible with normal femoral rollback. The "normal" rollback in the CR knees studied by Komistek et al. featured differing femoral condylar radii (Fig. 136.2). The differential radii allow the femoral component to roll posteriorly to a greater degree on the lateral side, as in the normal knee.[13,43] On the tibial side, a slightly flattened design in the sagittal plane takes advantage of the retained ligament, allowing the femur to both roll back and rotate in a relatively normal fashion. At the same time, significant congruence in the frontal plane allows stress in the polyethylene to be minimized, thus reducing long-term wear. It is clear that the geometry of articular surfaces affects motion-bearing surface strain and wear.[51,56]

[†]References 1, 8, 12, 13, 31, 54, and 64.

[‡]References 13, 14, 26-28, 43, 50, and 71.

FEMUR position on the tibia during a deep knee bend

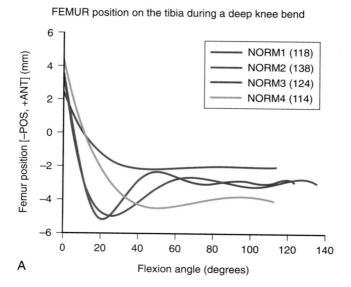

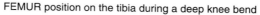

FEMUR position on the tibia during a deep knee bend

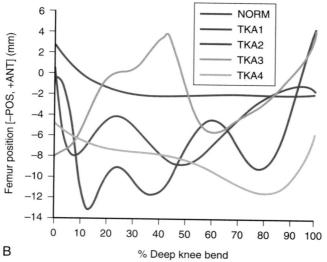

FIG 136.1 Paradoxical Anterior Motion of Many Cases of Posterior Cruciate–Retaining Total Knee Arthroplasty (A) Groups of normal knees demonstrating normal femoral rollback. (B) Groups of CR TKA demonstrating paradoxical anterior motion of femur on tibia in deep knee bend. *ANT,* Anterior; *NORM,* normal; *POS,* posterior; *TKA,* total knee arthroplasty.

POSTERIOR CRUCIATE LIGAMENT-RETAINING VERSUS POSTERIOR CRUCIATE LIGAMENT-SUBSTITUTING DESIGNS

Clinical Comparisons

Range of Motion. Numerous previous studies comparing CR and PS TKA have found no differences between the two in ultimate range of motion.[10,20,29] A recent Cochrane systematic review suggests that there may be an average of 2.4 degrees of flexion in favor of PS knees.[74]

Functional Studies. The theoretical advantage of improved proprioception attained by retaining the PCL was claimed by

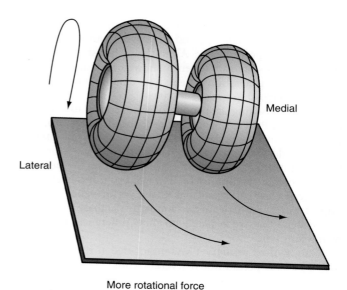

FIG 136.2 NexGen kinematics with a larger radius of curvature of the lateral condyle.

Warren et al.,[75] but most investigators have reported no difference in proprioception between the two types of TKA.[19,68] This may be due in part to the fact that the PCL in osteoarthritic knees has been shown to be more commonly histologically abnormal in comparison with control groups,[42] which may render the PCL less able to provide proprioception.

The question of "a normal feeling knee" has also been investigated using the forgotten joint score. Thippanna et al. investigated 169 CR knees and 178 PS knees, revealing no statistically significant differences between designs.[72]

Although early studies demonstrated more normal stair climbing patterns and improvement in CR TKA,[4] several studies have shown no difference.[29,67] Conditt et al.[24] found poorer functional scores on squatting, kneeling, and gardening in patients with PS knees. They suggested that retention of the PCL offers better functional capacity in higher-demand activities, especially those involving deep knee flexion. Unfortunately, like so many studies, this represents the results of one surgeon using one specific technique and one specific CR and PS implant system; thus it cannot be thought to validate the claim that these findings can be generalized to other implants, surgeons, or patient groups.

Bilateral Studies. Numerous studies have compared patients with a CR TKA on one side and a PS TKA on the other.[10,14,22,67] These studies have not demonstrated a persistent patient preference for one TKA type over another.

Polyethylene Wear. The earliest CR designs featured polyethylene of relatively poor quality, resulting in higher rates of wear. Problems included the use of excessively thin and heat-pressed plastic, as well as the addition of calcium stearate. Over time, other manufacturing and sterilization techniques were shown to affect wear. These problems have since been addressed, and increased wear rates have not been seen with newer designs. However, poor soft tissue balancing in a CR TKA can result in tightness of the PCL in flexion, which can lead to posterior polyethylene wear.[70,79] Problems of instability and post dislocation can be seen in PS TKA as well if the soft tissues are not balanced.[65] This delineates the importance of soft tissue balancing, no matter what type of TKA is performed.

Correction of Deformity. Proponents of PS TKA have argued that larger deformities present difficulty with soft tissue balancing and are more easily balanced with a PS TKA. Although this can certainly be the case, some authors have used CR TKA in the setting of significant preoperative deformity and have had good results.[12,32] If the deformity is severe enough, flexion/extension mismatches or collateral ligamentous insufficiency often necessitates that even PS TKA is insufficient, and that more constrained knee replacements or even hinged TKA is necessary (Figs. 136.3A and B and 136.4A to C).

Aseptic Loosening. Rates of aseptic loosening of both CR and PS TKA remain low in modern designs, implanted with good cement technique, soft tissue balance, and alignment. No advantage for either type of TKA is apparent with regard to aseptic loosening rates.

Inflammatory Arthritis. It has been suggested that PS TKA is the proper choice in patients with inflammatory arthritides such as rheumatoid arthritis because of perceived attenuation of the ligament often noted in these patients.[46] Many authors also feared that late rupture of the PCL could lead to late posterior instability.[44] However, Archibeck et al.[6] demonstrated 95% good or excellent results in 46 knees of rheumatoid patients treated with CR TKA at an average of 10.5 years. Of note, in only one patient did posterior instability develop as a late complication. Similar findings were noted by Dennis et al.[25] These studies suggest that treating rheumatoid patients with knee arthritis by CR TKA yields excellent results.

POTENTIAL ADVANTAGES OF POSTERIOR CRUCIATE RETENTION

Maintenance of a Central Stabilizer

It is often said that TKA is a soft tissue operation. It is the contention of the CR surgeon that it is inappropriate to remove an essential soft tissue structure when retaining it makes the soft tissue portion of the operation easier. How so? The intact PCL functions as an important secondary stabilizer. When the PCL is preserved, it not only resists posterior subluxation forces; it also serves as a secondary stabilizer that resists varus/valgus instability. As opposed to the standard PS technique, which requires maintaining a relatively tight flexion gap (to prevent cam-post subluxation), CR TKA provides a natural means of balancing the flexion space after collateral ligament release. When large collateral ligament releases are required, there is less flexion instability than in cases in which the cruciate is removed. Consequently, flexion/extension gap balancing is simplified.

Maintenance of Joint Line Position

Perhaps of equal importance, functioning of the preserved PCL requires strict maintenance of the joint line to allow for appropriate tensioning of the PCL through range of motion. One potential problem that has been noted with PS knees is elevation of the joint line. Elevation greater than 8 mm has been found to significantly affect knee kinematics and has been correlated with patellofemoral symptoms and the need for revision.[34] Retention of the PCL requires strict maintenance of the joint line;[30] thus rarely is joint line elevation a problem in CR TKA.

Patellar Clunk Syndrome

Traditional PS designs have included a rather abrupt transition from the patellofemoral groove to the intercondylar box.

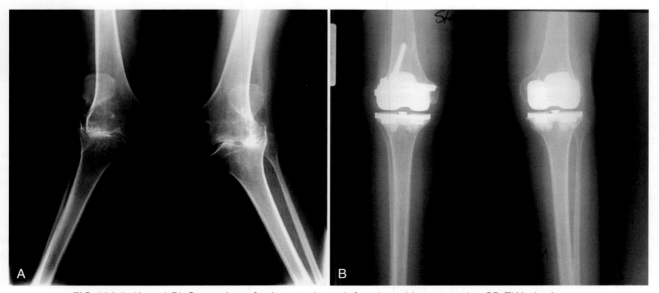

FIG 136.3 (A and B) Correction of a large valgus deformity with a posterior CR TKA. In A note severe bilateral valgus deformities. In B note correction of valgus deformity with cruciate-retaining total knee arthroplasty.

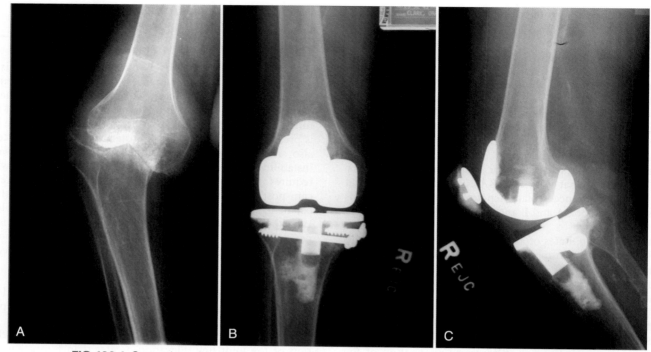

FIG 136.4 Correction of Large Varus Deformity With a Posterior Cruciate–Retaining Total Knee Arthroplasty (A) Large varus deformity. (B) Anteroposterior (AP) and (C) lateral films of correction of deformity with cruciate-retaining total knee arthroplasty.

Although recent designs minimize such transitions, PS TKA can still result in this complication. It generally is not seen in CR TKA.[1,45,56]

Avoidance of the Stress Inherent in Posterior Cruciate–Substituting Knees

In CR TKA, the PCL acts as a central stabilizer to absorb force and prevent posterior subluxation. Absorption of deforming force by the ligament may protect the fixation interface from such stress and prolong long-term fixation, in addition to eliminating the need for a mechanical structure (the cam-and-post mechanism) to absorb this force. In PS TKA, the spine/cam mechanism must resist posterior force, which can result in post wear.[18,58] O'Rourke et al.[53] noted relatively high rates of osteolysis in PS knees at intermediate follow-up and raised the question of increased polyethylene wear from the post. Wasielewski[76] raised the possibility that shear force can be higher in PS knees and in knee replacements with more conforming polyethylene inserts, also more commonly found in PS knees. Such shear force is noted at the modular articulation with the tibial baseplate; increases therefore could contribute to increased backside wear. Scott and Volatile similarly noted the possibility of increased loosening rates in PS TKA secondary to increased interface stress.[65] Post wear and post fracture can also occur with PS TKA and can lead to osteolysis and/or failure of the TKA.[23,52] A poorly balanced PS TKA can result in post dislocation. These problems are not encountered in CR TKA.

SURGICAL TECHNIQUE AND IMPLANT DESIGN

The primary focus of PCL retention in TKA is preservation of the PCL with recreation of an environment that maintains

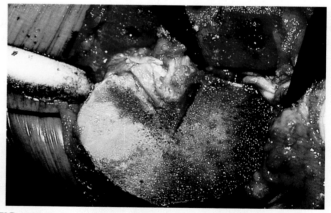

FIG 136.5 Bone block preserved for the posterior cruciate ligament.

appropriate ligament tension during function through the range of motion. To preserve the PCL, it must be recognized that the ligament inserts distal to the articular surface of the tibia by 5 to 10 mm, and during the tibial preparation, one should pay special attention to preserving the insertion. Some surgeons do this by placing an osteotome in front of the PCL insertion during the tibial cut. Another option includes leaving a small block of bone anterior to the PCL insertion (Fig. 136.5). The importance of this step has been highlighted by multiple recent studies. MRI-based studies have shown that a flat tibial cut of appropriate slope will disrupt all or some of the PCL insertion site.[5,66] Furthermore, a recent cadaveric study showed measurable anterior/posterior stability changes with a flat tibial cut. This study attributes this laxity to the violation of the posterior cortex adjacent to the PCL insertion. The authors recommend preservation of a bone island to protect the PCL insertion.[73]

Three important features of surgical technique lead to appropriate tensioning of the PCL. All of these involve accurate restoration of the flexion space in which the PCL functions. First, the femoral component size should be chosen to reproduce the anteroposterior (AP) dimension of the native posterior femoral condyles. Provision of a large number of femoral AP sizes makes PCL balancing through measured resection techniques easier. Having a choice of widths for every AP size makes selection of the appropriate implant easier.

Second, the joint line can be reproduced by attending to two details. The first involves resecting at least as much tibial bone from the healthy side of the tibia (lateral in the varus knee and medial in the valgus knee), as will be replaced by the smallest thickness of tibial component. This prevents inadvertent elevation of the joint line in two ways. If a maximum of 5 mm is taken from the healthy side of the tibia and is replaced with a 10 mm component, the joint line will have been moved proximally by 5 mm. The second technique is to be sure that full extension is achieved by appropriate soft tissue releases and not by taking excessive distal femur to enlarge the extension gap. The greater the amount of distal femoral resection, the more the joint line is relatively elevated, and the greater the likelihood that tension on the PCL will be inappropriate.

Third, it is equally important to re-create the natural degree of the patient's posterior tibial slope so as to avoid excessive tightness in flexion. If this slope is not re-established, the posterior aspect of the tibial component will be placed too far proximal relative to the patient's original joint line, which will result in excessive tightness in the PCL during flexion. This can cause excessive rollback with a "nutcracker" effect and high contact pressure in the posterior part of the tibial articulation. Polyethylene wear may be increased in this setting; perhaps equally important, the range of motion can be limited. Both of these situations are undesirable and can be eliminated by reproducing the normal tibial slope. If the prosthesis is designed to be inserted with a posterior inclination to the plane of resection, this must be surgically performed. Most tibial components are designed in this fashion.

After preparing the femur and the tibia, the surgeon must look for signs that the ligament may be too loose or too tight during the trial reduction.[21] This assessment is made with the knee in flexion—the position in which the ligament is placed under tension. Excessive tightness in flexion is evidenced by several signs: the trial base plate (if unrestricted by a post embedded in the tibia) may lift off from the tibial cut anteriorly; the femoral component may be pushed anteriorly off the distal femoral cut as the knee is brought into flexion; rollback of the femur on the tibia may be observed to be occurring too far posteriorly, with flexion indicating excessive tension in the PCL; and finally, the ligament tension can be palpated directly and assessed during the trial reduction (Fig. 136.6). An insufficiently tensioned ligament can also be assessed by palpation or by performing a posterior drawer test or observing a typical posterior sag.

Of course, tightness in flexion may simply indicate an unbalanced flexion/extension gap, and so correction of this tightness should be appraised with attention to appropriate filling of the extension gap as well. Assuming that the extension gap is well

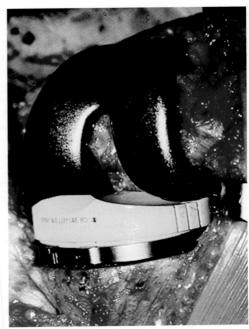

FIG 136.6 Tightness in flexion on this prosthesis can be checked at 90 degrees of flexion. Note the anterior lift-off of the polyethylene insert and the anterior position of the tibia, indicating excess posterior cruciate ligament tightness in flexion.

filled (there is no recurvatum or flexion contracture), one must actually assess the tension in the PCL to determine whether or not it is the sole contributor to flexion tightness. If the PCL is found to be too tight with the previously mentioned methods, this may reflect insufficient tibial slope; tightness should be checked before further attempts are made to alter PCL tension.

If the slope is appropriate and the implant system has a femoral downsizing capability (so-called minus sizing), this is where the smaller AP dimension of the femoral component will decrease tension on a tight PCL. Alternatively, when the PCL is found to be too tight with these methods of evaluation, the tibia can be moderately subluxed anteriorly, while the PCL is gradually released from the tibial insertion subperiosteally.

Occasionally, severe deformity may require release of the PCL, because contracture of the ligament is actually part of the pathology (generally moderate or severe sagittal plane alignment abnormalities combined with flexion contracture); in these cases and in the revision setting, substitution seems a most reasonable alternative. However, Worland et al.[77] demonstrated that patients' subjective and objective results were not compromised if flexion gap filling was appropriate as measured by acceptable KT-1000 measurements at follow-up in TKAs with PCL recession. The claimed advantages of this approach are that the patient's joint line is not changed and the rest of the knee kinematics are preserved. If "excessive recession" is observed, the surgeon must accurately assess the knee's AP stability and select an ultra-congruent (AP motion restricting) polyethylene or must convert to a PS knee. These ultra-congruent designs use the same CR femoral component and compensate for the deficient PCL using a more congruent poly insert. These have had good survival rates at an average of 5 years, and patient satisfaction is high.[40]

Several considerations must be kept in mind when the surgeon converts to a PS-substituting implant after initially preparing for a CR implant. Paradoxically, the most serious potential complication in converting to a PS knee is instability of the cam-and-post mechanism. This may occur through a combination of factors that produce a well-functioning CR knee but may sabotage the PS knee: a relatively excessive posterior tibial slope and the general principle of downsizing the femoral component when between sizes. Combined with relative flexion and collateral ligament instability, this may result in an underfilled flexion gap, and with flexion and varus or valgus stress (depending on the side of collateral instability), the post may slip under the cam. Increasing the filling of the flexion gap is likely to solve the problem, and the surgeon must keep this in mind when converting from the CR to the PS.

In cases in which the PCL is a part of the ligament contracture pathology (generally moderate or severe sagittal plane alignment abnormalities combined with flexion contracture) and in the revision setting, PCL substitution seems to be the most reasonable alternative. Additional settings in which PS designs are appropriate include a knee with complex deformity after proximal tibial osteotomy,[2] and a knee with severe inflammatory changes that have affected the integrity of the ligament itself.[6] A patellectomized knee was previously thought to be a contraindication to performing a CR knee.[9] This has been challenged in a recent paper by Reinhardt et al. that showed good results at a minimum of 2 years for CR knee designs in a previously patellectomized knee.[61]

CONCLUSION

The concept of simply resurfacing the joint and maintaining as much of the native structure as possible is a philosophically appealing one. However, retention of the PCL necessitates understanding the differences required in surgical technique and component design (and occasionally patient selection) for successful performance of this procedure. Multiple femoral sizes are needed to allow PCL balancing through measured resection techniques. The posterior slope must be reconstituted to allow a balanced PCL in flexion. Improvements in component design now allow improved kinematics with improved femoral rollback. These advances in design and surgical technique have led to great success in previous outcome studies and lend promise for ever-improving functional outcomes among patients in the future. In the near future, these improvements will help meet the increased demand for TKA in the younger, more active, more demanding patient with increased life expectancy.

KEY REFERENCES

8. Barrington JW, Sah A, Malchau H, et al: Contemporary cruciate retaining total knee arthroplasty with a pegged tibial baseplate: results at a minimum of ten years. *J Bone Joint Surg Am* 91:874–878, 2009.

11. Bellemans J, Robijns F, Duerinckx J, et al: The influence of tibial slope on maximal flexion after total knee arthroplasty. *Knee Surg Sports Traumatol Arthrosc* 13:193–196, 2005.

12. Berger RA, Rosenberg AG, Barden RM, et al: Long-term followup of the Miller-Galante total knee replacement. *Clin Orthop* 388:58–67, 2001.

15. Bozic KJ, Kinder J, Meneghini M, et al: Implant survivorship and complication rates after total knee arthroplasty with a third-generation cemented system: 5 to 8 years followup. *Clin Orthop* 430:117–124, 2005.

20. Chaudhary R, Beaupré LA, Johnston DW: Knee range of motion during the first two years after use of posterior cruciate-stabilizing or posterior cruciate-retaining total knee prostheses: a randomized clinical trial. *J Bone Joint Surg Am* 12:2579–2586, 2008.

23. Clarke HD, Math KR, Scuderi GR: Polyethylene post failure in posterior stabilized total knee arthroplasty. *J Arthroplasty* 19:652–657, 2004.

24. Conditt MA, Noble PC, Bertolusso R, et al: The PCL significantly affects the functional outcome of total knee arthroplasty. *J Arthroplasty* 19(7 Suppl 2):107–112, 2004.

37. Ginsel BL, Banks S, Verdonschot N, et al: Improving maximum flexion with a posterior cruciate retaining total knee arthroplasty: a fluoroscopic study. *Acta Orthop Belg* 75:801–807, 2009.

41. Jacobs WC, Clement DJ, Wymenga AB: Retention versus sacrifice of the posterior cruciate ligament in total knee replacement for treatment of osteoarthritis and rheumatoid arthritis. *Cochrane Database Syst Rev* (4):CD004803, 2005.

42. Kim YH, Choi Y, Kwon OR, et al: Functional outcome and range of motion of high-flexion posterior cruciate-retaining and high-flexion posterior cruciate-substituting total knee prostheses: a prospective, randomized study. *J Bone Joint Surg Am* 91:753–760, 2009.

44. Komistek RD, Mahfouz MK, Bertin KC, et al: In vivo determination of total knee arthroplasty kinematics: A multicenter analysis of an asymmetrical posterior cruciate retaining total knee arthroplasty. *J Arthroplasty* 23:41–50, 2008.

50. Niki Y, Mochizuki T, Momohara S, et al: Factors affecting anteroposterior instability following cruciate-retaining total knee arthroplasty in patients with rheumatoid arthritis. *Knee* 15:26–30, 2008.

52. Omori G, Onda N, Shimura M, et al: The effect of geometry of the tibial polyethylene insert on the tibiofemoral contact kinematics in advance medial pivot total knee arthroplasty. *J Orthop Sci* 14:754–760, 2009.

55. Pagnano M, Scuderi G: Rationale for posterior cruciate substituting knee arthroplasty. *J Orthop Surg* <FindArticles.com./p/articles/miqa3794/is200112/ain90007247/>, (Accessed 25.04.10.)

58. Ploegmakers MJ, Ginsel B, Meijerink HJ, et al: Physical examination and in vivo kinematics in two posterior cruciate ligament retaining total knee arthroplasty designs. *Knee* 17:204–209, 2010.

79. Wright RJ, Sledge CB, Poss R, et al: Patient-reported outcome and survivorship after Kinemax total knee arthroplasty. *J Bone Joint Surg Am* 86:2464–2470, 2004.

The references for this chapter can also be found on www.expertconsult.com.

137

Preserving the Posterior Cruciate Ligament

Ate Wymenga, Petra Heesterbeek

INTRODUCTION

Advocates for posterior cruciate ligament (PCL) substitution and PCL retention can point to excellent clinical and radiographic results in the literature. Furthermore, findings in the areas of biomechanics, histology, and gait analysis do not show convincing evidence for one technique above the other. However, a factor of major importance is PCL balancing. To function properly, the PCL must be accurately tensioned during knee replacement. It is crucial for a well-functioning total knee arthroplasty (TKA) that the PCL be placed under appropriate tension such that the kinetic benefits of its retention can be enhanced and the adverse effects of an excessively tight or a lax PCL can be avoided.

A recent meta-analysis reported that based on a systematic review of the currently published randomized controlled trials (RCTs), there are no clinically relevant differences between retention and sacrifice of the PCL in terms of clinical, functional, and radiologic outcome.[54] No information was available on patient-reported outcome measures, or on kinematics as antero-posterior (AP) stability or tibiofemoral contact position. Whether similar clinical and functional outcome translates into comparable implant survival remains to be investigated. An RCT is not the best design because they usually have a short follow-up period and small sample sizes, so no meta-analyses can be found on this topic. Survival analyses of large cohorts showed a 10-year and 15-year survival of 91% and 90% in PCL-retaining TKA.[1]

In this chapter the basics of kinematics after cruciate retaining (CR) TKA are summarized and key technical aspects concerning correct balancing of the PCL are discussed. Finally, a 10-step proposal for a surgical protocol is presented.

BASICS

Anatomy and Histology

The PCL is one of the four important ligaments that join the femur and the tibia. The PCL originates from the medial wall of the femoral intercondylar notch and inserts onto the posterior aspect of the tibia. The sagittal slope runs from anterior proximal to posterior distal. The origins of the anterior cruciate ligament (ACL) and PCL lie approximately on an axis through the centers of the femoral condyles: the condylar line. In extension, the PCL is curved around the posterior tibia, thereby being neither rigid nor taut.

As knee flexion increases from 0 to 120 degrees, the angle of the anterolateral bundle increased from 37 to 65 degrees and that of the posteromedial bundle from 47 to 60 degrees.[59] The PCL assists tibiofemoral positioning mainly in the medial compartment.

Although articular geometry is a more potent factor driving tibiofemoral positioning during knee kinematics than the ligaments, the PCL is the main restraint against posterior translation of the tibia, particularly so at about 90 degrees of flexion, and with little effect on knee kinematics in extension or high flexion. Most fibers of the PCL are under tension only at around 90 degrees of flexion and it controls the contact point (CP) of the medial femoral condyle on the tibia between approximately 60 and 120 degrees of flexion.

In histologic studies examining the quality of the PCL tissue in arthritic knee joints, the PCL was considered to be viable and sound for retaining.[41,45]

Contact Point and Step-Off in the Native Knee

In the native knee the medial CP lies a few millimeters posterior to the midline of the tibial plateau and is found to be relatively stable (±4 mm) from 20 to 120 degrees of flexion.[19,23,29,56] The lateral CP showed a variable rollback pattern, depending on the tibial rotation.[23]

The CP of the native knee in 90 degrees of flexion in a lateral radiograph is located at approximately the posterior one third of the AP dimension of the tibial plateau (Fig. 137.1A).[12] In this situation, the step-off of the tibia related to the distal femur joint surface is around 10 to 13 mm. If a PCL rupture occurs, the tibia will translate posteriorly and consequently, the femur will articulate more anterior on the tibia (see Fig. 137.1B). As a consequence, the (reduced) angle between the patellar tendon and quadriceps muscle reduces the moment arm (MA) of the extensor apparatus (see Fig. 137.1B). The patellofemoral contact forces will increase and more force is needed to extend the leg.[18,50] Evidently, the step-off between tibia and femur is clearly decreased and can therefore be helpful during clinical examination to diagnose PCL insufficiency.

Restoration Contact Point and Step-Off in Cruciate-Retaining Total Knee Arthroplasty

To restore tibiofemoral and patellofemoral function after CR total knee replacement, it is important to re-create a correct CP at 90 degrees of flexion.

To achieve this, it is important to precisely restore the joint surface and the surgeon should aim for *precise replacement of the resected bone cuts by the implant thickness*. Theoretically this will not change the lengths of the ligaments and the stability and laxity will be restored to a large extent.[7,24] This supports the

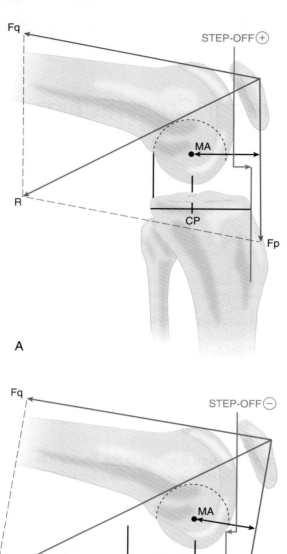

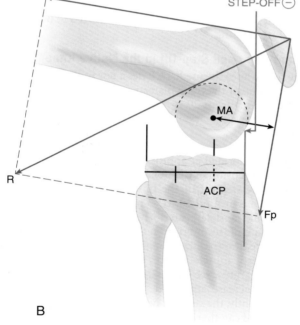

FIG 137.1 (A) Intact native knee with normal CP at posterior one third of tibia, normal step-off *(STEP-OFF+)*, which is approximately 10 to 13 mm; (B) posterior cruciate deficient knee with abnormal ACP, reduced step-off *(STEP-OFF−)*. The MA from the center of the femur condyle to the patellar tendon is reduced in this situation and the resultant patellofemoral force *(R)* is clearly increased. *ACP,* Anterior contact point; *CP,* contact point, *Fp,* patellar tendon force; *Fq,* quadriceps force; *MA,* moment arm.

concept that when joint surfaces are restored it is likely that the normal CP of the native knee will also be restored in CR TKA (Fig. 137.2)

The clinical importance of a functional PCL has been well described: patients with a TKA with PCL insufficiency reported persistent pain, effusion, and instability, and had poorer clinical results when compared to patients with a functional CR TKA.[44] All patients with a non-functional CR TKA had clinical signs of PCL insufficiency with a posterior sag of the tibia, and a positive Quadriceps Active Test.

A decreased patella tendon angle and an anterior patella position (indicating anterior sliding of the femur) are reported to correlate with lower clinical scores in CR TKA.[2] Churchill et al. and D'Lima et al. also stressed the importance of femoral rollback in relation to the MA and patellofemoral contact load, and reported an increase of patellofemoral load with reduced rollback.[10,11] Patients with a non-functional PCL after TKA need higher quadriceps muscle forces to extend the leg. This will raise the patellofemoral load and can consequently cause patellofemoral pain.

It is clear that the tibiofemoral CP in 90 degrees of flexion plays a major role in maintaining the MA. As is shown in the illustrations (Fig. 137.3A and B), the reduction of step-off and an anterior contact point (ACP) reduce the MA and increase patellar pressure. For a well-balanced and functional CR TKA, restoring the CP to enable a correct MA is necessary.

Kinematics and Balancing of the Posterior Cruciate Ligament in Cruciate-Retaining Total Knee Arthroplasty; in Vitro and in Vivo Results

As discussed previously, the PCL should be balanced to be functional. In the literature several authors have reported that this is challenging, but possible. Sorger confirmed in lab tests that the PCL prevented posterior translation and can maintain femoral rollback in CR TKA.[51] However, others had difficulty in balancing the PCL when performing in vitro tests.[26,36] In an in vitro study, Li et al. and Most et al. found only a partial restoration of the rollback of the medial condyle after CR TKA.[33,40] On the other hand, Heesterbeek et al. found similar kinematic patterns in a lab test in the native knee and after implantation of a CR TKA with an asymmetric anatomic implant design.[22] Here a precise spacer technique was used to measure the step-off between the femur and tibia after the bone cuts.

Several papers have reported difficulties in re-creating normal kinematics with a CR TKA in vivo. They found inconsistent restoration of rollback or paradoxical roll forward of the femur in flexion.*

However, others demonstrated better results and found normal and stable medial CPs for CR TKA with no paradoxical anterior slide of the femur.[4,8,30,32] Better mid-flexion sagittal stability in a CR TKA was also reported compared with posterior stabilized (PS) TKA in an in vivo fluoroscopic study during stair-climbing tasks, although some patients showed some anterior instability at low flexion angles.[20] In conclusion, it seems difficult but possible to create reproducible kinematics with a CR TKA. Although it has been reported that individual surgical technique does affect outcome,[30] rarely has a detailed and sound surgical technique been published.

---

*References 5, 13, 15, 31, 55, 57, and 58.

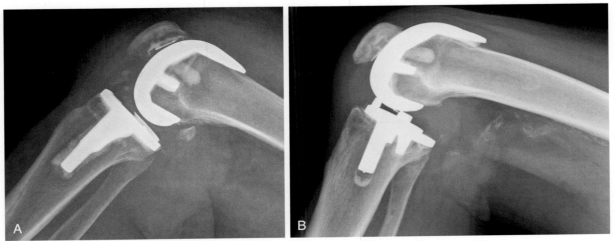

FIG 137.2 (A) The successful restoration of the contact point (CP) and step-off is shown in a case with a cruciate retaining total knee arthroplasty. (B) A non-functional posterior cruciate ligament (PCL) can be recognized by anterior sliding of the femur and the tibiofemoral CP is at the anterior one-third. There is also loss of step-off as a result of posterior sagging of the tibia because of a non-functional PCL.

Gap Dynamics and Effects of Tensioning of the Posterior Cruciate Ligament

Some recent insights into flexion gap dynamics can explain the difficulty of PCL balancing. During TKA, the PCL is balanced by distraction of the flexion gap through spacers, spreaders, tensors, and implant. The flexion gap is the three-dimensional space defined by the bony surfaces of the femur and tibia and by the surrounding soft tissue structures of the knee, and exists only under distraction. During flexion gap distraction, the tibia translates anteriorly with regard to the femur (Fig. 137.4) Anterior tibial translation is inevitable because of the oblique orientation of the PCL. With a mono-block tensor, a ratio between gap height increase and anterior tibial translation of 1 to 1.25 was found.[9] For a bi-compartmental tensor, a higher variable ratio was found: 1 to 1.9.[21] When the flexion gap is distracted with a bi-compartmental tensor, every extra millimeter that the flexion gap is distracted can be expected to move the tibia anteriorly by at least 1.7 mm (flat PCL) or even more if the PCL is oriented steeply relative to the transverse plane of the tibia.[21] So for a 2-mm-thicker insert or larger femur component, the tibia moves 3 to 4 mm anterior, which can easily make the PCL too tight.

KEY FACTORS FOR POSTERIOR CRUCIATE LIGAMENT BALANCING

Bone Cuts

The principal bone cuts needed to restore the native joint surfaces are shown in Fig. 137.5. The implant thickness of the distal and posterior femur component is usually 9 to 10 mm in most knee systems. Posterior referencing cutting guides are preferred to maintain the posterior condylar offset (PCO) and the surgeon should try to match the tibial implant to the native tibial slope.

The restoration of the medial femoral condyle joint surface is key in CR TKA and the bone cuts should match implant thickness in flexion and extension. To account for cartilage loss,

one can distalize the cutting jig 2 mm.[42] When checking the bone cuts, the loss of bone particles resulting from the cut made by sawing should be included in this check.

Tibial Slope

The posterior tibial slope has been reported to influence the flexion gap and the postoperative range of motion (ROM) after CR TKA. In in vitro and in vivo studies, it was found that more tibial slope was correlated with higher flexion and lower risk of a tight flexion gap.[6,17,25,35] Authors warned, however, against too much slope causing anterior instability and posterior loading of polyethylene causing wear. Fantozzi et al. adapted to the natural slope of the tibia and found in different motor tasks a more posterior CP, and in general, rollback kinematic patterns similar to the native knee.[15] Maintenance of the PCO and adapting the flexion gap by adjusting the slope has been advocated.[17] An additional 5 degrees of tibial slope resulted in a 4-mm increase in flexion gap space.[43]

Some knee systems have a built-in slope and surgeons should account for this slope. For example, in Fig. 137.5, the tibia cut has a slope of 3 degrees, and because this insert has a built-in 4 degrees slope, this makes a total slope of 7 degrees, which should match the slope of the patient. In this case cutting the tibia with the same slope as the native slope of the patient would remove too much posterior bone and create a loose flexion gap.

Increasing the tibial slope during surgery in case of a tight PCL leads to a decrease in PCL strain and helps prevent a PCL release and improper knee kinematics and reduced flexion (Fig. 137.6A and B).[49] Several authors advocated increase of tibial slope rather than a PCL release. Jojima et al. found in a lab study that increasing the slope in knees with a tight flexion gap gave a better restoration of the varus valgus and rotational laxity than a PCL release.[28]

Zelle and Heesterbeek recommended increasing the slope instead of releasing the PCL.[60] Releasing the PCL in a knee model with roughly 4 mm or increasing the posterior tibial slope to 7 degrees reduced the PCL force. The femoral rollback patterns during deep knee flexion were only marginally affected

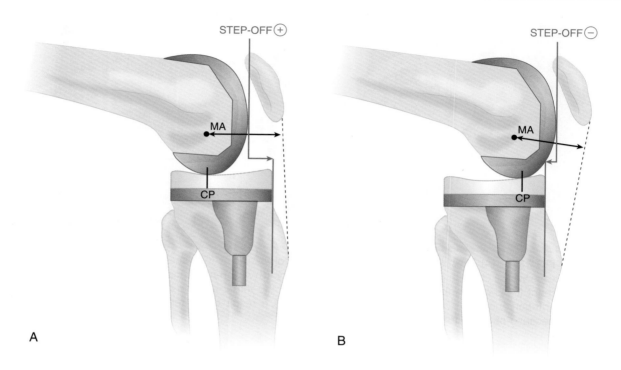

FIG 137.3 (A) Schematic drawing of a cruciate retaining total knee arthroplasty with correct *CP*, normal step-off *(STEP-OFF+)*, and correct *MA*. (B) As a result of a non-functional posterior cruciate ligament, there is an anterior contact point, a negative step-off *(STEP-OFF–)*, and a reduced *MA* of the extensor mechanism. *CP*, Contact point; *MA*, moment arm.

when extra posterior tibial slope was added, whereas additional PCL release resulted in paradoxical anterior movement of the femur. Straw et al. found worse clinical outcomes for patients after a CR TKA with a PCL release when compared with patients without a PCL release.[52]

Posterior Condylar Offset

Bellemans et al. proposed PCO restoration as a concept and found a correlation with PCO and flexion,[5] which was confirmed by Arabori et al. and Malviya et al.[3,37] On the other hand, Ishii et al. could not find a correlation between PCO and flexion in CR mobile bearing knees with PCO precisely measured on computed tomography (CT).[27] Changes in PCO can change the flexion gap. Fujimoto et al. found a clear relationship between the PCO and flexion gap change and that posterior slope increased the flexion gap, but posterior slope was correlated with flexion only at follow-up.[17]

Restoration of the PCO of the femur in CR TKA is an important factor in improving flexion[38] and preventing paradoxical rollback.[14] Some authors therefore propose using posterior referencing guides instead of anterior femur guides, which may cause variable bone cuts on the posterior condyle with the risk of reducing the tension in the PCL (Fig. 137.7A and B).

Target Step-Off

Based on the previously mentioned key factors, the spacer can be used during CR TKA to check the flexion gap and the expected step-off after final implantation. The goal of the surgery is to restore the patient's natural step-off. The target step-off during the CR TKA procedure with a spacer is a result of the patient's natural step-off and the thickness of the distal femoral component. In case of cemented components, one must take into account 1 mm of cement on both the posterior femur and proximal tibia, which will increase the flexion gap by 2 mm on average. Based on our findings that a 2-mm gap distraction causes 4 mm of anterior tibial translation (see "Gap Dynamics and Effects of Tensioning of the Posterior Cruciate Ligament"), surgeons need to correct the target step-off for this situation, otherwise the flexion gap will be too tight. For this reason, we advise to aim for a 4-mm smaller step-off than the sum of the natural step-off and the distal femur implant thickness. This results in the following formula:

TARGET STEP-OFF = NATURAL STEP-OFF + DISTAL FEMUR IMPLANT THICKNESS – 4 mm

For example, let us say that the natural step-off for the patient is 11 mm and the distal femur implant thickness is 9 mm. The 4-mm correction for cementing needs to be subtracted. For this patient, this will result in a target step-off of 11 + 9 – 4 = 16 mm.

OUR PREFERRED SURGICAL STEPS IN CRUCIATE-RETAINING TOTAL KNEE ARTHROPLASTY WITH EXTENSION GAP BALANCING FIRST AND SPACER TECHNIQUE (SURGEONS CAN USE OTHER SEQUENCES AS THEY PREFER)

Step 1. Measure Natural Step-Off

CR TKA is done routinely with a medial arthrotomy with resection of the ACL and menisci and preserving the PCL.

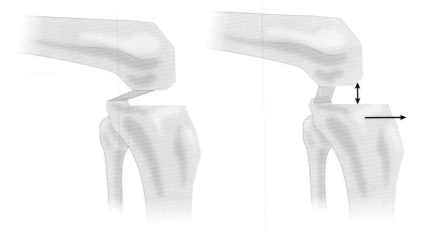

FIG 137.4 Schematic drawing showing the orientation of the posterior cruciate ligament (PCL) and the relative movement of the tibia in relation to the femur. As the flexion gap increases by distraction, the increase of tension in the PCL results in anterior translation of the tibia. (Reproduced with permission and copyright of the British Editorial Society of Bone and Joint Surgery, Christen B, Heesterbeek P, Wymenga A, Wehrli U: Posterior cruciate ligament balancing in total knee replacement: the quantitative relationship between tightness of the flexion gap and tibial translation. *J Bone Joint Surg Br* 89[8]:1046–1050, 2007, [Fig. 2].)

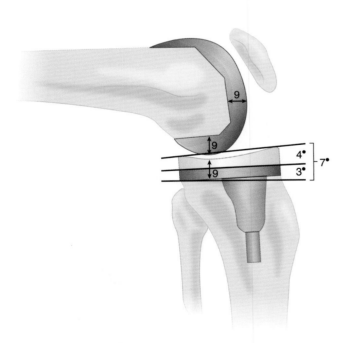

FIG 137.5 Principal bone cuts showing resections matching the implant thickness for the medial femur condyle and lateral tibia joint surface. The surgeon should adjust the tibial cut to the system; in this example the tibia cut is 3 degrees and 4 degrees built into the insert.

The natural step-off of the individual knee can be measured on the medial side from a marked point at the anterior edge of the tibia in 90 degrees of knee flexion to the distal surface of the femur with correction of cartilage loss on the distal femur (Fig. 137.8). For example, this could be 11 mm. At the end of

the surgery, this value should be restored, but certainly not be increased.

Step 2. Preserve the Bony Insertion of the Posterior Cruciate Ligament

Preservation of the PCL is important to maintain the ligament and its strength. With a simulated tibial bone cut in magnetic resonance imaging (MRI), more than 50% sacrifice of the PCL insertion was found together with a wide patient variation of the location of the PCL footprint.[34,39,47,48] Lab studies also showed a removal of 67% of the insertion site if a conventional tibial cut was made.[16] Van Opstal et al. found a 50% higher tensile strength of the PCL when the bony insertion of the PCL was preserved and proposed to leave a bony island in front of the PCL insertion when performing a CR TKA.[53] This can be done with a V-shaped bone cut with a pin as protection of the PCL in front of the ligament insertion (Fig. 137.9) After completing the tibia cut, splitting the tibia joint surface in two parts with a chisel facilitates removal without damaging the bony PCL insertion.

Step 3. Make a Tibial Cut With Conservative Slope

The tibia bone cut also aims for restoration of the joint surface, resecting the implant thickness from the lateral usually unworn side. Correction for cartilage wear and bone erosion should also be included. The tibial slope is adjusted to the natural slope of the patient, but correction must be made for the slope that is built into the inserts of some systems. It is preferable to start with a conservative slope of around 3 degrees to prevent a loose flexion gap.

Step 4. Make the Distal Femoral Bone Cut Match the Implant Thickness

The distal femur bone cut should aim to restore the joint surface. The thickness of the bone cut should equal the implant

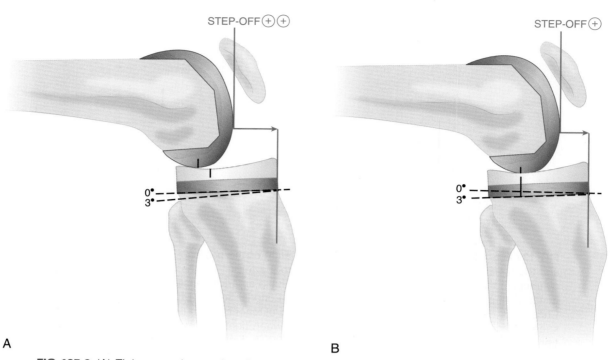

FIG 137.6 (A) Tight posterior cruciate ligament and posterior contact point (CP) and increased step-off because of limited slope in the tibia cut. (B) Correct CP in normal step-off after recut of the tibia with more slope.

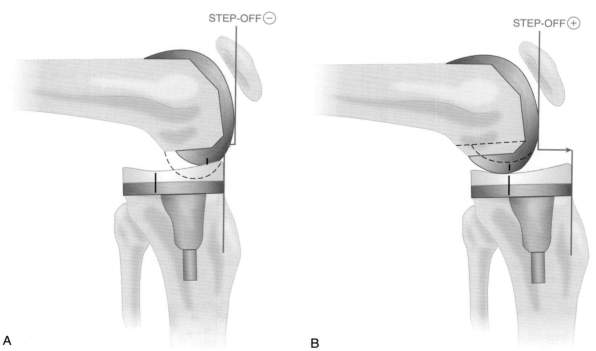

FIG 137.7 (A) Over-resection of the posterior condyle and subsequent loose posterior cruciate ligament and anterior contact point and reduced step-off. (B) Correct resection of the posterior condyle and restoration of the posterior condylar offset and correct flexion gap balancing.

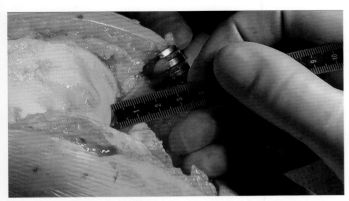

FIG 137.8 Measuring natural step-off after opening the joint. A correction should be made for the cartilage loss. In this case the natural step-off was 11 mm.

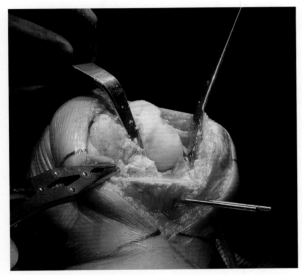

FIG 137.9 Intraoperative view on the anterior tibia where the posterior cruciate ligament insertion is preserved by leaving a bony island.

thickness minus the estimated cartilage and bone loss, in which case the jig should be distalized 1 to 2 mm.

Step 5. Balancing in Extension Plus Making the Anterior and Posterior Femur Bone Cuts

After balancing the knee in extension with a spacer and making the necessary releases if needed, the anterior and posterior femur bone cuts are made in flexion. Again, correction of the cartilage and bone wear should be incorporated to restore the PCO. Posterior referencing is preferred for this reason.

Step 6. Check Step-Off in Flexion

The knee step-off is checked in flexion by inserting the selected spacer on the anterior edge of the tibia. The target step-off is measured from the distal cut femur bone surface to the anterior edge of the spacer on the medial side. This is preferably done with repositioning of the patella. The surgeon then calculates the target step-off according to the formula: target step-off = natural step-off + implant thickness − 4 mm. For example, this can be 11 + 9 − 4 = 16 mm (Fig. 137.10).

Is the step-off correct? Proceed with Step 8.

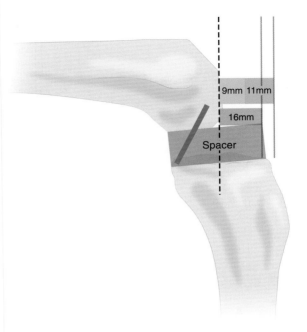

FIG 137.10 Correct target step-off as calculated with formula: Natural step-off 11 mm + 9-mm implant thickness − 4-mm correction for cementing = 16 mm.

Step 7A. Step-Off Too Large Means a Tight Posterior Cruciate Ligament: Increase the Tibial Slope

If the surgical step-off is too large (in Fig. 137.11A it is 19 mm instead of the desired 16 mm), indicating a tight PCL, we suggest increasing the tibial slope by 2 to 3 degrees. This does not change the extension gap and selectively increases the flexion gap by 2 mm, which will reduce the step-off by 4 mm on average (see Fig. 137.11A and B).

Step 7B. Step-Off Too Small Means a Loose Posterior Cruciate Ligament: Decrease the Tibial Slope

If the surgical step-off is too small, indicating a loose PCL and too large a flexion gap, one can decrease the slope 2 to 3 degrees and resect some more bone on the anterior part of the tibia but not posteriorly. This will increase the extension gap by 2 mm and a thicker insert can be used for re-tensioning the PCL. An additional distal femur cut is not needed with this technique (Fig. 137.12A and B).

Step 8. Trial Components and Extra Check Posterior Osteophytes

The trial components are inserted and care is taken to resect posterior osteophytes (if not already done). Additional bone on the posterior femur can impinge in the trial insert and simulate PCL tightness.

Step 9: Check Step-Off With Implant in Place

Check the step-off with the implant in place: this should be a few millimeters less than the patient's native step-off at the start of the surgery (Fig. 137.13). The AP-laxity should be preferably around 5 mm.

The pull-out lift-off (POLO) tests are performed and should be normal. Scott and Chmell proposed the POLO tests to check

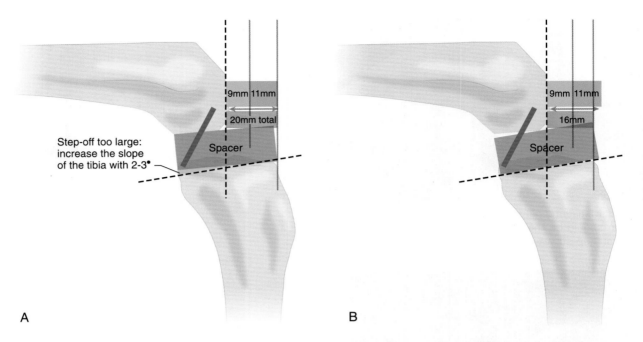

FIG 137.11 (A) The step-off with the spacer is 9 mm implant thickness + 11 mm natural step-off of the patient. Because cementing the implant could decrease the flexion gap space, one should have 4 mm less step-off during testing with the spacer to prevent stiffness. In this particular example, a recut of the tibia will create more space and the step-off will be reduced to 16 mm in (B), which is correct.

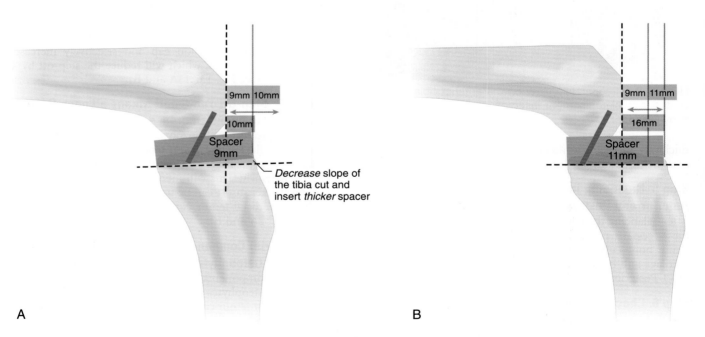

FIG 137.12 (A) In this example, the step-off is too small (10 mm instead of 16 mm). An additional cut of the anterior part of the tibia of 2 to 3 degrees will decrease of the slope of the tibia cut. Together with a thicker insert, this will increase the step-off to 16 mm in (B), which is correct.

the flexion stability and PCL tension.[46] They used an insert with a 3.5-mm posterior lip. The pull-out test was done with a non-stemmed baseplate with insert. If this baseplate could be pulled out of the joint, the flexion stability and PCL tension was insufficient and a thicker insert should be used. If the extension gap is too tight with this thicker insert, a tibia recut with decrease of the tibial slope by taking away some bone from the anterior side of the tibia will increase the extension gap. This will accommodate the thicker spacer.

The lift-off test was done with trial components and a reduced patella, and possible lift-off was observed in 90 to 100 degrees of flexion. Lift-off of the anterior tibial tray will occur in cases where the PCL is too tight and the femur component will force the tray down posteriorly together with elevation of the anterior part. In this situation, we would advise the surgeon to increase the slope of the tibial cut by 2 to 3 degrees. This will increase the flexion gap and decrease the PCL tension.

Step 10: Cementing and Closure

The implant is cemented and care is taken not to leave too thick a cement layer on the posterior part of the tibia because this could decrease the flexion gap and cause stiffness. In Fig. 137.14 the preoperative step-off is well restored on the postoperative radiogram after the CR TKA implantation. The final tests of the knee after cementation are measuring the final step-off with the definitive implants, which should be similar to the native step-off, and measuring the AP laxity, which should be around 5 mm.

KEY REFERENCES

4. Banks SA, Markovich GD, Hodge WA: In vivo kinematics of cruciate-retaining and -substituting knee arthroplasties. *J Arthroplasty* 12(3):297–304, 1997.
6. Bellemans J, Robijns F, Duerinckx J, et al: The influence of tibial slope on maximal flexion after total knee arthroplasty. *Knee Surg Sports Traumatol Arthrosc* 13(3):193–196, 2005.
9. Christen B, Heesterbeek P, Wymenga A, et al: Posterior cruciate ligament balancing in total knee replacement: the quantitative relationship between tightness of the flexion gap and tibial translation. *J Bone Joint Surg Br* 89(8):1046–1050, 2007.
11. D'Lima DD, Poole C, Chadha H, et al: Quadriceps moment arm and quadriceps forces after total knee arthroplasty. *Clin Orthop* 392:213–220, 2001.
15. Fantozzi S, Catani F, Ensini A, et al: Femoral rollback of cruciate-retaining and posterior-stabilized total knee replacements: in vivo fluoroscopic analysis during activities of daily living. *J Orthop Res* 24(12):2222–2229, 2006.
21. Heesterbeek P, Keijsers N, Jacobs W, et al: Posterior cruciate ligament recruitment affects antero-posterior translation during flexion gap

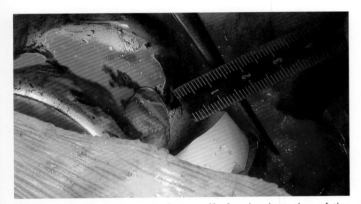

FIG 137.13 Measurement of step-off after implantation of the prosthesis referencing from the anterior side of the base plate to the distal surface of the femur in 90 degrees of flexion.

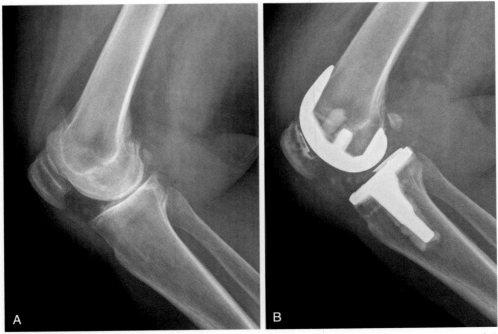

FIG 137.14 Preoperative (A) and postoperative (B) radiograph demonstrating a re-creation of the correct step-off and contact point.

distraction in total knee replacement. An intraoperative study involving 50 patients. *Acta Orthop* 81(4):471–477, 2010.

22. Heesterbeek PJ, Labey L, Wong P, et al: A new spacer-guided, PCL balancing technique for cruciate-retaining total knee replacement. *Knee Surg Sports Traumatol Arthrosc* 22(3):650–659, 2014.

23. Hill PF, Vedi V, Williams A, et al: Tibiofemoral movement 2: the loaded and unloaded living knee studied by MRI. *J Bone Joint Surg Br* 82(8):1196–1198, 2000.

29. Komistek RD, Dennis DA, Mahfouz M: In vivo fluoroscopic analysis of the normal human knee. *Clin Orthop* 410:69–81, 2003.

30. Komistek RD, Mahfouz MR, Bertin KC, et al: In vivo determination of total knee arthroplasty kinematics: a multicenter analysis of an asymmetrical posterior cruciate retaining total knee arthroplasty. *J Arthroplasty* 23(1):41–50, 2008.

32. Li G, Suggs J, Hanson G, et al: Three-dimensional tibiofemoral articular contact kinematics of a cruciate-retaining total knee arthroplasty. *J Bone Joint Surg Am* 88(2):395–402, 2006.

41. Mullaji AB, Marawar SV, Simha M, et al: Cruciate ligaments in arthritic knees: a histologic study with radiologic correlation. *J Arthroplasty* 23(4):567–572, 2008.

44. Pagnano MW, Hanssen AD, Lewallen DG, et al: Flexion instability after primary posterior cruciate retaining total knee arthroplasty. *Clin Orthop* 356:39–46, 1998. <http://www.ncbi.nlm.nih.gov/pubmed/9917666>. (Accessed 26.08.15).

53. Van Opstal N, Feyen H, Luyckx JP, et al: Mean tensile strength of the PCL in TKA depends on the preservation of the tibial insertion site. *Knee Surg Sports Traumatol Arthrosc* 24(1):273–278, 2014.

54. Verra WC, van den Boom LGH, Jacobs W, et al: Similar outcome after retention or sacrifice of the posterior cruciate ligament in total knee arthroplasty. *Acta Orthop* 86(2):195–201, 2015.

The references for this chapter can also be found on www.expertconsult.com.

138

Custom-Made Knee Replacements

Wolfgang Fitz, Frank A. Buttacavoli

Many studies have documented a significant percentage of dissatisfied patients with total knee arthroplasty (TKA).* The cause of patient dissatisfaction is debated, but patient selection, patient expectations, surgical technique, and surgical implants have been attributed to these patient outcomes. Many have shown with current "off-the-shelf" (OTS) implants that the knee's kinematics are changed and that OTS TKR fails to restore individual knee kinematics.[7,22,39,41]

Biomechanical studies have found that knee kinematics are highly variable,[13-15] individually different,[37] change with compromised soft tissue, such as a deficient anterior cruciate ligament, and vary depending upon activities, such as kneeling, squatting, and climbing stairs.[15,29,37] It is believed that the knee kinematics are driven by the individual surface geometry of the knee joint,[33] the three-dimensional (3D) location of the ligaments, and the physical constraints of the surrounding soft tissue.[5]

OTS TKR has symmetrical condyles and does not reproduce the individual surface geometry of the distal femur and proximal tibia. Basically, the art of total knee replacement consists of the placement of a nonfitting implant onto the distal femur and to the proximal tibia and the resulting management of ligament imbalances. Techniques of soft tissue releases have been described for a variety of conditions, such as varus and valgus deformities, tight posterior cruciate ligaments, and patellar maltracking. Such techniques as partial or total tendon releases, partial or complete tenotomies, and pie crusting or needling of tight soft tissue structures belong to the common armamentarium of a knee surgeon. Some of these releases are associated with increased risk of bleeding, higher infection risk, and increased morbidity, such as lateral releases. The nonanatomic shape of OTS implants lead to a loss of normal knee kinematics, including the tibial screw-home mechanism.

To mimic normal knee kinematics, engineers have designed surface geometries of the tibial insert that allow more rollback on the lateral side and a more static location of the medial condyle in the center of the medial tibia plateau (medial pivot knees). Some surface geometries on the tibia are more dished and increase the contact area, and others are less dished and less constraining. Other engineered structures include the post-cam mechanism in posterior-stabilized (PS) knees to facilitate rollback of both condyles with flexion greater than approximately 70 degrees. Kinematic studies have demonstrated that PS total knees have more reproducible knee kinematics with posterior rollback in flexion compared with cruciate-retaining (CR) TKA,[7,41] and PS knees have demonstrated better flexion of

approximately 10 additional degrees. CR TKA frequently show so-called paradoxical motion where the medial condyle slides forward in mid-flexion. On the femoral side, engineers have changed the geometry of the posterior condyles to improve flexion by decreasing the posterior condylar radius. The posterior condyles show a single radius,[27] and both condyles have a similar geometry. In so-called high-flexed designs the radii are decreased gradually somewhere between 120 degrees of flexion to facilitate lateral rollback of both condyles in deep flexion. It remains unclear how much additional implant stress forces could be reduced without these engineered surface modifications if total knee implants replicated the anatomic surfaces. It remains unclear to what extent these additional stress forces contribute to material or implant failure or impact clinical outcome.

Because the implants have an engineered fixed geometry and come in different sizes, it is difficult to place them on the asymmetrical femur and tibia. This appears not only in incomplete coverage or implant overhang but also in various malrotations, which impact clinical outcome.† It remains unclear to this date how big the soft spot is for appropriate femoral and tibial rotation without worsening of the clinical outcome. On the femur, external rotation is associated with better patella tracking, and Whiteside believes that up to 8 degrees of femoral external rotation is acceptable.[30] Internal rotation is associated with poor patella tracking and poor clinical outcome.[4] The femoral rotation is based upon anatomic landmarks that result in highly variable femoral rotation. Recent surgical techniques propose preoperative computed tomography (CT) to determine femoral component rotation using Berger method. This technique has shown high reliability, and the authors believe preoperative CT scanning is more favorable than traditional intraoperative landmark methods.[28,38]

On the tibial side it remains unclear whether 5, 10, or 15 degrees of internal rotation correlate with poor clinical outcome. This applies to both symmetrical and asymmetrical tibial components. We have shown that the anteroposterior (AP) length of medial and lateral tibial plateau is not fixed but varies,[16] and therefore even an asymmetrical tibial component may not match the misfit and may be placed internally rotated. On the other spectrum, maximizing coverage using symmetrical implants has also been shown to lead to malrotation of components and TKA failure.[25] It seems there is increasing consensus that the best tibial rotation is between the mediolateral (ML) axis[11] and the medial third of the tibial tubercle[21] for a symmetrical or asymmetrical component.

---

*References 1, 6, 8, 17, 18, 32, 35, and 40.

†References 2-4, 23, 24, and 31.

It appears that a tibial and femoral component replicating the anatomic surfaces would address these shortcomings. This anatomic implant may have the potential to improve knee kinematics, restore the individual knee kinematics, improve clinical outcomes, and increase patient satisfaction.

Well, this is not quite a new idea. Back in the 1970s in the times of early inventors of total knee replacement, several anatomic total knees were designed.[34] Large variances of individual patients' anatomies limited this approach, and ultimately it was abandoned: most anatomic knees had only a few sizes and would not match the large distribution of individual anatomy. It was the functional approach with sometimes only one available size that made total knee replacement successful (Insall-Burstein I, Zimmer, Warsaw, IN).

With current technology, combining CT and 3D reconstruction, each patient's knee (including the center of femoral head and talus) is scanned and individual 3D models of the distal femur and proximal tibia are created. Adding the center of the hip and ankle will allow to place the implants perpendicular to the mechanical axis and correct varus and valgus deformities. Special proprietary software is applied and virtual total knee implants are fitted to each patient's 3D models of distal femur and proximal tibia. Basic principles of total knee replacement are applied, such as the use of the same materials as conventional implants and the alignment of the components along the mechanical axis. Because the implants are based on the individual J-curves of the medial and lateral femoral condyles, potential flattening that may occur with wear in arthritic knees can be corrected, similar to fixing a bumper indentation on a car. The distal femoral condylar angle is individually reproduced. The tibial component is placed in surgery perpendicular to the mechanical axis as in traditional OTS implants, but the distal condylar angle is transferred to the tibial insert, which restores the individual distal femoral joint line (Fig. 138.1).

The lateral insert is higher compared with the medial, which allows a correction of the valgus or varus deformity because the distal femoral and the proximal tibia are cut perpendicular to the mechanical axis.

To correct potential trochlear dysplasia, a generic trochlear flange with similar dimension compared with OTS implants is added in the design process. However, the trochlear J-curve is approximated.

This system allows infinitive sizes, shapes, and geometries to match each individual patient's anatomy. From the individual virtual implants 3D wax models are printed and the implants casted as traditional implants. The design process for PS implants allows individual adjustments for the size of the box and virtual optimization of the cam-post placement (Fig. 138.2).

In addition, the individual 3D bony information is used to create individual 3D-printed, single-use instrumentation, replacing our current metal instrumentation to reduce the total number of instruments and trays and facilitate simplification of operating room (OR) processes and OR setup (Fig. 138.3).

AUTHOR'S SURGICAL PEARLS

With the reconstruction of the patient's specific anatomy, specifically the medial and lateral femoral J-curves, surgical technique is focused on the anatomic placement of the custom implant. The implants come with an individualized surgical plan, which defines the thickness of each bony resection to place the implant anatomically. Deviation from the surgical plan would place the implants in a nonanatomic position and could result in ligament imbalance.

There are six bony resections: four in the coronal plane and two for the femoral rotation flexion gap. With regard to coronal alignment, the distal femoral resections of the medial and lateral

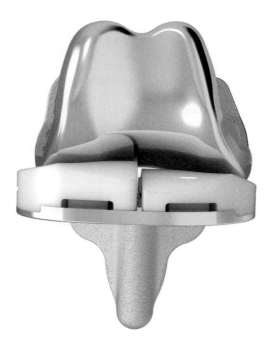

FIG 138.1 The distal femoral condylar angle is matched on the polyethylene insert side, increasing the lateral insert thickness accordingly. (Courtesy ConforMIS, Inc.)

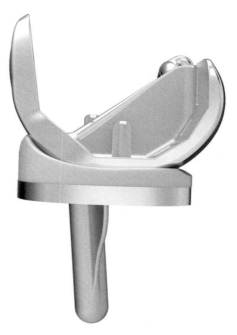

FIG 138.2 Shows a posterior-stabilized component. (Courtesy ConforMIS, Inc.)

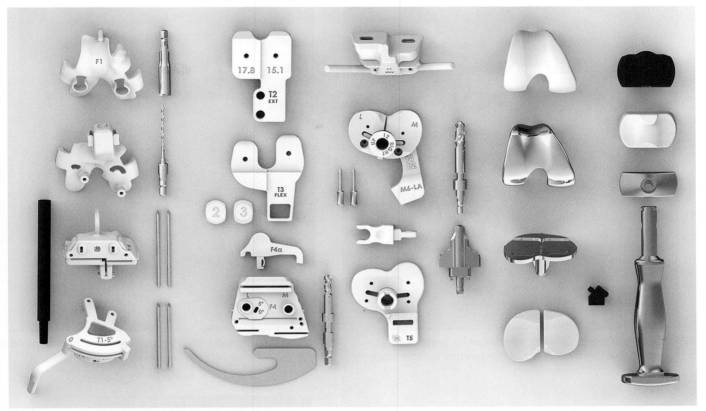

FIG 138.3 Instrumentation and implants for surgical case shown previously. (Confor-MIS, Inc.)

condyles and the resection of the medial and lateral tibial pla-teaus are described in the surgical plan and need to be matched intraoperatively. The surgical plan places the femoral and tibial components perpendicular to the mechanical femoral and tibial axis overall or mechanically neutral by default. For example, if resections are larger medially, the components would be in varus compared with the surgical plan. The same is true for the lateral side. Increased lateral resection resulted in more valgus. In general, approximately 1 mm equals approximately 1 degree. It is important to avoid over-resection; never place a varus knee in mechanical valgus and a valgus knee and mechanical varus. The author's advice is to try to slightly (1 to 2 degrees, but not more) undercorrect for both deformities. This is a slight devia-tion from the surgical plan provided by the manufacturer but prevents the surgeon from overcorrection because the surgical plan calls for neutral alignment. This illustrates the importance of measuring the bony resections to avoid overcorrection of deformity, which could result in a nonanatomic placement of the components.

The amount of posterior medial and lateral condylar resec-tion is important for correct femoral rotation and balancing of the flexion gap. If all bony resections match the planned amount, the implant is placed anatomically and no ligament imbalances need to be addressed. A deviation of more than 1 mm should be avoided. Measuring the resections with a feeler gauge prior to cutting is helpful.

Because the medial tibiofemoral joint is tighter than the lateral, accurate resections for the medial tibia, femoral condyle, and medial posterior condyle are of highest importance. In extension there is laxity of 1 to 2 mm that increases slightly to 2 to 3 mm in flexion. A tight flexion gap in CR TKR will result in less flexion. The resection in the center of the medial tibial plateau is by default 2 mm. The medial posterior condylar cut is the most important bony resection. Authors advise to recut the posterior medial condyle if the resection is less than planned. A 1-mm thicker bony resection is preferred to avoid any bony under-resection.

In severe varus or valgus knees, the authors advise to start under-resecting the distal femur and proximal tibia by 2 mm to avoid running out of thicker polyethylene inserts. The instru-ments allow these adjustments. The CR design comes in 6- and 8-mm thick inserts. Therefore the authors prefer to use the PS design in more advanced arthritic knees, which allows 6-, 8-, 10-, and 14-mm thick polyethylene inserts.

The surgical plan allows for both a measured resection and a gap-balancing technique. Both techniques can achieve an anatomically placed femoral component. Fig. 138.4 shows how the combined cutting jigs F2 and F3 allow the placement of the two pins, which are marked after the distal femoral resection is completed (Fig. 138.5) and placed (Fig. 138.6) to allow the placement of the distal femoral cutting block (Fig. 138.7). This block allows 5 degrees of additional external rotation (Fig. 138.8) if the flexion gap is too loose laterally or for cases in which patellar tracking has to be addressed.

The gap-balancing technique relies on the flexion spacer block placement onto the resected tibia. If the flexion gap is loose, there are 2- and 4-mm thick shims that can be added to the flexion spacer block and result in thicker polyethylene inserts. The extension gap needs to be matched. Then the exten-sion spacer block is placed with its 90-degree geometry on top

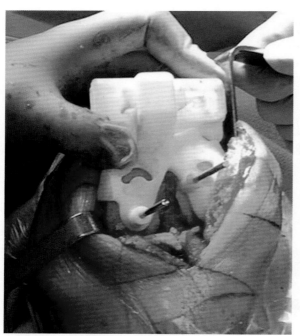

FIG 138.4 The first two pin holes are drilled for better stabilization and later used for placement of the femoral cutting block.

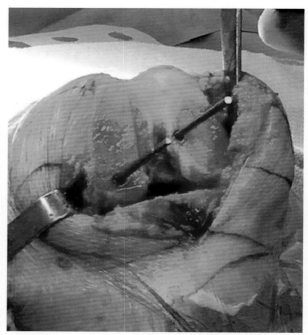

FIG 138.6 After cutting the tibia, two pins are placed into the marked pin holes drilled previously, as seen in Fig. 138.4.

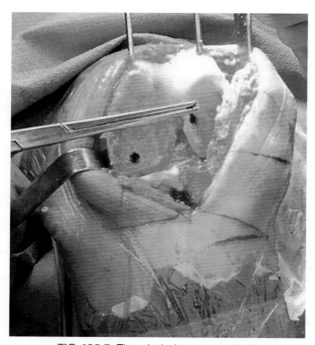

FIG 138.5 The pin holes are marked.

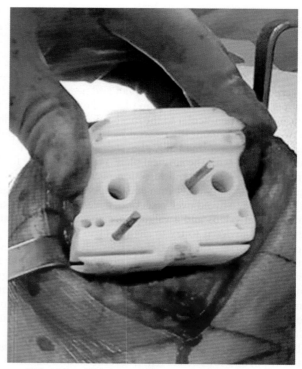

FIG 138.7 The femoral cutting block is placed.

of the flexion spacer block. The distal femoral cut is positioned 90 degrees relative to the tibia (Fig. 138.9). The femoral cutting block is then placed on top of the flexion spacer block, anatomically matching the medial lateral width, using the thumb and index finger to position (Fig. 138.10) and pin (Fig. 138.11) in place. The first cut is the medial posterior condyle, which is the

most important (Fig. 138.12). The resected bone is removed of any remaining cartilage (Fig. 138.13) and measured (Fig. 138.14). The saw blade thickness is added to the measurement. If the resection is not enough, the medial pin is removed. The cutting block is slightly externally rotated and repinned and additional posterior medial condyle resection is performed.

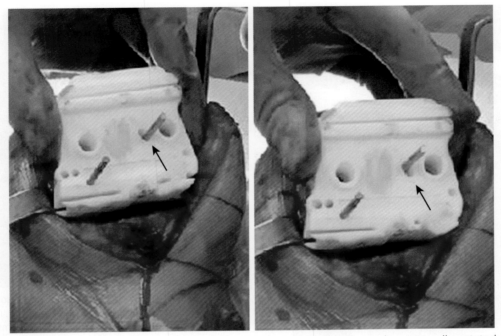

FIG 138.8 If the lateral flexion gap is too loose, the cutting block can be externally rotated 5 degrees.

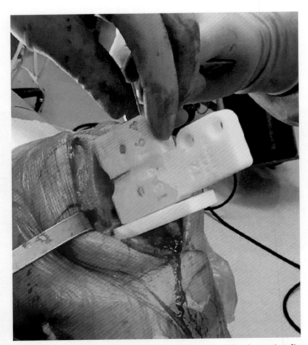

FIG 138.9 Gap balancing: place the extension block on the flexion spacer block and move the tibia until the angle between the flexion spacer block and distal femoral cut is exactly 90 degrees.

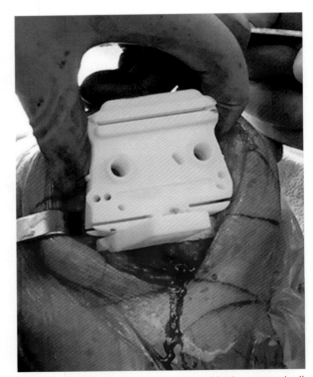

FIG 138.10 Place the femoral cutting block anatomically by feeling the mediolateral width with your fingers 90 degrees to the flexion spacer block.

Following placement of an anatomic femoral component, dynamic rotation of the tibial tray can be performed with the system. The patella was reduced, and the leg was taken through range of motion. The tibia is either internally or externally rotated until optimal patella tracking is achieved. The tibial position is then marked on the tibia (Fig. 138.15). The tibial component is slightly undersized to allow ±5 degrees of internal or external rotation for optimal patellar tracking.

Some argue that the technology is significantly more expensive, whereas others argue that potential gains from decreased

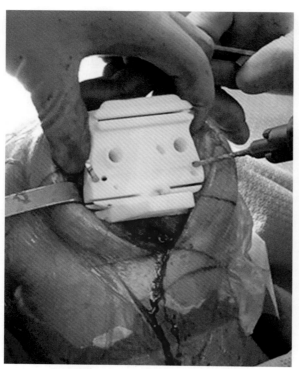

FIG 138.11 Pin the cutting block.

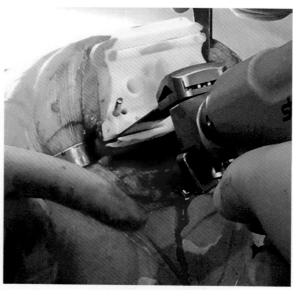

FIG 138.12 Always cut the medial posterior condyle first and verify the bony resection. If under-resected, remove fixation pin and move up cutting block medial 1 or 2 mm, repin and recut until resected amount matches the planned amount. With each cut, add the saw blade thickness.

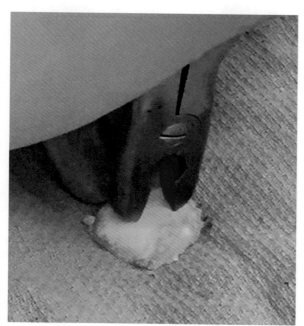

FIG 138.13 After removal of cartilage, the medial posterior condyle resected thickness is compared with surgical plan.

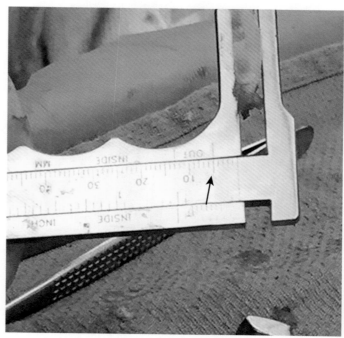

FIG 138.14 Measurement of bony resection, including saw blade thickness, to verify planned resection of medial posterior condyle using the caliper.

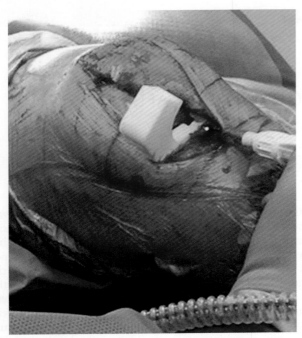

FIG 138.15 Dynamic rotation of tibial component: take the knee through range of motion with the patella reduced and see where the tibia settles. Mark the tibia.

inventory, reduced sterilization cost, and reduced adverse events could make this new knee system cost effective within the first 3 months.[12,26]

The proposed benefits of customized patient-specific implants (PSIs) are currently under investigation, and early studies have shown favorable results. Data show favorable outcomes with regard to kinematics and functional outcomes following PSI TKA. In vivo kinematics of the PSI versus OTS posterior CR implants was analyzed using mobile fluoroscopy. The authors found improved kinematics closer to that of a normal knee in the PSI group[9] (Cates). This is a similar finding to previous study of kinematics in cadaver limbs.[33] A multicenter study compared patients at seven centers and found PSI patients were more likely to perform high-demand activities without difficulty and performed regular activities of daily living significantly faster.[36] When comparing the radiographic outcomes of PSI to OTS implants, Ivie et al. found the PSI was 1.8 times more likely to be within the desired +3 degrees from the neutral mechanical axis when compared with the standard OTS control group. This study suggests that PSI can reliably reproduce the mechanical axis when compared with standard intramedullary femoral and extramedullary tibial instrumentation.[19]

Studies have also found promising results with regard to patient safety, intraoperative measures, and costs. Clyburn et al. analyzed short-term follow-up adverse events with the patient-specific knee and compared the results to current multicenter studies on OTS implants. Findings were favorable when reviewing adverse events and patient outcome scores. At 1 year postoperatively, the PSI demonstrated an excellent safety profile with a low transfusion rate, low manipulation rate, and low rate of revision for mechanical loosening.[10] Katthagen and

Chatziandreou prospectively studied matched pairs of 35 consecutive PSI and 35 OTC (Stryker Triathlon, Stryker, Mahwah, NJ) implants for TKA comparing intraoperative, postoperative, and patient satisfaction parameters.[20] Results indicate decreased surgical time and decreased hemoglobin level drops postoperatively. The PSI group also was able to return to activities of daily living faster than the OTS patients. At 1 year postoperatively the PSI group Knee Injury and Osteoarthritis Outcome Score (KOOS) scores and patient satisfaction scores were significantly higher compared with patients receiving OTS TKR. Martin et al. compared hospital outcome measures of PSI and OTS implants at a single institution. The PSI implant group showed decreased transfusion rates, decreased adverse event rate at discharge, decreased length of stay, and a decreased discharge rate to acute care facilities. The study also noted decreased costs of $832.59 per PSI patient in total in hospital costs of care. This figure included the cost of the CT scan needed for the PSI.[26]

Long-term data are necessary to evaluate if restoring more normal knee kinematics will improve function and increase patient satisfaction after TKA. Early reports of increased patient satisfaction in the 90% are encouraging, but more detail and longer follow-up are necessary to conclude whether a customized approach to anatomic knee replacement is superior to our standard functional approach, which we have been practicing for almost 40 years.

KEY REFERENCES

Cartier P, Sanouiller JL, Grelsamer RP: Unicompartmental knee arthroplasty surgery. *J Arthroplasty* 11:782, 1996.

Fitzpatrick C, Fitzpatrick D, Lee J, et al: Statistical design of unicompartmental tibial implants and comparison with current devices. *Knee* 14:138–144, 2007.

Hernigou P, Deschamps G: Posterior slope of the tibial implant and the outcome of unicompartmental knee arthroplasty. *J Bone Joint Surg Am* 86:506–511, 2004.

Kirkley A, Birmingham TB, Litchfield RB, et al: A randomized trial of arthroscopic surgery for osteoarthritis of the knee. *N Engl J Med* 359:1097–1107, 2008.

Kozinn SC, Scott RD: Current concepts review: unicompartmental total arthroplasty. *J Bone Joint Surg Am* 71:145, 1989.

Marmor L: Unicompartmental knee arthroplasty: ten to thirteen year follow-up study. *Clin Orthop* 226:24, 1987.

Moseley JB, O'Malley K, Petersen NJ, et al: A controlled trial of arthroscopic surgery for osteoarthritis of the knee. *N Engl J Med* 347:81, 2002.

Newman J, Pydisetty RV, Ackroyd C: Unicompartmental or total knee replacement: the 15-year results of a prospective randomised controlled trial. *J Bone Joint Surg Br* 91:52–57, 2009.

Pennington DW, Swienckowski JJ, Lutes WB, et al: Unicompartmental knee arthroplasty in patients sixty years of age or younger. *J Bone Joint Surg Am* 85:1968–1973, 2003.

Price AJ, Dodd CA, Svard UG, et al: Oxford medial unicompartmental knee arthroplasty in patients younger and older than 60 years of age. *J Bone Joint Surg Br* 87:1488–1492, 2005.

Riddle DL, Jiranek WA, McGlynn FJ: Yearly incidence of unicompartmental knee arthroplasty in the United States. *J Arthroplasty* 23:408–412, 2008.

Swienckowski JJ, Pennington DW: Unicompartmental arthroplasty in patients 60 years of age or younger: surgical technique. *J Bone Joint Surg Am* 86(Suppl 1):131–142, 2004.

Tabor OB, Jr, Tabor OB: Unicompartmental arthroplasty: a long-term follow-up study. *J Arthroplasty* 13(4):373–379, 1998.

The references for this chapter can also be found on www.expertconsult.com.

139

Posterior Cruciate Sacrificing Total Knee Arthroplasty

Aaron A. Hofmann, Brian P. Dahl

Debate continues regarding the posterior cruciate ligament (PCL) in total knee arthroplasty (TKA). Good long-term data exist both radiographically and clinically for PCL sparing and PCL substituting types of implants.[20,27] The decision to spare or sacrifice the PCL is largely surgeon preference, as a clear advantage in the literature has not been delineated. Many surgeons base the decision on intraoperative findings such as appearance of the PCL, bone quality, and integrity of the collateral stabilizers. National trends from the previous decades in which most knee arthroplasties were performed with PCL retaining–type implants have changed to a more recent trend of PCL substituting implants with a post and cam mechanism, or sacrificing and substituting with an ultracongruent polyethylene.[17]

This author represents the group of surgeons who routinely sacrifice the PCL, with the exception of younger athletic patients with early onset knee osteoarthritis. The algorithm followed closely matches that suggested by Lombardi et al.[12] Significant initial malalignment greater than 15 degrees in varus or valgus or significant flexion contracture precludes the ability to sufficiently balance soft tissues and expose the joint with PCL retention.[8,21] Inflammatory arthropathies are also known for late failure of PCL after initial retention.[1,9] Prior patellectomy disrupts the normal kinematics of the knee and yields inferior results if PCL retention is chosen.[13] Similarly, inferior results have been detected in prior high tibial osteotomy patients who do not have a PCL substituting implant.[28]

SPARING THE POSTERIOR CRUCIATE LIGAMENT

Salvage of the PCL provides possible kinematic and proprioceptive benefits. However, concerns with regard to salvage of the PCL have been raised. The kinematic benefit of cruciate retaining arthroplasty appears to be absent on fluoroscopic analysis.[26] One magnetic resonance imaging (MRI)–based study demonstrated that tibial bone cuts interrupted the PCL to a significant degree most of the time.[25] Late failure of a retained PCL leading to revision is described as occurring in up to 2% of cases in one series.[1,18] Histologically, the PCL is abnormal in a significant number of arthritic knees.[19] These findings and others show why this author recommends protecting the PCL (Fig. 139.1) with an osteotome if it is to be saved, and proving its stability before selecting PCL retaining or substituting final components.

SACRIFICING THE POSTERIOR CRUCIATE LIGAMENT

If a clinical indication for PCL sacrifice exists or if the PCL is proven not to be sufficiently stable, some form of sagittal plane motion stability is required. Currently, two techniques are available for stabilizing the sagittal motion of the tibia during flexion after PCL sacrificing primary TKA: (1) posterior stabilized polyethylene using a posterior middle intercondylar tibial post that articulates with a cam on the femoral component during flexion to reproduce femoral roll-back, and (2) stabilization using deeply dished polyethylene that has an anterior polyethylene buildup in a highly conforming fashion, which prevents posterior translation of the tibia on the femur. This author uses the highly congruent anterior buildup method if the PCL is to be sacrificed.

Posterior Stabilized Polyethylene Prosthesis

The posterior stabilized condylar prosthesis was introduced in 1978, with specific goals of preventing tibial subluxation, improving range of motion (ROM), and improving stair-climbing ability.[6] Design theory included lengthening the effective moment arm of the quadriceps by forcing the contact point of the femur more posterior, giving a mechanical advantage over previous designs.[6] Long-term results are adequate with the posterior stabilized design, but specific clinical problems are associated with this design.

Patellar clunk syndrome was a significant problem with early designs of posterior stabilized TKA. The long intercondylar notch of the femoral cam and post mechanism allows fibrous tissue overgrowth proximal to the patella. Impingement and occasional painful snapping occur upon extension of the knee.[5] Subsequent design changes to the femoral component have all but eliminated this problem.[15]

Post breakage and wear is another complication that occurs uniquely to posterior stabilized implants. The tibial post, which functions to keep femoral contact points posterior on the tibia, is impacted repetitively by the femoral cam through normal use. Loads of 8 to 10 times body weight have been recorded with chair rise. The small surface area of contact between cam and post yields a significant concentration of stress. Case reports have documented post breakage in both conventional polyethylene and highly cross-linked polyethylene.[2,23] The tibial post also serves as an additional source of wear contributing to osteolysis.[21]

Complications. Complications of posterior stabilized implants occur on the femoral side as well. The cam of the femur that articulates with the post requires more bone to be removed from the intercondylar notch than other designs. This results in bone loss that may complicate revision surgery. Case reports of fracture between the condyles as a result of intercondylar bone loss are a matter of concern.[14]

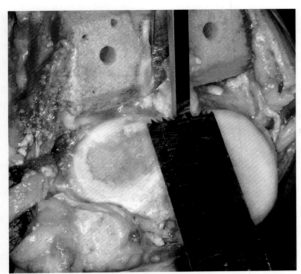

FIG 139.1 An osteotome is used to protect the PCL if it is to be spared.

The femoral cam of posterior stabilized implants can be dislocated and can become lodged anteriorly (Fig. 139.2). The tibial post engages the femoral cam at approximately 60 to 75 degrees of flexion. No contact or posterior stabilization occurs during this early ROM. Soft tissue imbalance may yield laxity that allows dislocation to occur.[13] If this occurs, closed reduction and/or revision may be required.

Anterior Polyethylene Buildup Alternative

The current highly congruent anterior buildup alternative to the cam and post form of stabilization was developed out of necessity. A particularly difficult case involving a long-stemmed revision was reported in 1991 in a patient with Parkinson's disease who had persistent dislocation of the standard congruent insert. Because his medical health would not allow a prolonged revision operation, an alternative solution was sought. A custom polyethylene insert of highly conforming nature with an anterior buildup of 12.5 mm was designed. This insert was subsequently placed in production for use with the Natural Knee system (Zimmer, Warsaw, Indiana) as the ultracongruent posterior stabilized polyethylene. Since that time, this concept has been incorporated into at least six other TKA systems.

The highly congruent anterior buildup alternative for PCL sacrificing TKA has several advantages. First, no additional femoral inventory is needed if the PCL is sacrificed or saved. Stabilization of the femur is maintained in flexion and stair climbing. The anterior buildup maintains the tibial and femoral anteroposterior relationship throughout the arc of motion. There is no need for a long intercondylar femoral notch for a cam mechanism that reduces bone loss at primary operation and reduces risk of iatrogenic femoral fracture. Additionally, lack of a long trochlear notch prevents abnormal fibrous tissue formation, with the theoretical advantage of preventing patellar clunk. To date, no case reports of patellar clunk in highly congruent anterior buildup components have been documented. Less stress concentration occurs on the tibial polyethylene than on the posts of posterior stabilized implants because of the highly conforming nature of the ultracongruent anterior lip stabilized polyethylene. No "forced" roll-back occurs via a cam

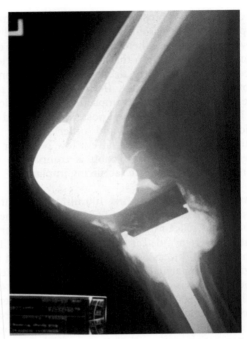

FIG 139.2 TKA with dislocated cam and post form of posterior stabilization.

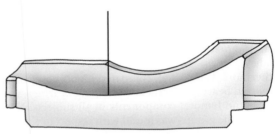

FIG 139.3 The null point, or femoral resting point, is 4 to 6 mm posterior to the midline.

and post mechanism; however, the null point or resting position of the femur on the tibia is posterior to midline by 4 to 6 mm (Fig. 139.3). Dislocation of this design has not been reported.

Disadvantages. Theoretical disadvantages of highly congruent anterior buildup polyethylene have been described.[14] In early flexion, less rotational laxity is noted than with cam and post posterior stabilization. This has been theorized to transmit greater shear stress to the tibia-bone interface and to create early loosening; however, this has not been our experience. Rotational freedom of the femur on the tibia is maintained with ±7.5 degrees of rotational freedom. A study of kinematics has demonstrated in cadaveric specimens an increase in quadriceps force (approximately 25 lb) to extend the knee with anterior buildup versus cam and post–type posterior stabilization.[14] This is most likely a result of the lack of full posterior translation that a post provides through deep flexion, giving the quadriceps lever arm maximal advantage. Preoperative and postoperative quadriceps rehabilitation negates this effect.

The wide acceptance of ultracongruent anterior buildup polyethylene inserts has suffered from initial design flaws. When the total condylar knee prosthesis was designed and implanted, lack of optimal flexion was noted with a deeply dished polyethylene. Several studies since then have published on the dramatic improvement in knee flexion that occurs with posterior stabilized knees. It is clear that the deeply dished tibial component on the total condylar knee was suffering from a high posterior lip of the polyethylene and was impacting the posterior femur at lower levels of flexion than the posterior stabilized component. Modern ultracongruent and other anterior buildup stabilization–type polyethylenes have a low posterior lip, and our experience suggests that flexion is comparable between cruciate retaining and cruciate sacrificing implants.

Study Results. Results of the first 100 ultracongruent inserts[4] compared with a control group of PCL sparing prostheses have been published. Goals of the study were to see whether patellar complications were avoided if the radiographic tibial interface was maintained, and to assess for differences in ROM between the two groups. No patellar complications were reported in this study group. Two revisions of the ultracongruent insert occurred during the average 60-month follow-up; these were likely because of cementless fixation of the modular tibial baseplate. No difference in ROM was noted between the two groups relative to preoperative motion.

Others have reported similar midterm results, with anterior buildup posterior stabilizing PCL sacrificing arthroplasty.[24] Laskin et al. performed a randomized prospective study comparing highly congruent anterior stabilization versus posterior stabilization with PCL sacrifice in all subjects. No difference between the two groups in terms of ROM, stair climbing, pain, knee scores, anterior knee pain, and stability was detected in that study.[10]

Furthermore, Peters et al. compared highly congruent anterior stabilized bearings to cruciate retaining bearings, using the same tibial and femoral components in all subjects. No difference between the groups was found with respect to Knee Society scores, component loosening, need for manipulation, radiographic alignment, or time to revision, except that there was a higher revision rate in the cruciate retaining bearing design.[22]

CONCLUSION

TKA enjoys excellent survivorship and functional outcomes, regardless of PCL status. There are clear indications to sacrifice the PCL to achieve the desired goal. Two ways of achieving stability of the tibiofemoral relationship after PCL sacrifice are known: posterior stabilized post and cam designs, and anterior buildup deeply dished highly congruent designs. Dished highly congruent stabilization may avoid some of the problems that post and cam–type posterior stabilized designs have encountered, with similar radiographic, functional, and clinical outcomes.

KEY REFERENCES

1. Archibeck MJ, Berger RA, Barden RM, et al: Posterior cruciate ligament-retaining total knee arthroplasty in patients with rheumatoid arthritis. *J Bone Joint Surg Am* 83:1231–1236, 2001.
4. Hofmann AA, Tkach TK, Evanich CJ, et al: Posterior stabilization in total knee arthroplasty with use of an ultracongruent polyethylene insert. *J Arthroplasty* 15:576–583, 2000.
10. Laskin RS, Maruyama Y, Villanueva M, et al: Deep-dish congruent tibial component use in total knee arthroplasty: a randomized prospective study. *Clin Orthop* 380:36–44, 2000.
12. Lombardi AV, Mallory T, Fada R, et al: An algorithm for the posterior cruciate ligament in total knee arthroplasty. *Clin Orthop* 392:75–87, 2001.
17. Mont M, Booth R, Laskin R, et al: The spectrum of prosthesis design for primary total knee arthroplasty. *Instr Course Lect* 52:397–407, 2003.
19. Mullaji A, Marawar S, Simha M, et al: Cruciate ligaments in arthritic knees: a histologic study with radiologic correlation. *J Arthroplasty* 23:567–572, 2008.
20. NIH Consensus Panel: NIH consensus statement on total knee replacement, December 8–10, 2003. *J Bone Joint Surg Am* 86:1328–1335, 2004.
21. Peters C, Mohr RA, Bachus K: Primary total knee arthroplasty in the valgus knee: creating a balanced soft tissue envelope. *J Arthroplasty* 16:721–729, 2001.
22. Peters C, Mulkey P, Erickson J, et al: Comparison of total knee arthroplasty with highly congruent anterior-stabilized bearings versus a cruciate-retaining design. *Clin Orthop* 472:175–180, 2014.
24. Sathappan S, Wasserman B, Jaffe W, et al: Midterm results of primary total knee arthroplasty using a dished polyethylene insert with a recessed or resected posterior cruciate ligament. *J Arthroplasty* 21:1012–1016, 2006.
25. Shannon F, Cronin J, Cleary M, et al: The posterior cruciate ligament preserving total knee replacement: do we "preserve" it? A radiological study. *J Bone Joint Surg Br* 89:766–771, 2007.

The references for this chapter can also be found on www.expertconsult.com.

Posterior Cruciate Ligament—Substituting Total Knee Arthroplasty

William J. Long, Justin B. Jones, Michael P. Nett, Gregory J. Roehrig, Giles R. Scuderi, W. Norman Scott

Posterior cruciate substitution in total knee arthroplasty (TKA) gathered momentum and popularity as the pioneering surgeons and design teams improved on their prototypes. Today, surgeons that prefer this principle and technique over cruciate retention believe that the anterior and posterior cruciate ligaments (ACL, PCL) are histologically abnormal and therefore compromised in arthritic knees.[4,16,39] Furthermore, these surgeons believe that it is difficult to balance the PCL appropriately while maintaining its functional integrity and ability to accomplish near-normal femoral rollback.[7]

An understanding of the history behind the current posterior-substituting prostheses on the market, key design concepts, and important surgical principles and techniques will aid surgeons in providing well-functioning, durable, total knee replacements (TKRs). This chapter first addresses the time line and progression of posterior-substituting components, from the earliest years to the currently available designs. The surgical technique and clinical results will then be reviewed.

The terms *posterior-substituting* and *posterior-stabilized* have been used interchangeably for many years. For clarity in this chapter, posterior-stabilized will be reserved to describe the Hospital for Special Surgery (HSS) implant that originally bore this name in 1978. Posterior-substituting will be used to reference this entire style of total knee design.

EVOLUTION OF POSTERIOR CRUCIATE LIGAMENT—SUBSTITUTING KNEE ARTHROPLASTY

The Insall Group

The early years of knee arthroplasty saw multiple designs and design modifications. The unicondylar design was applied, in fact doubled, to yield the duocondylar prosthesis. Other designs that were studied at that time at the HSS (1971–1973) included the geometric and the Gueper designs. These prostheses yielded good to excellent results in about 50% of patients. Problems included patellar pain, which led to the development of the duopatellar knee, and loosening of the components.

The next significant advancement was achieved with the original total condylar prosthesis, which was cruciate-sacrificing, but not PCL-substituting. It was a semiconstrained, nonlinked, cemented design that involved excising both cruciate ligaments. First implanted in 1974, this cobalt-chrome femoral component had a symmetrical anterior flange and groove, two symmetrical

condyles in the coronal plane, and a smaller radius of curvature posteriorly in the sagittal plane. The tibial component was a single piece of high-density polyethylene with biconcave articular surfaces, offering some stability.[54] It was fully conforming in extension and less conforming in flexion to allow for more rotation and gliding of the femur. The small intercondylar eminence helped prevent translation movement, and the 35×12.5-mm tibial peg helped achieve fixation. The patella was a dome-shaped, central peg, high-density polyethylene design.

Complete cruciate ligament excision accomplished greater exposure and allowed for easier correction of fixed deformities. Without an intact ACL and PCL, the knee design relied on the congruity of the articular surfaces and integrity and balance of the collateral ligaments for stability. With well-balanced flexion and extension gaps, the collateral ligaments will tighten as the femoral component translates anteriorly, up the conforming tibial well, preventing dislocation. This concept, designed with the input of engineer Peter Walker and surgeons John Insall and Chitranjan Ranawat, was termed the *uphill principle*. The femoral component was intended to articulate centrally on the tibial component surface, with no rollback built into the design. This original total condylar knee proved to be a durable, sound design,[33] but not without problems. Patients rarely achieved more than 90 degrees of flexion and, on occasion, the tibia would subluxate if the flexion gap was not adequately balanced, particularly during stair descent. Such issues could potentially be resolved with a new prosthetic design that spared or substituted for the PCL.

Insall-Burstein I Posterior-Stabilized Prosthesis. To address the posterior subluxation and instability that would sometimes occur with the total condylar prosthesis, a central tibial post was added. This modification, however, proved to be an imperfect solution because the specifics of the design and the hyperextension stop led to tibial edge loading and loosening.[69] In 1976, Al Burstein joined John Insall at the HSS, where they combined their experience, insight, and innovation to develop a posterior-stabilized knee that would substitute for the PCL, allow for complete correction of deformity, reproduce femoral rollback, improve flexion stability, and increase knee flexion.

The first-generation Insall-Burstein prosthesis (IB I) was first implanted in 1978. The tibiofemoral contact point was shifted from a more central location to a more posterior point,[34] resulting in a greater distance or hill to climb before the femur subluxates anteriorly. An intercondylar femoral cam was added to the design to replicate femoral rollback. It engaged the tibial post at approximately 70 degrees of flexion and, as the cam climbed the post, the tibiofemoral contact point shifted more posteriorly until approximately 115 degrees of flexion. These features, along with the increased conformity and 3-degree posterior slope of the all-polyethylene tibial component, helped the IB I achieve great success and durability.

Importantly, the Insall-Burstein prosthesis substituted for the PCL, not the collateral ligaments. Gap balancing was critical to prevent anterior tibial subluxation. The spine-cam mechanism did not articulate in extension and therefore provided no additional medial-lateral stability. Stability was dependent on the integrity and balance of the collateral ligaments and somewhat influenced by the conformity of the tibiofemoral surfaces. An insufficient collateral ligament would necessitate a design with more inherent constraint.

During the 1980s, the IB I went through some design modifications. Research on load transmission to the tibia concluded that metal backing of the tibial component would improve this factor and the all-polyethylene design was replaced at the HSS by 1981. Carbon reinforcement of the polyethylene was introduced with the hope of increasing its strength and durability, but it did not achieve the anticipated success, early failures were reported, and this alteration was abandoned. In the mid-1980s, the femoral component underwent a few improvements. The anterior flange was deepened and rounded to allow for better patellar tracking and a smoother transition as the patellofemoral contact point moved toward the distal runners with increasing flexion. Also, additional femoral component sizes became available, reducing the amount of mismatch between the prosthesis and distal femur.

Insall-Burstein II Posterior-Stabilized Prosthesis. The Insall-Burstein I posterior stabilized knee underwent more significant modifications in the late 1980s to yield the Insall-Burstein II. Intramedullary instruments assisted the surgeon in obtaining appropriate alignment in a reproducible and accurate manner. The original tension device for determining equal and rectangular flexion and extension gaps was replaced with a technique using spacer blocks. The concept of modularity was expanded to include multiple sizes for the femoral and tibial components, and different polyethylene thicknesses, intramedullary stems, and wedges to address defects.

Additional changes were made to enhance femoral rollback, thereby improving flexion. Reports of component dislocation arose, especially in knees with preoperative valgus alignment or those that achieved a high degree of postoperative flexion. Consequently, additional modifications of the tibial insert included positioning the tibial post more anteriorly and increasing its height. This posterior-substituting design proved to be a functionally sound concept that performed well for more than a decade before it evolved further (Fig. 140.1).

NexGen Legacy. The Zimmer NexGen Legacy (Zimmer, Warsaw, Indiana) prosthesis was the next generation in the line of posterior-stabilized knee components. This prosthesis and its new instrumentation became available in the mid-1990s. One of the key improvements in design was anatomic right and left femoral components. The tibial components were symmetrical and therefore universal. In addition, the lateral flange of the femur was enhanced and the trochlea deepened to further facilitate congruent patellofemoral tracking and kinematics.

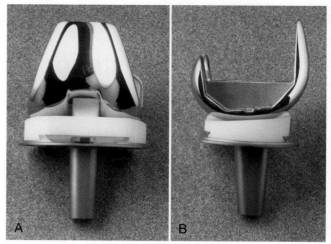

FIG 140.1 Insall-Burstein II prosthesis.

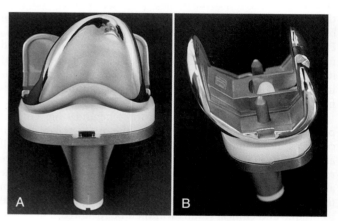

FIG 140.2 Zimmer NexGen prosthesis.

Previous posterior-stabilized designs, including the Insall-Burstein prostheses, occasionally experienced inadvertent flexion of the femoral component during implantation. This led to gapping between the anterior cortex of the femur and anterior flange of the component. Attempts to correct this intraoperatively, if noticed, could result in a gap between the posterior condyles of the native femur and posterior condyles of the component. The addition of femoral lugs to the NexGen design assisted the surgeon during cementation and helped prevent unwanted flexion of the femoral component.

An expanded array of instruments became available with the NexGen Legacy prosthesis. These include epicondylar instruments to assist with femoral component rotation, anterior and posterior referencing size guides, and instruments to prepare the femur and tibia using a milling technique instead of the traditional cutting blocks and oscillating saw (Fig. 140.2).

NexGen Legacy High-Flexion and Gender-Optimized Implants. The increased desire by patients to pursue activities associated with greater degrees of knee flexion, as well as acknowledgment of the important cultural requirements in certain Asian populations, have driven the development high-flexion knee prostheses. These implants are designed to exceed 140 to 150 degrees of flexion compared with the 120 degrees permitted by traditional designs. To accommodate higher flexion, these design modifications include enhanced posterior condylar geometry of the femoral component, which improves contact areas in high flexion, thereby reducing the risk of polyethylene wear.[6] In addition, modifications to the anterior aspect of the tibial polyethylene insert were made to reduce the potential for extensor mechanism impingement in high flexion. Finally the cam-post design of posterior-stabilizing (PS) variants was optimized to reduce the risk of dislocation in high flexion. To date, studies of high-flexion TKR prostheses have provided little data to support the theoretical advantages attributed to the optimized designs. In a recent meta-analysis, Ghandi et al.[26] noted that high-flexion designs were associated with improved range of motion (ROM) compared with traditional implants, but offered no clinical benefits. Meneghini et al.[56] have confirmed the lack of any functional benefit with flexion of more than 125 degrees after TKR.

An example of a high-flexion design is the Zimmer NexGen Flex-Fixed PS implant, a modification of the NexGen legacy prosthesis. Studies of the NexGen Flex-Fixed PS implant are inconclusive. Kim et al.[38] have reported on a prospective randomized study of 50 patients who underwent simultaneous bilateral TKR with a standard fixed-bearing Zimmer NexGen Legacy PS (LPS) knee prosthesis on one side and a high-flexion, fixed-bearing NexGen LPS-Flex knee prosthesis on the opposite side. The Knee Society and HSS scores were not significantly different for either knee, pre- or postoperatively. Moreover, there were no statistically significant differences in ROM at any time point pre- or postoperatively; at final follow-up, the standard prosthesis had a mean ROM of 135.8 degrees (range, 105 to 150 degrees) versus a mean of 135.8 degrees for the high-flexion prosthesis. A similar study was published by Nutton et al.,[60] who compared patients who had been randomized to receive a standard or high-flexion version of the Zimmer NexGen LPS fixed-bearing design. Again, no significant differences in outcomes or knee flexion were noted between the two groups of patients.

Shortly after the development of high-flexion designs, increased acknowledgment of the anthropomorphic variation that exists among humans of different genders, races, and ethnic origins led to the introduction of gender-optimized components.[28] These gender-specific components included modifications of the mediolateral-to-anteroposterior ratio of the femoral components, as well as the orientation and thickness of the trochlear groove and anterior flange. An example of a gender-specific implant is the Zimmer Gender Solutions NexGen High Flex LPS prosthesis. This implant is a further modification of the NexGen Legacy. Results examining the use of gender-optimized devices remain controversial. Although radiographic and anatomic studies have demonstrated the gender bias of standard implants toward white male anatomy, little data exist to date to support that this bias has adversely affected clinical outcomes in white females or patients of other races.[53]

Persona. The Zimmer Persona (Zimmer, Warsaw, Indiana) is the next advancement or evolution in this line of posterior-stabilized knee components. It was introduced in 2013 and advancements include laterality-specific tibial components designed to improve rotation and tibial coverage. Tibial inserts are also available in 1-mm increments to fine-tune ligamentous balance. The Persona offers multiple femoral component size options in the medial-lateral dimension for a specific anteroposterior (AP) size to accommodate anatomic variability between gender and ethnic groups. A recent study by Dai et al.[17] shows that having multiple medial-lateral options for a specific AP size femoral component reduces the incidence of femoral overhang. An additional study by Graceffa et al.[27] shows that the box osteotomy required for the Persona femoral component results in less volumetric bone removal than several other current femoral component designs.

Other Current Posterior Cruciate Ligament—Substituting Implants. The outstanding performance of the Insall-Burstein device prompted the other total knee prosthesis manufacturers and their engineers to incorporate a PCL-substituting design into their product lines.

PFC Sigma. DePuy (Raynham, Massachusetts) developed this comprehensive knee arthroplasty system with modularity in mind. The femoral component can be mated with a tibial tray of the same size, or one size larger or smaller, providing three choices for every femur size. This is meant to help optimize contact at the implant-implant interfaces and implant-bone interfaces.

The versatile tibial tray was designed to accept a PCL-retaining, PCL-supplementing, or PCL-substituting polyethylene insert of varying thicknesses. In addition, the tray can be augmented with wedges, blocks, and stems if bone loss or poor bone quality dictates. More recently, a tibial rotating platform design was released. The goals of this concept are improvement in rotational biomechanics (20 degrees of supported internal and external rotation in deep flexion), reduction of backside wear, and lower peak stresses on the condyles as a result of tibiofemoral self-alignment (Fig. 140.3).

Attune. Introduced in 2013, with the addition of a rotating platform option in 2014, the DePuy Synthes Attune knee incorporates innovations such as a gradually reducing radius of curvature to provide conformity throughout the ROM and an improved cam-engagement design. The tibial base plate can now accommodate up to two size variations in relation to the femoral component to optimize proximal tibial coverage. A total of 10 size options for the femoral and tibial components plus four additional narrow femoral components have been added. Improvements in patellofemoral design include a medial offset domed patella, which optimizes coverage and improves patellofemoral tracking.

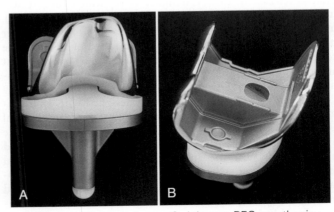

FIG 140.3 Depuy Johnson & Johnson PFC prosthesis.

Genesis II. The Genesis II total knee (Smith & Nephew, Andover, Massachusetts) was designed as a comprehensive knee system with a modern PCL-substituting option. The components are designed to be versatile and allow the femoral prosthesis to mate with four different-sized tibial components. An additional feature is the elongation and lateralization of the femoral component's trochlear groove to maximize contact with the patella throughout the arc of motion (full contact through 85 degrees of flexion).

The Genesis II design of the femoral component's posterior condyles is innovative. Most conventional knee system designs require external rotation of the femoral component to achieve a trapezoidal flexion gap. External rotation of the femoral cut results in more bone resected from the posterior medial femur than from the posterior lateral femur. The asymmetrical femoral bone resections help compensate for the traditional asymmetrical tibial resection that occurs with a perpendicular tibial cut. This traditional cut results in more bone resected from the lateral than from the medial tibial plateau. Thus, in the traditional method of component implantation, the bone cuts counterbalance each other and result in a rectangular flexion space. Traditional components are designed for this and have symmetrical posterior femoral condyles.

The Genesis II does not use external rotation of the femoral component and, consequently, the posteromedial femoral condyle is thinner than the posterolateral condyle. The designers hoped to minimize some of the theoretical limitations associated with traditional external femoral rotation including unnecessary anterolateral femoral bone removal, rotational malalignment of the femoral and tibial components, and excessive medial patellar tracking at high flexion angles. Conceptually, the flexion space remains balanced because the smaller medial posterior condyle compensates for the smaller posterior medial flexion space.

Stability of the Genesis II PCL-substituting knee depends on the component's articular geometry and the spine-cam interaction. The implants are designed to articulate freely through the first 60 degrees of flexion, with stability dependent on the surface geometry and soft tissue balance. Spine-cam engagement occurs at 60 to 70 degrees of knee flexion (Fig. 140.4).

Journey II. In an effort to reproduce more normal knee function, Smith & Nephew used analyses and comparisons of the geometry and kinematics of the normal knee and conventional TKA systems. The Journey II Bi-Cruciate Stabilized Knee System, released in 2012, is designed to replicate PCL and ACL function, accommodate deep flexion (up to 155 degrees), induce normal tibiofemoral axial rotation, and provide proper patellar tracking throughout the entire range of flexion. The combination of an oxidized zirconium femoral component articulating with highly cross-linked polyethylene offers potential enhanced durability.

The femoral component has been designed with an asymmetric flange anteriorly and an anatomic three-degree distal and posterior femoral joint line. Other design features include a tibial articular surface with a prominent posteromedial lip and medial sulcus near the anteroposterior midline. The lateral aspect of the tibial articular surface includes a smaller anterolateral lip to allow the screw home mechanism and an increased posterior slope to promote femoral rollback and external rotation (Fig. 140.5).

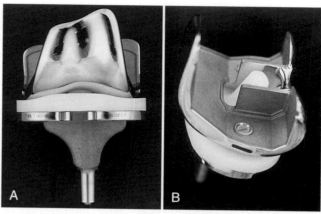

FIG 140.4 Smith & Nephew Genesis II prosthesis.

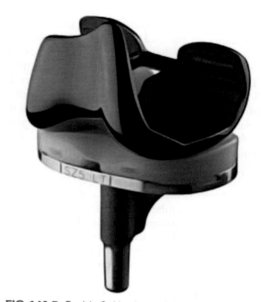

FIG 140.5 Smith & Nephew Journey prosthesis.

The anterior cam design replicates ACL function to reduce mid-flexion instability and paradoxical motion.

Vanguard. Vanguard, the newest complete knee system from Biomet (Warsaw, Indiana) offers 10 femoral component sizes and 9 tibial tray sizes. The femur comes in an open- or closed-box design and has a conservative bone resection for the intercondylar box. The posterior cam has been extended to minimize dislocation in deep flexion. The trochlear groove was deepened and lengthened in an effort to maximize patellar tracking and contact during deep flexion.

The tibial component is available in a monoblock design with a compression-molded polyethylene articular surface. If conversion to modularity is necessary, a removable bearing wedge allows for the polyethylene to be removed and the monoblock component to be rendered modular. The standard tibial tray has a locking clip that allows for compressive loading of the locking mechanism to minimize micromotion between the tray and the polyethylene.

The Vanguard system provides a spectrum of constraint from the standard PS insert, to the PS +, to the Super Stabilized

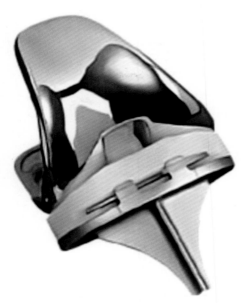

FIG 140.6 Biomet Vanguard prosthesis.

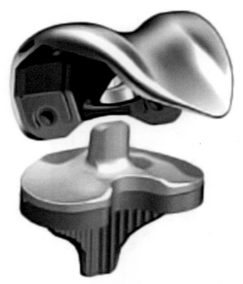

FIG 140.7 Stryker Triathlon prosthesis.

Knee (SSK), to the SSK Constrained. These different polyethylene inserts allow for varying degrees of rotation, post height, and varus-valgus constraint (Fig. 140.6).

Triathlon. The Stryker Triathlon TKA system (Stryker Orthopaedics, Mahwah, New Jersey) was designed with the common goals of improved motion, increased flexion, greater sizing options, and minimization of wear. The femoral component features a consistent radius of curvature centered at the transepicondylar axis and designed to be more anatomic between 10 and 110 degrees. The central edges of the posterior condyles were tapered and the articular surface of the polyethylene was precisely machined to allow for approximately 20 degrees of tibiofemoral rotation. An anthropometric study was used to optimize the tibial and femoral sizing options. A 7-degree flexion cut was built into the anterior flange so that the femoral component could be downsized when necessary, with a reduced chance of femoral notching. The tibial component was designed with a central inset island to improve the ease of insertion and stability of the polyethylene component. This feature, along with the surface geometry mentioned earlier, aim to minimize micromotion and backside wear (Fig. 140.7).

SURGICAL TECHNIQUE

The primary objectives of TKA are to relieve pain, improve function, correct deformity, and minimize the need for reoperation. The basic surgical technique for implanting PCL-substituting prostheses has been well documented.[32,34] The intraoperative goal is a well-aligned, well-fixed prosthesis with coronal balance, an equal flexion and extension gap, and constant collateral ligament stability throughout the full ROM. The postoperative mechanical axis is to be in the central portion of the knee. This will result in load sharing equally by the medial and the lateral compartments to minimize polyethylene wear and improve longevity.

As implant sizes expanded and instrumentation improved, Insall advocated a modified gap technique combining aspects of measured resection and the gap technique of TKA.[75] Tensors used to balance the collateral ligaments and align the knee were replaced with more sophisticated intramedullary instrumentation and spacer blocks. However, despite evolution of the technique and instrumentation, the basic concepts of the posterior-stabilized knee remain virtually unchanged.

The modern surgical technique begins with thorough preoperative planning. AP, lateral, and Merchant view radiographs are obtained. Templating for size is performed with traditional templates or with a digital templating system. A hip-to-ankle full-length radiograph provides additional critical information (Fig. 140.8) including the preoperative anatomic and mechanical axis, preoperative deformity, presence of hardware from prior surgery, and status of the ipsilateral hip. Ensuring that there is nothing to preclude the use of intramedullary instrumentation will help avoid intraoperative surprises. The surgeon may choose the angle of distal femoral resection from the measured difference between the anatomic and mechanical axes of the femur (Fig. 140.9). Other surgeons prefer using 6 degrees for varus knees and 5 degrees for valgus knees or patients with larger thighs. Finally, a line is drawn perpendicular to the mechanical axis of the tibia, noting the estimated amount of bone to be resected from the medial and lateral aspects of the tibia.

A bump is placed under the operative leg and secured to the operative table to help support the knee at 90 degrees of flexion. The contralateral leg is secured loosely to the operative table. A Foley catheter is placed. A tourniquet is placed high on the thigh and elevated after the limb is exsanguinated. The knee is exposed with a straight anterior skin incision extending from the medial aspect of the tibial tubercle to two finger breadths proximal to the superior patellar pole (Fig. 140.10). Full-thickness subcutaneous flaps are developed, and 30 mL of 1% lidocaine with epinephrine is injected along the planned arthrotomy site to reduce intraoperative blood loss. A straight medial parapatellar capsular incision is used for the arthrotomy. A portion of the fat pad and genu articularis is excised to improve exposure. The periosteum of the proximal medial tibia is raised in a

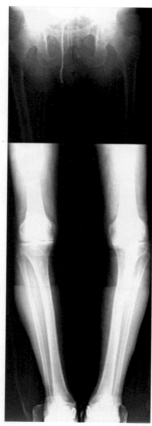

FIG 140.8 Full-length standing hip-to-ankle view is helpful in preoperative templating and in determining overall limb alignment.

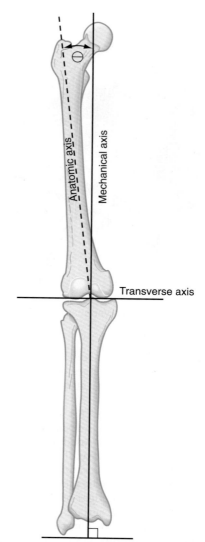

FIG 140.9 Calculating the angle between the anatomic and mechanical axes.

continuous layer from the tibia. Caution is used to avoid excessive medial dissection in the valgus knee. The knee is assessed for a coronal fixed deformity. In the varus knee with a fixed deformity, a medial release may be performed at this point using the ³⁄₄ -inch straight osteotome to elevate the superficial and deep fibers of the medial collateral ligament in continuity (Fig. 140.11).[37] The knee is flexed and the patella is allowed to sublux laterally (Fig. 140.12). Routine patellar eversion is not necessary.[70]

With the knee in the flexed position, the ACL is transected from the tibia surface, and the PCL is released from the medial aspect of the notch. The tibia is now rotationally subluxed anteriorly. It is sometimes necessary, especially on varus knees, to continue the release of the structures off the posteromedial aspect of the tibia, including a portion of the semimembranosus, to allow adequate exposure with tibial rotational subluxation.[37]

After adequate exposure has been achieved, attention is turned to the bone cuts. Proceeding with the tibial cut opens the flexion and extension gaps and further facilitates exposure. The tibia may be cut with an extramedullary or intramedullary guide, depending on the surgeon's preference and the knee anatomy. An extramedullary guide is more frequently used during primary TKA (Fig. 140.13). The ideal cut is 90 degrees to the mechanical axis of the tibia, with a slight posterior slope in the anteroposterior plane. A skim cut is performed on the side with more severe wear and only 5 to 9 mm of bone are

removed from the normal side. This is extremely important in patients with preoperative valgus deformity or obese females. In these patients, not only will excessive bone resection place the tibial component in a weaker cancellous bone bed, but it can lead to runway instability, requiring large polyethylene inserts or increased constraint. Additional tibial bone can easily be removed at a later stage of the procedure if the extension and flexion gaps are found to be too tight following the necessary ligament releases.

Attention is then turned to the femur. A small intramedullary hole is made to gain access to the femoral canal. This hole should be slightly (3 to 5 mm) medial to the center of the femoral groove and 10 mm anterior to the PCL insertion, to allow easy drilling of the intramedullary portion of the femur. The entry point can be more accurately determined using full-length radiographs and noting the point of intersection between the mechanical and anatomic axes of the femur. Because of concern regarding physiologic changes associated with intramedullary instrumentation, the hole is routinely vented by overdrilling the hole with a step drill and using a fluted intramedullary rod.[22] This helps reduce intramedullary pressure

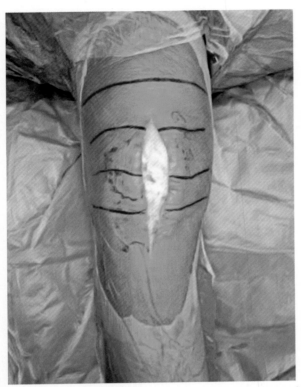

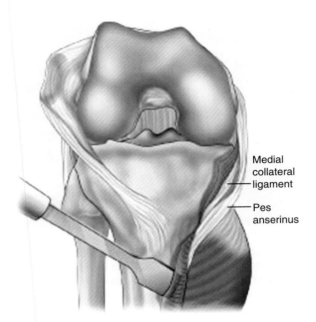

FIG 140.11 The correction of a fixed varus deformity may require subperiosteal release of the superficial medial collateral ligament. The preferred technique is elevation with a ¾-inch straight osteotome.

FIG 140.10 A straight anterior midline incision is made from just proximal to the superior pole of the patella, extending 10 to 14 cm distally to the medial aspect of the tibial tubercle.

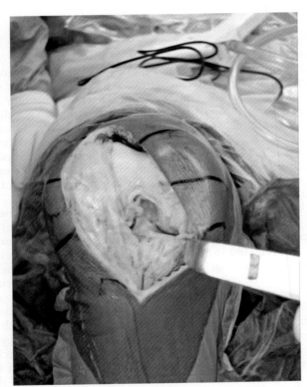

FIG 140.12 Excellent exposure can be obtained without routine patella eversion. The patella is allowed to sublux laterally as the knee is flexed to 90 degrees.

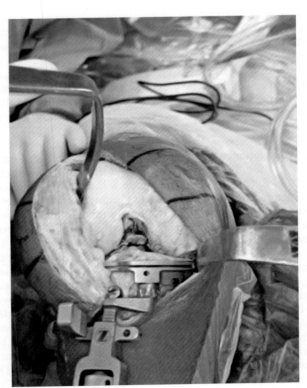

FIG 140.13 The extramedullary tibial cutting guide is placed perpendicular to the mechanical axis of the tibia. Medial offset tibial guides accommodate smaller incisions.

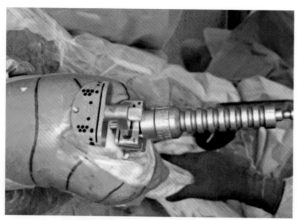

FIG 140.14 The femoral intramedullary guide is in place. A standard distal femoral cutting guide with 3 degrees of built-in flexion is used for the routine TKA. Additional femoral resection may be required in patients with a preoperative flexion contracture >20 degrees.

during the placement of subsequent intramedullary guides. The femoral alignment guide is inserted into this intramedullary channel. It should be set for the proper side and valgus angle (frequently 5 or 6 degrees) as determined by preoperative radiographs (Fig. 140.14).

For most knees, the standard cutting block is attached to the intramedullary femoral alignment guide before its insertion in the femoral canal. Most flexion contractures can be managed with standard bone cuts and soft tissue releases, and we do not routinely resect extra distal femoral bone at this point. Although this step does not set the final rotation of the femoral component, it is useful to place the guide carefully to achieve reasonable rotation of the distal femoral cut.

Two headed pins are placed in the femoral cutting block, the distal placement guide is loosened, and a slap hammer is used to remove the distal placement guide and intramedullary femoral alignment guide. The distal femur is cut through the cutting slot in the femoral cutting block (see Fig. 140.14).

The next step is sizing and establishing rotation of the femoral component. The AP sizing guide is used to determine which of the component sizes will yield the best reconstructive result. Ideally, the body of the guide will contact the resected distal femur. Both of the guide's feet should rest on the posterior femoral condyles. The guide is pinned to the distal femur with two short threaded pins (Fig. 140.15). The guide's anterior boom should contact the anterior cortex of the femur. The boom should be positioned so that it does not contact abnormal bony anatomy, such as an osteophyte or a depression. Occasionally, large anterior osteophytes must be removed to ensure accurate sizing. The ideal position to determine the size is with the boom at the beginning of the upslope of the lateral trochlear ridge. The femoral size should be read directly from the guide. If the guide falls between sizes, the closest size is chosen. The boom can be adjusted (normally by moving it medially or more proximally) until the guide directly aligns with a size. This maneuver essentially allows the AP sizing guide to be used in a posterior referencing manner. By adjusting the boom, the surgeon can optimize the AP position of the implant using strict anterior or posterior referencing, or a combination of both

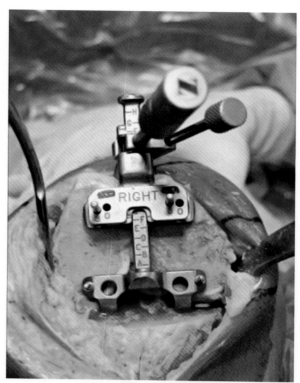

FIG 140.15 The anteroposterior sizing guide is pinned into place. For a varus knee, the femoral rotation is set at 3 degrees of external rotation. For the valgus knee with a deficient lateral femoral condyle, it may be necessary to increase the external rotation of the femoral component when referenced from the posterior femoral condyles.

techniques. Two headless holding pins are placed in the AP sizing guide's holes. These pins are used to establish the AP position of the femoral component and to place it in 3 degrees of external rotation (referenced from the posterior condyles; see Fig. 140.15). The pins should be checked to ensure that they are parallel to the epicondylar axis. If the headless pins do not align with the epicondylar axis, the pins should be fine-tuned (commonly, the lateral one is adjusted) so that the pins and axis correspond. With severe valgus deformity and a deficient posterolateral femoral condyle, the surgeon may choose to increase the external rotation to 5 degrees when referenced from the posterior condyles.

At this point, the correct size of four-in-one femoral finishing guide (as determined by the previous AP sizing guide) is placed onto the distal femur over the already positioned headless pins (Fig. 140.16). The four-in-one femoral finishing guide is pinned to the distal femur. The distal femur is cut in a sequential order. The collateral ligaments must be protected during this step to avoid iatrogenic injury.

A laminar spreader is inserted into the lateral joint space with the knee flexed to 90 degrees. The intercondylar notch is examined. Osteophytes are removed with a ¾-inch straight osteotome to expose the notch fully. The ACL is released directly from its femoral attachment. The PCL is released from its femoral attachment and followed to the posterior horn of the lateral meniscus. The medial meniscus is removed with care to avoid injury to the deep medial collateral ligament. Any remaining posterior osteophytes are removed from the posteromedial

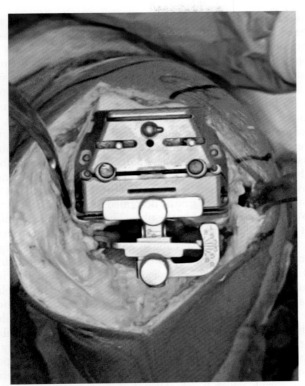

FIG 140.16 The four-in-one femoral guide corresponding to the appropriate size is pinned to the distal femur. The anterior, posterior, and chamfer femoral cuts are made.

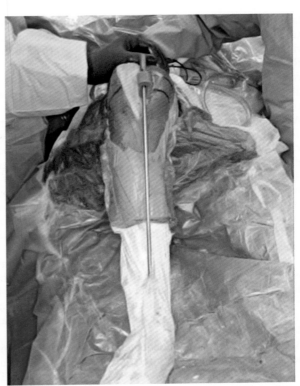

FIG 140.17 A spacer block and drop rod are inserted into the flexion space. Alignment of the tibia cut is confirmed. If the drop rod is not centered over the talus, the tibial cut is revisited to ensure appropriate alignment of the tibial component.

femoral condyle with a curved ¾-inch osteotome. A second laminar spreader is placed in the medial joint space and the lateral laminar spreader is removed. Remnants of lateral meniscus are removed with the PCL attached. Any remaining posterior osteophytes are removed from the posterolateral femoral condyle with a curved ¾-inch osteotome.

Next, the flexion and extension gaps are carefully measured and balanced. Various spacer blocks are used in the flexed knee until proper soft tissue balance is achieved. An alignment rod is placed through the end of a block and checked to ensure that its distal end aligns with the center of the ankle (Fig. 140.17). Malalignment of the rod is corrected by adjusting the proximal tibial bone cut. With the correct size block inserted to adequately balance soft tissue tension in flexion, the knee is brought into extension (Fig. 140.18).

At this point in the operative procedure, the collateral ligaments should be assessed to ensure correct knee balance. With the spacer block in place, a varus and valgus stress is applied. Spacing and collateral ligament tension must be symmetrical. In general, there are three situations that the surgeon will face:
1. Neutral knee: Knees with a preoperative alignment between 0 and 10 degrees are usually relatively easy to balance. In most cases, no releases are required other than those done initially to achieve adequate exposure.
2. Varus knee: In general, knees with a severe varus deformity require a more extensive medial release. An osteotome is used to strip the distal insertion of the superficial medial collateral ligament subperiosteally from the medial tibia. If necessary, particularly in combined varus and rotational deformities, the semimembranosus insertion on the tibia

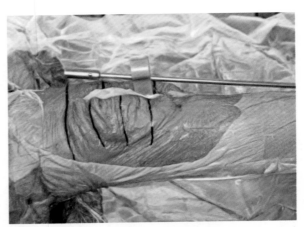

FIG 140.18 With the correct size of block inserted to balance soft tissue tension in flexion adequately, the knee is brought into extension. Collateral ligaments should be assessed to ensure correct knee balance. With the spacer block in place, a varus and valgus stress is applied. The appropriate soft tissue releases are performed to ensure symmetric collateral ligament tension.

and in some cases the pes anserinus tendon insertions are released while the foot is externally rotated.
3. Valgus knee: Knees with more than 10 degrees of anatomic valgus often require release of the lateral structures. There are multiple methods for performing the ligamentous releases necessary for balancing valgus knees. Currently, a

laminar spreader is used to tension the tight lateral structures. These structures are sequentially released using multiple stab wounds with a no. 15 blade in a "pie crust" manner. Rarely, it may be necessary to perform a lateral retinacular release in knees with a severe valgus deformity. This can also enhance ligamentous balance and improve patellar tracking.

After appropriate coronal soft tissue balancing is performed, flexion and extension gap balance is assessed with the spacer block in place. If the knee does not fully extend with the spacer block that is necessary to fill the flexion gap, the posterior capsule can be carefully released off the posterior aspect of the femur in a subperiosteal manner. Following posterior capsule release, if the knee still does not reach full extension, the optional distal femoral resector is used to remove additional bone until full extension is achieved. Bone from the distal femur can be resected back to the insertion of the collateral ligaments, but this is rarely indicated; it raises the joint line and is undesirable. However, it is imperative that additional femoral resection be undertaken if required to achieve full knee extension. The alternative choice of using a thinner tibial tray is unacceptable because it will result in laxity in flexion and increase the chance of flexion instability.

After the soft tissues are adequately balanced, the remaining bone cuts are completed. An intercondylar notch cutting guide that corresponds to the chosen size is used (Fig. 140.19). This determines the correct position of the femoral component mediolaterally. In general, the guide should be placed slightly lateral to the midpoint in the mediolateral plane, without any overhang. The intercondylar guide should not be placed medially. Lateral placement of the notch guide decreases the chances of intraoperative fracture of the medial femoral condyle and enhances patellar tracking by reducing the Q angle. Narrower components with reduced mediolateral dimensions may be more appropriate if the standard intercondylar guide demonstrates medial and lateral overhang. The appropriate decision to use a narrower component frequently becomes apparent during this step. Bone from the intercondylar notch can be removed with a mill, oscillating saw, reciprocating saw, or osteotome. If the chamfer cuts have not already been made, the anterior and posterior chamfer cuts can also be made through slots in the intercondylar notch guide. In addition, the femoral lugholes are now drilled. A number of instrumentation sets now allow these final cuts to be performed through the trial, but the principles remain the same as described previously.

Attention is returned to the tibia. The largest tibial template that fits on the resected proximal tibia with appropriate external rotation, and without overhang, is chosen (Fig. 140.20). Alignment of the tibial resection can be assessed again with a drop rod placed through the handle of the tibial template. Final adjustments to the tibial cut are made at this point. The template is carefully placed to ensure correct tibial component rotation. The template should align with the anterior aspect of the tibia, with the handle pointing to the medial third of the tibial tubercle. Care is taken to place the template as posteriorly as possible. Correct rotation of the template, coupled with a posterior placement, often causes slight overhang in the posterior lateral corner, which is acceptable, but the template should not overhang in other areas. Less overhang occurs with newer anatomic designs that feature a smaller AP dimension on the lateral side. After the template is positioned and pinned in place, the tibial stem hole is prepared. This is done by drilling through the tibial drill guide and completing tibial preparation with impaction of the appropriately sized tibial broach. The trial tibial component is gently impacted into place, or in some cases the cut guide may serve as the trial.

Attention is turned to the patella. Synovium around the patella is carefully debrided to minimize patellar clunk syndrome.[30,32] This is especially important in the region of the quadriceps tendon. The width of the patella is assessed with calipers; the aim is to restore the prosthesis-bone composite to the same width as the pre-resection patellar bone. Usually, the bone is prepared with an oscillating saw aligned with a patellar clamp or a patellar reaming system. The remaining patellar

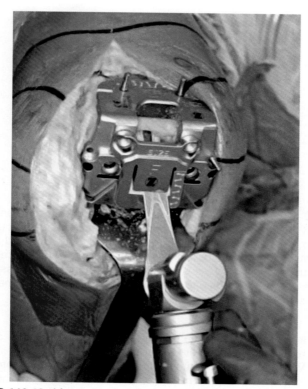

FIG 140.19 After balancing the knee, the final finishing cuts are made on the distal femur.

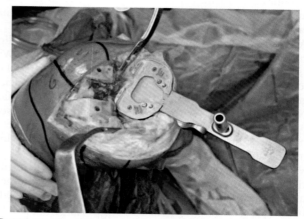

FIG 140.20 The tibia is sized and prepared to accept the final component.

bone should be more than 12 mm to minimize the risk of fracture.[74]

After preparation of the host patellar bone, the appropriate size and position of the patellar implant is chosen. The patellar component should be medialized to reduce the Q angle, but overhang must be avoided. Fixation holes are fashioned compatible with the prosthetic patellar design used. A trial component is put in place and thickness is once again assessed. This new thickness should be within 1 to 2 mm of the original width. If it is too thick, additional bone is resected.

At this point, the trial femoral component is put in place, as well as the trial insert. The knee is checked to ensure adequate balance of the collateral ligaments. The knee is inspected with regard to limb alignment. Finally, full ROM, without flexion contracture, excessive tightness, or laxity, is ensured.

Patellar tracking is assessed. The patella should track smoothly without lateral tilt or subluxation. The use of towel clips or thumb pressure should not be necessary in most cases. If the patella is noted to subluxate laterally, ensure that component rotation is appropriate. If subluxation persists despite appropriate component positioning and rotation, a retinacular release is performed. If a tourniquet is used, the tracking should be rechecked with the tourniquet down before considering lateral retinacular release. After the release is performed, the tracking of the patella is rechecked.

The trial components are removed. The bone surfaces are copiously irrigated and subsequently thoroughly dried. The components are cemented in place in one or two stages. The tibial component is cemented first. The femoral and patellar components are cemented with a second batch of cement (Fig. 140.21). Pressure is maintained on the components as the

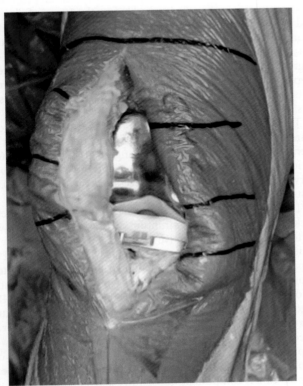

FIG 140.21 The final components are cemented in place with the final polyethylene insert.

cement polymerizes, and excess cement is trimmed away. The final tibial insert is snapped into place. Stability, alignment, and ROM are again confirmed. The knee is copiously irrigated and the arthrotomy carefully closed over an optional drain. After the skin is closed, a sterile dressing is applied and the patient is transferred to the recovery room.

CLINICAL RESULTS OF POSTERIOR CRUCIATE LIGAMENT—SUBSTITUTING DESIGNS

Insall-Burstein Posterior-Stabilized Prosthesis and Its Descendants

Insall Group Experience. The early cruciate-sacrificing design of the total condylar knee prosthesis provided excellent results. Insall et al.[36] reported on the 3- to 5-year results on the first consecutive 200 arthroplasties performed in 183 patients. Although 93% of knees were rated excellent or good, the complications, including four cases of posterior subluxation, highlighted the role for cruciate substitution. With evolution of design, the Insall-Burstein prosthesis incorporated posterior cruciate substitution.

Stern and Insall[72] have reported on the 9- to 12-year results of the original Insall-Burstein prosthesis with an all-polyethylene tibial component. Of 289 arthroplasties inserted at the HSS, 180 knees in 139 patients were available for review, with excellent or good results in 87%. Of the poor results, 14 knees required revision surgery; 9 knees were revised successfully for aseptic loosening of the femoral component (3 knees) or tibial component (6 knees), and 5 knees developed deep prosthetic infections and were treated with a two-stage procedure. The average annual rate of failure was 0.4%, with a 12-year cumulative success of 94% with an all-polyethylene tibial component.

Colizza et al.[15] reported on the long-term results of Insall-Burstein PS prosthesis with a metal-backed tibial component; 101 knees in 74 patients were examined at a mean follow-up time of 10.8 years. The HSS results were good to excellent in 96%. In this cohort, with a monoblock metal-backed tibial component, no cases of tibial component loosening were seen.

Long and Scott[50] recently reported on the longest-term follow-up of the Insall-Burstein PS prosthesis with the results of TKA in young patients (age 55 years or younger) at a minimum 20-year follow-up (mean follow-up 25.1 years). Of the original cohort of 114 total knee arthroplasties in 88 patients, follow-up data was obtained for 107 total knee arthroplasties in 84 patients (95%). Survival analysis revealed that survivorship with failure defined as aseptic revision of the tibial or femoral components was 82.5% at 30 years. Comparing the subgroups of this cohort, the monoblock Insall-Burstein I and the modular Insall-Burstein II prosthesis, there was a significant difference between survivorship for tibial and femoral aseptic revisions for the IB I component (92.3%) versus the IB II component (68.3%) at 30 years. This analysis reveals significantly increased survivorship for the monoblock IB I prosthesis. The Tegner and Lysholm activity scores improved overall from preoperative 1.3 to 3.5 at 8 years and 2.9 at an average of 25.1 years. In Knee Society Category A patients, the average Tegner and Lysholm activity score was significantly improved over the preoperative value from 1.9 to 3.9 at 8 years and remained identical at 25-year follow-up.

Modularity of the tibial component was introduced with the Insall-Burstein II prosthesis in 1987. The addition of modularity was attractive to surgeons because it simplified the procedure, allowed intraoperative fine-tuning, and isolated polyethylene revisions. However, concerns began to arise that polyethylene wear on the backside of the tibial component (backside wear) would lead to osteolysis. Brassard et al.[10] addressed the question of whether modularity affects clinical success with a long-term evaluation comparing the modular Insall-Burstein II prosthesis with the monoblock Insall-Burstein I. They compared the results over 10-year follow-up for 101 Insall-Burstein I knees with 117 Insall-Burstein II knees. Excellent or good results were seen in 96% and 95% of patients, respectively. The radiographic review demonstrated no cases of massive osteolysis, but the authors mentioned that three knees had local minimally progressive lesions, which were not clinically significant. This series of monoblock metal-backed tibial components had an overall incidence of tibial component radiolucent lines of 11%, compared with 26% seen with the modular tibial component. All radiolucent lines were nonprogressive and asymptomatic. Therefore, the introduction of modularity to this particular implant did not appear to raise concerns about osteolysis.

In other long-term studies of the Insall-Burstein posterior prosthesis with a metal-backed tibial component, best- and worst-case scenarios were noted.[10,15] The best-case scenario revealed a cumulative success of 96.4% at 11 years. In distinction, the worst-case scenario considered knees that were lost to follow-up time as failures; this yielded a cumulative success of 92.6% at 11 years. A further testimony to implant durability is a 94% survivorship at 18 years in an active patient population younger than 55 years with a PS prosthesis.[21]

The Insall-Burstein II prosthesis evolved into the NexGen LPS prosthesis in 1992. Modifications to patellofemoral geometry and the cam-and-post mechanism were made. In addition, left and right femoral components were introduced. The initial cohort of patients with the NexGen prosthesis has been reviewed.[23] In this study, 233 patients underwent 279 primary total knee arthroplasties between August 1997 and December 1999. Eleven patients (11 knees) subsequently died, and 22 patients (23 knees) were excluded because of severe medical disability. Patients with severe medical conditions included those known to be alive with the prosthesis still in place but for whom no meaningful assessment of knee scores could be made after communication with a family member. Inclusion of this group of 22 patients may have lowered the overall knee scores, but the incomplete data precluded adequate analysis. Telephone contact was able to determine that none of these patients required revision and the prosthesis seemed to be functioning well. An additional seven patients (seven knees) were lost to follow-up despite use of a professional search firm. Thus, 193 patients with 238 knees (85%) were available for analysis. The mean age at the time of surgery was 66 years. The mean duration of follow-up time was 48 months (range, 24 to 72 months).

Preoperatively, the mean arc of motion was 107 degrees, compared with 117 degrees at the latest follow-up examination. The mean preoperative Knee Society score was 48 points compared with 96 points at the latest follow-up examination. The mean Knee Society functional score was 83 points at the latest follow-up examination. Radiographic evaluation revealed an incidence of minor radiolucent lines of 4%, which was of no clinical significance. No evidence of loosening, osteolysis, or polyethylene wear was seen. Three patients (1%) developed late deep infections. Six patients (3%) required early manipulation

under anesthesia for arthrofibrosis. There were no cases of patellar dislocation, patellar clunk, or posterior dislocation.[23]

More recent modifications to the NexGen LPS prosthesis include a gender-specific prosthesis, high-flexion implants, and the addition of mobile bearings. The gender-specific prosthesis includes modification of the mediolateral-anteroposterior aspect ratio and the patellofemoral geometry. Long et al.[52] have demonstrated a significant decrease in lateral release rate with use of the gender-specific LPS femoral component. In 159 consecutive TKAs, the lateral release rate decreased from 16.5% to 4.3% when using the gender component compared with the standard femoral component in women. The high-flexion design includes modification to the cam-spine mechanism, deepening of the anterior patellar cutout on the tibial articulating surface, and extension of the posterior condyles on the femoral component. These changes make high flexion safe, if achieved.[51] In addition, high postoperative ROM has been shown to correlate with improved patient-rated outcomes. Interest, therefore, remains devoted to improving knee flexion.[5] Mobile bearings have been shown to improve knee kinematics and polyethylene wear in some studies, but clinical performance and longevity appear equivocal.[11,20] Highly crosslinked polyethylene inserts have been designed to decrease wear. Concerns exist regarding the mechanical strength of this new material, particularly when applied to the tibial post in a PS design. Long et al. noted no post failures and no wear at an early 2-year follow-up, but considerably longer follow-up observations are required with this novel material. Although all of these design changes likely improve clinical outcomes, further studies are needed.

Other Experiences. Aglietti et al.[2] reviewed their results at a minimum of 10 years with 99 IB posterior-stabilized prostheses; 39 knees were in patients who died before the 10-year follow-up and 4 were removed or revised, leaving 56 knees for evaluation at an average of 12 years. There were 58% excellent, 25% good, 7% fair, and 10% poor results. Knee flexion averaged 106 degrees. Of the six (10%) failures, four were attributable to aseptic component loosening; none was attributable to polyethylene wear. With revision as the end point, 10-year survivorship was 92%.

The same group reviewed their results at a minimum of 5 years with 92 IB II posterior-stabilized prostheses.[31] At an average follow-up of 7.5 years (range 5 to 9 years), 97% of patients demonstrated good to excellent Knee Society scores. Survivorship analysis showed a success rate of 98.9% and 90.9% best- and worst-case scenarios, respectively, at 8 years.

Thadani et al.[73] reviewed their results of the IB I metal-backed PS prosthesis at a minimum of 10 years; 100 TKAs were performed in 86 consecutive patients. Of these, 36 were in patients who died and 2 were in patients who were weak. Of the remaining 62 knees, 54 were evaluated directly and 8 by telephone at an average of 10.8 years. No patients were lost to follow-up. At latest follow-up, 64% were rated as excellent, 18% as good, 7% as fair, and 11% as poor, which included six failures. Flexion averaged 111 degrees. Excluding the failures, the average Knee Society clinical score was 91.6. Of the six failures, two were secondary to sepsis, two secondary to nonspecific pain, one secondary to patellar wear and fracture, and one because of aseptic tibial component loosening. Polyethylene wear was specifically examined in this study and no implant demonstrated significant polyethylene wear or failure. There were seven patellar fractures; four required additional surgery and the remaining three were asymptomatic and discovered incidentally at routine follow-up. Using revision as the end point, 12-year survivorship averaged 92%.

Abdeen et al.[1] published a 15- to 19-year follow-up of the same group of patients. Of this group, 55 patients (66 knees) had died and 29 patients were available for clinical or telephone follow-up. No additional knees required revision. With revision as the end point, the survival was 92.4% at 19 years. It was concluded that "the prosthesis is likely to outlive the patients when classic indications for age and activity are respected."

Vince et al.[77] also followed 100 IB II prostheses prospectively; 51 knees were evaluated at 10 or more years with Knee Society scores and radiographs and 14 were evaluated by telephone. An additional 6 knees required revision, and 29 were in patients who died. None were lost. Complete revision surgery was performed for instability (two knees), sepsis (two), loosening from osteolysis (one), and stiffness (one). Twelve patients required reoperation without revision of the tibia or femoral components: Patellar revision for loosening (one), patellectomy for fracture (one), polyethylene exchange for dislocation of the spine-cam mechanism (three) and for dissociation (one), and arthroscopic resection of scar from the quadriceps tendon in six (patellar clunk). One case of tibial osteolysis occurred in the IB II. The problem of patellar fractures was decreased significantly in the IB II group, probably as a result of smoothing the anterior trochlear groove. Tibiofemoral dislocation occurred in three IB II prostheses.

Li et al.[45] reported their experience with an IB II prosthesis in 1999. Of 146 knees, 94 were reviewed at a mean of 10 years. HSS scores were excellent or good in 79%, fair in 14%, and poor in 7%. The average Knee Society score was 87. Knee flexion improved from an average of 88 degrees preoperatively to 100 degrees after arthroplasty, considerably less than has been expected from this device. The 10-year survivorship was 92.35, using revision as the end point, and there were nine failures.

Lachiewicz and Soileau[42] performed a prospective consecutive study of 193 knees in 131 patients who were managed with the modular IB II PS total knee prosthesis by one surgeon. The mean age of the patients at the time of surgery was 68 years, and the mean duration of follow-up was 7 years (range, 5 to 14 years). Clinical evaluation was performed with the use of standard knee scoring systems. Radiographs were evaluated for the presence of radiolucent lines, osteolysis, and loosening. The overall result (as determined by HSS knee scores) was rated as excellent for 112 knees, good for 60, fair for 15, and poor for 6. The mean postoperative flexion was 112 degrees. No clinical or radiographic loosening of the tibial component was noted. Eight knees had osteolytic lesions of the tibia. Thin, incomplete, nonprogressive radiolucent lines were noted around 30 tibial components (16%). There were three reoperations.

Lachiewicz and Soileau reported results on the same cohort 5 years later.[43] With a mean follow-up of 12 years (range, 10 to 18 years), two additional knees were revised for mechanical failure. With mechanical failure as an end point, the 15-year survival was 96.8%. Overall survival rate was 90.6% at 15 years.

Oliver et al.[62] have reported the clinical and radiographic outcomes of a consecutive series of 138 hydroxyapatite-coated IB II TKRs, with a mean follow-up of 11 years (range, 10 to 13 years). The patients were entered in a prospective study and all living patients (76 knees) were evaluated. The HSS knee score was obtained for comparison with the preoperative situation.

No patient was lost to follow-up. Radiographic assessment revealed no loosening. Seven prostheses have been revised, giving a cumulative survival rate of 93% at 13 years.

Bozic et al.[9] have reviewed their experience with NexGen TKA system. Of 334 consecutive primary TKAs, 148 knees were NexGen Legacy posterior-stabilized prostheses. A minimum 5-year follow-up was available for 130 of these knees. The 5- and 8-year survivorships for the posterior-stabilized prosthesis were 100% and 94.6%, respectively. The revision rate was 1.5%, with only one knee being revised for aseptic failure. There were no cases of patellar dislocation, patellar clunk, or posterior dislocation.

Other Posterior Cruciate Ligament—Substituting Knee Results. There have been some reports on the results of PCL-substituting designs other than the Insall-Burstein posterior-stabilized prosthesis.

Press-Fit Condylar Posterior-Stabilized Design. Ranawat et al.[67] reviewed the results of 150 consecutive primary TKAs (118 patients) performed between 1988 and 1990. There were 16 bilateral procedures. All the knees in this study were PCL-substituting Press-Fit Condylar (PFC) modular knees implanted with the use of cement. The predominant diagnosis was osteoarthritis in 98 patients (83%). Mean age at the time of the index procedure was 70 years (range, 29 to 85 years); 125 knees were observed for a mean of 4.8 years (range, 3.8 to 6.2 years). The clinical results were excellent for 103 knees (82%), good for 13 (10%), fair for 3 (2%), and poor for 6 (5%). At the most recent follow-up, the Knee Society's average functional score was 78 points (range, 0 to 100 points), and the average knee score was 93 points (range, 57 to 100 points). The mean preoperative ROM increased from 107 to 111 degrees after arthroplasty. The rate of survival was 97% at 6 years. Three revision operations were necessary: two were for infection and one was for tibiofemoral instability. Patellofemoral symptoms were noted in 8% (10 knees). It was concluded that the PCL-substituting PFC modular knee system results in excellent relief of pain, excellent ROM, and restoration of function, with a low prevalence of patellofemoral problems.

The longer-term follow up to Ranawat's original article, previously published in 1997, follows these same patients to a mean duration of 12 years. The clinical results were good to excellent in 76 (90%) patients. The survival rate was 94% with an end point defined as failure for any reason and 98% with mechanical failure as the end point. Revision was required in five knees: Two for infection, one dislocation, and two for wear and femoral osteolysis.[68]

Kinematic Stabilizer Prosthesis. Hanssen and Rand[29] have reported on the Mayo Clinic experience with the Kinematic Stabilizer prosthesis. The Kinematic Stabilizer has a central tibial post in the femoral housing that restrains the anterior and posterior motion of the tibia between 0 and 30 degrees of flexion. Past 30 degrees of flexion, as in the Insall-Burstein prosthesis, the substituting mechanism replaces only the function of the PCL in enhancing femoral rollback. Neither design substitutes for the collateral ligament. In this study, 79 arthroplasties (66 patients) with an average follow-up of 37 months were reported. There were 53 revisions and 26 primary arthroplasties in the series. Postoperatively, of the entire group, 34 knees (43%) were rated excellent, 33 (42%) good, 7 (9%) fair, and 5 (6%) poor. However, in this group of arthroplasties, most underwent revision procedures. Separate analysis of the results of the 26 knees undergoing index procedures revealed 54% with excellent results, 38% good, 4% fair, and 4% poor. Postoperative motion averaged 101 degrees. Small (1- to 2-mm) tibial radiolucent lines were seen in 29% of the knees. Overall, five knees required removal, two for deep sepsis, two for instability, and one for tibial component malposition. Only one revision was required for instability in the group undergoing primary TKA.

Scorpio Prosthesis. Kolisek and Barnes[41] have reported on a series of 103 consecutive primary TKAs performed on 101 patients using the Scorpio PS knee system (Stryker Orthopaedics). The Scorpio knee was designed with a single sagittal radius and a more posterior center of rotation to reduce compressive forces across the patellofemoral joint. At a mean follow-up of 5.25 years, good to excellent HSS scores were exhibited in 96.1%. Mean ROM improved from a preoperative level of 96.5 to 124.5 degrees postoperatively. Four patients reported anterior knee pain. The complication rate was 4.9%. This included one postoperative patellar fracture, one deep infection, one wound complication, one case of excessive knee pain, and one transient peroneal nerve palsy.

Mahoney and Kinsey[54] have published results by a single surgeon on a series of 1030 consecutive cemented TKAs performed with the Scorpio PS prosthesis. At a mean follow-up of 7 years (range, 5 to 9.5 years), 32 knees required revision. The mean time to revision was 2.4 years (range, 0.1 to 8.2 years). The leading cause of failure was deep infection (11 of 32 knees). The Kaplan-Meier survivorship with revision as an end point was 95.8%. With aseptic loosening as the end point, the survivorship was 98.6%.

COMPLICATIONS OF POSTERIOR CRUCIATE LIGAMENT SUBSTITUTION

Certain complications have arisen with PCL-substituting total knee designs that can, at least in part, be attributed to this type of knee replacement. These include component dislocation, intercondylar fractures, patellar fractures, patellar clunk syndrome, and tibial spine wear and breakage.

Dislocations

As increasingly deep flexion was experienced with PCL-substituting designs, there were cases of the tibial spine riding underneath the femoral cam with subluxation of the flexed knee and painful locking of the joint.[35] A knee with a dislocated implant normally presents acutely with inability to extend. In many cases, the patients are unable to explain the exact mechanism, or the position of the knee, when the actual dislocation occurred. In fact, this problem can occur during sleep, causing the patient to awaken with an acute inability to extend the knee. On physical examination, an obvious knee deformity is commonly found. Radiographs reveal the femoral cam translated anterior to the polyethylene tibial spine. Often, the spine can be reduced by hyperflexion of the knee and application of an anterior drawer.

Reports of dislocations have included knees implanted with the Insall-Burstein Posterior-PS prosthesis,[24,35,46] IB II prosthesis,[14,46,59,78] Kinemax posterior substituting prosthesis[61] or Kinematic II Stabilizer prosthesis (Stryker Orthopaedics),[25] and other designs.[78] It is not surprising that this problem has been

seen most commonly with the Insall-Burstein and Kinematic II Stabilizer designs because they have the longest track record with the PCL-substituting concept.

Dislocations have been described in knees with a preoperative valgus alignment and in those after patellectomy.[14,24,25,47,61] Although preoperative valgus appears to increase the incidence of this problem, it can also occur in varus knees. There is some controversy over whether the actual component dislocation occurs with the knee in mild flexion with a straight posterior mechanism or at high flexion angles with a combination of posterior and rotatory stress.[46]

Lombardi et al.[47] analyzed the incidence of dislocations in 3032 primary knees implanted with the Insall-Burstein prosthesis series. The incidence of this problem was rare with the original Insall-Burstein PS prosthesis (0.2%, or 1 in 494). However, with the advent of the IB II prosthesis, the problem became more apparent (2.5%, or 1 in 40). Knees that dislocated were found to have achieved statistically significant higher average flexion (118 degrees) compared with control knees (105 degrees; $p < .001$). In addition, they tended to reach high flexion angles rapidly in the postoperative period. In response to this problem, the tibial plastic was modified by raising the tibial spine and moving it anteriorly. This increased the inherent stability of the component and decreased the incidence of dislocation (0.2%, or 1 in 656).

Combining two recent articles on a third-generation prosthesis, the NexGen Legacy posterior-stabilized implant, rates of dislocation continue to decrease.[9,23] In 323 knees with up to 8-year follow-up, no dislocations were reported. This likely represents an improvement in implant design and a better understanding of flexion instability and the role of soft tissue balance.

A computer analysis of this phenomenon analyzed the propensity of PCL-substituting knee components to dislocate in the sagittal plane.[19] Kocmond et al.[40] have defined a dislocation safety factor (DSF) as the jump distance between the bottom of the femoral cam and the top of the tibial spine. The DSF was found to vary with the knee flexion angle. For knees with the Insall-Burstein PCL-substitution mechanism, the DSF increases as knee flexion increases and peaks at about 70 degrees. Knee flexion beyond this angle causes the DSF to decrease and theoretically increases the risk of dislocation. Many contemporary designs have attempted to minimize the risk of dislocation by ensuring a DSF equal to or greater than that of the original Insall-Burstein Posterior-Stabilized prosthesis at high flexion angles.

The lesson with respect to arthroplasty design is simple. Sometimes, very small changes, on the order of millimeters, can result in catastrophic complications. Not all spine mechanisms are the same. In general, to prevent knee dislocations, it is imperative that the surgeon balance the knee in flexion and extension, with a special emphasis on knees with a preoperative valgus alignment. In addition, it may be undesirable to achieve large flexion angles (more than 115 degrees) in the first postoperative week.

Intercondylar Fractures

Femoral fractures, although a relatively rare occurrence, can occur at the time of knee arthroplasty. Because PCL-substituting components require the removal of extra bone from the intercondylar region, the possibility of distal femoral fracture with this technique is increased. Risk factors for fractures include inadequate, as well as excessive, intercondylar bone notch resection. Although it is self-evident that excessive bone removal results directly in stress risers and deficient bone, the risks associated with incomplete bone resection are not as clear-cut. Nonetheless, if insufficient notch bone is removed, the intercondylar region of the femoral component (or trial) can act like a wedge during insertion and induce a distal femoral fracture. It is imperative to remove enough bone to allow full seating of the cam. When placing the trial femoral component, forceful impaction should never be used. To ensure adequate bony resection, never undercut the femoral condyles. Although this complication has been reported, the exact incidence of this phenomenon has not been well defined. Lombardi et al.[48] have described the risk factors, which include osteopenic bone, improper bone cuts, an eccentric box cut for the posterior stabilized prosthesis, over-impaction of the femoral component, and misplacement of the trial component. They examined this complication by comparing two large series of PCL-substituting knees. In this report, 898 nonconsecutive primary knee arthroplasties performed with a PCL-substituting prosthesis were compared with a second nonconsecutive series of 532 PCL-substituting knee arthroplasties. In the second series, an intercondylar sizing guide was used to confirm the intercondylar resection size. In the initial series, 40 distal femoral fractures were noted (approximate rate, 1: 22; nondisplaced, 35; displaced, 5). This was in contrast to the second series, in which only one displaced fracture was noted (rate, 1:532). The rate difference between the two series was statistically significant. The authors advocated careful resection technique and intercondylar notch size verification to minimize this complication. Of note, no change in postoperative rehabilitation was required for patients identified with a nondisplaced intercondylar fracture or those with an intercondylar fracture treated with intraoperative stabilization.

Patellar Fractures

The initial follow-up of the original Insall-Burstein Posterior-Stabilized knee demonstrated a high patellar fracture prevalence. The AP dimensions and shape of the femoral component tended to be full to accommodate the spine-cam mechanism in the Insall-Burstein Posterior-Stabilized prosthesis. This pushed the patella anteriorly and presumably increased forces, which may have been responsible for a relatively higher rate of patellar fractures. In 10 cadaver knee specimens, Matsuda et al.[55] demonstrated significantly higher contact stresses in the un-resurfaced patella when compared with the normal knee throughout the flexion arc for several implants, including the Insall-Burstein Posterior-Stabilized prosthesis. They noted that in flexion exceeding 105 degrees, patellofemoral contact occurred in two small patches. They concluded that the forces could be normalized by extending the trochlear groove farther posteriorly and were less concerned with the anterior prominence of the component. The groove of the IB II was deepened potentially to decrease patella fractures and other patella problems. Other posterior-stabilized knees have been designed with a single sagittal radius and a more posterior center of rotation to reduce compressive forces across the patellofemoral joint.[41]

Larson and Lachiewicz[44] have concluded that many patellar complications with the IB Posterior-Stabilized prosthesis could be avoided by careful surgical technique. This includes appropriate rotation of the femur and tibia, adequate patellar resection, debridement of peripatellar synovium, and proper evaluation of patellar tracking before wound closure. They

studied 118 arthroplasties at 2 to 8 years and found that no knee required reoperation for the patellofemoral joint. Mean flexion of 112 degrees was comparable to other studies with this device, and they had no cases of patellar clunk syndrome and no subluxations. There were three patellar fractures (2.5%) treated without surgery. Even this small number of fractures might be expected to improve with changes to the femoral prosthesis. It was concluded that the total patellofemoral complication rate in the series was 4.2%. This was superior to the 11% that has generally been described, of which 7% were actually fractures.

With improved design, surgical technique, and more favorable patellofemoral geometry, it is likely that the incidence of patellar fracture will continue to decrease. Ortiguera and Berry[64] found an incidence of periprosthetic fracture of the patella to be only 0.68% following modern TKA. Additionally, when combining the two most recent articles on 323 knees treated with the NexGen Legacy posterior-stabilized implant, no patellar fractures were reported with up to 8-year follow-up.[9,23] Again, this likely represents an improvement in implant design and better surgical technique.

Patellar Clunk Syndrome and Synovial Entrapment

The deeper flexion provided by the initial Insall-Burstein stabilized design enabled the quadriceps tendon to extend beyond the trochlear groove of the femoral component. If the anterior edge of the femoral component terminates abruptly, synovium or scar residing on the tendon falls into the intercondylar groove. If this has occurred, the same tissue must ride up out of the intercondylar area and "jump" back up onto the femoral trochlea as the patient extends her or his knee. Within a few months after the arthroplasty, the offending (or offended) tissue hypertrophies and becomes rubbery. This creates the painful and noisy complication that has been described as patellar clunk. Historically, a case of patellar catching was mentioned by Insall in his original report on the posterior-stabilized knee. However, Hozack et al.[30] appear to be the first authors to define the term *patellar clunk syndrome*. They described a prominent fibrous nodule at the junction of the proximal patellar pole and quadriceps tendon. They believed that during flexion, this fibrous nodule would enter the femoral component's intercondylar notch but not restrict flexion. However, as the knee extended, the nodule would remain within the notch, while the rest of the extensor mechanism slid proximally. At 30 to 45 degrees of flexion, the tension on the fibrous nodule would be sufficient to cause the nodule to jerk out of the notch as it returned to its normal position. This sudden displacement would cause the audible and palpable clunk found with this entity.

Synovial entrapment or hyperplasia is a similar entity, but a less well-described syndrome.[65] It is caused by similar hypertrophy of soft tissue in the same location, but without a discrete nodule. Rather than a clunk or catch, the patient experiences pain and crepitus, typically with active knee extension from a 90-degree flexed position. This typically occurs during stair climbing or rising from a chair.

The original IB design had a high incidence of patellar clunk, up to 21%. This is likely related to the femoral trochlear geometry: a short trochlea with a sharp transition into the intercondylar notch.[3,13] Changes to the sagittal geometry of the femoral component in the IB II reduced the incidence to approximately 3% to 8%, but did not eliminate the problem. With the introduction of the NexGen Legacy prosthesis in 1997, one of the main areas of focus was the patellofemoral articulation and the reduction of patellofemoral complications. The side-specific components, with anatomically oriented trochlear grooves, lengthening and deepening of the femoral trochlea, and an increase in the number of femoral sizes, all helped reduce the incidence of patellar entrapment syndromes. In 238 knees reconstructed with the NexGen legacy prosthesis, no cases of patellar clunk or synovial entrapment were seen with 24- to 72-month follow-up.

Treatment recommendations for patellar clunk syndrome and synovial entrapment have included physical therapy, surgical removal of the nodule, patellar prosthesis revision, open resection through a limited lateral incision, and arthroscopic debridement.[8,30,57,76] Pollock et al.[65] have reviewed the prevalence of synovial entrapment with three different cam-post designs. Those with proximally positioned or wide femoral boxes were more likely to have a higher prevalence of this problem.

Beight et al.[8] have reported on 14 operative procedures (11 arthroscopic debridements and 3 patellar component revisions) performed in 12 patients. As in other reports, they found a suprapatellar fibrous nodule that wedged into the intercondylar notch during flexion and dislodged as the knee extended, causing the clunk. They noted that the symptoms resolved after nodule excision. However, four of the knees treated with arthroscopic debridement had recurrence of symptoms. None of the knees that underwent arthrotomy and patellar button revisions had recurrence. The authors recommended a treatment protocol that commenced with a short course of nonoperative physical therapy, although they acknowledged that the results were disappointing. Arthroscopic debridement was suggested for knees without radiographic component abnormalities. Arthrotomy was suggested for recurrent clunks or malpositioned or loose components.

The Mayo Clinic[18] reported on a series of 25 patients who underwent arthroscopic treatment of patellar clunk syndrome (15 knees) or patellofemoral synovial hyperplasia (10 knees). After surgery, patient-reported knee pain and crepitus as well as Knee Society knee and function scores improved in both groups. It was concluded that arthroscopic debridement of symptomatic patellofemoral synovium after TKA is a safe and effective procedure.

Tibial Spine Wear and Breakage

There has been a focus on the spine-cam mechanism in some posterior-stabilized prostheses as a source of wear debris. Mikulak et al.[58] have reported unanticipated aseptic loosening and osteolysis with the posterior-stabilized model of the Press-Fit Condylar implant. They found that 16 of 557 (2.9%) had been revised for osteolysis from 37 to 89 months after surgery. Retrieval analysis demonstrated damage to the lateral and medial walls of the tibial spine. There was also damage to the inferior surface of the articular polyethylene inserts.

Similar findings were reported by Puloski et al.[66] Their study, by contrast, was a retrieval analysis of a variety of failed posterior-stabilized implants. Wear was quantified on the tibial posts of all retrievals, including those revised for reinfection. They were unable to conclude that this wear mode was responsible for the failures, but cautioned that the interaction between the spine and the cam is not an "innocuous articulation."

Callaghan et al.[12,63] have studied this phenomenon extensively. When they recognized osteolysis around IB II modular components, as well as Press-Fit Condylar PS modular components, they began performing retrieval analyses. In their cases,

the patients were able to hyperextend slightly and most had bilateral implants. They hypothesized that impingement on the anterior post by the femoral cam causes wear damage to the post and transmits rotational stresses to the modular inserts, generating backside wear. Avoiding flexion of the femoral component and posterior slope in the proximal tibial resection should help eliminate the problem. In addition, cam-post designs should allow for hyperextension before impingement occurs.

CONCLUSION

The potential of the PCL-substituting type of knee design continues to evolve. In general, it has allowed the surgeon to perform a reproducible operation in almost all arthritic knees, no matter what the cause of the disease and how involved and complex the deformity of the knee. The recent modifications in prosthetic design and surgical technique have addressed most of the early concerns involving patellofemoral complication and tibiofemoral dislocation. Although many advancements have been made, there is still potential for functional and clinical improvements with newer designs.

KEY REFERENCES

1. Abdeen AR, Collen SB, Vince KG: Fifteen-year to 19-year follow-up of the Insall-Burstein-1 total knee arthroplasty. *J Arthroplasty* 25:173, 2010.
2. Aglietti P, Buzzi R, De Felice R, et al: The Insall-Burstein total knee replacement in osteoarthritis: a 10-year minimal follow-up. *J Arthroplasty* 14:560, 1999.
12. Callaghan JJ, O'Rourke MR, Goetz DD, et al: Tibial post impingement in posterior-stabilized total knee arthroplasty. *Clin Orthop* 404:83, 2002.
13. Clarke HD, Fuchs R, Scuderi GR, et al: The influence of femoral component design in the elimination of patellar clunk in posterior-stabilized total knee arthroplasty. *J Arthroplasty* 21:167, 2006.
23. Fuchs R, Mills EL, Clarke HD, et al: A third-generation, posterior stabilized knee prosthesis: early results after follow-up of 2 to 6 years. *J Arthroplasty* 21:821, 2006.
31. Indelli PF, Aglietti P, Buzzi R, et al: The Insall-Burstein II prosthesis: a 5- to 9-year follow-up study in osteoarthritic knees. *J Arthroplasty* 17:544, 2002.
32. Insall JN: Technique of total knee replacement. *Instr Course Lect* 30:324, 1981.
34. Insall JN, Lachiewicz PF, Burstein AH: The posterior stabilized condylar prosthesis: a modification of the total condylar design. Two to four-year clinical experience. *J Bone Joint Surg Am* 64:1317, 1982.
36. Insall J, Scott WN, Ranawat CS: The total condylar knee prosthesis. A report of two hundred and twenty cases. *J Bone Joint Surg Am* 61:173, 1979.
42. Lachiewicz PF, Soileau ES: The rates of osteolysis and loosening associated with a modular posterior stabilized knee replacement: results at five to fourteen years. *J Bone Joint Surg Am* 86:525, 2004.
43. Lachiewicz PF, Soileau ES: Fifteen-year survival and osteolysis associated with a modular posterior stabilized knee replacement. A concise follow-up of a previous report. *J Bone Joint Surg Am* 91:1419, 2009.
44. Larson CM, Lachiewicz PF: Patellofemoral complications with the Insall-Burstein II posterior-stabilized total knee arthroplasty. *J Arthroplasty* 14:288, 1999.
50. Long WJ, Bryce CD, Hollenbeak CS, et al: Total knee replacement in young, active patients: long-term follow-up and functional outcome. *J Bone Joint Surg Am* 96:e159, 2014.
68. Rasquinha VJ, Ranawat CS, Cervieri CL, et al: The press-fit condylar modular total knee system with a posterior cruciate-substituting design. *J Bone Joint Surg Am* 88(5):1006–1010, 2006.

The references for this chapter can also be found on www.expertconsult.com.

Posterior Cruciate Ligament Substituting Total Knee Arthroplasty: Considerations in the Middle East

Sam Tarabichi, Majd Tarabichi

INTRODUCTION

The goals of total knee arthroplasty (TKA) have always remained the same as pertains to restoring the native anatomy, relieving pain, and bringing patients back to an earlier level of functioning. However, different populations with variations in anatomy, physiology, and functional needs necessitate a different approach. These characteristics must be taken into account when performing TKA in Middle Eastern patients, and can be divided into systemic features, local anatomic features, severity of disease, and activities of daily living. We should stress that Asian and Middle Eastern patients are very similar because of culture and lifestyle, as well as anatomic features. We found that the features that we reported in our scientific exhibit at the American academy of orthopaedic surgeons 2012 annual meeting were endorsed by our Asian colleagues' literature.[27,47] We will also describe perioperative management of Middle Eastern patients. Our approach is based on the authors' experience of practicing both in the United States and the Middle East, as well as data from our registry of more than 8000 total knee replacements (TKRs). We will focus on our results with the posterior stabilized prosthesis because the demands of the Middle Eastern knee are better served by a posterior stabilized implant, and this is for multiple reasons. First of all, the activities of patients in the Middle East involve a great deal of kneeling. Komistek et al. demonstrated in a kinematic study that posterior stabilized knees exhibited greater roll-back of the femur on the tibia,[26] which plays a crucial role in facilitating high flexion in the knee. In contrast, the cruciate-retaining knee implants showed a "paradoxical movement" whereby the tibia rolls forward on the femur in high flexion. The femoral roll-back mechanism increases the leverage of the patellar tendon, allowing the patient to place greater forces on the patellar tendon and thus enabling him or her to tolerate more of the activities of daily living (Fig. 141.1). This principle was the driving force behind John Insall's design of the NexGen LPS Flex (Zimmer Biomet, Warsaw, Indiana) knee prosthesis designed to accommodate greater flexion at the knee because he believed that posterior stabilized prostheses would provide more physiologic roll-back and accommodate deeper flexion. Furthermore, flexion-varus deformity, which is extremely common in the Middle East, results in a contracted posterior cruciate ligament (PCL), and thus PCL resection is needed, especially with flexion deformity of greater than 20 degrees. A contracted PCL is dysfunctional, and this is observable intraoperatively with subluxation of the tibia despite an intact PCL. This is the rationale behind our extensive use of posterior stabilized prostheses in Middle Eastern patients.

FEATURES OF THE MIDDLE EASTERN KNEE

Systemic Features

The systemic features that set the Middle Eastern patient apart from other populations are osteopenia, ligamentous laxity, and metabolic syndrome. Osteopenia is quite prevalent in the Middle East despite the sunny climate. This may be because of vitamin D deficiency, particularly in females, because of low sun exposure. This has been studied extensively and has been demonstrated in the literature, with some rates reported as high as 30% of the population and with a higher proportion in females.[3,23] This plays a significant role in TKA in the Middle Eastern patient, therefore minimizing bone loss in these patients is even more significant than in other populations. A specific complication derived from this feature is periprosthetic insufficiency fracture, which can be seen with severe varus deformity where the lateral condyle becomes highly osteopenic because of unloading of the lateral condyle. When the deformity becomes corrected after TKA, the sudden increase in pressure on the lateral condyle can lead to a compression-type fracture of the lateral femoral condyle, which we have described in the literature.[38] This complication requires a revision procedure and should be kept in mind because it occurs because of the osteopenia and gross varus deformity, a combination frequently seen in Middle Eastern patients. The two main concerns of this complication are that this fracture is difficult to diagnose and is frequently missed on plain anteroposterior films (Fig. 141.2) and the extensive bone loss seen during the revision procedure because of adherence of the fractured bone to the femoral component when it is removed, further compounding the problem of bone loss (Fig. 141.3).

Another concern that must be addressed because of the osteopenia is adequate bone coverage. The senior author advocates the use of an anatomic tibial component versus a symmetric component (Fig. 141.4). With a symmetric component the surgeon is often forced to insert the plate in internal rotation to have a more complete coverage of the bony surface, and this may lead to the surgeon sacrificing the posterior edge of the tibia. The anatomic tibial component provides more coverage and gives the surgeon more freedom to place the tibial component in proper rotation.[17] This is especially important in the Middle East because the body mass index of these patients is especially high (Table 141.1). We should therefore try to cover the tibial surface perfectly to prevent subsidence of the tibial component.

The second feature is ligamentous laxity. This is seen in the broader Asian population and not just limited to the Middle

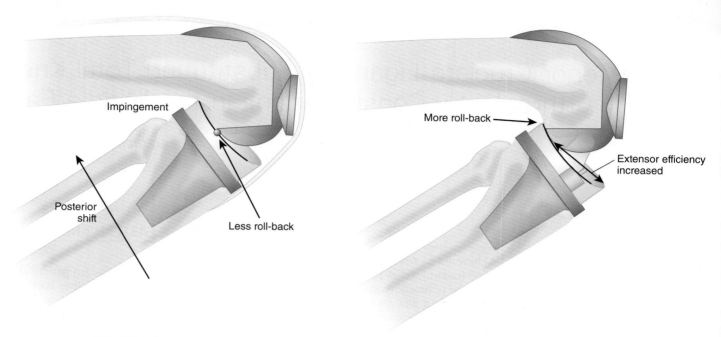

FIG 141.1 Comparison between kinematics of cruciate-retaining *(left)* and posterior stabilized *(right)* implants. With posterior stabilized prostheses, there is more posterior femoral rollback, increasing the leverage arm of the extensor mechanism. (Courtesy Zimmer Biomet.)

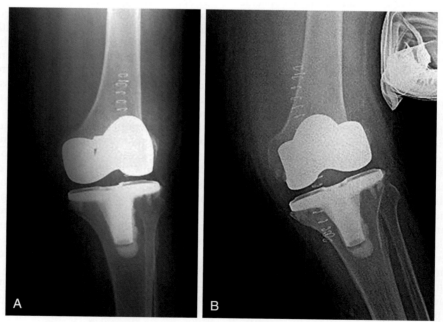

FIG 141.2 Insufficiency fracture not apparent on plain AP film (A) but seen on stress radiographs (B). (From Shahi A, Saleh UH, Tan TL, et al: A unique pattern of periprosthetic fracture following total knee arthroplasty: the insufficiency fracture. *J Arthroplasty* 30:1054–1057, 2015.)

East, with studies in the Far East and Southeast Asia showing significantly more anterior cruciate ligament (ACL) laxity in Asian populations when compared with white populations.[21,24] This laxity coupled with the advanced disease presentation makes the use of cruciate-retaining implants difficult because it may lead to instability. This laxity may dictate the use of more constrained implants, as seen with rheumatoid arthritis.[29,49] This concept also reinforces the need for the surgeon to be conservative with his or her bone cuts because aggressive resection of bone may result in the need for a thicker polyethylene

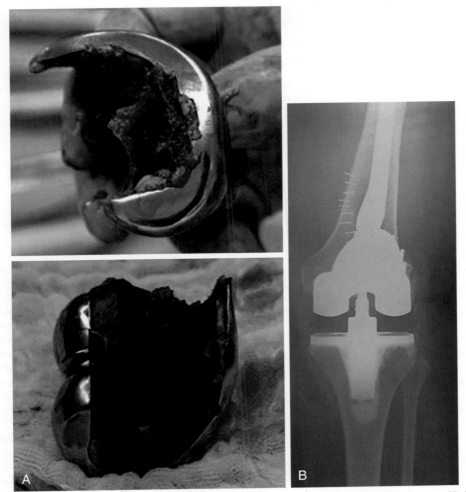

FIG 141.3 Bone adherent to femoral component after removal during revision for insufficiency fracture (A) along with postoperative radiograph (B). (From Shahi A, Saleh UH, Tan TL, et al: A unique pattern of peri-prosthetic fracture following total knee arthroplasty: the insufficiency fracture. *J Arthroplasty* 30:1054–1057, 2015.)

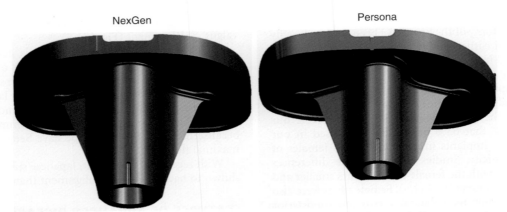

FIG 141.4 Comparison between tibial components between NexGen and Persona systems showing the asymmetrical tibial component in the Persona system, which is more anatomic. (Courtesy Zimmer Biomet.)

TABLE 141.1	**Body Mass Index of Senior Author's Patient Population**				
	BODY MASS				
	Under Weight	**Healthy Weight**	**Over Weight**	**Obesity**	*n*
Index	>18.5	18.50-24.99	25-29.99	>30	—
Joints	2	35	149	502	688
Bilateral	1	14	64	212	291
Single	0	7	21	76	104
Patients	1	21	85	288	395
%	0.25	5	20	75	1.0025

Courtesy Dr. Samih Tarabichi, MD.

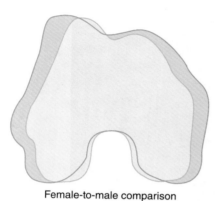

Female-to-male comparison

FIG 141.5 Comparison of distal femurs between males and females. (Courtesy Zimmer Biomet.)

spacer to fill the gap that has been made, and this may ultimately increase the risk of backside wear of the polyethylene component, which will decrease implant longevity.

Metabolic syndrome has a particularly high prevalence in the Middle East, with figures reported to be as high as 60%.[39] Our registry data show that 43% of our patients have diabetes. This indicates that the typical Middle Eastern patient has more co-morbidities preoperatively than a Western patient. This also has implications for the outcome of TKA as Amin et al. demonstrated, as when compared with nonobese patients showed lower mean knee society scores and had a lower rate of 5-year survivorship.[4]

Local Anatomic Features

Variations in the anatomy of the knee have been studied heavily in recent years, with earlier studies focusing on gender-based differences, followed by attention to differences across ethnicities. This first came to attention when it was realized that the female-specific implants were more compatible with Asian knees of both genders. The senior author used the NexGen system, and when the gender implant became available our registry data showed that 63% of the implants used in our patients were gender implants in both males and females of Middle Eastern ethnicity. Studies confirmed the differences between the genders, with the female distal femurs smaller and narrower than male femurs (Fig. 141.5). Female tibias were also smaller and had greater mediolateral versus anteroposterior ratios compared with male tibias.[6]

With regard to Asian anatomy, there are documented differences in the distal femur, the tibia, and the relationship between the tibia and the femur. Urabe et al. showed that Japanese women had smaller anteroposterior and metaphyseal widths of the femur, but the posterior condyle was longer in Japanese women.[47] Fig. 141.6 demonstrates the difference in the width of the metaphyses between Asian and Western populations, with the Asian metaphysis assuming a triangular shape as compared with the Western metaphysis, which is trapezoidal. The narrow metaphyses makes it difficult to accommodate large housing mechanisms for the stems. The longer posterior condyles demonstrate the posterior offset we see in Asian femurs, and this is most likely to accommodate deep flexion (Fig. 141.7). Distal femoral rotation is also markedly different, with Yip et al. demonstrating a posterior condylar angle of 5.1 degrees in Asian males compared with 3.5 degrees in a study by Berger et al., which was performed on whites, indicating external rotation of the femur is greater in Asians.[9,53]

Tibial differences should also be taken into account. Kwak et al. evaluated the proximal tibia and attempted to match the tibias to the most appropriate size of tibial implant. They found that implants with smaller anteroposterior dimensions were not large enough in the mediolateral dimension. On the other hand, the implants with larger anteroposterior dimensions showed mediolateral overhang.[27] Offset of the tibial shaft from the tibial plateau has also been noted in Asian populations. Yoo et al. have shown that the medial offset stem, which is based off anatomic studies in white patients, may not be appropriate in Korean patients.[54] Tang et al. performed magnetic resonance imaging scans on the tibial plateau and proximal part of the tibial shaft and found that the axis of the tibial shaft is anterolateral to the center of the tibial plateau in Chinese individuals.[41] With this variation in offset of the shaft form the plateau, if the offset is not predicted accurately it can lead to impingement or varus or valgus malalignment (Fig. 141.8).

Tibial slope in Asian populations is also greater than in Western populations, with the tibial slope of Western patients being 10 degrees. Chiu et al., found that the slope of the medial tibial plateau is 14.8 and 11.8 degrees in the lateral tibial plateau in Chinese populations (Fig. 141.9).[15] The increase in slope seen in Asian populations is most likely to accommodate high flexion because increases in tibial slope have been shown to increase maximal flexion.[7]

With regards to alignment, Japanese subjects have also been shown to have more varus alignment than white subjects.[17]

FEATURES OF ADVANCED DISEASE

This feature of Middle Eastern patients is because of the advanced presentation of disease. Patients in this region often

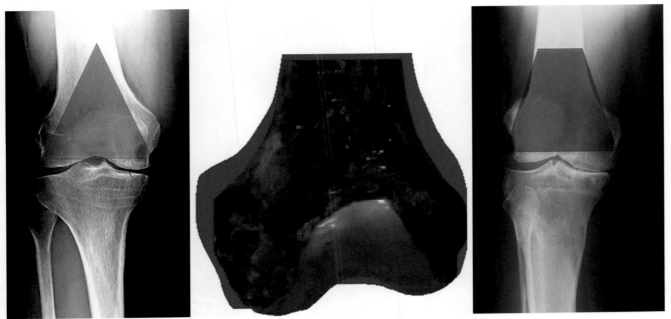

FIG 141.6 Width of metaphyses between Asians *(left)* and Westerners *(right)* with Asian knee superimposed on white knee *(center)*. (Courtesy Dr. Asit Shah, MD.)

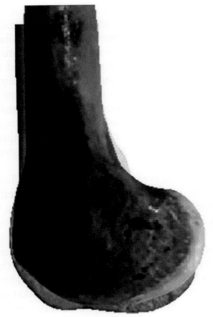

FIG 141.7 Asian knee superimposed on white knee, demonstrating posterior offset in Asians. (Courtesy Dr. Asit Shah, MD.)

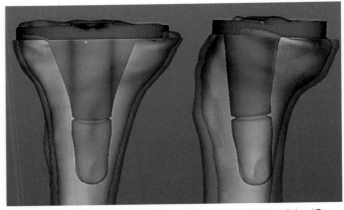

FIG 141.8 Use of a medial offset stem in an Asian tibia. (Courtesy Zimmer Biomet.)

present with gross varus deformity of 30 to 40 degrees (Figs. 141.10 and 141.11) and lateral thrust during gait, indicating instability.[13] This makes the procedure quite challenging. Advanced disease indicates there is some bone loss, as well as laxity and stretching, of the lateral side because of the severe varus deformity. Such severe deformity requires extensive release to balance the medial and lateral compartments, and this may lead to instability owing to the extensive release of the medial and lateral collateral ligaments. This makes the use of

cruciate-retaining implants almost impossible. This instability may require use of more constrained implants, such as the constrained condylar knee (CCK) (Zimmer Biomet). This can be problematic because it limits the surgeon's options for future revisions. We now have the constrained posterior stabilizer (CPS) insert (Zimmer Biomet), which has a higher and wider spine that locks into the intercondylar notch (Fig. 141.12). This is useful in cases of extensive release in which a simple posterior stabilizer will not suffice, and the CPS insert provides midlevel constraint between the CCK and simple posterior stabilizer.

ACTIVITIES OF DAILY LIVING

Asians perform a great deal of kneeling in their daily lives and in Middle Eastern patients even more so. Many patients lack conventional toilets and hence prefer to squat. Many patients

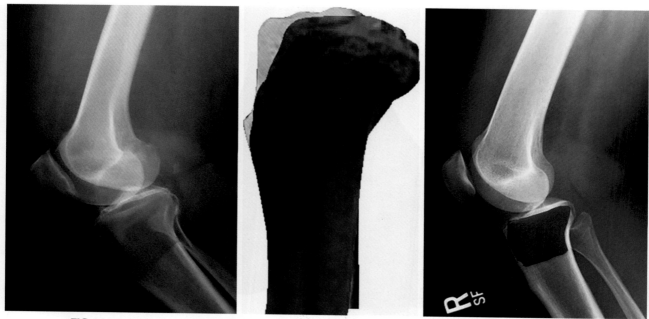

FIG 141.9 Differences in posterior tibial slope. Asian knee *(left)*. Western knee *(right)*. Asian knee superimposed on Western knee *(center)*. (Courtesy Dr. Asit Shah, MD.)

pray five times daily, with Saudi Arabian men flexing on average up to 159.6 degrees during prayer.[1] Fig. 141.13 displays positions commonly assumed by Asians, with kneeling and squatting featuring particularly in the Middle East. We have performed kinematic studies on frequent kneelers to study tibiofemoral movement in deep flexion using a three-dimensional (3D) C-arm (Siremobil Iso-C 3D, Siemens, Munich, Germany), and we showed that to kneel we need freedom of rotation of the tibia on the femur.[42] It is essential to understand the functional requirements of patients in the Middle East because many patients will refuse surgery out of fear that they will lose range of motion.[33] Thus we must bear in mind that high flexion past 130 degrees is important in these patients, and we will address how to achieve this in the operative section.

Surgical Considerations for the Middle Eastern Knee

This section will cover two aspects: choosing the right knee system and preoperative assessment.

Choosing the Right Knee System. The original knee systems were designed with mainly white patients in mind because it was based on averaging calculations for the white knee, which may not fit some Middle Eastern patients (as discussed previously). Preoperatively the surgeon should be very careful about his system selection, particularly in the small knee. Smaller Middle Eastern knees are quite challenging and unfortunately will not tolerate errors as compared with larger knees, which might be more forgiving. We are not in any way advocating any particular system, but we do believe that the surgeon should closely assess the system he or she intends to use on a smaller Middle Eastern knee.

Starting with the femur, we have discussed previously that the Asian knee has a posterior offset to accommodate deep flexion. This guides the surgeon to the use of a narrower implant. Use of the standard width implants made for white patients may lead to overhang of the components of the Asian

knee. The width of the box cut is another factor that must be taken into consideration. Significant variation exists between prostheses in the amount of intercondylar bone that is resected to accommodate the posterior stabilizer mechanism.[20] This is crucial because excessive bone resection can lead to periprosthetic fracture.[2] We also advocate the use of a system that allows freedom in setting the external rotation of the femoral component because, as has been reported in the literature, 3 degrees of external rotation is often not adequate in severe gross valgus deformity.[51] The system should allow more freedom in setting higher external rotation for the femur, which might reach up to 8 degrees.

On the tibial side, we have mentioned the utility of an anatomic tibial component, which will allow for better coverage and more precision in setting the rotation. This is preferred to obtain a balance between adequate coverage and proper rotation.[17]

An important aspect in keeping with the concept of the smaller dimensions of the Asian knee is looking at the difference in increments between the sizes in each system. The majority of systems that were initially available on the market had an increment of 4 mm. Some systems have 5-mm increments, and this is a great injustice to the Middle Eastern knees because it forces us to take much more bone to change from one size to another. We have a graph demonstrating the magnitude of the increments across different knee systems (Fig. 141.14). Another important point is that if you mismatch the flexion and extension gaps, a larger knee will be more forgiving in a posterior stabilized knee for larger sizes (Fig. 141.15). However, in smaller sizes a mismatch of the same size would be disastrous because the spine may disengage and dislocate. We advocate the use of systems that have 2-mm increments, particularly in the smaller sizes, because 2-mm increments are much more precise in balancing the flexion and extension gaps. Fortunately the industry has become more accommodating and has released systems with 2-mm increments (Fig. 141.16).

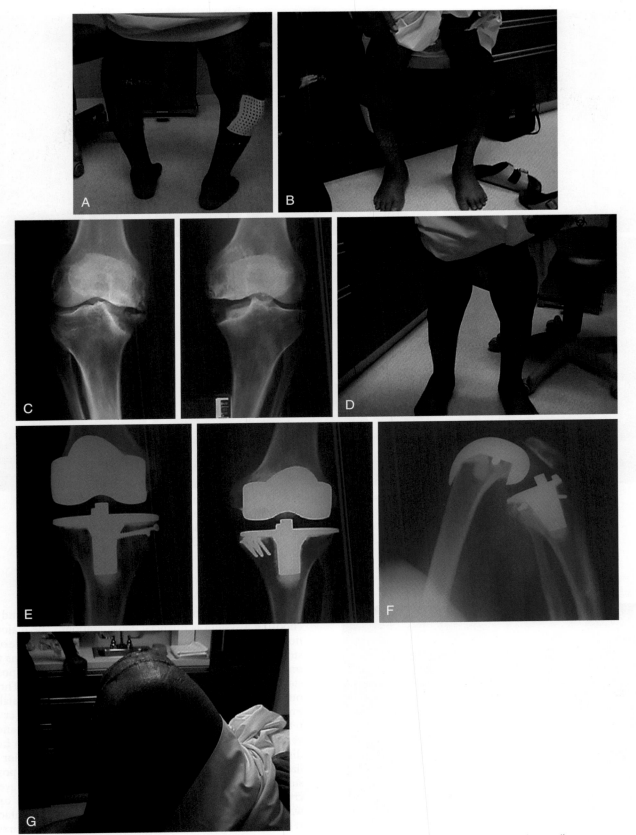

FIG 141.10 Sixty-four-year-old male with gross varus deformity, along with preoperative radiographs (A to C). Patient insists on kneeling postoperatively. Postoperative picture (D), as well as postoperative radiographs and full flexion (E to G). (Courtesy Dr. Samih Tarabichi, MD.)

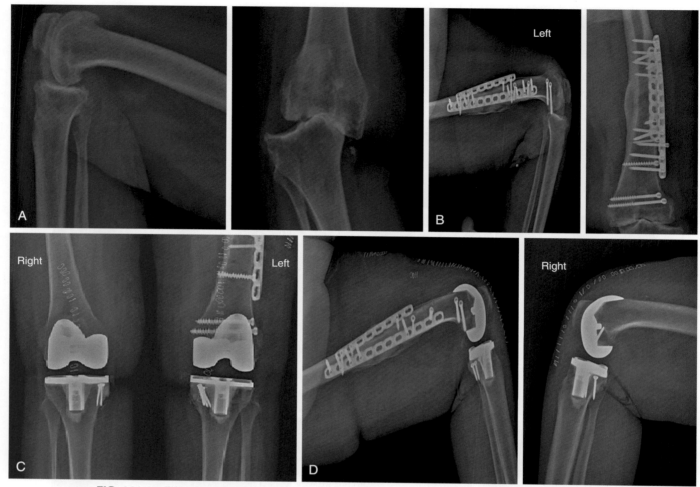

FIG 141.11 Fifty-three-year-old female with a history of open reduction and internal fixation because of left femur fracture presents with inability to walk for the past 5 months. Patient has gross varus deformity, along with gross mediolateral instability. Preoperative radiographs (A and B) and postoperative radiographs (C and D). (Courtesy Dr. Samih Tarabichi, MD.)

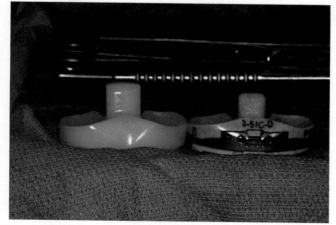

FIG 141.12 Constrained posterior stabilizer insert *(left)* versus simple posterior stabilizer *(right)* demonstrating thick and higher spine in the constrained posterior stabilizer. (Courtesy Zimmer Biomet.)

The second thought that we have to bear in mind when choosing a system is financial considerations. The majority of hospitals have limited budgets and cannot keep multiple options stored in the hospital, so they will force their surgeons to buy only one system and it is definitely safer to choose posterior stabilized rather than cruciate-retaining prostheses. Throughout this chapter we have made the case for a posterior stabilized implant. The senior author used to advocate for a cruciate-retaining implant until he moved to the Middle East and converted to posterior stabilized implant. We will not go into the discussion over whether cruciate-retaining or posterior stabilized is better; however, for the Middle Eastern knee the posterior stabilized prostheses is a much safer choice. We have used cruciate-retaining implants sporadically, but only in cases in which deformity was minimal and the ligament was intact. The relevance of this debate to finance is the inability to carry both systems at the same time because of monetary constraints, and this is an issue we faced in the Middle East. We believe posterior stabilized implants are a better choice for the full spectrum of Middle Eastern patients.

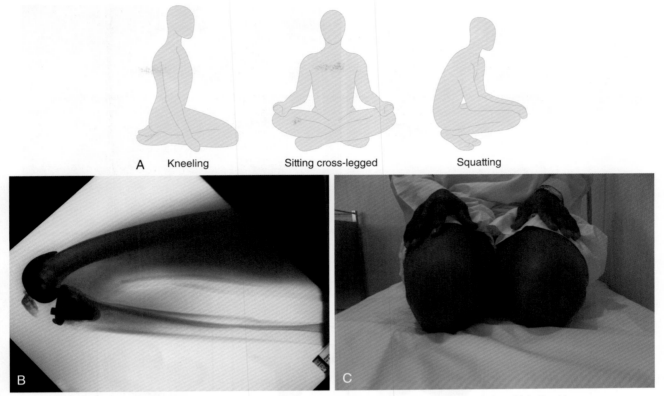

FIG 141.13 Activities of daily living in Middle Eastern individuals (A). (From Acker SM, Cockburn RA, Krevolin J, et al: Knee kinematics of high-flexion activities of daily living performed by Muslims in the middle east. *J Arthroplasty* 26:319–327, 2011.) (B and C) Full flexion in kneeling post TKA. (Courtesy Dr. Samih Tarabichi, MD.)

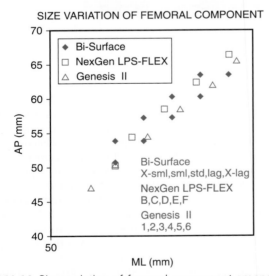

FIG 141.14 Size variation of femoral component among different systems. Most systems available have 4-mm increments between consecutive sizes. (Courtesy Zimmer Biomet.)

There are also implants that have given consideration to high flexion, and they should be used in Middle Eastern patients. However, it is key to know that the implants themselves do not provide high flexion but may be friendlier for deep flexion because many systems have not been assessed kinematically beyond 120 to 130 degrees of flexion.

Knee systems with higher constraint must also be available. In patients with complex deformity the initial instability coupled with the extensive release results in instability with a regular posterior stabilizer. As we discussed previously, this necessitates the use of a CCK, and we have used it in 5% of our primaries. The CCK provides medial and lateral stability. If there was any significant instability with the trial components because of the extensive release, then we proceeded to use a CCK implant. Thus in severe deformity a backup system should always be kept close by because the instability cannot be appreciated until after the bone cuts are made. We are now fortunate in that the CPS insert that has been released provides midlevel constraint between the regular posterior stabilizer and the CCK.

Another consideration is whether to choose mobile- or fixed-bearing implants. The principle behind mobile-bearing implants is to provide greater freedom of rotation. We have published work on the kinematics of the knee in daily activities and we have shown that in deep flexion there is significant rotation of the femur on the tibia (Fig. 141.17).

We have also presented at the American Academy of Orthopaedic Surgeons (AAOS) annual meeting,[43] comparing the

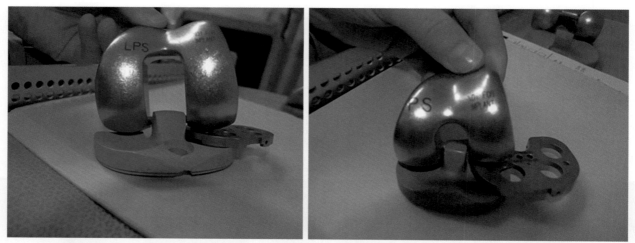

FIG 141.15 Figure demonstrating 3-mm mismatch in larger *(left)* versus smaller knee *(right)*. In smaller knees the spine can disengage easily because of the size of the spine itself. (Courtesy Dr. Samih Tarabichi, MD.)

Sizing/Identification Nomenclature:

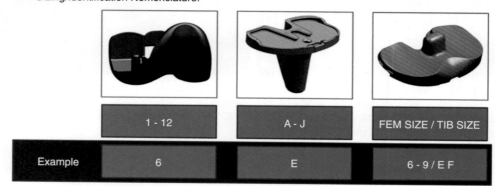

	1 - 12	A - J	FEM SIZE / TIB SIZE
Example	6	E	6 - 9 / E F

Standard width femurs shall be called 'Classic'

FIG 141.16 New sizing system in Persona System is more compatible with Asian knee. (Courtesy Zimmer Biomet.)

outcomes of mobile-and fixed-bearing knees in Middle Eastern patients. Although there was no significant difference in range of motion between mobile- and fixed-bearing knees, there was a higher percentage of frequent kneelers in the mobile-bearing group. Frequent kneelers were defined as those who kneel more than 5 times a day. This is most likely because of the increased rotation permitted by the mobile-bearing implant, making the patient more comfortable in deep flexion. We believe this is because of lack of rotation in the fixed-bearing knees. In other words, if the femur does not rotate to its normal position when kneeling, the patient will feel the ligaments around the knee to be tight and will be stretched, causing pain and discomfort, and so we recommend mobile-bearing prostheses in patients with low body mass index who are likely to achieve full flexion. However, the increased frequency in the mobile-bearing group came at a price, with the mobile-bearing group having a higher rate of dislocation. We should stress that mobile-bearing implants can dislocate even if the flexion and extension gaps are perfect. If the patient has severe deformity and after soft tissue balancing there is some instability, we prefer not to use mobile-bearing prostheses, out of fear that the knee might sublux.

Cemented Versus Cementless Total Knee Arthroplasty. Our discussion about choice of implant is not complete without going over the debate between cemented and cementless TKA. Our main indication is a younger patient, as has been shown in the literature as well.[52] We now perform only cementless TKA in patients younger than 55 years and/or a life expectancy of more than 20 years. Cementless TKA has gained popularity as more data emerges demonstrating the increased incidence of osteoarthritis in younger populations.[26a] We have now performed more than 1400 cementless TKA procedures, at an annual rate of 200 per year. Our series shows that the majority of patients with cementless TKA have been younger than 60 years of age. The reason for success is greater integration between the bone and the implant, with bone growing into the implant after cementless TKA (Fig. 141.18). The disadvantages associated with cemented implants were also a reason for the success of cementless TKA. In cemented TKA, we had greater bone loss after revision during removal of the prostheses (Fig. 141.19). Furthermore, in infected TKA, it is much easier to remove all of the foreign material in cementless TKA in a two-stage revision, and this will allow eradication of infection.

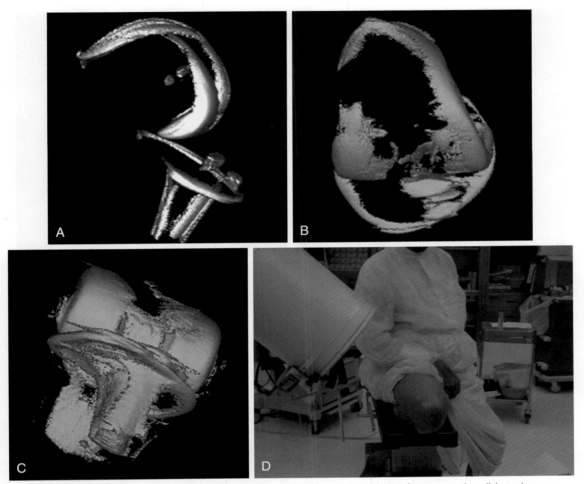

FIG 141.17 Three-dimensional (3D) images showing rotation of the femur on the tibia using a 3D C-arm (Siremobil Iso-C 3D, Siemens) (A to D). (Courtesy Dr. Samih Tarabichi, MD.)

However, in cemented TKA, it is very difficult to remove small pieces of cement that is interdigitated in the bone, and if even a small amount of bone cement residue is left it might be a reason for failure because of failure to remove all the foreign bodies in two-stage revisions.

One of the great advances in implant design that has encouraged the use of cementless implants is the advent of the metal tantalum. Tantalum has been used clinically for many years in pacemakers and cranioplasties, among other uses. Porous tantalum has a unique trabecular shape with pore sizes of 400 to 500 μm. Porous tantalum also has a stiffness similar to cortical bone. These properties make porous tantalum more physiologic, allowing it to move properly within the bone and become more integrated within the bone. The biocompatibility of tantalum can be observed during the revision of a cementless implant during removal of the components, and one will see significant bone growth on the implant.

The concern about cementless implants early during the 1980s was that we had multiple failed designs of the tibial component and great reluctance among surgeons to perform cementless TKA. Femoral components have never been an issue on review of the literature. Most of the literature has shown that cementless tibial components were problematic. Patella failures have also contributed to failure of cementless TKA.[8] Thus our practice has been to not resurface the patella. However, more recently, a cementless monoblock tibial component has demonstrated 96.8% survivorship at 20 years, which is quite impressive.[37]

Our clinical experience with cementless TKA has been excellent. We had the same clinical outcome in our series when compared to cemented. We had five cases of revision for femoral loosening and three cases of infection, which recovered completely. We also achieved similar range of motion in cementless TKA. We used a cementless posterior stabilized tibial monoblock. We previously used a tantalum tibia and titanium fever, but now with the release of the tantalum femur we use tantalum for both components.

PREOPERATIVE ASSESSMENT

At our institution we have a dedicated "knee day," when the patient's medical condition is thoroughly assessed. The physiotherapist also sees the patient, and we inform the patient what to expect postoperatively.

In our preoperative assessment, we normally flag cases which may be technically difficult. These cases include those with gross deformity, valgus deformity more than 20 degrees, flexion contracture, bone deformity proximal to the knee, osteoporosis,

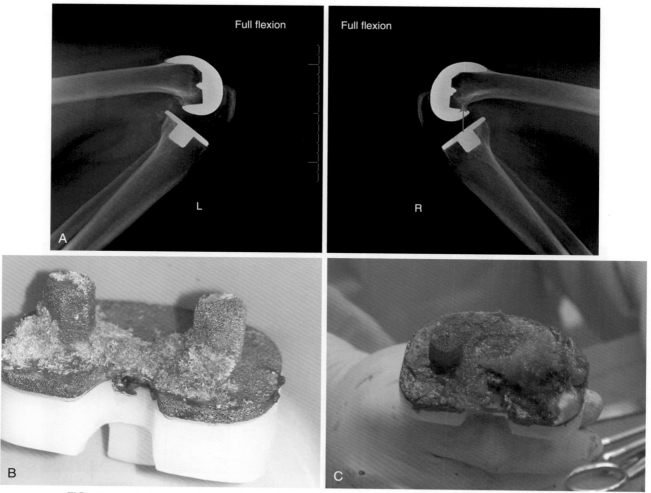

FIG 141.18 A, Bilateral lateral view radiographs of cementless TKA demonstrating full flexion and overgrowth of bone sealing off the femoral component *(arrow)*. Bone growth onto tantalum implants at 2 months (B) and 3 months (C) after primary cementless TKA. These cases were revised because of periprosthetic fracture. (Courtesy Dr. Samih Tarabichi, MD.)

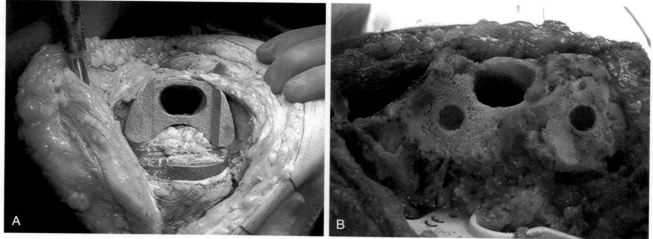

FIG 141.19 Greater bone loss seen with revision after primary cemented TKA requiring the use metaphyseal cones (A), as compared with revision of a primary cementless TKA (B). (Courtesy Dr. Samih Tarabichi, MD.)

and nonambulating patients. In these cases, we obtain standing alignment radiographs to assess their deformity and plan for their surgery. These flagged cases, such as a revision system, are readily available. We also prefer to perform simultaneous bilateral TKA in patients with severe deformity, and the logic behind this is that if we have a gross flexion contracture and we correct one side only then the contracture recurs on the operated knee. Furthermore, unilateral surgery can result in leg length discrepancies in patients with bilateral varus deformity.[48] Although initially there was great reluctance in the West to perform bilateral TKA, it has become routine in Asia. There is now a wealth of evidence to support bilateral TKA, with some studies showing a lower incidence of infection when comparing bilateral TKA with staged unilateral TKA.[32] It has also been shown that there is no significant difference in mortality between the two,[22] with bilateral TKA being more cost effective and having less overall hospitalization time.[34]

Simultaneous bilateral TKA is a necessity in some Middle Eastern patients. However, it is also a complex procedure, and our medical team must thoroughly assess the patients to see if they can tolerate bilateral TKA. We must advise surgeons against jumping into simultaneous bilateral TKA until they have an adequate medical team to support them. Furthermore, bilateral simultaneous TKA has been associated with higher rates of transfusion,[28] and we have found in a study we performed that tranexamic acid is useful in reducing blood loss after bilateral simultaneous TKA.[31]

We also perform bone density scans on our patients because of the prevalence of osteoporosis. We do not advocate delaying surgery to treat the osteoporosis because this in itself is a long process and many patients are quite disabled by their deformity; furthermore, the osteopenia arising from disuse might progress. We do it mainly to plan postoperative treatment and to draw the patient's attention to this problem and so that they can receive the appropriate treatment.

INTRAOPERATIVE CONSIDERATIONS

As mentioned earlier, most of our TKR procedures are done as simultaneous bilateral surgeries. We have discussed why we do simultaneous bilateral surgeries because of the gross deformity, and it is more economically feasible and there are now multiple studies in the literature, as revealed earlier, that show the efficacy of simultaneous bilateral TKA.

We have tried different modalities of simultaneous bilateral replacement using one team or two teams, and we have tried different ways based on the number of assistants. However, after multiple trials and seeing multiple surgeons performing simultaneous bilateral TKRs, we concluded that the best way is to have an operating team consisting of one senior surgeon, two assistants, and one scrub nurse. Our setup is demonstrated in Fig. 141.20 in a schematic diagram. This decreases the number of people in the room, making the procedure smoother. The diagram demonstrates how we recommend arranging the

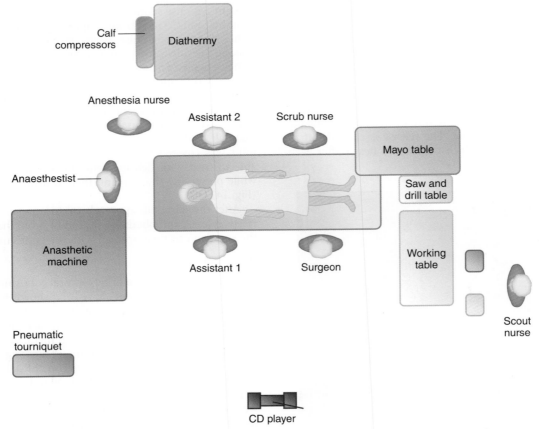

FIG 141.20 Diagram showing layout of operating room in simultaneous bilateral TKA. (Courtesy Dr. Samih Tarabichi, MD.)

operating room staff and equipment for the simultaneous bilateral TKR. Normally the operating surgeon starts on one side and the two assistants will be helping him or her, one across the table and one on the same side. After cementing the first side, then the other team will proceed with the left side. The tourniquet is inflated on the left side only after the first knee is cemented and the polyethylene insert has been placed. One assistant will start closing the operated side; the other assistant will start exposure along with the operating surgeon, and the procedure is finished as such. We found that increasing the number of assistants makes the procedure more difficult and more confusing. We normally prep both sides together (Fig. 141.21); however, we inflate first the first side, and on closure the tourniquet on the other side is inflated.

We have tried two teams operating independently; however, we found that there is a lot of confusion in the operating room. The instrumentation will be crossing both sides, and there is no advantage with regard to the length of the procedure. Normally, simultaneous bilateral TKA takes approximately 2 hours, skin to skin, in the majority of our cases. We also recommend organizing the operating theatre where we normally select only the instrumentation we are going to use and keep it in a tray, as illustrated in Fig. 141.20. We keep the set of instrumentation away from the field to clear the field and to have it available when certain instrumentation is required.

Subvastus Approach and Anterior Quadriceps Release

We use a modified subvastus approach. We proceed through a medial parapatellar incision while maintaining the attachment of the vastus medialis on the patella, thus leaving it intact. We dissect the vastus medialis until it is laterally mobilized. After the extensor mechanism is mobilized, the underlying suprapatellar pouch is identified and excised, along with any adhering bands or fibrotic tissue (Fig. 141.22A and B).[46] This provides access to the deep interface of the quadriceps muscle, allowing our anterior quadriceps release to be carried out (see Fig. 141.22C and D). Our release is performed bluntly by dissecting the deep surface of the quadriceps away from the anterior surface of the distal femur, as well as both medial and lateral intramuscular septa. The release is carried out in an incremental fashion in which the knee is flexed after each

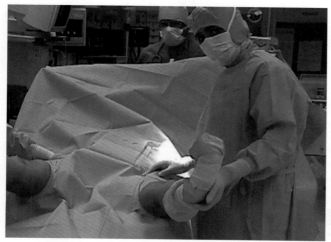

FIG 141.21 Both knees are prepared at the same time in bilateral simultaneous TKA. (Courtesy Dr. Samih Tarabichi, MD.)

release. If the range of motion is determined to be less than 130 degrees, the release is carried out more proximally along the anterior surface of the femur until a range of motion of more than 130 degrees is obtained. Fig. 141.23 illustrates the concept of the anterior quadriceps release. This approach allows greater excursion of the quadriceps and enables the surgeon to sublux the patella laterally without everting or dislocating it. This increased flexion will be helpful for the patient in his activity and aids the surgeon in performing his procedure by decreasing the tension on the soft tissue, decreasing the risk for avulsion of the patellar tendon or skin necrosis. This release is crucial in our patient population because of the importance of deep flexion to their activities of daily living. We previously thought that we could not achieve deep flexion in patients with restricted preoperative range of motion; the vast majority of literature reports that preoperative range is the strongest predictor of postoperative range of motion.[19,36] We performed a study in which we performed only the anterior quadriceps release, and bony resection, ligament releases, or lateral and medial retinacular releases were not performed at that point in surgery. The results of this study showed that, in all 42 patients, range of motion was significantly increased (Fig. 141.24).[45] This clearly demonstrates that inadequate excursion of the quadriceps muscle and tendon is the main limiting factor in better knee flexion. We have presented the results of our modified approach at the International Society for Technology in Arthroplasty in 2004 and concluded that minimally invasive techniques, such as midvastus and quad-sparing approaches, result in damage to the extensor mechanism. In our technique the extensor mechanism is maintained and patients were also shown to perform a straight-leg raise sooner than patients with a standard parapatellar incision.[18] The subvastus approach can even be performed in heavy patients because Asians have more relaxed soft tissue, making the subvastus approach easier. This approach is usually difficult in obese males in whom mobilization of the quadriceps is usually difficult. Another advantage of our approach is that if skin necrosis occurs in the proximal half of the incision, the intact muscle will prevent spread of sepsis into intra-articular spaces. We have had cases in which skin necrosis in the proximal half of the incision was quite deep. However, because the joint was covered with the vastus medialis muscle, we were able to treat with débridement and full-thickness skin grafts while preserving the implant, thereby avoiding deep infection (Fig. 141.25).

After the subvastus approach, performing an anterior quadriceps release, and obtaining flexion of more than 130 degrees, the surgeon can then proceed with the bone cuts.

Bone Cuts

We normally start with a distal femoral cut using the intramedullary guide. Asian patients have been shown to have a higher prevalence of anterior bowing in their femurs.[40] Thus the surgeon should raise his or her hands when entering the intramedullary canal so as to get better alignment. In smaller patients, it is sometimes more difficult to insert the long intramedullary guide used for white patients. Telescopic distal femoral guides can be used, which will help the surgeon to adjust the lengths of the rod accordingly. After performing the distal femoral cut, we normally measure the amount of bone taken from the distal femur and try to match it with the posterior condyles. Normally we try to finish the distal femoral cut and then focus on measuring the resected amount intraoperatively to match the bone

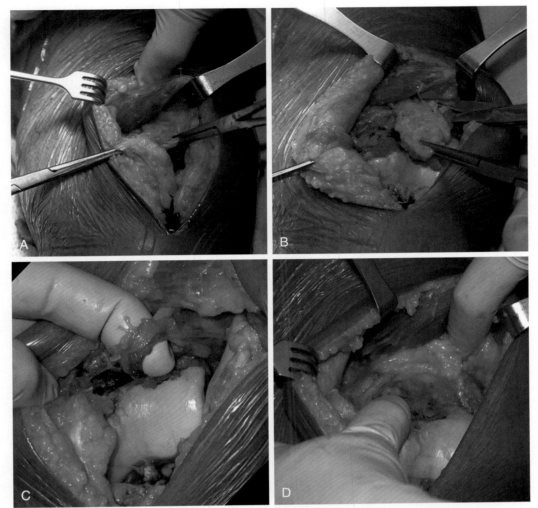

FIG 141.22 Photographs of the Left Knee While Performing Quadriceps Release A and B, The extensor mechanism being retracted laterally while the surgeon identifies and completely resects the suprapatellar pouch. C, A fibrotic band found tethering the deep surface of the quadriceps muscle to the distal femur, during the blunt release, which was subsequently excised. D, Clearing of the adhesions between the quadriceps and the femur. (From Tarabichi S, Tarabichi Y: Can an anterior quadriceps release improve range of motion in the stiff arthritic knee? *J Arthroplasty* 25:571–575, 2010.)

resected in flexion and extension. The guide for the distal femoral cut is used to perform the four bone cuts in one set. Most systems currently available allow you to do the anterior, posterior, and chamfer cuts using one guide.

The challenging thing normally is how to set the distal femoral rotation. As mentioned earlier, Asian populations tend to have an average of 5.1 degree of external rotation fit compared with 3.5 degree in white populations.[9,53] We prefer to use the transepicondylar axis, and determine our rotation using the medial and lateral epicondyles. This is quite important, especially in valgus knees in which the lateral femoral condyle is usually hypoplastic and posterior referencing to set the rotation might be quite misleading in the valgus knee[51] and in the patient who has had extensive posterior osteophyte formation. Thus we prefer a system that allows the surgeon to set the rotation based on the transepicondylar axis or the anteroposterior axis of the femur (Whiteside line).[51] We tend to try not to use the posterior

referencing for rotation because in gross deformity the osteophyte will prevent proper placement of the rotation guide on the posterior condyle (Fig. 141.26). If the deformity is mild then posterior referencing can be used to set the rotation. However, it should be remembered that in Asian patients the angle of external rotation if referenced to the posterior condyle is approximately 5 degrees.[9,53]

After performing the distal femoral cut, we proceed to the tibial cut. We must stress that sometimes our patients in this region have significant tibial bowing and that intramedullary guides may lead to malalignment, so we normally prefer the extramedullary guide. The extramedullary guide gives a better orientation for the tibia and the surface of the tibia, keeping it at 90 degrees regardless of the bowing.[14] A key element of performing bone cuts on Middle Eastern patients, which we have discussed previously, is minimizing the cuts because Middle Eastern patients have laxer soft tissues, as well as more

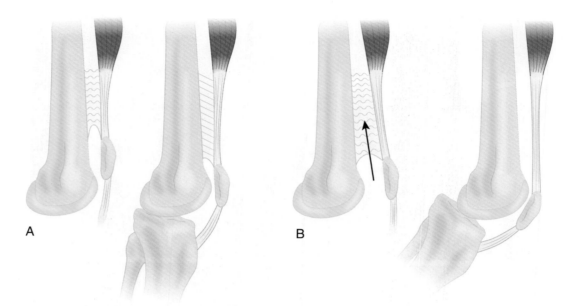

FIG 141.23 Illustration simplifying the anterior quadriceps release. (From Tarabichi S, Tarabichi Y: Can an anterior quadriceps release improve range of motion in the stiff arthritic knee? *J Arthroplasty* 25:571–575, 2010.)

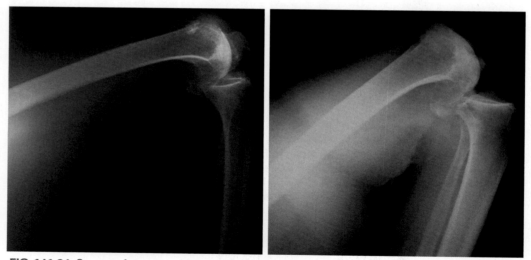

FIG 141.24 Seventy-four-year-old woman who underwent bilateral quadriceps release prior to TKA. Despite the large posterior osteophytes, we were able to increase flexion from 105 degrees *(left)* to 140 degrees *(right)*. (From Tarabichi S, Tarabichi Y: Can an anterior quadriceps release improve range of motion in the stiff arthritic knee? *J Arthroplasty* 25:571–575, 2010.)

severe deformity. This leads to a much wider gap than the bone cut itself, due to balancing of the collateral ligaments. This problem is amplified in a posterior stabilized implant when the contracted PCL is resected. Conventional wisdom in TKA dictates that the thickness we resect is equivalent to the thickness of implant. We have performed caliper measurements of the thickness of bone resection in 200 of our patients (Fig. 141.27). The average deformity was 16 degrees in varus knees and 12 degrees in valgus knees; 187 of the 200 knees had a varus deformity. We measured the proximal tibial cuts, distal femoral cuts, and posterior femoral cuts. We found that, in varus deformity, we consistently resected bone that was much thinner than the implant thickness (both components added to the thickness

of the polyethylene component). We also found that the lateral column cuts were much thicker than the medial because most of the bony erosion in our patients is on the medial side, due to the deformity (Fig. 141.28). Thus surgeons performing TKA in the Middle East should be careful not to follow the manufacturer recommendations of 8- to 10-mm bone cuts on the tibia and the femur because this will result in a large gap and the surgeon will have to resort to the use of a thick polyethylene component, which may ultimately lead to backside wear of polyethylene and decreased implant longevity. If the bony resection is generous, the surgeon may even generate a gap too large to be filled by a spacer. The recommendation for tibial bone cut in Western patients is to reach the bottom of the valley in the

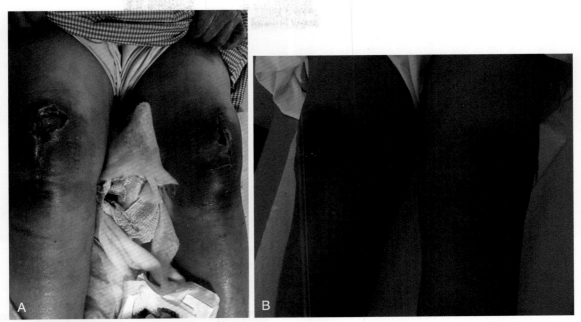

FIG 141.25 Eighty-six-year-old male who developed superficial skin necrosis post TKA (A). He was treated with débridement and full-thickness skin grafts. Wound was well healed at 4.5 months (B). (Courtesy Dr. Samih Tarabichi, MD.)

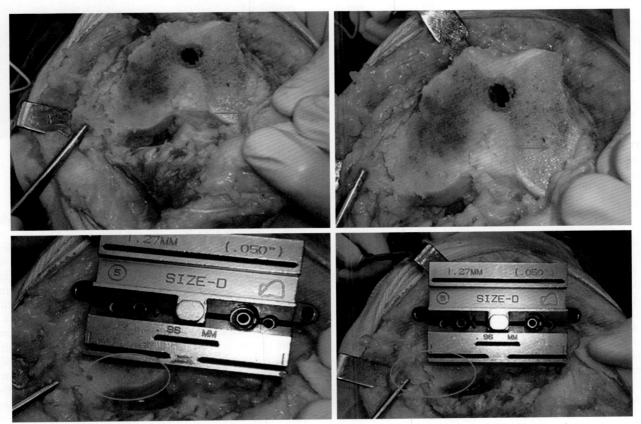

FIG 141.26 Posterior osteophytes distort the posterior condylar line *(red arrow)* and hence the posterior condylar angle, making posterior referencing difficult. The red circle demonstrates the bone protruding from the guide, distorting the surgeon's measurement of the posterior condylar angle. (Courtesy Dr. Samih Tarabichi, MD.)

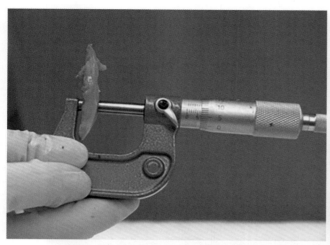
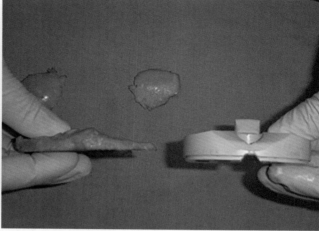

FIG 141.27 Caliper measurements of the resected bone *(left)* along with a comparison between the thickness of resected bone compared with the polyethylene, indicating that we resect much less bone than the total prosthesis thickness *(right)*. (Courtesy Dr. Samih Tarabichi, MD.)

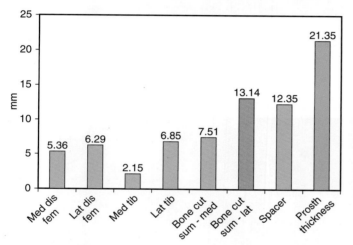

FIG 141.28 Bar graph showing the thickness of our bone cuts compared with the total prosthesis thickness. You can see the thickness of the lateral bone cuts *(red bar)* (the intact side in a varus knee) is much thinner than the overall prosthesis thickness *(green bar)*. (Courtesy Dr. Samih Tarabichi, MD.)

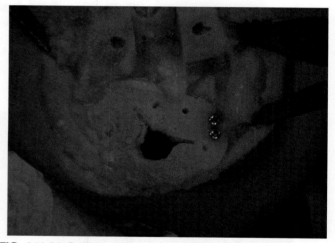

FIG 141.29 Drilling holes in the tibia and filling them with screws and cement to account for the concavity of the medial side of the tibia. (Courtesy Dr. Samih Tarabichi, MD.)

deficient side (ie, the medial side in varus knee). We strongly advise against this. We normally resect 5 mm from the lateral side, and we do not have any problem having a concave surface on the medial side of the bone. This concave surface is normally drilled with multiple holes and filled with cement and screws (Fig. 141.29). Trying to reach the bottom of the deficient bone with your bone cut on the medial side will lead to significant bone loss on the lateral side, which might lead to the use of a thicker bone component, and the deeper cut will lead to osteoporotic bone, increasing the risk of tibial subsidence, especially in obese patients.

In conclusion, it is advisable to take only 5 mm from the intact lateral condyle of the distal femur and 5 mm from the intact lateral tibial surface in a varus knee, even with mild deformity. It is quite easy for the surgeon to recut if after the release the gaps are still tight. However, in most cases, we found

that 5 mm is adequate and normally the release will widen the gaps, especially after resecting the pathologic PCL.

After performing the bone cuts, we proceed to check for symmetry between flexion and extension gaps and both medial and lateral compartments. Most of the time we will require extensive release to achieve symmetry. A varus deformity is present in the overwhelming majority of our patients, with only 7% of patients presenting with a valgus deformity. This varus deformity can exceed 30 degrees in some cases. Thus our soft tissue release is primarily done on medial structures, with our registry data showing the performance of a medial collateral ligament (MCL) release on 68% of our patients. We normally release in increments, meaning we initially release so that we have a reasonable opening and then fine tune the release after placement of a trial component. The stages of medial release are conventionally described as follows:
1. Superficial MCL
2. Deep MCL
3. Pes anserinus.

With the superficial release, we normally start with anterior part of the MCL with the use of a curved osteotome. We try to release the superficial part of the MCL from the metaphysis of the tibia. We should stress that in our release we try to preserve the anterior attachment of the pes anserinus, and we slide the osteotome deeper than the pes anserinus attachment. Hence we try to stay directly on the bone. This is challenging in obese patients because often the MCL is not clear, so we normally stress to just stay on the bone. We avoid releasing the pes anserinus because its release can render the MCL unstable because the MCL will not be pushed to the metaphyseal area of the bone. The pes anserinus is a dynamic stabilizer for the medial compartment; even if it is tight it will stretch because the tendon is attached to the muscle and it will later stretch in a gradual fashion.

The second degree of release is carried out on the deep ligament. We start releasing approximately an inch from the articular surface of the tibia. The surgeon can normally feel with his or her digit which part of the ligament is tight and precisely follow it up and detach it from the bone. We normally like to keep the MCL attached to the soft tissue sleeve as in one block. Failure to do that will weaken the MCL, and the surgeon can have instability. The third degree of MCL release is incising pes anserinus itself, which we rarely do in spite of severe deformity. This is a last resort and is mistakenly performed in cases in which there was actually inadequate release of the MCL.

With regard to release in valgus deformity, which is rarer in our population, we follow Whiteside's recommendation, which normally considers whether the valgus sleeve is tight in flexion or extension. If it is tight in extension, the iliotibial band is released. If it is tight in flexion, the lateral collateral ligament is released.[50] The point that should be stressed is that in any gross deformity the soft tissue release is carried out in an incremental fashion, meaning that after we perform our cuts we try to do some release to see if the gap balances medially and laterally. The release is not finished until we resect all the bony osteophytes and resected the PCL, and the last stage of the release is performed on the trial component. This is key because we have found that balancing on the trial component is more accurate with the trial component when compared with blocks. To aid in balancing the soft tissues, we have used a device labeled a dynamic spacer, which consists of two plates with two springs between the two plates on either side (Fig. 141.30). The purpose of the springs is to apply constant pressure, and we have found it quite useful in monitoring the amount of release, especially with MCL release.

The intramedullary notch is then made using a special guiding block, after which a trial component is placed. We test the stability, both in midflexion and extension and gap symmetry at this stage. If we have symmetry in the medial and lateral compartments and the knee is stable, then we proceed with a regular posterior stabilizer. If we get an opening of more than 4 mm in midflexion with the trial components with a regular posterior stabilizer we make sure to have a backup revision system, namely the CCK, which we use in 5% of our primary TKAs. We would consider using it if there was any significant medial and lateral instability with the trial components before cementing. This would usually happen in knees with severe deformity that were initially unstable and then with extensive release the instability increased. Surgeons should always have a backup revision system at hand because sometimes the instability is not obvious until the bone cuts are finished. More recently we have started using the CPS polyethylene insert. As we described previously, this insert has a higher and wider spine that locks into the normal implant. The advantage of this insert is that we can lock the spacer into the regular primary plate to stabilize the knee in flexion. This has proven to be quite beneficial in Middle Eastern patients, especially after extensive release of the MCL, which can lead to instability in flexion. Now the CPS insert is giving mediolateral stability and functions as an internal splint until the MCL heals.

The advent of the CPS insert has addressed the issue of instability with opening of the joint more than 2 to 4 mm that was noticed after cementing. Previously we would accept this instability as the price to be paid to have balance in the collateral ligaments or revise the primary knee that we had already placed. The latter choice of revising the primary knee is an unfortunate choice that we have been forced to make because of unacceptable instability post cementing. This prolongs the exposure time

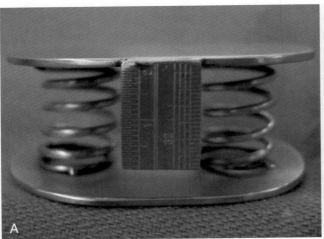
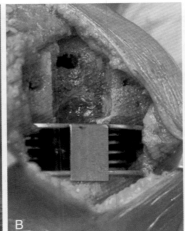
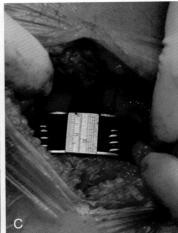

FIG 141.30 A, Dynamic spacer. Use of the dynamic spacer to detect an unbalanced flexion gap (B) or extension gap (C). (Courtesy Dr. Samih Tarabichi, MD.)

as well as incuring significant cost and trauma for the patient. The great advantage of the CPS insert is that decision about its use can be made after cementing when there is significant instability and locks into the same tibial tray, thus avoiding the use of a revision system. The only requirement for the CPS insert is that the surgeon deepen the intercondylar notch using a small osteotome. We normally hold the polyethylene and slide it onto the femur to make sure it is not hitting the roof of the intercondylar notch. Unfortunately there are no long-term data on the CPS insert, and we caution surgeons about using it until clinical trials can assess its longevity. We therefore advocate its use only in instances of instability post cementing.

Patella: To Resurface or Not to Resurface?

To resurface or not to resurface a patella has been a very controversial issue. Our preference is not to resurface the patella. This is based on Middle Eastern and Asian patients tending to have smaller and thinner patellas.[25] In addition, the patients are going to kneel on their knees, and the patient may have accidental trauma while they kneel on the ground. Our concern is that resurfacing the patella may weaken it, which may lead to patellar fracture. Patellar fracture is a very serious complication after TKA, especially if the patella has been resurfaced. Such fracture may require an allograft, and safe allografts in our region are difficult to acquire. There is also some literature showing that patellar resurfacing does not improve the outcome of TKA.[10,11] Based on these factors, we do not resurface our patella and we only trim the osteophytes of the patella to make sure that it will not catch on the edge of the femoral component. We normally smooth the sharp edges of the patella using an oscillating saw to round all the corners. We resurface the patella only if the patella is concave and we could not perform a patelloplasty and cannot restore the normal shape. In such rare occasions, we have resurfaced the patella and in only 2% of our procedures have we resurfaced the patella.

POSTOPERATIVE CARE

We encourage an active multidisciplinary approach to postoperative care. All the health care professionals that are involved in postoperative care routinely participate in meetings to discuss postoperative protocols and ways to improve them. We found that that these regular meetings for our staff, which includes pain management nurses, floor nurses, physiotherapists, and physicians, are quite helpful in establishing proper protocols to care for our patients. Among many factors, pain management is the most challenging problem in achieving full flexion following TKA.[35] Providing ineffective pain relief during the early postoperative period (7 to 10 days) can be detrimental in achieving full flexion. Effective management of pain during the early postoperative period can also prevent the development of chronic pain in the future. A multimodal approach to pain management is important to control postoperative pain. Attacking the pain pathway in different sites includes the following:

1. Local anesthesia
2. Nonsteroidal antiinflammatory medication
3. Narcotic analgesics
4. Nonnarcotic analgesics
5. Nonclassical pain medication.

Local anesthesia that includes central neuronal blockade and epidural anesthesia provides effective anesthesia for both legs.

This can provide prolonged pain management over a few days for postoperative pain. We have used peripheral nerve blocks, including femoral nerve blocks, especially in unilateral surgery. We also routinely use a local anesthetic infiltration before closure, consisting of 10 ml of 0.5% Bupivacaine. We also use the continuous infusion of local anesthetic intra-articularly using a catheter; we normally use the catheter for up to 3 days, after which it is removed. This has proven to be useful in patients who undergo unilateral TKR.

Nonsteroidal antiinflammatory medication is an important component of a multimodal approach to pain management. The choice is usually between cyclooxygenase (COX)-1 and COX-2 inhibitors, and we try to avoid it in patients with significant coronary heart disease. We normally prefer COX-2 inhibitors because we can also use our anticoagulant postoperatively. We have used an epidural catheter, which was kept in place for an average of 3 days postoperatively. We found this to be a good modality of pain control; however, it usually requires close monitoring on the floor. Naturally systemic narcotics delivered via parenteral or intramuscular routes are important for breakthrough pain or before physiotherapy. This will enable the physiotherapists to work harder on flexion for the patient. For oral narcotics, we normally use oxycodone on an as-needed basis.

Nonnarcotic analgesics include 1g of IV acetaminophen. It has been very effective for mild-to-moderate pain, without any sedation or respiratory depression. We have also used it orally on an as-needed basis. Nonclassic analgesics include anticonvulsant drugs, such as gabapentin and pregabalin. We normally start pregabalin 75 mg twice a day. There are studies supporting the effect of the anticonvulsants in preventing chronic pain.[12,16] We sometimes use antidepressant medication if we notice that our patients shows signs of postsurgical depression. On occasion we have used a short course of prednisone to prevent swelling and excessive pain. This has proven to be very effective, especially in patients who have generalized soft tissue swelling and those who wish to develop full flexion. We normally use oral prednisone 20 mg on a daily basis for 1 week. Studies have confirmed the effectiveness of steroids in controlling pain and improving recovery time postoperatively.[5,30]

The physiotherapy is quite aggressive in our patients to achieve full flexion. Preoperatively the physiotherapist evaluates the patient and documents range of motion and discusses with the patient the postoperative course. Those patients with good range of motion preoperatively and keen on achieving full flexion postoperatively are normally flagged to work with them aggressively postoperatively, and on some occasions, if the patient's general medical condition does not allow full flexion, we inform the patient that full flexion is not advisable for him or her because of either increased weight or a neurologic problem.

Postoperatively physiotherapy is started on day 1. It usually involves active ankle pumps and manual calf stretches and resisted plantarflexion and straight-leg raises. The patient is instructed how to do quadriceps isometric exercises and short arc quads. We normally do not use the continuous passive motion (CPM) machine, and we encourage the patient to do exercises on their own without the CPM machine.

On day 2, day 1 exercises are repeated. We start mobilization with a high frame walker. Two physiotherapists are normally required. We encourage the patient to ambulate with the walker.

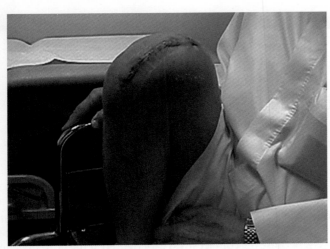

FIG 141.31 Full flexion in patient 2 to 4 weeks postoperatively. (Courtesy Dr. Samih Tarabichi, MD.)

Day 3 to 4 the patient is instructed to repeat exercises as before, we start mobilization with a regular frame, and we teach the patient the importance of deep flexion activity.

Day 5 to 7 we progress to ambulation with a lower frame walker for longer distances, and we teach the patient exercises he or she can perform independently and also encourage family participation. We also start stair training and investigating home facilities, and we get the family involved in discharge planning.

After 2 weeks, physiotherapy involves the stationary bicycle, quadriceps strengthening with light ankle weights, hamstrings and gastrocnemius stretches, and balance and proprioceptive exercises. Patients who achieve full flexion normally achieve it within the first month after surgery, and we try to encourage the patient to walk with a cane and gradually return to his or her functional activity. Our experience shows that patients who achieve full flexion normally achieve it in the first 6 weeks (Fig. 141.31). If they do not achieve it within this time, it is quite difficult to achieve it later. After 1 month, we allow the patient to kneel on his knee in full flexion with the calves touching the hamstrings, and we encourage him to do water-based exercises if the wound is dry. We have organized a small group for our postoperative patients; this group includes five patients per group, and the exercises are carried out for this group together. We have found this to be quite helpful and the patients tend to encourage each other. However, we must stress that all these patients should be of similar body mass indices, objectives, and age, to the greatest degree possible.

CONCLUSION

Patients who present for TKA in the Middle East have special needs, and the anatomy of the knee has some unique features when compared with Western patients. These features are not limited to Middle Eastern patients but also found in the Asian population at large. This will dictate some considerations when TKA is performed in Middle Eastern patients. The surgeon should be aware that special considerations should be taken into account regarding the implant. Some implants may not be appropriate because of the anatomy and pathologic features of Middle Eastern and Asian patients. For example, cruciate-retaining implants may not work in some of our patients. In addition, the severity of the disease will force the surgeon to perform simultaneous bilateral TKA more often than in Western populations. The activities of daily living force the patient into activities involving deep flexion. We believe that full flexion can be achieved to meet the specific needs of the patients. The subvastus approach and anterior quadriceps release have worked well for us and enabled us to achieve better flexion than reported in most of the Western literature. In spite of all these challenges, we have managed to achieve results that meet the patient's expectations in our region. We still believe that industry has to give more consideration to specific needs of Middle Eastern patients so that they can produce more compatible designs for our patients.

KEY REFERENCES

14. Chiu KY, Yau WP, Ng TP, et al: The accuracy of extramedullary guides for tibial component placement in total knee arthroplasty. *Int Orthop* 32:467–471, 2008.

15. Chiu KY, Zhang SD, Zhang GH: Posterior slope of tibial plateau in Chinese. *J Arthroplasty* 15:224–227, 2000.

17. Dai Y, Scuderi GR, Bischoff JE, et al: Anatomic tibial component design can increase tibial component coverage and rotational alignment accuracy: a comparison of six contemporary designs. *Knee Surg Sports Traumatol Arthrosc* 22:2911–2923, 2014.

18. Gado I, Tarabichi S: Subvastus approach: the only true MIS approach in total knee. *J Bone Joint Surg Br* 94-B:66, 2012.

22. Huotari K, Lyytikainen O, Seitsalo S, et al: Patient outcomes after simultaneous bilateral total hip and knee joint replacements. *J Hosp Infect* 65:219–225, 2007.

25. Kim TK, Chung BJ, Kang YG, et al: Clinical implications of anthropometric patellar dimensions for TKA in Asians. *Clin Orthop* 467:1007–1014, 2009.

26. Komistek RD, Scott RD, Dennis DA, et al: In vivo comparison of femorotibial contact positions for press-fit posterior stabilized and posterior cruciate retaining total knee arthroplasties. *J Arthroplasty* 17:209–216, 2002.

31. MacGillivray RG, Tarabichi SB, Hawari MF, et al: Tranexamic acid to reduce blood loss after bilateral total knee arthroplasty. A prospective, randomized, double blind study. *J Arthroplasty* 26:24–28, 2011.

37. Ritter MA, Meneghini RM: Twenty-year survivorship of cementless anatomic graduated component total knee arthroplasty. *J Arthroplasty* 25:507–513, 2010.

38. Shahi A, Saleh UH, Tan TL, et al: A unique pattern of periprosthetic fracture following total knee arthroplasty: the insufficiency fracture. *J Arthroplasty* 30:1054–1057, 2015.

41. Tang Q, Zhou Y, Yang D, et al: The offset of the tibial shaft from the tibial plateau in Chinese people. *J Bone Joint Surg Am* 92:1981–1987, 2010.

45. Tarabichi S, Tarabichi Y: Can an anterior quadriceps release improve range of motion in the stiff arthritic knee? *J Arthroplasty* 25:571–575, 2010.

46. Tarabichi S, Tarabichi Y, Hawari M: Achieving deep flexion after primary total knee arthroplasty. *J Arthroplasty* 25:219–224, 2010.

48. Vaidya SV, Patel MR, Panghate AN, et al: Total knee arthroplasty: limb length discrepancy and functional outcome. *Indian J Orthop* 44:300–307, 2010.

53. Yip DK, Zhu YH, Chiu KY, et al: Distal rotational alignment of the Chinese femur and its relevance in total knee arthroplasty. *J Arthroplasty* 19:613–619, 2004.

The references for this chapter can also be found on www.expertconsult.com.

142

Mobile-Bearing Total Knee Arthroplasty

Jason M. Jennings, David C. McNabb, Raymond H. Kim

INTRODUCTION

Indications for total knee arthroplasty (TKA) have expanded as prosthetic designs, implant materials, and surgical techniques have improved. Although early total knee designs were generally reserved for elderly and sedentary patients with debilitating pain and loss of function, excellent clinical results with 10- to 15-year outcomes[12,13,18,60,62] have encouraged many surgeons to consider performing TKA on younger patients who have higher activity demands. The mobile-bearing (MB) TKA was introduced to potentially reduce the risk of aseptic loosening and wear of the polyethylene insert by having an increase in conformity and reducing the stress across the bone-implant interface.[23,32] The careful integration of clinical and laboratory studies has led to advances in development of MB TKA systems over the past several decades.

DESIGN RATIONALE OF MOBILE-BEARING TOTAL KNEE ARTHROPLASTY

Studies have shown that highly conforming fixed-bearing (FB) TKA designs are intolerant of higher rotational and anteroposterior translational kinematic motion patterns that are commonly encountered after TKA, with increased polyethylene wear frequently observed.[15,25,44,48,70] Subsurface polyethylene stresses experienced in situations of malalignment have also been shown to be significantly increased in highly conforming FB TKA systems, compared with less conforming fixed or highly conforming MB TKA designs.[15,48,70]

Understanding that the highly constrained implant designs of the 1970s increased the risk of early aseptic loosening, the next generation of implant designs were subsequently developed that relied more on the load-sharing and stabilizing roles of the native soft tissue structures. This was accomplished by reducing articular conformity constraint, which typically incorporated the use of round-on-flat or flat-on-flat articular geometries. These designs allowed for rotation and multiplane translation to occur at the articulating interface and relied more on the surrounding soft tissue structures than conformity of the articular surfaces for stability and dispersion of the applied loads.

Although these low conformity TKA designs significantly reduced stresses transmitted to the fixation interface, this also decreased the contact area between the femoral component and the polyethylene-bearing surface. Decreased articular congruity increases detrimental subsurface contact stresses experienced by the polyethylene and also increases the amount of cross-shear stresses that risk accelerated polyethylene wear. Use of round-on-flat and flat-on-flat bearings produces elevated point and line loading conditions at the articular interface, respectively. Because the contact stress experienced at the polyethylene surface is inversely proportional to the degree of conformity between the femoral condyles and the tibial polyethylene insert, low conformity designs led to accelerated polyethylene wear and subsequent premature TKA failure.[45,64]

Fluoroscopic kinematic evaluations of round-on-flat and flat-on-flat articulations have also demonstrated an increased incidence of both paradoxical anterior femoral translation during deep flexion (instead of controlled posterior femoral rollback) and reverse axial rotation patterns. These abnormal kinematic patterns are likely secondary to a reduction in articular conformity with resulting instability.*

This paradoxical motion produces detrimental cyclical tensile shear stresses at the articulating surface, further increasing the risk of accelerated polyethylene wear.[4,8]

In summary, the higher the conformity of the articular surfaces, the lower the amount of cross-shear stresses. Also, greater articular surface contact area means less subsurface polyethylene contact stress per unit area, and subsequently less polyethylene wear is seen. In contrast to total hip arthroplasty where conformity may be achieved in all planes, the focus in TKA is primarily on achieving sagittal and coronal plane conformity. It has been demonstrated that increasing coronal plane conformity is the most critical plane to reduce peak polyethylene stresses,[4,44] particularly in the presence of femoral condylar lift-off.[4,44,63]

PROPOSED BIOMECHANICAL ADVANTAGES OF A MOBILE-BEARING TOTAL KNEE ARTHROPLASTY

The increased sagittal plane conformity typically present in most MB TKA designs provides the opportunity of improved control of anteroposterior translation with reduced paradoxical anterior femoral translation, particularly when tested during gait.[22,68] The increased coronal plane conformity in most MB TKA designs increases the contact area and lessens the increased contact stresses, which are present if femoral condylar lift-off occurs.[4,44,63,65]

Numerous studies have shown the increased conformity in MB designs substantially increases the contact area and reduces contact stresses, which may reduce the rate of polyethylene wear.† Greenwald and Heim[34] has demonstrated contact areas

---

*References 3, 19, 21, 22, 24, and 25.
†References 4, 8, 34, 49, 55, 65, and 70.

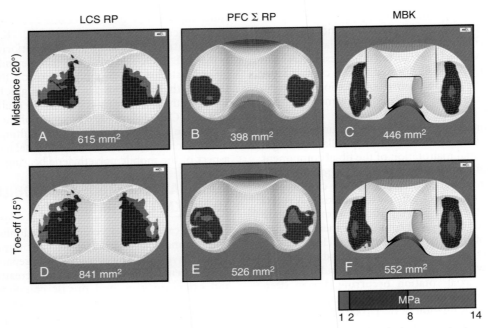

FIG 142.1 Contact area and stress analysis demonstrating high polyethylene contact areas (mm²) and low peak stresses (MPa) of three mobile-bearing TKA designs. *LCS RP,* Low Contact Stress Rotating Platform; *PFC Σ RP,* Press Fit Condylar Sigma Rotating Platform; *MBK,* Mobile Bearing Knee. (Reprinted with permission from AAOS, Greenwald AS, Heim CS: Mobile-bearing knee systems: ultra-high molecular weight polyethylene wear and design issues. *Instr Course Lect* 54:195–205, 2005.)

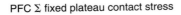

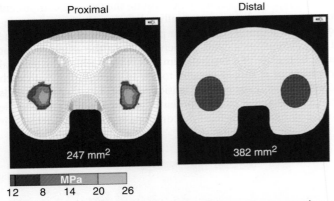

FIG 142.2 Contact area and stress analysis demonstrating a lower polyethylene contact area (mm²) and higher peak stress (MPa) in a fixed-bearing TKA design. (Reprinted with permission from AAOS, Greenwald AS, Heim CS: Mobile-bearing knee systems: ultra-high molecular weight polyethylene wear and design issues. *Instr Course Lect* 54:195–205, 2005.)

of MB TKA during gait range from approximately 400 to 800 mm², which minimizes contact stresses to 14 MPa or less (Fig. 142.1). This magnitude of contact area is substantially greater than what is typically seen in most FB TKA designs (200 to 250 mm²) (Fig. 142.2). Other finite element evaluations have similarly demonstrated reduced polyethylene contact stresses as a direct result of increased contact area, further supporting these observations.[5,54,55] The advantage of this increase in

contact area is reflected in knee simulator wear studies of FB versus MB TKA.[49]

Most rotating platform systems use a flat tibial tray-polyethylene counter-surface that allows freedom of the polyethylene insert to rotate around a central post on a highly polished, cobalt-chrome surface with a very low surface roughness. In vivo fluoroscopic kinematic studies conducted with two commonly implanted rotating platform designs have confirmed that polyethylene-bearing rotation predictably occurred in all subjects tested.[23,43] These data have demonstrated that most axial rotation in these rotating platform designs occurs at the polyethylene-bearing-tibial tray interface as the polyethylene bearing "follows" the rotation of the femoral component.[23,25,43]

All rotating platform knee designs, however, are not the same kinematically. Garling et al.[31] performed a similar fluoroscopic kinematic evaluation of 10 rheumatoid patients implanted with a different rotating platform TKA and found that the femoral component underwent greater axial rotation than the mobile polyethylene-bearing insert, suggesting that the femoral component was sliding on the top of the insert. They concluded that this finding was possibly attributed to the limited articular conformity in this design, an anterior pivot point for the rotating platform, insert impingement, or fibrous tissue caught between the insert and the tibial tray. Therefore the kinematic finding of polyethylene-bearing rotation in conjunction with the femoral component may be a design-specific condition.

Rotation of the polyethylene insert with the femoral component, independent of the rotation of the firmly fixed tibial tray, creates the potential for self-alignment[53] of the polyethylene bearing with the femoral component. Self-alignment is advantageous both for optimizing the kinematics of the prosthesis and reducing cross-shear stresses experienced by the polyethylene-bearing surface, as well as maintenance of acceptable stresses on posterior cruciate substituting tibial posts. This self-aligning behavior with a highly conforming design has been shown to maintain large, centrally located surface contact areas at the femorotibial articulation during both flexion-extension and axial rotation of the knee,[70] which is much more difficult to achieve in FB TKA designs.

An additional advantage of the self-aligning feature of rotating platform TKA systems is facilitation of central patellar tracking.[76] In a FB TKA, if substantial malrotation of the tibial component relative to the femoral component is present (especially tibial component internal rotation), the tibial tubercle can become lateralized, enhancing the risk of patellar maltracking. A rotating platform design, through bearing rotation, may provide greater self-correction of the component malalignment, allowing better centralization of the extensor mechanism. However, the prevalence of lateral retinacular release or patellar subluxation in a prospective cohort was the same between MB and FB TKA.[56]

The magnitude of axial rotation occurring during deep flexion activities is an important factor in knee implant design. An in vivo fluoroscopic evaluation of over 1000 TKAs incorporating 33 different FB and MB TKA designs has demonstrated that most TKAs will experience less than 10 degrees of axial rotation with normal postoperative activities. However, in this large multicenter analysis, a number of subjects experienced either normal or reverse axial rotational magnitudes greater than 20 degrees during these same activities, which are beyond the rotational boundaries of most FB TKA designs.[24] Therefore MB TKA designs that provide more freedom of rotation may reduce rotational polyethylene impingement, with the potential for reduction of polyethylene wear. In addition, studies examining the contribution of posterior cruciate substituting (PS) polyethylene post wear to TKA failure have shown that excessive axial rotation in PS FB designs can predispose to premature polyethylene wear and compromise the integrity of the central post because of lateral and medial post impingement with attempted excessive rotation of a fixed square tibial polyethylene post in a fixed femoral intercondylar housing.[59,79] The freedom of rotation present in MB designs may prevent this complication.

The additional polyethylene-metal interface at the undersurface of the polyethylene bearing has raised concerns about the generation of additional polyethylene particles and accelerated polyethylene wear. With FB TKA systems, "backside" polyethylene motion against a rough tibial tray that is not designed to accommodate motion has shown significant polyethylene wear and subsequent periprosthetic osteolysis with certain TKA designs.[26,61,73] In MB systems, a rotating yet flat polyethylene bearing is matched against a highly polished, cobalt chromium surface with extremely low surface roughness. To date, backside polyethylene wear has not emerged as a clinically significant issue in MB designs. Retrieval studies that have physically examined the backside-bearing surface of rotating platform polyethylene inserts have reported only limited evidence of significant undersurface wear.[37,38]

Concern that polyethylene wear microparticulate debris created in MB designs will result in increased osteolysis has yet to be observed. Fisher et al.[30] analyzed wear debris created in both FB and MB TKA designs in a knee simulator analysis under high kinematic conditions, attempting to simulate the activity patterns of the younger patient. They observed no differences in microparticulate size but thought the osteolytic potential was

much higher in FB designs because of substantially more debris particle generation observed in the FB TKA subgroup.

In contrast to a purely rotating platform TKA design, additional MB TKA systems exist that permit both rotation and anteroposterior translation to occur on the inferior aspect of the polyethylene bearing. In these designs, the inferior aspect of the polyethylene bearing is exposed to multidirectional motion patterns. Close follow-up evaluation of this type of MB TKA is merited to see if premature failure resulting from backside wear occurs secondary to the multidirectional motion on the inferior aspect of the mobile polyethylene bearing.

SURGICAL TECHNIQUE FOR MOBILE-BEARING TOTAL KNEE ARTHROPLASTY

The surgical goals and techniques used (alignment, bone resection, ligamentous balancing, etc.) for implantation of an MB TKA are typically no different from preparations used with FB TKA systems. Soft-tissue balancing, creation of equal flexion and extension gaps, and precise component positioning are extremely important in both of these TKA systems. Extension and flexion gap balance is of particular importance in use of an MB TKA. Bearing dislocation or "spin-out" can occur when there is an imbalance in the flexion gap and the polyethylene bearing is no longer congruous with the femoral component. Gap balance can be achieved by several methods. The authors use a spacer block to initially evaluate and balance the extension gap prior to addressing the flexion gap and the directly related femoral component rotation. Proper rotation of the femoral component is essential to obtain a balanced flexion gap. Numerous methods are available to assist in gaining correct rotation of the femoral component.[1,2,27,58,77] These include the use of cutting jigs, which automatically rotate the femoral component three or more degrees externally relative to the posterior condylar axis; femoral component placement either parallel to the transepicondylar axis or perpendicular to the anteroposterior axis; or the use of a gap balancing method in which the femoral component is placed parallel to the tibial resection with each collateral ligament equally tensioned (Fig. 142.3). All methods have been shown to have potential shortcomings, and the use of a combination of femoral component rotational methods is

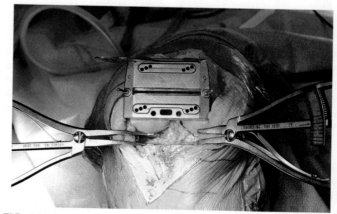

FIG 142.3 Intraoperative photograph of an equalized flexion gap achieved by placement of the anteroposterior femoral cutting jig parallel to the tibial resection with each collateral ligament equally tensioned using laminar spreaders.

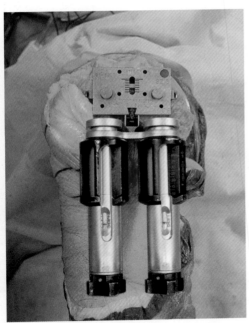

FIG 142.4 Intraoperative photograph of a flexion-extension gap balancer (Knee Balancer, DePuy Orthopaedics, Warsaw, Indiana) placed into the flexion gap to determine gap symmetry, width, and tension.

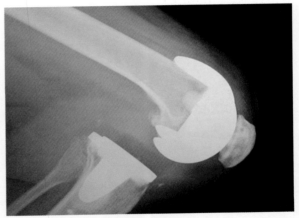

FIG 142.5 Lateral radiograph demonstrating a polyethylene-bearing "spin-out" of a rotating platform TKA.

wise. With the use of MB TKA systems, the authors have found that the use of a gap balancing method with some type of tensioning device (laminar spreaders, spacer blocks, or a specific gap tensioning device) to tension the flexion gap while femoral component rotation is determined provides the most reliable and reproducible balance and tension of the flexion gap.[20] Specific gap tensioning devices provide an additional advantage of facilitating equalization of the flexion gap width to the previously established extension gap (Fig. 142.4). These tensioning devices have been specifically designed to allow measurements (width and tension) obtained from a balanced extension gap to determine and direct flexion gap resections and femoral component rotation. Obtaining 1 to 2 mm of medial and lateral laxity in flexion is desired. Inability to obtain flexion-extension gap balance or substantial incompetence of the collateral ligamentous structures should prompt consideration of using a more constraint TKA system to lessen the risk of polyethylene-bearing instability. When using constraint, the authors will consider using an MB versus FB TKA individualized to that particular patient's knee.

CLINICAL RESULTS OF MOBILE-BEARING TOTAL KNEE ARTHROPLASTY

MB TKA was introduced to potentially reduce the risk of aseptic loosening and wear of polyethylene inserts, particularly in the younger population. However, to date, most studies with direct comparison of MB and FB TKAs have not shown consistent clinical advantages between the two designs.[‡] In addition,

multiple systematic reviews and meta-analyses[§] have also revealed no clinical differences. The typical comparisons in these studies have included outcomes such as aseptic loosening, wear rate, revision rates for any reason, range of motion, functional outcomes, radiographic parameters, and patellar tracking—all of which have been proposed benefits of the MB over the FB designs. The anticipated benefits between MB and FB TKR may manifest themselves with longer follow-ups. It is important for future studies to continue to explore this possibility.

Reports of polyethylene-bearing "spin-out" in rotating platform TKA have traditionally described this phenomenon as occurring during deep knee flexion (Fig. 142.5). Most commonly, the polyethylene bearing rotates 90 degrees around its central axis in the tibial tray as the posterolateral polyethylene lip slips posteriorly and the anteromedial polyethylene lip slips anteriorly. This complication is usually reducible via a closed reduction but may require operative reduction in rare cases. Although there is a legitimate concern with use of rotating platform designs, the highest incidence of bearing spin-out (3.3% [5 of 149] to 12% [2 of 17])[6,12] has been associated with early outcome evaluations of rotating platform TKA, when attention to flexion gap tension and balance was less emphasized. Advances in component design, surgical implantation instrumentation, and an increased understanding of the importance of flexion and extension gap tension and balance, accurate ligamentous balancing, and proper femoral component rotation have decreased the incidence of bearing instability following MB TKA.[16] Several recent outcome evaluations have reported a nominal incidence of bearing spin-out in primary TKA at up to 20 years following the operative procedure.[12,14,16,37]

MOBILE-BEARING USE IN REVISION TOTAL KNEE ARTHROPLASTY

Revision TKA (Figs. 142.6A to D) presents numerous additional challenges beyond those in the primary arthroplasty setting. Significant bone loss secondary to osteolysis or iatrogenic removal is commonly encountered. As a result, fixation naturally becomes increasingly difficult in the context of diminished bone stock. Disrupted or unbalanced soft tissue supporting structures may also be encountered, which often requires the use of revision components with increased prosthetic constraint. Although increased constraint can substitute for ligamentous

‡References 7, 10, 11, 17, 28, 29, 35, 39-42, 46, 47, 51, 52, 57, 66, 69, 71, and 75.
§References 9, 36, 50, 67, 72, 74, and 78.

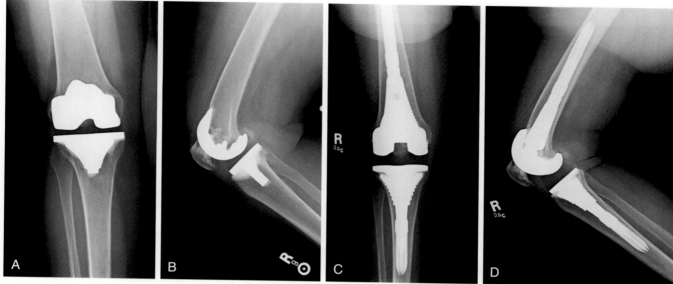

FIG 142.6 (A and B) Preoperative anteroposterior (A) and lateral (B) radiographs of a failed total knee resulting from disabling instability. (C and D) Postoperative anteroposterior (C) and lateral (D) radiographs following revision TKA with posterior stabilized MB components.

instability, it often increases stresses at the fixation interface that may lead to premature component loosening and increased polyethylene postwear secondary to increased torque on the constraining mechanism. Potential advantages of the use of MB in the revision TKA setting include reduction in polyethylene wear, decreasing fixation stresses, and protection of the constraining mechanisms. Additionally, the rotating platform construct permits the surgeon to align the tray for fixation and not compromise the rotation of the tibial insert.[33] Prospective studies with longer follow-ups are necessary to see if the theoretical benefits of MB use in revision TKA are clinically observed.

CONCLUSION

The long-term outcomes of MB TKA remain excellent, however; the exact indications for MB TKA designs remain unclear. Studies continue to be published in the orthopedic literature comparing outcomes of MB and FB, but there appears to be no clinical advantage to support the use of one design over the other. The proposed advantages of MB designs may still be of value, but these clinical results may not be noticed until longer follow-up is obtained in a large cohort. Because of the potential for reduced polyethylene wear and enhanced fixation longevity, MB TKA designs are to be considered particularly for younger and higher demand patients with longer life expectancies. Rotational polyethylene post wear seen in FB posterior stabilized systems should be minimized in rotating platform designs and may be another indication for MB TKA use. Lastly, rotating platform TKA systems should be considered in revision or extremely complicated primary TKA situations where constrained or hinged components are needed. Rotating platform designs may help reduce the high torque stresses typically seen at the fixation and hinge interfaces when using an FB TKA system. Future research should be directed in these areas to justify their use.

Although MB TKA designs demonstrate a number of potentially favorable features when compared to FB systems, it is important to remember that not all MB systems are the same. Differences exist both in the condylar geometry and as well as the bearing mobility patterns. To date, the purely rotating platform design appears to be the most clinically successful, reliable, and predictable among mobile-bearing designs. Future studies are indicated to determine and compare the kinematic and clinical effects associated with multidirectional (anteroposterior translation and bearing rotation) versus unidirectional (rotation only) MB TKA systems.

KEY REFERENCES

7. Bistolfi A, Massazza G, Lee GC, et al: Comparison of fixed and mobile-bearing total knee arthroplasty at a mean follow-up of 116 months. *J Bone Joint Surg Am* 95:e83, 2013.
10. Breeman S, Campbell MK, Dakin H, et al: Five-year results of a randomised controlled trial comparing mobile and fixed bearings in total knee replacement. *Bone Joint J* 95-B:486–492, 2013.
13. Callaghan JJ, O'Rourke MR, Iossi MF, et al: Cemented rotating-platform total knee replacement. a concise follow-up, at a minimum of fifteen years, of a previous report. *J Bone Joint Surg Am* 87:1995–1998, 2005.
40. Kelly NH, Fu RH, Wright TM, et al: Wear damage in mobile-bearing TKA is as severe as that in fixed-bearing TKA. *Clin Orthop* 469:123–130, 2011.
41. Kim YH, Kim JS, Choe JW, et al: Long-term comparison of fixed-bearing and mobile-bearing total knee replacements in patients younger than fifty-one years of age with osteoarthritis. *J Bone Joint Surg Am* 94:866–873, 2012.
42. Kim YH, Park JW, Kim JS, et al: Long-term clinical outcomes and survivorship of press-fit condylar sigma fixed-bearing and mobile-bearing total knee prostheses in the same patients. *J Bone Joint Surg Am* 96:e168, 2014.
43. Komistek RD, Dennis DA, Mahfouz MR, et al: In vivo polyethylene bearing mobility is maintained in posterior stabilized total knee arthroplasty. *Clin Orthop* 428:207–213, 2004.
46. Mahoney OM, Kinsey TL, D'Errico TJ, et al: The John Insall Award: no functional advantage of a mobile bearing posterior stabilized TKA. *Clin Orthop* 470:33–44, 2012.

53. Okamoto N, Nakamura E, Nishioka H, et al: In vivo kinematic comparison between mobile-bearing and fixed-bearing total knee arthroplasty during step-up activity. *J Arthroplasty* 29:2393–2396, 2014.

56. Pagnano MW, Trousdale RT, Stuart MJ, et al: Rotating platform knees did not improve patellar tracking: a prospective, randomized study of 240 primary total knee arthroplasties. *Clin Orthop* 221–227, 2004.

57. Pijls BG, Valstar ER, Kaptein BL, et al: Differences in long-term fixation between mobile-bearing and fixed-bearing knee prostheses at ten to 12 years' follow-up: a single-blinded randomised controlled radiostereometric trial. *J Bone Joint Surg Br* 94:1366–1371, 2012.

68. Stiehl JB, Dennis DA, Komistek RD, et al: In vivo kinematic analysis of a mobile bearing total knee prosthesis. *Clin Orthop* 345:60–66, 1997.

69. Stoner K, Jerabek SA, Tow S, et al: Rotating-platform has no surface damage advantage over fixed-bearing TKA. *Clin Qrthop* 471:76–85, 2013.

75. Woolson ST, Epstein NJ, Huddleston JI: Long-term comparison of mobile-bearing vs fixed-bearing total knee arthroplasty. *J Arthroplasty* 26:1219–1223, 2011.

76. Yang CC, McFadden LA, Dennis DA, et al: Lateral retinacular release rates in mobile- versus fixed-bearing TKA. *Clin Orthop* 466:2656–2661, 2008.

The references for this chapter can also be found on www.expertconsult.com.

143

Cemented Total Knee Arthroplasty: The Gold Standard

Nicholas T. Ting, Bryan D. Springer

INTRODUCTION

Total knee arthroplasty (TKA) is one of the most successful surgical procedures in medical history. A condylar design with good cementing technique is considered the gold standard in TKA. Many implants today should reasonably be expected to function well for the remaining life of the patient.

Despite the success of cemented condylar knee replacements, many surgeons have advocated a change to cementless fixation for their total knee patients. The impetus for this change is to try to improve on the current results, particularly as they relate to longevity in young patients. The purpose of this chapter is to look critically at the available evidence to determine what type of fixation is best for our total knee patients. An evidence-based analysis of the current literature regarding knee fixation should help define the role for cemented and cementless knee fixation.

EVOLUTION OF CEMENTLESS FIXATION

Cementless fixation was developed as a response to the early failures of total hip arthroplasty (THA) in young patients. Cemented total hips did poorly in this subset of patients. Dorr et al. reported a 67% revision rate in patients undergoing cemented total hips in patients less than 45 years old.[8] Ranawat et al. reported a 30% radiographic loosening rate in patients who had cemented total hips between ages 40 and 60.[31] Sullivan et al. looked at 90 patients with an 18-year follow-up, all of whom were less than 50 years old, and found that 50% of the acetabular components loosened, while 8% of the stems loosened.[39] In an effort to improve the long-term results of hip replacement, cementless fixation was offered as a potential solution. The transition from cemented THA to cementless THA in young patients has been a true success. Tapered or extensively coated cementless femoral hip implants have demonstrated outstanding clinical results at long-term follow-up. In addition, the success and durability of modern cementless femoral components in young patients is well documented.[38] At this point in time, many authors would suggest that total hip fixation is a solved problem.

The success of cementless hip fixation in young patients led to increased interest in cementless fixation in knee replacement. Proponents of cementless fixation in TKA believe that biologic fixation has the potential to achieve a more durable bond of the implant to the bone and hence improved success over cemented fixation. In addition, the introduction of newer porous metals for fixation in TKA has the potential to provide more reliable ingrowth than has previously been achieved with cementless total knee arthroplasty.

RATIONALE FOR THE USE OF CEMENTLESS TOTAL KNEE ARTHROPLASTY

With the success of cemented condylar TKA, one must critically look at the potential advantages of a cementless TKA design prior to widespread introduction of this technology. What advantages does it offer, and what potential problems with cemented TKA are we trying to improve upon? The purported advantages of cementless total knee fixation include shorter operative time, elimination of cement as a cause of third body polyethylene wear, ease of revision should failure occur, and improved longevity for our younger patients.

Reduced operative time is probably the most seductive reason for a surgeon to use this technology. By eliminating the 15 to 20 minutes per case for polymerization of the cement, the surgeon can complete the procedure in a more timely manner. In the age of diminishing reimbursement, certainly this is enticing. In addition, the elimination of cement from the surgical procedure removes a possible source of third body wear. Retained cement has been shown to leading factor in the damage of retrieved polyethylene inserts. This has the potential to be a source of increased polyethylene wear and osteolysis.[6,22,28,41]

Another potential advantage of cementless knee fixation is ease of revision. In the absence of cement interdigitation, component removal is simplified. The interface between the host bone and the prosthesis is divided, and there is no need to remove imbedded cement fragments. Additionally, where porous implants have failed to ingrow, removal is easily accomplished with disruption of the fibrous membrane. The resultant bone is usually a sclerotic bed that can be prepared for revision implants with only a few millimeters of bone resection. Data has shown, however, that the results of revision of a failed cementless implant to a cemented construct is similar to that of a failed cemented knee revised with cement.[12]

The main advantage of cementless fixation in young patients is the potential for improved longevity. With the improved success of TKA, indications are being expanded to younger patients. Concern remains regarding the durability and longevity of a cemented TKA in the young, more physically demanding patient population. In addition, recent demographic data suggest that by 2011, almost 50% of all TKAs will be performed in patients younger than age 65.[26] These factors are the driving force behind the evolution to cementless total knee fixation.

Once a cementless implant becomes osseous integrated, it is extremely rare for it to subsequently loosen. This outcome certainly is attractive for our younger patients. In contrast, there is concern that the bone cement interface has the potential for late deterioration, especially in young active patients. While this failure mechanism is possible, it occurs infrequently. It must be recognized that a cemented knee replacement is loaded primarily in compression—a force well tolerated at the bone cement interface. This is distinctly different from that of hip replacement, in which the forces on the cement bone interface are a combination of tension, compression, and shear. While such forces can lead to early failure in young active hip patients, there is little evidence in the literature to substantiate that deterioration of this interface is a significant problem in young cemented knee replacement patients.

RESULTS OF CEMENTED TOTAL KNEE ARTHROPLASTY

To justify this change to a cementless design, we first must analyze the currently available data on cemented TKA to determine if in fact change is necessary. Secondly, we must determine if the cementless designs solve concerns of cemented TKA. An evidenced-based approach of the current literature offers the best opportunity to do so. To date, true long-term prospective studies comparing the result of cemented versus cementless TKA are scarce and fail to show the advantage of a cementless design.[1]

If we look at the long-term results of cemented total knee arthroplasty in all age groups, the results are outstanding (Fig. 143.1). Without stratifying for age, multiple articles that have been published cite a greater than 90% success rate. Scuderi et al., looking at 1200 posterior stabilized knees, had 98% good

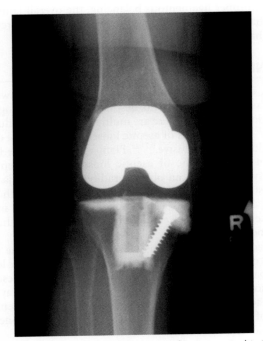

FIG 143.1 Twenty-two-year follow-up of a cemented total knee arthroplasty with pristine interfaces and no evidence of polyethylene wear or osteolysis.

or excellent results.[36] Ranawat et al., looking at a 14-year survivorship of cemented total knee replacement, had a 95% success rate.[32] Font-Rodriguez et al., looking at over 2000 posterior stabilized metal-backed knees at 14-year follow-up, noted a success rate of 98%.[15]

Thus a cemented TKA performed in an elderly patient should have a service life longer than the life of the patient, barring technical failure or infection. However, the true test of longevity comes from examining the results of cemented total knee replacement in studies stratified for age.

CEMENTED TOTAL KNEE ARTHROPLASTY IN YOUNG PATIENTS

The initial reports of mid- to long-term results of cemented condylar knee design in young patients have been encouraging. Ranawat et al. reported a 94% 10-year survivorship in patients less than 55 years old using cemented fixation.[33] Gill et al. reported a 98% good or excellent result at 10 years in his cemented total knee patients less than 55 years old.[19] Diduch et al., in evaluating 118 patients less than 55 years old, had a 94% good or excellent result at 8 years using cemented fixation.[7]

More recent reports have also echoed these results, indicating the continued durability of a cemented condylar knee design in a young, high-demand patient population. Ritter et al. reported on 207 cemented cruciate retaining TKA in patients younger than age 55.[35] The survival rate at 12 years was 94.8%. Duffy et al. reported a 96% survivorship at 10 years using a Press-Fit Condylar prosthesis (Depuy, Warsaw, Indiana) on patient younger than 55 years of age.[11] There were no revisions for aseptic loosening. Similarly, Long et al. demonstrated in their review of 114 cemented posterior stabilized total knees in patients 55 years old and younger that at 30 years, survivorship without revision for any cause was 70.1% (25 revisions) and survivorship with failure defined as aseptic revision of the tibial or femoral components was 82.5%.[27]

The results of cemented fixation in this demanding patient subset is encouraging and fails to substantiate the theory of cement interface deterioration over time. Therefore, the rationale that there is a mandate for change because of poor results of cemented fixation in young total knee patients is not substantiated by long-term data.

COMPARATIVE LITERATURE: CEMENT VERSUS CEMENTLESS

There are a number of studies available in the literature that directly compare cemented fixation to cementless fixation in TKA.[10,17] Rand et al. looked at over 11,000 TKAs and performed a survivorship analysis at 10 years. Ninety-two percent of TKAs were successful when cemented fixation was used, while only 61% were successful without cement ($p < 0.001$).[34] Barrack et al. looked at 82 cementless rotating platform knees and compared them to 76 cemented rotating platform mobile-bearing knees.[2] Eight percent of the cementless knees were revised, while no cemented knees were revised. The cementless knees also had significantly lower Knee Society scores. Gioe et al. evaluated 5760 knees, looking at various implants and methods of fixation, and found that cementless total knees had the lowest survival rate of all implants reviewed.[20] Berger et al., in evaluating 131 cementless total knees at a mean follow-up of 11 years, found that 8% of the tibial components never achieved ingrowth.[3] The authors of this article and designers of this implant commented that they have abandoned cementless fixation in TKA. Duffy et al. reported the results in a community-based registry on TKA in patients less than 55 years of age.[21] This community joint registry was comprised of 1047 total joints representing three predominant implant designs, 48 surgeons and four hospitals. The mean age for this cohort was 49.8 years, and 62.8% (657/1047) of the patients were female. There were a total of 73 revisions performed, 5.6% (37/653) in women and 9.2% (36/394) in men. Cemented TKAs performed best, with a cumulative revision rate of 15.5%, compared to 34.1% in cementless designs. Eighty-five percent of cemented TKA implants survived at 14 years in the population under 55 years, and cementless designs were an independent risk factor for revision.

More recent studies have suggested more comparable durability when fixation techniques alone are compared. Park et al. compared identical cemented or cementless TKAs implanted bilaterally in the same patient in their series of sequential simultaneous bilateral total knee replacements in 50 patients (100 knees).[29] The rates of survival of the femoral components were 100% in both groups at 14 years. The rates of survival of the cemented tibial component were 100% and 98% in the cementless tibial components. No osteolysis was identified in either group. Similarly, in their meta-analysis, Wang et al. showed no difference between cemented and uncemented TKAs for odds of aseptic loosening when design-related failures were excluded.[40] Finally, in their prospective, randomized study comparing cemented and cementless fixation in 100 TKA patients, Fricka et al. found that while more radiolucencies were seen in cementless knees ($p < 0.001$), they had equivalent survivorship (revision for any reason as the endpoint) compared to cemented TKA at 2 years of follow-up.[16]

HYBRID FIXATON TECHNIQUES

Two so-called hybrid techniques are currently used clinically:
1. Cementing the tibial component while leaving the femoral component cementless
2. Partial cementation of the tibial component—that is, cementing the baseplate and leaving the tibial stem cementless

Neither of these hybrid fixation methods have supporting evidence-based literature. Campbell et al. looked at 74 hybrid total knees where the tibia was cemented and the femur was left cementless.[5] They found the femoral components' survivorship to be only 87%. They concluded that cementless femoral fixation is unreliable and that this type of hybrid fixation should be abandoned. Gioe evaluated 5760 knees and found that cemented metal backed components had a 96% survival, while hybrid total knee replacements had only an 89% success rate.[20] Gao et al. performed a small prospective randomized study of cementless femoral components.[18] At short-term follow-up, the cementless design offered no advantage over a cemented femoral component. The magnitude and pattern of migration as measured by RSA did not differ significantly between the cemented and uncemented fixation during the 2-year follow-up, nor were there any differences between the groups in clinical outcomes.

In addition, biomechanical studies do not support the use of partial cementation of the tibial stem. Bert and McShane found that tibial trays treated with partial cementation had significantly more micromotion compared with a fully cemented construct.[4] Jazrawi et al. confirmed this in their laboratory

finding that cemented metaphyseal engaging stems had significantly less tray motion than a cementless construct of the same length.[24] More recently, however, in their review of the Norwegian Arthroplasty Registry, Petursson et al. showed an estimated 94.3% survival at 11 years (95% CI, 93.9 to 94.7) in the cemented TKR group and 96.3% (95% CI, 95.3 to 97.3) in the hybrid TKR group.[30] The adjusted Cox regression analysis showed a lower risk of revision in the hybrid group (relative risk, 0.58; 95% CI, 0.48 to 0.72, $p < 0.001$).

FAILURES MODES IN TOTAL KNEE ARTHROPLASTY

The rationale for cementless total knee arthroplasty fixation hinges on more reliable fixation and a decreased risk of aseptic loosening. Patients who have undergone total knee replacement expect at least 10 to 15 years of in-service life before subsequent revision surgery becomes necessary. If one looks critically at the modes of failure in cemented TKA, aseptic loosening is an uncommon mode of failure and thus may not justify the use of a cementless design.

Fehring et al. analyzed the mechanisms of failure in patients requiring revision surgery within 5 years of their index arthroplasty.[14] From a revision TKA dataset of 440 knees, the authors found that 63% of patients were revised within 5 years of their index arthroplasty. The key reasons for these revisions were infection, poor surgical technique, or poor surgeon judgment. Thirty-seven percent of the early failures of those patients revised within 5 years failed because of infection. Twenty-six percent failed because of instability. Thirteen percent of patients were revised within 5 years because of failure of cementless fixation. In contrast, only 3% of the early failures failed because of aseptic loosening of a cemented implant. The dominant modes of failure within the first 5 years were infection, instability, and fibrous ingrowth of cementless implants. If all patients in this early failure group would have been routinely cemented and had proper ligamentous balancing, the overall failure rate would have decreased 40% and the overall number of revisions would have decreased 25%.

DIAGNOSIS OF FAILED CEMENTLESS KNEES

Results of TKA are generally positive. There is, however, a certain subset of patients who, despite an excellent radiographic result, do not do well. There are multiple reasons for failure of a TKA.[14,37] The diagnosis of aseptic loosening as a source of pain and failure can be elusive.[9,23,25] Plain radiographs are helpful and can be diagnostic of aseptic loosening, but even slight obliquity of the film can obscure radiolucent lines adjacent to the prosthesis.[9] Plain radiographs with a divergence of the beam of only 3 degrees from a plane parallel to the bone implant interface will not detect a 2-mm lucent line beneath the tibial component.

To facilitate the diagnosis of aseptic loosening, the use of fluoroscopic radiographs of the knee to evaluate aseptic loosening in patients with cementless total knees has been described. Fluoroscopic guidance allows one to position the x-ray beam parallel to the bone prosthetic interface so that the presence and extent of radiolucent lines beneath a cementless component can be measured (Fig. 143.2).[13]

In contrast to failed cemented TKA, where cement fragmentation may be evident and the cement-bone interface is not as close to the obscuring metal of the implant, the interface

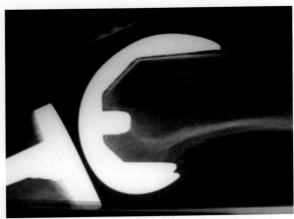

FIG 143.2 Fluoroscopic view of a cementless total knee depicting failure of ingrowth.

beneath a cementless implant may be more difficult to assess. The porous surface may obscure a demarcation line, and sclerosis beneath a fixed porous implant can be confused with consolidation and spot welds.

In cementless knee arthroplasty, the presence of any line between the implant and bone shows a lack of bony incorporation in that area. If such lines are extensive or progressive, this implant is loose and may be the source of symptoms.[13] Undoubtedly there are patients who lack bony ingrowth yet function well with a fibrously ingrown implant. However, if a patient presents with a painful TKA, normal-appearing x-rays, and has start-up pain, fluoroscopic views are indicated. If fluoroscopic radiographs corroborate a problem with the interfaces, chances for successful revision are high.[12]

CONCLUSION

Much interest is being generated in the arena of cementless TKA fixation. With the purported advantages of less operative time, easier revision, and the potential for improved survivorship, especially in younger patients, this approach has some theoretical appeal. In addition, the advent of new porous surfaces to allow for more rapid and reliable bony ingrowth has the potential to improve the current results and address some of the concerns with previous cementless designs.

We have presented in this chapter a systematic review of the current available literature on cemented and cementless TKA. It is clear that the results of cemented TKA are excellent, and

durable long-term results can be achieved in all patient populations. In addition, the issue of aseptic loosening in cemented TKA design is minimal, therefore undermining the rationale for the use of a cementless design. While continued research efforts are important to evaluate cementless designs and their application in arthroplasty, a cemented TKA must still be considered the gold standard.

KEY REFERENCES

1. Baker PN, Khaw FM, Kirk LM: A randomised controlled trial of cemented versus cementless press-fit condylar total knee replacement: 15-year survival analysis. *J Bone Joint Surg Br* 89:1608–1614, 2007.
2. Barrack RL, Nakamura SJ, Hopkins SG, et al: Winner of the 2003 James A. Rand Young Investigator's Award: early failure of cementless mobile-bearing total knee arthroplasty. *J Arthroplasty* 19(7 Suppl 2):101–106, 2004.
3. Berger RA, Lyon JH, Jacobs JJ, et al: Problems with cementless total knee arthroplasty at 11 years followup. *Clin Orthop* 392:196–207, 2001.
5. Campbell MD, Duffy GP, Trousdale RT: Femoral component failure in hybrid total knee arthroplasty. *Clin Orthop* 356:58–65, 1998.
12. Fehring TK, Griffin WL: Revision of failed cementless total knee implants with cement. *Clin Orthop* 356:34–38, 1998.
13. Fehring TK, McAvoy G: Fluoroscopic evaluation of the painful total knee arthroplasty. *Clin Orthop* 331:226–233, 1996.
14. Fehring TK, Odum S, Griffin WL, et al: Early failures in total knee arthroplasty. *Clin Orthop* 392:315–318, 2001.
15. Font-Rodriguez DE, Scuderi GR, Insall JN: Survivorship of cemented total knee arthroplasty. *Clin Orthop* 345:79–86, 1997.
17. Furnes O, Espehaug B, Lie SA, et al: Early failures among 7,174 primary total knee replacements: a follow-up study from the Norwegian Arthroplasty Register 1994-2000. *Acta Orthop Scand* 73:117–129, 2002.
18. Gao F, Henricson A, Nilsson KG: Cemented versus uncemented fixation of the femoral component of the NexGen CR total knee replacement in patients younger than 60 years: a prospective randomised controlled RSA study. *Knee* 16:200–206, 2009.
19. Gill GS, Chan KC, Mills DM: 5- to 18-year follow-up study of cemented total knee arthroplasty for patients 55 years old or younger. *J Arthroplasty* 12:49–55, 1997.
20. Gioe TJ, Killeen KK, Grimm K, et al: Why are total knee replacements revised? Analysis of early revision in a community knee implant registry. *Clin Orthop* 428:100–106, 2004.
21. Gioe TJ, Novak C, Sinner P, et al: Knee arthroplasty in the young patient: survival in a community registry. *Clin Orthop* 464:83–87, 2007.
34. Rand JA, Trousdale RT, Ilstrup DM, et al: Factors affecting the durability of primary total knee prostheses. *J Bone Joint Surg Am* 85:259–265, 2003.
37. Sharkey PF, Hozack WJ, Rothman RH, et al: Insall Award paper: why are total knee arthroplasties failing today? *Clin Orthop* 404:7–13, 2002.

The references for this chapter can also be found on www.expertconsult.com.

144

Cementless Total Knee Arthroplasty

R. Michael Meneghini, Lucian C. Warth

INTRODUCTION

Cementless fixation for total knee arthroplasty (TKA) was initially popularized in the 1980s[39,40] and has enjoyed variable rates of success over the three decades since then. Historical registry data demonstrate a relatively small percentage of usage internationally for cementless fixation in TKA, with slightly higher failure rate consistently observed with uncemented fixation.[63] Although historically the orthopedic community has been slow to embrace cementless fixation in TKA, particularly in the United States, interest has been rekindled in large part because of the increasing incidence of TKAs performed in younger,[37] more active, and more demanding patients. In addition, improvements in biomaterials (which may enhance osseointegration and initial component stability), improved polyethylene, and a better understanding of the failure mechanisms of past designs portend a bright future for cementless fixation in TKA. Although cemented fixation has a well-established track record and remains the gold standard,* aseptic loosening with fragmentation and debonding of the cement interface continues to be a major failure mechanism.[18,22,45,53] This is particularly concerning with TKA in the increasing population of young patients[46,47] with whom a more durable biologic fixation method holds the promise of improved longevity.

The modern economics of total joint arthroplasty in an increasingly cost-conscientious health care system is also a major driver leading many to re-evaluate cementless TKA options. There are several potential benefits that may offset implant costs. Improved efficiency and decreased idle time in the operating room during cement curing can yield improved operating room efficiency and translate directly into health care dollars saved.[16] It is documented that decreasing surgical procedure duration has a positive impact on postoperative infection rate, and this may be a potential advantage to cementless fixation in TKA.[60] In addition, the longevity of a biologic ingrowth interface may yield decreased long-term revision burden in patients who would have outlived traditional cemented fixation.

Despite potential advantages, improved materials, and design changes, cementless fixation remains controversial. Past failures in the early cementless implant designs are well documented and are often directly attributable to various design flaws or inferior biomaterials.[6,20,35,55,69] Poor-quality polyethylene, inferior polyethylene locking mechanisms, tibial patch porous coating,[74,77] tibial screw augmentation, fatigue fracture of the femoral component,[78] and patellar failures[3,4,41] have all contributed to poor outcomes. Despite these early failures, certain cementless TKA designs have yielded excellent long-term results on par with those of cemented TKA.[12,29,66,75,76] With the emergence of porous ingrowth metals and improved polyethylene, the current generation of modern cementless designs is an enticing option for fixation in total knee arthroplasty.

EARLY CEMENTLESS DESIGNS: A MIXED BAG

As with early generations of cementless total hip arthroplasty (THA), close clinical follow-up has identified several design-related failures associated with early cementless TKA systems. These unanticipated shortcomings of early designs underscore the significance of close clinical follow-up as new technologies and cementless TKA designs are introduced into the marketplace. The somewhat checkered history of cementless TKA has left us with a cache of knowledge that can be implemented to enhance future designs. In most systems the femoral component has achieved reliable long-term fixation to bone in both hybrid and cementless TKA constructs,[29,30] whereas the tibial and patellar components remained problematic in many series[3,4,41,74,77] and are considered the "Achilles heel" of successful uncemented TKA.

Fixation success seen on the femoral side is likely related to the inherent mechanical stability of the geometrical press fit obtained with multiplanar bone preparation. Although fixation was not an issue, some early-generation cementless femoral component designs demonstrated catastrophic failures because of fatigue fracture of the thin regions of the implant (Figs. 144.1 and 144.2).[14,78] In addition, designs with porous-coated femoral pegs supplement early mechanical stability and facilitate osseointegration but have been shown to cause stress shielding, which can lead to loss of anterior femoral bone stock at revision surgery for cementless TKA systems. Early-generation femoral components, both cemented and cementless, were not designed to optimize patellar tracking[17,73] and likely contributed to polyethylene wear and metal-backed patellar component failure.

Tibial component fixation and design in cementless TKA continues to be a main area of focus. Early designs achieved fixation with short pegs, which did not attain adequate mechanical stability for osseointegration, instead allowing lift-off and subsidence. Moran et al. reported on a series of cementless porous coated anatomic (PCA; Howmedica, Rutherford, New Jersey) TKAs and found a 19% failure rate at an average 64-month follow-up. All failures in this cohort were found on the tibial side, with collapse of the anteromedial tibia, subsidence, aseptic loosening, and severe polyethylene wear.

---

*References 7, 25, 50, 62, 64, 65, and 68.

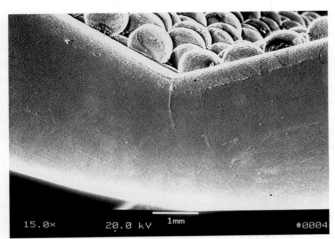

FIG 144.1 A crack originated from the inner beaded surface at the junction between the posterior bevel and distal surface of the nonfractured lateral side in a femoral condyle. The references for this chapter can also be found on www .expertconsult.com (From Whiteside LA, Fosco DR, Brooks JG Jr: Fracture of the femoral component in cementless total knee arthroplasty. *Clin Orthop* 286:75, 1993.)

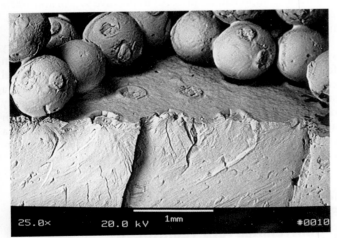

FIG 144.2 Scanning electron micrograph of the inner beaded surface. The fracture joint remnants of several bead craters can be seen. (From Whiteside LA, Fosco DR, Brooks JG Jr: Fracture of the femoral component in cementless total knee arthroplasty. *Clin Orthop* 286:75, 1993.)

The addition of stems or screws to augment initial tibial component stability has been shown in biomechanical studies to minimize micromotion and provide toggle control to prevent tray lift-off. Although supplemental screw fixation can enhance initial stability, there has been reported failure of ingrowth and metaphyseal osteolytic lesions predominating around tibial screw tracks. Berger et al. reported results in a series of 131 consecutive cementless Miller-Galante-1 (Zimmer, Warsaw, Indiana) with an ingrowth tibial interface and screw augmentation, finding an 8% tibial aseptic loosening rate because of failure of ingrowth and a 12% incidence of osteolytic lesions around screw holes at a mean 11-year follow-up. The incidence of screw hole osteolysis is reported to be greater than 30% in some cementless tibial component designs and has been

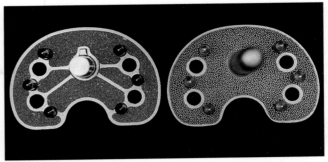

FIG 144.3 Undersurfaces of the Ortholoc Modular (*left*) and Ortholoc II (*right*) tibial components. The Ortholoc Modular has smooth metal bridges around the pegs and screw holes that converge on the central stem. Porous coating covers the entire undersurface of the Ortholoc II component. No bridges of smooth metal connect the joint cavity or screw holes to the smooth stem. (From Whiteside LA: Effect of porous-coating configuration on tibial osteolysis after total knee arthroplasty. *Clin Orthop* 321:93, 1995.)

attributed to the screw holes acting as access channels for particulate debris to the proximal tibial metaphysis.

Although screw holes provide access, the osteolytic process is likely multifactorial and tied to the polyethylene quality, polyethylene thickness, and integrity of the polyethylene locking mechanism. Hoffman et al. reported no cases of screw track osteolysis in a series of 176 cementless Natural-Knee prostheses (Zimmer) at minimum 10-year clinical follow-up. In the next iteration of this design, the Natural-Knee II (Zimmer) screw augmentation was found to be unnecessary by Ferguson et al. This study evaluating 116 consecutive TKA studies demonstrated equivalent stability and ingrowth at average 67-month follow-up in cementless TKA both with and without screw fixation. Therefore one of the factors inherent in osteolysis in uncemented tibial fixation is likely implant design.

Tibial baseplates that contain patch porous coating and/or smooth metal tracks separating pads of porous coating on the undersurface of the tibial tray allow a path of minimal resistance for egress of particulate wear debris and the subsequent development of osteolysis in the proximal tibia.[74,77] Whiteside et al. reported a high rate of osteolysis in the first-generation Ortholoc Modular tibial component (Wright Medical Technology, Arlington, Tennessee), which contained such a configuration (Fig. 144.3). When compared with the next-generation Ortholoc II tibial component (Wright Medical Technology) that used continuous porous coating, no cases of osteolysis in 675 cementless TKAs were identified. These clinical findings support that maintaining a circumferential and fully porous coated cementless tibial tray is important to effectively seal off the tibial metaphysis from particulate debris and can prevent particulate egress and subsequent tibial lysis in cementless TKA tibial designs.

The most commonly reported complication in early cementless total knee arthroplasty designs was failure of cementless metal-backed patellar components.[6,36,44,69] Failure mechanisms included dissociation of the metal-polyethylene interface,[44] dissociation of the peg-baseplate junction because of lack of osseointegration of the baseplate,[69] and excessive polyethylene wear with subsequent metal-metal articulation,[36] proliferative synovitis and pain. These complications were linked to both component design, as well as errant surgical technique, such as excessive femoral component internal rotation. Berger et al.[6] reported a 48% failure rate requiring reoperation for failed Miller-Galante (Zimmer) cementless patellar components, with the two failure mechanisms being failure of ingrowth and excessive polyethylene wear and metallosis.

EARLY CEMENTLESS DESIGNS: SUCCESS STORIES

Despite the early design failures and complications reported with cementless TKA, there are a number of designs that have obtained successful long-term results similar to cemented TKA, with 10-year survival rates greater than 95% (Table 144.1). Hoffman et al. reported on the cruciate-retaining (CR) cementless Natural Knee system (Zimmer), which used a tibial tray with a stem and screw augmentation and a countersunk metal-backed patella, and reported 99.1%, 99.6%, and 95.1% 14-year survivorship for the femoral, tibial, and patellar components, respectively.[29] As with most cementless systems, the majority of failures were attributed to patellar edge wear, and the authors attributed the excellent long-term results to the asymmetric tibial component, augmentation of the bone surfaces with autograft bone slurry, and a countersunk patella component.[29]

Whiteside reported the 10-year results of 163 CR Ortholoc I (Wright Medical Technology) cementless tibial and femoral components.[76] The tibial component had a fully porous coated undersurface with a smooth central stem and smooth pegs, whereas the femoral component had porous coating on the distal three surfaces with smooth anterior and posterior condylar flanges to avoid transmitting axial forces to those bone regions. Considering loosening and infection as failure criteria, Whiteside reported 97% survivorship at 10-year follow-up. However 91 of the original 256 knees were lost to follow-up or had died prior to follow-up in this series.[76] Buechel et al. reported the 20-year results of the Low Contact Stress (LCS; Depuy, Warsaw, Indiana) cementless CR meniscal bearing and rotating platform designs with a rotating-bearing cementless metal-backed patellar component.[11] Using revision for any mechanical reason, including bearing wear, survivorship of the cementless CR meniscal bearing knee was 97% at 10 years and 83% at 16-year follow-up. Survivorship of the cementless rotating platform knee group was 98% at both 10- and 16-year follow-up. The tibial component was fully porous coated, stabilized with a stem and, was without screw augmentation. In

the total 309 cementless tibial and femoral components, there was only one reported tibial component loosening, at 0.9 years in a patient with a failed prior high tibial osteotomy, and no femoral component loosening.[11] A report of 76 CR cementless Osteonics series 3000 (Osteonics, Allendale, New Jersey) TKAs documented a 100% survival rate at 10 years and 97% at 13 years.[75] The femoral and tibial components were both made of cobalt-chrome with cobalt-chrome beads on the undersurface and the tibial components were stemmed and secured with supplemental screw fixation.[75]

The cementless Anatomic Graduated Component (AGC) knee system (Biomet, Warsaw, Indiana) has demonstrated excellent long-term results. The system consists of a CR, nonmodular tibial component with a porous coated undersurface and a grit-blasted central stem without screw fixation. In an update of a previously reported cohort,[34] a series of 73 cementless AGC total knee arthroplasties were reviewed at a minimum of 10 years by the original designer. The investigators discovered a 97% cumulative survivorship at 20 years, with only two cases of tibial component loosening at 1 and 9 years. There were 12 cases of metal-backed patellar failure and metallosis requiring revision.[66] Eriksen et al. also reported on the AGC knee system (Biomet), finding an 84.4% all-component survivorship at 20 years for this system, with the majority of failures attributable to patellar component failures. An impressive 97.2% and 100% 20-year survival was found for the tibial and femoral components, respectively.[21]

It is clear that certain cementless total knee arthroplasty systems provide durable long-term results. The implant design features common in these successful systems include a tibial component that achieved initial implant stability with either a stem, supplemental screw fixation or both. High-quality compression-molded polyethylene in a nonmodular design appears to avoid the problem of osteolysis and using either a countersunk or mobile-bearing patellar component yields satisfactory long-term results if patellar resurfacing is indicated.

MODERN CEMENTLESS TOTAL KNEE REPLACEMENT DESIGNS: IMPROVED BIOMATERIALS AND TECHNOLOGY

Recently developed biomaterials, including hydroxyapatite (HA), and highly porous metals, and improved polyethylene, have demonstrated enhanced wear characteristics and improved biologic fixation. These biomaterials have achieved acceptance

TABLE 144.1 **Long-Term Follow-Up of Traditional Cementless Total Knee Replacement Designs**

Authors	Patient Number	Knee System	Tibial Fixation	10-Year Survivorship (%)	Comments
Buechel et al.	309	LCS	Stem	97	One tibial component aseptic loosening at 0.9 years
Hoffman et al.	176	Natural	Stem and screws	95.10	No screw-associated osteolysis
Ritter et al.	73	AGC	Stem	98.60	Two tibial component failures, 98.6% 20-year survivorship
Eriksen et al.	114	AGC	Stem	97	84.4% 20-year survivorship
Watanabe et al.	54	Osteonics	Stem and screws	100	—
Whiteside	163	Ortholoc	Stem and smooth pegs	94.10	23% lost to follow-up

AGC, Anatomic graduated component; *LCS*, low contact stress.

through clinical success in a wide variety of hip and knee arthroplasty applications, which can hopefully be translated to improve primary cementless TKA designs and outcomes.

HA has emerged as excellent surface coating to facilitate osseointegration of prosthetic components. Soballe et al. documented three times greater interface shear strength with implants coated with HA when compared with titanium alloy without HA.[70] Gejo et al. examined a prospective cohort of patients who underwent CR TKA using the cementless NexGen (Zimmer) knee system with either a titanium porous coated tibial component and supplemental screw fixation or a HA-coated tibial tray without screws.[27] At 12-month follow-up of the 92 knees the authors documented clear zones radiographically under 32% of the tibial components in the non-HA group, whereas the HA-coated tibial components demonstrated only a single clear zone underneath the medial aspect of one tibial tray. The authors suggest the HA provides additional interface strength and bone ingrowth that allows for tibial fixation without screws.[27]

Porous metals, most notably porous tantalum (Fig. 144.4), have emerged as biologically and mechanically friendly options that have a number of applications in knee replacement surgery. In addition to rapid bone ingrowth and increased interface strength,[10] porous tantalum provides improved material elasticity and an increased surface coefficient of friction. The coefficient of friction for porous-tantalum on cancellous bone (0.88 to 0.98) is significantly greater than that previously reported for traditional porous coated and sintered-bead materials (0.50 to 0.66).[15] Furthermore, the modulus of elasticity of porous-tantalum is in between cortical and cancellous bone, significantly less than titanium and chromium cobalt materials. This elasticity of porous tantalum may create a more physiologic stress transfer to the periprosthetic bone, which may affect initial mechanical stability and adaptive bone response, while minimizing stress shielding in the longer term.

Highly porous titanium has also been developed to improve fixation strength to bone through a more biologically friendly macrostructure and microstructure. A canine study was conducted to determine the fixation strength of traditional titanium beads (porosity 30% to 35%), cobalt chrome beads (porosity 35% to 40%), and the newly developed Tritanium Dimensionalized Metal (Fig. 144.5) (Stryker, Mahwah, New Jersey), which is a highly porous titanium surface treatment that has a porosity of 65% to 70%.[26] The authors reported a far greater amount of bone ingrowth and mechanical strength with the Tritanium highly porous titanium over the other two traditional porous surfaces.[26] Ultimately, the advantage of these newly developed biomaterials, such as porous metals, will likely improve cementless fixation and long-term patient outcomes in knee replacement through greater initial mechanical prosthesis fixation and more rapid osseointegration.

If new porous metals enhance the biologic osseointegration of TKA components, the rate-limiting factor to indefinite longevity of these implants will likely become the bearing surface. Crosslinked polyethylene (XLPE) has significantly reduced wear-related failures and osteolysis in THA[58,59,71] yet is less well characterized in knee arthroplasty. Because the cross-linking process changes the mechanical properties of the polyethylene, there has been some trepidation in adopting this technology in TKA because of concerns with fatigue resistance and oxidation, particularly in posterior-stabilized (PS) designs. Several studies have demonstrated equivalent outcomes when comparing XLPE to conventional polyethylene in TKA without catastrophic mechanical failures at early follow-up.[28,38,51] Further follow-up of XLPE is necessary to determine if there will be sufficient benefit to offset increased cost and potential mechanical failures at long-term follow-up; however, XLPE as a bearing surface holds promise in TKA applications. In addition, second-generation locking mechanisms and tibia preparation improved backside wear characteristics in modular tibial designs to reduce particulate debris and associated osteolysis from backside wear.[1,24]

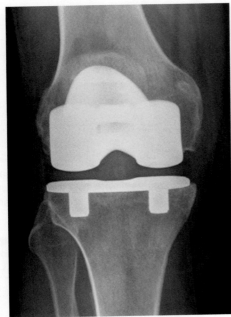

FIG 144.4 Anteroposterior radiograph of Zimmer trabecular metal femoral component with monoblock trabecular metal tibial component (Zimmer, Warsaw, Indiana).

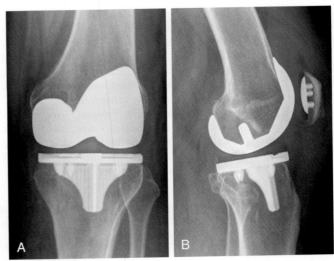

FIG 144.5 (A) Anteroposterior radiograph of Stryker Triathalon TKA. (B) Lateral radiograph, note careful attention was paid to posterior slope of tibial component approximating native posterior slope of tibial plateau to enhance ligament balancing in PS design (Stryker, Mahwah, New Jersey).

MODERN CEMENTLESS TOTAL KNEE REPLACEMENT: EARLY CLINICAL PERFORMANCE

The future of cementless fixation in TKA is very promising. Using the newly developed biomaterials discussed previously, the next generation of implants will ideally preserve bone while providing the necessary mechanical stability to obtain rapid and long-lasting osseointegration. In addition, the fixation strength of the newer materials will likely obviate the need for supplemental screw fixation and the potential for screw track osteolysis that has been observed in some previous designs. Improved wear characteristics associated with new polyethylene and more robust locking mechanisms may minimize the production of biologically active wear particles. Modern tibial components have adopted circumferential ingrowth coating at the bone-implant interface and abandoned supplemental screw fixation to minimize effective joint space and eliminate egress channels for biologically active polyethylene particles to ensure that the bone-implant interface remains stable over time.

Although there are a number of modern designs using porous metals currently available on the market, there is little literature evaluating short- and mid-term clinical outcomes of these implants. An exception is the cementless, monoblock porous Trabecular Metal tibial component (see Fig. 144.4) (Zimmer), which has been shown to exhibit excellent initial mechanical stability[24] with two hex pegs for fixation without screws (Fig. 144.6) and has emerged with encouraging early clinical outcomes (Table 144.2).[23,33,61,72]

In a randomized controlled trial Fernandez-Fairen et al. compared 74 cementless TKAs using the Trabecular Metal monoblock tibial component against the 71 hybrid TKAs using cemented tibial components.[23] Patients receiving the cementless tibiae had slightly improved Knee Society scores (KSSs), as well as Western Ontario & McMaster Universities Osteoarthritis Index (WOMAC) scores, and were found to have no increased frequency of complications, reoperations, or tibial loosening at average 5-year follow-up. Kamath et al. reported on a series of 100 patients younger than 55 years of age who received a cementless TKA with the Trabecular Metal monoblock tibial component.[33] At minimum 5-year follow-up in this cohort, there were no component-related failures, significant radiographic lucencies, osteolysis, or changes in component positioning. In a randomized clinical trial, Pulido et al. compared 106 cementless Trabecular Metal monoblock tibial components against 115 cemented Trabecular Metal monoblock tibial components and a 126 traditional modular cemented tibial components.[61] At minimum of 2 years (mean 5 years), survivorship with revision for all causes as the endpoint was not different among the groups, and the 5-year cumulative risk of aseptic loosening of the tibia was greater in the traditional cemented modular tibia group than in the uncemented cohort (3.1% vs.

0%, respectively). Unger reported average 4.5-year follow-up data on a cohort of 108 cementless TKAs with the Trabecular Metal monoblock tibial component, noting no tibial revision and no progressive lucencies.[72]

These early successes are tempered by the findings of Meneghini et al.[49] in a study of 106 consecutive cementless TKAs using Trabecular Metal monoblock tibial components. In this cohort, nine tibial failures occurred at a mean of 18 months postoperatively and were predominantly identified in tall, heavy, male patients. Although not statistically significant, the authors identified a trend toward the failure group having a greater postoperative varus tibiofemoral angle. Refinements in patient selection, implant design, and surgical technique remain to be made. The early success and acceptance of porous tantalum materials in primary knee replacement[42] has ushered in a new era of cementless TKA designs and strategies. However, mid- and long-term results are required to assess the outcomes of these new designs and compare them with the gold standard of cemented TKA and the excellent long-term results that have been obtained to date.

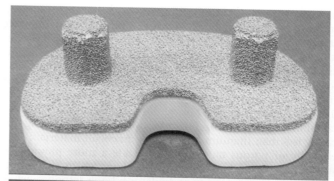
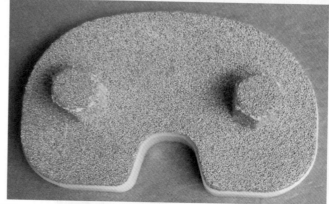

FIG 144.6 Monoblock Zimmer Trabecular Metal tibial component. Initial fixation is achieved with two trabecular metal hexagonal pegs without screws (Zimmer, Warsaw, Indiana).

TABLE 144.2	**Short-Term Follow-Up of Modern Cementless Total Knee Replacement Designs**				
Authors	**Patient Number**	**Knee System**	**PS/CR**	**Mean Follow-Up**	**Tibial Component Survivorship (%)**
Fernandez-Fairen et al.	74	NexGen (Zimmer)	CR	5 years	100.0
Kamanth et al.	100	NexGen (Zimmer)	PS	5 years	100.0
Meneghini et al.	106	NexGen (Zimmer)	PS	3.4 years	84.9
Pulido et al.	106	NexGen (Zimmer)	PS	5 years	100.0
Unger et al.	108	NexGen (Zimmer)	CR	4.5 years	100.0

CR, Cruciate retaining; *PS*, posterior stabilized.

SURGICAL CONSIDERATIONS AND PREFERRED TECHNIQUE

When compared with cemented designs, cementless TKA is a more technically demanding procedure, with less room for error, which can be compounded with each consecutive cut. Cemented fixation is forgiving and achieves maximal fixation strength immediately and can be used as a grout to accommodate bony defects, imperfect surgical cuts, and varying levels of bone porosity. With cementless TKA, optimal cut orientation, cut quality, ligament balance, and limb alignment can minimize micromotion from eccentric loading during knee motion and weight bearing and will improve the biomechanical milieu of the joint, maximizing potential for osseointegration. This is considered an essential surgical principle inherent in the success of cementless TKA, and the performing surgeon should accept very little imperfection in achieving planar cuts and intimate bone-implant apposition.

There is currently little clinical evidence to guide patient selection and determine the optimal candidate for cementless TKA. However it is the contention of the authors that bone quality and viability are essential for mechanical stability and subsequent osseointegration. Furthermore there is biomechanical evidence that supports this notion. Meneghini et al. reported decreased mechanical stability of uncemented tibial components in an osteoporotic bone model, compared with normal controls.[48] The authors further reported that using a keeled design conferred enhanced stability in the osteoporotic model compared with a smaller two-peg designed tibial component and that mechanical stability is dependent on implant design and host bone quality. It is therefore reasonable to reserve cementless fixation in TKA for patients with sufficient bone quality. However, objectively quantifying sufficient bone quality remains a challenge. The authors' current preference is to offer cementless TKA to those patients under the age of 65 who do not have radiographic osteopenia, clinical osteoporosis, or any medical condition that could potentially compromise bone quality such as nicotine addiction, long-term immunosuppression, or autoimmune arthropathy. However, this conservative approach has expanded with success of modern cementless designs to include healthy, active individuals over the age of 65, who are more commonly male and have robust radiodense bone quality radiographically. The final confirmation of sufficient bone quality occurs intraoperatively with a critical visual inspection of the cancellous and cortical bone, along with confirmation of final implant stability with manual assessment.

Component Selection: Cruciate Retaining versus Posterior Stabilized, Fixed Bearing versus Mobile Bearing

The majority of cementless TKA designs with reported long-term results have been of the CR variety. There has been some hesitancy in the adoption of PS implants with cementless tibial fixation because the post mechanism transfers substantial stress through the tibial component to the component-bone interface, where early stability is crucial to osseointegration. Although PS cementless options are currently on the market, there is a dearth of literature regarding the efficacy of these designs at this time. Mobile-bearing implants have been available in some iteration for many years in cementless TKA designs and theoretically

decouple rotational stress from axial and bending forces which may decrease stress transferred to the component bone interface. Although good results have been observed with mobile-bearing designs, the current literature does not support a clinical benefit with respect to ingrowth or longevity over fixed-bearing options. It is currently the senior author's preferred technique to use a CR, fixed-bearing implant. With improved biomaterials for ingrowth and optimized, geometrically forgiving polyethylene, close attention to leg alignment, bone cut alignment, and ligament balance may prove to be more consequential to patient outcomes, irrespective of how the posterior cruciate ligament (PCL) is managed.

Alignment

Overall limb alignment and deformity correction in TKA has been demonstrated to be important to outcomes and patient satisfaction.[19,49,63] Traditional intramedullary femoral guides and extramedullary tibial guides have been the gold standard and had provided adequate deformity correction and long-term clinical success, especially in cemented TKA. Navigation in TKA for the distal femoral and proximal tibial cuts has been shown to reduce outliers,[56,57] although little long-term clinical benefit has been demonstrated to date. Although there is a lack of literature supporting superiority of advanced navigation in TKA, because of the demanding technical nature of cementless TKA, it is the practice of the senior author to use eNdtrack Articular Surface Mounted (ASM) Navigation (Stryker, Kalamazoo, MI). This system allows for navigation of both the femoral and tibial cuts in the coronal plane and sagittal plane and can assist with depth of resection. The senior author has also reported that navigation reduces blood loss in cemented TKA,[43] which may be advantageous in cementless TKA.

Femur

As mentioned previously, cementless femur fixation has been shown to be successful in multiple designs and has shown demonstrated excellent results in both cementless and hybrid constructs. The femur is prepared in standard manner for a cemented PCL-retaining component, with particular attention to accurate planar cuts (Fig. 144.7). After the distal femoral cut is made, the senior author will use a straight osteotome or saw blade to ensure a level and accurate cut because the chamfer and condylar cuts are based off the distal cut via a traditional 4-in-1 guide. In the senior author's current practice the distal femoral cut is navigated to ensure a cut perpendicular to the mechanical axis of the femur without violating the femoral canal, which has been demonstrated minimize blood loss.[43] Blood loss and postoperative hematoma and swelling are of additional concern with cementless implants because there is no cement to tamponade bleeding from fresh metaphyseal bone cuts. Topical or intravenous tranexamic acid and a postoperative drain are routinely used.[31,54]

Tibia

In cementless TKA, achieving rigid initial fixation is a necessity to promote osseointegration, and this has been most vexing to surgeons on the tibial construct. Component design and proximal tibial preparation are important to ensure adequate early stability. Careful consideration should be given to several intraoperative variables, which are technique related. Small surface incongruities may contribute to component lift-off with weight bearing and lead to unacceptable amounts of micromotion at

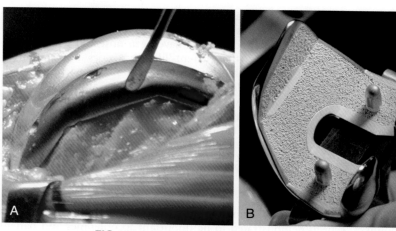
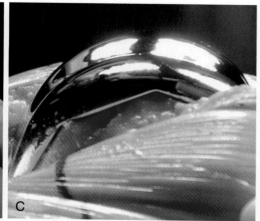

FIG 144.7 (A) Intimate apposition of femoral cuts with trial components. (B) Triathalon HA-coated PS femoral component (Stryker, Mahwah, New Jersey). (C) Intimate apposition of femoral cuts with final femoral implant.

the component-bone interface, which is incompatible with ingrowth. This can be evaluated with the "four corners" technique described by Whiteside (digital impaction of each corner of a flat tibial baseplate trial to ensure no lift-off, which would indicate an irregular cut surface) and is demonstrated in the video supplement provided. It is most common for the saw blade to skive over the hard sclerotic subchondral bone of the diseased compartment, whereas there is a tendency for the saw blade to cut a greater depth of bone off the uninvolved compartment because of the softer bone. Surgeons should be aware of this tendency when cutting the tibia and be vigilant in ensuring an accurate and level tibial planar resection. Care should also be taken to achieve a neutral tibial cut in the coronal plane to minimize shear forces across the bone implant interface with axial load. Irrespective of a gap-balance or measured resection technique, symmetric ligament balance in both flexion and extension will prevent asymmetric loading during motion, which can cause lift-off. Approximating native tibial slope in CR designs will minimize risk of flexion-extension ligament balance mismatch, which may contribute to anterior tibial component lift-off with flexion. The depth of tibial cut is also a potentially important variable when using cementless designs. An aggressive tibial resection with a standard cemented component is often inconsequential and can be ameliorated by increasing polyethylene thickness. In a cementless design a large tibial resection will expose softer bone in the tibial metaphysis, which may be a less ideal substrate for initial rigid cementless fixation, in addition to increasing the proximal tibial strain, which some have postulated to cause medial tibial overload and collapse.[5]

Our preferred technique on the tibial side includes a navigated cut at 90 degrees to the tibial axis in the coronal plane and paralleling the anatomic slope of the tibia in the sagittal plane. A minimal cut is taken to prevent over-resection into soft metaphyseal tibial bone. The four-corner technique is used to evaluate each quadrant of the tibial tray for lift-off, and any irregularities are addressed. A symmetric tibial component with circumferential porous titanium undersurface, a central ongrowth keel, and supplemental crucifix fixation pegs is used (Fig. 144.8). This configuration has been demonstrated to have greater resistance to rocking and lift-off compared with a porous tantalum baseplate with dual-hex peg fixation.[9]

Patella

Viable options for addressing the patella in cementless TKA include nonresurfacing,[13] a cemented all-polyethylene component,[32] or a metal-backed cementless component. As described earlier, most metal-backed cementless components in traditional designs have had a poor track record and have been associated with early polyethylene failure and metallosis. Standard surgical techniques that have evolved to enhance patellar tracking should be used in all cases, irrespective of how the patella is addressing intraoperatively. These include attention to appropriate femoral rotation, tibial rotation, medialization of the patellar component, lateralization of the tibial component, and soft tissue release when necessary. If the surgeon considers resurfacing the patella with a cementless patella, particular attention should be paid to the implant design. Most modern designs incorporate modern tenets of maximizing high-quality polyethylene, highly porous metal ingrowth surface and an optimized robust polyethylene-metal interface to minimize risk of dissociation. Further enhancing the modern cementless patellofemoral articulations are patella-friendly trochlear designs of modern femoral components.

In current practice the senior author discusses all three options with the patient during preoperative counseling; however, a definitive choice is determined after intraoperative assessment for presence of arthritis and evaluation of patellar tracking when trialing components (Fig. 144.9). If there is minimal to no arthritic change of the patella in a young patient and the patella tracks well intraoperatively, then it is left unresurfaced, which has the advantage of preserving patellar bone stock in young patients typically under the age of 60 and is supported with data on selective patella resurfacing.[67] If there is moderate or significant arthritic change, the patella is resurfaced with a cemented component in older patients with less optimal bone quality, as well as patients with borderline patellar tracking. If patellar tracking is excellent and there is significant arthritic change of the patella, a metal-backed cementless component is selectively used in the younger patient typically under the age of 60 (Fig. 144.10). Collectively, the modern advancements in implant designs and biomaterials in conjunction with the improved surgical techniques to optimize patellar tracking provide cautious optimism that cementless patella

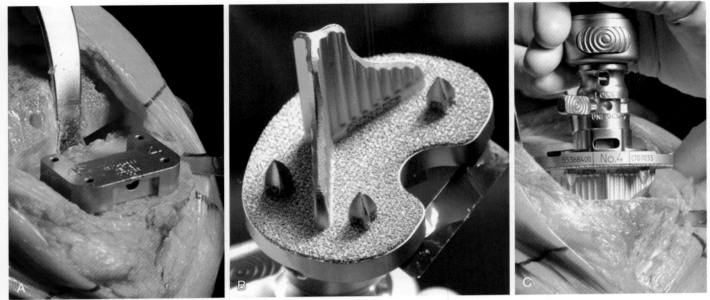

FIG 144.8 (A) Tibial pilot hole guide for cruciform pegs sitting flush on tibial cut. (B) Triathlon tibial component with circumferential porous titanium (Tritanium) undersurface, a central ongrowth keel, and supplemental crucifix fixation pegs (Stryker, Mahwah, New Jersey). (C) Care is taken to impact tibial component parallel to 90-degree tibial cut.

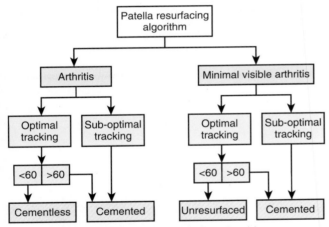

FIG 144.9 Patella resurfacing algorithm.

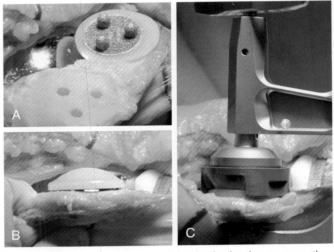

FIG 144.10 (A) Triathlon metal backed tritanium cementless patella, flush freehand patella cut. (B) Care is taken to impact patella component parallel to cut bone surface. (C) Compression device used to ensure uniform bony apposition.

components will enhance patient outcomes with durable and long-lasting fixation.

CLINICAL AND PERIOPERATIVE CONSIDERATIONS

Postoperative management of modern cementless total knee arthroplasty patients is nearly identical to those of cement fixation. Patients are allowed to be full weight bearing and progress in their activity level as tolerated. Intra-articular drains are used to prevent an acute hemarthrosis and are removed the morning the day after surgery. It is the senior author's experience that cementless TKA patients have greater drain output; however, the use of tranexamic acid has been instrumental in minimizing this blood loss in uncemented fixation and is used routinely in all patients.[31,54] Some patients may experience a slight delay in pain resolution during the first 4 to 8 weeks after surgery compared with cemented TKA, which may be attributable to the documented early motion and settling that occurs with cementless tibial components.[2]

Patients are seen in follow-up at regular intervals, and radiographic evaluation is performed with attention to visualizing the bone-implant interface. This requires diligence on the part of the technologist to direct the x-ray beam perpendicular to the implant, so that the prosthesis-bone interface is visualized in line with the planar cut. This methodology is well described in the updated Knee Society Radiographic Methodology.[52]

CONCLUSIONS

The long-term results of cementless total knee arthroplasty designs, combined with examination of early failure of some designs, support the notion that after osseointegration is achieved, fixation and the structural integrity of the bone-prosthesis interface are maintained into the long term. Fixation will likely be enhanced and improved though newly developed biomaterials, such as highly porous tantalum and titanium. If osteolysis is prevented through improved quality polyethylene and minimization of backside wear through modern tibial tray locking mechanisms and nonmodular tibial components, need for revision surgery should be minimal out past 20 years. The bone-preserving nature of cementless TKA, combined with previously mentioned benefits, suggest that cementless total knee arthroplasty is likely the future of knee replacement, particularly in the young patient with an active lifestyle.

KEY REFERENCES

5. Berend ME, Small SR, Ritter MA, et al: The effects of bone resection depth and malalignment on strain in the proximal tibia after total knee arthroplasty. *J Arthroplasty* 25(2):314–318, 2010.

6. Berger RA, Lyon JH, Jacobs JJ, et al: Problems with cementless total knee arthroplasty at 11 years followup. *Clin Orthop* 392:196–207, 2001.

9. Bhimji S, Meneghini RM: Micromotion of cementless tibial baseplates: keels with adjuvant pegs offer more stability than pegs alone. *J Arthroplasty* 29(7):1503–1506, 2014.

10. Bobyn JD, Stackpool GJ, Hacking SA, et al: Characteristics of bone ingrowth and interface mechanics of a new porous tantalum biomaterial. *J Bone Joint Surg Br* 81(5):907–914, 1999.

21. Eriksen J, Christensen J, Solgaard S, et al: The cementless AGC 2000 knee prosthesis: 20-year results in a consecutive series. *Acta Orthop Belg* 75(2):225–233, 2009.

33. Kamath AF, Lee GC, Sheth NP, et al: Prospective results of uncemented tantalum monoblock tibia in total knee arthroplasty: minimum 5-year follow-up in patients younger than 55 years. *J Arthroplasty* 26(8):1390–1395, 2011.

37. Kurtz SM, Lau E, Ong K, et al: Future young patient demand for primary and revision joint replacement: national projections from 2010 to 2030. *Clin Orthop* 467(10):2606–2612, 2009.

43. Licini DJ, Meneghini RM: Modern abbreviated computer navigation of the femur reduces blood loss in total knee arthroplasty. *J Arthroplasty* 30(10):1729–1732, 2015.

47. Meehan JP, Danielsen B, Kim SH, et al: Younger age is associated with a higher risk of early periprosthetic joint infection and aseptic mechanical failure after total knee arthroplasty. *J Bone Joint Surg Am* 96(7):529–535, 2014.

49. Meneghini RM, de Beaubien BC: Early failure of cementless porous tantalum monoblock tibial components. *J Arthroplasty* 28(9):1505–1508, 2013.

50. Meneghini RM, Hanssen AD: Cementless fixation in total knee arthroplasty: past, present, and future. *J Knee Surg* 21(4):307–314, 2008.

51. Meneghini RM, Lovro LR, Smits SA, et al: Highly cross-linked versus conventional polyethylene in posterior-stabilized total knee arthroplasty at a mean 5-year follow-up. *J Arthroplasty* 30(10):1736–1739, 2015.

61. Pulido L, Abdel MP, Lewallen DG, et al: The Mark Coventry award: trabecular metal tibial components were durable and reliable in primary total knee arthroplasty: a randomized clinical trial. *Clin Orthop* 473(1):34–42, 2015.

66. Ritter MA, Meneghini RM: Twenty-year survivorship of cementless anatomic graduated component total knee arthroplasty. *J Arthroplasty* 25(4):507–513, 2010.

67. Roberts DW, Hayes TD, Tate CT, et al: Selective patellar resurfacing in total knee arthroplasty: a prospective, randomized, double-blind study. *J Arthroplasty* 30(2):216–222, 2015.

77. Whiteside LA: Effect of porous-coating configuration on tibial osteolysis after total knee arthroplasty. *Clin Orthop* 321:92–97, 1995.

The references for this chapter can also be found on www.expertconsult.com.

145

Patellar Resurfacing in Total Knee Arthroplasty

Oliver S. Schindler

INTRODUCTION

For a long time, the patella was wrongfully marginalized and merely considered an afterthought during total knee arthroplasty (TKA). Although awareness of the importance of this "somewhat mysterious bone" has gradually removed the patella from its wrongful "Cinderella" status, patellar resurfacing nevertheless remains a procedure all too often thrown in for good measure without a proper understanding of the functional interplay among arthroplasty components. The patella however, whether resurfaced or not, represents an integral part of any TKA, and clinicians must recognize that judicious surgical management of the patella occupies a pivotal role in success or failure of TKA.

Clinicians should therefore possess principle knowledge of patellofemoral anatomy, biomechanics, and kinematics as surgically imposed changes following joint arthroplasty may have significant effects on the clinical performance of the patella. The recognition of the consequences of the mechanical environment on patellar behavior are of particular importance when contemplating patellar resurfacing, because the addition of a third component will invariably add certain complexities to the procedure. However, clinicians are often blasé in their attitude towards technical issues of patellar resurfacing, despite mounting evidence that surgical precision may be crucial for the long-term survival of the implant.

Whether the patella should be resurfaced during primary TKA remains an argument that has deeply divided the orthopedic community for decades and one that has become synonymous to topics of religion or politics. The key element in this debate is embodied by our lack of understanding why irrespective of the management of the patella some patients may suffer pain following TKA and others may not. The fact that neither primary nor secondary resurfacing (SR) is able to predictably reduce anterior knee pain (AKP) is strongly suggestive that more obscure functional or structural pathologies may be responsible for its development other than the patella itself. Despite improvements in surgical technique and implant design, which admittedly have helped to reduce the incidence of patella-related complications, persistent AKP nonetheless remains the largest single source of postoperative patient dissatisfaction. Although symptoms are rarely severe enough to justify revision, they are often sufficient to spoil an otherwise satisfactory result. AKP hence continues to remain the enigma that is fueling the argument for and against patellar resurfacing, and one that has so far stifled our efforts to define a reliable treatment strategy.

With the following chapter the author has tried to provide an overview of the available evidence on a variety of aspects pertaining to the patellofemoral joint and its surgical management in the hope that it may provide clinicians with appropriate insight and guidance.

HISTORY OF PATELLAR RESURFACING

The earliest types of TKAs were pure tibiofemoral replacements, primarily designed to treat severe axial deformities and intractable knee pain in patients affected by tuberculosis or rheumatoid arthritis.[9,161,411,468] The procedure was seen as an alternative to arthrodesis and performed in patients of extremely low demand, for whom any improvement in pain relief or mobility level was considered a success.[470] Patients not infrequently suffered disabling AKP, but rather than addressing the problem by improving the design, the initial response was to promote patellectomy as part of the arthroplasty procedure.[276,411,489] In those days there was a general consensus on the appropriateness of patellectomy, conceived as a procedure of innocuous nature and heralded by many as the treatment of choice for AKP, patellar dislocation, and fracture.[63,66,133,471] Some surgeons even went as far as removing, what Bruce and Walsmley in 1942 described as this *"somewhat mysterious bone,"* as part of a suitable alternative to displacing it during arthrotomy of the knee;[276] it is fair to say that especially those cases not affected by fracture or degenerative disease of the patella often ended up being worse.[6,66,388] Insall et al. reported on four different prosthetic models used in the early 1970s, none of which made any provision to accommodate the patella.[216] Out of 178 patients, 35 received a patellectomy at the time of arthroplasty, and complaints of pain after patellectomy were as frequent as were complaints from those patients in whom patellectomy had not been performed.

Soon clinicians began to recognize the shortcomings of available knee implants, and subsequent design changes focused on proximal extension of the femoral component and creation of a trochlear groove.[101,301,393,406,438] A case in point was the Duocondylar prosthesis, which did not cater for the patellofemoral joint (PFJ), thus yielding mixed results. Changes in the design through the addition of a trochlear flange, allowing the natural patella to articulate with the femoral component throughout the entire range of flexion, significantly reduced the incidence of patellofemoral complications.[351] According to Greenberg et al., this was an era when *"knee arthroplasty was in great part an art as well as a science"* and *"performed with minimal instrumentation and considerable eyeballing."*[170] Arthroplasty surgery in the 1960s and 1970s remained compromised by inadequacy not just in prosthetic design but instrumentation, making it impossible for the surgeon to perform accurate, reproducible TKAs that would yield predictable results. In an attempt to improve outcome, clinicians started to experiment with replacement of the retropatellar surface.[6,175,183]

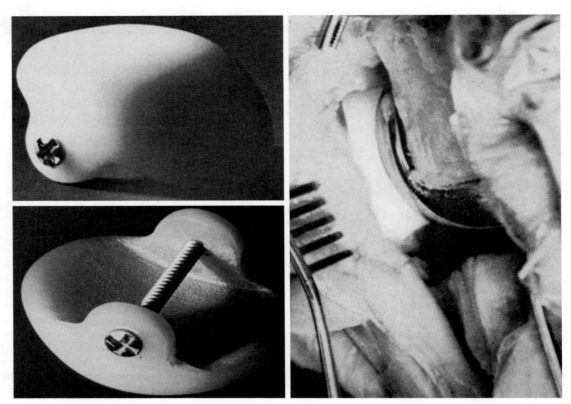

FIG 145.1 Polyethylene patellar component used by Hanslik in 1969 in conjunction with the hinge arthroplasty by Young. (From Hanslik L: Das patellofemorale Gleitlager beim totalen Kniegelenksersatz. *Z Orthop* 109:435–440, 1971.)

In 1969 Lothar Hanslik of Berlin reported the use of a modified version of the McKeever patellar prosthesis made of high-density polyethylene, which he combined with the hinged arthroplasty by Young (Fig. 145.1).[183,184,489] Hanslik was critical of the replacement designs available at that time and argued against patellectomy, stressing the importance of patellar preservation for enhancing the functional outcome. Between 1969 and 1973 he performed 46 procedures, mostly for end-stage osteoarthritis. Results were encouraging, with the great majority of patients walking unaidedly, with only slight or no pain, and attributed to the addition of the patellar implant.[184] The first recorded patellar resurfacing combined with a nonhinged, condylar-type replacement arthroplasty was performed by Groeneveld et al. in 1970.[173-175] The Münster TKA combined a femoral mold arthroplasty with tibial polyethylene disks and a three-pegged polyethylene patellar component with a surface geometry described as "*carina shaped*" (Fig. 145.2). At 2-year follow-up, 64% of patients with a replaced patella had excellent or good results, compared with 46% in whom the patella was left unresurfaced. The authors, however, expressed uncertainty about the long-term survival of the patellar implant and thought that patellar resurfacing should be reserved for cases of persistent pain and used only in combination with a patella-friendly femoral component.

Gunston and MacKenzie developed a patellofemoral arthroplasty designed to work in conjunction with the polycentric knee system in response to the inability to alleviate AKP.[177] A stainless steel patellar button articulating with a grooved polyethylene track placed into the trochlea was used between 1973 and 1976 in several knees, with satisfactory initial results.

However, Gunston was aware that the additional prosthetic components would increase the possibility of complications and therefore urged it not to be used indiscriminately.

Charles Townley of Michigan, who had launched the "Anatomic Total Knee" system in 1972, recognized the importance "*to include an articulating surface for the patella on the femoral component [in order to] eliminate a major source of chronic pain inherent in an arthritic patello-femoral compartment, and to minimise anterior compartment fibrosis and limitation in joint motion*".[438] He later added a polyethylene patellar component, which he first implanted in 1973 (Fig. 145.3).[379,440] For the patella to be placed in its optimum position Townley suggested a self-alignment technique: "*While the cement is still malleable the patella is reduced and the prosthesis is rotated into its accurate articular position with the femoral component and is maintained firmly in this position until the cement has hardened*".[439] In the same year, Eftekhar and a group of clinicians from the Hospital for Special Surgery in New York started work independently on designing a dome-shaped, single-peg patellar implant.[6,122]

Peter Walker recalls that "*in early 1973 contact area studies of the intact knee joint were carried out, and it was decided that for an artificial knee, a dome shape would give the most reproducible contact areas in that it would form 2 contact points in every shape of patella groove whether juxtaposed to a native or artificial knee*" (Peter Walker, personal communication, 2015). The initial patellar implants were made of Co-Cr-Mo and used in isolation for the treatment of localized patellofemoral arthritis, with variable results.[219] The material choice aimed to increase

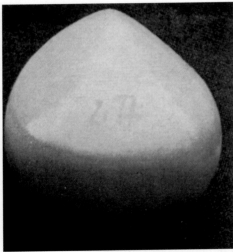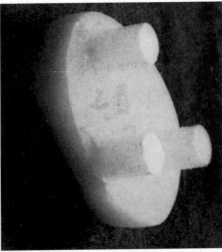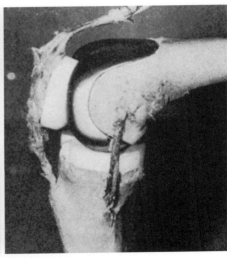

FIG 145.2 Three-peg patellar component used by Groeneveld et al. in 1970 as part of the cruciate-retaining Münster total knee arthroplasty. (From Groeneveld HB: Combined femoro-tibial-patellar endoprosthesis of the knee joint preserving the ligaments. *Acta Orthop Belg* 39:210–215, 1973; Groeneveld HB, Schöllner D, Bantjes A, Feijen J: Eine Kniegelenkstotalendo-prothese unter Erhalt der Kreuz und Seitenbänder. *Z Orthop* 109:599–607, 1971.)

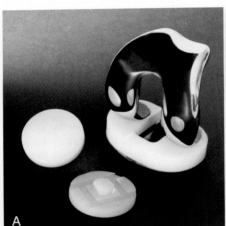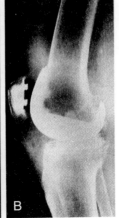

FIG 145.3 Charles Townley's cruciate retaining "Anatomic Total Knee" became the first total knee arthroplasty systems which allowed for optional resurfacing of the patella (A). The cone shaped polyethylene patellar component was first implanted by Townley at Port Huron Hospital/MI in 1973 (B). (Implant courtesy BioPro, Port Huron, Michigan.)

biologic tolerance because polyethylene was feared to wear when articulating with cartilage and bone.[219] Coventry was critical upon such use of a patellar implant because he believed that *"the patella should not be surfaced without a comparable surfacing of the juxtaposing femur."*[101]

The group of Insall subsequently created a variant of their dome-shaped patella, made of high-density polyethylene, designed to be used in conjunction with the total condylar knee. According to Walker the prefix "total" was chosen *"to reflect the fact that all 3 bearing surfaces of the knee joint were replaced"* (Peter Walker, personal communication, 2015). Based on anatomic studies the patella component was offered in two sizes, measuring 30 and 35 mm, respectively, and was first implanted

by Insall and Scott in February 1974 (W Norman Scott, personal communication, 2015). Soon the dome patella was also made available for use with the posterior cruciate ligament retaining Duopatella knee.[218,352,463] The design rationale behind the dome shape was based on its simplicity and tolerance to surgical malpositioning and to prevent binding in the femoral groove at higher flexion angles. Scuderi, Insall, and Scott later described the "central-dome component" as the most adaptive with the least congruency that eliminates concerns about rotational alignment while maintaining contact throughout the flexion arc.[393] Other implant manufacturers followed, and by the beginning of the 1980s almost all available knee replacement systems offered provisions for patellar resurfacing.[172,204,251,463]

In the early stages, patella preparation was by and large performed freehand with an oscillating saw, using an "eyeball technique." Resection guides did not become available until the latter part of the 1980s and were thought to make patellar resection more reliable and reproducible, particularly for the low-volume surgeon. Peterson of San Diego filed the first application for a patella cutting guide at the US Patent Office in May 1985 (U.S. Patent No. 4,633,862), which offered posterior referencing to estimate residual patellar thickness. This was followed by Dunn and Bertin from Salt Lake City and Whitlock and Brown of Austin, Texas, who launched anterior referencing guides in 1987 and 1991, respectively (US Patent No. 4,759,350 and 5,147,365, respectively). However, the use of resection guides has not been without its controversy, and many of the more experienced surgeons continue to prefer freehand preparation combined with haptic assessment.[267,399]

Following on from encouraging results achieved through the addition of a patellar button, a number of different patellar surface designs became established. Hungerford in Baltimore and Walker in Boston started working on developing anatomic saddle–shaped patellae in the late 1970s (Fig. 145.4).[134,204,465] Both believed that an asymmetric, facetted design of an anatomic patella would offer not only superior biomechanical

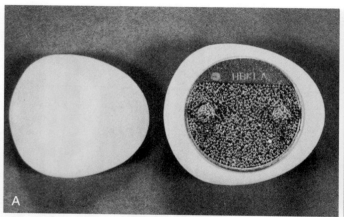
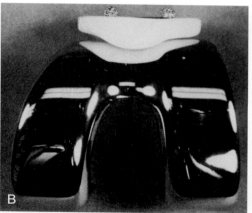

FIG 145.4 Asymmetric anatomic patellar component of the porous coated anatomic (PCA) TKA system designed by Hungerford and Kenna for use without cement and first implanted in 1980 (A). Rotating the patella by 180 degrees allowed it to serve as a left or right implant. The retropatellar surface geometry provided a high level of conformity with the femoral component especially in the early flexion range (B). (From Hungerford DS, Krackow KA, Kenna RV: Total knee arthroplasty. A comprehensive approach, Baltimore, MD, 1984, Williams & Wilkins.)

properties but also improved stability and kinematics (David Hungerford and Peter Walker, personal communication, 2015). Peter Walker, who was working on the kinematic knee at that time, recalls that in *"the femoral component was a geometrical analogue of the anatomic shape of the femur ill-suited for a dome patella. For the patella a saddle shape type was chosen as the ideal geometry, since it provided a much larger surface area of contact on the patella flange. It was asymmetric so the surgeon had to be sure the orientation was correct, which was not immediately obvious when the patella was flipped during surgery"* (Peter Walker, personal communication, 2015).

Buechel et al. of New Jersey designed the first rotating platform patellar implant for either cementless or cemented use.[72] The surface geometry of the polyethylene component was saddle-shaped, asymmetric, and facetted and attached to a metallic anchoring plate. It was designed as part of the mobile bearing New Jersey knee system to articulate with an anatomic femoral component. The device, which was first implanted by Buechel in July 1979, has remained available in its original design within the Low Contact Stress (LCS) and the Buechel-Pappas (BP) knee systems. (Frederick Buechel, personal communication, 2006).

Despite the relative clinical success of cemented, all-polyethylene patellar components, metal-backed patellar implants were introduced in the early 1980s. Metal backing was initially applied to polyethylene acetabular and tibial components to improve load transfer and bending resistance, in addition to allowing for the application of porous metal surfaces for biologic anchoring.[29,361,464] Concerns about the failure of cemented prosthesis through loosening and bone resorption, erroneously thought to be caused by an adverse biologic response to methylmethacrylate, added to the enthusiasm for cementless fixation and the use of porous-coated patellar implants.[204,476] However, the principal advantages of metal backing were applied to the patella without clinical justification.[354]

Hungerford and Kenna developed the Porous Coated Anatomic (PCA), the first uncemented total knee system, which also included a metal-backed patellar implant, featuring 1.5-mm-thick sintered porous coating made of cobalt-chrome beads (see Fig. 145.4).[203,204] It was first implanted by Hungerford in January 1980 at John Hopkins Hospital in Baltimore. Hungerford later conceded that *"we were convinced that cementless fixation at the knee was essential, but which turned out to be less important as we once thought"* (David Hungerford, personal communication, 2015). Problems of polyethylene deformation and wear, fatigue fracture, and component dissociation through locking mechanism failure led to the rapid demise of the metal-backed patella, which by the end of the decade was almost universally abandoned.[31,354,382,430]

Over the past two decades all-polyethylene patellar components have experienced a renaissance and are currently available for the majority of contemporary knee arthroplasty systems. Nonetheless, some niche products, such as the Trabecular Metal Augmentation Patella (NexGen, Zimmer) and anatomic rotating platform patellae (LCS, DePuy; BP-Knee, Endotec), continue to have their place.

BASIC SCIENCE

The articulation between patella and femur is relatively complex and displays intricate biomechanical behavior. Concerns exist with regard to the treatment of the patella in TKA because surgically imposed changes may have significant effects on kinematic performance and transfer of forces within the patellofemoral joint.[117] Patellar tracking, contact area, and pressure distribution are known to differ quite significantly between native and prosthetic knee.[132,209,210,428] The understanding of the mechanical environment of the PFJ is therefore of particular importance when developing knee replacement systems that provide low levels of complications, a high level of patient satisfaction and clinical long-term success.

Matthews et al., who investigated the load-bearing characteristics of the patellofemoral joint, remarked, *"High patello-femoral load values, small patello-femoral contact areas, and resultant high stress magnitudes indicate the need for caution in the design and development of a patello-femoral component for total joint replacement prostheses."*[286] Analysis of retrieved patellar components and the significant failure rate of metal-backed

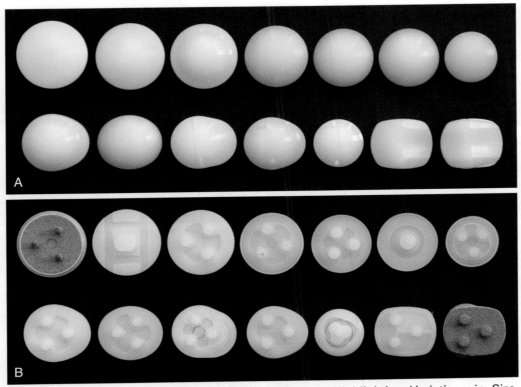

FIG 145.5 Selection of Different Patellar Components Highlighting Variations in Size, Surface Geometry, and Fixation Methods A, Uncemented Townley TKO, Biopro; cemented Townley TKO, BioPro; Triathlon, Stryker; AGC, Biomet; Evolution, Wright Medical; Advance, Wright Medical; Vanguard, Biomet. B, Triathlon offset, Stryker; PFC-Sigma, DePuy; Journey offset, Smith & Nephew; Stryker medialized dome, Stryker; Genesis biconvex, Smith & Nephew; fixed bearing LCS, DePuy; uncemented mobile bearing LCS, DePuy.

patellar designs underscored the extreme mechanical environment in which these implants are expected to perform.*

A successful patellofemoral articulation must henceforth be designed to function under high-stress conditions and over a long period of time because ground reaction, gravitational, ligamentous, and muscular forces all act to produce significant compressive, shear, and torsional loads.[172,307,407] Thus both design and materials used must be at least compatible with the mechanical forces of up to 5× body weight (BW), as encountered during activities of daily living.[390]

Patellar Component Design

The multitude of patellar components currently available reflects the lack of consensus with respect to the ideal design (Fig. 145.5). Although articular surface geometries of patellar components vary greatly, they can be classified into five basic shapes: convex or dome shaped; modified dome shaped or Gaussian; anatomically or saddle shaped; cylindrical; and mobile bearing (Figs. 145.6 and 145.7).[242] Every implant design bears particular advantages regarding conformity, stability, forgiveness, and wear pattern, with none being ultimately superior. However, advantages attributed to a particular design should not be generalized to all designs of similar shape because the behavior of a particular patellar component is directly

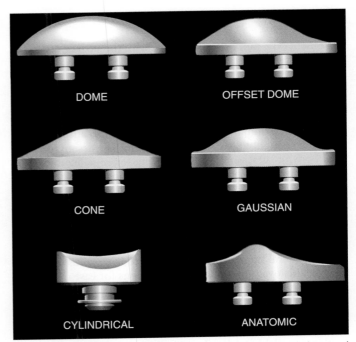

FIG 145.6 Principle surface geometries of commonly used patellar component types.

*References 10, 31, 95, 99, 200, 266, and 392.

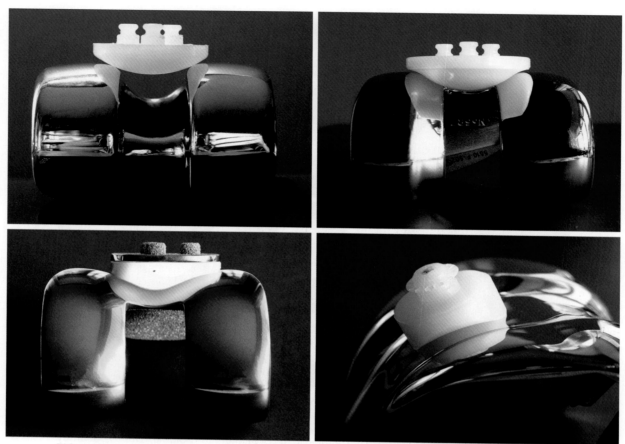

FIG 145.7 The four principle patella surface geometries of *(clockwise)* dome, Gaussian, cylindrical, and anatomic, articulating with their designated femoral component (Scorpio, Stryker; Triathlon, Stryker; Medial Rotation Knee (MRK), MatOrth; BP-Knee, Endotec).

dependent on a number of variables, with the surface geometry of the juxtaposing femoral component probably being the most important.†

Although Insall pointed out that *"in an articulation, the softer material should be concave,"*[213] traditionally most patellar components have been dome shaped. Based on engineering principles such a configuration is far from ideal because a convex surface is thought to wear poorly. However, the design offers an axial body of rotation, thereby allowing for considerable tolerance in component placement. Anatomic and cylindrical patellar component address this issue by providing a more desirable surface configuration with larger contact areas that delivers better wear characteristics. Such implants are inherently more stable but require careful positioning because potential advantages can easily be offset by component malalignment.

As a general trend, clinicians appear to favor spherical patellar implants over anatomic patellar designs for ease of application because they are less prone to surgical malalignment.[213,356,371] Whether this trend is truly based on surgeons' choice or driven by manufacturers remains debatable, especially if one considers the relatively small number of anatomically shaped patellar implants available to date (see Fig. 145.5).

Dome-Shaped Patella. The majority of currently available patellar components belong to the dome-shaped type, which as a result of their spherical surface geometry have also been referred to as axisymmetric.[6,242] In the dome patella the mating geometries between patella and femur are simple spherical shapes, which usually provide congruency only in the early flexion range up to 70 degrees. At higher flexion angles the patella rests against the inner surface's convexities of the femoral condyles, exposing the patella to high stresses and point contact (see Fig. 145.7). Some of these problems have been addressed successfully through design adaptation of femoral condylar and trochlear geometries. Extension of the trochlear groove concavity onto the inner portion of the femoral condyles has provided for an increase of patellofemoral congruency in flexion.

The principal advantage of dome-shaped components compared with all other designs is their ability to allow for flexion and rotation to occur in various planes, without binding of the implant against the femoral component (Fig. 145.8).[213,482] Rotatory alignment is thus less critical, highlighting the relative forgiveness of dome-shaped patellae regarding minor degrees of malpositioning. Its current prevalence is therefore in itself an offshoot of its practicality. However, despite their excellent clinical results, failure of cemented, all-polyethylene, dome-shaped patellar components is not uncommon, particularly

---

†References 89, 115, 291, 434, 435, and 488.

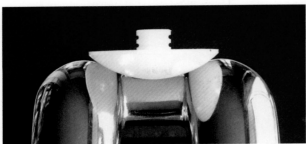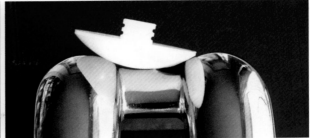

FIG 145.8 Axisymmetric spherical patellar implant designs can compensate for a limited degree of patellar tilt and rotation by maintaining contact with the juxtaposing femoral component. (Insall-Burstein II, Zimmer.)

after prolonged periods in service and attributed to the exposure to high contact stresses.‡

Modified Dome-Shaped or Gaussian Patella. The "Gaussian patella" or "sombrero hat" is a modification of the dome patella, designed to improve the articulation with the convexities of the femoral condyles, especially at higher flexion angles. The component is characterized by a central projection surrounded by a transitional concavity that develops into a circumferential flat region, thus emulating a Gaussian graph. Its surface geometry allows for a closer match with the inner curvature of the femoral condyles in the axial plane (see Fig. 145.7).[62,457]

The increased material thickness at the sides reduces the risk of deformation, especially in activities of high flexion. Singerman et al. showed that patella shear forces for Gaussian types are significantly lower when compared with simple dome-shaped designs.[413] Thus it is not surprising that wear simulator studies have confirmed increased durability of such components when tested against standard dome types.[199]

Anatomically Shaped Patella. Prostheses with anatomic surface profile have distinct lateral and medial facets and are referred to as "one-plane symmetric."[242] They provide a more conforming articulation with an increased contact area and reduced contact stresses between patellar flanges and femoral component, thereby decreasing the risk of subluxation (see Fig. 145.7).[70-72,164,186,203] Walker showed that an anatomically shaped patella, articulating in an anatomic groove, is stable at all angles of flexion without tilting, as long as the Q angle is no greater than 14 degrees.[466]

A variety of anatomically shaped patellar implants have been available over the years, including mobile bearing variants. Although anatomic patellar implants make the most sense theoretically, they have introduced a number of complexities into the instrumentation and surgical technique. Because of their high-level congruency, they are more sensitive to malpositioning, and appropriate orientation toward the juxtaposing trochlea is essential for their proper function.[275]

Cylindrical Patella. The cylindrical patellar component occupies a fringe position in TKA.[148,487] The initial idea was developed by Freeman and Swanson in the late 1970s, who attempted to combine a high level of congruency with relatively large contact areas throughout flexion of up to 110 degrees.[149-151] Because of design specifics, the patella becomes highly dependent on a close matching geometry of the femoral component in both coronal and the sagittal plane, requiring a femoral trochlea of single radius (see Fig. 145.7).[150,248] The diameter of the patellar component is reduced to 25 to 30 mm, allowing the implant to be recessed into the patella, similar to an inlay technique. Subsequently, the remaining patellar rim participates in articulating with the femoral component and in further assisting stress dissipation. The patellar implant possesses a central peg with a collar and can be used with or without cement. If left uncemented the implant retains some ability to self-align, although fibrous ingrowth may eventually halt this process.[21,248,446] Despite concerns of being rotationally constrained, the design concept has provided for satisfactory function and pain relief, with 10-year survival rates of 96% to 98.4%.[150,248,279,448]

Mobile Bearing Patella. A different biomechanical concept has been conceived with the anatomically shaped, mobile bearing, metal-backed patella (see Figs. 145.5 and 145.7).[69,71,72] The design is based on the same principle as rotating platform tibial components. It allows for the articulating part of the component to rotate up to 30 degrees clockwise and counterclockwise, thereby maintaining optimal alignment within the trochlea groove. Laboratory testing has shown that contact areas remain relatively high compared with the native patella, whereas contact stresses remain well below those of dome-shape types.[226,306] The absence of significant backside wear in mobile patellar bearings has led some clinicians to believe that these devices may not actually rotate in service. Therefore, it has been speculated that the advantages of mobile bearing patellae may be their ability to compensate for variations in surgical alignment by rotating into a preferential position after engagement with the femoral component and simply to stay there.[79,291]

Although not generally affected by complications otherwise associated with metal-backed prostheses, failures caused by fracture, wear, and dissociation of the polyethylene element have been described.[201] Overall, the clinical performance record of mobile bearing patellae has been relatively good, with reported survival rates of up to 99.5% at 12 years in single surgeon series.[223] However, some registry data have shown lower survival rates for resurfaced compared with unresurfaced LCS TKA.[273]

‡References 31, 99, 113, 144, 147, 200, 392, and 483.

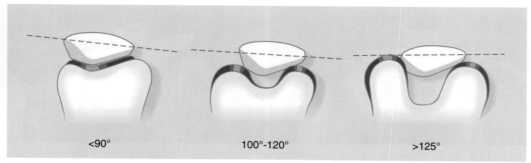

FIG 145.9 Patellofemoral contact areas at various degrees of knee flexion. Bifurcation of patellofemoral contact beyond 100 degrees of knee flexion. Odd facet of patella engages with the medial femoral condyle between 125 and 135 degrees of knee flexion. Red dotted lines indicate changes in patellar tilt angle in the coronal plane during flexion. (Adapted from Schindler OS, Scott WN: Basic kinematics and biomechanics of the patello-femoral joint. Part 1: the native patella. *Acta Orthop Belg* 77:421–431, 2011.)

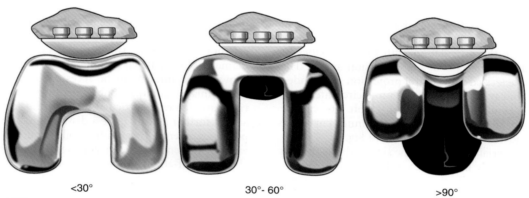

FIG 145.10 Patellofemoral relationship in resurfaced TKA. Point contact in extension and early flexion, because of limited conformity between patellar implant and femoral flange; line contact in mid-flexion (30 to 60 degrees), due to increasing conformity between patellar implant and trochlea; bifurcation of contact area beyond 90 degrees. (Adapted from Schindler OS: Basic kinematics and biomechanics of the patellofemoral joint part 2: the patella in total knee arthroplasty. *Acta Orthop Belg* 78:11–29, 2012.)

Patellar Contact Area

In the native knee the size of the contact areas is highly dependent on knee position and proceeds from the distal pole in full extension to the proximal pole in full flexion (Fig. 145.9). From 20 to 60 degrees of flexion the average contact area increases linearly from approximately 150 to 480 mm^2.[6,286,442] It then remains almost constant up to approximately 90 degrees of flexion, after which a linear reduction occurs.[168,202] Because of the drastically changed contact pattern beyond 100 degrees, when the patella leaves the trochlea straddling the intercondylar notch, contact areas may fall well below 100 mm^2.[168]

The mechanical environment of the replaced PFJ differs significantly from the natural knee. The contact area in the prosthetic patellofemoral joint measures, at best, no more than 40% of that of the native knee.[§] Measurements obtained experimentally vary widely and depend on the technical setup and the level of compression force applied during testing. For dome-shaped designs, contact areas range from 13 to 162 mm^2, with highest values usually observed between 30 and 90 degrees of

knee flexion (Fig. 145.10).[306] Values for modified dome-shaped, anatomic, and cylindrical patellar components are generally higher because of the increased level of conformity, with contact areas of up to 325 mm^2.[226,283,306,425,459] Kim, Rand, and Chao assessed contact areas of eight different patellar designs articulating with their designated femoral component. The largest contact area was identified for the rotating patella of the DePuy LCS and the smallest for the two-plane symmetric dome of the DePuy PFC, with a difference between the two of more than 125%.[242] Although the contact area in anatomic implants is characterized by area contact on both facets, those of dome or cone shape type generally present line contact (Fig. 145.11).

Up to 75 degrees of flexion, the contact area between prosthetic patella and femur is relatively large and contact pressures generally low. As with the native patella the area of contact on the patellar component moves proximally with increasing flexion, reaching the superior patellar pole between 60 and 90 degrees, depending on trochlea design (Fig. 145.12). Beyond this point the patella leaves the trochlea in most arthroplasty designs, leading to bifurcation of the patellofemoral contact area (see Figs. 145.10 and 145.13).[388] The transition from a one-area to a two-area contact is associated with a significant

§References 188, 242, 283, 306, 433, and 486.

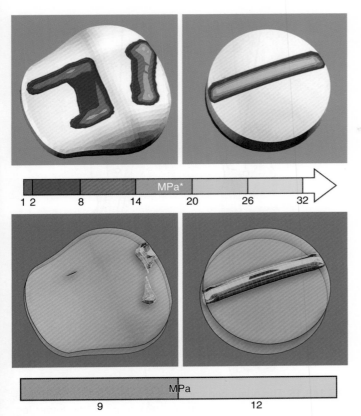

FIG 145.11 *Top row:* Surface contact stress distribution for anatomic and dome patellar implants simulating stair ascend (45 degrees knee flexion, PRF = 1760 N). Area contact and lower average stress values for anatomic compared with line contact and increased contact stresses for the dome implant. *Bottom row:* Equivalent images showing distribution of von Mises subsurface stress, illustrating the volume of polymer stressed above 9 MPa.

decrease in contact surface, whereas patellofemoral compressive force continues to rise. The direct influence of this transition in contact area on wear pattern can be observed in retrieved patellar components, which demonstrate deformation and development of characteristic facets at the margin of the polyethylene patellar surface (Fig. 145.14).[123,199,289,291,483]

Patellofemoral Kinematics in Total Knee Arthroplasty

Kinematics of the knee joint characterize the relative motion that exists between femur, tibia, and patella.[423] The patella is a sesamoid bone implanted within the tendon of the extensor mechanism. Arguably its most important property is its role in facilitating extension of the knee by increasing the efficacy of the quadriceps muscle.[189] To achieve this, the patella functions as a fulcrum, thus anteriorly displacing the line of pull and increasing the moment arm of the quadriceps muscle force in relation to the center of rotation (COR) of the knee. The patella has been shown to enhance the force of extension by as much as 50% throughout the entire range of motion.[423] The patella also facilitates improved distribution of patellofemoral reaction force (PRF) through an increase in contact area during flexion. In addition, the patella acts as a guide for the extensor mechanism by centralizing the divergent pull from the four muscles of the quadriceps and transmitting these forces to the patella tendon. Together with the anatomic shape of the patellofemoral articulation, this protects the extensor apparatus from dislocating.

As with the native patella the motion path of the resurfaced patella is complex and influenced by extrinsic stability, provided by muscle and soft tissue support, and intrinsic stability, provided by implant design. Extrinsic stability is based on the interplay between relatively static retinacular structures, which mainly provide guidance to the patella, and the dynamic stabilizing function provided by the extensor muscles. When contracted, the quadriceps apparatus, being oblique in its angulation towards the patella and patella tendon, creates a line of pull with

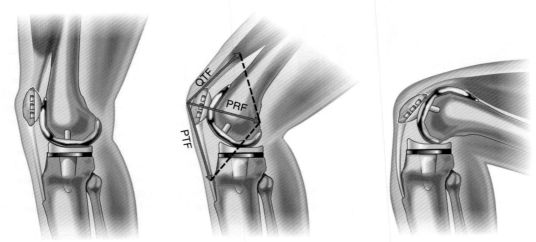

FIG 145.12 Changes of patellar position in the sagittal plane in relation to the femoral component. With increasing flexion the patella rotates around a transverse axis and moves in a posterior direction with the femur, whereas the patella contact area progresses proximally. Simplified free-body diagram (parallelogram of forces) is shown in the central image, depicting the force vectors acting on the patella. The patellofemoral reaction force *(PRF)* is the resultant vector of the quadriceps tendon force *(QTF)* and the patella tendon force *(PTF)*. (Adapted from Schindler OS: Basic kinematics and biomechanics of the patellofemoral joint part 2: the patella in total knee arthroplasty. *Acta Orthop Belg* 78:11–29, 2012.)

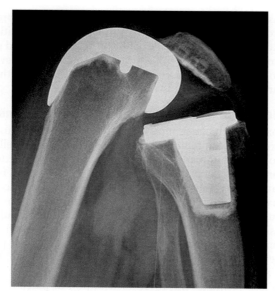

FIG 145.13 Lateral roentgenogram showing the position of the patella in a cruciate-retaining TKA at approximately 150 degrees of flexion when kneeling. The proximal portion of the patella component maintains minimal contact with the femoral component by straddling its condyles, thereby drastically reducing contact area.

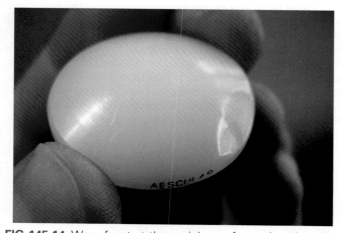

FIG 145.14 Wear facet at the periphery of a retrieved patellar component, created through point contact with inner margins of femoral condyles at higher flexion angles. This is typically observed with dome-shaped implants and considered part of a wearing-in process in partially congruent patellofemoral articulations and described as "conforming deformation."

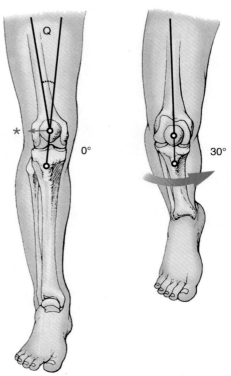

FIG 145.15 The quadriceps or Q angle (average 5 to 7 degrees), a measure of the overall rotational alignment of the lower leg, is affected by the knee flexion angle. As the knee progresses from full extension into flexion the tibia rotates internally, reversing the screw-home mechanism. This neutralizes the Q angle and assists in centralizing the extensor mechanism. Please note the lateral force vector (*) which may influence patellar stability in early flexion. (Adapted from Tria AJ Jr, Klein KS: An illustrated guide to the knee, New York, NY, 1992, Churchill Livingstone.)

an outward directed horizontal component. The angle between the line of pull and the patella tendon is often referred to as the Q angle, which is responsible for a tendency of the patella to shift outward onto the lateral femoral condyle, creating a lateral force vector (Fig. 145.15).[140] To offset this propensity, the lateral condyle projects farther forward while the fibers of vastus medialis, which secure the patella medially, extend farther distally.[423]

The patella is drawn into the trochlea groove during the initial 30 degrees of knee flexion. This process is aided by the reversal of the "screw-home mechanism," which essentially derotates the tibia, leading to a reduction in Q angle (see Fig. 145.15).[51,141,167,297,299] The patella is most vulnerable in early flexion up to 30 degrees because of a lack of mechanical engagement into the trochlea while the effect of the Q angle, albeit reduced, has not yet neutralized (see Fig. 145.10).

Intrinsic design stability is defined as the capacity of the implant alone, with or without patellar resurfacing, to resist interaction between implant and muscular, capsular, or ligamentous structures. The geometry of the prosthetic components, as well as surgically imposed changes, will bring with them a plethora of variables, which all have the potential to influence patellar tracking. However, even in a well-aligned and balanced total knee prosthesis the resurfaced patella will present a complex three-dimensional movement pattern broadly similar to the native knee, and predominantly consisting of translation, rotation, and tilt in sagittal, axial, and coronal planes.[228,256,313,366]

Stiehl et al. assessed patellar kinematic patterns with fluoroscopy.[429] The authors demonstrated that patellar axis rotation, which compares the angle between the patellar tendon and the sagittal axis of the patella, increases with flexion in TKA beyond the levels observed in normal knees. Contact position of dome-shaped and anatomically shaped patellar components showed greater variability compared with the normal knee, with the average contact position for the resurfaced patellae lying more superior, while tilt angles are increased. However, the kinematic behavior of an anatomically shaped or an unresurfaced patella more closely resembled normal knee kinematics, compared with those observed with dome-shaped designs.

The complexities of the patellofemoral movement pattern highlight the difficulties in reproducing natural patellar kinematics when resurfacing the patellofemoral joint.[453] Although an unconstrained patellofemoral articulation would allow the patella to move relatively unrestrictedly, it requires a low level of conformity between the mating surfaces, which in turn would lead to an increase in contact stresses. In contrast, a highly conforming articulation will constrain patellar movement, imparting unwanted shear forces, which may increase the risk of patellar subluxation and component loosening.

In a cadaver study, Kim et al. assessed the effect of patellar kinematics on the contact area of dome, modified dome, anatomic, and rotating patellar designs.[242] Under optimal tracking conditions the contact areas of the dome-shaped patella were significantly smaller compared with the modified dome and anatomic designs. However, when exposed to three-dimensional movements, the contact area of the dome-shaped patella was significantly greater, indicating enhanced forgiveness regarding patellar malpositioning, whereas modified dome and anatomic components appeared more sensitive to patellar malalignment.

Patellofemoral Biomechanics in Total Knee Arthroplasty

The mechanical environment of the replaced patellofemoral joint differs quite significantly from the natural knee and is biomechanically disadvantaged by having smaller contact areas through which high contact stresses are transferred.[337,388,390] Anterior patellar strain, a measure of the effect of external forces on the geometric configuration of the patella, shows a threefold increase following TKA.[289]

The forces transmitted by the patella originate from the pull of the quadriceps, resulting in a tension force in the patellar tendon and a contact pressure force between the patella and the trochlea. The patellofemoral reaction or compressive force is acting perpendicular to the articulating surface of the patella and is equal and opposite to the resultant of the patella tendon

and quadriceps force (see Fig. 145.12). In addition, a tangential or sideways component of force may occur in coronal and axial plane, which is referred to as the lateral force vector (see Fig. 145.15). It is a function of the directional forces of the quadriceps and the Q angle. It diminishes with knee flexion and reductions in Q angle and is balanced by the reaction occurring on the slope of the femoral trochlea.[462] "In the midrange of flexion, the condition for lateral stability of the patella is that the angle of inclination of the lateral trochlear groove is larger than the Q-angle" (Peter Walker, personal communication, 2010). The lateral force vector is generally small but may be sufficient to create patella subluxation especially if amplified through increases in Q angle.

The term patellofemoral compressive force, representing the sole load acting on the patella, and PRF may be used interchangeably, although it is conceivable that the resultant (reaction) force produced by the quadriceps mechanism at different angles of flexion may be broken into normal (compressive) and tangential force components (Seth Greenwald, personal correspondence 2011). In a simplified model, these forces act coplanar (in the sagittal plane) and even concurrent, in such a way that it is permissible to consider them as a single resultant force. In vitro studies have shown that these forces can be quite considerable, with PRF values of $1.2 \times BW$ for simple activities, such as walking on level ground, $5.7 \times BW$ for descending stairs or rising from a chair, and $7.7 \times BW$ for jogging (Table 145.1). In vivo studies have so far looked only at peak forces generated within the replaced tibiofemoral joint, confirming values of $1.3 \times BW$ for biking, $2.7 \times BW$ for walking, $3.8 \times BW$ for tennis, and up to $4.5 \times BW$ for golf, and those for the patellofemoral joint are assumed to be even higher.[97]

The level of contact stress is directly influenced by the magnitude of the contact force (PRF). Contact stress, measured in megapascal ($1 MPa = 1 N/mm^2$), is defined as force divided by the area over which the force is applied. It will increase with a rise in reaction force but decrease with an increase in contact area. When considering the magnitude of the PRF, it has to be remembered that this force acts through an area that varies with knee flexion.[280,441,462] Thus an increase in PRF does not necessarily assume an increase in patellofemoral pressure. As we know from the native knee, the increase in patellofemoral

TABLE 145.1   Patellofemoral Joint Reaction Forces for Various Activities

Author	Activity	Body Weight (kg)	Knee Flexion Angle (Degree)	Peak PRF (N)	Peak PRF (BW)
Reilly and Martens[360]	Level walking	70	10	334	0.5
Morra and Greenwald[306]	Walking gait	—	15	420	0.6
Bresler and Frankel[57]	Level walking	71	20	840	1.2
Ericson and Nisell[131]	Cycling	71	83	905	1.3
Morra and Greenwald[306]	Stair ascent	—	45	1760	2.5
Kaufman et al.[231]	Isokinetic exercise	81	70	—	5.1
Kelley et al.[237]	Rising from a chair	—	90	3800	5.5
Andriacchi et al.[15]	Stair descent	71	60	4000	5.7
Huberti and Hayes[202]	Isometric extension		90	4600	6.5
Reilly and Martens[360]	Squatting	85	130	6375	7.6
Winter[479]	Jogging	72	50	—	7.7
Wahrenberg et al.[461]	Kicking	76	100	5800	7.8
Smith[415]	Jumping	—	—	—	20
Nisell[319]	Quads tendon rupture	—	—	10,900-18,300	14.4-24.2
Zernicke et al.[490]	Patellar tendon rupture	—	90	—	25

BW, Body weight; PRF, patellofemoral reaction force.

contact area with flexion up to 90 degrees, together with the "turn-round" phenomenon of the quadriceps tendon beyond 90 degrees, helps to dissipate the PRF.[168,172] However, despite these compensatory mechanisms, we observe a net increase in patellar contact stress during flexion in TKA as reaction forces increase disproportionately compared with the contact area.

The magnitude of PRF is a function of implant design. It is important to ensure that the combined articulating surfaces of patella and femoral components allow rotation about the transverse axis, thereby accommodating the changing angle between quadriceps mechanism and patellar tendon (see Fig. 145.12). This maintains the PRF not only to the articulating surface but also to the fixation interface of the patella. Thus allowing shear stresses at the fixation interface and loading at the patellofemoral surface to be kept at tolerable levels.

Force transmission in the patellofemoral joint is dependent on the relationship between the center of gravity (CG), its distance to the COR of the knee and the knee flexion angle.[25,106] Changes of posture in the sagittal plane (leaning forward or backward) will alter the distance between CG and COR, thereby leading to substantial differences in static force transmission.[25] Patients with quadriceps weakness can rise from a chair by leaning forward, bringing the CG closer to the knee. Similarly there are significant differences between ascending and descending stairs, with predicted PRF values for stair ascending of up to 2.3 × BW, compared with up to 6 × BW for descending.[15,337] In ascending stairs, the lever arm is reduced through leaning forward, whereas the opposite is true for descending, when the CG is moved further backward behind the patellofemoral joint to maintain balance (Fig. 145.16).[390]

Following TKA, patients are more likely to experience difficulties on descending rather than ascending stairs, which is not simply an equation of increased PRF values.[386] Ascending a standard step requires knee flexion to approximately 65 degrees, whereas the tibial plateau maintains an almost horizontal alignment. On descending, approximately 85 degrees of flexion is necessary and the tibial plateau becomes almost vertically inclined, thereby allowing the downward force of the BW to drive the femur anteriorly (see Fig. 145.16). This anterior subluxation potential of the femur is primarily resisted by the patellofemoral mechanism. However, some of the forces are absorbed by either the PCL in cruciate-retaining implants or cam-post engagement in posterior stabilized implants, both of which function as checkreins. In an attempt to reduce such forces, Hungerford has suggested that patients suffering AKP may want to consider "*descending stairs either sideways or backward, which is biomechanically equivalent to ascending stairs with its decreased mechanical and range of motion demands.*"[205]

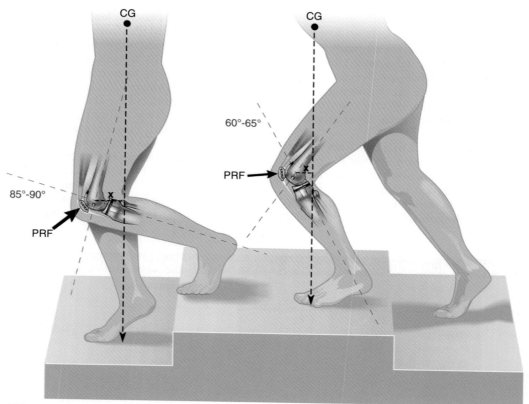

FIG 145.16 Biomechanical differences between ascending and descending stairs. On stair descend, both the distance *(X)* between the center of gravity *(CG)* and the center of rotation, and the knee flexion angle are increased, thereby creating longer moment arms and a rise in the patellofemoral reaction force (PRF) (*). At the same time, the tibial plateau becomes more vertically aligned, thus enabling the force of body weight to impart an anterior subluxation force onto the distal femur, which is likely to further increase PRF. (Adapted from Schindler OS, Scott WN: Basic kinematics and biomechanics of the patello-femoral joint. Part 1: the native patella. *Acta Orthop Belg* 77:421–431, 2011.)

Research has shown that certain patient demographics, such as younger age, above average body mass index (BMI), and increased postoperative flexion, especially in those patients of high demand, are likely to further increase the level of compressive and shear forces on the patellar component during knee flexion.[123,292,324] In addition, the particular geometry of the patellar component and the moving center of loading produced by knee mechanics and interaction with the femoral trochlea impose peculiar stresses on the patellar fixation site. The resulting strains are compressive, shear, and tensile in character and presumed to be relatively small. They are often referred to as "micromotion" and implicated as a mechanical contribution to loosening.[45]

The fixation surface of all-polyethylene onlay patellar components has also been subject to biomechanical investigations. Large, single central fixation pegs, which were particularly popular in the 1970s and 1980s, require significant bone removal, leaving only a relatively shallow bone bridge below the peg (see Fig. 145.3).[6] This creates focal stress raisers, which have been implicated with increasing the risk of patellar fracture.[62,92] However, despite such concerns, some single peg designs have performed particularly well, even over the long term.[234] Single peg designs have nevertheless been largely superseded by those in which three smaller fixation pegs are placed peripherally onto the retro surface of the implant. Such an arrangement is subject to less stress compared with pegs placed centrally, especially if pegs are oriented in a transverse direction.[88] The construct of three pegs has been shown to avoid precarious bone weakening and provides better resistance against tilt and rotational forces.[250,282] However, inlay patellar components of convex, biconvex, or cylindrical configuration continue to use single peg fixation (see Fig. 145.5). These pegs are usually quite small in size, and the low rate of complication with this technique may be because of the additional strength gained through peripheral bone preservation.[130,279]

Material Science and Performance of Patellar Implants

Patellar component wear because of force concentration remains a major concern in TKA (Fig. 145.17).[10,95,113,199,392]

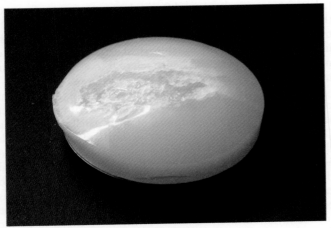

FIG 145.17 Retrieved metal-backed patellar component affected by a variety of different modes of wear, including cold-flow, pitting, delamination, abrasion, and burnishing.

Owing to the great disparity between moduli and strength of cobalt-chrome alloys on the one hand and ultra–high-molecular-weight polyethylene (UHMWPE) on the other, *wear* is primarily observed on the polymeric side of the prosthetic patellofemoral articulation. Wear is known to be particularly rapid when stress is concentrated on areas in the periphery of the implant where polyethylene is relatively thin. This has been well illustrated through excessive wear recorded in metal-backed patellae where the polyethylene thickness in the periphery was seriously compromised because of design requirements. Wear may be further accelerated if the implant is maltracking. Allen et al. observed significant surface damage in 59 out of 69 patellar components retrieved during revision surgery, with burnishing, abrasion, and pitting being the most prevalent modes of wear (see Fig. 145.17).[10] The severity of damage was directly associated to the time the implant had spent in situ, with a significant increase being noted if the implant had been in service beyond 2 years. Dome-shaped components generally exhibited more severe wear than conforming implants of Gaussian or saddle shape. The authors also noted that patellar implants articulating with an asymmetric femoral component showed decreased levels of creep, presumed to be because of improved patellar tracking.

Notwithstanding its limitations, UHMWPE has evolved as the material of choice for the patellar component, based on the low friction principle.[87] Mechanical properties of UHMWPE are far from ideal, with *yield* strength affected by the level of molecular weight, degree of cross linking, and sterilization method (Seth Greenwald, personal communication, 2012). Uniaxial yield strength of UHMWPE, which equals the lowest stress at which the material undergoes plastic deformation, is estimated at approximately 23 MPa.[28,95,369,422] Concerns have been raised if such stresses are applied continually. For industrial applications, repeated maximum contact stresses of 10 MPa have been recommended, a value which incidentally is identical to the yield strength estimated for articular cartilage.[364] Buechel et al. have even suggested that, for long-term human use, maximum contact stresses of 5 MPa may be more appropriate because body temperature may further reduce the strength of UHMWPE by up to 25%.[71] In vitro contact stress analysis has confirmed that all-polyethylene, dome-shaped patellar components produced contact pressures between 20 and 30 MPa in extension, rising to between 36 and 100 MPa at 90 to 120 degrees of knee flexion, therefore exceeding the yield strength of UHMWPE by up to 400%.[95,209,242,291,486] Anatomically shaped, rotating platform patellar components produced significantly lower values, mostly staying below the yield strength of UHMWPE.[95,291] Wear simulator studies further confirmed that congruent patellar components (Gaussian and anatomic) exhibited significantly lower rates of creep and wear than dome-shaped designs, again indicating that conformity is critical to wear resistance and protection against post-yield deformation.[95,197,199,466] Polyethylene damage is also correlated with the design of the femoral component.[10] Symmetric femoral components and those that exhibit a relatively small radius of curvature on the edge of the femoral condyles have been shown to inflict significantly more damage to patella implants than asymmetrical implants and those with a larger radius of curvature (see Fig. 145.7).[10,482]

Xu et al. demonstrated the effect of patellar resurfacing on contact area and pressure in cadaveric knees.[486] The mean contact area between 30 and 120 degrees of flexion in the nonresurfaced patellofemoral joint ranged from 70 to 150 mm², whereas peak patellar contact pressures did not exceed 12 MPa. After being resurfaced, the mean contact area decreased almost 10 fold to 10 to 15 mm², creating a dramatic increase in patellar contact pressure values of 50 to 100 MPa. Greenwald et al. performed biomechanical studies assessing patellar surface contact area, compression force, and contact pressure, using a variety of different prosthetic models (see Fig. 145.11).[85,306,426] The authors found that patellofemoral contact pressure values at knee flexion angles beyond 45 degrees exceeded polyethylene yield strength in all tested components, with peak measurement of up to 75 N/mm² (=75 MPa).[85,306]

Steubben et al. measured the distribution of patellofemoral surface stresses by mapping areas above and below the tensile *yield* strength of polyethylene.[425,426] All implants, whether of dome, modified dome, or anatomic shape, demonstrated material yielding throughout the range of flexion. Their results indicated the importance in appreciating the location of the yield areas within a given patellar component because rim loaded contact areas above yield are more likely to deform and *wear*. According to Greenwald *"polymer integrity does not rest primarily with the size of the contact area, but rather with the extent of the surface within this region which exceeds yield condition"* (Seth Greenwald, personal communication, 2011).

Subsequently, contact stresses above the *yield* strength do not necessarily lead to catastrophic failure as has been demonstrated by the not infrequent finding of relatively undamaged retrievals. Because highest values of contact stress are experienced during flexion, variations in patients' activity may not expose the patellar component to large cyclic loads frequently enough to accumulate damage. McNamara et al. considered the constraining effect of surrounding polyethylene responsible for this phenomenon.[291]

Viscoelastic properties of surface cartilage allow for its deformation under load and subsequent increase in pressure transmitting area. Because of differences in elastic modulus between cartilage and UHMWPE, the prosthetic patella has limited ability to change its surface contact area through variations in patellofemoral load.[37,192,199,291]

However, yield in polyethylene is characterized by plastic deformation, also known as "creep" or "cold-flow," rather than brittle failure, which explains why nonconforming patellar components are capable of "wearing-in."[37] Retrieval studies have shown that creep of polyethylene occurs independent of *wear*, which permits adaptation to the tracking position.[99,142,482] Unlike other modes of polyethylene damage, plastic deformation does not result in material removal and, as such, does not represent true wear. However, in most circumstances, creep often occurs in conjunction with burnishing, a form of "wear polishing" characterized by localized surface abrasion.[10]

Over a period of time this process can lead to typical surface adaptations at the margin of spherical patellar implant often described as facets (see Fig. 145.14).[92,199,291] Flattening of the polymer geometry at high-stress locations is thought to be of benefit in reducing surface stress by increasing component conformity. Although it is unclear whether this process may lead to detrimental alterations in patellar kinematics, it has so far not been associated with obvious clinical problems. Scuderi, Insall, and Scott described this phenomenon, which has been noticed almost universally on retrievals of prosthetic domes as *"conforming deformation."*[404,433]

Although reductions in contact stresses of 23% to 58% through increased conformity have been reported, contact stress values generally remain above the UHMWP yield strength.[95,123,188] Elbert et al. were surprised that, despite artificial *"wearing in"* of a polyethylene patellar surface into a concave shape, the von Mises stress (a criterion used in predicting the onset of yield in ductile materials) was at or near the polyethylene yield stress in most of the contact areas, an indication that deformation might continue.[123] Williams found, via analysis of von Mises stress, that most stresses above yield strength occurred 1 to 2 mm below the articulating surface area in the newly manufactured component (see Fig. 145.11).[477] However, in retrieved components, von Mises stress remained near yielding through the depth of the implant. Because of subsurface stresses, permanent deformation may henceforth be expected to continue even when the component has "worn-in."[123] Although Collier et al. conceded that *"all-polyethylene patellar components are not the answer as an ideal bearing surface,"* in the absence of a suitable alternative, UHMWPE is likely to remain the material of choice at least in the foreseeable future.[95]

Implant Design Issues: Femoral Component Design

The patella, whether native or prosthetic, cannot be considered in separation, because it works in direct partnership with the femoral component (see Fig. 145.7). Motion constraints of the patella are determined by the surface geometry of the femoral component, which is referred to as "intrinsic stability," and by the balance of soft-tissue forces, which is referred to as "extrinsic stability." Bartel et al. highlighted the importance of conformity in prosthetic design by demonstrating that contact area and contact stress are highly dependent on the congruency of the patellofemoral joint articulation.[28,29]

Following on from the disappointing results of early arthroplasty designs, which frankly ignored the patellofemoral joint, an array of design changes to the femoral component were suggested to improve patellofemoral function.[406,438] It is generally believed that a more congruent patellofemoral articulation with a deepened trochlear groove that extends both proximally and distally together with a built-up lateral trochlear wall is likely to provide for improved patellar tracking and enhance patella stability (Fig. 145.18).[89,406,488] Current femoral implant designs display a wide variation in length, depth, and orientation of the trochlear groove, sagittal radius, and axial geometry.[115,435] Anatomically shaped femoral components conform to the native trochlea and intercondylar notch topography, which take the geometry of the native patella into account.[474] Such implants are particularly suitable when articulating against the nonresurfaced patella, and hence referred to as being "patellar friendly" or "conforming" (Fig. 145.19).

The increased conformity between native patella and femoral component maximizes surface contact and minimizes contact stress, thereby facilitating minimal biologic patellar remodeling (Fig. 145.20).[71,134,235] Nonanatomic designs are those in which the trochlear groove is concave spherical and designed to accommodate a nonanatomic patella usually of dome-shaped design. Proximal extension of the femoral flange will help to capture the patellar implant during early flexion, whereas extension of the concave shape of the trochlear groove onto the intercondylar surface will allow for increased metal-to-plastic contact at higher flexion angles.[378,394,488]

Freeman believes that the design of the trochlea is the key feature in providing satisfactory clinical results.[124,148,248] He has

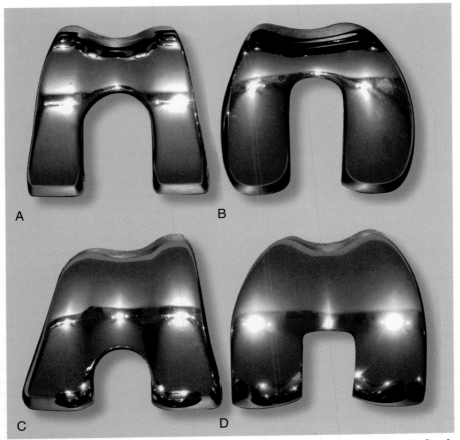

FIG 145.18 Femoral Component Designs Displaying Various Degrees of Patella Conformity and Subluxation Resistance (A and B) Relatively nonconforming universal design, featuring a symmetric, short trochlear groove and a wide intercondylar notch. Abrupt transition of the inner convexity of condyles in (A) and shallow trochlea sulcus in (B). (C and D) Relatively conforming and side-specific femoral design, featuring an asymmetric, deepened, and extended trochlea groove with an elevated lateral flange. Implant (D) more closely emulates the anatomic analog of the native femur. (Implant A and C courtesy of Leo Whiteside of the Missouri Bone & Joint Research Foundation, St. Louis, Missouri.)

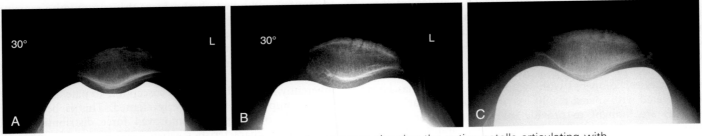

FIG 145.19 Postoperative skyline roentgenograms showing the native patella articulating with three different prosthetic femoral components displaying varying degrees of conformity. (A) Optetrak, Exactech, USA; (B) AGC Biomet, USA; (C) LCS, DePuy, USA.

postulated that the floor of the prosthetic trochlea, viewed from the side, should be circular (single radius), similar to the native knee, extending from 0 to 110 degrees of flexion (see Fig. 145.7). Furthermore, it should be recessed to an anatomical extent to restore the patellofemoral joint line, a feature not to be confused with the height of the patella in relation to the tibiofemoral joint. In a large cohort study using such a design, Kulkarni et al. found no clinical differences between resurfaced and native

patellae at a mean follow-up of 10 years.[248] Based on this observation, it has generally been accepted that increasing the radius of curvature and deepening of the trochlear groove reduces patellofemoral shear and compressive forces.[85,89,343,435]

Biomechanical studies have looked at the potential merits of single-radius femoral components and suggested that a more posterior flexion–extension axis would lengthen the extensor mechanism moment arms, thereby improving extensor

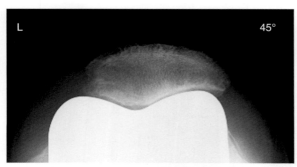

FIG 145.20 Skyline roentgenogram obtained 3 years following total knee arthroplasty, demonstrating increasing conformity between patella and femoral component through a process known as biologic remodeling or stress contouring. (From Schindler OS: The controversy of patellar resurfacing in total knee arthroplasty: Ibisne in medio tutissimus? *Knee Surg Sports Traumatol Arthrosc* 20:1227–1244, 2012.)

mechanism function. Browne et al. showed a reduction of up to 18% in patellofemoral compressive force and 14% in quadriceps tension at knee flexion angles between 50 and 90 degrees when comparing a single to a multi-radius femoral component.[64] Whether such theoretical advantages can be replicated in vivo remain uncertain because they may be offset against paradoxical sliding and rotational pattern known to affect cruciate-retaining implants.[427,429]

The importance of femoral component design and its influence on the clinical performance of the patellofemoral has been highlighted by Theiss et al. based on outcome results of two arthroplasty designs with distinct differences in trochlear geometry.[435] A 14-fold decrease in patellar-related complications was observed when using a patellar-friendly design with an extended anterior flange, and a deeper and wider trochlea groove. The authors concluded that more proximal capture of the patella in a deeper groove with more gradual proximal-to-distal transition appeared advantageous in reducing patella morbidity. Similar results have been reported by Kavolus et al., who analyzed patellar complications using two different posterior-stabilized TKA systems. Avascular necrosis, patellar fracture, and patella clunk syndrome were significantly less frequent when using the asymmetric and conforming NexGen TKA compared with the symmetric and nonconforming IB-II design.[232]

The effect of valgus alignment of the trochlear groove on shear stresses, compared with symmetrical designs, has been investigated with mixed results. Asymmetric trochlear groove designs are thought to provide for earlier patellar capture through prominence of the lateral flange and to decrease the predominant valgus force vector, thus reducing patellar shear.[114] In some reports, reduction in lateral shear forces of up to 10% was observed, whereas others saw either no effect or even a shift towards the generation of medial shear forces.[89,114,343,435] However, potential clinical advantages of asymmetric designs are still lacking compelling clinical proof.[43,89,464]

Compressive and lateral forces acting at the patellofemoral articulation increase with knee flexion.[464] The magnitude of the lateral forces, which are dependent on valgus alignment, Q angle, and soft tissue balance may, if excessive, cause patellar subluxation and contribute to component failure. Steubben et al. investigated the resistance offered to lateral subluxation of

the resurfaced patella by defining the intrinsic lateral stability of various patellofemoral designs.[425,426] They disregarded surgical variables, such as component placement, alignment, and correction of varus and valgus deformity but recognized their importance in assisting this process. They found that the mediolateral component of force was highly dependent on the interaction of condylar and patellar surface geometry. All tested implants presented force values required to produce lateral subluxation at or above those measured for the native knee. Force values of up to 2250 N at 90 degrees were generated by some designs, representing a sixfold increase compared with the native patella, highlighting that appropriate design changes (eg, deepening of the trochlear groove) can significantly increase resistance to patellar subluxation.[425,426]

Some experimental evidence also exists that the depth of the trochlear groove may be a more important variable in the prevention of patellar subluxation than the shape of the articulating surface itself.[85] However, excessive deepening of the trochlea groove will decrease the moment arm of the quadriceps muscle force as the patella is brought closer to the COR of the knee. In an experimental study, Yoshii et al. demonstrated that specific femoral design changes, including deepening and distal extension of the trochlea groove and elevation of the lateral trochlear flange, improved patellar tracking compared with an unmodified femoral component (see Fig. 145.18).[488]

The question on conformity or nonconformity between femoral and patellar components has engaged bioengineers and clinicians since the advent of patellar resurfacing.[366,428,429,452,453] The level of conformity between femoral and patellar prosthetics influences the joint's ability to tolerate natural variations in motion, potentially limiting the patella's ability to follow its natural movement path.[366,428,453] Conformity increases contact area and stability, whereas nonconformity allows the patella to establish an "equilibrium of forces" and avoids excessive shear forces from arising. Potential advantages of conforming designs may hence be offset by an increase in constraint, potentially resulting in deleterious effects on patellar tracking and fixation. This typically leads to a compromise, whereby conformity and subsequently contact areas are reduced to avoid overconstraining the joint. However, the question of how much contact area to sacrifice and how to best achieve this compromise remains unanswered.

From a biomechanical point of view a femoral component with an anatomic trochlea articulating with an asymmetric anatomic patella of matching conformity would appear, at least theoretically, to be a very suitable combination because it is inherently more stable and less susceptible to patellar tilt, provided components are properly aligned. This is because of enhanced contact profile, improved force distribution, and better wear characteristics when compared with spherical designs.[306,466,482] A dome-shaped patella placed against a circular trochlea of matching radius would be similarly stable, even if rotated. However, juxtaposing the native patella against a non-anatomic trochlea will cause the patella to tilt laterally, whereas a dome in an anatomical groove would be liable to excessive wear and deformation.[289]

A number of studies assessing the effect of patella-friendly implant designs on functional outcome suggested improvements after TKA without resurfacing.[50,76,134,273] On the other hand, evidence exists that is suggestive of non–patella-friendly spherical designs achieving better functional outcomes with resurfacing.[83,334,469,481] Whatever the surgeon's preference may be, it would appear prudent not to underestimate the importance of the choice of implant and its potential effect on the performance of the patellofemoral joint.

Effect of Patellar Retention

If the patella is retained during TKA, its retropatellar surface becomes exposed to the metallic trochlea of the femoral component. Because of differences in the modulus of elasticity, the articular surface of the patella must adapt to the geometry of the opposing surface by bedding-in. This process of remodeling, also known as "stress contouring," produces gradual adaptation of the retropatellar surface and subchondral bone plate to the trochlear shape (see Fig. 145.20).[211,417] Keblish et al. observed that minimal remodeling was required if the patella was exposed to an anatomic design with constant radius of curvature and uniform femoral geometry, whilst remodelling appeared to be excessive in nonanatomic designs.[236] The remodeling process is time dependent and not displayed on axial radiographs much before 2 years after implantation.

Matsuda et al. assessed patellofemoral contact stress and contact area following TKA by comparing a nonconforming dome patella, a conforming anatomic patella, and an unresurfaced patella with those values obtained in the native knee.[283] In the unresurfaced patella, peak contact stress and contact area remained almost at the level of the native knee. Following patellar resurfacing, patellofemoral contact stress rose beyond yield strength for UHMWPE, with an average increase of 200%, whereas patellofemoral contact area decreased on average by 60%. The authors concluded that, although the effect of metal action on cartilage was uncertain, the option of leaving the patella without a prosthetic component remains an attractive one. This is thought to apply especially to those cases in which the patella is not severely worn, because peak stresses are known to be closer to normal if the patella is left unresurfaced.

The choice of prosthetic design has proven even more critical when the patella is left unresurfaced.** Most current femoral components present a surface geometry intended to articulate with a designated patellar component but are ill equipped to accommodate the native patella (see Fig. 145.19).[274,284,466]

Tanzer et al. looked at the effect of femoral component designs on contact and tracking characteristics of the unresurfaced patella in TKA.[434] The authors noted substantial alterations in patellofemoral contact areas, contact pressures, and tracking at higher flexion angles when the native patella was articulating with a prosthetic femoral component. The percentage of patellofemoral contact area compared with the native knee reduced markedly with increasing knee flexion, with measured values of 79%, 69%, and 65% at 60, 90, and 105 degrees, respectively.

The surface geometries of some prosthetic femoral components, particularly those of posterior-stabilized design, often appear incompatible with the native patella because the apex of the retropatellar ridge may impinge on the roof of the intercondylar housing at high flexion angles. Patellar deformation and wear are likely consequences, and, in the case of significant patellar tilt, displacement of the patella into the notch becomes possible.[289] Whiteside's group showed that distal extension of the trochlea and shortening of the intercondylar notch safeguarded patellar support beyond 90 degrees of knee flexion (see

Fig. 145.18).[488] Such design modifications are thus important if one considers leaving the patella unresurfaced.

Effect of Cruciate Retention or Substitution

Moment arms affecting the patella are dependent on the distance between the patellofemoral joint to the axis of rotation (flexion and extension) of the femoral component. They are increased if the axis is deviated posteriorly from its physiologic position. Femoral rollback facilitates this process and represents a characteristic feature of normal knee kinematics. Increased rollback effectively lengthens the patellar moment arm, thus increasing the efficacy of the extensor mechanism.

D'Lima et al. investigated the influence of various degrees of posterior femoral rollback on patellofemoral compressive force.[115] Posterior substituting (PS) designs add an intercondylar cam-post mechanism to prevent anterior femoral subluxation and posterior femoral displacement in high flexion.[467] The sagittal and frontal geometrics are typically defined by connecting radii generally resembling the total condylar, whereas the intercondylar cam-post is designed separately, usually contacting from mid-flexion to maximum flexion. In such designs the lateral and medial condyles are often symmetric, providing no lateral or medial bias to the motion. Femoral rollback resulting from cruciate retention (CR) produces reductions in patellofemoral compressive force of up to 7% throughout knee flexion, whereas the effect in PS devices only becomes noticeable after cam-post engagement, with maximum effect recorded at 85 degrees of knee flexion.

Miller et al., comparing CR with PS designs, failed to note femoral rollback when the PCL was retained.[300] They stipulated that the absence of the anterior cruciate ligament may render the PCL ineffective, which may explain the appearance of paradoxical movements (reverse rollback) observed on fluoroscopic investigation.[109,110,115] Although PCL substitution kept patellofemoral forces close to the level of the native knee, a lateral release became necessary in 50% of knees, raising potential concerns about an increase in patellofemoral stress through ligamentous tension.[300] This notion has also been expressed by Ranawat and Sculco, who raised concern that femoral rollback through cam and post engagement may increase tensile forces across the patella in flexion.[350,352] Overall, patellar thickness following resurfacing should therefore not exceed preoperative values, particularly in PS designs because this may tighten the extensor mechanism, create loss of flexion, and increase both anterior patellar strain and PRF.[118,298,365,421,443]

Clinical results in some series not only indicated increased requirements for lateral retinacular release but also a higher than normal proportion of patellofemoral complications.[94,215,249,443] In 1982 Insall et al. reported an overall incidence of patellofemoral complications, with the original PS condylar prosthesis of 11%, the great majority of which were the result of patellar fractures and soft tissue impingement.[215] After appropriate modifications to the femoral component, issues associated with patellar fracture became less prevalent, whereas impingement continued to be present in up to 20% of patients.[4,424] However, such problems have not been reported universally, and some TKA systems appear to fare better than others, suggesting that performance of this type of implant may be design specific.[5,91,232]

Some concerns have been raised with regard to potential impingement of the tibial post against the patellar component in deep flexion. Verborgt and Victor found that post

---

**References 49, 207, 274, 283, 284, 321, 434, and 435.

impingement was associated with raising the joint line, patella baja, anterior placement of the tibial component, and smaller femoral component size.[454] However, the clinical significance of this remains unclear.

SURGICAL TECHNIQUE

Satisfactory TKA can be defined in terms of clinical and technical objectives. Basic clinical objectives are to relieve pain and to improve function, but to achieve this goal technical objectives have to be met. Despite major contributions exerted by the specific geometry of the arthroplasty itself, proper patellofemoral function is ultimately dependent on good, reproducible surgical technique and an understanding of the principles of biomechanics of the PFJ.[245,332,353,354] Surgical decisions may compensate to some extent for implant design limitations but conversely may also exacerbate them.[116] The patella functions in a complex arrangement between the extensor mechanism and tibiofemoral articulation, and the ultimate goal is to centralize the quadriceps muscle force and thereby maintain the patella at its ideal position. Re-creation of physiologic leg alignment, Q angle, and joint line, appropriate component rotation, and balancing of the extensor mechanism are all key ingredients in achieving this goal irrespective of whether or not the patella is resurfaced in the process. The surgeon is thus required to adhere to the following surgical principles.[245,330,381]

1. Restoration of physiologic patellofemoral spacing (composite thickness)
2. Re-creation of retropatellar high point through correct placement of the patellar implant
3. Restoration of the patellofemoral relationship (joint level)
4. Restoration of the rotational alignment of the femoral and tibial components
5. Balancing of the patellofemoral soft tissues

Mistakes that are known to detrimentally affect patellar tracking are manifold and relate to component mismatch and sizing errors (eg, undersized patella, overstuffing), component malpositioning (eg, lateralization of patellar component, internal rotation and medialization of femoral component, internal rotation of tibial component, excessive joint line elevation >8 mm), overall leg malalignment (eg, excessive valgus or varus), and ligamentous imbalance.[††]

In all of this the Q angle remains the most significant factor influencing patellar tracking. Any increase of the Q angle beyond normal limits will lateralize patellar tracking and if severe enough will lead to patellar subluxation or even dislocation. Deviation from the ideal patellar tracking pattern is often the manifestation of a technical error or a combination of minor errors and, according to Pagnano and Kelly, should be considered a *"red flag."*[330] Proceeding directly with a lateral retinacular release may improve patellar tracking but should only be considered after the surgeon is satisfied that there are no errors in rotational, translational, or angular alignment of the arthroplasty components. It should be remembered that surgical improprieties may exert a cumulative effect on patellar tracking and stability, potentially leading to disastrous results. If maltracking is not corrected, it may increase shear stresses at the fixation site, which are likely to increase the risk of implant loosening and wear and thus affect the long-term survival of the patellar component.[235,446]

††References 16, 34, 300, 312, 356, 365, and 378.

The surgeon should bear in mind that intraoperative assessment of component positioning is unable to account for the effect of muscles and tendons on the kinematic behavior of the patella. Thus it is not surprising that, despite careful surgical technique, postoperative patellar tilt often occurs, because intraoperative tests may underestimate the effect of the dynamic function of the extensor mechanism.[42,213,330] Scott has described this phenomenon *"dynamic patellar instability,"* which is occasionally seen in patients who present with significant preoperative swelling and stretching of the medial retinacular structures.[394] It rarely causes functional disability but may potentially contribute to accelerated patellar component wear.

Femoral Positioning

In resecting the distal femur, care must be taken to maintain the articular surface relative to the attachments of the collateral ligaments. In addition, any mismatch between anteroposterior depth of the native knee and the prosthesis has to be avoided because it alters patellofemoral spacing and extensor mechanism offset, thereby preventing the patella from maintaining its ideal position in relation to the femur (Fig. 145.21).

The patella is particularly sensitive to malrotation of the prosthetic implants of the femur and tibia.[17,162,413] Internal rotation of the femoral component is known to create an unfavorable mechanical environment for patellar tracking because it lateralizes the direction of pull of the extensor mechanism. Furthermore, it will force the lower leg into valgus malalignment during flexion and create gross alteration of the foot progression angle during gait (Fig. 145.22). The situation is often compounded because the internally rotated femur necessitates subsequent internal rotation of the tibial component to establish rotational congruency (Fig. 145.23).

Placing the femoral component in 3 to 5 degrees of external rotation relative to the posterior condylar axis and parallel towards the transepicondylar axis (TEA), improves patellar tracking, and proximal patellar engagement (Fig. 145.24).[36,213,347,381] The basis for this evolved from Insall's "gap" theory designed to correct any mismatch in flexion gap created through cutting the proximal tibia perpendicularly to its long axis, rather than emulating its natural varus alignment.[100,305,333,381] Whiteside et al. found patellar tracking pattern and contact areas to be closer to normal when the femoral implant was externally rotated by approximately 5 degrees in relation to the PCA (Fig. 145.25).[17,19,312] Singerman et al. recorded a 17% increase in patellofemoral contact force when the femoral component was internally rotated by 10 degrees, whereas external rotation by the same amount reduced contact force by 8%.[413] Miller et al. have shown improved patellar kinematics and significant reduction of patellofemoral shear forces when the femoral component was placed in neutral rotation with respect to both TEA and "Whiteside line."[300]

It should be remembered that the position of the femoral component cannot be considered in isolation when assessing the effect it may exert on patellar tracking. As Hungerford et al. has pointed out, *"simply rotating the femoral component externally will, to the degree that the tibial component still mates properly with the femur, serve to rotate the tibial component and the tibia itself, with the tibial tubercle in a corresponding amount of external rotation as the knee comes into extension."*[205,246] Therefore any effect on patellar stability in extension would seem to be canceled out by the amount of femoral component external rotation being immediately transferred to the tibia and tibial

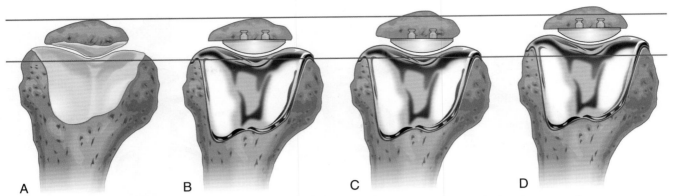

FIG 145.21 Re-creation of physiologic patellofemor spacing requires bone resection according to implant thickness (A and B). Overstuffing of the patellofemoral joint through under-resection of patella (C) or distal femur (D) is to be avoided because it increases patellar strain and may exacerbate minor degrees of patellar tilt or maltracking particularly during knee flexion.

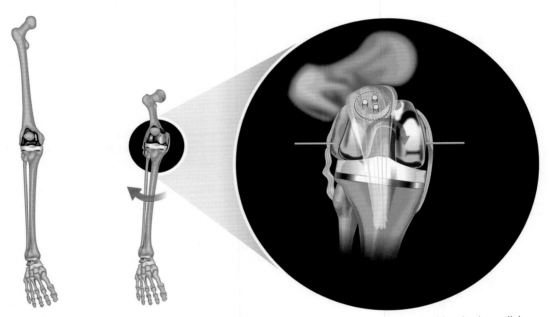

FIG 145.22 Internal rotation of the femoral component will affect patellar tracking by lateralizing the direction of pull of the extensor mechanism. It further creates excessive valgus alignment of the lower leg in flexion and changes to the foot progression angle.

tubercle. At the same time the effect on patellar stability in flexion is equally uncertain and may be influenced more by the configuration of the prosthetic trochlea groove and lateral condylar extension rather than small degrees of component rotation.

Alignment of the femoral component in the sagittal plane also requires attention. Placing the femoral component in flexion creates liftoff of the anterior flange and patellar impingement with the proximal lip of the trochlear groove at lower knee flexion angles. Patellar component wear, loosening, subluxation, and catastrophic failure may be the consequence. Excessive extension of the femoral implant will displace the extensor mechanism anteriorly, increasing retinacular tension and patellofemoral compressive force. The result is a potential decrease in range of motion and an increased risk of patellar fracture.

Slight lateralization of the femoral component in the coronal plane has been shown to improve patellar kinematics (see Fig. 145.25).[228,366] Rhoads et al. have found that laterally translated femoral implants demonstrate improved patellar tracking compared with those placed centrally or medially.[366] The ideal position can be achieved by placing the center of the femoral component immediately lateral to the midline of the intercondylar notch. Excessive lateral translation must be avoided because it enhances the risk of implant overhang and impingement with the lateral retinaculum, PCL, and popliteus tendon.

Tibial Positioning

Accurate rotational alignment of the tibial component is equally critical in preventing patellar maltracking and instability.[313] According to Insall the center of the anterior portion of the tibial baseplate should be aligned with the tibial crest, which is equivalent to the medial third of the tibial tubercle (see Fig. 145.23).[213] This will create relative external rotation and lateral translation of the tibial component, improving extensor

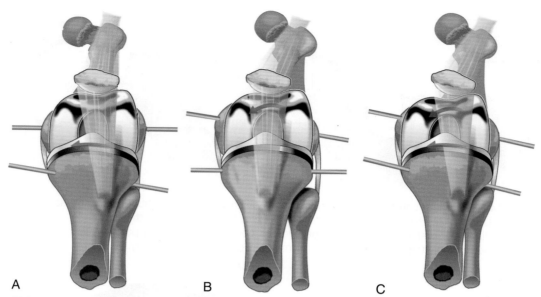

FIG 145.23 Internal rotation of the tibial (A) or femoral (B) arthroplasty component will increase the Q angle and lateral force vector and may lead to patellar maltracking and instability. Combined internal rotation will exacerbate the effect on the patella (C).

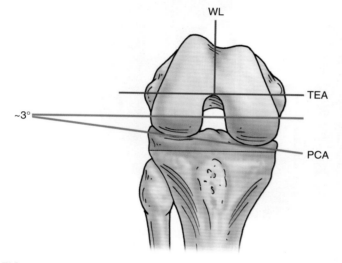

FIG 145.24 The transepicondylar axis *(TEA)* and the anteroposterior axis or Whiteside line *(WL)* are used as reference guides for femoral component rotation and have shown to be more reliable than the posterior condylar axis *(PCA)*. (Adapted from Krackow KA: The technique of total knee arthroplasty, St. Louis, MO, 1990, Mosby.)

mechanism stability by internally rotating the tibial tubercle and decreasing the Q angle. Appropriate rotation can also be determined with the so-called self-seeking method by using a stemless tibial trial component, which will rotate the tibial component in alignment with the chosen femoral component rotation after the knee has been brought into full extension.[257] According to Scott this method yields a rotationally congruent articulation during weight bearing and minimizes the torsional forces being transferred through a conforming tibial surface.[395] Tibiofemoral compression is to be avoided during this maneuver because it inhibits free rotation of the tibial baseplate. The

clinician must be aware that if dynamic positioning suggests excessive internal or external rotation, reassessment of femoral component orientation is required.

Internal rotation of the tibial component has been implicated as the leading cause of patellar instability and may occur as a result of inadequate exposure of the lateral tibial plateau, particularly if the knee is approached through a minimally invasive medial incision.[34] Barrack et al. found that in patients suffering AKP after TKA, the tibial component measured on average 6.2 degrees of internal rotation, compared with 0.4 degrees in the control group.[26] Berger et al. assessed 30 knee arthroplasties affected by patellar tracking abnormalities by relating the level of lateralized patellar tracking to the degree of combined internal rotation of the femoral and tibial components.[34] Combined internal rotation of 1 to 4 degrees resulted in lateralized patellar tracking and tilt, 3 to 8 degrees in patellar subluxation, and 7 to 17 degrees in frank patellar dislocation.

The degree of conformity of the articulating surfaces between the tibial and femoral components may determine the rotational position of the tibia. This is particularly evident in fully conforming prostheses, in which condylar geometry drives kinematic function, forcing the tibia to rotate in unison with the femoral component during the terminal degrees of extension. However, if the articular surfaces are nonconforming, the tibial rotational position is far less dependent on component position and instead is guided by ligament tension.[473] Therefore it is not surprising that Nagamine et al. showed that up to 15 degrees of malrotation of an unconstrained tibial tray did not affect patella tracking compared with a semiconstrained implant.[313] However, the potential benefits on the PFJ may be negated by detrimental tibiofemoral kinematics displayed in fluoroscopic investigations of flat-on-flat condylar arthroplasty designs.[427]

Some uncertainty surrounds the potential benefits of mobile-bearing total knee designs in compensating for malalignment of the extensor mechanism resulting from implant malrotation.[314,332] Improvements in patellar tracking, reduction in patellofemoral contact stresses, and a decrease in

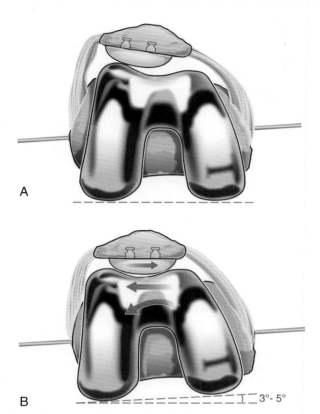

FIG 145.25 Measures to improve patellar tracking: Lateral positioning of the patellar implant will tighten the lateral retinacular structures and may provoke lateral patellar tilt and subluxation (A). Moderate medialization of the patellar component in conjunction with slight external rotation and lateralization of the femoral component will balance medial and lateral retinaculum, assist in centralizing the extensor mechanism, and improve patellar tracking (B). Red dotted line refers to the femoral component alignment relative to the position of the posterior femoral condyles. Blue rod indicates the TEA.

the rate of lateral retinacular release have been observed in some clinical studies and attributed to the self-aligning properties of mobile compared with fixed bearing implants.[77,383] However, others have failed to confirm such clinical advantages.[314,332] Altogether the effect such implants may exert in reducing patellofemoral maltracking is at best moderate and should thus not be seen as a carte blanche for surgical imperfections.[239]

If positional deviations of any of the prosthetic components are suspected, radiographs are often too crude an assessment tool, whereas computed tomography has become the investigation of choice, particularly in determining subtle degrees of rotational abnormalities (Fig. 145.26).[34,447]

Axial Leg Alignment

The key is to reestablish physiologic leg alignment, which varies between 5 and 7 degrees of anatomic valgus.[333,444] Any increase in valgus angle beyond 7 degrees will increase the Q angle and therefore contribute to patellar maltracking. Long-term follow-up studies have shown that prosthetic survival is not compromised if leg alignment is restored within 2.4 to 7.2 degrees of anatomic valgus.[136] There is a higher probability of placing the femoral component in excessive valgus if the knee is affected by preoperative valgus malalignment, especially if the lateral femoral condyle is deficient.[330] Even if compensated for by a tibial component placed into varus, this is still likely to create abnormal patellofemoral kinematics.

Patellar Preparation

The normal patella has an asymmetrical shape with the prominent articular ridge located toward its medial aspect, which separates medial and lateral facets. The patellar bone should be resected parallel to its anterior surface to create a uniformly thick remnant (Fig. 145.27). According to Insall the resection of the articular surface is *"done by eye running the saw blade from the margin of the medial articular surface to the margin of the lateral articular surface"* (Fig. 145.28).[213] Dorr and Boiardo emphasized that, to achieve a symmetrical cut, considerably more bone is usually required to be removed from the medial aspect of the patella.[118]

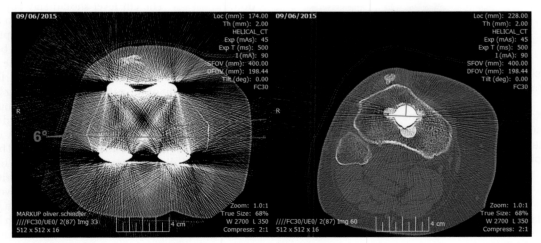

FIG 145.26 Computed tomography sequences showing axial cuts through the femoral and tibial component of a total knee arthroplasty. The femoral component is internally rotated by 6 degrees in relation to the transepicondylar axis. The tibial component is aligned with the medial third of the tibial tuberosity.

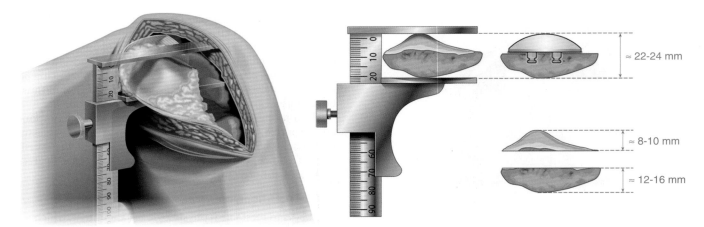

FIG 145.27 The overall patella thickness (average: 22 to 24 mm) should be established using a caliper, along with the dimension of the selected implant to be subtracted. The remainder equals the target dimension of the bony patellar remnant following resection. Care should be taken to preserve a minimum of 12 mm of bone. Composite height of patella should not exceed preresection levels unless the patella was affected by significant deformation or bone/cartilage erosion, in which case its predisease height needs to be estimated.

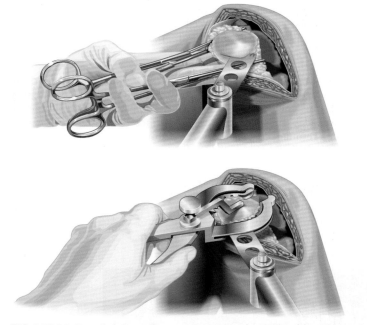

FIG 145.28 Patellar resection can be performed "freehand" by keeping the cut surface just above the attachment of patellar and quadriceps tendon. Patellar and quadriceps tendon are captured with Kocher clamps, while the patella is supported by upward pressure from index and middle finger. Alternatively, commercial resection guides that include a stylus to allow for presetting of the cutting level are available from most manufacturers.

Proper patellar exposure and appropriate removal of surrounding soft tissues will allow for better visualization and judgment of the cutting level. Failure to appreciate the asymmetry of the patella may lead to the removal of equal amounts of bone from the medial and lateral facets, creating an oblique cutting surface (Fig. 145.29). Such errors in preparation have

been shown to increase the risk of patellar tilt and maltracking, while also leading to increases in patellar strain.[107,353] In a series of 300 TKAs, Pagnano and Trousdale encountered 21 patellae with an asymmetrical cutting surface, 52% of which either developed debilitating AKP or presented with patellofemoral complications requiring revision.[331]

Achieving accurate patellar resection can be accomplished with a "freehand" technique or by using a designated resection guide or clamp (see Fig. 145.28). Although resection guides produce a smooth and even cut surface, they are position dependent and relying on the surgeon's ability to apply the guide at the appropriate depth and obliquity. Asymmetric resurfacing is hence not uncommon. However, if used correctly, resection guides can achieve accurate and reproducible postre-construction patellar thickness.[30] Freehand preparation on the other hand has been particularly popular with experienced arthroplasty surgeons who use attachments of patellar and quadriceps tendon as reference points to guide patellar resection.[69,118,205,267,399] The cut level should stay approximately 1 to 2 mm above the tendon insertion and needs to be co-planar to prevent rocking and to produce close coaptation between implant and bone surface. After the patella has been cut and the desired thickness confirmed using a caliper, the remnant patellar bone is examined between thumb and forefinger. This manual palpation of the patellar remnant using haptic feedback has shown to be an excellent means of assessing the symmetry of the resection. With this technique, Lombardi et al. reported restoration of patellar thickness within 1 mm of preoperative values in 91% of their cases, a finding confirmed by others.[81,111,267]

Camp et al. directly compared the precision of patellar resection achieved through using a resection guide with two different freehand preparation techniques. The latter involved a preliminary cut 1 to 2 mm above the desired resection level before the retropatellar surface was either assessed through haptic feedback or divided into four quadrants that were measured individually using a caliper. The patella was then recut until symmetry was achieved. The authors showed that their "four-quadrant" technique was the most accurate in achieving symmetric resection, with a mean asymmetry of 0.85 mm compared with 1.40 mm

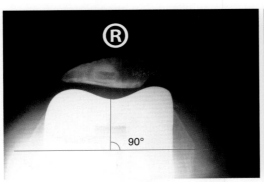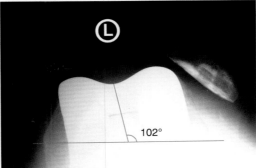

FIG 145.29 Laurin roentgenogram of bilateral knee arthroplasties highlighting numerous surgical improprieties. The patella in the right knee shows asymmetric patellar resection, lateralization of the patellar implant, and associated medial tilt. The patella in the left knee is dislocated as a result of lateralization of the patellar implant and excessive internal rotation of the femoral component in relation to the transepicondylar axis (TEA).

for haptic assessment and 1.73 mm when using a cutting guide.[82]

Patellar Component Placement

Hungerford has raised the point that *"the central ridge on the patella, separating the medial and lateral facets is not equidistant between the medial and lateral margins of the patella and a symmetrical dome, implanted in the middle of the cut surface of the patella, will have the effect of medializing the articular surfaces of the patella, increasing the Q-angle and leading to increased patellar subluxation"* (David Hungerford, personal communication, 2015). Coapting the medial margin of the dome patella with the medial margin of the cut surface of the patella would come closer to re-creating the natural high point (Fig. 145.30). An anatomic patellar implant (or offset dome), with its shorter medial facet, would overcome such problems and at the same time provide better coverage of the retropatellar surface (see Fig. 145.30). However, correct rotational position of an asymmetric patellar implant is critical to its function because the retropatellar ridge needs to be aligned with the trochlea groove (Fig. 145.31).

Because the majority of patellar components currently in use are dome shaped and axisymmetric, it is widely accepted that placing them in a more superomedial position relative to the center of the retropatellar surface is considered beneficial because it emulates the location of the native retropatellar eminence (see Fig. 145.30).[386] Medialization of the patellar component by 2 mm reduces peak lateral shear force by 10 to 15 N, but a corresponding medial shear force was noted at knee flexion angles below 25 degrees.[115] Radiographic results of medialized insertion of patellar prosthesis have confirmed the effect on lateralization of the bony structure of the patella, which is thought to decrease lateral shear forces and decrease the likelihood of patellar subluxation.[488] In clinical series the rate of lateral retinacular release was 13% to 17% when the patellar component was placed medially compared with 46% to 48% when placed centrally onto the retropatellar surface.[196,262] Anglin et al. have measured the impact of various levels of patellar component medialization on patellar kinematics and force distribution in a cadaver model.[16] A significant reduction of patellofemoral contact force above 60 degrees of knee flexion occurred with increasing medialization of the patellar component. However, at the same time, the researchers noted that the

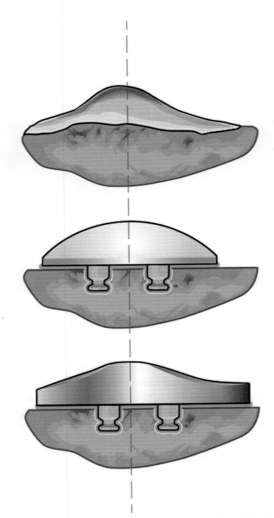

FIG 145.30 Recreation of the native patellar "high point" through appropriate positioning of patellar component. Because of its surface geometry, an anatomic component can be placed centrally, whereas a dome variant requires to be positioned off-center towards the medial patellar border. Red dotted line indicates the location of the high point of the retro-patellar ridge.

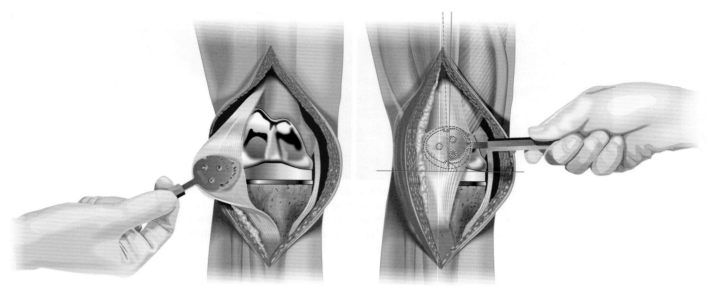

FIG 145.31 Positioning of the patellar component onto the retro-patellar cut surface. Correct alignment is critical to unimpeded patellar tracking particularly when using an asymmetric, anatomic implant. The sizing spoon is aligned perpendicular to the patellar tendon and placed in a slight superolateral position onto the everted retropatellar surface. When the patella is reduced, the spoon handle needs to attain perpendicularity with the trochlea groove and should be approximately 3 degrees off parallel to the joint line *(external rotation)* to enhance proximal patellar capture.

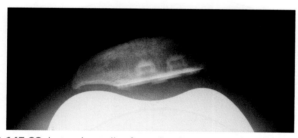

FIG 145.32 Lateral patellar facet impingement and erosion can occur as a result of excessive medialization of the patellar implant, inappropriate soft tissue balancing, or failure to perform partial lateral facetectomy.

more the patellar was medialized, the more it tended to tilt laterally relative to the femur.

Biomechanically the tendency to lateral tilt is thought to result from the mediolateral moment created when the extensor mechanism, positioned centrally on the patella and acting posteriorly, becomes off-center from the patellar implant after medialization. To take advantage of reduced contact force while containing the level of lateral patellar tilt, Anglin et al. recommended medializing the patella by no more than 2.5 mm.[16] In addition, overzealous medialization has been shown to leave excessive bone on the exposed lateral patellar facet, potentially creating painful contact with the femoral condyle (Fig. 145.32).[116] Thus it has been recommended to chamfer the patellar rim to reduce risk of bony impingement.[268]

An equivalent effect to medialization of the patella implant may, in many respects, be achievable by lateralizing the femoral component in terms of both reducing tension in the lateral retinaculum and reducing the Q angle (see Fig. 145.25). The principal advantage of changing the femoral rather than

patellar component position lies in reducing the risk of patellar tilt, because the extensor mechanism would remain centered on the patella. The final decision on which measures to choose should rest with the intraoperative assessment prior to the definitive placement of the implants.

It is important to realize that intraoperative assessment of patellar tracking following patellar resurfacing is merely static. As such, it is unable to predict with any degree of certainty the functional effects of the quadriceps on patellar tracking during activities. This may in many respects explain the discrepancy between satisfactory intraoperative alignment and variations in postoperative tracking and tilt and gives a distinct advantage to nonconforming spherical implants. One may speculate that the underlying reason for this may be that any intraoperative assessment potentially underestimates the clinical need for soft tissue balancing and retinacular release.

Patellar Composite Thickness

When resurfacing the patella, it is important to re-create physiologic patella thickness (see Fig. 145.27). Estimating normal patellar height may be difficult if the surface anatomy is distorted through advanced degeneration, deformation, or erosion. Under those circumstances it is appropriate to aim at reestablishing average patellar height, which in men and women is surprisingly constant, with values ranging from 22 to 24 mm.[90]

Some have recommended keeping the composite height of the patella (total height of patellar shell plus patellar implant) slightly below the level of the native patella. Pagnano and Kelly observed improved patellar tracking when reducing the composite thickness by 1 to 2 mm.[330] Greenfield et al. reduced the incidence of lateral retinacular release from 55% to 12% by ensuring that the overall patellar thickness was less than or equal to that of the native patella.[171] Reithmeier and Plitz have been providing biomechanical data in support of this concept.

The authors showed that lowering the effective patellar component height allows for the load-sharing effect of the quadriceps tendon (turn-round phenomenon) to commence at lower knee flexion angles, resulting in a linear reduction in force ratio between patellofemoral and quadriceps forces.[363]

Care should be taken not to compromise the structural integrity of the remaining patellar bone shell because removal of excessive bone during the resurfacing procedure will weaken the patella, making it prone to fracture.[224,365] Fitzpatrick et al. defined the critical thickness of residual patellar bone at no less than 11 mm, below which patellar surface strain increased exponentially.[145] In their experimental setup a mere reduction to 9 mm in patellar bone thickness led to a fivefold increase in surface strain levels, which was most notable in the midrange of flexion. Although one should aim to preserve approximately 15 mm, as has been suggested by Reuben et al, most surgeons are willing to accept a minimum of 12 mm as the cutoff point below which they consider leaving the patella unresurfaced.[39,365]

Particular problems have been observed when patellar composite thickness exceeds preoperative values (see Fig. 145.21). This will create overstuffing of the PFJ, with subsequent increases in retinacular tension, anterior patellar strain, and PRF, leading to patellar tilt and subluxation. An increase in the overall patellar composite thickness of just 10% has been shown to significantly increase patellofemoral forces with knee flexion greater than 70 degrees.[421] In such circumstances, overall flexion is generally reduced and the risk of patellar component failure and fracture increased.[118,298,365]

Joint Line

Maintenance of the joint line and patellar height has been shown to be an important factor in re-creating normal patellofemoral kinematics.[4] This is of particular importance when using a posterior cruciate-retaining arthroplasty design, because ligaments must be balanced properly to achieve satisfactory range of motion. Raising or lowering the joint line will create secondary patella baja or alta, respectively. In cases of patella baja, the patellofemoral compressive forces will be increased during early knee flexion and overall range of motion is often compromised. In addition, if joint-line elevation is excessive, the patella will become prone to impinge on the anterior margin of the tibial articular surface. Patella alta is generally less common and often developmental rather than secondary to surgery. It is primarily associated with patellar instability and subluxation.

Inlay versus Onlay Patellar Implant

The great majority of currently available patellar components are of the onlay type whereby the implant is placed onto the cut retropatellar surface. Inlay patellae are inserted into a reamed cavity, which, to provide adequate stability, requires the preservation of a certain amount of surrounding bone. Such implants are hence generally smaller than their onlay counterparts. The technique of using an inlay patella was initially described by Gschwend in 1978.[176] It has been suggested that inlay patellar components provide greater composite strength between the implant and patella and may decrease the amount of patellar tilt and shift.[150,253,254] However, insetting the patellar component is not without risks because overzealous removal of subchondral cancellous bone may weaken the patella, increasing its susceptibility to fracture. Therefore the preservation of a minimum of

15 mm of bone has been recommended to minimize surface strain on the patella.[224,365] In a biomechanical analysis, Wulff and Incavo recorded increased patellar surface strains in inlay compared with onlay designs. In addition, onlay patellae were noted to be more tolerant to excess cutting. Overcutting the patella by 2 mm created a 22% increase in surface strain compared with a 42% increase when the patella was overreamed by the same amount.[484]

Critics of inlay designs have raised concerns regarding potential detrimental effects caused through the contact between remaining cartilage, bone, and soft tissues with the femoral component.[214] In a cadaver study, Ezzet et al. observed similarities in patellar kinematics among implant types, although inlay components showed a higher tendency to lateral shift and tilt.[135] However, some in vivo studies revealed less patellar tilt and better overall patellar alignment in patients with inlay implants.[165,358] Rand and Gustilo compared 135 onlay and 116 inlay patellar components using an identical total knee system, recording a lateral release rate of 79% and 28%, respectively.[358] Thus the authors concluded that using an inlay implant would result in better ability to centralize the extensor mechanism. Despite such reports, benefits of inlay patellae have remained largely theoretical and have not been converted into improved clinical outcomes.

Lateral Release

Krakow suggested releasing the lateral patellofemoral ligament when performing a medial parapatellar approach, because it assists with exposure and eversion of the patella, allows for correction of minor tracking abnormalities, and may render a more formal lateral release unnecessary.[245,330,393] A formal lateral release may become necessary if, after placement of all implants, the patella shows a tendency to lateral tracking or subluxation. Although the reasons for such tracking abnormalities often remain obscure, it is paramount to assess the arthroplasty components for potential malalignment before proceeding with any soft tissue release. Patellar tracking should be assessed at a point when trial components are assembled, because at this stage minor adjustments are still relatively easy to perform. In an otherwise well-aligned knee, often simply reducing the patellar thickness by 1 to 2 mm can diminish the need for more extensive soft tissue release, provided a minimum thickness of 12 mm residual patellar bone is maintained.[404]

Scott's *"rule of no thumb"* is widely used in the assessment of patellar tracking.[393] The test is performed before closure of the medial capsule. If the patella tracks well throughout the full flexion arc without the surgeon's thumb holding the patella located in the trochlear groove, no release is necessary. If the patella subluxes without counteracting pressure from the thumb, the lateral retinaculum should be released in a staged fashion until the patella is stabilized. This technique has been criticized by some who believe that it may overestimate the need for lateral release if a medial parapatellar approach is used.[44,323,330] Other techniques, such as the towel clip test and one-stitch or single-suture test, have been described, claiming certain advantages, but essentially represent no more than a variation on a theme.[18,349] Briard has described the kissing rule, implying that, if in deep flexion the medial surface of the patella does not touch the medial condyle of the femoral component, a lateral retinacular release is indicated.[61] Tourniquet release is thought to provide a more realistic appreciation of patellar tracking and has been shown to reduce the number of lateral releases

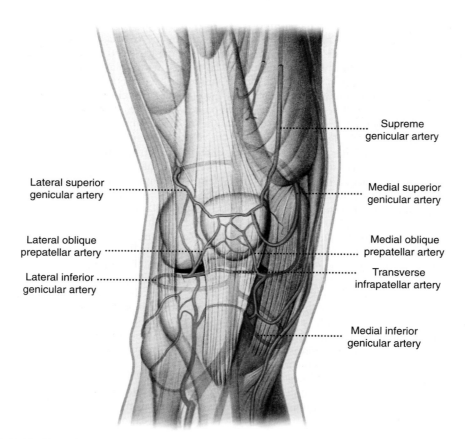

FIG 145.33 Blood supply to the patella. (Adapted from Lanz T, Wachsmuth W: Praktische Anato-mie, Bd.1, Part 4. Bein und Statik, Berlin, 1938, Julius Springer.)

otherwise performed by up to 31%.[206,252] Dynamic forces may also favor lateral patellar tracking, but unfortunately these are outside the realm of clinical assessment during surgery.[42]

Although the technique of performing a lateral release is simple, much debate exists about the potential morbidity associated with it. The all-inside technique is favored by the great majority of surgeons because it avoids the creation of a cutaneous flap and with it, potential wound-healing problems. The knee should be extended during the maneuver and the patella retracted anteriorly or everted halfway. Keeping the retinaculum under tension helps to define the various soft tissue planes and may assist in identifying the genicular arteries (Fig. 145.33). The incision is made approximately 1 to 2 cm lateral to the patellar margin, dividing the synovium, capsule, and retinacular fibers up to the subcutaneous fat. The release is performed in stages, with the clinician assessing patellar tracking regularly and therefore tailoring the amount of tissue released to the requirements. An extensive release may start distal to the joint line close to the fascia lata attachment onto Gerdy's tubercle, reaching up proximally to the junction of the vastus lateralis. Care should be taken not to buttonhole the incision through the skin, a problem associated with the use of electrocautery especially in thin patients. The procedure itself carries some morbidity, including postoperative swelling, bruising, and hemarthrosis, most of which is related to inadequate hemostasis.

Much has been written about the importance of preserving the patellar blood supply, in particular the superior genicular

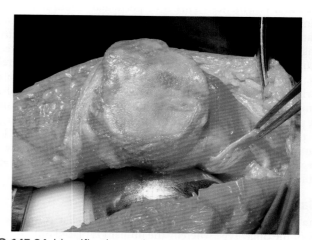

FIG 145.34 Identification and protection of the lateral superior genicular artery prior to performing a lateral retinacular release will help to preserve blood supply to the patella and reduce the risk of avascular necrosis.

artery, when performing a lateral release.[400,472] The medial genicular vessels are obviously sacrificed as part of the medial parapatellar approach to the knee, whereas the lateral inferior genicular artery is often compromised during excision of the lateral meniscus, leaving the lateral superior genicular artery as the main source of circulation to the patella (Fig. 145.34).[445] The vessel can be found close to the superior pole of the patella and,

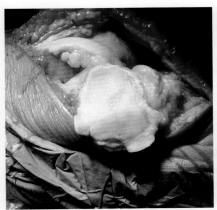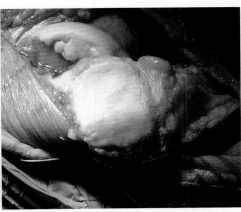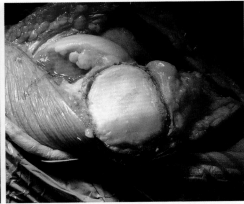

FIG 145.35 Patelloplasty is advisable if the patella is left unresurfaced. Marginal osteophytes are excised *(center image)*, and circumferential thermocoagulation of the surrounding synovium performed *(right image)*. If necessary, enlarged or overhanging facets may be reshaped or a facetectomy performed.

if identified, should be isolated through blunt dissection and protected during the release procedure (see Fig. 145.33).[405] However, it is not always possible to preserve the lateral superior genicular artery and provide adequate release at the same time. Under those circumstances, it may be advantageous to leave the lateral skin flap intact without separating skin from subcutaneous tissue; this is thought to preserve superficial vessels and ensure nourishment to the patellar bone from the overlying skin.[370]

The importance of the preservation of the lateral superior genicular artery remains open to debate. Accessory blood supply through the anterior vascular plexus, Hoffa fat pad, and patellar and quadriceps tendon may be sufficient to maintain patellar viability, but there is evidence of temporary devascularization of the patellar bone after surgery.[290,349,472] Pawar et al. demonstrated transient patellar hypovascularity following lateral release using scintigraphy, which resolved within 2 months.[339] Although most of the consequences arising from the sacrifice of the lateral genicular vessels are theoretical in nature, direct clinical complications, including avascular necrosis, patellar fracture, and wound-healing problems, have been reported.[292] In a series of 1146 TKAs, Ritter et al. observed patella fractures in 5.4% of patients who had undergone lateral release, compared with 2.4% in those who had not.[372]

The surgical approach may also influence patellar tracking. A reduced incidence of lateral release has been shown with the midvastus and subvastus approach compared with a standard medial parapatellar incision.[44,128,285] However, this should be viewed against an increase in medial patellar tilt associated with a muscle-splitting approach.[44] Keating et al. observed no difference in the rate of lateral release or patellar function when using a modified medial parapatellar approach in which the cut was directed into the musculotendinous junction of the vastus medialis, leaving the quadriceps tendon intact.[233]

Wachtl and Jakob have described a lateral patellar osteotomy as an alternative surgical procedure to the traditional retinacular release.[460] The lateral patellar facet is exposed through eversion of the patella, and a portion of it is resected, thereby relaxing the lateral retinaculum and making a formal release unnecessary. Although none of their 76 patients required retinacular release, 15% nonetheless developed lateral patellar tilt.

Overall, the potential complications of a lateral retinacular release should be viewed in the light of the detrimental long-term effects of patellar maltracking and subluxation on patellar component survival and the development of AKP. Most clinicians hence would agree that the potential advantages by far outweigh the consequences of those complications.

Patelloplasty

Patelloplasty is recommended if the clinician decides not to resurface the patella. The procedure is essentially designed to re-create a patellar shape and surface configuration similar to the native patella. It involves the removal of any marginal osteophytes from the periphery and, in case of significant patellar deformation, a lateral facetectomy (Fig. 145.35). Areas of eburnization are shaved or exposed to transcortical Pridie drilling to encourage fibrocartilage ingrowth.[212,235,236] The surrounding patellar meniscus and excessive synovial tissue are generally excised to avoid soft tissue impingement. Some surgeons promote circumferential thermocoagulation, thought to create a level of sensory denervation, in an attempt to combat the occurrence of postoperative AKP.[235]

PROS AND CONS OF PATELLA RESURFACING

In 1836 Malgaigne of Paris wrote, *"When one searches among the past or present authors for the origins of doctrines generally accepted today concerning dislocation of the patella, one is surprised to find among them such disagreement and such a dearth of facts with such an abundance of opinions."*[278] Although focusing on a slightly different subject matter, Malgaigne's views very much characterize the diversity of opinions expressed in the debate about the value of patella resurfacing in TKA, which according to Krackow "has become synonymous to topics of religion and politics."[245]

The discussion on the merits of patellar resurfacing is focused on the potential benefits a patellar implant can offer a patient undergoing TKA and whether such benefits may outweigh possible risks and complications attached to the procedure.[78,387] The key questions one has to address are (1) can resurfacing improve patellofemoral performance and function (eg, stair climbing ability)? (2) Can it provide a reduction in the incidence of AKP? (3) Can it enhance patients' overall satisfaction? And (4) is it cost effective?

Resurfacing Strategies

Three basic treatment strategies pertaining to the use of patellar components have evolved so far: "always to resurface," "never to resurface," or to "selectively resurface." Clinicians who prefer to always resurface claim reduced incidence of postoperative AKP, avoidance of SR, higher patient satisfaction, better overall function, a low complication rate, and that the procedure is relatively inexpensive and not time consuming.[244,260,350,396,398,469] Some have also argued that the addition of a patellar implant assists in centralizing the extensor mechanism, thereby compensating for minor degrees of maltracking.[83,318,338] To the proponents of "always to resurface," the articulation between cartilage and metal is considered un-physiologic, and prolonged exposure to high compressive forces is believed to cause cartilage erosion.[146] The prevalence of patellofemoral complications following primary resurfacing has decreased significantly and currently remains at around 4% to 5% when using contemporary implant designs,[‡‡] whereas the proportion of revisions attributable to the resurfaced patella has dropped over the past 25 years from over 70% in the 1980s to less than 15% today.[§§] Finally, there has also been an economic argument in favor of primary resurfacing.[295,310] This is based on the increased level of SR procedures recorded in this patient group, which are generally classified as revisions and thus a substantial burden to health care providers.[299] Supporters of "always to resurface" believe that primary resurfacing offers both cost and health utility advantages, given the high costs of a revision surgery and that fewer than half the patients appear to benefit from SR.[194,310]

Clinicians in support of patellar retention argue that clinical results between patients with and without resurfacing are broadly similar and that patellar resurfacing therefore represents an unnecessary step in performing a TKA.[272] Other claims pertain to shorter operating time, conservation of patellar bone, reduced likelihood of patellar osteonecrosis, more physiologic patellofemoral kinematics, ability to withstand high patellofemoral forces especially in younger and more active patients without the concern of prosthetic wear or failure, and ease of resurfacing in case of recalcitrant AKP.[1,80,138,236] Not using a patellar implant is also seen as avoiding an additional source of polyethylene particulate debris and associated consequences.[273] One major argument brought forward in the discussion on the merits of patellar retention is the avoidance of intraoperative and postoperative complications associated with patellar resurfacing.[31,107,108,235]

Advocates of "never to resurface" emphasize that no conclusive evidence exists that patellae articulating with a metallic surface are likely to become symptomatic even after prolonged periods in service.[260,436] However they emphasize the importance of deploying femoral components of anatomically shaped trochlear configuration, which provide matching articulating surfaces to better accommodate the native patella, as such implants are believed to reduce the incidence of postsurgical AKP.[49,418,474]

Goodfellow argued that "*routine resurfacing exposes over 90% of patients to the unnecessary risks associated with adding a patellar implant*" (John Goodfellow, personal communication, 1998). According to Barrack "*the major determinants of clinical results and anterior knee pain after TKA are surgical technique and component design, and not whether or not the patella is resurfaced*" (Robert Barrack, personal communication, 2015). For Robertsson "*the usefulness (or not) of the patellar button is mostly a matter of belief, and opinion builders (surgeons and representatives) have a good opportunity to influence this*" (Robertsson, personal communication, 2012).

Selective Patellar Resurfacing

Contrary to common belief, the concept of selective resurfacing is not simply based on resurfacing patellae presenting with significant retropatellar cartilage degeneration but aims to identify those individuals who are thought to have an improved clinical outcome with patellar resurfacing while at the same time avoiding potential complications associated with unnecessary resurfacing.[***] With this approach, 10-year survival rates of 90% to 98% have been reported.[241,373,397]

Selective patellar resurfacing was first advocated by Scott and Reilly in 1980.[397] Although they recommended routine resurfacing in all patients with rheumatoid arthritis, they proposed selective resurfacing in patients with osteoarthritis who present with a deformed patella, absent retropatellar cartilage, and imperfect patellar tracking. Their rationale was based on the belief that advanced patella wear would invariably equate to a poorer outcome if the patella was left unresurfaced and provided Scott and Reilly with a 97.5% survival rate at 10 years, using a single TKA design.

Nowadays supporters of selective patellar resurfacing base their decision on the presence of certain prerequisites pertaining to a number of patient and knee-specific factors. Patellar retention is favored in patients below the age of 65, who are not affected by rheumatoid or crystalline disease, whose retropatellar cartilage is reasonably well preserved, who have no significant anatomic abnormality (eg, adequate patellofemoral congruence, normally shaped patella of adequate thickness), normal patellar mechanics (eg, central patellar tracking), and do not suffer localized AKP. Vince et al. suggested that the archetypal patient who does not need patellar resurfacing should be "*short and relatively thin, with a congruous patello-femoral joint and less than grade III arthritic changes.*"[404,457]

The decision to resurface is generally based on the presence of preoperative patellofemoral symptoms (eg, localized AKP), radiologic evidence of patellofemoral arthritis, the intraoperative assessment of the state of the retropatellar cartilage and patellar tracking.[318,345,380] Few would argue about the indication of primary resurfacing in patients with symptomatic patellofemoral disease in which patellar degeneration is coupled with preexisting AKP.[345] In this situation, which Barrack describes as the "*primary patellofemoral arthritis scenario,*" the majority of surgeons would consider patellar resurfacing, provided that there is enough bone stock to safely support a patellar component.[255] However, most proponents of selective resurfacing would also favor primary resurfacing in the presence of full-thickness cartilage damage irrespective of preexisting AKP, even though evidence to support such action is not unequivocal.[138,207,215,436]

Some uncertainty exists about the indication of patellar resurfacing in patients affected by inflammatory arthropathies.

---

‡‡References 26, 52, 249, 273, 296, and 481.
§§References 53, 62, 273, 373, 409, and 456.

***References 1, 187, 236, 241, 261, 345, 373, 397, and 436.

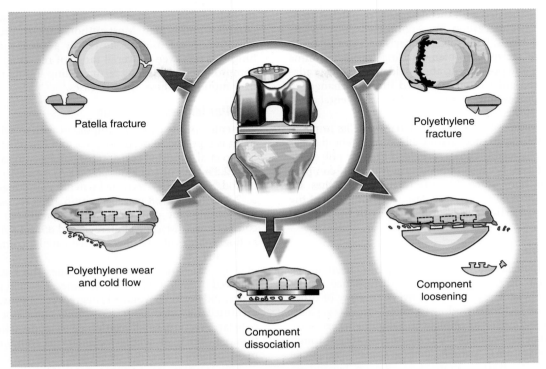

FIG 145.36 Pathomechanics of common modes of failure associated with patellar resurfacing. (Adapted from Schindler OS: The controversy of patella resurfacing in total knee arthroplasty: Ibisne in medio tutissimus? *Knee Surg Sports Traumatol Arthosc* 20: 1227–1244, 2012.)

Sledge and Ewald suggested that failure to resurface the patellar in rheumatoid arthritis may allow continued release of sequestered antigen from the retained cartilage, resulting in recurrent inflammation.[414] However, concerns about an ongoing inflammatory process have remained largely theoretical, and although various studies have recommended routine resurfacing on all patients with rheumatoid arthritis,[26,261,345,393] others have failed to notice any ill effects despite patellar retention.[†††]

PATELLA-RELATED COMPLICATIONS IN TOTAL KNEE ARTHROPLASTY

The advent of patellar resurfacing introduced a new and different set of complications to the surgical community (Fig. 145.36).[62,304] Soon patella-related complications became the most common mode of failure reported in TKA.[31,62,107,301,354] However, over time clinicians recognized that inadequacies in prosthesis design and surgical improprieties, such as component malrotation and overzealous soft tissue releases, were partially to be blamed for this.[137,309] Although improvements in surgical precision and advances in implant design have led to an overall reduction in the rate of complications, patellofemoral problems still account for up to one-third of all revisions performed within the first 10 to 15 years.[‡‡‡]

Although the great majority of patella-related revisions in unresurfaced TKAs merely concern the addition of a patellar implant (SR), those performed in previously resurfaced TKAs, although relatively rare, are generally of a different magnitude of complexity.[40,222,264,292] Subsequently, the long-term outcome of the latter group is often less predictable and the physical long-term impact and associated morbidity on the patient potentially not inconsiderable.[40] Data from the Swedish Arthroplasty Registry suggest that patients with primary patellar resurfacing are three times more likely to undergo revision for any cause other than pain when compared with patients in whom the patella was retained.[264,273] Out of all revisions performed in patients with resurfaced patellae, 17% were performed for patellar dislocation, 13% for patellar implant loosening, 6% for patellar implant wear, and 2.5% for patellar fracture. Secondary patellar resurfacing is mostly performed for recalcitrant AKP in what often appears to be an otherwise well-performing TKA. However, the procedure carries limited success with no more than 50% of patients eventually becoming symptom free.[26,84,302]

Failures associated with the patellar resurfacing are multifactorial and may relate to patient selection (eg, age, BMI), surgical technique (eg, component mal-rotation), implant design (eg, metal backing), and biologic factors (eg, avascular or heat necrosis).[354,355] One of the most common reasons for premature patellar failure is surgical mismanagement and the consequences thereof. Subsequent complications include postoperative patellar maltracking and instability, patellar fracture, polyethylene wear, component loosening and dissociation, soft tissue impingement, and extensor mechanism disruption.[281] Component design, material choice, and the manufacturing process also appear to have a significant effect on performance, longevity, and potential complications. A case in point is the

---

†††References 1, 52, 104, 129, 187, 270, 321, and 412.
‡‡‡References 95, 130, 232, 264, 273, and 408.

high failure rate associated with metal backing of patellar components and the use of carbon fiber–reinforced polyethylene in the 1980s and 1990s, with reported revision rates of up to 48%.[35,266,430] More recently, problems arising through gamma sterilization in air and post-sterilization oxidation and degradation have been recognized and addressed through changes in the sterilization process and awareness of the detrimental effect of prolonged shelf life.[96,288,368]

In cases of revision not directly related to the patellar implant, retention of a well-positioned, stable, all-polyethylene patellar component is a reasonable choice, provided that the polyethylene has not oxidized, because implant removal often compromises remaining bone stock. Manufacturing mismatches are acceptable with most contemporary designs as long as that the patellar component articulates appropriately with the femoral implant.[271]

Patellar Fracture

Fractures of the patella following resurfacing have been attributed to avascular necrosis secondary to disturbance of the patellar blood supply. The literature conveys an array of other potential causative factors, including technical errors (eg, patellar maltracking secondary to implant malalignment, excessive or asymmetric patellar bone resection, thermal necrosis through cement polymerization), patient demographics (eg, male gender, obesity with BMI > 35 m², knee flexion beyond 95 degrees, high activity level), and implant design (eg, large patellar component ≥37 mm, inlay patellar design, large central fixation peg, PS implant).[§§§]

The overall risk of patella fracture following patellar resurfacing is generally low, with reported figures ranging from 0.2% to 5.2%.[****] Although fractures may result from trauma,[287] the majority are either iatrogenic or occur spontaneously.[215,292,400] A compromise in patellar vascularity through medial arthrotomy combined with lateral retinacular release is thought to be a major factor in the etiology of patellar fractures, but its clinical significance remains unclear.[33,287,472,478] Some series have demonstrated a relationship between avascularity and fracture,[33,80,218,400] whereas others have failed to do so.[142,328,370]

Fortunately a large proportion of patellar fractures are asymptomatic. Ortiguera and Berry diagnosed 78 fractures (0.6%) in 12,464 TKAs, 44 of which were asymptomatic and discovered incidentally during postoperative follow-up.[324] Surgical intervention may be necessary when the patellar component is loose or dislodged, provided that the patient is sufficiently symptomatic, but becomes essential in cases of extensor mechanism disruption. In the view of the authors, reconstitution of the latter should always take precedence over patellar reconstruction, and patellectomy may have to be considered if implant fixation is difficult. The complication rate in this series was less than 10% in patients treated conservatively but rose to 56% in patients treated operatively, 90% of whom required a further surgical procedure.

In the management of patellar fractures, the clinician must evaluate the underlying cause and eradicate any associated pathology. Malalignment of the femoral or tibial component should be rectified at the time of patellar fixation or component revision to avoid recurrence. However, conservative management

should be considered whenever possible because the risk of complications is high. Most authors support prolonged immobilization in extension, followed by gradual mobilization in a hinged brace. Even if overall range of movement is likely to be compromised in the long term, healing should take precedence over motion in these difficult cases.[108,324,355]

Patellar Implant Loosening

Loosening of the patellar component with or without displacement is reported to occur in 0.6% to 4.8% of cases.[62,107,130,292,408] Sextro et al. reported revision for patella component loosening in 4 (2.3%) out of 168 kinematic TKAs over a 10-year follow-up period.[408] Erak et al. recorded patellar component loosening in 5 (2.9%) out of 168 patients within 10 years using a biconvex patellar implant combined with a patellar-friendly femoral component.[130] Meding et al. reviewed 8531 TKAs and recorded radiographic evidence of cemented patellar component loosening in 409 (4.8%) cases, at a mean of 7 years.[292] In this series, obesity placed the patella at 6.3 times the risk of loosening, followed by lateral release at 3.8 times, elevated joint line at 2.2 times, and flexion beyond 100 degrees at 2.1 times. Other factors identified included poor remaining bone stock, asymmetric patellar resection, small fixation pegs, inadequate implant fixation, patellar maltracking secondary to component malalignment, osteonecrosis, and osteolysis.[33,271]

There appears to be a consensus that patellar implant loosening is most commonly associated with the biologic pathway of osteonecrosis, although other causes, such as patellar fracture, implant/cement dissociation, and traumatic peg fracture, are recognized (see Fig. 145.36).[235] Characteristic radiologic features show a natural progression starting with increased bone density, followed by subchondral bone resorption and progressive radiolucency, and culminating in patellar fracture and fragmentation. Berend et al. recorded a total of 180 failed patellar components, of which 81% progressed to the stage of fragmentation and lateral subluxation.[33] The authors noted that 73% of knees with loose patellar implants had received lateral retinacular release, compared with 59% in which the implant was stable.

Patellar Implant Wear

Wear is a common feature in patellar implants because of the unfavorable mechanical environment of the patellofemoral articulation (see Figs. 145.15, 145.17, and 145.36).[10,99,113,199] The in vivo wear pattern is highly dependent on the inherent mechanical properties of the materials used, the interaction between patella and femoral component, and the external forces acting on them. The mechanical performance of the various designs is best assessed from observations made on retrieval components, which have shown considerable degree of wear and deformation.[10,99,113,144,291] The level of wear damage appears to increase with the patient's weight, postoperative range of motion, and length of time the component has been in service.[144] It is of interest to note, that despite patellofemoral compression forces exceeding the yield strength of UHMWPE, catastrophic failure or component fracture are seen infrequently and have not become an endemic problem.[433]

Patellar Instability and Dislocation

Patellar instability represents a serious problem and is responsible for a number of associated complications, making it the second most common reason for revision surgery following

---

§§§References 59, 117, 292, 324, 410, and 443.
****References 130, 163, 169, 222, 292, and 372.

primary patellar resurfacing (see Fig. 145.29).[62,84,264] Although less common, the condition may also occur in cases of patellar retention. Patients often present with a plethora of symptoms, ranging from mild discomfort to pain, weakness, giving way, and locking. Some have suggested patellar resurfacing in all cases in which satisfactory soft tissue balance cannot be achieved, based on the assumption that resurfacing as such might overcome minor degrees of maltracking.[83,318,338] Others feel that the resurfaced patella, most probably carries a higher propensity to emphasize any maltracking, whereas the native patella offers at least a limited ability to adapt to adverse conditions over time.[236]

The effect of implant design on patellofemoral stability is well recognized.[426,473] Femoral components featuring a shallow and symmetric trochlea groove with abrupt changes in sagittal radius have been shown to create abnormal patellar kinematics and increase the risk of patellar maltracking.[84,343,435,488] Campbell et al. reviewed 289 knee arthroplasties with a shallow and narrow trochlea and found that out of 20 revisions 14 were required for patellar maltracking.[84]

Surgical improprieties during patellar resurfacing are common reasons for patellar instability and include residual valgus limb malalignment, patella alta, increased internal rotation of femoral or tibial component, medial translation of the femoral component, excessive valgus alignment of the femoral component (even if the overall limb alignment appears neutral), asymmetric patellar resection, lateral placement of the patellar button, excessive patellar composite thickness, improper soft tissue balancing, and failure to perform a lateral release when required (see Figs. 145.23 and 145.25).[††††]

Soft Tissue Impingement and Patellar Clunk Syndrome

Any redundant or proliferative synovial, fibrotic, or fat tissue may become impinged between patella and femoral component and act as a mechanical impediment.[389] Patients may experience minor clicking but, if severe, mechanical symptoms of locking, catching, popping, and giving way, associated with various degrees of discomfort, can occur. Late-onset patellar maltracking may be caused by the proliferation of granulation tissue or the development of fibrous adhesions tethering the patella during joint movement. Such tissue growth is thought to originate from exposed cancellous bone at the margins of the components or proliferating synovium caused by chronic synovial irritation through rubbing against prosthetic prominences.

In 1982 Insall et al. first described peripatellar synovial hypertrophy as a cause of symptomatic patellar clicking and catching in posterior-stabilized TKAs during knee flexion.[215] Hozack et al. later coined the term "Patellar Clunk Syndrome" (PCS), referring to a painful catching sensation on knee extension.[198] The cause of this syndrome was found to be a prominent fibrous nodule at the junction between the proximal patellar pole and distal quadriceps tendon, which becomes entrapped in the intercondylar housing of a PS femoral component between 30 and 45 degrees of knee flexion (Fig. 145.37). An impingement problem of a similar type was described by Pettine and Bryan, who observed entrapment of infrapatellar fibrous tissue in the intercondylar notch.[344] This "reverse" PCS often creates pain during knee extension as tissue entrapment prevents smooth proximal transition of the patella (see Fig. 145.37).

PCS usually occurs within 6 to 18 months following arthroplasty surgery. It is known to be associated with PS TKAs but may also occur with CR implants, especially if femoral components present sharp transition zones between the trochlear groove and intercondylar notch. The reported incidence of PCS ranges from 0% to 16% and appears higher with certain knee arthroplasty systems.[91,155,181,269,279] Choi et al. recorded significant differences in incidence of PCS between various implant designs, ranging from 0% for the Scorpio PS to 9.7% for the PFC-Sigma RP.[91] The authors also noted an increased probability of PCS if the patella remained unresurfaced. Lonner et al. assessed 300 knees of 2 PS designs and found an incidence of 6% for the Insall-BursteinII, compared with 0% for the NexGen-Legacy.[269] Frye et al. showed that with appropriate design changes to the PFC-Sigma PS femoral component, including deepening of the trochlear groove and creation of a less abrupt transition toward the intercondylar box, complications arising from soft tissue impingement reduced from 13% to 0%.[152]

The initial treatment of any painful soft tissue impingement following TKA is geared towards conservative measures, and should include ultrasound application and deep friction massage.[404] If the condition is diagnosed early, patients may respond to an exercise program that concentrates on repetitive flexion and extension. Quadriceps strengthening using the stationary bike may prove beneficial because it mechanically softens and autodébrides the lesion through repetitive motion. If nonoperative management fails, open or arthroscopic excision of the tissue growth is usually curative.[102,114,437,455]

Extensor Mechanism Disruption

Rupture of the patellar or quadriceps tendon is an unlikely complication following patellar resurfacing and not infrequently iatrogenic. The reported incidence for quadriceps tendon rupture is 0.1% and for patellar tendon rupture between 0.2% and 2.5%.[62,107,275,354,355] Factors associated with tendon ruptures are significant preoperative flexion contracture and angular deformities, difficult surgical exposure, obese patients, revision surgery, arthrofibrosis, quadriceps release (quadriceps snip), and extensive lateral retinacular release.[328,359] Systemic diseases, such as diabetes mellitus, chronic renal insufficiency, Parkinson disease, gout, morbid obesity, and multiple intra-articular steroid injections, will predispose patients and should be thought of, particularly if the rupture occurs spontaneously.

Quadriceps tendon ruptures may be amenable to conservative management, especially in low-demand patients using prolonged brace immobilization.[46,47] Repair of patellar tendon ruptures is extremely challenging, and treatment results are often discouraging and fraught with peril. Rand et al. reported a failure rate of 75% and infection rate of 25% after primary suture repair.[355] To improve fixation strength, the use of cortical EndoButtons has been suggested, especially if the tear is located close to its bony attachment near the inferior patella pole.[322] If tendon adaptation appears difficult or if tendon reinforcement is desired, either "Codvilla quadriceps lengthening" or the "Scuderi turndown" technique should be considered.[46,47,401,402] Additional augmentation using autogenous semitendinosus tendon graft, patellar tendon or Achilles tendon allograft, or rerouting of a fascia lata strip may be added to the repair.[328] If necessary, the repair is secured with a figure-of-eight tension band wire loop. Should the viability of the repair tissue be compromised, a medial gastrocnemius flap may be

†††† References 61, 62, 84, 163, 298, 343, and 356.

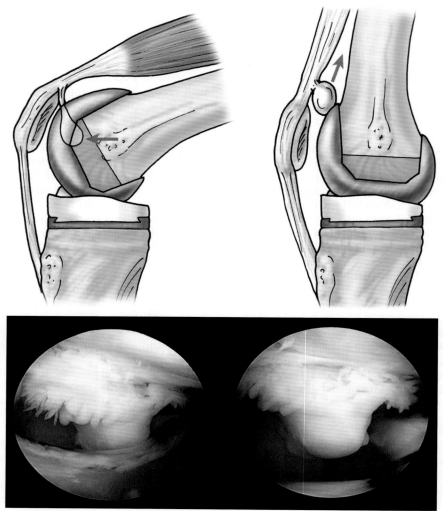

FIG 145.37 Patellar clunk syndrome: A nodule of fibrous tissue becomes entrapped in the housing of a posterior stabilized total knee arthroplasty during flexion *(red arrow top left)*. The nodule is subsequently released with an audible clunk *(red arrow top right)*. Arthroscopic image showing a "reverse" patellar clunk syndrome with an infrapatellar nodule commonly impeding knee extension. The patient experienced painful locking sensation before the nodule was surgically excised.

advantageous but carries the disadvantage of poor cosmetic appearance and weakness of plantar flexion.

The literature supports a prolonged period of bracing and protection from extremes of motion and impact activities for 3 to 6 months following surgery. Functional outcomes are often disappointing, with a residual extensor lag to be expected in most cases. Allograft reconstruction of the extensor mechanism, as popularized by Emerson et al., remains controversial.[126] In a series of 36 patients receiving an extensor allograft, Nazarian and Booth reported 8 graft ruptures, 15 patients with extensor lag, and 2 functional failures.[316]

More recently Browne and Hanssen introduced a technique using a knitted monofilament polypropylene mesh graft to reconstruct the patellar tendon and reported good results in 13 patients with subacute or chronic patellar tendon disruption.[65]

Patellectomy and Its Alternatives

AKP was a common complication associated with early knee arthroplasties, but instead of addressing the problem by improving the design, the initial response was to promote patellectomy as part of the arthroplasty procedure.[411,489] For Insall, patellectomy represented the *"end-of-the-road solution"* to the problem of AKP because it failed to alleviate AKP reliably.[219] Nowadays, patellectomy has largely been abandoned as a routine measure and is reserved for the treatment of severe comminuted fractures, advanced osteonecrosis, and tumors.[3,356]

Removal of the patella creates a biomechanical disadvantage by decreasing the lever arm and extensor torque of the quadriceps mechanism, leaving most patients with measurable weakness.[‡‡‡‡] Haxton demonstrated that this decrease in lever arm is

‡‡‡‡References 3, 112, 216, 230, 258, and 431.

particularly noticeable in the more extended knee positions, when the patella would normally move out of the intercondylar fossa onto the femoral trochlea.[189] Although patellectomy improves the efficiency of the extensor mechanism at higher flexion angles, in the daily flexion range between 0 and 90 degrees, extensor power is greatly reduced.[153,179] Increases in tibiofemoral reaction force and subsequent joint degeneration have also been reported following patellectomy.[154]

The surgeon contemplating patellectomy must thus be aware that the biomechanical effect of the loss of the fulcrum is the increased strength requirement of the quadriceps to provide extensor stability. Seriously disabled patients may not be able to develop sufficient quadriceps strength to provide this necessary extensor force.[13]

The general consensus has been to preserve the patella, even when severe bone loss may compromise its integrity. If less than 10 mm of bone remain the so-called "gullwing" osteotomy, according to Vince et al., is a useful salvage procedure because it helps to retain some residual lever arm.[127,160,458] Buechel and Hanssen developed patellar augmenting techniques to either enhance a severely compromised patellar remnant or to recreate a de novo patella following prior patellectomy.[68,185]

Alternative measures are the use of biconvex, all-polyethylene patellar components, trabecular metal inlays, or bone grafting of the patellar defect.[130,185,317] The biconvex patella requires at least 10 mm of bone stock and a 70% circumferential rim of bone equal to the thickness of the peripheral edge to provide for adequate cement fixation.[130] Trabecular metal components made of tantalum allow for cementless fixation because of their osteoconductive properties. (Fig. 145.38).[314,317] Medium-term results, despite a reported incidence of fracture through the patella remnant in up to 15% of cases, have been promising. Trabecular metal facilitates excellent bonding to the patellar shell, even with less than 10 mm of bone remaining but, as with cancellous bone grafting, sufficient peripatellar blood supply is required to promote bone ingrowth.[314] As Ries et al. pointed out, the use of the implant is not recommended if most of the fixation surface is composed of soft tissue and if patellar blood supply is poor.[367] If patellectomy is unavoidable, the technique

by Compere has proven popular, with longitudinal shelling out of bone fragments and formation of a tube by suturing the medial and lateral edges of the rectus tendon together.[98]

ANTERIOR KNEE PAIN AND CAUSES THEREOF

AKP represents a most challenging and often unfathomable clinical entity, in large part because of the highly subjective nature of the condition and because the search for reliable objective indicators of a presumed underlying pathologic process that may account for the symptoms is ongoing. Our inability to determine with any degree of certainty, whether a patient may develop AKP irrespective of the management of the patella, remains a surgical conundrum and one that demands further investigations.[26,340,481]

AKP was initially thought to be a design-related complication because it commonly occurred in early hinge arthroplasties, which failed to make provision for normal patellar tacking.[195,384,411,468,489] However, even nowadays, AKP remains the most common complication associated with TKA and, although rarely severe enough to justify revision, it is often sufficient enough to spoil an otherwise satisfactory result.

In 1980 Mark Coventry raised the question, of *"just how great is the problem of patello-femoral pain after total knee arthroplasty?"*[101] However, efforts to qualify and quantify AKP remain dwarfed by the absence of reliable and reproducible assessment tools, making its prevalence primarily dependent on the importance the clinician places on patients' symptoms.

Etiology and Pathophysiology of Anterior Knee Pain

AKP is a rather ill-defined entity pertaining to the subjective nature of a condition that is characterized by pain perceived to be located in and around the patella. Although occasionally sharp or lancinating in character, AKP is generally dull and toothache-like and often lingers on following physical activities. It may be activity-related or troublesome at rest but rarely presents as nocturnal discomfort. AKP is most commonly associated with activities that involve patellofemoral loading, such as rising from a chair or descending stairs, or may simply occur after prolonged sitting with the knee held in a flexed position, thus suggestive of the patella being ultimately responsible for the creation of it.

In 1906 Bundinger first implicated traumatic fissuring of patellar articular cartilage as a source of AKP, a condition later described by Aleman as chondromalazia.[8,67] In 1926 Heine presented evidence that patellar cartilage degradation may be associated with aging when he noted a prevalence of 88% in the eldery.[193] Using the term "chondromalacia patellae," Owre believed that degenerative changes in articular cartilage are the key causative factor in causing AKP.[327] However, in 1956 Wiles et al. started to cast doubt on Owre's theory.[475] Although the authors described chondromalacia as a precursor of osteoarthritis, they were unable to estimate how often the condition gave rise to symptoms. Outerbridge gave credence to this view when he discovered that chondromalacia was not only far more common than generally believed but also mostly asymptomatic when present.[325,326] More recently Kelly and Insall reported that the natural history of this condition remains unclear and, although according to Goodfellow and Hungerford *"chondromalacia almost becomes the rule in old age,"* the degree of chondromalacia rarely correlates with symptoms.[166,238]

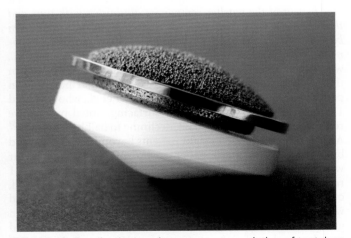

FIG 145.38 Patellar composite construct consisting of tantalum metal base unit that is sutured against the patellar bone remnant. The cone-shaped polyethylene patellar component requires to be cemented onto the base unit. (NexGen Trabecular Metal patella, Zimmer.)

One explanation for this may be that the retropatellar surface cartilage is deprived of any neural innervation and hence thought to be insensate.[121] Conversely, subchondral bone possesses an extensive nerve supply, which explains why increases in intraosseous pressure can cause the perception of substantial pain.[120,362] It is indisputable that subchondral nerve fibers may be activated in the presence of cartilage degradation either through subtle increases in intraosseous pressure or through partial exposure of sensory nerve endings. However if one made the assumption that AKP is solely caused by the patella, then simple resurfacing would be expected to solve any such problems. The fact that neither primary nor SR has been able to predictably reduce AKP is strongly suggestive of other sources of pain beyond the condition of the retropatellar cartilage.[26,143,208,219]

In particular the soft tissue envelope surrounding the patellofemoral joint has been implicated in the etiology of AKP, because of the high density of free nerve endings and nociceptors found in quadriceps and patellar tendon, retinaculi, fat pad, and synovial membrane.[41] Free nerve endings may be activated through mechanical, thermal, or chemical stimuli or a combination thereof. In defining the pathophysiology of patellofemoral pain, Dye has spoken about the variable mosaic of possible pathophysiologic processes.[119] In his view the etiology of patellofemoral pain is based on simple joint overload which may trigger inflammation of the synovial tissues, creation of retinacular neuromas, and increases in intraosseous pressure.

A variety of more obscure functional and structural pathologies have been implicated as potential causes of AKP. These include a number of soft tissue abnormalities (eg, peripatellar tendinopathy, bursitis, impinging synovial folds and scar tissue bands, neuromas, Sudeck dystrophy, complex regional pain syndrome), bony abnormalities (eg, Sinding-Larsen-Johansson syndrome, stress fracture, retained osteophytes, impinging loose bodies), and those directly associated with patellar maltracking.[58,75,76,102,389] Muscle weakness and imbalance, especially when affecting hip abductors, glutei, and extensor mechanism, have also been implicated as causative because they may force the knee into a valgus position on load bearing.[342] On the background of already heightened patellofemoral compressive force in flexion, this in turn will increase the Q angle and the lateral patellar force vector, thereby creating a form of dynamic patellar maltracking.[341] This situation may be further exacerbated by any apparent instability, especially if present in mid-flexion.[329]

Even though many clinicians believe that the presence of preoperative symptoms may be holding the key when suggesting patellar resurfacing,[76] the scientific basis for such action is missing. In a randomized controlled trial (RCT), Barrack et al. found that 28% of patients without AKP before resurfacing suffered AKP after surgery.[26] Similarly 9% of patients with preoperative AKP continued having pain postoperatively despite resurfacing. In the group in which the patella was retained, 23% continued suffering pain, whereas new pain developed in 14%. Similar observations were conveyed by Peng et al. in a comparative study of bilateral TKAs.[340] Twenty percent of resurfaced patellae suffered postoperative AKP, of which 6% had been present preoperatively. In the nonresurfaced patellae, 20% had postoperative AKP, of which 9% were present preoperatively.

Incidence of Anterior Knee Pain

The incidence of AKP differs widely, with reported figures ranging from 0% to 47% following primary patellar resurfacing,[52,76,83,469] and 0% to 43% when the patella is retained.[139,187,227,321,345] These variations are likely because of a lack of reproducible classification systems and validated outcome tools with which to assess patellofemoral pain and function. They may also be influenced by patient selection, surgical technique, and implant design. However, overall the occurrence of significant AKP seems to have lessened over the past decade, with a currently reported incidence of around 10% irrespective of the treatment of the patella.[§§§§]

Scott and Kim[396] indicated that regardless of the management of the patella, clinicians can expect approximately 10% to 20% of patients to be affected by nondisabling AKP following TKA, a finding confirmed through numerous prospective, observational studies.[*****] Meftah et al. tried to define the natural history of AKP by following 250 patients with primary resurfaced TKA over a 10-year period.[294] The authors noted that one-third of patients were suffering mild-to-moderate nondisabling AKP at 1 year, which persisted in approximately 30% at 10 years. During the same time period, new AKP developed in 10% of previously asymptomatic patients, resulting in the presence of nondisabling AKP in approximately 20% of patients at 10 years.

Temporal Development of Anterior Knee Pain

Patient satisfaction is directly linked to the level of pain experienced following TKA, and patient suffering AKP are thus generally less satisfied.[9,14,26] Evidence is emerging that suggests that both patient satisfaction and AKP following TKA have a tendency to improve over time irrespective of the initial management of the patella.[32,54,375,474] Inoue et al. recorded mild AKP in 14.6% of rheumatoid and 24.4% of osteoarthritis patients following TKA with patellar retention.[211] AKP gradually subsided in the osteoarthritis (OA) group over a period of 3 to 4 years, whereas the proportion of symptomatic rheumatoid arthritis (RA) patients remained static.

Robertsson et al. reviewed data of 27,372 patients from the Swedish Knee Register and found that 15% of patients with resurfaced patellae were generally dissatisfied, compared with 19% in which the patella had been retained.[375] However, patients with patellar resurfacing became less satisfied with their knee over time, whereas the satisfaction rating in those without resurfacing remained unchanged. The authors concluded that *"the benefit of the patellar component diminishes with time and that the need for secondary resurfacing may in the longer term be balanced by the need for revision of failed patellar components."*[375,376] Similar findings were reported by Roberts et al., who observed improved satisfaction ratings and reduction in the levels of AKP at rest over a 10-year period but only in patients with unresurfaced TKA.[373] Brander et al., who reviewed 116 patients following primary resurfacing, noted progressive reduction in postoperative pain, declining to half by 3 months.[55] AKP continued in one in eight patients beyond 12 months, and by 5 years 65% of those patients who suffered pain at 1 year were all but pain free and satisfied.[54] Beaupre et al. reviewed 21 resurfaced and 17 nonresurfaced TKAs over a 10-year period, observing significantly improved pain scores when compared with the baseline, with no significant differences between groups.[32] Contrary to the aforementioned, Wood et al. noted that the number of patients affected by AKP increased with time but remained lower if the patella was resurfaced initially.[481] It

---

has since been argued that these results may be a reflection of the relatively patellar-unfriendly design of the Miller-Galante prosthesis used in this study.

Effect of Patellar Tilt and Subluxation on Anterior Knee Pain

The effect patellar tilt and subluxation may have on the development of AKP following TKA is debatable.[385] Although some have noted an increased incidence of AKP in patients with patellar tilt or subluxation,[211,229,385] others have failed to observe any such correlation.[27,42,83,187] In a series of 178 unresurfaced TKAs, Inoune et al. reported a direct association between levels of lateral patellar shift, as viewed on tangential radiographs, and the incidence and severity of AKP.[211] Newman et al. also looked at the influence of patellar malalignment on knee performance and outcome scores.[318] Although malalignment exerted an overall adverse effect on clinical outcome measures, moderate degrees of malalignment were better tolerated when the patella had been resurfaced. The latter observation was shared by Campbell et al., who observed no cases of patellar subluxation in 36 resurfaced patients but 5 in the 46 in which the patella had been retained.[83] However, the incidence of AKP was not influenced by the presence of patellar tilt or subluxation in either group. Hasegawa and Ohashi followed 78 unresurfaced TKAs for 12 years. Seventeen knees developed patella subluxation and lateral facet erosion, but only four of these (30%) experienced pain.[187]

Influence of Component Design on Anterior Knee Pain

Implant design is known to influence patella kinematics and may thus induce a significant effect on the development of AKP.[187,277,343,434,488] Townley already recognized this fact in 1974 when he wrote *"It is particularly important to include an articulating surface for the patella on the femoral component [as] this eliminates a major source of chronic pain inherent in an arthritic patello-femoral compartment".*[439] Although one may be inclined to believe that the effect of design is more influential when the patella is retained, there is evidence to suggest that the same may apply in resurfaced TKAs.[64,148,277] This is not entirely surprising if one considers that the natural motion path of the patella is independent of the resurfacing procedure and structurally reliant on the surface geometry of the trochlea.[453] It would also explain the great variation in the incidence of AKP between different arthroplasty systems, regardless of the treatment of the patella, and which is likely to be influenced by design properties. Mahoney et al. compared a multiradius femoral component to one with a single flexion–extension axis in patients following primary resurfacing and recorded significantly less AKP on rising from a chair when using a single radius design.[277] Hwang et al., who compared 7-year results of two groups of patients who received a femoral component with patella-friendly design features, recorded low levels of AKP between resurfaced and unresurfaced knees, with values of 4.2% and 6.1%, respectively.[207] In a study of similar design, Kulkarni et al. recorded AKP in 7% (7 of 96 patients) following resurfacing compared with 10% (12 of 115 patients) when the patella was retained, with only 1 patient in each group having pain severe enough to require medication.[248]

In case of patellar retention, abnormal contact and tracking characteristics may ensue, especially if the femoral component is primarily designed to juxtapose with a designated patellar prosthesis of spherical type.[248,434,435,474] Thus it has been speculated that AKP following patellar retention may be secondary to altered patellar biomechanics and incongruence of surface geometries[††††††] (see Fig. 145.19).

How important design issues are has been highlighted by a group of researchers from the University of Western Australia who conducted two randomized controlled studies with almost identical study design in which the only major variable was the type of prosthesis used.[418,481] In the first study the authors used a relatively unfriendly patellar design, featuring flat-shaped condyles with a shallow and angular trochlea groove.[481] In their second study a relatively patellar-friendly design, characterized by a deepened trochlea groove with curved transition towards the femoral condyles, was used.[418] Comparing the outcome of nonresurfaced patients between both studies revealed a drop in the rate of postoperative AKP from 31% to 21%, a reduction in the reoperation rate for patellofemoral complications from 12% to 1.2%, and an increase in Knee Society Rating Score by 11 points. Whiteside and Nakamura arrived at a similar conclusion when they compared the prevalence of AKP following patellar retention in three different femoral component designs of varying degrees of patellar friendliness.[474] Severe AKP on stair climbing occurred in 63% at 1 year when using an implant whose trochlea surface did not conform closely to the shape of the patella. In the comparison groups using a design characterized by deepened trochlear groove and improved lateral patellar support, none of the patients suffered severe AKP. However, at 2 years mild AKP on stair climbing was recorded in 18% in the former and 10% in the latter patient cohort, with a general tendency to further improvement with time.

Although a review study failed to observe an association between clinical outcome and prosthetic design, inclusion criteria for qualifying as "patellar friendly" were used indiscriminately.[338] This resulted in most implants, including those generally considered "patella unfriendly," such as the IB-II, to fall into this category, thereby clouding interpretation of the data. Lygre et al, on reviewing data from the Norwegian Arthroplasty Register, noted a continuing reduction in the risk of revision for pain in TKA since the first observation period of 1994–2001. These changes coincided with the introduction of the newer and more patellar-friendly implants (eg, NexGen), whereas older designs (eg, Genesis I and Tricon-C) had been phased out, prompting the authors to surmise that the occurrence of AKP may be design related.[273]

Manufacturers are clearly trying to address some of the design issues raised in relation to so-called patellar unfriendliness. Although differences between implant types still exist, variations in femoral component designs have become much more subtle, which may explain the general reduction in AKP seen when contemporary implants are used.[180,221,265,273,373]

Influence of Component Positioning on Anterior Knee Pain

It has long been recognized that component malrotation of both femoral and tibial implant are a significant contributing factor in the development of AKP following TKA.[27,34,449] Barrack et al., who assessed a group of patients suffering AKP following TKA, with computed tomography, found that patients with combined component internal rotation were more than five times more likely to experience AKP compared to those with

---

[††††††]References 50, 52, 76, 283, 284, 417, and 418.

combined component external rotation (see Figs. 145.23 and 145.26).[27] Figgie et al. showed that AKP was present in 23 of 75 TKAs in which the implants were positioned outside ideal alignment parameters, compared with no cases of AKP in the group of 41 knees in which components were positioned correctly.[143]

Influence of Mobile versus Fixed Bearing TKA on Anterior Knee Pain

Some evidence exists suggesting that the use of a mobile bearing TKA may, at least in the initial postoperative period, influence the rate of postoperative AKP.[480] Kim et al. compared results of 92 patients who received a fixed bearing TKA in 1 knee and a mobile bearing one in the other. At a mean follow-up of 2.6 years the authors reported reduced levels of pain and increased satisfaction in patients treated with a mobile implant.[243] Breugem et al. recorded persistent AKP in 4.3% patients who received a mobile bearing implant compared with 18.9% in which a fixed bearing implant had been used.[59] The same group of patients was reviewed again at 6 to 10 years, when it became apparent that the differences in AKP had not been sustained.[58,60]

Influence of Patellar Denervation on Anterior Knee Pain

In an attempt to reduce the likelihood of postoperative AKP when retaining the native patella, Keblish et al. suggested circumferential thermocoagulation of the patellar rim using electrocautery.[235,236] The procedure is thought to create a level of sensory deprivation and was used by Keblish in conjunction with patellar débridement and occasional transcortical Pridie drilling to areas of cartilage loss (see Fig. 145.35). Rand suggested that, because of the detrimental effect electrocautery may have on articular cartilage, treatment should be restricted to the peripatellar rim.[357] Although some studies have reported improved clinical outcomes when circumferential electrocautery is used,[11,348,451] others have failed to do so.[24,178,450] Most studies nonetheless show a reduced incidence of AKP, at least during the initial postoperative period.[450,451,485] However, the potential long-term merits of such surgical intervention, whether used in conjunction with patellar resurfacing or not, remain unclear.

Influence of Retinacular Release on Anterior Knee Pain

There is evidence to suggest that performing retinacular release may lead to a reduction in postoperative AKP.[491] However, any such benefit must be balanced against increased likelihood of avascular necrosis (AVN), patellar fracture, and patellar component loosening.[292,405] Zha et al. enrolled 148 patients, half of which were randomly assigned to receive lateral release.[491] At 18 months, 5.6% in the release group and 20.6% in the control group suffered AKP. However, the fact that retinacular release was performed indiscriminately and not based on actual needs suggests that a number of patients in the control group may have been affected by postoperative patellar maltracking, thereby artificially increasing the number of AKP sufferers in this cohort.

PREDICTORS OF ANTERIOR KNEE PAIN

A variety of predictors of postoperative AKP have been suggested but few, such as obesity and flexion contracture, have been reliably identified.[190,345,418,419] Most clinical studies have been unable to depict a specific cause that may explain why some knees are affected by AKP and others are not.[26,83,418,469] Results from RCTs have failed to show any reliable association between BMI, gender, preoperative AKP, degree of chondromalacia or chondrolysis, lateral release, and the occurrence of AKP.[26,83,418] Elson and Brenkel prospectively assessed 602 primary TKAs, of which 13% were affected by AKP.[125] The authors discovered that age was the only reliable predictor of pain, with patients below the age of 60 being more than twice as likely to be affected. It may be speculated that the positive effect of increasing age may be because of lower expectations and reduced activity levels in the elderly. Wood et al. found BW to be a significant predictor of AKP but only in patients in whom the patella was retained.[481] However, Waters and Bentley, who assessed 514 knees randomized for patellar resurfacing, found no difference regarding age and weight between knees with AKP and those without.[469] Furthermore, no association concerning gender, lateral release, cruciate retention or sacrifice and whether the knees were affected by osteoarthritis or rheumatoid arthritis was noted. Other studies have shown that height and weight but not BMI are implicated as being predictive of AKP and of revision following primary resurfacing.[76,292,481] This is thought to be because of increased lever arms and raised patellofemoral forces displayed in taller and heavier individuals.

Although many clinicians may believe that the presence of preoperative AKP is predictive of postoperative AKP, evidence in support of such notion is missing. Conversely, Burnett et al. noted that patients free of AKP prior to surgery remained pain free during the entire follow-up period of 10 years, whether they were resurfaced or not.[76] Although the authors concluded that the absence of AKP before surgery was predictive of remaining pain free, their findings are disputed by others.[26,83,340,418,440]

The state of the retropatellar surface is commonly implicated as one of the key factors in the prediction of postoperative AKP; however, data are mostly anecdotal and often based on presumption rather than clear evidence.[345] Han et al., who assessed the severity of the retropatellar surface damage at the time of TKA surgery, found only a weak correlation to preexisting AKP, and none to the functional parameters of chair rising, stair climbing, and quadriceps strength.[182] We are all aware of the somewhat incomprehensible fact that some patients may suffer extreme AKP in the absence of notable cartilage damage, whereas others in whom cartilage degradation is severe are relatively pain free.[86,182] A biologic explanation for such discrepancy remains illusive, and the paradigm of a pure structural or biomechanical explanation of the genesis of patellofemoral pain is thus not sustainable. Isolated patellofemoral OA should therefore not be considered a proxy for AKP.

In 1985 Townley, on looking back at his experience with TKA over a 13-year period, revealed that *"neither the occurrence nor the degree of the symptoms appears to be related to the preoperative condition of the patella."*[440] His view was shared by Insall et al, who were also unable to define a correlation between the degree of cartilage damage and the level of pain or outcome result in patients who had been left unresurfaced.[217,218,419] A plethora of studies have since tried to address the relationship between the level of patellar arthritis and the emergence of postoperative AKP but have failed to draw a clear conclusion.[‡‡‡‡‡] In a prospective trial, Feller et al. noted a lack of correlation between the state of the patellar articular cartilage and either Hospital of Special Surgery (HSS) or Patellar Score in patients

---

‡‡‡‡‡References 26, 76, 83, 138, 207, 318, and 474.

TABLE 145.2 Bristol Patella Wear Score[318]

Bristol Patella Wear Score
The retropatellar surface is divided into four zones and graded:

0 = normal cartilage
1 = softened cartilage
2 = fibrillated/fissured cartilage
3 = exposed bone
Maximum total score 12

From Newman JH, Ackroyd CE, Shah NA, Karachalios T: Should the patella be resurfaced during total knee replacement? *Knee* 7:17–23, 2000.

in whom the patella was retained.[138] These results were echoed by Hwang et al., who reviewed 132 unresurfaced and 143 resurfaced TKAs at a mean follow-up of 7.8 years. Feller's Patellar Score, Knee Society Score (KSS), and the presence of AKP were unaffected by the degree of cartilage damage in either group.[207] In a series of 100 patients, Campbell et al. found no relationship between the grade of chondromalacia and preoperative or postoperative AKP, irrespective of whether the patellar was retained or resurfaced.[83]

Newman et al. assessed the patellar status through formulating a patella wear score, by dividing the retropatellar surface into 4 quadrants, grading each from 0 (representing normal cartilage) to 3 (for exposed bone), giving a maximum score of 12 (Table 145.2).[318] Although at 5 years the subgroup of unresurfaced TKAs with well-preserved retropatellar cartilage at the outset showed a trend toward better performance than those with poor cartilage, results were nonetheless quite unpredictable. Newman hence concluded that patellar wear does not prove to be a reliable guide when considering selective resurfacing (John Newman, personal communication, 2015). Rodriguez et al. came to a different conclusion in a study in which patients were stratified according to the Outerbridge classification.[380] After a minimum follow-up of 5 years, 11.6% of patients with grade IV changes, compared with 0.6% with grade I to III, required SR, leading the authors to conclude that patients with advanced levels of cartilage degradation should be resurfaced at index procedure. However this study evaluated only the risk of reoperation and failed to assess AKP and patellofemoral function and hence carries limited validity.

If one accepts that retropatellar wear and AKP considered in isolation may be less of a predictor regarding clinical outcome, then the circumstances are generally viewed to be different if patellar degeneration is coupled with preexisting AKP.[105] The majority of surgeons would contemplate patellar resurfacing on the background of symptomatic patellofemoral disease, provided that there is enough bone stock to safely support a patellar component.[345] The good results achieved with patellofemoral arthroplasties or TKAs in the *"primary patellofemoral arthritis"* scenario have given credibility to such action.[2,293,303] As Picetti et al. have pointed out, *"there appears to be a strong association between preoperative patellofemoral symptoms, a class-IV patellar surface, and postoperative patellofemoral pain."*[345] However, if the patella is small and porotic, the risk of resurfacing may outweigh potential benefits, because of an increase in the risk of patellar fracture, AVN, and component loosening. In such circumstances, patellar retention is favorable and outcome results may still be acceptable, especially if an anatomic femoral component is used (Robert Barrack, personal communication, 2015).[436]

SECONDARY RESURFACING

SR, despite its limited success, remains a viable option and potential remedy in patients with retained patella, who are affected by persistent AKP that has been recalcitrant to conservative treatment measures. SR is performed in 0.7% to 12% of cases,[26,129,335,385,419] but can be curtailed to approximately 2.5% if appropriate criteria for selective resurfacing are applied.[241,318] Especially older and nonconforming TKA designs have been implemented with higher rates of SR. Insall recalled having performed SR in approximately 8% of cases in his initial series of several hundred IB-II TKAs and attributed this to the implant's patellar-unfriendly design features of juxtaposing convexities in knee flexion (John Insall, personal communication, 1998) (see Fig. 145.8).

In countries where patella retention represents the primary mode of management, SR appears to be surprisingly uncommon, with rates of 1.8% in Norway, 0.9% in New Zealand, and 0.7% in Sweden.

The great majority of SR procedures are performed within the first 2 years following TKA.[52,264,345] However, the long-term outcome is often disappointing, with almost half the patient base failing to improve or suffering recurrence of symptoms.[26,84,302] The decision whether or not to offer a patient such a procedure rests with the surgeon, his or her appreciation of the severity of the patient's suffering, and his or her general attitude towards the potential benefits SR may be able to offer. Thus it is strongly open for bias, a fact reflected by the large variation in the level of SR reported in the literature. It has been argued that the increased revision rates in unresurfaced TKAs may not necessarily be because of patients suffering more severe pain but because surgeons are more likely to revise a painful patella in an unresurfaced TKA than in a knee in which the patella had already been resurfaced at the index procedure.[93] In a meta-analysis of 7075 cases, Pavlou et al. found no difference regarding the incidence of AKP between resurfacing and nonresurfacing groups. This invited the authors to the conclusion that the rate of reoperations in nonresurfaced patients is a mere indicator that SR provides the only viable surgical option in this group of patients, thereby artificially increasing the primary revision rate.[338]

Even if the SR procedure appears successful at first, recurrence of symptoms has been reported to occur in 30% to 80% of patients.[§§§§§] Parvizi et al. reviewed 41 knees at an average of 4.5 years following SR for AKP.[335] The mean time delay between primary TKA and SR was 29 months (range: 24 to 92). The authors considered 40% as failures, either because of patients' dissatisfaction, absence of improvement, or the need for further revision because of patellar maltracking. Barrack et al. performed SR in 7 of 60 knees, 6 of which presented with clinical improvement initially.[26] However AKP recurred in four out of five patients available for review 5 years later.

Mouneke et al. reported on 20 out of 623 TKAs who underwent SR.[308] At a mean follow-up period of 3 years, 6 patients (30%) showed a significant improvement, whereas 14 (70%) either did not improve or became worse. Khatod et al. reviewed 28 knees at a mean of 2.9 years (range: 1 to 12) following SR, with 52% of patients indicating that they would undergo revision surgery again, suggesting that 48% were dissatisfied.[240] Spencer et al. reviewed 28 patients who had undergone SR for

---

§§§§§References 26, 84, 158, 248, 286, 302, 308, 335, 375, and 420.

persistent AKP.[420] Patient satisfaction was assessed at a mean of 28 months, resulting in 59% feeling improved, 34% feeling the same, and 7% feeling worse.

Some uncertainty remains about the potential effect of time lapse between index procedure and SR on clinical outcome. Karnezis et al. reported on 14 patients who received SR at an average of 4.9 years (range: 1.7 to 10.7 years) post TKA.[229] Patients were reviewed between 2 and 5 years following SR, with 64% achieving significant reduction in AKP, whereas other parameters, such as "pain on stairs" and "patella tenderness," failed to improve significantly. The authors showed that the time delay between the original surgery and the SR procedure was inversely related to the level of clinical improvement. However these results are in contradiction to a more recent study by Scheurer et al., who reviewed 58 cases at an average of 2.6 years following SR. A total of 26% of patients remained dissatisfied, and the author noted that the time interval between index procedure and SR in these patients was often shorter compared with patients who were satisfied.[385]

The poor results often encountered with SR may to a large extent be because of unrecognized component malpositioning (see Fig. 145.26). Common reasons for this are rotational malalignment of femoral and/or tibial component, changes in the height of the joint line, or overstuffing of the patellofemoral joint, either through under-resection of distal femur or patella or a combination thereof (see Fig. 145.23). If such underlying abnormalities are not corrected at the time of SR, symptoms are likely to recur.[40] Even in the well-aligned arthroplasty, SR is simply not always able to address the apparent pathology and pain pathways effectively. Thus, it would appear reasonable to suggest that failure to improve patients' AKP following SR may point either to a multifactorial etiology or a different cause other than a problem pertaining to the PFJ. Parvizi et al. has hence coined the term *presumed patellar-related AKP* in an attempt to emphasize the current lack of understanding surrounding this clinical entity.[335]

Results of using three-phase bone scintigraphy as an assessment tool to distinguish patients who are likely to benefit from SR has been contradictory.[7,385] In a study by Ahmad et al., 21 out of 22 patients suffering AKP presented an increased tracer uptake of the patella, compared with 7 out of 33 affected by diffuse pain.[7] All of the 20 patients with a "hot patella" who went on to receive SR had relief of their symptoms. However, none of the "cold patellae" underwent simple SR hence limiting the validity of the study. Scheurer et al. recorded 35 'hot patellae' in 50 patients affected by AKP.[385] All patients subsequently underwent SR and were reviewed at an average of 2.5 years post surgery. Of the patients with a hot patella, 63% were satisfied, compared with 93% if the patella was cold, leaving the authors to call into question the usefulness of bone scanning as an indicator for SR.

Ultimately the decision whether or not to offer SR to the symptomatic patient remains with the clinician. It is his or her experience and judgment that holds the key in the decision-making process. To improve outcomes after SR, clinicians have emphasized the importance of patient selection. Barrack has suggested that if the pain is extremely well localized and consistent with pain of patellar origin (classically occurring during patellofemoral-loading activities), then the results of SR are relatively good. However if the pain is more diffuse in location and occurrence, one should exercise caution when suggesting SR (Robert Barrack, personal communication, 2015).

If a patient following primary patellar resurfacing presents with AKP, few options are available to the surgeon, short of a formal patellar revision. Isolated patella component revision for pain is generally not recommended because the clinical outcome is at best uncertain.[40] Furthermore, patella revision is far from being an innocuous procedure and should be approached with utmost caution because complications are frequent and outcomes are often poor.[40,259,314] Therefore, it could be argued that if this clinical situation occurs in which a patient is affected by AKP following primary patellar resurfacing, it would be prudent for the surgeon not to proceed with a revision procedure, unless a specific underlying cause (eg, maltracking) or component malrotation can be delineated and remedied.

PATELLAR SCORING SYSTEMS

Most clinical outcome scores either fail to address joint-specific aspects concerning the clinical performance of the patellofemoral joint or to detect minimum perceived clinical differences.[48] Common scoring systems, such as the Hospital of Special Surgery Knee Score, KSS, Oxford Knee Score, Bristol Knee Score, and Western Ontario McMasters Universities Arthritis Index, all contain references to aspects of patellofemoral joint function; however they are not provided in the context of assessing the PF joint but rather the overall performance of patients following TKA. These scores tend to underestimate the problem in patients predominately affected by patellofemoral disease, besides not being validated for a subset of data referring to PF function to be extracted and assessed independently.

In the case of the Knee Society Clinical Score the main component focuses on pain when weight-bearing, which is generally understood to relate to pain when walking on level ground. However most patients with patellofemoral disease have little pain on level walking but suffer marked pain when descending stairs or rising from a chair. Although the Knee Society Function Score extracts information on the way patients negotiate stairs, it does not assess whether such activity is painful. In its updated version of the KSS, some of these shortcomings have been addressed by including questions more specific to patellofemoral function.[403] These refer to the level of pain with stairs and inclines, problems when getting up from a low chair, or when climbing up or down a flight of stairs; however no reference is made to the location of discomfort or the presence of AKP.

Because the majority of general knee scores do not allow for the detection of subtle changes concerning patellofemoral function or pain, specific patella scores have hence been introduced, including the Feller Patella Score, Kujala Function Score, Bristol Patellar Score, and Fulkerson Patellofemoral Joint Evaluation Score.[138,156,247,318] The Fulkerson Score was derived from the Lysholm Knee Ligament score and assesses seven key components of patellofemoral function.[156] The maximum possible score is 100 and compiled of 45 points for pain, 10 points each for limp, support, stair climbing ability, instability, and swelling and 5 points for squatting.

The two most popular scoring systems currently in use are the Feller Patella Score and Bristol Patella Score, which is in part because of their simplicity and ease of use (Tables 145.3 and 145.4). The Bristol Patella Score consists of two parts, the "Clinical Score" and the "Wear Score" (see Tables 145.2 and 145.3).[318] The Clinical Score allocates 2 points each for AKP,

TABLE 145.3 Bristol Clinical Patella Score[318]

BRISTOL CLINICAL PATELLA SCORE				
	Severe	Moderate	None	Score
Anterior knee pain	0	1	2	
Pain on stairs	0	1	2	
Patella tenderness	0	1	2	
Crepitus/catching	0	1	2	
Clinical maltracking	0	1	2	
Total				Max. 10

Adapted from Newman JH, Ackroyd CE, Shah NA, Karachalios T: Should the patella be resurfaced during total knee replacement? *Knee* 7:17–23, 2000.

TABLE 145.4 Feller Patellar Score[138]

Feller Patellar Score	
Anterior Knee Pain	
None	15
Mild	10
Moderate	5
Severe	0
Quadriceps Strength	
Good (5/5)	5
Fair (4/5)	3
Poor (<4)	1
Ability to Rise From a Chair	
With ease (no arms)	5
With ease (with arms)	3
With difficulty	1
Unable	0
Stair Climbing	
1 foot/stair, no support	5
1 foot/stair, with support	4
2 feet/stair, no support	3
2 feet/stair, with support	2
Total score	**Max. 30**

Adapted from Feller JA, Bartlett RJ, Lang DM: Patellar resurfacing versus retention in total knee arthroplasty. *Bone Joint J* 78:226–228, 1996.

TABLE 145.5 Anterior Knee Pain Rating Score According to Waters and Bentley[469]

Stanmore Anterior Knee Pain Rating Score	
No pain	0
Mild pain that does not intrude on daily activities	1
Moderate pain that is a nuisance; patient not considering further surgery	2
Severe pain; patient considering further surgery	3

From Waters TS, Bentley G: Patellar resurfacing in total knee arthroplasty. *J Bone Joint Surg Am* 85:212–217, 2003.

in nature. Unfortunately, follow-up periods are often relatively short and may thus fail to capture AKP, which, according to Insall, often occurs in the unresurfaced TKA as late as 5 years after the index procedure (John Insall, personal communication, 1998). Studies on the subject often combine a variety of implant designs, based on the assumption that they are "all the same," whereas some of the older studies use implants that are simply redundant today. Whether the findings of these studies can be generalized to contemporary implants is debatable. Studies are not infrequently affected by observer bias, and their methodologic limitations prevent a direct comparison of like for like. One major weakness associated with the majority of RCTs is that they asses only the "always resurface" versus the "never resurface" operative approaches, without addressing selective resurfacing. These studies have henceforth done little to reduce the insurmountable divide between clinicians who promote resurfacing and those who do not. Randomized, controlled, prospective trials have tried to address these shortcomings, but variations in patient assessment and study design remain and continue to impair their comparability (see Patellar Scoring Systems).

In addition, defining reliable outcome measures when assessing failure and complications following TKA, with or without primary resurfacing, is not without its own controversy. Revision surgery is widely considered to be the most objective endpoint in defining failure. This may be applicable in tricompartmental TKA, in which revision, surgery is often unavoidable because of the nature of the complication (eg, fracture, implant loosening). However, in patients with bicompartmental TKA SR for presumed patellar related AKP, the most common indication for revision, is generally discretional and potentially distorted by surgeons' experience and attitude.

Analysis of 18 RCTs revealed a total of 1704 knees that were treated with patellar resurfacing at the time of TKA, compared with 1717 knees in which the patella had been retained (Table 145.6). The average follow-up period was 5.9 years (range: 1 to 10.8 years). Postoperative AKP was present in 18.8% of unresurfaced and 18.0% of resurfaced patients. Combined Knee Society Scores of 152 in unresurfaced and 154 in resurfaced arthroplasties were recorded. Patellar complications led to a reoperation rate of 4.8% in all unresurfaced and of 2.3% in all resurfaced knees. Overall, 11 studies were unable to define a clinically significant difference between resurfacing and nonresurfacing in patients' function and their perception of pain. Two studies showed preference towards nonresurfacing, whereas in five studies resurfacing appeared superior over nonresurfacing. These results are echoed by recent meta-analyses that found equivalence in patient satisfaction, proportion of patients suffering AKP, and clinical outcome results between treatment groups, although patients with primary resurfacing underwent fewer additional surgical procedures.[56,338,346]

pain on stairs, tenderness, crepitus/catching, and maltracking, giving a maximum score of 10. The Wear Score defines the level of retropatellar degeneration by assessing the status of the articular cartilage (Tab. 145.2). The Feller Patella Score allows for a maximum possible score of 30 and assigns 15 points for AKP and 5 points each for quadriceps strength, ability to rise from a chair, and stair climbing (see Table 145.4).[138] Apart from the Visual Analog Score traditionally used in the assessment of pain, the Stanmore Anterior Knee Pain Rating Score tries to define an association between the level of pain and the patient's willingness to undergo further surgery (Table 145.5).[469] Although none of the above patellar scores have been officially validated, they nevertheless represent a welcome addition to the general knee scores currently available.

PROSPECTIVE AND RANDOMIZED CONTROLLED TRIALS

The controversy surrounding the need for patellar resurfacing at the time of TKA has been fueled by differing results derived from clinical studies and historic data, most of which are retrospective

TABLE 145.6   Randomized Controlled Trials Published Between 1995 and 2015 Comparing the Outcome of Total Knee Arthroplasty With and Without Patellar Resurfacing

	TKA Implant Type	Patellar Implant Type	Number of Cases NR/RS	Mean Follow-Up (Years)	NRS AKP (%)	RS AKP (%)	NRS ROP (%)	RS ROP (%)	NRS KSS	RS KSS	Comments
Partio and Wirz[334]	PFC CR	Modified dome	50/50	2.5	22	2	0	0	169	170	RS better
Feller et al.[138]	PCA	Offset dome	20/20	3	—	—	0	5	(89)[a]	(86)[a]	NRS better
Schroeder-Boersch et al.[391]	Duracon	Onlay	20/20	4.8	20	10	10	5	150	163	RS better
Barrack et al.[26]	MG-II CR	Modified dome	60/58	5	17	19	12	0	169	162	No difference
Fengler[139]	PFC	Dome (inlay)	68/68	1	0	0	0	0	147	138	NRS better
Wood et al.[481]	MG-II CR	Not specified	128/92	4	31	16	12	10	152	157	RS better
Mayman et al.[287]	AMK	Dome	50/50	9	10	47	10	4	156.5	146.8	No difference
Waters and Bentley[469]	PFC CR/PS	Dome	231/243	5.3	25.1	5.3	4.8	1.2	162	167	RS better
Burnett et al.[76]	AMK CR	Dome	48/42	10.8	25	37	6	2	146	145	No difference
Gildone et al.[159]	NexGen PS	Dome	28/28	2	21	0	0	0	178	178	RS better
Myles et al.[311]	LCS RP	Anatomic	25/25	1.75	—	—	0	0	162	147	No difference
Campbell et al.[83]	MG-II CR	Modified dome	54/46	10	43	47	3.7	2.2	136[b]	138[b]	No difference
Burnett et al.[73]	MG-II CR	Modified dome	32/32	10	17.3	16.5	6.2	3.1	148	146	No difference
Smith et al.[418]	Profix	Dome (inlay)	86/73	4.4	21	30	1.2	1.4	163	152	No difference
Burnett et al.[74]	MG-II CR	Modified dome	60/58	10	16	21	12	3	155	146	No difference
Breugem and Haverkamp[58,c]	Variable	Variable	646/664	5	—	—	2.4	1.3	(34.0)[d]	(35.1)[d]	No difference
Liu et al.[265]	PFC-PS	Modified dome	64/68	7	12.5	14.7	0	0	125	121	No difference
Roberts et al.[373]	PFC-Sigma CR	Dome	47/67	10	2.1	3.0	5.8	2.8	146	153	No difference
Totals			1717/1704	5.9	18.8	18.0	4.8	2.3	154	152	

[a]Hospital for Special Surgery Score (0-100).
[b]Four-year follow-up data only.
[c]Multicenter trial.
[d]Oxford Knee Score (0-48).

AKP, Anterior knee pain; *AMK*, anatomic medullary knee; *CR*, cruciate-retaining; *CS*, cruciate-sacrificing; *KSS*, Knee Society Score (knee score 0-100 + function score 0-100); *LCS*, low-contact stress; *MG*, Miller-Galante; *NRS*, nonresurfacing; *PCA*, porous-coated anatomic; *PFC*, press-fit condylar; *PS*, posterior-stabilized; *ROP*, reoperation rate; *RP*, rotating platform; *RS*, resurfacing; *s/s*, statistically significant.

In the Knee Arthroplasty Trial involving a number of centers in the United Kingdom, 1715 patients were randomly allocated into resurfacing or nonresurfacing groups and followed for a period of 5 years.[56] Data analysis revealed no significant effect on patient functional status, revision rate, and quality of life. However the authors noted that patellar-related revisions occurred more frequently in unresurfaced compared with resurfaced TKA, with recorded values of 2.4% and 1.3%, respectively. The same group of patients were reviewed again at 10 years, at which point the authors recognized that, although clinical difference between groups remained insignificant, a trend had emerged suggesting that primary resurfacing was superior with regard to cost effectiveness.[310]

In 2015 Roberts et al. presented a 10-year follow-up study looking at potential merits of selective patellar resurfacing.[373] In their study they excluded all patellae that presented with exposed bone, leaving 350 patients who were followed for a minimum of 2 years and a subset of 114 for a minimum of 10 years. Cumulative revision rate, stair climbing ability, AKP, KSS, and active range of motion measured equal values for both groups. Patient satisfaction reached statistical significance in favor of resurfacing at 2 years but failed to do so at 10 years. The authors concluded that the *"vast majority of patients with remaining patellar articular cartilage do very well with TKA regardless of patellar resurfacing."* In this series, no patellar-related complications or revisions were encountered over the entire observation period, which the authors attributed to improvements in implant design and use of a surgical technique that focused on appropriate patellar tracking and restoring patellar thickness.

Stair Climbing Ability

Some studies have examined knee function in more detail by assessing the patient's ability to climb stairs.****** Bourne et al., who devised a 30-second stair climbing test, found no statistically significant difference at 2-year follow-up between patients with and without patellar resurfacing.[50] The same groups of patients were again reviewed at 10 years, by which time those with patella resurfacing climbed on average 20 stairs, compared with 31 stairs in the nonresurfaced group, a difference which reached statistical significance.[76] Similar findings were reported by Feller et al., who found that the stair-climbing ability in the nonresurfaced patient group was significantly better compared with those with patella resurfacing.[138] Two RCTs found no significant difference regarding the performance of functional tasks between resurfaced and nonresurfaced patients,[159,418] whereas two other RCTs showed a trend toward increased pain with stair ascend and descend if the patella was retained, although values failed to reach statistical significance.[83,481]

Wood et al. recorded AKP during stair ascend in 25% of patients with retained patella, compared with 17% with patellar resurfacing.[481] In addition, 33% of patients without patellar resurfacing and 19% with patellar resurfacing descended stairs

******References 76, 83, 138, 159, 340, 412, 418, and 481.

TABLE 145.7 Randomized and Prospective Trials Published Between 1989 and 2011 in Which Patients Received Bilateral Total Knee Arthroplasties With the Patella Being Resurfaced One Side Only

	TKA Type	Patellar Implant Type	Type of Trial	Number of Cases	Mean Follow-Up (Years)	RS Preferred (%)	NRS Preferred (%)	No Preference (%)	Author's Comments
Shoji et al.[412]	Yoshino-Shoji total condylar CS	Not specified	Prospective	35	2	23	29	48	Routine resurfacing not advisable
Enis et al.[129]	Townley	Dome metal backed	Prospective	20	3.3	45	15	40	Better pain relief with resurfacing
Levitsky et al.[261]	Not specified	Not specified	Retrospective	13	7.5	46	8	46	Patellar retention acceptable if selection criteria applied
Keblish et al.[236]	LCS RP	Anatomic RP	Prospective	30	5.2	30	23	47	Patellar retention acceptable with patella-friendly implant
Barrack et al.[26]	MG-II CR	Modified dome	Randomized	23	5	21	29	50	Anterior knee pain unrelated to patellar resurfacing
Waters and Bentley[469]	PFC CR/CS	Dome	Randomized	35	5.3	51	11	37	Patellar resurfacing preferred
Peng et al.[340]	NexGen/MG-II	Dome	Prospective	35	3.2	28	26	46	No difference
Burnett et al.[73]	MG-II CR	Modified dome	Randomized	32	10	37	22	41	Equivalent clinical results
Smith et al.[418]	Profix	Dome (Inlay)	Randomized	16	4.4	—	—	100	No benefit of patellar resurfacing over nonresurfacing
Patel and Raut[336]	PFC	Modified dome	Prospective (staged)	60	4.5	68	15	17	Resurfacing recommended. Secondary resurfacing in four patients
Total				299	5	35	18	47	

CR, Cruciate-retaining; *CS*, cruciate-sacrificing; *LCS*, low-contact stress; *MG*, Miller-Galante; *NRS*, nonresurfacing; *PFC*, press-fit condylar; *PS*, posterior-stabilized; *RP*, rotating platform; *RS*, resurfacing.

one at a time, leading with the involved limb, indicating a reluctance or an inability to load the affected knee. Ewald et al., who prospectively reviewed 124 patients following kinematic TKA at 2 to 4 years postoperatively, found that restriction of stair-climbing ability appeared to be a function of involvement of multiple joints rather than of patellar replacement.[134] In their series, rheumatoid patients with resurfaced patellae performed the worst, whereas osteoarthritic patients with involvement of a single joint performed best, regardless of whether the patella was resurfaced or not. Shoji et al. examined 35 patients with RA who underwent bilateral TKA with one side receiving patellar resurfacing.[412] Because stair-climbing ability did not allow a functional comparison between the two knees, the researchers asked the patients which knee they considered to be more dependable functionally. Of those who could climb stairs, 27% preferred the knee that had been resurfaced, 31% preferred the knee that had not, and 42% had no preference. In an almost identical trial, Peng et al. found that out of 30 patients 31% preferred the resurfaced side when climbing stairs, 29% the nonresurfaced side, and 20% expressed no preference.[340]

Two randomized controlled biomechanical studies looked at functional range of movement and walking gait pattern.[311,416]

Both studies were unable to delineate any clinically relevant differences between resurfaced and nonresurfaced knees but highlighted discrepancies in kinematics compared with normal individuals.

Bilateral Comparative Trials

A total of 10 studies (prospective or randomized controlled) incorporating a comparative assessment of patients who received bilateral TKAs, with patellar resurfacing performed on one side only, were identified (Table 145.7). A meta-analysis of these studies revealed a total of 299 patients who had been followed up between 2 and 10 years (average: 5 years). Satisfaction was assessed by asking patients which knee they prefer. The resurfaced side was favored by 35% of all patients, the nonresurfaced side was favored by 18%, and 47% expressed no preference for either knee.

REGIONAL AND NATIONAL ARTHROPLASTY REGISTRIES

National joint registries are a valuable source of information because they pool data from a large number of patients, which

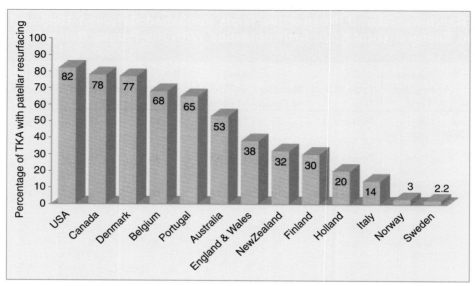

FIG 145.39 Percentage of patellar resurfacing in primary TKA in countries featuring a national joint arthroplasty registry. (Data extracted from the most recent registry report available [range 2007–2016].)

allows for comparison of differing surgical practices and outcome data within and between nations.[220] Given the difficulties in assessing rare incidences, such as arthroplasty revisions by way of high-powered RCTs, registry data provide an appealing alternative. However as a result of the observational nature of data obtained, causality cannot generally be inferred. Data collection within registries is often of variable quality and not immune to selection bias. Furthermore, registry data does not necessarily cover all aspects of treatment and complications surrounding the management of the PFJ in TKA and may be affected by selective under-reporting with regard to complications or revision procedure, such as secondary patellar resurfacing.[376,377]

The frequency of implanting a patellar component during primary TKA varies greatly between countries and based on 2015–2016 registry data ranges from 2.5% in Sweden to 77% in Denmark (Fig. 145.39). In the United States, information on the rate of patellar resurfacing is presently still relying mainly on survey data, which suggest that approximately 85% of all TKA cases receive a patellar implant.[††††††]

The Swedish Knee Arthroplasty Registry has been providing long-term data on the use of patellar components since 1975.[377,432] Following a peak in patellar resurfacing during the 1980s, with rates greater than 70%, overall numbers have steadily declined. In the most recent report published in 2015, patella resurfacing was performed in only 2.2% of cases. Lindstrand et al. carried out a subgroup analysis between patients with retained and resurfaced patellae and recorded an overall revision rate of 1.55% for both groups.[264] In patients with retained patella, 46% of revisions were performed for AKP and 12.5% for patellar instability, making patella the most common reason for revision surgery in this group. In patients with tricompartmental TKA, 43% of revisions were performed for patellofemoral problems. Of those, 17% were revised because of patellar instability and dislocation, 13% for patellar implant

loosening, 6% for material failure, 5% for pain, and 2.5% for patellar fracture. Although patients with retained patella were 1.3 times more likely to undergo revision for any reason, compared with patients with primary patellar resurfacing, the latter group was three times more likely to undergo revision for any cause other than pain when compared with patients in whom the patella had been retained.

Data from the 2016 arthroplasty registry report in Norway indicated that, out of a total of 5276 primary TKAs, 3% received a patellar component.[157,320] Lygre et al., who reviewed 972 patients from the registry, failed to observe any perceptible clinical differences between resurfaced and nonresurfaced patients.[272] The authors nonetheless noticed a tendency toward better results, regardless of patellar management, for the relatively patellar-friendly NexGen TKA design, when compared with the reference brand (AGC TKA).

According to the 2016 Annual Report of the Danish Knee Arthroplasty Registry, it was estimated that the use of patellar resurfacing in TKA had increased from 68% in 2000 to 77% in 2016.[103] The report further revealed that of all revision procedures performed in Denmark, 5.0% are performed for secondary patellar resurfacing and 2.6% for polyethylene wear of patellar components.

Robertsson et al. analyzed 10-year data from the Nordic Arthroplasty Association obtained between 1997 and 2007.[374] To the authors, it remained unclear why the use of patellar components increased in Denmark but decreased in Norway and Sweden in the given time frame and why surgical practice in these counties differs so significantly. It is unlikely that the variations in the proportion of primary resurfaced TKAs between national joint registers can be attributed to cultural differences alone. Thus it may be assumed that surgeon's choices must have been affected by clinical evidence, experience, education, tradition, and manufacturers' marketing politics or a combination thereof.

The American Joint Replacement Registry was established in 2008.[12] It is currently run as a voluntary and fee-based registry endorsed by the American Academy of Orthopaedic Surgeons

---

[††††††]References 12, 22, 23, 38, 103, 225, 315, 320, and 432.

(AAOS), American Association of Hip and Knee Surgeons (AAHKS), and both the Hip and the Knee Society, respectively. In the first year, two institutions provided information on approximately 1000 hip and knee arthroplasties but without details on patellar resurfacing. By 2014 the number of participating hospitals had risen to 417 providing data of 109.829 total knee arthroplasties of which 81.8% received a patellar component. It is of interest to note that the proportion of primary patellar resurfacing in TKA has remained static since 2012.[12]

A 2009 survey by AAHKS revealed that approximately 76% of members resurface virtually all of their TKA cases, 16% resurface more than 90% of the time, and 5% resurface fewer than 10% of their TKA cases.[38] Johnson et al. reported on a community-based register in Minnesota, where the rate of patellar resurfacing increased from 84% in 1991 to 98% in 2009.[222] Data analysis of 9348 resurfaced and 655 unresurfaced TKAs revealed a cumulative revision rate for "patella-only" revision of 0.8% and 4.8%, respectively. SR accounted for almost 90% of revisions in the retention group. Unfortunately the registry data did not capture the incidence of AKP and its association with patellar component revision or SR.

Most registries use revisions as the preferred end point because it represents a definitive event. However, the process of revision is not universally defined, and what may classify as a revision in one registry may not be considered a revision in another. A case in point is the later addition of a patellar implant otherwise classified as SR that is not classified as a revision procedure in two out of eight registers.[263] However, Robertsson et al. pointed out that one should be aware of the relative indication for revision, which may be dependent on the surgeon's attitude and ease of revision, and which applies in particular for the threshold of SR.[377]

The Swedish Knee Arthroplasty Register revealed that, during the 1990s, arthroplasty patients with retained patella had a higher risk of revision than those in whom the patella had been resurfaced. This increased frequency was caused by the need for secondary patellar resurfacing because of persistent AKP. In 2007 the benefit of the patellar component began to diminish and in their most recent report released in 2013, this difference in revision rate has become nonsignificant. These changes are a direct reflection of the relatively low rate of SRs in countries with preponderance of patella retention. During the period of 2002 to 2011, Swedish surgeons performed 85,774 primary TKAs without patellar resurfacing, whereas at the same time 723 patients (0.85%) were revised to receive a patellar component. Results compare favorably with those from the New Zealand registry, in which between 2005 and 2014 a total of 48,542 TKAs remained unresurfaced, whereas SR was performed in 465 patients (0.9%). Figures from Norway for the time period 1994 to 2009 revealed a proportion of 29,532 unresurfaced TKAs to 537 SRs (1.8%). The authors of the Swedish registry report surmised that the reduction in the rate of SRs "*may be that the femoral components have become more 'patellar friendly' or if the surgeons have discovered that a patellar addition is not always successful and thus are performing fewer such revisions.*"[432] Robertsson believes that the reason for the change in overall revision rate may be because of the "*reluctance of surgeons to offer patients secondary patellar resurfacing given the poor predictions but also because those with resurfacing may have increasing problems given the length of the observation period*" (Otto Robertsson, personal communication, 2015).

CONCLUSION

Early arthroplasty designs were associated with a high level of AKP because they failed to cater to the patellofemoral joint. Patellar resurfacing was heralded as the savior, but complications specific to the patellofemoral joint have continued to affect clinical results, whereas AKP, albeit reduced, has remained the largest single source of postoperative patient dissatisfaction. Therefore it is not surprising that the great debate about the pros and cons of patellar resurfacing continues to revolve around our lack of understanding why, irrespective of preoperative symptoms and patellar resurfacing, some patients may suffer AKP and others may not.

The fact that neither primary nor SR have been able to predictably reduce AKP has not only stifled our efforts in defining a more dependable treatment strategy but made us realize that we have to look beyond the patella for pathologic causes of the genesis of patellofemoral pain. Although many such causes have been identified, not enough emphasis has been placed on surgical improprieties, in particular with regard to component malrotation, which has a strong association with patellofemoral complications. Clinicians have a tendency to underestimate such problems, which in part may be because of sheer ignorance or simply the result of one's reluctance to accept mistakes.

The scientific literature, which is hampered by methodologic limitations and observer bias, has been unable to provide clinicians with clear guidance and appears to provide as much evidence in support of resurfacing as it does of patellar retention. Older, nonrandomized retrospective studies have commonly given preference to patellar resurfacing, which critics believe is associated with the use of nonconforming, patellar unfriendly femoral implant designs. Recent evidence-based research and meta-analyses have failed to draw clear conclusions, while blinded satisfaction studies comparing resurfaced and nonresurfaced knees generally reveal equivalent results. The level of confusion is echoed by national arthroplasty registry data that show wide variations in the proportion of patellar resurfacings that cannot be explained by cultural differences alone (see Fig. 145.39). Our endeavor to obtain reliable evidence remains hampered by a paucity of validated outcome tools with which to assess the patellofemoral joint, as most scoring systems are not sensitive enough to detect differences in patellofemoral pain and function between resurfaced and unresurfaced patients. Although some specific patellofemoral scores exist, they have not found widespread acceptance (see Tables 145.3 and 145.4).

The past decade has seen significant improvements in clinical results, with overall reduction in both postoperative AKP and patellar-related complications. The reasons for this are likely to be multifactorial and may include diverse aspects, such as improved surgical technique, based upon awareness of the detriments of component malpositioning and overzealous soft tissue release, advances in implant design that accommodates both resurfaced and unresurfaced patellae, judicious patient selection, and better patient education. Despite such positive developments, we need to avoid becoming complacent because the proportion of unsatisfied patients following TKA still remains too high.

Meanwhile, the different management strategies to always, never, or selectively resurface the patella continue to be a reflection of the deep divisions within the orthopedic community on how best to treat the patella. Opponents of resurfacing contend that the native patella provides better patellar tracking, improved clinical function, and avoids implant-related complications, whereas proponents of resurfacing argue that patients have less pain, are overall more satisfied, and avert the need for SR. Both groups will happily argue the respective merits of resurfacing versus patellar retention without making a real effort to ascertain the facts upon which their case might rest. This is not entirely surprising if one considers that our established knowledge on the subject merely represents a tiny foothold of fact in a quagmire of misinformation, prejudice, and guesswork.

Currently clinicians are required to weigh the increased probability of complications arising from patellar resurfacing and future implant revision against the risk of SR for persistent AKP. Although the potential need for SR is a known downside in patients with retained patellae, it would be a fallacy to consider the proportion of SR a true indicator for a heightened frequency of persistent AKP compared with resurfaced patients. It is essentially a mere reflection of the fact that this surgical option is available only to patients without patellar implant, and the overall differences in the incidence of AKP between resurfaced and unresurfaced patients are relatively small. However, few would argue that there appears to be at least initially a reduced likelihood of patients suffering AKP following primary resurfacing. Combined with the relatively poor success rate of SR and the additional health care costs thereof, it is seen by some as justification to offer routine primary resurfacing at least to the elderly who are less likely to encounter long-term complications associated with the patellar implant.

Clinical trials have mainly considered the "all-or-nothing" approach of always or never to resurface, while paying little attention to "selective resurfacing" as a possible treatment arm. Advocates who always resurface or never resurface indiscriminately expose the patella to a random choice, whereas the paradigm of selective resurfacing attempts to identify those individuals who are likely to benefit from patellar resurfacing and at the same time avoid potential complications associated with unnecessary additions of a patellar component. Although evidence regarding the validity of selection criteria is still under debate and the decision when to resurface is not infrequently based on intuitive reasoning, clinical long-term results using selective resurfacing strategies have nevertheless been excellent.

"Whether all patellae should be resurfaced, regardless of their appearance at surgery, the age of the patient, and the demands on the knee, is still a moot question and must be left to the discretion of the orthopedic surgeon." Despite the passage of time, this question raised by Coventry in 1980, remains as valid today as it was then. The fact that the topic of patellar resurfacing has engaged clinicians for almost half a century without a consensus being attained could be an indicator that either way of treating the patella may be acceptable. Surely if one school of thought had proved superior, clinical outcome results would have revealed a more noticeable difference between treatment strategies by now. Thus it may not be improbable that the decision whether or not to resurface the patella may in time become more a matter of surgeon's choice rather than one dependent on specific indications or certain variables.

ACKNOWLEDGMENTS

The author would like to offer many thanks to Norman Scott, John Newman, Bob Barrack, Dick Scott, David Hungerford, Peter Walker, Gil Scuderi, Seth Greenwald, Fred Buechel, Otto Robertsson, and Leo Whiteside for their support and advice and for sharing the common interest of improving the care for our patients. Sylvia Louise Davies deserves a special thank you for her indefatigable patience, dedication and editorial support, and John Lawson for his excellent art work. Finally, special gratitude is conveyed to John Insall who has been an inspiration to us all.

KEY REFERENCES

23. Baker PN, Petheram T, Dowen D, et al: Early PROMs following total knee arthroplasty—functional outcome dependent on patella resurfacing. *J Arthroplasty* 29:314–319, 2014.
26. Barrack RL, Bertot AJ, Wolfe MW, et al: Patellar resurfacing in total knee arthroplasty. A prospective, randomised, double-blind study with five to seven years of follow-up. *J Bone Joint Surg Am* 83:1376–1381, 2001.
34. Berger RA, Crossett LS, Jacobs JJ, et al: Malrotation causing patellofemoral complications after total knee arthroplasty. *Clin Orthop* 356:144–153, 1998.
41. Biedert RM, Sanchis-Alfonso V: Sources of anterior knee pain. *Clin Sports Med* 21:335–347, 2002.
49. Bourne RB, Burnett RSJ: The consequences of not resurfacing the patella. *Clin Orthop* 428:166–169, 2004.
56. Breeman S, Campbell M, Dakin H, et al: Patellar resurfacing in total knee replacement: five-year clinical and economic results of a large randomized controlled trial. *J Bone Joint Surg Am* 93:1473–1481, 2011.
74. Burnett RSJ, Boone JL, Rosenzweig SD, et al: Patellar resurfacing compared with nonresurfacing in total knee arthroplasty. A concise follow-up of a randomized trial. *J Bone Joint Surg Am* 91:2562–2567, 2009.
95. Collier JP, McNamara JL, Suprenant VA, et al: All-polyethylene components are not the answer. *Clin Orthop* 273:198–203, 1991.
115. D'Lima D, Chen PC, Kester MA, et al: Impact on patellofemoral design on patellofemoral forces and polyethylene stresses. *J Bone Joint Surg Am* 85:85–93, 2003.
214. Insall J: The patella in total knee replacement: does it matter? *Knee Surg Sports Traumatol Arthrosc* 9(Suppl 1):S2, 2001.
241. Kim BS, Reitman RD, Schai PA, et al: Selective patellar nonresurfacing in total knee arthroplasty. 10 year results. *Clin Orthop* 367:81–88, 1999.
273. Lygre SH, Espehaug B, Havelin LI, et al: Failure of total knee arthroplasty with or without patella resurfacing. *Acta Orthop* 82:282–292, 2011.
294. Meftah M, Ranawat AS, Ranawat CS: The natural history of anterior knee pain in 2 posterior-stabilised, modular total knee arthroplasty designs. *J Arthroplasty* 26:1145–1148, 2011.
335. Parvizi J, Mortazavi SM, Devulapalli C, et al: Secondary resurfacing of the patella after primary total knee arthroplasty does the anterior knee pain resolve? *J Arthroplasty* 27:21–26, 2012.
346. Pilling RW, Moulder E, Allgar V, et al: Patellar resurfacing in primary total knee replacement: a meta-analysis. *J Bone Joint Surg Am* 94:2270–2278, 2012.
373. Roberts DW, Hayes TD, Tate CT, et al: Selective patellar resurfacing in total knee arthroplasty: a prospective, randomized, double-blind study. *J Arthroplasty* 30:216–222, 2015.
375. Robertsson O, Dunbar M, Phersson T, et al: Patient satisfaction after knee arthroplasty: a report on 27,372 knees operated on between 1981 and 1995 in Sweden. *Acta Orthop Scand* 71:262–267, 2000.
387. Schindler OS: The controversy of patellar resurfacing in total knee arthroplasty: Ibisne in medio tutissimus? *Knee Surg Sports Traumatol Arthrosc* 20:1227–1244, 2012.
388. Schindler OS: Basic kinematics and biomechanics of the patellofemoral joint part 2: the patella in total knee arthroplasty. *Acta Orthop Belg* 78:11–29, 2012.
404. Scuderi GR, Insall JN, Scott NW: Patellofemoral pain after total knee arthroplasty. *J Am Acad Orthop Surg* 2:239–246, 1994.
418. Smith AJ, Wood DJ, Li MG: Total knee replacement with and without Patellar resurfacing: a prospective, randomised trial using the Profix total knee system. *J Bone Joint Surg Br* 90:43–49, 2008.

435. Theiss SM, Kitziger KJ, Lotke PS, et al: Component design affecting patellofemoral complications after total knee replacement. *Clin Orthop* 326:183–187, 1996.

449. van Jonbergen HP, Reuver JM, Mutsaerts EL, et al: Determinants of anterior knee pain following total knee replacement: a systematic review. *Knee Surg Sports Traumatol Arthrosc* 22:478–499, 2014.

488. Yoshii I, Whiteside LA, Anouchi YS: The effect of patella button placement and femoral design on patellar tracking in total knee arthroplasty. *Clin Orthop* 275:211–219, 1992.

The references for this chapter can also be found on www.expertconsult.com.

146

Patella Resurfacing—Never

Tomoyuki Matsumoto, Hirotsugu Muratsu

INTRODUCTION

Whether the patella should be resurfaced or not during primary total knee arthroplasty (TKA) is still controversial. On the basis of the philosophy of TKA, there are three types of surgeons: those who always, those who selectively, and those who never resurface the patella during TKA. Recent literature reports tend to focus on advances in the patella-femoral prosthetic design and indicate that resurfacing of the patella reduces the complication rate if the patella is resurfaced. Nevertheless, when complications of the resurfaced patella do occur, they can be potentially catastrophic.

In this chapter, evidence-based data from the national arthroplasty registers of many countries and a meta-analysis with strict selection of randomized studies are introduced. In addition, this chapter will focus on the disadvantages of resurfacing the patella, according to recently published studies. The authors report that patellar resurfacing in primary TKA is only done in knees with rheumatoid arthritis, severe patellofemoral arthritis, patellar dislocation, and patellar bone defect, based on rare cases with anterior knee pain associated with an unresurfaced patella and the experience of catastrophic failure after patellar resurfacing. Thus, in this chapter, some cases in which patellar resurfacing was absolutely needed and some cases of catastrophic failure associated with patellar resurfacing are also introduced, and thus the surgical procedure of trimming and reshaping of the patella is presented.

NATIONAL ARTHROPLASTY REGISTERS

National joint registers pool a large volume data in each country, providing surgeons with useful information. The frequency of patellar resurfacing, or that of not resurfacing, varies greatly across countries. The Swedish Knee Arthroplasty Register, since 1975, has shown a steady decline in the number of TKA procedures with patellar resurfacing, from greater than 70% to greater than 3% of cases in 2010.[32] Although the register revealed a higher rate of revision in unresurfaced TKAs, there was no statistically significant difference. In comparison, the Norway Arthroplasty Register reported in 2010 that of a total of 3965 TKAs, only 96 (2.4%) involved resurfacing, whereas secondary resurfacing for anterior knee pain was performed in 1.8% of all arthroplasty cases.[20] The Danish Knee Arthroplasty Register in 2010 estimated that the use of patellar resurfacing in TKA had increased from 68% in 1997–2000 to 80% in 2009.[6] The report further revealed that of all revision procedures performed in Denmark, 9.1% were done for secondary patellar resurfacing and 5.1% for polyethylene wear of patellar components. A report with combined data from three Nordic knee arthroplasty registers (Sweden, Norway, and Denmark) suggested that the difference in performing patellar resurfacing or not among the countries may be affected by scientific evidence, surgeon's experience, educational environment, tradition, and manufacturer-dictated marketing policies.[28]

A report of the Australian National Joint Replacement Registry in 2011 confirmed an increase in the rate of resurfacing from 41.5% in 2005 to 49.5% in 2010.[2] If the patella was left unresurfaced, the cumulative revision rate for posterior stabilized implants at 10 years was calculated to be 8.1%, compared with 5.8% for all others. Patellofemoral pain was listed as the reason for revision in about 13.5% of all primary TKAs. Similarly, a pilot project of the Japanese Arthroplasty Association, started on 2006 with 16,647 knees, reported that 50.8% of the knees were to receive patellar replacement and 49.0% would be left unresurfaced.[1]

A report comparing Norwegian and US arthroplasty registers showed a different tendency in the choice between patellar resurfacing or not resurfacing.[25] While 94.7% of 25,004 TKAs were performed without patellar resurfacing in Norway, 98.3% of 56,208 TKAs were performed with patellar resurfacing at Kaiser Permanente in the United States. Many of the revision procedures in the Norwegian cohort were performed for anterior knee pain in patients who had undergone TKAs without initial patellar resurfacing; in these limbs, the femoral and tibial implants were not revised. Although surgeons in Norway and Sweden have a similar tendency to not perform patellar resurfacing, as described previously, in Denmark, similar to the United States, surgeons tend to practice patellar resurfacing.[28] In Norway, the functional status and revision rate associated with patellar resurfacing and unresurfacing in TKA was investigated, and no difference was found, which may explain the low use of patellar resurfacing in this country.[16,17] A slightly higher revision rate in unresurfaced knees might be explained by the option of adding a patellar component in unresurfaced knees.[17]

PROSPECTIVE AND RANDOMIZED CONTROLLED TRIALS

Many prospective and randomized studies have compared the clinical scores, anterior knee pain, complication rate, and revision rate among patients receiving TKAs with and without patellar resurfacing. Relatively old references on meta-analyses by Parvizi et al.,[24] Pakos et al.,[23] and Nizard et al.[19] all concluded that resurfacing the patella decreases the incidence of anterior knee pain and reduces the risk of revision surgery. However, following these meta-analyses, several studies reported contrasting conclusions. Seo et al. randomly performed patellar resurfacing in a group of 277 patients undergoing TKA.[29] At an average follow-up of 74.6 months, the functional and radiographic results as well as complication rates showed no difference between patients who received resurfacing of the patella and those who did not, leading to the conclusion that patellar cartilage defect, which was previously considered an important determinant for patellar resurfacing, had no influence on clinical and radiologic outcomes.[29] Similarly, Liu conducted a prospective study on 133 patients with osteoarthritis, randomizing them into a patellar resurfacing group and a retention group. He could not find a significant difference in the Knee Society score, anterior knee pain, and radiographic assessment at a minimum 7-year follow-up.[15]

These contradictory results may be the consequence of several confounding variables, such as surgeon's experience, differences in prosthetic designs, different surgical options for the retained patella, severity of patellar degeneration, or preoperative extensor mechanism imbalance. The most recent meta-analyses, however, allow more precise conclusions. In a meta-analysis that included 16 randomized controlled trials with 1710 resurfaced patella and 1755 unresurfaced patella in primary TKA, Pilling demonstrated that patellar resurfacing had no significant effect on patient satisfaction, infection rate, anterior knee pain, or most of the knee scoring systems. However, the Knee Society score was superior in cases with resurfacing.[27] He concluded that patients with patellar resurfacing had equivalent anterior knee pain and satisfaction to patients with patellar retention. However, patients who received resurfacing were significantly less likely to need subsequent surgery. In the meta-analysis by Fu et al.[9] and He et al.,[11] no differences were found between the resurfacing and unresurfacing groups in terms of the anterior knee pain rate. They only found a significant difference in reoperation risk between the two groups. The systematic review by Li et al. had a similar conclusion—that patellar resurfacing could reduce the risk of reoperation, but could not improve postoperative anterior knee pain, knee function, or patient satisfaction.[14] Chen et al., in his meta-analysis, also concluded that patellar resurfacing reduces the risk of reoperation.[4] Moreover, this option was associated with a high Knee Society score at long-term follow-up (≥5 years). Concerning other aspects such as anterior knee pain, patient satisfaction, or radiologic outcomes, the benefit of patellar resurfacing was limited.[4]

CASES NEEDING PATELLAR RESURFACING

In some cases such as severe patellofemoral arthritis, patellar permanent dislocation, and patellar bone defect, surgeons have no choice but to resurface the patella. For example, a 76-year-old female patient with severe patellofemoral arthritis (Fig. 146.1A) was compelled to undergo replacement of the patellofemoral joint because of severe patellofemoral pain (see Fig. 146.1B). Another example is that of a 72-year-old female patient with permanent patellar dislocation (see Fig. 146.2A), who had no other option but to undergo patellar resurfacing to avoid patellar maltracking and instability (Fig. 146.2B). One more important example for which patellar resurfacing is unavoidable is patellar bone defect. Fig. 146.3 shows an example of patellar bone defect in a patient with severe arthritis in the lateral facet (see Fig. 146.3A) that also needed patellar resurfacing (see Fig. 146.3B).

Rheumatoid arthritis has also been traditionally reported to be an indication for patellar resurfacing during TKA.[3,26] Retaining the patella in patients with rheumatoid arthritis was reported to allow continued release of sequestered antigen from the retained cartilage, resulting in recurrent inflammation.[31] However, Deehan et al. recently examined the anterior knee function in two patient groups who had undergone primary TKA without patellar resurfacing, to identify differences between osteoarthrosis and rheumatoid disease.[7] The results indicated no difference in the Hospital for Special Surgery score, Western Ontario and McMaster University score, patellar score, visual analogue scale, and reoperation rate between the two groups. Similarly, some surgeons recently reported no clinical disadvantage, even when the patella was retained in patients with rheumatoid arthritis.[12,21] Taken together, the decision to retain or resurface the patella in patients with rheumatoid arthritis could also be controversial.

COMPLICATIONS ASSOCIATED WITH PATELLAR RESURFACING

Some surgeons prefer resurfacing the patella because of the increasing rate of revision surgery and anterior knee pain without patellar resurfacing, whereas others routinely do not resurface the patella to avoid the complications associated with patellar resurfacing. These complications include patellar fracture, polyethylene wear, aseptic patellar component loosening and dissociation, maltracking and instability, extensor mechanism disruption, and patellar clunk syndrome (Fig. 146.4), which usually result in revision surgery and sometimes cause catastrophic outcomes. Meding et al. reported patellar complications at an average of 7-years' follow-up in a series of 8530 cases with the same posterior-cruciate-retaining TKA with all-polyethylene patellar components.[18] Patellar fracture was

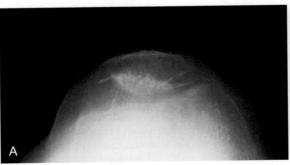
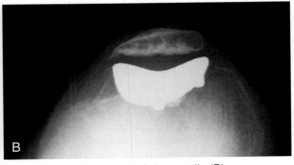

FIG 146.1 Severe patellofemoral arthritis (A) needing replacement of the patella (B).

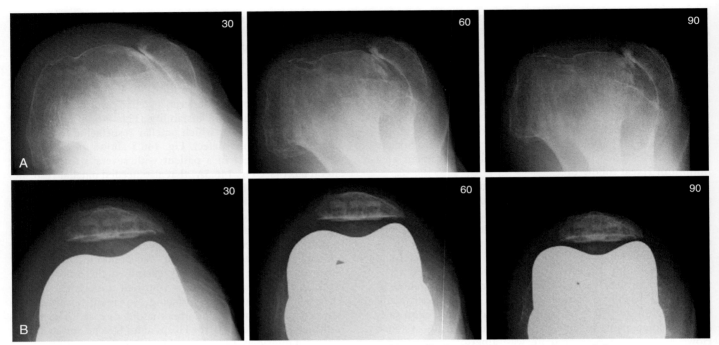

FIG 146.2 Patellar dislocation (A, 30°, 60°, and 90° of knee flexion) needing replacement of the patella (B, 30°, 60°, and 90° of knee flexion).

reported to be identified in 5.2% of TKA cases (444 knees), and patellar component loosening was observed in 4.8% (409 knees), in which 25 patellae were revised (0.3%).

Patellar fractures after patellar resurfacing are some of the most problematic complications after TKA. A 64-year-old female patient who had bilateral TKAs with patellar resurfacing (Fig. 146.5A) experienced gradual component loosening without any apparent cause (see Fig. 146.5B). Five years after the surgeries, she had bilateral patellar complicated fractures and component dissociations as a result of a falling accident (see Fig. 146.5C and D). She underwent open reduction and internal fixation with multiple pinning, wiring, and bone grafting from the iliac spine. Although her bone mass index was 35.1 kg/m², which may be one of the causes of fractures, her fractures resulted in catastrophic outcomes. The factors inducing patellar fracture were reported to include technical errors, patient demographics (eg, obesity, high activity level), and implant design (eg, large patellar component, inlay patellar design, large central fixation peg, and posterior stabilizing implant).[18,30] Considering these multifactorial issues related to patellar fractures, great care should be taken if the patella is to be replaced.

Patellar maltracking and instabilities are also among the most problematic complications after TKA. An 82-year-old female patient who had TKA with some extent of remaining maltracking 4 years ago (Fig. 146.6A) gradually developed severe patellar maltracking and lateral shift (see Fig. 146.6B), which was associated with anterior knee pain. Another example is that of a 73-year-old female patient who had TKA with good patellar tracking 5 years ago (Fig. 146.7A) but also exhibited patellar maltracking with lateral patellofemoral facet pain (see Fig. 146.7B), resulting in the need for revision surgery. These conditions led to polyethylene wear and needed patellar revision (Fig. 146.8C) and lateral facetectomy (see Fig. 146.8D).

Patellar clunk syndrome, which is characterized by painful catching, grinding, or jumping of the patella when the knee is moving from a flexed to an extended position, is also related to patellar resurfacing, especially after a posterior-stabilized TKA. This condition is caused by overgrowth of a fibrous nodule on the superior aspect of the patellar button. For example, a 68-year-old female who had posterior-stabilized TKA with patellar resurfacing experienced painful patellar clunk syndrome 7 months after the surgery, resulting in the need for arthroscopic synovectomy. Fukunaga et al. reported a case of design (intercondylar box ratio)–induced patellar clunk syndrome after mobile-bearing posterior-stabilized TKA.[10] Fifteen of 113 knees (13.3%) that received the same implant were found to have patellar clunk syndrome, suggesting that great care should be taken in patellar resurfacing during surgery. However, the advancement of the box shape on the same prosthesis is reported to reduce the incidence of patellar clunk syndrome.[8] These findings indicate that patellar clunk syndrome is associated with implant design, especially in posterior-stabilized TKA; however, technical-based patellar tilt during patellar resection is reported to have a significant relation with the incidence of patellar clunk syndrome.[10]

Considering these complications associated with patellar dislocations, even if patellar resurfacing has some merits as previously mentioned, some surgeons may recognize that patellar resurfacing has little benefit over not resurfacing.

SURGICAL APPROACH: RESHAPING THE PATELLA

When the patella is not resurfaced in TKA, a portion of the lateral facet of the patella and the osteophytes surrounding the patella should be resected, and the patella should also be trimmed and reshaped to better match the trochlea of the femoral component (see Fig. 146.5). Partial lateral facetectomy

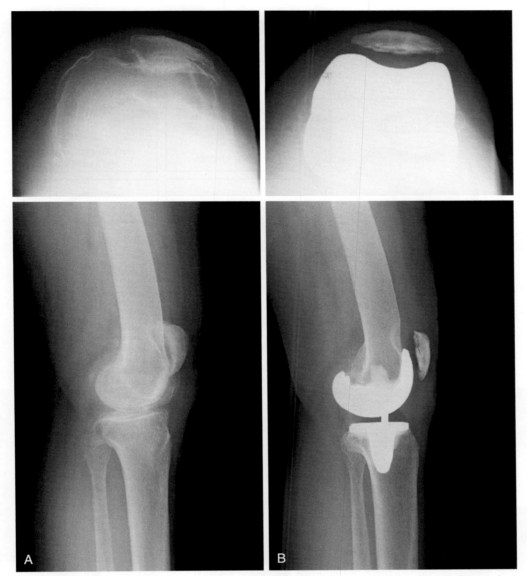

FIG 146.3 Patellar bone defect in a patient with arthritis in the lateral facet (A) needing replacement of the patella (B).

is reported to have better clinical outcomes and fewer lateral patellar osteophytes in radiographs than procedures without facetectomy.[33] Pagenstert et al. recently compared the clinical outcomes in patients with lateral patellar facet syndrome between partial lateral patellar facetectomy and secondary patellar resurfacing.[22] In their study, partial lateral patellar facetectomy was found to result in higher scores and less pain than patellar resurfacing.[22] Circumpatellar electrocautery, which is thought to alleviate pain in the patellofemoral area after TKA through desensitization or denervation of the pain receptors in the anterior knee, is also one of the techniques for managing the patella (see Fig. 146.5). A recent meta-analysis assessing the effect of patellar denervation with electrocautery indicated no significant difference in complications or incidence of anterior knee pain between the electrocautery and nonelectrocautery groups.[5] However, in terms of patellar score and Knee Society score, circumpatellar electrocautery improved clinical outcomes compared with nonelectrocautery.[5] Optimal patellar tracking should also be ensured by appropriate soft-tissue balancing, and a lateral release is to be performed if the patella is subluxed during the no-thumb test.

Because there have been no final conclusions about resurfacing of the patella or not during TKA, more studies need to be conducted in the future. In a retrospective study comparing 132 patellar retention and 143 resurfacing cases with a minimum of 7-year follow-up, Hwang et al. concluded that if soft tissue balancing and a patella-friendly prosthetic design are properly used, patellar retention with patelloplasty might be viable, even in knees with significant patellofemoral arthritis.[13]

CONCLUSION

Recent meta-analyses, including advanced prosthesis designs, showed no difference in the clinical scores and anterior knee

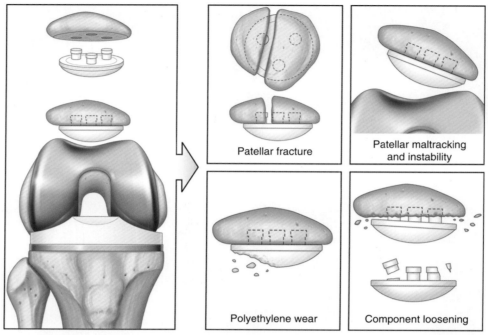

FIG 146.4 Schema of the complications associated with patellar resurfacing.

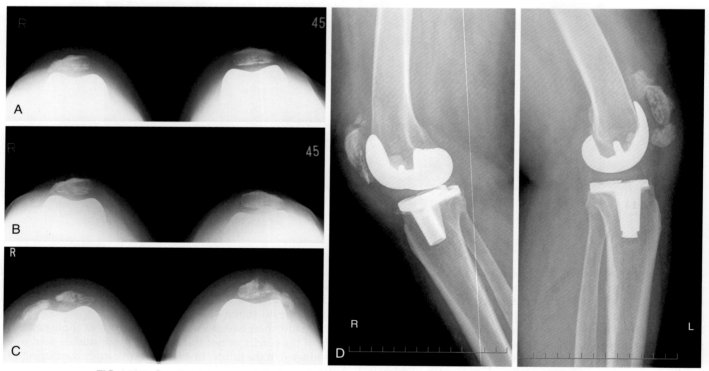

FIG 146.5 Patellar component that gradually loosened 5 years after TKA (A, B). Bilateral complicated patellar fractures occurred as a result of a falling accident (C, D).

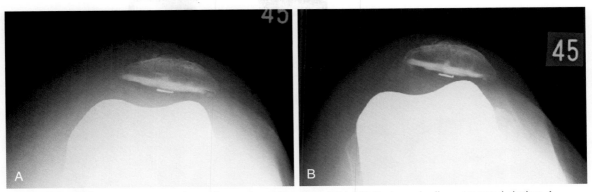

FIG 146.6 Some extent of patellar maltracking after TKA (A) that gradually worsened during 4 years (B).

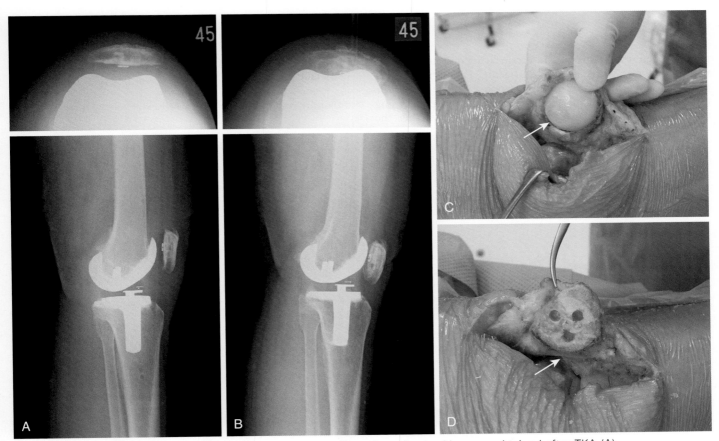

FIG 146.7 An example showing that even if good patellar tracking was obtained after TKA (A), maltracking and lateral facet syndrome gradually occurred without any apparent cause (B), leading to polyethylene wear (C, *arrow*) and resulting in the need for patellar revision with lateral facetectomy (D, *arrow*).

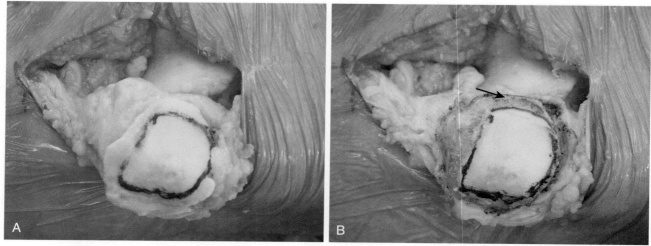

FIG 146.8 In reshaping the patella for the lateral flat facet (A), trimming around the patella and resection of the lateral facet *(arrow)* is performed with circumpatellar electrocautery (B).

pain between resurfacing over not resurfacing despite the lower reoperation rate with patellar resurfacing. Furthermore, surgeons should recognize that catastrophic failure could be avoided by not resurfacing the patella and instead performing appropriate trimming and reshaping. However, whether the patella should be resurfaced or not is indeed multifactorial and still controversial.

The references for this chapter can also be found on www.expertconsult.com.

147

Patella Resurfacing—Always

Khalid Odeh, Stephen Yu, Daniel J. Kaplan, Claudette Lajam, Richard Iorio

Surgical techniques and component designs in total knee arthroplasty (TKA) have undergone evolutionary advancement in recent decades. As the patellofemoral (PF) joint plays a critical role in the function and transmission of forces in the lower extremity, it is important understand the impact of patella resurfacing on clinical outcomes following TKA. The advent of patella resurfacing has been reported to reduce the rate of reoperation for anterior knee pain and improve patient satisfaction following TKA.[60,78,99] The decision to resurface the patella during a TKA should be made after a thorough analysis of modern implant design, biomechanics, surgical technique, and clinical outcomes. Orthopedic surgeons today who perform TKA generally fall into three categories: those who never, those who selectively, and those who always resurface the patella. Although patella resurfacing does have its own complications, the benefits of a properly performed procedure, including a lower risk of reoperation, ultimately outweigh the associated risks.

HISTORICAL TRENDS OF PATELLA RESURFACING

The history of patella replacement can be traced back to 1955, when the McKeever prosthesis was introduced. It was composed of a Vitallium shell that was used in cases of isolated patella resurfacing; however, this procedure was eventually discarded because of native trochlear wear.[56] The earliest designs for TKA did not include a patella component and may have contributed to high rates of anterior knee pain of 40% to 58%.[37,100] Eventually, it was theorized that the PF joint was a major source of residual anterior knee pain following TKA. Historical treatments included patellectomy with or without soft tissue realignment, which often failed to resolve the residual anterior knee pain and in some cases even increased anterior knee pain by increasing the amount of force required by the quadriceps muscle following patellectomy.[44,48] This prompted the novel solution to resurface the underside of the patella and implant a component to complete a true tri-compartmental prosthetic design.

The first widely used patella resurfacing implants for TKA came about in the 1970s with the development of the total condylar knee prosthesis.[46] By the 1980s, most systems had incorporated patella components. As patella resurfacing became popularized, some designer surgeons began to recommend universal implantation.[16,45,80] During this time period, there came about a reduced incidence of anterior knee pain following TKA. However, the introduction of patellar components gave rise to a new spectrum of complications at the PF joint, including patella fracture, component wear and loosening, patella instability, and extensor mechanism damage. As a greater

understanding of the biomechanics and function of the PF joint became more disseminated, there were improvements in design and surgical technique. The decision of whether or not to resurface the patella continues to be debated with no clear consensus, which has led to wide variations in practice.

There are data to suggest that the use of patella resurfacing is increasing in countries where the practice is already widespread. Data from the Danish joint replacement registry show an increase from 68% in 1997–2000 to 80% in 2009.[25] A similar increase in the Australian registry was observed, with an increase from 41% in 2005 to 56% in 2013.[5] This contrasts with low use nations such as Norway and Sweden, where the rate has decreased to around only 2%.[70,95] Data from a nationwide registry is unavailable for the United States, but a database of mainly community hospitals and some academic centers in the United States estimates the patella resurfacing rate at 96% in 2012.[67] In a moderate usage country like the United Kingdom, where 37% of patients undergoing TKA receive patella resurfacing, a study was conducted that surveyed surgeon preference and found that there was a tendency for more experienced and high volume surgeons to always resurface.[88]

IMPLANT CHOICE AND DESIGN

The design of patellar components is an area of continued evolution. There is a lack of consensus regarding the ideal patella design for the greatest stability, conformity, and minimization of wear patterns. The standard component today is a cemented, all-polyethylene, dome-shaped patella, although various shapes of the articular surface of the patella implant have been introduced as an attempt to restore native patella-femoral biomechanics (Fig. 147.1). The first polyethylene dome-shaped patella was developed and used by Aglietti et al. after an anatomical study of 80 arthritic knees.[2] The modified dome-shaped patella was designed to conform to the femoral condyles by offering a concavity that increased contact area between the components, especially when the knee is in flexion. This design has been shown to be particularly resistant to wear and deformation when compared to the standard dome because of lower magnitudes of contact pressures across the PF joint.[43] Other designs, including anatomic, offset dome, cylindrical, and mobile bearing types, have each been studied and marketed for distinct biomechanical advantages; however, these designs do not represent a significant portion of used implants. Despite the theoretical improvement of biomechanical properties of the modified dome or offset dome patella, the clinical performance of these implant designs compared to the traditional dome-shaped patella are equivalent. Dome-shaped components also

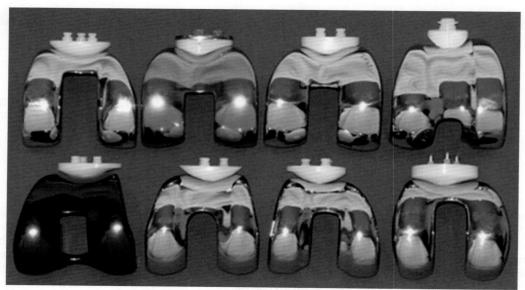

FIG 147.1 Various femoral arthroplasty components with their respective, designated patellar implant. *Top row, left to right*: AGC (dome patella), Biomet, Warsaw, USA; Buechel-Pappas (uncemented anatomic rotating platform patella), Endotec, Orlando, USA; LCS (anatomic fixed bearing patella), DePuy, Warsaw, USA; Medial rotating knee (cylindrical patella), Finsbury, England. *Bottom row, left to right*: Journey (offset dome patella), Smith and Nephew, Andover, USA; PFC-Sigma (modified dome patella), DePuy; Triathlon (offset dome patella), Stryker, Kalamazoo, USA; BioPro Townley Total Knee Original (uncemented metal-backed dome patella), Biopro, Port Huron, USA. (Illustration by kind permission of Oliver Schindler and reproduced from Schindler OS: The controversy of patellar resurfacing in total knee arthroplasty: Ibisne in medio tutissimus? *Knee Surg Sports Traumatol Arthrosc* 20:1227–1244, 2012.)

possess the advantage of a uniform shape that does not require specific orientation during implantation. This make makes the insertion of the component less technically demanding and reduces the potential for error.

Patellar components have also differed in the way that they are fixed to the native patella with both inlay and onlay designs. Inlay components are designed to be placed in a recessed hole that is reamed into the patella, whereas onlay designs lie flush onto the cut patella surface and holes are drilled to insert the pegs. Theoretically, the inlay patella has increased resistance to sheer stress and less tilt at the cost of potentially removing an excess amount of bone, predisposing the patient to an increased patella fracture risk.[53] The onlay design has a longer history of clinical use and has been shown to have noninferior resistance to tilt and similar kinematic properties.[27] A prospective trial comparing 135 knees with an onlay patella component to 116 knees with an inlay design found no clinical differences in patient outcomes. Although a decreased need for lateral retinacular release was observed with the inlayed components, there was also a significantly higher incidence of radiolucent lines.[83]

Peg design has also been improved to reduce patella complications. Most implants currently use three small pegs rather than one large central peg of early designs. The increased number of peripheral pegs help better distribute the stresses that the component is subjected to during motion.[14,55] Another proposed advantage of the three peg design includes potentially less interference with patella blood supply, thus reducing fracture risk. Although rare, there have been reports of peg breakage,

but this has been improved by the introduction of beveled peg-plate junctions as opposed to a sharp angled interface.[53]

The use of metal backed patella components experienced a brief period of popularity in the 1980s as a result of a belief that they would offer superior fixation through bony ingrowth. However, early designs did not incorporate a thick enough layer of polyethylene and were prone to catastrophic failure.[23,76] This led the orthopedic community to largely abandon the metal backed patella in favor of the all-polyethylene design. In revision cases where there is a severe bony deficit, the use of a trabecular metal baseplate made of porous tantalum has emerged as a viable option to restore patella height.[11] Recently, more biologic friendly designs, including a hydroxyapatite coated metal backed patella, have been shown to have equitable short term outcomes when compared to a standard polyethylene one.[69]

BIOMECHANICS OF A RESURFACED PATELLA

The biomechanical environment of the PF joint is drastically changed when the femoral and tibial prostheses are implanted (Fig. 147.2). The dynamic forces across the prosthetic trochlear groove are implant dependent and vary between femoral and patella designs. As such, to normalize the PF joint reaction forces and restore adequate patella tracking, a prosthetic patellar component is required to sync successfully with the implanted femoral component. Careful consideration must be given when selecting and implanting a specific patella component design to create a biomechanically favorable environment.

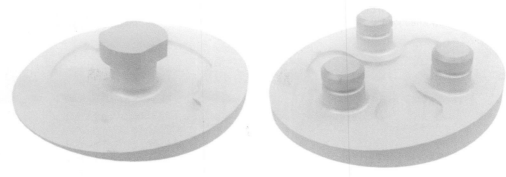

FIG 147.2 Three peg patella compared to central peg patella. (Courtesy DePuy Synthes Companies.)

Otherwise, the advantages of resurfacing the patella may be lost and can lead to detrimental results.

The design of the femoral component plays an integral role in the function of the PF joint following TKA. When the patella is not resurfaced, contact surfaces are altered as the native patella cartilage contacts with a metal femoral component, instead of the native femoral trochlear cartilage. The biomechanical advantages of a compressible cartilaginous trochlea are lost, which causes contact stress across the PF joint to rise considerably. This may lead to accelerated patella chondrolysis and degeneration, especially if there is malrotation of the femoral component.[92] As femoral implant designs have evolved, femoral components have become increasingly "patella friendly." Some favorable changes include a deepened patella groove to allow for deep flexion, a more distal extent of the trochlear groove, conformity of the anterior flange groove, and a more valgus orientation of the trochlear groove.[12,57,74] It is thought that these design elements would improve extensor mechanism function by increasing the length of the moment arm, which in turn decreases the joint reaction forces and contact stresses that may cause pain.[6,58,98]

In a TKA with an unresurfaced patella, PF joint reaction forces are strongly influenced by the placement, alignment, and rotation of the femoral and tibial components. The goal of normal PF tracking is to maintain a congruent and center-line axis along the trochlear groove of the prosthesis. It is hypothesized that over time the patella may conform to the congruency of the implanted femoral prosthesis as a result of a stress countering effect on the native undersurface of the patella.[8] The degree and effectiveness of this phenomenon, although conceptually sound, occurs to an unknown degree and is difficult to quantify.

TECHNICAL PEARLS FOR PATELLA RESURFACING

Adequate surgical exposure is the first step of proper surgical technique. Exposure of the patella is achieved when the surgeon can consistently and accurately measure the native patella thickness (Fig. 147.3). This includes resection of surrounding synovial soft tissue and peripatellar osteophytes. Sufficient working space is necessary to properly resect and prepare the patella for component implantation. In the horizontal plane, the chondro-osseous junction of the patella must be visualized to provide a target and appropriate starting point for the oscillating saw.

In addition to adequate exposure, attention to the peripatella soft tissues is necessary to yield an asymptomatic post prosthetic anterior knee. Sensory fibers, which may contribute to patella pain, may be denervated by using electrocautery to outline the lateral soft tissue around the patella.[97] Moreover, fibrosynovial overgrowth at the superior and inferior poles of the patella may be present. Careful resection of this tissue, without disruption of the extensor mechanism, can lead to a reduction in a reactive fibrosynovial hyperplasia that occurs postoperatively.[21] The exposed lateral facet must be addressed and minimized to avoid lateralization of trochlear contact forces. Careful resection, without encroaching upon the outline of the patella component, helps reduce osseous contact on the lateral facet and decreases symptomatic lateralization of patellar tracking (Fig. 147.4).[32,59] Adequate restoration of patella composite thickness is critical to maximize efficiency of the patella femoral mechanism and ensure adequate offset, which prevents irritation of the proximal extensor mechanism on the femoral flange and is important to avoid crepitus. Patellar crepitus is also associated with shortened patellar tendon length, smaller patellar components, and increased posterior femoral condylar offset.[26]

Medial/lateral constraint primarily affects patella tracking and can significantly influence the outcome of the TKA.[59,85] To ensure proper patella tracking, the patella component must congruently engage along the center of the prosthetic trochlea. When considering placement of the patella component, the apex of the dome can be offset medially in reference to the center of the patella, using the medial crest of the native patella as an anatomical landmark (Fig. 147.5). Centering the patella component over the native center of the patella functionally lateralizes the component and encourages lateral patellar tracking. A biomechanical study examining the effect of patella medialization recommended 2.5 mm of medialization.[3] Excessive medialization of the component should also be avoided, as this can increase lateral patella tilt and induce high contact stresses.[85]

Patella tilt in the axial plane is important when resurfacing the patella. The medial facet thickness in the native patella is typically thicker than the lateral side, and the surgeon must account for this increased thickness when resecting the subchondral bone. A common mistake is to resurface the patella in the plane of the native undersurface, which would induce patella tilt and could lead to significant patellar maltracking. The subchondral bone at the lateral facet should be referenced,

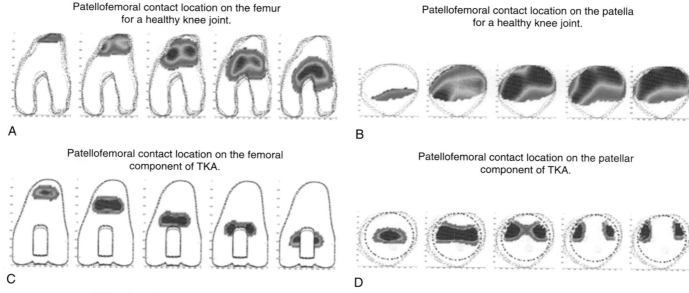

Patellofemoral contact location on the femur for a healthy knee joint.

A

Patellofemoral contact location on the patella for a healthy knee joint.

B

Patellofemoral contact location on the femoral component of TKA.

C

Patellofemoral contact location on the patellar component of TKA.

D

FIG 147.3 Normalized distance maps showing most frequent locations of patellofemoral contact for healthy (A and B) and TKA (C and D) knees at full extension, and at 30, 60, 90, and 120 degrees. *Red* represents the most probable area of the contact location. *TKA,* Total knee arthroplasty. (From Leszko F: Biomechanics and vibroarthrography of the patellofemoral joint. In Scott WN, ed: *Insall & Scott surgery of the knee*, ed 5, Philadelphia, 2011, Churchill Livingstone, pp 129–147.)

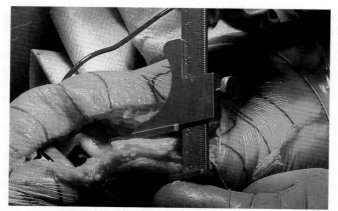

FIG 147.4 Adequate exposure of the patella allows easy placement of the caliper for thickness measurement.

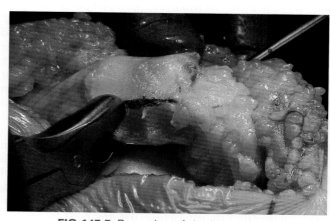

FIG 147.5 Resection of the lateral facet.

and both medial and lateral facets should be resected to a similar thickness. Patella tilt during assessment of tracking must also be analyzed during trialing to avoid any excessive dynamic patella tilt.

A careful balance must be struck to maximize the overall contact area of the prosthetic patella with the trochlear groove and to minimize lateral tracking/tilt of the patella. This is achieved through patella component positioning, femoral and tibial component rotational alignment, and balancing of the extensor mechanism. In general, relative lateralization and external rotation of both the tibial and femoral components can contribute to improving patellar tracking. After ensuring proper placement of all components, a release of the lateral retinacular soft tissues may also be necessary if the patella still continues to

maltrack. This technique must be used with caution, however, because a lateral retinacular release can have negative consequences (hematoma, soft tissue herniation or entrapment, pain, medial PF instability).

A lateral retinacular release may be considered if there is significant lateral tracking/subluxation of the patella and all other possible contributing factors have been addressed (eg, proper rotation of components and extra-articular contributions to the quadriceps angle). It is important to note that an inflated tourniquet can have an effect on PF tracking. The tourniquet decreases the forgiveness of the soft tissues and can falsely induce lateral tilt and tracking of the patella. It has been shown that a maltracking patella may correct itself following deflation of the tourniquet.[42] Therefore before performing a lateral release for a maltracking patella, one should consider deflating the tourniquet and reassessment of PF tracking. It is critical to use a proper PF tracking assessment technique, such as the "rule of no thumbs."[89] This test is performed by flexing the knee from 0 to 90 degrees with no lateral force applied to the patellar component to prevent it from subluxating laterally. The surgeon should observe the component to see that it maintains contact with the medial femoral condyle throughout the range of motion. Any noticeable elevation of the medial edge, subluxation, or dislocation could be considered a positive test suggestive of a tight lateral retinaculum, and a release should be considered.[36] It is also important to note that during surgery when the patella is everted, the extensor mechanism is lateralized, thus artificially increasing the lateral compartment native joint loads by acting as a tether.[90] This should be considered to avoid potential overrelease of the lateral soft tissue.

Proper placement of the patella component in the sagittal plane must be performed to achieve a good outcome. Superior placement of the patella component can contribute to postoperative patella crepitus. Uneven resection of the undersurface of the patella that results in caudal tilt can also mimic this condition. Conversely, placement of the component in an inferior position, or cephalic tilt from uneven resection, can cause a relative patella baja condition, which may limit flexion.[21,35] Generally, correct sagittal tilt can be approximated by using the quadriceps and patellar tendon insertion plane as an anatomic landmark. There are other extra-patella factors that contribute to patella positioning in relation to the trochlear in the sagittal plane, such as tibial tray height and joint line positioning, which can play a significant role in the development of a PF issue in postoperative TKA.[10,29,66]

The degree of resection of the undersurface of the patella has important significance for eventual outcomes. Over-resection decreases the integrity of the bone and increases the risk of patella fracture. A goal of at least 15 mm of postresection native patella thickness has been shown to minimize patellar strain.[84] Other risk factors of patellar fracture include asymmetrical resection of the patella, central single peg patellar implant design, uncemented patella components, metal-backed patellar components, and inlay type patellar components.[61,93,96,101] Conversely, under-resection of the patella leads to an increase in joint reaction force across the prosthetic patella-femoral joint and can lead to a loss in range of motion, pain, and overstuffing of the PF joint.[1,13] Therefore, a careful balance must be struck, with the goal of recreating the native patella thickness with a composite of remaining patella and prosthetic patella. Frequent and accurate measurement of the patella during resection will help eliminate error in appropriately resecting the patella. The average thickness of arthritic patella has been reported to be 26.1 mm for males and 22.6 mm for females.[1] The surgeon should be aware that a severely arthritic patella may be unusually thin, and resection and goal prosthetic thickness should be adjusted accordingly. At least 12 to 15 mm of native bone is necessary for adequate fixation of the patellar component and minimizing fracture risk.[84]

Cementation of the patella component is required for adequate fixation and satisfactory outcome of TKR. Careful attention to detail to ensure complete cement coverage of the component while removing excess cement from the bone prosthetic interface must be accomplished (Fig. 147.6). Additionally, the patella peg holes must be cleared of debris to

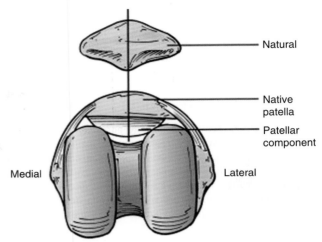

FIG 147.6 Medial placement of the patellar component. (From Hansen EN: Patella instability. In Scuderi GR, ed: *Techniques in revision hip and knee arthroplasty*, ed 1, Philadelphia, 2015, Saunders, pp 176–186.)

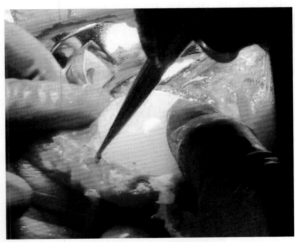

FIG 147.7 Removal of excess cement around the patellar component.

achieve the best fixation of the component through interdigitation of the cement. A small caliber drill (1.5 mm) may be used to increase the available surface area of the subchondral undersurface of the patella, typically favoring the lateral facet, to increase cement interdigitation. Drilling should be performed with care so as not to create stress risers leading to patella fracture. Finger (digital) pressure into peg holes and throughout the patella undersurface enhances cement fixation, and application of a compression clamp until cement hardening is necessary to ensure adequate component fixation. It is also important to note that excess cement must not only be removed to prevent impingement, but particulate debris must be cleared from the joint to avoid third-body wear (Fig. 147.7).

A technically sound resurfacing is imperative to achieving optimal outcomes after TKA. Failure to adhere to these technical pearls may result in outcomes worse than when resurfacing is not performed. General aims are to duplicate native patella thickness, decrease joint reaction forces, and maximize range of motion. Pre- and postresection measurement is important to the success and reproducibility of resurfacing techniques. Staying within 2 mm of the native patella thickness is recommended to avoid the aforementioned issues of over- or under-resection of the patella.

SPECIFIC SURGICAL TECHNIQUES

Several established techniques exist to accurately and precisely resurface the patella, such as freehand cuts, milling, and use of saw guides. Ultimately, the chosen surgical technique is surgeon-dependent. Few studies have prospectively compared resection techniques, although whichever technique is chosen, the principles remain the same: restore native patella height/thickness and produce patellar symmetry while avoiding excessive patellar tilt and poor tracking.

The freehand technique involves the surgeon resecting the patella without cutting guides (Fig. 147.8). Anatomic landmarks, such as the quadriceps and the patellar tendon, are used for starting point references, and frequent measurements across the undersurface are made to ensure the desired thickness is achieved. This approach has advantages and disadvantages resulting from the fact that no cutting guides are used. The surgeon has control over the resection depth and pitch of the oscillating saw. Although cutting guides assist in producing reliably consistent cuts in the plane of the jig, the accuracy of the cuts are entirely dependent on the measurements and the placement of the guide. Thus, many surgeons who choose to freehand the patella enjoy the freedom of having full control with resecting all areas of the patella. Frequent measurements

of standardized reference points, medial/lateral facets, or even a "four-quadrant technique" can be used to ensure that the resection is adequate in a reproducible manner.[17] The four quadrant technique is performed by dividing the patella into four quadrants and measuring the thickness at the center of each quadrant using a caliper. Resection can be repeated until symmetry is achieved using these measurements. A prospective randomized study examining the differences in patella asymmetry compared the use of freehand, saw guide, and freehand in combination with the four quadrant technique found that use of the four quadrant measurements produced the least asymmetry.[17]

Saw guides are commonly used to resect the patella (Fig. 147.9). Several saw guide variations exist. Pre-resection measurements are crucial to aligning the guide to the proper resection depth. Additionally, the pitch of the guide needs to be adjusted so the resultant tilt of the patella is acceptable. The saw blade can follow a more controlled path and cut the patella in a reproducible plane according to the guide. One must bear in mind that the resection is only as accurate as placement of the guide, and faulty placement, even to slight degree, can result in patellar tilt or over-resection. The guides are generally large and have aggressive teeth to maintain fixation during resection. Care must be taken to avoid extensor mechanism damage.

Another resection tool option is the patella reamer (Fig. 147.10). A recessed cavity is reamed to a desired thickness. This allows an inlay technique, where the native rim is left intact, and also an onlay technique, where the rim is removed using a saw. Proponents of the inlayed patella component describe several advantages, including increased fixation of the component, a

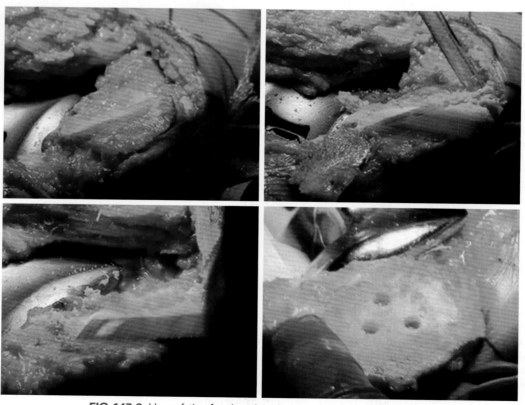

FIG 147.8 Use of the freehand technique to resect the patella.

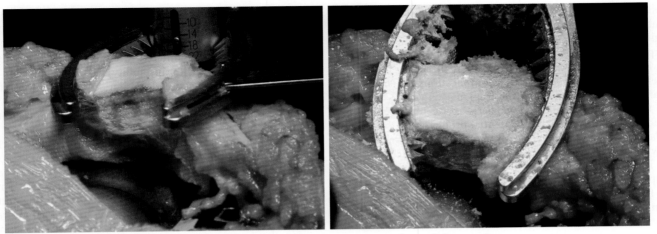

FIG 147.9 Use of a saw guide to cut the surface of the patella.

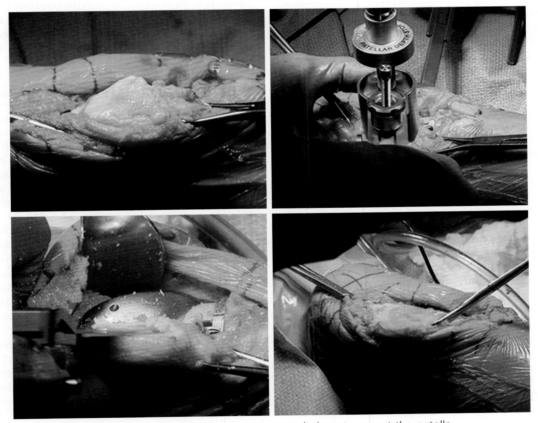

FIG 147.10 Use of a patella reamer technique to resect the patella.

more planar preparation of the patella, and ease of centralizing patella tracking.[27,34,83] However, reaming is not without its risks, as the guide must be appropriately positioned and pre-reaming measurements must be accurate to avoid over-resection and excessive patella tilt. Several studies have determined that inlay components have a tendency to excessively resect native patella bone thickness, leading to postoperative patella complications such as fracture.

There is a wide array of surgical techniques for resurfacing the patella. If a guide is used, proper placement and accurate measurements must be taken to ensure appropriate resection.

If a freehand technique is used, frequent measurements at more than one area of resection are recommended. The approach is surgeon-dependent, and each technique has its own advantages and disadvantages.

ADDRESSING THE COMPLICATIONS OF PATELLA RESURFACING

There is a subset of specific complications that occur at the PF joint, which a surgeon must consider when performing patella resurfacing. These include patella fracture, osteonecrosis of the patella, component wear and loosening, patella crepitus, patella instability, and extensor tendon damage. With improvements in surgical technique and implant design, the rate of patella-related complications after TKA has decreased in recent decades.[28,78,81,80] It is has been hypothesized that patella maltracking may ultimately be the cause of most patella complications.[9,59] Continued advances in the design of patella implants, as well as femoral and trochlear articulation, have been made in an effort to reduce the incidence of these potential problems.

Patella fractures after TKA are infrequent but have been shown to occur at a greater frequency with a resurfaced patella. The incidence is reported to be twice as high in males when compared to females, possibly as a result of greater force generation from the quadriceps and higher body mass index (BMI).[71] Rheumatoid arthritis, osteopenia, osteonecrosis, and malalignment are all risk factors for patella fracture, but proper surgical technique can help mitigate fracture risk.[33,101] Lateral retinacular releases can cause transient patellar hypovascularity but has not been shown to have a clear link with fracture.[52,75] As discussed previously, an over-resected patella can make the bone more prone to fracture, whereas an under-resected patella can increase implant thickness, causing excessive force and traction on the extensor mechanism as well as a decreased flexion arc.[33,71,101] Historic patella implant designs, particularly those using central fixation pegs, were associated with twice the rate of patella fracture when compared to the peripheral peg design.[14,55] A study of 12,464 patients who underwent TKA found a prevalence of patella fracture to be 0.68%, with a rate of 1.01% among men and 0.40% among women. Almost half of these were asymptomatic or minimally symptomatic at the time of diagnosis.[71]

The Danish knee registry reports that 2.1% of revision TKA procedures were performed for patella polyethylene wear.[25] Polyethylene wear is commonly a cause of late failure in TKA and is influenced by a multitude of factors, including implant design, patient characteristics, and technical factors. More modern component designs use highly cross-linked patella polyethylene, which has been shown to have a marked improvement in wear properties but has not yet been proven to be clinically superior.[20,30,54] There have not been any retrieval wear studies with regard to patella performance in vivo to demonstrate the potential improvements and properties of the highly cross-linked polyethylene patella.

Following TKA, the entrapment of hyperplastic fibrous nodules of scar or granulation on the posterior, supra-patella quadriceps tendon can be a source of mechanical symptoms and pain. Patellar crepitus is characterized by a palpable continued grinding sensation best detected during terminal knee extension; it can occur in up to 14% of patients, although only a subset will experience significant pain or symptoms.[26] Transient entrapment of the fibrosynovial hyperplasia in the intercondylar box, limiting the movement of the patella until the hyperplasia escapes in a sudden superior motion, is known as patella clunk syndrome, first described by Hozack in 1989.[26,41] It is more commonly encountered in posterior-stabilized (PS) rather than cruciate-retaining (CR) designs. The advent of design changes to femoral components—including the removal of sharp ridges at the intercondylar groove, which creates a smooth transition that allows for greater clearance during soft tissue tracking—has decreased the incidence of this syndrome.[31,79]

Patella instability following TKA is a potentially serious problem that may lead to reoperation. It can be avoided by proper component placement, patella preparation, and soft tissue balancing. The incidence for symptomatic instability requiring revision is reported to be between 0.5% and 0.8%.[82,91] This issue may be encountered, whether or not the patella is resurfaced. Patients with instability will often present with discomfort, pain, functional limitation, subluxation of the patella, and rarely dislocation. As mentioned previously, the main contributor to maltracking leading to instability is improper placement of components.

Improvements in patella resurfacing and femoral trochlear design have minimized the risk of complication from historical rates when less emphasis was placed on restoration of patella thickness and patellar tracking. A meta-analysis of randomized controlled trials reported PF complications excluding anterior pain at a rate of 1.3% in resurfaced knees and 1.1% in unresurfaced knees.[78] The most recent study by Roberts et al. examined 327 knees in a prospective randomized controlled trial comparing TKA with and without patella resurfacing. There were no patella specific complications in the resurfaced cohort at a mean follow-up of 7.8 years and one patella fracture in the nonresurfaced group.[86] As with any surgical procedure, potential complications should factor into deciding which treatment is the most ideal for each patient.

OUTCOMES OF PATELLA RESURFACING

Several high quality randomized prospective trials have examined the clinical outcomes of resurfaced versus unresurfaced patella in TKA. Much of the literature has examined differences in anterior knee pain, functional outcomes, and reoperation rate.* There are reports of lower incidence of anterior knee pain in the past with resurfacing, but most recent studies show no difference. Determining the cause and ideal treatment for anterior knee pain following a TKA can be a complex and challenging problem. Patients seek out TKA for relief of pain and improvement of function. Persistent pain is negatively correlated with patient satisfaction and quality of life.[7,73] Anterior knee pain has been attributed to both functional causes (muscle weakness or imbalance) that lead to incorrect loading of the patella and mechanical causes (oversizing, instability, rotational errors, maltracking, chondrolysis, or aseptic loosening) that may cause pain.[77]

Most of the randomized prospective studies lack adequate sample size and power to adequately detect differences in patient outcomes. Pilling et al. conducted a meta-analysis of 16 prospective randomized controlled trials to assess reoperation rates following TKA in 1710 procedures that included patella resurfacing and 1755 that did not. Anterior knee pain was reported in 23.5% of the unresurfaced cohort and 13.4% of the resurfaced group, but this difference was not significant and was attributed to high heterogeneity. There was a significant ($p < .0001$) difference in the reoperation rate for anterior knee pain, with reoperation in 6% of the unresurfaced group compared to 1% of the resurfaced group. There were no significant differences in functional knee scores, patient satisfaction, infection rate, or operative time identified.[78]

Previous meta-analyses have also concluded that patella resurfacing reduces the risk of revision surgery.[39,68,72,73] In the

---

*References 15, 60, 86, 94, 99, and 102.

United States, Khatod et al. studied 39,286 TKA from the Kaiser Permanente National Total Joint Replacement Registry. They report a significant difference in the revision rates, with 1.7% in resurfaced and 3.6% in unresurfaced knees.[49] An estimated 2.5% to 10% of patients with an unresurfaced patella will undergo a secondary resurfacing procedure.[45] The success rates for patella resurfacing after index knee replacement are reported to be only 50% to 60%.[22,24,63,64] Even in patients who did experience subsequent improvements in Hospital for Special Surgery knee scores, a much higher risk for complications and subsequent failure were reported.[18]

There is a clear link between not resurfacing the patella during a TKA and an increased likelihood of a revision operation despite similar pain and function scores. Orthopedic surgeons whose patients have anterior knee pain following a TKA will consider secondary resurfacing if it was not performed in the initial operation because the unresurfaced patella can be a pain generator. A similar patient with a resurfaced patella is less likely to be offered a revision if there are no radiographic or clinical findings to warrant a reoperation.

ECONOMICS OF PATELLA RESURFACING

In 2010 an estimated 719,000 patients underwent TKAs in the United States (Centers for Disease Control and Prevention [CDC]). With this number expected to increase to over 1 million annually by 2020, 3 million by 2030, and similarly in other countries around the world, the economic implications of patella resurfacing should be considered as a cost-effectiveness issue.[40,51] There are increased costs associated with patella resurfacing, including the patella component, cement, and a longer operative time during a primary TKA. Although the initial cost may be higher, the projected total health care costs 10 years following surgery of patients with unresurfaced patella exceed those with patella resurfacing.[65] The cost disparity is related to a higher rate of reoperation to treat persistent anterior knee pain with secondary resurfacing. Meijer and Dasa conducted an expected value decision tree analysis and also projected increased health care costs at 5 years following the initial surgery without resurfacing. This model remains valid so long as revision rates after patella resurfacing remain below 3.54% and revision rates for an unresurfaced patella remain above 0.77%.[62] Despite no strong clinical evidence in support of secondary resurfacing, surgeons continue to offer patients with persistent anterior knee pain this operation, which ultimately increases the health care cost burden.

SELECTIVE RESURFACING

Some surgeons have advocated the practice of selective patella resurfacing. Specific selection criteria include minimal articular changes, congruent patellar tracking, a normal patella anatomy, younger age, and no known inflammatory arthritis.[50] However, these selection criteria have not been validated as predictors of avoiding anterior pain following TKA. Gross examination of the patella can often be misleading and may underestimate articular degeneration.[4] Han et al. studied 87 knees in 57 patients by taking intraoperative photos during TKA to evaluate the status of the patellar cartilage and comparing it with postoperative PF pain and function scores. They found a weak correlation with anterior knee pain, no association with functional parameters, and cautioned against using cartilage status as a determinant of

patella resurfacing.[38] Patients with Grade IV Outerbridge patellae at the time of primary TKA surgery are predictive of secondary resurfacing.[87] All patients with severely damaged patellar articular cartilage should undergo resurfacing, as currently there are no indications to counter this recommendation.

CONCLUSION

Orthopedic surgeons must carefully consider the PF joint during TKA. Although initial cost savings may be attractive for nonresurfacing of the patella, improvements in patellar and femoral implants, operative techniques, and understanding of the patella-femoral articulation allow reproducible, biomechanically sound patella resurfacing with minimal complications. To avoid the unnecessary burden to patients and society of secondary resurfacing, we recommend routine patella resurfacing during primary TKA.

KEY REFERENCES

4. Athiviraham A, Fechisin J, Hartman A, et al: The normal patella—does it exist? A histologic analysis. *Am J Orthop* 43:370–373, 2014.
7. Barrack RL, Bertot AJ, Wolfe MW, et al: Patellar resurfacing in total knee arthroplasty. A prospective, randomized, double-blind study with five to seven years of follow-up. *J Bone Joint Surg Am* 83:1376–1381, 2001.
9. Berger RA, Crossett LS, Jacobs JJ, et al: Malrotation causing patellofemoral complications after total knee arthroplasty. *Clin Orthop* 356:144–153, 1998.
14. Brick GW, Scott RD: The patellofemoral component of total knee arthroplasty. *Clin Orthop* 231:163–178, 1988.
15. Burnett RS, Boone JL, Rosenzweig SD, et al: Patellar resurfacing compared with nonresurfacing in total knee arthroplasty. A concise follow-up of a randomized trial. *J Bone Joint Surg Am* 91:2562–2567, 2009.
18. Campbell DG, Mintz AD, Stevenson TM: Early patellofemoral revision following total knee arthroplasty. *J Arthroplasty* 10:287–291, 1995.
26. Dennis DA, Kim RH, Johnson DR, et al: The John Insall award: control-matched evaluation of painful patellar crepitus after total knee arthroplasty. *Clin Orthop* 469:10–17, 2011.
28. Feller JA, Bartlett RJ, Lang DM: Patellar resurfacing versus retention in total knee arthroplasty. *J Bone Joint Surg Br* 78:226–228, 1996.
39. He JY, Jiang LS, Dai LY: Is patellar resurfacing superior than nonresurfacing in total knee arthroplasty? A meta-analysis of randomized trials. *Knee* 18:137–144, 2011.
41. Hozack WJ, Rothman RJ, Booth RE, et al: The patellar clunk syndrome. A complication of posterior stabilised total knee arthroplasty. *Clin Orthop* 241:203–208, 1989.
45. Insall J, Tria AJ, Aglietti P: Resurfacing of the patella. *J Bone Joint Surg Am* 62:933–936, 1980.
47. Karnezis IA, Vossinakis IC, Rex C, et al: Secondary patellar resurfacing in total knee arthroplasty: results of multivariate analysis in two case-matched groups. *J Arthroplasty* 18:993–998, 2003.
48. Kaufer H: Mechanical function of the patella. *J Bone Joint Surg Am* 53:1551–1560, 1971.
59. Malo M, Vince KG: The unstable patella after total knee arthroplasty: etiology, prevention, and management. *J Am Acad Orthop Surg* 11:364–371, 2003.
60. Mayman D, Bourne RB, Rorabeck CH, et al: Resurfacing versus not resurfacing the patella in total knee arthroplasty: 8- to 10-year results. *J Arthroplasty* 18(5):541–545, 2003.
68. Nizard RS, Biau D, Porcher R, et al: A meta-analysis of patellar replacement in total knee arthroplasty. *Clin Orthop* 432:196–203, 2005.
71. Ortiguera CJ, Berry DJ: Patellar fracture after total knee arthroplasty. *J Bone Joint Surg Am* 84:532–540, 2002.
72. Pakos EE, Ntzani EE, Trikalinos TA: Patellar resurfacing in total knee arthroplasty. A meta-analysis. *J Bone Joint Surg Am* 87:1438–1445, 2005.

73. Parvizi J, Rapuri VR, Saleh KJ, et al: Failure to resurface the patella during total knee arthroplasty may result in more knee pain and secondary surgery. *Clin Orthop* 438:191–196, 2005.

81. Rand JA: Patellar resurfacing in total knee arthroplasty. *Clin Orthop* 260:110–117, 1990.

86. Roberts DW, Hayes TD, Tate CT, et al: Selective patellar resurfacing in total knee arthroplasty: a prospective, randomized, double-blind study. *J Arthroplasty* 30:216–222, 2015.

91. Scuderi GR, Insall JN, Scott NW: Patellofemoral pain after total knee arthroplasty. *J Am Acad Orthop Surg* 2:239–246, 1994.

99. Waters TS, Bentley G: Patellar resurfacing in total knee arthroplasty. A prospective, randomized study. *J Bone Joint Surg Am* 85:212–217, 2003.

The references for this chapter can also be found on www.expertconsult.com.

148

Alignment in Total Knee Arthroplasty

Johan Bellemans

The main purpose of either partial or total knee arthroplasty (TKA) has always been to replace the eroded cartilage and bone by an artificial implant, which is usually made out of metal and plastic and compensates for the erosion or damage. When doing so, restoration of neutral mechanical alignment has traditionally been considered as the most important factor with respect to the durability of the implant.

When neutral mechanical alignment is restored, the mechanical axis of the leg passes through the center of the knee, which leads to an even mediolateral load distribution and a minimized risk for implant wear and component loosening.

In past literature, several reports have indeed been published, demonstrating the adverse effect of inadequate restoration of neutral leg alignment on implant survivorship.* Knees that had been implanted with mechanical alignment deviating from neutral were associated with increased failure rates because of accelerated polyethylene wear, implant loosening, osteolysis, bone collapse, and implant subsidence.*

It is generally accepted that these adverse events occur because of deviations from neutral mechanical alignment leading to increased mechanical loads on the implant, as well as the bone-prosthesis interface, leading to subsequent implant and/or fixation failure.

Therefore the current general consensus is that an overall mechanical femorotibial alignment (FTMA) of 0 ± 3 degrees should be the target to aim for to avoid implant failure at medium or long term.[8,19,23]

For this reason, several techniques to obtain intraoperative restoration of mechanical alignment have been used in the past, usually by referencing from intramedullary or extramedullary alignment rods, or using more sophisticated computerized navigation methods.[4,18,22,25,32]

TRADITIONAL ALIGNMENT PRINCIPLES

The most common strategy to achieve neutral alignment was popularized by Insall and Freeman[9,16] and has since been referred to as the "classical alignment" philosophy.

In this approach the surgeon aims at obtaining a perpendicular implant position in reference to the mechanical axis of both the femur and tibia in the coronal plane (Fig. 148.1). As such, a minor deviation from the natural anatomy is induced because the physiologic (natural) joint line is oriented on

average 3 degrees instead of perpendicular (0 degrees) to the overall mechanical leg axis (Fig. 148.2).

In the classical alignment philosophy the proximal tibial joint line is therefore converted from an average of 87 degrees (3 degrees varus) to 90 degrees (neutral) and the distal femoral joint line from 87 degrees (3 degrees valgus) to 90 degrees (neutral).

Therefore Hungerford, Kenna, and Krackow proposed an alternative strategy, which became known as the "anatomic alignment" school.[15] In this approach the obliquity of the joint line was restored by resecting parallel to the tibial and femoral surfaces, matching the prosthetic implant thickness ("matched resection"). As such, a 3-degree varus position of the tibial component combined with a 3-degree valgus position of the femoral component led to an overall neutral mechanical alignment.

Despite the obvious theoretical advantages of being more physiologic in restitution, for several reasons the anatomic alignment philosophy did not become generally adopted. One of the main reasons being that the implant system with which the philosophy was associated (posterior condylar axis [PCA] knee, Howmedica, Rutherford, New Jersey) turned out to be associated with accelerated polyethylene wear characteristics, and, although in later years it became obvious that these were the consequence of intrinsically poor polyethylene quality, the general concern at the time was that the underlying alignment philosophy played an important role. The fact that occasionally excessive varus tibial cuts occurred (because of surgeon's and instrument variability) further impeded the widespread adoption of the "anatomic" alignment philosophy, and it gradually faded out.

However, interestingly, the recent insights on constitutional knee joint alignment and orientation, together with the availability of modern implant materials and fixation, have induced a renewed interest in some of its underlying principles.

In addition, current results after TKA are somewhat disappointing when compared with the outcome after hip replacement; this has made some surgeons question the dogmatic acceptance of classical neutral alignment restoration.

NEWER INSIGHTS

The classical model of restoring neutral mechanical—with perpendicular cuts on the mechanical axes of the femur and tibia—leads to systematic **distalization of the lateral joint line** (see Fig. 148.1). A perpendicular mechanical cut on the femur will indeed remove approximately 7 mm in the unworn knee,

*References 2, 6, 14, 17, 27, 29, and 33.

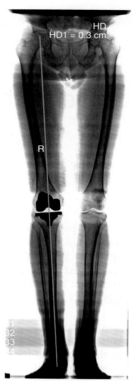

FIG 148.1 Restoration of neutral mechanical alignment according to the "classical" alignment philosophy. However, as a consequence, the physiologic joint obliquity is lost, with distalization on the lateral side (see contralateral knee for comparison).

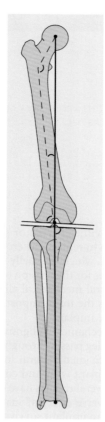

FIG 148.2 The normal joint line is on average 3 degrees inclined to the mechanical axis of the leg. In the traditional way of performing TKA with perpendicular mechanical cuts on both the femur and tibia, this inclination is lost and becomes perpendicular.

which is replaced by a 9-mm-thick metal component, thereby distalizing the lateral femoral joint line with 2 mm. This is compensated by the perpendicular tibial resection, which removes an equal amount of additional bone that is replaced by the tibial implant, compensating for the femoral side. The result is an unphysiologic obliquity of the joint line, with distalization on the lateral side (see Figs. 148.1 and 148.2).

As a consequence, patellofemoral mechanics may become distorted, potentially leading to pain or discomfort with a sensation of anterior tightness in flexion (Fig. 148.3).

Another area of concern with traditional mechanical alignment restoration is the lack of an individual, **patient-specific strategy.** The relatively poor performance of current TKA designs, which lack the ability to reproduce physiologic knee kinematics, has led to an increased interest towards patient-specific, anatomic restoration[10,12,29]

Given this philosophy, the natural anatomy of the knee is restored by using implants that selectively or completely resurface the eroded or damaged parts of the knee back to its original anatomic contours. This approach would not necessarily restore the alignment to neutral but rather to the natural alignment of the knee before the disease or damage occurred.

CONSTITUTIONAL ALIGNMENT

Indeed, a number of patients exist for whom neutral mechanical alignment is abnormal. Patients with so-called constitutional varus knees have had varus alignment since their end of growth.

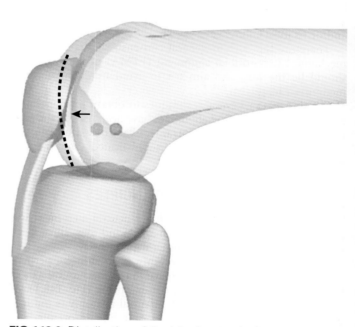

FIG 148.3 Distalization of the joint line on the lateral side leads to distorted patellofemoral mechanics, which can be a cause of pain or discomfort with a sensation of anterior tightness in flexion.

Restoring neutral alignment in these cases would be abnormal for them and would almost per definition require some degree of medial soft tissue release (Fig. 148.4).

At the same time, anatomic restoration of these knees would lead to a mechanical alignment in varus, which could jeopardize the long-term survivorship of the procedure. The surgeon is therefore confronted with a strategic dilemma in these patients with constitutional varus: to opt for either neutral mechanical alignment restoration while realizing that this is abnormal for that specific patient or anatomic restoration and accepting varus mechanical alignment.

Unfortunately, until recently no data were available on the question whether constitutional varus (or valgus) really exists in the normal population, and if so in what percentage of healthy individuals it occurs. It was also unclear how these patients could be identified during surgery. Therefore we performed an interesting study to investigate this.[1]

A cohort of 250 asymptomatic adult volunteers between 20 and 27 years old was recruited, and all of them underwent full leg, standing digital radiography, on which 19 different alignment parameters were analyzed. The incidence of constitutional varus alignment was determined and contributing factors were analyzed using multivariant prediction models.

Interestingly, as high as 32% of males and 17% of females had constitutional varus knees with a natural mechanical alignment ≥3 degrees varus.[1]

Constitutional varus was associated with increased sports activity during growth, increased femoral varus bowing, an increased femoral neck shaft angle, and an increased femoral anatomic-mechanical angle.

The average mechanical hip and knee angle (HKA) in the male knees was 1.9 degrees varus (standard deviation [SD] 2.1), and in the female knees it was 0.8 degrees varus (SD: 2.4) (Figs. 148.5 and 148.6); 165 (66%) of the male knees and 200 (80%) of the female knees had an HKA between −3 and +3 degrees. Five (2%) of the male and seven (2.8%) of the female knees had an HKA ≥ +3 degrees.

The number of patients with constitutional varus in our study (32% of males; 17% of females) may at first sight seem relatively high.

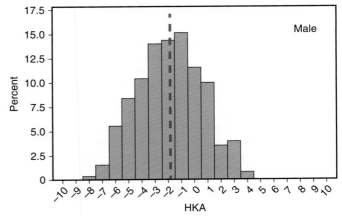

FIG 148.5 Histogram depicting the large variability in natural alignment in healthy male individuals, which contradicts the general belief that normal alignment is zero. Large variability exists between individuals. *HKA*, Hip and knee angle. (From Bellemans J, Colyn W, Vandenneucker H, Victor J: The Chitranjan Ranawat Award: is neutral mechanical alignment normal for all patients? The concept of constitutional varus. *Clin Orthop* 470:45–53, 2012.)

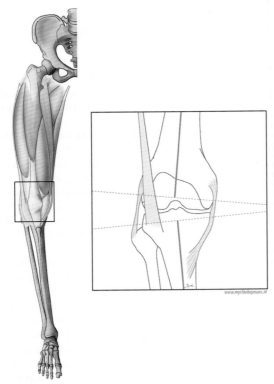

FIG 148.4 Patients with constitutional varus knees have varus alignment since they reached skeletal maturity. Restoring neutral alignment in these cases may indeed be abnormal and undesirable and would almost per definition require some degree of medial soft tissue release. (From Bellemans J, Colyn W, Vandenneucker H, Victor J: The Chitranjan Ranawat Award: is neutral mechanical alignment normal for all patients? The concept of constitutional varus. *Clin Orthop* 470:45–53, 2012.)

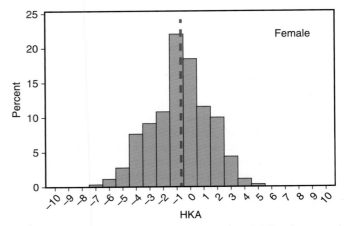

FIG 148.6 Histogram depicting the large variability in natural alignment in healthy female individuals. *HKA*, Hip and knee angle. (From Bellemans J, Colyn W, Vandenneucker H, Victor J: The Chitranjan Ranawat Award: is neutral mechanical alignment normal for all patients? The concept of constitutional varus. *Clin Orthop* 470:45–53, 2012.)

Indeed, although many authors have studied normal lower leg alignment in humans before, this finding has been unrecognized so far. Some of the reasons for this are because many classic alignment studies have been flawed with a number of shortcomings, such as a limited number of participants, a large variability in the subjects' age, recruitment in a hospital setting, lack of stratification, and selection bias of the subjects.

The association of constitutional varus alignment with increased physical activity during growth has been raised by other authors before. Witvrouw et al. have noted that intense sports activity during growth leads to the development of varus knees, and this phenomenon occurs especially towards the end of the growth spurt.[35]

We believe that such is the consequence of Hueter-Volkmann law, which states that growth at the physes is retarded by increased compression, whereas reduced loading accelerates growth.[28,30,34] The increased loads caused by the adduction moment on the knee during ambulation and physical activity leads to the development of varus alignment secondary to delayed growth on the medial side and accelerated growth on the lateral physes. Cook and Lavernia have in the past already alluded to this theory in a biomechanical study on the etiology of pediatric tibia vara.[5]

The observations from our study indicate that an important variability in natural alignment exists among individuals. One should therefore question the dogma that 0-degree mechanical alignment should be the goal in every patient undergoing TKA.

Restoring the alignment to neutral in patients with constitutional varus would indeed be abnormal and unnatural for them because it would implicate an overcorrection towards their natural situation in which they had spent their life since skeletal maturity.

A strategy where the natural "constitutional" alignment of the patient is determined and subsequently reproduced seems therefore much more logical (Fig. 148.7).

Modern TKA implant designs with better material characteristics, combined with improved implant fixation and surgical technique (compared with the past), may allow this strategy to be followed successfully.

MODERN OUTCOME STUDIES

Recent literature seems to confirm this.[7,11,13,31] In 2013 Vanlommel et al. published the outcome of a cohort of 132 consecutively operated patients with preoperative varus alignment that were evaluated at 5- to 9-year follow-up.[31]

Knees that were restored to their constitutional alignment had significantly better Knee Society and Western Ontario and McMaster Universities Arthritis Index (WOMAC) scores compared with knees that were corrected to mechanically neutral, as well as compared with knees that were left in severe varus exceeding 6 degrees. After a midterm follow-up in none of these groups, a revision occurred.

In 2014 Dossett et al. published the results of a randomized controlled trial comparing kinematically (ie, constitutionally) aligned versus mechanically aligned knees, again demonstrating better outcome scores for the kinematically aligned knees. The odds ratio of having a pain-free knee with the kinematically aligned knee (Oxford and WOMAC pain scores) was 3.2 (*P* = .020) and 4.9 (*P* = .001), respectively, compared with the mechanically aligned technique.[7]

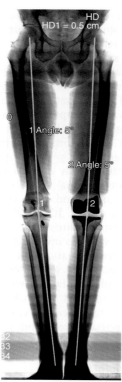

FIG 148.7 Restoration of "constitutional" alignment. The knee is restored to its natural 3-degree varus alignment for this patient (see contralateral knee for comparison).

Howell et al. have repeatedly reported equally satisfactory results in isolated series of kinematically (or constitutionally) aligned knees.[11,13]

Although the previously quoted authors have used the term "kinematic alignment" instead of "constitutional alignment," we believe the latter is a better and intuitively more understandable terminology to address the same principles.

In addition to the previously mentioned reports, several studies have failed to demonstrate an inferior outcome for so-called malaligned versus mechanically neutrally aligned knees, when modern implants and a contemporary surgical technique were used.[3,20,21,24,26]

Surgeons from the Mayo Clinic reported in 2010 the 15-year survivorship data of 398 knees, of which most were preoperatively in mechanical varus.[24] At time of the latest follow-up, 15.4% in the mechanically neutrally aligned group had been revised for any reason, versus 13% in the so-called outlier group (*P* = .88); 9.2% in the mechanically aligned group had been revised for aseptic loosening, mechanical failure, wear, or patellar problems, compared with 7.5% in the outlier group (*P* = .88); and 5.8% % in the mechanically aligned group had been revised for aseptic loosening, mechanical failure, or wear, compared with 3.8% in the outlier group (*P* = .49). Therefore the authors concluded that restoration of the mechanical axis to 0 ± 3 degrees did not improve the 15-year implant survival in these modern TKAs.

Similar findings were reported by Matziolis et al. who followed a group of 218 TKAs for a minimum of 5 years and could not detect any correlation between varus malalignment and a bad medium-term radiologic or clinical outcome. Indeed, they noted even slightly better Knee Society (KS) scores for knees that were left in varus compared with those that were restored to normal, although not statistically significant.[21]

Bonner et al. reported on 501 total knee replacements (TKRs) and could not detect a significant difference in 15-year survivorship between so-called malaligned knees and those that were restored to neutral within 3 degrees. Morgan et al. came to the same conclusion when studying 197 TKAs at 9-year follow-up.[3]

Other authors have additionally looked into the influence of individual component positioning. Interestingly, Magnussen et al. noted similar survivorship and International Knee Society (IKS) scores for preoperative varus knees that were left in varus (constitutional alignment) compared with those that were restored to neutral, although varus tibial alignment was associated with lower scores.[20]

Probably the most convincing study on this matter was published by Ritter et al., who reviewed 6070 knees with a minimum follow-up of 2 years. Knees that were restored to residual varus with the tibial component neutral had the lowest aseptic failure rate (0 degrees), followed by the knees in which both the overall alignment and tibial component alignment was restored to neutral (0.2% aseptic failure rate). However when the tibial component was implanted in varus, the aseptic failures rate was always significantly higher; 3.3% when overall alignment was restored to neutral, 4.4% when overall alignment was in varus, and 4.7% when overall alignment was valgus.

Although these latter reports therefore seem to indicate that restoration of constitutional alignment should be accomplished while maintaining a neutral tibial cut, further evidence to support this finding should be awaited before definite conclusions can be drawn.

SUMMARY

Restoration of neutral mechanical limb alignment is traditionally considered one of the prerequisites for successful total knee replacement and is currently for most surgeons still the gold standard.

However, newer insights have taught us that, for a significant proportion of the population, neutral alignment is not normal, and restoring these patients to neutral may not be the best available option.

As a consequence, the concept of restoring constitutional rather than mechanical alignment has gained interest. In this philosophy the natural alignment of the knee is restored to its original state that was reached at skeletal maturity, before the disease or damage had occurred. The author has defined this as the patient's constitutional alignment.[6] Growing evidence exists that such strategy could lead to better patient outcome without jeopardizing implant longevity. However, excessive varus inclination of the tibial implant remains of concern, even when combined with compensatory valgus inclination on the femoral component and overall neutral alignment.

The references for this chapter can also be found on www.expertconsult.com.

149

Surgical Approaches in Total Knee Arthroplasty: Standard and Minimally Invasive Surgery Techniques

William J. Long, Jason P. Hochfelder, Michael P. Nett, Alfred J. Tria, Jr., Giles R. Scuderi

Critical to exposing the knee during total knee arthroplasty (TKA) is a complete understanding of the local anatomy, which is described in Chapter 1. With such knowledge, the pathologic condition, anatomy, and planned surgery can be correlated. Although well-defined soft tissue layers provide reproducible planes of dissection,[37,51,67] the blood supply to the skin should be respected, especially when previous incisions are present or multiple incisions are planned. Most of the blood supply to the skin arises from the saphenous artery and the descending geniculate artery on the medial side of the knee (Fig. 149.1).[21,70] The vessels perforate the deep fascia and form an anastomosis superficial to the deep fascia. Continuing through the subcutaneous fat to supply the epidermis, little communication occurs in the superficial layer. Therefore, dissection should be deep to the fascia to maintain the blood supply to the skin.[69]

Many incisions and approaches to the knee joint were originally designed for open meniscectomy and reconstructive procedures before the advent of arthroscopy and are mainly of historical value.[1] The intent of this chapter is to detail the surgical approaches that are useful for TKA. Many planned approaches are extensile but have been modified for performing minimally invasive surgery (MIS).[23]

APPROACHES

Skin Incisions

A longitudinal midline straight anterior skin incision is extensile and can be extended proximally and distally to expose the distal end of the femur, the patella, and the proximal end of the tibia. This anterior incision allows exposure of the medial and lateral supporting structures and can be reopened or extended if a revision is necessary. Through this skin incision, a medial parapatellar arthrotomy can be performed; this is the most versatile approach in that it allows the broadest exposure to the knee joint. Other arthrotomies, such as midvastus and subvastus approaches, are also performed through this skin incision and are detailed in the following sections.

The anterior midline skin incision has provided a utilitarian extensile approach to the knee (Fig. 149.2). With proximal and distal extension of the skin incision, large flaps can be developed to expose the anterior, medial, and lateral supporting structures.[30] If the midline skin incision is moved medially, it will be parallel to Langer cleavage lines and subject to less tension and disrupting force than an anterior midline incision.[65] Incisions parallel to the cleavage lines heal faster, gain strength more quickly, and result in a finer scar; however, this approach does not offer a versatile exposure to the knee, and so a midline incision is used.[35] No evidence indicates that this position creates any more hypoxia in the lateral skin margin than an anterior midline incision does.

The anterior Kocher U incision[35] and the Putti inverted U incision[48] have become obsolete, primarily because of complications associated with vascular compromise to the surrounding skin. The anterior transverse incision may be cosmetically pleasing, but it does not allow extensile exposure (see Fig. 149.2).[65]

ARTHROTOMY

The medial parapatellar arthrotomy, or anteromedial approach, has been the most used approach for exposure of the knee joint. It provides extensive exposure and is useful for open anterior cruciate ligament reconstruction, TKA, cartilage preservation or restoration procedures, and fixation of intraarticular fractures. Because this approach has been implicated in compromise of the patellar circulation (see Fig. 149.1C),[59,60] some authors have advocated the subvastus, midvastus, and trivector approaches for exposure of the knee joint. Alternatively, the anterolateral approach exposes the knee joint from the lateral side, although it is more difficult. With careful planning and arthrotomy selection, the anterior aspect of the joint can be fully exposed in most cases with each of these arthrotomies.

MEDIAL PARAPATELLAR ARTHROTOMY

A medial parapatellar arthrotomy allows excellent exposure to most structures of the knee joint (Fig. 149.3). Von Langenbeck[65] originally described dissection of the vastus medialis from the quadriceps tendon with distal extension through the medial patellar retinaculum and along the patellar ligament. The synovium is divided in line with the capsular incision, and the fat pad is often retracted or incised. Pinsornsak and colleagues[47] found a lower incidence of anterior knee pain (0% vs 8%) in patients who did not have their fat pads excised. They found no other clinical or radiographic differences and no difference in incidence of complications. Because dissection continues to the joint line, one must be aware of the anterior horn of the medial meniscus as well as the transverse ligament between the medial and lateral menisci. Completion of this arthrotomy permits the patella to be everted or subluxated laterally. When the patella is dislocated and the knee is flexed, care should be taken to avoid avulsing the patellar tendon from the tibial tubercle. In a randomized study of 68 patients, Reid and associates[50] showed no early to midterm benefit to subluxation rather than eversion of the patella. If it is difficult to dislocate the patella laterally, the proximal quadriceps tendon incision should be

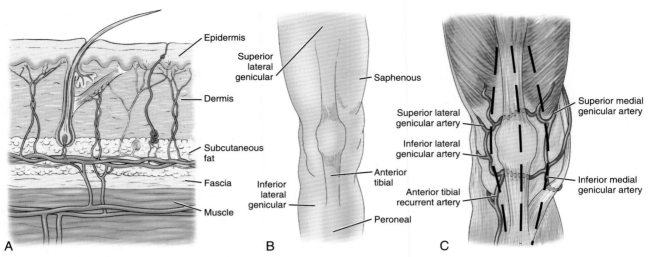

FIG 149.1 Blood supply to the knee. (A) Microcirculation to the skin. (B) Vessels contributing to the blood supply to the skin. (C) Patellar blood supply. (A and B, Redrawn from Younger AS et al: Surgical exposures in revision total knee arthroplasty. *J Am Acad Orthop Surg* 6:55, 1998; C, redrawn from Scott WN: *The knee,* vol 1, St Louis, 1994, Mosby-Year Book, p 56.)

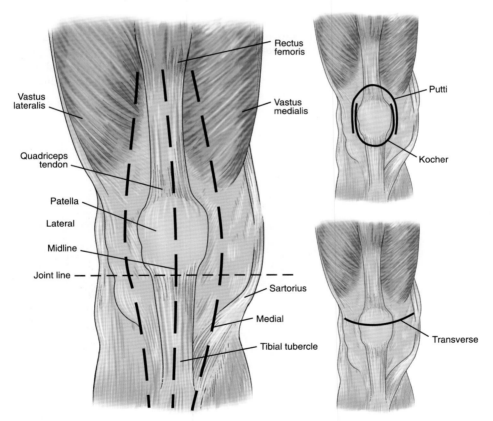

FIG 149.2 Anterior approaches to the knee. (Redrawn from Scott WN: *The knee,* vol 1, St Louis, 1994, Mosby-Year Book, p 56.)

extended superiorly or the patellar tendon carefully reflected subperiosteally along the medial border of the tibial tubercle to its crest similar to a banana peel. Chareancholvanich and Pornarattanamaneewong[10] showed that an incision into the quadriceps tendon up to 4 cm does not affect recovery. The patellar tendon must not be avulsed from the tibial tubercle.

Insall[26] modified the split patella approach, as described by Sir Robert Jones, because of damage to the patellar articular surface (Fig. 149.4). The extensor mechanism is exposed through a midline skin incision, the quadriceps tendon is divided 8 to 10 cm above the patella, and the incision is continued distally in a straight line over the patella and along the

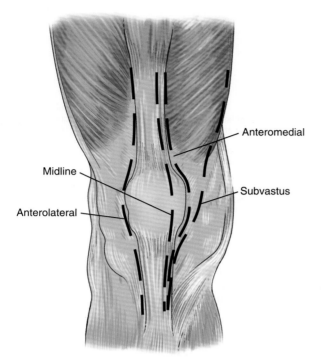

FIG 149.3 Preferred anterior approaches to the knee. (Redrawn from Scott WN: *The knee,* vol 1, St Louis, 1994, Mosby-Year Book, p 57.)

medial border of the patellar tendon. The quadriceps expansion is peeled from the anterior surface of the patella by sharp dissection until the medial border of the patella is visualized. The synovium is divided, and the fat pad is split in line with the arthrotomy. The patella is then subluxated laterally. Rather than going over the patella, the arthrotomy can alternatively be carried medial to the patella after dividing the quadriceps tendon. No internervous plane is used with this approach. Both the rectus femoris and the vastus medialis are supplied by the femoral nerve proximal to this incision.

When the midline approach is performed, the infrapatellar branch of the saphenous nerve comes into view (see Fig. 149.4, center). The saphenous nerve travels posterior to the sartorius muscle and pierces the fascia between the tendons of the sartorius and gracilis muscles, where it becomes superficial to the medial aspect of the knee. At this level, the infrapatellar branch of the saphenous nerve arises to supply the skin over the anterior and anteromedial aspect of the knee. Kummel and Zazanis[36] and Chambers[8] noted variation of this infrapatellar branch and recommended protecting it at the time of surgery to avoid painful neuromas. Insall and colleagues[28] believed that neuroma formation is more related to the patient's temperament than to an actual pathologic condition.

SUBVASTUS APPROACH

The subvastus approach, which allows direct access to the anterior knee joint, has been heralded as being more anatomic than the medial parapatellar arthrotomy (Fig. 149.5).[24,43] The

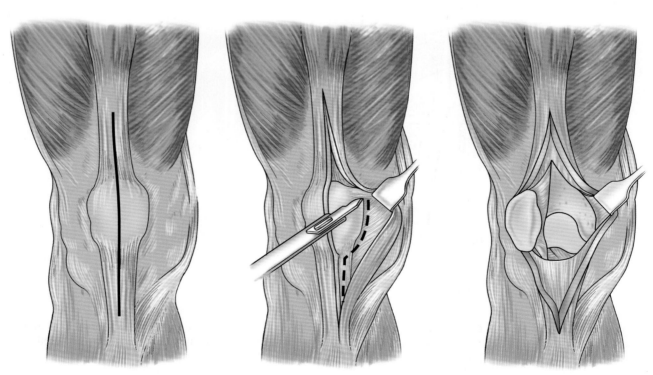

FIG 149.4 Insall's anterior approach. (Redrawn from Scott WN: *The knee,* vol 1, St Louis, 1994, Mosby-Year Book, p 57.)

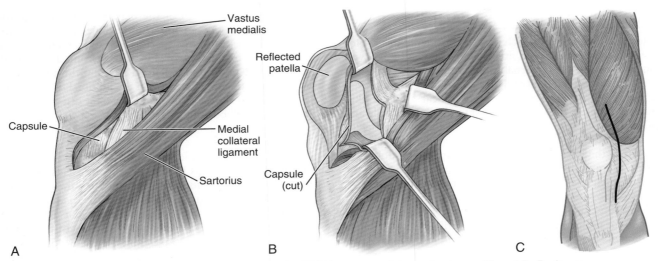

FIG 149.5 (A and B) Subvastus approach. (C) Trivector-retaining arthrotomy. (A and B, Redrawn from Scott WN: *The knee*, vol 1, St Louis, 1994, Mosby-Year Book, p 58; C, redrawn from Scuderi GR, Tria AJ: *Surgical techniques in total knee arthroplasty*, New York, 2002, Springer Verlag.)

subvastus approach is applicable to most primary reconstructive procedures of the knee.

This approach uses a straight midline skin incision that is extended above and below the patella. After development of a medial subcutaneous flap, the lower border of the vastus medialis is visualized. Because the vastus medialis inserts into the superior medial aspect of the patella, the fascial sheath along the inferior border of the vastus medialis is incised from the patella to the intermuscular septum.[46] This incision separates the vastus medialis from the intermuscular septum. The arthrotomy continues distally along the medial margin of the patella, with the medial retinaculum incised along the medial border of the patellar tendon and down onto the tibia. The vastus medialis then is peeled proximally, with blunt dissection, from the intermuscular septum. Care should be taken at this point to avoid injury to the neurovascular contents of Hunter canal. To gain access to the joint, the capsule of the suprapatellar pouch should be divided to release the patella, which is everted or subluxated laterally as the knee is flexed.

Tomek and coworkers[63] found minimal differences when comparing patients who had quadriceps-sparing subvastus approaches with patients who had medial parapatellar arthrotomies. The only statistically significant differences between the groups were that the patients who had a subvastus approach had slightly less pain at rest on postoperative day 1 and slightly less pain with activity on postoperative day 3. There were no significant differences in all other parameters.

MIDVASTUS APPROACH

The midvastus muscle-splitting approach is performed through a standard anterior midline skin incision. The incision is carried down through subcutaneous tissue and deep fascia to expose the quadriceps musculature. The vastus medialis is identified and split parallel to its muscle fibers. The quadriceps tendon is not incised. The incision is extended to the superior medial corner of the patella and then is continued distally along the medial patella and the patellar tendon to the level of the tibial tubercle. As with the subvastus approach, the capsule of

the suprapatellar pouch is divided so that the patella can be everted or subluxated laterally. Advocates of this approach believe that it is easier to evert the patella with the midvastus approach than with the subvastus approach because of the reduced bulk of the vastus medialis. This approach splits the muscle well away from its neurovascular supply.[17] Basarir and associates[3] described the course of the descending geniculate artery in relation to the midvastus approach. They described its insertion into the superior patella and suggested blunt dissection of the vastus medialis starting 13.5 mm medial to the superior pole.

TRIVECTOR-RETAINING ARTHROTOMY

The quadriceps musculature is exposed through an anterior midline skin incision. The trivector-retaining arthrotomy begins with transection of the vastus medialis obliquus muscle fibers 1.5 to 2 cm medial to the quadriceps tendon. Because the quadriceps tendon is not incised with this approach, the incision is extended distally 1 cm medial to the patella and the patellar tendon to the level of the tibial tubercle. It is recommended that this approach be performed with the knee flexed 90 to 110 degrees so that the quadriceps musculature is under maximal tension during the incision. To evert the patella or subluxate it laterally, the capsule of the suprapatellar pouch must be divided.[6]

ANTEROLATERAL APPROACH

The anterolateral approach, as described by Kocher,[35] consists of a lateral capsular incision that begins approximately 8 cm proximal to the patella at the insertion of the vastus lateralis muscle into the quadriceps tendon and continues distally along the lateral retinaculum (see Fig. 149.3). The incision can be extended distally through the fat pad for visualization of the lateral compartment and ends just distal to the tibial tuberosity. This approach is less favorable than the anteromedial approach because it is more difficult to subluxate the patella medially than laterally.

LATERAL PARAPATELLAR APPROACH

The lateral parapatellar approach may be considered in TKA for fixed valgus deformities that are isolated or combined with flexion contracture or external tibial rotation. Fixed varus deformity represents the only relative contraindication.

In performing this approach, a curvilinear midline skin incision or a laterally placed anterior skin incision is made and extended distally over the lateral border of the tibial tubercle. The joint is entered through a lateral parapatellar incision that extends from the lateral border of the quadriceps tendon, over the lateral margin of the patella, and continues distally into the anterior compartment fascia, 3 cm distal to the tibial tubercle. To dislocate the patella medially and expose the joint, osteotomy of a thin segment of the tubercle with the attached patellar tendon can be performed if necessary. A medial periosteal hinge is maintained along with the infrapatellar fat pad, which is used for later closure of the lateral retinacular defect. If necessary, the lateral arthrotomy can be left open to act as a lateral release to assist with patellar tracking.[7,32]

EXTENDED APPROACHES

Quadriceps Turndown

Coonse and Adams[14] originally described a quadriceps turndown. They used a paramedian skin incision that begins at the lower end of the quadriceps tendon along the patella and extends along the medial border of the patellar tendon. Skin flaps are developed; the quadriceps tendon is split down the middle; and approximately 1 cm above the patella, the incision is swung both medially and laterally and continues along the patella and the patellar tendon. The patella and the patellar tendon can be turned down to allow complete exposure of the joint (Fig. 149.6).

Further modification of the patellar turndown approach[27] involves the use of an anterior midline incision. A medial parapatellar arthrotomy is performed, and a second incision is made at an inclination of 45 degrees from the apex of the quadriceps tendon and extended laterally through the vastus lateralis and the upper portion of the iliotibial tract. This lateral incision stops short of the inferior lateral geniculate artery to preserve the blood supply (Fig. 149.7).

Quadriceps Snip

The full patellar turndown is now rarely necessary because cutting the quadriceps tendon proximally yields excellent soft tissue exposure, and functional reconstruction is possible (Fig. 149.8). This technique has been called the *quadriceps snip* by Insall.[27] Following a long medial parapatellar arthrotomy, an oblique incision is made at the proximal apex of the quadriceps tendon. This incision is approximately at a 45-degree angle across the quadriceps tendon and directly in line with the fibers of the vastus lateralis. This extended approach relieves tension on the extensor mechanism and the tibial tubercle. As the tibia is externally rotated and the patella subluxated laterally, the joint is exposed.

Tibial Tubercle Osteotomy

In cases where adequate exposure cannot be achieved with a quadriceps snip, a tibial tubercle osteotomy can be performed. A tibial tubercle osteotomy can also be used to assist in the extraction of a well-fixed tibial stem or to realign the extensor mechanism if necessary. A longer osteotomy can be performed if a tibial stem is well fixed distally.

An anterior midline incision is made that extends 8 to 10 cm below the tibial tubercle. The medial parapatellar arthrotomy extends from 6 cm above the patella and distally along the tibial tubercle and anterior tibial crest (Fig. 149.9). Whiteside and

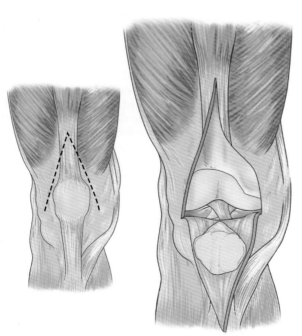

FIG 149.6 Coonse-Adams quadriceps turndown. (Redrawn from Scott WN: *The knee,* vol 1, St Louis, 1994, Mosby-Year Book, p 66.)

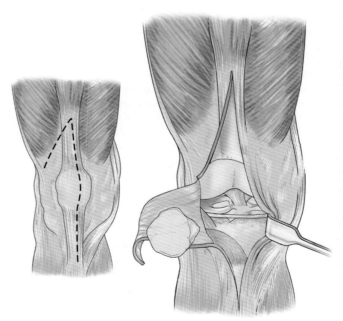

FIG 149.7 Modified Coonse-Adams quadriceps turndown. (Redrawn from Scott WN: *The knee,* vol 1, St Louis, 1994, Mosby-Year Book, p 66.)

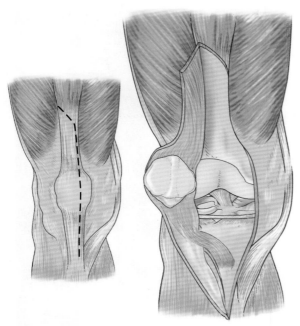

FIG 149.8 Insall's quadriceps snip. (Redrawn from Scott WN: *The knee,* vol 1, St Louis, 1994, Mosby-Year Book, p 67.)

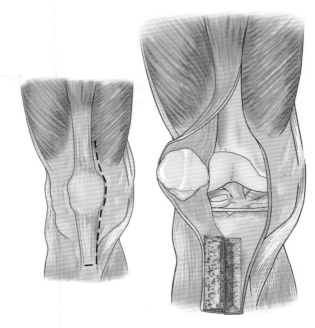

FIG 149.9 Anterior approach to the knee with osteotomy of the tibial tubercle. (Redrawn from Scott WN: *The knee,* vol 1, St Louis, 1994, Mosby-Year Book, p 67.)

Ohl[67] used this exposure for difficult TKA, and they recommended using an oscillating saw to transect the tibial crest 8 to 10 cm below the tibial tubercle while elevating the tibial crest from the tibia. The lateral periosteum and musculature structures are left attached, as is the lateral aspect of the quadriceps mechanism. Fernandez[18] recommended tibial tubercle osteotomy for bicondylar tibial fractures. He used a straight anterolateral parapatellar incision. Large medial and lateral subcutaneous flaps are developed. The lateral musculature must be elevated and protected. The osteotomy of the tibial tubercle is performed with an oscillating saw and osteotomes. The osteotomy must be beveled anteriorly proximally to avoid a fracture propagating to the joint line. The osteotomy is trapezoidal, 5 to 8 cm long, 2 cm wide proximally, and 1.5 cm wide distally. Once the tibial tubercle and the anterior tibial crest are freed, the entire extensor mechanism is elevated laterally, and the retropatellar fat pad is divided to expose the entire joint. The osteotomy is usually fixed with fully threaded screws or cerclage wires. The major risk of this approach is nonunion of the tibial tubercle, which can be a devastating result. If a tibial tubercle osteotomy is performed, the postoperative rehabilitation protocol must be modified to include a period of partial weight bearing.

Minimally Invasive Surgery Total Knee Arthroplasty

TKA has been performed for decades by using a traditional extensile approach. Historically, surgical exposure was achieved through an 8- to 10-inch skin incision and a long medial parapatellar arthrotomy, although some authors used a midvastus[17] or a subvastus approach.[24] This was followed by extensive soft tissue dissection and eversion of the patella. With improvement in the techniques of ligament balancing, adjustments in the overall alignment, and flexion-extension gap equalization techniques, good to excellent clinical outcomes have been reported in long-term follow-up studies for TKA completed using an extensile approach.*

The introduction of MIS for unicondylar knee replacement[52,54] encouraged interest in applying a similar approach to standard TKA. Various MIS approaches, including limited medial parapatellar, limited midvastus, limited subvastus, and quadriceps-sparing approach, are considered a continuum of traditional extensile approaches. The surgeon can shorten the skin incision as he or she becomes more familiar with the surgical technique, progressing along on the scale of complexity, and finally can become competent in performing quadriceps-sparing MIS TKA. The MIS approach can be easily converted to a traditional approach if required. Potential benefits of less invasive surgery include reduced blood loss, reduced pain, less morbidity, and faster recovery.[38,58,62] The primary objective in MIS TKA is to limit surgical dissection without compromising component position, ligament balancing, or overall limb alignment. Although some studies show improved early outcomes with no increase in complications with MIS techniques, in their John Insall Award–winning article, Wegrzyn and colleagues[66] showed no benefits of MIS TKA on gait or strength outcomes. Modification of TKA instrumentation, including the addition of robotic assistance, which has been shown in some studies to improve the precision of component positioning, has facilitated the procedure, but appropriate patient selection remains critical for a successful outcome.[33] The ideal candidate for MIS TKA is a patient of small to average stature with minimal deformity and good preoperative motion. Our patient selection preference has evolved to include patients with less than 15-degree varus, 20-degree valgus, or 10-degree flexion contracture, with a minimum of 90-degree range of motion. Scuderi[58] and

---

*References 12, 28-30, 41, 49, 53, 57, and 61.

Tenholder and colleagues[62] reported that short, thin women with low body mass index and narrow femurs are good candidates for this approach. Muscular men with prominent vastus medialis and wider femurs often are better served by a more traditional approach. Patients with a compromised soft tissue envelope or a short patellar tendon and patients with severe deformities requiring extensive release should undergo a standard approach to avoid excessive soft tissue tension and wound healing difficulties. Moreover, patients with diabetes mellitus, rheumatoid arthritis, or inflammatory arthritis, and patients who are obese tend to be less favorable candidates for MIS TKA.[62]

Limited Medial Parapatellar Arthrotomy

A limited parapatellar approach is useful in most cases because it involves little deviation from the traditional approach. This approach is popular because of its familiarity, simplicity, and excellent exposure of all three compartments of the knee. Additionally, it can be easily extended if a more extensile exposure is required, with little risk of skin or patellar tendon complications. This approach has four characteristic features: a small skin incision, a limited medial parapatellar arthrotomy, the use of a mobile window, and patellar subluxation instead of eversion.

A straight anterior midline skin incision of approximately 10 to 14 cm in length is made, extending from the superior pole of the patella to the tibial tubercle. Limited medial and lateral full-thickness flaps are created to expose the extensor mechanism. Release of the deep fascia proximally beneath the skin aids mobilization of the skin throughout the procedure. Because of the elasticity of the skin, the skin incision usually stretches by 2 to 4 cm with knee flexion; this can be used to permit broader exposure. The planned arthrotomy path and the fat pad can be injected with 30 mL 1% lidocaine with epinephrine. This has been shown to reduce perioperative blood loss when combined with an MIS technique.[16]

The limited parapatellar arthrotomy is performed extending 2 to 4 cm into the quadriceps tendon proximal to the superior pole of patella, then curving around the medial border of the patella or straight over the medial aspect of the patella, and extending distally along the medial border of the patellar tendon (Fig. 149.10). The deep medial collateral ligament, the posteromedial capsule, and the semimembranosus tendon are elevated subperiosteally from the proximal tibia. The knee is flexed, and the patella is subluxated laterally. The arthrotomy can be gradually extended proximally if difficulty is encountered in displacing the patella laterally. The supporting soft tissues are protected by careful placement of the retractors. The mobile window created by arthrotomy can be moved from medial to lateral and from superior to inferior as necessary to enable optimal exposure of the joint without application of undue pressure on the skin or the capsular tissues. It is recommended to extend the skin incision by 1 to 2 cm proximally or distally if excessive stretching of soft tissues is done to gain exposure without compromising wound healing. Skin under appropriate tension takes the shape of the letter "V" at the proximal and distal pole of the incision, whereas skin under excessive tension takes the shape of the letter "U."

Bone resection can be performed according to surgeon preference. We recommend cutting the tibia first because this enlarges the soft tissue envelope of the knee in flexion and extension, which provides better visualization of the knee (Fig.

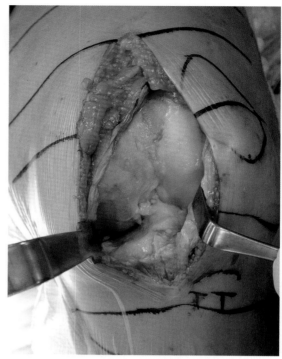

FIG 149.10 Limited medial parapatellar arthrotomy (minimally invasive surgery total knee arthroplasty).

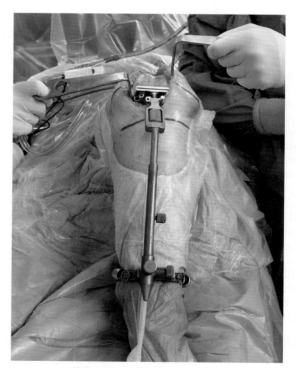

FIG 149.11 Tibial resection.

149.11). Modified instrumentation, including alignment guides and cutting blocks, is used. Their altered geometry facilitates placement within a smaller soft tissue envelope. The mobile window is moved medially and laterally during resection of the medial and lateral aspects of the tibia, respectively. The bone is

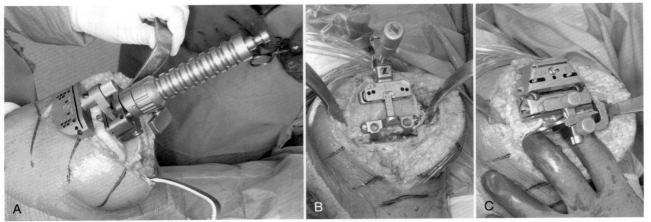

FIG 149.12 (A) Distal femoral cutting guide. (B) Femoral sizing guide. (C) Femoral cutting block.

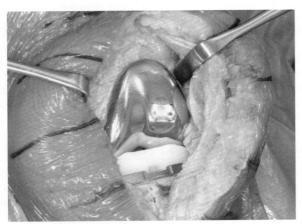

FIG 149.13 Final components implanted through a limited medial arthrotomy.

removed after the roots of the medial and lateral menisci and the anterior and possibly posterior cruciate ligaments have been cut, depending on the implant design. The resected tibial bone is externally rotated as the soft tissues are released.

Attention is then directed toward the femur where a limited amount of synovial tissue and fat is resected from the anterior cortex. (Fig. 149.12A). After the bone has been removed from the femur, the size and rotation of the femoral component are determined with a guide (Fig. 149.12B and C). Although some authors showed higher failure rates, Yoo and coworkers[68] described the use of a mini-keel tibial component to facilitate MIS approaches and showed high survival rates and excellent clinical and radiographic results. Finally, the patella is prepared in a standard fashion.

The additional laxity and space in the knee joint cavity after tibial and distal femoral resections allow patellar preparation with minimal disruption of the extensor mechanism. With the knee in extension or slight flexion, the patella is everted and resected to the appropriate depth. After the cement has hardened, the final tibial polyethylene component is inserted (Fig. 149.13). The arthrotomy is closed with or without a suction drain with figure-of-eight absorbable polyglactin 910 (Vicryl) sutures. The sutures in the arthrotomy are placed in a slightly oblique fashion to use the vector pull of the vastus medialis

muscle. The subcutaneous layer and the skin are closed in a routine manner.

Ample evidence indicates that MIS TKA is associated with decreased blood loss, leading to reduced transfusion requirements and improved postoperative motion.[38,58,62] The MIS approach reduces the average length of incision by approximately 50% to an average length of 10 to 14 cm without adversely affecting the clinical outcome.[13] Tenholder and colleagues[62] reported a consecutive series of 118 TKAs that included 69 patients with reconstruction using an MIS approach and 49 patients with reconstruction using a conventional approach. Better knee flexion and lower transfusion rates were observed in the MIS group. No differences in radiographic alignment and complication rates were noted between the two groups.

Han and coworkers[22] prospectively followed 30 patients undergoing simultaneous bilateral TKA. Patients were randomly assigned to an MIS group (mini–medial parapatellar approach) or a conventional group. Functional recovery was faster in the MIS group for rehabilitation milestones such as walking without assistance and for improvement in range of motion. Bonutti and associates[5] reviewed clinical outcomes of 25 staged bilateral TKAs (50 knees) in which conventional TKA was performed on one knee, and MIS TKA was later performed on the contralateral side. Knee flexion and Knee Society objective scores were significantly greater in the MIS group. Quadriceps muscle strength was statistically better in the MIS group at 12 weeks and at 1 year postoperatively, as demonstrated by isokinetic testing. No difference in alignment was noted on radiographic analysis between the two approaches. Similar to any other surgical procedure, a learning curve is associated with MIS TKA. King and colleagues[34] quantified the number of surgeries required to become proficient in MIS TKA. They noted that the learning curve for MIS TKA was approximately 50 TKA procedures in the hands of high-volume arthroplasty surgeons, making this procedure a less desirable option for low-volume surgeons.

LIMITED SUBVASTUS APPROACH

The limited subvastus approach takes advantage of the natural planes of dissection and minimizes patellofemoral instability by avoiding disruption of the extensor mechanism. The vastus medialis obliquus (VMO) inserts at a 50-degree angle relative to the long axis of the femur and extends to the midpole of the patella on the medial side.[45] It is imperative to clearly identify the inferior border of the VMO to preserve the entire quadriceps.

The arthrotomy is made along the inferior edge of the VMO down to the midpole of the patella. The arthrotomy is then extended straight distally along the medial border of the patella and the patellar tendon (Fig. 149.14). The VMO tendon and the patella are retracted laterally with a right-angled Hohmann retractor placed in the lateral gutter. The knee is flexed to 90 degrees, providing good exposure of both distal femoral condyles. The TKA is performed in a similar fashion, as described earlier for limited medial parapatellar arthrotomy. Closure begins by reapproximating the corner of the capsular flap to the extensor mechanism at the midpole of the patella. Interrupted sutures are placed along the proximal limb of the arthrotomy. Care is taken to place the sutures through the fibrous tissue or the synovium attached to the distal surface or the undersurface of the VMO. Then the distal or vertical limb of the arthrotomy is closed with multiple interrupted sutures.

The indications for the MIS subvastus approach are similar to indications for other MIS approaches.[44] In addition, patients with patella baja and poor patellar mobility are poor candidates for the subvastus approach because of difficulty in translating the patella laterally. When this approach is performed, care must be taken while working in the subvastus region adjacent to the adductor tubercle because it contains the descending genicular artery and its branches, the intermuscular septal arteries, and the saphenous nerve.

In a prospective randomized study, Roysam and Oakley[55] compared 46 MIS subvastus TKAs with 43 TKAs performed through a traditional medial parapatellar approach. Clinical assessment revealed significantly earlier return of straight-leg raising (3.2 days vs 5.8 days; $P < .001$), lower consumption of narcotics in the first week (78 mg vs 102 mg; $P < .001$), less blood loss (527 mL vs 748 mL; $P < .001$), and greater knee

flexion at 1 week (78 degrees vs 55 degrees; $P < .001$) in group II (subvastus approach). In another study, Varela-Egocheaga and associates[64] compared MIS subvastus TKA with conventional TKA performed by the parapatellar approach. They noted superior Knee Society scores and range of motion at a minimum follow-up of 36 months in the MIS group. Functional recovery has been observed to be faster after a subvastus approach than after a medial parapatellar approach, as measured by isometric and isokinetic muscle strength.[9,56] Chang and colleagues[9] noted greater peak torque in quadriceps strength at 6 months postoperatively and earlier normalization of hamstrings to quadriceps peak torque ratio after a subvastus approach compared with a medial parapatellar approach. In a matched retrospective analysis of 120 patients, the mini-subvastus approach was associated with prolonged tourniquet time (average 15 min) and two intraoperative complications. It was thought to be technically more challenging than a standard medial parapatellar approach. However, the mini-subvastus approach was associated with less blood loss, less postoperative pain, faster straight-leg raising, and better knee flexion. All patients, including patients with complications, had good limb alignment and implant positioning.[4] In a randomized study, Aglietti and coworkers[2] noted earlier straight-leg raising and better knee flexion at 10 days and 30 days postoperatively with a mini-subvastus approach compared with a quadriceps-sparing technique. No difference in knee flexion was observed at 3 months of follow-up.

LIMITED MIDVASTUS APPROACH

Following an anterior midline skin incision, a medial arthrotomy is performed beginning at the superior pole of the patella to the tibial tubercle distally. The VMO is identified, and an oblique 2- to 4-cm split is made in line with the fibers at the level of the superior pole of the patella (Fig. 149.15). Sharp proximal dissection should be avoided because this can lead to VMO

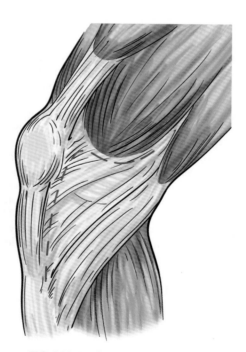

FIG 149.14 Subvastus approach.

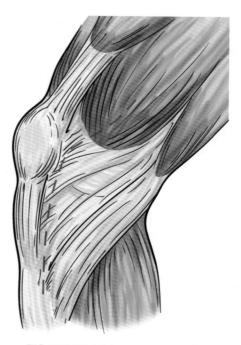

FIG 149.15 Midvastus approach.

denervation.[15] The patella is subluxated laterally as the knee is brought into flexion. The fascia and the muscle fibers tend to split further as the knee is flexed upward; this has no adverse effect on outcome.

Exclusion criteria for the limited midvastus approach are similar to exclusion criteria for limited parapatellar arthrotomy. The midvastus approach preserves vascularity. Additionally, some reports have described improved patellar tracking.[39] Reported benefits of the limited midvastus approach include decreased postoperative pain, better quadriceps function, decreased blood loss, and shorter hospital stay.[19,20,39] Laskin and colleagues[39] compared 32 MIS midvastus TKAs with 26 TKAs done through a standard medial parapatellar approach. Improvements in knee scores were statistically greater in the MIS group at 6 weeks postoperatively. Additionally, the average visual analog scale (VAS) pain score and the total amount of pain medication required were lower in the MIS group. Radiographic alignment and implant positioning were equally accurate in the two groups. Similar encouraging clinical outcomes were noted in a retrospective analysis of 335 consecutive patients (391 TKAs). Range of motion was 111 degrees at 6 weeks, 121 degrees at 3 months, and 125 degrees at 1 year and 2 years. Postoperative knee scores were greater than 95 in all patients. No increase in the complication rate was noted with this approach.[20] Karachalios and coworkers[31] reported superior Oxford Knee Scores and knee function scores after MIS midvastus TKA compared with conventional TKA up to 9 months postoperatively. Patients in the MIS group had greater early knee flexion ($P = .04$) postoperatively compared with the conventional group.[30,31]

QUADRICEPS-SPARING SURGICAL APPROACH

In the quadriceps-sparing surgical approach, a curvilinear medial skin incision is made in a varus knee, extending from the superior pole of the patella to the tibial joint line (Fig. 149.16). The arthrotomy is made in line with the skin incision and may extend beneath the vastus medialis to improve exposure of the medial femoral condyle (Fig. 149.17). In the valgus knee, the incision can be made along the lateral aspect of the patella to the tibial joint line (Fig. 149.18). A vertical lateral parapatellar arthrotomy is performed, and the iliotibial band is dissected from the tibial joint line in an anteroposterior direction (Fig. 149.19). After satisfactory exposure is achieved, the patella is resected using a free-hand technique to assist with

exposure (Fig. 149.20). The patellar preparation can be completed at this stage.

Specialized instrumentation customized for side cutting is required for execution of this approach. These instruments can be used to cut in a medial-to-lateral direction, which allows incisions 6 to 10 cm in length. Moreover, these instruments can be used with a limited parapatellar, mini-midvastus, or mini-subvastus approach. Knee position must be varied between 30 degrees and 80 degrees of flexion during the procedure. The patella is subluxated laterally for implantation of the components (Figs. 149.21 through 149.28).

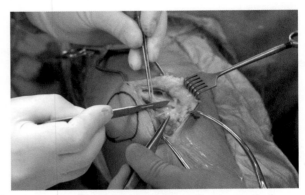

FIG 149.17 Surgical knife blade dissection beneath the vastus medialis.

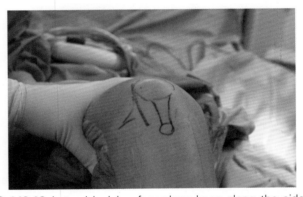

FIG 149.18 Lateral incision for valgus knee along the side of the patella to the tibial joint line.

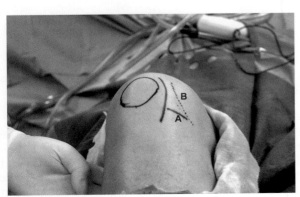

FIG 149.16 Medial incision in a varus knee. Line *A* represents the tibiofemoral joint line, and *B* outlines the margin of the medial femoral condyle.

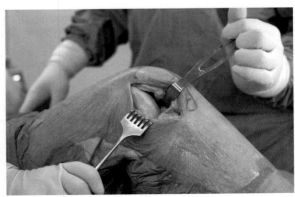

FIG 149.19 The iliotibial band is sharply elevated from the lateral aspect of the patella.

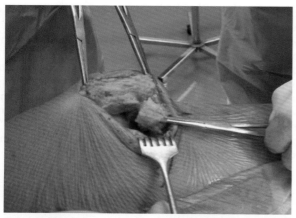

FIG 149.20 The fad pad is excised and the patellar surface is resected with a free-hand oscillating saw.

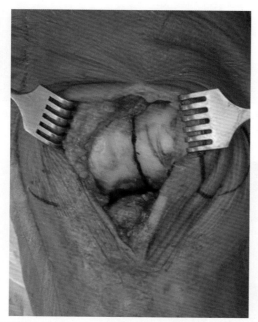

FIG 149.21 The anteroposterior axis (Whiteside line) is drawn along the uncut femoral surface.

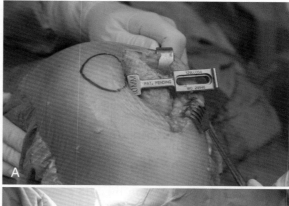

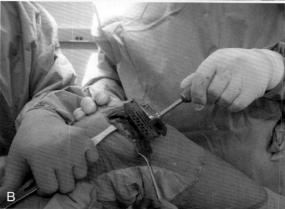

FIG 149.22 (A) The intramedullary (IM) guide rests on the medial femoral condyle. (B) The cutting block is attached to the IM guide, and distal femoral resection is performed from the medial side.

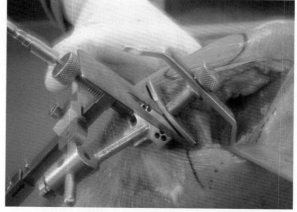

FIG 149.23 Extramedullary cutting guide with depth gauge sets the cutting block for proximal tibial resection.

Although the potential benefits of MIS TKA are realized with the quadriceps-sparing MIS approach using side-cutting instrumentation, this technique has been associated with relatively more complications compared with the other three MIS approaches.[11] Huang and associates[25] reported on 2-year follow-up of quadriceps-sparing MIS TKA. The quadriceps-sparing MIS group had significantly faster recovery of quadriceps strength and knee flexion and had less pain during the first 2 postoperative weeks compared with the traditional group. However, nine radiographic outliers were identified in the MIS group, and no radiographic outliers were identified in the standard group. Similarly, in a randomized study, Martin and colleagues[42] compared MIS TKA using side-cutting implant instrumentation and standard anteroposterior mini-incision instrumentation. In each cohort, 50% of TKAs were performed with computer-assisted navigation. Investigators found greater accuracy for limb and component alignment with standard mini-incision instrumentation compared with quadriceps-sparing side-cutting instrumentation. The navigation technique could not compensate for shortcomings of the side-cutting instrumentation. In another study, Lin and coworkers[40] noted a greater number of outliers for tibial and femoral component alignment in the quadriceps-sparing MIS TKA group compared with the MIS medial parapatellar TKA group. However, no differences in short-term isokinetic peak muscle torque,

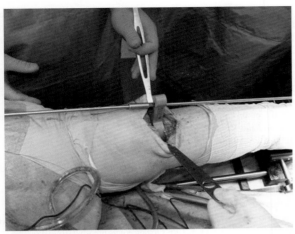

FIG 149.24 Extension space measured with a spacer block and an extramedullary rod.

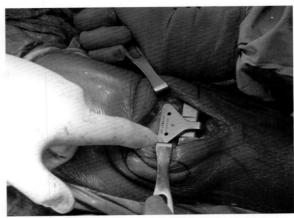

FIG 149.27 The femoral finishing block is attached to the plate that references the anterior femoral cut and is positioned in a medial-lateral direction in full extension.

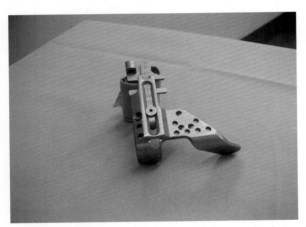

FIG 149.25 The femoral tower has two foot pads that reference the posterior aspect of the femoral condyles.

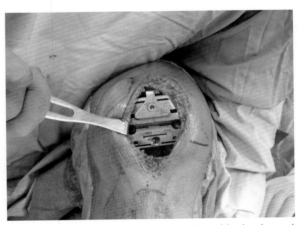

FIG 149.28 Femoral finishing cuts made with the knee in 90 degrees of flexion.

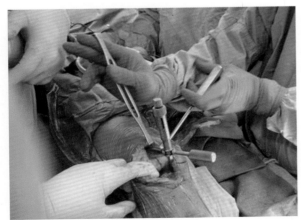

FIG 149.26 The probe identifies the size of the femur and the location of the anterior surface cut.

postoperative pain, and functional outcomes were noted between the two approaches.

CONCLUSION

MIS TKA is not defined by the length of the incision or by the cosmetic result. True MIS TKA is defined by limited violation of anatomic structures around the knee. The goal of MIS TKA is to reduce postoperative pain and promote faster recovery. To be successful, MIS TKA must not compromise surgical technique, accurate limb alignment, component positioning, soft tissue balancing, or longevity of the reconstruction. Appropriate patient selection as outlined previously is critical for the successful and safe execution of these approaches. The optimal MIS technique is expandable or can be extended for situations in which the surgeon encounters difficulty and requires additional exposure. Extension of the arthrotomy into the quadriceps tendon and the vastus medialis produces variations of the quadriceps-sparing approach and can be considered part of the continuum of MIS TKA surgery. The best way to become adept with less invasive TKA exposures is to start by using MIS instrumentation during traditional TKA and gradually progressing to a mini-incision approach with increasing surgical experience.

KEY REFERENCES

1. Abbott LC, Carpenter WF: Surgical approaches to the knee joint. *J Bone Joint Surg Am* 27:277, 1945.

6. Bramlett KW: *The trivector arthrotomy approach,* AAOS Instructional Videotape, Rosemont, IL, 1994, American Academy of Orthopaedic Surgeons.

11. Chen AF, et al: Quadriceps sparing total knee replacement: the initial experience with results at two to four years. *J Bone Joint Surg Br* 88:1448–1453, 2006.

12. Colizza WA, et al: The posterior stabilized total knee prosthesis: assessment of polyethylene damage and osteolysis after a ten-year-minimum follow-up. *J Bone Joint Surg Am* 77:1713–1720, 1995.

14. Coonse KD, Adams JD: A new operative approach to the knee joint. *Surg Gynecol Obstet* 77:344, 1943.

17. Engh GA, et al: A midvastus muscle-splitting approach for total knee arthroplasty. *J Arthroplasty* 12:322–331, 1997.

20. Haas SB, et al: Minimally invasive total knee arthroplasty: the mini midvastus approach. *Clin Orthop Relat Res* 452:112–116, 2006.

23. Henry AK: *Extensile exposure,* ed 2, Baltimore, 1970, Williams & Wilkins.

24. Hofmann AA, et al: Subvastus (Southern) approach for primary total knee arthroplasty. *Clin Orthop Relat Res* 269:70–77, 1991.

26. Insall J: A midline approach to the knee. *J Bone Joint Surg Am* 53:1584, 1971.

27. Insall JN, editor: *Surgery of the knee,* New York, 1984, Churchill Livingstone, pp 41–54.

28. Insall J, et al: Total condylar knee replacement: preliminary report. *Clin Orthop Relat Res* 120:149–154, 1976.

29. Insall J, et al: The total condylar knee prosthesis: the first 5 years. *Clin Orthop Relat Res* 145:68–77, 1979.

32. Keblish PA: Valgus deformity in total knee arthroplasty: the lateral retinacular approach. *Orthop Trans* 9:28, 1985.

35. Kocher T: *Textbook of operative surgery,* Stiles HJ, Paul CB (trans), ed 3, London, 1911, Adam & Charles Black.

43. Mullen M: The subvastus approach for total knee arthroplasty. *Tech Orthop* 6:64, 1991.

45. Pagnano MW, et al: Anatomy of the extensor mechanism in reference to quadriceps-sparing TKA. *Clin Orthop Relat Res* 452:102–105, 2006.

58. Scuderi GR: Minimally invasive total knee arthroplasty with limited medial parapatellar arthrotomy. *Oper Tech Orthop* 16:145–152, 2006.

61. Stern SH, Insall JN: Posterior stabilized prosthesis: results after follow-up of nine to twelve years. *J Bone Joint Surg Am* 74:980–986, 1992.

62. Tenholder M, et al: Minimal-incision total knee arthroplasty: the early clinical experience. *Clin Orthop Relat Res* 440:67–76, 2005.

67. Whiteside LA, Ohl MD: Tibial tubercle osteotomy for exposure of the difficult total knee arthroplasty. *Clin Orthop Relat Res* 206:6–9, 1990.

The references for this chapter can also be found on www.expertconsult.com.

150

Surgical Techniques and Instrumentation in Total Knee Arthroplasty

Thomas Parker Vail, Jason E. Lang

In this updated chapter, we are reminded of the vision, clarity of thought, and enduring concepts that are attributable to John Insall. In the years since he personally authored the original version of this foundational chapter, many new concepts have emerged. However, as the reader will discover, there is very little in our latest understanding of knee surgery that does not have roots that trace to John Insall. Thus, with eternal respect and gratitude to Dr. Insall, Jason Lang and I dedicate the 6th edition of this chapter on surgical techniques and instrumentation.

RELEVANT KNEE ANATOMY AND ALIGNMENT

Medicine is moving simultaneously toward less variability in care and personalization of care. Personalized medicine extends to total knee replacement from the standpoint of using accepted techniques to create an appropriately balanced and sized knee arthroplasty that functions in concert with each patient's own anatomy and knee mechanics. The latest techniques and implant designs create some separation from prior iterations, with emphasis on nuances of limb alignment, ligamentous support, and skeletal anatomy. In addition, limb alignment is increasingly set into the larger context of the interplay between the knee, hip, and ankle joints. To understand these nuances, it is important to examine a patient in three positions: weightless, standing, and when walking. The weightless exam, either with the patient seated or supine, allows a careful assessment of ligament competence, range of motion, passive patellar tracking, and the anatomic origin of pain. When the patient is standing, one can assess the overall axial alignment of the leg, the angle of the joint line in dual stance, and the static position of the patella. Walking the patient allows one to add a dynamic component to the exam, observing the presence of antalgic movement, pathologic patella movement, soft tissue impingement, and varus or valgus thrust during active single-leg stance. There increased recognition of the considerable variation in body habitus, natural femoral anteversion, foot and ankle alignment, and patterns of gait, resulting in less emphasis on what is "normal"[73,98] and more emphasis on what is the best reconstruction for the individual patient with anatomic uniqueness being considered.

Static Alignment

The mechanical axis of the leg (Fig. 150.1) is formed by a line that passes from the center of the hip through the center of the knee into the center of the ankle joint. The offset of the hip joint contributes to the definition of the limb alignment and is measured by the distance between the femoral shaft axis and the center of rotation of the hip. The offset is in turn determined by the angle of the femoral neck, the length of the neck, and the distance to the shaft of the femur. A valgus angle of 5 to 9 degrees between the femoral and tibial shafts allows the transverse axis of the knee joint to be perpendicular to the midline vertical axis of the body during stance. Because the proximal-to-distal mechanical axis forms an angle of 3 degrees with the midline vertical axis of the body, there typically exists a 3-degree angle between the knee joint line and the axis of the tibial shaft and a 10-degree angle between the joint line axis and the axis of the femoral shaft. Hungerford and Krackow[96] and Townley[209] have pointed out that the "normal" angle of proximal tibial varus is variable because of inherited and developmental anatomic factors, such as pelvic width, femoral neck varus, femoral and tibial bowing, physeal growth, and femoral length. Because the mechanical axis passes through the medial compartment and the transverse knee joint axis is in slight varus, the distribution of body weight when standing is more medial than lateral in most knees.[94,101,148,209] The debate as to the best position of tibial and femoral total knee components relative to the mechanical axis remains unresolved, with disparate perspectives based upon anatomic, kinematic, and gap balancing considerations.

Dynamic Alignment

During normal walking, the supporting leg moves toward the body center of gravity in the swing phase of gait. The distribution of contact forces across the knee joint in stance is not symmetric; it is estimated that between 60% and 75% of the knee joint contact forces are carried by the medial compartment of the knee due to the femoral anatomy that causes the mechanical axis to pass through the medial compartment of the knee.[63,78,110] In addition, a greater medial load can be explained by the laterally directed ground reaction force.[78] Another important anatomic feature that is relevant to the resultant mechanical loading of the knee joint is the 2 to 10 degrees posterior and distal slope of the tibial plateau. However, when the menisci are taken into account, the cartilaginous articulation is not posteriorly sloped; only the bony surfaces give the appearance of posterior slope. Furthermore, the medial tibial subchondral bone is concave ("dished") relative to the more convex lateral tibial subchondral surface. Combined with the 3-degree angle of the tibial anatomic axis relative to the transverse knee axis, a varus moment is imparted during normal gait. This varus moment creates a lateral "thrust" to varying degrees from person to person, which is resisted by the lateral stabilizing force arising from the lateral capsule, lateral collateral ligament (LCL), cruciate ligaments, ligamentum patellae, popliteus, posterior oblique ligament, and iliotibial band (ITB).[98]

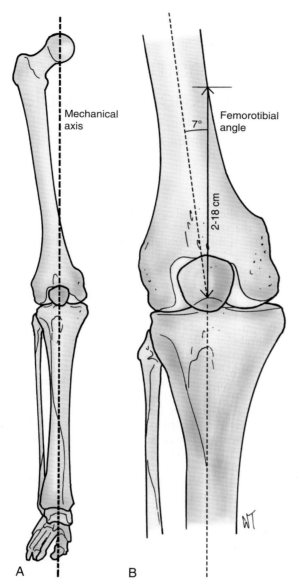

FIG 150.1 The mechanical axis (A) usually corresponds to a femorotibial angle of approximately 7 degrees (B), and the mechanical axis intersects the medial femoral cortex 12 to 18 cm proximal to the knee.

Abnormal patterns of gait because of alignment or other factors can change the resultant loading of the knee joint. For example, muscle imbalance caused by deconditioning or obesity can accentuate a varus thrust during the stance phase of gait. Gait studies performed on obese patients and patients with high degrees of varus thrust have demonstrated locomotor adaptations, such as slower speed, shorter steps, external rotation, increased double support time, and decreased knee range of motion. In addition, Sharma et al.[194] reported on a correlation between body mass index (BMI) and osteoarthritis (OA) severity in knees with varus malalignment that was not seen in knees with valgus malalignment. Compensatory external rotation of the foot is a mechanism of unloading a painful medial compartment during stance. An extension moment moving the center of gravity anterior to the knee joint is a

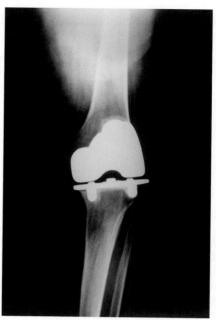

FIG 150.2 Radiograph of a prosthesis with a varus tibial cut. The instrument system designed for this prosthesis recommended a 3-degree tibial cut because this slope more closely duplicates normal anatomy. In practice, it often led to a greater and undesirable sloping cut to the tibia.

compensatory mechanism for quadriceps weakness that eventually can lead to laxity in the posterior capsule and posterior cruciate ligament (PCL).

OBJECTIVES OF PROSTHETIC REPLACEMENT

Insall held the opinion that the objective of prosthetic replacement is to distribute contact stresses across the artificial joint symmetrically, avoiding overloading of one compartment. Debate continues as to how correction of deformity and optimal loading of the knee joint is achieved with respect to an individual's prearthritic and postarthritic anatomy. For example, it is likely that many patients who develop medial compartment arthritis in the absence of acute injury have walked with some degree of a varus thrust since childhood, some have tibia vara, and others have more or less obliquity of the joint line. Restoration of the prearthritic alignment, although "normal" for high adductor moment individuals, could result in a component position that is in varus relative to the mechanical axis. Varus angulation of the joint line can create higher medial compartment loads, which may be detrimental to long-term implant fixation (Fig. 150.2). However, the counter to that concern is that small amounts of varus position could facilitate better balance of the knee and a more conservative bone resection. Thus the debate about what is "best" continues unresolved.

Although debate may continue about the nuances of the optimal implant alignment, the most important end result of surgical technique is to achieve the desired implant position with the smallest amount of variability away from the planned goal (Fig. 150.3). The surgical workflow can be carried out using standard instruments, computer navigation, or custom-fitted cutting blocks. However, to date, there is no conclusive evidence to support the superiority of navigation or custom blocks over

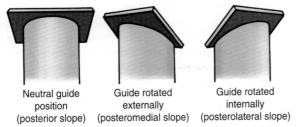

Neutral guide position (posterior slope) Guide rotated externally (posteromedial slope) Guide rotated internally (posterolateral slope)

FIG 150.3 Care must be taken when making a 10-degree posterior slope on the tibial cut. The guide must be placed in the neutral position. When it is externally rotated, a posteromedial slope (varus) will be produced. When the guide is internally rotated, a posterolateral slope (valgus) will result.

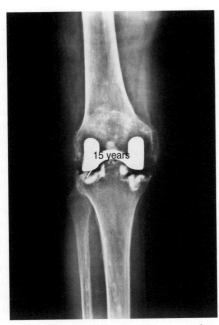

FIG 150.4 Radiograph of a 15-year follow-up of a duocondylar prosthesis with two separate tibial components. Osteopenia is apparent around the femoral component runners. The knee continued to function well.

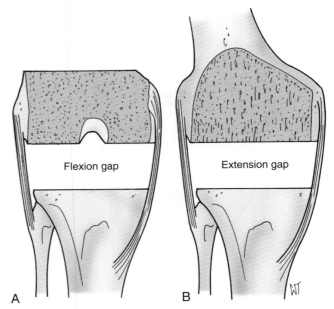

Flexion gap   Extension gap

A   B

FIG 150.5 The flexion gap (A) must exactly equal the extension gap (B).

standard techniques and instruments. Insall believed that restoration of "normal" anatomy was not often achieved, and perhaps was not of paramount importance to success of a prosthetic knee replacement. Reflection on the reality of early total knee replacement surgery reveals that early models of knee prostheses were often mismatched in size, because of a limited inventory of sizes, and incompatible with ligamentous structures, suggesting that some compromises had to be accepted in the early days. Nevertheless, a surprising number of knee replacements from the 1970s and 1980s functioned for many years (Fig. 150.4). As clinical experience increased, surgical expertise improved, instruments improved, and prosthetic design came to more closely resemble natural knee articular contours. Along with the improvement of surgical process and the expansion of indications to more active patients, patient expectations have risen. Patients report a desire to achieve normality of feel and a high level of function. Yet, despite tremendous success in restoring function and relieving human suffering, total knee replacement is not universally successful in restoring original knee function or universal patient satisfaction as measured by patient-reported outcome.[110a]

THEORIES OF SURGICAL TECHNIQUE

The evolution of knee implants and instruments led to two distinct surgical techniques or "workflows" during the development of knee arthroplasty: the gap balancing technique and the measured resection technique.[53] Over time, instrument systems and surgical techniques have adopted aspects of both philosophies, blurring the distinctions in technique but placing emphasis on achieving optimized knee kinematics, balance, and alignment.

Gap Balancing Technique

The gap balancing technique[73,98,100] focuses upon achieving a balanced flexion and extension gap. The workflow consists of performing the proximal tibial and distal femoral cut first, thereby establishing the extension gap. The next step immediately following these bone cuts is balancing the medial and lateral ligaments in extension. Ligament releases (see later discussion) are performed to correct fixed deformity, bringing the limb into approximate alignment before the final femoral bone cuts are made (Fig. 150.5). After the desired alignment is achieved in extension, the knee is flexed and the soft tissue envelope and tibial cut are used to set the femoral component size, rotation, and translation. One important goal of the gap balancing technique is to create a rectangular flexion gap (Fig. 150.6) by creating the appropriate rotational position of the femoral component. In the gap balancing workflow, the rotational position of the femoral component is created by referencing the cut tibial plateau and tensioning the balanced collateral ligaments. Implant systems currently offer a wide array of component sizes and polyethylene thicknesses that allow the surgeon to more accurately match the femoral component dimensions with the relevant bone anatomy in the coronal and sagittal planes.

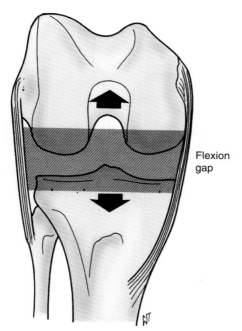

FIG 150.6 The flexion gap is created first by removing bone from the tibial plateaus and the posterior femoral condyles.

Flexion gap

In practice, one can create either the extension space or the flexion space first and then match the space remaining with the known thickness of the first space created. Insall would traditionally perform the tibial cut first, measure the flexion gap before cutting the femur, and then make the distal femoral cut at a point such that the extension gap would match the flexion gap. Insall would then proceed to balance the flexion gap by positioning the anteroposterior (AP) femoral cutting block on the distal femur set in rotation parallel to the tibial cut surface, often in line with the transepicondylar axis (TEA). The criticism that some have leveled at this sequence is that there is risk of elevating the joint line (thereby decreasing flexion) if matching the flexion gap requires cutting the distal femur above the material thickness of the femoral component. Because the distal femoral cut establishes the distal femoral joint line, which is especially important for stability in extension and patellar tracking, many surgeons prefer to establish the extension space first. If one establishes the extension space first, it is possible to prioritize the preservation of distal femoral bone and thereby minimize the risk of over-resection of the distal femur, which would cause elevation of the joint line. In addition, multiple variables, such as the size of the femoral component, translation of the femoral component, and thickness of the polyethylene articulation surface, can be manipulated to properly fill the flexion gap after the extension gap is established. The gap balancing method ensures soft tissue balance and correct tensioning in full extension and at 90 degrees of flexion, but midrange laxity may occur when a tight posterior capsule is not corrected. When the posterior contracture is not addressed, the extension gap balance is hinged upon the posterior capsule rather than the collateral ligaments. Thus the collateral ligaments are not balanced throughout the range of motion, particularly in midflexion. Patients with midflexion laxity may report a loose knee or lack of confidence when descending stairs or walking on inclines.

Measured Resection Technique

The second theory of surgical technique, the measured resection theory, begins with the philosophy of maintaining joint line position. This theory is predicated on the observation that a properly positioned joint line is essential to proper collateral ligament and cruciate ligament function and consequently posterior cruciate retention.[139] Hungerford and Krackow developed the method of measured resection. This technique has been used in conjunction with principles of anatomic alignment, as well as the neutral tibial cut.[19,96]

The bone cuts in the measured resection technique are created using the same instruments as one would use in the gap balance workflow, but the order of cuts is different. In addition, ligament balancing is complete after all of the bone cuts are made, rather than after the extension cuts are made. Thus the essential workflow in measured resection is as follows: distal femoral cut, femoral sizing, femoral anterior and posterior and chamfer cuts, proximal tibial cut, and ligament balancing. The patella can be prepared or not, either before or after the tibiofemoral cuts.

The bone cuts in measured resection are made largely by referencing the bone surface anatomy and by cutting away the exact amount of bone that will be replaced by the components. Thus the distal femur is generally cut at 9 to 10 mm above the distal femoral joint line, with referencing that accommodates for any bone loss so as not to over-resect. Most implants are 9 to 10 mm in thickness distally, and there is a small accommodation of the bone resection for the cement mantle of 1 to 2 mm. Femoral rotation is set by referencing the TEA as described previously, or Whiteside line. In many instrument systems the posterior condylar bone is used to secure the sizing guide, which also is used to set the rotational position of the AP cutting block. It is critical to recognize that the posterior condylar axis (PCA) is typically internally rotated relative to the desired AP cutting plane that sets the femoral component position. The proximal tibial cut is made using an intramedullary or extramedullary cutting guide, again resecting the amount of bone from the joint line that equals the composite thickness of the tibial component.

After the bone cuts are completed, trial implants are placed and ligament balance is checked. If preferred, spacer blocks can also be used to measure the flexion and extension gaps and assess the ligament balance before making all of the distal femoral cuts that would be required to position the trial prosthesis. Soft tissue contractures leading to condylar lift-off, imbalance, or laxity are corrected with appropriate releases, and polyethylene thickness is adjusted until the appropriate balance of the knee is restored throughout the range of motion.

Current Practice in Knee Balancing

From the previous discussion of gap balancing and measured resection, it is apparent that philosophical differences exist. The classic gap method emphasizes preservation of tibial bone and conforming joint surfaces and accepts, when required, proximal migration of the joint surface to balance the gaps. More modern gap balancing in primary joint replacement prioritizes the joint line, creates the extension gap first, and uses the array of implant sizes and instrumentation to control more variables that allow optimization of the flexion gap. The measured resection workflow emphasizes preservation of the joint line level. The differing philosophies are also reflected in technique and instrument systems. Although the instruments used for making bone cuts are generally similar, gap systems depend on a tensor or a series of spacers. Despite differences in philosophy, the distinctions between the gap and measured resection techniques have blurred with the evolution of surgical techniques. The recent emphasis in total knee replacement surgery is on restoration of kinematics, not simply on the presence or absence of the PCL, or the sequence of steps performed.

The current practice in knee ligament balancing has elements of both gap and measured resection methods. Insall advocated a blend of techniques whereby measured resections of both the distal femur and the proximal tibia are performed, avoiding the need for a variable distal femoral cut. Posterior referencing of the femoral condyles with some accommodation to a balanced flexion gap at the same time allows measured resection and balancing of the flexion gap as well. In addition, modern instruments allow ligament tensioning, implant sizing, and implant positioning with measurement prior to making the cuts. This enhanced control of variables in sizing and position, as well as the ability to measure and assess balance before making the bone resections allows the potential for a more reliable and planned outcome. Clearly, instrumentation is complemented by a larger inventory of femoral component sizes than existed when gap balancing was described, as well as a femoral component designed with a divergent anterior cut to minimize the risk of anterior femoral notching. Femoral component sizing and positioning remain critical to proper balancing. One should avoid allowing the femoral component to sit proud of the anterior femoral cortex, even to a minor degree (Fig. 150.7). Finally, with instrument systems that link component position, ligament balancing, and spacer thickness, the kinematics surgeon is able to opt for a joint line that aligned according to preference.

Summary of Modern Technique

1. Cut the distal femur in valgus relative to the anatomic axis (usually 4 to 6 degrees) at a predetermined level (usually 9

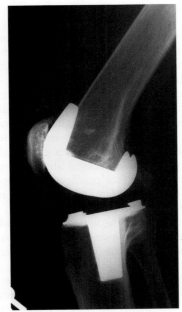

FIG 150.7 Lateral radiograph demonstrating the femoral component cemented in 3 degrees of flexion to avoid anterior notching of the femur.

to 10 mm above the medial condyle, accommodating for bone deficiency).
2. Make a proximal tibial cut perpendicular to the anatomic axis.
3. Balance ligaments in extension.
4. Establish femoral rotation in flexion using the epicondylar axis, ligament tension, and the proximal tibial cut surface.
5. Cut the anterior and posterior femur.
   a. Posterior referencing: perform (1) 3-degree flexion cut (or divergent anterior cut) and (2) correct preoperative flexion contractures by posterior release.
   b. Anterior referencing: avoid over-resection of the posterior condyles of the femur.
6. Choose femoral component (downsize for in-between sizing) that allows for a polyethylene thickness that matches the desired extension gap thickness.
7. Reassess ligament balance, midflexion balance, and posterior capsular tightness.
8. Adjust distal femoral cut to deal with extension gap tightness. (Note that under-resection of the distal femur is seldom needed with the possible exception of certain knees with preexisting recurvatum.)

Performing Bone Resection in Total Knee Arthroplasty

Proximal Tibial Resection. The depth of the proximal tibial resection contributes to the size of both the flexion and extension gap. The proximal tibial osteotomy is generally performed 9 to 10 mm below the least compromised articular cartilage (Fig. 150.8). This resection depth is chosen because it represents the minimum composite thickness of the tibial implant (polyethylene and metal substrate thickness combined). A perpendicular tibial cut establishes limb alignment perpendicular to the mechanical axis of the tibia. Harada et al.[85] suggested that the proximal tibia bone strength weakens below a depth of 5 mm, prompting many surgeons to resect as little bone as possible and requiring the use of thinner polyethylene inserts at the risk of stress-related wear.[229] Clinical experience and later research on tibial bone strength[78] have supported a 9- to 10-mm cut below the joint line, obviating the need to use excessively thin polyethylene components. Another practical matter is that over-resection of the tibia will require the use of a smaller tibial tray to avoid component overhang because of the tapering of the tibial bone. A large size mismatch between tibia and femur can potentially put articular conformity between the femoral and tibial components at risk.

A consideration in joint balancing is whether the PCL is sacrificed or not. When the PCL is resected, the flexion gap increases a few millimeters, usually necessitating an additional millimeter or two of distal femoral bone resection that would slightly elevate the joint line and thereby match the flexion and extension gap. When the gap theory is applied to cruciate retaining designs, the PCL may be retained if it is appropriately balanced and the joint line position is restored with modular tibial inserts.

Extension Gap. The extension gap is created by the distal femoral and proximal tibial resection. The distal femoral osteotomy may be performed before or after the proximal tibial cut is completed. With this concept in mind, the distal femoral resection is made to accommodate the thickness of the femoral component, and the proximal tibial cut is made to accommodate the combined thickness of the tibial component

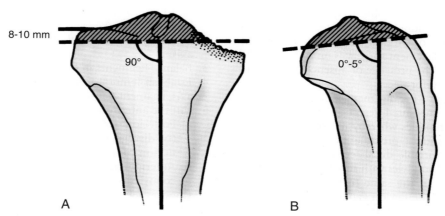

FIG 150.8 The correct cut on the tibia ignores defects and removes 10 mm from the normal side, cut at right angles to the long axis in the coronal plane (A) and sloped posteriorly no more than 5 degrees in the sagittal plane (B).

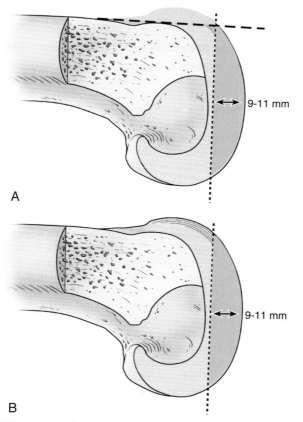

FIG 150.9 The thickness of the prosthesis, normally somewhere between 9 and 11 mm, is removed from the distal femur.

(polyethylene and substrate metal). One approach to creating the proper distal femoral resection depth is to cut the distal femur at a predetermined level (usually 10 mm above the joint line) corresponding to the thickness of the femoral component (Fig. 150.9). The valgus cut on the distal femur relative to the anatomic axis is the difference between anatomic and mechanical axes, which can be measured using long cassette radiographs.

The extension space so formed is then assessed with a spacer block or tensiometer, and the distal femur may be recut later if necessary to match the flexion gap or to accommodate a residual flexion contracture (Fig. 150.10). Cutting away more distal femur than the femoral component will ultimately replace should be minimized because it will elevate the joint line. When a preoperative flexion contracture contributes to gap imbalance, appropriate soft tissue balancing and posterior release should be performed before additional bone resection is considered.

An alternative to using a predetermined distal femoral resection is to cut the extension gap based on the measured height of the flexion gap. With the soft tissue under proper tension, the level of distal femoral osteotomy is determined by the thickness of spacer blocks that fit the flexion gap. A distal femoral osteotomy is performed at this level perpendicular to the mechanical axis and at a measured valgus angle relative to the anatomic axis of the femur (Figs. 150.11 to 150.13).

Rotational Alignment of the Femur. The proper rotational alignment of the femoral component is determined by the anatomy of the femur and is also influenced by the length and tension of medial and lateral ligaments and tissues. In a standard varus knee, some external rotation of the femoral AP cutting block is needed to account for the normal medial inclination of the tibial plateau and the flexion laxity of the lateral ligamentous structures (Fig. 150.14). By creating a small amount of external rotation a rectangular "flexion gap" is produced (Figs. 150.15 and 150.16). This proper rotational alignment also places the patellar trochlea in optimal position to support the proper tracking of the patella. The femoral component rotation can be created by using a balanced gap technique that references the cut tibial surface and sets the femoral resection block through ligament tensioning, or by using anatomic landmarks, such as the epicondylar axis when using the measured resection technique.

Proper femoral rotation is essential because inappropriate femoral component rotation may result in many downstream biomechanical issues, such as flexion instability and patellofemoral maltracking problems.[9,16,167] Although an arbitrary external rotation of 3 degrees with respect to the PCA is often satisfactory,[70,168] several methods have been developed in an

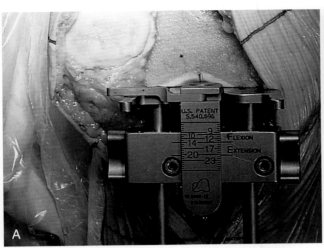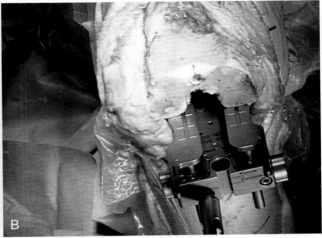

FIG 150.10 Close-up Intraoperative View of a Tensor (A) In extension. (B) In flexion.

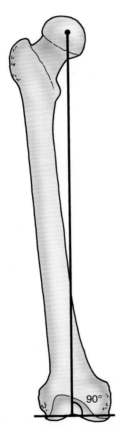

FIG 150.11 The distal femoral cut should be templated by measuring from the center of the femoral head to the center of the knee on a full-length radiograph of the femur. A second line passing into the intramedullary canal of the femur will indicate the angulation of the distal femoral cut.

effort to accurately determine appropriate femoral rotation (Fig. 150.17):
1. Medial and lateral epicondyles[18,163]
2. Posterior femoral condyles[83]
3. AP femoral axis ("Whiteside line")[10,223]

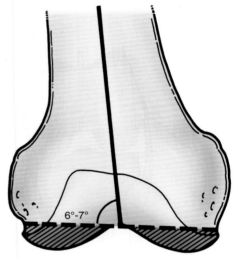

FIG 150.12 The distal femoral cut is normally aligned at 6 to 7 degrees of valgus from the intramedullary alignment rod.

4. Tibial shaft axis[201]
5. Ligament tension

Femoral rotation is difficult to instrument precisely because of surface landmark variability and topography, such as the epicondyles that are hard to palpate. Consequently, the surgeon must take many factors into account, making sure to create the desired rectangular flexion gap and patellar tracking. This goal typically requires slight external rotation relative to the PCA.[9,16,167] The PCA is frequently used as an anchor point for pin guides that set the position of the distal femoral AP and chamfer cutting blocks. Although an excellent anchor point and reference for the distal femoral component size, the PCA cannot be used as a reliable reference for component position. In most circumstances, the PCA is internally rotated relative to the TEA. Furthermore, posterior condylar erosion as part of the arthritic process, particularly in the valgus knee, often distorts this reference angle even further.[83,201] The AP axis of the femoral sulcus, described by Whiteside and Arima,[10,223] has also been shown to be an accurate reference point for determining femoral rotation; however, it has been shown to be less reliable in cases

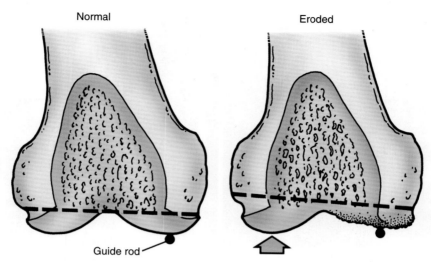

Normal

Eroded

Guide rod

FIG 150.13 Ideally the amount of distal femoral resection should be judged from the normal side. When measurement is made from the medial femoral condyle, regardless of the pathology, extra-distal femoral resection will occur.

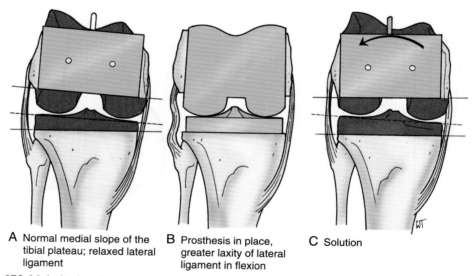

A Normal medial slope of the tibial plateau; relaxed lateral ligament

B Prosthesis in place, greater laxity of lateral ligament in flexion

C Solution

FIG 150.14 Imitating the normal anatomy results in lateral laxity in flexion. (A) Femoral cutting block placed parallel to the normal medial slope of the tibia results in relaxed lateral ligaments. (B) Placing a femoral prosthesis with this rotation will result in greater laxity of the lateral ligament in flexion. (C) In order to avoid the situation in B, the femoral block should be externally rotated relative to the native medial slope of the tibia and parallel to the tibial resection.

of trochlear dysplasia and valgus deformity.[163] The tibial shaft axis has been described as an effective reference axis for defining femoral rotation.[201] Using the anatomic axis of the tibia is particularly useful because it should facilitate balancing the flexion space when perpendicular proximal tibial cuts are created and subsequently used as a reference for femoral component rotation.

Insall preferred the epicondylar axis as the reference that would most closely re-create the patient's natural femoral rotation.[18,163] The center of the medial epicondyle is located in a sulcus that lies between the proximal origin of the superficial deep medial collateral ligament (MCL) and the distal origin of the deep MCL. The medial epicondylar ridge at the origin of

the superficial MCL can be identified by isolating the condylar vessels that lie proximal and anterior to the medial epicondylar ridge. From these vessels the epicondylar ridge can be readily outlined; the center of this outline is the sulcus, which typically can be palpated without dissection (Fig. 150.18). The lateral epicondyle is the most prominent point on the lateral aspect of the distal femur. Following the lateral condylar vessels (similar to the medial side) confirms the exact location of the lateral epicondyle, lying immediately distal to the vessels (Fig. 150.19). The line across the distal femur connecting the epicondyles with the knee flexed to 90 degrees is the epicondylar axis.

The benefit of having several different methods of assessing femoral rotation is that one or more can be used to confirm the

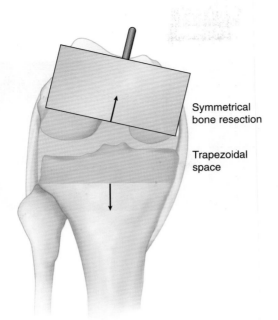

FIG 150.15 In the osteoarthritic knee, lateral laxity is accentuated; when symmetrical bone is excised from the posterior femoral condyles, the resulting space on distraction is trapezoidal.

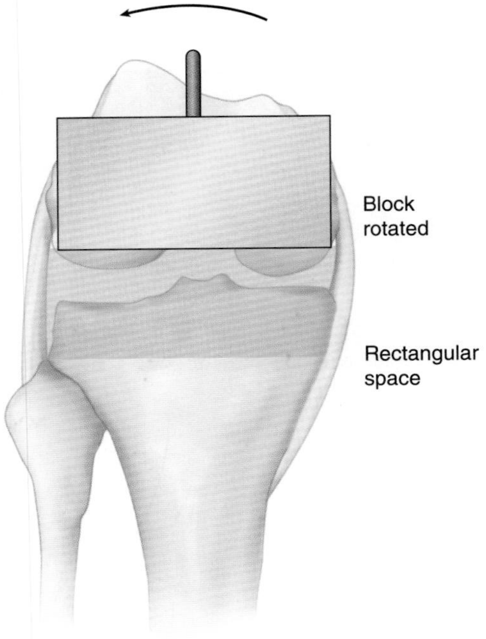

FIG 150.16 By externally rotating the femoral component and removing an asymmetrical amount of bone from the posterior femoral condyles, soft tissue length is equalized and the resulting space is rectangular.

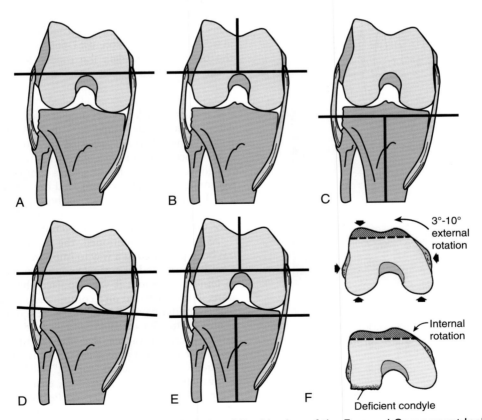

FIG 150.17 Reference Points for Rotational Positioning of the Femoral Component Include the Epicondyles, Trochlear Surface, Tibial Shaft, and Posterior Condyles (A) Transepicondylar axis. (B) Anteroposterior trochlear sulcus ("Whiteside line"). (C) Tibial shaft axis. (D) Posterior condylar angle. (E) Transepicondylar axis is perpendicular to the anteroposterior sulcus line and the tibial shaft axis. (F) When the posterior condyles are used for rotational reference, one must beware of erosion of the condyles. For example, in valgus knees, posterior erosion of the lateral femoral condyle is often present, which may result in internal rotation of the femoral component.

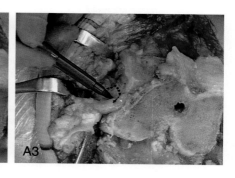

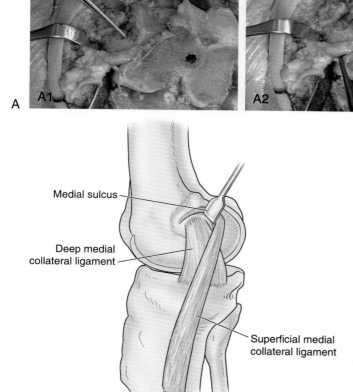

FIG 150.18 (A) Intraoperative photos of the medial epicondyle. (A1) Leash of vessels over the insertion of the superficial MCL. (A2) Instrument placed to define the insertion of the deep MCL. (A3) Between the two MCL insertions, at the medial sulcus, the medial epicondyle is marked in a "bull's eye" fashion. (B) Deep to the superficial MCL, the deep MCL overlies the medial sulcus, the palpable focus of the medial epicondyle.

that using the TEA was less predictable and resulted in excessive external rotation as compared with the AP axis and the balanced tension line. Fehring[67] reported rotational errors of at least 3 degrees occurring in 45% of patients when rotation was determined by fixed bony landmarks as compared with the balanced tension line. One study compared the use of the PCA and TEA and demonstrated a decrease in the requirement for lateral retinacular release when the TEA was used: 56.9% with PCA reference versus 12.3% with TEA reference.[155]

As previously mentioned, the use of computer navigation has been proposed as a way to improve component position. In a study conducted to evaluate computer navigation as it relates to femoral rotation, it was reported that intraoperative decisions should be based on a combination of reference points and that computer navigation alone suggested the incorrect femoral size in up to 50% of the cases reviewed. Furthermore, 34% of cases required intraoperative adjustments in rotation from the computer-modeled placement.[15] Ultimately, the determination of whether the rotation is "correct" will be made by considering all available anatomic references, ensuring proper tracking of the patella, creating a balanced flexion gap without condylar lift-off, and confirming unconstrained movement of the tibiofemoral articulation.

Flexion Gap—Anterior Versus Posterior Referencing. In contrast to early knee replacement designs, there exists now a larger range of femoral component sizes, with combinations of width and depth of the component allowing better matching of the

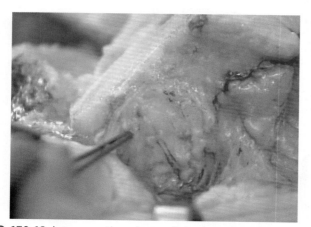

FIG 150.19 Intraoperative photo of the lateral epicondyle, the most prominent point on the distal lateral femur.

surgeon's preferred method (Fig. 150.20). Several investigators have compared these various methods. Poilvache et al.[163] correlated the transepicondylar, AP, and PCA. Berger et al.[18] and Griffin et al.[82] described the relationship of the epicondylar axis to the PCA. Whiteside and Arima[10,223] defined the relationship of the AP and PCA. Stiehl and Cherveny[201] demonstrated that referencing from the tibial shaft axis is more accurate than referencing from the PCA. More recently, Katz et al.[109] found

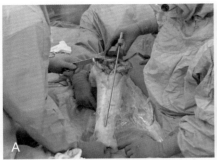 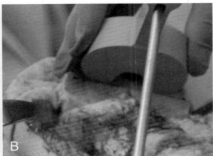 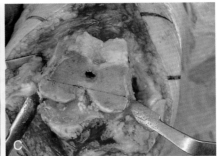

FIG 150.20 Confirming Proper Femoral Rotation (A) Tibial shaft axis. (B) Comparison of transepicondylar and tibial shaft axes. (C) Transepicondylar axis.

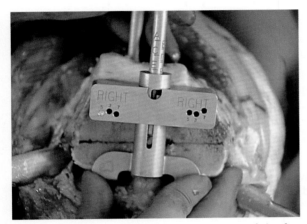

FIG 150.21 Instrument used for sagittal sizing of the femur.

patient's dimensions. Nevertheless, there will seldom be an exact match between the sagittal dimension of the femoral component and the actual size of the bone, necessitating some choices to create a balanced knee. With anterior referencing, the placement of the anterior flange of the femoral component on the anterior femoral cortex is prioritized, and the size of the femoral component is determined by the amount of the posterior femoral condyle that is removed. Thus the size of the flexion gap after the posterior condylar resection will differ from anatomic if the exact amount of resected condyle does not equal the amount replaced by the femoral implant. To create equal flexion and extension gaps, adjustments in the posterior condylar resection and size of the femoral component is a useful variable to control. Over-resection of the posterior condyles can cause flexion instability, and under-resection can lead to excessive tightness in flexion, particularly when the PCL is preserved. Conversely, with posterior referencing (Fig. 150.21), the flexion gap is constant, and variability in sagittal size is determined by the anterior femoral cut. This type of referencing is very useful when prioritizing the flexion gap but creates a risk of "notching" the anterior femoral cortex with an aggressive resection of bone or of having the femoral flange sit anterior to the anterior femoral cortex when the component is larger than the bone. To compensate for in-between sizing when using anterior referencing, Insall recommended downsizing components and placing the femoral component in slight flexion (typically 3 degrees) to lessen the risk of anterior notching (see Fig. 150.7). The same effect can be achieved if the instrument system creates a slightly

divergent (as opposed to parallel to the anterior cortex) anterior cut, also minimizing the risk of anterior femoral notching.

In the classic Insall technique of posterior referencing and flexion-gap-first workflow, after the posterior condylar cut is made, the flexion gap is measured. Spacer blocks are then used to determine the gap size (Fig. 150.22). An increasingly popular alternative to static blocks is to use ligament tensor devices, ranging from something as simple as a lamina spreader to a more complicated sensor with a digitally calibrated read-out. The tensor technique balances the flexion gap by allowing one to set the position of the AP cutting block such that it creates a desired soft tissue tension on the medial and lateral sides of the flexion gap (Fig. 150.23; see also Fig. 150.10). To review, the workflow using the gap balance technique using a tensor would be as follows: distal femoral cut, proximal tibia cut, balance ligaments in extension, measure extension gap, flex the knee, and use the tension guide to position the femoral AP cutting block choosing the size, AP cut position, and rotation to create a rectangular flexion gap with an articular size that equals the extension gap. The role for the tensors is to allow the surgeon to properly tension the flexion space and create a corresponding posterior condylar cut (Fig. 150.24). The size of the flexion space corresponds to the combined thickness of tibial and femoral components.

Posterior Cruciate Ligament

Preservation of the PCL in primary total knee arthroplasty (TKA) offers many potential advantages because this ligament is an important varus/valgus stabilizer of the knee; it is a strong structure that can absorb stresses that might otherwise be transmitted to the prosthesis-bone interface, can control the roll-back of the femur on the tibia that occurs with flexion, may be important for stair-climbing activities, and may have a proprioceptive function (although abnormal proprioception will not return to normal after knee replacement).

To function properly, the PCL must be accurately tensioned during knee replacement. If the PCL is too tight, this will promote excessive tibial roll-back, thereby impeding knee flexion, causing increased posterior stresses, and risking posterior polyethylene overload and anterior femoral component displacement. A tight PCL may also cause the knee to hinge "open like a book" (Fig. 150.25). Recognition of excess PCL tightness is possible by observing anterior tibial component "lift-off" with trial components (Fig. 150.26). Conversely, when the PCL is too loose, it does not control the gradual posterior roll-back of the femoral condyles on the tibial plateau as the

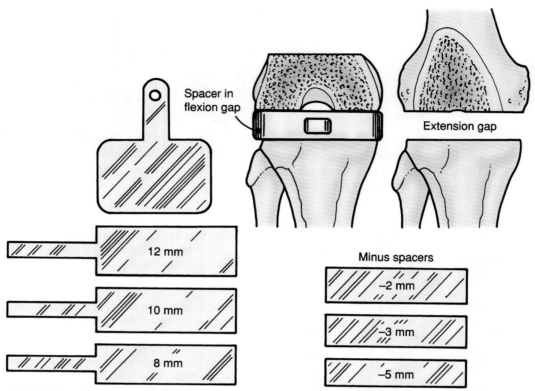

FIG 150.22 Flexion and extension gaps are assessed by a series of spacers. When the extension gap is smaller than the flexion gap, it must be equalized by resection of extra distal femoral bone. The amount needed is assessed using the spacer system. Minus spacers are available when the flexion gap requires the thinnest (8 mm) spacer.

knee flexes (Fig. 150.27). Lack of PCL function allows the femur to roll forward paradoxically (opposite of normal roll-back) in flexion, potentially limiting flexion by impingement of the posterior femoral cortex on the posterior tibial plateau. The "slide-back" test has been described to assess for proper PCL tension following component positioning in rotating platform systems. The trial insert (without stabilizing post) is inserted and the knee flexed to 90 degrees. If the PCL is too tight, the insert moves posteriorly. Conversely, a PCL with excessive laxity will allow anterior migration of the insert. Best results have been reported with PCL tension adjusted to provide for 1 to 3 mm of posterior insert translation.[189]

Proper PCL tension is dependent upon maintaining the level of the joint line and the spatial relationship between the femur and the tibia. The ideal posterior cruciate retaining knee replacement would meet the following criteria:

1. The joint line or axis is restored to its prearthritic condition.
2. The shape and size of the femoral condyles are restored to re-create the natural distal and posterior femoral cam effect.
3. The tibial plateau surface is sloped approximately 10 degrees posterior and approximately 3 degrees medial.
4. The tibial surface offers no impedance to rotation and gliding movements.

In practice, techniques that are aimed at preserving the PCL meet these requirements to varying degrees. The balance of the PCL remains a subjective assessment. Proper balancing even in

the hands of experienced surgeons does not guarantee normal knee kinematics and tibial roll-back. A few systems mimic the medial slope of the normal tibia, and some cut the tibia at right angles to its shaft. However, all measured resection knee systems share the objective of closely preserving or restoring the anatomic joint line by referencing the distal femur. If this joint line preservation is achieved and the PCL is retained, the arc of motion should also be close to normal with correct ligament tensioning and optimal patellar tracking throughout the range of motion. Because patellofemoral dysfunction remains the cause of many unsatisfactory knee arthroplasties, maintenance of the anatomic joint line is potentially valuable. An optimal joint line avoids patella infera (Fig. 150.28). Further evidence comes from Figgie et al.[70] who demonstrated that if the patella is not within a defined sagittal neutral zone (10 to 30 mm above the joint line), a greater number of patellar problems are observed (Fig. 150.29).

Successful PCL retention in TKA requires proper initial balancing and sustained function. Ligament balancing techniques have been developed that permit PCL retention when the ligament is contracted but remains competent.[174,184,191] The technique is similar to the medial release performed for balancing varus deformity. A graduated PCL release (Fig. 150.30A) is performed from the posterior aspect of the tibia, using a periosteal elevator until the PCL tension is deemed appropriate (see Fig. 150.30B). However, even for an experienced surgeon, it may be difficult to achieve the aims of successful PCL retention.[40]

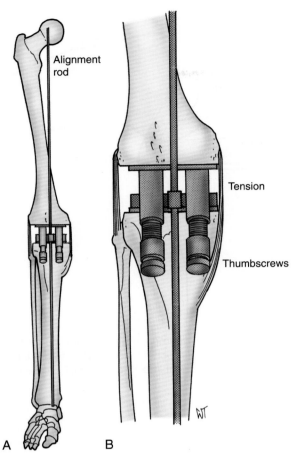

FIG 150.23 By adjusting the medial and lateral thumbscrews of the tensor, the alignment rod is brought into the mechanical axis. (A) Long-leg representation of an operative limb with tensor in place achieving a neutral mechanical alignment. (B) Close-in view of the tensor and thumbscrews.

Although the PCL is typically intact in most arthritic knees,[188,192] the PCL can also degenerate and contract as part of the arthritic process,[6,114] rendering the ligament nonfunctional and making PCL retention not applicable in some arthritic knee deformities.[123,192] Similarly, the PCL occasionally becomes incompetent in the months or years after knee replacement, rendering the prosthesis unstable.[159,217] Using cine-radiography, Dennis et al. demonstrated paradoxical roll-forward of the femur on the tibia as the knee flexes in apparently well-functioning knees with a retained PCL.[47] Follow-up studies by these investigators have reported improved and more consistent kinematics with an intact PCL when combined with an asymmetrical femoral component. More recent studies have demonstrated reliable femoral roll-back with PCL retention in newer posterior-stabilized designs.[28,115]

Anterior Cruciate Ligament

The anterior cruciate ligament (ACL) is an important functional element in the normal knee; its absence causes not only instability but an abnormal pattern of motion, including rotational and sliding movements (eg, pivot shift). Together with the PCL, the ACL forms a "four-bar linkage"[149] at the center of the knee, and the absence of either component destroys this mechanism. Abnormal sliding movements, in particular, can be expected when only the PCL is preserved.[45,46,111,202] The ACL is sacrificed in most modern bicondylar total knee systems. Only a few knee prostheses are designed to preserve both cruciate ligaments. There are new bicruciate retaining designs in clinical trial at this time, but little data on performance of these devices are available.

PREOPERATIVE PLANNING

Full-length radiographs that show hip, knee, and ankle joints are desirable for preoperative planning. Standard radiographs showing the distal femoral and proximal tibial anatomic axis serve as an acceptable alternative to long films when there is no

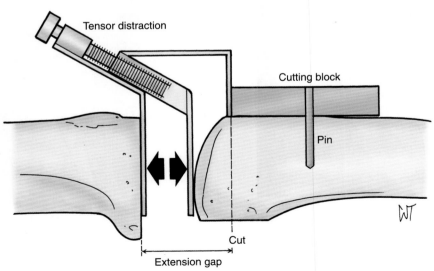

FIG 150.24 The distal femoral cutting guide is controlled by the tensor and is positioned to create an extension gap of the correct dimensions.

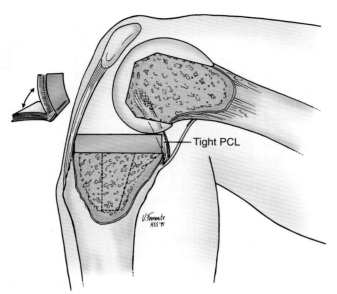

FIG 150.25 An overtight PCL causes "booking." Excessive roll-back of the femur occurs, and the knee hinges open. *PCL,* Posterior cruciate ligament.

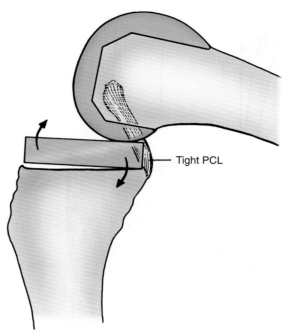

FIG 150.26 Method of demonstrating a tight PCL intraoperatively. The tibial trial component does not have undersurface fixation, and the component lifts anteriorly. *PCL,* Posterior cruciate ligament.

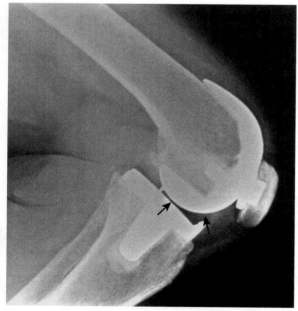

FIG 150.27 Sagittal radiograph of a "nonfunctional" PCL. "Roll-forward" rather than "roll-back" is seen with knee flexion. The anterior margin of the femoral component abuts the anterior margin of the tibial component as it does in a total condylar-type design. *Arrows* indicate an anterior position of the femur component on the tibia as well as the anterior margin of the femur abutting the anterior margin of the tibial component.

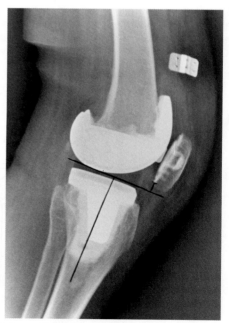

FIG 150.28 Lateral radiograph of a posterior-stabilized prosthesis shows a patella infera. The distal pole of the patella lies just proximal to a projection of the joint line. Patella infera may be associated with increased frequency of patellar symptoms.

history of prior bone instrumentation or trauma, or clinical suspicion of excessive tibial bowing. Radiographs are position sensitive, requiring care to obtain the films in neutral rotation (Figs. 150.31 and 150.32).[104] Information concerning the angle of femoral and tibial cuts and the desired entry hole position (which may not be in the bone center) is obtained. Unusual shaft bowing is noted (Fig. 150.33). Unusual anatomic variations, such as unusual canal size, angular malalignment, or previous surgery, that could cause intraoperative difficulty are noted (Fig. 150.34). Templating is helpful and can be quite elaborate with advanced imaging, such as computed tomography (CT) or magnetic resonance imaging (MRI), when custom cutting blocks are used.

EXPOSURE

Medial Parapatellar Approach

The medial parapatellar approach is the most common approach for TKA. A midline skin incision centered over the patella extends from the level of the tibial tuberosity to just above the patella. The incision is made sufficiently long to avoid traction on the skin edges during the procedure. Distally, the incision is placed approximately 1 cm medial to the prominence of the tibial tubercle. A paramedian skin incision may be elected if a straight anterior incision is deemed undesirable by the patient who desires more comfortable kneeling after surgery. The medial parapatellar arthrotomy may cross the medial border of the patella to avoid transecting longitudinal fibers of the extensor mechanism. Proximally, the capsular incision is positioned along the medial margin of the vastus medialis within 6 to 8 mm of its edge; distally, the distal arthrotomy may include a small portion of the infrapatellar ligament or may parallel the patellar tendon medial to the tibial tubercle. Standard exposure includes a medial periosteal sleeve that includes the deep MCL, which is elevated from the tibia to allow the proximal tibia to be translated anteriorly and rotated externally. When the ACL is present, it is divided to improve the ease of this translation. In general, the lateral patellofemoral ligament is divided, the menisci are removed, and the joint line is exposed.

Techniques to Enhance Exposure in Standard Medial Parapatellar Approach

1. Elevation of the deep fibers of the MCL just below the tibial surface with posterior extension reflecting the medial

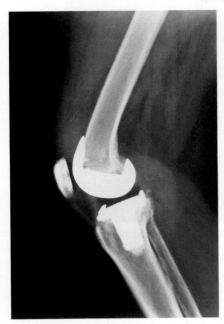

FIG 150.29 Lateral radiograph shows a satisfactory patellar position postoperatively. The patella lies in its normal position in relation to the joint line. The patellar prosthesis composite is of the correct thickness. Note the sclerosis that has developed in the remaining patellar bone. This is a common finding that develops several years postoperatively and is an example of Wolff's law.

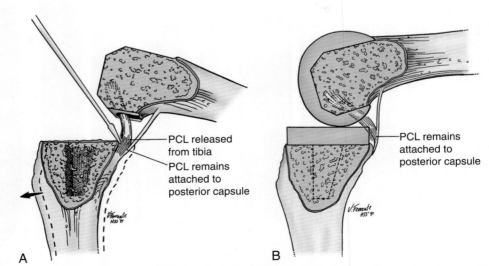

PCL released from tibia

PCL remains attached to posterior capsule

PCL remains attached to posterior capsule

A   B

FIG 150.30 Posterior Cruciate Ligament Release from the Posterior Tibia Lengthens a Tight PCL (A) The release can be done progressively until correct tension is obtained. (B) The PCL remains attached to the posterior capsule. *PCL,* Posterior cruciate ligament.

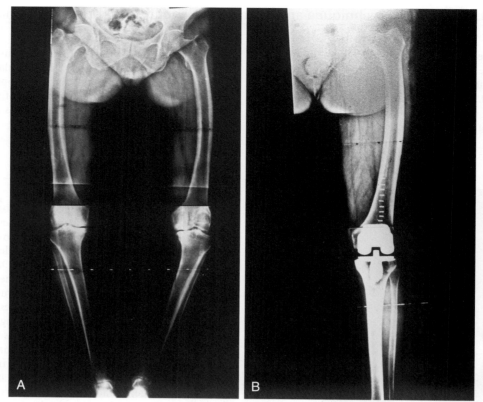

FIG 150.31 (A) Long, 52-inch radiograph of a preoperative patient with varus osteoarthritis. From preoperative planning, a 14-degree valgus cut on the femur was predicted. (B) Postoperative radiograph of the same patient. Extramedullary alignment check showed that the 14-degree prediction was grossly incorrect; in fact, the femur was resected at 7 degrees of valgus. Apparent lateral bowing was, in fact, excessive anterior bowing of the femur seen in a position of some external rotation.

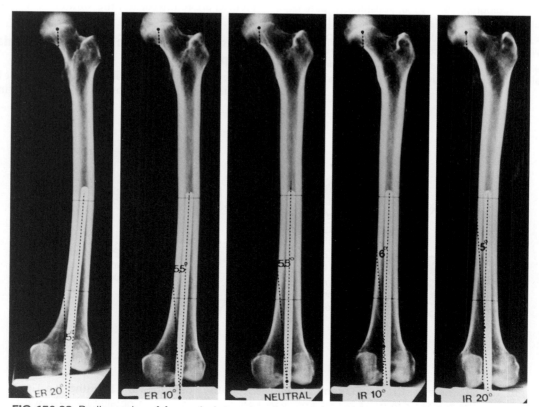

FIG 150.32 Radiographs of femur in internal and external rotation. It can be seen that internal rotation is perceived as medial bowing and external rotation as lateral bowing. This is a normal femur, and the effect would be accentuated if the femur had excessive anterior bowing.

capsule, the deep MCL, and the semimembranosus (Fig. 150.35). Extension of the posteromedial release allows hyperflexion and external rotation of the tibia, thereby enhancing exposure by rotating the tibia out from under the femur and moving the patella and extensor mechanism laterally.

2. Elevation of a small cuff of periosteum immediately adjacent to the patellar tendon insertion at the tibial tubercle. This diminishes the risk of patellar tendon avulsion during exposure.
3. Division of the lateral patellofemoral ligament, which permits slightly greater patellar eversion.
4. Excision of the fat pad. Although some surgeons perform a longitudinal split of the fat pad, excision of the fat pad can improve mobilization of the patella and minimize the potential for postoperative infrapatellar scar formation.
5. Separation of the capsule from the patella at the lateral osteochondral border of the patella.

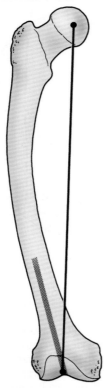

FIG 150.33 When the femur is bowed, the angle of the distal femoral cut will be increased. When templating the femur, beware of excessive valgus cuts because bowing may represent external rotation of the femoral bone on the radiograph. An external alignment check is advisable.

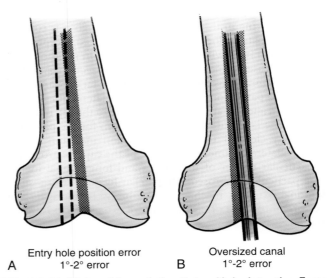

A   Entry hole position error   1°-2° error

B   Oversized canal   1°-2° error

FIG 150.34 Malposition of the Entry Hole into the Femur Introduces an Error into the Valgus Cut (A) Lateral entry hole increases the valgus of the cut. (B) Oversized canal allows the intramedullary rod to toggle, and a 1- to 2-degree error in both varus and valgus can be produced.

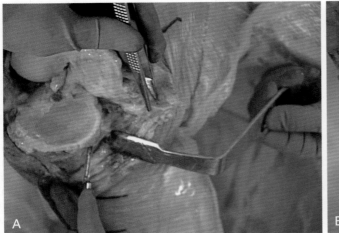

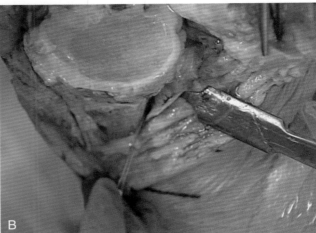

FIG 150.35 Routine exposure includes release of all soft tissues from the medial tibia at the joint line. A medial release involves distal stripping of the superficial MCL, which was not performed in this case. (A) Exposure to the posteromedial proximal tibia. (B) Close-up view.

6. Extension of the incision proximally will also facilitate mobilization of the extensor mechanism and relieve skin tension in tight knees.

Other accepted methods of exposing the knee, such as the subvastus, vastus splitting, trivector, and lateral parapatellar methods are discussed elsewhere.

Difficult Exposures

When a stiff or ankylosed knee is exposed, there is risk of avulsing the patellar tendon attachment to the tibial tubercle. If all aspects of the standard exposure are used, with additional specific attention to areas of contracture, it is possible to minimize the risk of avulsion or damage to the extensor mechanism. When mobilizing the patella, it is important to perform releases to allow external rotation of the tibia, so that the patella can be subluxated laterally rather than everted. This may entail creating a pocket in the lateral gutter for the patella if there is extensive scarring in the lateral gutter. Although it is common practice, the patella does not need to be everted except during patellar preparation with the knee extended. In addition to the standard releases, which include medial dissection around to the semimembranosus bursa, excision of the fat pad, and lateral release of the patella, one should expose the lateral tibial plateau, remove scar, and elevate the lateral capsule to the top of Gerdy's tubercle. The lateral dissection makes room for the patella but should stay clear of the popliteal tendon insertion and the fibular collateral ligament. Elevation of the capsule around the osteoarticular border of the patella and longitudinal incision into a particularly fibrosed infrapatellar ligament can result in additional extensor mechanism flexibility. In more resistant cases of contracture or stiffness, more extensile exposures are required.

Rectus Snip. The rectus snip is the extensile proximal exposure described by Insall for the medial parapatellar approach.[75] The snip is performed (Fig. 150.36) as needed after other methods of patellar mobilization already described have been used. The medial incision for the quad snip is the same as that described for the standard midline approach. At the apex of the quadriceps tendon, the arthrotomy is continued laterally across the thin proximal portion of the tendon into the vastus lateralis, dividing the rectus tendon superficially and the trilaminar tendon extensions of the vastus muscles deeply. More distally, a lateral retinacular patellar release may also be done at this stage if it is determined that the lateral retinaculum is sufficiently tight so as to pull the patella laterally or restrict knee bending. The superior lateral genicular vessels need to be identified and isolated as they run at the lower border of the vastus lateralis muscle. These vessels can sometimes be saved when identified and protected during the lateral release. An important feature of this approach is that none of the structures contributing to knee extension are transversely divided.

Tibial Tubercle Osteotomy. A tibial tubercle osteotomy can facilitate exposure of a stiff knee.[224] This technique requires that the fragment of bone osteotomized should be sufficiently large to enhance the potential for later healing back to the tibia (Fig. 150.37). The tibial fragment is opened on a lateral soft tissue hinge. A tibial fragment of sufficient size (generally 8 to 12 cm in length and 1 to 2 cm thick) may be securely reattached by wires or screws at the conclusion of the operation, whereas small fragments in osteoporotic bone afford insufficient

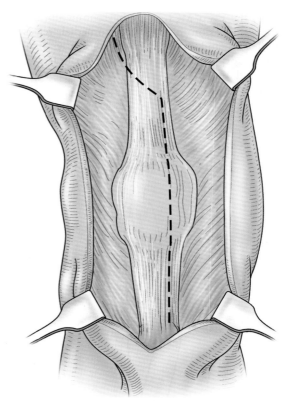

FIG 150.36 The Rectus Snip The medial parapatellar incision is continued proximally across the apex of the rectus femoris tendon into the fibers of the vastus lateralis. Division of the rectus tendon in and of itself allows elasticity and takes stress off the patellar ligament insertion into the tibial tubercle. When combined with a lateral patellar release, but when a bridge of tissue consisting of the vastus lateralis insertion into the quadriceps tendon is retained, the result is equivalent to a quadriceps turndown.

substance for successful reattachment. Whiteside[222] reported on use of this technique in 136 knees—both primary and revision TKAs. Complications were few, and no further release of the quadriceps mechanism was necessary in any procedure. However, Wolff et al.[227] reported a 23% complication rate when using a similar technique.

Subperiosteal Peel. In ankylosed knees or knees with severe angular deformity, it may be necessary to perform a subperiosteal exposure of the femur or tibia. It is advisable to begin with a subperiosteal exposure of the medial tibia to mid-diaphysis while attempting to flex and externally rotate the knee, being careful not to avulse the femoral attachment of the MCL. If medial peel is not successful in creating adequate motion, the periosteum of the lower femur is incised by subperiosteal dissection (Fig. 150.38). The soft tissue envelope is peeled from the bone as a continuous sleeve and is retracted posteriorly, allowing the distal femur to be buttonholed forward. This exposure, combined with medial subperiosteal dissection of the upper tibia, allows the knee to be flexed without danger of damaging or tearing important soft tissue structures, which are often very fragile in an ankylosed knee because of prolonged lack of movement and physiologic stress. When the incision is closed, the

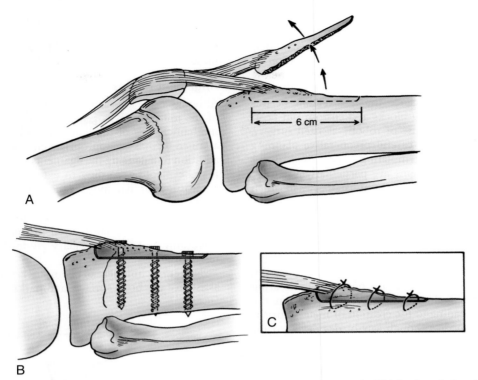

FIG 150.37 **Method of Exposure for Difficult or Ankylosed Knees** (A) Tibial tubercle is osteotomized by taking a large fragment of bone, at least 6 cm long. This allows firm reattachment with screws (B) or wire sutures (C).

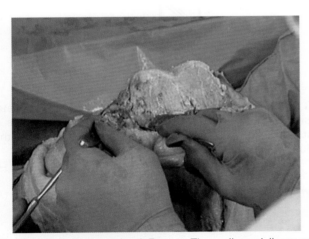

FIG 150.38 **A Skeletonized Femur** The collateral ligaments, together with the adjacent periosteum of the distal femur, have been stripped posteriorly, allowing the distal femur to be buttonholed anteriorly. The soft tissues remain in continuity, and after the operation has been completed, the soft tissue sleeve remains intact, providing stability. This type of exposure, combined with subperiosteal stripping of the proximal tibia and quadriceps turndown or modification thereof, is very useful in dealing with ankylosed knees or reimplantation after infection.

soft tissue envelope falls back around the bones. This technique is useful for long-standing ankylosis of the knee and for reimplantation after infection.[145] Extensive exposures that result in medial-lateral instability patterns may occasionally require the use of increased articular constraint or a hinged prosthesis. The risk of extensive subperiosteal exposure is devascularization with subsequent osteonecrosis of the condyle. As such, extensive releases should be reserved for only the most extreme cases.

Closure. Closure should be anatomic, with effort made to restore the longitudinal alignment of the medial and lateral soft tissues along the incision. Tissues should be approximated without being excessively tightened or imbricated. Closure of the knee in 45 degrees of flexion or greater will help to align the capsular incision, using the shape of the incision or a transverse ink or cautery mark as a guide to alignment.[60,140] Insall routinely performed a modified vastus medialis obliquus (VMO) advancement, in which the medial soft tissue envelope is advanced several millimeters distal relative to the lateral soft tissues. Because the VMO is important in terminal extension, this advancement was meant to reduce the risk of a postoperative extension lag.

TECHNIQUES AND INSTRUMENTATION

Implant systems on the market today have similarities, differing according to the two philosophies described previously. Thus many of the instruments used in total knee replacement are similar. The interest in minimally invasive and computer-navigated approaches has led to the downsizing of standard instrumentation and the development of alternative approaches, such as making the distal femoral cut from a lateral approach. Such innovative ideas and concepts have not been widely adopted and still require clinical testing and evaluation to determine accuracy, reproducibility, and performance before widespread adoption can be advocated. The newest addition to the inventory of instruments since the last version of this chapter includes custom cutting blocks and custom pin positioning devices, as well as the use of robotic-assisted surgery. These systems are based upon careful preoperative planning with advanced imaging and templating. These instrument systems and cutting block systems are particularly useful in cases of deformity, retained hardware, or unusual cases in which standard systems may be difficult or impossible to use.

Cutting Blocks

Bone cuts may be made from the free edge of the cutting block or through slotted capture guides. The slots may afford some degree of safety by limiting the excursion of saw blades; however, in practice they obscure the saw blade tip, potentially increasing the risk of compromising important structures, such as the MCL, and sometimes leading to the creation of metal debris if the saw becomes confined. Although saw blades designed for the capture guides function well in the cutting slots, their cutting teeth are less efficient because the teeth are designed with less offset to allow the blade to pass through the cutting slot (Fig. 150.39). When capture guides are used, it is important to lubricate surfaces and not to lever the saw blade against the guide to minimize the generation of metallic debris from the saw rubbing the cutting block. Milling frames are particularly useful in patellar preparation and notch preparation. Rotary blades have been shown to generate less heat than standard saw blades, thereby creating less damage to the cut bony surface.

Efficiency in femoral and tibial preparation has been advanced through improved instrumentation. Traditionally, multiple femoral cuts were made with individual cutting blocks. Newer universal cutting blocks allow multiple steps of ligament tensioning, sizing, and bone surface preparation to be performed using a single block (Fig. 150.40) or instrument. Modern femoral cutting blocks provide slots for the anterior, posterior, and chamfer cuts, as well as guides for creation of the distal femoral lug holes. New technology has allowed introduction of

cutting blocks prefabricated for an individual patient based on preoperative imaging and preplanned cuts (custom cutting blocks). The accuracy, reliability, and economic feasibility of these designs for widespread use have yet to be determined.

Alignment Guides

Although there is debate about the optimal coronal orientation of the joint line, it is generally agreed that restoration of the mechanical axis of the limb should be achieved. Alignment is attained by making appropriate cuts on the femur and tibia, in addition to balancing the ligaments. Standard alignment guides may be placed according to external landmarks, such as the anterosuperior iliac spine or the center of the hip joint[170] proximally and the ankle mortise distally (Fig. 150.41). Because these landmarks can sometimes be hard to identify, intramedullary guides are predominantly used for making the distal femoral osteotomy and extramedullary guides for the proximal tibial resection.

Newer techniques of computer navigation or robotic-assistance use bone surface landmarks, which are registered in

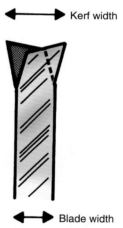

Kerf width

Blade width

FIG 150.39 Saws with cutting slots must use appropriately designed blades with reduced offset to the cutting tips so that kerf width and slot width are nearly the same, thus reducing "slot."

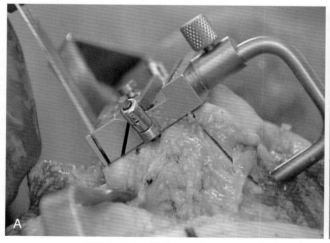
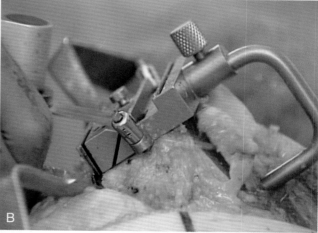

FIG 150.40 Universal Femoral Cutting Block (A) Anteroposterior cuts. (B) Chamfer cuts.

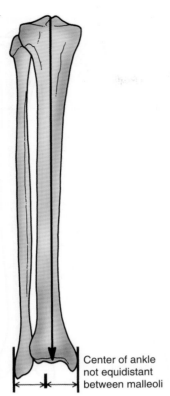

FIG 150.41 Center of the Knee Center of the talus axis lies a few millimeters medial to the center point between the malleoli.

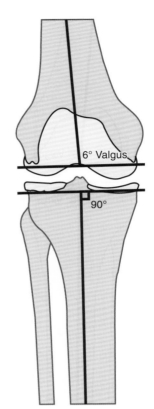

FIG 150.42 Classic alignment.

the computer using a navigated stylus or a gyroscopic instrument that locates the center of rotation of the hip joint. An advantage of navigation is the potential to obviate the need to cannulate the medullary canal to achieve the desired mechanical alignment. Alignment is created by feeding data on surface topography into the computer, using an instrumented stylus to map the bone surface. After the bone contour is established by entering certain key points into the computer, the data are combined with data stored in the computer on standard tibial or femoral anatomy. This process of combining individual patient-derived data with stored data is called *morphing*. Computer morphing generates an image or likeness of the knee on the computer screen during surgery. From this hybrid of real data and stored data, the computer will proceed to direct the surgeon regarding accuracy of alignment.

Method of Alignment

Classic Method. Either the tibial or the femoral osteotomy may be performed first (Fig. 150.42). The valgus cut at the distal femur in theory is the difference between the anatomic and mechanical axes, created using the intramedullary femoral canal as the anatomic reference. The distal femoral valgus can vary depending on the patient's body habitus, generally falling around 5 to 6 degrees of valgus. A long-leg preoperative x-ray can be used to plan this cut based on the patient's particular anatomy. The distal femur in a valgus knee is generally cut in 4 to 5 degrees of valgus, whereas a varus or normally aligned knee is cut at 5 to 6 degrees of valgus. In obese patients, it is important to limit the amount of valgus to 5 degrees to avoid contact between the medial knee soft tissues. The tibial cut is always

made neutral to the tibial anatomic axis.[132] Hsu et al.[93] confirmed that 7 degrees of femoral valgus matched with 0 degrees of proximal tibial alignment resulted in the most even load distribution across a total condylar knee prosthesis. Evidence suggests that a varus tibial cut not only results in uneven stress distribution in the proximal tibia[81] but also leads to premature clinical failure.[175] Nevertheless, the optimal orientation of the joint line in the coronal plane remains a topic of debate, with some still favoring proximal tibial anatomic varus.

Anatomic Method. In an attempt to re-create natural knee kinematics with a PCL retaining prosthesis, Hungerford and Kenna used an anatomic method (Fig. 150.43) of lower limb alignment for TKA.[95] Femoral valgus is set at an anatomic 9 to 10 degrees, and the tibial cut is made in 2 to 3 degrees of varus, thereby creating an anatomic 6 to 7 degrees of lower extremity valgus. Hsu et al.[93] demonstrated that these angles produce even load distribution across the knee joint in a cruciate-retaining design. As noted previously, if the surgeon is not experienced in this technique, intentional varus tibial cuts can easily result in excessive tibial varus, creating uneven load distribution and ligament imbalance.

Tibial Guides

Background. Most systems will offer either intramedullary or extramedullary guides for the upper tibial osteotomy. Advocates of intramedullary tibial guides maintain that a rod of sufficient length reaching well into the tibial diaphysis will reliably align the tibial-cutting guide when there is no bow or offset to the tibial shaft. One potential pitfall of the intramedullary technique

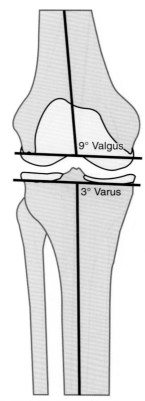

FIG 150.43 Anatomic alignment.

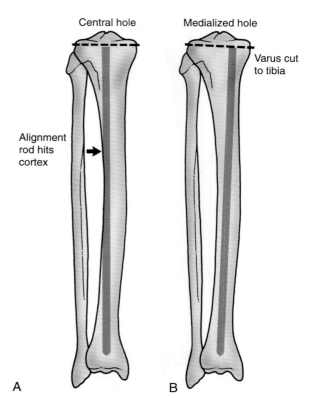

FIG 150.44 **Intramedullary Guides Are Not Satisfactory When the Tibia Is Bowed** (A) The guide passed through a central hole abuts the lateral cortex. (B) To pass the guide down the shaft to the ankle, the entry hole has to be medialized. This produces a varus cut to the tibia.

is that the shape of the tibia is inconsistent. In addition, as for any intramedullary guide, the entry point is critical to alignment. Templating to determine the proper entry point for the tibial guide on the tibial surface will minimize the risk of creating a varus tibial cut based on a medial entry point and a bowed tibia. A central entry hole often will cause the intramedullary rod to impact against the tibial cortex (usually lateral), and placing the entry hole so that this does not happen alters the angle of the proximal guide (Fig. 150.44).

The extramedullary tibial guide is placed on the leg, using surface landmarks. The distal end of the guide attaches above the ankle, while the proximal end is pinned to the center of the proximal tibia, generally at the medial one-third of the tibial tubercle. Most guides allow adjustment at the ankle in both mediolateral and AP directions. The center of the ankle does not exactly correspond to the midpoint between the malleoli but instead is slightly medial to this point (5 to 10 mm) (see Fig. 150.41). The AP distal guide adjustment controls the posterior slope of the proximal tibial cut. The posterior slope of the proximal tibia may also be incorporated into the tibial osteotomy. Some systems, especially cruciate-retaining designs and some mobile-bearing knee designs, function more effectively with posterior slope. The 7 degrees of posterior slope is anatomic when the subchondral bone is considered, but when the posterior menisci are taken into consideration, the proximal tibial surface is actually perpendicular to the shaft (Fig. 150.45).

In obese patients, AP guide adjustment at the ankle may be necessary to make the guide parallel to the tibial shaft. Locating the proper proximal position of the extramedullary guide may be difficult; the natural tendency is to place the guide medially, producing a varus cut. Mobilization of the

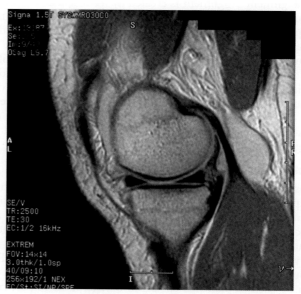

FIG 150.45 Lateral magnetic resonance image of the knee demonstrating that the posterior slope is present when the subchondral surface is considered; however, with the menisci intact, the 5 to 7 degrees of "physiologic posterior slope" is reduced to essentially neutral.

infrapatellar ligament combined with a lower profile lateral plateau cutting surface will facilitate placement of the tibial guide. By referencing off the tibial plateau center, the tibial shaft axis, and the center of the ankle, proper alignment for the proximal tibial osteotomy is usually possible. Several investigators have demonstrated that extramedullary and intramedullary systems are equally accurate in establishing tibial alignment.[44,125] However, intramedullary instrumentation forfeits some of its accuracy in the face of tibial bowing or offset of the tibial shaft, especially when used for valgus knees. Simmons et al.[197] noted that accuracy for intramedullary tibial alignment systems was 83% for varus knees versus 37% for valgus knees; they attributed the poor accuracy to tibial bowing observed in two thirds of valgus knees.

Authors' Preferred Technique of Tibial Preparation.

The upper tibial osteotomy is made at right angles to the tibial shaft, both in the coronal plane and sloped posterior approximately 3 to 5 degrees in the sagittal plane. The extramedullary guide is provisionally secured to the tibia in alignment with the medial third of the tibial tubercle, the tibial shaft, the center of the tibial plateau, and the middle of the ankle. Adjustments to the tibial cutting block are then performed at the ankle. The depth of proximal tibial resection is determined such that enough bone is removed to accommodate the tibial component (with a 10-mm polyethylene insert being the desired lower limit in modular tibial components, and 8 mm being the lower limit with all polyethylene components). Given the few additional millimeters of laxity produced following PCL excision, 1 cm of proximal tibia is excised to accommodate at least a 10-mm tibial component when a cruciate-substituting knee is performed. The 10 mm of resection is typically measured using a stylus placed on the articular surface with the most residual cartilage; alternatively, the stylus can measure 2 mm of resection from the most eroded articular surface (Fig. 150.46). The concept is really to restore the tibial joint line to its proper height so that the collateral ligaments are balanced throughout the range of motion. Although studies have shown that resection of up to 20 mm from the least involved side of the joint is acceptable,[78]

excessive tibial resection can create tibial and femoral component size mismatches and excessively thick articular surfaces that might compromise ligament attachments on the tibia.

Femoral Guides

Background. Multiple investigations have demonstrated that both intramedullary and extramedullary alignment systems are accurate; however, most studies suggest that intramedullary femoral alignment systems are more commonly used because of limitations of extramedullary alignment as noted previously.[136] Femoral alignment can be determined using intramedullary methods and confirmed with extramedullary methods if any uncertainty exists (eg, unusual femoral bowing, wide or obstructed intramedullary canal).

Preoperative radiographic evaluation with a three-joint view allows identification of extra-articular deformity, such as abnormal femoral bowing. A strong correlation has been noted between the mechanical axis and the anatomic axis obtained with standard radiographs in the absence of extra-articular deformity.[119] Rotation of the femur in the preoperative full-length radiograph can create a false impression of varus or valgus bowing (Fig. 150.47). With extra-articular deformity, the starting position for femoral canal access can be altered slightly to properly position the intramedullary guide. However, when an extra-articular deformity prevents passage of a standard femoral guide, then a modified (shorter) intramedullary alignment rod may be used, provided that the distal segment of the femoral canal that serves as a reference is oriented to achieve proper component alignment. A disadvantage of intramedullary guides is that if the angle of entry or the starting point into the canal is incorrect, the intramedullary rod may contact the femoral cortices rather than pass directly into the center of the diaphysis (see Fig. 150.34). If the rod contacts the lateral cortex, the valgus angle may be reduced, and if the medial cortex is contacted, the valgus angle may be increased.

Depending on the particular instrument system and arthritic pattern, an intramedullary rod may cause the distal femoral cutting block to contact the medial (valgus knee) or the lateral (varus knee) condyle first. If attempts are made to fully seat the

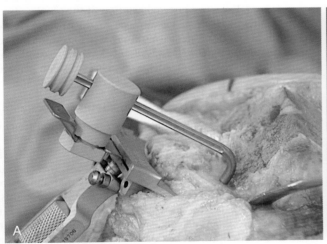
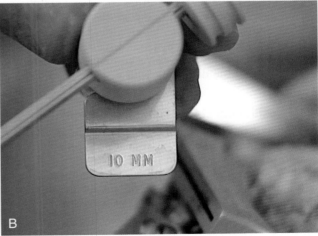

FIG 150.46 (A) Intraoperative photo of the stylus used to determine the amount of proximal tibial bone resection. (B) In this case a 10-mm resection is measured off the least affected articular surface.

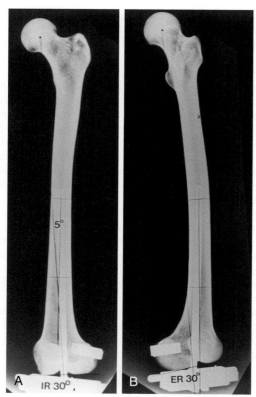

FIG 150.47 Radiographs of femur in (A) internal and (B) external rotation. It can be seen that internal rotation is perceived as medial bowing, and external rotation as lateral bowing. This is a normal femur, and the effect would be accentuated if the femur had excessive anterior bowing.

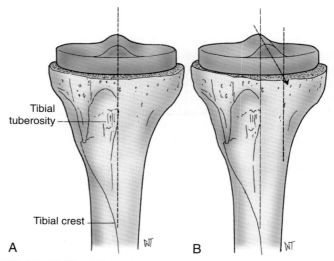

FIG 150.48 The Tibial Component Should Be Aligned With the Tibial Tubercle (A) Correct position. (B) Tibial component internally rotated on the tibia.

instrumentation on both condyles, errors in the distal femoral cut may occur. For example, in valgus knees (associated with lateral femoral condylar erosion), the distal femoral cutting block attachment typically contacts the medial femoral condyle first. If the surgeon allows the instrumentation to contact both condyles in this situation, the valgus angle of the distal femoral cut will be exaggerated. To avoid such errors, the surgeon must be aware of the arthritic pattern and use the intramedullary guide to establish proper positioning of the distal femoral cutting block, even if the instrumentation contacts only a single condyle (see Fig. 150.13). Asymmetrical distal femoral resections are very common, serving to correct the angular deformity rather than re-create the deformity with a symmetrical bone resection.

Rotational Positioning of Prosthetic Components

Rotational alignment of the femoral component is based most reliably on the epicondylar axis. Rotational positioning of the tibial component can be based on the posterior surface of the cut tibia, the anterior surface of the tibia, the tibial tubercle, and the ankle mortise. Assessment can be done with the knee in flexion, in extension, or in both as the knee is passed through a range of movement with trial components in place.

When the tibial component rotation is determined with the knee flexed, the rotation can be related to the anterior surface of the tibia and to the position of the tibial tubercle, which should lie slightly lateral to the midposition of the component (Fig. 150.48). Reference is then made to the ankle and to the position of the malleoli, which should lie approximately 30 degrees externally rotated to the tibial component position. An alignment rod can be suspended from the tibial guide to view the relationship between the tibial component and the ankle joint. When a symmetrical tibial component is used, some overhang may be noted posterolaterally (Fig. 150.49) because the medial tibial plateau is larger than the lateral; for this reason, we do not favor using the posterior margins of the tibial plateau as alignment landmarks.

Rotational alignment can also be assessed in extension, allowing the tibial component position to be related to the patellar groove of the femoral component, the tibial tubercle, and the ankle mortise. With the femoral trial prosthesis in position, a range of motion is performed and patellar tracking is observed before the final fixation holes for the tibial component are made. Tibial tray malrotation is detrimental to patellar tracking, especially with excessive internal rotation of the tibial component. Excessive internal rotation of the tibial component increases the risk of patellar subluxation.[16] Conversely, excessive external tibial component rotation may also result in abnormal tracking of the patella,[153] as well as a kinematic conflict in the femorotibial articulation, such as notch-cam impingement in a cruciate-substituting design.

Mediolateral Positioning of Prosthetic Components

The mediolateral positioning of both femoral and tibial components is important. In general, components should be positioned anatomically on their respective bones without overhang. Overhang can create pain and predispose to stiffness because of capsular stretching. For prosthesis systems that allow separate sizing of the femur and tibia (interchangeable components), the tibial component selected will normally and precisely coincide with the resected tibial plateau. However, for some cruciate-substituting designs, the option exists for some medial or lateral translation of the tibial component. This option is useful when marginal bony defects exist, to reduce the size of the bony defect (Fig. 150.50). On the femoral side the component ideally should

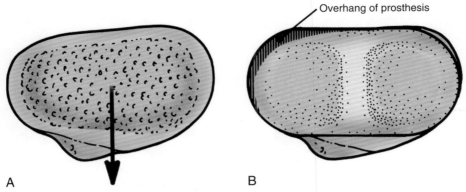

FIG 150.49 (A and B) With a symmetrical component, some degree of posterolateral overhang of the prosthesis is expected.

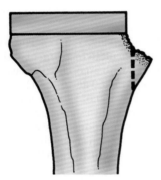

FIG 150.50 Lateralization of the tibial component can be done with cruciate-substituting designs. The tibia is deliberately undersized and is placed at the lateral margin of the tibia. The medial defect is reduced, and overhanging bone can be excised vertically.

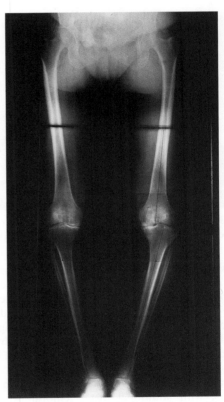

FIG 150.51 A 52-inch radiograph shows the positions of entry holes from preoperative templating. Note that the femoral entry hole is slightly medial, and that the tibial entry hole is slightly lateral.

coincide with the resected margin of the lateral femoral condyle. The femoral components should not be placed medially because of consequent stress on the lateral patellar retinaculum. Many component systems allow for standard and narrow options to match the coronal and sagittal dimensions more exactly.

Authors' Preferred Technique of Femoral Preparation. The entering hole for a femoral intramedullary guide is made approximately 1 cm anterior to the origin of the PCL, although this position can be adjusted to accommodate any abnormalities noted on preoperative radiographs; usually the entry hole is directed slightly medially toward the top of the intercondylar notch (Fig. 150.51). Overdrilling the entry to 12 mm is recommended because of increased intramedullary pressure during intramedullary rod insertion; use of a fluted rather than a round intramedullary rod has also been shown to diminish intramedullary pressure during rod insertion.[169] The distal femoral osteotomy guide is attached to the intramedullary guide at an angle derived from the preoperative radiograph; this is normally 5 to 7 degrees, representing the difference between the mechanical and anatomic axes of thefemur. When intramedullary assessment appears unreliable, an extramedullary rod should be used to confirm that the proposed osteotomy is appropriate. When this step provides conflicting information,

the preoperative radiographs should be re-evaluated; intraoperative radiographic determination of the proper femoral valgus angle is rarely necessary.

The distal femoral osteotomy is made by removing precisely the amount of bone that will be replaced by the femoral prosthesis. Some systems measure this amount from the uninvolved condyle, whereas others key off the medial femoral condyle, regardless of the knee pathology (see Fig. 150.24). In general, the surgeon can make a choice regarding the depth of the distal femoral resection. It is important to keep in mind that any

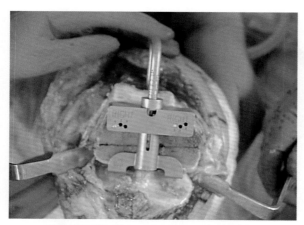

FIG 150.52 Sizing the femoral condyle.

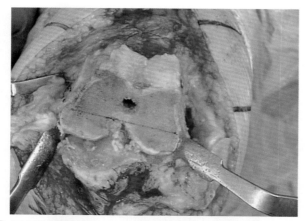

FIG 150.53 Intraoperative photograph demonstrating the epicondylar axis drawn across the cut distal femoral surface.

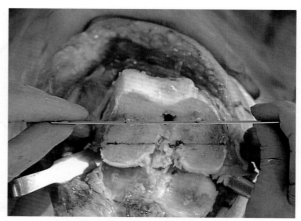

FIG 150.54 The instrumentation is aligned with the epicondylar axis (pins are parallel to the epicondylar axis, as indicated by a ruler placed across them).

resection above that which is replaced by the prosthesis will result in a corresponding elevation of the joint line. After the distal osteotomy is completed, appropriate templates are used to size the distal femur and perform anterior and posterior femoral resections (Fig. 150.52). Rotational alignment is adjusted when the femoral template is positioned by marking the epicondylar axis on the distal femoral surface (Figs. 150.53 and 150.54).

Flexion and extension gaps can be measured with spacers or tensiometers, with additional distal femoral bone removal performed when the extension gap is tighter than the flexion gap (Fig. 150.55A and B). Measured resection of the distal femur will rarely warrant readjustment (typically only with severe flexion contractures). Adjustment cuts should be made before the chamfer cuts (see Fig. 150.55B and C). Chamfer, notch, and fixation holes are made on the distal femur (Fig. 150.56) and the proximal tibia (Fig. 150.57). A flexion contracture due to posterior capsular contracture or a narrow extension gap should be corrected in favor of accepting an overly thin polyethylene liner (Fig. 150.58). Flexion of the femoral component will more readily lead to anterior impingement, and a thinner tibial insert can lead to accelerated polyethylene wear.

Patellar Cuts and Cutting Guides

The goal of the patellar osteotomy is a patellar cut that facilitates central tracking of the patella and minimal tilt while accurately

restoring patellar height (Fig. 150.59). The patellar osteotomy is perhaps the most difficult to instrument and still is often done by freehand technique with an oscillating saw used to resect the articular surface (Figs. 150.60 and 150.61).[131] Reaming or patellar milling devices (Fig. 150.62)[79] used for inset patellar components are also effective in establishing the proper resection level for onset patellar components. Caliper measurements of the patellar size after resection should be equal to or slightly less than the original thickness of the patellar bone (Fig. 150.63).

Patellar resurfacing is generally recommended in patients with osteoarthrosis involving the patellofemoral joint, crystalline disease, or inflammatory arthropathy[166]; however, the patella does not have to be resurfaced. Investigators have reported acceptable results without patellar resurfacing,* especially when the patellar articular cartilage has limited articular wear. On the other hand, extreme patellar articular erosion makes use of a patellar component difficult or impossible in some cases. In these cases, contouring of the residual patellar bone (*patelloplasty*) is performed. TKA without patellar resurfacing in these patients has been reported with satisfactory results on short-term follow-up.[138,166] However, a study with follow-up at 8.5 years on nonresurfaced patellae showed progressive patellofemoral arthritis and maltracking in 40% of patients studied.[195]

Prospective, randomized trials have supported patellar resurfacing. Waters and Bentley[218] randomized 514 primary TKAs to have the patella resurfaced or retained. The incidence of anterior knee pain was significantly higher in the nonresurfacing group (25.1%) as compared with the resurfaced group (5.3%), and 10 of 11 patients undergoing secondary resurfacing for anterior knee pain experienced complete relief. A prospective randomized study by Wood et al.[228] also showed a significant difference in anterior knee pain between resurfaced and nonresurfaced groups, although 10% of patients in the resurfacing group underwent a revision or reoperation involving the patellofemoral joint, as compared with 12% in the nonresurfacing group.

Lug or fixation holes are made into the patella. Most designs currently favor 3- to 4-mm holes placed in a triangular fashion

*References 11, 12, 19, 20, and 138.

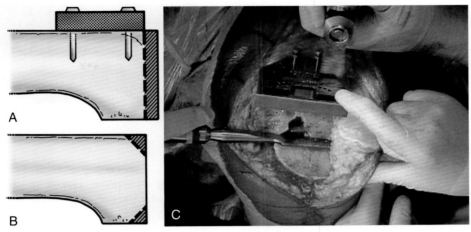

FIG 150.55 (A) Femoral recutting should be done before the chamfer cuts are made—an important reason for incorporating spacers into the system. It is simple to remove 2 to 3 mm from the end of the distal femur. (B) When the femur has been sculpted to receive the prosthesis, recutting is much more complex. (C) The distal femoral recutter, allowing 2, 3, and 5 mm of additional resection. (The cut tibial surface should be protected.)

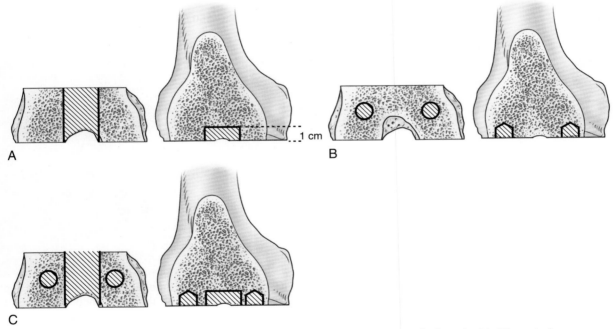

FIG 150.56 Femoral fixation can be enhanced by a central box usually found with (A) posterior-stabilized designs, (B) medial and lateral fixation lugs, or (C) both.

rather than at a larger, centrally placed fixation point (Fig. 150.64). A small, centralized single-peg inset design has also functioned well.[121] A round, dome patellar prosthesis should be positioned to the medial side of the oblong patellar osteotomy and sized by the superoinferior dimension of the bone (Fig. 150.65). The median ridge of the patella is a useful reference point for centering the component, given that the medial facet is shorter and more acutely sloped than the lateral patellar facet. Insetting designs of 28 or 32 mm in diameter have been tried with some success (Fig. 150.66). These designs require central reaming of the patella, leaving the periphery intact. Studies focused on appropriate sizing of patellar inserts have identified

a relationship between patellar thickness and knee flexion in cases where increasing thickness by 2-mm increments led to a 3-degree decrease in intraoperative flexion but did not affect patellar subluxation or tilt.[14] Inadvertent patellar fracture can be avoided by adequately lubricating the reamer, firmly grasping the patella during reaming, and not resecting an excessive amount of patellar bone.

FITTING OF TRIAL COMPONENTS

Fitting of trial components is done when all of the initial bone cuts are completed. Stability and alignment are checked in both

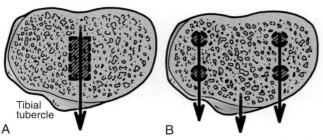

FIG 150.57 (A) Alignment of the tibial component is projected at a point slightly medial to the tibial tubercle. (B) Alignment of a symmetrical component with the posterior margin of the tibial plateau usually will result in some internal rotation of the tibial component. One should err on the side of external rotation.

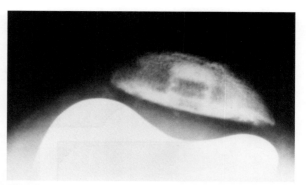

FIG 150.59 Radiograph shows a patellar component with "ideal" patellar tracking, orientation, and thickness.

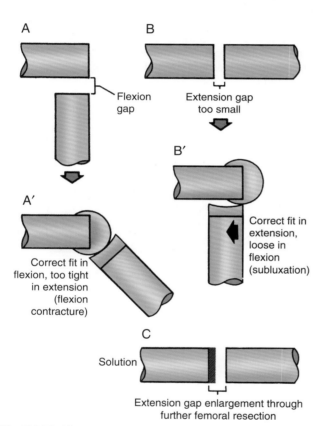

FIG 150.58 Unequal gap size is a frequent technical error. When the extension gap is too small, the knee will not fully extend; if a thinner tibial component is used, the prosthesis will be too loose in flexion. The solution is to excise more bone from the distal femur.

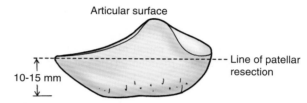

FIG 150.60 The line of patellar resection.

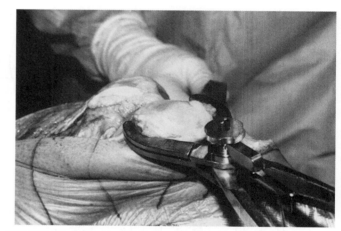

FIG 150.61 A Slotted Patellar Cutting Guide The depth of the resection is selected by the knurl knob. The jaws grasp the patella, and the slots direct the cutting blade.

flexion and extension. For cruciate-substituting designs with balanced gaps, little further adjustment should be required. For cruciate-retaining and measured resection workflows, ligament balancing is done at this stage, using different thicknesses of tibial trial components until satisfactory stability is obtained. When the PCL is spared, particular attention must be paid to the PCL balance. Excessive tightness of the PCL can be detected by noting a tight flexion gap with excessive femoral roll-back. On the contrary, a loose PCL will allow roll-forward of the femur on the tibia as the knee is flexed, resulting in posterior

impingement. PCL recession can be performed by completing intrasubstance ligament lengthening or by elevating the ligament off the tibial insertion. At this stage, if optimal balance cannot be obtained, it is wise to make an intraoperative change to a PCL-substituting design.

Patellar Tracking and Position

When the correct tibial component thickness has been selected, patellar tracking is observed with the patellar component in place. The "no thumb" test is applied: the patella should track with its medial border in contact with the femoral component throughout the range of motion without the surgeon maintaining it in this position manually (Fig. 150.67). It is permissible to take the slack out of the quadriceps tendon by applying

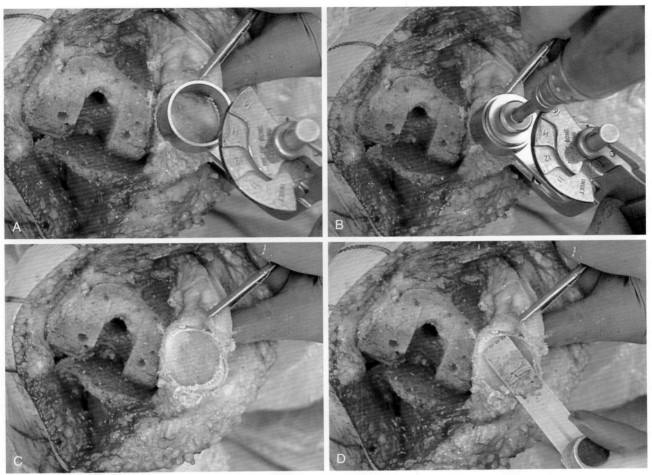

FIG 150.62 Although the reamer is traditionally used for insetting patellar components, it may also be used in creating an accurate flat cut for an onset component. (A) Patellar clamp balanced on the patella. (B) Reamer positioned within the clamp. (C) Patella reamed to desired resection level. (D) Resection completed with the saw blade.

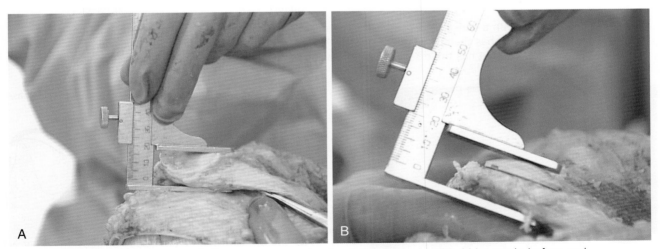

FIG 150.63 (A and B) Caliber measurements of patellar thickness should be made before and after patellar osteotomy. The thickness of the patellar composite should not be increased; rather, a thickness of 2 to 3 mm less is preferred. Between 10 and 15 mm of patellar bone should remain.

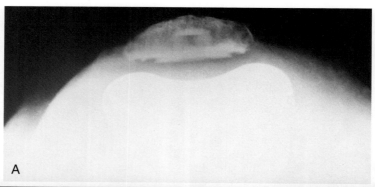

FIG 150.64 (A) Merchant's view radiograph of a well-aligned and well-positioned polyethylene patellar implant. The thickness of the bone polyethylene composite restores the original thickness of the patellar bone. (B) Patellar implants done some years apart. On the left, the patellar cut was made by eye and a single-peg patellar implant was used. The patella is too thick, and the patellar osteotomy is not quite symmetrical. On the right, the arthroplasty was done more recently, a slotted patellar cutting guide was used, and a three-peg patellar implant was inserted. Although there is a slight tilt, the patellar cut is symmetrical, and the patellar thickness is correct.

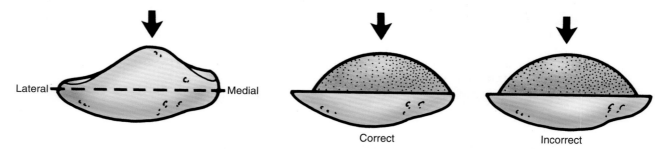

FIG 150.65 With a conventional patellar dome onset on the patella, the component should be medialized. This has the advantage of placing the apex of the dome in the correct position for patellar tracking but has the disadvantage of leaving peripheral lateral bone exposed.

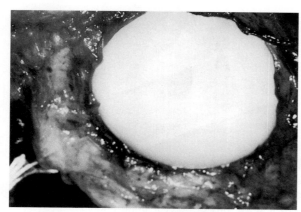

FIG 150.66 Insetting the patella allows greater thickness of polyethylene and use of metal backing. A rim of peripheral exposed bone can impinge against the femur.

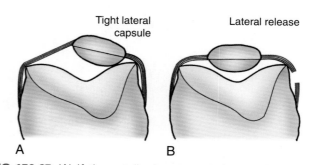

FIG 150.67 (A) If the patella does not track smoothly without a tendency to displace, a lateral release is done (B).

longitudinal tension (Fig. 150.68) or by using a single stitch or towel clip to reapproximate the vastus medialis to the proximal patellar margin. If this suture ruptures or if there is any doubt about patellar tracking, a lateral retinacular release is considered. Because the "no thumb" technique may be a particularly stringent test of patellar tracking, one should consider the status of the tourniquet and other factors that might impact patellar movement during trial testing.

Testing of patellar tracking with the tourniquet deflated will give a better assessment of patellar tracking and may decrease the number of lateral releases performed.[129] Another method of checking lateral retinacular tightness is to subluxate the patellar component over the medial femoral condyle with the knee in extension. If the patella can be subluxated one half of its diameter over the medial femoral condyle, then the retinaculum likely is not too tight. If it is determined that the patella will not track properly when the assessments already mentioned are used, a lateral retinacular release is performed. After the lateral

superior genicular vessels (Fig. 150.69), which can be found distal to the lower border of the vastus lateralis, have been isolated and protected, a lateral retinacular release is done from inside out approximately 1 to 2 cm from the lateral patellar margin (Fig. 150.70).

It should be noted that proper tracking of the patella is dependent upon proper femoral and tibial component position, in addition to soft tissue balance of the patellar retinaculum. If adjustment of the retinacular tension does not improve the patellar balance, then the surgeon should recheck the femoral and tibial component size and position. The patellar position in the sagittal plane is also important, but it is for the most part determined by the bone cuts of the femur and tibia. There is a tendency toward producing patella infera when the joint line is elevated or a thick tibial component is required. Observation of a postoperative patella infera may also be related to fibrosis around the infrapatellar ligament.[116] In the end, tracking of the patella is impacted by every step in the knee

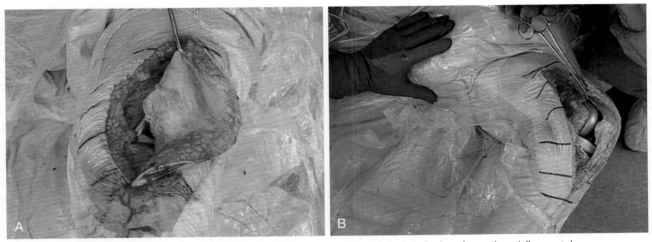

FIG 150.68 (A and B) When patellar traction is assessed, the "rule of no thumb" must be observed, but it is advisable to take longitudinal slack out of the extensor mechanism because, on bringing the knee from flexion into extension, the patellar ligament tends to buckle and can cause a misleading lateral tilt to the patella.

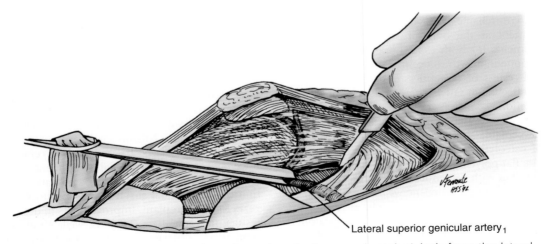

Lateral superior genicular artery₁

FIG 150.69 The patellar release is performed vertically approximately 1 inch from the lateral border of the patella from inside out while the lateral genicular vessels are retracted and preserved. The release may include the lower fibers of the vastus lateralis.

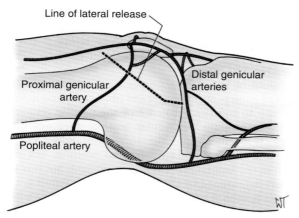

FIG 150.70 The lateral release is done obliquely to preserve the distal genicular arteries.

replacement procedure. If the patella does not track properly, the size, rotation, translation, and balance of every component must be considered and reassessed.

CEMENTED VERSUS UNCEMENTED FIXATION

Interest in cementless total knee implants remains. However, the expense and lack of convincing data on performance has limited widespread adoption of cementless total knee implants to date. In contrast, long-term follow-up studies of cemented TKA have consistently demonstrated successful clinical results and survivorship, particularly when used in combination with a posterior-stabilized design (Fig. 150.71A).[37,48,190,199] Cemented designs afford the benefit that slight incongruities of the bone-prosthesis interface can be eliminated with the cement, whereas cementless prostheses require almost perfect bone cut congruency to optimize bony ingrowth with available materials for cementless fixation. Failure of early cemented TKA designs was most likely a result of excessive prosthetic tibiofemoral constraint, concerns over polymethylmethacrylate degradation, bone-cement interface deterioration, and resultant third-body wear. This experience led to the development of minimally constrained, PCL-retaining TKA designs that featured cementless fixation.[95] The limitation of cementless total knee design has been related to unreliable bone ingrowth secondary to incongruity, movement at the bone-prosthesis interface, or heightened requirements for both exact bone cuts and prosthetic stability for bone ingrowth to occur on the tibial side.

Although initial results of cementless and cemented TKA were comparable, a decline in satisfactory results was observed with cementless fixation.[5,146,152] Berger et al.[17] published in 2001 that his group was abandoning cementless fixation in TKA because of an unacceptable aseptic loosening rate (8%) and a 12% incidence of osteolytic lesions around screw holes. PCL retention with thin, flat polyethylene inserts frequently used in the past in combination with cementless designs created high-contact stresses, resulting in polyethylene wear and osteolysis.[†] However, all failures of cementless TKA cannot be attributed to PCL retention and nonconforming polyethylene inserts alone. Cement fixation appears to provide an advantage in durability

over currently available press-fit techniques. In a prospective comparison of cemented and cementless fixation using the same implant, Duffy et al.[56] demonstrated better durability of femoral and tibial fixation with cemented techniques. At an average follow-up of 10 years, survival rates of cemented prostheses were 94% versus 72% for the uncemented group. Although these results suggest that cementless fixation alone is responsible for a higher failure rate, failure of cementless TKA is probably multifactorial. Knee implants designed for cementless use will require not only rethinking of design and instrumentation but also new materials to improve the chances for bone ingrowth. Highly porous metals may offer this possibility, with recent data suggesting better durability and reliability of bone ingrowth into cementless tibial components.

Retrieval studies of cementless components revealed minimal bone ingrowth, resulting in component loosening and migration. To enhance fixation, pegs were added to the distal femoral component and screws to the tibial component. Although femoral component fixation improved, screw osteolysis was observed under the tibial component, resulting in proximal tibial bone resorption without enhancing bone ingrowth.[63,128] Smooth tracks on the undersurface of the tibial baseplate, screw holes in the tibial baseplate itself, and drill holes in bone serve as conduits that permit polyethylene debris to reach the cancellous tibial surface.[221] Despite dramatic cases of osteolysis with some cementless knee designs, the use of cement in TKA does not eliminate the risk of osteolysis. Cases of severe osteolysis have been observed in cemented TKA.[‡] Osteolysis has been related to polyethylene quality and backside wear issues accelerated by poor polyethylene locking mechanisms in cemented TKA.

Renewed efforts in cementless total knee design have resulted in the development of methods to improve bony ingrowth, including uniform porous coating of the tibial baseplate that is not recessed,[221] use of highly porous tantalum tibial baseplate, and fixation enhanced by hydroxyapatite (HA).[158,159] O'Keefe et al. reported excellent 5-year follow-up results in 125 knees implanted with a partially cemented porus tantalum monoblock implant with uncemented pegs. In this series, no patients were lost to follow-up, and the implant demonstrated 100% survivorship with regard to loosening and no observed osteolysis.[157] Akizuki et al.[4] reported on a series of 32 HA-coated TKAs at 7-year follow-up. By 6 months after implantation, no radiographic clear zones surrounded the prostheses. Patients were doing well clinically, with no reported revisions. One patient died 2 years after implantation of her prosthesis, and autopsy showed bone tissue at 77.7% of the interface. Results reported by Murty et al.[151] on HA-coated femoral components showed 94% survivorship at 7- and 10-year follow-up. Ritter et al's[177] cemented cruciate-retaining total condylar knees and the series of cemented cruciate retaining TKAs described by Scott[188] approached results with cemented posterior-stabilized designs.

More recently, Nilsson et al.[156] reported 2-year follow-up data for a randomized trial comparing cement fixation versus uncemented HA-coated tibial components and recommended the use of uncemented HA-coated implants without screw fixation based on equal survivorship and implant migration at 2 years for each implant. Improvements in design have enhanced results in cementless TKA as well; Whiteside's[220] series of cementless, cruciate-retaining prostheses with conforming

†References 22, 69, 106, 185, and 203.

‡References 32, 82, 162, 167, and 180.

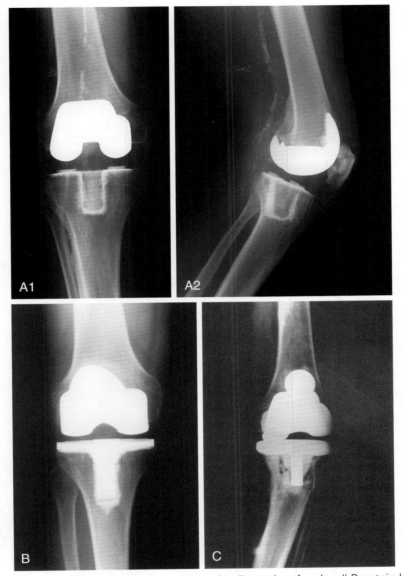

FIG 150.71 (A1 and A2) Anteroposterior and lateral radiographs of an Insall-Burstein I prosthesis at 19-year follow-up. (B) Radiograph of a knee prosthesis that has been correctly cemented. The amount of cement is minimal. This type of cement fixation is obtained by using cement in the doughy stage. (C) Radiograph of a knee prosthesis showing undesirable cement technique. In addition to varus positioning, excessive cement is noted in the proximal tibia and around the stem.

articular surfaces and intramedullary alignment techniques common to posterior-stabilized cemented designs demonstrated outcomes matching those of cemented cruciate-substituting prostheses. Buechel et al.[24] also reported excellent results at 18 years using a cementless mobile-bearing knee design. Although these and more recent articles report promising results with new uncemented implants,[7,37,89] the literature continues to support improved survival of cemented components,[77] and this will be the gold standard by which other techniques are measured.

Cement Technique

Cement fixation is achieved as polymethylmethacrylate penetrates the porous cancellous bony surfaces, creating a mechanical interlock. Pulsatile lavage is used to remove blood, fat, and debris, and proper cleaning of the cancellous bone permits uninhibited penetration of cement.[178] Cement should be applied to bone digitally in the doughy tactile state, which allows for easy handling and manual pressurization (see Fig. 150.71B and C). Insall believed that centrifugation is unnecessary in TKA because the cement layer is thin and air bubbles escape readily. Walker et al.[212] determined that the ideal cement penetration into bone is 3 to 4 mm; however, caution should be exercised in softer rheumatoid bone, where deeper penetration may occur. In contrast, sclerotic surfaces frequently encountered in OA may be drilled. Drilling of bone surfaces is performed with a 2-mm drill and should be limited to no more than 3 to 4 mm in drill depth because deeper cement penetration transfers the bone-cement interface away from the tibial surface into the cancellous bone, where tibial bone strength tends to be less.

MANAGEMENT OF INSTABILITY OR DEFORMITY

Principles

In most arthritic knees, some degree of instability, deformity, contracture, or a combination of these elements is present.[35,102] Deformity and instability can be created by a variety of circumstances resulting in asymmetrical loss of articular cartilage and bone, resulting in collateral, capsular, and cruciate imbalance. Contracture of soft tissues is a secondary change that generally arises as a consequence of trauma or long-standing and severe angular malalignment. Variations in anatomy, such as tibia vara or a diminutive lateral femoral condyle, can also contribute to angular abnormalities that should be corrected at the time of total knee replacement. Although some minor degree of postoperative ligament asymmetry may be tolerated, it is ideal to obtain near-perfect stability, avoiding persistent contracture while accepting only small amounts of laxity through surgical technique.

Although some experts have suggested that residual malalignment is not detrimental to the outcome of TKA,[41,65,179,198] other authors have demonstrated that malalignment has a negative influence on long-term results of TKA.[§] These investigations suggest that the most important factor for maintaining satisfactory long-term outcome in TKA is anatomic alignment, which depends significantly on ligamentous balance and accurate bone resection. Although bone cuts can be made to establish anatomic alignment, proper ligamentous balance is required to maintain alignment throughout the range of motion and dynamic stability under loading conditions. In a polyethylene retrieval study, Wasielewski et al.[215] noted that increased wear occurred when preoperative varus or valgus was present. Polyethylene wear and cold flow tended to be greater in the tightest prearthroplasty compartment, most frequently when ligament releases were inadequate.

Instability of the arthritic knee may be viewed as a fixed deformity or correctable deformity. A correctable deformity is a result of erosion of cartilage or bone without associated adaptive ligamentous changes. This type of deformity is common in early arthritis of the knee and can be corrected under active reciprocal stress during physical examination. Standard surgical techniques that create symmetrical flexion and extension gaps are typically adequate to restore ligamentous balance (Fig. 150.72) in a correctable deformity. Asymmetrical instability with a fixed deformity is more common in advanced knee arthritis, occurring when bone and cartilage loss is associated with adaptive ligamentous change (Figs. 150.73 and 150.74). These adaptive changes present as a continuum of deformity and may include contracture on the concave side of the joint with or without associated ligament laxity on the convex side of the deformed joint. Standard surgical technique and prosthesis spacing may prove inadequate in balancing fixed ligament changes or ligament deficiency. Ligament release and ligament balancing are required to address contractures, and ligament reconstruction or increased articular constraint may be needed to manage advanced deformity.

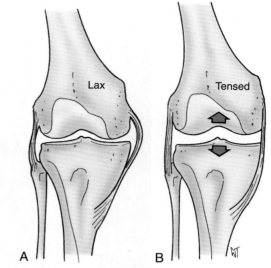

FIG 150.72 Symmetrical Instability (A) The ligaments, although lax, are of equal length. (B) Both alignment and stability are restored by tensioning the ligaments.

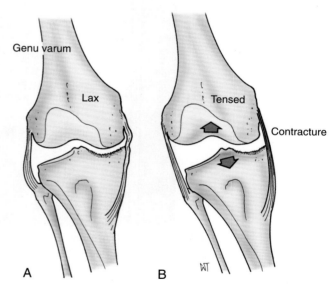

FIG 150.73 Asymmetrical instability in varus. The medial ligament is shorter than the lateral ligament. Varus knee with fixed deformity. (A) Knee in varus with lax medial ligament. (B) Varus knee with fixed contracture under tension demonstrates asymmetric opening of the joint due to a contracted medial ligament.

Operative management of a contracture cannot be accomplished by bone cuts alone. Although postoperative bracing has been described for the management of instability following TKA, it is seldom optimal. Bracing is a treatment for ligament instability, not a treatment for ligament contracture. Two surgical methods have been described for correction of a fixed deformity. The first technique is a controlled ligament release from the contracted concave side of the deformity; the second technique consists of ligament advancement on the attenuated convex side. Ligament release of the contracted structures is adequate for correction of most deformities, although there are

---

§References 25, 81, 92, 93, 103, 127, 147, 175, 209, and 226.

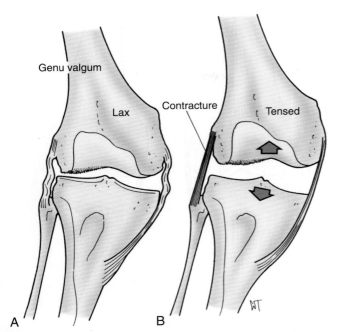

FIG 150.74 Asymmetrical instability in valgus. (A) Knee in valgus with lax ligament. (B) Under tension, the knee opens asymmetrically due to the contracted lateral ligament structures.

limits to the amount of correction that can be gained with ligament release. The challenge is that one cannot balance a knee simply by releasing the contracted side of the knee when the opposing ligaments are stretched to the point of being incompetent. When a ligament is incompetent, repair of the incompetent ligament or use of a more constrained knee design will be required. When extreme deformity cannot be balanced with controlled ligament release, options for treatment include bracing of instability, reconstruction of the incompetent ligament, and adding increased articular constraint (such as a constrained condylar knee or hinged implant) that provides for collateral ligament substitution (Figs. 150.75 to 150.77).

Varus Deformity

Pathophysiology. Varus deformity is defined as any preoperative femorotibial angle less than naturally occurring anatomic valgus. This definition is not absolute because of the variability of human limb alignment; in patients with habitual genu varum, this malalignment is typically exaggerated. In general, TKA in patients with arthritis and habitual genu varum involves realignment to physiologic valgus. Moderate-to-severe varus has been arbitrarily defined as greater than 15 to 20 degrees of varus deviation from the mechanical axis.[123,205]

Development of varus instability typically follows a sequence with loss of medial compartment bone and cartilage imparting

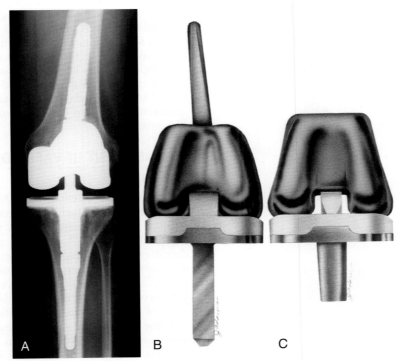

FIG 150.75 Constrained Condylar Knee Prosthesis (A) Radiograph. (B) The constrained condylar device uses an unlinked constrained design that places limitations on varus/valgus deflection, anteroposterior displacement, and rotation within the flexion-extension axis of the knee. Restriction of varus/valgus deflection and rotation is provided by a large tibial spine within an intracondylar femoral box, while posterior subluxation is prevented by engagement of the spine on the femoral cam. (C) Posterior-stabilized device. Nonlinked, semiconstrained posterior-stabilized devices prevent posterior subluxation via a tibial spine that engages a femoral cam. Slight rotational constraint is afforded by the degree of conformity of the femorotibial articulation. (B and C, From Scott WN (ed): *The knee,* vol 2, St Louis, MO, 1994, Mosby–Year Book, p 1308.)

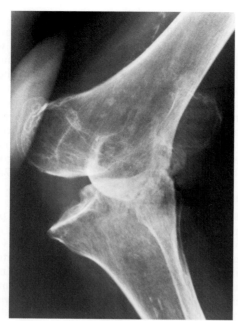

FIG 150.76 Radiograph of a Very Unstable Valgus Knee This degree of ligamentous instability cannot be managed by any type of ligament release. Reconstruction will involve a medial ligament tightening procedure or a constrained prosthesis.

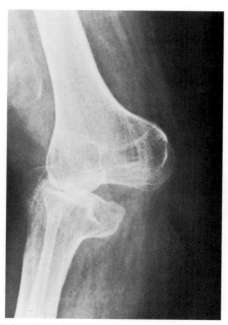

FIG 150.77 In this valgus knee, although the medial ligament is not absent, it is so elongated that soft tissue balancing by lateral release is impractical. This is an indication for a constrained prosthesis.

a varus moment to the joint. The varus moment combined with the attendant periarticular inflammation associated with the arthritic process ultimately results in pathologic fibrosis and contracture of the MCL. Bony deficits in a varus knee typically occur on the medial tibial plateau, although both the medial tibia and the femur may develop deficits in advanced disease.

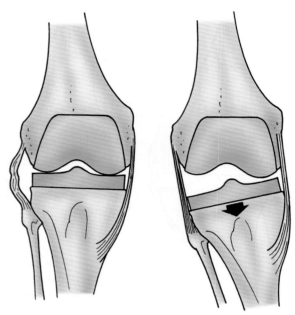

FIG 150.78 The medial ligament was not released; hence, asymmetrical instability remains.

The MCL contracture is worsened by medial osteoarthritic overgrowth pressing outward from the joint on the ligament, thereby causing relative shortening of the MCL. Eventually, the effect of contracture of the MCL is a fixed varus deformity (Fig. 150.78; see also Fig. 150.73). Simultaneously, adaptive elongation may occur in the LCL and lateral capsule, resulting in attenuation of these lateral soft tissue structures. This combination of elements results in a *lateral thrust* or *varus thrust* of the knee that is observed during the stance phase of walking. Varus contracture may also be associated with a flexion contracture (described later).

MANAGEMENT OF VARUS DEFORMITY

Principles

MCL release is essential to achieve soft balance in TKA with fixed varus deformity. Several authors have shown that residual varus deformity in TKA increases the failure rate.** Sambatakakis et al.[183] described a radiographic *wedge sign* characteristic of incompletely corrected varus deformity hinging on a tight medial ligament; this finding has been confirmed by Laskin[123] and correlates with Insall's observation that most TKA failures occur because of medial tibial collapse related to recurrence of the preoperative deformity.

Some studies have suggested that moderate-to-severe varus deformity warrants PCL resection because of its contribution to varus malalignment. Alexiades et al.[6] showed that without the counterbalance of the ACL, the PCL tends to contract. Dennis et al.[47] demonstrated that retaining the PCL may not result in the desired femoral roll-back, nor does it prevent condylar lift-off during knee flexion. Laskin et al.[123,124] (Fig. 150.79) reported that for fixed varus deformities exceeding 15 degrees, the best results in terms of pain relief, correction, and

---

**References 25, 92, 93, 103, 127, 147, 209, 215, and 226.

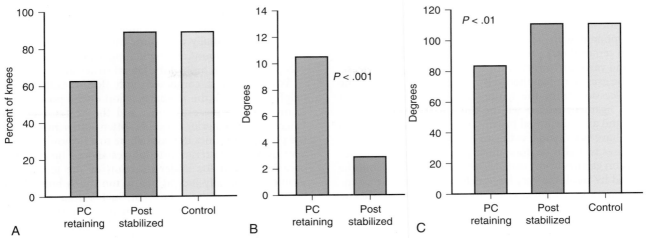

FIG 150.79 Bar graphs showing (A) percentage of knees accurately aligned, (B) residual flexion contracture (average), and (C) average range of motion in knees with greater than 15 degrees of fixed varus deformity. The parameters studied were equivalent to those for a group of control knees (without significant deformity) in which a cruciate-retaining prosthesis was used. Cruciate retention in deformed knees led to a less satisfactory correction of alignment and flexion contracture and an inferior range of motion. *PC*, Posterior cruciate.

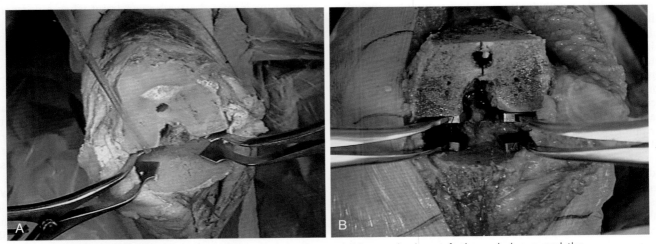

FIG 150.80 (A and B) Laminar spreaders are useful in monitoring soft tissue balance and the performance of ligament releases.

range of motion are obtained by excision of the PCL and use of a cruciate-substituting prosthesis. Teeny et al.[205] noted that 40% of knees with preoperative varus tended to remain in varus; their series included more than 50% of knees with cruciate-retaining prostheses. Both Laskin[123] and Teeny et al.[205] observed that functional outcomes of varus knees approached but did not equal the results of nondeformed knees.

Conversely, Ritter et al.[173] reported on his group's series of 82 patients undergoing PCL-retaining TKA with greater than or equal to 20 degrees of preoperative deformity, both varus and valgus. Their results showed no difference in knee score, postoperative alignment, or revision rate as compared with a group of patients with smaller preoperative deformity. However, longer follow-up did correlate the risk of failure with the presence of preoperative deformity. Similarly, Kubiak et al.[120] reported on a series of cruciate-retaining TKAs with at least 15 degrees of preoperative coronal plane deformity that showed

93% revision-free survival at 10 years. Both of these studies conclude that with proper balancing of the soft tissues, a PCL-retaining TKA provides very good long-term outcomes, whereas not achieving the best outcomes reported in cohorts of patients with lesser deformity.

Technique

Ligament balance is achieved by progressively releasing the medial soft tissues until they reach the length of the lateral ligamentous structures. The extent of the release can be monitored by periodically inserting lamina spreaders (Fig. 150.80), spacer blocks, or using a ligament tensiometer to judge alignment with the aligning rod or plumb line. The endpoint of the release is a stable position in which a plumb line will extend from the hip through the center of the knee to the ankle joint. Computer navigation of TKA also allows the possibility of a real-time assessment of knee alignment and balance during the course of a ligament release. Component placement can also affect angular deformity. Scott has described the use of a downsized tibial component with lateral translation of the component, along with removal of a portion of the medial tibial plateau to correct rigid varus deformity. If the PCL is tethering the release, it should be excised or lengthened by posterior release from the tibia or recession from the femur. In a measured resection technique, ligament release will be done partially during the approach and after the initial proximal tibial and distal femoral bone cuts have been made; with gap balancing technique, ligament releases will also be done during the approach and after the extension gap has been created. The gap balancing technique was favored by Insall for very large deformities because extension laxity in the knee joint after release may occasionally dictate an under-resection of the distal femur to accurately balance the knee (Fig. 150.81). A full MCL release not only will correct fixed varus but also will open the medial space in flexion (whereas the normal knee in flexion has more lateral than medial laxity). Flexion gap symmetry is influenced by medial release. Attention to the importance of gap balancing and joint line preservation dictates that femoral component rotational alignment should be determined relative to both femoral anatomy and ligament balance.

The medial release (Fig. 150.82) is done in steps by first removing medial osteophytes from the femur and tibia, including the protruding flare of the tibial plateau, and raising a sleeve of soft tissue from the upper medial tibia that is allowed to slide proximally. The sleeve consists of periosteum, deep medial ligament, superficial medial ligament, and insertion of the pes anserinus tendons. More posterior, at the joint surface, the sleeve is continuous with the semimembranosus insertion and the posterior capsule. Distally, the release may include the deep fascia investing soleus and popliteus muscles. The sleeve is made by stripping the periosteum medially from the tibia 10 to 15 cm distal to the standard arthrotomy. The knee is flexed, and the tibia is progressively externally rotated to gain posterior access. The distal attachment of the superficial medial ligament can be left intact in moderate deformities. When this is not enough, the release is continued posteriorly and distally by further subperiosteal stripping of the superficial fibers of the MCL. Thereby, correction of deformity occurs in a graduated manner and is aided by the intermittent stretching action of a medial laminar spreader. With progressive release, no discontinuity between the medial soft tissue structures is noted, but rather a progressive

separation of the periosteal layer from the tibia at a point distal to the MCL attachment to the tibia (Fig. 150.83). The result is balancing, potentially with some minor overall lengthening of the limb (the amount of lengthening depends on the degree of preoperative stretching of the lateral structures).

When varus is combined with flexion contracture, it is helpful to elevate the medial portion of the posterior capsule from both the posterior tibia and the posteromedial femur. Laterally, the posterior capsule is often sufficiently stretched to the point that it does not contribute to a flexion contracture in a varus knee. Posterior osteophytes should be removed. The occasional need for under-resection of the femur and tibia should be carefully judged before too much bone is removed because bone can always be recut. Such a situation may arise in a varus knee when the lateral structures are stretched and the medial structures are released to balance those structures, thereby increasing the height of the extension gap. When proper release and balancing is performed, mobilization can be started immediately.

Ligament advancement procedures have also been described to correct varus deformity.[205] In the rare case when varus knees cannot be fully corrected with medial release and are associated with lateral laxity, consideration may be given to lateral ligament reconstruction. This is a rare situation, with most surgeons opting for increased articular constraint when a degenerative ligament is chronically incompetent.

ASYMMETRICAL VALGUS INSTABILITY

Pathophysiology

Valgus deformity is defined as malalignment exceeding natural femorotibial valgus orientation, typically greater than 7 to 10 degrees.[144,200,219] Krackow et al. classified valgus deformity into three distinct types.[118] Type I involves lateral femoral bone loss, lateral soft tissue contracture, and intact medial soft tissues. Type II is type I with lengthened medial soft tissues. Type III is severe valgus deformity with malpositioning of the proximal tibial joint line (eg, secondary to high tibial osteotomy).

In the valgus knee the lateral soft tissue structures, including the LCL, ITB, and lateral capsule, contract, while the medial soft tissues become stretched. The lateral femoral condyle has been shown to be frequently dysplastic in the valgus deformity; therefore most of the bony deficit occurs on the femoral side.[200]

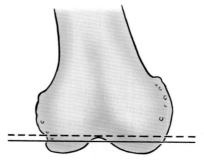 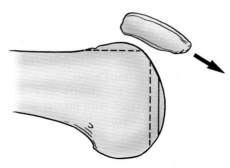

FIG 150.81 In cases with considerable ligamentous laxity, an under-resection of the distal femur may be preferable. The standard femoral resection will necessitate a thicker tibial component to take up the slack in the soft tissues and may cause distal migration of the patella. By under-resecting the femur, desirable patellar position is maintained.

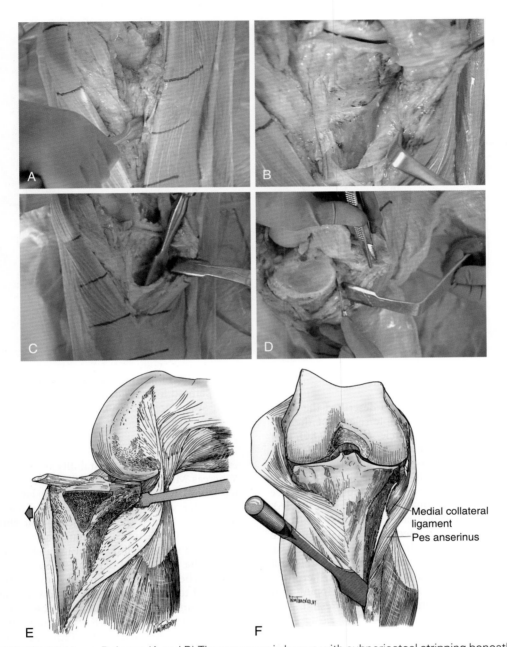

FIG 150.82 Varus Release (A and B) The exposure is begun with subperiosteal stripping beneath the superficial MCL. (C) Completed release. Only the superficial MCL remains intact, but this too can become detached if necessary. (D) The tibia is externally rotated with a complete posteromedial release. (E) Graphic illustration demonstrating complete release of the deep and superficial MCL, and the semimembranous. (F) Subperiosteal elevation of the MCL and pes anserinus tendon completes the full medial release.

However, in advanced disease, cartilage and bone erosion may also be observed on the tibial side. In long-standing deformity, lateral contracture and medial lengthening become permanent (see Fig. 150.74). This combination of pathologies may result in a *medial thrust* or scissoring during gait. Similar to varus deformities, valgus contractures may be associated with a flexion contracture or occasionally recurvatum in paralytic cases. A fixed external rotation deformity often accompanies valgus instability, particularly in patients with inflammatory arthritis.

Management

Principles. Valgus release traditionally has been performed by elevating the lateral capsule, LCL, arcuate ligament, popliteus tendon, lateral femoral periosteum, distal ITB, and adjacent lateral intermuscular septum from their bony attachments. Except for the ITB, release is performed from the lateral femoral condyle; the ITB is released from Gerdy's tubercle. Because desired postoperative alignment is physiologic valgus, some degree of lateral laxity after an extensive lateral release is typically well tolerated. The sequence of lateral release is still guided

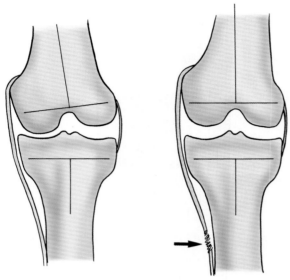

FIG 150.83 The ideal MCL release occurs distal to the insertion of the ligament into the tibia through the periosteum and in continuity with the MCL. At this level a controlled release is obtained. *Arrow* indicates the level of the MCL release described.

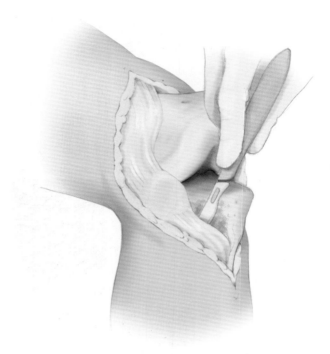

FIG 150.84 First Stage of a Lateral Release The iliotibial band is separated from its attachment to Gerdy's tubercle and capsular attachments from the lateral margin of the tibia.

by individual surgeon preference.[††] Insall described the management of lesser deformities with simple release of the ITB from its insertion on Gerdy's tubercle (Fig. 150.84). For moderate-to-severe fixed deformities, the lateral femoral condyle would be stripped of its soft tissue attachments proximally for about 9 cm, and at this level the periosteum, the iliotibial tract, and the lateral intramuscular septum would be transversely divided from inside out (Figs. 150.85 and 150.86). Any part of the lateral intramuscular septum that remained attached to the distal femur was divided longitudinally until the entire flap was free to slide. Although such an extensive release generally corrects any severity of deformity, posterolateral flexion instability may occur postoperatively.[101,144] Furthermore, case reports have described extensive soft tissue stripping that has devascularized the lateral femoral condyle, resulting in osteonecrosis.

Because of the risk of posterolateral instability (and osteonecrosis) following extensive soft tissue stripping from the lateral femoral condyle, stab-incision[144] and pie-crusting techniques were developed and have become the methods of choice. These techniques permit a graduated intra-articular release of the posterolateral capsule and ITB. Although both techniques involve transverse punctures (pie-crusting) of the ITB well above the joint line and some degree of transverse release of the posterolateral capsule, the stab-incision technique includes a more extensive transverse release of the arcuate complex immediately above the joint line and posterior to the ITB (Fig. 150.87). Releasing at the joint line leaves only the LCL for lateral restraint; perforations of the lateral capsule and ITB above the joint line in combination with a limited transverse posterolateral capsular release maintain greater soft tissue continuity. Both techniques typically allow for preservation of the popliteus

tendon, affording greater stability to the posterolateral corner. Whereas Miyasaka et al.[144] observed a 24% incidence of posterolateral instability with extensive lateral femoral condylar release for valgus deformity, by using the stab-incision technique they limited the incidence to 6%, similar to what Insall described. Correction of valgus deformity in TKA has been associated with patellofemoral instability due to lateral tethering of the patella and peroneal palsy due to stretching of the nerve. The incidence of patellofemoral instability has been reported to be as high as 4%[126]; however, the incidence using the stab-incision technique and preserving the popliteus has been reported as low as 0%.[144] Although the overall incidence of peroneal nerve palsy after TKA has been estimated as less than 1%, the incidence in valgus knees has been reported at 3% to 4%.[118,200] In a recent investigation using the stab-incision technique, no cases of peroneal nerve compromise were observed.[144] Clinical outcomes in patient series in which the pie-crusting technique has been used to correct valgus deformity in TKA have shown positive results. Clarke et al.[34] reported excellent Knee Society scores and range of motion and no cases of postoperative instability in a series of 24 patients who underwent TKA with a valgus preoperative deformity corrected with the pie-crusting technique. Aglietti et al.[2] reported the 5-year follow-up on 53 patients who underwent correction of valgus deformity at the time of TKA using the pie-crusting technique. Coronal alignment was within 5 degrees of neutral in 96% of knees; one patient had transient peroneal nerve palsy, one patient had varus instability, and no revisions were reported.

In older patients and in those with low physical demands, the use of articular constraint may avoid postoperative morbidity. In Insall's series of primary constrained implants (with up

[††]References 1, 22, 110, 126, 144, 200, and 219.

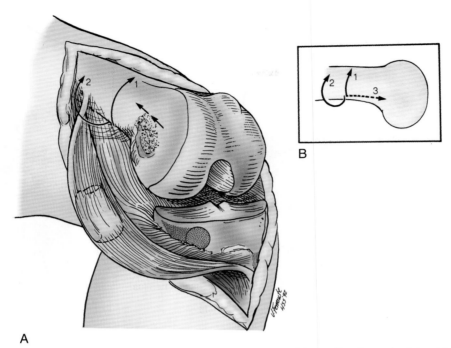

FIG 150.85 (A) Additional stages of lateral release include raising a flap from the lateral femoral condyle to a point 3 inches proximal to the joint. (B) The periosteum is incised transversely *(1)*; the lateral intramuscular septum and the proximal iliotibial tract are divided transversely at the same level *(2)*; and the remaining distal attachment of the lateral intramuscular septum is divided vertically and separated from the femur *(3)*.

to 10 years of follow-up), uniform success has been reported without prosthetic loosening, indicating that this approach may be a reasonable option in selected cases.

Technique

Pie-crusting method (Insall). The knee is approached through a standard midline incision and a standard medial parapatellar capsular approach. Femoral and tibial bone cuts are made to gain access and to create congruent surfaces to assess gap symmetry. Because erosion occurs on the lateral femoral condyle in long-standing valgus malalignment, bone resection from the lateral condyle is often minimal. Appropriate femoral rotation is imperative to ensure proper balancing in flexion. Referencing from the posterior condyles often is not reliable because of posterior condylar erosion. Insall believed that the PCL often contributed to the deformity, which led him to recommend a posterior-stabilized design for valgus knees.[101,144] Other studies have reported good outcome in valgus TKA with preservation of the PCL and appropriate soft tissue balancing. The posterolateral capsule and arcuate complex lateral to the popliteus are cut transversely at the level of the tibial cut or just below and parallel to the popliteus tendon, and titrated with intra-articular and extra-articular releases of the lateral capsule at the tibial insertion and the ITB at Gerdy's tubercle are performed using a knife blade. This technique is performed with a moderate amount of stress in the lateral compartment, using a laminar spreader or ligament tensiometer. Multiple stab incisions are made in the contracted lateral soft tissues (particularly the ITB and the portion of the arcuate complex below the popliteus that tends to tether the popliteus tendon) within and above the joint until the deformity is corrected (see Fig. 150.87A and B). Spacer

blocks are frequently used to check the balance to avoid overcorrection. As noted previously, the popliteus and the LCL are preserved if possible to limit posterolateral instability in flexion. A cadaver study by Mihalko and Krackow[142] highlights the risk of injury to the peroneal nerve during this technique. In their study the peroneal nerve was found to be between 6 and 12 mm (less than the depth of a no. 11 blade [16 mm]) from the surface of the posterolateral corner in full extension.

Ligament advancement or tightening. Ligament advancement or tightening is rare in TKA. Krackow[117] has described techniques for ligament tightening for both medial and lateral soft tissues and estimates that he has performed them in 1% to 2% of knee replacements. In the correction of a valgus knee, a lateral ligament release may allow overlengthening of perhaps 5 mm to compensate for 5 mm of stretching of the MCL (Fig. 150.88). However, when MCL elongation is 10 mm or greater, it simply is not possible to achieve this much stretching by lateral release alone. The same argument can be applied to varus deformities, although there are differences (notably that there is no counterpart to the peroneal nerve). It is possible to overlengthen the medial side a greater extent and, provided axial alignment is correct, some degree of lateral laxity is tolerable. As a rule of thumb, lateral laxity is acceptable provided the knee alignment cannot be passively brought into varus with the knee extended. The MCL can be tightened by proximal or distal advancement. This type of soft tissue reconstruction may have merit as an alternative to using increased articular constraint in younger patients. In support of Krackow's methods, Healy et al.[88] reported success with lateral soft tissue release and proximal MCL advancement with bone plug recession into the medial femoral condyle to correct valgus deformity in a small

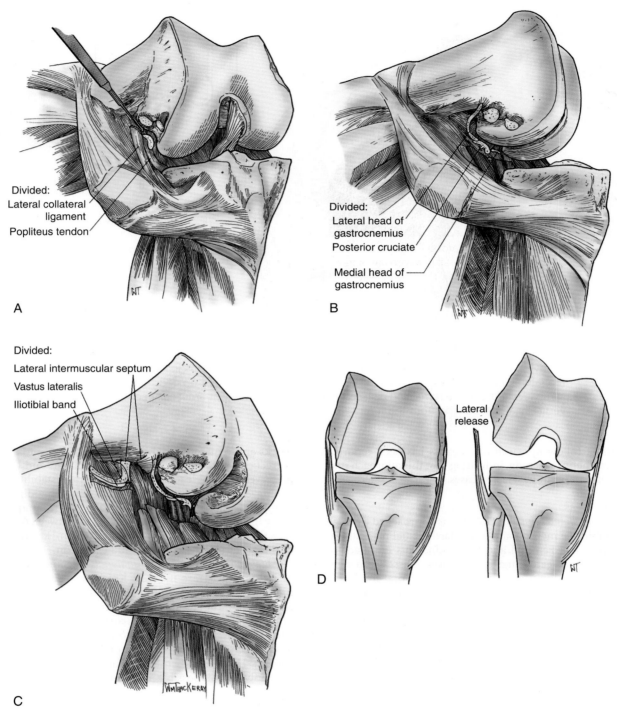

FIG 150.86 (A to C) Valgus release is done on the femur, completely releasing the soft tissues from the lateral femoral condyle and, if necessary, transversely dividing the iliotibial band. (D) After lateral release for the correction of valgus, the knee is always inherently unstable in flexion. A lateral rotary instability may develop that will be exacerbated if any malrotation of the tibial component occurs.

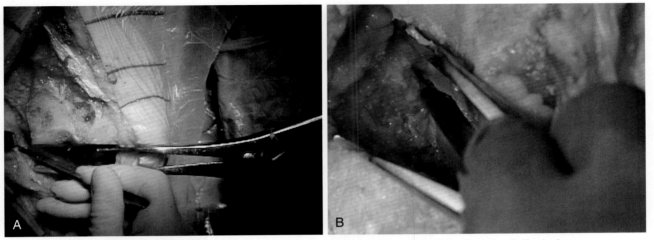

FIG 150.87 Intraoperative Photo of Lateral Release Using the "Pie-Crusting" Technique (A) Joint distracted using a laminar spreader placed medially. (B) Close-up view of multiple intra-articular punctures in the contracted lateral soft tissues proximal to the joint line.

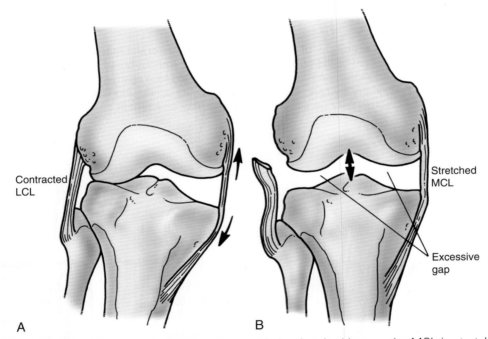

FIG 150.88 (A and B) There are limits to ligament balancing. In this case the MCL is stretched beyond its normal length, and after lateral release, the knee will be distracted abnormally. Stabilizing this knee with thicker components involves actual lengthening of the limb, and there are clearly limits to how much lengthening can be tolerated without damage to the neurovascular structures. *LCL,* Lateral collateral ligament; *MCL,* medial collateral ligament.

group of patients. In lower-demand patients, for whom long-term concerns for articular surface breakdown is less, the use of increased articular constraint is also an option.

   Medial and lateral proximal advancement. Krackow[117] has described a method whereby the proximal attachment of the MCL to the medial femoral epicondyle is detached from the bone over a fairly wide area (Fig. 150.89). The flap of tissue is advanced to a more proximal and slightly anterior position. It is secured by passing an interlocking stitch through the flap and tying this tightly over a proximally placed screw and washer,

with further augmentation using a staple placed into the area of the original femoral condyle (Fig. 150.90). Engh and Ammeen[61] have described the use of an epicondylar osteotomy with advancement of a ligament and bone block for correction of varus deformities; Healy's method[88] involves recession of the MCL attachment in its anatomic position at the medial femoral condyle rather than translocation of the proximal ligament (Fig. 150.91). The recessed proximal bone plug is secured over a bony bridge or button on the lateral side. For lax lateral structures, Krackow's method has been described for the varus knee;

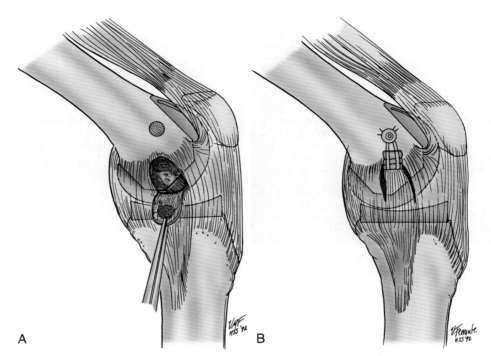

FIG 150.89 Krackow Technique of Proximal Medial Collateral Ligament Advancement
(A) The proximal attachment of the MCL is removed en bloc without bone. A screw and washer
are placed proximal and slightly anterior. (B) Using the locking loop ligament fixation suture, the
MCL is tightened proximally by tying the sutures around the screw and washer, which is then
tightened. A second screw may be placed through the new attachment of the MCL.

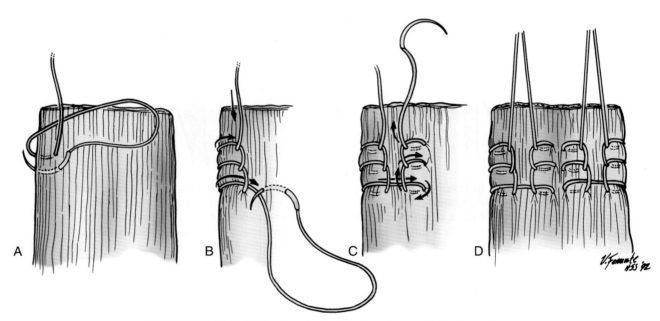

FIG 150.90 (A to D) Krackow's locking loop ligament fixation suture.

reports describing Healy's method of proximal recession of the LCL are not available.

FLEXION CONTRACTURE

Pathophysiology

Flexion contractures involve the posterior capsule, the PCL, and the musculotendinous units crossing the posterior aspect of the knee joint. In OA the deformity is typically limited to soft tissue

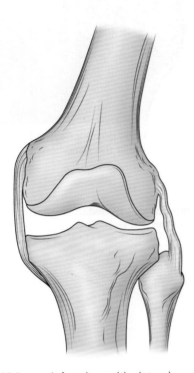

FIG 150.91 Valgus deformity with lateral contracture and medial laxity. (Illustration redrawn from Lahey Clinic, Burlington, Massachusetts.)

contracture associated with posterior compartment osteophytes (Fig. 150.92), whereas in inflammatory arthritis, flexion contracture may result in significant posterior femoral condylar erosion (Fig. 150.93). Extreme posterior femoral condylar erosion generally occurs in patients who have been unable to walk and have developed fixed flexion deformities that may exceed 90 degrees. Because of posterior condylar erosion, in addition to posterior capsular contracture, flexion contracture may be paradoxically associated with flexion instability. This situation represents a considerable technical challenge and typically warrants application of revision TKA principles.

Several authors have suggested that full intraoperative correction of flexion contractures in TKA is not essential because postoperative correction is possible[72,141,204] and clinical outcome is not affected by residual flexion contractures of up to 30 degrees.[141,206] In contrast, Firestone et al.[72] reported that if a flexion contracture remains at the completion of TKA, then the residual deformity will persist and worsen with time, especially if the PCL is preserved. Ritter et al. similarly found that a postoperative flexion contracture was associated with poorer postoperative outcomes. The current consensus among knee surgeons is that flexion contractures should be corrected to the maximum extent possible at the time of TKA.

Technique for Release of Flexion Contracture

Posterior capsular release should be done after the bone cuts. Until the bone cuts are made, posterior visualization is impeded by the posterior femoral condyles. Initially, distal femoral and proximal tibial bone cuts should be conservative. Small flexion contractures can be reduced by removal of posterior osteophytes and elevation of the posterior capsule (Fig. 150.94).[204,206] Correction by bone resection from the distal femur alone unbalances the collateral ligaments so that stability in extension is provided by the tight posterior capsule, resulting in kinematic abnormalities. Posterior capsulotomy is the preferred method for moderate-to-severe contractures and should be performed with the knee flexed. First, the shortened posterior capsule is elevated from the central posterior aspect of the femur at the top of the intercondylar notch. Next, the medial and lateral capsule is elevated in a subperiosteal plane off the back of the

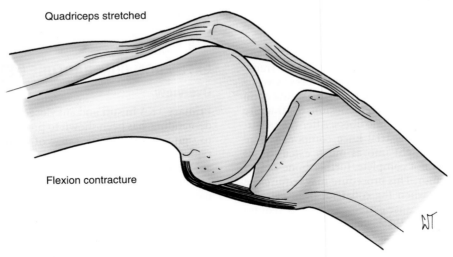

Quadriceps stretched

Flexion contracture

FIG 150.92 In a flexion contracture, the posterior capsule is shortened and adherent.

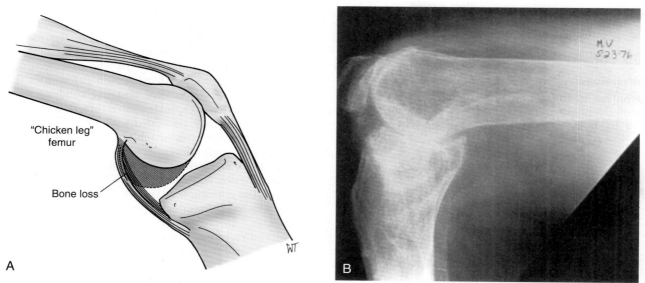

FIG 150.93 (A) In rheumatoid arthritis, excessive loss of bone is evident on the posterior aspect of the femoral condyles. (B) Lateral radiograph showing this condition. Unless the condition is recognized and the technique adjusted for it, flexion instability will result.

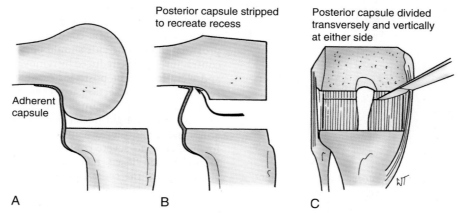

FIG 150.94 Posterior Capsulotomy for Flexion Contracture (A) The posterior capsule is adherent. (B) The original recess is re-established. (C) The cruciate ligaments have already been excised; only the medial and lateral parts of the posterior capsule need division. Often the underlying gastrocnemii are adherent and must be divided as well. At the margin of the collateral ligaments, vertical incisions must be made in the capsule.

femur. In more resistant cases the capsule may be cut transversely and may be separated from collateral structures by vertical incisions made at the medial and lateral corners. Resection of the PCL may be necessary in severe flexion contracture cases and aids in division of the midline fibers. After the capsulotomy and posterior release, the trial knee components are inserted, and the knee is brought into as much extension as possible. If extension is still not complete, further bone can be removed from the distal femur. This procedure may require use of a constrained prosthesis when the collateral ligaments are removed from their origins because extreme cases may require resection of so much bone that the knee becomes completely unbalanced. Surgery is followed by aggressive range of motion with an emphasis on extension in the immediate postoperative period.

EXTENSION CONTRACTURE ("STIFF KNEE")

Overview

Primary TKA in stiff and ankylosed knees, although technically demanding, has been shown to provide excellent pain relief and to significantly improve range of motion.[3,145,150] Stiff knees are typically defined as having less than 50 degrees of motion; ankylosed knees have essentially no motion (Fig. 150.95). Montgomery et al.[145] studied 82 stiff or ankylosed knees in 71 patients at an average follow-up of 5.3 years. Investigators noted an average Hospital for Special Surgery (HSS) knee score improvement of from 38 to 80 points and an average arc of motion improvement of from 36 to 93 degrees. All prostheses were posterior stabilized, with most being nonconstrained. Only one quadricepsplasty was necessary. Two patients with

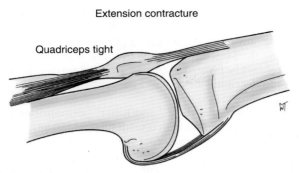

FIG 150.95 In an extension contracture, not only are intraarticular adhesions present, but the quadriceps muscle itself is shortened and tight.

flexion-valgus deformities developed peroneal nerve palsies that resolved spontaneously, and one patient had an inferior pole of the patellar fracture managed conservatively. This investigation is reflective of previous, smaller series,[3,150] although one series reported that quadricepsplasty was required in 42% of cases. More recently, Kim et al.[112] presented a series of 86 stiff knees undergoing TKA. This group also showed improvement in range of motion and in knee ratings, along with a 12% complication rate, most commonly related to skin necrosis.

Technique

The approach, as described by Montgomery et al., is made using a midline longitudinal incision and a medial parapatellar arthrotomy. Typically, the techniques described in the section "Difficult Exposures" are necessary. Eversion of the patella is generally challenging and may not be possible or necessary. Early release of the lateral retinaculum and lateral patellofemoral ligaments is commonly performed. Soft tissue releases are performed in the same fashion as they are for the varus, valgus, and flexion deformities described earlier; however, extensive soft tissue releases are routinely required. In varus knees, an extensile proximal medial tibial release is performed, whereas valgus knees are managed with lateral release, occasionally including elevation of the LCL off the femoral side. Flexion contractures require posterior capsule release; because of its contribution to contractures, Insall favored excision of the PCL. Complete subperiosteal reflection of the soft tissues from the distal femur (femoral peel) is occasionally necessary (see Fig. 150.38). Adequate bone cuts are then made to create balanced flexion and extension gaps. Despite extensive releases, constrained prostheses typically are not required unless ligament stability is forfeited.

CORRECTION OF GENU RECURVATUM

Genu recurvatum is an uncommon deformity that is seldom severe, except in paralytic conditions, such as poliomyelitis, or certain soft tissue abnormalities, such as Ehlers-Danlos. Operative correction is obtained by under-resection of the bone ends (particularly the distal femur) and use of thicker components. However, paralytic types tend to recur. Krackow[117] has described a technique whereby the proximal ligament insertions are transferred proximally and posteriorly; this repositioning causes the collateral ligaments to tighten in extension. Postoperative bracing or the use of a heel wedge to promote a flexion moment

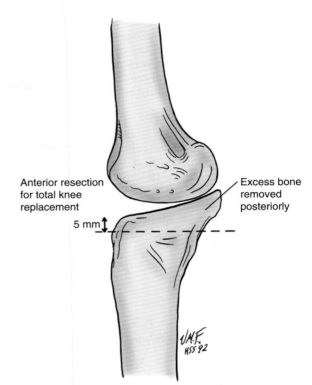

FIG 150.96 Tibial Recurvatum After High Tibial Osteotomy The osteotomy has healed with the distal fragment extended on the proximal, resulting in an anterior tilt to the anterior surface. Unless care is taken in performing the tibial resection for total knee replacement, excessive bone may be removed.

may enhance chances for success. Recurrent cases of recurvatum may constitute one of the few indications for the use of a hinged implant or a similarly constrained prosthesis. Occasionally after a previous tibial osteotomy, recurvatum will be noted because of deformity of the tibia itself (tibial recurvatum) (Fig. 150.96). The anterior cortices have impacted, and the result is an anterior slope to the tibia. This should be evident from a study of the radiographs, and the level of the tibial cut should be adjusted accordingly.

MANAGEMENT OF BONE DEFECTS

Principles

Although bone defects are more common in revision TKA, they do occur in primary TKA. Causes of bone defects in primary TKA include erosion secondary to angular arthritic change, inflammatory arthritis, osteonecrosis, and fracture. Bone defects in primary TKA are typically asymmetrical and peripheral, although contained deficiencies caused by cyst formation may occur. The base of contained and peripheral defects in primary TKA typically comprises condensed sclerotic bone, in contrast to revision surgery, in which removal of components often leaves osteopenic surfaces. A major concern with tibial defects is that subchondral bone strength diminishes substantially distal to the subchondral plate.[13,95]

Management

Various techniques are available to compensate for bone defects in primary TKA, including (1) translation of the component away from a defect, (2) lower tibial resection, (3) cement filling, (4) autologous bone graft, (5) allograft, (6) wedges or augments, and (7) custom implants. Use of stems in primary TKA is necessary when bone grafting is required or when the bone defect compromises fixation and renders the resurfacing component unstable without the added support of intramedullary fixation.

Lower Tibial Resection. A lower tibial resection is often effective in elimination of bony defects (Fig. 150.97). The limit of a lower tibial resection is the insertion of the ITB and infrapatellar ligament. When more than 10 mm of bone is removed, the resection must be proximal to Gerdy's tubercle, or else ITB function may be compromised. In addition, a lower tibial resection will complicate component fit because of the natural taper of the tibia, necessitating the use of a smaller tibial component or tapered tibial augments.

Lateral Translation. Lateralizing a smaller tibial component may effectively eliminate a bony defect (see Fig. 150.50) by removing any contact of the implant with the defect.[99,132] However, the largest tibial tray size and polyethylene insert should always be favored to create the largest reasonable contact surface to distribute load.

Cement Filling. Lotke et al.[134] and Ritter[171] demonstrated satisfactory long-term results with cement fill (Fig. 150.98), provided tibial bone defects are no deeper than 20 mm and involve less than 50% of either plateau. Despite these results, other authors recommend that use of cement should be limited to smaller peripheral defects that do not compromise tibial component support because biomechanical testing suggests that cement fill with or without screw reinforcement is an inferior method of defect management.[22] Clinical results have demonstrated that radiolucent lines are commonly observed under defects filled with cement.[52,102] Furthermore, larger volumes of cement introduce the risk of thermal necrosis of the cement-bone interface, and net cement shrinkage during polymerization may diminish the cement-prosthesis and cement-bone interface contact areas[22] (Fig. 150.99).

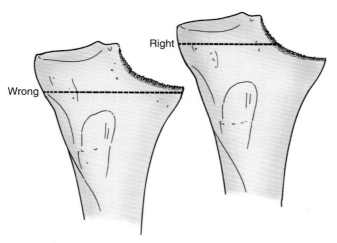

FIG 150.97 When asymmetrical bone loss occurs from the upper tibia, the tibial resection must not be too distal, but rather must be at the usual level.

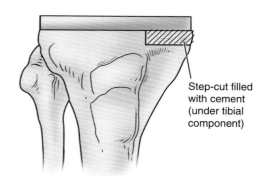

FIG 150.99 Step-cut technique for cement filling of a peripheral proximal tibial defect.

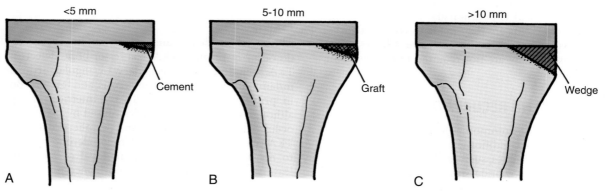

FIG 150.98 Bone Defects Are Frequently Seen in the Medial Tibia It is incorrect to make the tibial cut at the base of the defect. It is correct to resect a normal amount from the upper tibia and fill the remaining defect. (A) Defects smaller than 5 mm can be filled with cement. (B) Defects between 5 and 10 mm are suitable for bone grafting. (C) Defects larger than 10 mm are best treated with a metal wedge or augment.

Bone Grafting. Autologous bone and allograft (Figs. 150.100 to 150.102) are readily available in primary TKA. Both have demonstrated high rates of incorporation that are particularly important in re-establishing proximal tibial bone strength and restoring bone stock, should revision surgery be required. Autografting generally is favored because of its osteoinductive properties and lack of potential disease transmission. Bone graft is typically used when the size criteria for cement fill are exceeded. Dorr et al.[55] identified criteria that promote improved outcome, as follows: (1) creation of a viable/bleeding bed of host bone, (2) proper fit and finish of graft in host bed, (3) complete coverage of graft by the component to avoid graft resorption secondary to stress shielding, (4) optimal alignment of components for even load distribution, (5) limited weight bearing when larger grafts are used to allow for graft union, and (6) grafts protected with stems when required. Advantages of bone graft include its availability, its adaptability to size or shape of defect, and its biologic compatibility.[193]

Although contained defects are easily filled with bone graft, peripheral defects are more challenging. Several techniques have been developed using bone available during surgery from other areas of the knee to address peripheral defects. Dorr et al.[55] described success with a technique in which the peripheral defect is converted into a single oblique cut at the base of the deficiency and is filled using bone from the larger distal femoral condylar resection. The graft is secured to the oblique surface using screw fixation (see Fig. 150.101). Altcheck et al.[8] reported good-to-excellent results at an average follow-up of 4 years in 14 patients with severe angular deformity managed with this technique. All grafts had consolidated without evidence of collapse, resorption, or prosthetic subsidence. In contrast, Laskin[122] used the resected posterior femoral condyles as bone graft to fill tibial defects and concluded after a 5-year

follow-up review that the long-term prognosis for this method of bone grafting was not satisfactory.

Insall originally described the inlay autogeneic bone-grafting technique. An interference fit for a contoured bone graft is created by converting the dish-shaped peripheral defect into a trapezoidal shape (see Fig. 150.102). Because of the interlocking fit, this method of bone grafting does not require fixation. Windsor et al.[225] and later Scuderi et al.[193] reviewed 26 primary TKAs treated using this technique, reporting 96% good-to-excellent results at an average follow-up of 3 years. Graft position medially or laterally did not influence the results. With restoration of anatomic knee alignment, no tibial component loosened and one medial bone graft collapsed.

Custom Prostheses and Metal Wedge Augmentation. Metal wedge augmentation permits intraoperative construction of a custom implant to address a bone defect, affording load transfer from the implant to the bone.[160] Custom prostheses (Figs. 150.103 to 150.106) are an option for dealing with larger defects[22]; however, custom prostheses have limitations of practicality and cost. Defects of less than 25 mm can be managed effectively with metal wedge augmentation.[21] Custom prostheses may be required for larger defects. Brooks et al.[22] demonstrated that metal wedge augmentation of tibial trays provided support similar to that provided by custom prostheses. Augments are available in triangular and rectangular shapes, in both cemented and cementless options. Although the mechanical support afforded by triangular[29] and rectangular wedges has been shown to be similar,[208] load transfer across a larger defect probably is best managed with a rectangular block[68] and stem augmentation[23,208] (see Fig. 150.104). Modular augments do introduce the potential for interface fretting; however, reports have described good results using wedges attached with screw

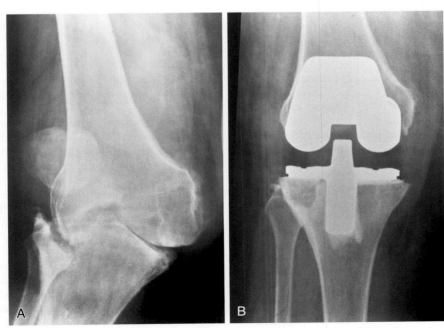

FIG 150.100 (A) Radiograph showing large defect in lateral tibial plateau. (B) Radiograph showing appearance after packing defect with cancellous bone graft. The graft can be autologous or homologous.

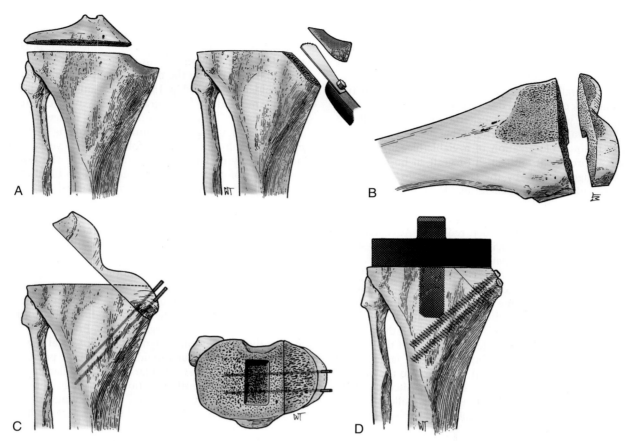

FIG 150.101 Bone Graft Technique (A) The tibia is resected at the usual level, leaving a medial defect. The sclerotic bone at the base of the defect is removed with a saw, exposing cancellous bone. (B) The bone graft is obtained from the distal femoral resection. (C) The femoral condyle is applied to the defect temporarily with Kirschner wires. The graft is resected at the level of the tibial cut. (D) Kirschner wires are replaced by screws, and the tibial component is in place. (From Behrens JC, Walker PS, Shoji H: Variation in strength and structure of cancellous bone at the knee. *J Biomech* 7:201, 1974.)

fixation.[186] In the series of Pagnano et al. of 24 primary cemented TKAs performed using metal wedge augmentation for tibial bone deficiency, clinical results were 96% good to excellent at an average follow-up of approximately 5 years.[160] Radiolucent lines at the cement-bone interface beneath the metal wedge were noted in 13 of 24 knees. Longer-term consequences of the radiolucencies are not known.

Authors' Preferred Method in the Management of Bone Defects

Tibial defects

Contained defects. When the bony defect, cavity, or cyst is enclosed within the bone, it is known as a contained defect. The treatment of choice is bone grafting using local bone graft from the osteotomies. In the rare event that local autograft is insufficient, supplementary allograft may be added.

Peripheral defects. Peripheral defects typically are located in the posteromedial aspect of the tibial plateau. Although small- and intermediate-size defects are relatively shallow and elliptical and are bound anteriorly, medially, and posteriorly by a solid

rim of cortical bone, severe defects have a steeper pitch and may involve the entire medial plateau. Several management options are available:

1. If possible, translate the tibial tray away from the location of the peripheral defect. Although simple and attractive, this method results in use of a smaller polyethylene tray that may not distribute load as effectively as a larger tibial tray (see Fig. 150.58).[96,99]
2. If not deeper than 10 mm, the defect can be eliminated by resecting the tibia at a lower level. However, when a larger defect is present, the tibial resection can be increased up to 12 to 14 mm (see Fig. 150.97).
3. Defects smaller than 5 mm can be managed with cement. Cement performance can be enhanced by converting the dished defect into a rectangular shape with a horizontal base and three vertical borders. The defect base should be cleaned to permit cement interdigitation (see Fig. 150.98).
4. For defects measuring between 6 and 10 mm after the proximal tibial osteotomy is performed, bone graft is used through the technique described by Dorr et al.[55] The inlay

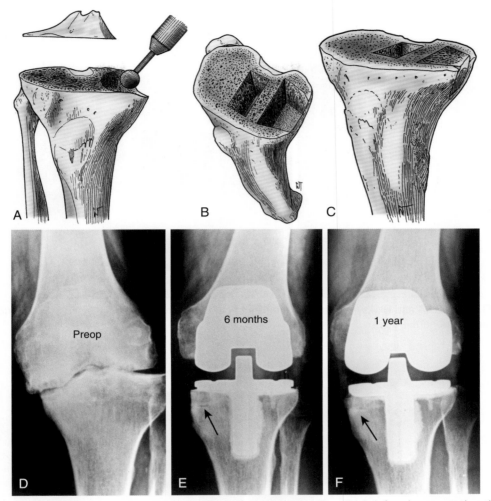

FIG 150.102 Autogenous Tibial Bone Graft Technique (A) The tibial defect is resected at the standard level. The remaining medial defect is reshaped with a burr. (B) A trapezoidal defect is formed medially; usually, intact bone is present anteriorly and posteriorly to make this possible. (C) A self-locking bone graft is fashioned to fit into the trapezoidal defect. The bone graft can be obtained through local resection in the knee; in the case of the posterior stabilized prosthesis, bone removed from the intercondylar notch serves as an ideal source. (D) Preoperative radiograph of a medial defect. (E) Radiograph taken 6 months after medial bone grafting using the interlocking technique. (F) Bone graft after 1 year; arthroplasty appears to be fully incorporated. *Arrow* indicates location of bone grafting. *Preop,* Preoperative.

bone-grafting method[193] is preferred because it allows for an interference fit of the graft and does not require fixation that may interfere with tibial stem placement (see Fig. 150.102).

In situations with massive defects, alternative sources of bone graft (allograft) or metal augmentation are used. When bone can be used, the bone block is tapped into place and should fit snugly into the defect to prevent cement from entering the graft-tibia interface. In the technique of Dorr et al. the anterior and posterior margins of the defect are excised to create a single oblique cut to the base of the tibial deficiency.[55] The base of the cut should comprise a bleeding cancellous surface. To fill this defect, local autograft is obtained from the larger condyle of the distal femoral resection that is rotated so that its cancellous surface is matched to the cancellous surface of the tibial defect. The junction of intact tibia and graft is occluded with supplemental bone graft to prevent cement from entering the space between the graft and the tibia.

5. When inlay bone grafting with autogenous graft is not feasible, modular wedges or blocks attached to resurfacing prostheses may be used. To diminish shear forces, an intramedullary stem is added to the tibial component when a full or half oblique wedge is used.

Distal femoral defects

Contained defects. Contained femoral defects are managed in the same manner as contained tibial defects.

Peripheral defects. Surface or peripheral defects of the femur are categorized as (1) affecting the chamfer cuts, (2) affecting the distal surface, or (3) causing major bone loss. Loss of femoral condylar bone is most frequently observed in valgus deformities when the lateral femoral condyle is dysplastic. As

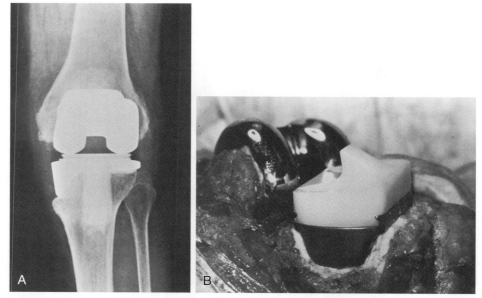

FIG 150.103 (A and B) Asymmetrical bone loss should be compensated for by an asymmetrical tibial component.

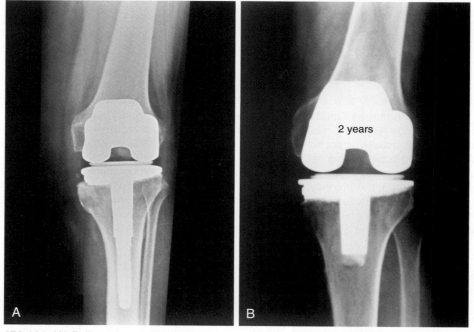

FIG 150.104 (A) Full wedge applied to a tibial component for a medial tibial defect. In this case an uncemented stem has been added. (B) Full wedge applied to a tibial component. No stem extension has been added. It is not known at present whether a stem extension is necessary to resist possible shearing effects.

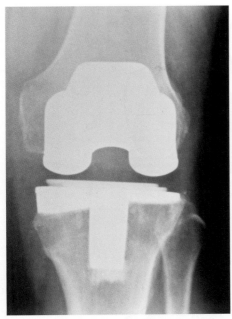

FIG 150.105 A modular medial wedge is attached to the prosthesis to fill a medial defect in the tibia.

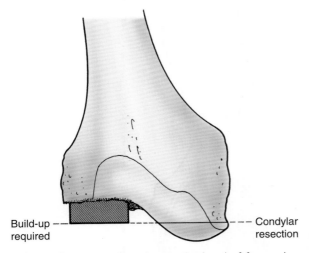

Build-up required — — — Condylar resection

FIG 150.106 In some valgus knees the level of femoral resection may pass distal to the lateral femoral condyle. Lateral augmentation of the femoral component is required.

with the tibia, defects can be managed with cement, bone graft, and metal augments.

Femoral deficiencies can be viewed in increasing stages of bone loss.

- Stage 1

Stage 1 is observed when the femoral osteotomy includes a portion of the lateral distal femur, but contouring to accommodate the femoral component results in chamfer "air cuts" anteriorly and posteriorly. In our experience, cement fill is acceptable for filling anterior and posterior spaces between bone and prosthesis. The sclerotic bone surface should be prepared to accept cement interdigitation.

- Stage 2

Stage 2 occurs when the level of the femoral osteotomy passes distal to the lateral femoral condyle even without chamfer cuts. In this situation, cement fill typically is unsatisfactory unless combined with a femoral stem extension. Even in this instance, a metal augment to the distal femur is preferred.

- Stage 3

Stage 3 refers to massive bone loss of one femoral condyle. Substantial bone loss can be managed with allograft or metal block augmentation, which has been shown to incorporate well but requires a period of non-weight bearing postoperatively and a femoral stem extension. The advantage of allograft is that if a revision is required, bone stock may be partially restored. Metal augments allow quicker rehabilitation without restricted weight bearing. Posterior augmentation without distal augmentation is required in cases of posterolateral deficiency. This unusual situation is encountered in the rheumatoid patient with long-standing flexion contracture that results in posterior condylar erosion, and in cases of combined valgus and flexion deformity. Most cases requiring posterior augmentation are also deficient distally. In general, optimized collateral ligament stability and restoration of normal anatomy is preferable to the use of constrained prostheses.

INTRAOPERATIVE PROBLEMS AND THEIR SOLUTIONS (INSALL)

Many of the basic elements of technique, bone cutting, soft tissue balancing, and overall alignment have already been addressed. A few intraoperative situations remain to be discussed (Fig. 150.107):

1. The flexion gap is too small to admit the thinnest tibial component. If spacers are used, this error will be identified early on. It may be caused by under-resection of the proximal tibia or oversizing of the femoral component. Therefore the size of the tibial fragment should be measured, and if 7 to 8 mm has already been removed from the normal side, then the problem lies in oversizing of the femur, and it will be necessary to recut the posterior femoral condyles so that one size smaller can be used.

2. The flexion gap is unequal (ie, tighter medially or laterally). The cause is an error in the tibial cut into varus or valgus, malrotation of the femoral component, or excessive ligament release. If the cause is either of the first two or insufficient release of a contracted structure, it should be corrected. However, sometimes the necessary medial or lateral release will cause an asymmetrical flexion gap that must be accepted. A larger than normal medial gap is not of clinical consequence, but an excessive lateral gap can lead to posterolateral subluxation. The soft tissues must be given time to adhere, which means pursuing postoperative flexion rehabilitation less vigorously than normal.

3. The extension gap is larger than the flexion gap (Fig. 150.108). This unusual situation is created by standard bone resection in a knee with excessive ligamentous laxity. A tensor obviates this occurrence because the need for femoral under-resection will be indicated; if one has committed to a standard femoral cut, the solution is to augment the distal femur (a thicker tibial component cannot be used because the flexion gap will not admit it). Augments on the distal femur usually require the use of a stemmed femoral component to get proper fixation. The laxity must be symmetrical and limited to a few

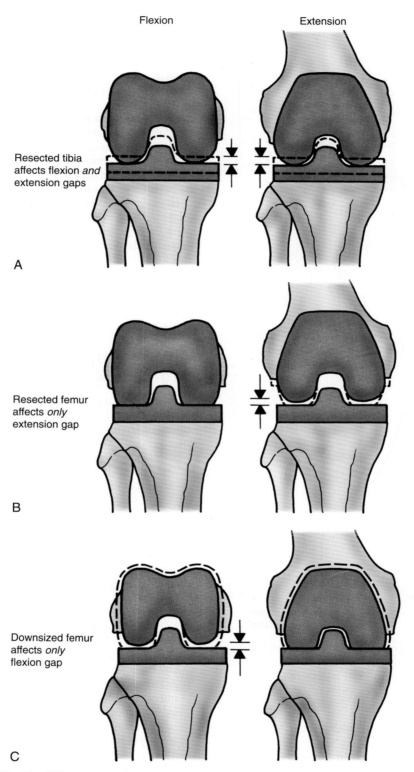

Flexion   Extension

Resected tibia affects flexion *and* extension gaps

A

Resected femur affects *only* extension gap

B

Downsized femur affects *only* flexion gap

C

FIG 150.107 The Effect of Bone Cuts on Prosthetic Fit (A) The level of tibial resection affects flexion and extension gaps equally. Under-resection of the tibia will make the joint tight in both positions. Over-resection of the tibia can be compensated for by using a thicker tibial component. (B) Distal resection of the femur affects only the extension gap, which may cause instability in extension. If the knee is too tight in flexion to admit a thicker tibial component, distal femoral buildup is the solution. (C) Over-resection of the femur in the sagittal plane affects only the flexion gap, causing laxity in flexion. This cannot be overcome by a thicker tibial component because the knee will be too tight in extension. A solution is (1) to restore the proper sagittal dimension of the femur by using a larger femoral component with a posterior buildup, or (2) to resect additional distal femur. The former is preferred.

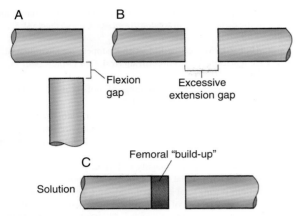

FIG 150.108 When the extension gap is too large, equalization cannot be attained by further bone resection. The prosthesis must be built up on the femoral side. (A) Femur and tibia cut surfaces demonstrating the flexion space. (B) Femur and tibia cut surfaces demonstrating the extension space, larger than the flexion space in A. (C) Solution to this problem with a build-up on the distal femur to equalize the spaces.

millimeters of passive motion. No "thrust" on weight bearing is permissible. Conversely, the components should not be so tight as to produce a flexion contracture.

4. The patella cannot be made to track in spite of an extensive lateral retinacular release. Causes include (1) femoral malrotation, (2) tibial malrotation, and (3) an overly thick patella. The latter two causes are readily correctable, but the first is more difficult and will result in a poor fit of the femoral component. Recutting the femur in additional external rotation and adding a posterolateral augment can remedy the first situation. A stemmed component and cement are needed to attain adequate fixation.

5. Alignment, fit, and motion with the trial components are satisfactory, but this is not so when the final components are inserted. There are several reasons for this:

   a. The knee does not reach full extension. The probable explanation is that the femoral component has been put on flexed, so it is sitting proud of the bone. This problem has been virtually eliminated with the use of pegs that engage the femur, ensuring proper sagittal position of the femoral component. Careful placement of the final component is required when pegs are not available.

   b. The knee is too loose in extension after satisfactory trial reduction. This can happen even with a proper fit because the finished components are polished and become slightly less bulky than the trials; adjustment to the thickness of the tibial component will remedy the situation. A more serious occurrence is when the femoral component has been driven into soft rheumatoid or osteoporotic bone. A thicker tibial component may upset the flexion-extension balance, and a stemmed femoral component, possibly with augments, may be needed to restore the proper femoral position.

   c. Varus/valgus alignment and balance are incorrect. This is also because of compacting of one or the other of the components (usually the femoral component)

asymmetrically into soft bone. The correction is the same as previously described. When the final cementation is performed, it is important to hold the leg so it does not fall into the preoperative deformity or create component lift-off while the cement hardens.

   d. Patellar tracking is unsatisfactory. The cause is insertion of the final components in a different position to the trials. This usually happens when the bone is soft, and it is most likely to happen when a central stem tibial design is used and the tibial component is allowed to spin into internal rotation. It is, of course, correctable but can be prevented if the position of the tibial trial on the tibia is marked with methylene blue, so that the surgeon can be certain that both the trial and the final components are correctly inserted.

   e. Excessive bleeding occurs. Opinions differ about the timing of tourniquet release or even on whether to use it at all. Studies have showed blood loss to be similar with and without tourniquet release. Tourniquet release serves two purposes: (1) occasional profuse bleeding, usually from the lateral genicular artery, can be secured (see Fig. 150.48), and (2) blood flow may not return through an arteriosclerotic femoral artery when the tourniquet is let down. According to Insall, this is usually because of clotting in the femoral artery and, if treated early, has an uneventful outcome. Release of the tourniquet alerts the surgeon to this possibility, whereas identification of this potentially catastrophic event may be delayed in the recovery room. Blood loss has become much less of a concern in TKA in recent years as a result of the advent of better blood management protocols and the routine use of tranexamic acid in eligible patients.

AFTERCARE OF TOTAL KNEE ARTHROPLASTY

At the conclusion of the operation, a bulky cotton dressing or compression stocking is applied to limit extremity swelling. The bulky dressing is removed on the first postoperative day. Some surgeons prefer to apply a lighter dressing and to initiate continuous passive motion in the recovery room, with use of simultaneous continuous passive motion machines in bilateral cases. The patient is encouraged to flex the knee as much as is tolerated; investigations suggest that high flexion in the immediate postoperative period accelerates postoperative rehabilitation and is not associated with wound complications.[107]

With a cemented knee, full weight bearing under the supervision of a therapist is allowed immediately. Some surgeons recommend protected weight bearing even when cement is used from the perspective of patient comfort. Progression of walking is variable and age dependent and walking is initially done with a walker until the patient is steady enough to use canes. General muscle exercises are for the feet and ankles, and isometric exercises are for the thigh and buttock muscles. Bicycle exercises are most useful as soon as the patient has sufficient flexion. Motivated patients are placed on a "fast track" and will initiate ambulation on the afternoon of surgery, with some centers even moving to outpatient total knee replacement in selected patients. Regional anesthesia and local infiltration of longer-acting anesthetic agents and drug cocktails have improved pain management. Care must be taken to protect patients from falls when femoral nerve blocks and other peripheral nerve blocks are used.

KEY REFERENCES

16. Berger RA, Crossett LS, Jacobs JJ, et al: Malrotation causing patellofemoral complications after total knee arthroplasty. *Clin Orthop* 356:144, 1998.

18. Berger RA, Rubash HE, Seel MJ, et al: Determining the rotational alignment of the femoral component in total knee arthroplasty using the epicondylar axis. *Clin Orthop* 286:40, 1993.

31. Chen F, Krackow KA: Management of tibial defects in total knee arthroplasty: a biomechanical study. *Clin Orthop* 305:249, 1994.

47. Dennis DA, Komistek RD, Mahfouz MR: In vivo fluoroscopic analysis of fixed-bearing total knee replacements. *Clin Orthop* 410:114, 2003.

68. Fehring TK, Peindl RD, Humble RS, et al: Modular tibial augmentations in total knee arthroplasty. *Clin Orthop* 327:207, 1996.

112. Kim YH, Kim JS, Choi Y, et al: Computer-assisted surgical navigation does not improve the alignment and orientation of the components in total knee arthroplasty. *J Bone Joint Surg Am* 91:14, 2009.

153. Nagamine R, Whiteside LA, White SE, et al: Patellar tracking after total knee arthroplasty: the effect of tibial tray malrotation and articular surface configuration. *Clin Orthop* 304:262, 1994.

159. Pagnano MW, Hanssen AD, Lewallen DG, et al: Flexion instability after primary posterior cruciate retaining total knee arthroplasty. *Clin Orthop* 356:39, 1998.

163. Poilvache PL, Insall HN, Scuderi GR, et al: Rotational landmarks and sizing of the distal femur in total arthroplasty. *Clin Orthop* 331:35, 1996.

175. Ritter MA, Faris PM, Keating EM, et al: Postoperative alignment of total knee replacement: its effect on survival. *Clin Orthop* 299:153, 1994.

179. Ritter MA, Stringer EA: Predictive range of motion after total knee replacement. *Clin Orthop* 143:115, 1979.

189. Scott RD, Chmell MJ: Balancing the posterior cruciate ligament during cruciate-retaining fixed and mobile-bearing total knee arthroplasty: description of the pull-out lift-off and slide-back tests. *J Arthroplasty* 23:605, 2008.

215. Wasielewski RC, Galante JO, Leighty RM, et al: Wear patterns on retrieved polyethylene tibial inserts and their relationship to technical considerations during total knee arthroplasty. *Clin Orthop* 299:31, 1994.

219. Whiteside LA: Correction of ligament and bone defects in total arthroplasty of the severely valgus knee. *Clin Orthop* 288:234, 1993.

224. Whiteside LA, Ohl MD: Tibial tubercle osteotomy for exposure of the difficult total knee arthroplasty. *Clin Orthop* 260:6, 1990.

The references for this chapter can also be found on www.expertconsult.com.

151

Gap-Balancing Techniques in Total Knee Arthroplasty

Jason M. Jennings, Douglas A. Dennis

INTRODUCTION

Creation of symmetrical and balanced flexion and extension gaps is a surgical goal of a total knee arthroplasty (TKA).[15] Multiple differing surgical techniques are currently used to achieve this balance, but controversy remains regarding the single best method. Some favor a measured resection technique in which bony landmarks (transepicondylar axis [TEA], posterior condylar axis [PCA], or the anteroposterior [AP] axis) are the primary determinants used for determination of femoral component rotational position.* Others recommend a gap-balancing methodology in which the femoral component is positioned parallel to the resected tibia, with each collateral ligament equally tensioned.[4,5,9,13] The authors believe this technique results in a more precise and reproducible flexion gap and improved flexion stability. This chapter will review gap-balancing techniques, emphasizing key surgical strategies to achieve a reproducible method of obtaining correct femoral component rotation.

SURGICAL TECHNIQUE

Gap-balancing techniques consist of ligament releases prior to completing all of the bone resections. These releases will correct preoperative fixed deformities, allowing the surgeon to restore neutral axial mechanical alignment prior to the determination of femoral component rotation. Two gap-balancing techniques have been used to achieve this goal. One relies on balancing the flexion gap first, whereas the other initially performs balancing techniques in extension. The authors favor the "extension gap first" method of gap balancing (matching the flexion gap to the initially established extension gap), because of the precision of soft tissue balancing in extension, which provides more reproducible gap balance.

Extension Gap First Surgical Technique

The knee is exposed with a subperiosteal release of the deep medial collateral ligament (MCL) to the midcoronal plane of the tibia to provide initial surgical exposure. The articular surface of the distal femur is then resected with use of an intramedullary guide. This cut is typically made between 4 and 7 degrees of valgus, which is based on the preoperative measurement of the angle formed by the intersection of the patient's femoral anatomic versus mechanical axes on hip-to-ankle

radiographs. Resection of the proximal tibia is then performed perpendicular to its mechanical axis. Over- or under-resection of the femoral or tibial bone resections can lead to a mismatch of flexion and extension gap dimensions. The authors recommend distal femoral and proximal tibia resections that approximate the implant thickness. Resected bone fragments should be measured with a caliper to ensure resections are precise. All osteophytes, including posterior femoral and tibial osteophytes, must then be removed before any additional soft tissue releases are performed, due to their tensioning of adjacent ligamentous structures. This step is crucial because these osteophytes can mislead the surgeon into thinking a supporting soft tissue structure is too tight, resulting in a surgical release of that "tight" structure. If the osteophytes are removed late, after soft tissue releases have been performed, unwanted laxity of the released structures is incurred that results in asymmetry of the flexion and extension gaps leading to potential malrotation of the femoral component. It is typically difficult to gain access to the posterior femoral condylar osteophytes in most cases. The authors recommend making a preliminary 4-mm resection of one or both of the posterior femoral condyles with the knee flexed at 90 degrees (Fig. 151.1). A laminar spreader is then introduced to open the flexion gap an allow access to the posterior osteophytes. A curved osteotome is then used to remove the posterior femoral osteophytes (Fig. 151.2A and B). A spacer block is placed to fill the newly created extensor gap to assess lower limb alignment and coronal plane soft tissue balance in extension. If imbalance is present, tight soft tissue structures are released in a sequential fashion until alignment of the limb is neutral and the extension gap is symmetrical.[10] Occasionally, further bone resection in the form of a medial tibial reduction ostectomy (Fig. 151.3) is needed to obtain symmetry.[17]

Attention is then directed to the flexion gap, with the goal of duplicating the dimensions of the extension gap. The knee is flexed to 90 degrees, and each collateral ligament is equally tensioned with either laminar spreaders or implant-specific tensioners. Care should be taken to avoid overtensioning of the medial laminar spreader. This can have numerous adverse effects, including under-resection of the posterior aspect of the medial condyle, which results in increased superficial MCL tension and subsequent knee stiffness. In addition, excessive tensioning of the medial laminar spreader can result in internal rotation of the femoral component relative to the TEA if the AP cutting block is then positioned parallel to the resected proximal tibia. Subluxation of a *tight* extensor mechanism laterally can increase lateral flexion gap tension by pulling the posterior aspect of the lateral femoral condyle towards the resected proximal tibial surface. In this situation, tightening the lateral

*References 1, 8, 16, 18, 21, 22, and 24.

laminar spreader a bit tighter than medially can negate the effect of lateral patellar subluxation and enhance obtaining a rectangular flexion gap.

The authors then identify and outline the TEA and AP axes as secondary determinants of femoral component rotation. If the knee is well balanced in extension, the resected proximal tibial should align parallel with the TEA and the AP axis will align perpendicular to the tibia (Fig. 151.4). If there is a substantial divergence of the TEA from the proximal tibial resection with each collateral ligament appropriately tensioned, one must perform secondary checks to ensure an error in surgical technique has not occurred (Table 151.1). An appropriately sized AP cutting block is then positioned parallel to the resected proximal tibia to create a rectangular flexion gap. The width of the resection is determined from the width of the extension gap that was previously created to ensure balance between the gaps (Fig. 151.5). The tensioning devices are then removed. To ensure flexion-extension gap symmetry, a spacer block of identical width to that selected for the extension gap is placed beneath the posterior aspect of the AP cutting block and the resected proximal tibial surface and flexion gap tension is again assessed before resection of the posterior femoral condyles (Fig. 151.6A and B). If imbalance of the flexion gap is identified at this point, the AP cutting block is appropriately repositioned. Remaining

femoral bone resections are then completed, trial components are inserted, and gap symmetry is confirmed before final component implantation.

Flexion Gap First Surgical Technique

After initial exposure, a perpendicular proximal tibial resection is made relative to the longitudinal axis of the tibia. Accuracy of this cut is crucial because it will serve as a base and reference for the remaining femoral bone resections. As with the "extension gap first" gap-balancing technique, a varus proximal tibial resection will result in femoral component internal rotation when a tensioned, rectangular flexion gap is created. Conversely, a valgus tibial resection will result in excessive femoral component external rotation. After the appropriate tibial resection has been performed, it is crucial to remove all osteophytes before soft tissue release or further bone resection is performed. The joint is then accurately tensioned in flexion with a tensioning device, and the tibial cut should align perpendicular to the AP axis and parallel to the TEA. Corrective soft tissue releases are performed if these landmarks do not align appropriately. After this is performed, the anterior and posterior condylar cuts are made using an anterior referencing AP cutting block. Usually spacer blocks are inserted into the flexion gap to ensure symmetry.

The extension gap is then addressed based on the dimensions of the balanced flexion gap. Tensioning devices are used with the knee in extension, which are set to a similar tension level that was set for the balancing of the flexion gap. An intramedullary or extramedullary guide is attached to the tensioning jig, and the lower limb alignment is critically assessed. Additional soft tissue releases may be performed to achieve appropriate alignment and balance. After a symmetric gap is obtained,

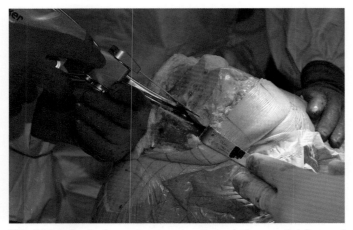

FIG 151.1 Preliminary 4-mm resection of the medial femoral condyle to allow access to the posterior osteophyte.

TABLE 151.1   **Reasons for Divergence of the Relationship of Transepicondylar Axis and Proximal Tibia Resection**
Error in resection of the proximal tibia (varus or valgus)
Error in precise determination of the TEA
Flexion gap stabilization structures being tensioned are incompetent
• Medial—superficial medial collateral ligament
• Lateral—lateral collateral ligament–popliteus tendon complex

TEA, Transepicondylar axis.

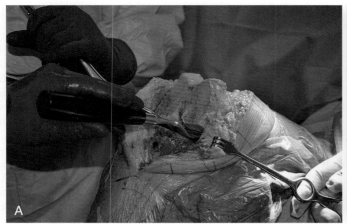
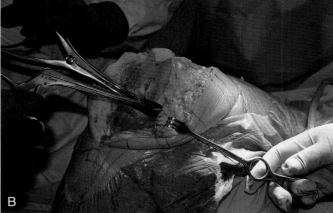

FIG 151.2 (A and B) Removal of the posterior osteophyte with a curved type osteotome and pituitary rongeur.

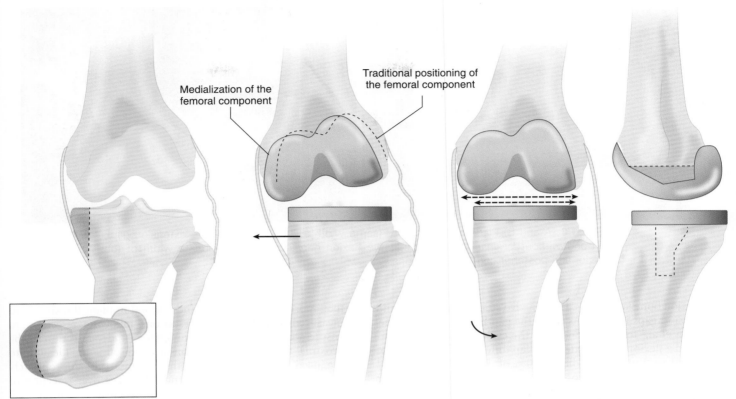

Medialization of the femoral component

Traditional positioning of the femoral component

FIG 151.3 Medial tibial reduction osteotomy to assist with gap balancing in a knee with significant varus deformity. (From Krackow KA, Raju S, Puttaswamy MK: Medial over-resection of the tibia in total knee arthroplasty for varus deformity using computer navigation. *J Arthroplasty* 30:766–769, 2015)

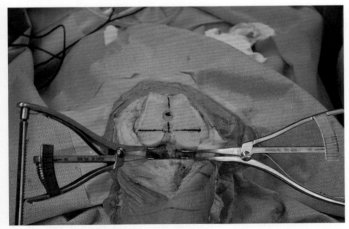

FIG 151.4 Collateral ligaments equally tensioned using laminar spreaders. Note the TEA is parallel and the AP axis is perpendicular to the resected proximal tibia.

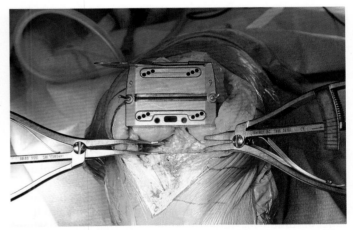

FIG 151.5 Placement of the anteroposterior femoral cutting block parallel to the resected proximal tibia with each collateral ligament tensioned to create a rectangular flexion gap.

the distal femoral cut is performed with the assistance of a cutting jig. A spacer block is placed to ensure the equality of balance in both flexion and extension.

GAP-BALANCING ADVANTAGES AND DISADVANTAGES

Improved flexion stability may be obtained using the gap-balancing technique by creating a rectangular flexion gap.[9,13]

Katz et al.[13] compared the reliability of use of the TEA, AP axis, and gap-balancing techniques in eight cadaveric knees to determine femoral component rotational alignment. These data demonstrated the TEA was less predictable and significantly resulted in more femoral component external rotation than the AP axis or the gap-balancing methods. Because of its independence from obscured or poorly defined bony anatomic landmarks, these authors suggested the gap-balancing method may be more reproducible than use of the typical measured

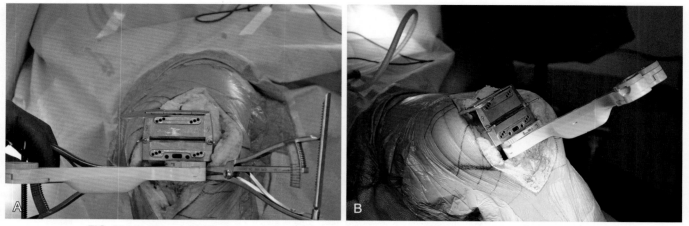

FIG 151.6 (A and B) Placement of spacer (same width as used to create the extension gap), with and without laminar spreaders, into the flexion gap to assure appropriate width of the anterior and posterior condylar resections.

resection bone landmarks. In an in vivo study of the flexion and extension gaps in 84 TKAs using the gap-balancing technique, Griffin et al.[2] found that none of the evaluated knees demonstrated a flexion versus extension gap difference (mismatch) of more than 3 mm. In addition, 90% of 38 randomly selected gap-balanced TKAs demonstrated that the posterior condylar angle was within 3 degrees of the surgical TEA when measured using a computed tomography (CT) scan.[2]

A consequence of flexion gap asymmetry is midflexion instability, evidenced by the presence of femoral condylar liftoff. Femoral condylar liftoff has been thought to lead to (1) eccentric loading; (2) premature wear of polyethylene; (3) excessive load of the subchondral bone; and (4) premature prosthetic loosening.[6] Dennis et al.[5] compared the stability of 40 TKAs performed using a measured resection technique (20 posterior cruciate ligament (PCL) retaining and 20 posterior stabilized) versus 20 posterior-stabilized knees implanted using a gap-balancing method. The presence and magnitude of femoral condylar liftoff was evaluated for each technique at 0, 30, 60, and 90 degrees of flexion using an automated three-dimensional (3D) model-fitting kinematic analysis. The presence and magnitude of liftoff greater than 1.0 mm was significantly less with the gap-balancing technique ($p < .0001$). Sixty percent of the PCL-retaining and 45% of the posterior-stabilized TKAs implanted using a measured resection technique demonstrated condylar liftoff greater than 1.0 mm versus none (0%) of the knees in the gap-balanced cohort. The gap-balanced TKA group also had a lower maximum magnitude of femoral condylar liftoff (0.9 mm) than either of the two measured resection group (PCL-retaining, 3.1 mm; posterior stabilized, 2.5 mm; $p = .0002$).

Errors with use of a gap-balancing technique can occur if precise surgical performance is not maintained. A critical step in the gap-balancing technique is an accurate proximal tibial resection. A varus or valgus tibial cut will result in internal or excessive external rotation of the femoral component, respectively, when the AP cutting block is placed parallel to the resected proximal tibia. Over- or under-resection of the distal femur or proximal tibia will result in potential changes in the native joint line and may lead to excessive patellar alta or baja, as well as difficulties obtaining good gap balance throughout the entire flexion range. The authors recommend resections

that approximate the tibial and femoral implant thickness and measurement of all bone resections following resection, to ensure accuracy. Bone resection errors (under-resection of the proximal tibia or over-resection of the distal femur) leading to the need for a thicker polyethylene insert to appropriately tension the extension gap will necessitate an over-resection of the posterior condyles of the femur to create a symmetrical flexion gap. This will lead to a subsequent reduction of the posterior femoral offset and a potential loss of knee flexion.

The integrity of the collateral ligaments and precise soft tissue balancing are unique and critical components of the gap-balancing technique. Because gap-balancing methodologies involve tensioning of ligamentous structures, deficiencies in the primary ligamentous stabilizers have consequences and must be recognized to avoid critical errors in operative technique. The superficial MCL is the primary stabilizer of the medial aspect of the flexion gap. The lateral aspect of the flexion gap is primarily stabilized by the lateral collateral ligament and popliteal tendon complex. If the superficial MCL is incompetent, tensioning the medial flexion gap will result in an excessive medial flexion gap and lead to excessive internal rotation if the femoral component is placed parallel to the resected tibia. When the lateral complex is deficient, the femoral component will be externally rotated excessively when placed parallel to the proximal tibial resection.

Lastly, as previously mentioned, subluxation of a tight extensor mechanism laterally can result in flexion gap asymmetry because subluxation can cause the lateral flexion gap to be excessively tensioned.[19,23] In this situation, if the AP cutting block is positioned parallel to the tibia, too much bone would be resected from the posterior aspect of the lateral condyle, resulting in flexion gap laxity after the extensor mechanism is reduced. This can be compensated for by tightening the lateral laminar spreader slightly tighter to accommodate for the extensor mechanism tension.

MEASURED RESECTION ADVANTAGES AND DISADVANTAGES

Advantages of using a measured resection technique are intraoperative simplicity. Most TKA systems have well-developed instrumentation to guide bone resections, and satisfactory results are obtained in most patients. Bony landmarks, such as the TEA,[1,8] AP axis,[21,24] and PCA,[16,22] are used to set femoral component rotation when using this technique. Bone cuts are initially made independent of soft tissue tension, unlike the gap-balancing techniques.

Reports with use of measured resection techniques have demonstrated that precise flexion gap stability is often not obtained.[3,5,9] Fehring[9] reported a 45% (45 of 100) incidence of a trapezoidal flexion gap when using traditional bony landmarks (TEA, AP axis, PCA). In addition, Clatworthy et al.[3] analyzed 212 TKAs performed with computer navigation that placed the femoral component to obtain a rectangular flexion gap and then compared that femoral component rotational position with flexion gap symmetry obtained with use of the TEA, AP axis, and PCA. *On average*, the femoral component position chosen using gap balancing was similar to that selected from the use of each of the three bony landmarks. However, a wide divergence of femoral component rotation was seen with use of each of the bony landmarks. They reported that creation of a rectangular flexion gap was not reproducible with use of any of the bone landmark axes. If the TEA was used, a rectangular flexion gap to within ±3 degrees was obtained in only 41.5% of cases. When the AP axis was used, a rectangular gap was created in only 39.6% of subjects and in 51.9% of cases when the PCA was selected. Lastly, Yau et al.[25] similarly showed gap balancing was more reproducible. In this study, postoperative CT scans were used to detail the true TEA. Outliers in rotation of greater than ±5 degrees occurred in 20% for gap balancing, 52% for TEA, 60% for use of the AP axis, and in 72% when the PCA was selected.

Placement of the femoral component parallel to the TEA has been shown to lessen the incidence and magnitude of femoral condylar liftoff.[11] Unfortunately, numerous studies report that surgeons may be unable to accurately and reproducibly identify the TEA.[12,14] Kinzel et al.[14] intraoperatively placed pins to identify the femoral epicondyles and construct the TEA. Postoperative CT scans revealed the surgeons identified the TEA to within ±3 degrees in only 75% (55 of 74) of the knees, with a wide range of error (6 degrees of external rotation to 11 degrees of internal rotation). Jerosch et al.[12] compared accuracy of surgeon identification of the femoral epicondyles under experimental conditions. The range of position chosen in identifying the medial epicondyle varied by 22.3 mm, and the lateral epicondylar location varied by 13.8 mm.

The AP axis has been advocated for appropriate femoral component rotation.[24] It is dependent on normal anatomy of the trochlear groove and intercondylar notch of the distal femur.[13] Therefore the identification is less reliable in cases of trochlear dysplasia or severe patellofemoral arthrosis, and this landmark is absent in the revision TKA setting. Patients with either severe trochlear dysplasia[21] or medial femorotibial osteoarthritis[20] may be at risk of femoral component placement in excessive external rotation leading to subsequent coronal plane instability in flexion when this landmark is used to determine component rotation. Lastly, a wide range of error in femoral component rotation with of range of up to 32 degrees (15 degrees of external rotation and 17 degrees of internal rotation) has been reported with use of this measured resection bone landmark.[25]

When the posterior condylar anatomy is normal, external rotation of 3 to 4 degrees relative to the PCA will orient the AP

femoral bone resections perpendicular to the resected proximal tibial surface in most cases. Despite the apparent simplicity of using instrumentation based on the PCA to set femoral component rotation, errors are common due to anatomic variability. The decision to externally rotate the cutting guide relative to the PCA to set femoral rotation was derived from mean data. The posterior condylar twist angle has substantial variability anatomically, ranging from −1 degree to 7 degrees (range, 8 degrees) of external rotation[21] and from 0.1 degree to 9.7 degrees (range, 9.6 degrees) of external rotation[16] in two separate studies. If a knee has a posterior condylar twist angle of 9 degrees and the cutting guide is set to 3 degrees of external rotation versus the PCA, the femoral component will be internally rotated 6 degrees.

The PCA is difficult to rely on in the setting of significant arthritic deformities, particularly those patients with lateral femoral condyle hypoplasia or erosion commonly seen in knees with valgus gonarthrosis. If the PCA is used in this setting to determine femoral component rotation, this will lead to erroneous femoral component internal rotation.[7] In the varus knee with chronic insufficiency of the anterior cruciate ligament (ACL), the posterior aspect of the medial femoral condyle may be eroded. In this scenario the femoral component may be placed in excessive external rotation if the PCA is used. Lastly, in the revision TKA, the PCA is wholly absent.

CONCLUSIONS

Controversy continues regarding the best surgical technique to use to obtain gap balance during TKA. Currently, measured resection and gap-balancing techniques can be used to establish appropriate femoral component rotation and a rectangular flexion gap. Although measured resection techniques may be accurate in a majority of the cases, use of this technique exclusively appears to lead to more outliers, resulting in flexion gap asymmetry and increased femoral condylar liftoff. Fundamentally the anatomy of each femur is different. As such, using bone landmarks as a way to achieve reproducible femoral component rotation may prove challenging. For the aforementioned reasons, the authors use the gap-balancing technique, with bony landmarks as a "secondary check" in TKA.

KEY REFERENCES

1. Berger RA, Rubash HE, Seel MJ, et al: Determining the rotational alignment of the femoral component in total knee arthroplasty using the epicondylar axis. *Clin Orthop* 286:40–47, 1993.
2. Boldt JG, Stiehl JB, Munzinger U, et al: Femoral component rotation in mobile-bearing total knee arthroplasty. *Knee* 13:284–289, 2006. doi: 10.1016/j.knee.2006.01.007.
3. Clatworthy MG, Lindberg K, Harrill W, et al: Rotational alignment of the femoral component in computer-assisted total knee arthroplasty. *Reconstr Rev Joint Implant Surg Res Found* 2:37–42, 2012.
5. Dennis DA, Komistek RD, Kim RH, et al: Gap balancing versus measured resection technique for total knee arthroplasty. *Clin Orthop* 468:102–107, 2010. doi: 10.1007/s11999-009-1112-3.
6. Dennis DA, Komistek RD, Walker SA, et al: Femoral condylar lift-off in vivo in total knee arthroplasty. *J Bone Joint Surg Br* 83:33–39, 2001.
7. Griffin FM, Insall JN, Scuderi GR: The posterior condylar angle in osteoarthritic knees. *J Arthroplasty* 13:812–815, 1998. doi: 10.1016/S0883-5403(98)90036-5.
8. Griffin FM, Math K, Scuderi GR, et al: Anatomy of the epicondyles of the distal femur: MRI analysis of normal knees. *J Arthroplasty* 15:354–359, 2000.

9. Fehring TK: Rotational malalignment of the femoral component in total knee arthroplasty. *Clin Orthop* 380:72–79, 2000.

10. Heesterbeek PJC, Jacobs WCH, Wymenga AB: Effects of the balanced gap technique on femoral component rotation in TKA. *Clin Orthop* 467:1015–1022, 2009. doi: 10.1007/s11999-008-0539-2.

11. Insall JN, Scuderi GR, Komistek RD, et al: Correlation between condylar lift-off and femoral component alignment. *Clin Orthop* 403:143–152, 2002.

13. Katz MA, Beck TD, Silber JS, et al: Determining femoral rotational alignment in total knee arthroplasty: reliability of techniques. *J Arthroplasty* 16:301–305, 2001. doi: 10.1054/arth.2001.21456.

21. Poilvache PL, Insall JN, Scuderi GR, et al: Rotational landmarks and sizing of the distal femur in total knee arthroplasty. *Clin Orthop* 331:35–46, 1996.

23. Springer BD, Parratte S, Abdel MP: Measured resection versus gap balancing for total knee arthroplasty. *Clin Orthop* 472:2016–2022, 2014. doi: 10.1007/s11999-014-3524-y.

24. Whiteside LA, Arima J: The anteroposterior axis for femoral rotational alignment in valgus total knee arthroplasty. *Clin Orthop* 321:168–172, 1995.

25. Yau WP, Chiu KY, Tang WM: How precise is the determination of rotational alignment of the femoral prosthesis in total knee arthroplasty. An in vivo study. *J Arthroplasty* 22:1042–1048, 2007. doi: 10.1016/j.arth.2006.12.043.

The references for this chapter can also be found on www.expertconsult.com.

152

Modern Measured Resection Technique

Andrea Baldini, Giovanni Balato, Vincenzo Franceschini, Alfredo Lamberti

"Never internally rotate the femoral component relative to the posterior condyles even if the ligaments told you to do so."

John N. Insall

INTRODUCTION

Total knee arthroplasty (TKA) procedure has been historically instrumented using two distinct techniques: the "gap-balancing (GB) technique," popularized by Freeman and Insall,[22,31] and the "measured resection (MR) technique," popularized by Hungerford-Krackow.[30] These represented two completely distinct philosophies developed as a result of two approaches toward implants and instruments during the early days of knee arthroplasty. Although these techniques originated from fundamentally two different schools of thought, over time the instruments developed for implantation have incorporated aspects from both philosophies, thus obscuring the main distinctions. The differences between these two techniques are represented by three peculiarities (Table 152.1).

Tibia first: The GB technique, also called the "dependent-cut" technique, starts with a tibial resection to create a platform where the femoral cuts can be adjusted. For the MR technique, also called the "independent-cut" technique, either the femur or the tibia can be resected first and these bone resections are independent of each other. Achieving an accurate tibial resection is fundamental to any technique in total knee replacement (TKR), but for the gap technique it is particularly important. In fact, a varus tibial resection will automatically result in an increased internal rotation of the femoral component when the femoral component is placed parallel to the resected proximal tibia. Correspondingly, a valgus tibial cut will lead to excessive external rotation of the femoral component. In the MR technique, bone cuts are fixed and are initially made prior to the final soft tissue balancing, which can be done at the end of the procedure, even after trial component implantation.

Ligament release: Ligament release should be minimal or absent in the GB technique because all the main adjustments are done on the bony side. The extension gap is created by the distal femur and proximal tibia resections. Equal medial and lateral gaps are created in extension by a stepwise release of tight structures on the concave side, so surgeons must understand the structures that affect extension, flexion, and both to create proper balance. In the MR technique, ligament releases are done as needed throughout the procedure in a progressive manner after all bone resections have been made according to the planned axis of correction. Residual imbalances are adjusted by additional ligament release.

Bone resections: Bone resections are, of course, variable in the GB technique because the ligament balance in the gap configuration is created by a bone resection on the femoral site. In the MR technique, bone resections are fixed and based on bony landmarks and according to implant dimensions and patient anatomy. Bony landmarks may provide accurate rotation of the femoral component as long as the surgeon is able to accurately and reproducibly find them intraoperatively. In contrast, the GB technique, also called the "soft tissue tension in flexion" technique, relies on symmetric tension placed on the ligaments in flexion to set femoral component rotation. Therefore, the rotation and anteroposterior (AP) placement of the femoral component are used to create flexion gap symmetry.

RATIONALE OF THE GAP-BALANCING TECHNIQUE

Insall and Freeman first introduced the GB technique in the 1970s,[22,31] and were aiming for a functional knee replacement that resected the posterior cruciate ligament (PCL).[53] This technique was developed at a time when a limited number of implant sizes were commercially available. Consequently, a relatively small femoral component was frequently fitted onto a larger distal femur, a procedure that typically required over-resection of the posterior femoral condyles. Furthermore, to appropriately balance the flexion gap and avoid flexion instability, less proximal tibial resection was performed, thereby increasing the risk of creating a tight extension gap.

The gap technique relied on creation of equal and symmetric flexion and extension gaps resulting from bone cuts and ligament balancing during the initial part of the procedure.[32] These ligament releases corrected fixed deformities and brought the limb into correct approximate alignment before the rotation of the femoral component was determined. Three essential features characterized the gap technique as originally described. The first feature entailed a section of the tibia perpendicular to the long axis of the bone. The second entailed two gap sequences: a first gap resection in the flexed knee, with the posterior femoral and proximal tibial cuts positioned to provide balanced soft tissue tension and a second gap between the bones of a

TABLE 152.1 **Main Technical Differences Between Gap-Balancing and Measured Resection Techniques**

	Gap-Balancing	Measured Resection
Tibia first	Yes	Independent
Ligament release	No/minimal	As needed
Bone resections	Variable	Fixed

width equal to the thickness of the prosthesis. The third feature consisted of a resection of the distal femur in a plane, and at a distance from the resected tibia, to provide appropriate alignment in extension with balanced soft tissue tension.[21]

The GB technique starts with the creation of the flexion gap, which must be done before the corresponding gap is cut in extension so that the surgeon can make the extension gap the same size as the flexion gap. If the extension gap is made first by resecting the distal end of the femur, it may not be possible to resect the tibia at the optimal level without sacrificing excessive tibia bone, or without further resection of the distal femur.[31] In the description of the classic GB technique, the proximal tibia should be resected 6 to 8 mm below the unworn compartment perpendicular to the mechanical axis, and after osteophyte removal, a bicompartmental tensor is inserted into the knee in extension. Frontal alignment of the leg is extramedullary and is controlled by ligament tension. Releases of the collateral ligaments are performed when necessary to achieve correct leg alignment. The soft tissues are tensioned with laminar spreaders or tensors and determine the rotation of the femoral component. Once the joint is accurately tensioned in flexion, anterior and posterior femoral condylar resections are made using an anterior referencing AP cutting block. The femur rotates irrespective of bony landmarks guided by the ligaments to create flexion gap symmetry. The anterior surface of the femur should be resected at a distance from the posterior resection that is equal to the size of a femoral prosthesis. With the knee in extension, tensioning devices, set at a tension level similar to the flexion gap, establish the extension gap, referencing from the resected tibia. An intramedullary or extramedullary guide is attached to the tensioning jig and the lower extremity alignment versus the mechanical axis is carefully evaluated. Additional soft tissue balancing can be done to correct alignment. Once symmetric flexion and extension gaps are obtained, the distal femoral cutting jig is applied and the distal femoral cut is made. Again, a spacer block is inserted into the extension gap to check extension gap symmetry and equality with the flexion gap.

The GB technique has been adopted and further popularized by surgeons who introduced the use of rotating platform implants.[9,11,61]

With mobile-bearing implants, there is a definite risk of "spin-out" and bearing dislocation when the flexion gap is unbalanced or asymmetric. The GB technique prioritizes the flexion gap configuration, thereby providing a safe surgical technique flow for mobile-bearing TKA users.[11,59]

ADVANTAGES OF THE GAP BALANCING TECHNIQUE

Theoretically, this technique results in stable and balanced (ie, rectangular) extension and flexion gaps.[18,37] Dennis et al.[15]

compared the stability of 40 MR TKAs and 20 GB TKAs. The presence and magnitude of femoral condylar lift-off was evaluated for each technique at 0, 30, 60, and 90 degrees of flexion using an automated 3-dimensional model fitting kinematic analysis. The GB technique exhibited a much lower incidence of condylar lift-off greater than 1.0 mm ($p < .0001$). In particular, a lift-off greater than 1 mm was found in 60% (cruciate-retaining [CR] prosthesis) and 45% (posterior-stabilized [PS] prosthesis) of the MR group versus none in the GB group. The presence of femoral condylar lift-off may have adverse effects on the clinical results of TKA and represents a possible factor for polyethylene wear because of condylar edge loading. This is supported by the in vitro work of Jennings et al.,[34] who studied the effect of femoral condylar lift-off on wear of ultra-high-molecular-weight polyethylene in fixed-bearing and rotating-platform TKAs using a physiologic knee simulator. The presence of femoral condylar lift-off substantially accelerated (greater than twofold) the wear of the fixed-bearing and rotating-platform knees. A number of authors believe that the GB technique is able to provide greater accuracy in achieving the proper rotational alignment of the femoral component compared to the MR technique, which relies on obscured bony landmarks.[14,37] In a cadaveric study, Katz et al. compared the reliability of the transepicondylar axis (TEA), AP axis, and GB techniques to determine femoral rotational alignment. They showed that the TEA was less predictable and significantly more externally rotated than the AP axis and the GB technique. They concluded that the balanced flexion gap tension technique showed more accuracy and reliability in determining femoral rotational alignment in relationship to the flexion-extension axis.[37]

DISADVANTAGES OF THE GAP BALANCING TECHNIQUE

There are three possible primary negative consequences of the GB technique described in the literature: femoral internal rotation, asymmetric overload in flexion, and change in joint line position. Malrotation of the femoral component has been associated with patellofemoral and tibiofemoral instability, arthrofibrosis, knee pain, and abnormal knee kinematics.[7,55] In the pure GB technique, the femoral component internal rotation may occur in three possible scenarios: a valgus knee, a varus knee treated by over-release of medial soft tissue structures, and in the metaphyseal varus deformity characterized by a hyperplastic medial femoral condyle. After the tibial resection is performed and tension is applied on both sides of the medial and lateral compartment in flexion, if the medial side has a larger gap than the lateral, this will create the need to resect more lateral femoral condyle than medial condyle to attain parallelism of the resected planes of the femur and tibia.[28] This larger gap might result from a preexisting valgus deformity with medial laxity or from an over-release of the medial compartment for a varus deformity. To create a rectangular gap in flexion when the medial site has a larger gap than the lateral site, the surgeon, using a pure gap technique, must internally rotate the femoral component. This action has obvious negative consequences on patellar-femoral tracking with residual valgus limb alignment in flexion and lateral patellar subluxation.[8] High interpatient variability in femoral component rotation was found regardless of whether ligament releases were necessary (range −3 to 12 degrees for knees that did not need ligament releases and −4 to 13 degrees for knees that needed ligament releases). However, as expected, the type of release influenced femoral component rotation; knees with major medial releases showed the least mean external rotation (2 ± 4.2 degrees) compared with knees with minor lateral releases that had the most mean external rotation (7 ± 3.8 degrees).[28] This wide variation of intraoperative femoral component rotation is also described by Fehring.[18] Matziolis et al. described the role of the GB technique in determining the rotational alignment of the femoral component using computed tomography (CT) analysis in 67 patients undergoing CR computer-navigated TKA. They showed that, even when the gap technique is performed correctly, it results in a relevant deviation (7.4 degrees internal rotation to 5.9 degrees external rotation) of the femoral component from the surgical epicondylar axis (SEA).[45] In contrast, Babazadeh et al.[2] and Nikolaides et al.[49] showed no differences in terms of femoral component rotation between the GB and MR techniques.

Yau et al.'s[69] sample group included 25 TKAs in 14 patients. Yau et al. reported that the "pure gap technique" for determining the rotation of the femoral prosthesis seemed to be the most precise method in terms of having the least variability and the lowest percentage of surgical outliers of more than 5° (20%), when comparison was made with a reference TEA determined by CT.[69]

Another possible complication of the GB technique described in the literature is asymmetric overload in flexion. As described by Whiteside et al., correction of a varus knee with the GB technique may result in residual varus limb alignment in flexion.[27,68] A 90-degree resection of the tibia, with or without medial collateral ligament (MCL) release, is followed by soft tissue tension in flexion using tensiometers, which internally rotate the femur (Fig. 152.1A and B). A rectangular flexion gap is obtained with an externally rotated femoral bone resection parallel to the tibia (see Fig. 152.1B). When the femur derotates in its original position, the knee joint in flexion will be malaligned again in varus (see Fig. 152.1C).[67] Lee et al. evaluated the femoral component rotation and varus-valgus laxity at 0 and 90 degrees of flexion in 44 patients undergoing a CR computer-assisted TKA. They concluded that the GB technique provides good intraoperative alignment and laxity of knees at 0 and 90 degrees. However, increased femoral component external rotation was found to be correlated with increased varus alignment at 90 degrees of knee flexion. Furthermore, the more the femoral component was rotated externally, the greater the varus alignment at 90 degrees of flexion.[41]

The third disadvantage reported in the literature is the change of joint line position. The objective to obtain symmetric flexion and extension gaps may not respect the joint line position because of the possibility of performing a greater distal femoral resection. If the joint line is elevated more than 3 to 4 mm, it may cause the so-called mid-flexion instability problem.[43] In a prospective blinded randomized controlled trial, Babazadeh et al. compared 103 patients randomized to GB or MR computer-navigated TKA. The GB technique resulted in a significantly raised joint line compared to the MR technique (2.18 mm vs. 0.63 mm, respectively).[2] In addition, Lee et al. reported that mean polyethylene liner thickness and flexion/extension gaps were significantly greater in the GB group as compared to the MR group.[40]

Finally, a recognized bias for the GB technique has been the precision and accuracy of the instruments provided to assess the soft tissue tension, particularly in flexion, with the knee exposed and the patella most often laterally displaced or everted.[48] For this reason, different types of tensioning devices have been developed by different authors, and recently force sensor devices have been added to the surgical instruments required for the GB phase of the procedure (Fig. 152.2).[10,19]

RATIONALE OF THE MEASURED RESECTION TECHNIQUE

The MR technique was first introduced by Hungerford, Kenna, and Krackow in the early 1980s.[30] The aim was to resect an amount of bone equal in thickness to the prosthesis to be implanted and thus maintain the joint-line position. This technique was developed based on the observation that a properly positioned joint line is essential to proper collateral ligament and cruciate ligament function.[43] This is the reason that the MR technique was initially associated with a CR philosophy. When using a CR implant, balancing of flexion and extension gaps cannot be achieved by modifying bone cuts (which must be limited to maintain proper tension of the PCL), but instead relies on soft tissue releases. Proper PCL tension is dependent upon maintaining the level of the joint line and the spatial relationship between the femur and the tibia, which is often guaranteed by the MR technique. In the early phases, the MR technique was used in association with principles of anatomic alignment as described by Hungerford et al.[30] In the following decades, the use of the MR technique was extended to PS implants and to classic mechanical alignment.

Unlike the GB technique, bone cuts are fixed and are made independent of soft tissue release, which is performed progressively throughout the procedure. The femur or the tibia can be resected first and each bone resection is independent of the other. Bone landmarks are used to guide resections, which are equal to the distal and posterior thicknesses of the femoral component. The distal femoral and posterior femoral condyles are used to determine the amount of bone to resect to restore the distal and the posterior joint lines to their original anatomic positions. The femoral component rotation relies on accurate intraoperative identification of different reference axes derived from bony landmarks. Of these, the surgical transepicondylar axis (sTEA), the anatomic transepicondylar axis (aTEA), the posterior condylar axis (PCA), and the AP trochlear axis (AP or Whiteside line) are the most popular. The sTEA is a line connecting the prominence of the lateral epicondyle to the medial epicondylar sulcus, where the deep fibers of the MCL are inserted. The sTEA is positioned perpendicular to the tibial mechanical axis with the knee in 90 degrees of flexion, and therefore represents a good reference for femoral component rotation.[6,33,47,50] Better central patellofemoral tracking and better coronal stability can be achieved by placing the femoral component parallel to the TEA.[33] Placement of the femoral component parallel to the TEA also assisted in obtaining a rectangular flexion gap (90% using the TEA, 83% using the AP axis, and 70% using the PCA) in an analysis performed by Olcott and Scott.[50] The AP axis or Whiteside line connects the deepest point of the trochlea anteriorly to the center of the intercondylar notch posteriorly and is perpendicular to the sTEA. This axis depends on the normal anatomy of the trochlear groove and intercondylar notch of the distal femur, and is easily identified intraoperatively with the knee flexed. The femoral surfaces are resected in a line perpendicular to the Whiteside line to establish

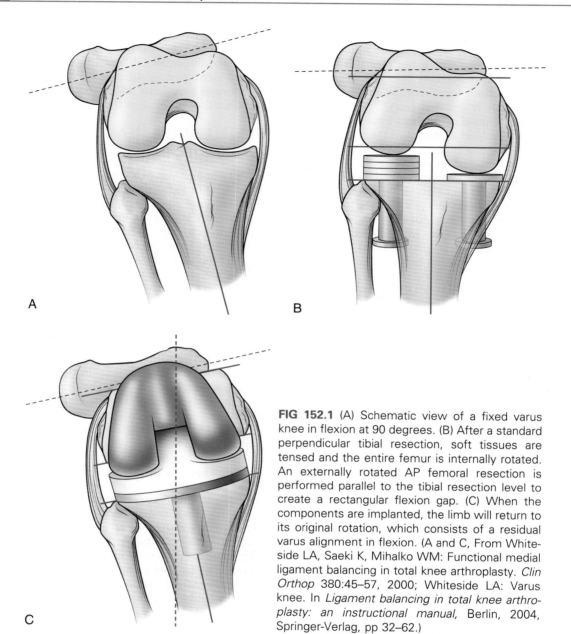

FIG 152.1 (A) Schematic view of a fixed varus knee in flexion at 90 degrees. (B) After a standard perpendicular tibial resection, soft tissues are tensed and the entire femur is internally rotated. An externally rotated AP femoral resection is performed parallel to the tibial resection level to create a rectangular flexion gap. (C) When the components are implanted, the limb will return to its original rotation, which consists of a residual varus alignment in flexion. (A and C, From White-side LA, Saeki K, Mihalko WM: Functional medial ligament balancing in total knee arthroplasty. *Clin Orthop* 380:45–57, 2000; Whiteside LA: Varus knee. In *Ligament balancing in total knee arthroplasty: an instructional manual,* Berlin, 2004, Springer-Verlag, pp 32–62.)

rotational alignment of the femoral component. This line results in approximately 3 to 5 degrees of external rotation with respect to the PCA. When the femoral component is placed perpendicular to the AP axis, enhancement of stability and patellar tracking has been observed.[66] The PCA refers to a line along the posterior aspect of the femoral condyles. The angular relationship between the PCA and the TEA is externally rotated approximately 3 to 4 degrees.[1] It is important to emphasize that in a severely valgus knee, there is commonly hypoplasia or erosion of the posterior aspect of the lateral femoral condyle. In this case, if the PCA is used as the primary determinant of femoral component rotation without adding corrections, erroneous femoral component placement in internal rotation will occur.

In summary, with the MR technique, the recommendation is to implant the femoral component parallel to the sTEA, perpendicular to the Whiteside line, or 3 to 5 degrees externally

rotated with respect to the PCA. Generally, the resection of the posterior femoral condyles results in slightly more resection of the medial condyle than of the lateral condyle in normal knees; in valgus knees, there is more extensive resection of the medial condyle than of the lateral condyle.[17]

The tibial cut is done independently, and the amount of tibial resection varies depending on tibial bone loss, but must, at a minimum, be the thickness of the thinnest tibial prosthesis on the unworn compartment (if collaterals are not stretched out by a severe deformity).[29] Once the distal femur and proximal tibia bony resections have been performed, the knee stability is tested in extension with spacer blocks. At this point, preliminary ligament balancing is performed if necessary. Because flexion and extension gaps cannot be balanced by modifying bone cuts, soft tissue release plays a key role.[29] Whiteside and other authors have emphasized the concept of selective rather than global release of tight soft tissue structures and the resultant independent effect

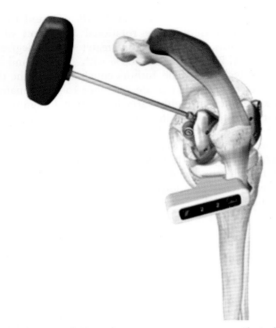

FIG 152.2 This picture shows a pressure sensor that electronically measures the relative pressures within the medial and lateral compartments before bony cuts are performed. eLibra Dynamic Knee Balancing System (ZimmerBiomet Inc., Warsaw, Indiana).

TABLE 152.2 Studies Demonstrating a More Physiologic Preservation of the Joint Line With the Measured Resection Technique as Compared to the Gap-Balancing Technique			
		JOINT-LINE ELEVATION (MM)	
Study	Number of Patients	MR	GB
Tigani et al.[62]	126	3.0 ± 2.3	4.1 ± 2.3
Lee et al.[40]	30	2.2 ± 1.5	3.8 ± 1.2
Sabbioni et al.[56]	67	3.5	4.0
Babazadeh et al.[2]	103	0.63 ± 1.2	2.18 ± 2.3

GB, Gap-balancing; *MR*, measured resection.

on the flexion and extension spaces to achieve a balanced TKA.[65] Stability of the knee involves ligaments that behave differently in flexion and extension. The contracture and stretching that occur because of deformity and osteophytes affect these ligament structures unequally and often cause different degrees of tightness or laxity in flexion and extension after the bone surfaces are resected correctly. Only ligaments that are tight need to be released, minimizing trauma and maximizing stability of the knee.[65] The anatomic flexion gap may not be exactly quadrilateral with the MR technique, but may instead be larger on the lateral side than on the medial side. In the normal knee, the collateral ligaments are more lax laterally, especially during flexion. This residual lateral ligament laxity tends to be allowed, and some authors suggest that it favors normal kinematics of the knee in permitting a greater degree of rotational freedom on the lateral side than on the medial side.[44,57,63] They also believe that the lateral compartment has more inherent laxity than the medial side in the normal knee, and that it is dynamically stabilized by the musculotendinous units, which include the popliteus, the iliotibial band, the biceps femoris, and the lateral head of the gastrocnemius.[29]

ADVANTAGES OF THE MEASURED RESECTION TECHNIQUE

Four main advantages are usually attributed to the MR technique: preservation of the joint line, enhanced patellar tracking, preservation of proper alignment in flexion and extension, and easy recovery from minor mistakes in surgical technique.

Preservation of the joint line is one of the key factors for a satisfactory outcome favoring normal knee kinematics and appropriate ligamentous balance. Failing to preserve the preoperative joint line position can have detrimental effects on PCL

function, collateral ligament function, the patellofemoral joint mechanism, and eventually compromise clinical outcomes.[58,70] In particular, an elevation of more than 3 to 4 mm can increase PCL strain. This makes the joint line position particularly important in CR designs. Moreover, an elevation of more than 4 mm of the joint line can also lead to mid-flexion instability.[43] Several studies have demonstrated that MR technique maintains a more physiologic joint line than the GB technique[2,40,56,62] (Table 152.2). In a prospective blinded randomized controlled trial, Babazadeh et al.[2] compared 103 patients randomized to GB or MR computer-navigated TKA using a total condylar prosthesis. Although no difference in functional and clinical outcomes were found 24 months after surgery, the GB technique resulted in a significantly raised joint line compared to the MR technique (0.63 mm vs. 2.18 mm, respectively) because of a greater distal femoral resection (9.6 mm vs. 11.2 mm) and larger tibial insert thickness. Although there is no published evidence showing that minor changes of the joint line position in primary TKA have an effect on the clinical outcome, in cases of preoperative shortening of the patellar tendon or clear patella infera, the MR technique should be considered a better choice.

Patellofemoral dysfunction remains the cause of many unsatisfactory TKAs. As patellofemoral mechanics is adversely affected by elevation of the joint line resulting in impingement of the patella and the patellar tendon on the tibial component, maintenance of the anatomic joint line is valuable.[2,16,51] Further evidence comes from Figgie et al.,[20] who demonstrated that if the patella is not within a defined sagittal neutral zone (10 to 30 mm above the joint line), a greater number of patellar problems are observed.[20]

Maintaining proper alignment of the knee in flexion and extension is essential for the survivorship of an implant. Different authors demonstrated that the MR technique creates a better alignment in flexion compared with GB.[27,42] Hanada et al.[27] showed that the GB technique can cause the knee to shift into a varus malalignment in flexion, causing overload on the medial side, whereas the MR technique results in a well-balanced and aligned knee in extension and flexion. Specifically, because the GB technique does not take into account the natural laxity on the lateral side of the knee, especially during flexion, more joint space opening will result on the lateral side if equal tension is applied to the medial and lateral collateral ligaments, creating a balanced but more externally rotated flexion gap. This external rotation will cause the knee to shift to varus in flexion, causing overload on the medial side.[27,41,42]

Finally, because femoral and tibial cuts are independent of one another, it is easier to recover from a slight error in surgical technique, such as an imperfectly aligned tibial cut. On the contrary, because the resected proximal tibia is used as a reference to balance the flexion space at 90 degrees, a precise proximal tibial resection is critical when using the GB technique. A varus tibial resection will result in increased internal rotation of the femoral component when the femoral component is placed parallel to the resected proximal tibia. Correspondingly, a valgus tibial cut will lead to excessive external rotation of the femoral component.[13,15]

DISADVANTAGES OF THE MEASURED RESECTION TECHNIQUE

There are three main disadvantages of the MR technique: risk of flexion gap imbalance, risk of iatrogenic ligament injury, and interindividual variability and poor reliability of bone landmarks.

Obtaining a symmetrically balanced knee in flexion and in extension by creating rectangular flexion and extension gaps has historically been one of the basic principles of knee arthroplasty because asymmetric flexion gaps are associated with poorer postoperative outcomes and an increased incidence of postoperative tibial radiolucent lines.[12,55] An asymmetric flexion gap and the presence of increased mediolateral laxity have been reported to result in asymmetric pressure under the medial and lateral aspects of the tibial component and a greater risk of condylar lift-off, potentially placing the polyethylene liner at greater risk of surface damage or uneven wear patterns.[12,15,60]

One of the main differences between the MR and GB techniques is the rate of ligament releases. Although they should be minimal or absent in the GB technique because flexion gap balance is mainly obtained by modifying the femoral bone cut, the MR technique requires ligament releases because bone cuts are fixed and cannot be modified to obtain better balance. For this reason, it is easier to create iatrogenic injury of the collateral ligaments with the MR technique.

Another problem of a classic MR technique is interindividual inconsistency of the reference axis. Several studies show the wide variability of distal femoral anatomic landmarks. Arima et al.[1] reported an average AP axis of 3.8 ± 2 degrees of external rotation, whereas the TEA was statistically more externally rotated with an average of 4.4 ± 2.9 degrees.[1] Poilvache et al.[52] found, in a study of 100 knees undergoing TKA, an epicondylar axis relative to the posterior condylar line of 3.51 ± 2.03 degrees in varus or neutral knees and 4.41 ± 1.83 degrees in valgus knees; regarding the AP axis, the external rotation relative to the posterior condyles was 2.73 ± 2.57 degrees and 5.91 ± 2.21 degrees in varus or neutral knees and valgus knees, respectively.[52] Berger et al.[6] found, in a group of 40 cadaver femurs, a mean aTEA of 4.7 ± 3.5 degrees for males and 5.2 ± 4.1 degrees for females. The mean sTEA measured 3.5 ± 1.2 degrees for males and 0.3 ± 1.2 degrees for females.[6]

Although the AP axis is not reliable in the presence of severe trochlear dysplasia and PCA is not reliable in a valgus knee with lateral femoral condyle hypoplasia, TEA is considered to be the most accurate of the bony landmarks. However, different studies reported that surgeons may be unable to accurately and reproducibly identify this landmark. Locating the medial and lateral epicondyles precisely is often difficult to reproduce intraoperatively as demonstrated by Jerosch[35] and Katz.[37] Yau et al.,[69] who

compared the precision of TEA, PCA, AP axis, and the GB technique in determining the rotational alignment of the femoral prosthesis, found an error greater than 5 degrees in 56% with TEA, 72% with PCA, 60% with AP axis, and 20% with the GB technique. The authors concluded that the three alignment techniques that made reference to fixed anatomic landmarks resulted in highly variable rotational alignment of the femoral prosthesis and that the GB technique seemed to be the most precise method.[69] These results are in contrast with those from the work of Matziolis et al.,[45] who demonstrated that, even when the gap technique was performed correctly, it resulted in a relevant deviation (7.4 degrees internal rotation to 5.9 degrees external rotation) of the femoral component from the referenced TEA.[45]

AUTHOR'S PREFERRED TECHNIQUE: EXTENSION GAP FIRST WITH HYBRID (COMBINED MEASURED RESECTION AND GAP BALANCING) TECHNIQUE

Our technique of choice for primary TKA is a combination of elements of the GB and the MR techniques. The classic MR technique has been implemented with multiple double checks on flexion and extension gap configurations using different measurement tools while tensing the soft tissues or filling the gaps before and after the bone resections are performed. John Insall described this technique first in 2000.[23] The same author, using the early version of this technique in 104 consecutive TKAs, found that none of the evaluated knees demonstrated a flexion-versus-extension gap difference of more than 3 mm. This result created a symmetrical rectangular flexion and extension gap that translated into good clinical and radiographic outcomes at long-term follow-up.[23] Fluoroscopic kinematic in vivo analysis of 25 patients operated with an MR technique blended with GB rules showed a very limited amount of lift-off during gait (maximum of 2 mm), less than the reported values in the literature evaluating TKA operated with a pure MR or GB technique.[33] With this hybrid technique, standard bone resections are performed considering different bony landmarks in extension and in flexion, whereas contracted ligaments are released incrementally. Gap equalization is checked before and after the bone resections using laminar spreaders, different types of spacer blocks, and trial components (classic or "smart") throughout the entire procedure. The surgical steps are summarized in Box 152.1.

1. Some minimal ligament releases are performed during the surgical approach. With the knee joint in slight flexion, incision of the anterior horn of the medial meniscus allows subperiosteal elevation of a medial flap of tissue, which includes the meniscotibial fibers of the deep MCL (for the varus knees). Proximal tibial insertion of the superficial MCL is often involved in the subperiosteal elevation of the medial soft tissue flap as part of the exposure. The tibia is carefully subluxed forward in flexion and external rotation (called the *RanSall maneuver*, after its originators Ranawat and Insall).

2. Using an extramedullary guide, a proximal tibial osteotomy is performed perpendicular to the mechanical axis of the tibia, 8 to 10 mm (or less, in case of severe angular deformity) below the least-compromised articular cartilage. Accuracy in execution of the proximal tibial cut is mandatory because it also acts as a reference for femoral bone resections. In this

BOX 152.1 Surgical Steps of the Extension Gap First With Hybrid (Combined Measured Resection and Gap-Balancing) Technique

1. Perform minimal ligament releases during the surgical approach.
2. Perform a proximal tibial cut 8-10 mm below the least-compromised articular cartilage.
3. Perform a distal femoral cut of 8-10 mm on the most prominent condyle with a planned valgus angle.
4. Balance the extension gap with release of ligaments as required
5. Position the AP femoral cutting jig with posterior reference aiming for a stable flexion gap
6. Double-check the flexion gap configuration before the AP resection with a dedicated spacer block.
7. Fine tune the ligament balance and posterior capsular tension with trial components.

AP, Anteroposterior.

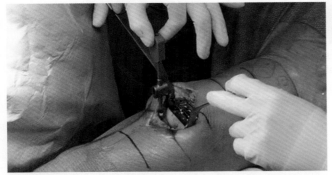

FIG 152.3 Intraoperative picture of the evaluation of the extension gap using a unicompartmental spacer block in a varus knee after a proximal tibial bone osteotomy is performed.

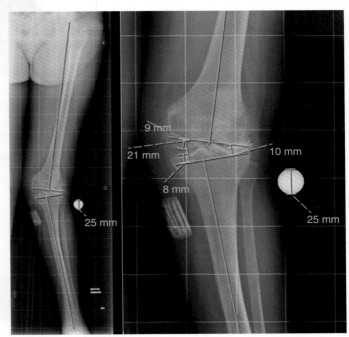

FIG 152.4 Evaluation of a full limb weight-bearing film of the lower limb with a magnification marker. This film enables the surgeon to plan the configuration of the extension gap, which will be created by standard femoral and tibial resections that are perpendicularly aligned along the mechanical axis of the single bones.

phase, a preliminary assessment of the extension gap symmetry or asymmetry could be done with a unicompartmental spacer (equal to the tibial baseplate plus polyethylene liner combined thickness) to carefully evaluate extension and flexion gaps in medial and lateral compartments (Fig. 152.3).

3. A distal femoral osteotomy of 8 to 10 mm (or less, in case of hyperextension deformity) on the most prominent condyle, with the planned valgus angle, is performed. Accurate preoperative planning based on AP full limb weight-bearing x-rays can be useful to anticipate the gap configuration (Fig. 152.4).

4. The extension gap can be assessed with spacer blocks and preliminary selective releases, mainly on the deep MCL, posteromedial capsule, and semimembranosus, can be performed (iliotibial band and eventually posterolateral capsule for valgus knees).

5. With the knee flexed at 90 degrees, the AP cutting jig is positioned after proper component sizing with a posterior referencing jig. The flexion gap is usually created according to the MR technique, using all available information from the bony landmarks (TEA, PCA, and AP axis). However, given the variability of anatomic bony landmarks, a preliminary assessment of the femoral AP resections can be done including the evaluations adopted from the GB technique.

6. Using a dedicated spacer block or just a simple "minus 3-mm" spacer block between the posterior aspect of the AP

guide and the tibial resected plateau, the flexion gap configuration can be anticipated before performing the AP resections (Fig. 152.5A and B). If a discrepancy in this double-check occurs, one of the following two surgical tips can be used to avoid a gap imbalance: in the GB technique, the femoral cutting jig can be internally or externally rotated as needed, whereas in the MR resection technique, a selective ligamentous release can be performed. If the first solution is preferred, it should be kept in mind that the classical central pivoting of the distal femur would create an over-resection of the posterior medial or lateral femoral condyle, which may lead to excessive "paradoxical" opening of the corresponding flexion gap in the subsequent surgical phases. In this scenario, the pivot point of rotation of the AP cutting jig can be switched from the center of the knee to the medial or lateral condyle. Anterior femoral notching can be avoided by applying few degrees of flexion in the distal femoral cut. When performing an extension-gap-first technique, the risk of creating a wider flexion gap exists, in particular with cruciate-substituting implants.[36,46] This can occur in two circumstances: when a release of the superficial MCL is performed and in cases of important flexion contracture in which the PCL is part of the deformity. In a study of 50 osteoarthritic knees, a PCL release created only a slight symmetrical increase in flexion gap, averaging 1.3 mm medially and laterally, and a significant increase was found only in cases with preoperative flexion contracture.[3] This tendency in flexion/extension gap discrepancy (with a bigger flexion gap) can be more common in PS implants, and can be limited with a number of measures: by adding 2 to 3 degrees

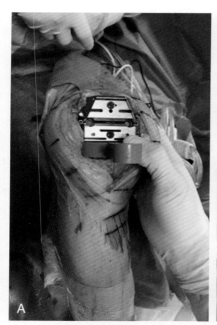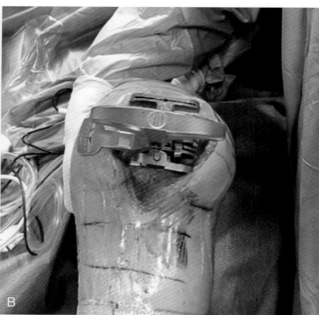

FIG 152.5 Intraoperative picture of two different spacer blocks in flexion (A, classic and B, mobile) to evaluate the flexion gap configuration before the AP resections are performed.

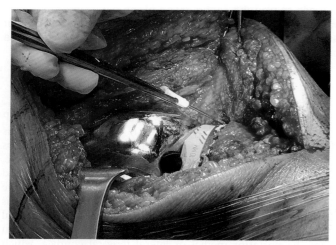

FIG 152.6 Additional MCL release is achieved by puncturing the ligament with a 16-gauge needle at various levels under valgus stress.

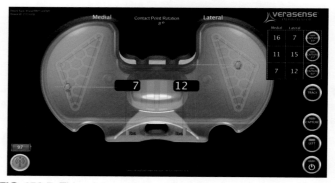

FIG 152.7 This picture shows the Verasense monitor (Ortho-Sensor Inc., Dania Beach, FL) monitor with different loads for the two compartments of the knee joint.

of flexion to the distal femoral cut[64]; by reducing the tibial sagittal slope by 2 to 3 degrees; by switching the femoral component rotational pivot point from central to medial to avoid an over-resection of the medial posterior condyle. The risk of mediolateral overhang, which may occur if a larger femoral component is needed, can be avoided given the availability of gender-specific implants or narrow mediolateral implants.

7. With the trial components in place, a fine-tuning of flexion-extension balance is performed.[65] If some medial tension persists, the MCL can be "pie-crusted" with multiple punctures by a 16-, 18-, or 19-gauge needle[5] (Fig. 152.6). Puncturing should be done at different levels of the MCL proximodistally and anteroposteriorly. On average, 12 to 15 punctures are needed to observe a 1- to 2-mm "opening"

effect. Using the needle instead of the small blade is safer, and even if the compartment opening is achieved with small sudden openings, there is no risk of complete ligament disruption.[4,38,39]

Recently, new intraoperative devices have been developed to provide a quantitative and more objective assessment of gap balance and to help surgeons with soft tissue releases (Fig. 152.7). These systems provide a quantitative way to measure the compressive forces across the knee joint in the medial and lateral compartments. The geometry and the shape of this sensor correspond to that of the standard tibial trial insert, so it can be adapted for use in different total knee systems.[26] By using the sensor in combination with graded shims, the appropriate thickness of the trial component can be constructed. The device replaces the standard tibial trial insert during surgery and can be used in the MR or GB technique. The "smart" tibial tray is composed of a microprocessor and an integrated nanosensor system that transmits real-time data to a portable graphic display unit through a wireless connection. The sensor measures and localizes peak load in the medial and lateral compartments. Loads can be captured intraoperatively through a full range of motion (ROM) so that balance of the knee can be dynamically assessed in full extension, at mid-flexion (45 degrees), and in 90 degrees of flexion. Subjective varus-valgus stress testing can also be performed to assess stability of the knee. Soft tissue releases can be performed sequentially while visualizing their effect on balancing the compartment pressures.[24] The smart tibial tray can also assess the rotation of the tibial and femoral components. Contact points at the tibiofemoral interface are shown as point markers in the medial and lateral compartments of the virtually displayed tibial tray. A nonparallel position of the contact points indicates incongruence in tibiofemoral rotation. The surgeon can dynamically modify tibial tray rotation until the contact points appear parallel in the graphic display, indicating rotational congruency between the components.[54] Although the use of this new technology seems promising,[25] more independent studies are needed to effectively evaluate the accuracy and cost-effectiveness of these devices in current practice.

KEY REFERENCES

2. Babazadeh S, Dowsey MM, Stoney JD, et al: Gap balancing sacrifices joint-line maintenance to improve gap symmetry: a randomized controlled trial comparing gap balancing and measured resection. *J Arthroplasty* 29(5):950–954, 2014.
3. Baldini A, Scuderi GR, Aglietti P, et al: Flexion-extension gap changes during total knee arthroplasty: effect of posterior cruciate ligament and posterior osteophytes removal. *J Knee Surg* 17(2):69–72, 2004.
5. Bellemans J, Vandenneucker H, Van Lauwe J, et al: A new surgical technique for medial collateral ligament balancing: multiple needle puncturing. *J Arthroplasty* 25(7):1151–1156, 2010.
7. Boldt JG, Stiehl JB, Hodler J, et al: Femoral component rotation and arthrofibrosis following mobile-bearing total knee arthroplasty. *Int Orthop* 30(5):420–425, 2006.
14. Dennis DA: Measured resection: an outdated technique in total knee arthroplasty. *Orthopedics* 31(9):940, 943–944, 2008.
15. Dennis DA, Komistek RD, Kim RH, et al: Gap balancing versus measured resection technique for total knee arthroplasty. *Clin Orthop* 468(1):102–107, 2010.
18. Fehring TK: Rotational malalignment of the femoral component in total knee arthroplasty. *Clin Orthop* 380:72–79, 2000.
23. Griffin FM, Insall JN, Scuderi GR: Accuracy of soft tissue balancing in total knee arthroplasty. *J Arthroplasty* 15(8):970–973, 2000.
27. Hanada H, Whiteside LA, Steiger J, et al: Bone landmarks are more reliable than tensioned gaps in TKA component alignment. *Clin Orthop* 462:137–142, 2007.
28. Heesterbeek PJ, Jacobs WC, Wymenga AB: Effects of the balanced gap technique on femoral component rotation in TKA. *Clin Orthop* 467(4):1015–1022, 2009.
32. Insall JN, Scott WN: *Insall & Scott surgery of the knee*, ed 4, Philadelphia, PA, 2006, Churchill Livingstone/Elsevier.
41. Lee DS, Song EK, Seon JK, et al: Effect of balanced gap total knee arthroplasty on intraoperative laxities and femoral component rotation. *J Arthroplasty* 26(5):699–704, 2011.
45. Matziolis G, Boenicke H, Pfiel S, et al: The gap technique does not rotate the femur parallel to the epicondylar axis. *Arch Orthop Trauma Surg* 131(2):163–166, 2011.
50. Olcott CW, Scott RD: A comparison of 4 intraoperative methods to determine femoral component rotation during total knee arthroplasty. *J Arthroplasty* 15(1):22–26, 2000.
55. Romero J, Stahelin T, Binkert C, et al: The clinical consequences of flexion gap asymmetry in total knee arthroplasty. *J Arthroplasty* 22(2):235–240, 2007.

The references for this chapter can also be found on www.expertconsult.com.

153

Is the Understanding of Gap Balancing and Measured Resection Techniques Necessary to Understand Image-Guided Surgical Techniques for Knee Arthroplasty?

Dana Lycans, Ali Oliashirazi

INTRODUCTION

As the development of total knee implants has progressed, there has been a divide among surgeons regarding surgical technique into two main categories: those who are gap balancers and those who perform measured resection. Regardless of technique, the goal of any knee arthroplasty is to recreate a balanced and aligned knee as this has been demonstrated to be associated with reduced wear and longer implant survival.[17,25,33] In addition, numerous studies have shown rotational malalignment of the femoral to be associated with higher incidence of patellofemoral and tibiofemoral instability, knee pain, arthrofibrosis, and overall abnormal knee kinematics.[3,6,9,34,37]

Although the overall goal of alignment and component rotation in the total knee arthroplasty (TKA) is more or less agreed upon, the means to this end are often debated with both sides citing valid pros for their technique with cons of the alternative. The details of each technique, gap-balancing and measured resection, are discussed at length in previous chapters. This chapter will discuss the pros and cons of each of these techniques and will briefly discuss the use of these techniques in relation to imaging techniques in TKA such as computed-assisted surgery.

GAP BALANCING TECHNIQUE

Gap balancing refers to a surgical technique where ligaments around the knee are released to correct gross knee malalignment prior to completion of all bony resections. In this technique the extension gap is altered and balanced by the extent of ligament releases, whereas the flexion gap is primarily balanced with proper sizing and rotation of the femoral component.[13] The goal of gap balancing is to create equal, rectangular gaps in both flexion (at 90 degrees) and extension (at 0 degrees). Laskin demonstrated that rectangular flexion gaps had superior clinical results when compared to those left with a trapezoidal gap.[21] Most commonly the extension gap is balanced first, after the distal femoral and proximal tibial resections are made. Osteophytes are removed next in either of these sequences, and finally corrective soft tissue releases are made to make a symmetric, rectangular extension gap.[10] With a rectangular gap in extension, the femoral component's rotation is set in flexion to lead to a rectangular extension gap without any more soft tissue releases.

Pros of Gap Balancing

Several studies have demonstrated better wear characteristics with a properly balanced and aligned knee.[3,6,9,34,37] Katz et al. showed in their cadaveric study that gap balancing technique gave more predictable rotation than using the transepicondylar or anteroposterior axes. In their study, the transepicondylar axis (TEA) was significantly more externally rotated than both gap balancing and the anteroposterior (AP) axis.[18]

Pang et al. used a computer-assisted gap balancing technique in their study comparing 140 patients randomized into either gap balancing or measured resection. The gap balancing group had more precise soft tissue balance compared to the measured resection group. With short follow-up, they found better knee scores in this group as well.[30]

Dennis et al.'s study examining 40 TKAs performed by measured resection and comparing them to the 20 gap balanced knees showed less coronal plane instability in the gap balanced group. This was measured using femoral condylar lift-off greater than 0.75 mm at any flexion interval. None of the patients who underwent gap balancing technique had lift-off greater than 1 mm, whereas the measured resection group had 25 patients with greater than 1 mm of lift-off.[12] It should be noted here that 1 to 1.5 mm of lift-off has been associated with significantly increased wear. Jennings et al. found statistically significant increases in wear in both mobile and fixed-bearing knees.[17]

Advocates of gap balanced technique cite numerous studies already discussed that show inconsistencies with the bony landmarks often used solely to determine femoral rotation in the measured resection technique and argue that using soft tissue tensioning to form a perfect rectangular space in flexion and extension more consistently reproduced a stable knee throughout motion.[10,13,18,31]

These data are further corroborated by Dennis, who performed computer navigation–assisted TKAs comparing gap balancing and measured resection. He found higher variability of the femoral component rotation when using the TEA and posterior condylar axis (PCA) when compared to the gap balanced knees. He recommended using all available methods to accurately assess TKA alignment.[11]

Cons of Gap Balancing

Despite various studies revealing good results with the use of gap balancing in TKA, there are several potential pitfalls that must be taken into consideration. These include careful attention to the accuracy of the tibia resection. If the resection is in varus, the femoral component will have increased internal rotation. In contrast, a valgus tibial resection could result in increased external rotation giving the potential for increased wear.[10,40]

If a large flexion gap requires increasing the amount of distal femur that must be removed, then the joint line can be moved proximally. The altered mechanics can alter the collateral ligament balance as well as the PCL in cruciate retaining prostheses, all of which can ultimately influence satisfaction with the procedure.[23]

Gap balancing looks at the flexion gap (at 90 degrees) as well as the extension gap (at 0 degrees), but this leaves the potential for midrange laxity. This most likely occurs when the posterior capsule is difficult to release with the posterior condyles still intact.[36,40] This laxity results mainly in complaints of instability, mainly when the patient descends stairs. Blunn et al. pointed out that this midflexion instability may accelerate wear of the prosthesis.[5]

Excessively loose medial structures cause excessive opening of the medial side and can result in internal rotation of the femoral component, whereas insufficient lateral structures can result in an externally rotated femoral component when placed parallel to the tibial surface, as is done in gap balancing.[10]

MEASURED RESECTION TECHNIQUE

Measured resection refers to a technique where bony resections equal the depth of the components and bony landmarks are used to determine femoral component rotation. Many authors favor this approach to arthroplasty rather than gap balancing.* In measured resection, bone cuts are made prior to any significant soft tissue releases. The femoral rotation is the set based on fixed bony landmarks, such as the TEA, anteroposterior axis (Whiteside's line), or the PCA. Soft tissue releases in flexion and extension are done after all osteophytes are removed and bony resections made.

Femoral Rotation

Rotational malalignment of the femoral component is associated with complications such as patellofemoral instability, pain, arthrofibrosis, and abnormal kinematics.[3,6,9,34,37]

The primary methods used for determining and checking rotation are the TEA, posterior femoral condyles, and the anteroposterior femoral axis (Whiteside's line). Each of these methods has its drawbacks, which can cause a malrotation of the femoral component potentially leading to problems, as outlined previously. Generally, the surgeon should take multiple axes and landmarks into account when determining the rotational alignment of the femoral component and, when possible, should err on the side of external rotation, given that a combined internal rotation of the components has shown a direct correlation with the severity of patellofemoral complications.[3,14,32,36]

Posterior Condylar Axis

One of the most common methods for referencing femoral rotation is to use the PCA. In this technique, a referencing guide is abutted up against the condyles after the menisci and any other obstructing soft tissues are removed. One of the main problems arising from the sole use of this method is in the case of a valgus knee, which typically accompanies a hypoplastic lateral condyle, or in any other case where there is posterior condylar erosion; this can cause a distortion in the reference axis and malrotation (internal rotation) of the component.

Nagamine et al.[28] performed a CT study of 84 knees examining the relationship between the TEA and AP axis (described later) as well as the PCA. Their results showed that the PCA was internally rotated approximately 6 degrees relative to the TEA. This matched the control knees in their study and led them to determine that the PCA could be used in knees with medial tibiofemoral arthritis to consistently reproduce natural rotation. Several other studies have been performed and indicate that the PCA can be used to effectively determine femoral rotation, especially if checked against another axis such as the TEA.[16,22]

A report by Schnurr et al., however, disputed this conclusion. He and his colleagues found that if the PCA technique had been used independently, the femoral rotation would only have been correct 51% of the time.[35] Typically, if using the PCA to determine rotation of the femoral component, the component will be positioned approximately 3 degrees in external rotation. Fehring reported from his study of 100 PS knees that if 3 degrees of external rotation was used, as high as 44% of patients would be outliers, which he defined as greater than 3 degrees of rotational error.[13]

Transepicondylar Axis

Insall, as well as many other authors, thought that using the TEA most closely re-created the patient's natural femoral rotation when performing TKA.[4,36] Some authors, however feel that the landmarks used for referencing this axis can be difficult to find without more extensive soft tissue dissection.[18,31] The medial epicondyle has been described as a horseshoe shaped ridge with a sulcus in the central part of the ridge. This sulcus can be used as a landmark for the medial epicondyle and can be found approximately 27 mm from the joint line. Across the femur on the lateral side, the epicondyle is described as a peak approximately 24 mm from the lateral joint line.[15]

Poilvache et al.[31] demonstrated in their study of 100 knees undergoing TKA that the TEA is a reliable landmark for proper rotation of the femur. They also noted it was easier to locate than the AP axis at the time of surgery. This is especially true in cases of trochlear dysplasia or valgus knees where relying on the AP axis can induce excessive external rotation of the femoral component leading to patellar maltracking.

As with the PCA, there are studies showing potential errors with the TEA as well. Siston et al. and Yau et al. demonstrated significant error ranges with all axes of reference including the TEA.[39,44] Katz et al. studies fresh-frozen cadaver knees and found the TEA to be more externally rotated compared to the AP axis and balanced tension line.[18] Another study found that only 75% of knees using the TEA solely as the method of alignment were within 3 degrees of the target alignment. The range for this study was 6 degrees external rotation to 11 degrees internal rotation.[20]

Anteroposterior Axis (Whiteside's Line)

The AP axis has been described as an accurate method for determining the correct alignment of the femoral component. A line 90 degrees to the AP axis has been shown to consistently

---

*References 1, 4, 15, 27, 31, 35, and 43.

approximate 4 degrees of external rotation when compared to the PCA, even in a valgus knee.[1,43] Problems with using this axis can arise in cases of trochlear dysplasia where the typical intercondylar notch is obliterated and accuracy of the landmarks used for this axis is decreased.[31]

Although many authors agree that the TEA is one of the most reliable methods for establishing rotation, the AP axis as well as the PCA are more easily identified during surgery, as there is no soft tissue coverage of the landmarks required.[1,4,28,31,45] Katz et al. found the AP axis to be less externally rotated than the TEA and better approximate the balanced tension line in their cadaveric study.[18]

It is important to remember that each of these axes described previously should not be used alone, but instead, multiple reference points should be used whenever possible to confirm correct rotation. Yau et al.[44] examined the precision of several methods of determining alignment. Their study of 25 TKAs using computer navigation looked at the TEA, PCA, and AP axis of the femur and compared them after performing their cuts. The range of error for the TEA was 28 degrees, with a range of 17 degrees internal rotation to 11 degrees external rotation. For PCA, the range was 27 degrees with 13 of internal rotation to 14 of external rotation. The error for the AP axis was a 32-degree range from 17 degrees internal to 15 degrees external rotation, and the range of using collateral ligament tension and flexion gap was 26 degrees with 14 internal to 12 external rotation. This study is similar to that of Siston et al., who used cadavers in their study to examine the error ranges. These studies found similar error ranges, but the Siston study was not able to reach a statistically significant difference in the error ranges of the different bony references, leading the authors to a conclusion that no specific technique was better than the others. Overall, only 17% of the cases using only bony references resulted in a femoral rotation within 5 degrees of the TEA.[39,44]

Pros of Measured Resection

Good long-term outcomes have been obtained from gap balancing technique. Studies show that similar results can be obtained from measured resection methodology. Nikolaides et al. showed comparable rotational alignment with both measured resection and gap balancing in their evaluation of CT scans taken 7 days after TKA. No significant differences were found.[29]

Cons of Measured Resection

The disadvantages of measured resection arise from inconsistencies in referencing for femoral rotation. This has been discussed previously and will not be repeated here. In summary, variability in bony anatomy can alter the rotation of the femur. This is illustrated in valgus knees where the lateral condyle is hypoplastic and worn more so than the typical varus knee. This can result in excessive internal rotation.

Similarly, the actual bony landmarks used for typical referencing can be difficult to find in the setting of surgery, where exposure may be limited. For example, if using the TEA, a surgeon needs adequate exposure of the epicondyles to ensure they are easily palpated or viewed. The intercondylar notch can also be hard to identify, particularly in cases of trochlear dysplasia, which can throw off rotation.

Lastly, in the setting of revision TKA, bony landmarks may be obliterated. For example, the PCA and AP axis landmarks are resected in the primary surgery. In this setting, gap balancing or TEA axis must be used to establish proper femoral rotation and give good knee kinematics.

Use of Imaging Techniques and Computer-Assisted Techniques in Total Knee Arthroplasty. Throughout the years, medicine has made many advancements in pharmacology, understanding of both anatomy and pathophysiology of diseases, surgical techniques, and imaging techniques/modalities. These innovations have allowed us to provide exponentially better care and surgical outcomes. Some have argued that the use of advanced imaging techniques and computer-assisted techniques in surgery are the next big step in improving patient care.

Computed tomography (CT) scans have been used to evaluate rotational alignment of the femoral component postoperatively; however its use is not limited to post hoc evaluation. CT scanning protocols have been designed by several manufacturers that assist in the production of patient-specific cutting blocks or implants.

Preoperative CT scans were used in a study by Luyckx et al. Here, 96 patients underwent "adapted measured resection," where preoperative CT scans were used to help determine external rotation. When this group was compared to a "gap balanced" group, no differences in femoral rotation between the groups was found.[26]

Several studies have evaluated computer-assisted navigation to determine if this improves surgical outcomes, and variable results have been reported.[19,24,38,41,42] Proponents of computer-assisted technology cite improved accuracy of the tibial cut alignment in particular.[7,30] Additionally, the overall alignment correction has been reported to be better with computer-assisted technology.[2,8,30]

Singh et al. found improvements in function of 52 TKA patients who underwent computer-assisted navigation. In this study, half the patients were randomized to undergo gap balancing and the rest were randomized to measured resection. Although both groups had significantly improved function following TKA, the gap balancing group was slightly better. This difference did not reach significance.[38]

Recommendations. This chapter has discussed pros and cons of both gap balancing and measure resection technique. Each technique has been used by many surgeons to reconstruct normal alignment and rotation in the knee during arthroplasty. Although research continues to be performed, currently the authors believe that a combination of techniques should be used by checking multiple axes in addition to ligament balance. We believe this will help the surgeon establish appropriate rotation and stability, thus giving the patient an excellent outcome, which is the ultimate goal of TKA.

KEY REFERENCES

1. Arima J, Whiteside LA, McCarthy DS, et al: Femoral rotational alignment, based on the anteroposterior axis, in total knee arthroplasty in a valgus knee. A technical note. *J Bone Joint Surg* 77(9):1331–1334, 1995.
3. Berger RA, Crossett LS, Jacobs JJ, et al: Malrotation causing patellofemoral complications after total knee arthroplasty. *Clin Orthop* 356:144–153, 1998.
6. Boldt JG, Stiehl JB, Hodler J, et al: Femoral component rotation and arthrofibrosis following mobile-bearing total knee arthroplasty. *Int Orthop* 30(5):420–425, 2006.

10. Daines BK, Dennis DA: Gap balancing vs. measured resection technique in total knee arthroplasty. *Clin Orthop Surg* 6(1):1–8, 2014.

11. Dennis DA: Measured resection: an outdated technique in total knee arthroplasty. *Orthopedics* 31(9):940, 943–944, 2008.

12. Dennis DA, Komistek RD, Kim RH, et al: Gap balancing versus measured resection technique for total knee arthroplasty. *Clin Orthop* 468(1):102–107, 2010.

18. Katz MA, Beck TD, Silber JS, et al: Determining femoral rotational alignment in total knee arthroplasty: reliability of techniques. *J Arthroplasty* 16(3):301–305, 2001.

29. Nikolaides AP, Kenanidis EI, Papavasiliou KA, et al: Measured resection versus gap balancing technique for femoral rotational alignment: a prospective study. *J Orthop Surg (Hong Kong)* 22(2):158–162, 2014.

31. Poilvache PL, Insall JN, Scuderi GR, et al: Rotational landmarks and sizing of the distal femur in total knee arthroplasty. *Clin Orthop* 331:35–46, 1996.

36. Scott WN: *Surgery of the knee*, ed 5, Philadelphia, PA, 2012, Elsevier.

37. Scuderi GR, Komistek RD, Dennis DA, et al: The impact of femoral component rotational alignment on condylar lift-off. *Clin Orthop* 410:148–154, 2003.

38. Singh VK, Varkey R, Trehan R, et al: Functional outcome after computer-assisted total knee arthroplasty using measured resection versus gap balancing techniques: a randomised controlled study. *J Orthop Surg (Hong Kong)* 20(3):344–347, 2012.

40. Springer BD, Parratte S, Abdel MP: Measured resection versus gap balancing for total knee arthroplasty. *Clin Orthop* 472(7):2016–2022, 2014.

43. Whiteside LA, Arima J: The anteroposterior axis for femoral rotational alignment in valgus total knee arthroplasty. *Clin Orthop* 321:168–172, 1995.

44. Yau WP, Chiu KY, Tang WM: How precise is the determination of rotational alignment of the femoral prosthesis in total knee arthroplasty: an in vivo study? *J Arthroplasty* 22(7):1042–1048, 2007.

The references for this chapter can also be found on www.expertconsult.com.

154

Mid-Flexion Instability After Total Knee Arthroplasty

Jan Victor, Thomas Luyckx

INTRODUCTION

Instability has long been recognized as a major cause of early total knee arthroplasty (TKA) failure[23,25] and has recently been reported as the most prevalent pathology leading to early revision after TKA.[24] This disturbing fact is not an unexpected surprise because the surgical workflow of TKA includes the resection of important knee joint stabilizers such as the menisci and the cruciate ligaments. In addition, subtle surgical damage to the collateral ligaments, popliteal tendon, and knee capsule can further decrease the natural defense against instability of the joint.[1,21] This significant loss of stabilizing structures must be mitigated by the implant, a very difficult and maybe impossible engineering mission. One of the best-known, well-recognized, and successful features contributing to increased stability after TKA was the introduction of the posterior stabilized (PS) TKA,[15] where the function of the posterior cruciate ligament was replaced by a cam-and-post mechanism that provided posterior stability of the tibia relative to the femur. This PS system also helped to restore the native knee kinematics, by pushing the femur backward with increasing flexion.

Types of Instability

Instability after TKA can be described in three planes:
- **Coronal plane instability:** This type of instability can be symmetric, and is related to an excessive extension gap or a polyethylene insert that is too thin. In that case, hyperextension will be a typical symptom. Asymmetric coronal plane instability is caused by a deficient medial or lateral collateral ligament, or by errors in implant positioning that leave the joint too loose or too tight on the medial or lateral side. It is crucial to understand that knee stability can be normal in *full* extension, even if there is a deficient medial or lateral collateral ligament, because of the stabilizing action of the posteromedial and posterolateral corner. As soon as the fully extended position is abandoned, coronal plane stability will rely on competent medial and lateral collateral ligament function.
- **Sagittal plane instability:** Increased anteroposterior laxity as compared to the native knee is a significant challenge for TKA. The loss of cruciate ligament function and the posterior horn of the medial meniscus destabilizes the joint in the sagittal plane. Stability can be improved with a meticulous fill-in of the so-called flexion gap, a cam-post mechanism, or increased tibiofemoral congruency. The latter solution is not as powerful and carries the intrinsic risk of inducing kinematic conflicts. An anterior build-up will mimic posterior cruciate ligament function; a posterior build-up will mimic anterior cruciate ligament function. Traditionally, sagittal plane stability has been described with the knee at 90 degrees of flexion, with important consequences for the assessment of stability intra- and postoperatively.
- **Horizontal plane stability:** Instability in the horizontal plane has received little attention, but kinematic studies based upon fluoroscopic imaging[5] show a significant range of rotational laxity after TKA. The "spin-out" that has been described with some types of rotating platforms is another symptom of horizontal plane instability.

We previously mentioned the close relationship in the surgeon's mind between coronal stability and the extension position, versus sagittal stability and the 90-degree flexion position. This is, in part, a result of the surgical concept of the flexion and extension gap, but it does not reflect reality for the following reasons:
1. As pointed out earlier, there is a significant difference between coronal stability at full extension (posterior capsular structures) and at 10 degrees of flexion (collateral ligaments).
2. At 90 degrees of flexion, instability often occurs in the three planes. A typical example is the (rare) dislocation of a posterior stabilized implant. It is often the combination of increased sagittal instability at 90 degrees of flexion with varus instability and excessive opening of the joint on the lateral side.

Consequently, the traditional *true flexion instability* as a consequence of an "excessive" flexion gap and *true extension instability* as a consequence of an "excessive" extension gap rarely present as isolated clinical events and are often complicated with three-dimensional instability patterns.

What Is Mid-Flexion Instability?

There seems to be significant semantic confusion in the literature when it comes to the term *mid-flexion instability*. This terminology is somehow a misnomer. The naming originated from the concept of stability in full extension and at 90 degrees of flexion. Instability at positions between these two reference positions was called mid-flexion instability. As we discussed previously, every form of instability in full extension and 90-degree flexion is associated with some form of instability in the mid-flexion range. We define *true* mid-flexion instability as a coronal and sagittal plane instability occurring in the mid-flexion range (15 to 60 degrees) despite an *equal* flexion and extension gap.

Why Is Mid-Flexion Stability So Important?

During most activities of daily living, the knee is not loaded at full extension, but in the early and mid-flexion range of the arc of motion.[18,19] Therefore, stability in the mid-flexion range is critical for a good functional outcome after TKA. Mid-flexion instability is characterized by the inability to descend stairs without the support of a handrail, sudden giving way during single stance loading as occurs in getting in and out of a car, chronic effusion, and synovitis. In the native knee, mid-flexion stability in the sagittal plane is secured by the cruciate ligaments. It is easy to understand the technical difficulty of achieving this stability in the absence of the cruciate ligaments. In addition, most surgeons evaluate stability of the knee at 0 and 90 degrees only and frequently overlook excessive laxity in the mid-flexion range.

The following section explains how changes in the joint line position, induced by TKA, can lead to true mid-flexion instability.

SURGICAL TECHNIQUE OF TKA INDUCES JOINT LINE ELEVATION

The traditional TKA surgical technique using cutting blocks induces a more cranial joint line in many cases. Traditional jigs use a valgus angle of 5 to 7 degrees relative to the femoral anatomic axis in the coronal plane for positioning of the distal femoral cutting block, because surgeons aim for a perpendicular cut relative to the femoral mechanical axis. This cut changes the natural joint line orientation. In the knee with a structurally undamaged medial condyle, the instrument will hit the distal part of the medial condyle and a similar thickness of bone (usually 9 mm) will be removed and replaced by the implant (Fig. 154.1A). This will restore the original medial joint line level after TKA. Many arthritic knees obviously display cartilage and even bone loss on the medial condyle, leading to a more proximal position of the cutting block that now abuts the lateral condyle (see Fig. 154.1B). The volumetric compensation by the femoral implant on the medial side will not compensate for the cumulative resected thickness and worn cartilage-bone unit. As a consequence, the joint line will be raised in extension.

The cuts that will determine the position of the femoral implant in anteroposterior position (often called the *flexion cuts*) are subjected to a different erroneous mechanism, leading

to a similar result. The perpendicular joint line orientation that the surgeon is trying to accomplish in the coronal plane requires rotation compensation in the axial plane. Many systems rotate the femoral cutting block around a central pivot, thereby taking out more bone on the medial side than on the lateral side (Fig. 154.2A and B). Again, a raise of the joint line on the medial side of the knee is the result.

This more proximal and anterior position of the femoral component on the medial side will be compensated by an increase in polyethylene thickness. Because the medial side of the knee is the isometric and stable side of the knee,[29] good stability in full extension and 90 degrees of flexion will follow. The lateral side of the knee will stretch out slightly to accommodate the raised joint line level. Because the lateral side of the knee is mainly dynamically stabilized, this does not cause significant soft tissue problems.[30]

EXPERIMENTAL EVIDENCE: JOINT LINE ELEVATION CAUSES MID-FLEXION INSTABILITY

In an experimental setup, a knee prosthesis was implanted in 10 fresh frozen cadaveric knees with the use of computer navigation. The target of the implantation was a restoration of the medial joint line both distal and posterior. This was done by making sure that both the distal and posterior medial resections exactly equaled the implant thickness (Fig. 154.3). Afterward, the joint line was raised in two steps of 2 mm (4 mm in total) by increasing the distal and posterior resections. By doing this, the flexion and extension gap remained equal and stability of the joint at 0 and 90 degrees was maintained by increasing the thickness of the insert by 2 and 4 mm respectively (Fig. 154.4).

Coronal Plane Laxity

Native Knee. The mean coronal plane laxity in full extension for the native knee was 2.2 degrees (standard deviation [SD] 1.3 degrees). At 30 degrees of flexion, the laxity was 5.7 degrees (SD 1.8 degrees); at 60 degrees of flexion, 5.7 degrees (SD 2.2 degrees); at 90 degrees of flexion, 8.0 degrees (SD 2.3 degrees); and at 120 degrees of flexion, 10.0 degrees (SD 3.1 degrees) (Fig. 154.5). This proportional increase in laxity versus flexion was

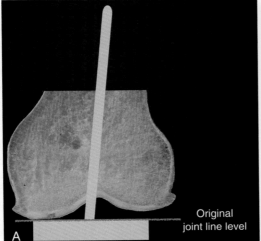
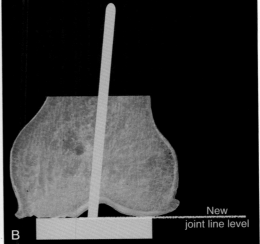

FIG 154.1 (A) Illustration of the distal referencing instrument against the intact distal medial condyle. (B) In case of medial cartilage and bone loss, the instrument will be positioned more cranial, leading to a change in joint line position.

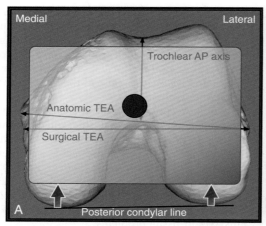
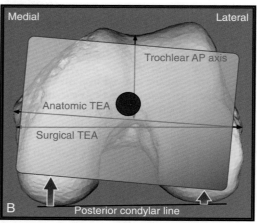

FIG 154.2 (A) Femoral cutting block in neutral rotation. (B) Femoral cutting block in external rotation, rotating around a central pivot point with excessive bone resection on the posteromedial condyle as a consequence. *AP*, Antero-posterior axis; *TEA*, trans-epicondylar axis.

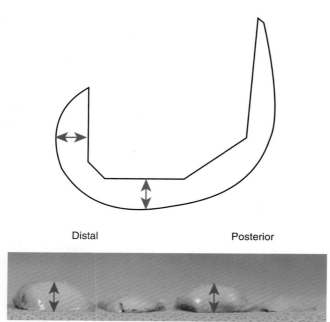

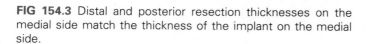

FIG 154.3 Distal and posterior resection thicknesses on the medial side match the thickness of the implant on the medial side.

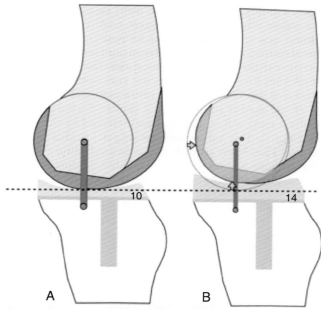

FIG 154.4 The increased resection and resulting greater flexion and extension gap is filled in with a thicker polyethylene insert. A shows the femoral implant with exactly the same size and position as the original distal femur. B shows a smaller femoral implant, positioned more proximally. The *yellow arrows* show the geometric difference in the sagittal plane. The increased resection and resulting greater flexion and extension gap is filled in with a thicker polyethylene insert.

statistically significant with $P < .05$ for all positions except the 30-degree versus 60-degree position and the 90-degree versus 120-degree position. These results are in line with previous studies.[4]

Total Knee Arthroplasty. The mean coronal plane laxity throughout the range of motion after implantation of a TKA prosthesis with restoration of the medial joint line level (TKA0) showed no significant differences with the native knee (see Fig. 154.5).

After raising the joint line, no significant differences were observed between the three TKA positions (TKA0, TKA2, TKA4) in extension for coronal plane stability. In mid-flexion position (30 and 60 degrees), however, a significant increase in

coronal plane laxity was observed for the TKA2 and TKA4 positions (Fig. 154.6). The first distal recut of 2 mm (TKA2) increased overall coronal plane laxity by an average of 64% (3.1 degrees) at 30 degrees of flexion ($P < .01$) and 51% (3.0 degrees) at 60 degrees of flexion ($P = .02$). Performing a second 2-mm recut (TKA4) of the distal femur increased the mid-flexion laxity by 111% (5.4 degrees) ($P < .01$) at 30 degrees and 95% (5.5 degrees) at 60 degrees of flexion ($P < .01$), compared to the 9-mm baseline resection (TKA0). At 90 degrees and 120 degrees, no significant differences were observed among the three groups.

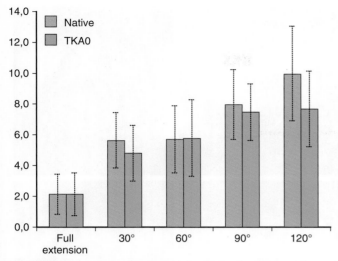

FIG 154.5 Mean coronal plane joint laxity in degrees is presented for each flexion angle. Results for the native knee and the TKA with the restored medial joint line are shown (TKA0). No statistically significant differences were noted between the native knee and the TKA0 position. Error bars indicate the standard deviation. *TKA,* Total knee arthroplasty.

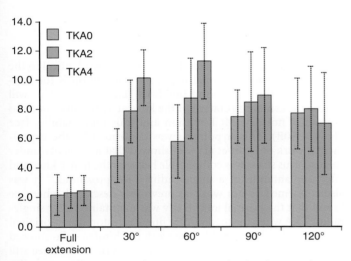

FIG 154.6 Mean coronal plane joint laxity in degrees is presented for each flexion angle. Results for the TKA with the restored joint line (TKA0), the 2-mm (TKA2), and the 4-mm (TKA4) raised joint line are shown. No statistically significant differences were noted among the three groups in extension or at 90 and 120 degrees of flexion. However, a significant increase in coronal plane laxity was noted at 30 and 60 degrees of flexion. *TKA,* Total knee arthroplasty.

An almost-perfect linear correlation between the level of the joint line and the coronal plane stability was found ($R^2 = 0.99$). From the linear regression model, it was calculated that for every millimeter rise in joint line level, a 31% increase in coronal plane laxity at 30 degrees and a 25% increase at 60 degrees can be expected.

These results confirm the clinical findings of Martin et al. and those of Cross et al. who also found significant instability in the mid-flexion range after raising the joint line.[3,22]

GEOMETRICAL EXPLANATION OF THE RELATION BETWEEN RAISING THE JOINT LINE AND MID-FLEXION INSTABILITY

The link between the level of the joint line and the coronal plane laxity was recognized by previous authors[3,22] and confirmed by our experimental data. A proper explanation for the relation between the two findings is still lacking. It cannot be explained by the classic flexion-extension space paradigm because the instability occurred despite a well-balanced flexion and extension gap. In an attempt to provide more profound insight in the association between the level of the medial joint line and joint stability, we developed a geometrical model of the knee.

Development of a Simplified Geometrical Model for the Knee

A simplified model of the knee can help in understanding the observed phenomena and explain the experimental and clinical findings. We chose to describe sagittal stability of the knee based on a two-dimensional model of the medial compartment. In contrast to the lateral side of the knee, the medial side is geometrically more conforming, has a more stable meniscus, and displays less translation during the motion arc than the lateral side. In addition, the superficial medial collateral ligament (sMCL) is isometric in its central fibers, in contrast to the lateral collateral ligament, which slackens with increasing flexion.[9,10,30,32] With these arguments, a stability model based on the medial compartment seems logical, despite of the obvious limitations that follow reduction of an intricate three-dimensional system to a simple two-dimensional model. However, the model can be defended if one accepts the following three theorems:

a. The sMCL is isometric in its central fibers, with minimal length changes (order of magnitude 1 mm) during the motion arc. There are sufficient data in the literature to support this statement.[9,10,30]

b. From a morphologic point of view, the shape of the posterior femoral condyles in the sagittal plane can be described as a circle. This knowledge goes back as far as 1836 when the Weber brothers were the first ones to describe the shape of the posterior condyles as a circle.[31] There are numerous more recent studies showing that with the use of sophisticated 3D imaging techniques, the shape of the femoral condyles can be described by best-fitting a circle, sphere, or cylinder in the posterior medial and lateral condyle (Figs. 154.7 and 154.8).[2,6,7,12,13] Achieving the best fit possible to the articular surface in the posterior condyles corresponds to a flexion range of 10 to 160 degrees.[6,13,31]

c. Within small mathematical errors, knee motion can be described as rotation around two axes that cross at the center of the medial condyle.[12] Other kinematic descriptions also use a flexion axis that runs very close to the center of the medial condyle.[2,12] Consequently, from a kinematic standpoint, the medial compartment can reasonably be considered as the stable compartment of the knee joint.*

Application to the Native Knee

Based on these three theorems, we created a simplified geometric model of the medial side of the knee in the sagittal plane.

*References 7, 11, 16, 17, 28, and 29.

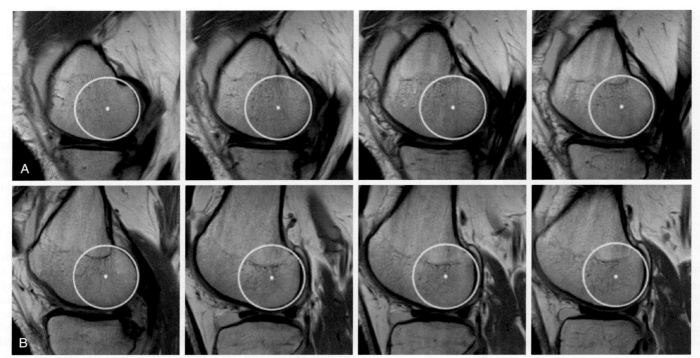

FIG 154.7 Sagittal MRI of a normal left knee. A best-fit *circle* to the subchondral-cancellous bone interface of the medial (A) and lateral (B) femoral condyle is shown. The radius of the *circle* was identical for all images.

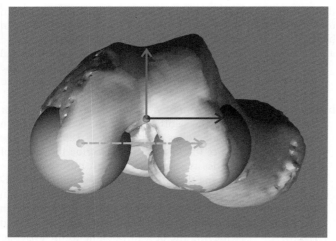

FIG 154.8 3D reconstruction image from a computed tomography (CT) scan of the left knee. The *grey spheres* represent the best-fit spheres to the medial and lateral condyle. The *blue arrow* is parallel to the line connecting the centres of the spheres, the *green arrow* represents the anteroposterior axis.

The sagittal cross section of the posterior medial condyle was represented as a circle. The center of rotation throughout the range of motion was considered fixed and coincided with the center of the circle, and the sMCL was considered isometric throughout the range of motion with its insertion site on the femur at the center of rotation of the knee (Fig. 154.9).

Application for Total Knee Arthroplasty

Assuming the insertion of a TKA prosthesis with exactly the same size and geometry as the native knee, strain patterns and tension in the medial collateral ligament will be identical to the native knee. One additional necessary assumption is the conservation of the initial joint line level (Fig. 154.10). This will restore the center of rotation of the knee at its original spot and reproduce normal sMCL tension and thus joint stability (see Fig. 154.10B). This hypothesis was confirmed by the experimental work of Hunt et al., who showed that joint laxity under valgus/varus stress was comparable between the native knee and after implantation of a single-radius TKA prosthesis.[14] It was also confirmed by our work, as previously described, where we found that the normal joint laxity was maintained after single-radius TKA when the medial joint line was restored at its original level. It is also supported by the work of Shimizu, who showed that after a single-radius TKA, the medial side of the knee still moves with a stable center of rotation with virtually no translation between 10 and 110 degrees of flexion.[26]

Predicting the Effect of Joint Line Changes

Changes in joint line position with a TKA will change the tibiofemoral center of rotation from its original position (Fig. 154.11). As the femoral insertion site of the sMCL is not altered, it will pivot around the new center of rotation during knee flexion and its isometric behavior will be changed (Fig. 154.12).[20] The precise effect on the length change of the sMCL depends on the direction of the joint line change. From the geometric model, the length changes of the sMCL induced by changing the joint line were calculated.

Joint Line Elevation. First, the effect of elevating the joint line by 4 mm was modeled. This was done by shifting the femoral component 4 mm proximal (see Fig. 154.11). To maintain joint stability in extension, a 4-mm thicker insert is used. The proximal shift of the distal joint line will cause a 4-mm proximal shift

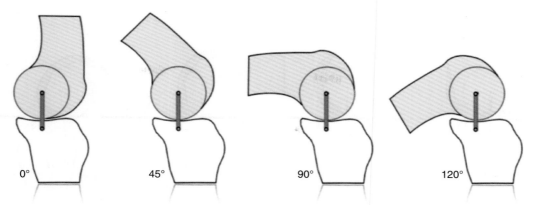

FIG 154.9 Simplified geometric model of the medial side of the native knee in the sagittal plane. A circle represents the curvature of the posterior medial condyle. The center of this circle coincides with the center of rotation and the femoral insertion site of the sMCL. During the range of motion, no change in length in the sMCL is observed. The *red dots* represent the center of insertion of the medial collateral ligament on the femur and the tibia.

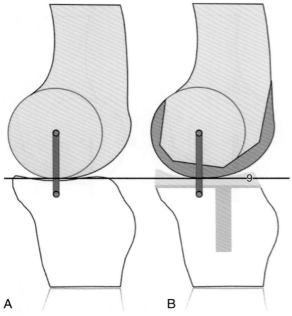

FIG 154.10 Geometric model of the medial side of the knee representing the posterior medial condyle as a circle with the sMCL insertion site at the center of this circle (A). A TKA with exactly the same surface geometry (ie, single radius) and size as the native knee restores the natural situation if the distal and posterior joint line are maintained at their original level (B). The *red dots* represent the center of insertion of the medial collateral ligament on the femur and the tibia.

of the tibiofemoral center of rotation. The effect of this shift on the length of the sMCL is shown in Figs. 154.12 and 154.13. A progressive lengthening is expected with a maximum change in length of 7.2 mm at 140 degrees of knee flexion. This observation is obvious and can also be explained by the flexion-extension gap theory. Because only the extension space was enlarged by raising the joint line, the flexion space is too tight for the 4-mm thicker insert. According to our model, the length change will be mild in early flexion, and progress linearly from 40 to 140 degrees of flexion.

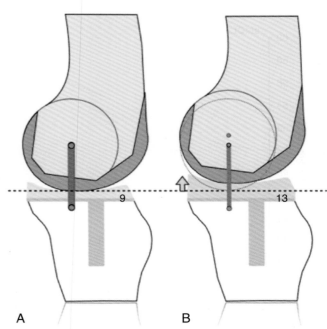

FIG 154.11 Schematic representation of the effect of a proximal shift of the joint line on the sMCL isometry. A new center of rotation *(blue dot)* is created as a result of the joint line shift. Because the insertion site of the sMCL is unchanged *(red dot)*, it will pivot around this new center of rotation during the range of motion. A shows the femoral implant with exactly the same size and position as the original distal femur. B shows the femoral implant, positioned more proximally, the *yellow arrow* represents the proximal displacement.

Femoral Downsizing. Next, the effect of placing the femoral component more anterior, and consequently raising the joint line by 4 mm, was modeled. This was done by increasing the posterior resection by 4 mm and fitting a 4-mm smaller component on the same knee (Fig. 154.14). The anterior shift of the posterior joint line will cause a 4-mm anterior shift of the tibiofemoral center of rotation. The effect of this shift on the length of the sMCL is shown in Figs. 154.15 and 154.16. A progressive slackening is predicted with a maximum change in

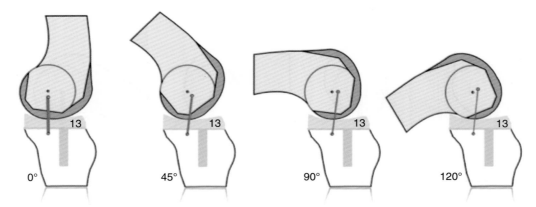

FIG 154.12 Schematic representation of the effect of a proximal shift of the joint line on the sMCL isometry. A new center of rotation *(blue dot)* is created as a result of the joint line shift. Because the insertion site of the sMCL is unchanged *(red dot)*, it will pivot around this new center of rotation during the range of motion. A proximal movement of the sMCL insertion site during the range of motion will cause progressive elongation of the sMCL.

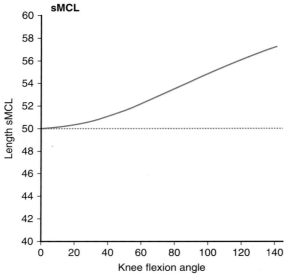

FIG 154.13 A graph plot of the sMCL length against the knee flexion based on the geometric model. The *dotted line* represents the isometric sMCL with the native joint line. The *blue line* represents the change in length after a proximal shift of the *joint line*. *sMCL,* Superficial medial collateral ligament.

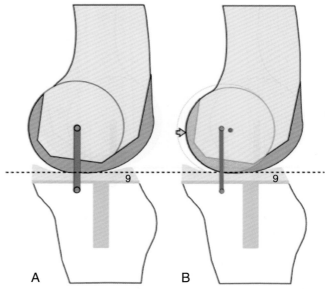

FIG 154.14 Schematic representation of the effect of an anterior shift of the joint line on the sMCL isometry. A new center of rotation *(blue dot)* is created as a result of the joint line shift. Because the insertion site of the sMCL is unchanged *(red dot)*, it will pivot around this new center of rotation during the range of motion. The *yellow arrow* represents the anterior shift of the femoral component.

length of 3.8 mm at 85 degrees of knee flexion. This observation is again obvious and can also be explained by the flexion-extension gap theory. Because only the flexion space is enlarged by anteriorizing the joint line, the flexion space is too loose for the 4-mm thicker insert. According to our model, the length will progress linearly from 0 to 70 degrees of flexion. Between 70 and 100 degrees, the length changes remain small. The sMCL is tensioned again toward deeper flexion. However, it never reaches its original length.

Combined Downsizing of the Femoral Component and Elevation. Next, the experimental setting of anteriorizing and raising the joint line by 4 mm (TKA4) was modeled by fitting a 4-mm smaller femoral component in a 4-mm more proximal position on the same knee. Stability in flexion and extension was maintained by using a 4-mm thicker insert. As such, the joint line was raised by 4 mm (Fig. 154.17). The effect of this shift on the length of the sMCL is shown in Figs. 154.13 and 154.14. A progressive slackening is predicted in the mid-flexion range with a maximum slackening of 1.8 mm at 45 degrees of knee flexion. At 90 degrees, a length equal to that at 0 degrees was predicted, and further elongation was observed in deeper flexion.

These observations cannot be explained by the flexion-extension gap paradigm, because the flexion and extension gaps were equal and balanced. However, our geometric mode shows that the anterior and proximal shift of the joint line will cause

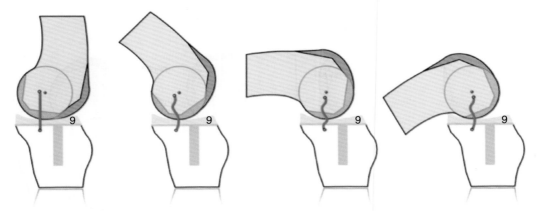

FIG 154.15 Schematic representation of the effect of an anterior shift of the joint line on the sMCL isometry. A new center of rotation *(blue dot)* is created as a result of the joint line shift. Because the insertion site of the sMCL is unchanged *(red dot)*, it will pivot around this new center of rotation during the range of motion. A distal movement of the sMCL insertion site will cause laxity in mid-flexion and at 90 degrees. In deep flexion, limited lengthening of the sMCL occurs because of a mild proximal shift of the insertion site.

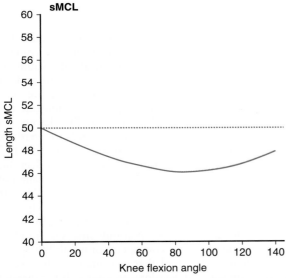

FIG 154.16 A graph plot of the sMCL length against the knee flexion based on the geometric model. The *dotted line* represents the isometric sMCL with the native joint line. The *blue line* represents the change in length after an anterior shift of the *joint line*. *sMCL,* Superficial medial collateral ligament.

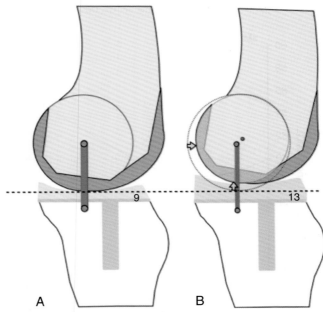

FIG 154.17 Schematic representation of the effect of a proximal and anterior shift of the joint line on the sMCL isometry. A new center of rotation *(blue dot)* is created as a result of the joint line shift. Because the insertion site of the sMCL is unchanged *(red dot)*, it will pivot around this new center of rotation during the range of motion. The *yellow arrows* represent the anterior and proximal shift of the femoral component.

a 4-mm anterior and proximal shift of the tibiofemoral center of rotation. Consequently, a new center of rotation will be defined (see Fig. 154.17B, *blue dot*). The slackening in mid-flexion is a consequence of the fact that in mid-flexion, the sMCL insertion site was moved distally relative to the center of rotation (Figs. 154.18 and 154.19). This is consistent with our data in publication and is supported by the data of others.[3,20,22] At 90 degrees, a length equal to that at 0 degrees was shown. The knee would therefore be considered balanced by most surgeons. In deeper flexion, a proximal movement of the sMCL insertion site relative to the center of rotation causes elongation. This is again consistent with our own data on strain in the sMCL after joint line elevation and is also consistent with the reports of others.[8,20,32]

DISCUSSION

The value of our geometric model is not the prediction of absolute length changes of the sMCL caused by joint line changes, but the qualitative explanation for the effect that joint line changes have on sMCL isometry and thus joint stability. In contrast to the classic flexion-extension gap paradigm, it provides a new paradigm to understand knee stability throughout the full motion arc.

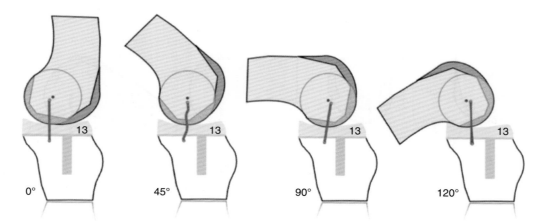

FIG 154.18 Schematic representation of the effect of a proximal and anterior shift of the joint line on the sMCL isometry. A new center of rotation *(blue dot)* is created as a result of the joint line shift. Because the insertion site of the sMCL is unchanged *(red dot)*, it will pivot around this new center of rotation during the range of motion. A distal movement of the sMCL insertion site will cause laxity in mid-flexion. At 90 degrees, an sMCL length equal to the length at 0 degrees is observed. The knee is therefore considered balanced. In deep flexion, progressive lengthening of the sMCL occurs because of a relative proximal shift of the insertion site.

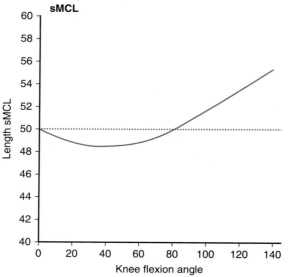

FIG 154.19 Schematic representation of the effect of a proximal and anterior shift of the joint line on the length changes in the sMCL. The *dotted line* represents the isometric sMCL with the native joint line. The *blue line* represents the length change after a proximal and anterior shift of the joint line.

The strength of the model is that, despite its simplicity, it is perfectly compatible with previous workflows. As for the explanation for the observations done in the setting of the isolated elevation or isolated anteriorization, the model is compatible with the classic flexion-extension gap thinking.

Second, it adds a new perspective to the understanding of joint stability by enabling the surgeon to predict the effect on knee stability not only at 0 and 90 degrees of flexion, but throughout the whole motion arc.

Third, it provides an explanation for our previously unexplained experimental observations and previous findings by other authors. If the joint line is raised and the femoral component downsized, bringing the posterior condylar contact area 4 mm anterior, the flexion-extension gap theory would predict equal tension on the flexion and extension gap and thus a balanced knee. However, in an experimental setup, we were able to show that raising the distal and posterior joint line in TKA introduced significant mid-flexion instability despite a well-balanced flexion and extension gap. Second, we were able to show that raising the distal and posterior joint line in TKA significantly increased the strain in the sMCL in deep flexion (unpublished data). The model provides an explanation for these observations, based on the movement of the sMCL insertion site relative to the new center of rotation (see Fig. 154.18).

It has become obvious that stability in the mid-flexion range is important for a good functional outcome. Our model adds to the understanding of the concept of joint stability by providing the surgeon with a tool that can qualitatively predict the effect of certain surgical decisions on joint stability throughout the range of motion.

The model has several limitations. First, our model is based on some theorems that are open to discussion. However, those theorems are widely supported in the literature and by our own data. Nevertheless, they should be kept in mind while interpreting these results. Predictions made by the model in the range of motion greater than 120 degrees of flexion should be interpreted with caution for the same reason. Second, the tibiofemoral movement in the medial compartment is simplified and reduced to two dimensions. It does not account for the rotational movement that takes place in the axial plane near terminal extension and in deep flexion. Nevertheless, this rotation is limited between 10 and 120 degrees of knee flexion. Because the center of this rotation is also located in the medial condyle, the excursions on the medial side are small compared to the lateral side. Third, the model predicts the length of the sMCL and not joint laxity. Whether the relationship between the sMCL length and the joint laxity is a linear one, still needs to be determined. The predictions that are made are therefore qualitative and not quantitative. Nevertheless, we were able to show that the relationship between the level of the medial joint line and the joint laxity is a linear one. Fourth, it only takes into account the medial side of the knee. One can also expect an effect of the level of the lateral joint line on joint stability. However, our data showed that in a well-balanced knee, there was no effect of the level of the lateral joint line on knee joint stability. Fifth, the TKA modeled was a single-radius design. The extent to which these findings can be applied to other TKA designs (ie, dual radius, J-curve) depends on the difference in geometry in the sagittal plane between such a design and a single radius. The study of the geometry of different TKA designs in the sagittal plane is an exhaustive and difficult one. However, the difference between the different TKA designs is smaller than one would expect. Amis et al. showed that the difference in contour in the sagittal plane between a single radius design and an old obsolete J-curve design was 0 mm at 0 and 90 degrees of flexion and 1.8 mm at 45 degrees of flexion.[27] This difference would probably be even smaller with more recent J-curve designs. A 110% increase in joint laxity at 30 degrees was observed by raising and anteriorizing the joint line by 4 mm. It is therefore unlikely that such a small difference of sagittal plane contour could eliminate the observed instability. We therefore believe that the effect will be similar with other TKA designs.

CONCLUSION

The medial side of the knee is the stable and isometric side. Changes in medial joint line position can induce mid-flexion instability and limitation of deep flexion. This can be predicted in a simplified mathematical model and has been confirmed in experimental setup. The surgeon should be meticulous in restoring the native joint line level on the medial side of the knee joint.

KEY REFERENCES

3. Cross MB, Nam D, Plaskos C, et al: Recutting the distal femur to increase maximal knee extension during TKA causes coronal plane laxity in mid-flexion. *Knee* 19(6):875–879, 2012.
7. Eckhoff D, Hogan C, DiMatteo L, et al: Difference between the epicondylar and cylindrical axis of the knee. *Clin Orthop* 461(461):238–244, 2007.
13. Howell SM, Howell SJ, Hull ML: Assessment of the radii of the medial and lateral femoral condyles in varus and valgus knees with osteoarthritis. *J Bone Joint Surg Am* 92(1):98–104, 2010.
15. Insall JN, Lachiewicz PF, Burstein AH: The posterior stabilized condylar prosthesis: a modification of the total condylar design. Two to four-year clinical experience. *J Bone Joint Surg Am* 64(9):1317–1323, 1982.
20. Luyckx T, Verstraete M, De Roo K, et al: The effect of single radius TKA implantation and joint line proximalisation on the strain pattern in the sMCL of the knee. *Bone Joint J* 95(Suppl 34):401, 2013.
22. Martin JW, Whiteside LA: The influence of joint line position on knee stability after condylar knee arthroplasty. *Clin Orthop* 259(259):146–156, 1990.
24. Schroer WC, Berend KR, Lombardi AV, et al: Why are total knees failing today? Etiology of total knee revision in 2010 and 2011. *J Arthroplasty* 28(Suppl 8):116–119, 2013.
25. Sharkey PF, Hozack WJ, Rothman RH, et al: Insall Award paper. Why are total knee arthroplasties failing today? *Clin Orthop* 404:7–13, 2002.
28. Victor J, Van Glabbeek F, Vander Sloten J, et al: An experimental model for kinematic analysis of the knee. *J Bone Joint Surg Am* 91(Suppl 6):150–163, 2009.
29. Victor J, Labey L, Wong P, et al: The influence of muscle load on tibiofemoral knee kinematics. *J Orthop Res* 28(4):419–428, 2010.
32. Whiteside L, Summers R: The effect of the level of the distal femoral resection on ligament balance in total knee arthroplasty. Annual Meeting of the Knee Society, Atlanta, 1984.

The references for this chapter can also be found on www.expertconsult.com.

155

Correction of Fixed Deformities With Total Knee Arthroplasty

Andrea Baldini, Giovanni Balato, Alfredo Lamberti

Correction of deformity is a main goal after total knee arthroplasty (TKA). Full correction means re-establishment of a neutral mechanical axis with a balanced ligamentous envelope of the joint. When deformity is fixed and nonreducible, correction is more difficult to achieve. In arthritic knees, deformity becomes fixed when the disease is at a late stage of its natural history. Some degree of bone erosion is often present at the concave side of the deformity, where ligaments and knee capsule are contracted. Bone erosion or condylar dysplasia usually involves one knee compartment, leading to an asymmetrical configuration of the joint relative to the flexion-extension axis of the knee. The opposite, convex side of the joint is affected by tension forces and may be stretched to varying degrees. Fixed deformities are rarely limited to a single plane. Significant varus or valgus malalignment on the coronal plane is very often associated with sagittal plane (eg, flexion contracture) and torsional deformities. Correction of the deformity with the TKA procedure should be done as completely as possible because no residual degree of a fixed deformity will be successfully addressed by postoperative means.

PREOPERATIVE PLANNING

Clinical Assessment

It is helpful to recognize preoperatively the abnormal gait patterns of patients with fixed deformities of the knee. Patients with varus knees and high adduction moments without flexion contracture, experiencing an evident lateral thrust at heel strike, will show elongated lateral soft tissues intraoperatively. The medial release that these deformities need to match the elongated lateral side will generate automatic opening of the flexion and extension gaps. Standard tibial bone resection in this scenario will result in larger gaps, which need to be filled by thicker polyethylene inserts.

Patients with valgus knees and a planovalgus foot walking with a high abduction moment at the knee are prone to stretch the medial collateral ligament (MCL) after TKA if not overcorrected and if the foot deformity is not addressed by surgery or insoles.[26] In bilateral fixed valgus deformity after one side is corrected with TKA, the other valgus nonoperated knee may push the operated leg in a high adduction moment. If a nonconstrained implant was used and an extensive lateral release was performed, the adduction moment created by the contralateral limb may predispose to a varus angulation, as in a windswept deformity. In bilateral significant fixed flexion contracture deformity, when one side is addressed by TKA, the other flexed and shortened limb will drive the operated leg in

flexion again. Careful planning with bilateral simultaneous or short-term staged procedures, when possible, and precautions against flexion contracture recurrence are mandatory. Neuromuscular disorders with low or absent quadriceps activity remain a relative contraindication to TKA; if a patient with this disorder undergoes a TKA procedure, the surgeon will have to address the patient's need to walk with some residual recurvatum while working with the biomechanical properties of the implant.

Radiographic Assessment

The surgeon should identify the presence and magnitude of osteophytes. If prominent, they may tent capsule and ligaments enough to avoid correctability of the deformity. Osteophyte removal may sometimes be sufficient to achieve balance. Beware of significant fixed flexion deformities without associated hypertrophic osteophytes. In this scenario the surgeon may need more extensile soft tissue work on the posterior capsule and gastrocnemius insertions. In a radiographic study by Moon et al. the amount of preoperative varus deformity and the presence of a proximal tibia vara correlated with the reducibility of the varus deformity under a stress view.[29] According to Sim et al., the use of preoperative stress radiographs can predict the extent of medial release when performing TKA.[42] We believe that the reducibility of the deformity can be assessed with enough accuracy by a physical examination and varus-valgus stress maneuvers.

Extra-articular diaphyseal or metadiaphyseal deformities are often associated with the development of fixed deformities at the knee joint. Preoperative planning should analyze the possibility of correcting the deformity at the joint level with generous bone resections and ligament releases, or whether a combined osteotomy is needed.

Intra-articular bone deformities can be recognized preoperatively. Hypoplasia of the lateral femoral condyle in valgus knees and the possible need for augmentation should be identified. With hypertrophic medial femoral condyles in knees with a metaphyseal varus deformity, a preoperative kneeling view or computed tomography (CT) scan may prove beneficial to establish the amount of rotational correction needed to achieve a stable and rectangular flexion gap.[36,45]

The femoral entry point for intramedullary instruments should be planned on both coronal and sagittal x-ray views to avoid mistakes in the amount of angular correction achieved. A common mistake in large canals is to use a low entry point and the wrong reaming direction in the sagittal plane, resulting in a flexed position of the femoral component.

FIXED VARUS DEFORMITY

Our technique of choice is a combination of the gap balancing technique and the measured resection technique as described by Insall and Easley.[16] Standard bone resections are performed with different bone landmarks in extension and flexion, whereas contracted ligaments are released incrementally. Gap equalization is then checked with laminar spreaders, blocks, and trial components.[16]

Bone resections are performed according to the preoperative template on the long weight-bearing films. Tibial cutting jig positioning should be done according to the talus center distally and the plateau-to-anatomic axis intersection proximally. In constitutional metaphyseal varus deformities, the proximal center of the tibial cutting jig is usually facing the lateral tibial plateau spine (Fig. 155.1). On the femoral side, angulation of the intramedullary cutting guide for valgus correction is established by measuring the divergence between the anatomic and mechanical femoral axes. Failure in achieving varus correction to neutral ±3 degrees is related to a greater incidence of loosening at medium- to long-term follow-up.[6]

As part of the approach, some initial medial release is performed. With the knee joint in slight flexion, incision of the anterior horn of the medial meniscus allows subperiosteal elevation of a medial flap of tissue, which includes the meniscotibial fibers of the deep MCL. Proximal tibial insertion of the superficial MCL is often involved in the subperiosteal elevation of the medial soft tissue flap as part of the exposure.[23] The second step is to sublux the tibia forward in flexion and external rotation (the so-called RanSall maneuver, from its originators Ranawat and Insall) (Fig. 155.2). In advanced deformities the worn tibial medial plateau develops a concave "pagoda" shape in which the femoral condyle is embedded, leading to a difficult tibial

dislocation maneuver that may harm the MCL. In these cases, we suggest violating the posterior tibial osteophyte with the tibia still in situ by using a straight osteotome between femur and tibia at 90 degrees of flexion (Fig. 155.3). After joint exposure, both tibial and femoral osteophytes are removed. Proximal tibial and distal femoral cuts are performed. Anteroposterior (AP) femoral resections are performed with a rotational position of the cutting jig, according to multiple bone landmarks, such as the Whiteside line, transepicondylar axis, and posterior condylar line. In cases in which more than 3 degrees of external rotation with respect to the posterior condylar line is required, we suggest switching the pivot point of the cutting guide from the center of the knee, as usual, to the medial condyle.[40] Pivoting the femoral guide at the center of the femur would create an over-resection of the posterior medial femoral condyle, which may lead to excessive "paradoxical" opening of the medial gap in flexion in a varus knee (Fig. 155.4A and B). The stretched lateral compartment will be better filled in flexion, and anterolateral notching will be avoided if few degrees of flexion in the distal femoral cut are applied.

We prefer to remove the posterior cruciate ligament (PCL) and to use a posterior-substituting implant for these advanced deformities. We believe that the PCL is part of these deformities. By removing the PCL, it is easier to address complex ligament balancing and to guarantee a reproducible, nonerratic postoperative pattern of kinematics.[24] Only in advanced flexion contracture will PCL removal selectively open the flexion gap farther. This 2- to 3-mm gap opening can be filled by adding a few degrees of flexion to the femoral component and by switching the femoral component rotational pivot point from central to medial.[4]

Calibrated laminar spreaders and spacer blocks can now be used to check gap symmetry both in flexion and in extension.

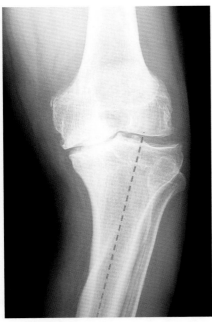

FIG 155.1 In metaphyseal varus deformed knees, anatomic and mechanical axes of the tibia have their proximal centers at the lateral tibial spine level *(dashed line)*.

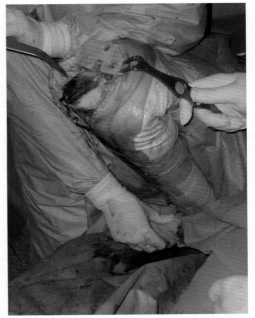

FIG 155.2 The RanSall maneuver: the assistant is keeping full flexion and maximal external rotation of the limb while pushing the tibia forward with the pressure of his elbow on the patient's thigh.

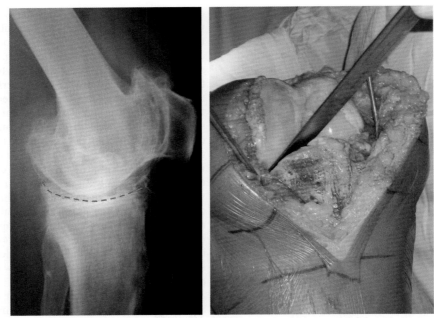

FIG 155.3 Advanced medial wear in varus knees may produce a sagittal "pagoda-shaped" deformity, with the medial femoral condyle embedded in the worn medial tibial plateau *(dashed line)*. Posterior tibial osteophytes, which constrain anterior tibial dislocation, can be violated using a straight osteotome with the tibia still in situ.

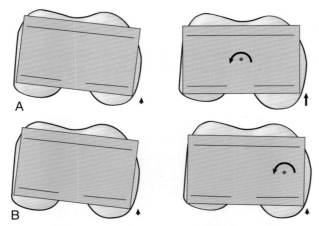

FIG 155.4 (A) Femoral external rotation with a central pivot decreases the amount of posterior lateral condyle resection and increases the amount of posterior medial condyle resection. (B) If the femoral resection guide pivot point is medially based, the posterior medial resection will not change with external rotation.

TABLE 155.1 Medial and Lateral Soft Tissue Structures of the Knee and Their Involvement in Flexion and Extension Gap Tension		
	Extension Gap	**Flexion Gap**
Medial Structures		
Superficial MCL (anterior fibers)	–	+
Superficial MCL (posterior fibers)	+	–
Deep MCL	+	+
Posterior oblique ligament	+	–
Semimembranosus tendon	+	–
Pes anserinus tendons	+	–
Posteromedial capsule	+	–
Medial gastrocnemius head	+	–
Lateral Structures		
Iliotibial band	+	–
Anterior iliotibial band fibers + Lateral retinaculum	–	+
Popliteal tendon	–	+
Lateral collateral ligament	+	+
Biceps tendon	+	–
Posterolateral capsule	+	–
Lateral gastrocnemius head	+	–

MCL, Medial collateral ligament.

In fixed deformities, it is common in this phase of the procedure to face the need for additional medial release for residual varus in extension. This is particularly evident if a combined fixed flexion deformity is present. The following soft tissue structures will be involved in the incremental medial release to balance the extension gap: the posterior capsule, posteromedial corner with the posterior oblique ligament (POL), semimembranosus (SM) direct tibial insertion, and posterior fibers of the superficial MCL (Table 155.1).[48] All these structures can be released with the knee in flexion. Using laminar spreaders, the posterior capsule can be addressed by a periosteal elevator from the femoral side. By holding the knee in deep flexion and applying a posterior drawer to the proximal tibia, it is possible to access the femoral insertion of the posterior capsule with a periosteal elevator. The posteromedial corner of the knee is safely exposed

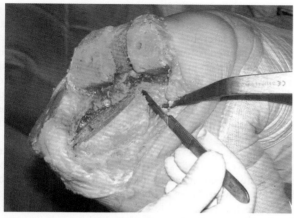

FIG 155.5 SM tendon subperiosteal release with the knee joint in "figure-of-four," with combined flexion, adduction, and external rotation.

while the joint is held in the "figure-of-four" position, with the foot externally rotated (Fig. 155.5). All of the tibial medial metaphysis is easily exposed, progressively involving the POL and SM insertions up to the posterior midline. If some residual medial tension remains, the distal insertion of the superficial MCL can be released from its posterior aspect in flexion or in extension. To reach this distal broad insertion, the elevator should be deepened distally on the tibial diaphysis at least 8 to 10 cm from the joint line. Alternatively, the MCL could be "pie-crusted" with a 16-gauge needle with multiple punctures, but progression of this type of release is not always achievable.[5,12] In advanced fixed varus deformities, it is helpful to select a relatively small tibial size to lateralize the tibial component and remove the exposed medial sclerotic bone, which is tenting the medial structures both in extension and in flexion (Fig. 155.6A and B).[10] The resultant effect is similar to osteophyte removal, with a reduced need for ligamentous release.[21] Krackow et al., in 35 consecutive navigated total knee replacement (TKR), found that every millimeter of medial tibial bone over-resection resulted in 0.5 degrees of coronal axis correction. They did not observe any varus collapse or instability.[21] This result is in agreement with the results of a larger cohort of 71 TKA described by Mullaji and Shetty. They found that for a mean reduction osteotomy of 7.5 ± 2 mm, a mean correction of 3.5 ± 1 degree was achieved.[34] A comparative study of soft tissue medial release versus tibial medial over-resection to balance varus deformities showed the same clinical results at 6 months but shorter operative time and better ligamentous balance in deep flexion in the tibial over-resection group.[2] The effect of tibial undersizing after a tibial "reduction" osteotomy in severe varus knees has been evaluated by Niki et al.[35] Cementless trabecular metal tibial trays showed good clinical results at short term with a limited nonprogressive subsidence in 9 out of 39 TKAs.[35]

With trial components inserted, a final flexion-extension balance check is performed. Cases with preoperative advanced disease showing lateral tibiofemoral subluxation and rotational deformity may experience popliteal tendon retraction, which snaps over the lateral femoral component condyle during flexion-extension. The popliteal tendon insertion can be partially released from its femoral attachment to avoid postoperative painful lateral snapping symptoms.[17] When the femoral

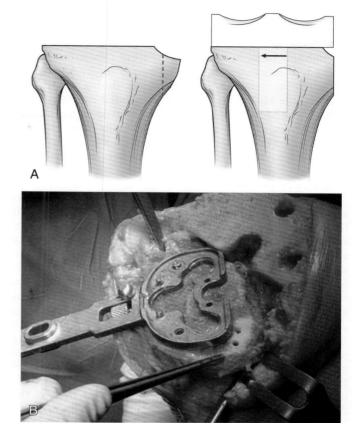

FIG 155.6 (A) Tibial component undersizing and lateralization. The resultant effect is to reduce the amount of medial bone defect while decreasing tension on the medial soft tissue sleeve. (B) Surgical view of undersizing the tibial component to reduce the medial aspect of the tibia. (From Dixon MC, Parsch D, Brown RR, Scott RD: The correction of severe varus deformity in total knee arthroplasty by tibial component downsizing and resection of uncapped proximal medial bone. *J Arthroplasty* 19:19–22, 2004).

insertion of the popliteus tendon has to be released, we prefer to maintain some function of this muscle-tendon unit by performing a tenodesis to the lateral collateral ligament (LCL).

A number of cases with severe varus deformities may require extensive soft tissue releases, including the need to subperiosteally elevate the tibial attachment of the MCL.[12,31,41,46] This carries the risk of mediolateral instability (if there is overrelease or inadvertent total detachment of the superficial MCL) and results in the flexion gap exceeding the extension gap, both of which increase the potential need for a constrained prosthesis.[30] On the other hand, leaving the knee with mediolateral imbalance because of inadequate medial release may lead to long-term instability, polyethylene wear, and potential loosening of tibial component from persistent adductor thrust.[37]

Meftah et al. described an "inside-out" release technique to balance severe varus and flexion deformity of the knee joint without risking MCL over-release or hematoma formation in extensive subperiosteal release.[27] This technique involves performing a posteromedial capsulotomy at the tibial cut level and perforating the superficial MCL in a pie-crust manner in extension followed by serial manipulations with valgus stress. The authors reported excellent results using the "inside-out" technique in a series of 31 consecutive varus TKR at an average 3 year follow-up.[27]

Engh and Ammeen[13] described the use of a wafer-thin medial epicondylar osteotomy (MEO) in conventional TKA to correct soft tissue contractures in varus knees during TKA. They detached the MCL with a slice of the medial epicondyle that included the adductor magnus tendon insertion; it was allowed to find its own position and was not internally fixed.[13] It is our belief that for those patients in whom full correction of alignment and mediolateral soft tissue balance have failed despite an extensive release of medial soft tissue structure, a sliding MEO should be performed.

Osteotomy of the medial epicondyle has been reported to aid in balancing and providing exposure of the varus knee with flexion contraction. This technique may be useful in the knee with severe combined varus and flexion contracture deformity and may be worthy of consideration when managing the severely contracted varus knee.[13,32,33] In a retrospective comparative study, Sim et al. concluded that epicondylar osteotomy achieve a better balance in TKR for severely deformed varus knee compared with a standard soft tissue release.[43] Mihalko et al. evaluated the biomechanical effect of an MEO on 10 specimens and found that coronal and transverse plane laxity increased significantly at 60 and 90 degrees after MEO compared with the classic subperiosteal MCL release technique.[28] For this reason emi-epicondylar osteotomy could be preferable to control the isometric position of the MCL relatively to the flexion space (deformity in the coronal plane affect ligamentous balance for extension gap only) (Fig. 155.7). Osteotomy should

be performed in the sagittal plane using a reciprocating saw, with the knee in 90 degrees flexion (Fig. 155.8A to E). The cut is started 5 mm lateral to the medial edge of the bony medial condyle, continued proximally and slightly obliquely in a superomedial direction, and exited distal to the adductor tubercle. Therefore surgeons can create a track in which only the extension gap can be changed by distalizing the epicondyle, thereby preventing it from sliding posteriorly. When choosing the correct position for the epicondyle, the block is then fixed to cortical fixation of the opposite condyle (Fig. 155.9A to C).

When dealing with severe varus deformities, it is not uncommon to observe a "paradoxical" medial gap opening in flexion after the bone resections and the ligament balancing have been made. This may indicate a technical mistake. The surgeon should recheck for a possible excessive external femoral rotation, a varus tibial resection, or full-thickness damage to the superficial MCL (Fig. 155.10). If this is not the case, a biomechanical reason can explain the residual medial laxity in flexion. When a severe varus deformity is corrected with extensive release, the medial sleeve usually tends to slide behind the isometric point in flexion, causing a paradoxical medial laxity in flexion (Fig. 155.11A and B). The surgeon can limit and control this phenomenon by attaching the capsule back on the anteromedial tibial surface using transosseus bony suture (Fig. 155.12A and B). As a result the paradoxical medial opening in flexion will be eliminated without the need for a constrained implant.

FIXED VALGUS DEFORMITY

Classification of deformity for valgus knees considers a fixed noncorrectable deformity with some medial soft tissue stretching as type II.[22] Type III valgus deformity is severe osseous deformity seen after a prior osteotomy with an incompetent medial soft tissue sleeve. We believe it is possible to safely address all valgus deformities with a medial parapatellar approach. Some surgeons advocate the need for a lateral approach to these deformities to directly access contracted structures and to preserve the blood supply to the patella.[18] We do not support the use of a lateral approach because the surgeon is facing the joint with an unusual view, which can be misleading. Extensile approaches, such as tibial tubercle osteotomy, are needed to expose difficult cases without damaging the patellar tendon. Distal capsular closure difficulties are frequent and may predispose to postoperative skin problems, even when the fat pad tissue is used as a capsular patch. From the lateral side, it is not possible to perform a medial soft tissue retensioning procedure if needed. Moreover, in cases of failure requiring revision, the knee would receive a parallel medial capsulotomy. A review of all the literature on valgus deformities approached through a medial parapatellar capsulotomy reveals only one paper reporting a significant occurrence (2 of 25 cases) of patellar necrosis.[25] In this study, a lateral retinacular release was performed in all 25 cases without preserving the superior lateral geniculate artery.[47]

Bone resection levels and directions should be planned preoperatively. A distal femoral bone cut is performed with a slight overcorrection to avoid recurrence of medial soft tissue stretching. We suggest planning the degree of correction, but most often we select the option of 4 degrees of valgus for the distal femoral cut. Attention is paid to entering the femoral canal from the appropriate entry point, which is often more medial than usual in cases with femoral diaphyseal valgus

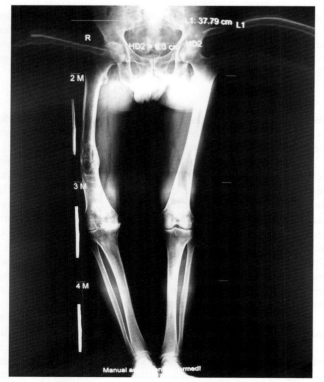

FIG 155.7 Full-limb x-ray showing severe varus with femoral extra-articular deformity of the right knee.

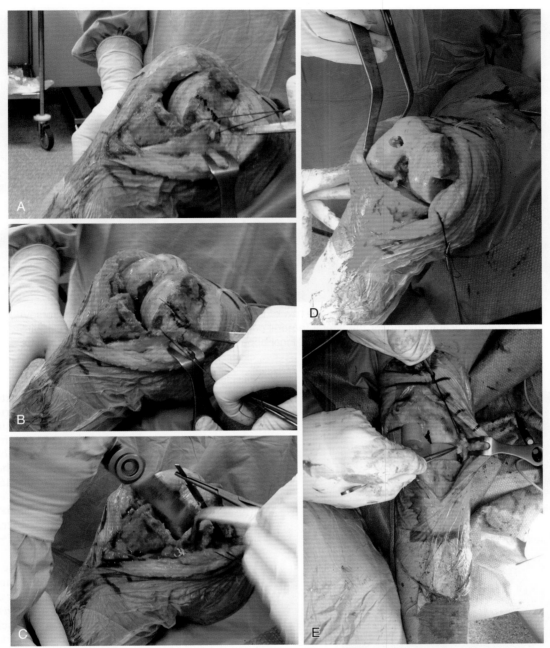

FIG 155.8 (A) Isolation of femoral MCL insertion and markings on the epicondylar line just above the ridge of the medial epicondyle. (B) Sagittal partial osteotomy performed with the reciprocating saw on the marked line. (C) Coronal osteotomy using the oscillating saw blade and producing an emi-epicondylar fragment 5 to 6 mm thick. (D) Frontal view of the osteotomized medial condyle after emi-MEO has been performed. Note the lateral entry point of the intramedullary (IM) rod to achieve adequate valgus correction. (E) With the spacer block opening the extension gap the osteotomized epicondyle migrates distally (here approximately 1.5 cm) driven by the coronal correction of the deformity. Isometry in flexion is guaranteed by the engagement of the fragment in the L-shaped osteotomy.

bowing (Fig. 155.13). Because of hypoplasia of the lateral femoral condyle, distal and posterior lateral resections usually remove a minimal amount of bone or no bone at all. We suggest starting bone resections from the femoral side in valgus deformities. Through a medial capsulotomy, the knee joint should be exposed without the need to perform the usual subperiosteal peel of the deep MCL around the medial tibial metaphysis. Once the distal and posterior femoral condyles are resected, the tibia can be easily exposed with less risk for MCL disruption caused by the RanSall maneuver.

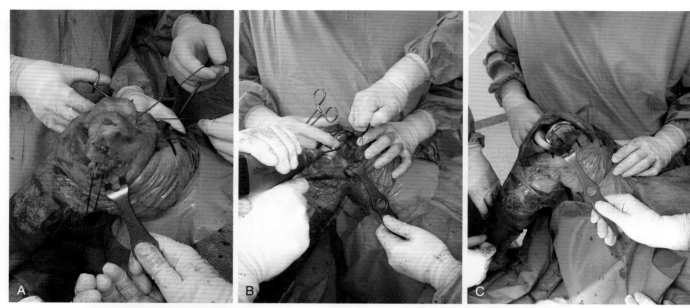

FIG 155.9 (A) MEO fixation using a double row of Ethibond #5 (Ethicon, Somerville, New Jersey) with transcortical fixation over the lateral femoral cortex. (B) Additional fixation is provided with a screw in the medial femoral condyle. (C) Final appearance of the emi-MEO with appropriate length and MCL tension in flexion.

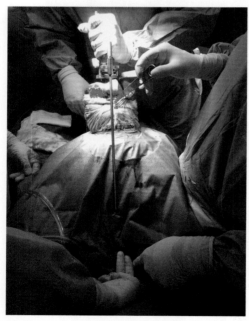

FIG 155.10 Extramedullary double check showing correct IM instrument position medial to the anterosuperior iliac spine.

Tibial resection is performed perpendicular to the mechanical axis, as usual. Conservative femoral and tibial resections are performed in cases of recurvatum or medial soft tissue stretching to allow soft tissue balancing without elevating the joint line or creating an extension gap that is too large.

AP femoral bone resections are performed using all available rotational landmarks, with a special focus on the epicondyles, which are not affected by the disease. The posterior condylar angle is increased as the result of lateral condyle hypoplasia and

wear, thus requiring additional degrees of external rotation related to the posterior condylar line. This correction, if performed using a central pivot of the AP resection guide, will generate a greater resection of the posterior medial femoral condyle, which may lead to medial laxity in flexion. Medializing the pivot point of the cutting guide, as described earlier, will limit the amount of medial resection (see Fig. 155.4A and B).

Valgus knees usually are more deformed in extension than in flexion. This makes the posterior capsule and the iliotibial band (ITB) the most frequently contracted structures.[47] The LCL is also contracted in more than 50% of cases, and the popliteal tendon is less commonly involved.[25]

Our preferred lateral release technique is the so-called pie-crusting technique, performed with multiple punctures.[38] With the knee in extension and the laminar spreader distracting the femorotibial joint space, the contracted structures are palpated. A no. 15 small blade is used to perform a capsular incision at the level of the tibial bone cut of the posterior capsule, following the lateral corner anterior to the popliteal tendon (Fig. 155.14). Care is taken at this time to avoid cutting the popliteal tendon, which is always preserved. Resection of the popliteal tendon in valgus deformity leads to uncontrolled knee instability in flexion. A cadaveric study with incremental lateral soft tissue sectioning clearly showed the sudden flexion gap increase after the popliteal tendon was involved.[20]

The pie-crusting release is then performed in a progressive manner with multiple horizontal stab incisions involving the ITB at the tibial resection level and continuing proximally as needed, with the aim of reaching a rectangular gap (Fig. 155.15). The LCL is sometimes involved in the pie-crusting (for the LCL we recommend a puncturing technique using a 16-gauge needle and not the small blade), if needed. The transverse incision and multiple stab incisions through the lateral structures should be made with only the tip of the knife blade (no. 15), and soft tissue penetration should be limited to 5 mm or less, particularly in

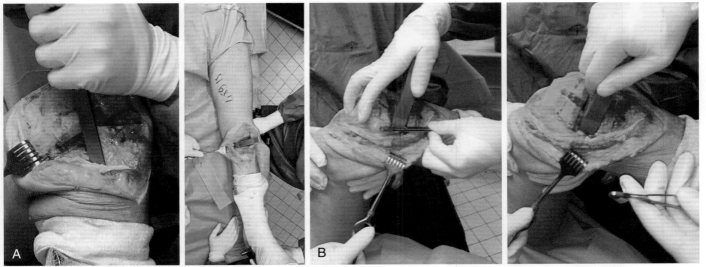

FIG 155.11 (A) Knee specimen with a 20-degree varus deformity simulated. Complete MCL release has been performed *(left)* and extension gap has been balanced *(right)*. (B) At 90 degrees of flexion the MCL is posterior to the sagittal midline *(left)*, resulting in residual paradoxical medial laxity in flexion *(right)*.

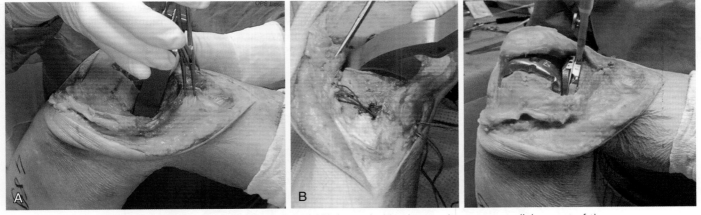

FIG 155.12 (A) The released superficial MCL is settled back over the anteromedial aspect of the tibia and isometry is checked with towel clips. (B) Transosseous suture of a pair of Ethibond #5 using Krackow stitches on the superficial MCL guarantees stability both in extension *(left)* and flexion *(right)* under valgus stresses.

patients with small legs, to avoid direct peroneal nerve damage, as has been revealed by magnetic resonance and cadaveric studies.[8,9]

Results with this technique were analyzed by Aglietti et al. in 48 patients with 53 valgus knees who underwent TKA and were followed a minimum of 5 years (mean: 8 years; range: 5 to 12 years).[1] A fixed-bearing posterior-stabilized implant or an ultracongruent mobile-bearing implant was used. A lateral patellofemoral retinacular release was performed in 67% of cases. One transient postoperative peroneal nerve palsy, which spontaneously recovered, was observed. In 51 of 53 knees (96%), alignment within 5 degrees from neutral was achieved. One patient had varus instability in extension. None of the components were revised. In this series the pie-crusting technique reliably corrected moderate-to-severe fixed valgus deformity, with a low complication rate and reasonable midterm results. Multiple punctures allowed gradual stretching of the

lateral soft tissues and preservation of the popliteal tendon, reducing the risk of posterolateral instability.[1]

Very rarely, when substantial soft tissue release laterally fails to correct deformity or achieve mediolateral soft tissue balance, a sliding lateral epicondylar osteotomy (LEO) may be indicated.[7,32] Some authors reported excellent outcome in patients undergoing total knee replacement in the presence of severe valgus deformity using computer navigation. With this technique, it was possible to restore femorotibial balance throughout the entire range of motion, as well as exact coronal and sagittal alignment. The navigation technique helps to exactly calculate the amount of sliding distance needed before the osteotomy is performed, to measure the difference between the medial and lateral gaps, and therefore reduces the number of attempts to reach a completely balanced knee.[14,32,44]

The medial convex side of the deformity needs to be addressed when medial soft tissue stretching is significant, with

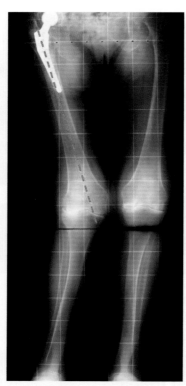

FIG 155.13 Femoral entry point in valgus deformity may be more medial *(dashed line)* than usual if lateral diaphyseal bowing occurs.

a medial compartment opening in extension of 15 mm or more. In this scenario, even minimal bone resection creates a medial gap larger than 25 mm, which would require an extensive lateral release and raising the joint line with the use of a thick polyethylene insert. Possible solutions include medial soft tissue retensioning and the use of a varus-valgus constrained (VVC) implant. Krackow et al. described MCL advancement off the tibial side, and the same authors described MCL midsubstance division and imbrication to equalize the joint gaps.[19,22] Healy et al. described recessing the origin of the MCL with a bone block from the femoral epicondyles.[15] Although these procedures are technically demanding and may affect ligament strength and isometricity, they may be necessary to equalize joint gaps to achieve stability without the use of a VVC implant, particularly in a young, active patient.

Use of a stemmed VVC condylar implant for fixed valgus deformities has produced excellent results at mid- to long-term follow-up.[11] Biomechanical analysis of VVC implants showed no difference in stresses at the bone-implant interface between stemmed and nonstemmed VVCs, given adequate metaphyseal bone stock.[39] We reviewed our midterm clinical results with 70 consecutive primary nonstemmed VVC implants for severe valgus deformity (Fig. 155.16).[3] From 1998 to 2001, 70 non-stemmed constrained TKAs were performed in 61 patients with knees in 15 degrees valgus or greater. Forty-nine patients (55 knees) were followed for 44.5 months (range: 2 to 6 years). Outcome was assessed using the Knee Society scoring system. Knee Society scores and functional scores improved from 34

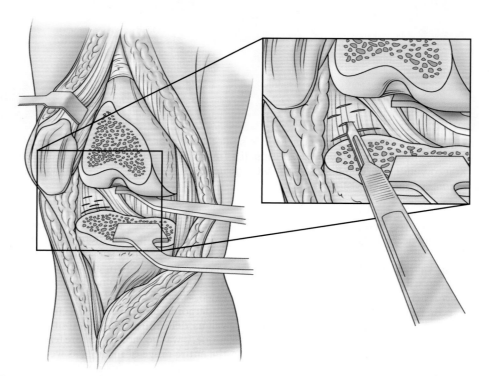

FIG 155.14 Illustration of the "Pie-Crusting" Technique for Valgus Deformity Although the laminar spreader is distracting the knee joint in extension, a longitudinal incision is made in the posterolateral capsule, along with multiple punctures, with a small blade in the iliotibial band. (From Clarke HD, Schwartz JB, Math KR, Scuderi GR: Anatomic risk of peroneal nerve injury with the "pie crust" technique for valgus release in total knee arthroplasty. *J Arthroplasty* 19:40–44, 2004).

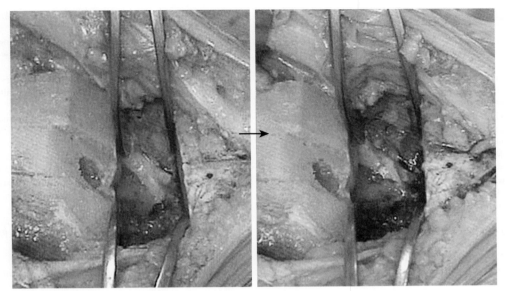

FIG 155.15 Intraoperative picture shows the extension gap of a valgus knee before *(left)* and after *(right)* lateral release is performed with multiple punctures. Gap symmetry is attained, and the popliteal tendon is preserved.

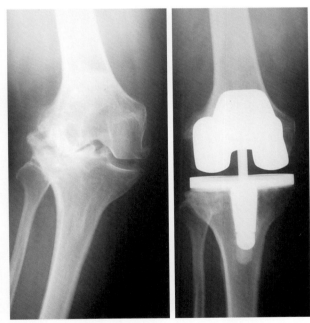

FIG 155.16 Preoperative *(left)* and postoperative *(right)* AP x-ray views of a severe valgus deformity treated by TKA with a nonstemmed VVC implant at 6-year follow-up. (From Anderson JA, Baldini A, MacDonald JH, et al: Primary constrained condylar knee arthroplasty without stem extensions for the valgus knee. *Clin Orthop* 442:199–203, 2006).

points and 40 points to 93 points and 74 points, respectively. No radiographic loosening or wear was found. No peroneal nerve palsies were noted, and no patients had flexion or medial instability. One patient with a preoperative chronically dislocated patella had a postoperative recurrence of the dislocation.

Constrained condylar knee implants in patients with severe valgus deformity resulted in excellent pain relief and improved function, without substantial complications at midterm follow-up and without diaphyseal–engaging stem extensions.[3]

CONCLUSIONS

The need to balance the soft tissue sleeve of the knee to create rectangular gaps is well recognized as a critical step in TKA. Multiple techniques are available for use in addressing the soft tissue imbalance that arises in fixed deformities during primary TKA. Correction of angular deformity with ligament release is done variably by different techniques, with little scientific evidence to support any of them. The few scientific studies that have been done have examined the influence on knees from cadavers without fixed deformity, or they have reported clinical outcomes of TKA cases following correction of fixed deformity. Correction of fixed deformity by separate bone resection and ligamentous release requires a thorough understanding of the underlying pathology. Extensive ligamentous releases are often required, but they should be performed in a progressive manner with recognition of which of the contracted structures is responsible for extension or flexion gap tensions. When extensive ligamentous releases are performed, resection of the PCL and implantation of a PCL-substituting prosthesis may be advisable to obtain more reproducible kinematics. The deformity should be completely corrected intraoperatively, and the knee should be balanced with an unconstrained implant most of the time. If residual ligamentous laxity is present by the end of the procedure, a VVC implant type with a relatively low threshold for older patients should be selected. Advanced fixed deformities with a combined flexion contracture may develop postoperative complications at a higher rate than minor deformities usually do. Careful surgical technique and postoperative monitoring are mandatory in these demanding cases.

KEY REFERENCES

1. Aglietti P, Lup D, Cuomo P, et al: Total knee arthroplasty using a pie-crusting technique for valgus deformity. *Clin Orthop* 464:73–77, 2007.

3. Anderson JA, Baldini A, MacDonald JH, et al: Primary constrained condylar knee arthroplasty without stem extensions for the valgus knee. *Clin Orthop* 442:199–203, 2006.

4. Baldini A, Scuderi GR, Aglietti P, et al: Flexion-extension gap changes during total knee arthroplasty: effect of posterior cruciate ligament and posterior osteophytes removal. *J Knee Surg* 17:69–72, 2004.

6. Berend ME, Ritter MA, Meding JB, et al: Tibial component failure mechanisms in total knee arthroplasty. *Clin Orthop* 428:26–34, 2004.

8. Bruzzone M, Ranawat A, Castoldi F, et al: The risk of direct peroneal nerve injury using the Ranawat "inside-out" lateral release technique in valgus total knee arthroplasty. *J Arthroplasty* 25:161–165, 2010.

9. Clarke HD, Schwartz JB, Math KR, et al: Anatomic risk of peroneal nerve injury with the "pie crust" technique for valgus release in total knee arthroplasty. *J Arthroplasty* 19:40–44, 2004.

10. Dixon MC, Parsch D, Brown RR, et al: The correction of severe varus deformity in total knee arthroplasty by tibial component downsizing and resection of uncapped proximal medial bone. *J Arthroplasty* 19:19–22, 2004.

18. Keblish PA: The lateral approach to the valgus knee: surgical technique and analysis of 53 cases with over two-year follow-up evaluation. *Clin Orthop* 271:52–62, 1991.

22. Krackow KA, Jones MM, Teeny SM, et al: Primary total knee arthroplasty in patients with fixed valgus deformity. *Clin Orthop* 273:9–18, 1991.

23. LaPrade RF, Engebretsen AH, Ly TV, et al: The anatomy of the medial part of the knee. *J Bone Joint Surg Am* 89:2000–2010, 2007.

25. Laurencin CT, Scott RD, Volatile TB, et al: Total knee replacement in severe valgus deformity. *Am J Knee Surg* 5:135–139, 1992.

38. Ranawat AS, Ranawat CS, Elkus M, et al: Total knee arthroplasty for severe valgus deformity: surgical technique. *J Bone Joint Surg Am* 87(Suppl 1 Pt 2):271–284, 2005.

40. Scott RD: Primary total knee arthroplasty surgical technique. In Scott RD, editor: *Total knee arthroplasty*, Philadelphia, PA, 2006, Saunders Elsevier, pp 20–38.

The references for this chapter can also be found on www.expertconsult.com.

156

Correction of Deformities With Total Knee Arthroplasty: An Asian Approach

Shuichi Matsuda, Shinichi Kuriyama

OUTLINE

During total knee arthroplasty (TKA), surgeons correct knee deformities to improve postoperative function and longevity of the implant. Many studies have shown that ethnic differences exist in anthropometric variables, and considerable differences are also found in the femur and tibial anatomy between Caucasian and Asian patients. These differences are very important and should be considered when performing TKA. Understanding the characteristics of these deformities would increase the success of TKA for Asian patients. Generally, most Asian patients have varus deformities, and few have valgus deformities. Although controversy remains regarding appropriate postoperative alignment, this chapter focuses on the correction of varus deformities to neutral alignment during TKA. To achieve appropriate coronal, sagittal, and rotational alignment in Asian patients, many characteristics should be considered compared with Caucasian patients. Femoral and tibial sizing is an important issue to be discussed. Finally, correcting deformities to neutral alignment might affect ligament balancing, but to date, how ligament balancing improves patient function, symptoms, and implant longevity remains unclear. Recent studies on the effects of ligament balance on knee kinematics have also been introduced.

CORONAL ALIGNMENT

Femoral Alignment

Patients with varus deformities in Asia tend to have lateral bowing of the femur. Nagamine et al.[24] investigated the anatomy of the femur in 133 Japanese patients with medial osteoarthritis and found that the bowing angle of the femoral shaft was 2.2 degrees (−3.5 to 11 degrees), and the distal femoral valgus angle (the angle between the mechanical axis and the distal anatomic axis) was 7.7 degrees (4 to 13 degrees) (Fig. 156.1). Usually, lateral bowing is found at the mid-shaft of the femur. On the other hand, the distal femoral valgus angle was 5.8 degrees (4.5 to 7.0 degrees) in the patients in the United States.[21] It was reported[3] that a fixed valgus angle can reach acceptable femoral alignment in femoral resection during TKA, but this is not applicable in Asian patients. Some studies[14,23] have reported that the distal femoral valgus angle was greater than 5 ± 2 degrees in 32% to 55.8% of Asian patients with varus deformities. Considering the wide range of femoral valgus angles in Asian patients, the fixed valgus angle using the intramedullary guide would create a certain amount of malalignment. A study showed that individual valgus correction angle improves the accuracy of postoperative limb alignment in Asian patients.[36] Preopera-

tive planning for the distal femur resection is especially important for Asian patients.

When a large extra-articular deformity exists in the femur, the extent to which the deformity can be corrected intra-articularly has yet to be determined. An anatomic study from Korea[13] showed that the femoral condylar orientation angle (the angle between the condylar line and the mechanical axis, see Fig. 156.1) was 2.6 degrees in varus (14 degrees varus to 7 degrees valgus) in patients undergoing TKA. Therefore with an aim to achieve neutral alignment for these femoral varus patients, the bone resection line should be 2.6 degrees of valgus relative to the joint surface on an average, and should be up to 14 degrees of valgus to the joint surface in patients with severe varus deformity. This bone resection would compromise the attachment of the lateral collateral ligament and popliteus tendon, or would at least cause a large ligamentous imbalance. If resection of more than 15 mm of the lateral distal part of the femur is needed, there is a possibility of injury at the attachment of the lateral stabilizing structure.[8] In these cases, extra-articular correction should be considered. When the lateral soft tissue attachment is secured, ligament imbalance caused by unequal bone resection should be treated from the medial and lateral condyles. Usually, it is difficult to correct more than 5 degrees of ligamentous imbalance in extension by using medial release.[32] Although a couple of degrees of instability and varus alignment is allowed, correction of more than 10 degrees from the articular surface of the femur is difficult.

Tibial Alignment

Most patients with varus knee deformities in Asia have tibia vara. In contrast to the mid-shaft deformities at the femur, tibial deformities are limited to the proximal part of the tibia. An anatomic study of the tibia using 3D computed tomography (CT) showed that the line between the medial third of the tibial tuberosity to the anterior border at the distal fourth of the tibia is parallel to the tibial mechanical axis and shows a small variation in 101 Japanese patients with varus deformities before TKA.[4] This finding suggests that tibial varus deformity exists mainly proximal to the tibial tuberosity. These proximal deformities indicate that the anatomic axis (tibial shaft axis) and postoperative mechanical axes are different in varus knees of Asians (Fig. 156.2).[19] To achieve neutral alignment of the tibia, the tibial component should be aligned perpendicular to the postoperative mechanical axis (the line connecting the center of the cut surface and the center of the ankle), not to the tibial shaft axis. Precise preoperative planning is necessary to ensure that the line of tibial resection is perpendicular to the postoperative mechanical axis.[19] Because anatomic landmarks do not

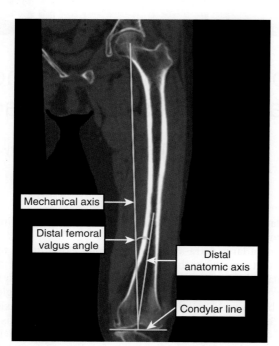

FIG 156.1 Mechanical and anatomic axes of the femur.

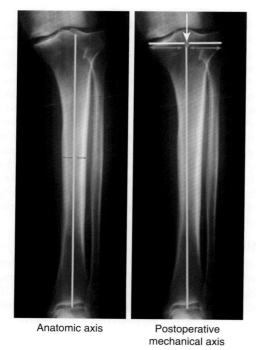

Anatomic axis   Postoperative
                       mechanical axis

FIG 156.2 The anatomical axis of the tibia (tibial shaft axis) does not pass the center of the articular surface because of proximal tibial deformity *(left)*. The postoperative mechanical axis connects the center of the resected surface of the tibia *(white arrow)* and the center of the ankle *(right)*.

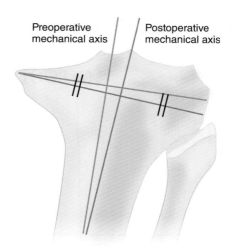

FIG 156.3 When the tibia is cut perpendicular to the preoperative mechanical axis *(red line)* in cases of proximal varus deformity of the tibia, the cut surface becomes varus relative to the mechanical axis of the tibia *(blue line)*. Preoperative planning should be done to ensure that the planned cut surface is perpendicular to the postoperative mechanical axis.

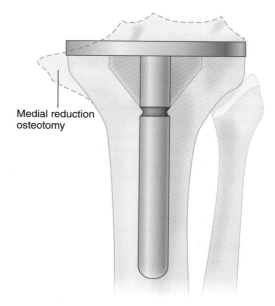

FIG 156.4 Medial reduction osteotomy resects the medial edge of the tibia, which the implant does not cover. The *red dotted line* shows the contour of the preoperative proximal tibia.

always reliably correct postoperative alignment, the proximal reference point on the tibia should be determined at preoperative planning. Preoperative planning for the reference point should be performed using navigation, if needed. If the proximal reference point is selected as the center of the articular surface, the tibia can be cut in varus because preoperative and

postoperative mechanical axes are different in tibia vara (Fig. 156.3).[38] On the other hand, in cases of severe varus knee deformity with a bone defect or ligamentous insufficiency, the extended stem is used for the tibial component. In such cases, the tibial component would be laterally implanted relative to the center of the articular surface (Fig. 156.4). Medial reduction osteotomy can be used to manage these problems and is effective to treat soft tissue contracture on the medial side. Ligament imbalance can be corrected by approximately 0.4 degrees for every millimeter of medial bone resection.[9,27] One of the drawbacks of medial reduction osteotomy is the risk of loosening the tibial component because this technique would involve the placement of the medial part of the tibial component on the cancellous bone of the tibia, but not on the cortical bone. Therefore this technique is not recommended for routine application, but can be performed in severely deformed knees because the medial bone is usually sclerotic in severe varus knees and the use of the extended stem enhances implant fixation.

SAGITTAL ALIGNMENT

Femoral Alignment

Controversy still exists on the appropriate sagittal alignment of the femoral component. However, aligning the femoral component to the distal anatomic axis is recommended to avoid dramatically changing the articular surface geometry and to avoid an anterior notch. The intramedullary guide theoretically aligns the femoral component perpendicular to the distal anatomic axis, but insertion of the guide is not very accurate. Care should also be taken even when the computer navigation system is used, because many such systems have default settings for sagittal alignment of the femoral component perpendicular to the sagittal mechanical axis, which places the implant in extension relative to the distal anatomic axis because the femur has anterior bowing. To date, few studies have directly compared anterior bowing of the femur between the Asian and Caucasian patients, but anterior bowing is more significant at the middle to the distal part of the femur in Asian patients (see Fig. 156.4). Tang et al.[39] investigated 85 Chinese patients before TKA and reported that the distal one-third of the femur is significantly more bowed than the middle and proximal portions. Seo et al.[34] evaluated 76 Korean patients undergoing TKA and found that the axis of the distal femoral anterior cortex was 4.1 degrees more flexed than the sagittal mechanical axis. Therefore care should be taken for determining the insertion point and direction of the intramedullary guide for Asian patients (Fig. 156.5).

It is well known that extension of the femoral component will cause anterior notching,[15] but cutting in extension would also affect femoral anteroposterior (AP) sizing. A simulation study[26] showed that the AP dimension of the prepared femur increased by 2 mm and 3 mm with 3 degrees and 5 degrees extension in bone resection, respectively (Fig. 156.6). This could be one of the reasons for the discrepancy between preoperative

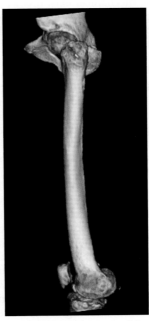

FIG 156.5 3D bone image reconstructed from a CT scan of a Japanese patient. The distal part of the femur shows anterior bowing.

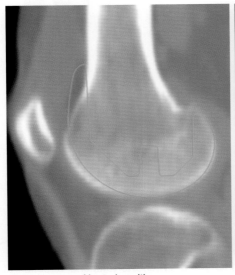

Neutral position

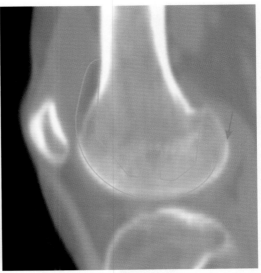

5 degrees in extension

FIG 156.6 Preoperative templating. In the neutral position, the femoral component is perpendicular to the distal anatomic axis of the femur *(left)*. When the femoral component is at 5 degrees extension, the femoral component moves anteriorly to avoid an anterior notch, requiring a larger AP dimension component to maintain the flexion gap *(red arrow, right)*.

planning and intraoperative measurement. Sagittal cutting error in extension would make surgeons choose a larger component, which might cause symptomatic overhanging[17] of the femoral component. Another concern is the relationship with the tibial component. Using a cruciate-retaining implant, surgeons can align the femoral component to the distal anatomy, but care should be taken when using the posterior-stabilized implant. Anatomic replacement with the femoral component might align the femoral component in an excessive flexed position relative to the mechanical axis; this would cause anterior impingement of the post, increasing wear and tear of the post. For posterior-stabilized knees, preoperative planning should be performed to include this issue.

Tibial Alignment

Some studies[2,12] have found that Asian people have a steep posterior tibial slope, but a direct comparison study[41] between Asian and Caucasian populations did not show a significant difference in the posterior tibial slope. For posterior-stabilized knees, the postoperative posterior tibial slope should be smaller than the preoperative slope to control a flexion gap,[31] which may have increased because of resection of the posterior cruciate ligament (PCL).[7] In addition, decreasing the posterior slope is recommended to avoid anterior impingement of the post.[28] For cruciate-retaining knees, the postoperative tibial slope should be adjusted to the preoperative slope to maintain the PCL tension.[10,33] However, the posterior tibial slope is highly variable, and some Asian patients have more than 10 degrees of tibial slope (Fig. 156.7). In such cases, it is difficult to maintain the preoperative posterior slope. Thus far, we do not have a definite upper limit of the tibial slope, but some studies[35,40] have suggested that more than 10 degrees of slope would be a risk for increased contact stress and wear of the posterior part of the polyethylene. From these findings, it is difficult that proper tension of the PCL cannot be maintained by the cruciate-retaining total knee in patients with more than 10 degrees preoperative tibial posterior slope.

ROTATIONAL ALIGNMENT

In the resection technique, rotation of the femoral component causes its alignment to the transepicondylar axis or the Whiteside line. The surgical epicondylar axis is externally rotated from the posterior condylar axis in about 3 degrees, and there is no significant difference in this posterior condylar angle between Asian and Caucasian patients.[5,18] Therefore surgeons do not have to change their strategy of rotational alignment of the femoral component for Asian patients. For the tibial alignment, to avoid rotational mismatch between the femoral and tibial components, the tibial AP axis, such as the Akagi line,[1] can be used in the Asian population. The rotational relationship between the tibia and femur of Asian patients is not significantly different from that of Caucasians. However, care should be taken to avoid distal torsion of the tibia. The angle between the malleolar line of the ankle and the AP axis of the tibia varies among individuals and one study reported that the range was more than 40 degrees in 52 Japanese subjects.[25] Therefore care should be taken when using the extramedullary guide for the tibia. The rotational direction of the guide should be aligned to the AP axis of the proximal tibia, not to the AP axis of the ankle[20] (Fig. 156.8). If the rotational position of the guide is adjusted to the ankle or foot, this procedure would cause coronal malalignment of the tibial component. In addition, excessive external rotation of the tibial component would cause internal rotation of the foot postoperatively. If preoperative internal torsion of the tibia exists, postoperative internal

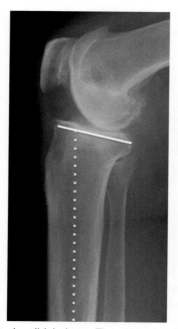

FIG 156.7 Posterior tibial slope. The posterior tibial slope was 12 degrees in this Japanese patient.

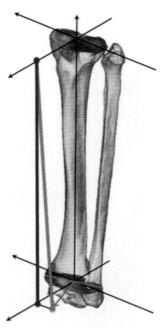

FIG 156.8 When the rotational direction of the extramedullary guide is adjusted to the AP axis of the ankle *(red arrow)*, the distal end of the guide is shifted laterally *(red line)*, resulting in varus alignment when the distal part of the tibia is externally rotated. The rotational direction of the guide should be aligned to the AP axis of the proximal tibia *(blue line)*.

rotation would be more significant. This is not recommended from the cosmetic standpoint, and toe-in gate would increase the adduction moment of the knee. Care should be taken to determine the rotational position of the tibial component, especially in Asian patients with internal torsion of the tibia.

FEMORAL AND TIBIAL MORPHOLOGY

Many studies have shown race-based differences in knee morphology.[16,41] Studies of Asian patients showed that Asian female patients tend to have narrower distal femurs. A Chinese study[41] showed that the medial-lateral (ML)/AP ratio is significantly smaller in the Chinese female population than in the Caucasian female population. Gender-specific implants are especially useful for Asian female patients. A tibial shape analysis[41] showed that Chinese male patients had wider tibias than Caucasian male patients. Many studies support the existence of some differences in the shape of the femur and the tibia among ethnic groups, but there is also a large amount of variation within individual ethnicities, and such differences also exist between genders. Therefore this issue may not be related solely to ethnicity. Recently, knee designs have become available in more sizes. This development will help the surgeon choose an implant based on bone dimensions in individual patients and decrease the risks of significant overhang or underhang of the knee prosthesis in patients of all ethnic groups.

LIGAMENT BALANCING

As mentioned previously, most Asian patients have varus deformities. Therefore achieving neutral coronal alignment can possibly cause ligamentous imbalance in knee extension. Okazaki et al.[30] evaluated 50 normal knees and found that the lateral side was 2.5 degrees laxer than the medial side. Therefore a couple of degrees of lateral laxity would not be symptomatic. Okamoto et al.[29] investigated laxity of osteoarthritic knees during TKA. In that study, lateral soft tissue laxity increased with an increase in severity of knee deformities, but the medial side did not contract with an increase in varus deformity. These results suggest that release on the medial side is unnecessary and is only needed to allow for implant replacement, even in severely deformed knees. However, that study also showed that the mean ligamentous imbalance was 4.9 mm in cases with more than 20 degrees of varus deformity, suggesting the need for solutions to treat this imbalance. One of the classical methods to treat this situation is medial release, but many studies have indicated difficulty managing extension imbalance by medial release alone[22]; medial release would cause flexion instability in such cases. Another important point is the extent to which ligament imbalance can be allowed. Some studies have focused on the effect of ligament imbalance on knee kinematics. A fluoroscopic analysis by Hamai et al.[6] showed that the static varus-valgus imbalance on stress radiographs did not influence lift-off motion of the femoral component. Furthermore, a computer simulation study[11] using KneeSIM software (LifeMOD/

KneeSIM 2010; LifeModeler Inc., San Clemente, California) showed that no lift-off motion was detected in the knee with neutral to 1 degree of varus malalignment even when the knees had 5 mm of lateral laxity. Lateral laxity, theoretically, increases the risk of lift-off motion, but these risks would decrease with neutral alignment. These studies suggest that lateral laxity up to 5 degrees extension would be acceptable when neutral alignment is achieved. In addition, the role of ethnic differences in normal soft tissue laxity remains unresolved. A previous study[37] reported ethnic differences in knee-joint laxity. If such differences exist, our methods of ligament balancing should be modified, because adequate tension when assessing joint gaps is different among ethnic groups.

KEY REFERENCES

2. Chiu KY, Zhang SD, Zhang GH: Posterior slope of tibial plateau in Chinese. *J Arthroplasty* 15:224, 2000.
4. Fukagawa S, Matsuda S, Mitsuyasu H, et al: Anterior border of the tibia as a landmark for extramedullary alignment guide in total knee arthroplasty for varus knees. *J Orthop Res* 29:919, 2011.
5. Griffin FM, Math K, Scuderi GR, et al: Anatomy of the epicondyles of the distal femur: MRI analysis of normal knees. *J Arthroplasty* 15:354, 2000.
7. Kadoya Y, Kobayashi A, Komatsu T, et al: Effects of posterior cruciate ligament resection on the tibiofemoral joint gap. *Clin Orthop* 391:210, 2001.
19. Matsuda S, Mizu-uchi H, Miura H, et al: Tibial shaft axis does not always serve as a correct coronal landmark in total knee arthroplasty for varus knees. *J Arthroplasty* 18:56, 2003.
20. Mizu-uchi H, Matsuda S, Miura H, et al: The effect of ankle rotation on cutting of the tibia in total knee arthroplasty. *J Bone Joint Surg Am* 88:2632, 2006.
21. Moreland JR, Bassett LW, Hanker GJ: Radiographic analysis of the axial alignment of the lower extremity. *J Bone Joint Surg Am* 69:745, 1987.
24. Nagamine R, Miura H, Bravo CV, et al: Anatomic variations should be considered in total knee arthroplasty. *J Orthop Sci* 5:232, 2000.
25. Nagamine R, Miyanishi K, Miura H, et al: Medial torsion of the tibia in Japanese patients with osteoarthritis of the knee. *Clin Orthop* 408:218, 2003.
26. Nakahara H, Matsuda S, Okazaki K, et al: Sagittal cutting error changes femoral anteroposterior sizing in total knee arthroplasty. *Clin Orthop* 470:3560, 2012.
27. Niki Y, Harato K, Nagai K, et al: Effects of reduction osteotomy on gap balancing during total knee arthroplasty for severe varus deformity. *J Arthroplasty* 30(12):2116–2120, 2015.
32. Saeki K, Mihalko WM, Patel V, et al: Stability after medial collateral ligament release in total knee arthroplasty. *Clin Orthop* 392:184, 2001.
38. Takasaki M, Matsuda S, Fukagawa S, et al: Accuracy of image-free navigation for severely deformed knees. *Knee Surg Sports Traumatol Arthrosc* 18:763, 2010.
39. Tang WM, Chiu KY, Kwan MF, et al: Sagittal bowing of the distal femur in Chinese patients who require total knee arthroplasty. *J Orthop Res* 23:41, 2005.
40. Wasielewski RC, Galante JO, Leighty RM, et al: Wear patterns on retrieved polyethylene tibial inserts and their relationship to technical considerations during total knee arthroplasty. *Clin Orthop* 299:31, 1994.

The references for this chapter can also be found on www.expertconsult.com.

157

Pressure Sensors and Soft Tissue Balancing

Patrick A. Meere

BACKGROUND

The overall patient satisfaction with knee arthroplasty has not improved significantly over the last decade.* This is despite technological advances in design, innovative instrumentation, computer-assisted surgery (CAS), patient-specific instrumentation (PSI), refinement in muscle-sparing surgery, and ancillary pain management. Meta-analyses place the satisfaction rate below 85%.[14,15,30,36,51]

Instability has become a major recognized cause of early failure, leading to early revision surgery.† Soft tissue imbalance of the collateral ligaments has been implicated as a direct source of instability, albeit subclinical, and may well be the source of patient dissatisfaction and fair performance in many cases.[5,6,26,46,57]

Alignment alone is no longer deemed sufficient to ensure long-term implant survival or improved patient satisfaction and functional performance.‡ CAS experience has demonstrated a reduction in outliers in alignment but no significant difference in scores, with the notable exception of recent data from the Australian registry, which demonstrates a reduction in revision rates in patients younger than 65 years.[19] Furthermore, there is much controversy as to what constitutes the optimal target alignment. Constitutional varus, kinematic axis, and joint line obliquity have added complexity to the debate.[7,41,61,80]

There is nonetheless a general consensus that measured resection or gap balancing is not absolute and has intrinsic limitations. Most experienced surgeons adjust their technique to stay within established boundaries and thus, in effect, use hybrid models with variable degrees of soft tissue balancing, often in an empirical fashion.

CLASSICAL SOFT TISSUE BALANCING

Soft tissue balancing is known to have a direct impact on patient function and satisfaction. Incomplete balancing may not be adequately detected as abnormal kinematics by the surgeon, but may cause sufficient kinetic dysfunction to be the source of pain, stiffness, and delayed instability.[71,83] The established norm for balancing has been algorithmic sequences championed by expert surgeons.§ Two philosophies have emerged to systematize this very subjective component of knee arthroplasty

instrumentation: measured resection and gap balancing.[22,69,70] The dedicated instrumentation includes static passive spacer blocks, dynamic ligament tensioners, and sophisticated navigation. The historical goal of perfect gap balance at 0 and 90 degrees has been challenged by the complexity of mid-flexion instability.[33,81] The development of modern investigational tools and instrumentation, such as fluoroscopy, computer-assisted navigation, and sensors, have brought some quantitative objectivity. There is nonetheless still no clear target zones for kinematic trajectories, laxity envelopes, or kinetic loading and distribution throughout the flexion range of motion (ROM).[78,85,89] Interobserver variance in the testing method and perceived ligamentous laxity remains an inherent obstacle.[16,54] Matsuda et al. concluded that coronal laxity, especially balanced laxity, is important for achieving an improved ROM in mobile-bearing total knee arthroplasty.[52] Heesterbeek et al. cite published ranges within 4 degrees in each direction of varus and valgus upon standard testing.[40] Several authors have also shown that the ratio of varus to valgus laxity is closer to 0.55, reflecting a stiffer medial soft tissue envelope, despite comparable stiffness values for medial and lateral collateral ligaments.[40,68,88] Bellemans et al. have warned against the potential change in stiffness caused by surgical instrumentation.[8,21] Walker et al. recently demonstrated the compartmental asymmetry in relative anteroposterior (AP) motion of the femur onto the tibia.[82] Instability and failure studies have recommended restricting AP laxity to less than 5 mm.[66,77] Fluoroscopy and gait analysis have become a validated method of detection of post facto clinical instability based on the presence or absence of more than 1 mm lift-off in flexion.[84] Several kinematic studies have documented ranges of relative motions for different knee designs and instrumentation techniques. In contrast to CAS and alignment, there has been a paucity of meta-analyses of clinical outcome studies to validate the superiority of any specific soft tissue balancing method,[13,14,22,30,41] as a result of the heterogeneity of methods and devices and the lack of validated outcome ranges needed for any power analysis. Of note, several studies revealed a patient preference for increased moderate laxity over stiffness.[47,52]

PRESSURE SENSORS: AN INTRODUCTION

Pressure is defined as force over unit area. In the context of the knee joint, the force is the contact load exerted by the femoral condyle on the tibial plateau. In knee arthroplasties, the tibial surface varies based on design morphology and degree of constraint. Cadaveric studies of native knees have predominantly used pressure film technology to study topographical distribution of intensity.[82] The wired and fragile films are, however, ill-suited for dynamic or in vivo studies. Commercially available

---

*References 11, 12, 25, 26, 36, 63, 64, and 79.
†References 25, 26, 36, 63, 65, 66, 77, and 79.
‡References 14, 15, 30, 36, 64, and 66.
§References 24, 33, 52, 59, 60, 66, 86, and 87.

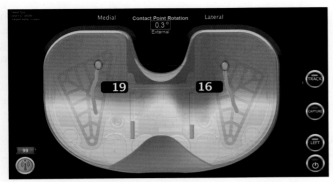

FIG 157.1 GUI display of a pressure sensor matrix embedded in a commercially available tibial liner insert. The magnitude of the compartmental contact loads appears in numerical and columnar formats. The contact load central points are seen here in tracking mode. The relative tibial rotation is noted as a CP rotation numerical value.

implant sensors can be static or dynamic. The former class is popular for gap balancing.** Dynamic balancing generally displays compartmental loads as singular contact points (CPs). These represent the resultant vectorial sum of individual loads captured by peripheral sensors, typically three, strategically based at the perimeter of the mapped tibial contact surface area (Fig. 157.1). There are several versions of pressure sensors in various stages of development. Alternative load-capture methods have included standard strain gauges, polyimide-based microelectromechanical systems (MEMS) strain sensors, magnetic and piezo-electric sensors, as well as pneumatic technology.[††]

Implantable sensor technology for the knee was introduced to quantify joint reactive loads with activity. In seminal studies by D'Lima et al., ranges of contact loads, expressed as a multiple of body weight, were produced using in vivo telemetry of imbedded sensors on the tibial surface of a few patients.[10,17,18] The range was between 0.9×BW (stationary bicycle) to 4.4×BW (golf swing). Bergmann et al. produced telemetry kinetic reference ranges for recreational activities. Slow jogging reached peak values of 5165 N and the maximal torque at the implant stem was 10.5 Nm with walking.[10] Wasielewski et al. were the first to establish a correlation between kinetic load application and kinematic motion through fluoroscopic analysis. They found that "abnormal compartment pressures and distributions as recorded by the intraoperative pressure sensor were correlated with inappropriate or paradoxical postoperative kinematics." Balanced compartmental loads did not generate a lift-off greater than 1 mm as seen by fluoroscopy.[84]

Modern application of pressure sensors has been restricted to the intraoperative load-balancing event. Few types are currently clinically available, however, more are in the developmental stages.[28,45,72,90] A common design consists of a matrix of contact load sensors imbedded into manufacturer-specific tibial trial trays. The contact load information is wirelessly transmitted from the surgical field to the adjacent computer processing unit (CPU) and visualized on a screen in a general user interface (GUI) display. Sensors provide the surgeon with real-time

compartmental tibiofemoral contact load information in magnitude and geographical position. The latter provides critical kinematic data that enables optimization of tibial component rotation through CP coronal symmetry and relative AP displacement. The collateral ligamentous tension is influenced by liner thickness and potential gap space and can be assessed by AP drawer laxity, differential load deltas, and lift-off points under standardized varus-valgus torque testing.

BALANCING WITH SENSORS

The objective of soft tissue balancing by means of pressure sensors is to achieve a distribution of compartment loads that are compatible with the physiological demands of the native knee. Because this pioneering clinical field has no validated standards, certain working definitions have to be established. These are working hypotheses to be refined with time and scientific evidence. Given the relative absence of large-scale data on in vivo load distribution, an acceptable consensus is to define balance as equal loads or an even load distribution between the medial and lateral compartments. Wasielewski et al. found that comparable loads led to no lift-off greater than 1 mm on fluoroscopy.[84] Walker et al., in a cadaveric testing series, hypothesized that a threshold of 15 pounds is considered reasonable to qualify as a balanced state.[83]

The practical goal of knee balancing with sensors is to bring the medial and lateral compartmental loads to a magnitude that is equal or comparable (i.e., with a differential that is less than or equal to 15 pounds). This is achieved through corrective action steps from an imbalanced-state starting point through specific strategic moves, known collectively as single surgical variable (SSV) corrections. These can be catalogued as bony cuts (mechanical axis, joint line obliquity, sagittal slope), components (sizing, shifting), or soft tissue releases or dynamization.[83] In contrast with historical soft tissue balancing, which was largely empirical, balancing with sensors provides quantified information that leads to a best-fit correction. The authors demonstrated, in a series of 105 patients, that a balanced state could be achieved with an average of two targeted moves (range = [0, 5]).[56] Because it prevents unintended destabilization and inflammatory response associated with excessive release, load sensor–based balancing is considered tissue preserving.

The authors' preferred instrumentation surgical sequence is as follows:

1. Distal femoral resection and proximal tibial neutral resection with verification of restoration of the mechanical axis and sufficient extension gap (on the looser compartment if the load differential is asymmetrical).
2. Measured resection of the distal femoral posterior cut with patient-specific adjustments for wear or dysplasia.
3. Verification of the gross parallelism (visual) of the distal femoral and proximal tibial cuts (rectangular flexion gap).
4. Insertion of trial components and sensor-instrumented trial tibial liner.
5. Macro-rotational positioning of tibial baseplate based on peripheral fit and anatomical referencing.
6. Balancing testing sequence:
   a. Leg in unsupported extension (sag)
   b. Leg in supported extension at 10 degrees
   c. Gradual flexion through heel push and thigh pull with interval measurements (30, 45, 60, and 90 degrees). All steps are captured on the GUI screen for analysis.

**References 4, 13, 23, 38, 39, and 53.
[††]References 1-3, 17, 18, 28, 32, 34, 45, 49, 50, and 90.

d. AP drawer and reverse drawer testing in tracking mode (crumb trace)

e. Repositioning in 10 degrees to test varus-valgus laxity with a calibrated applied force in the range of 20 to 30 N, corresponding to a torque in the range of 8 to 12 Nm at the joint line for most patients.

7. Analysis of the GUI results. The magnitude of the loads at the various stages of flexion reflects compartmental gap compression. Load differentials between compartments greater than 40 pounds are best handled by tibial or occasionally femoral minor (less than 2 mm) bone trimming. Walker et al. have demonstrated the importance of 2 mm or 2 degrees on load reduction in a controlled cadaveric setting.[83] Load differentials under 40 pounds can usually be balanced with soft tissue SSV corrections (see below).

8. Performance of the best fit selected SSV correction. The exact sequence of release or bone trimming depends on the load distribution pattern. As a general rule the tightest compartment is addressed first. Extension balance precedes flexion balance. Overload in extension points to the posterior soft tissue structures of the affected compartment. The popliteus can be dynamized but should be spared if possible. The posterolateral corner is complex. Excessive loads can be successfully normalized by variable release of the popliteofibular ligament, the arcuate ligament, and the capsule. The iliotibial band does not limit the overall extension but may contribute to excessive lateral force and must be inspected and partially released if necessary. The posteromedial corner release includes the elevation of the posterior two thirds of the medial collateral ligament and occasionally the attachment of the semimembranosus. The medial fibers of the posterior cruciate ligament (PCL) can lead to excessive flexion load. The dominant reason for excessive medial load in mid and late flexion, however, remains the anterior one third of the medial collateral ligament. After classical limited releases have been performed and assuming the relative overload does not exceed 40 pounds, a controlled pie-crusting may be performed.[9,42,43,58,62]

9. Reiterative testing (step 6) using the standard sequence until balance in the coronal plane has been achieved.

10. Validation or adjustment of the tibial component rotation. The line segment between the CPs and the neutral coronal axis of the tibia should be parallel.[73]

11. Assessment of the kinematic tracking of the CPs for compartmental rollback or paradoxical motion in cruciate-retaining designs. Excessive posteriorization with flexion indicates PCL tightness or flexion gap crowding. Excessive anteriorization in sag extension indicates recurvatum or an insufficient liner thickness.

12. Patella resurfacing with reiterative testing (step 6). The patella thickness and a closed arthrotomy will influence the loads in flexion as demonstrated by Schnaser et al.[76]

13. Final verification of gap balancing by comparing the balanced values in extension and flexion. Classical gap theory applies at this stage.

14. Validation of the soft tissue laxity envelope. The knee is placed at 10 degrees and a varus-valgus torque test is performed. A compartmental joint line separation or lift-off is desirable as demonstrated by several authors. In addition, this author recommends a supplemental rise in pressure to a delta of 20+ pounds per compartment (compression load rise above baseline on the compartment opposite to the tested ligament). This ensures that the ligamentous tension is engaged beyond the toe zone of the elasticity curve. Heesterbeek et al. have demonstrated a similar effect using tensiometers and have qualified the stiffness transition point.[39]

15. Cementing of the final implants and reverification of optimal liner thickness. Roche et al. has demonstrated the significant effect of joint line elevation by cementing.[74]

CLINICAL EVIDENCE

There are few studies that have reported on the clinical outcomes of pressure sensor balancing. Gustke et al. reported significant improvement in patient satisfaction and function in a series of 135 patients, with patient satisfaction scores reaching 96.7%.[36] In a follow-up study, the average activity level scores of quantitatively balanced patients were 68.6 (corresponding to tennis, light jogging, and heavy yard work), whereas the average activity level of unbalanced patients was 46.7 (corresponding to light housework and limited walking distances) ($p = .015$). The authors concluded that balance was the most highly significant factor in improving patient activity level.[35,36]

DISCUSSION

Soft tissue balancing is a critical component of the surgical technique of knee arthroplasty. It should complement the established and essential restoration of the mechanical axis alignment. Although there is still much debate about what constitutes the ideal axis,[‡‡] it appears reasonable that any balancing algorithm should respect the boundaries of 3 degrees from neutral or risk premature clinical failure.

A common criticism of a quantified balancing technique has been the skepticism of load values under anesthesia. In real life, the resultant forces across the joint line are presumed to be far greater as a result of compressive axial ground reaction forces and the interplay of agonist and antagonist active muscular forces across the knee joint. The quantification of live compression forces relies on telemetry from imbedded joint sensors. To date, only few cases are available to study this.[10,17,18] Kutzner et al. comment that peak loads are high (1 to 4×BW), yet "resultant contact forces during dynamic activities were lower than the ones predicted by many mathematical models."[47] Pianigiani et al. used such a validated numerical physiological knee model and studied the effects of deliberate surgical errors using different knee implants. They concluded that contact forces are more heavily (67%) influenced by malconfigurations than kinematics.[71] This supports the findings of Walker et al., who demonstrated the importance of minute surgical deviations on resultant individual compartment loads.[83] The essential assumption is that optimizing relative compartment load ratios at the time of surgery under anesthesia still improves the clinical behavior of the knee. This was originally demonstrated by fluoroscopy in one of the few studies comparing kinetic balance at the time of surgery with kinematic postoperative control. Wasielewski et al. observed that balanced compartments did not generate lift-offs greater than 1 mm, emphasizing that surgical factors "influence the magnitude and distribution of forces at the articulation, postoperative kinematics, and likely, implant longevity."[84]

---

‡‡References 7, 37, 41, 61, 67, and 80.

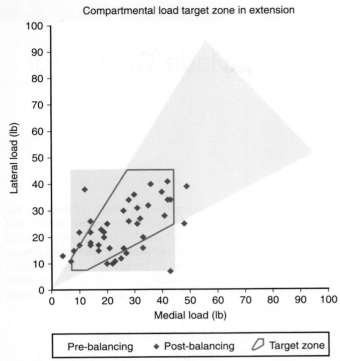

FIG 157.2 Target Zone Concept for Compartmental Load Balancing The limits are set by the intersection of two sectors: an adjustable range in absolute magnitude *(green area)* and relative compartmental load ratio *(blue zone)*.

FUTURE DEVELOPMENTS

The authors have recommended the concept of balancing target zones, which can be derived directly at the time of the instrumentation. In a retrospective series of 105 patients and a subsequent prospective series of 200 patients, significant clustering on the scatter plot graphs can be seen (Fig. 157.2). Based on the clinical scores for each data point, safe balancing zones can be derived.[55] The integration of the captured perioperative data and patient-reported outcome measures into large registries will allow for critical analysis and correlation among loads, kinematics, ligamentous tension, and specific corrective strategies. These will consequently strengthen or force adjustments to the current theories about how to best use load sensor technology to achieve knee function that is as natural as possible.

In vivo telemetry and numerical or mathematical modeling of the knee are two supplemental areas of ongoing development.[27,31,75] Quantified in vivo objective outcomes from impartial sensors will provide the data sets needed for numerical models to be tested and confirmed as accurate, as initiated by the Grand Challenge Competition to Predict In-Vivo Knee Loads.[29] Undoubtedly, validated models will strongly influence, if not direct, future knee designs and surgical protocols including soft tissue balancing algorithms.

The references for this chapter can also be found on www.expertconsult.com.

158

The Clinical Effectiveness of Custom-Made Guides for Total Knee Arthroplasty

Emmanuel Thienpont

Custom-made guides (CMGs) are, like many things in orthopedic surgery, a recurring phenomenon. Radermacher initially used them in the late 1990s to help surgeons to position pedicular screws during spine surgery.[26] However, this technique went out of fashion, and only few people continued to work with guides. The cycle of innovation brought the technology back to our attention when software programs were developed to convert two-dimensional radiographic images into three-dimensional (3D) clinical images. This allowed surgeons both to perform 3D surgical planning and to simulate the final component size and position.

The first instruments for total knee arthroplasty (TKA) were called patient-specific instruments (PSIs). However, this name became closely linked to a specific manufacturer, and the name changed to patient-matched instruments (PMIs) or patient-matched guides (PMGs). Designed to optimize the surgical workflow, PSIs were, in the first instance, pin-positioning guides. These evolved into patient-specific cutting guides (PSCGs), which allowed cuts to be made through slots in the guides. The latest evolution of the technology allows surgeons to combine PSCGs with single-use disposable instruments.

CMGs are made from resin powder that is built up layer by layer to match the individual joint geometry of each patient. The 3D plan can be derived from computed tomography (CT) scan, magnetic resonance imaging (MRI), or a combination of one of those two alongside standing full-leg radiographs. Many clinical advantages were promised at the birth of this technology. These included: surgical accuracy in all three component planes, precise 180-degree hip-knee-ankle (HKA) angle limb alignment without outliers; reductions in blood loss leading to zero transfusion; a reduction in venous thromboembolisms because the femoral canal would not need to be opened; better clinical outcomes thanks to reductions in surgical time and improvements in rotational alignment; and, finally, the ability to perform an extra case per day because of improved surgical effectiveness.[18,20,23,41]

However, in process management, the first step in becoming efficient is to "do things right." The next step is to become effective, which means "doing the right things right." In this chapter, we will discuss the effectiveness of CMGs in achieving accurate component and lower limb alignment, reductions in blood loss and the need for transfusion, reductions in surgical time, better clinical outcomes and cost effectiveness. Finally, we discuss whether there are differences in effectiveness between CT- and MRI-based systems.

A number of extensive investigations have already been carried out to assess differences in alignment between CMGs and conventional instrumentation. To reflect that, we collated nine meta-analyses comparing the alignment achieved by the two approaches (Table 158.1) and three review papers that assessed surgical time and blood loss.[30-32] Data from case series and original publications were used to assess whether there were any clinical or health economic differences. Because of differences in methodologic approach and measured outcomes between the studies, the information provided is primarily descriptive/narrative.

LIMB ALIGNMENT AND COMPONENT POSITIONING ACCURACY

In TKA malalignment leads to polyethylene wear, pain, and early implant failure, with coronal plane malalignment greater than 3 degrees increasing the likelihood of implant failure and medial bone collapse approximately 17-fold.[28,38] Despite the current debate among clinicians and researchers as to whether coronal alignment should be mechanically neutral, defined as an HKA angle of 180 degrees on full-leg standing radiographs, or should be in slight varus,[7,37] there is little dispute that the objective of TKA is to avoid component placement outside the accepted range of ±3 degrees of error from neutral alignment.[2,37]

Hip-Knee-Ankle Angle

None of the meta-analyses included in this chapter identified any differences between CMGs and conventional instrumentation in the risk of malalignment greater than 3 degrees from the neutral mechanical axis (Table 158.2).*

Coronal Plane

All meta-analyses that reported on coronal alignment for the femoral and tibial components found that the risk estimate of coronal femoral malalignment favored CMGs over conventional instrumentation.† However, the differences reached statistical significance in only three of the seven studies.[10,31,41] For tibial coronal alignment, four studies identified a significantly increased risk of tibial coronal plane malalignment with CMGs,[16,32,41,45] whereas three did not find any significant differences.[10,19,31]

Sagittal Plane

No significant differences were found between CMGs and conventional instrumentation in the sagittal plane for the

---

*References 10, 16, 19, 21, 31, 32, 41, 42, and 45.
†References 10, 16, 19, 31, 32, 41, and 45.

TABLE 158.1   **Meta-Analyses Comparing Alignment Achieved by Custom-Made Guides and Conventional Instrumentation**

	Year of Publication	Included Studies	Randomized Clinical Trials	Total Study Population
Sharareh et al.[31]	2015	12	5	1446
Jiang et al.[19]	2015	18	7	2471
Mannan et al.[21]	2015	26	4	1792
Shen et al.[32]	2015	14	7	1906
Zhang et al.[45]	2015	24	12	2739
Cavaignac et al.[10]	2014	15	6	1914
Thienpont et al.[41]	2014	16	8	1755
Fu et al.[16]	2014	10	10	837
Voleti et al.[42]	2014	9	n/a	957

n/a, Not available.
All values *n,* unless otherwise stated.

femur.[‡] In contrast, four meta-analyses found an increased risk of tibial sagittal plane malalignment.[16,32,41,45] In the remaining studies, the difference was not significant.[10,19]

Rotational Plane

None of the meta-analyses found a significant difference in femoral rotational malalignment between CMGs and conventional instrumentation.[10,16,32,41,45]

FUNCTIONAL OUTCOME

A number of clinical parameters have been analyzed to identify any clinical advantages from using CMGs. Both patient-reported outcome measurement scores and surgeon-reported outcomes have been reported.

No significant differences in Knee Society score (KSS); Oxford Knee Score (OKS); Short Form Health Survey (SF-36); Western Ontario and McMaster Universities (WOMAC) Arthritis Index; visual analog scale (VAS); and University of California, Los Angeles (UCLA) activity scores between CMGs and conventional instrumentation have been reported. Furthermore, no differences in range of motion have been observed between patients operated on using the two techniques.

Sassoon et al. found only 2 studies, including a total of 184 patients, that compared CMGs and conventional instrumentation on the basis of clinical data.[30] The consensus was that the use of patient-specific cutting blocks did not confer any functional gains when compared with traditional instrumentation.[30] Chen et al. compared PSI and conventional instrumentation in 60 patients undergoing TKA.[12] Two years after surgery, KSS, OKS, and SF-36 scores were comparable between the two groups. Although the KSS was 9 ± 3 points higher with CMGs ($p = .008$), the improvement in KSS at follow-up was comparable between the two technologies.[12] Another study assessed whether CMGs improve clinical outcomes, as determined by UCLA activity, SF-12, and OKS scores, versus conventional instrumentation.[22] The researchers found that, alongside comparable alignment, there were no differences at final follow-up between the two technologies in terms of range of motion (114 ± 14 degrees with CMG vs. 115 ± 15 degrees for conventional instrumentation; $p = .7$), UCLA activity scores (6 ± 2 vs. 6 ± 2; $p = .7$), SF-12 physical scores (44 ± 12 vs. 41 ± 12; $p = .07$), and

OKS (39 ± 9 vs. 37 ± 10; $p = .1$). There were also no differences in the incremental improvement in UCLA activity scores (1 ± 4 with CMG vs. 1 ± 3 with conventional instrumentation; $p = .5$), SF-12 physical scores (12 ± 20 vs. 11 ± 21; $p = .8$), and OKS (16 ± 9 vs. 19 ± 10; $p = .1$) between preoperative and postoperative assessments.[22]

Anderl et al. examined KSSs and VAS pain scores in a cohort study of 150 TKA patients operated on using CMGs and the same number who received conventional instrumentation.[3] OKSs and WOMAC scores were also collected at follow-up. At a mean follow-up of 28.6 ± 5.2 months, clinical outcomes were comparable between the two patient groups. Interestingly, there were significant outliers in terms of 3D component positioning with CMGs versus conventional instrumentation. Non-outliers, defined as an HKA angle of 180 ± 3 degrees, had better clinical results than outliers at 2-year follow-up.[3]

Another study found no differences between CMGs and conventional instrumentation in terms of postoperative VAS pain scores, patient satisfaction, or functional outcomes, based on Knee Injury and Osteoarthritis Outcome Score and Lysholm scores, after a mean follow-up of just longer than 6 months.[43] A study by Yaffe et al. also failed to reveal any differences in KSS, range of motion, or improvements in pain scores between custom-made and conventional jigs.[44] However, these authors did note that there were greater improvements in Knee Society function scores with CMGs at 6-month follow-up. Firm conclusions on the purported benefits of CMGs nevertheless remain elusive, as the preoperative function scores were higher in the CMG group than in patients assigned to conventional instrumentation.[44]

Pietsch et al. measured KSS at week 2, 6, and 12 in 80 patients undergoing TKA, finding no significant difference between those who were operated on using CMGs and those who received conventional instrumentation.[25] Knee flexion, measured on days 7 and 10 and at weeks 6 and 12, and knee swelling and pain, measured on days 1, 3, and 10 and at weeks 6 and 12, also revealed no significant differences between the groups.[25]

None of the studies we identified addressed the survival of components implanted using CMGs versus those placed with standard instrumentation.

BLOOD LOSS

It has been claimed that CMGs reduce blood loss because of both shorter surgical times and the extramedullary approach used. However, Fu et al. were unable to perform a meta-analysis

‡References 10, 16, 19, 32, 41, and 45.

TABLE 158.2   Risk of Malalignment Greater Than 3 Degrees With Custom-Made Guides and Conventional Instrumentation

	PATIENT-SPECIFIC INSTRUMENTS (A)		CONVENTIONAL INSTRUMENTATION (B)		A VERSUS B		
	Sample Size	Malaligned	Sample Size	Malaligned	Risk Ratio of Outliers*	95% Confidence Interval[a]	p Value
Mechanical Axis Malalignment Greater Than 3 Degrees							
Sharareh et al.[a,31]	669	119	631	136	0.8	0.60-1.06	.11
Jiang et al.[19]	1149	200	1124	217	0.84	0.61-1.11	n/a
Mannan et al.[a,21]	901	184	175	946	0.9	0.72-1.14	n/a
Shen et al.[a,32]	880	154	932	168	0.99	0.65-1.49	.94
Zhang et al.[a,45]	1068	237	1001	212	1.04	0.35-3.53	.81
Cavaignac et al.[10]	872	155	958	198	0.88	0.68-1.13	.3
Thienpont et al.[41]	833	151	783	165	0.84	0.60-1.18	.3
Fu et al.[16]	330	62	334	56	1.12	0.81-1.54	.5
Voleti et al.[42]	302	23	402	24	n/a	n/a	.70
Tibial Component Coronal Plane Malalignment Greater Than 3 Degrees							
Sharareh et al.[a,31]	207	17	212	16	0.83	0.24-2.88	.77
Jiang et al.[19]	492	27	536	32	0.84	0.52-1.35	n/a
Shen et al.[a,32]	399	28	475	14	2.29	1.20-4.35	.01
Zhang et al.[a,45]	499	69	614	40	2.22	1.36-3.63	<.01
Cavaignac et al.[10]	508	36	566	36	1.09	0.54-2.19	.81
Thienpont et al.[41]	427	42	379	20	1.75	1.06-2.88	.03
Fu et al.[16]	255	21	260	8	2.5	1.16-5.36	.02
Femoral Component Coronal Plane Malalignment Greater Than 3 Degrees							
Sharareh et al.[a,31]	207	12	212	30	0.38	0.19-0.74	.01
Jiang et al.[19]	569	33	613	65	0.56	0.32-1.05	n/a
Shen et al.[a,32]	399	27	475	44	0.64	0.39-1.06	.08
Zhang et al.[a,45]	479	40	517	65	0.72	0.46-1.14	.16
Cavaignac et al.[10]	508	28	566	63	0.55	0.36-0.86	.01
Thienpont et al.[41]	427	48	379	59	0.65	0.45-0.94	.02
Fu et al.[16]	255	21	260	31	0.64	0.38-1.07	.09
Tibial Component Sagittal Plane Malalignment Greater Than 3 Degrees							
Jiang et al.[19]	430	102	401	87	1.04	0.69-1.55	n/a
Shen et al.[a,32]	360	90	436	71	1.67	1.16-2.42	<.01
Zhang et al. (Slope)[a,45]	263	84	347	66	1.97	1.30-2.99	<.01
Zhang et al. (LTC)[a,45]	236	70	231	55	1.46	0.58-3.66	.42
Cavaignac et al.[10]	508	36	566	36	1.33	0.85-2.07	.21
Thienpont et al.[41]	283	91	288	67	1.34	1.05-1.71	.02
Fu et al.[16]	216	61	221	41	1.47	1.07-2.03	.02
Femoral Component Sagittal Plane Malalignment Greater Than 3 Degrees							
Jiang et al.[19]	459	122	434	145	0.83	0.60-1.14	n/a
Shen et al.[a,32]	360	109	436	119	0.94	0.67-1.33	.74
Zhang et al. (LFC)[a,45]	236	112	231	140	0.52	0.23-1.20	.13
Zhang et al. (FEM Flexion)[a,45]	183	27	259	26	1.44	0.79-2.64	.23
Cavaignac et al.[10]	426	89	480	108	0.88	0.58-1.33	.54
Thienpont et al.[41]	283	81	288	94	0.87	0.70-1.09	.237
Fu et al.[16]	216	90	221	96	0.93	0.76-1.14	.51
Femoral Component Axial Plane Malalignment 3 Degrees							
Jiang et al.[19]	381	45	436	51	1.02	0.57-1.83	n/a
Shen et al.[a,32]	264	33	345	44	0.84	0.33-2.11	.7
Zhang et al.[a,45]	346	50	431	70	0.75	0.39-1.44	.38
Cavaignac et al.[10]	375	50	435	53	1.08	0.76-1.54	.67
Thienpont et al.[41]	231	20	243	32	0.67	0.40-1.12	.13
Fu et al.[16]	163	18	172	20	0.96	0.54-1.72	.9

[a]Odds ratios.
FEM, Flexion-extension motion; *LFC*, lateral femoral component; *LTC*, lateral tibial component; *n/a*, not available.
All values *n*, unless stated otherwise.

on blood loss because of a lack of useable data in the studies they identified.[16] They nevertheless reported that, of the five individual studies they included, three found no significant difference in blood loss,[11,14,23] whereas two found a significant difference.[8,25]

Pietsch et al. reported a reduction in blood loss with the use of CMGs, measured as a mean blood drainage of 391 mL versus 603 mL with conventional instrumentation ($p < .001$).[25] There were no significant differences in the estimated hemoglobin (Hb) loss, at 3.6 g/dL versus 4.1 g/dL, and in the need for transfusion, with 7.5% and 10% of patients, respectively, requiring a transfusion.[25] Thienpont et al. could not confirm these findings and observed no difference in visible or hidden blood loss, and no difference in transfusion rates.[39] In contrast to Pietsch et al.,[25] Thienpont et al. performed surgery with a tourniquet, and the femoral entry hole was plugged with a cortical bone plug, sealing the canal completely.[39]

Shen et al. evaluated blood loss as a secondary endpoint in their meta-analysis of seven randomized controlled trials (RCTs) and seven non-RCTs,[32] as four of the studies reported on blood loss.[8,11,14,29] Of those, Boonen et al. reported that blood loss was significantly reduced with CMGs versus conventional instrumentation,[8] whereas the other three studies detected no differences between the groups.[3,5,11] However, Shen et al. were unable to pool the data because the original studies reported only the mean, and not the variance, in blood loss.[32]

Turning to more recent studies, it was reported by Ferrara et al. in a prospective comparative randomized study of 30 TKA patients that CMGs were associated with less intraoperative bleeding than conventional instrumentation group, at 149 mL versus 290 mL, respectively, ($p < .01$).[15] Postoperative blood loss was also significantly lower, at 968 mL versus 1084 mL, respectively, ($p = .03$).[15] Rathod et al.[27] noticed a nonsignificant reduction in Hb loss with CMGs compared with conventional instrumentation, at a mean of 2.87 ± 1.5 versus 4.03 ± 2.0, respectively, ($p = .07$). The average units of allogeneic blood transfused was also lower with CMGs, although, again, the difference was not statistically significant, at 0.5 units versus 1.2 units, respectively, ($p = .10$). In a comparison of PSCG and conventional instrumentation in 140 TKA patients, Abane et al. did not identify any differences in blood loss ($p = .58$).[1] Finally, in a comparison of outcomes with CMGs in 75 TKA patients and a matched group operated on using conventional instrumentation, we found that there were no statistically differences in calculated blood loss, maximal drop in Hb or hematocrit, or the number of transfusions required.[39]

It is clear from the literature that CMG does not offer benefits over conventional instrumentation in terms of blood loss. However, the ability of meta-analyses to determine blood loss is hampered by inconsistent reporting of between studies.

TOURNIQUET AND SURGICAL TIME

Sassoon et al.[30] reported that a number of individual studies have examined the impact of CMGs on operative time, several of which have concluded that CMGs have no impact on the length of TKA compared with conventional instrumentation.[4,6,13,35] Other studies have found that CMGs decrease operative time or total time in the operative room by up to 20 minutes,[5,9,11,23,24] whereas some authors reported that the procedure was slightly longer when using CMGs versus conventional instrumentation.[17]

Shen et al.[32] pooled data from seven studies for a meta-analysis, finding no significant differences in operative time between CMGs and conventional instrumentation, at a weighted mean difference of -1.78 (95% confidence interval: -4.45 to 0.90; $p = .19$). It was also noted that there was a high degree of heterogeneity between the studies ($I^2 = 89\%$).[32] For their meta-analysis, Sharareh et al. examined 12 studies, of which 5 reported operative times.[31] The mean reduction in procedure length with CMGs was 2.2 minutes, at a mean of 65.5 minutes versus 67.7 minutes with conventional instrumentation. The difference was not significant ($p = .22$).[31]

COST EFFECTIVENESS OF CUSTOM-MADE GUIDE

It is conceivable that CMGs could offer cost benefits over conventional instrumentation through increased operative efficiency. However, as noted previously, the majority of studies have not found marked reductions in operative times with CMGs, and the reported reduction in the number of surgical trays required, compared with conventional instrumentation, is offset by the number of cases in which the preoperative plan for the CMG needs to be altered during the procedure.[30]

Siegel et al. examined whether single-use instruments would lead to cost benefits through reduced total operating room time and reductions in the number of surgical site infections (SSIs).[33] In 449 TKAs performed with single-use instruments and 169 carried out with traditional instrumentation trays they found that total operating room time was reduced by a mean of 30 minutes with single-use instrumentation, although surgical time was not found to be statistically different ($p = .09$). However, single-use instruments were associated with a significant reduction in the number of SSIs, at one versus five with traditional instrumentation ($p = .006$). Although single-use instrumentation added US$490 in acquisition costs, it saved between US$480 and US$600 in operative efficiency, leading the authors to conclude that such instrumentation may be of benefit both to patients and in terms of overall hospital costs.[33]

COMPUTED TOMOGRAPHY–VERSUS MAGNETIC RESONANCE IMAGING–BASED CUSTOM-MADE GUIDE

The debate as to whether CT or MRI is preferable for the creation of CMGs is ongoing. On the one hand, CT is relatively inexpensive but has the obvious disadvantage of exposure to radiation. On the other hand, MRI does not expose patients to radiation but is markedly more expensive than CT and has longer waiting lists. The majority of CT-based CMG systems use only scans of the hip, knee, and ankle joint to minimize radiation exposure. Nevertheless, the radiation dose required for CMG is equivalent to a standard yearly background radiation dose, or approximately 70 chest x-rays.[34]

In terms of accuracy a meta-analysis examined seven studies that compared MRI- and CT-based CMG. The pooled incidence of outliers greater than 3% was 12.5% for CT-based systems versus 16.9% for MRI-based systems. The difference was not found to be statistically significant.[34]

Furthermore, CT does not have the possibilities of MRI of cartilage and soft tissue imaging. The next generation of CMG will have to provide accurate information about the ligaments, trochlear anatomy, and alignment, as well as the thickness of residual cartilage. Therefore the use of CT-based CMGs could lead to over-resection of the posterior condyles as such what could lead to flexion gap instability and decreased posterior condylar offset.[3]

DISCUSSION AND CONCLUSION

CMGs did not deliver the promises made at the beginning of this new hype.[36] No significant differences were observed for blood loss, transfusion, clinical outcome, and patient reported outcome measures (PROMs) data. Except for the coronal femoral alignment, the observed angles are inferior to those of conventional instruments. For the important rotational plane no sufficient data are currently available to come to conclusions after having implanted huge numbers of TKAs with CMGs. The economical importance for the implant manufacturers if they are able to eliminate loaner sets of instruments in the hospitals and just-in-time delivery of components, reducing inventory costs, will keep this surgical trend alive.[37] The important questions about lower limb mechanical alignment precision and three plane component accuracy combined with outlier reduction should be answered as soon as possible by level I studies. With the data available currently about the clinical effectiveness of CMG-assisted TKA and the total cost of this technology, it cannot be defended to continue using it systematically for standard primary TKA cases.[40]

KEY REFERENCES

2. Abdel MP, Oussedik S, Parratte S, et al: Coronal alignment in total knee replacement: historical review, contemporary analysis, and future direction. *Bone Joint J* 96-B:857–862, 2014.

7. Bellemans J, Colyn W, Vandenneucker H, et al: The Chitranjan Ranawat award: is neutral mechanical alignment normal for all patients? The concept of constitutional varus. *Clin Orthop* 470:45–53, 2012.

10. Cavaignac E, Pailhe R, Laumond G, et al: Evaluation of the accuracy of patient-specific cutting blocks for total knee arthroplasty: a meta-analysis. *Int Orthop* 39:1541–1552, 2015.

12. Chen JY, Chin PL, Tay DK, et al: Functional outcome and quality of life after patient-specific instrumentation in total knee arthroplasty. *J Arthroplasty* 30(10):1724–1728, 2015.

22. Nam D, Park A, Stambough JB, et al: The mark coventry award: custom cutting guides do not improve total knee arthroplasty clinical outcomes at 2 years followup. *Clin Orthop* 474(1):40–46, 2016.

37. Thienpont E, Bellemans J, Victor J, et al: Alignment in total knee arthroplasty, still more questions than answers. *Knee Surg Sports Traumatol Arthrosc* 21:2191–2193, 2013.

38. Thienpont E, Fennema P, Price A: Can technology improve alignment during knee arthroplasty? *Knee* 20(Suppl 1):S21–S28, 2013.

39. Thienpont E, Grosu I, Paternostre F, et al: The use of patient-specific instruments does not reduce blood loss during minimally invasive total knee arthroplasty. *Knee Surg Sports Traumatol Arthrosc* 23(7):2055–2060, 2015.

40. Thienpont E, Paternostre F, Van Wymeersch C: The indirect cost of patient-specific instruments. *Acta Orthop Belg* 81:462–470, 2015.

41. Thienpont E, Schwab PE, Fennema P: A systematic review and meta-analysis of patient-specific instrumentation for improving alignment of the components in total knee replacement. *Bone Joint J* 96-B:1052–1061, 2014.

The references for this chapter can also be found on www.expertconsult.com.

159

Computer Navigation in Primary Total Knee Arthroplasty

James Brown Stiehl

INTRODUCTION

Computer navigation was pioneered in the early 1990s by Stephane Lavallee, PhD, at the University of Grenoble, France, with the first navigated total knee replacement being performed in 1996 by Saragalia.[72] The improvements possible in mechanical alignment of total knee replacement over the use of conventional instrumentation were immediately apparent.* Until recently, outcome data have not been able to demonstrate significant improvements in overall revision rates and general outcomes. However, a review of a large national total knee registry was able to show statistical improvements in the occurrence of implant loosening and osteolysis with the use of computer navigation.[17]

The pushbacks for conversion to navigation have considered overall costs, added time expenditure, and the complexity of navigation systems as reasons not to adopt these systems. However, these issues have gradually fallen away with the evolution of current technology in the field. The cost problem has been solved by the effect of technology evolution, where over time, the high numbers of product sales decrease the costs of components by reducing production costs. The technologies currently applied in total knee replacement are markedly streamlined with fewer "bells and whistles" and targeted applications. Patient-specific cutting guides are another example of simplicity, where the guide is created in advance by a vendor, using preoperative computed tomography (CT) or magnetic resonance imaging (MRI) scan data to model a cutting guide that is created as a custom device that is then applied intraoperative to the specific patient's geometry.[27,51] Accelerometer-based guides offer similar accuracy to conventional computer navigation with a restricted menu of measurements.[61] Time efficiency has dramatically improved, even for the standard navigational systems, and this comes from the ability of the navigational software protocol to perform only those maneuvers that the surgeon is specifically requiring.[84] This is in great contrast to the early systems that provided a "standard" method of registration, basic surgical technique, and order of the surgical procedure.

Digital imaging has been a part of robotics and computer navigation from the outset and has been characterized by the need of a preoperative CT scan or MRI. Early on with the Robodoc system, the digital image described the bone dimensions that could be used to create custom prosthetic implants and could guide the milling process of the bone down to submillimeter levels. The Mako robotic system (Stryker, Inc, Mahwah, NJ) relies on preoperative CT Digital Imaging and Communications in Medicine (DICOM) files that are loaded into the Mako computer at the time of surgery. Conventional anatomic registration methods are used to guide a haptic robotic that directs the patient's bone preparation from a predetermined software protocol. These systems have been shown to have better precision than conventional instrumentation but require a preoperative CT scan. With the availability of intraoperative three-dimensional (3D) CT, such as the Medtronic O-arm, the surgeon will be able to capture the appropriate digital images at the time of surgery, eliminating the preoperative imaging for navigation.[67] I would highlight the concept of "complete" intervention because intraoperative digital imaging allows all of the steps to be completed at the time of the intervention, in addition to the steps that are currently performed by imageless computer navigation in total knee replacement.

LITERATURE REVIEW

Early data on the use of these image-free optical tracking systems appeared positive, with improved mechanical alignment, frontal and sagittal femoral axis alignment, and frontal tibial axis alignment. We are now approaching the 20th year mark from the original introduction of this technology, and clinical experience is beginning to show some favorable improvements. Several meta-analysis studies have shown the advantage of computer-assisted surgery over conventional techniques for component alignment, blood loss, the Knee Society and Western Ontario and McMaster (WOMAC) scores and a tendency for fewer overall adverse events.[8,12,43,48,68] Multiple randomized control trials were able to demonstrate a statistically significant improvement in terms of placing the final mechanical alignment of the knee within 3 degrees of the ideal mechanical axis.† We note that 93% of the overall cases from these studies reach this level of precision with computer navigation compared with 74% in which conventional methods are used (Table 159.1). Zhang et al. performed a comparison study with bilateral total knees showing that conventional technique resulted in 28% outside of the 3-degree mechanical outlier, with no cases outlying in the navigation group.[98]

---

*References 1, 2, 5, 10, 11, 22, 23, 32, 33, 35, 48, 63, 64, 66, 72, 74, 78, and 79.

†References 16, 18, 19, 23, 25, 33, 36, 40, 45, 58, 63, 64, 67, 78, 88, and 91.

TABLE 159.1   Clinical Studies That Compare the Ability of Conventional Manual Surgical Techniques With Computer Navigation for Placing the Limb Alignment Within ±3 Degrees of the Mechanical Axis of the Lower Extremity

Author	N	Navigated (%)	Conventional (%)	% Diff.
Haaker et al.[22]	100	96	75	21
Sparmann et al.[79]	120	98	78	20
Victor and Hoste[91]	50	100	74	27
Jenny et al.[36]	235	97	74	23
Jenny and Boeri[33]	30, 30	83	70	17
Kim et al.[45]	69, 78	78	58	20
Perlick et al.[64]	40	93	75	28
Song et al.[78]	47, 50	96	76	20
Bathis et al.[2]	159	96	78	18
Perlick et al.[63,64]	50	92	72	20
Hart et al.[23]	60	88	70	18
Anderson et al.[1]	51, 116	95	84	11
		93 (average)	**74 (p < .001)**	**20**

Blood loss has been significantly reduced with the use of computer navigation and avoidance of intramedullary rods.[56,73,98] Kalairajah et al. were able to reduce the mean blood loss from 1747 mL to 1351 mL by using the pin-placed trackers instead of intramedullary guided femur and tibia jigs, which was a significant difference in 60 patients.[41] McConnell et al. similarly showed the reduction of mean blood loss from 1362 mL to 1137 mL, with an even larger study including 130 patients.[54] A number of studies have been able to demonstrate early improvements in functional outcome with computer assisted over conventional.[32,50] Gothesien et al. showed that the Knee Injury and Osteoarthritis Outcome Score was significantly better for sports and symptoms categories at 1-year follow-up.[21] Hoffart et al. found that navigation resulted in better mean Knee Society Scores (p = .008) compared with conventional instruments at 5-year follow-up.[29]

Imageless navigation referencing suffers from inherent inaccuracy of the surgeon picking the correct proscribed anatomic reference points.[‡] Yau et al. compared the combined intraobserver error for image-free acquisition of reference landmarks during total knee arthroplasty, finding that the maximum combined error for the coronal plane mechanical axis alignment was 1.32 degrees.[95,96] However, Davis et al. found that the mechanical axis of the femur in the coronal plane could vary from 5.2 degrees valgus to 2.9 degrees varus.[15] They point out that the clinical scenario must consider all possible errors, in this case the movement of the pelvis with hip registration that is assumed to be fixed in space. Other errors can arise from various steps during a total knee replacement, including for example the placement of pins for cutting blocks, actual variation of the sawcut with subsequent bone resection errors, and errors from cementing the implants into place. These errors can be additive, and the surgeon should be constantly evaluating these effects using a navigated surface block.[14,20]

The results for the assessment of the transepicondylar axis (TEA) or the anterior/posterior (AP) axis of Whiteside are inconsistent as compared with mechanical axis alignment.[34] This most likely reflects the difficulty in reproducibly picking the epicondylar or AP axis landmarks. The problem with the AP axis for computer navigation referencing can easily be understood by the distances for landmarking being very short. Slight errors in judgment can be off by several degrees. This contrast with the mechanical axis landmarking, in which an error of only 1 degree will require a point matching mistake of at least 5 mm. Yau et al. found that errors in the TEA could be as high as 9 degrees.[96] Davis et al. found the TEA error could range from 11.1 degrees of external to 6.3 degrees of internal rotation.[15] Restrepo et al. found that the fixed posterior condylar axis reference could result in malalignment of more than 5 degrees in 17% of cases, as compared with other rotational axes.[69] Siston et al. has shown that femoral rotation errors could easily exceed 5 degrees in the hands of multiple surgeons with imageless navigation referencing.[76,77]

For femoral and tibial prosthesis rotation errors, combining computer navigation and digital registration offers the potential for improving the precision, both of the implant position and ligament balancing techniques.[57,81,87,90] Heyse et al. demonstrated the potential of preoperative digital registration with the creation of patient-specific cutting blocks.[27] They were able to show that the outliers of greater than 3 degrees from the neutral TEA axis using MRI for femoral component rotation were reduced from 22.9% with conventional instrumentation and direct resection anatomical references to 2.2% with patient-specific guides. The ability to assess axial images from preoperative MRI and computed tomography scans clearly exceeds the ability to pick visual landmarks in the intraoperative setting.[26,92] Tibial rotation alignment of the tibial tray can normally be quite difficult even with navigation of the AP axis of the tibia or other landmarks, such as the medial one-third of tibial tubercle. Numerous authors have used CT images to assess these landmarks postoperatively. Roper et al. were able to show interobserver reliability of 0.9 for assessing the position of the medial one-third of the tibial tubercle in relation to the tibial tray postoperatively.[71] Kuriyama et al. have shown that tibial tray position can be markedly improved using a CT-based navigation system.[47] Those authors used the intraoperative registration that was CT based to define the anteroposterior axis of the tibia and then used a navigation-assisted placement of the tibial tray to demonstrate a precision of ±3 degrees for rotational alignment as compared with Akagi line.

An important advantage of using computer-aided surgery (CAS) is the ability to carefully measure gap balance through the range of motion.[37,62,82] This measurement relies on the

‡References 7, 14, 19, 42, 70, 83, and 94.

inherent precision of measuring the gap distances, and a recent study would suggest that this measure is clearly in the submillimeter range. Walde et al. have used computer navigation to assist the process of femoral rotation determination, noting that the best results were obtained using a tenor ligament balancing method.[93] They found that using direct-measured resection referencing, the resulting femoral rotation varied from 12 degrees of internal rotation to 15 degrees of external rotation. Using tensors with ligament balancing, this was reduced to 3 degrees of internal rotation to 2.5 degrees of external rotation. Hino et al. found significant midflexion laxity when measuring the gaps at 10 degrees intervals from 0 degree to 90 degrees of flexion.[28] This laxity was not apparent at 0 degree and 90 degrees and was found to be exaggerated in the posterior-stabilized techniques over the posterior cruciate-retaining total knees. A number of studies have shown the ability of CAS to improve outcomes by aiding the surgeon in the ligament release and balancing methods.[89]

Several authors have studied the ability of the computer to capture intraoperative kinematic data, with passive range of motion of the knee before and after prosthesis placement.[13,53,75,97] It is likely that these data could be analyzed with comparison to intraoperative CT data.[92] This may offer some predictive preimplant scenarios in which the surgeon may optimize various choices of the bone resection steps and even choices of prosthetic geometry. Siston et al. suggested that collecting this type of data could be combined with direct referencing of femur for improved determination of femoral component rotation. Matziolis et al. used navigation to calculate the flexion axis through the range of motion and with the help of a tensor during the assessment and noted that the measured axis more correctly paralleled the surgical epicondylar axis as compared with direct referenced cuts using the TEA or Whiteside line.[53]

There are a number of anecdotal reports of stress fracture from pin placement for navigated trackers.[§] These reports have demonstrated the larger 5-mm pins are problematic when placed bicortical in the shaft areas of the femur and tibial. Following the suggestion of Mihalko, the maximum pin thickness should be no more than 3 mm and probably should be placed unicortical in the tibia.[55] For the femoral side, I favor placement of a pin percutaneously through the TEA, palpating the placement and orientation from inside the knee wound. A second pin is placed more proximal but still remains in the metaphyseal distal femur area. The trackers are well out of the surgical exposure, yet quite accessible to the navigation cameras. I have not seen a single complication with this method in several hundred cases. More recently, I have obviated this problem with the guided personal surgery (eGPS) system (Exactech, Inc.), in which optical trackers are anchored to base plates, to which navigated cutting blocks are fixed for bone resection. This eliminates the need for separate tracker pod placement.

Several authors have been able to demonstrate the ability of computer navigation to guide implant placement in situations in which conventional instruments are not applicable. This could include cases of extra-articular deformity and old traumatic cases in which prior plates and rods impair the use of intramedullary guides.[**] I would consider these cases to be of higher complexity, and the surgeon must be fastidious and confident that referencing will be accurate. However, the capability to perform these techniques is obvious and enabling for the experienced surgeon (Fig. 159.1).

A recent publication from the Australian Orthopaedic Association National Joint Replacement Registry has demonstrated that long-term revision rates in patients under the age of 65 have been significantly reduced by the use of computer navigation.[17] That study covered a period from 2003 to 2012 and considered more than 44,000 navigated total knees of a cohort that represented 14% of all total knees performed. The cumulative rate of revision at 9 years for younger patients was 7.8% for conventional, with a rate of 6.3% with the use of navigation (hazard ratio, 1.38; 95% confidence interval [CI], 1.13 to 1.67, $p = .001$). The most common cause of revision was implant loosening and chronic osteolysis. The conclusion was that computer navigation could be shown to improve implant survivorship in younger patients and could be shown to be cost effective over the long term on this basis. In 2012 computer navigation had grown to include approximately 22% of all cases in Australia.

CONTEMPORARY NAVIGATION SYSTEM FEATURES

Computer imageless navigation requires three basic components: the computer, tracking technology, and trackers. For imageless navigation, the optical charge-coupled device (CCD) cameras from Northern Digital Incorporated (NDI) have been the industry standard for years and are highly accurate to the near micron level. Trackers have been pods of reflective balls or other devices that the camera tracks from the light beams that are created. The computer then tracks these trackers, and ultimately the free body that they represent, using software algorithms to create a "live" or virtual rendering of the instantaneous spatial orientation. Of course, a modern feature has been the remarkable advance of computer technology that allows current systems to have powerful computers that approximate the dimensions of the iPad.

The eGPS navigation system (Exactech, Inc., Gainesville, FL) is an evolutionary optical image-free system that incorporates many upgrades of the standard computer technologies (Fig. 159.2). The camera system has a field of view of less than 6 feet. This places the camera system in the surgical field, and the current technology of the camera upgrade has a precision an order of magnitude greater than older systems.[82] The trackers are active with battery-powered light-emitting diode (LED) lights that are attached to the base plates, which also serve as the attachments for the navigated cut guides (Fig. 159.3). The computer is now in the field with the camera system and has the dimension of a personal tablet. The screen of the system is covered with a sterile plastic cover, allowing the surgeon to engage the system by simply touching screen commands (Fig. 159.4). Of course the other digital control comes from a manual finger button on the touch probe. The immediate benefit of the increased field of view is that the line of sight camera function is not a factor for assistants, making the navigation function seamless without having to constantly adjust for the screen data going away. The functionality is also improved by active LED trackers because they are not easily foiled by blood splash or other contamination. Finally, surgeons enjoy the ability to interact with the computer for small adjustments that can be performed by simply touching the screen.

---

§References 3, 30, 38, 39, 43, 49, 52, and 80.
**References 6, 9, 24, 44, 46, 59, and 60.

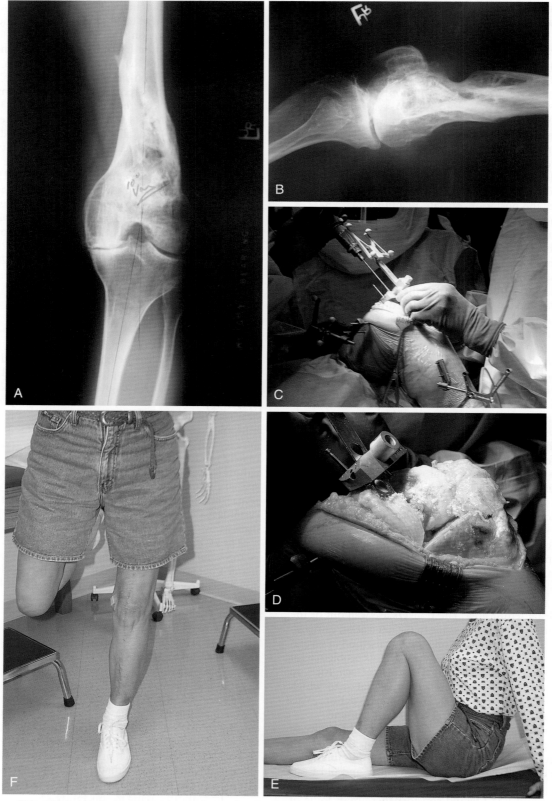

FIG 159.1 (A) Anteroposterior radiograph of a 52-year-old with severe posttraumatic arthritis following femoral fracture treated in traction 30 years before. (B) Lateral radiograph demonstrates loss of the intramedullary canal. (C) Navigation of the femoral distal cut block after registration. (D) Distal femoral cut after block is secured. (E) Twelve-month follow-up shows neutral alignment with single limb stance. (F) Flexion of 120 degrees.

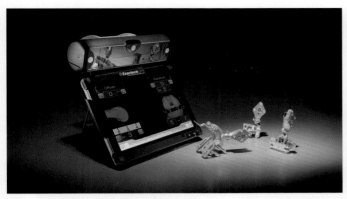

FIG 159.2 Exactech GPS computer navigation system performed with navigable cut blocks.

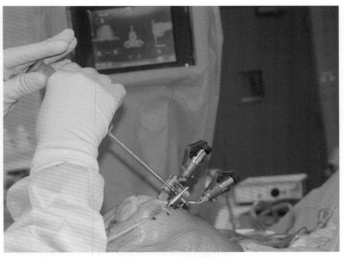

FIG 159.4 The base plate for the cut block has an LED tracker for registration of the femur. The attachment for the cut block is navigated by turning three set screws into the appropriate position for the appropriate femoral cut. These screws are shown on the computer screen and turn green when the position is correct.

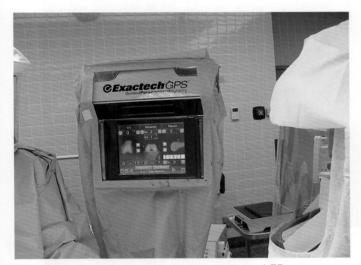

FIG 159.3 Computer camera and computer LED screen are placed on pole within 6 feet of the operative field. Sterile cover allows manipulation by the surgeon.

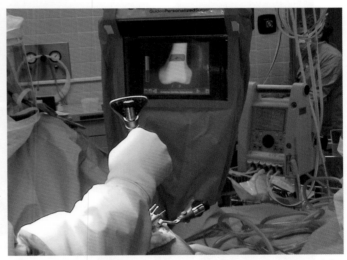

FIG 159.5 Registration of the distal femur is performed by touch pointing an area on the anterior femoral cortex using the "bone morphing" algorithm.

Another advance of the system is the ability to use a "bone morphing" to determine precise anatomic points.[85,86] Although this technology has been around for more than 15 years, the application is currently specific, with limited areas of surface painting with an active probe to determine to exact location of the anterior femoral cortex or the deepest dimension of the posterior femoral condyle (Fig. 159.5). The computer automatically captures the optimal single point. Similarly ligament balancing uses an algorithm that automatically captures the greatest dimension of the joint gap from two known points on the tibia and femur and can do this at each degree of flexion through the entire range of motion.

The computer software planning module for this system is highly sophisticated, yet has a simple interactive pull-down menu that allows the surgeon to personalize the entire procedure. This can range from simply registering and navigating the proximal tibial and distal femoral cuts to an elaborate scheme that considers steps, including bone resection, ligament balancing, and final documentation of the operation. For example, I prefer a tibial cut first approach and use the anterior cortex of the distal femur as the primary reference point (Fig. 159.6). The

flexion space cuts are made after a ligament tensor has spread and measured the flexion space (Fig. 159.7). Adjustments can be made on a screen for sizing the implants, which alters the flexion space or changes the femoral rotation, which will alter the symmetry of the flexion space. Again, adjustments are made in real time, and the surgeon can determine exactly what the final joints spaces and prosthetic dimensions will look like. The surgeon then completes the intervention by making the planned bone resections with the expectation that bone resections and ligament gaps will be correct (Fig. 159.8). Another advance of the system has been to store all anonymized or patient deidentified data from a procedure on the hard drive and to make copies

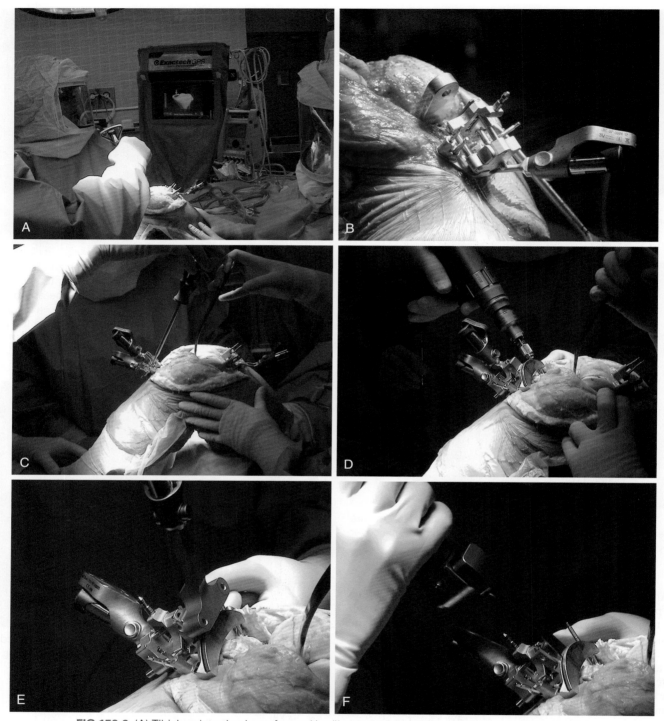

FIG 159.6 (A) Tibial registration is performed by "bone morphing" the lowest point on the medial femoral condyle. (B) Tibial base plate with cut block attachment jig is placed on proximal tibial. (C) Tibial cut block position is determined by navigating the set screws of the jig. (D) Tibial cut block is secured with pins. (E) Block position confirmed by navigating a block guide. (F) Tibia surface resection done with saw.

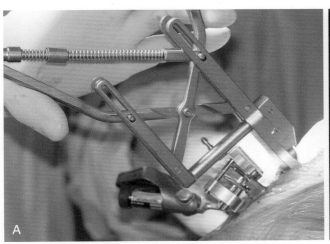
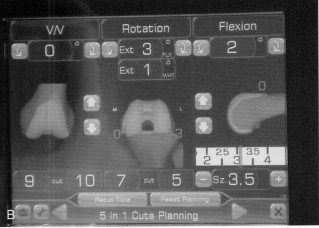

FIG 159.7 (A) Simple tensor distracts the flexion space that is navigated precisely to 90 degrees of flexion. (B) Planning of the "five-in-one" position of the femoral component is performed at this step, adjusting varus/valgus alignment, anterior offset, component flexion, femoral implant rotation, distal femoral resection, posterior condyle resection, and optimum prosthetic size.

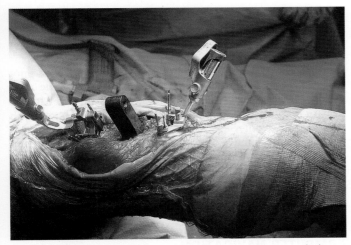

FIG 159.8 Femoral and tibial resections and ligament balance are assessed with extension block in place.

that can be placed on a "flash" drive. This allows for retrieval of large numbers of cases over a time period, and surgeons can go back and assess the techniques that were performed in patients who have had postoperative problems.

Another improvement of this system has been to combine the function of the tracker pods and the cutting guides. Most navigation systems must still create a "free body" based on the application of fiducials to bones, such as the femur and tibia, and then registering the dimensions of the free body into the computer. Fiducials have been pods or trackers that are fixed to bone in a separate site. With the eGPS system, the fiducials are the cut guide base plates that have attachments for the active trackers. Cut guides can then be attached to the base plate, and the cut guide will have its own active tracker. This system eliminates the need for a separate pod that has the tracking balls. The potential for fracture or infection from the separate pin placements is eliminated.

The most recent version of the eGPS system is the use of a "five-in-one" cutting block guide that allows for virtually all cuts of the distal femur to be made in the same step (Fig. 159.9). This functions much like a patient-specific block, with the added improvement that the block placement is planned and controlled during the intraoperative procedure, with the additional element of ligament balancing being a controlled step. That makes the intervention more "complete" as compared with the patient-specific instrumentation (PSI) that does not offer the surgeon planning features nor the ability to assess the ligament gaps.

METROLOGY AND CLINICAL EVALUATION OF THE EGPS

The eGPS system was assessed with a 3D surface scanner that could precisely register a plastic lower extremity model to the 25-μm level. A board-certified orthopedic knee surgeon performed a simulated total knee replacement on 28 lower extremity synthetic knee models. The population of plastic knees included 12 models with a 5-degree varus deformity, 12 models with a neutral mechanical axis, and 4 models with a valgus alignment of 5 degrees. The implant used was the Exactech Optetrak Logic PS system, assessing primarily the extension gap resections and the ultimate mechanical axis alignment and positions of the prosthetic implants. The registration process was specific to each limb model and the surgeon used the same dimples that were used to create the original 3D surface model. This is an important consideration because the registration error produced by surgeon variation is removed, basically testing the true precision of the computer navigation system. The result of reassessing the bone resections on the plastic bones was that the maximum errors were submillimeter for the resection depth (<0.68 mm) or subdegree for the angle measurements (<0.90 degrees). No statistical difference was apparent between error indexes for the various groups comparing femur or tibia, nor between the various deformity groups. This study demonstrated that the errors produced by the computer navigation system in the actual process of registering the lower

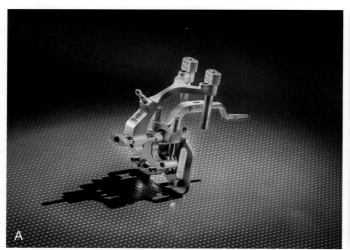
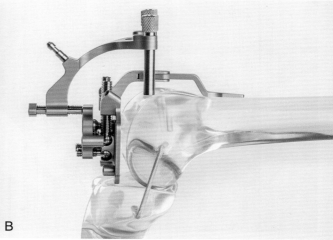

FIG 159.9 (A) Exactech GPS "five-in-one" cut block (B) performs all femoral cuts after a single navigation step adjusting all resections and ligament balance.

extremity, creating the bone resections, and then remeasuring the extremity were minimal at the submillimeter range. This study did not factor the potential of error created by poor registration nor was the possibility of poor tracker fixation with inadvertent movement considered. The surgeon must make every effort to control these unknown variables in the in vivo setting.

I performed an extensive study using multiple cadaver extremities to assess the precision of ligament-balancing measurements.[82] That study considered eight cadaver limbs and compared the ligament gaps created after the proximal tibial resection had been made using a computer navigated resection. Uniquely, variables considered included multiple surgeon reregistration, ligament gaps of the medial and lateral compartments, and the assessment of the gaps from full extension to 120 degrees of flexion at 5-degree intervals. The maximum error considered was submillimeter, with a distance of 0.75 millimeters for any measurement for 0 to 90 degrees. Repeated measures revealed that the gaps tended to permanently strain with time. Bellemans et al. made a similar finding in the clinical setting, in which permanent relaxation of ligaments could be observed after 30 minutes.[4] My study demonstrated that precision assessment of ligaments through the range of motion was possible and that the measurement of ligament gaps through the full range may be a more representative assessment for a specific knee, than just looking at gaps created at 0 and 90 degrees of flexion. As noted, recent authors have documented the mismatch of the gaps that may be occurring in midflexion even with appropriate technique. By understanding these gaps during the ligament release phase, one may refine the overall result for technical precision.

A clinical evaluation of the eGPS was performed to assess time efficiency from the early learning period to typical usage after the surgeon was considered experienced.[65] An orthopedic surgeon studied three cohorts of patients over a longitudinal period of time in which the control group consisted of 21 consecutive total knees using conventional methods, 21 total knees within the initial learning experience, and 21 total knees after the surgeon had performed at least 30 navigated total knee.

The finding, though not statistically significant, was that the mean time during the learning curve had increased by 7 minutes, whereas the time after experience had decreased by 2 minutes over the control. The result optimistically supported the conclusion that contemporary computer navigation protocols do not necessarily add, and may in some cases diminish, the time commitment. I performed a similar study several years ago with the Praxim computer navigation system that was compared with the older Medtronic Stealth station and was able to demonstrate a significant difference of 10 minutes on average in reduction operating procedure time. The Praxim software had a similar attempt to customize the surgical flow and steps for the surgeon, and that became a software design objective for the eGPS original creation in 2009.[84]

FUTURE EVOLUTION OF DIGITAL IMAGING AND COMPUTER NAVIGATION

Just 5 years ago, my review for this text included the preliminary evaluation of the eGPS system that was considered the "future" in those days. That system has now fairly extensive clinical experience and has lived up to the design expectations. So the question is, What new technology advances loom on the horizon? I believe the most important will be the possibility of combining new digital imaging options into the registration process, allowing for greater precision and efficiency.[27] We know for example that one of the significant benefits of the patient-specific implant cutting blocks is the ability to improve the precision of femoral rotation over imageless registration or conventional methods, which rely on simple direct point picking. This is accomplished by the use of CT scans that improve the "visualization."[92]

In spinal surgery, the ability to use 3D CT imaging and navigation with such systems as the Medtronic O-arm have substantially improved the precision of pedicle screw orientation over two-dimensional (2D) fluoroscopy or 3D fluoroscopy.[67] Adequate CT can be performed in the operating room during the operative procedure with existing technologies. The CT scans can be dumped into DICOM files that can be transferred to a procedure and before the cuts are completed. The surgeon will able to assess the potential shape of an implant to match basic normal anatomy of the patient. We know from current literature that midflexion laxity possibly may result from variations in optimal prosthetic shape and joint line alteration, as well as limitations with appropriate ligament balancing.[28,31] These concerns may be addressed with future technologies.

KEY REFERENCES

15. Davis ET, Pagkalos J, Gallie PA, et al: Defining the errors in the registration process during imageless computer navigation in total knee arthroplasty: a cadaveric study. *J Arthroplasty* 29(4):698–701, 2014.

17. De Steiger RN, Liu Y-L, Graves SE: Computer navigation for total knee arthroplasty reduces revision rate for patients less than sixty-five years of age. *J Bone Joint Surg Am* 97:635–642, 2015.

26. Heyse TJ, Chong LR, Davis J, et al: MRI analysis for rotation of total knee components. *Knee* 19:571–575, 2012.

28. Hino K, Ishimaru M, Iseki Y, et al: Mid-flexion laxity is greater after posterior-stabilised total knee replacement than with cruciate-retaining procedures: a computer navigation study. *Bone Joint J* 95-B(4):493–497, 2013.

47. Kuriyama S, Hyakuna K, Inoue S, et al: Tibial rotational alignment was significantly improved by use of a CT-navigated control device in total knee arthroplasty. *J Arthroplasty* 29(12):2352–2356, 2014.

59. Mullaji A, Lingaraju AP, Shetty GM: Computer-assisted total knee replacement in patients with arthritis and a recurvatum deformity. *J Bone Joint Surg Br* 94(5):642–647, 2012.

61. Nam D, Weeks KD, Reinhardt KR, et al: Accelerometer-based, portable navigation vs imageless, large-console computer-assisted navigation in total knee arthroplasty: a comparison of radiographic results. *J Arthroplasty* 28(2):255–261, 2013.

71. Roper GE, Bloemke AD, Roberts CC, et al: Analysis of tibial component rotation following total knee arthroplasty using 3D high definition computed tomography. *J Arthroplasty* 28(8 Suppl):106–111, 2013.

75. Siston RA, Cromie MJ, Gold GE, et al: Averaging different alignment axes improves femoral rotational alignment in computer-navigated total knee arthroplasty. *J Bone Joint Surg Am* 90:2098–2104, 2008.

82. Stiehl JB, Heck DA: How precise is computer assisted gap assessment in navigated total knee replacement. *Clin Orthop* 473:115–118, 2015.

98. Zhang GQ, Chen JY, Chai W, et al: Comparison between computer-assisted-navigation and conventional total knee arthroplasties in patients undergoing simultaneous bilateral procedures: a randomized clinical trial. *J Bone Joint Surg Am* 93(13):1190–1196, 2011.

The references for this chapter can also be found on www.expertconsult.com.

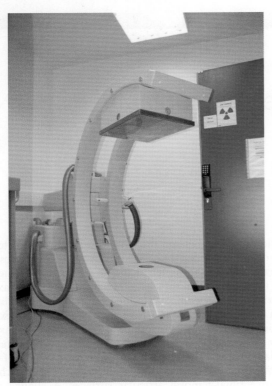

FIG 159.10 Intraoperative 3D CT that uses a flat panel detector for image acquisition and fully integrated computer navigation system for "image-based" navigation (University of Grenoble Robotics Laboratory, Grenoble, France).

computer navigation system, or the scans can be directed into an integrated navigation system (Prototype, University of Grenoble Robotics Laboratory, Grenoble, France) (Fig. 159.10). Ultimately the surgeon will have control of all variables of the surgical procedure, including the appropriate placement of implants for optimal axial plane rotation and the final ligament balancing of the flexion space. For surgeons who prefer the use of flexion space tensors to guide the femoral anteroposterior cuts, this may be planned and assessed during the operative

160

Kinematically Aligned Total Knee Arthroplasty

Stephen M. Howell, Maury L. Hull, Mohamed R. Mahfouz

OVERVIEW

Kinematically aligned total knee arthroplasty (TKA) has gained interest because two randomized trials and a national multi-center study showed that patients treated with kinematic alignment reported significantly better pain relief, function, flexion, and a more normal feeling knee than mechanical alignment with a similar implant survivorship at 2, 3, and 6 years.[4,8,17,18,26] This chapter introduces the three goals of kinematically aligned TKA: (1) restore the native tibial-femoral articular surfaces, (2) restore the native knee and limb alignments, and (3) restore the native laxities of the knee. Because kinematically aligned TKA is relatively new and is not as well understood as mechanically aligned TKA, the technique and quality assurance steps for kinematically aligning the femoral and tibial components to the native tibial-femoral articular surface are detailed. Examples of patients with severe varus and valgus deformity and flexion contractures treated with kinematically aligned TKA are shown. Surgical considerations for performing kinematically aligned TKA in the knee with an incompetent posterior cruciate ligament and fixed valgus deformity are discussed. Finally, studies describing the similarities and differences of the function, limb, knee, and tibial component alignment, and survivorship between the kinematically and mechanically aligned TKA are presented.

GOAL ONE: RESTORE THE NATIVE TIBIAL-FEMORAL ARTICULAR SURFACES

One goal of kinematically aligned TKA is to set the anterior-posterior, proximal-distal, and medial-lateral translation and flexion-extension, varus-valgus, internal-external rotation (6 degrees-of-freedom) of the femoral and tibial components to restore the native tibial-femoral articular surface of the knee. Setting the femoral and tibial components on the native tibial-femoral articular surface coaligns the axes of the components as close as possible with the three kinematic axes of the normal knee[8,10,19] (Fig. 160.1). One kinematic axis is the flexion axis of the tibia. This axis penetrates the two centers of the circular portion of the posterior femoral condyles from about 20 to 120 degrees, like an axle passing through two wheels, and determines the native arc of flexion and extension of the tibia on the femur.[10,14,22,30,35] The second kinematic axis is the flexion axis of the patella. This axis lies parallel to the flexion axis of the tibia, averages 10 mm anterior and 12 mm proximal to the flexion axis of the tibia, and determines the native arc of flexion and

extension of the patella on the femur.[6,21] The flexion-extension plane of the extended knee lies perpendicular to these two kinematic axes in the center of the knee. The third kinematic axis is the longitudinal rotational axis of the tibia. This axis lies approximately perpendicular to the flexion axes of the tibia and patella and determines the native arc of internal and external rotation of the tibia on the femur.[6,14] These kinematic axes are closely parallel or perpendicular to the native tibial-femoral articular surface.* Therefore, a change in the position of either component in one or more of the 6 degrees of freedom changes the native tibial-femoral articular surfaces. A change in the native articular surface malaligns the rotational axes of the components with the three kinematic axes of the knee, which changes the native resting length of the collateral, retinacular, and posterior cruciate ligaments. Changing the native resting length of these ligaments causes unnatural tightening and/or slackening of the ligaments and unnatural tibial-femoral and patella-femoral motions that patients may perceive as pain, binding, stiffness, or instability.[10,13,14,31]

GOAL TWO: RESTORE THE NATIVE KNEE AND LIMB ALIGNMENTS

The second goal of kinematically aligned TKA is to restore the native knee and limb alignments.[13,18-20] Several studies support correction to the native or "constitutional" alignment when performing TKA as opposed to restoring mechanical alignment to neutral (Fig. 160.2).[13,23,33,34] Restoring mechanical alignment to native in patients with constitutional varus and valgus alignment is unnatural, and causes greater strain deviations in the medial and lateral collateral ligaments from the native knee.[1,7,13,23] Patients with preoperative varus have better clinical and functional outcome scores and the same implant survivorship at 7 years when the alignment is left in mild varus, as compared with patients overcorrected to neutral.[33] At a mean of 6 years after kinematically aligned TKA, restoration of the native alignments of the knee, limb, and tibia did not adversely affect implant survival and resulted in high function, which supports the consideration of kinematic alignment as an alternative to mechanical alignment when performing primary TKA.[18]

Current evidence suggests that the native alignment of the limb does not cause osteoarthritis of the knee. The clinical findings of bilateral osteoarthritis with a varus deformity in one

---

*References 6, 10, 11, 14, 16, and 21.

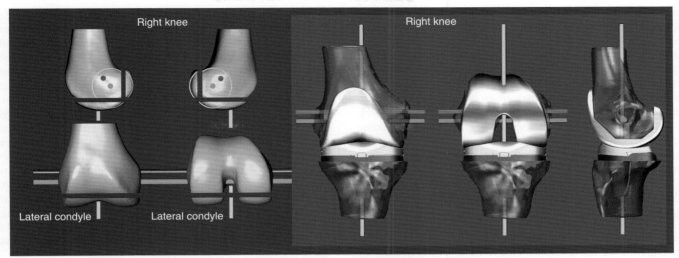

FIG 160.1 A right femur *(left)* and kinematically aligned TKA *(right)* shows the relationships between the three kinematic axes of the knee and the joint lines of the distal and posterior femoral resections and the 6 degrees-of-freedom position of the components. The flexion axis of the tibia is the *green line*, the flexion axis of the patella is the *magenta line*, and the longitudinal rotational axis of the tibia is the *yellow line*. All three axes are closely parallel or perpendicular to the joint lines. The flexion-extension plane of the extended knee is perpendicular to the flexion axes of the tibia and patella and is centered in the knee. Compensating for wear and kerf and resecting bone from the distal and posterior femur condyles by an amount equal in thickness to the condyles of the femoral component kinematically aligns the femoral component by coaligning the axis of the femoral component with the flexion axis of the tibia, assuming that the condyles of the femoral component are symmetric in the flexion-extension plane of the tibia. (From Howell SM, Papadopoulos S, Kuznik KT, Hull ML: Accurate alignment and high function after kinematically aligned TKA performed with generic instruments. *Knee Surg Sports Traumatol Arthrosc* 21(10):2271–2280, 2013.)

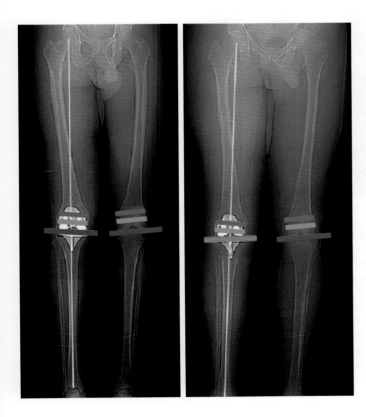

FIG 160.2 This composite shows that (1) the kinematically aligned TKA *(left patient)* restores the native tibial-femoral joint surface *(blue line)* and the native limb alignment *(white line)*. The axes of the femoral component are coaligned with the flexion axes of the tibia *(green line)* and patella *(magenta line)*. (2) The mechanically aligned TKA *(right patient)* changes the native tibial-femoral joint surface *(red line)*, the native limb alignment, and malaligns the axes of the femoral component oblique to the flexion axes of the tibia and patella. Studies have shown that kinematic alignment creates fewer varus limb and varus knee outliers and has the same average limb and knee alignment as mechanical alignment. (From Dossett HG, Estrada NA, Swartz GJ, et al: A randomised controlled trial of kinematically and mechanically aligned total knee replacements: two-year clinical results. *Bone Joint J* 96-B(7):907–913, 2014; Dossett HG, Swartz GJ, Estrada NA, et al: Kinematically versus mechanically aligned total knee arthroplasty. *Orthopedics* 35(2):e160–e169, 2012; Nunley RM, Ellison BS, Zhu J, et al: Do patient-specific guides improve coronal alignment in total knee arthroplasty? *Clin Orthop* 470(3):895–902, 2012.)

knee and a valgus deformity in the other ("wind-swept"), and the lack of osteoarthritis in most older adult Asian patients with severe constitutional varus, suggest that native alignment plays little role in the development of osteoarthritis. Instead, the onset of osteoarthritis is associated with known changes in cartilage metabolism that occur with aging. Articular cartilage is a mechanosensitive tissue that, when healthy, increases anabolic activity and thickens when loaded. Chondrocytes experience age-related declines in their anabolic activity and thickening response and cause osteoarthritis because the ability to respond to and compensate for high loads from activity and obesity is gradually lost.[2]

GOAL THREE: RESTORE THE NATIVE LAXITIES OF THE KNEE

The third goal of kinematically aligned TKA is to restore the native laxities of the knee, which are tighter at 0 degrees of flexion than at 45 and 90 degrees of flexion (Fig. 160.3).[31,32] At 0 degrees of flexion, the native tibia-femoral joint behaves as a rigid body because the average varus (0.7 degrees), valgus (0.5 degrees), internal (4.6 degrees), and external (4.4 degrees) rotations of the tibia on the femur are negligible under applied loads that just engage the soft tissue restraints.[12,31,32] At 45 degrees and 90 degrees of flexion, the mean laxity is fivefold greater in varus (3.1 degrees) rotation; fourfold greater in distraction; threefold greater in valgus (1.4 degrees), internal (14.6 degrees), and external (14.7 degrees) rotation; and twofold greater in anterior translation than at 0 degrees of flexion.[31,32] The maintenance of these native differences in laxities between positions of knee flexion requires the maintenance of the native resting lengths of the collateral ligaments, posterior cruciate ligament, and retinacular ligaments. The alignment goal of gap balancing a TKA overtightens the laxities of the flexion gaps at 45 and 90 degrees of flexion to match those at 0 degrees of flexion, which patients may perceive as pain, stiffness, and/or limited flexion.[10,31]

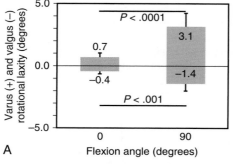
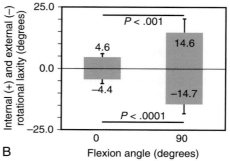
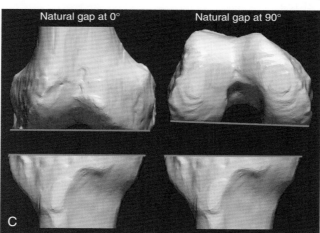

FIG 160.3 This composite shows column graphs of the native varus (+), valgus (−), internal (+), and external (−) rotational laxities of the normal knee at 0 and 90 degrees of flexion (A and B), and the native gaps of a right knee at 0 and 90 degrees of flexion after making the resections using kinematic alignment (C). The paired columns connected by a *P*-value of less than 0.05 indicate that the laxity at 90 degrees is greater than at 0 degrees of flexion. The resected right knee shows a symmetrically shaped gap that is equal medially and laterally at 0 degrees of flexion, and an asymmetrically shaped gap that is smaller medially than laterally at 90 degrees of flexion. Therefore, the surgical goal of gap balancing a TKA overtightens the flexion gap. Error bars show ±1 standard deviation. (From Roth JD, Howell SM, Hull ML: Native knee laxities at 0 degrees, 45 degrees, and 90 degrees of flexion and their relationship to the goal of the gap-balancing alignment method of total knee arthroplasty. *J Bone Joint Surg Am* 97(20):1678–1684, 2015; Roth JD, Hull ML, Howell SM: Rotational and translational limits of passive motion are both variable between and unrelated within normal tibiofemoral joints. *J Orthop Res* 33(11):1594–1602, 2015.)

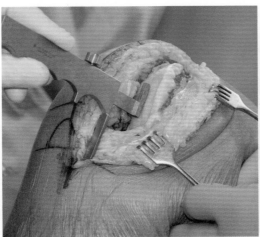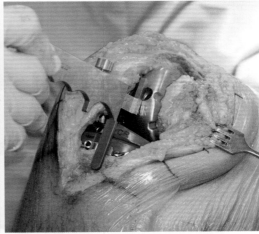

FIG 160.4 Intraoperative photographs of a right knee with a varus deformity in 90 degrees of flexion shows the measurement of the native anterior offset of the tibia from the worn distal medial articular surface of the femur in a knee at the time of exposure *(left)* and at the time of reduction with the trial components *(right).* The laxities of the knee in 90 degrees of flexion are restored by first compensating 2 mm for cartilage wear on the distal medial femur. The anterior-posterior slope and the thickness of the tibial component are adjusted until the offset of the anterior tibia from the distal medial femoral condyle with the trial components matches that of the knee at the time of exposure. Finally, the internal and external rotations of the tibia are set to approximately 14 degrees.

Restoring the native knee laxities at 0 degrees of flexion requires removal of all osteophytes, extending the knee to 0 degrees, and adjusting the varus-valgus angle and thickness of the tibial component until the varus, valgus, internal, and external rotational laxities are negligible.[19] To restore the native laxities of the knee at 90 degrees of flexion, begin by flexing the knee to 90 degrees. Adjust the anterior-posterior slope and thickness of the tibial component until the offset of the anterior tibia from the distal medial femoral condyle, measured at the time of exposure, matches the knee with the trial components, and the internal and external rotation of the tibia approximate 14 degrees (Fig. 160.4).[19] The kinematically aligned TKA can restore native knee and limb alignments and resolve knee laxity issues. A randomized clinical trial and a national multicenter study showed patients with a kinematically aligned TKA reported better pain relief, better function, better flexion, and a more normal feeling knee than patients with a mechanically aligned TKA.[8,26]

TECHNIQUE AND QUALITY ASSURANCE STEPS FOR MINIMIZING FLEXION AND KINEMATICALLY ALIGNING THE FEMORAL COMPONENT TO THE NATIVE ARTICULAR SURFACE

Kinematic alignment sets the femoral component at the native angle and the level of the distal (0 degrees) and posterior (90 degrees) joint line. The surgical technique begins by using an offset caliper to measure the anterior-posterior offset of the anterior tibia from the distal medial femur with the knee in 90 degrees of flexion (see Fig. 160.4). Two millimeters are subtracted from the offset measurement cartilage that is missing on the distal medial femoral condyle. Once the knee is fully exposed, the locations of cartilage wear are assessed on the distal

femur. A ring curette is used to remove any partially worn cartilage to bone. The flexion-extension position of the femoral component is set by the insertion of a positioning rod 8 to 10 cm through a drill hole placed parallel to the anterior surface of the distal femur and perpendicular to the distal articular surface (Fig. 160.5). The varus-valgus rotation and proximal-distal translation of the femoral component are set by using a disposable distal referencing guide that compensates 2 mm when there is cartilage wear on the distal medial femoral condyle in the varus knee, and 2 mm when there is cartilage wear on the distal lateral femoral condyle in the valgus knee. The anterior-posterior translation and internal-external rotation of the femoral component are set by placing a 0-degree rotation posterior referencing guide in contact with the posterior femoral condyles (Fig. 160.6). The positioning of the posterior referencing guide rarely requires correction because complete cartilage loss is uncommon on the posterior medial and posterior lateral femoral condyles in most varus and valgus osteoarthritic knees. Correction for bone wear is rarely needed at 0 and 90 degrees of flexion, even in the most arthritic knees.[19,25]

The first intraoperative quality assurance step checks that flexion of the femoral component is minimized by positioning the starting hole for the positioning rod midway between the top of the intercondylar notch and aligning the positioning rod parallel to the anterior cortex of the femur (see Fig. 160.5). The second intraoperative quality assurance step checks that the femoral component is kinematically aligned to the native femoral articular surface. A caliper measurement of the thickness of the distal and posterior femoral resections that adjust the thicknesses within ±0.5 mm of the thickness of the condyles of the femoral component is performed after compensating for cartilage wear and kerf (see Fig. 160.6). Alignment references used to position the femoral component in mechanically aligned TKA, such as the femoral mechanical axis, intramedullary canal,

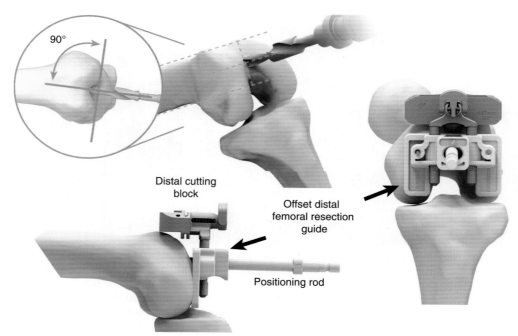

FIG 160.5 This composite shows the method of setting the flexion-extension and varus-valgus rotations and the proximal-distal translation of the kinematically aligned femoral component with disposable instruments *(blue)*. The insertion of a positioning rod 8 to 10 cm through a hole drilled midway between the top of the intercondylar notch and the anterior cortex, parallel to the anterior surface, and perpendicular to the distal articular surface of the distal femur sets the flexion-extension rotation of the femoral component. The distal cutting block is inserted into the offset distal femoral resection guide. This assembly compensates for 2 mm of cartilage wear on the worn condyle(s) and is placed over the positioning rod, in contact with the distal femur, and sets varus-valgus rotation and proximal-distal translation of the femoral component.

transepicondylar axis, and anterior-posterior axis, are not of interest or of use when performing kinematically aligned TKA.[10,11,13,18,19]

TECHNIQUE AND QUALITY ASSURANCE STEPS FOR ALIGNING THE TIBIAL COMPONENT TO THE NATIVE ARTICULAR SURFACE

Kinematically aligned TKA sets the tibial component at the native internal-external, varus-valgus, flexion-extension, and proximal-distal positions of the articular surface of the tibia. The internal-external rotation can be set to the major axis of the lateral tibial condyle or by using a kinematic tibial baseplate method.[19,27,28] The varus-valgus, flexion-extension, and proximal-distal positions are set using an extramedullary tibial guide (Figs. 160.7 to 160.9).[19] The preferred method for setting the internal-external rotation of the tibial component is chosen. When the major axis of the lateral tibial condyle method is used, the elliptically shaped boundary of the articular surface of the lateral tibial condyle is identified and the major axis is drawn (see Fig. 160.7).[19,27,28] A guide is used to drill two holes into the medial articular surface, parallel to the major axis drawn on the lateral tibial condyle. After the tibial resection is made, the anterior-posterior axis of the tibial component is aligned parallel to these two holes using a rationale similar to the Cobb method, which finds the flexion-extension plane of the knee by

fitting circles to the medial and lateral tibial condyles.[5] In mechanically aligned TKA, the medial border and medial one-third of the tibial tubercle are considered useful landmarks. In contrast, a study of a case series of kinematically aligned TKAs showed that aligning the tibial component to the medial border or medial one-third of the tibial tubercle would have malrotated the tibial component 5 degrees or more from the flexion-extension plane of the knee in 70% and 86% of the knees, respectively.[3,15,19] The use of the major axis of the lateral tibial condyle is a reproducible method, as shown by negligible bias (−1 degree internal) and acceptable precision (±5.4 degrees) between the anterior-posterior axis of the tibial component and the flexion-extension plane of the knee, and minimal malrotation of the tibial component on the femoral component.[27,28] Next, a conventional extramedullary tibial resection guide is applied to the ankle and an angel wing is placed in the saw slot of the guide (see Fig. 160.8). The varus-valgus position of the tibial component is set by medially translating the slider at the ankle of the guide until the saw slot is parallel to the tibial articular surface after visual compensation for cartilage and bone wear. The flexion-extension or slope of the tibial component is set by adjusting the inclination of an angel wing placed in the saw slot until it is parallel to the slope of the medial joint line. The proximal-distal translation of the tibial component is set by adjusting the level of the saw slot until the 10-mm tibial resection gauge contacts the center of the unworn tibial condyle.[19] A conservative tibial resection is made while

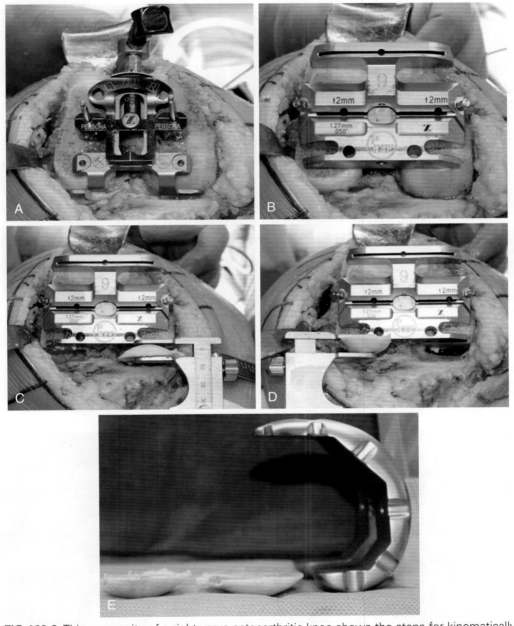

FIG 160.6 This composite of a right varus osteoarthritic knee shows the steps for kinematically aligning the femoral component at 90 degrees of flexion. A 0-degree rotation posterior referencing guide is inserted in contact with the posterior femoral condyles and pinned (A). The correct size chamfer guide is inserted into the pinhole (B). A caliper measures the thickness of the posterior medial femoral condyle (C) and posterior lateral femoral condyle (D). These steps set internal-external rotation and anterior-posterior translation of the femoral component to the native articular surface of the posterior femur (E).

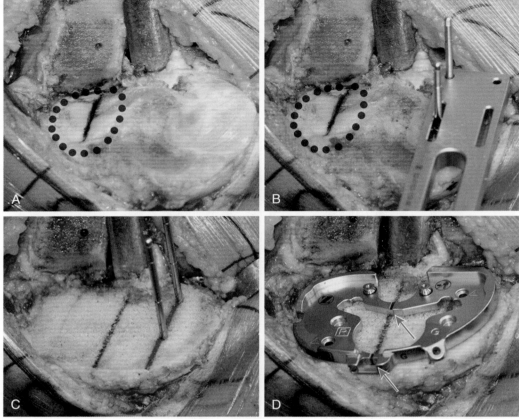

FIG 160.7 This composite of a right knee shows the major axis of the lateral tibial condyle method for kinematically aligning the internal-external rotation of the trial tibial component to the anterior-posterior axis *(blue line)* of the almost elliptically shaped boundary of the articular surface of the lateral tibial condyle *(black dots)* (A). A guide is used to drill two pins through the medial tibial articular surface and parallel to the major axis (B). The tibial articular surface is resected and removed, the two drill holes are identified (pins), and lines parallel to the drill holes are drawn (C). The score marks *(green arrows)* indicate that the anterior-posterior axis of the trial tibial baseplate is aligned parallel to these lines (D).

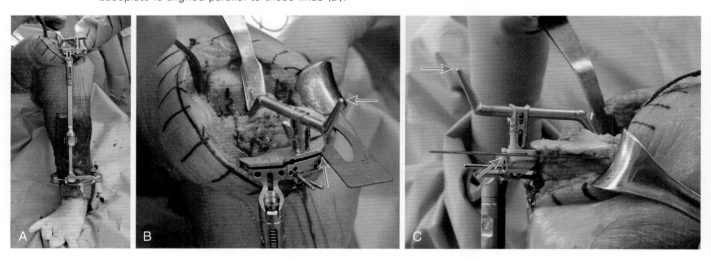

FIG 160.8 This composite of a right knee shows the steps for kinematically aligning the tibial component. A conventional extramedullary tibial resection guide with a 10-mm offset tibial resection gauge *(magenta arrow)* and angel wing *(green arrow)* is applied to the ankle (A, B, and C). The varus-valgus position of the tibial resection is set by adjusting the medial-lateral position of the slider at the ankle end of the guide until the saw slot is parallel to the tibial articular surface after visually compensating for cartilage and bone wear. The proximal-distal translation of the tibial component is set by adjusting the level of the saw slot until there is contact between the 10-mm offset tibial resection gauge and the center of the unworn tibial condyle (B). The flexion-extension rotation of the tibial component is set by adjusting the inclination of the angel wing parallel to the slope of the medial joint line (C). These steps set the proximal-distal translation and the varus-valgus and flexion-extension rotations of the tibial component parallel to the native articular surface of the tibia.

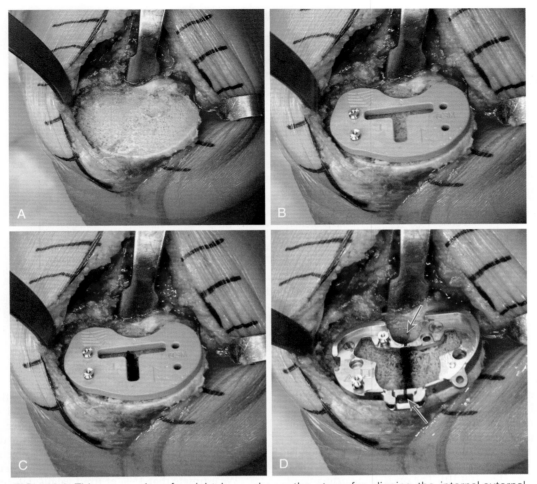

FIG 160.9 This composite of a right knee shows the steps for aligning the internal-external rotation of the trial tibial component parallel to the flexion-extension plane of the knee with a kinematic tibial baseplate *(gray)*. The cortical contour of the anatomic resection of the tibia is shown (A). The largest size kinematic tibial baseplate that fits within the contour is selected from the seven kinematic tibial baseplates and is fit within the cortical contour (B). The anterior-posterior axis of the kinematic tibial baseplate is marked *(blue line)* (C). The score marks *(green arrows)* indicate that the anterior-posterior axis of the trial tibial baseplate is aligned parallel to the *blue line* (D).

protecting the insertion of the posterior cruciate ligament. When the kinematic tibial baseplate is used to set internal-external rotation of the tibial component, the largest of the seven available sizes that fits within the cortical contour of the tibial resection is selected and best fit to the anterior and medial cortical edge (see Fig. 160.9). The in vitro reproducibility of the kinematic tibial baseplate was evaluated on 166 tibial resections by five arthroplasty surgeons, three orthopedic surgery fellows/residents, and three students, and showed a negligible bias (0.7 degrees external) and acceptable precision (±4.6 degrees) between the anterior-posterior axis of the kinematic tibial baseplate and the flexion-extension plane of the knee. The in vivo reproducibility was evaluated in 63 kinematically aligned TKAs by one arthroplasty surgeon and showed a negligible bias (0.2 degrees external) and an acceptable precision (±3.6 degrees) between the anterior-posterior axes of the tibial and the femoral components (unpublished study).

The third intraoperative quality assurance step checks that the internal-external rotation of the tibial component is parallel to the flexion-extension plane of the knee by using the major axis of the lateral tibial condyle or the kinematic tibial baseplate method.

The fourth intraoperative quality assurance step checks that the varus-valgus rotation of the tibial component restores the native tibial joint line by adjusting the varus-valgus of the tibial resection to minimize varus-valgus laxity and to restore the native knee and limb alignments with the knee at 0 degrees of flexion.[19,27,28,31]

The fifth and final quality assurance step checks that the flexion-extension or slope of the tibial component restores the native tibial joint line. The flexion-extension of the tibial resection is adjusted to restore the anterior offset of the anterior tibia from the distal medial femoral condyle. This adjustment is accomplished with trial components that are comparable to that of the knee at the time of exposure and that restore approximately 14 degrees of internal-external rotation of the tibia on the femur with the knee in 90 degrees of flexion (see Fig. 160.4).[19,28,31] Alignment references used to position the

Step-wise algorithm for balancing
KA TKA

Tight in flexion and extension	Tight in flexion and well-balanced in extension	Tight in extension and well-balanced in flexion	Well-balanced in extension and loose in flexion	Tight medial and loose lateral in extension	Tight lateral and loose medial in extension
Use thinner liner Recut tibia and remove more bone	Increase posterior slope until natural A-P offset is restored at 90° of flexion	Remove posterior osteophytes Reassess Strip posterior capsule	Add thicker liner and recheck knee extends fully When knee does not fully extend check PCL tension When PCL is incompetent consider PS implants or UC liner	Remove medial osteophytes Reassess Recut tibia in 2° more varus Insert 2 mm thicker liner	Remove lateral osteophytes Reassess Recut tibia in 2° more valgus Insert 2 mm thicker liner

FIG 160.10 The table shows a stepwise algorithm for balancing the kinematically aligned TKA. The top row lists six malalignments, and the bottom lists the corresponding corrective actions. Notice that the corrections that require a recut of bone are performed by fine-tuning the proximal-distal translation and the varus-valgus and flexion-extension (slope) rotations of the tibial resection and not by recutting the femur. *A-P,* Anterior-posterior; *KA,* kinematic alignment; *PCL,* posterior cruciate ligament; *PS,* posterior stabilized; *TKA,* total knee arthroplasty; *UC,* ultra congruent.

tibial component in mechanically aligned TKA, such as the tibial mechanical axis, intramedullary canal, posterior condylar axis, and tibial tubercle, are not of interest or of use when performing kinematically aligned TKA.[†]

When any of these conditions is not met, a stepwise alignment algorithm determines the corrective actions to achieve kinematic alignment (Fig. 160.10). The underlying principle of this algorithm is that the corrections requiring a recut of bone are performed by fine-tuning the varus-valgus, flexion-extension or slope, and proximal-distal positions of the tibial resection, and not by recutting the femur.

MANAGING THE KNEE WITH AN INSUFFICIENT POSTERIOR LIGAMENT OR SEVERE FIXED VALGUS DEFORMITY

There are special considerations when performing kinematically aligned TKA in the patient with an insufficient posterior cruciate ligament (Fig. 160.11) and severe fixed valgus deformity (Fig. 160.12). There are three potential corrective actions when there is a chronic posterior cruciate ligament tear or an insufficiency is discovered after resecting the femur (see Fig. 160.11). One corrective action is to use a narrow version of a 2-mm larger posterior stabilized femoral component when the implant design permits this adjustment. The larger posterior stabilized femoral component is cemented contacting the anterior resection of the femur and the 2-mm gaps between the posterior resections and femoral component are filled with cement. This maintains the level of the distal joint line and compensates for the 2- to 3-mm increase in the flexion gap caused by the insufficiency of the posterior cruciate ligament. The second action is

to use an ultracongruent tibial liner when the flexion gap is not excessive. The third is to resect an additional 2 mm from the distal femur and use a 2-mm thicker liner. This approach requires the surgeon to accept that raising the distal and posterior femoral joint line 2 mm violates the kinematic alignment goal of restoring the native tibial-femoral articular surfaces.

We estimate that 15% of fixed valgus deformities remain in 2 to 3 degrees of excessive valgus deformity after adjusting the varus-valgus angle and thickness of the tibial component until the varus-valgus laxity is negligible with the knee to 0 degrees of flexion (see Fig. 160.12). In this small subset of valgus knees, we perform a careful lengthening of the lateral collateral ligament 2 to 3 mm via the pie-crusting technique with a spinal needle, with distraction applied with a laminar spreader to the lateral compartment with the knee in 90 degrees of flexion (Fig. 160.13). After completing the lengthening, a recut guide is used to cut the tibia in 2 to 3 degrees more varus, and a 2-mm thicker liner is inserted. For a tibia of normal length, each degree of varus or valgus correction at the knee joint causes a 6- to 7-mm medial or lateral translation of the ankle. Therefore, a 3-degree varus correction at the knee causes an 18- to 21-mm medial translation at the ankle, which corrects the valgus deformity of the limb and knee. On the rare occasion that these corrective actions do not reduce a chronic lateral patella subluxation or dislocation, a lateral release is performed.

ALIGNMENT AND 3- AND 6-YEAR SURVIVORSHIP OF KINEMATICALLY ALIGNED TOTAL KNEE ARTHROPLASTY

Kinematically aligned TKA can restore the native alignment of the limb, knee, and joint line, provide an acceptable angle in patients with severe varus and valgus deformities with flexion contracture, and rarely requires release of the collateral,

[†]References 3, 13, 15, 19, 27, and 28.

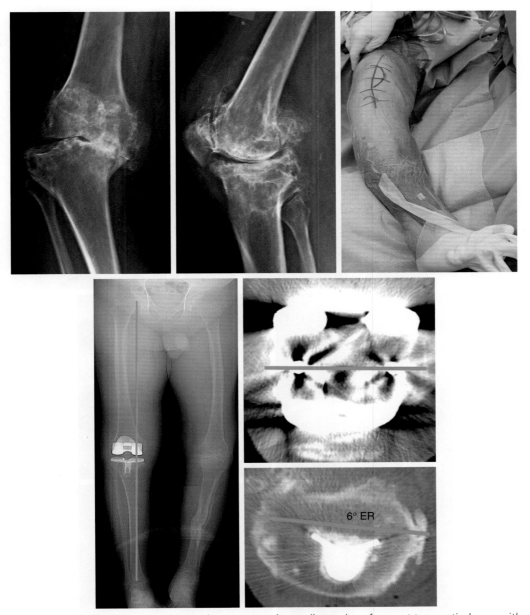

FIG 160.11 This composite shows the preoperative radiographs of a post-traumatic knee with a severe varus deformity, flexion contracture, and chronic posterior cruciate ligament insufficiency; an intraoperative photograph of the varus deformity; and a postoperative computer tomographic scanogram of the limb and axial views of the femoral and tibial components. The kinematically aligned TKA restored the native alignment and laxities of the knee without a release of the medial collateral ligament. This TKA was performed with posterior cruciate ligament–substituting implants because of the torn posterior cruciate ligament. The tibial component is 6° externally rotated on the femoral component, which is acceptable *(green lines)*.

retinacular, or posterior cruciate ligaments (see Figs. 160.11 and 160.12). A multicenter comparison of three case series showed that mechanically aligned TKAs performed with patient-specific and conventional instrumentation had more varus limb and knee outliers than kinematically aligned TKAs performed with patient-specific instrumentation.[29] A Level 1 randomized trial showed that the hip-knee-ankle angle (0.3 degrees difference; P = .693) and anatomic angle of the knee (0.8 degrees difference; P = .131) were similar for kinematically and mechanically

aligned groups. In the kinematically aligned group, the angle of the femoral component was natively aligned 2.4 degrees more valgus ($P < .0001$) and the angle of the tibial component was natively aligned 2.3 degrees more varus ($P < .0001$) than the mechanically aligned group.[9]

Several studies suggest that the 2-degree average varus alignment (range 7 degrees varus to 7 degrees valgus) of the kinematically aligned tibial component relative to the mechanical axis of the tibia in the coronal plane should not have an adverse

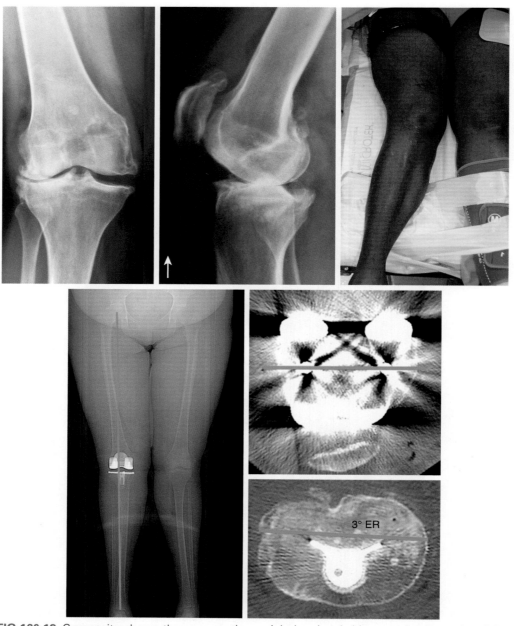

FIG 160.12 Composite shows the preoperative weight-bearing *(white arrow)* radiographs of the knee with severe valgus deformity, intraoperative photograph of the severe valgus deformity and flexion contracture, and postoperative computer tomographic scanogram of the limb and axial views of the femoral and tibial components. The kinematically aligned TKA restored the native alignment of the limb *(vertical green line)*, set the rotation of the tibial component 3° externally rotated on the femur *(transverse green lines)*, and restored the laxities of the native knee without a release of the lateral collateral ligament in this patient with an intact posterior cruciate ligament.

effect on implant survivorship. A study of mechanically aligned TKAs reported that a 3-degree varus average alignment (range >7 degrees varus to 5 degrees valgus) was associated with a high implant survivorship of 96% at 10 years.[24] Two case series, each consisting of more than 200 kinematically aligned TKAs, reported a low incidence of catastrophic failure regardless of the alignment category at 3- and 6-year follow-up and high restoration of function as measured by the self-reported Oxford Knee Score. At 3 and 6 years, 75% and 80% of tibial components,

33% and 31% of knees, and 6% and 7% of limbs were categorized as varus outliers. These outliers were associated with a low 0% and 0.5% incidence of catastrophic failure of the femoral or tibial component and a high average Oxford Knee Score (48 best) of 42 and 43 points.[13,17] Another study opined that the reason for the good implant survivorship of kinematically aligned TKA is that 89% of kinematically aligned tibial components are aligned parallel within 0 ± 3 degrees relative to the floor in a weight-bearing film, which is more akin to how the

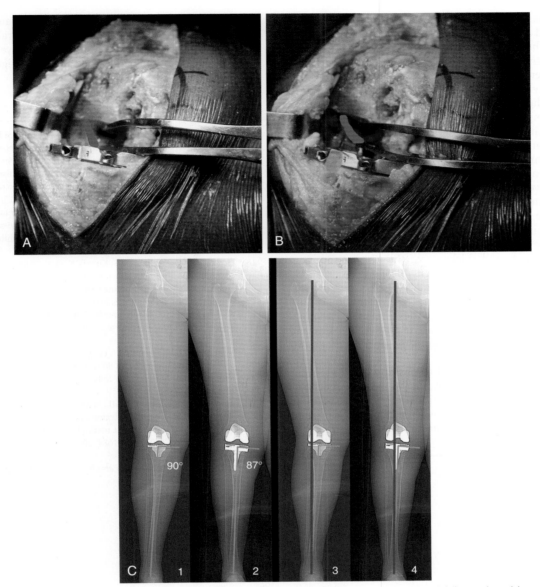

FIG 160.13 Composite shows the laminar spreader and the length of the gap *(oblique short blue lines)* in the lateral side of a right knee before (A) and after a 3 mm incremental lengthening of the lateral collateral ligament with use of the pie-crusting technique (B), and the use of the pie-crusting technique in another patient to correct the alignment of the knee and limb left too valgus at the time of primary kinematically aligned TKA (C). The tibial component in the primary surgery was originally set at 90° to the mechanical axis of the tibia (angle formed by *green lines)* *(1)*, which left the leg too valgus *(3)*. The revision followed the step-wise algorithm for correcting the valgus deformity by adjusting the varus-valgus alignment of the tibial component and leaving the original femoral component alone (Fig. 160.10). At revision, the varus-valgus alignment of the tibial component was set at 87° to the mechanical axis of the tibia by lengthening the lateral collateral ligament 3 mm *(2)*, and the insertion of a thicker liner moved the ankle 20 mm more medial, which realigned the limb to neutral *(vertical long blue lines)* *(4)*.

prosthesis is functionally loaded in mechanically aligned TKA with good survivorship.[20] Therefore, the concern that kinematic alignment places the components at a high risk for catastrophic failure and compromises function is allayed. This result should be of interest to surgeons who are committed to cutting the tibia perpendicular to the mechanical axis of the tibia.[17]

SUMMARY

Kinematically aligned TKA has gained interest because two randomized trials and a national multicenter study showed that patients treated with kinematic alignment reported significantly better pain relief, function, flexion, and a more normal feeling knee than mechanical alignment with similar implant survivorship at 2, 3, and 6 years.[4,8,17,18,26] A caliper measurement of the thicknesses of the distal and posterior femoral resections that equals the thicknesses of the condylar regions of the femoral component after compensating for cartilage wear and kerf provides quality assurance that the femoral component is kinematically aligned. Alignment references used to position the femoral component in mechanically aligned TKA, such as the femoral mechanical axis, intramedullary canal, transepicondylar axis, and anterior-posterior axis, are not of interest or of use when performing kinematically aligned TKA. Ensuring that the native alignment and laxities of the knee are closely restored to normal involves the following tasks:

1. Setting the internal-external rotation of the tibial component based on the major axis of the lateral tibial condyle or a kinematic tibial baseplate;
2. Extending the knee to 0 degrees of flexion and adjusting the varus-valgus angle and thickness of the tibial component until the varus-valgus laxity is negligible; and
3. Flexing the knee to 90 degrees and adjusting the anterior-posterior slope and thickness of the tibial component until the offset of the anterior tibia from the distal medial femoral condyle matches that of the knee at the time of exposure and the internal and external rotation of the tibia on the femur approximates 14 degrees.

Alignment references that are used to position the tibial component in mechanically aligned TKA, such as the tibial mechanical axis, intramedullary canal, posterior condylar axis, and tibial tubercle are not of interest or of use when performing kinematically aligned TKA.[‡] Aligning the femoral and tibial components

---

[‡]References 3, 13, 15, 19, 27, and 28.

kinematically, removing osteophytes, and retaining the native lengths of the medial collateral, lateral collateral, and posterior cruciate ligaments closely restore the native tibial-femoral articular surfaces, the native knee and limb alignment, and the native laxities of the knee.

KEY REFERENCES

4. Calliess T, Bauer K, Stukenborg-Colsman C, et al: PSI kinematic versus non-PSI mechanical alignment in total knee arthroplasty: a prospective, randomized study. *Knee Surg Sports Traumatol Arthrosc* 27:1–6, 2016.
8. Dossett HG, Estrada NA, Swartz GJ, et al: A randomised controlled trial of kinematically and mechanically aligned total knee replacements: two-year clinical results. *Bone Joint J* 96-B(7):907–913, 2014.
13. Gu Y, Roth JD, Howell SM, et al: How frequently do four methods for mechanically aligning a total knee arthroplasty cause collateral ligament imbalance and change alignment from normal in white patients? *J Bone Joint Surg* 96(12):e101, 2014.
18. Howell SM, Papadopoulos S, Kuznik K, et al: Does varus alignment adversely affect implant survival and function six years after kinematically aligned total knee arthroplasty? *Int Orthop* 1–8, 2015.
19. Howell SM, Papadopoulos S, Kuznik KT, et al: Accurate alignment and high function after kinematically aligned TKA performed with generic instruments. *Knee Surg Sports Traumatol Arthrosc* 21(10):2271–2280, 2013.
25. Nam D, Lin KM, Howell SM, et al: Femoral bone and cartilage wear is predictable at 0 degrees and 90 degrees in the osteoarthritic knee treated with total knee arthroplasty. *Knee Surg Sports Traumatol Arthrosc* 22(12):2975–2981, 2014.
31. Roth JD, Howell SM, Hull ML: Native knee laxities at 0 degrees, 45 degrees, and 90 degrees of flexion and their relationship to the goal of the gap-balancing alignment method of total knee arthroplasty. *J Bone Joint Surg Am* 97(20):1678–1684, 2015.

The references for this chapter can also be found on www.expertconsult.com.

161

Computer-Assisted Navigation: Minimally Invasive Surgery for Total Knee Replacement

David R. Lionberger

After 10 years of minimally invasive surgery (MIS) and computer-assisted surgery (CAS) use, there is little evidence supporting functional benefits of either technology.[12,32,40] However, there are a number of objective differences in both, which have been brought to bear in the recent years. CAS has continued to be proven indisputably more accurate than traditional instrumentation.[8,15] Although there was a brief period when patient-specific instrumentation (PSI) promised improvements in efficiency and accuracy,* there appears still great debate as to its benefits in terms of reduction of surgical time or in its improving accuracy enhancement.[13,18,19]

Recently, several important findings have been brought to bear with regard to using CAS. First are its proven benefits in several studies by reducing blood loss and/or transfusion rates.[28,34,36] Secondly, as a result of not violating the femoral cortex through large intermedullary guides, there is a reduction of fat emboli, presumably through lessening the intermedullary pressure.[27] Finally, one of the more telling long-term outcomes in favor of CAS has been the reduction and revision risks in the younger than 65-year age group.[38]

By comparison, MIS results are far less impressive in terms of advantages over traditional incisional exposures. Although there are a few reports of lessened pain or subtle subjective improvements, it is the patient's perceived benefits that continue to drive the surgical community to perform this less invasive exposure. Whether psychological or not, patient's desires for limited exposure makes CAS more appealing if it can reduce outliers and documentation of results continue to influence surgical technique and decision making on the part of the surgeon.[14,37] Thus it is unlikely we will abandon MIS, likewise making other assistive technologies, such as CAS, an attractive venue to embellish accuracy to its utmost.

Much of the hesitation in using MIS in total knee replacement (TKR) evolves from coping with the complexities of a smaller incision without visual cues. Reliance on instruments rather than direct visual reference is paramount when using a constrained exposure.[11] Secondly, sequencing to augment exposure has become important to afford better access. If one adds deformity or increased body mass to the equation, the traditional visual references are, at the very least, compromised. As such, dependence on traditional instruments, which rely on some degree of eyeballing cuts, may result in less dependable accuracy.[1,4,5,7]

Just as instruments are crucial to pilots flying through inclement weather in which clouds obscure runways, *CAS has become indispensible because it reclaims lost visual reference and accuracy in MIS*. Some surgeons avoid the use of small incisions because of lost accuracy. The addition of CAS serves to calm the concerns of this deficiency. Although doubt still exists regarding the efficiency of CAS to improve performance or even more accuracy, the extra step of enhanced accuracy with precision provides merit for extra time used.

CAS has gained a reputation of excellence in accuracy and documentation while providing the surgeon proof with archival documentation. Although this may overcome any reticence of the learning curve necessary for the adoption of this technology, it is important to assess where time losses occur in CAS (Fig. 161.1).[23] By separating the divisions of CAS time use into three basic categories, it is easier to discern causes for time expenditures. Phase 1 is insertion and way point acquisitions, phase 2 involves two segments of cutting block positioning and resection followed by the second portion of checking cuts and corrective measures to assure accuracy. Phase 3 is: testing of provisional implants and data recording (see Fig. 161.1). In a series of 50 patients investigated for time use, phase 1 was found to be significantly improved by 6 minutes by software upgrades and enhanced computational speeds.[24] Taken a step further, the first part of the second phase, in which jig positioning and cuts are made, may be abbreviated by the use of a conjoined cutting block, saving an additional 1 minute. Simply put, the surgeon uses the femoral navigation block to first navigate the femur (Fig. 161.2). An attached set distance gap block set for 22 mm is pinned before detachment and disconnect (described in detail later). This allows for navigation of the femur without the need of navigating the tibia, resulting in aligning the knee joint in the correct mechanical alignment (MA) and gap distanced from the opposing femoral resection. In essence, this would create its own "poor man's" PSI cutting jig by using the measured resection rectangular alignment of the correct MA of the lower extremity. However, there still remains the final frontier of data collection and individual surgeon's personal limits of acceptable accuracy. For instance, some surgeons will chase numbers to the last degree, whereas other surgeons are willing to accept the plus or minus 3 degrees of accuracy for the sake of expediency. No matter what the surgeon's personal goals are, these types of applications in CAS use can serve to shorten time to a point at which the CAS merely becomes an alternative means of instrumentation. However, other factors in addition to the time required to learn the system are at work. Confidence in believing what the instruments are reading can also stymie surgical progress.[9,17] Although some readings are often not

---

*References 2, 22, 26, 29, 30, and 42.

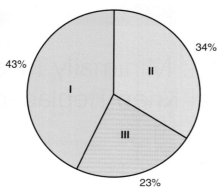

FIG 161.1 There are three phases of time use during typical CAS operations. The first phase *(green)* is insertion and way-point acquisition dependent on both surgical dexterity and software capabilities. The second phase *(blue)* is cutting block positioning and, in some surgeon's hands, a second check of accuracy of the cut by improvement of the measured check of accuracy. Phase three *(red)* is the data recording testing of trial implants.

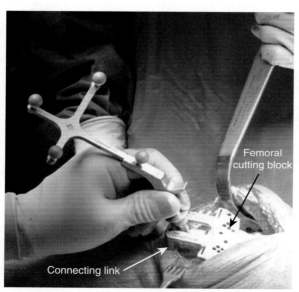

FIG 161.2 Attached to the lower portion of the femoral cutting block is a conjoined cutting block, which provides for distance separation of implant replacement hardware. If the femoral cutting block is positioned correctly and the appropriate releases are done to correctly orient the femoral tibial angle to approximate the mechanical access desired, the tibia resection will be appropriate in a measured resection distance in relationship to the femur.

realistic or believable, the majority of the time the computer is smarter than the surgeon. After reliance and confidence in CAS is achieved, less time is spent using the traditional instruments to align the CAS-driven instruments, making CAS a "primary" means of guidance.

I have reviewed every system on the market in an effort to give a new perspective on relative advantages and disadvantages of all the systems currently available (see end of chapter). Although many vendors have put high priorities on the development of CAS and improving the software packages, many others have left this technology to flounder and have all but

abandoned its development. Nonetheless, there are still numerous systems on the market that are excellent choices, given the particular surgical demands and desires of the implant being used (Table 161.1). Although CAS use continues to decline in the United States, the recent articles out of Australia and Asia drive the world market toward continued use, which will further refine this technology.

CHOICES IN SYSTEMS

Accelerometer-Based Computer-Assisted Surgery

This newest addition to CAS was derived directly from the aerospace industry. These basic navigation units supply information on changes of trajectory, which then account for angular degrees and distance of translation. With the improvement in technology, these systems have now achieved a capacity to virtually navigate an entire TKR.[33] Most systems navigate a single jig application or discreet resection maneuver, if one even has the ability to perform post checks. Although somewhat rudimentary in application, they provide at least as much accuracy without the invasive use of pins, arrays, or reflective active and passive transmissions to have real time updates in positioning. Several systems now offered are compatible with generic use of navigating one or both of the tibia and femoral sides independently.

Infrared Computer-Assisted Surgery

Infrared (IR) CAS continues to hold the competitive edge for acceptance not only in the bulk of available products but also the versatility worldwide for multiple system implementations. IR still remains the gold standard by which all other systems are judged and compared. It offers an abundance of proprietary choices, as well as software versatility and signal stability.

Electromagnetic Computer-Assisted Surgery

Although on a decline in the majority of the world, electromagnetic (EM) was a technology that was probably abandoned prematurely. The beauty that it offers is the absence of direct line of sight limitations, much like radiofrequency signal generation, that IR simply cannot provide. The downside to EM is its sensitivity to external EM fields and metal sensitivity.[25] The advantages include a smaller dynamic reference frame, which is the same as a tracker array in IR navigation. These small active transmitters are hardwired to a fixed point on the tibia and femur. They are small sized (less than a dime in diameter) and afford use of insertion and virtually disappear in the case short of the wire that exits from the incision. Given the absence of availability and lack of continued technologic attention, this chapter will not deal with this technology.

SURGICAL TECHNIQUE: TRACKER MOUNTING OPTIONS

All systems (except Aesculap) have now gone to a dual or multiple thin pin fixation formats for the tracker arrays. Pins are placed at a dedicated distance such that they will accommodate a tracker mounting block. For the majority of systems, a parallel mounting configuration on a $\frac{1}{8}$-inch, 3.2-mm self-tapping threaded screw is the norm. Because the fixation is superior with dual pin fixation, many surgeons have opted for a unicortical fixation to lessen fracture risks. Depending on the bone quality, fixation of the pin can use a single cortical

TABLE 161.1 Computer-Assisted Surgery System Evaluation

Company	BB Braun, Aesculap	Brain Lab	Stryker	Zimmer ORTHOsoft	Zimmer iASSIST Knee	Exactech
Universal or implant-specific	Both	Both	Open	Universal	Universal	Open for exactor knee size
Control	Foot, screen	Gesture-driven foot control	Trigger, screen, cumbersome	Touchscreen registration pinter[a]	Automatic triggers on instruments on screen	Touch screen only, probe air mouse
Pin mount	Single pin	Pinless[b]	Pinless[c]	Yes	No	2 pins on inst option
Reception range	1.4-2.4 m	1-3 m	1-2 m	6 feet is optimal	No range, wireless	0.3-1.5 m
Reception Azimuth	0-90°	Info not provided	180°	135° for trackers, 127° for spheres	135°	145°
Screen realization ease	Good	Best	"u" joint confusing curve 1st 2 plane screen	Easy to read	On iPad no screen	Good but cluttered
GAP (femoral-tibial) capable	Yes (mm)	Yes (mm)	Yes (degrees)	Yes (degrees: 0, 30, 60, 90)	No	Yes (∞ mm Aug.)
GAP presentation speed	Requires tensometer, mm, degrees instant, no preplan	Instant	Instant	4 preset angles only	Angular measurements only No preplan	Preplan easiest to perform
Ball debris resistance	10%[d]	15%	Immune to debris[f]	Least sensitive to debris	Immune to debris[f]	Active, never rem. very resisted
Archive instant recall	No	Yes	Yes	Yes	No	Yes
Acquisition speed	4.3 min	2.1 min	2.9 min	3.2 min	3.8 min	3.1 min
Picture capture	Automatic	Manual, yes	Yes	Yes	Yes	Yes
Picture file ease	Yes, touch screen	3 clicks to cloud, 5 clicks to USB	Slow, cumbersome	Yes, touch screen or pointer	No	Instant, fastest, most complete, on screen forced
Chart note capability	Yes	No	No	No	No	Yes
Hip center RMS throw out	~2 cm	±0.5 cm	0.5 mm	2 cm	N/A	2 mm

[a]Slow and cumbersome.
[b]Can provide recheck of resection.
[c]Recheck angles only at distance.
[d]Spheres do not work if any small amount of debris is present.
[e]The trackers recover almost 100% of their accuracy, whereas spheres cannot recuperate adequately.
[f]The system is not affected by debris because there are no trackers.[23]
[g]All models reviewed are ambidextrous and capable of keeping archives.
RMS, Root mean square.[23]

penetration rather than exiting the opposed cortex to achieve bicortical fixation. Eliminating thread strippage on contact to the opposite cortex and without risk of penetration, which may endanger soft tissue structures. Tracker mounts are generally inserted on the medial portion of the femur.

Despite variability of certain hardware applications, the insertion of arrays for the femur and tibia are very similar. If you are a surgeon who stands on the same side as the extremity with which you are operating, the array that you will use for the femoral tracker will most often be on the distal femur in the soft tissue quadriceps musculature. If your incisions are large enough, you can use an optional intra-incisional array mount along the medial epicondyle region of the femur (Fig. 161.3). This varies in conjunction with the type of exposure and type of TKR being used (Fig. 161.4). For example, if using a subvastus or medial type of approach versus a standard midline quadriceps incision, there is ample room to mount the array on the anteriomedial portion of the femur and slide the pins into the crease posterior to the VMO, thereby avoiding the quadriceps. One word of caution in regard to the medial femoral pin placement in an intra-incisional location must be made with regard

to shrinking incisions too small. With an effort to lessen the size of the incision, it is common to see soft tissue tethering on the tracker arrays, and one must be certain that through the range of motion of the knee that the pins do not become tethered by the quadriceps or the posterior medial skin edge so as to alter the accuracy of the tracker array. If a cruciate-substituting knee is used, the pins must be inserted 2 cm proximal to the joint line because the tibial cam articulation in the intracondyle notch will violate the pin trajectory and cause complications in terms of preparing the femur. On the other hand, the cruciate-retaining knee allows the pin placement to be at a more distal level closer to the joint line.

Some surgeons may use a VMO exposure and stand on the opposite side of the table to perform a TKR. For instance, a left TKR would place the surgeon on the right-hand side of the field and pin placements would be variable in terms of reflection to the opposite side of the field. Although tibial pins are not generally a problem, the femoral side can be a potential source of vascular injury. The femoral vessels coursing into the adductor canal have not reached the posterior position of the lower femur until the lower one-third of the extremity. Mounting trackers

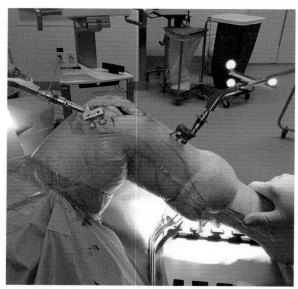

FIG 161.3 Traditional positioning of the tracker arrays for a typical left total knee. Whether a surgeon is standing on the opposite or the same side as the operative extremity, the arrays are mounted in the same fashion unless a preference for a percutaneous femoral stab wound through the extensor mechanism is preferred.

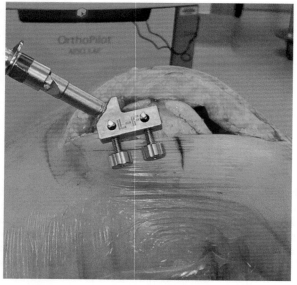

FIG 161.4 In close-up view of the infra vastus medialis positioning of two pin fixations for the femoral tracking when using a cruciate-substituting knee. The lower pin needs to be placed slightly higher to accommodate the notch resection.

using bicortical fixation can jeopardize the femoral artery on a lateral approach, so care must be exercised in placement in both angulation and extension beyond the cortical edge—yet another reason for single cortical fixation.

When it comes to the tibial mounts, the preferred position would be along the medial upper crest of the tibia. The higher this pin placement can be, the better in terms of reducing the likelihood of skin irritation, thermal necrosis, injury, or fracture.

Again, I would encourage surgeons to try to use single cortical fixation as often as possible so as to reduce additional stress risers on the tibia. Because the arrays naturally crowd the operative field, a yoke is incorporated to distance the airway away from the incision to provide more space when the knee is in extension and keeps the arrays free of the operation field while the pins remain in the larger dimensional metaphaseal area of bone less prone to thermal necrosis.

Some older systems have no provision for medial mounting of tracker arrays on the tibia, and therefore the surgeon is compelled to affix them to the lateral side.

SEQUENCE CHANGES IN COMPUTER-ASSISTED SURGERY

If one talks to three surgeons who do TKRs, you will probably get three different sequences with which they prefer to perform TKR. Although some software packages mandate a certain flow in terms of the order, most modern systems now can force a sequence change through manual overrides. For most surgeons, the debulking of a tight knee incision begins with removal of osteophytes and soft tissue releases. Having done that, I feel that performing the patellar resection can extend the soft tissue envelope and lessen incisional tension by first removing excessive unused portions of the patella, thereby releasing the extensor hood pressure and providing better flexion. Secondly, most implant companies provide a post-resection patellar protector insert to prevent damage from retraction and allow for better retraction of the patella off to the lateral side.

I have also found that the femur-first seems to be the logical sequence to perform in terms of the osteotomy sequence. By removal of the distal femur followed by the 4-in-1 cutting block to allow posterior condyle resections, the joint tends to collapse on itself and gives the surgeon better viewing of the tibial surface, as well as the ability to translate the tibia anteriorly with a posterior tibial retractor. When performing the posterior femoral resection, remember to remove the osteophytes and free up the posterior capsule to maximize the range of motion in flexion. This is especially true in higher flexion conditions in which posterior roll-back is forced by the cam mechanism and minimization of soft tissue tensioning is paramount to achieve the best flexion capability.

CONJOINT CUTTING JIG TECHNIQUE

One of the most impressive improvements that has been used in recent years is in minimally deformed knees; the use of one way to make the CAS system work to save steps in TKR is using a measured resection block to place femur and tibia cutting blocks at the same time. This is only applicable when using a conjoint cutting block technique. Simply put, if the joint is correctable to a satisfactory MA (7 degrees or less deformity) either with minimal soft tissue releases or osteophyte removals, it would seem logical to navigate the femur with the previously mentioned co-linked tibial resection block, using measured resection distance to place it. By aligning the knee in the correct MA and pinning the femoral cutting block with a detachable tibial pin assembly, a single navigational waypoint cutting block move can turn into a dual cutting block insertion maneuver (Fig. 161.5; also see Fig. 161.2). Again, this is like a poor man's PSI in which pins are placed using CAS to be used later for cutting block insertions based on a measured predetermined

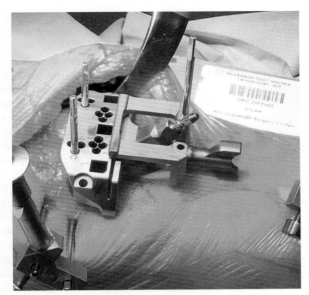

FIG 161.5 The femoral block is placed into position such that it is appropriately anatomically aligned to the distal femur, and the conjoint cutting block affixed to the lower portion is then pinned with co-parallel pins. After the block is removed, the pins will remain in place on the tibia, thereby allowing a tibial cutting block to be placed at a measured resection distance from the femur.

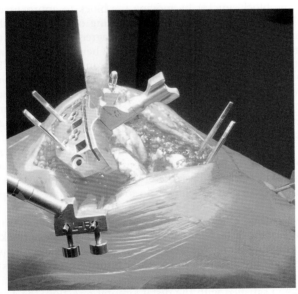

FIG 161.6 The femoral cutting block is in position and ready for resection. The lower tibial pins, now detached from the conjoint cutting block, will allow for the tibial cutting block to be positioned so the tibia resection can be performed without renavigating.

resection level (Fig. 161.6). Often resections done using this technique are within 3 inches of the desired MA; because of the fortunate difference in this case, if you are off, you will find out because you can correct it by checking it with CAS! The accuracy is maintained while using less time. No matter what your

aspirations are for navigation, to be more exacting in placing the 4-in-1 cutting block for rotational perfection will prevent downstream flexion, which is very complex to correct. Complex angles in rotation, especially femoral, are not only the least accurate in CAS but can also be the most difficult to correct if inaccurately performed. Using Whiteside posterior condyles or kinematic arcs and any previous bone excoriation to reference will be helpful.

PATIENT-SPECIFIC INSTRUMENTATION AND COMPUTER-ASSISTED SURGERY

Unless you make it a habit of using CAS with PSI, you are not likely to be able to check finished resection results. We investigated a series of 50 patients, 25 using CAS with PSI and 25 using only PSI, to see if it made any measurable improvement in MA accuracy by catching outliers compared with the cost of the time used to achieve this. Our accuracy improvement was not significantly better, and it cost us another 7 minutes of navigation time over a fairly respectable short PSI without navigation time in the control group. The results from this series suggest using CAS in conjunction with PSI to improve even MA accuracy alone provides no benefit.

PROCEDURAL NOTES IN DETAIL

The preoperative preparation of patients is probably as important as the procedure itself. All my patients use a polypharmacy preemptive of 400 mg celecoxib or diclofenac epolamine patches along with scopolamine preemptive nausea medications before incision 20 mL of ropivacaine (5 mg/mL) is injected in the knee. We are also advocating clear liquids up to 2 hours prior to surgery. Although anesthesia preference varies from country to country, our local community is very adept at single-shot spinals using Duramore with a general anesthetic. epidurals more than regional blocks. After the routine antibiotic administration, we also add Tranexamic 10 mg/kg intravenous (IV) (one ampule), followed by one more ampule (diluted with 10 mL NS intra-articular) at closure. My incision of preference is a sub-vastics incision with options for quadriceps "snip" extension. In approximately 5% to 10% of the males, I perform a slight lateralizing snip to ease the quadriceps retraction. There is less importance of the size of incision and preserving the vastus bulk of the medialis than preventing skin stretching on the superior incision, which can be unsightly and a constant reminder of the procedure. It is rare that patients complain that they have lost strength in their vastus medialis, but they will often complain about a stretch mark from overzealous retraction and undersized incision. Other exposure enhancements include removal of the fat pad and early ACL removal, followed by a posterior capsule stretch by performing an anterior drawer using retractors and medial periosteum stripped at the tibial level to afford anterior medial subluxation at the tibia later in the procedure. In addition, osteophyte removal and early MCL release in nonarredable varus deformities can aid in better exposures and less time spent balancing gaps when provisional implants are trialed. Where prominent osteophytes and loose bodies are removed but I do not spend a lot of time on this unless it constrains exposure. The knee is flexed into 95 degrees of flexion. The patella is retracted laterally. If not performing a bicruciate-preserving a posterior cruciate retained implant, the ACL ligament is rongeured free with a posterior joint retractor, forcing the tibia forward to free the pcl and posterior capsule structures. The knee joint is then extended, whereby the medial patella is clipped with a towel clip and everted, in which either instrumented patellar preparation is used or an oscillating saw is used to remove measured levels of patella to afford patellar resurfacing. I remove excess lateral patellar osteophyte formation to both afford better tracking. This tends to lessen flexion tension and enhance flexibility by decreasing tethering of the extensor hood of the patella quadriceps mechanism.

Tracker pins are now inserted in the incision medial femoral metaphasis lubricate (with adipose fatty tissue from the incision) prior to insertion to minimize friction. Tibial pins are inserted percutaneously starting with an 11-inch blade so as to not damage the skin. These transcutaneous pin fixation points disappear within the first week to 10 days of the procedure, especially if thermal necrosis does not occur from excessive heating during bone penetration.

Femoral preparation, performed next, is through waypoint acquisition to confirm the accuracy of joint level resection with regard to any fixed flexion contractions and preoperative varus/valgus inadequacies. It has been said in a number of different ways that the accuracy of CAS is highly dependent on waypoint acquisition. Critics of CAS will commonly term it as "garbage in, garbage out." That being said, I would put any CAS user who occasionally creates some "garbage in" way beyond the expertise and excellence of a non-CAS user who erroneously thinks that he or she is not subject to error and inaccuracies of the traditionally held belief of 30% off target.[3] However, several key issues need to be considered in acquisition of accurate targeting in CAS. First, the femoral waypoint acquisition on most systems are set to a root mean square (RMS) value that provides for plus or minus 2 degrees or less inaccuracy. This is far better than an intermedullary rod could ever hope to achieve in terms of centering the head of the femur, assuming you have an anatomic femoral angle. Especially if one considers that the intermedullary steel rods do not know the anatomic variances in angulation at the hip neck junction. However, some (high body mass index [BMI]) patients are hard to get acceptable RMS values due to hip motion such that satisfactory hip centers can be calculated. Several tricks can be helpful in this area. If the patient is excessively obese, they tend to roll with internal rotation and external rotation, thereby making the RMS value creep higher than acceptable. Secondly, if the patient has an arthritic hip, it may force the pelvis to roll, causing the exclusion of the femoral acceptable waypoint acquisition. To help to dampen the effects of both of these to be minimized, I have found it helpful to check the range of motion of the hip initially and see where there is a sweet spot for obtaining range of motion in a functional arc without high joint resistance. It is rare that by using this technique, one cannot eventually acquire a usable hip center RMS value.

The other second major pitfall is a posterior femoral condyle acquisition. This is critical in that it has a lot to do with rotation of the femur, gap distance balancing, and femoral sizing in many software applications. If this is off, it tends to have a downstream effect on the size of femoral endplates, as well as rotation, as mentioned before. It is rotation that is the least accurate in CAS, and it is probably from this acquisition point that the failure occurs rather than by the software deficiencies of CAS.[6,31] I found it helpful to roll the patient into a very high flexion position so that I can actually see the point that I am touching rather than trying to feel in between the femoral to tibial articulation. The guesswork is lessened by this maneuver, and you will eventually have to have this kind of exposure anyway so you might as well gain that early on by soft tissue débridement and forcible anterior tibial excursion, described previously in this chapter, to lessen the soft tissue tensions. After these waypoints are acquired, the remaining tibial eminence, tibial plateau, and ankle centers are easily acquired and of less magnitude of importance to spend much time on. Before I place the femoral cutting block, I know in my mind what potential joint line elevation I will use to retain full extension with closure of the procedure. Although still debated (do releases for extension lag versus moving the joint line?), I feel there is a place for both and using only one method is not sufficient.[21,41] I use the formula of 9 mm (the tightness of the implant) plus 1 mm more resection for every 4-degree lag of extension noted preoperatively in the CAS-derived preoperative range-of-motion screen. For instance, if you found a 12-degree flexion contracture in full extension on your preparation CAS measurement, 12 divided by 4 would equal 3 more mm of extra resection (for a total of 12 mm) to allow for full leg extension with closure of the procedure. Incidentally, if joint laxity exists prior to surgery, the same calculation exists for lowering the joint line to make up for laxity of ligament or post injury scenarios. The only instance in which this formula may not be applicable is in the highly osteophyte-invaded joints with posterior loose bodies and osteophytes present.

A note is made as to the freehand navigation of the femoral cutting block in terms of your end goals. I find that I can navigate the block quicker by moving the block to approximately the height that I want and then working on varus or valgus alignment. My ideal target value is 2 degrees varus and 0 to 1 degree of flexion with precalculated joint height elevation based off the most prominent or uninvolved condyle. Although it is important to keep a 2-degree window of accuracy in all of these resections, this is an excellent place at which to speed the process along as to not chase numbers. Remember, although varus/valgus is less important than joint height over-resection and more easily corrected than excessive femoral resection, rotation is a much more difficult thing to correct and even harder to recognize due to the limited exposure. I pay attention to preoperative skid marks and wear or erosion trajectory grooves in the femoral condyle as much as I do to Whiteside line to prepare for the future femoral external rotation positioning of the 4-in-1 cutting block. So before you remove all of the articular surface of the distal femur, take note of any evidence of tracking or troughing along the articular femoral condyle and put a marker on the direction of travel for future cross references for femoral rotation.

When satisfied with the distal femoral resection, the 4-in-1 cutting block can be applied. While zero degree if usingIn the aligned knee without angular deformities a choice of Whiteside's line is a good target. especially However, if you have deformities, rotation must be considered to correct for unequal flexion gaps. on the femoral condyle with which to judge, you need to always bear in mind an excessively varus knee will likely have excessive tight medial flexion gaps. At this point, extra external rotation of the femoral component is likely to be required to get balanced flexion and extension gaps because of preexisting medial contraction from varus deformity. By rolling the femoral component externally, you will effectively widen the flexion gap that is already contracted in a varus knee. For the same reason, externally under-rotating for a valgus knee is a wise idea to keep in mind to widen the lateral joint in flexion where lateral joint contractures exist. I do not navigate my patient knees with tensometers nor gapped distance measuring for this reason gap balancing by hand, use traditional posterior referencing instruments. Whether you use tensometers or CAS to balance flexion gaps, adherence to these concepts makes the final tuning much closer to balanced than if one ignores varus/valgus deformity when deciding on femoral rotation.

Next is the tibial preparation. For minimally invasive exposure, the aim in tibial preparation is to insert a 12- to 14-mm polethylene insert not a 10-mm poly. There are two reasons for this. First, this is the midrange for what is provided by the vendors, and it is able to put you in the mid-target range of what is available without undoing over-resection of the tibia. Secondly, if postoperatively a fibrotic issue occurs where a downsizing of poly is necessary one has "a way out of jail," so to speak. Thirdly, and probably most important for the MIS surgeon, it affords more movement and room for inserting the tibial tray without damaging the posterior condyles of the femur and minimizes stress to soft tissues. Although I understand the implications for weakening the tibial matrix of bone strength the lower one goes, I think there is a place for a mid-range poly of 12 mm to provide for an upsizing or downsizing depending on stress testing and tensioning.

A useful trick that I have used in removal of the proximal osteotomy of the tibia is to use a large osteotome, which I place across the osteotomy after the completion of the saw cut has been made (Fig. 161.7). I then place a second osteotome on top of the large osteotome to prevent deformity while prying the tibial osteotomy free. Often I have seen surgeons try to pry on the proximal tibia only to leave a permanent deformity on the osteotomy from excessive force. This double support mechanism of using an osteotome to pry loose this fragment provides for preservation of the tibia and is a quicker method to remove the tibial fragment. The instrument I prefer to use on the upper side is a handle from a rib splitter affixed to a 0.75-inch straight osteotome, better known as a Hector. These can be fabricated by one's own ingenuity or working with a creative instrument maker to provide for a torsional handle, as well as a pry bar use. This multiply adaptive instrument is commonly used in other applications throughout the joint, including clearing debris from the knee when in extension and in removal of incomplete resection osteophytes from the posterior condyle. After all of the resections have been completed with posterior osteophytes removed, the knee is placed in full extension, where upon a laminar retractor is inserted and the knee joint is débrided.

BALANCING GAP

Much has been written on obtaining proper balance of ligaments in TKR. The majority of authors suggest that balancing the flexion and extension gap in an equilateral rectangle is the preferred method.[20,21,39,41,43] Articles have been appearing that may not be the proper thinking.[13,16,22,35,40] If one subscribes to the belief that lateral roll-back occurs in deep flexion, an equilateral rectangle simply will not allow for this to happen, especially in using some of the more constrained designs of implants. Something has to give. Either the ligaments have to become more compliant, the articular surface allows more rollback, or both. That being said, my preference has been to be less constrained in the majority of posterior cruciate sacrificing designs during deep flexion to allow for rollbacks. This provides slightly larger gap distances laterally than medially. In 10 to 15 degrees off of full extension, the gap distance preference is 2 to 3 mm either side, with lateral distances approaching a maximum of 4 to 5 mm before moving to the next size poly (Fig. 161.8). In flexion, as long as midflexion stability or excessive laxity does not occur because of articular disparity, a 90- to 100-degree flexion liftoff of 6 laterally and 4 medially is not in my experience a correctable distance for which I would move to the next size poly. These balancing techniques become very difficult in a valgus knee because the knee tends to become tight laterally

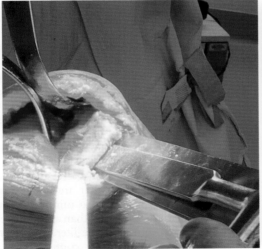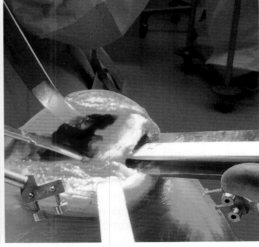

FIG 161.7 This two-picture sequence shows a typical resection maneuver, protecting the tibia from indentation or damage from prying by using a large osteotome or a second osteotome is applied superiorly and twisted in such a manner to force the tibia up and out of the joint capsule. By using a similar retraction posteriorly, an easier removal of the bone is afforded without damaging the tibial surface.

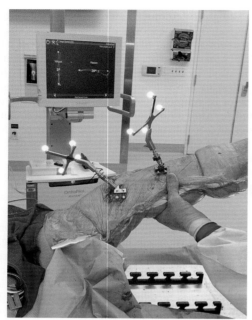

FIG 161.8 The image shows valgus stress being applied to the knee in slight flexion so as to ascertain the amount of angular displacement and angular deviation of 1 degree. One millimeter of gap displacement is present on the joint under force.

after the MA is re-established. Much more vigilance is necessary to achieve laxity in these more deformed knees, thereby explaining the relative ease of a varus knee even if it happens to be highly deformed. It just naturally adapts to a loose lateral, tighter medial scenario, which is the resultant goal.

Some systems provide for eloquent balancing techniques done intraoperatively with computer guidance. While these are phenomenal and provide the surgeon some objective data on the specific distances at any given angle, my preference is a manual technique while visualizing the screen. The common belief of 1 mm of toggle equals 1 degree of freedom is the method I use for purposes of speed, while not sacrificing accuracy.

The knee replacement incision is subject to bleeding while still being without tourniquet insufflation; therefore, take special note to look for lateral recurrent arterial vessels just anterior to the popliteal tendon. This is a common source of bleeding, and if one can cauterize this it minimizes postoperative morbidity. A second area is commonly the medial meniscus; as mentioned above, I do a second injection of the joint. Pay close attention to a very large load of approximately 30 mL of naropin or ropivacaine (5 mg/mL) on the medial pes bursal tissues as a time-release for local analgesia. I spend less time placing injections on the posterior capsule or medial joint space as I have found that that is not the most sensitive area of tenderness. A 5-mL volume of the remaining injection is placed on in the VMO musculature so as to have a second depot of time-release lidocaine Naropin for the postoperative phase. This mixture in 30 20 mL volume is 0.5% bupivacaine. Naropin with one-half epinephrine. We have recently abandoned using Toradol and morphine. I then irrigate the knee with a commercially available solution of chlorhexidine, where upon the trials are inserted and the patient's knee is placed through range

of motion to center the tibia in rotation. Checks of alignment, MA, and gap distance testing are done in slight flexion and deep flexion. I like taking five snapshots of the knee. The first is the full extended, unforced extension MA, the second is a hyperextended forced extension to make sure secure stability is achieved, the third and fourth are a varus/valgus stress test in medium flexion, and the fifth is a full flexion, maximum range of motion, all of which are recorded for data collection purposes. The tibial rotation is marked in full extension so as to verify component mating and congruence of femoral to tibial rotation and give a secondary measure of the tibial tray rotation prior to tibial preparation. Finally, the implants are removed, the tibial preparation is completed, and the first and only insufflation of the tourniquet is performed after 2 minutes of elevation, using one more round of the chlorhexidine solution for antimicrobial purposes. During this time, I also remove tracker pins and irrigate sites because I do not retest MA after cementing. We irrigate with 3 L of normal saline, of which the final irrigation of chlorhexidine is allowed to remain in the knee for one more minute before washout, and then meticulous drying is performed before cement is forcibly injected under low pressure on the proximal tibia prior to insertion of implants. I have found that a beveled cut on the injector gun is preferable to the roughened squared edge that is difficult to insufflate cement under pressure to hard to reach areas. We use low-viscosity cement without antibiotics in the absence of any real objective data to support antibiotic use in cements.

Closure of the knee joint is done in flexion while the cement is setting. This is subject to some degree of risk. The knee must be in an Alvarado knee holder and be held firmly in place. Secondly, excessive flexion can tend to rock the tibial tray into the anterior lift-off position. However, to be fair, a full extension closure carries with it the risk of excessive tightening of the now lax extensile tissues, causing reduced range of motion postoperatively and can potentially rock the posterior tibia into a lift-off position. Somewhere in the middle is an ideal sweet spot for tensioning, and I find that a bend of 45 to 60 degrees gives that neutral tension point for the tibial tray and makes the surgical team honest about how much tension they apply across the extensile mechanism. Available on the market is a new self-locking monofilament, which we have had extensive experience with and written about with regard to its speed and efficiency of closure. We have found a tendency for the suture to self-strangulate or creep on itself causing necrosis and local skin irritation. As a result, we have abandoned this to the more traditional monofilament interrupted polyglyconate suture and no longer use Quill (Surgical Specialties Corporation, Wyomissing, PA). We are advocates of subcutaneous skin closure without staples; it offers meticulous wound closure and the absence of unsightly staples while minimizing postoperative care and follow-up. Finally, we have adapted the use of silver nitrate–impregnated occlusive dressings (MepilexAG, Mölnlycke, Göteborg, Sweden) that are not changed until 1 week postoperatively in an effort to minimize postoperative infections. Although no data other than anecdotes exist, silver nitrate dressings hold promise in the literature to improve infection incidence; however, we cannot confirm this as yet.[10]

ACKNOWLEDGMENTS

I would like to give a special thanks to Chelsea Serrano and Lou Shields PhD for their assistance in editing this manuscript.

KEY REFERENCES

4. Bengs BC, Scott RD: The effect of distal femoral resection on passive knee extension in posterior cruciate ligament retaining total knee arthroplasty. *J Arthroplasty* 21:161–166, 2006.

9. Carter RE, Rush PF, Smid JA, et al: Experience with computer-assisted navigation for total knee arthroplasty in a community setting. *J Arthroplasty* 23:707–713, 2008.

15. Hetaimish BM, Khan MM, Simounovic N, et al: Meta-analysis of navigation versus conventional total knee arthroplasty. *J Arthroplasty* 27(6):1177–1181, 2012.

19. Kim YO, Park JW, Kim JS: Computer-navigated versus conventional total knee arthroplasty a prospective randomized trial. *J Bone Joint Surg Am* 94:2017–2024, 2012.

22. Lionberger DR, Crocker CL, Chen V: Patient specific instrumentation. *J Arthorplasty* 29:1699–1704, 2014.

23. Lionberger DR, Crocker CL, Rahbar MH: Is computer-assisted surgery in total knee arthroplasty as accurate as it can be? *Comput Aided Surg* 17(4):198–204, 2012.

25. Lionberger DR, Weise J, Ho DM, et al: How does electromagnetic navigation stack up against infrared avigation in minimally-invasive total knee replacement? *J Arthroplasty* 23:573–580, 2008.

27. Malhotra R, Singla A, Lekha C, et al: A prospective randomized study to compare systemic emboli using the computer-assisted and conventional techniques of total knee arthroplasty. *J Bone Joint Surg Am* 97:889–894, 2015.

28. Merz MK, Bohnenkamp FC, Sulo S, et al: Perioperative differences in conventional and computer-assisted surgery in bilateral total knee arthroplasty. *Am J Orthop* 43:260–261, 2014.

30. Mont MA, McElroy MJ, Johnson AJ, et al: Single use instruments, cutting blocks, and trials increase efficiency in the operating room during knee arthroplasty: a prospective comparison in navigated and non-navigated cases. *J Arthroplasty* 28:1135–1140, 2013.

32. Moskal JT, Capps SG, Mann JW, et al: Navigated versus conventional total knee arthroplasty. *J Knee Surg* 27:235–248, 2014.

33. Nam D, Nawabi DH, Cross MB, et al: Accelerometer-based computer navigation for performing the distal femoral resection in total knee arthroplasty. *J Arthroplasty* 27:1717–1722, 2012.

35. Ritter MA, Davis KE, Davis P, et al: Preoperative malalignment increases risk of failure after total knee arthroplasty. *J Bone Joint Surg Am* 95:126–131, 2013.

38. Steiger RN, Liu YL, Graves SE: Computer navigation for total knee arthroplasty reduces revision rate for patients less than sixty-five years of age. *J Bone Joint Surg Am* 97:635–642, 2015.

43. Yoon JR, Jeong HI, Oh KJ, et al: In vivo gap analysis in various knee flexion angles during navigation-assisted total knee arthroplasty. *J Arthroplasty* 28:1796–1800, 2013.

The references for this chapter can also be found on www.expertconsult.com.

162

Robotics in Total Knee Arthroplasty: Development, Outcomes, and Current Techniques

William L. Bargar, Nathan A. Netravali

INTRODUCTION

Primary reconstructive knee surgery can consist of unicompartmental knee arthroplasty (UKA), multicompartmental knee arthroplasty (MCKA), or total knee arthroplasty (TKA) and is commonly performed to relieve pain and restore function in patients with end-stage osteoarthritis of the affected knee. Currently there are approximately 600,000 primary TKA procedures and 45,000 primary UKA procedures performed annually in the United States.[28,70] The number of procedures is growing rapidly, with TKA growing at a rate of 9.4% per annum and UKA growing at a rate of 32.5% per annum in the United States[55] with potentially more than 3 million primary TKAs by 2030.[29] The goal of a knee arthroplasty is to restore the knee joint to a functional and pain-free state. In terms of clinical outcomes, TKA is a successful procedure when looking at pain relief and restoration of patient mobility with 10- to 15-year implant survival rates of greater than 90%.[15,40,60,74] UKA has a slightly lower survival rate of more than 85% at 7 years.[75]

However, patients are far from fully satisfied, especially in the case of younger patients. Patient satisfaction remains at only 82% to 89% after TKA,[1,3,7] and patients who received UKA are satisfied only 80% to 83% of the time.[58] In addition, younger patients are increasingly demanding an active lifestyle and require an increased longevity of their implants. Both implant survival and patient satisfaction are dependent on multiple factors, including patient selection, implant design, the preoperative condition of the joint, surgical technique, and rehabilitation.

When looking to improve implant survival and patient satisfaction, surgeons may choose from a variety of implants and surgical techniques. The first factor is implant design. It includes component geometry, materials, and manufacturing processes and has changed since TKA first came about. However, patient satisfaction does not seem to have improved with these contemporary implants.[7] Although the majority of implants used nowadays are generic, there are now custom implants based on a patient's individual anatomy (ConforMIS; Burlington, MA). These implants are too new to draw any conclusions regarding their effects on implant survival and long-term patient satisfaction. The other factor is surgical technique, which includes access to the joint, implant sizing, implant alignment and positioning relative to anatomic features, implant fixation to the bone, soft tissue balancing, and wound closure.[35,60] It has been suggested that errors in surgical technique may be the most common reason for failure of TKAs.[60,63,68] Thus

many recent developments in knee reconstructive surgery have focused on improvements in surgical technique.

The traditional surgical technique involves making bone cuts and soft tissue balancing. Bone cuts are typically performed with reference to anatomic landmarks and available implant geometry. Ideal implant sizing involves reproducing the native dimensions of the knee with those of the implant. Conventional TKA instruments typically use intraoperative sizing guides to help the surgeon to determine the appropriate implant size. In terms of implant to bone fixation, most knee replacement implants are fixed to the host bone using bone cement (polymethylmethacrylate). In the alternative, cementless fixation, the implants have a porous backside that allows for bony ingrowth. Although bone cement provides good initial fixation even with poor quality bone, cementless fixation provides direct bone-to-metal attachment, which reduces migration after an initial period, and thus may lead to a potentially longer implant life.[42] To achieve reliable cementless fixation, precise bone cuts must be made so that the implants achieve stable initial fixation with little to no gaps. Conventional techniques result in cuts that are made using bone attached cutting guides and an oscillating saw. As demonstrated by Plaskos et al.,[52] these cutting guides combined with an oscillating saw resulted in errors in cuts ranging from 0.6 to 1.1 degrees in varus–valgus and 1.8 degrees in flexion–extension. These cutting errors can result in gaps that delay bone ingrowth into the implant[44] or may require bone cement to ensure initial stability.

The postoperative alignment of the knee has a large effect on the load transferred through the implant. Implant design has traditionally assumed that the "ideal" mechanical axis of the leg is restored. This mechanical axis is defined as a straight line passing from the center of the femoral head to the center of the talus.[25,49] The implants also typically attempt to preserve the anatomic joint line and remove minimal bone. Many studies have shown that restoring a neutral postoperative mechanical axis, defined by the center of the hip, center of the knee, and center of the ankle within ±3 degrees of the mechanical axis, may result in improved postoperative pain, biomechanics, function, and an increased implant longevity.[8,25,56,57] However, there are a few studies that have found little relationship between a neutral mechanical axis and implant longevity.[39,46]

Planning for TKA has traditionally involved the use of acetate implant overlays on appropriately magnified radiographs of the knee.[67] Intraoperatively, mechanical alignment jigs are used to assist in making the bone cuts. These jigs typically reference the long axis of the bone either by estimating it externally or internally entering the intramedullary canal. Cutting guides are then attached to the bones, and a handheld oscillating saw is used to perform the bony cuts.

With respect to achieving balanced soft tissues within the knee postoperatively, there are two main techniques used by surgeons: "gap balancing" and "measured resection." Gap balancing determines the rotational and anteroposterior (AP) position of the femoral component intraoperatively in an attempt to achieve a rectangular flexion gap equal to or close to the extension gap. This can achieve ligament balance but may result in a nonanatomic alignment of the femoral component. The measured resection technique relies on the intraoperatively determined location of the transepicondylar axis (TEA). The TEA has been shown[9,41] to be the best indicator of a patient's true anatomic flexion axis. However, locating the TEA intraoperatively can be difficult due to osteophytes and limited exposure. Thus several other alignment measures are often used instead of the TEA, such as the Whiteside line. Although the Whiteside line is likely easier to locate, it is also prone to error. As such, many surgeons will simply place the femoral component in a fixed position of external rotation (typically 3 degrees) relative to the posterior condylar axis as an estimation of the TEA. Although this position is easy to find repeatedly, the posterior condyles relationship to the TEA is variable between patients and can result in unequal ligament balance.[26,43]

Numerous peer-reviewed published papers have identified knee alignment as the most important factor in achieving good long-term clinical results.* As such, computer-assisted surgical systems have been developed to address the challenges associated with knee arthroplasty. Surgical navigation systems typically provide the surgeon with information including bone orientations and limb alignments through a display. In addition, patient-specific instrumentation and implants are now being used.[18,20] These systems typically require computer-assisted planning and design of custom instrumentation that can be rapidly manufactured using such methods as three-dimensional (3D) printing. These computer-assisted passive systems may be classified outside of the robotic realm.

Robotic assistive systems are robotic devices that perform specific tasks according to preoperative or intraoperative data. These systems can be classified into three main categories: passive, semiactive robotic systems, and active robotic systems.[50] Passive systems perform part of the surgical procedure under continuous and direct control of the surgeon. An example of a passive system is one in which a robot holds a guide or jig in a predetermined location and the surgeon uses manual tools to prepare the bony surfaces. A semiactive robotic system is a tactile feedback system that augments the surgeon's ability to control the tool, typically by restricting the cut volume by defining constraints of the cut motion in space; however, it still requires the surgeon to manipulate the cutter. Finally, an active robotic system performs a surgical task without direct intervention of the surgeon, such as allowing the robotic arm to cut the bone without direct manipulation of the cutter by the surgeon.

Although navigation systems have been shown to reduce the number of mechanical axis alignment outliers,[37] these systems still rely on manual tools to make the cuts, which limits their accuracy.[4] For this reason, surgeons and engineers successfully integrated robotically controlled surgical instruments into joint replacement surgery.[71] In addition to the computer-controlled cutting instrument, robotic systems typically use computed tomography (CT)-based 3D visualization and templating to plan the cuts. This allows easier accurate preoperative identification of anatomic landmarks, such as the TEA. Most robotic systems consist of very similar components. The steps to a robotically assisted surgery typically involve (1) creation of a patient-specific model and surgical plan; (2) intraoperative registration of the model and plan to the patient's anatomy; and (3) robotic assistance to make bone cuts and carry out the preoperative plan on the patient.

HISTORY

The first active robotic system for use in orthopedic procedures was ROBODOC (THINK Surgical, Inc., Fremont, CA) and was developed jointly between the University of California–Davis and IBM's Thomas Watson Research Labs in New York from 1986 to 1992. Howard A. Paul, DVM, and William L. Bargar, MD, invented the system as a method to improve the ingrowth of early cementless femoral components in total hip arthroplasty (THA). Based on a traditional computer-aided design (CAD)–computer-aided manufacturing (CAM) system, ROBODOC consists of a CT-based computer-aided robotic device that enables accurate preparation and anatomic placement of the components in primary cementless THA. Since the initial version, the application has been expanded to accommodate primary TKA and revision THA.[2]

Matsen et al.[38] were the first to describe a robotic system for knee arthroplasty. Their passive system was based on a robot that positioned saw and drill guides with respect to the bony geometry. Kienzle et al.[27] developed another passive system that used a preoperative CT scan and a pin-based registration technique. The preoperative CT allowed the surgeon to plan and accurately execute implant placement based on 3D reconstructions of the bones. Van Hamm et al.[73] presented a semiactive system in which the robot constrained the motion of the cutting tool as it was guided by the surgeon. This system used an intraoperative registration method using an intramedullary rod. Martelli et al.[36] presented a passive robotic system for use in TKA based on preoperative CT. Intraoperative registration was performed using a surface-matching technique based on the surface models created from the CT scans. Glozman et al.,[19] La Palombara et al.[30] and Fadda et al.[17] used similar surface matching techniques to register bones without fiducial markers. These registration methods were then combined with active or semiactive robots that provided precision bone milling according to the preoperative plan.

In addition to these larger robots, there has been development of smaller bone-mounted robots. For example, PiGalileo (Plus Orthopedics AG, Smith & Nephew, Switzerland) is a passive system using a hybrid navigated-robotic device that clamps on to the mediolateral aspects of the distal femoral shaft. The Mini Bone-Attached Robotic System (MBARS) was an active system developed for patellofemoral joint replacement procedures.[76] Plaskos et al.[51] presented Praxiteles in 2005 as a passive system that is a miniature bone-mounted robot for TKA. Song et al.[64] have developed an active system consisting of a hybrid bone-attached robot for joint arthroplasty (HyBAR) that uses hinged prismatic joints to provide a structurally rigid robot for minimally invasive joint arthroplasty.

*References 4, 6, 8, 25, 34, and 72.

Although many of these systems have been developed and prototyped, only a handful have been used successfully in clinical settings throughout the world. These include the ROBODOC System (THINK Surgical, Inc., Fremont, CA), the Computer-Assisted Surgical Planning and Robotics (CASPAR) system (URS Ortho, Rastatt, Germany), the Robotic Arm Interactive Orthopedic System (RIO; Stryker Orthopaedics, Mahwah, NJ), The Navio PFS (Blue Belt Technologies, Plymouth, MN), APEX Robotic Technology (OMNIlife science, Inc., East Taunton, MA), and the Stanmore Sculptor Robotic Guidance Arm (RGA) System (Stanmore Implants, Elstree, UK), formerly known as the Acrobot System. OMNIlife science's APEX Robotic Technology is a passive system, whereas MAKO's RIO, Blue Belt's Navio PFS, and the Stanmore Sculptor RGA System are semiactive systems, and the CASPAR and ROBODOC systems are active robotic systems. The surgical technique for ROBODOC is described next in some detail.

SURGICAL TECHNIQUE

Preoperative Preparation

The ROBODOC System consists of Orthodoc, a preoperative planning workstation, and ROBODOC, an electromechanical arm, electronic control cabinet with display monitor, operating software, tools, and accessories. Each ROBODOC procedure requires a preoperative CT scan. A motion rod is scanned with the joint that enables the Orthodoc software to detect if any patient motion occurred during the scan. Any movement adversely affects the ability to perform intraoperative registration due to image quality, decreasing the accuracy of implant placement.

After the scan is complete, the CT data are used as input into Orthodoc, which combines the individual slices to produce a series of two-dimensional (2D) images for templating. A 3D surface model of the operative bone is also created in Orthodoc for intraoperative registration purposes. Orthodoc contains a library of 510(k) cleared hip or knee replacement implants, depending on the application installed. The surgeon selects an implant model from this library and manipulates the 3D representation of the implant in relation to the bone to optimally place the implant. After the surgeon is satisfied with the implant location, the data are written to a transfer media file for use with ROBODOC during surgery.

Operating Room Setting

In the operating room (OR), surgical exposure during a ROBODOC surgery is the same as is performed during a normal TKA. After the joint is exposed, fixation is required to ensure that the distal femur and proximal tibia are immobilized with respect to the ROBODOC base. After fixation has been established, bone motion recovery markers are placed on the bone. Recovery markers are used to recover the 3D location and orientation of the bone in the event that the bone moves after it has been registered. Bone motion monitors (BMMs) are directly attached to the operative bones and can determine if a bone motion occurs. If a bone motion occurs during registration or cutting, the procedure is immediately paused. This requires the bone to be reregistered before the procedure may continue.

After the BMMs have been attached, the operative bone is then registered within ROBODOC's workspace. ROBODOC uses a widely accepted method of registration used in computer vision, based on a point-to-surface technique. It requires the

creation of a surface model of the bone from the preoperative CT scan using a semiautomated process in Orthodoc and collecting, or digitizing, bone surface points on the patient intraoperatively.

During surgery, the surgeon uses a digitizer located on the ROBODOC system to collect points on the bone with respect to the ROBODOC arm-coordinate system. The software directs the surgeon towards areas on the surface of the bone where points need to be collected. This method does not require the collection of specific anatomic points, but rather the algorithm is designed to match the surface of the bone based on a variety of points over broader anatomic regions. If the points are not well distributed, a software check will require the points to be recollected until they are sufficiently spread apart. If the calculated registration meets the accuracy requirements, the surgeon is asked to verify the results of the registration by digitizing specific points. The graphic display then indicates where each collected point lies relative to the CT surface model. If the collected points are acceptable to the surgeon, he or she can accept the registration and proceed with the surgery.

Technique—Execution

The next step of a ROBODOC procedure is the milling of the bone. The surgeon must ensure that the soft tissue is properly retracted prior to allowing ROBODOC to begin cutting the bone (Fig. 162.1). During the entire bone preparation procedure by ROBODOC the surgeon is in control of the process and is in direct view of the operative site. The surgeon has the ability to pause, stop, or abort the use of ROBODOC at any point of the process with the use of a handheld controller, or pendant. In addition, during cutting, the OR monitor shows a continuously updated graphical representation of the cutting progress superimposed on top of the CT data.

After ROBODOC has finished preparing the bone, the software will prompt the surgeon to move ROBODOC away from the operating table. At this point the surgeon removes the recovery markers and fixation system and proceeds with implant

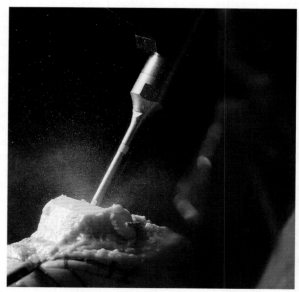

FIG 162.1 ROBODOC actively milling the distal femur during a total knee arthroplasty procedure. (Reproduced with permission from THINK Surgical, Inc., Fremont, California.)

TABLE 162.1   Summary of Clinical Studies Using Robotic Assistance for Unicompartmental or Total Knee Arthroplasty

Study	System	Procedure	# Robotic Cases	# Conventional Cases
Clark et al.[10]	OmniNav/Praxiteles	TKA	52	29
Börner et al.[76]	ROBODOC	TKA	100	N/A
Song et al.[65]	ROBODOC	TKA	30	30
Song et al.[66]	ROBODOC	TKA	50	50
Yim et al.[77]	ROBODOC	TKA	117	N/A
Liow et al.[31]	ROBODOC	TKA	31	29
Siebert et al.[61]	CASPAR	TKA	70	52
Bellemans et al.[5]	CASPAR	TKA	25	N/A
Cobb et al.[11]	Sculptor RGA	UKA	13	15
Coon et al.[12]	MAKO	UKA	36	45
Coon et al.[13]	MAKO	UKA	33	44
Sinha et al.[62]	MAKO	UKA	20	N/A
Pearle et al.[47]	MAKO	UKA	10	N/A
Lonner et al.[33]	MAKO	UKA	31	27
Dunbar et al.[14]	MAKO	UKA	50	N/A
Hansen et al.[21]	MAKO	UKA	30	32

CASPAR, Computer-assisted surgical planning and robotics; *N/A,* not available; *RGA,* robotic guidance arm; *TKA,* total knee arthroplasty; *UKA,* unicompartmental knee arthroplasty.

fitting and insertion in the same manner as a manual knee arthroplasty. Finally, the exposed joint can be closed per standard procedures.

PUBLISHED RESULTS

A summary of published clinical studies in which robotic-assistance systems are used for TKA is presented in Table 162.1. The studies and their primary findings are described in the sections below for each individual system.

OmniNav

The OmniNav iBlock, part of the APEX Robotic Technology system, is an imageless navigation-based robotic cutting jig. It evolved from Praxiteles, which was developed by PRAXIM Medivision S.A. (La Tronche, France) and guides the surgeon's saw blade when making femoral osteotomy cuts. The robotic guide is mounted on the bone and moves to a new position to locate each of the five osteotomies performed on the femur during a TKA. There have been limited published data on its clinical use, but improvements have been shown in terms of time required, malalignment, and hospitalization length when compared to a computer-assisted navigation system.[10]

Computer-Assisted Surgical Planning and Robotics

The CASPAR system, although no longer on the market, was used clinically and has some published results. The principles of operation and procedure were very similar to the first version of ROBODOC. The system required placement of fiducial markers in the patient's bone prior to a CT scan that was used for planning the TKA. Siebert et al.[61] performed a study using CASPAR for TKA in which 70 CASPAR-assisted surgeries were compared with 52 control surgeries performed in Kassel, Germany. Postoperative standing long-leg radiographs showed that the CASPAR group had a higher accuracy in achieving the planned femorotibial alignment, with an average error of 0.8 degrees (range, 0 to 3 degrees) compared with the control group's average error of 2.6 degrees (range, 0 to 7 degrees). Another study looked at 25 TKA cases that were consecutively performed using the CASPAR system[5] with follow-up from 5.1

to 5.8 years. The results demonstrated that all angular measurements for the tibial and femoral components in this study were within 1 degree of the target as defined in the preoperative plan. Operating time for these first 70 cases averaged 135 minutes but toward the end of the study achieved a steady state of approximately 90 minutes, which was nearly equivalent to the control group. No major adverse events related to the CASPAR system were found, but one minor complication was recorded. One TKA in one patient was successfully converted to a manual technique after femoral milling could not be completed due to a defective registration marker. In addition, three patients had superficial skin irritations at the pin sites that were resolved using conservative treatment.

ROBODOC

The ROBODOC system has been used clinically for TKA since 2000. The first 100 ROBODOC TKA procedures were performed by Professor Martin Börner at the Trauma Clinical of Trade Associations (BGU) in Frankfurt, Germany.[6] All of the patients received the Duracon Total Knee (DePuy Orthopedics Inc., Warsaw, IN). The ROBODOC system made cuts that allowed cementless implantation for both the tibia and femur in 76 of the first 100 patients. Sixteen of the remaining cases needed cement for the tibial component, and eight cases needed cement for both components due to poor bone quality. In 97% of the cases the alignment of the knee was restored to the planned ideal mechanical axis (0-degree error). The remaining three cases resulted in knee alignment being restored to within 1 degree of the ideal mechanical axis. The operating time decreased from 130 minutes for the first case to a typical time of 90 to 100 minutes by the end of the study. Of the first 100 cases, five were successfully converted to a manual procedure due to technical issues with the ROBODOC system.

A more recent study by Song et al.[65] directly compared between a ROBODOC-assisted TKA and a manual TKA in the same patient using a prospective randomized study. Thirty patients underwent simultaneous bilateral TKA with a ROBODOC-assisted procedure in one knee and a manual procedure in the contralateral knee. Knee alignment and individual component alignment were determined postoperatively, along with clinical outcome measures, including the Hospital for Special Surgery (HSS) and Western Ontario and McMaster (WOMAC) scores. The results showed significantly fewer outliers in terms of alignment errors and nearly equivalent clinical outcome results for both HSS and WOMAC scores. The postoperative mechanical axis was improved to 0.2 ± 1.6 degrees (mean ± SD) in the ROBODOC group and only 1.2 ± 2.1 degrees (mean ± SD) in the manual group. Furthermore, the ROBODOC group had no outliers in mechanical axis, defined as an error greater than or equal to ±3 degrees, whereas the manual group had seven outliers. However, the ROBODOC-assisted surgeries took, on average, 25 minutes longer than the manual cases but resulted in significantly less postoperative bleeding. There were no major adverse events related to the use of the robotic system reported.

Song et al.[66] also published another prospective randomized study comparing ROBODOC-assisted and manual TKAs. One hundred total subjects that were randomly divided into 50 receiving ROBODOC-assisted TKA and 50 receiving manual TKA. Again, the goal was to improve the mechanical axis alignment to neutral (0 degree). The results showed that the postoperative mechanical axis was improved to 0.5 ± 1.4 degrees (mean ± SD) in the ROBODOC-assisted group and 1.2 ± 2.9 degrees (mean ± SD) in the manual group. The ROBODOC group had significantly fewer outliers (0), again defined as error greater than or equal to ±3 degrees, compared with the manual group (12). Again, the operative time was 25 minutes longer in the ROBODOC cases, but they again resulted in significantly less blood loss. The clinical results (range of motion, HSS scores, and WOMAC scores) showed no differences between the two groups. In addition, this study compared the ability to balance the flexion and extension gaps after the bony cuts and soft tissue balancing were completed. The ROBODOC group resulted in only three outliers (defined as a difference in flexion and extension gap outside of 2 ± 2 mm [mean ± SD]), which were significantly fewer than the 10 outliers found in the manual group. Finally, PCL tension was measured intraoperatively. The ROBODOC group resulted in 96% of the knees having excellent tension and 4% having poor tension, whereas the manual group had only 76% of the knees with excellent tension and the remaining 24% with poor tension. This difference between groups was statistically significant. The ROBODOC group experienced six local and five systemic complications compared with the manual group, which experienced three local and eight systemic complications. These complications rates were not statistically different.

Yim et al.,[77] using the ROBODOC system with a cohort of 117 subjects, performed a comparison of alignment methods. They compared clinical outcomes using both a classical (56 subjects) and anatomic (61 subjects) alignment method for implant positioning to determine if there were any clinical or radiologic differences in outcome. The classical method, as defined by Insall et al.,[23] suggests making tibial and femoral cuts perpendicular to the mechanical axis of the tibia and femur, resulting in a joint line that is perpendicular to the mechanical axis. The anatomic method, described by Hungerford et al.,[22] suggested cutting the tibia in varus and the femur in valgus to create a joint line that is parallel with respect to the ground. Yim et al. compared postoperative varus and valgus laxities, ROM, HSS and WOMAC scores, and radiologic outcomes. There were no differences between the groups in any of the outcome measures they considered, including mechanical alignment of the

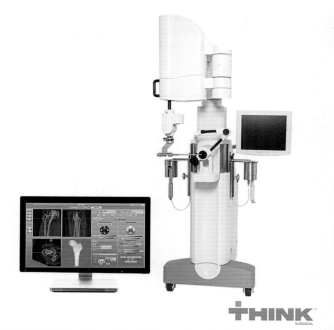

FIG 162.2 TSolution One. (Reproduced with permission from THINK Surgical, Inc., Fremont, California.)

lower limb. They concluded that the ROBODOC system eliminated any surgeon variability in technique and showed that both the classical and anatomic alignment methods result in comparable outcomes.

A prospective randomized study by Liow et al.[31] compared 31 ROBODOC-assisted TKAs with 29 manual TKAs. They looked at how accurately each technique can restore the joint line and mechanical axis and also looked at clinical outcome measures. There were no outliers (>3 degrees) in postoperative mechanical axis in the ROBODOC-assisted group compared with 19.4% of the subjects in the manual group. In addition, there was a shift in joint line greater than 5 mm in 3.2% of the ROBODOC group compared with a shift in joint line greater than 5 mm in 20.6% of the manual group. With regard to clinical outcome, there were no significant differences between the groups in ROM, Oxford Knee Scores, Knee Society Scores (KSS), or SF-36 scores. They concluded that the ROBODOC system reduces the number of implant placement outliers but has no effect on short-term clinical outcomes. They believed that until an intermediate or long-term benefit is shown, conventional techniques might remain more cost effective.

Although the ROBODOC system is still being used throughout the world, it is not currently cleared for use for TKA by the US Food and Drug Administration (FDA). However, its current manufacturer, THINK Surgical, Inc. (Fremont, California) has recently developed a new generation robotic system based on the same principles, called TSolution One (Fig. 162.2). It received 510(k) clearance for THA in the United States, and the TKA application is currently under development.

Stanmore Sculptor Robotic Guidance Arm

The Stanmore Sculptor RGA system, previously known as the Acrobot System, is no longer commercially available but was a semiactive system using CT-based preoperative planning. During cutting, Acrobot uses a type of active constraint control in which the surgeon pushes the robot end effector to move the cutting tool, and the system gradually increases the stiffness of the robot as it approaches the predefined boundaries. This approach is quite different from an automated system, such as an active robot, in that all robot movements are initiated and performed by the surgeon. Acrobot used a clamp-based fixation system to ensure that the operative bone was fixed relative to the robot.

It was used in a randomized study performing UKA.[11,59] This study included 13 patients undergoing Acrobot-assisted surgery and 15 patients undergoing UKA using conventional techniques. Postoperative CT scans showed that the femorotibial alignment for all 13 patients in the Acrobot-assisted group was less than 2 degrees from the goal, whereas only 6 of the 15 patients in the conventional group had femorotibial alignments in this range. The functionality scores (American Knee Society) measured at 6 months postoperatively were also better for the patients operated using Acrobot. The operative time was typically approximately 10 minutes longer than conventional cases.

MAKO RIO

The MAKO RIO is another semiactive system using CT-based preoperative planning. Its principles of operation are very similar to that of Acrobot in that the system provides a haptic boundary while the surgeon manipulates a tool attached to the robot end effector. However, it differs because the bones do not have to be rigidly fixed to the robot because it uses optical trackers placed on the bone. If the bone moves, the motion is captured by a tracking system, and the system compensates for the bone motion and adjusts the haptic boundary in near real time. The surgeon still manipulates the cutting tool, but the RIO system provides audible and tactile feedback to keep the tool within the predefined margins. The RIO system was developed for UKA and has received clearance for TKA application, although the results reported below are only for the UKA application.

It was used in a pilot study for UKA at Pennsylvania Hospital, Philadelphia,[33] that included 31 consecutive patients who underwent UKA using MAKO robotic arm-assistance and 27 consecutive patients who underwent UKA performed with conventional manual instrumentation. Postoperative radiographs showed that the root mean square (RMS) error of the posterior tibial slope was 3.1 degrees using manual techniques and 1.9 degrees using robotic arm assistance. The average error of tibial alignment in the coronal plane was 2.7 ± 2.1 degrees (mean ± SD) using the conventional instruments compared with 0.2 ± 1.8 degrees (mean ± SD) using robotic arm assistance. Varus-valgus RMS error was 3.4 degrees manually compared with 1.8 degrees robotically.

Pearle et al.[47] reported on a feasibility study in which 10 subjects needing a UKA were included. The results of this study showed that all of the patients had tibiofemoral angles in the coronal plane that were within 1 degree of what had been planned. There were no complications with the system, and the wounds healed successfully.

Sinha[62] reported on their first 20 cases and stated that all were successfully completed as planned, and the results showed a good ability to recreate individual patient anatomy. Prior to surgery, 62.5% of the knees were in varus and 37.5% were in valgus. The surgeries were planned to maintain this alignment and after surgery, all of the knees succeeded in matching their preoperative alignment. There were no outliers in terms of flexion. With respect to the tibiae, they were all varus prior to surgery, and this was maintained as preoperatively planned. The mean tibial slope prior to surgery was 5.00 ± 2.37 degrees (mean ± SD) with 25% outliers (defined as <0 degree or >7 degrees) and after surgery the mean slope was 4.29 ± 3.24 degrees (mean ± SD) with 19% outliers. Sinha reported no failures using the system in their first 20 patients but reported one failure of tibial registration in their next 17 patients. This patient was successfully converted to a manual technique.

Coon et al.[12] compared 45 minimally invasive UKAs performed using manual instrumentation with 36 UKAs performed with RIO. A comparison of postoperative KSS showed was no significant difference in terms of average KSS, change in KSS, or Marmor ratings between the two groups. This suggested that the RIO provides comparable clinical results to manual techniques for UKA. Coon et al.[13] also compared a group of 44 UKAs performed using manual instrumentation with 33 UKAs using the RIO. The goal using both techniques was to match the natural tibial posterior slope. The results showed that the RMS error using the manual technique was 3.5 degrees and the error using the robotic system was 1.4 degrees. In the coronal plane the manual instruments resulted in an average error of 3.3 ± 1.8 degrees (SD) of varus compared with 0.1 ± 2.4 degrees (SD) for the robotic system. Thus the RIO resulted in improved accuracy in terms of implant placement during UKA when compared with manual instrumentation.

Hansen et al.[21] published a retrospective review of patients who had undergone robotic-assisted UKA (30 patients) using the MAKO system versus conventional UKA (32 patients). They found that both techniques resulted in excellent consistent outcomes with few complications. However, they found that there was little to no clinical or radiographic differences between the two groups and furthermore that the robotic-assisted UKA group took significantly longer (20 minutes). They suggested that for a high-volume surgeon who is well trained, the benefits may be limited and that an economical study may be warranted.

THE FUTURE

At this point, there is limited long-term data demonstrating the benefits of robotics for total knee replacement. However, it is clear that these systems improve the surgeon's ability to position an implant accurately based on his or her preoperative plan. Although each individual will likely have his or her "ideal position" for the implants, which may still need to be determined, it is clear that robotics can improve the surgeon's ability to achieve these targets. Each case must be individually planned preoperatively and the robotic system can execute the plan with precision that is not possible with conventional, manual techniques. Indeed, robotics may serve as the research tool to help to determine ideal implant position because its use can help to eliminate surgeon variability and enable true comparisons between various alignment techniques. In any case, surgical robots have demonstrated that current technology is capable of assisting in orthopedics, and it is likely that their use will continue to grow within the OR and the area of research.

The key to future acceptance of new technologies such as robotics is to demonstrate their benefits. Systems such as these may require substantial initial cost, in addition to recurring costs for disposables. However, if the improved precision and accuracy reduces the complications or improves long-term outcomes, these added costs may be justified. Currently these systems add time to the procedure. However, with increased development and acceptance, these times will be reduced such that robots can eventually become time neutral or perhaps even faster than the conventional techniques.

Furthermore, because a robot has significantly more versatility in terms of its ability to cut various geometries, the possibilities for new implant designs is tremendous. Current femoral implants rely on jigs to help to achieve five or six planar cuts. However, with a robot, the bone can be prepared such that less bone is removed and implants can truly be designed to only resurface the bone with curved backsides that match the patient's condyles. Furthermore, advances in 3D printing have made patient-specific implants a reality, and thus each patient's individual anatomy can be recreated exactly.

It is clear that robotic surgery seems to offer some definite benefits in terms of accuracy, precision, and reproducibility. The overall utility of these systems will be clarified over time as it is determined whether these benefits outweigh the associated costs. However, with time, these systems will become cheaper, smaller, faster, and easier to use and may eventually provide clinical benefits that cannot be attained with conventional instrumentation.

KEY REFERENCES

2. Bargar WL: Robots in orthopaedic surgery: past, present, and future. *Clin Orthop* 463:31–36, 2007.

5. Bellemans J, Vandenneucker H, Vanlauwe J: Robot-assisted total knee arthroplasty. *Clin Orthop* 464:111–116, 2007.

7. Bourne RB, Chesworth BM, Davis AM, et al: Patient satisfaction after total knee arthroplasty: who is satisfied and who is not? *Clin Orthop* 468:57–63, 2010.

8. Choong P, Dowsey MM, Stoney JD: Does accurate anatomical alignment result in better function and quality of life? Comparing conventional and computer-assisted total knee arthroplasty. *J Arthroplasty* 24(4):560–569, 2009.

10. Clark TC, Schmidt FH: Robot-assisted navigation versus computer-assisted navigation in primary total knee arthroplasty: efficiency and accuracy. *ISRN Orthop* 2013:1–6, 2013.

11. Cobb J, Henckel J, Gomes P, et al: Hands-on robotic unicompartmental knee replacement: a prospective, randomized controlled study of the acrobot system. *J Bone Joint Surg Br* 88-B:188–197, 2006.

14. Dunbar NJ, Roche MW, Park BH, et al: Accuracy of dynamic tactile-guided unicompartmental knee arthroplasty. *J Arthoplasty* 27:803–808, 2012.

21. Hansen DC, Kusuma SK, Palmer RM, et al: Robotic guidance does not improve component position or short-term outcome in medial unicompartmental knee arthroplasty. *J Arthroplasty* 29:1784–1789, 2014.

28. Kurtz SM, Ong KL, Lau E, et al: Impact of the economic downturn on total joint replacement demand in the United States. *J Bone Joint Surg Am* 96:624–630, 2014.

31. Liow MHL, Xia Z, Wong MK, et al: Robot-assisted total knee arthroplasty accurately restores the joint line and mechanical axis. A prospective randomised study. *J Arthroplasty* 29(12):2373–2377, 2014.

33. Lonner JH, John TK, Conditt MA: Robotic arm-assisted UKA improves tibial component alignment: a pilot study. *Clin Orthop* 468(1):141–146, 2010.

46. Parratte S, Pagnano MW, Trousdale RT, et al: Effect of postoperative mechanical axis alignment on the fifteen-year survival of modern, cemented total knee replacements. *J Bone Joint Surg Am* 92:2143–2149, 2010.

50. Picard F, Moody J, DiGioia IIIAM, et al: Clinical classifications of CAOS systems. In DiGioia IIIAM, Jaramaz B, Picard F, et al, editors: *Computer and robotic assisted hip and knee surgery*, New York, 2004, Oxford University Press, pp 43–48.

65. Song EK, Seon JK, Park SJ, et al: Simultaneous bilateral total knee replacement with robotic and conventional techniques: a prospective, randomized, comparative study. *Knee Surg Sports Traumatol Arthrosc* 19(7):1069–1076, 2011.

66. Song EK, Seon JK, Yim JH, et al: Robotic-assisted TKA reduces postoperative alignment outliers and improves gap balance compared to conventional TKA. *Clin Orthop* 471:118–126, 2013.

70. Swank ML, Alkire M, Conditt M, et al: Technology and cost-effectiveness in knee arthroplasty: computer navigation and robotics. *Am J Orthop* 38(Suppl 2):32–36, 2009.

The references for this chapter can also be found on www.expertconsult.com.

163

Robotic Unicompartmental Knee Arthroplasty

Aaron Althaus, William J. Long, Jonathan M. Vigdorchik

INTRODUCTION

Unicompartmental knee arthroplasty (UKA) has been shown to be a successful operation in appropriately selected patients.[1,3] Proponents cite bone and ligament preservation, adaptability to less invasive surgery, and improved biomechanics as advantages when comparing functional outcomes to total knee arthroplasty (TKA). Concerns remain because multiple studies have shown an increased revision rate when compared with TKA.[20,23] Theories for the increased revision rate include poor patient selection but also may be the result of technical factors, such as malpositioning of implants.[7,10,17] Robotic-assisted surgery was developed, in part, to improve the accuracy and precision of component placement, with the goal of improving clinical outcomes and decreasing revision rates.

Robotic technology for use in orthopedic surgery was first used by Dr. William Bargar in the late 1980s. His team developed the Robodoc system, with its first application designed to improve the placement of femoral stems in total hip arthroplasty.[24] The robot was physically attached to the femur by an external fixator and milled the femoral canal using three-dimensional (3D) data obtained from a computed tomography (CT) scan (Fig. 163.1). It was shown to improve the radiographic fit and fill of the stem in a precise manner and to limit the risk for fracture.[2] The technology was adapted for use in TKA to improve accuracy of bone cuts.[28] Precision and accuracy were indeed improved, yet widespread use in TKA has not been attained. Other applications of robotic technology have engendered considerable interest, specifically for use in UKA.

Haptics,[12] from the Greek *haptikos*, meaning able to touch or grasp, is a robotic technology designed to give human users the sensation of touch, either through changes in texture or production of a force to provide tactile feedback. Its first application was for safe handling of radioactive materials in the 1940s. Early designs used a mechanical linkage between the controller, who was behind a barrier, and the haptic arm. Currently computers have become the interface and no longer require physical connection between the human operator and the robotic arm.[13] The medical application of this technology began with interest in telemedicine and remote site surgery and has been used broadly in many surgical specialties. The typical use of the haptic device in the medical setting is as a semiactive robot, meaning that the robot does not perform surgical tasks but rather places limits on the surgeon's ability to deviate from the surgical plan.

Haptic robotic technology was first developed for use in UKA by Professor Justin Cobb and his team at Imperial College in London. The device was named Acrobot and was initially designed for use in TKA with application for use in UKA. A similar device, the RIO, Robotic Arm Interactive Orthopaedic System by Mako Surgical Corp (now Stryker Corp), was developed independently and has been used clinically in the United States since 2006 (Fig. 163.2). Both systems rely on preoperative CT scans and stereotactic boundary robotic arm, with Mako being a dynamic referencing system allowing the ability to change limb position during the procedure, whereas the Acrobot is a static referencing system in which the leg is required to be in one position. A newer system, Navio by Blue Belt Technologies, uses a handheld burring device and has the advantage of not requiring a preoperative CT scan (Fig. 163.3). Significant advances in robotic technology have allowed early clinical success but require further outcome studies.

ACROBOT

The Acrobot (Active Constraint Robot) haptic device was designed to improve the accuracy of bone cuts and restoration of mechanical axis for use in TKA. It was an alternative to some of the earlier robots used in orthopedic surgery, which were essentially modified industrial robots. It used a novel concept of "active constraint," which was defined as a synergy between the surgeon and the robot. The surgeon used his or her superior human tactile sensation with the advantage of using a robotic tool that was able to provide accuracy by use of preoperative CT scan for planning of the precise location of bone resection. The bone cutting was performed in a safe manner by a predefined 3D safe zone, which constrained the surgeon from straying off course from the surgical plan. Initial studies first on cadaver and plastic bone models showed accurate production of bone cuts reproducing the mechanical axis. Human trials were performed and confirmed the ability to produce accurate cuts but showed increased operative time.[15]

The Acrobot system was sold to Stanmore Implants, Worldwide in 2010. The Stanmore Sculptor Robotic Guidance Arm (RGA) obtained US Food and Drug Administration (FDA) clearance for use in the United States in 2013. Shortly afterwards Mako surgical purchased the robotic division of Stanmore and acquired the patents and technology of the Acrobot system. The Mako system has been in clinical use since 2006.[4]

MAKO

The Mako Surgical Corporation, now a part of Stryker Corporation, initially developed the Mako RIO for use in UKA.

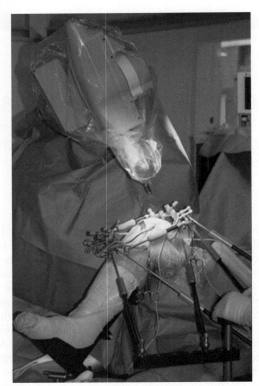

FIG 163.1 Intraoperative photo of the Acrobot robotic arm with the lower extremity secured to the table. (From Cobb J, Henckel J, Gomes P, et al: Hands-on robotic unicompartmental knee replacement. A prospective, randomized controlled study of the acrobot system. *J Bone Joint Surg Br* 88:188–197, 2006.)

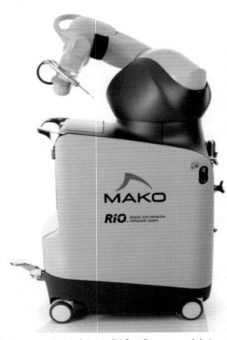

FIG 163.2 Image of the Mako RIO. (Courtesy Mako. Makoplasty partial knee arthroplasty. makosurgical.com. nd, Web, July 25, 2015.)

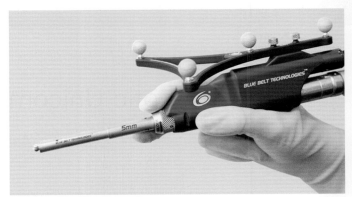

FIG 163.3 The Navio handheld burr with the tracking array attached. (Courtesy Navio Blue Belt Technologies, Inc.)

The first case was performed by Dr. Martin Roche in 2006. It has seen considerable growth since that time and is currently one of the most popular systems used in the United States. The platform consists of a robotic arm, optical infrared camera, and guidance module housing the planning software. RIO, Robotic Arm Interactive Orthopaedic Systems, uses stereotactic feedback for direct surgeon control. The infrared camera provides data on the 3D location of the involved knee by tracking the position of arrays placed on the femur and tibia. The computer system is able to combine preoperative and intraoperative data to create a 3D model to allow for precise planning of the resection of the bone required for optimal implant placement. For this to be possible, the patient must obtain a preoperative CT scan for planning purposes, with 5-mm slices through the hip and ankle and 1-mm slices through the knee joint.[8]

BLUE BELT TECHNOLOGIES

Navio PFS (Precision Freehand Sculptor) is a "semiactive" robot used for unicondylar knee arthroplasty. These robots combine the advantages of robots—repeatability and accuracy—with the flexibility, adaptability, and intelligence of a surgeon. Semiactive robots work in collaborative fashion, allowing the surgeon to make adjustments in real time.

Compared with a conventional robot, this is an intelligent tool that allows accuracy and precision in bone preparation. A major difference between the Navio PFS and the Mako RIO platform is that no preoperative CT imaging is needed. Instead of a CT scan, the PFS relies on a surface mapping or registration of the bone during the operation. Surgical planning is then performed in the same fashion as with conventional navigation systems, and after an appropriate plan is created, the bone is prepared with a handheld burr that is tied into real-time control loop that enables or disables the bone cutting relative to the surgical plan.[16]

OPERATIVE TECHNIQUE FOR MEDIAL UNICOMPARTMENTAL KNEE ARTHROPLASTY

3D data from the preoperative CT (Mako) or surface registration (Navio) are uploaded into the computer system, and a plan is created for implant placement. Overlapping computer-generated models of the femoral and tibial implants are

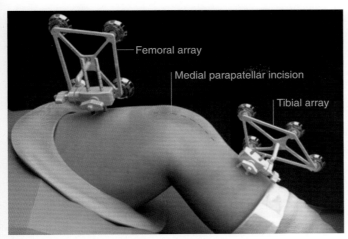

FIG 163.4 Representation of a lower extremity with the femoral and tibial arrays in place providing enough room for a medial parapatellar incision. (Courtesy Mako. Makoplasty partial knee arthroplasty. makosurgical.com. nd, Web, July 25, 2015.)

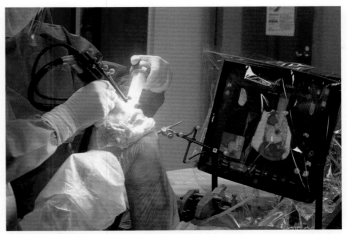

FIG 163.5 The Navio device during a cadaveric demonstration. The screen showing the progress of bone resection. (Courtesy Blue Belt Technologies, Inc., now acquired by Smith & Nephew Orthopaedics (Memphis, TN). From Jamamaz A, Nikou C, Simone A: Naviopfs for unicondylar knee replacement: early cadaver validation. *Bone Joint J* 95-B(Suppl 28):73, 2013.)

displayed and can be adjusted for optimal fit based on maximum implant coverage on bone, overall limb alignment, and presence of anatomic irregularities (periarticular cysts, etc.).

The procedure is performed on a standard operating table with a special leg holder attached to the bed. A limited incision technique may be performed, allowing for adequate exposure to the medial joint. Next, arrays are placed on the femur and tibia, allowing for freedom of motion of the limb to optimally access the joint (Fig. 163.4). Checkpoint pins are inserted, one on the femur and one of the tibia, achieving good bone purchase as these are used throughout the procedure for position reference and safety checks for the arrays.

Registration of landmarks is initiated by locating the hip center (by circumducting the hip) and the center of the tibial plafond (by using the blunt handheld probe and locating the medial and lateral malleoli). The femoral and tibial arrays are then verified, allowing the computer to generate various virtual landmarks based on the surface registration or CT plan. The sharp handheld probe is then used to localize these landmarks and create a map of the actual bone geometry, which corresponds to the digital data obtained from the preoperative CT scan (Mako) or the surface registration (Navio). It is important to note that osteophytes are left in place during the registration process.

After the femur and tibial registration is complete, the next step involves identifying the appropriate amount of correction for ideal soft tissue balancing. The osteophytes are now removed, relieving tension on the medial collateral ligament (MCL). The knee is taken through a range of motion while applying a valgus load to tension the MCL to assess the corrected flexion and extension gaps. At least four positions in the arc of motion are required to assess the gaps throughout the range of motion of the knee. The computer is able to account for the positioning of the implants and provides a graph showing the relative tightness and looseness in the arc of motion. With the implant positions determined, the next step involves using the robotic arm to resect the appropriate amount of bone needed to place the implants.

The robotic-arm mounted burr or the robotic arm is then moved into the operative field and registration is performed. The predefined volume of bone for resection is represented on the 3D model of the knee on the screen. The burring is performed safely either by the closed-loop feedback system of the Navio PFS or with stereotactic boundaries created by the Mako RIO, which creates a virtual wall that prevents resection outside of the boundaries. Resection of the femoral and tibial bone is performed along with peg holes that allow for accurate placement of the implants (Figs. 163.5 to 163.7). Following bone resection the remaining meniscus and cartilage is removed to allow for placement of the trial components. The trials are taken through a range of motion, allowing real-time evaluation of limb alignment and flexion and extension gaps. The final components are then cemented in place and the femoral and tibial arrays are removed. The skin is closed in a standard fashion, completing the procedure[8,16,21] (Fig. 163.8).

LITERATURE REVIEW

Robotic-assisted surgery is a new technology with relatively few studies available for review. Multiple bone model and cadaveric studies have shown reproducible accuracy in implant placement.[5,14,19,27] However, there are few clinical outcome studies, with most evaluating accuracy of implant placement versus conventional technique. At this time there is no clear evidence for improved patient satisfaction or decreased revision rates when comparing robotic technology to standard technique.

A prospective, randomized controlled trial by Cobb et al. compared the Acrobot system with conventional surgery. The authors randomized 27 patients indicated for medial compartment UKA to undergo either robotic-assisted or conventional surgery. They hypothesized that the Acrobot system would achieve more consistent angular alignment of the prosthesis and corresponding tibiofemoral alignment in the coronal plane than conventional instrumentation. All of the patients underwent preoperative CT scans, and surgical planning was made based on the findings. Following the procedure, all patients had a

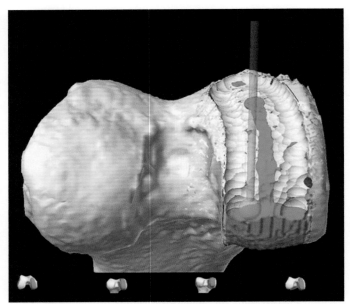

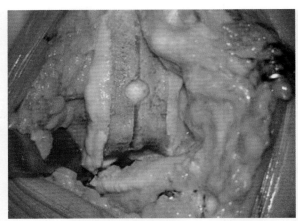

FIG 163.7 Image of the prepared femur following bone resection during a Makoplasty. (From Conditt MA, Roche MW: Minimally invasive robotic-arm-guided unicompartmental knee arthroplasty. *J Bone Joint Surg Am* 91:S63–S68, 2009.)

FIG 163.6 Image of the progress of bone resection while performing a Makoplasty medial unicompartmental knee arthroplasty. The green represents the remaining bone posteriorly planned for resection. (From Roche MW: Robotic-assisted unicompartmental knee arthroplasty: the MAKO experience. *Clin Sports Med* 33(1):123–132, 2014.)

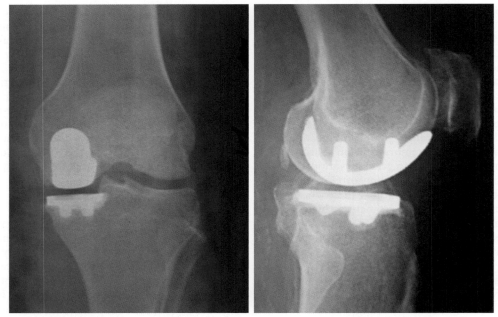

FIG 163.8 Anteroposterior (AP) and lateral films following Makoplasty with well-aligned components. (From Roche MW: Robotic-assisted unicompartmental knee arthroplasty: the MAKO experience. *Clin Sports Med* 33(1):123–132, 2014.)

second CT scan for confirmation of implant placement. The authors found that all of the patients in the Acrobot group had tibiofemoral alignment in the coronal plane within 2 degrees of the planned position, whereas only 40% of the conventional group achieved this level of accuracy. Operative times in the Acrobot group were found to be longer but did not result in increased complication rate. There was a trend toward improved Western Ontario, McMaster Universities Osteoarthritis Index and American Knee Society scores at 6 weeks and 3 months.[6]

Dunbar et al.[9] evaluated 20 of the first 50 cases using the Mako robotic-arm assisted UKA with dynamic referencing comparing the results with the paper written by Cobb et al., who used the

Acrobot, which used a static referencing system. The proposed advantage of the dynamic referencing system is the ability to use optical motion capture technology to dynamically track marker arrays fixed to the femur and tibia, allowing for freedom of limb positioning for ease of exposure and implant placement. The findings of the study showed that implant placement errors were comparable with the results seen from Cobb et al. One area of difference was noted with the proximal/distal placement of the femoral component, which showed slightly more error in the dynamically referenced group.

Lonner et al.[18] in a retrospective study evaluated the accuracy of tibial implant positioning on his first 31 cases using the Mako robotic-arm assisted UKA compared with 27 consecutive patients who underwent conventional technique. Preoperative radiographs were used to identify the ideal sagittal and coronal implant placement, which was compared with the postoperative radiographic results. The findings showed that with conventional technique the average error was 2.7 ± 2.1 more varus of the tibial component relative to the mechanical axis compared with 0.2 ± 1.8 with the robotic-arm assisted ($p < .00001$). The appropriate tibial slope was also shown to be more accurate in the robotic-arm assisted group. A limitation of the study was the short-term follow-up and that plain radiographs were used for measurement as opposed to the superior accuracy of CT scans.

Pearle et al.[25] showed excellent correlation between preoperative planning and postoperative outcomes with respect to tibiofemoral angle, which was within 1 degree, and long-leg axis radiographs, which was within 2 degrees. Plate et al.[26] showed that robotic-assisted UKA was able to accurately balance the knee to within 1 mL of medial opening in the vast majority of cases throughout the range of motion. Mofidi et al.[22] confirmed accuracy in placement of implants by comparing intraoperative planned measurements to postoperative radiographic measurements and further evaluated the cases that were less accurately placed. They concluded that the inaccurately placed implants were likely due to poor cementation technique and stressed the importance of ensuring that the implants are seated perfectly and pressurized during implantation.

Despite the promising aspects of robotic-arm assisted surgery, some evidence suggests that there is no meaningful improvement in the accuracy of implant placement or short-term clinical benefit. In a retrospective review of a matched group of patients, Hansen et al.[11] compared the use of robotic-arm assisted UKA to a standard operative technique and found only minimal radiographic differences. Notably there was no significant difference in postoperative tibial coronal alignment. However, the authors did note improvement in recreating the femoral axis, as well as less medial overhang of the tibial component, in the robotic-arm assisted group. The operative time in the robot-arm assisted group was significantly greater, with an average increase of 20 minutes. In addition, there was a significant reduction in average time to physical therapy clearance (10.3 hours less), and the average length of stay was 9 hours less in the robotic-arm assisted group. The authors concluded that there is minimal clinical benefit to using robot-arm assisted UKA compared with conventional technique, especially when performed by a high-volume surgeon.

CONCLUSION

There are currently no long-term outcome studies documenting improvements in outcome scores or revision rates when using robotic UKA versus conventional technique. Several studies document an improvement in accuracy of implantation both in cadaveric and in clinical series. It is reasonable to hypothesize that an improvement in accuracy of implant placement would result in improved longevity, but there is no evidence at present to support this hypothesis, and the ideal position for implants has not been determined. Future robot-assisted UKA studies should focus on attempts to document clear benefit of using robotic technology over conventional technique.

KEY REFERENCES

1. Baker P, Jameson S, Critchley R, et al: Center and surgeon volume influence the revision rate following unicondylar knee replacement: an analysis of 23,400 medial cemented unicondylar knee replacements. *J Bone Joint Surg Am* 95:702–709, 2013.
5. Citak M, Suero EM, Citak M, et al: Unicompartmental knee arthroplasty: is robotic technology more accurate than conventional technique? *Knee* 20:268–271, 2013.
6. Cobb J, Henckel J, Gomes P, et al: Hands-on robotic unicompartmental knee replacement. A prospective, randomized controlled study of the acrobot system. *J Bone Joint Surg Br* 88:188–197, 2006.
7. Collier MB, Eickmann TH, Sukezaki F, et al: Patient, implant, and alignment factors associated with revision of medial compartment unicondylar arthroplasty. *J Arthroplasty* 21:108–115, 2006.
8. Conditt MA, Roche MW: Minimally invasive robotic-arm-guided unicompartmental knee arthroplasty. *J Bone Joint Surg Am* 91:S63–S68, 2009.
9. Dunbar NJ, Roche MW, Park BH, et al: Accuracy of dynamic tactile-guided unicompartmental knee arthroplasty. *J Arthroplasty* 27:803–808. e1, 2012.
10. Epinette JA, Brunschweiler B, Mertl P, et al: Unicompartmental knee arthroplasty modes of failure: wear is not the main reason for failure: a multicentre study of 418 failed knees. *Orthop Traumatol Surg Res* 98:S124–S130, 2012.
11. Hansen DC, Kusuma SK, Palmer RM, et al: Robotic guidance does not improve component position or short-term outcome in medial unicompartmental knee arthroplasty. *J Arthroplasty* 29:1784–1789, 2014.
18. Lonner J, John TK, Conditt MA: Robotic arm-assisted UKA improves tibial component alignment: a pilot study. *Clin Orthop* 468:141–146, 2010.
19. Lonner JH, Smith JR, Picard F, et al: High degree of accuracy of a novel image-free handheld robot for unicondylar knee arthroplasty in a cadaveric study. *Clin Orthop* 473:206–212, 2015.
23. Niinimaki T, Eskelinen A, Makela K, et al: Unicompartmental knee arthroplasty survivorship is lower than TKA survivorship: a 27-year Finnish registry study. *Clin Orthop* 472:1496–1501, 2014.
24. Paul HA, Bargar WL, Mittlestadt B, et al: Development of a surgical robot for cementless total hip arthroplasty. *Clin Orthop* 285:57–66, 1992.
25. Pearle AD, O'Loughlin PF, Kendoff DO: Robot-assisted unicompartmental knee arthroplasty. *J Arthroplasty* 25:230–237, 2010.
26. Plate JF, Mofidi A, Mannava S: Achieving accurate ligament balancing using robotic-assisted unicompartmental knee arthroplasty. *Adv Orthop* 2013:837167, 2013.
28. Song EK, Seon JK, Yim JH, et al: Robotic-assisted TKA reduces postoperative alignment outliers and improves gap balance compared to conventional TKA. *Clin Orthop* 471:118–126, 2013.

The references for this chapter can also be found on www.expertconsult.com.

164

Management of Extra-Articular Deformity in Total Knee Arthroplasty With Navigation

Clint Wooten, J. Bohannon Mason

Total knee arthroplasty (TKA) is challenging in the presence of extra-articular deformity because the anatomic landmarks may be altered, traditional instrumentation may not be applicable, and ligament balance may be compromised. In addition, with prior surgery, complicating hardware may be present. The ability to obtain a neutral mechanical axis is reported to be central to the long-term survival of total knee replacements.[18,34,51,54] In most TKAs performed for arthritic knees with intra-articular varus or valgus deformity, the surgeon is able to obtain appropriate alignment and ligament balancing through bone cuts and soft tissue releases. Extra-articular deformities, particularly of the femur, require placement of implants often at odds with the usual referenced bone landmarks to achieve a summed mechanical axis that is neutral and perpendicular to the ground at the joint line.[11,33] The intramedullary canal used to assist with femoral component alignment instrumentation may be blocked by callus from a malunited fracture or obstructed with previously placed hardware. The diaphyseal canal additionally may be offset from the metaphysis, resulting in sagittal or coronal plane deformities.

These deformities are not new, and surgeons for the past 35 years have attempted to compensate for them with "best guess" measure and cut techniques or with more sophisticated alignment systems.[3,27,44] In recent years, imageless computer-assisted navigation systems have been developed that allow surgeons to accurately plan and execute bone resections in TKA based on a virtual mechanical axis, which is calculated by using the center of the femoral head, the center of the knee joint, and the center of the ankle.[19,29,31] Numerous studies have shown the accuracy of this navigation technology, often reporting fewer outliers in sagittal and coronal plane alignment compared with manual conventional total knee instrumentation.* Although debate over the utility of computer-assisted total knee for routine total knee surgery continues, focusing on the cost of the technology, surgical time investment, and the impact of error reduction on revision rates,[32,36,47,48,55] one distinct area of benefit of computer-assisted navigation is help with the management of extra-articular deformity.

EXTRA-ARTICULAR DEFORMITIES: INTRA-ARTICULAR VERSUS EXTRA-ARTICULAR CORRECTION

Painful arthritis resulting in the need for total knee replacement may occur in association with extra-articular deformity of the

femur or tibia. These deformities are typically the result of prior trauma with malunited fractures, but they can result from other conditions, such as prior corrective osteotomies and metabolic conditions, such as Blount or Paget disease, tertiary syphilis, or rickets.[53] Often the surgeon is forced to consider the possible presence of confounding hardware or a tortuous relationship of the diaphysis to the metaphysis, which may prevent the passage of intramedullary guide instrumentation or may complicate the placement of stems required for secondary stabilization of the implant (Fig. 164.1).

Strategies for management of extra-articular deformity include performing simultaneous corrective osteotomies at the time of total knee, with restoration of the diaphyseal to metaphyseal relationship,[12,26,38,39] or correction of the deformity within the joint via corrective bone resections and subsequent soft tissue balancing to allow implant stability throughout the motion arc of the knee.[53] However, realignment in such limbs can require extensive soft tissue release, and achieving coronal balance can be challenging. The strategy of intra-articular correction with soft tissue balancing is appealing because it is more efficient for the surgeon. It does not require creating an osteotomy that needs to be stabilized and healed. However, if the degree of deformity would require a bone resection that extends to the epicondylar attachment of the collateral ligaments, ligament integrity may be compromised and constrained implants may be required.[14,38] Extra-articular deformities that are close to the joint line are challenging because the local bony morphology may be distorted and can make optimal component positioning and alignment difficult to achieve. In some cases a better strategy is a corrective osteotomy, which can be performed either simultaneously or in a staged fashion (Fig. 164.2A to C).

Some authors have argued that when deformities of the distal femur or proximal tibia exceed 15 degrees, because of the difficulty associated with simultaneous osteotomy and total knee replacement, corrective osteotomies should be performed and allowed to heal before total knee replacement surgery is performed.[8,32,34,43] Wang and Wang[53] reported on 15 patients with extra-articular deformities and arthritis treated with total knee replacement using intra-articular bone resections and soft tissue releases to achieve correction of mechanical alignment. The authors stressed the importance of long-standing films to outline the deformity. Using line drawings, they determined whether the intra-articular bone resection necessary to correct the mechanical axis of the extremity would pass through the insertion of the collateral ligaments. Successful intra-articular correction was attained when coronal plane resections were less than 20 degrees and/or sagittal plane resections less than 25

---

*References 2, 9, 10, 16, 30, and 53.

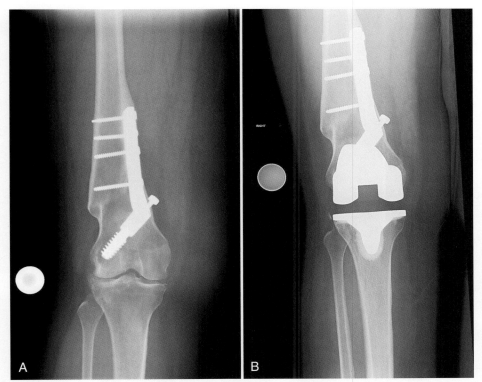

FIG 164.1 (A) Anteroposterior (AP) radiograph of a patient with translational deformity status post osteotomy of the distal femur. (B) Using intraoperative navigation, the axial alignment was corrected to neutral. Traditional instrumentation would be difficult to use because of the femoral deformity and the retained hardware.

degrees in the femur, or less than 30 degrees in coronal plane alignment of the tibia and when the deformity was an adequate distance from the joint line.

Wolff et al.[56] stressed the relationship between degree of deformity and distance from the joint line. The closer the deformity apex is to the joint line, the greater the impact is on soft tissue releases necessary for balancing. In addition, the authors noted that deformities of the tibia are easier to correct at the time of total joint replacement than those of the femur before the ligaments are balanced. Compensatory wedge resections necessary for axial correction of femoral deformities result in an asymmetrical extension space, with reduced impact on flexion balance. In contrast, correction of tibial deformity by compensatory wedge resection equally impacts flexion and extension spaces. Finally, varus deformities that cannot be completely balanced via intra-articular correction and soft tissue releases produce subtle lateral laxity that can be tolerated if the alignment is proper. In contrast, valgus deformity that cannot be completely balanced leads to medial laxity, which is much less tolerated.[56] These authors also concluded that in cases of extreme deformity wherein intra-articular resection is unlikely to yield satisfactory ligament balance, extra-articular osteotomy is indicated. Severe femoral bowing and severe lateral laxity in varus arthritic knees with or without medial soft tissue contracture should alert the surgeon that realignment and balancing may be difficult via intra-articular resection.

With coronal plane deformity of less than 20 degrees in the femur or less than 30 degrees in the tibia, intra-articular correction with total knee replacement is advantageous.[26,28,56]

One-stage correction of these deformities eliminates the risks associated with a possible second incision for the osteotomy, nonunion of the osteotomy, the need for osteotomy-stabilizing hardware, and potential delay in rehabilitation related to the osteotomy. For these reasons, when possible, one-stage intra-articular correction is preferable to performing a corrective osteotomy.

RATIONALE FOR TOTAL KNEE ARTHROPLASTY WITH NAVIGATION IN THE MANAGEMENT OF EXTRA-ARTICULAR DEFORMITIES ABOUT THE KNEE

Optimal component alignment and positioning are critical to the long-term clinical success of total knee replacement.[4,18,41,42,45] Failure to achieve optimal positioning of prosthetic knee implants can result in instability, increased pain, decreased range of motion, increased polyethylene wear, and implant loosening.[5,14,17,22,51] The challenges of alignment and positioning in routine total knee replacement surgery and its association with compromised results when these goals are not achieved have led to the development of numerous systems and alignment guides designed to achieve neutral mechanical alignment and correct component rotation. These mechanical alignment systems include intramedullary and extramedullary guide rod systems that have inherent limitations in accuracy.[24,50] Despite surgical experience and improved mechanical alignment devices, errors in postoperative alignment in total knee surgery

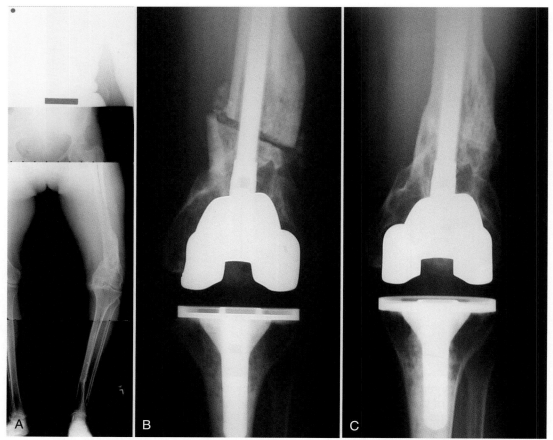

FIG 164.2 (A) AP radiograph showing coronal plane deformity because of a malunited distal femoral fracture. Intra-articular correction would sacrifice the integrity of the lateral collateral ligament. (B) Navigation-assisted distal femoral osteotomy is stabilized with a fluted press-fit stem. (C) Three-year postoperative AP radiograph showing union of the osteotomy.

still occur.[49] Optical navigation systems—so-called imageless navigation—have become readily available in operating theaters around the world. Endorsement in multiple centers has allowed evaluation of the accuracy of the navigation systems, as well as comparative assessment versus manual instrumentation. Meta-analysis of available data suggests that these systems can deliver coronal and sagittal plane alignment that is superior to that attained with manual instrumentation.[29]

Although adoption of computer-assisted navigation for routine total knee replacement is hampered by the cost of the instrumentation, operative time requirements, and the paucity of literature linking its use to improved clinical outcomes,[46] the value of this technology is uniquely leveraged when patients present with extra-articular deformity, retained hardware, or both (Fig. 164.3A and B). With computer-assisted navigation systems, the mechanical axis for the femur is determined irrespective of the bone between the femoral head and the central portion of the distal femur and similarly between the central aspect of the tibia and the ankle. By virtually linking these points through imageless navigation, a mechanical axis is automatically calculated. In contrast, conventional instrumentation in the presence of obstructing hardware, a tortuous medullary canal, or complete occlusion of the medullary canal would require extramedullary alignment devices, osteotomy, or removal of the obstructing hardware. Digital mapping of the

hip center of rotation, articular portions of the knee, and the ankle center offers the surgeon a clinical solution to the obstacles associated with extra-articular deformity.

In the relatively common presentation of patients with arthritis of the knee and retained hardware, the advantage of navigation is unique (Fig. 164.4A and B). Two scenarios may present. The first is hardware that for structural reasons may not be removed and that obstructs the use of conventional intramedullary instrumentation. In the second presentation, removal of the hardware is structurally feasible but requires greater surgical exposure, operative time, and risk to the patient. In these cases, navigation may represent a better option for the surgeon.

SURGICAL TECHNIQUE: NAVIGATION FOR EXTRA-ARTICULAR DEFORMITIES NOT REQUIRING OSTEOTOMY

Standard midline incision and medial parapatellar arthrotomy are recommended to facilitate any extensile approaches required. Imageless navigation requires placement of reference arrays, either active emitting or passive reflective (manufacturer dependent), which present a stereographic series of at least three points that the computer can record. Biopic cameras

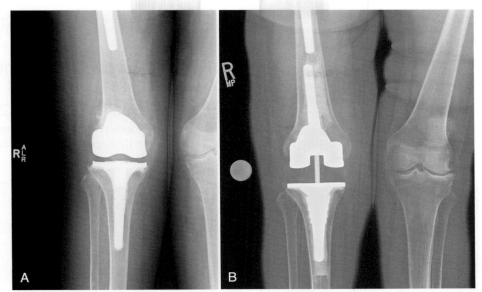

FIG 164.3 (A) AP radiograph of a patient with a failed TKA because of valgus instability. (B) Navigation was helpful in this revision situation because the femoral canal was blocked by a femoral hip stem.

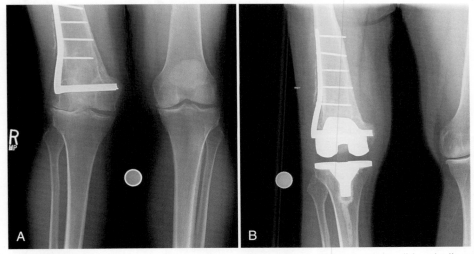

FIG 164.4 (A) Hardware from prior surgery can present a challenge to traditional alignment instrumentation. (B) Computer-assisted navigation was used, obviating the need for increased surgical exposure and hardware removal.

record the location of the position of the array, and using trigonometric algorithms can fix and follow the points, and hence the bone, in space. The bone model is created by registering the center of the femoral head as the central rotation point when the femur is taken through a range of motion and a series of distal points are collected with a stylus, which is also visible to the computer. The center of the distal femur, the condylar morphology, and the epicondylar axis are typically collected. The tibia is modeled in a similar fashion; after collecting the central axis point within the footprint of the anterior cruciate ligament and surface points defining the medial and lateral tibial plateaus, the surgeon estimates the anterior to posterior axis of the proximal tibia and uses the malleoli to establish the ankle center.

The mechanical axis of the extremity prior to bone resection can then be recorded. Standard navigation cutting guides are used to perform a distal femoral resection perpendicular to the mechanical axis of the femur; the proximal tibial resection is performed at 90 degrees to the long axis of the tibia. Soft tissue releases are governed by the residual soft tissue tension, which can be assessed with a tensioning device, with lamina spreaders, or manually. Releases proceed until a rectangular extension gap is obtained.

In cases with deformity primarily in the coronal plane, rotational alignment of the femoral component may be based on routine landmarks, such as the transverse epicondylar axis. Unfortunately, in patients with extra-articular deformities, simple coronal deformity is uncommon and is often associated with rotational deformities. The correct rotational position of the femoral implant is perpendicular to the resected surface of the proximal tibia when the knee is flexed and the ligaments are tensed. Consequently, after sufficient releases are obtained in extension to create a rectangular extension space, classic gap balancing techniques are used to obtain femoral rotation in flexion, while tensioning the collateral ligaments at 90 degrees of flexion and making anterior and posterior femoral cuts parallel to the tibial cut. Most navigation balancing algorithms assist the surgeon in referencing the femoral rotation to the resected tibial plane. After femoral rotation is determined, femoral bone resections are completed (Fig. 164.5).

SURGICAL TECHNIQUE: NAVIGATION FOR EXTRA-ARTICULAR DEFORMITIES REQUIRING OSTEOTOMY

As discussed previously, the amount of bone resection necessary to correct extremity alignment to a neutral mechanical axis is

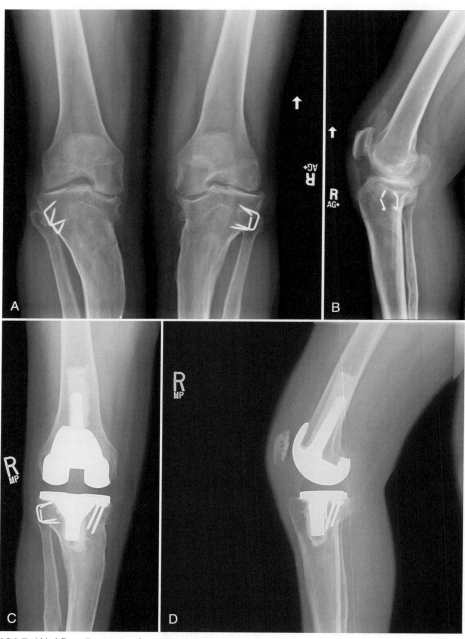

FIG 164.5 (A) AP radiograph of a 68-year-old male with profound deformity of the proximal tibia post osteotomy and prior fracture. (B) Lateral radiograph showing sagittal plane deformity of the proximal tibia. (C) AP postoperative film of the same patient. Navigation was helpful to establish neutral axial alignment despite the significant tibial deformity. (D) Lateral postoperative radiograph.

positively related to the degree of deformity and is inversely related to the distance of the deformity from the joint line.[56] In instances in which preoperative planning indicates that the scale of bone resection required to correct femoral coronal plane alignment would result in resection of the origin of either collateral ligament, or exceeds 30 degrees of correction within the tibia, an associated osteotomy should be considered.[53] The surgical technique used for navigation in these cases varies from that used in intra-articular correction because the optical tracking reference to the osteotomized bone segment can be lost after the osteotomy is performed.

When an osteotomy of the femur is anticipated, the femoral array should be placed proximal to the planned osteotomy. Pins generally should be unicortical to avoid interference with stabilizing intramedullary stems, if used. The surgical approach and registration of the bone are identical to those of navigation techniques used for deformity when no osteotomy is required. Soft tissue releases are minimized because alignment correction is achieved via the osteotomy proximal to capsular and collateral ligament origins. First, the navigated tibial resection is performed perpendicular to the long axis of the tibia (Fig. 164.6A to D). Next, with the extremity in extension, the collateral ligaments are tensed with lamina spreaders or a commercial tensioning device. With equal tension medially and laterally, the mechanical axis of the extremity is recorded by the navigation system. The degree of mechanical axis error from neutral is

noted, and a corresponding resection of the distal femur is performed parallel to the proximal tibial resection (coplanar if the tibia is resected at 0 degrees of slope). In appropriate circumstances, biplanar correction through the osteotomy is facilitated by the bone model created from registration of the bone anatomy. In such cases the anterior cortex of the distal femur is referenced to the sagittal axis of the femur, and this angular difference is considered in the osteotomy. After being performed, the osteotomy is collapsed and stabilized with medullary reamers and/or bone clamps, while the remaining femoral resections are completed. Rotational alignment should be clearly marked on the femoral bone traversing the osteotomy before the osteotomy is performed. The correct mechanical axis can be confirmed with trial components in place.

Navigated alignment correction when a tibial osteotomy is anticipated for extra-articular deformity is similar to the technique for the femur but differs in the sequence of resections. In these cases, minimal soft tissue releases are again required. The tibial array is secured to the tibia in the diaphyseal region, below the osteotomy site, which is at the metaphyseal-diaphyseal junction, distal to the medial collateral ligament insertion and the tubercle. After completion of the femoral bone cuts, the extremity again is brought to full extension, and the collateral ligaments are tensioned. Axial alignment of the distorted extremity is recorded with the navigation system. The proximal tibial resection is performed with the navigated cutting guides at the "angle

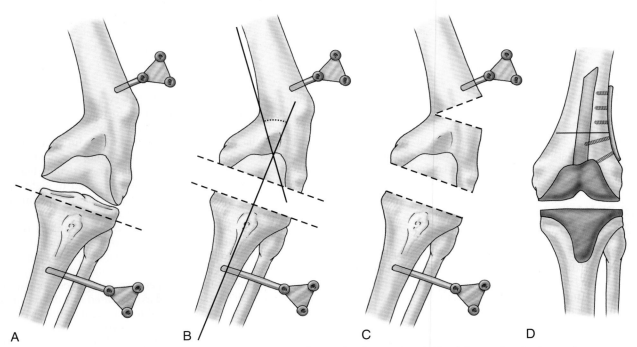

A   B   C   D

FIG 164.6 (A) Sequence of surgical steps for navigation-assisted distal femoral osteotomy for severe extra-articular deformity. The array of the femur is positioned proximal to the planned osteotomy. The proximal tibial resection is performed at 90 degrees to the long axis of the tibia. (B) The collateral ligaments are tensioned in extension, and the overall limb alignment is recorded. A distal femoral resection of appropriate depth was navigated and made parallel to the proximal tibial resection. (C) The difference between the overall limb alignment and a neutral mechanical axis is the angle of the corrective osteotomy. The plane orientation tool in most navigation systems is used to navigate the angle for the osteotomy. (D) The osteotomy is collapsed and stabilized. The surgeon should note the rotational alignment of the femur before performing the osteotomy.

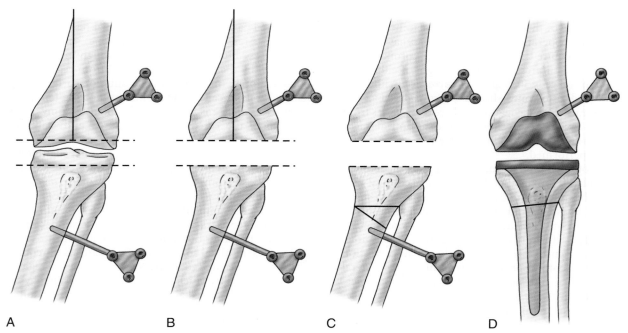

A   B   C   D

FIG 164.7 (A) Navigation arrays are placed distal to the anticipated osteotomy. (B) Distal femoral resection is performed as usual. The proximal tibial resection is performed parallel to the distal femoral resection after tensioning of the collateral ligament structures in extension. (C) The resultant angle of "error" between extremity positions in extension, with collateral ligament tension equilibrated, is the angle of the wedge osteotomy. (Technical note: Spacer blocks are useful in stabilizing the extremity while the osteotomy is navigated.) (D) The osteotomy is performed distal to the tibial tubercle and collateral insertions and is transfixed with a tight diaphyseal fitting stem. (Technical note: The distal navigation array may need to be removed before the stem is placed.)

of error" of the extremity (Fig. 164.7A to D). This resection plane is parallel to the distal resected femur, creating a rectangular extension space. A wedge osteotomy of equal angle is removed from the tibia at the metaphyseal-diaphyseal junction. The osteotomy is collapsed and stabilized with a tightly reamed, fluted tibial stem. In cases of extreme tibial correction a fibular osteotomy additionally may be required.

RESULTS OF NAVIGATION FOR EXTRA-ARTICULAR DEFORMITY

Klein et al.[21] first reported on the use of navigation-assisted TKA in patients with extra-articular deformity, retained hardware preventing standard intramedullary alignment instrumentation, or intramedullary implants. In this case series of five patients, collected from the senior author's experience with more than 500 primary and revision total knees over 2 years, TKA was successfully completed with navigation. The mechanical axis was restored to within 1 degree of neutral in four of five patients and to within 2 degrees in the fifth. Klein et al. recognized that the risks associated with hardware removal, including multiple surgeries, multiple incisions or elevation of larger flaps to gain access to remove hardware, and creation of stress risers in the bone after removal of screws (which potentially requires additional support, such as addition of stems, struts, or intramedullary (IM) rods), were obviated with the use of navigation.

We reported on 16 patients requiring TKA for advanced osteoarthritis, in whom navigation was used to achieve alignment.[14] Standard intramedullary alignment guides could not be used because of angular deformity, obliteration of the canal, or use of intramedullary hardware or when standard intramedullary guides were believed to be clinically contraindicated (prior osteomyelitis or severe cardiopulmonary compromise). Nine of 16 patients had severe extra-articular deformities. The mechanical axis was accurately restored in eight of these nine. We concluded that in such patients, navigation was of direct benefit for both the surgeon and patient.

Chou et al.[11] reported a single case of femoral deformity because of a malunited distal femur with a coronal plane angulation of 15 degrees of varus and a sagittal plane angulation of 8.7 degrees. Navigation was "feasible and satisfactory" in this patient; however, the postoperative component position was not reported. The mechanical axis resulted in 1 degree of varus. Kim et al.[20] reported a series of four patients with severe extra-articular femoral deformities managed with navigation-assisted minimally invasive knee arthroplasty. The authors argued that the advantages of minimally invasive knee surgery (MIS), namely, decreased pain, faster recovery, and improved function,[1,6,23,25] justified the potential reported disadvantages, including improper component alignment and orientation because of inadequate exposure.[1,13] Investigators postulated that the increased accuracy of computer-assisted surgery may compensate for the possible alignment complications associated with MIS. Mean mechanical axis alignment improved from 15.1 degrees to 0.3 degrees (range: −1.2 to 0.5 degrees), and no complications were related to the MIS technique or the use of navigation. In addition, significant improvement in function, Knee Society score, and SF-36 score was reported.

Bottros et al.[7] reported a series of nine knees (seven patients) with femoral extra-articular deformities severe enough to prevent the use of standard intramedullary alignment rods and advanced osteoarthritis necessitating total knee replacement. With the use of imageless navigation, the mean mechanical axis deviation postoperatively was 1.3 degrees (range: −0.2 to 2.5 degrees). The authors reported clinical outcomes, noting improvement in Knee Society score from a mean of 62 preoperatively to 92 postoperatively and in function scores (from 52 to 83; $p < .05$) and range of motion (from a mean of 4 to 74 degrees to 0.6 to 98 degrees; $p < .05$) at 12-month follow-up. Despite distorted anatomic landmarks and extra-articular femoral deformity, navigation was a useful and accurate tool for patients.

Tigani et al.[52] reported on a series of 14 cases in which ideal mechanical and prosthetic alignment were achieved with computer-assisted navigation systems because of extra-articular deformity (nine patients) or retained hardware (five patients). Of the nine patients with extra-articular deformity, the deformity followed a fracture in five cases, three involving the femur and two on the tibia. In one patient it was secondary to a supracondylar femoral osteotomy, and in the other case the deformity involved both the femur (10 degrees valgus) and tibia (15 degrees of valgus). The last two had posttraumatic deformities with an ipsilateral hip stem. Clinical outcomes were reported with a mean follow-up of 28 months, noting Knee Society score improvement from a mean of 33 preoperatively to 78 postoperatively and in functional scores (from 32 to 72; $p < .05$). Postoperative mechanical axis ranged between 3 degrees of varus and 3 degrees of valgus.

The largest reported series to date of extra-articular deformities about the knee corrected with the assistance of computer navigation was reported by Mullaji and Shetty,[33] who managed 40 severe extra-articular deformities in 34 patients. Twenty-two were femoral deformities, and 18 were tibial. The mean deformity was 9.3 degrees. Three of the 40 patients required simultaneous corrective osteotomy. In addition to reporting sagittal plane correction to a mean mechanical axis deviation of 1 degree (standard deviation, 1.4 degrees), the authors described similarly accurate results for coronal plane alignment postoperatively, noting that this is the only report on excessive coronal plane alignment complicating TKA managed with computer-assisted navigation. Papadopoulos et al.[37] reported on a series of patients who were treated with simultaneous corrective osteotomy and saw increased risk of restricted motion and 50% of patients without optimal component position or axial alignment in the absence of computer navigation assistance; in contrast, Mullaji noted no complications in patients treated with an osteotomy. Other authors have highlighted the challenges of simultaneous corrective osteotomy at the time of total knee replacement, including risks of nonunion, arthrofibrosis, infection, and pulmonary embolism.[26] Consequently, Mullaji notes that surgeons undertaking simultaneous corrective osteotomies with navigation assistance should be well versed in navigation before they apply combined techniques.

A recent study by Rajgopal et al.[40] looked at 36 knees in 32 patients with arthritis associated with extra-articular deformity. All patients had intra-articular resection with soft tissue balancing to correct the deformity. Mean follow-up was 85 months. Amenable deformities were coronal plane deformities of the femur 11 to 18 degrees, sagittal plane deformities 0 to 15 degrees, and tibial deformities in the coronal plane 12 to 24 degrees. There was an improvement in range of motion from a mean of 54 degrees preoperatively to 114 degrees postoperatively ($p < .05$). The Knee Society score improved from 37 points to 85 points postoperatively ($p < .05$). The functional score improved from a mean value of 19 to a mean of 69.5 at follow-up ($p < .01$). The preoperative hip-knee-ankle angle in the coronal plane improved from a mean of 14 ± 2 degrees varus to a mean of 2 ± 0.6 degrees varus. Computer navigation was considered only in severe multiplaner or rotational deformities or in knees where intramedullary instrumentation could not be used ($n = 4$).

CONCLUSIONS

TKA in the presence of extra-articular deformity has always been a challenge because the typical alignment references are frequently absent or distorted and traditional alignment guides cannot be used accurately because of hardware, malunion, or metabolic conditions. Computer-assisted surgical navigation offers a new tool for surgeons who undertake these difficult cases, allowing intraoperative spatial feedback to the operating surgeon that can be used to orient bone resections and occasionally osteotomies. Emerging data suggest that computer navigation in the clinical setting of total knee replacement surgery can be used to accurately align implants with the mechanical axis in the coronal and sagittal planes. Extension of these navigation techniques to difficult cases with extra-articular deformity is only logical because traditional tools for alignment are often precluded by the deformity itself. As clinical data are accumulated via case series and more rigorous studies, intraoperative computer-assisted navigation will remain a useful adjunctive technique in these difficult cases.

KEY REFERENCES

7. Bottros J, Klika AK, Lee HH, et al: The use of navigation in total knee arthroplasty for patients with extra-articular deformity. *J Arthroplasty* 23:74, 2008.

11. Chou WY, Ko JY, Wang CJ, et al: Navigation-assisted total knee arthroplasty for a knee with malunion of the distal femur. *J Arthroplasty* 23:8, 2008.

14. Fehring TK, Mason JB, Moskal J, et al: When computer-assisted knee replacement is the best alternative. *Clin Orthop* 452:132, 2006.

20. Kim K, Ramteke AA, Bae DK: Navigation-assisted minimal invasive total knee arthroplasty in patients with extra-articular femoral deformity. *J Arthroplasty* 25:658, 2010.

26. Lonner JH, Siliski JM, Lotke PA: Simultaneous femoral osteotomy and total knee arthroplasty for treatment of osteoarthritis associated with severe extra-articular deformity. *J Bone Joint Surg Am* 82:342, 2000.

27. Mann JW, III: Total knee replacement with associated extra-articular angular deformity of the femur. In Scuderi GR, Tria AJ, Jr, editors: *Surgical techniques in total knee arthroplasty*, New York, NY, 2002, Springer-Verlag, p 636.

29. Mason JB, Fehring TK, Estok R, et al: Meta-analysis of alignment outcomes in computer-assisted total knee arthroplasty surgery. *J Arthroplasty* 22:1097, 2007.

30. Matziolis G, Krocker D, Weiss U, et al: A prospective, randomized study of computer-assisted and conventional total knee arthroplasty: three-dimensional evaluation of implant alignment and rotation. *J Bone Joint Surg Am* 89:236, 2007.

33. Mullaji A, Shetty GM: Computer-assisted total knee arthroplasty for arthritis with extra-articular deformity. *J Arthroplasty* 24:8, 2009.

37. Papadopoulos EC, Parvizi J, Lai CH, et al: Total knee arthroplasty following prior distal femoral fracture. *Knee* 9:267, 2002.

38. Papagelopoulos PJ, Karachalios T, Themistocleous GS, et al: Total knee arthroplasty in patients with pre-existing fracture deformity. *Orthopedics* 30:373, 2007.

39. Radke S, Radke J: Total knee arthroplasty in combination with a one-stage tibial osteotomy: a technique for correction of a gonarthrosis with a severe (>15 degrees) tibial extra-articular deformity. *J Arthroplasty* 17:533, 2002.

47. Slover JD, Tosteson A, Bozic KJ, et al: Impact of hospital volume on the economic value of computer navigation for total knee replacement. *J Bone Joint Surg Am* 90:1492, 2008.

48. Sparmann M, Wolke B, Czupalla H, et al: Positioning of total knee arthroplasty with and without navigation support: a prospective, randomized study. *J Bone Joint Surg Br* 85:830, 2003.

53. Wang JW, Wang CJ: Total knee arthroplasty for arthritis of the knee with extra-articular deformity. *J Bone Joint Surg Am* 84:1769, 2002.

The references for this chapter can also be found on www.expertconsult.com.

165

Computer-Assisted Total Knee Arthroplasty for Extramedullary Deformity

Peter Pyrko, Matthew S. Austin

INTRODUCTION

In 1977, Lotke and Ecker demonstrated that malalignment of total knee arthroplasty (TKA) components resulted in an increased risk of early failure.[11] Subsequently, several studies have demonstrated that achieving alignment to within 3 degrees of a neutral mechanical axis improves outcome scores and is associated with lower aseptic failure rates.[2,5,14,15] There is considerable debate over the merits of computer assisted orthopedic surgery (CAOS) for uncomplicated TKA.[7] The majority of the literature has demonstrated that CAOS can reduce the number of "outliers" from acceptable coronal plane alignment.[10,16-19] "Outliers" are cases that fall outside the accepted range from neutral alignment. The goal of restoring alignment to a neutral mechanical axis can be made more challenging in patients with excessive bowing, congenital deformity, posttraumatic deformity with medullary discontinuity or intramedullary ossification, and/or the presence of intramedullary hardware from prior surgical procedures. CAOS in such situations may be a good tool in the knee arthroplasty surgeon's armamentarium.

Rationale for Computer Assisted Orthopedic Surgery

A CAOS navigation system obviates the need for intramedullary and extramedullary guides by calculating the prearthroplasty mechanical axis from the center of the femoral head, the center of the knee, and the center of the ankle. This calculation can be performed preoperatively using advanced imaging modalities (computed tomography [CT]) or intraoperatively using tracking devices and bony landmarks. CAOS is a tool the surgeon can use to position the components in relation to the mechanical axis without the need for intramedullary or extramedullary guides. The surgeon also receives "real-time" feedback while placing instrumentation and during the trialing and implantation process.

Alternatives to Computer Assisted Orthopedic Surgery

Traditionally, a patient with significant extra-articular deformity in the setting of degenerative joint disease was treated with corrective osteotomy, addressed either in a staged fashion or during the TKA.[10,19] Another approach involves intra-articular deformity correction of the extra-articular deformity during the TKA. Wang and Wang established the limits of deformity correction achievable with intra-articular correction alone as less than 20 degrees of femoral varus and less than 30 degrees varus or valgus of the tibia.[18] In general, these recommendations

seem reasonable, and it would be prudent for the surgeon consider the use of corrective osteotomy for larger deformities. The osteotomy can be performed in a staged fashion or at the time of TKA. Shao et al. have shown that a simultaneous osteotomy and TKA can be performed with the use of the computer assisted navigation system.[16] Recently, patient specific instrumentation (PSI) has been developed. PSI tibial and femoral cutting blocks are prepared from preoperative CT or magnetic resonance imaging (MRI) studies. PSI has been shown to be capable of facilitating correction of extra-articular deformities during TKA.[17]

LITERATURE REVIEW

The results of the published literature are summarized in Table 165.1. Klein et al., in 2006, presented five cases of knee degenerative joint disease with extra-articular femoral and/or tibial deformity or retained hardware. All cases had restoration of the mechanical axis to within 2 degrees (range, 1.8 degrees varus to 0.4 degrees valgus) on standing full-length radiographs.[7] Removal of hardware was not necessary, femoral intramedullary guides were not used, and all knees were well-balanced according to the authors. Fehring et al. used CAOS in a case series of 18 knees in 16 patients for whom traditional instrumentation was not feasible or desirable.[4] The criteria for the inability to use standard instrumentation included presence of deformity preventing passage of intramedullary guides, hardware that was difficult to remove, and history of osteomyelitis and cardiopulmonary disease. The rationale for using CAOS in cardiopulmonary disease was to reduce the risk of fat embolus by avoiding instrumentation of the intramedullary canal. CAOS was abandoned in one patient with a body mass index of 43, for whom the registration process for navigation failed. This technique was successful in restoration of acceptable alignment in 16 of 17 knees.

Several other reports followed, mostly involving femoral deformities.[3,6,8,12] Chou et al. presented a case report where CAOS was used in a patient with distal femur malunion.[3] The tibia was cut using a standard extramedullary guide. At 14 months follow-up, the patient was pain free, without leg length discrepancy, and had normal alignment; range of motion (ROM) was 0 to 95 degrees. A German language article described two cases, one involving a long intramedullary femoral nail, which was retained, and a second with femoral extra-articular malunion.[12] Bottros et al. described femoral deformity

TABLE 165.1   Summary of Literature

Authors	Journal	Year	Number of Cases	Indication for Computer Assisted Orthopedic Surgery	Outcomes
Klein et al.[7]	*Journal of Arthroplasty*	2006	5	Retained hardware and significant deformity of femur and tibia	Within 2 degrees of neutral mechanical axis
Fehring et al.[4]	*Clinical Orthopaedics and Related Research*	2006	17	Retained hardware, deformity of tibia or femur, cardiopulmonary issues	Acceptable alignment in 16 of 17 knees
Chou et al.[3]	*Journal of Arthroplasty*	2008	1	Severe extra-articular femoral deformity	Pain-free knee and normal alignment
Bottros et al.[1]	*Journal of Arthroplasty*	2008	9	Femoral extra-articular deformity	Improved Knee Society Scores, function scores, and ROM
Kuo et al.[8]	*Journal of Arthroplasty*	2011	1	Severe posttraumatic femoral deformity	0 degrees varus valgus of the femur, 0.2 degrees of valgus tibia
Kim et al.[6]	*Journal of Arthroplasty*	2010	4	Posttraumatic femoral deformity (minimally invasive approach)	−0.3 degrees from mechanical axis
Mullaji et al.[13]	*Journal of Arthroplasty*	2009	40	Femoral and/or tibial deformity, three requiring simultaneous osteotomy	Mean postop limb alignment 179.1 degrees, improved knee society scores and function scores
Lee et al.[9]	*Journal of Orthopaedic Surgery and Research*	2014	137 patients	Asian patients with physiologic femoral bow preventing intramedullary rod use	Reconstruction of the mechanical axis significantly better in CAOS group

CAOS, Computer assisted orthopedic surgery.

correction using a navigation system and provided pre- and postoperative Knee Society Scores, function scores, and range of motion.[1] All three parameters increased from pre- to postoperative evaluation.

Kuo et al. presented a single patient who underwent computer assisted TKA in a setting of severe posttraumatic femoral deformity.[8] In another study, femoral deformity was successfully corrected with TKA through a minimally invasive approach (mid-vastus arthrotomy and 10-centimeter average incision) using computer assisted navigation.[6]

Mullaji et al. retrospectively reviewed the records of 34 patients with femoral and/or tibial deformity who underwent computer assisted TKA at their institution.[13] Three patients who required corrective osteotomies were excluded. The patients underwent corrective osteotomy for coronal deformity greater than 20 degrees for the femur and greater than 30 degrees for the tibia or if the proposed cuts potentially compromised the collateral ligament insertion site. Functional outcomes scores increased significantly from prior to surgery to an average follow-up of 26 months after surgery. There were no nonunions of osteotomy sites at latest follow-up.

Recently, a study used computer assisted TKA for Asian patients with and without severe femoral bowing.[9] More than 5 degrees of femoral bowing was considered significant. Such bowing may prevent the use of a rigid intramedullary rod or create exaggerated cut angles when flexible intramedullary rod is to be used. Fifty-nine percent of patients in this study had marked femoral bowing. Patients with significant femoral bowing who underwent computer assisted TKA had better component alignment than patients who underwent conventional TKA. When using greater than 3 degrees deviation from a neutral mechanical axis, only 3.7% of CAOS TKAs were outliers versus 50% of conventionally instrumented TKAs.

In conclusion, these studies were all retrospective, and all except one study were case reports or series. None had control groups or compared outcomes of patients in whom surgery was performed with or without computer navigation, with the exception of the study by Lee et al.[9] Given the relative dearth of deformity cases, studies with a higher level of evidence may be difficult to generate. Despite their shortcomings, these studies highlight the fact that computer assisted navigation can be successfully used as a tool for TKA in the setting of extramedullary deformity.

CASE PRESENTATION AND SURGICAL TECHNIQUE

A 48-year-old male sustained a right femur fracture 15 years prior to presentation. He underwent open reduction and internal fixation (ORIF) with subsequent nonunion. Revision ORIF with iliac crest bone grafting was performed, and fracture union was achieved. His radiographs prior to arthroplasty are shown in Fig. 165.1. The femur was noted to have an angular deformity, and the use of standard intramedullary instrumentation of the femur would have been challenging because of the retained hardware and ossification of the intramedullary canal.

PREOPERATIVE PLANNING

The use of CAOS, custom PSI, extramedullary femoral guides, and removal of hardware with recanalization of the femur were considered during preoperative planning. CAOS is readily available at our institution, and the senior author had considerable experience with the system. Therefore, we chose a CAOS system that would allow us to perform the femoral cuts without removal of the hardware and without the need for recanalization of the femoral canal.

TECHNIQUE

Setup and Surgical Approach

The central unit of the navigation system is placed on the contralateral side of the table, making sure that the infrared array is not obstructed by any equipment or operating room staff (Fig. 165.2A).

A posterior cruciate substituting design was selected for this patient. A standard medial parapatellar approach under

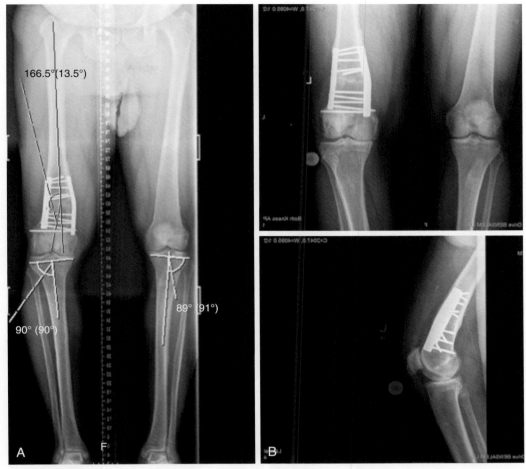

FIG 165.1 Preoperative Radiographs of the Patient (A) Long-standing radiograph. (B) Anteroposterior (AP)/lateral of the right knee.

tourniquet control was used. The surgical approach and resulting exposure did not differ secondary to the use of CAOS. A medial retinacular release was performed, but the cruciate ligaments and menisci are not yet resected to allow for the kinematics of the knee to be assessed prior to resection of these structures.

Tracker Pin Placement

The system used requires that threaded pins (to secure the wireless trackers) be placed in the femur and tibia. The pins have self-tapping threads and are placed with bicortical fixation, taking care not to overpenetrate the posterior cortices. Fixation must be secure, or the accuracy of the system will be compromised. The femoral pin is placed in the distal and medial aspect of the anterior femur, and the tibial pin is placed at the distal margin of the medial exposure (see Fig. 165.2B and C). The pins were placed within the surgical approach in this case but also may be placed outside of the main incision through small, separate stab incisions. The pins must be placed in such a fashion to avoid interference with cutting jigs, trials, and final components. This requires that the femoral tracking pin be placed medial to the midline of the femur, clear of the anterior flange of the trial and final component, and allow for approximation of the arthrotomy to assess for patella tracking. The tibial tracking pin should not interfere with placement of the tibial cutting guide,

be distal to the keel of the component, and allow for approximation of the arthrotomy to assess for patella tracking.

Registration

Once the pins are inserted, the femoral and tibial trackers are placed (see Fig. 165.2D). The trackers send wireless signals to the CAOS system, allowing three-dimensional positioning to be interpreted by the computer and visualized by the surgical team. Proper registration of mechanical alignment and anatomic landmarks is paramount to the success of the surgery. The colloquialism "garbage-in, garbage-out" accurately describes poor registration technique. Poor information provided to the CAOS system will result in poor feedback from the system. One must remember that CAOS is a tool, just as traditional jigs are tools, used to accomplish the aforementioned goals of TKA.

Preoperative mechanical axis is calculated using the femoral head center of rotation, the center of the knee, and center of the ankle. Femoral head center of rotation is calculated by the computer from the movement of the trackers as the surgeon rotates the hip (Fig. 165.3A). The pelvis must be stabilized to allow for the center of rotation of the hip to remain static. The center of the femur and tibia (as determined by preoperative templating) are digitally marked (see Fig. 165.3B and C). The center of the ankle is determined by the computer after digitally

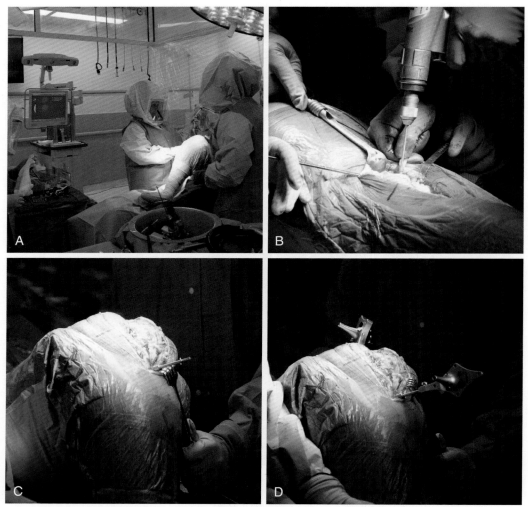

FIG 165.2. Application of the Trackers (A) Orientation of the equipment; note the clear path from the tracker to the computer. (B) Femoral tracker pin placement. (C) Tibial tracker pin placement. (D) Trackers placed on tracker pins.

marking the medial and lateral malleoli (see Fig. 165.3D). After registering the center of rotation of the femoral head, the process continues in a stepwise fashion. The following femoral anatomic landmarks are digitally marked: the medial and lateral epicondyles, center of the femur, Whiteside's line, and the contour of the medial and lateral condyles.

Attention is then turned to the tibia. The center of the tibia, contour of the medial and lateral plateaus, and anteroposterior axis are digitally marked.

The knee is then put through an alignment, range of motion, and stability (kinematic) verification check (Fig. 165.4A-C). The information provided by the computer should be correlated with the clinical exam. Any discordance should be addressed, always checking to make sure that the trackers are fully secured to the pins and that the pins are firmly fixed to the bone. Re-registration should be performed if the accuracy of the initial data provided by the CAOS system is in doubt.

After the initial verification process is accepted, the surgeon proceeds with the remainder of the surgical dissection. The

cruciate ligaments are resected and the knee is dislocated. The menisci are removed and the proximal tibia is exposed.

The tibial or femoral cuts may be performed first. In the absence of tibial deformity, the tibia is addressed primarily with the use of a standard extramedullary cutting guide (Fig. 165.5A). However, if preferred, a CAOS guide can be used. The accuracy of the tibial cut is verified with the CAOS tracker (see Fig. 165.5B). The remainder of the tibial preparation is then completed. One can use the CAOS system to determine tibial component rotational alignment, or the surgeon can use their standard technique.

The distal femur is then exposed. The CAOS jig is used for the distal femoral resection (Fig. 165.6A). The jig for the distal femoral cutting guide is affixed to the femur, and the cutting position is guided by the computer system. The tracker on the cutting guide and the tracker on the femur send wireless signals providing the surgical team with a three-dimensional image of the cutting guide's position in space relative to the distal femur. The central unit then displays that position on the screen,

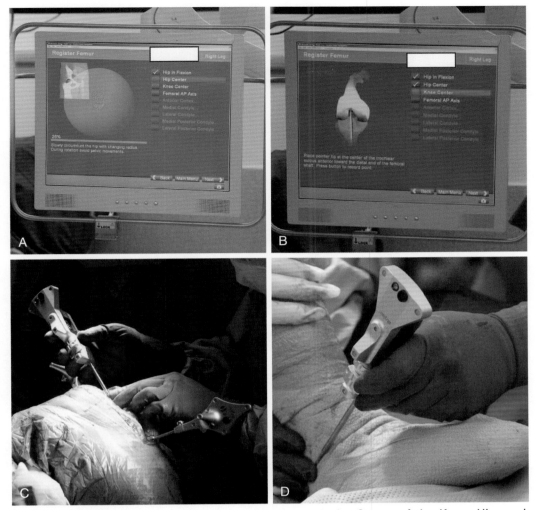

FIG 165.3 Establishment of Mechanical Axis Through the Center of the Knee, Hip, and Ankle (A) Hip center determination. (B) Registering the center of the femur. (C) Registering the center of the tibia. (D) Registering the medial and lateral malleoli to determine the center of the ankle.

overlying it onto the model of the registered knee. The surgeon can then make real-time adjustments of the distal resection depth and alignment (see Fig. 165.6B). The thickness of the bone resections should correlate with the clinical picture. For example, to correct a valgus deformity, one would expect the medial condylar resection to be thicker than the lateral condylar resection. One can measure the thickness prior to resection if the feedback from CAOS does not correlate with the surgical plan. Any discordance should be addressed, always checking to make sure that the trackers are fully secured to the pins and that the pins are firmly fixed to bone. Once the cutting guide is in the desired position, the cut is made in standard fashion (see Fig. 165.6C). The accuracy of the femoral cut is verified with the CAOS tracker (see Fig. 165.6D). The femoral finishing guide can be placed at this point with or without the use of the CAOS system. Because the rotation of the femoral component is based on the landmarks chosen by the surgeon during the registration process (transepicondylar axis and Whiteside's line), one can use CAOS or use standard instrumentation to determine the desired rotational alignment (Fig. 165.7A and B). The remainder

of the bony portion of the surgery is performed in a standard manner (see Fig. 165.7C and D). Following placement of spacer blocks or trial components, soft-tissue releases are performed. Once soft-tissue balancing is deemed satisfactory, the trial components are then put through an alignment, range of motion, and stability check (Fig. 165.8A-D). The information provided by the computer should be correlated with the clinical exam. Any discordance should be addressed, always checking to make sure that the trackers are fully secured to the pins and that the pins are firmly fixed to bone. Further soft tissue or bony adjustments can then be made according to feedback from both the CAOS system and clinical inspection of the trial TKA. Once the surgeon is satisfied with the trial components and soft tissue balancing, the tracking pins can then be removed. If so desired, the tracking pins may be retained and the alignment and soft tissue balancing can be tested with the final components implanted. The knee is irrigated, the final components are inserted, and the incision is closed. Postoperative radiographs are shown in Fig. 165.9.

Text continued on p. 1836

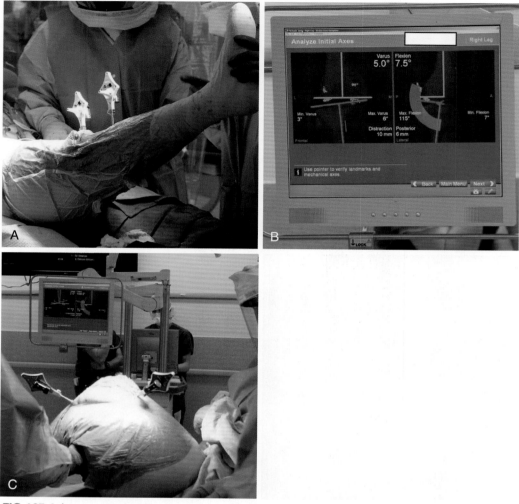

FIG 165.4 Intraoperative Evaluation of the Knee, After Initial Registration, Using Computer Navigation (A) Evaluating extension, coronal plane alignment. (B) Screenshot quantifying coronal plane alignment, range of motion, and translation of the tibia relative the femur. (C) Evaluating flexion, coronal plane alignment in flexion.

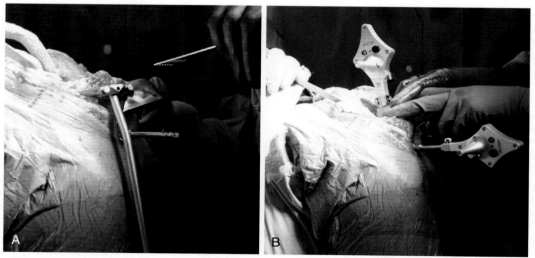

FIG 165.5 Tibia Cut and Evaluation of the Cut With Computer Assisted Orthopedic Surgery (A) Tibial cut using standard extramedullary guide. (B) Checking the tibial cut using CAOS.

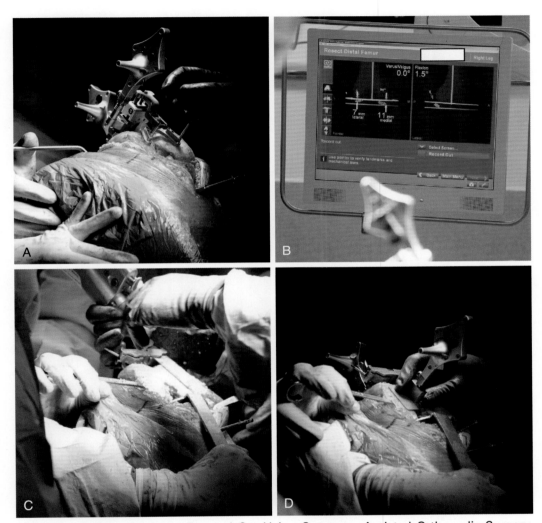

FIG 165.6 Performing Distal Femoral Cut Using Computer Assisted Orthopedic Surgery
(A) CAOS femoral cutting guide. (B) Screenshot quantifying femoral coronal plane alignment, flexion, and resection depth. (C) Distal femoral resection using the CAOS guide. (D) Checking the femoral cut using CAOS.

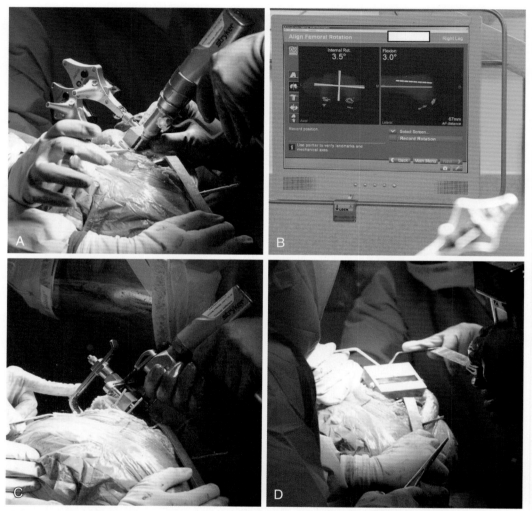

FIG 165.7 Establishment of Femoral Component Rotation, Anterior, Posterior, and Chamfer Cuts Using Computer Assisted Orthopedic Surgery (A) CAOS femoral rotation guide. (B) Screenshot quantifying femoral component rotation and flexion. (C) Anterior femoral resection using CAOS guide. (D) Placement of the femoral finishing guide.

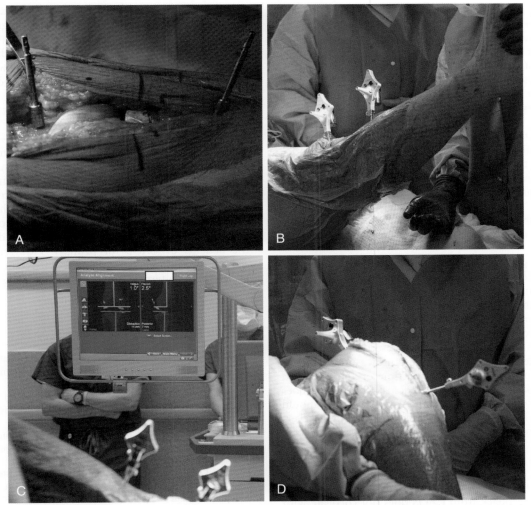

FIG 165.8 Evaluation of the Knee Using Computer Assisted Orthopedic Surgery With Trial Components (A) Trial components in place. (B) Evaluating extension, coronal plane alignment. (C) Screenshot quantifying extension, coronal plane alignment. (D) Evaluating flexion, coronal plane alignment.

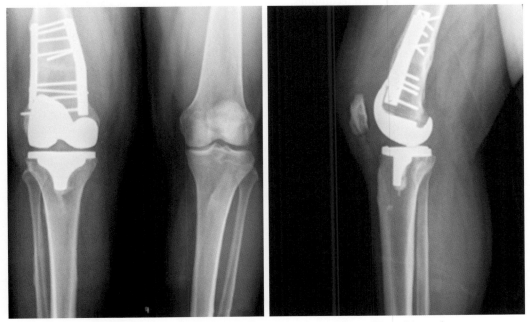

FIG 165.9 Postoperative radiographs of the patient. AP and lateral.

PEARLS AND PITFALLS

- Make sure that the infrared array is not obstructed by any equipment or operating room staff.
- Fixation must be secure or the accuracy of the system may be compromised.
- Care must be taken to stop advancing the pins when the second cortex is reached to avoid injury to posterior structures.
- The pins for the trackers must be placed in a way to avoid trackers interfering with cutting jigs, trial, and final components during the operation.
- Proper registration of anatomic landmarks and determination of mechanical alignment is paramount to the success of the surgery.
- One must remember that CAOS is a tool just as traditional jigs are tools used to accomplish the aforementioned goals of TKA.
- "Garbage-in, garbage-out" accurately describes poor registration technique.
- The information provided by the computer should be correlated with the clinical exam.
- Re-registration should be performed if the accuracy of the initial data provided by the CAOS system is in doubt.
- The thickness and slope of the tibial resection should correlate with the clinical picture. One can measure the thickness of the medial and lateral portion of the proposed resection prior to cutting if the feedback from CAOS does not correlate with the surgical plan. Any discordance should be addressed, always checking to make sure that the trackers are fully secured to the pins and that the pins are firmly fixed to bone.
- The thickness of the medial and lateral femoral bone resections should correlate with the clinical picture. One can measure the thickness of the proposed resection prior to cutting if the feedback from CAOS does not correlate with the surgical plan. Any discordance should be addressed, always checking to make sure that the trackers are fully secured to the pins and that the pins are firmly fixed to bone.
- Certain steps, such as femoral and tibial component rotation, can be performed with either CAOS or standard techniques.

- Once soft tissue balancing is deemed satisfactory, the trial components are then put through an alignment, range of motion, and stability check. The information provided by the computer should be correlated with the clinical exam. Any discordance should be addressed, always checking to make sure that the trackers are fully secured to the pins and that the pins are firmly fixed to bone.

CONCLUSION

The use of CAOS for situations when intramedullary guides are difficult or impossible to use offers the surgeon a reliable tool to establish acceptable mechanical alignment and assess soft tissue balancing. The surgery can be performed without the need to remove hardware. This obviates the need for more extensive surgical dissection, additional incisions, and the creation of stress risers from removed hardware. Although the benefits of CAOS for primary TKA remain controversial, this technique has established itself in the last decade as the good alternative technique for TKA in a setting of deformity.

KEY REFERENCES

1. Bottros J, Klika AK, Lee HH, et al: The use of navigation in total knee arthroplasty for patients with extra-articular deformity. *J Arthroplasty* 23:74–78, 2008.
3. Chou WY, Ko JY, Wang CJ, et al: Navigation-assisted total knee arthroplasty for a knee with malunion of the distal femur. *J Arthroplasty* 23:1239.e13–1239.e17, 2008.
6. Kim KI, Ramteke AA, Bae DK: Navigation-assisted minimal invasive total knee arthroplasty in patients with extra-articular femoral deformity. *J Arthroplasty* 25:658.e17–658.e22, 2010.
8. Kuo CC, Bosque J, Meehan JP, et al: Computer-assisted navigation of total knee arthroplasty for osteoarthritis in a patient with severe posttraumatic femoral deformity. *J Arthroplasty* 26:976.e17–976.e20, 2011.
10. Lonner JH, Siliski JM, Lotke PA: Simultaneous femoral osteotomy and total knee arthroplasty for treatment of osteoarthritis associated with severe extra-articular deformity. *J Bone Joint Surg Am* 82:342–348, 2000.

The references for this chapter can also be found on www.expertconsult.com.

166

Impact of the Cavus Foot and Ankle on the Painful Knee

Michael P. Clare

INTRODUCTION

The cavus foot and ankle, whether the lifelong "normal" for the patient or the result of a prior injury, can significantly influence shock absorption and body weight distribution during normal gait. Sangeorzan et al. showed in a study of asymptomatic volunteers that up to 24% of the population had pre-existing pes cavus alignment.[6] Although some patients with cavus alignment remain relatively pain free throughout their lifetime, others experience the deleterious mechanical effects of the cavus foot and ankle throughout the lower extremity. Although the severe, neurologic cavus deformity, such as with Charcot-Marie-Tooth disease or post-polio syndrome, can be obvious, the subtle cavus deformity can often be considerably more difficult to diagnose and subsequently treat.

PATHOMECHANICS OF THE CAVUS FOOT AND ANKLE

Normal Gait

During normal gait, the transverse tarsal joints are aligned in a parallel, flexible, and unlocked position so as to absorb body weight stresses at heel strike. As the foot transitions to foot flat, the posterior tibial tendon actively inverts the hindfoot, whereby the transverse tarsal joints convert to a nonparallel, rigid, and locked position in anticipation of push-off. As this occurs, the Achilles insertion shifts medial to the subtalar joint axis in terminal stance phase, contributing plantarflexion power to the now rigid midfoot.

Gait in the Cavus Foot and Ankle

During gait with the cavus foot and ankle, the transverse tarsal joints remain in a nonparallel, rigid, and locked position throughout the entirety of the gait cycle, which substantially limits the shock absorption and distribution of body weight stresses. These stresses are absorbed in adjacent joints, particularly the ankle joint.[7]

Cavus alignment produces a varus thrust on the ankle joint, which substantially increases the workload of the peroneal muscles, which act as dynamic stabilizers of the lateral ankle and hindfoot. This varus thrust clearly impacts the development of lateral ankle problems, such as lateral ankle instability and peroneal tendon pathology.[1] The peroneus longus additionally acts as a dynamic stabilizer of the first ray, such that "peroneal overdrive" plantarflexes the first ray, and increases the so-called kickstand effect of the first ray. The combination of varus thrust and the plantarflexed first ray contribute to overload of the lateral column of the foot, often resulting in stress reaction or stress fractures in the lateral midfoot.

Varus thrust on the ankle also produces vertical shear forces on the medial malleolus and the medial column of the tibia, which can result in similar stress reaction or stress fracture. These same vertical shear forces may also transmit proximally to the medial compartment of the knee, contributing to varus gonarthrosis.[10] These mechanical effects, if not addressed and neutralized, produce an often vicious, perpetuating cycle of mechanical overload and subsequent structural deterioration.

Posttraumatic varus deformities in the tibia can produce similar mechanical effects in the foot and ankle and, depending on the extent of the deformity, can lead to secondary cavus adaptations in the foot and ankle.

CLINICAL EVALUATION

Standing Examination

As with any foot and ankle problem, a standing examination is a key component to identification of the suspected cavus foot and ankle. It is imperative that the extremities be exposed to at least the midthigh, so as to facilitate evaluation of the mechanical alignment of the entire lower limb. The patient is assessed both from front to back, and back to front, assessing for symmetry and comparing the alignment of the knee, tibia, ankle, and foot of each leg (Fig. 166.1A and B).

The patient with pes cavus will typically exhibit a "peak-a-boo" heel, as described by Manoli,[8] whereby the medial heel pad prominently protrudes relative to the remainder of the medial ankle and foot (Fig. 166.2).

Coleman Block Test

If pes cavus alignment is identified, it is then critical to perform a Coleman block test to discern whether the cavus deformity is being driven by the forefoot or by the hindfoot.[2] The test involves the patient standing on a block of wood perhaps $\frac{3}{4}$ to 1 inch thick, with the first ray and medial column of the foot off the inside edge of the block, which in effect eliminates the influence of the first ray on foot alignment. The patient is viewed from back to front, and hindfoot alignment is assessed (Fig. 166.3A and B).

If the hindfoot alignment corrects on the block, then the deformity is forefoot driven, likely as a result of the plantarflexed first ray or overdrive of the peroneus longus. If the hindfoot alignment does not correct on the block, then the deformity is hindfoot driven. These results are invaluable in preoperative planning of surgical correction of a cavus deformity.

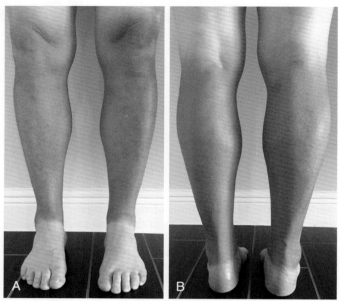

FIG 166.1 Standing Examination The patient's lower extremities are examined from (A) front to back, and (B) back to front. Note the varus deformity through the knee and the secondary subtle cavus through the ankle and foot.

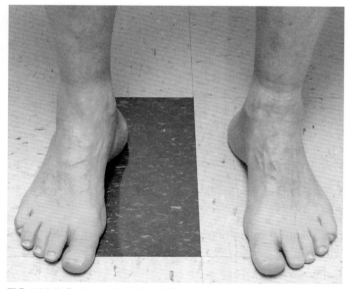

FIG 166.2 Peak-A-Boo Heel Sign Note the prominence of the medial heel pad relative to the medial foot and ankle.

Assessment of Tenderness, Stability, Strength, and Range of Motion

With the patient now seated, the involved limb must be assessed for areas of tenderness, as well as stability, strength, and range of motion. With respect to pes cavus, particular attention is directed to ligamentous stability of the lateral ankle, eversion strength, and hindfoot motion. The patient with cavus alignment, depending on extent of deformity, will typically have a stable lateral ligamentous complex in the ankle, strong peroneal muscles, and supple hindfoot range of motion, which should be symmetric to the contralateral limb. Typically as the hindfoot

is manually brought into maximum eversion through the subtalar joint, the relative plantarflexion of medial column of the foot is accentuated, further demonstrating the deforming power of the first ray.

RADIOGRAPHIC EVALUATION

Just as with physical examination, standing radiographic evaluation is critical in the assessment of the suspected cavus foot and ankle. Full-length, long-leg standing radiographs that include the distal femur, knee, tibia, ankle, and foot are ideal but may not be possible with some digital radiographic systems. Otherwise, weight-bearing anteroposterior (AP) and mortise views of the ankle and weight-bearing AP, oblique, and lateral views of the foot (including the ankle) should be obtained, as well as similar views of the tibia where necessary.

Radiographic Findings in Pes Cavus

Compared with the neutral foot and ankle, the cavus foot and ankle typically exhibits certain radiographic characteristics, which are reflective of the deformity and allow quantification of the extent of the deformity.

Full-Length Long-Leg Anteroposterior; Anteroposterior and Lateral Views of Tibia

The full-length, long-leg AP, and the AP and lateral views of the tibia reveal deformity in the coronal and/or sagittal planes, which is often posttraumatic in origin (Fig. 166.4). The extent of the deformity can be defined by the Center of Rotation of Angulation angle.[9]

Anteroposterior and Mortise Views of Ankle

The AP and mortise views of the ankle demonstrate the extent of symmetry of the ankle mortise. Although the subtle cavus deformity may have a symmetric ankle mortise, the more severe cavus deformity may have actual varus tilt of the talus. These views also reveal varus thrust through the ankle, which is demonstrated through a line down the long axis of the tibia through the ankle and hindfoot. This line will pass relatively more lateral in the ankle and hindfoot, such that relatively more of the midfoot and forefoot is seen on profile medial to this line (Fig. 166.5).

Lateral View of Ankle and Foot

The lateral view of the ankle and foot typically demonstrates an increased calcaneal pitch angle and an increased talo-first metatarsal (Meary) angle. The relative external rotation of the limb is such that the fibula will typically be more posterior relative to the tibia and the subtalar joint will appear more "on profile" rather than the typical oblique projection (Fig. 166.6).

Anteroposterior and Oblique Views of Foot

The AP and oblique views of the foot show "metatarsal stacking," in which the lateral metatarsal bones appear stacked on one another, and which results from supination through the lateral column of the midfoot (Fig. 166.7). There may also be adductus through the midfoot to some degree, which accentuates the lateral column overload clinically. Midfoot adductus is further defined by a line down the long axis of the talus, extending to the metatarsals, which will often intersect the second or third metatarsal; in a neutral foot, this line will usually intersect the first metatarsal (Fig. 166.8).

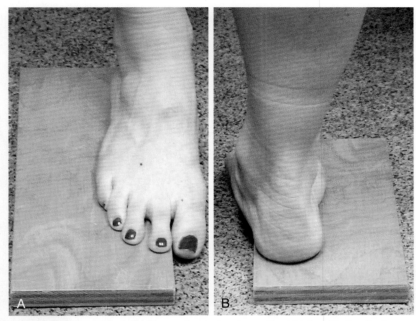

FIG 166.3 Coleman Block Test (A) The patient stands on the block with the first ray and medial column of the foot off the edge of the block, neutralizing the effect of the first ray. (B) If the hindfoot corrects into valgus, the test is positive, meaning that the forefoot is driving the deformity.

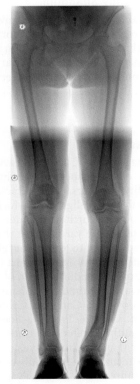

FIG 166.4 Full-Length, Long-Leg Anteroposterior View Note the varus gonarthrosis, and posttraumatic varus deformity through the distal tibia.

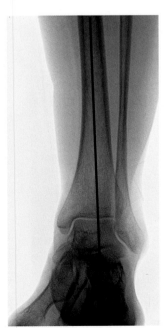

FIG 166.5 Weight-Bearing Anteroposterior View of the Ankle Varus thrust: the *black line* along the long axis of the tibia crosses relatively more lateral in the ankle and hindfoot.

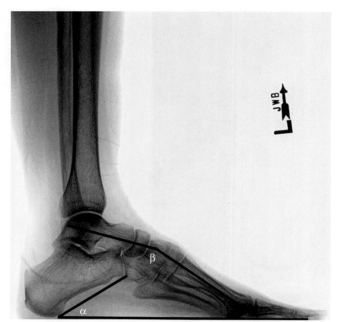

FIG 166.6 Weight-Bearing Lateral of the Ankle and Foot Note the increased calcaneal pitch angle *(α)*, and *(β)* increased Meary angle.

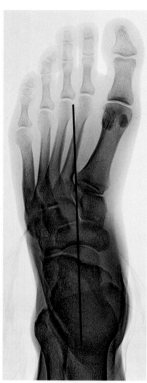

FIG 166.8 Subtle Cavus With Metatarsus Adductus Note that the talometatarsal angle *(black line)* intersects the forefoot between the second and third metatarsal.

Computed Tomography Scanning

Computed tomography scanning can be invaluable in further defining and evaluating cavus or varus deformities in the limb, particularly those that are posttraumatic in origin. The three-dimensional information provided can be particularly beneficial in preoperative planning of deformity correction in a varus- or cavus-aligned limb.

TREATMENT

Nonoperative Management

Nonoperative management of a subtle cavus foot and ankle includes treatment of the associated condition (medial knee pain, ankle instability, metatarsal stress fracture, etc.), in addition to treatment of the cavus alignment, which typically consists of a cavus orthotic. A cavus orthotic includes a lateral heel and sole wedge to counteract the varus thrust through the ankle, a first metatarsal head recess to offset the effect of the plantarflexed first ray, and minimal arch support to roll body weight toward the weight-bearing medial column of the foot. There are two commercially available brands of noncustom cavus orthotics (ArchRival, DonJoy, Inc., Carlsbad, California; and Arches Orthotic-Supination Control-Type 3, Foot Scientific, Inc., Draper, Utah). The author prefers use of one of these noncustom orthotics rather than a custom cavus orthotic.

In more severe deformities, a more substantial and restrictive orthosis may be required. Typically such a device will extend across the ankle and provide immobilization and support to the ankle, hindfoot, and midfoot. Options would include a prefabricated lace-up style ankle brace, U-shaped ankle stirrup brace,

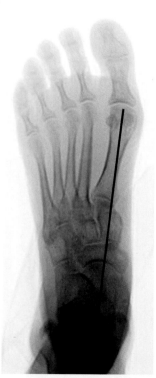

FIG 166.7 Weight-Bearing Anteroposterior of Foot Note the metatarsal stacking, in which the lateral metatarsals appear relatively stacked on one another. Note also that the talometatarsal angle intersects the forefoot through the first ray *(black line)*.

or possibly a custom Arizona-type brace. In the latter instance, a lateral heel and sole wedge and lateral post can be built in to the device for additional support where necessary.

Operative Management

In the event of concomitant knee and ankle/foot deformities, the limb is corrected in staged fashion. Although controversial, the ankle and foot should ideally be corrected before the knee, so as to facilitate more accurate deformity correction in the knee and re-establishment of the mechanical axis of the limb. In the instance of a cavus foot and ankle, addressing the knee first would (1) theoretically increase polyethylene wear due continued loss of shock absorption with gait until the foot and ankle is corrected, and (2) possibly lead to overcorrection of the knee into excessive valgus.

Forefoot-Driven Subtle Cavus. With a forefoot-driven deformity, the plantarflexed first ray and/or overdrive of the peroneus longus is the source of the deformity, such that neutralizing these deforming factors will correct the deformity. Therefore treatment consists of a dorsiflexion osteotomy of the first ray and a peroneus longus to peroneus brevis transfer. The osteotomy is typically done as a dorsal closing wedge approximately 1 cm from the first tarsometatarsal joint. Depending on the extent of the deformity, a 1- to 2-mm wedge is removed dorsally, which when added to the 1 mm from each of the cuts, produces significant corrective power. The osteotomy is stabilized with either a mini-fragment plate and screws, or a single small fragment screw (Fig. 166.9). If additional correction is required, a lateralizing calcaneal osteotomy may be added.

The peroneus longus to peroneus brevis transfer consists of a tenodesis of the two tendons, so as to preserve eversion strength while eliminating the plantarflexion pull of the peroneus longus on the first ray. The hindfoot is held in slight equinus and maximum eversion, to shorten the peroneus brevis, and the first ray is positioned in maximum dorsiflexion at the first tarsometatarsal joint, to tension the peroneus longus, and figure-of-eight sutures are passed between the two tendons. The peroneus longus is released distal to the tenodesis to complete the transfer.

In the instance of concomitant metatarsus adductus, the first ray may be supinated through the osteotomy site for additional rotational correction (Fig. 166.10). A plantar fascia release and fractional lengthening of the abductor hallucis muscle may also be added.

Hindfoot-Driven Pes Cavus. With a hindfoot-driven deformity, treatment typically at the least includes a lateralizing calcaneal osteotomy, dorsiflexion first metatarsal osteotomy, and peroneus longus to peroneus brevis transfer.

The calcaneal osteotomy, which is typically completed as the first step, might consist of a simple oblique sliding osteotomy for less significant deformities, or an oblique lateral closing wedge osteotomy for more significant deformities. For severe deformities, a calcaneal scarf osteotomy can be used, which allows a combination of translation, rotation, and/or closing wedge to facilitate multiplanar correction.[3]

The first metatarsal osteotomy is next completed, typically as a dorsal closing wedge osteotomy, followed by a peroneus longus to peroneus brevis transfer, as previously described. A plantar fascia release may also be added.

In severe, neurologic cavus deformities, a dorsal closing wedge osteotomy at the apex of the deformity, typically at the level of the cuneiforms, may be required. In the instance of more of a transverse plane deformity, such as an undercorrected congenital clubfoot, an opening wedge medial column lengthening osteotomy, with or without a closing wedge lateral column shortening osteotomy may be necessary. These transverse plane osteotomies may be truncated in to provide additional sagittal plane correction.

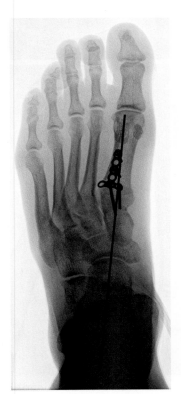

FIG 166.10 Correction of Subtle Cavus With Metatarsus Adductus The first ray (distal fragment) is supinated to provide simultaneous correction of the adductus. The talometatarsal angle now intersects the forefoot at the first ray (*black line*).

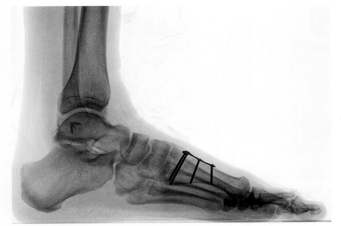

FIG 166.9 Dorsiflexion Osteotomy of the First Ray The osteotomy is stabilized with a mini-fragment T-plate and screws.

Varus Deformities of the Distal Tibia and Ankle. If the varus deformity derives from the distal tibia, corrective osteotomies of the distal tibia and fibula are performed (Fig. 166.11A to F). These osteotomies may consist of a medial opening wedge osteotomy; lateral closing wedge osteotomy; or crescentic type osteotomy in the tibia.[4,5] Similarly, these instances will often require further corrective procedures for additional corrective power.

In the instance of a varus deformity through the ankle, deformity correction may be completed through the ankle joint by either an ankle arthrodesis or ankle arthroplasty. Further corrective procedures, as described above, are usually required for additional corrective power.

Postoperative Protocols. Metatarsal and calcaneal osteotomies typically require cast immobilization and non–weight-bearing restrictions for approximately 6 weeks postoperatively. Tibial osteotomies and ankle arthrodeses require up to 3 months of non–weight-bearing restrictions. After the structural corrections are satisfactorily healed, the patient is converted to a

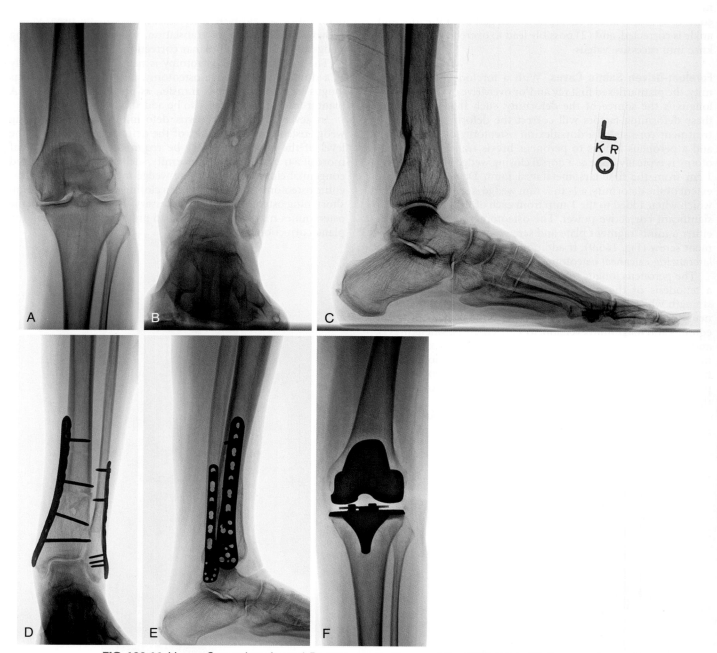

FIG 166.11 Varus Gonarthrosis and Posttraumatic Varus of the Tibia (A to C) Preoperative weight-bearing (A) AP of the knee; (B) A/P of the ankle; and (C) lateral of the ankle and foot. (D to F) Postoperative weight-bearing (D) AP of ankle; (E) lateral of ankle following distal tibial opening wedge and oblique fibular osteotomies; and (F) weight-bearing AP of knee following staged total knee arthroplasty.

removable walking boot and weight bearing is advanced. The patient then transitions to regular shoe wear thereafter. Physical therapy may be instituted to assist with range of motion, strengthening, and gait training. Full recovery from these procedures typically requires approximately 6 months.

CONCLUSIONS

The cavus ankle and foot can have a significant impact on the painful knee, primarily because of the loss of shock absorption through the hindfoot, which places vertical shear forces on the medial distal tibia and extends proximally to the medial compartment of the knee. By performing a thorough physical examination, including a standing examination and Coleman block testing, and weight-bearing radiographic examination, the physician can determine the appropriate method of treatment, including nonoperative and operative options.

KEY REFERENCES

1. Chilvers M, Manoli A, 2nd: The subtle cavus foot and association with ankle instability and lateral foot overload. *Foot Ankle Clin* 13(2):315–324, 2008.
2. Coleman SS, Chesnut WJ: A simple test for hindfoot flexibility in the cavovarus foot. *Clin Orthop Relat Res* 123:60–62, 1977.
6. Ledoux WR, Shofer JB, Ahroni JH, et al: Biomechanical differences among pes cavus, neutrally aligned, and pes planus feet in subjects with diabetes. *Foot Ankle Int* 24(11):845–850, 2003.
8. Manoli A, 2nd, Graham B: The subtle cavus foot, "the underpronator". *Foot Ankle Int* 26(3):256–263, 2005.

The references for this chapter can also be found on www.expertconsult.com.

167

Flat Foot and Its Effect on the Knee

Justin Greisberg

"The foot bone is connected to the leg bone. The leg bone is connected to the knee bone…"

Despite the wonderful simplicity of that catchy tune, the relationship of arch height and knee pathology is not quite so straightforward. For decades, doctors and patients have suggested that flat feet are a common cause of knee pain, but is there really good evidence to support the claim? Both flat feet and painful knees are very common, so the presence of both could be coincidence, not causation.

WHAT IS A FLAT FOOT?

The term "flat foot" is used commonly, so much so that many insurers will not reimburse for procedures with flat foot as the diagnosis code. Arch height varies along a bell curve. A flat foot is simply someone at the lower side of the curve. It can be considered within the spectrum of normal, just as someone who has short stature or even just dark hair.

Just as people vary in their normal knee alignment, the shape and alignment of individuals' hindfoot bones vary. On a lateral weight-bearing x-ray, the talus should be mostly in line with the first metatarsal. Although the height of the arch may vary from one individual to another, so long as the talo-metatarsal relationship is straight, then both feet are "normal," despite the visible differences (Fig. 167.1). It probably is better to refer to someone with a low arch but normal hindfoot alignment as a low-arched individual, instead of the generic term "flat foot."

Although we refer to arches as high or low, arch height is not at all a two-dimensional deformity. In the coronal plane, the hindfoot can be in valgus or varus; the heel will be lateral to the long axis of the leg in valgus. A slight bit of heel or hindfoot valgus is considered normal when standing still. In the sagittal plane, the medial column of the foot makes up what we normally refer to as arch height. In the axial plane the foot moves around the talus; the midfoot and forefoot moves laterally relative to the talus with eversion.

But it is really not possible to separate sagittal plane arch height from axial plane forefoot abduction or heel valgus. Rather, the entire hindfoot rotates around the talus, in a complex spiral (or screw) motion. The navicular and calcaneus move mostly together, through the talonavicular (TN) and subtalar (ST) joints. Hindfoot inversion includes forefoot adduction in the axial plane, heel varus in the coronal plane, and an increase in arch height sagitally. Hindfoot eversion leads to the components of the collapsed arch: heel valgus, sagittal plane collapse, and forefoot abduction.

When standing, there is no muscle/tendon activity in the foot. Integrity of the arch is maintained by the ligaments connecting the hindfoot bones. If the ligaments are attenuated or ruptured, then the hindfoot bones are able to fall into excessive valgus/eversion relative to the talus. This should be considered a collapsed arch. This is usually not normal. The heel will be in excessive valgus. The arch will look broken on an x-ray, with the talus pointing much lower than the first metatarsal (Fig. 167.2). To emphasize the three-dimensional nature of this deformity, Dr. Hansen has coined the phrase "dorsilateral peritalar subluxation"; the foot is rotating dorsally and laterally relative to the talus, which is fixed in the ankle mortise.[7]

THE PAINLESS LOW-ARCHED FOOT AND THE PAINFUL KNEE

A person with a low-arched foot will have some degree of hindfoot valgus. With the heel lateral to the long axis of the tibia in the coronal plane, a valgus force is then applied to the knee. This alignment would increase pressures in the lateral compartment of the knee when the person is standing still (Fig. 167.3).

The unfortunate individual with a valgus hindfoot and a valgus knee will have increased pressures in the lateral compartment and would be expected to be at increased risk of developing lateral knee arthritis. There is no evidence-based medicine to support this claim, but it certainly seems reasonable to try to decrease hindfoot valgus in a patient with a painful valgus knee and hindfoot valgus.

A hindfoot orthotic can be used to decrease hindfoot valgus. The key concept is that we are not trying to lift up or support the arch; rather we want to decrease hindfoot valgus. This is accomplished by adding a medial heel post or wedge, to tilt the heel into some varus. The orthotic prescription might read, "custom orthotic with some arch support and medial heel posting." There probably is not any benefit in extending the orthotic up around the ankle, despite the popularity of those designs.

Treatment tactics are less straightforward in the patient with a valgus hindfoot and a painful varus knee. This combination is quite common, although it is not clear if the alignment of the knee and foot are related. Hindfoot valgus will complement knee varus, so the net effect will be a knee joint that is parallel to the floor (see Fig. 167.3). Perhaps the varus knee results in compensatory hindfoot valgus, or maybe hindfoot valgus leads to knee varus. Although the relationship here is hard to know with any certainty, there is at least some evidence that patients

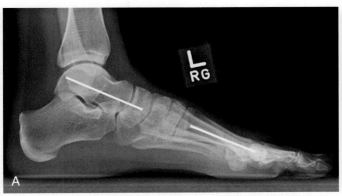
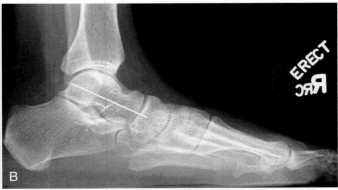

FIG 167.1 High and Low Arches Both of these feet are "normal" with no arch-related symptoms. The *white lines* represent the axis of the talus and first metatarsal. They should be fairly parallel. (A) Foot with a higher arch (calcaneal pitch is steeper, and the medial cuneiform is higher off the floor). (B) Foot with a lower arch, but the talus remains lined up with the first metatarsal.

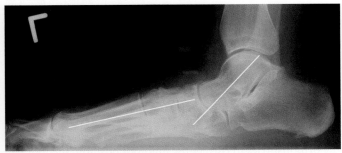

FIG 167.2 Collapsed Arch Here the talus is pointing plantar to the long axis of the first metatarsal. This is generally not "normal" alignment.

with hindfoot valgus may have a slightly higher prevalence of medial knee pathology.[6]

If the hindfoot valgus is compensatory for knee varus, should we even try to correct it? Will adding a medial heel post worsen anatomic alignment? Although there may be individuals who swear by their foot orthotics in improving their knee symptoms, there is insufficient clinical evidence to support widespread use. Custom foot orthotics are very expensive, but the vast majority of over-the-counter foot orthotics do not have medial heel posting. A simple "arch support" probably is no better than a well-made walking shoe or sneaker.

Many patients with a low-arch foot will have tightness in the gastrocnemius. The question of the tight gastrocnemius has caused much debate in foot orthopedic circles for decades. When a patient is standing, any tightness in the gastrocnemius will cause a hyperextension force on the knee. An elevated heel will decrease this hyperextension force, so it seems sensible to recommend a low heel for these patients, and to discourage the use of completely flat shoes.

THE COLLAPSED ARCH AND ITS EFFECT ON THE KNEE

In most cases a low-arch foot will be symmetric on both legs. The patient will state they have always had these "flat feet," but a collapsed arch (acquired flat foot) is a different entity, with

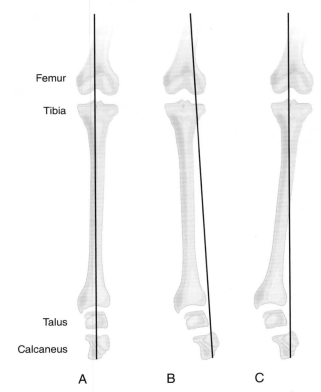

FIG 167.3 Alignment Diagrams In each diagram the *solid black line* travels from the center of the hip (not shown) to the heel and is the axis of weight bearing. (A) In the "normally" aligned leg, the heel is in slight valgus relative to the talus. The weight-bearing axis runs mostly through the center of the knee and the ankle. (B) With valgus in the knee and excess valgus in the hindfoot, the weight-bearing axis falls laterally within both the knee and ankle, increasing joint stresses. (C) In the common scenario of a varus knee with increased hindfoot valgus (the pronated foot or flatfoot), the weight-bearing axis ends up passing more or less through the center of the knee but is far off center in the ankle.

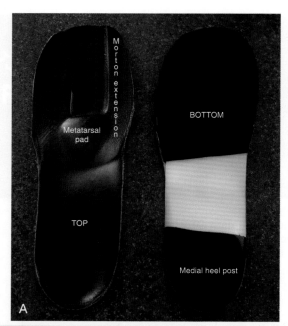

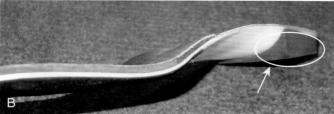

FIG 167.4 Custom Foot Orthotics (A) The image on the left is the upper view, and the one on the right shows the lower surface of this foot orthotic. The metatarsal pad and Morton extension are not needed for the collapsed arch but may be helpful when treating forefoot complaints. (B) This view shows the medial heel post *(circled)*.

The knee will feel an increased valgus stress from a collapsing arch. It is common for a patient with a collapsed arch to complain of pain in the ipsilateral knee. Even if a patient does not feel pain in the collapsed foot, it is appropriate to offer mechanical support to minimize eccentric forces on the ankle and the knee. Of course, many patients with a collapsed arch will feel pain in the foot, often along the posterior tibial tendon medially and the hindfoot laterally.

When ordering an orthotic for a collapsed arch, it is important to determine how flexible the arch is. With the patient sitting on the exam table, can the hindfoot be inverted back into reasonably normal position? The hindfoot usually retains flexibility, but the arch collapses under weight-bearing forces. Less commonly, the hindfoot will be fixed in valgus, even with the patient sitting on the exam table.

For the collapsed arch with retained flexibility (the flexible flat foot), a custom foot orthotic with moderate arch support and a medial heel post should be ordered (Fig. 167.4). (Most prefabricated orthotics will not have this support.) For these patients, several studies have shown that the majority of patients will feel marked improvement in pain with a custom orthotic, usually over 1 to 2 months.[4] There are also several styles of ankle-foot orthoses that can be used. An Arizona brace is a custom lace-up brace; it may not be as popular with patients because it is bulky and may require a larger shoe. A Richie brace consists of a foot orthotic with hinged double uprights around the ankle. There are no clinical data to suggest an ankle-foot orthosis is more effective than a simple foot orthosis.

For the patient with a collapsed arch and a fixed deformity (no hindfoot flexibility), corrective orthotics cannot be used. If the orthotist tries to correct the hindfoot position, the foot will not move. Instead, the orthotic will just put pressure on the foot. In this case a custom, softer accommodative orthotic can be used, mostly as a supportive cushion. For this patient the surgeon may want to try an Arizona brace. In general, orthotics for a rigid deformity may be less successful.

For any foot with marked arch collapse, an orthotic is able to only improve alignment in the leg, not completely correct it. If symptoms are persisting or deformity is progressing, it is wise to consider surgery. The goal of surgery is both to reduce patient's symptoms and to restore alignment (to decrease abnormal stresses on the ankle and knee). Thus an in situ hindfoot fusion (in which the hindfoot is fused in valgus) is not an effective solution for most patients.

Realignment surgery can be performed either through fusion of hindfoot joints, or realignment around the hindfoot joints. The most logical surgery would restore the integrity of the "stretched out" hindfoot ligaments, such as the spring ligament. Unfortunately, surgeons are only beginning to explore the outcomes of such ligament reconstructions.[1,2]

Realignment and arthrodesis of the TN and ST joints will correct hindfoot position. Traditionally the calcaneocuboid joint is included in the fusion, although most cases do not really need it. In some patients the collapsed arch has resulted in an elevated first ray (compensatory forefoot supination), so realignment and fusion through the first metatarsocuneiform joint is often part of the procedure. Arthrodesis of these essential hindfoot joints eliminates all hindfoot motion, so fusions are favored in those with feet that are already stiff, or in less active patients.

For the flexible collapsed arch, especially in a more active patient, the surgeon may choose to avoid fusing essential

progressive collapse over time. Most of the time the feet will not look symmetric; the affected foot will show increased arch collapse, heel valgus, and forefoot abduction.

The adult acquired flat foot is most commonly caused by failure of the posterior tibial tendon. This tendon normally inverts the heel and locks the hindfoot just before the heel rise portion of the gait cycle. If the tendon begins to fail (elongates, ruptures, or just does not work as well), then the hindfoot will slowly fall into a collapsed position of increasing eversion over time. The hindfoot ligaments will attenuate or rupture.

The cause of posterior tibial tendon failure is not clear. Some cases may be because of primary failure of the tendon in a middle-aged individual. Other cases might be secondary to the increased stress imposed on the hindfoot by a tight gastrocnemius muscle. Regardless of cause, the condition can be progressive.

Other causes of an acquired flat foot deformity include rare cases of spring ligament rupture in the hindfoot, as well as posttraumatic midfoot deformity. As the hindfoot falls into increasing valgus over time, the ankle will feel increasing valgus stress. Indeed, the final stage of a collapsing arch deformity is when the ankle collapses into severe valgus deformity from lateral plafond degeneration and deltoid ligament rupture.

hindfoot joints. Perhaps the most popular solution is the medial sliding calcaneal tuberosity osteotomy. By sliding the tuberosity medially, the weight-bearing axis is moved medially as well, along with the Achilles tendon insertion. Theoretically this translation would help alignment and knee mechanics. In reality, even though the clinical results of the procedure show excellent relief of pain in the foot, the magnitude of arch realignment is partial at best.[3,8]

The Evans procedure, often referred to as lateral column lengthening, is an opening osteotomy of the anterior process of the calcaneus. This procedure is very effective at restoring normal hindfoot alignment, more so than the tuberosity osteotomy. Unfortunately, the procedure sometimes leads to chronic lateral hindfoot pain that is difficult to resolve. Either of these calcaneal osteotomies may be combined with a procedure to plantarflex the medial column, such as an opening wedge osteotomy of the medial cuneiform (Cotton procedure), or a fusion of the first tarsometatarsal joint.[5]

Whichever procedures are chosen, the surgeon's goal is to improve alignment of the hindfoot to restore the foundation for the ankle and knee.

The references for this chapter can also be found on www.expertconsult.com.

168

The Impact of the Foot and Ankle on Total Knee Replacement

Craig S. Radnay

Total knee arthroplasty has been a very successful procedure designed to relieve pain and improve patient function. In the United States, as baby boomers mature, and as life expectancy increases, more people are becoming disabled by the pain of knee arthritis. In the United States, knee osteoarthritis is reaching almost epidemic proportions, with one in three adults expected to have this diagnosis by 2030.[45] Consequently, the annual number of lower extremity total joint procedures is expected to double by the year 2016.[36] Projections for 2016 include more than 1,046,000 total knee replacements (TKRs), with 3,500,000 replacements expected to be performed in 2030.[33] Fortunately, TKR has proved to be a durable procedure as well, with multiple studies demonstrating patient satisfaction rates of 90% to 95% and over 90% implant survival over 15-year follow-up.* The patient population younger than 55 years of age is also enjoying similar benefits.[20]

Although total knee arthroplasty has been very successful and durable in terms of relieving pain and returning patients to function, complications occur. A recent analysis noted that 38,300 revision knee replacements were performed in 2005, this number is projected to reach close to 268,200 by 2030 (a 600% increase).[36] Equally concerning is that although the number of primary and revision total joint procedures is increasing, the number of adult reconstruction surgeons is decreasing.[44]

For various reasons, substantial dysfunction develops in 15% to 20% of TKR patients, renders them unresponsive to standard physical therapy modalities, and may require them to have revision surgery.[6,27] Recent studies have shown that an important proportion of TKR patients are dissatisfied with the procedure and have not had their expectations met.[7] Sharkey et al. noted that more than half of revisions were done less than 2 years after the index operation.[70] In their series, 50% of early revision surgeries were related to malalignment or malposition, instability, and failure of fixation. Prodromes of failure following total knee arthroplasty can include pain, swelling, stiffness, deformity, and instability. Radiographic findings may include loosening, polyethylene wear, and osteolysis.[66,70,89]

Much of the literature has not considered lower extremity alignment as a mode of failure. Pain that was present prior to the surgery and persists without change suggests an extrinsic cause, such as persistent lower extremity deformity.[37] The large number of knee replacements done annually makes even a small percentage of revision surgery a large absolute number. Design and surgical innovation will continue to help eliminate the

potential for surgical errors. Management of foot and ankle deformity and restoring overall limb alignment will improve implant survival and patient outcomes.

PHYSICAL EXAMINATION

Clinical examination should begin with a complete history of symptoms, mechanism of injury or progression, and postoperative course. In addition to the patient history, physical examination should note where the pain is located and if there is any associated instability. The surgeon should evaluate active and passive ranges of knee motion, check patellar tracking, evaluate the integrity of the extensor mechanism, and perform a thorough neuromuscular examination of the knee and adjacent joints. Careful assessment of quadriceps and gastrocnemius strength and flexibility should be performed as well, with the knee flexed and extended. Both limbs should be examined with the patient standing and with the entire limb visible to assess overall alignment. One can estimate limb varus or valgus by placing a goniometer to the anterior aspect of the thigh and lower part of the leg, centered on the patella. A limb length discrepancy may also result in a varus or valgus deformity about the knee. The patient's gait should also be observed while walking down the hall, as will be discussed in the next section. The standing anteroposterior (AP) knee radiograph is usually the most important study for evaluating the preoperative status of the knee. Serial radiographs are helpful in assessing changes in implant position or progression of intra-articular deformity. Lateral and patella Merchant or sunrise views are also relevant in assessing the pre- and postoperative knee. Dedicated foot and ankle films are useful in the patient with ankle or hindfoot pain and deformity. Radiologic osteoarthritis of the ankle has been observed in 35% of patients with knee osteoarthritis before TKA was performed.[47,75]

In addition, hip-to-ankle weight-bearing films will help assess malalignment and concomitant lower extremity deformity, which is also helpful with potential deformities that might interfere with the use of stemmed components (Fig. 168.1). The clinical alignment of the lower part of the leg—the anatomic axis—measures the femorotibial angle. This axis is measured by drawing lines parallel to the long axis of the femur and the tibia and then measuring the intercepting angle. The normal femorotibial angle is 6 degrees valgus, which distributes 60% of the load to the medial knee and 40% laterally.[77] The anatomic axis is differentiated from the load-bearing mechanical axis of the limb, which is measured from the center of the femoral head through the knee to the center of the talus on a standing x-ray. The mechanical axis angular measurement gives the best

---

*References 5, 11, 17, 22, 26, 44, 52, 60, 65, 69, 70, and 89.

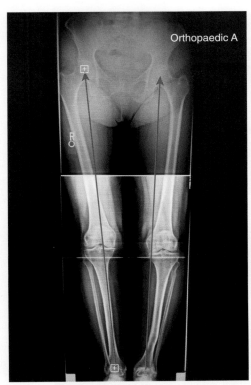

FIG 168.1 Hip-to-ankle weight-bearing films are essential for the assessment of lower extremity alignment.

functional evaluation of lower extremity alignment, and is considered the gold standard method for assessing knee alignment.[23,35,38,65,85]

Correct limb alignment proportionately distributes load across the medial and lateral articular surfaces.[35] In neutrally aligned limbs (0 to 2 degrees of varus), the medial compartment bears 60% to 70% of the force during weight bearing, and the mechanical axis line passes through a midpoint between the tibial spines.[1,12,42] In a varus knee, the load-bearing axis passes medial to the knee and a moment arm is created, further increasing the force across the medial compartment.[35] In contrast, in a valgus knee, the load-bearing axis passes lateral to the knee, and the resulting moment arm increases force across the lateral compartment.[78]

Close observation of a patient's gait will yield insight as to how foot and ankle deformity might result in TKR failure. The normal human walking cycle is divided into stance and swing phases as they affect each limb. A single cycle is the motion between the heel strikes of two successive steps of the same foot. One cycle consists of a stance and swing phase of the same leg (Fig. 168.2). The stance phase, which represents the weight-bearing portion of the cycle, is approximately 62% of the cycle, and lasts from initial heel strike until toe-off. The swing or recovery phase represents approximately 38% of the cycle, and lasts from toe-off to heel strike. The stance phase is divided into three segments: heel strike, flat foot (midstance and terminal stance), and heel rise.[88] There are two periods of double limb support with both feet on the ground (from 0% to 12% and 50% to 62% in the gait cycle), which are split by a period of single limb support (12% to 50%). Foot flat should be observed by 7% of the cycle, opposite toe-off at 12%, heel rise beginning at 34% as the swing leg passes the stance foot, and opposite heel strike at 50%.[51]

In general, normal weight bearing progresses from the lateral heel at strike to the great toe at push-off. The foot is a shock absorber at heel strike and adapts to uneven surfaces during stance. When the foot absorbs the body's weight when first striking the ground, the hindfoot moves into valgus as the calcaneus passively everts and the longitudinal arch flattens, both of which help to unlock the transverse tarsal joint.[56,59] During the swing phase, the patient requires adequate hip and knee flexion to clear the foot, and the lower extremity everts in part because of the swinging contralateral limb. At this point, the subtalar joint inverts, and the transverse tarsal joint begins to stiffen and stabilize.[56,59] The final period of the stance phase will see most of the body weight transferred to the other foot. At this time, the subtalar joint further inverts, the longitudinal arch is maximally elevated, and the transverse tarsal joints become rigid in preparation for toe-off. A healthy posterior tibial tendon also assists with subtalar inversion and with heel lift. At push-off, the foot becomes a rigid lever to provide a propulsive forward force.

Shoe wear will affect the way a person walks, so shoes should also be inspected. The character of wear on the soles, in addition to the presence of supports or pads in the shoes, can indicate gait difficulties. For example, patients with a varus hindfoot deformity, which can cause increased medial tibiofemoral joint stresses, have shoes that show marked lateral wear. With genu valgum, more load may be placed on the medial ankle, and shoes may reveal more posteromedial wear.[28] Patients can be advised to consider modifying their shoe wear internally (orthotics, arch supports) and externally (lifts, resoling), in addition to addressing chronic foot and ankle complaints, such as pain, swelling, and instability.

FOOT AND ANKLE DEFORMITY AND KNEE ALIGNMENT

Malalignment is a potent predictor of disease progression in patients with osteoarthritis of the knee; postoperative limb alignment also plays a crucial role in the long-term survival of TKR.[4,9,35,65] Excessive medial or lateral tibial loading, secondary to component alignment, limb malalignment, or ligamentous imbalance is found to be associated with edge loading, bone collapse, and component failure.[2,4,49,71,79] Berend et al. found that posterolateral subluxation was highly associated with preoperative valgus alignment.[4] Extra-articular planovalgus foot deformity along with a valgus knee creates a rotational imbalance in the knee that can lead to failure.[4,14,25]

Bhave et al. noted that 6% of functional problems following TKR were secondary to ipsilateral foot malalignment.[6] These deformities can include pes planovalgus (flatfoot), hindfoot cavovarus, muscle tightness, gastrocnemius contracture, fracture malunion, ipsilateral distal arthritis, and neuroarthropathy (diabetes, Charcot). Foot and ankle deformity can lead to knee malalignment, progressive knee deformity, maltracking, and increased wear and loosening, which result in pain and difficulty ambulating.[9,24,64] Varus malalignment has been shown to predispose the medial compartment of the knee to a fourfold amplification of forces loaded, whereas valgus malalignment has been shown to predispose the lateral compartment of the knee to a two- to fivefold increase in loading.[12,35,72] For these reasons, restoring the mechanical limb is paramount during

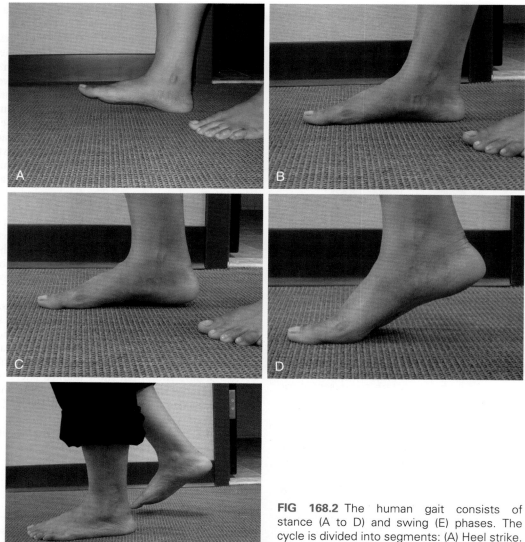

FIG 168.2 The human gait consists of stance (A to D) and swing (E) phases. The cycle is divided into segments: (A) Heel strike. (B) Flatfoot. (C) Heel rise. (D) Toe off. (E) Push off.

knee arthroplasty. Placing components within 3 degrees of freedom (negative or positive) of the mechanical axis is advocated to prevent premature implant failure and to improve prosthesis survival times.[2,3,49,79] In patients with altered lower extremity kinematics, the use of a knee prosthesis with increased conformity and constraint might lead to increased rates of loosening, increased polyethylene wear, and osteolysis.[4,14,53]

Norton et al.[57] looked at the pre- and postoperative long-leg radiographs of 401 TKAs. They found that as the mechanical axis becomes more varus or valgus, the hindfoot orients in a more valgus or varus alignment, respectively. For every degree increase in the valgus mechanical axis angle, the hindfoot shifts into varus by −0.43; for every degree increase in the varus mechanical axis angle, the hindfoot shifts into valgus by −0.49 degrees. They noted that 72% of the variance in overall hindfoot angle was secondary to changes in subtalar joint orientation. Mullaji and Shetty[55] noted similar findings that restoration of limb alignment with TKA may be associated with persistent hindfoot valgus and lateral deviation of the weight-bearing axis.

TREATMENT OF FOOT AND ANKLE DEFORMITY

Malalignment is associated with disease progression, and it is also susceptible to the effects of other risk factors, including obesity, quadriceps strength, and laxity.[35] Consequently, nonoperative treatment includes a combination of weight loss, shoe-wear modification, and physical therapy focusing on quadriceps and foot and ankle stretching, strengthening, and stabilization. Initially, a total contact arch support made of a semi-rigid material supporting the longitudinal arch and providing appropriate heel posting should help correct the flexible component of the deformity and decrease the load in the affected compartment. Orthotics can help slow progression of the disease and augment surgical and exercise treatments. Should the deformity progress and/or become more rigid, an ankle joint–spanning or more rigid brace or casting might be required. According to the American Academy of Orthopaedic Surgeons (AAOS) Clinical Practice Guideline Summary for the Nonarthroplasty Treatment of Osteoarthritis of the Knee, published in 2013,[40] patients with symptomatic arthritis of the knee should be encouraged to lose weight and to engage in exercise and quadriceps strengthening.[62] However, the guidelines did not recommend lateral heel wedges for patients with symptomatic medial compartmental osteoarthritis of the knee. This conclusion was based on the limited evidence for effectiveness of these inserts as addressed by one level II systematic review of three level II randomized controlled trials that examined the use of lateral heel wedges in patients with symptomatic varus arthritis knees.[50,58,73-76,81-84]

If nonoperative measures fail, numerous surgical options are available to address lower extremity deformities in the foot and ankle, including synovectomy, tendon transfer, osteotomy, reconstruction, medial and/or lateral column stabilization, arthrodesis, and arthroplasty.[8,62,81] The goal of surgery is to restore a painless, well-aligned, plantigrade foot that will allow a return to activities of daily living. Treatment should be tailored to the specific deformity. These procedures are technically demanding, and soft tissue reconstruction alone usually fails to correct alignment and provide long-lasting pain relief. Good outcomes require the use of sufficient hardware to maintain alignment and to optimize healing. These procedures require a long recovery and extended periods of non–weight bearing for sufficient healing.

POSTERIOR TIBIAL TENDON DYSFUNCTION

There are multiple causes described for posterior tibial tendon dysfunction or insufficiency including chronic soft tissue degeneration, rheumatoid arthritis, degenerative joint disease, posttraumatic arthritis, or Charcot neuropathy. Most patients develop deformity gradually, initially without pain. Occasionally trauma can be the cause of acute disability. Posterior tibial tendon dysfunction occurs more commonly in white, obese, hypertensive women in the fourth to sixth decade.[15,21,34,59] Sharkey et al. reviewed a series of revision knee arthroplasties, and noted that although the prevalence of posterior tibial tendon insufficiency in the general population is unknown, its 25% prevalence in a population of revision total knee arthroplasty patients was very high.[70] Valgus deformity of the hindfoot is a notably common and disabling defect in patients who have rheumatoid arthritis. It has been estimated that 89% of patients who have rheumatoid arthritis have problems with their feet.[42] Of these patients, 13% to 64% later develop posterior tibial tendon insufficiency, and disability increases with duration of the disease.[42,53] A study of United States Marine recruits also found that flat, pronated feet were associated with knee pain.[39,64] Brouwer et al. compared patients with osteoarthritis of the knee and age-matched healthy subjects and found that patients with osteoarthritis of the knee had a more inverted subtalar joint neutral position on the affected side.[9,64] Genu valgum has also been shown to accentuate a flatfoot deformity.[86]

Because the posterior tibial tendon lies posterior to the axis of the ankle and medial to the axis of the subtalar joint, its function is to plantar flex the ankle, invert the midfoot, and elevate the medial longitudinal arch.[86] In normal feet, contraction of the posterior tibial tendon locks the midtarsal joints in a varus position so that, during gait, the forefoot functions as a rocker while body weight progresses anteriorly during the stance phase.[40] The rigid midfoot conformation facilitates the push-off required to propel the body through the last aspect of gait.

Over time, an attenuated posterior tibial tendon loses strength and the arch collapses. The relative strength of the posterior tibial tendon is more than twice that of the peroneus brevis, its primary antagonist because of its large cross-sectional area.[86] However, because of its short excursion, elongation of the tendon by only 1 cm makes it ineffective as the primary restraint to the longitudinal arch.[73,86] Weakness is seen with failure to perform single leg heel rise on the affected side, as well as limited resistance against an inverted and plantarflexed foot.[56] In the stance position, the posterior tibial tendon is unable to initiate hindfoot inversion. Meanwhile, the antagonist peroneus brevis muscle maintains heel eversion, which further prevents locking of the transverse tarsal (midfoot) through late stance and push-off.

The deformity will progress to heel equinovalgus, pes planus and pronation, excessive external foot progression, relative internal rotation of the talus and tibia, and forefoot abduction, yielding the classic "too many toes" sign (Fig. 168.3). When subtalar pronation persists through midstance, while contralateral pelvic advancement produces an external rotation moment on the femur, the knee is placed under significant axial torsion.[86] This results in increased valgus stress and internal rotation at the knee, patellar maltracking with an increased Q angle, and painful lateral tibiofemoral stress syndrome. With the hindfoot in valgus, the Achilles insertion is also lateralized and effectively shortened, reinforcing the deformity and weakening other supporting ligaments, resulting in ligamentous imbalance and medial ankle instability. The gastrocnemius contracture also increases tension in the posterior calf, potentially causing a postoperative knee flexion contracture (lack of extension ≥10 degrees) which causes anterior knee pain.[6]

In addition, the abducted forefoot overloads the metatarsal heads, leading to painful metatarsalgia. To manage, the patient tries to shorten the effective lever arm provided by the painful foot and further externally rotates the weight-bearing limb during gait. This position exacerbates the stresses on the ipsilateral knee. This results in the mechanical axis shifting laterally through the knee and ankle joints, and stiffness increasing with the severity of the hindfoot deformity.[29,53] Eventually degenerative arthritis develops in the hindfoot, forefoot, and possibly the ankle joint as well.[21] Increased rigidity of the foot and ankle leads to greater stresses across the knee and periarticular joints in the foot, further exacerbating deformity on the TKR.

The classification of posterior tibial tendon dysfunction includes four stages.[56,59] Stage 1 involves pain and swelling along the tendon with minimal foot deformity. Stage 2 indicates the onset of a flexible flatfoot deformity, with inadequate passive arch support. This stage is marked by hindfoot valgus and forefoot abduction with a loss in medial longitudinal arch height. Stage 3 disease is a rigid hindfoot deformity, typically with degenerative changes and a flattened arch that is not passively correctable. Stage 4 disease, which occurs with longstanding tendon dysfunction, affects the ankle joint and is marked by the involvement of the deltoid ligament and valgus tibiotalar tilt.

The stage and progression of the flatfoot deformity generally determines the degree and duration of the treatment.[28] If shoewear modification, lifestyle changes, and physical therapy fail, surgical options are available. Painful tendonitis (Stage 1) can be treated with debridement alone in limited cases. More advanced flexible deformity (Stage 2) typically requires a flexor

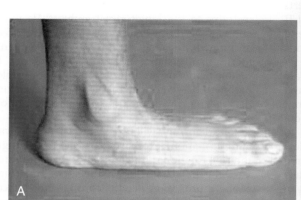
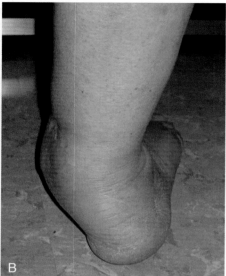

FIG 168.3 Pes planovalgus deformity with (A) flattened arch, pronation, and (B) hindfoot abductovalgus.

tendon transfer, spring ligament reconstruction, and some combination of hindfoot osteotomy such as a medializing calcaneus osteotomy and/or a lateral column lengthening. Additional tendon transfers or midfoot osteotomies or fusion may also be required to maintain correction. More rigid deformities (Stage 3 and 4) typically require an arthrodesis, classically a double or triple arthrodesis of the subtalar, talonavicular, and/or calcaneocuboid joints. Additional procedures might also include a Strayer gastrocnemius recession, selective naviculocuneiform or tarsometatarsal fusion, deltoid ligament reconstruction, and concomitant or staged ankle correction with arthrodesis or total ankle replacement (Fig. 168.4).

CAVOVARUS DEFORMITY

When the ankle and foot are in excess supination or varus, the weight-bearing line passes medially. This in turn increases the lateral ankle and foot stresses, and increases tension on the peroneus longus, causing additional first ray plantar flexion, which contributes to an increased calcaneal pitch.[29,72] This muscle imbalance creates a more rigid forefoot, which results in increased weight absorption on the first and fifth metatarsals and inefficient ground reaction force absorption. This weight absorption limits internal rotation of the foot and can lead to inversion sprains, peroneal tendonitis, iliotibial band friction syndrome, varus stress on the knee, and trochanteric bursitis. This can cause varus malalignment of the TKR.

When shoe-wear modification fails, surgical correction is based on whether the deformity is forefoot- or hindfoot-driven, which can be determined by Coleman block testing. The patient stands on a ¾-inch wooden block under the lateral column of the forefoot, leaving the medial column and first ray unsupported. If the heel can be forced into valgus, the subtalar joint remains flexible and the cavus can be corrected by addressing the forefoot deformity alone.[31] If the hindfoot remains rigid during Coleman block testing, then both the hindfoot and forefoot are involved and require correction. Surgery for cavovarus deformity can include a combination of procedures, including

but not limited to, partial plantar fasciectomy, peroneus longus-to-brevis transfer, lateral ligament reconstruction, lateralizing and/or closing wedge calcaneus osteotomy, dorsiflexion closing wedge first metatarsal osteotomy, first ray Jones procedure, and claw toe corrections.

POSTTRAUMATIC DEFORMITY

In other cases, patients may have a history of lower extremity trauma with resultant deformity that can adversely affect the knee. Fractures that heal with a malunion or nonunion with coronal and/or sagittal plane malalignment can overload the knee and/or ankle. This is certainly best evaluated with clinical evaluation and 3-joint standing radiographs. Deformity should be corrected to unload the joint above and below, which should slow the progression of degenerative changes. This deformity will typically be noted prior to the primary knee arthroplasty, and the decision can be made whether to perform correction simultaneously or in staged fashion.

NEUROARTHROPATHY

Charcot arthropathy is a devastating bone and joint disease. Although it most commonly occurs in those with diabetes and neuropathy, it has been known to occur with other nondiabetic neuropathies as well.[67] Patients can initially present with subtle pain and instability. Initial treatment should include bracing or casting and frequent skin checks to monitor for development of ulcerations or other skin lesions. Neuropathic osteoarthropathy, otherwise known as Charcot neuroarthropathy, is a chronic, degenerative arthropathy and is associated with decreased sensory innervation. Typical findings include joint destruction, disorganization, and effusion with osseous debris. Progression of Charcot neuroarthropathy can follow a predictable clinical and radiographic pattern described by the Eichenholtz classification.[87] Although not an absolute contraindication, lower extremity neuroarthropathy can lead to severe deformity that can compromise the success of total knee arthroplasty.

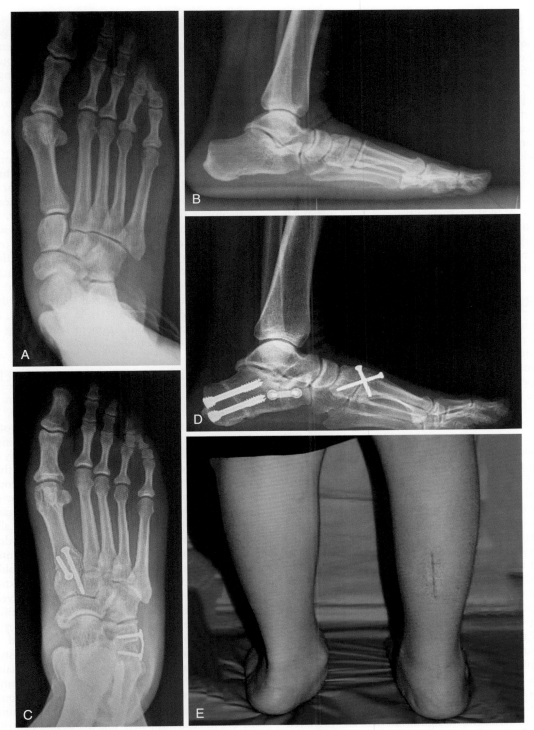

FIG 168.4 Correction of a Flexible Pes Planovalgus Deformity (A and B) Note the flattened arch with decreased lateral talo-first metatarsal angle and increased talar head uncoverage. (C and D) Correction achieved with flexor tendon transfer, spring ligament reconstruction, lateral column lengthening with bone graft and plate fixation, medializing calcaneus osteotomy, gastrocnemius recession, and first tarsometatarsal arthrodesis to correct residual forefoot varus. (E) Note the difference between corrected and uncorrected sides.

Many of these patients are still active and working full-time, and they cannot afford to be disabled with painful deformity and arthritis. Consequently, bracing is not always tolerated for long periods. The profound loss of bone density also makes these patients difficult to treat with standard techniques of fixation. When knee arthroplasty is performed, it must be well balanced and well fixed, with cement and stem fixation. Foot and ankle deformity often requires extensive corrective and stabilization procedures that entail salvaging the lower extremity beneath the arthroplasty. The choice of treatment must be determined by what is best for the patient, not what is best for the ankle or foot.[67] Treatments that can be considered include a combination of procedures involving bone resection, osteotomies, arthrodeses, and wound care, typically using supplements to the usual means of fixation, such as plates, screws, intramedullary nail, and/or multiplanar external fixation (Fig. 168.5). The risks of surgical reconstruction and the difficulties of postoperative convalescence are considerable in this patient population and should not be underestimated.[67]

ANKLE ARTHRITIS

Although most hip and knee arthritis is degenerative, over 70% of ankle arthritis results from a traumatic event.[66] Ankle arthritis is disabling, with the ankle having one-third the contact area but 3 times the forces compared with the hip and knee.[67] With failure of nonoperative treatment, ankle arthrodesis has historically been the gold standard surgical treatment for painful, end-stage ankle arthritis, especially in the younger, more active patient. The ankle should be fused preferentially in 5 degrees of valgus and external rotation, and in a plantigrade position with the talus positioned under the tibia to reduce the lever arm. This position maximizes the compensatory potential of the subtalar and Chopart joints and allows the closest approximation to normal gait patterns for the knee, foot, and ankle. In this position, the weight-bearing line of the body passes medial to the calcaneus, which unloads the lateral collateral ligaments of the ankle. The transverse tarsal joint is also unlocked, and the forefoot falls into slight pronation and valgus for an even weight distribution throughout the gait cycle. Excess external rotation should be avoided in the fused ankle because it can cause medial knee laxity.[13] If there is a short lower extremity or an unstable knee joint as a result of quadriceps weakness or a compromised extensor mechanism, the ankle joint should be fused in slight plantar flexion (7 to 10 degrees) to help give stability to the knee joint, without causing a back-knee thrust on the knee joint.[51] However, excess plantar flexion (>10 degrees) is associated with genu recurvatum.[13]

Recent studies have demonstrated concerns about the long-term durability of ankle arthrodesis; development of ipsilateral hindfoot osteoarthritis leading to significant pain and impaired function is of special concern.[16,80] In the appropriate patient, total ankle replacement is another treatment option. With improved implant designs, surgical techniques, and instrumentation, recent studies have found that intermediate and long-term functional outcomes, pain relief, and survival of total ankle replacement are comparable and superior to those of ankle fusion.[9-18,33,68,76] The preservation of motion significantly decreases stresses on the surrounding joints, which should decrease the likelihood that they will progress toward painful arthritis. Total ankle arthroplasty has been shown to reproduce a more normal gait and cadence compared to ankle

fusion (Fig. 168.6). A recent presentation at the American Orthopaedic Foot and Ankle Society studied gait mechanics in patients who underwent total ankle replacement and found improvement in pain, gait, and function through 2 years postoperatively and maintenance of ankle range of motion.[18] According to the authors, there is a significant reduction in pain, and improved stability and balance following total ankle replacement. Patients are able to decrease dependence on double-leg support, and increase surgical-side single-leg support time, stride length, and walking speed.

Experienced surgeons can safely perform concurrent realignment procedures at the time of total ankle arthroplasty without an increased rate of complications.[10,19,43] For a valgus ankle, these procedures may include medial displacement calcaneus osteotomy, flexor digitorum longus transfer, spring ligament reconstruction, lateral column lengthening, subtalar or triple arthrodesis, deltoid reconstruction, Achilles tendon lengthening, or tibia or fibula osteotomy.[10] For patients with varus deformity, corrective procedures may also include lateralizing (Dwyer) calcaneus osteotomy, dorsiflexion first metatarsal osteotomy, first tarsometatarsal (Lapidus) arthrodesis, plantar fascia release, subtalar or triple arthrodesis, lateral ligament reconstruction, deltoid ligament lengthening or release, or a lengthening medial malleolar osteotomy.[43]

KNEE ARTHROPLASTY WITH FOOT DEFORMITY

Sobel et al. reported that valgus knee alignment is associated with increased stresses at the medial hindfoot.[13,73] Kennan et al. also noted an association between valgus foot deformity and valgus knee deformity in patients with rheumatoid arthritis.[42] They concluded that valgus hindfoot deformity in these patients is a result of exaggerated pronation forces on the weakened and inflamed subtalar joint, which results in a compensatory gait secondary to pain and weakness. This deformity resulted in increased valgus stresses on the knee during gait. Radiographic findings supported the concept that valgus alignment of the knee is commonly associated with valgus deformity of the hindfoot. The authors suggested that prevention of a valgus hindfoot deformity in patients with rheumatoid arthritis might slow or avert deterioration of the ipsilateral knee.

Chandler and Moskal looked prospectively at a single-surgeon series of patients suffering from painful knee arthritis with coexistent hindfoot malalignment.[13] They compared knee and hindfoot alignment preoperatively and postoperatively. Although the authors did not find a consistent relationship between knee malalignment and hindfoot malalignment, they found that hindfoot alignment was significantly changed by knee arthroplasty, with up to 50% of hindfoot malalignment corrected by TKR. They concluded that alignment of the foot before knee arthroplasty was the largest contributing factor to the hindfoot alignment after knee arthroplasty. They also noted that patients with larger preoperative deformities had the most postoperative improvement of their hindfoot deformity after arthroplasty. Overall, valgus deformities remained in valgus, and varus deformities remained in varus, although the angular amount was reduced by half by knee arthroplasty.

Meding et al. reported on the outcomes of 9475 cruciate-retaining cemented total knee arthroplasties.[53] In this group, 48 tibias required revision, but none were because of infection or extensor mechanism dysfunction. Sixteen required revision secondary to ligamentous instability. Twelve of these 16 unstable

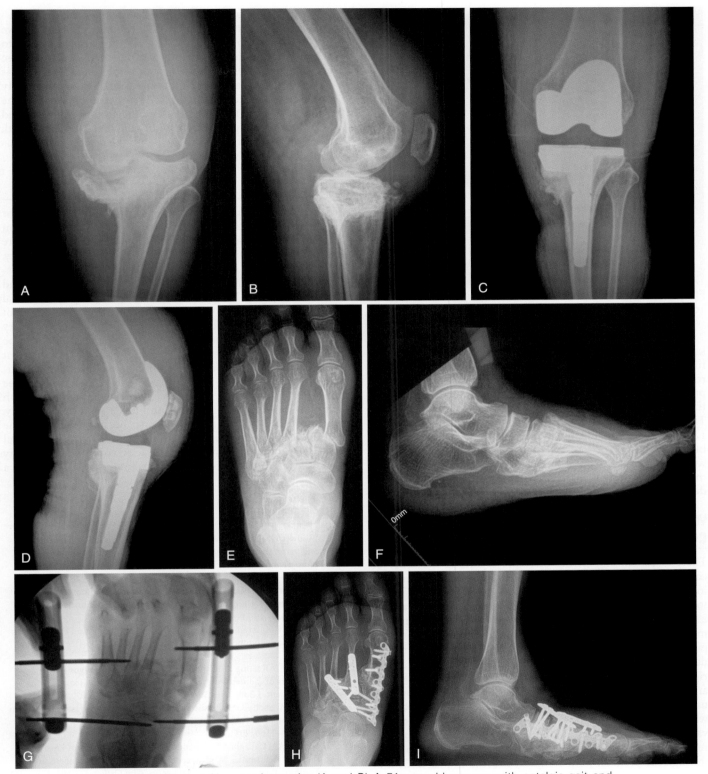

FIG 168.5 Charcot Neuroarthropathy (A and B) A 51-year-old woman with antalgic gait and neuropathic degenerative changes and significant bone loss. (C and D) Total knee arthroplasty with cemented, stemmed fixation with tibial augments. Six months postoperatively she complained of foot swelling and compromised gait, but not pain. (E and F) Chronic complete divergent Lisfranc fracture dislocation. (G to I) Provisional intraoperative external fixation was required to aid reduction. Extended arthrodesis provided stability and allowed the patient to return to regular weight bearing and full activities.

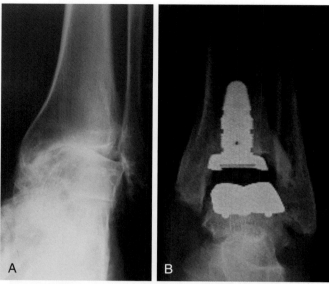

FIG 168.6 (A) Painful ankle arthritis with valgus deformity. (B) Total ankle arthroplasty.

knees had their tibias revised secondary to ipsilateral posterior tibial tendon insufficiency, with noted posterolateral femoral rollback and subluxation, and resultant posterolateral and posteromedial wear. Eight of the 12 had documented posterior tibial tendon insufficiency at the time of the index operation. The average time to revision was 6 years 4 months (range 3 to 12 years). They concluded that increased relative tibia and talus internal rotation (or foot external rotation) leads to increased valgus knee stress. In addition, the offset of the lower extremity mechanical axis will increase with the severity of hindfoot deformity.

WHICH DEFORMITY SHOULD BE CORRECTED FIRST?

There is controversy in the literature regarding the order of correction of lower extremity deformity affecting multiple joints. Figgie et al. recommended addressing the more symptomatic joint first.[13] Kennan et al. recommended correcting any hindfoot malalignment prior to total knee arthroplasty to minimize the stresses on the implant.[42] They believed that if progression of the deformity of the foot was prevented, then deterioration of the knee might be slowed or averted. Severe rigid foot and ankle deformity is likely responsible for early pain and failures in patients who had severe knee deformity prior to undergoing TKA. Norton et al. recommended that patients with varus arthritis of the knee be examined for fixed hindfoot valgus deformity.[57] The inability of a rigid subtalar joint to reorient itself after knee realignment, with failure to compensate through the peritalar joint complex, can lead to post-TKA foot and ankle pain, disability, and premature failure of the TKA because of an inability to offload malaligned forces.

Most of the current literature suggests that the TKA be performed first.[13,53,74,86] Correction of lower extremity alignment with total knee arthroplasty leads to changes in alignment

of the ankle joint as well as the intended changes in knee joints.[39] Mullaji and Shetty[55] noted a 31% change in postoperative hindfoot alignment after TKA. Chandler et al. noted that up to 50% of the hindfoot deformity can be corrected with knee replacement alone.[13] It is the author's opinion that, if pain is similar at the knee and the foot/ankle, total knee arthroplasty should be performed before the foot reconstruction because the alignment between the hindfoot and the ground will be altered once the knee is aligned. If foot and/or ankle surgery is required, the reconstruction can be aligned with the corrected mechanical alignment of the TKR.

CONCLUSIONS

TKR has proven to be a successful and durable treatment for knee arthritis. With improved instrumentation and navigation technology, we can perform knee replacement and restore physiologic alignment with higher precision and accuracy. Outcomes can be further improved with appropriate assessment and management of foot and ankle deformity before and after arthroplasty. Postoperative limb alignment plays a crucial role in the long-term survival of a TKR. Understanding gait mechanics and the effect on the limb is important for every arthroplasty surgeon because foot and ankle deformity can be a common reason for failure. Should nonoperative treatment fail, surgical correction and restoration of overall limb mechanical alignment should provide pain relief and improve knee implant survival and patient satisfaction. For patients with painful knee arthritis and foot and ankle pain or deformity, the knee should be addressed first because much of the hindfoot deformity can be corrected with a well-aligned total knee arthroplasty. If symptomatic foot and ankle deformity persists, appropriate reconstruction should be performed at a later date.

KEY REFERENCES

9. Brouwer GM, van Tol AW, Bergink AP, et al: Association between valgus and varus alignment and the development and progression of radiographic osteoarthritis of the knee. *Arthritis Rheum* 56:1204–1211, 2007.

13. Chandler JT, Moskal JT: Evaluation of knee and hindfoot alignment before and after total knee arthroplasty: a prospective analysis. *J Arthroplasty* 19:211–216, 2004.

29. Guichet J-M, Javed A, Russell J, et al: Effect of the foot on the mechanical alignment of the lower limbs. *Clin Orthop* 415:193–201, 2003.

53. Meding JB, Keating EM, Ritter MA, et al: The planovalgus foot: a harbinger of failure of posterior cruciate-retaining total knee replacement. *J Bone Joint Surg* 87A(Suppl 2):59–62, 2005.

55. Mullaji A, Shetty GM: Persistent hindfoot valgus causes lateral deviation of weightbearing axis after total knee arthroplasty. *Clin Orthop* 469:1154–1160, 2011.

57. Norton AA, Callaghan JJ, Amendola A, et al: Correction of knee and hindfoot deformities in advanced knee osteoarthritis: compensatory hindfoot alignment and where it occurs. *Clin Orthop* 473:166–174, 2015.

73. Sobel M, Stern SH, Manoli A II, et al: The association of posterior tibial tendon insufficiency with valgus osteoarthritis of the knee. *Am J Knee Surg* 5:59, 1992.

The references for this chapter can also be found on www.expertconsult.com.

Revision and Complex Knee Arthroplasty

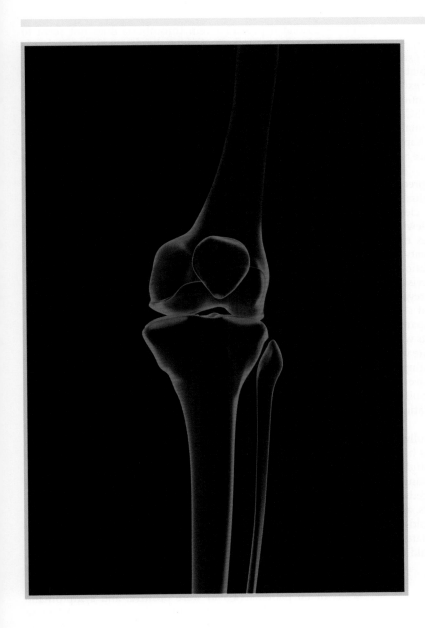

169

Complications of Total Knee Arthroplasty

Saurabh Khakharia, Michael P. Nett, Christopher A. Hajnik, Giles R. Scuderi

GENERAL COMPLICATIONS

The results following total knee arthroplasty (TKA) are excellent. The literature demonstrates over 90% survivorship at 20 years with a well-performed arthroplasty. Despite routine excellent outcomes, as with any substantial surgery, complications occur. With the Surgical Care Improvement Project (SCIP) initiative, emphasis has been placed on avoiding preventable complications during the perioperative period. This chapter will focus on management of complications, but avoidance and prevention will also be discussed.

Prevention of medical complications begins with the preoperative evaluation. Prior to TKA, the patient should be evaluated by the primary care physician for preoperative medical clearance. The orthopedic surgeon is also responsible for reviewing the medical history and should note the comorbidities that must be addressed to minimize the chance of complication. Memtsoudis et al.[152] reported on in-hospital complications, including mortality, following unilateral, bilateral, and revision TKA. Over 4 million discharges were evaluated with regard to patient demographics, comorbidities, and in-hospital stay. Complications and mortality of each procedure were compared. In this series, in-hospital mortality was highest for patients who had bilateral TKA (0.5%), whereas the lowest mortality rate was associated with unicompartmental TKA (0.3%). Interestingly, TKAs had a similarly low mortality rate of 0.3%. The overall complication rate during hospitalization was highest for bilateral TKAs, 12.2%, but the rate for in-hospital complications following unicompartmental TKA was still 8.2%.

A patient's medical history should be reviewed carefully if bilateral TKA is contemplated. Although several studies have demonstrated success in bilateral procedures, numerous studies have demonstrated the higher risk of complication.[29,52] Younger patients in good health seem to tolerate a bilateral procedure with little increased risk. However, older or obese patients, and those with an extensive medical or cardiac history, should be discouraged from considering a bilateral procedure. If a bilateral procedure is performed, postoperative monitoring should be considered.

SYSTEMIC COMPLICATIONS

Thromboembolism

Deep venous thrombosis (DVT) occurs in approximately 50% of unilateral cases and in 75% of bilateral cases when no prophylaxis is used. Although DVT occurs mainly in the calf veins (Fig. 169.1), life-threatening emboli do not arise from this region. In contrast to the situation after total hip arthroplasty (THA), isolated proximal vein thrombosis does not seem to occur after knee surgery, despite the possible trauma of a pneumatic tourniquet.

Some have argued that distal thrombosis can be ignored, provided that the patient convalesces normally and is not confined to bed for a lengthy period. We believe that this view is too optimistic, although we concede that the risk of a fatal thromboembolus is small and is lower than that after THA. In a prospective review of 527 TKAs in 499 patients, Khaw et al.[119] using no prophylaxis other than antithrombotic stockings and relatively early (48 hours) mobilization, found only one death in 3 months from pulmonary embolism (0.19%). This patient had bilateral TKA and had a myocardial infarction 1 day postoperatively, with the subsequent pulmonary embolus occurring 22 days postoperatively. Seven other patients (1.3%) developed symptomatic pulmonary embolism and were treated with anticoagulation, without sequelae. This low incidence of fatal pulmonary embolism has been supported in other studies by Stulberg et al. (0%),[215] Stringer et al. (0%),[214] Khaw et al. (0.2%),[119] and Ansari et al. (0.4%).[4] Fatal emboli do occur, however, and three patients died as a result of emboli in the first 400 arthroplasties performed at the Hospital for Special Surgery. No specific prophylaxis was used at that time; the cause of death was confirmed by autopsy in all cases. In addition, we believe that the incidence of fatal pulmonary emboli is underestimated. A certain proportion of calf clots propagate proximally to form the more dangerous clots in the popliteal and femoral veins. This process takes time, however, and the major risk period for a fatal pulmonary embolism after TKA may be in weeks 3 and 4 postsurgery; this is in contrast to what occurs after THA, in which a clot in the proximal veins may be found in 20% of cases after the first week. Because most TKA patients now are discharged after hospitalization of 2 to 3 days, sudden death at home in a patient having no clinical evidence of venous thrombosis may be attributed to myocardial infarction.

Calf clots may not in themselves be important but should be regarded as a harbinger of more proximal clotting. Haas et al.[86] have studied 1329 patients with 1697 TKAs. Thrombosis was found in 808 patients (61%); 53% had thrombosis of the calf vein and 8% had thrombosis of the proximal veins. The lung scans of 60 patients (4.5%) were positive, and symptomatic pulmonary emboli occurred in 14 patients (1.1%). All these patients received aspirin as prophylaxis. Venography was performed between postoperative days 4 and 6. A perfusion lung scan obtained on postoperative day 5 to 7 was compared with a preoperative baseline perfusion lung scan. Thrombosis of the calf vein was treated with warfarin (Coumadin); the dosage was adjusted to maintain a prothrombin time at approximately

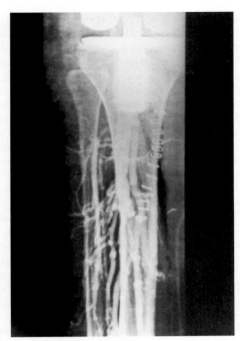

FIG 169.1 Venogram showing clots in the calf veins.

1.5 times control. Only patients with symptomatic proximal thrombi or symptomatic pulmonary emboli were fully anticoagulated with intravenous heparin. Although the natural history of thromboembolic disease was altered by prophylaxis and treatment, 6.5% of patients with calf thrombi had a positive lung scan and 1.6% had symptomatic pulmonary emboli. This finding was compared with patients who had no venographic evidence of DVT, of whom 1.9% had a positive lung scan and 0.2% had symptomatic pulmonary emboli. Statistical significances for the difference in lung scan and pulmonary embolus results were $p = 0.001$ and $p = 0.034$, respectively. Patients with calf or proximal thrombi were found to have similar rates of positive lung scans and symptomatic pulmonary emboli.

The risk of symptomatic and fatal pulmonary embolism is of greatest concern. Without prophylaxis, the rates of pulmonary embolism and fatal pulmonary embolism range from 1% to 28% and 0.1% to 2.0%, respectively.[75] From six randomized studies comparing low-molecular-weight heparin (LMWH) with warfarin, the total rate of DVT was 33% for patients who received LMWH, compared with 48% for patients who received warfarin. Similarly, the rate of proximal DVT was 7.1% and 10.4% for patients who received LMWH and warfarin, respectively. Barrett et al.[11] have reviewed 122,385 US Medicare enrollees who had a TKA in 2000. Pulmonary embolism developed in the first 3 months in 0.81% of patients who had a unilateral TKA, compared with 1.44% of patients who had undergone a simultaneous bilateral TKA.

The discussion of appropriate DVT prophylaxis is covered elsewhere in this text and is beyond the scope of this chapter. Many questions concerning how best to effect thromboprophylaxis in the orthopedic setting remain unanswered, and our (likely unobtainable) need for an ideal strategy combining complete efficacy with absolute safety remains unmet. However, we should not permit such questions and needs from obscuring fundamental truths made clear by intense research over the past several decades: (1) venous thromboembolism (VTE) is a known and serious complication of total joint arthroplasty; (2) evidence-based thromboprophylaxis works; (3) the orthopedic community needs to improve compliance with available guidelines and work on reaching a consensus.

Protocol for Patients With Documented Thromboembolic Disease

Positive venography or ultrasound. Patients with calf, popliteal, or femoral thrombi are treated with warfarin for 6 weeks. Asymptomatic pulmonary emboli are treated in the same manner. Symptomatic proximal thrombi and symptomatic pulmonary emboli are treated with heparin until the effect of the warfarin is established.[226] Based on the discretion of the individual medical consultant, intravenous heparin treatment may be continued for 1 week. Intravenous heparin carries an extreme risk of local bleeding complications and, in our opinion, should be used only in potentially life-threatening situations. This policy sometimes may cause conflict among medical advisors, who often may wish to use heparin in less threatening circumstances. Orthopedic surgeons should preemptively discuss and establish a policy and guidelines within their own institution on which surgeons and medical consultants can agree.

Greenfield filter. A Greenfield filter should be considered when pulmonary embolism occurs despite therapeutic warfarin prophylaxis, when warfarin is contraindicated in a high-risk patient, or when complications develop as a result of anticoagulation. Vaughn et al.[223] have reported on its use in 66 patients and found the technique to be safe, easy, and effective. They inserted the filter preoperatively in 42 patients who were considered at high risk for pulmonary embolus (group I) and postoperatively in 24 patients (group II). The preferred site of insertion was by way of the right internal jugular vein, and a vascular surgeon carried out the implantations. One patient in group II died of a massive pulmonary embolism 3 days after implantation. At follow-up, none of the remaining patients experienced migration of the filter, and there was no evidence of postphlebitic syndrome or chronic symptomatic edema of the lower extremity.

Fat Embolism Syndrome

The diagnosis of fat embolism can be elusive,[21,33,57,65,161] and we suspect that the condition often may pass unrecognized as the cause of transient confusional states after surgery. The syndrome results from the embolization of fat and other debris from the femur or tibia that travels mostly to the lungs. The initial effects in the lungs are mechanical, with an increase in perfusion pressure, engorgement of the vessels in the lungs, and secondary right-sided heart strain. In the presence of hypovolemic shock, the patient may die from acute right-sided heart failure. The delayed effects of fat embolism occur after 48 to 72 hours because of the chemical effects of fat. The pulmonary tissue secretes lipase, which hydrolyzes fat into free fatty acids and glycerol. These free fatty acids increase capillary permeability, cause destruction of alveolar architecture, and damage lung surfactant. The end result of all these changes is hypoxia.[185]

Clinical findings of fat embolism syndrome include tachypnea, dyspnea, profuse tracheobronchial secretions, apprehension, anxiety, delirium, confusion, unconsciousness, and petechial hemorrhage. Laboratory findings are hypoxemia on arterial blood gas testing and thrombocytopenia lower than 150,000 mm^3. Treatment is supportive. Mechanical ventilation may be required in advanced cases. Corticosteroids may be beneficial in diminishing the inflammatory response from the chemical effects of fat emboli.[175]

Monto et al.,[161] in a review of the literature, reported 19 cases with 9 deaths. Of the 19 cases, 15 were associated with long-stem cemented prostheses, such as the Guepar hinge. Four cases were associated with total condylar arthroplasty. One case was associated with intramedullary instrumentation. Fahmy et al.[65] have shown human intramedullary (IM) femoral canal pressures of 500 to 1000 mm Hg generated by using standard alignment rod techniques. Venting the canal did not lower the canal pressure significantly. IM pressures were maintained within normal limits only by overdrilling the femoral canal and gently placing the guide rod. Copious irrigation of the IM canal with pulsatile lavage, suction of marrow contents after irrigation, and use of fluted rods to assist the egress of bone marrow elements may reduce the intramedullary pressure. The use of a pneumatic tourniquet does not protect against fat embolism and, with the popularity of IM guidance systems for femoral and tibial components, an increase in the incidence of fat embolism syndrome may be expected. The surgeon should consider avoiding routine instrumentation of the IM canals of the femur and tibia in bilateral cases.

Kim et al.[121] have compared the prevalence of fat embolism after TKA in 160 patients (210 knees) with navigation and 160 patients (210 knees) without navigation. They found no significant difference in the intraoperative and postoperative hemodynamic values between the groups. A higher prevalence of fat embolism was seen (60% versus 41%) in patients with higher triglyceride levels. However, in contrast, Kalairajah et al.[114] have demonstrated a significant reduction in the number of cranial fat emboli in a group treated with computer-assisted TKA, compared with a group treated with TKA using standard IM instrumentation.

LOCAL COMPLICATIONS

Wound Drainage and Delayed Wound Healing

Soft tissue considerations must always be at the forefront when planning surgical intervention. This is especially true for high-risk patients, including those with prior incisions. Although several plastic surgery techniques are available to treat wound complications, much of the damage is already done once the complication occurs. Even the best outcomes of salvage techniques following wound failure result in functional loss and cosmetic deficit. Therefore, the surgeon's primary goal should be to avoid postoperative wound complications. Despite appropriate planning and meticulous technique, however, wound complications will occur. The orthopedic surgeon must work in conjunction with the plastic surgeon and be aware of the nonsurgical and surgical techniques available to minimize functional loss. Inappropriate management of postoperative skin problems can result in failure of the reconstruction, deep infection, a nonfunctioning extremity, amputation, and/or a potentially life-threatening situation.

Preoperative Considerations

General overview. The knee has a thin, overlying soft tissue envelope that must be protective, well vascularized, and supple enough to allow for the large degrees of stretch and shear required for a functional range of motion (ROM). Although most TKAs can be performed with standard protocols, an

understanding of when to apply specific soft tissue management principles is required. Preoperative evaluation for TKA should include not only a complete history and physical examination, including radiographic and clinical assessment of the degree of deformity and joint space narrowing, but also a thorough history and evaluation of the skin. Systemic concerns include vascular compromise, obesity, malnutrition, prolonged corticosteroid or nonsteroidal anti-inflammatory drug use, diabetes mellitus, an immunocompromised state, and a history of smoking.[*] Local factors that affect wound healing include the inability to incorporate a previous incision into the planned incision, a small skin bridge between the previous incision and the planned incision, local radiation or burns, and dense or adherent scar tissue. Other local factors may play a role as well. The correction of severe deformity may make subsequent closure difficult. Special caution should be used in patients with severe varus and rotational deformity because, as the deformity is corrected, there may not be enough skin to close the inferior aspect of the wound over the subcutaneous surface of tibia. Prior trauma may also play a role because of previously placed skin incisions, significant scarring, and loss of skin mobility.

Preoperative consultation regarding medical optimization and early plastic surgery consultation for soft tissue management should be considered in any complex case. Not only will this help minimize complication, but it will also help ensure comprehensive involvement, should complications be encountered.

Planning the skin incision. Previous anterior incisions present a concern regarding both the planned approach and healing potential of the skin and underlying tissue. A balance must be achieved between the ability to expose the knee through a prior incision and avoiding extensive undermining of the subcutaneous flaps. A clear history of the previous incision should be obtained, including the age of the wound, subcutaneous dissection and procedure performed, and any wound complications encountered. The previous surgical reports often provide critical information.

Understanding of the local anatomy and blood supply is also necessary. Terminal branches of the peripatellar anastomotic ring of arteries are responsible for most of the blood supply to the anterior skin and subcutaneous tissues. This occurs through a subdermal plexus supplied by arterioles in the subcutaneous fascia. Thus, flap formation over the anterior aspect of the knee must be limited and performed deep to the subcutaneous fascia. A midline skin incision is optimal and should be used whenever possible. This approach reduces the dimensions of the lateral skin flap, at which lower skin oxygen tension is noted. Previous longitudinal incisions can be used safely. Some degree of modification is often required to incorporate previous paramedian incisions. If multiple parallel longitudinal incisions exist, the most lateral incision is chosen, because the predominant blood supply enters medially. Johnson[109] has shown a reduction in oxygenation of the skin in the lateral region after skin incisions about the knee by the measurement of transcutaneous oxygen. Clarke et al.[39] have also described decreased oxygen tension in the incisional skin margins when using tourniquets. This hypoxia increased with tourniquet tightness. The recommended pressure is 125 mm Hg above the mean blood pressure.

---

*References 51, 55, 85, 111, 192, 235, and 238.

Transverse skin incisions, such as those from previous patellar surgery or osteotomy, can be safely approached at a 90-degree angle. Short oblique incisions, such as from previous meniscectomies, can often be ignored. Caution should be exercised when crossing longer oblique incisions or oblique incisions that cross the midline, because crossing these incisions may result in a narrow point at which the incisions intersect. When the planned surgical incision and prior incision create an angle of less than 60 degrees, alternative techniques should be considered.

Alternative techniques. If the previous skin incision cannot be incorporated and there are other concerns, several techniques can be considered. One option is the sham incision. This technique has limited applications today; we mention it here mainly for historic reasons. A sham incision involves making the planned skin incision, performing the necessary subcutaneous dissection, developing flaps, closing the wound, and then waiting a period of time to observe how the wound heals. This provides information regarding the ability of the tissues to heal and creates a so-called delay phenomenon, with increased local perfusion. If the sham incision heals, then the TKA can proceed as planned 1 to 3 weeks later. Disadvantages to this approach include the need for two procedures and, in patients in whom the sham incision does not heal, the need for further prearthroplasty management but with more limited options.

Another option is prophylactic flap coverage. The best candidates for prophylactic flap coverage are patients with prior skin graft, local irradiation, or densely adherent scar tissue. The choice of flap depends on the location of the lesion, extent of coverage required, and status of the limb. Most lesions can be covered adequately with a medial or lateral gastrocnemius muscle flap or myocutaneous flap. Lesions proximal to the superior pole of the patella may require a free flap. The principles involve excision of the area of concern followed by soft tissue coverage. A minimum of 12 weeks should be allowed between coverage and subsequent arthroplasty. Available data demonstrate successful outcomes in most patients. However, because the indications for this procedure are few, results are extremely limited.

Indications for soft tissue expansion. Our preferred technique is soft tissue expansion. Soft tissue expanders are indicated when insufficient or inadequate soft tissue is present for wound healing. This may occur with multiple crossing and combined incisions, previous skin grafts or flaps, or severe preoperative deformity, or when expanded soft tissue coverage is required. For example, when an extensor mechanism allograft as well as a TKA is to be performed, the added bulk of the extensor mechanism reconstruction may necessitate soft tissue expansion, and 8 to 10 weeks must be allocated for this procedure. Good long-term results have been reported from our institution. Soft tissue expansion is discussed elsewhere in this text.

Postoperative Considerations. Appropriate postoperative wound management depends on the severity and timing of the complication. The failure of the soft tissues to heal following TKA has serious effects. Careful examination at the time of the first dressing change can often alert the clinician to a potentially problematic wound. Early indications may include ecchymosis, blistering, and persistent or large amounts of wound drainage. The goal is early intervention, when possible, to prevent further wound breakdown and complication.

Serosanguineous drainage from the incision is common and is a cause for concern only when the drainage is profuse and persistent. If there is no purulence or erythema, initial management should be a compression dressing, immobilization, and observation. Wound healing takes precedence over motion. When there is drainage, antibiotic therapy is controversial because it may mask a deep infection, making it difficult to identify the causative organism. We recommend consulting with an infectious disease specialist and administering intravenous antibiotics only in select cases. This is a matter of clinical judgment, but we do not consider antibiotics in these circumstances wrong if clinical suspicion for a deep infection is low. Prolonged and persistent serosanguineous drainage raises the issue of a capsular defect, which should be surgically repaired. Some authors recommend that if drainage does not stop after 5 days of appropriate treatment, an open débridement should be performed.

Local care. Local care measures begin with frequent dressing changes, elevation of the extremity, and limiting mobilization, including ROM activities. When a wound is identified to be at risk in the early postoperative period, we routinely discontinue continuous passive motion, apply a compressive or incisional negative pressure dressing, place the knee in an immobilizer, and institute physical therapy without ROM exercises. When superficial epidermal loss occurs in an area smaller than 2 to 3 cm^2, several modified dressing protocols can be instituted to protect the underlying tissues and allow for secondary healing (Fig. 169.2). These include antibacterial ointments or gels and enzymatic débriding agents. During this phase, we may consider temporary discontinuation of the anticoagulant agent, because a hematoma related to overaggressive anticoagulation can be devastating at this stage of healing. The use of mechanical devices for DVT prophylaxis should be considered until the wound stabilizes.

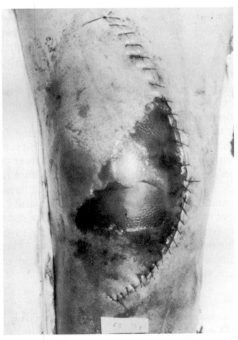

FIG 169.2 Because of its subcutaneous position, skin necrosis is a particular hazard in knee joint replacement. Overaggressive débridement can lead to deep infection. When necrosis occurs, the knee should be immobilized until the eschar separates.

Irrigation and débridement. Early surgical intervention may be helpful and is indicated in certain situations. In cases of imminent wound compromise caused by a large or expanding hematoma or prolonged wound drainage beyond 1 week postoperatively, early surgical interventions should be considered. The goal of irrigation and débridement (I&D) is to prevent further wound breakdown and deep infection. Studies have shown that each day of persistent drainage greatly increases the risk of wound infection. In addition, other studies have shown a lower incidence of deep infection when postoperative hematoma or persistent drainage is treated with I&D versus nonsurgical management.

Burnett et al.[31] have reported that the rates of surgical site complications necessitating readmission, irrigation and débridement of hematoma and the wound, or prolonged hospitalization for wound drainage are 4.7%, 3.4%, and 5.1%, respectively. Wound drainage occurred for 4 to 7 days after 9.3% of the procedures and for more than 7 days after 9.3% of the procedures, with more than 7 days of drainage being highly predictive of readmission and wound reoperation.

Once the decision is made to proceed with surgery, the patient is taken to the operating room (OR) expediently. The setup is the same as with the index arthroplasty. Thorough I&D is performed. Deep cultures should be obtained to direct antibiotic therapy, if indicated. If an opening in the arthrotomy exists, or if the hematoma is deep to the arthrotomy, then the entire prosthesis should be exposed and irrigated and a polyethylene liner exchange is performed. It is best to assume that deep infection is present and perform a thorough I&D with antibiotic irrigation. After hemostasis is obtained, the wound is closed in a layered fashion over a drain. A compressive dressing is applied. Occasionally, when a tension-free closure cannot be obtained, a gastrocnemius muscle flap may be necessary. This should be anticipated before surgery. Appropriate accommodations should be made preoperatively, including the involvement of a plastic surgeon.

Postoperatively, the limb is elevated while ROM and chemical DVT prophylaxis are initially held. Broad-spectrum antibiotics are given until pending cultures are final. An infectious disease consultation is obtained for patients in whom infection is suspected or whose cultures return positive. Decisions regarding ROM, DVT prophylaxis, and continued antibiotic therapy are made on an individual basis.

Galat et al.,[73] in their study of 17,784 primary TKAs, have reported that the rate of early return to surgery for wound complication is 0.33%. They found that the 2-year cumulative probabilities of major subsequent surgery (component resection, muscle flap coverage, or amputation) and deep infection were 5.3% and 6.0%, respectively, in the knees with early surgical treatment of wound complications, as compared with 0.6% and 0.8%, respectively, for knees without early surgical intervention. The overall prosthesis salvage rate was 98%, but obviously results are inferior compared with those of patients without early wound complication.

Hematoma

A current debate exists between appropriate VTE guidelines following TKA. Although discussed elsewhere in this text, the debate centers on the incidence of postoperative hematoma. Given the nature of a TKA with numerous bone cuts, intramedullary canal violation, and soft tissue releases, it is no surprise that postoperative hematomas can occur. Symptoms include not only intense palpable hemarthrosis around the knee but can also be accompanied by skin discoloration, bruising, increased pain, decreased ROM, and wound drainage.

Wound drainage is of particular concern. Weiss and Krackow[229] have described an increased rate of knee infection with prolonged wound drainage. Patel et al.[174] have evaluated factors that lead to prolonged drainage in the postoperative period. The authors have demonstrated that an increase in the initial postoperative drainage in the recovery room was most indicative for further drainage on days 2, 3, 4, and 5. In other words, better control in the immediate postoperative period, with less postoperative recovery room drainage, led to less wound drainage on subsequent hospitalization days. Limiting blood loss in the recovery room begins in the OR. Plugging of the intramedullary canal can help decrease initial blood loss, as can cauterization of known sources of bleeding, such as genicular vessels and the posterior capsule[50] (Fig. 169.3). Intraoperative tourniquet deflation has not been shown to decrease blood loss; in fact, some studies have shown an increase in blood loss when this is performed.[183] The appropriate timing of tourniquet release remains debated, even among surgeons at our institution. The improved designs of TKA and improved surgical techniques have led to improved patellar tracking, resulting in less wound drainage when the lateral release is avoided. At our institution, we use a multimodal approach to minimizing intraoperative bleeding, including a smaller quadriceps-sparing incision, meticulous surgical technique, a periarticular injection cocktail with epinephrine, bipolar sealer device, and intravenous tranexamic acid.

When postoperative hematoma occurs, a period of immobilization and observation is permissible, and many hematomas subside spontaneously. If bleeding continues, as evidenced by tense and painful swelling, the knee must be reopened and the source of the bleeding identified (an argument for intraoperative tourniquet release). Probing and squeezing the wound to evacuate a hematoma are not recommended, because this could lead to retrograde contamination. Indications for surgical evacuation of a hematoma include skin compromise, wound dehiscence, impending skin necrosis, leakage through the incision, persistent sanguineous drainage, and pain. Galat et al.[72] have studied 42 TKA patients matched with 42 control subjects.

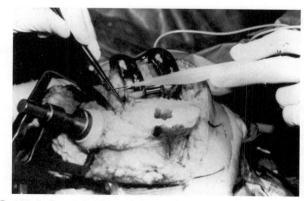

FIG 169.3 Cauterization of the lateral genicular artery. Unless this artery is visible, it is advisable to release the tourniquet before closure so that the vessel can be clearly identified. It is the major source of dangerous postoperative bleeding.

They found that the rate of return to surgery within 30 days for evacuation of a postoperative hematoma was 0.24%. The 2-year rates of a subsequent major operation or deep periprosthetic infection in the study group were 12.3% and 13.6%, respectively, and 0.9% and 1.4%, respectively, in the control group.

Skin Necrosis

Postoperative soft tissue and skin necrosis should be handled early and aggressively. Treatment options for small areas (<4 cm), especially over the patella or more proximal, include healing by secondary intention, split-thickness skin grafts, or local fasciocutaneous flaps. Small areas (<4 cm), especially over the patella or proximal, may be treated by secondary intention healing, split-thickness skin grafts, or local fasciocutaneous flaps. Skin loss over the patellar tendon or tibial tubercle is best treated with muscle flap coverage; usually, the medial head of the gastrocnemius rotator flap is adequate.

VASCULAR COMPLICATIONS

Arterial complications are rare,[131,184] and the preoperative absence of peripheral pulses has not been regarded as a contraindication to surgery, provided that the capillary circulation was adequate. Vascular complication has been reported in 0.03% to 0.2% of cases.[49] Injury to the popliteal artery can occur during resection of the proximal tibia or posterior femoral condyles and while releasing the posterior capsule or posterior collateral ligament (PCL). Failure to remove protruding cement from the back of the tibia can also cause direct damage or thermal injury.

Da Silva and Sobel[54] have reported on 19 patients with TKA-related popliteal artery injury. Of these, 84% (16/19) of patients had full recoveries. Limb loss occurred in 2 of 19 patients (10.5%). Parvizi et al.[173] collected data on 13,517 patients undergoing total joint arthroplasty and reported 16 vascular injuries (0.1%). Eleven injuries occurred after TKA and five after THA. Of the 16 patients, 8 (50%) had launched a legal suit against the operating surgeon. Abularrage et al.,[1] in their prospective study of 41,633 patients, evaluated the predictors of lower extremity arterial injury after TKA or THA. They found that the revision procedures and African American race were statistically significant predictors of arterial injury.

Numerous studies have reported arteriovenous fistula formation, arterial aneurysm, and pseudoaneurysm following TKA. A possible reason may be an unrecognized injury to the perigenicular vessels, leading to hemarthrosis. Most present within 6 months of surgery, but some may be delayed. In a case reported by Sharma et al.,[211] three large hemorrhagic effusions occurred 4 weeks after total knee replacement (TKR). An arteriogram revealed a pseudoaneurysm filling from the inferior medial genicular artery. Ibrahim et al.[103] have reported two cases of pseudoaneurysm after TKR, presenting after 5 days and 1 month, respectively. The first patient was successfully embolized and the second patient was treated by injecting a solution of thrombin into the pseudoaneurysm to produce immediate thrombosis without impairing flow across the vessel. Sandoval et al.[203] have reported a case of popliteal pseudoaneurysm following TKA. Open vascular surgery with resection of the pseudoaneurysm and end-to-end bypass of contralateral saphenous vein graft was successfully performed. Their possible explanation was perforation of the anterior wall of the popliteal artery during the TKA. Haddad et al.[87] have reported a case of recurrent hemarthrosis following TKR after a previous dome

tibial osteotomy for medial compartment osteoarthritis. Recurrent hemarthrosis in this case was secondary to arteriovenous (AV) fistula of the peroneal artery at the site of the previous fibular osteotomy. Thomas et al.[219] have reported an iatrogenic popliteal AV fistula 3 years after TKA. This was successfully treated by resection of the fistula and direct repair of the artery and vein.

Acute arterial occlusion can be seen after TKA. Rates in the literature have been reported from 0.03% to 0.17%.[126] Possible causes include manual manipulation to reduce a flexion contracture[59,148] and the use of tourniquet. Pressure on a preexisting atheromatous plaque may cause release of the plaque, which is then lodged into a more distal artery. Gregory et al.[82] have reported a case of an 81-year-old patient with acute arterial occlusion 9 days after TKA. This was successfully treated by urgent surgical embolectomy.

It is important to determine and document the presence of peripheral vascular disease, arterial calcifications, and popliteal aneurysm preoperatively (Fig. 169.4). Absolute vascular contraindications for performing a TKA include the presence of verified vascular claudication with minimal or no activity, active skin ulcerations secondary to arterial insufficiency or venous stasis, and ischemia or frank necrosis in the toes. Others have cautioned against the use of a tourniquet after previous bypass surgery.

When there is concern about the circulation, we recommend preoperative evaluation by a vascular surgeon. The operation should be scheduled at a time of day when consultant advice is available postoperatively, so that prompt investigation with arteriography can be done if the state of the circulation is in

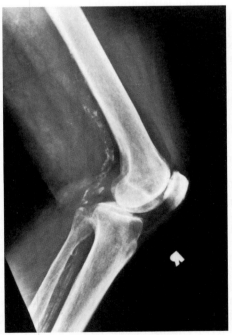

FIG 169.4 Lateral radiograph showing extensive calcification in the femoral, popliteal, posterotibial, posterior tibial, and peroneal arteries. Although this patient had palpable peripheral pulses, knee surgery may result in arterial occlusion by a dislodged clot. Some investigators recommend avoiding a tourniquet. The patient should be watched closely after surgery for evidence of arterial insufficiency.

doubt. Prompt embolectomy usually restores the circulation. Prolonged observation of postoperative vascular insufficiency is justified only in a setting of extreme vigilance and under the guidance of a vascular surgeon.

NERVE PALSY AND NEUROLOGIC COMPLICATIONS

Anatomy of the Peroneal Nerve

The peroneal nerve is composed of fibers from the dorsal portion of the L4 and L5 and S1 and S2 nerves. As the nerve courses down from the thigh, it curves laterally behind the head of the fibula to reach the two heads of the peroneus longus. The nerve flattens as it passes between these two heads, separating the bundles and exposing unprotected nutrient vessels. The nerve then curves around the neck of the fibula and divides into deep and superficial branches. The deep peroneal nerve continues under the extensor digitorum longus, along the anterior aspect of the intraosseous membrane. It sends motor branches to the tibialis anterior, extensor digitorum longus, extensor hallucis longus, and peroneus tertius. The nerve continues distally, ending in the medial and lateral terminal branches, which, among other functions, supply sensation to the first web space of the foot.

The superficial peroneal nerve passes distally between the peronei and extensor digitorum longus. Motor branches are given off to the peroneus longus and peroneus brevis. In the lower third of the leg, the nerve branches into the medial and intermediate dorsal cutaneous nerves. These terminal branches complete the sensory innervation of the feet. Bruzzone et al.[27] identified anatomic landmarks after 20 cadaveric knee dissections and defined a danger zone and a safe zone to avoid common peroneal nerve injury when performing the inside-out release technique of the posterior-lateral corner during TKA. During the release of the posterior-lateral capsule, the nerve was identified to be at risk in the triangle defined by the popliteus tendon, tibial cut surface, and most posterior fibers of the iliotibial band (danger zone), but not during "pie-crusting" of the iliotibial band (safe zone). They also defined the average distance from the nerve to the posterior-lateral corner of the tibia and to the posterior border of the iliotibial band as 13.5 and 35.8 mm, respectively.

Postoperative Clinical Findings

Peroneal nerve palsy is an infrequent but worrisome complication after TKA. The incidence is higher in revision cases than primary TKA. The prevalence of peroneal nerve palsy has been reported many times in the literature. Mont et al.[158] have reviewed the literature and found the cumulative prevalence to be 0.58% (74 of 12,784). Asp and Rand[6] reported an incidence of 0.3% in 8754 TKAs performed at the Mayo Clinic. Yacub et al.,[241] in their retrospective study of 14,979 patients, reported a 0.01% incidence of nerve injury after TKA. They noted a 10-fold difference in nerve injury rates between diabetic and nondiabetic patients, 0.11% versus 0.01%, respectively.

Numerous causes for nerve palsy have been described, but they are most commonly associated with the correction of severe flexion and valgus deformity or a combination of the two. The following factors contribute to the development of peroneal nerve palsy: (1) stretching of the nerve in valgus and flexion contractures, (2) fascial compression of the nerve and

its vascular supply, (3) direct pressure from the postoperative dressing, and (4) epidural anesthesia. In rare idiopathic cases, none of the mechanisms listed seem to apply. Factors that have not been found to be associated with peroneal nerve palsy include age, gender, type of arthritis, and duration of tourniquet. Idusuyi and Morrey[104] performed 10,321 TKAs from 1979 to 1992 at the Mayo Clinic and reported 32 postoperative peroneal nerve palsies. The factors associated with peroneal nerve palsies in this series were epidural anesthesia for postoperative pain control, previous laminectomy, and preoperative valgus deformity. The relative risk for patients who had previous proximal tibial osteotomy was doubled but was not statistically significant.

In patients with severe combined deformities, the large soft tissue dissections required to balance the deformities may be responsible for increased traction or vascular compromise to the nerve. The alternative method of bone sacrifice to correct large deformities, although appealing because of elimination of the need for obtaining soft tissue balance, does not entirely avoid peroneal nerve palsy. The bone-sacrificing method also leaves a residual, permanent, leg-length discrepancy that may be associated with an extensor lag because of relative lengthening of the quadriceps mechanism. When ligament balance is not attempted, a constrained prosthesis is needed. In younger patients, this may lead to eventual loosening, although, with the constrained condylar prosthesis, this has not yet been seen in our practice. In older patients at high risk for peroneal nerve palsy, the use of the constrained condylar knee is a suitable alternative. These patients recover much more rapidly than after major release procedures and, because of their age, the risk of ultimate loosening is less concerning.

Although it is sometimes necessary to splint the knee in extension after correction of a severe flexion contracture, evidence of nerve palsy demands immediate removal of the splints and flexion of the knee. If this is done promptly, complete recovery can be expected. In the case of varus deformities, splinting is not necessary. For severe valgus deformity (>20 degrees), one may consider splinting the patient with the knee in 30 degrees of flexion. Nerve function is then monitored closely when the surgical dressing is removed on postoperative day 2. Tight dressings that might press directly on the peroneal nerve should also be avoided.

Postoperative dressings that are too tight or improperly padded can cause direct pressure on the peroneal nerve, causing nerve palsy. In their study, Beller et al.[16] described a double crush syndrome, which includes unrecognized pressure on the peroneal nerve caused by continuous epidural anesthesia and an axonal lesion from the pressure of the pneumatic tourniquet. To prevent a peroneal lesion after TKA while using continuous epidural anesthesia, they recommended limiting the pneumatic tourniquet pressure to 320 mm Hg and ensuring pressure-free positioning of the operated leg.

Asp and Rand[6] performed 8998 arthroplasties and reported 26 nerve palsies. They noted that complete recovery was more likely when the palsy was initially incomplete. Dressing removal and flexion of the knee on diagnosis did not always help. The time of presentation of the problem varied from discovery in the recovery room to postoperative day 6. The motor fibers of the tibialis anterior and extensor hallucis longus muscles were affected in all cases; a sensory deficit was noticed in 20 patients (87%). The peroneus longus muscle was affected in nine patients (39%). Electromyographic evaluation showed a diffuse motor neuropathy in the mild cases and denervation potentials in muscles supplied by the deep branch of the common peroneal nerve in the more severely involved cases. The treatment rendered on discovery of these findings varied according to the discretion of the surgeon involved. The most frequent therapeutic measure was to loosen the Robert Jones dressing and place the knee in a more flexed position. In two cases, this maneuver brought immediate improvement of motor and sensory deficits. The time interval between discovery and the beginning of the return of function ranged from immediately in the two cases mentioned to 6 months. Motor improvement occurred first, with sensory return lagging behind.

Omeroglu et al.[167] have reported the case of a 46-year-old rheumatoid patient with bilateral peroneal nerve palsy on the second postoperative day after simultaneous bilateral TKA. Electromyographic studies revealed bilateral axonotmesis. Complete motor recovery was seen on both sides within 6 months, although sensory deficit was present on one side at 2 years postoperatively. They reported preoperative severe flexion contracture and epidural anesthesia as the risk factors for the development of the nerve palsy in this patient.

Treatment and Results

The treatment of chronic peroneal nerve palsy usually consists of an ankle-foot orthosis for a footdrop and passive ankle ROM to prevent an equinus deformity. Complete recovery of a peroneal palsy is rare. The recovery seen is usually partial, with sensory deficits that may be permanent; residual motor deficits are not usually of clinical significance. Occasional marked weakness, especially of the great toe extensor, may be seen. In Asp and Rand's study[6] of 26 postoperative peroneal palsies, palsies were complete in 18 and incomplete in 8. Of these patients, 23 had motor and sensory deficits and 3 had only motor deficits. At 5-year follow-up, recovery was complete for 13 palsies and partial for 12. Complete recovery was more likely in palsies that were initially incomplete.

Although most investigators support nonoperative treatment of this complication, others disagree. Krackow et al.[130] treated five patients with operative exploration and decompression of the peroneal nerve for a postoperative palsy. The procedure was performed 5 to 45 months after the index TKA. All patients have shown improved nerve function, and 4 of 5 patients had full peroneal nerve recovery. All patients were able to discontinue their ankle-foot orthosis.

MECHANICAL COMPLICATIONS

Instability

Instability is a common cause of mechanical failure of TKA. Instability accounts for 10% to 22% of TKA failures requiring revision.[†] The direction of instability at the tibiofemoral articulation can occur in the coronal (varus-valgus) plane, sagittal (anteroposterior) plane, or as a combination of planes. Early instability may be a result of malalignment of the components, failure to restore the mechanical axis of the limb, imbalance of the flexion-extension space, intraoperative or postoperative rupture of the medial collateral ligament (MCL), or PCL rupture with cruciate-retaining designs. Commonly, late instability is secondary to polyethylene wear. Asymmetrical

polyethylene wear related to malalignment can result in relative lengthening of the collateral ligament on the involved side and subsequent coronal instability. In patients with cruciate-retaining knees, it is not uncommon for the PCL to elongate or attenuate. This can lead to progressive polyethylene wear and late sagittal plane instability. However, late sagittal plane instability is not only seen with cruciate-retaining designs; significant wear or fracture of the tibial polyethylene post in posterior-stabilized knees may also result in late sagittal plane instability.[208] Instability after knee arthroplasty can be subdivided into three types—extension instability, flexion instability, and genu recurvatum.

Extension Instability

Symmetrical instability. Symmetrical extension instability occurs when the extension space is not filled by the thickness of the components. This can be caused by overresection of the tibia or the distal femur.[25] Although overresection of the tibia results in equally large flexion and extensions gaps, excessive resection from the distal femur results in asymmetrical flexion and extension gaps. If overresection of the tibia is recognized intraoperatively, it can be easily managed by increasing the size of the polyethylene insert. Similarly, if a postoperative TKA is noted to be equally loose in flexion and extension, one option is revision surgery with a polyethylene exchange to a larger insert. Overresection of the distal femur creates a much different scenario. With overresection of the distal femur, the joint line is elevated. This creates a larger extension gap, compared with the flexion gap. By simply increasing the size of the tibial insert, the result will be a knee that is too tight in flexion. The elevated joint line will also affect patellar tracking and limit flexion, and may result in midflexion instability[171] (Fig. 169.5). It is best in these cases to restore the joint line by adding distal femoral augmentation.

Asymmetrical instability. Asymmetrical extension instability is frequently encountered. Following the femoral and tibial preparation, the extension and flexion gaps must be assessed. An asymmetrical extension gap in the face of appropriate bony resection is most often caused by inadequate correction of the preoperative deformity.[25,171] Preoperative varus deformity is the most common soft tissue deformity. The shortening or tightening of the medial structures, including the superficial MCL, must be recognized. Often, these tightened structures are not sufficiently released, and the deformity is not completely corrected (Fig. 169.6). This will lead to progressing varus deformity with increased medial joint line stresses, accelerated polyethylene wear, and stretching out of the soft tissue structures on the lateral side. The asymmetrical extension gap must be recognized intraoperatively and an appropriate subperiosteal elevated of the superficial MCL performed, as described by Insall et al.[106] They thought that valgus instability from overrelease of the medial structures during correction of a fixed varus deformity was rare.

Knees with asymmetrical extension instability may also result from undercorrection of a preoperative valgus deformity.[171] Excessively tight lateral structures, including the lateral collateral ligament (LCL) and iliotibial band (ITB), if left uncorrected, will lead to recurrence of the valgus deformity and increased lateral joint line forces. Currently, the most commonly used technique to correct preoperative valgus deformity without causing lateral instability has been described by Insall et al.[106] as the "pie-crust" technique. This is recommended for

---

†References 25, 168, 171, 225, 242, and 243.

patients with a preoperative valgus deformity of less than 20 degrees.[3] Clarke et al.[37] have published the results of 24 TKAs with preoperative valgus deformity, ranging from 9 to 30 degrees. The deformity was corrected using the "pie-crust" technique, and the knee was reconstructed with a posterior-stabilized prosthesis. This series reported complete correction

of the deformity and no instability in all cases. In patients with more than 20 degrees of valgus deformity, the risks of iatrogenic peroneal nerve injury must be considered.[60] The surgeon may consider the use of a constrained condylar design in much older patients, whereas increased constraint in younger patients should be avoided unless absolutely necessary.

Extension instability can result secondary to iatrogenic injury of the collateral ligaments (Fig. 169.7). The excursion of

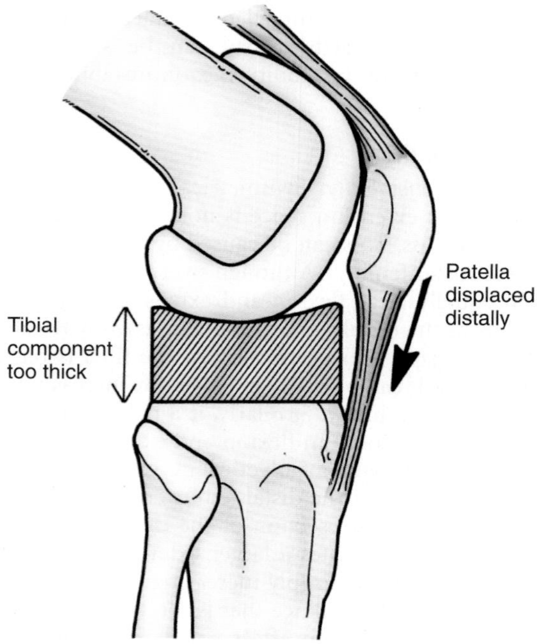

FIG 169.5 If an extra thick tibial component is needed to stabilize the knee, the patella is displaced distally, causing a patella infra. Undersizing of the femoral component in the sagittal plane and anterior malpositioning are possible causes. Excessive distal resection of the femur moving the joint line proximally is another cause.

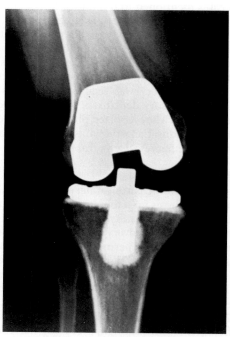

FIG 169.7 Radiograph showing the instability that results from a transected medial collateral ligament. This is not the result of an overzealous medial release.

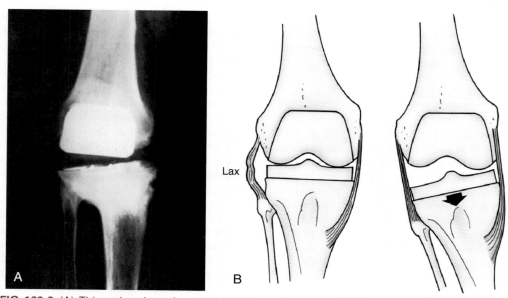

FIG 169.6 (A) This arthroplasty is unstable, but not because of a ligament deficiency. (B) The medial ligament was not released; an asymmetrical instability remains.

large oscillating saw blades was studied and found to be greater than the width of the medial and lateral femoral condyles in the female knee.[60] Meticulous attention must be paid to the position of retractors during femoral and tibial resection. Also, iatrogenic collateral ligament injury can be produced during aggressive testing of varus-valgus stability or with attempts to reduce the polyethylene insert in an excessively tight knee. With iatrogenic injury to the MCL, most authors advocate a direct repair with Krackow-pattern suturing. If primary repair is insufficient, augmentation can be performed using the hamstring tendons. Finally, a constrained condylar design can be used to provide additional stability while the repair heals. Several studies have demonstrated good outcomes without the use of increased constraint or tissue augmentation. Leopold et al.[138] have demonstrated good to excellent results in 100% of 16 TKAs treated with direct repair of an iatrogenically injured MCL, reconstruction using a cruciate-retaining implant, and postoperative bracing for 6 weeks. More recently, Koo and Choi[127] performed a retrospective review of 15 TKAs treated conservatively for intraoperative iatrogenic detachment of the MCL from the tibia. Specifically, no increased constraint, bracing, or ligament reconstruction was performed. No significant difference was seen between MCL-intact TKAs and the knees with iatrogenic MCL injury, with a minimum of 2-year follow-up.

Flexion Instability. Flexion instability results from inadequate filling of the flexion gap or attenuation of the PCL following cruciate-retaining TKA. Flexion instability is now a well-recognized cause of TKA failure (Fig. 169.8). Early flexion instability is likely secondary to gap imbalance, with or without laxity of a collateral ligament[171] (Fig. 169.9). Late flexion instability can occur in cruciate-retaining and posterior-stabilized TKAs, but the cause is different. In patients with cruciate-retaining knees, it is not uncommon for the PCL to elongate or attenuate. This can lead to progressive polyethylene wear and late flexion instability.[168] Late flexion instability in posterior-stabilized knees may result from significant wear or fracture of the tibial polyethylene post.[208] Symptoms can range from a vague sense of instability and recurrent effusions to frank dislocation. Flexion instability is best assessed with the knee in 90 degrees of flexion while the patient sits on the end of the examination table.

Frank dislocation following posterior-stabilized TKA is a rare complication[205] (Fig. 169.10). Improved prosthetic design with increased jump distances have reduced this complication to well below 0.5%.[171] Although the posterior-stabilized prosthesis can resist direct posterior translation, deep flexion combined with a varus or valgus stress can lead to posterior dislocation of the tibia. Patients who are at highest risk are those who have had the correction of a large valgus deformity and quickly regained their ROM during the postoperative period. The dislocated TKA can continue to function well following closed reduction under anesthesia; however, subsequent dislocation may occur. Recurrent dislocation requires revision to a

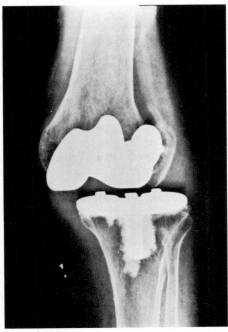

FIG 169.8. AP radiograph of a knee with flexion instability. With the knee in flexion, a posterolateral dislocation is observed. This dislocation is caused by inequality between the flexion and extension gaps, and the PCL is not sufficient to provide stability, particularly when the prosthesis is unconstrained.

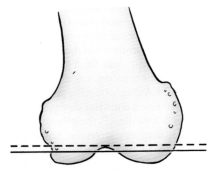

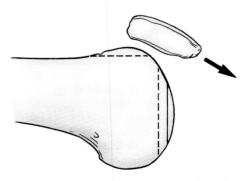

FIG 169.9 In cases with considerable ligamentous laxity, an underresection of the distal femur may be preferable. The standard femoral resection necessitates a thicker tibial component to take up the slack in the soft tissues and may cause distal migration of the patella. By underresecting the femur, a desirable patellar position is maintained.

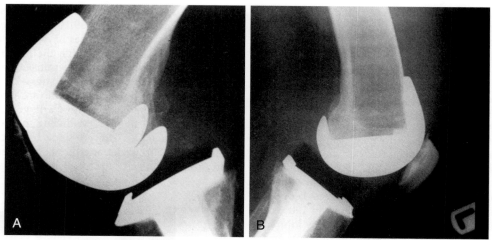

FIG 169.10 (A) Posterior dislocation of a PS prosthesis. (B) After reduction.

larger polyethylene insert, if the extension gap permits, or component revision to a constrained condylar design.

More commonly, posterior stabilized knees may be symptomatic because of flexion instability but not demonstrate dislocation.[205] Patients report a sense of instability, recurrent effusion, periarticular tenderness, and difficulty ambulating on stairs. The diagnosis is made on clinical examination with the knee flexed at 90 degrees. Schwab et al.[205] have reviewed 1370 revision TKAs performed at the Mayo Clinic (Rochester, MN). Ten revisions were performed for flexion instability. Eight (80%) had successful outcomes following revision of both components and appropriate balancing of the flexion and extension gaps. The excessively large flexion gap was frequently managed by upsizing the femoral component following posterior femoral augmentation.

Similarly, cruciate-retaining (CR) knees can be symptomatic because of flexion instability without dislocation. Patients again report a sense of instability, recurrent effusion, periarticular tenderness, pes anserine tenderness, and difficulty ambulating on stairs. Additionally, on physical examination, a posterior sag and positive posterior drawer may be readily apparent. Pagnano et al.[168] have reported two types of causes for flexion instability following CR TKA. The first type creates an excessive flexion gap by surgical error. This can occur by undersizing the femoral component, which results in overresection of the posterior femoral condyles and a reduction in the femoral offset. Alternatively, the creation of excessive tibial slope can result in a knee that is well balanced in extension but remains loose in flexion. The second type involves late failure of the PCL and late instability. Other causes may include polyethylene wear, synovitis, iatrogenic PCL injury, traumatic PCL rupture, and an excessively tight flexion gap and PCL rupture following aggressive ROM exercises.

Treatment of CR knees with flexion instability most often involves revision arthroplasty to a posterior-stabilized (PS) design.[171] At the time of revision, a larger femoral component is frequently used following posterior femoral augmentation. This improves posterior femoral offset and reduces the size of the flexion gap. Attention must also be paid to the tibial slope. If excessive posterior slope is present preoperatively, this must be addressed with revision of the tibial resection. Careful balancing of the flexion and extension gaps is then performed.

Pagnano et al.[168] have demonstrated successful outcomes following revision of a CR knee with flexion instability to a well-balanced PS design in 19 of 22 knees (86%).

Genu Recurvatum. Genu recurvatum, or hyperextension, is difficult to manage and therefore is best prevented during primary TKA. Because genu recurvatum is known to recur in patients with certain neuromuscular disorders, the cause of the hyperextension deformity must be elucidated thoroughly before surgery. In the absence of neuromuscular disease, however, hyperextension deformities tend not to recur after TKA. In the remainder of cases, recurvatum was likely present at the end of the index procedure as a result of excessively loose collateral ligaments and failure to fill the extension gap.[150]

Recurvatum before TKA is rare and is most often associated with neuromuscular diseases, including poliomyelitis.[150] Patients with neuromuscular disease and significant quadriceps weakness rely on hyperextension of the knee to prevent limb collapse during the stance phase of gait. In the absence of neuromuscular disease, recurvatum may develop in patients with a fixed valgus deformity associated with a contracted ITB or in patients with rheumatoid arthritis. Patients at risk and those with preoperative hyperextension must be recognized so that appropriate considerations can be made.

Several options have been described to prevent the recurrence of recurvatum when performing a TKA in a patient with preoperative recurvatum. One option is to use a rotating hinged component with an extension stop. Giori and Lewallen[77] reviewed the Mayo Clinic experience performing TKA in patients with poliomyelitis. They recommended the use of a rotating hinged prosthesis in patients with less than antigravity quadriceps strength. Jordan et al.[112] more recently demonstrated 95% good to excellent results in 15 TKAs performed in patients with poliomyelitis using a PS or constrained condylar design. Unlike the results published by Giori and Lewallen,[77] their results did not deteriorate with worsening quadriceps strength. Anterior-posterior stability was restored in all 15 patients. Only one patient required a hinged implant for reconstruction. The discrepancy in results remains unclear. Caution should remain when treating patients with less than antigravity quadriceps function.

A second alternative for patients with preoperative recurvatum is to underresect the distal femur. This will result in a relatively smaller extension gap. Then, by filling the flexion gap with the largest polyethylene insert possible, the knee will have a slight flexion contracture,[171] which will prevent hyperextension. Finally, others have recommended repositioning the collateral ligaments more posteriorly to re-create the normal tightening action as full extension of the knee is achieved. The largest series available of patients with preoperative recurvatum without neuromuscular disorder has suggested that increased constraint, thicker components, and collateral ligament transfer are not necessary. Meding et al.[149] published results of 57 TKAs performed on patients with at least 5 degrees of flexion contracture in the absence of neuromuscular disease. Using a CR design, they corrected the hyperextension deformity in 98% of knees. All but two knees (5%) reached full extension at the end of the procedure. With an average 4.5-year follow-up, only two knees had a hyperextension deformity. Both these knees demonstrated residual medial instability immediately following insertion of the prosthesis.

Inadequate Motion

Arthrofibrosis is the most common cause of stiffness following TKA. The incidence ranges from 1.2% to 17%. Inadequate motion has several causes, including patient-related factors, surgical factors, and postoperative complications. Patient factors include preoperative ROM (most important risk factor), preoperative diagnosis (eg, juvenile rheumatoid arthritis, ankylosing spondylitis, post-traumatic arthrosis, previous septic arthritis), body habits, and patient personality factors, such as depression or a low threshold for pain.[165,209,210] Fisher et al.,[71] in their study of 1024 TKAs, identified patient-related factors contributing to poor results. The authors identified female gender, higher body mass index (BMI), previous knee surgery, disability status, diabetes mellitus, pulmonary disease, and depression as being significantly associated with the risk of having stiffness or pain at 1 year after surgery, despite the presence of well-aligned, well-fixed components.

Stiffness not only limits the patient's function but also predisposes the patient to pain. The cause is often unclear. Correct component position is critical, and the internal rotation of the femoral component and patellar maltracking must be avoided because they can contribute to a painful knee with limited ROM. It is also thought that certain factors may predispose an individual to the formation of abundant scar tissue, resulting in arthrofibrosis and limited motion. Pereira et al.[176] compared those patients with those with an acceptable ROM following arthroplasty procedures. No kinematic factors could be identified as the cause of stiffness in these patients. Lang et al.[135] recently looked at preoperative and postoperative ROMs for a contralateral TKA in patients with a history of a stiff TKA. They found that the ROM was not significantly different than a control group at 2-year follow-up, but the rate of manipulation was 26.7% in the study group compared with 8% in the control group. They demonstrated that good results could be obtained in the contralateral knee of patients with a history of arthrofibrosis but that there is a predisposition for the need of manipulation. Some patients may be more prone to keloid formation and may also be prone to arthrofibrosis. Abundant keloid or scar tissue results in decreased ROM. Another risk factor is an abnormal response to pain or poorly controlled pain, which limits postoperative rehabilitation. A new emphasis on intraoperative injections and multimodal anesthesia may help make progress toward avoidance of a stiff knee because of poorly controlled pain.

Scott[206] reviewed stiffness associated with TKA and discussed factors such as patient diagnosis, preoperative ROM, prosthetic geometry, surgical technique, intraoperative ROM, capsular closure, postoperative rehabilitation, and wound healing factors, which he considered as all playing a role in the development of a stiff knee. Ipsilateral hip degenerative joint disease (DJD) can also lead to the stiffness through persistent pain and limitations with regard to participation in therapy.

If the stiff knee fails to resolve after adjustments in pain medication and physical therapy, manipulations can be considered. This is done usually at the 6-week period, when adequate wound healing has occurred. The hip is gently flexed to 90 degrees and gentle flexion is applied. Manipulations tend to be more successful for poor flexion, although mild improvement can be made in extension. Yercan et al.[244] have evaluated 1188 knee arthroplasties with a prevalence of stiffness of 5.3%. The average premanipulation ROM was 67 degrees and improved to 117 degrees after manipulation. It should be noted that motion at follow-up was better for those who had manipulation early compared with those who had it done later. Kim et al.[123] have evaluated stiffness after TKA. In their series, stiffness was associated with knees having a preoperative flexion contracture of 15 degrees or less than 75 degrees of flexion. The prevalence of stiffness was 1.3%. Recently, Rubinstein and DeHaan[198] reported the results and incidence of manipulation for primary knee arthroplasty. In this study, 37 of 800 TKAs were manipulated, with a 4.6% incidence of stiffness; the ROM improved from 68 to 109 degrees postmanipulation. Keating et al.[118] found no difference between patients who had undergone manipulation before and after 12 weeks in 113 knees, with an average flexion of 70 degrees. Namba and Inacio[163] studied 102 patients who had undergone manipulation under anesthesia within 90 days after TKA and 93 patients who had undergone manipulation more than 90 days after TKA. Manipulation was found to improve the ROM and function in both groups, although greater gains were observed in the early-manipulation group. The authors recommended manipulation for the treatment of stiffness after TKA, even if it was delayed beyond 90 days.

In cases of a stiff knee that does not respond to manipulation, the results of arthroscopic lysis of adhesions have been reported. These findings are rather controversial in the literature. Numerous authors have reported significant improvement, but some have reported poor results.[207] Court et al.[48] have described the results of arthroscopic arthrolysis after a TKR procedure. In this procedure, retinacular releases were performed medially and laterally, and patella mobility was restored. Regional anesthesia was continued postarthroscopy to allow for intensive mobilization and early ROM. They recommended that this arthroscopic arthrolysis be done from 3 to 6 months after the knee replacement for better results. Best results are obtained in the case of isolated patellofemoral fibrosis. Bocell et al.[23] reported an increase in postoperative ROM in 43% of patients. Williams et al.[234] reported an average increase in ROM of 30.6 degrees, whereas Mont et al.[160] reported an average improvement of 31 degrees in 94% of patients. In the case of severe ROM limitation, arthroscopic treatment alone is less effective. Cates and Schmidt have evaluated the stiff TKA.[34] They found that manipulation is most successful in patients within 8 weeks with full extension and at least 90 degrees of flexion prior to manipulation. Patients with large flexion contractures were less successfully treated with manipulation.

For those with significant flexion contracture who did not respond to more conservative management, open lysis is a final option before revision arthroplasty. However, open arthrolysis and isolated tibial insert exchange have not been successful in the Mayo Clinic series. Babis et al. reported on a series of severely stiff knees treated between 1992 and 1998, and seven knees were identified that underwent isolated tibial insert exchange and open arthrolysis.[8] Unfortunately, isolated tibial insert exchange with arthrolysis and débridement did not yield significant improvement in this group of patients. Hutchinson et al.[100] reported an increase in ROM from 55 to 91 degrees 6 months after open arthrolysis, and Pretzsch and Dippold[180] showed an increase in knee flexion from 46 to 90 degrees and a decrease in flexion contracture from 11 to 7 degrees. In contrast, Babis et al.[8] have reported poor results with open arthrolysis and polyethylene exchange for stiff knees with fixed and well-aligned prosthetic components. More recently, Della Valle et al.[14] described their results with open arthrolysis with lysis of adhesions. Their emphasis was on access to the posterior capsule to regain full extension. With this technique, significant increases in ROM were noted.

Prosthetic Loosening

Aseptic loosening of knee implants is multifactorial in regard to cause. The causes include but are not limited to malalignment of the prosthesis, higher BMI, small tibial components, higher potential stresses, polyethylene wear, and osteolysis.[17] Recently, a rapid increase in loosening of total knee components has been seen. Hossain et al.[93] reviewed 349 revision TKAs (343 patients) and reported aseptic loosening in 14.9% patients undergoing revision TKA and 1.4% in patients undergoing re-revision TKA. Piedade et al.[178] have compared 944 primary TKAs without surgical revision (890 patients) and 22 primary TKAs (22 patients) that had revision TKA secondary to aseptic failure. They reported that component loosening was one of the most common causes (50%) for revision in their study.

Tibial Component. There is reason to believe that the high failure rate caused by tibial component loosening (Fig. 169.11) represents a design problem that is now on the way to being solved (Fig. 169.12). High rates of loosening have been reported with polycentric, geometric, and early Freeman-Swanson designs. In addition to loosening, plastic deformation and cold flow were reported with the original University of California at Irvine (UCI) prosthesis, indicating that the rigidity of polyethylene can be compromised by excessively thin components and generous cruciate cutouts. Modifications to the tibial components were made in subsequent designs. The total condylar prosthesis had a one-piece tibial component and a central fixation peg, and no component loosening was seen in 220 knees monitored for 3 to 5 years. Reports from the Brigham and Women's Hospital in Boston[239] on the PCL-retaining, but otherwise similar, Kinematic prosthesis also have shown aseptic loosening to be negligible.

Malalignment and malposition should be related to mechanical loosening and are perhaps the leading cause (Figs. 169.13 and 169.14). There is some evidence for this. Lotke and Ecker[144] have shown a correlation between malalignment and radiolucent lines and Hvid and Nielsen[102] confirmed these findings. Dorr and Boiardo[56] stated that "prosthetic alignment is the most important factor influencing postoperative loosening and instability." Hsu et al.[95] and Hsu et al.[96] were unable to show an

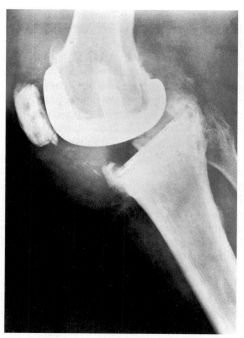

FIG 169.11 Flat tibial components, although of one piece, are inadequately supported by the cancellous bone of the upper tibia and are susceptible to sinkage, usually in an anterior or medial direction.

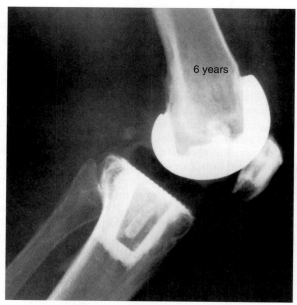

6 years

FIG 169.12 The addition of a central fixation peg to the tibial component almost eliminates tibial component loosening.

association between varus positioning and component loosening, however, and Smith et al.,[212] using a cemented total condylar prosthesis, could find no relationship between radiolucent lines or loosening and component position. Cornell et al.,[47] also using the total condylar prosthesis, did find a correlation between radiolucency (although not loosening) and varus positioning. Tew and Waugh[218] found the association between positioning and loosening to be inconclusive. There are possible

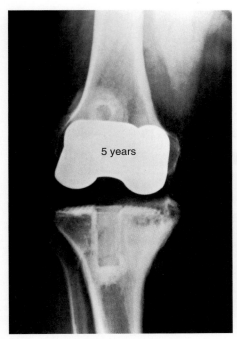

FIG 169.13 The importance of axial alignment. This total condylar knee prosthesis was positioned at surgery in slight varus, which gradually increased over a 5-year period. Collapse of the medial bone support with distortion of the polyethylene can be seen.

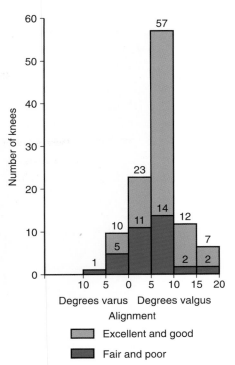

FIG 169.14 Bar graph showing the relationship between postoperative alignment and the clinical rating. The best results were obtained in knees aligned between 5 and 15 degrees of valgus. However, the relationship between alignment and the clinical result is by no means absolute. (From Insall J, Hood RW, Vanni M: The correction of knee alignment in 225 consecutive total condylar knee replacements. *Clin Orthop Relat Res* 160:94, 1981.)

explanations for these discrepancies. Loosening rates for modern prostheses are low, and not all prostheses that are positioned in varus loosen. The identification and interpretation of radiolucent lines are confusing to the point that their analysis is probably meaningless (Fig. 169.15) unless the radiolucency is complete and progressive, a circumstance usually accompanied by clinical symptoms (Fig. 169.16). Analyzing the modes of failure in revision TKA, Mulhall et al.[162] identified polyethylene wear as a late mode of failure that may occur after an 11-year mean TKA revision interval. In addition, implant malalignment was reported in 9% of TKA loosening cases.

The use of metal-backed tibial components has further reduced the incidence of tibial loosening, presumably by more evenly distributing stress. The earliest version of the posterior stabilized knee had an all-polyethylene tibial component, and at 9- to 12-year follow-up, a 3% tibial loosening rate was recorded.[213] More recently, a minimum 10-year study[40] of the same prosthesis with a metal-backed tibial component indicated no tibial loosening and no complete radiolucent lines. Partial radiolucent lines were seen in 50% of the all-polyethylene components, compared with 10% of the metal-backed components. Faris et al.[66] have described an unacceptably high failure rate of 30% at 10 years in all-polyethylene tibial components with a coronal flat on flat design. All components failed beneath the medial tibial plateau, with bony collapse and medial tibial subsidence. It was thought that all-polyethylene tibial component success rates are highly design-specific and should be used with more conforming designs. Gioe et al.[76] reported the 8- to 12-year follow-up of congruent all-polyethylene tibial components with a modular metal-backed tibial component of the same design. Ten-year survivorship of the all-polyethylene tibial

component was 91.6% with revision for any reason and 100% for aseptic loosening. The metal-backed tibial component survivorship was 88.9% with revision for any reason and 94.3% for aseptic loosening. Lachiewicz and Soileau[133] in their study of 193 knees (131 patients) with the modular Insall-Burstein II PS total knee prosthesis, noted thin, incomplete, nonprogressive radiolucent lines around 30 tibial components (16%). No clinical or radiographic loosening of the tibial component was noted. Parsch et al.[172] reported on long-term survivorship and clinical outcomes for the Sigma PFC TKA (PFC-TKA; DePuy Orthopaedics, Warsaw, IN) in a series of 141 TKAs with a mean follow-up of 13 years. With aseptic loosening of the implant as the end point, the 10- and 14-year survival rates were 97%.

The underlying mechanism of loosening is also of interest. Miller[155] has indicated that the process is initiated by micromotion between the component and bone, postulating that micromotion could be reduced or eliminated by improving the interlock between cement and cancellous bone. This argument, similar to others in joint arthroplasty, may apply more to hip prostheses than to knee prostheses. Another possible mechanism of loosening is that the components sink or subside into the bone. Seitz et al.,[210] using computed tomography (CT), noted a loss of bone density for several months after knee arthroplasty, coupled with a tendency for the implant to migrate in a mediolateral direction. Periprosthetic osteolysis is another cause of component loosening (Fig. 169.17). The tibia is the

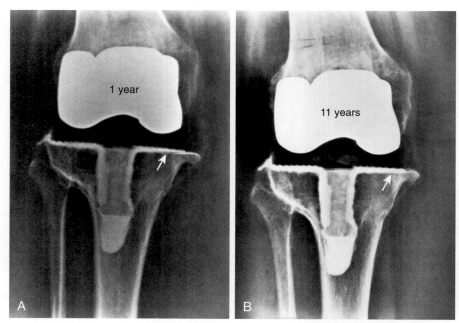

FIG 169.15 (A) Small partial radiolucency beneath the medial tibial plateau. (B) The radiolucency is barely perceptible 10 years later, probably because of a slight difference in projection.

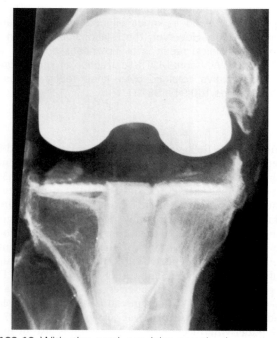

FIG 169.16 With the total condylar prosthesis, a complete radiolucency is attributed to low-grade infection until proven otherwise.

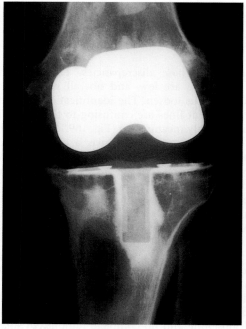

FIG 169.17 Radiograph showing an example of osteolysis involving a prosthesis.

more common site, but there have been documented cases in the literature involving femoral and tibial components. Osteolysis is discussed in more detail in the next section.

Ryd et al.[199-202,221] have extensively studied fixation of knee prostheses in vivo using roentgenographic stereogrammetric analysis. This technique was developed in Lund, Sweden, in 1974 and applied to various orthopedic problems, such as

spinal fusion stability, healing of tibial osteotomy, and skeletal growth patterns. It has also been used for assessing hip joint prosthetic loosening. In the knee, three or more tantalum balls of 0.8-mm diameter are implanted into the tibial metaphysis, using a special instrument with a needle and piston. Markers also are introduced approximately 3 mm into the polyethylene tibial component from underneath, using holes made with a

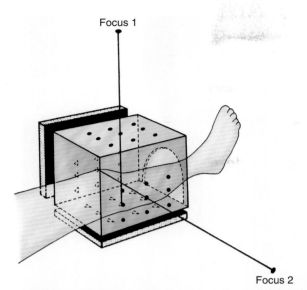

FIG 169.18 Biplanar radiographic setup for roentgenographic stereogrammetric analysis of the knee joint. (From Ryd L, Boegård T, Egund N, et al: Migration of the tibial component in successful unicompartmental knee arthroplasty: a clinical, radiographic, and roentgen stereophotogrammetric study. *Acta Orthop Scand* 54:408, 1983.)

dentist's drill. The postoperative reference examination, using a biplanar radiographic technique (Fig. 169.18), is carried out on the supine patient before the operated leg has become weight bearing. The follow-up examination is carried out with the patient standing on the operated leg only. Rotations about the transverse and sagittal axes were the only movements determined. The initial study was performed on Marmor unicondylar replacements, all of which were clinically successful. The study indicated that none of the prostheses were rigidly fixed to the skeleton, and a degree of micromotion and migration occurred. There was some pattern to migration. Of the six patients studied, five showed posterior and downward migration and four showed medial tilting away from the central axis of the knee.

Subsequent studies have been performed with cemented and uncemented prostheses, with similar results. Migration was greatest in the first year, after which it tended to stabilize; the direction tended to be medial, posterior, and downward. The mode of fixation was important, and migration was greater for uncemented prostheses. The magnitude was approximately 1 mm for a cemented total condylar prosthesis and 2.6 mm for an uncemented porous-coated anatomic (PCA) prosthesis. In another study, the same authors examined 26 patients randomized to cemented or cementless TKA.[221] Using a similar study design, they found the migration between the two groups to be similar. At 1 year, the cemented tibial migration was 1 ± 0.2 mm compared with 1.4 ± 0.22 mm for the cementless TKA. Ryd and Linder[201] have published a description of the bone-cement interface in three well-functioning unicondylar replacements that initially had been shown to migrate by roentgenographic stereogrammetric analysis. The three prostheses were removed for reasons other than fixation. The tibial components were solidly fixed to the bone. The three interfaces had a similar distribution of fibrous tissue and fibrocartilage. The peripheral

5 to 10 mm consisted of fibrous tissue, whereas the remainder of the supporting tissue was fibrocartilage. This layer of cartilage always rested on bone, sometimes with a seam of osteoid sandwiched between the bone and cartilage. The bone underneath the cartilage was vital. There was a total absence of any cellular reaction in the fibrocartilage.

Studies by Ryd et al.[199-202,221] have shown that there is no such thing as rigid fixation between prosthesis and bone and that the normal situation allows some degree of micromotion. Prostheses move or migrate a certain amount early on and then, in most cases, stabilize into a state of equilibrium, which is compatible with satisfactory long-term function. The normal interface between cement and bone consists of fibrocartilage and fibrous tissue, with little cellular reaction. This interface probably corresponds with thin stable radiolucencies that can be identified in long-term studies of well-functioning knee arthroplasties. Hvid and Nielsen[101,102] have concluded that bone strength may be crucial from the point of view of fatigue. Consequently, it can be argued that excessive penetration of cement into the cancellous bone of the knee may be undesirable. It is unlikely that bone trabeculae enclosed within a massive amount of cement remain viable; although the initial mechanical interlock may be improved, the long-term effect may be to transfer the interface to a more distal area of the tibia and into an area in which the strength of the bone is weaker. If one believes this argument, cement penetration should be minimal; 2 to 3 mm is ideal.[227] The theoretical argument coincides with clinical observations. Long-term studies of prostheses using old-fashioned cement techniques that gave little bone penetration have shown extremely good survival. For about 2 years, roughly encompassing 1984 and 1985, we sought greater cement penetration using low-viscosity cement[155]; however, after realizing that our earlier patients continued to function well, we returned to the earlier cement techniques. Most of our metal-backed tibial components have been fixed, using a thin layer of cement with little attempt to penetrate the cancellous bone.

Alignment is more crucial in cementless knees because cement fixation is not present to help protect against excessive point loading, which may occur with malalignment. With cement fixation, the load is distributed more evenly across the tibia, even when malalignment is present. Without cement fixation, this even distribution of the load is not present, and a point-load situation is created, which causes necrosis of bone under the overloaded tibial component. Also, without the protective effect of cement fixation, failure of fixation at the opposite condyle occurs from excessive tension at the interface.[58] Ritter and Meneghini[195] have reviewed 73 cementless TKAs (AGC; Biomet, Warsaw, IN). They found that survivorship for aseptic loosening of any component was 76.4% at 20 years, and two tibial components failed because of aseptic loosening at 1.1 and 2.2 years.

Femoral Component. Loosening of femoral components is uncommon, whether cemented or uncemented. When it does occur, however, it follows a particular pattern in which the bone resorbs posteriorly, allowing the femur to migrate anteriorly and rotate into flexion (Fig. 169.19). King and Scott[124] described a series of 15 loose, cemented, duopatellar femoral prostheses. The incidence of femoral loosening was not stated, but in one series at the Hospital for Special Surgery, there were 6 femoral loosenings in 430 cemented arthroplasties (1.4%) over a 15-year follow-up period. The mechanism of loosening was similar to

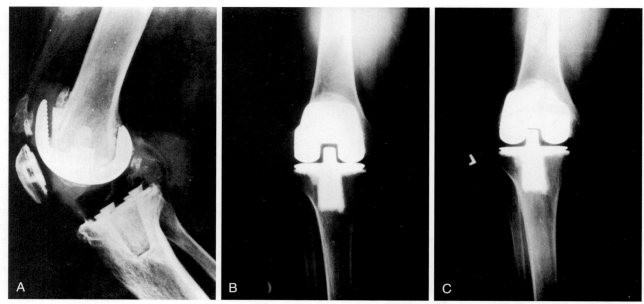

FIG 169.19 (A) Radiograph showing a typical example of femoral loosening. In the lateral view, the femur has migrated anteriorly and moved into a flexed position as a result of resorption of posterior bone. (B and C) The diagnosis of femoral loosening in the AP view is not always easy to make. The femur tends to migrate proximally so that there is the appearance of bone overgrowth medially or laterally. In this case, the diagnosis of loosening was made because a change in position into varus was noted and was confirmed by overlapping the radiographs.

that described by King and Scott, who thought that the lack of posterior femoral support as a result of osteoporotic bone or poor technique was the cause. In this region, cancellous bone hypertrophy was reported by Whiteside and Pafford[233]; this region of the femur is most likely to be highly stressed.

Patellar Component. Loosening of the patellar component is associated most often with patellar fractures or with dissociation of polyethylene and metal-backed components. Loosening of cemented all-polyethylene patellae in other circumstances is infrequent. The incidence of patellar component loosening is approximately 1% but has been reported to be as high as 3%.[239] Loosening of the patella was more common with the small central lug, but more recently, the tripod configuration of three small peripheral lugs has become popular. Mason et al.[147] have reported no loose patellar components among 577 tripod configuration patellae at an average of 3 years.

Firestone et al.[70] found loosening rates of 0.6% to 11.1% in several cementless patellar component designs. Factors associated with loosening include insertion of the prosthesis with cement into worn or sclerotic bone, malpositioning of the patellar component, subluxation, fracture or avascular necrosis of the patella, osteoporosis, asymmetrical resection, loosening of other prosthetic components, and lack of osseous growth into the porous coating.[189,229] Reduction in the rate of loosening of the patellar component requires improved bone preparation and cementing techniques, proper patellar resection, avoidance of asymmetrical or excessive bone removal, and central patellar tracking.[7]

Osteolysis

Osteolysis is well documented in the THA literature in response to particulate debris, and it has shown a rapid increase more recently in the TKA literature. The cause of osteolysis in the knee is the same as in the hip—inflammatory response to particulate debris.

Osteolysis has been reported to be associated with the polyethylene stock and sterilization method, tibial modularity and backside wear, design of the PS tibial post, patient factors (eg, age, activity level), and surgical factors.[19,61,164,228] Lachiewicz and Soileau[133] at a mean of 12 years (range, 10 to 18 years), reported 7% osteolysis. This study indicated an association between younger patient age and radiographic evidence of osteolysis.

Collier et al.[44] reviewed 365 PCR-TKAs and found that the prevalence of osteolysis at 5 to 10 years was 34% when polyethylene sterilized with gamma radiation in air was used on a grit-blasted titanium base; the prevalence was 9% when polyethylene sterilized with gamma radiation in air or polyethylene that had been sterilized with gas plasma was used on a polished cobalt-chromium (Co-Cr) base. Their analysis has shown that osteolysis is associated with male gender, the use of a grit-blasted titanium tibial base, three polyethylene-related factors (the variety from which it was machined, sterilization method, and shelf age), and femoral component hyperextension.

The incidence of osteolysis around a knee replacement is difficult to assess for many reasons. First, obtaining an accurate radiographic assessment at the interface is difficult. For example, if there is tibial osteolysis below the tray, and the x-ray angle is from slightly above the joint, this lysis may be missed. Engh et al.[62] indicated that femoral lesions are more difficult to recognize. Femoral lesions are often hidden by the femoral component on the radiograph. Posterior femoral condyle overlap and the central box of PS components limit complete evaluation of femoral condyles on lateral radiographs. Whereas the anterior flange of the component may hide lesions on the anteroposterior (AP) image, Miura et al.[157] have reported that the oblique posterior femoral condylar radiographic view is significantly better than a true lateral view for the detection of radiolucencies.

Reish et al.[190] have determined the accuracy of plain radiography in detecting osteolytic lesions around total knee prostheses, compared with multidetector CT. They studied 31 patients diagnosed with periprosthetic osteolysis by plain radiography and multidetector CT after TKA. They reported that plain radiographs are inadequate for evaluating periprosthetic osteolysis in TKA, with only 8 of 48 lesions (17%) detected by multidetector CT visible on the standard radiographs.

Another reason for the difficulty in assessing the incidence of osteolysis is the length of follow-up. Ezzet et al.[64] reported a strong correlation between length of follow-up and the prevalence of osteolysis. Before 24 months, no cases of osteolysis were identified; between 24 and 60 months, the incidence was 15%, and at follow-up longer than 60 months, the incidence was 39%.[182]

The cause of the particulate debris, which contributes to osteolysis, remains controversial. Small particles are generated from the articular surface, tibial post impingement in PS knees, backside wear in all modular designs, and backside wear in mobile-bearing knees. It is apparent, however, that osteolysis is extremely rare in monoblock tibial designs, especially with net shape–molded components. Particulate debris displaced from the articular and backside surfaces of tibial polyethylene inserts is considered to be a predominant cause. Polishing the tibial baseplate counterface, polyethylene sterilization by gamma radiation in an inert gas environment and nonradiation sterilization methods have reduced loss of polyethylene debris and may yield a more fatigue-resistant bearing surface. Collier et al.[43] also investigated the factors of the backside interface and polyethylene sterilization method in a study of 365 CR TKAs (anatomic modular knee; DePuy Orthopaedics, Warsaw, IN) with minimum 5-year follow-up. They reported a significant reduction in the prevalence of osteolysis, from 24% to 2%, when transition was made to a polished baseplate and away from gamma irradiation in air.

Histologic analysis of synovial tissue and osteolytic tissue has been performed. The synovial tissue of knees associated with osteolysis shows subsynovial infiltrates consisting of histiocytes and giant cells.[177] Polyethylene and metal particulate debris have been found in specimens. The size of the debris and type of material are both important. Polyethylene particles smaller than 3 μm are usually engulfed by giant cells. Polyethylene particles larger than 3 μm are found in the cytoplasm of histiocytes and occasionally within giant cells. Larger particles of metal (≈5 μm) usually elicit little cellular response. Histologic examinations of osteolytic tissue have revealed a hypercellular membrane consisting of sheets of histiocytes and occasional giant cells. There is no necrosis and little associated vascularity.

The presentation of a patient with osteolysis varies. Most patients with well-fixed components are asymptomatic. Others present with symptoms of boggy synovitis. Mild or moderate diffuse pain may occur with activity, especially in patients in whom the tibial component is unstable. The radiographic criteria for diagnosis of osteolysis, as proposed by Peters et al.,[177] included a lytic osseous defect that extends beyond the limits of that potentially caused by loosening of the implant alone, absence of cancellous bone trabeculae, and geographic demarcation by a shell of bone. Accelerated polyethylene wear and the subsequent osteolysis can give rise to aseptic loosening,

periprosthetic fracture, recurrent painful effusions, and polyethylene fractures, which can necessitate or complicate revision surgery.

TKA produces greater wear of the polyethylene surface than THA, yet less osteolysis is seen compared with THA. Engh et al.[62] have described four factors that could explain this phenomenon. First is the size of the particles produced, which is related to the type of wear (ie, delamination and abrasion in TKA); this releases large fragments of polyethylene, rarely seen in THA. Large particles produced in the TKA are relatively bioinert. Second, the synovial cavity of the knee is the most extensive of any synovial joint in the body and has greater capacity to engulf and digest wear debris (ie, greater resistance to osteolysis). Third, the fixation interface with polymethylmethacrylate (PMMA) is a better seal to potential debris than PMMA in a THA. Fourth, the shear and tensile stresses on PMMA may be less at the knee than at the hip. The modulus of elasticity of PMMA is relatively close to that of the cancellous bone of the upper tibia and tibial component. The decreased amount of stress and fatigue means decreased fracture of the cement mantle, which leads to decreased access for debris to the bone-cement interface.

When osteolysis appears around a TKA, it usually appears on the tibial side; this is probably a multifactorial event. Peters et al.[177] have suggested three possible causative factors for this:
1. Gravity and weight bearing through the medial side of the knee tend to localize the particulate polyethylene on the tibial side.
2. On the femoral side, if the osteolytic process is initiated along the implant-bone interface, the flanges of the femoral implant tend to obscure a radiographic diagnosis.
3. The addition of screws to the tibial implant provides avenues for the migration of debris into metaphyseal bone.

The treatment of osteolysis around a TKA is controversial. If the implant is stable, and the patient is asymptomatic, one can observe the patient with serial x-ray films on a yearly basis. If the patient is symptomatic or the prosthesis is grossly loose, there are several different options. For patients who are symptomatic with a well-fixed modular prosthesis and excessive polyethylene, one can débride the lesion with a curette, pack the defect with a morcellized bone graft, and exchange the polyethylene. Exchange of the bearing surface in TKA offers several potential benefits compared with complete component revision, including the preservation of bone stock, reduced complexity, reduced cost, and potentially easier patient recovery. Because polyethylene wear and osteolysis are increasingly indicated as reasons for revision, the prospect of less complicated isolated insert exchange is an attractive option. Griffin et al.[84] have evaluated the results of isolated polyethylene exchange for wear and/or osteolysis in 68 press-fit condylar TKAs at the mean 44 months and had 11 failures (16.2%). Failures included aseptic loosening in 10 knees and infection in 1. They reported an 84% success rate with modular polyethylene exchange and the lack of progression of osteolytic lesions in the 97% of knees. O'Brien et al.[166] reported that osteolytic lesions resolved in the 17 of 18 hips studied at a mean of 3 years after the postexchange procedure. Similarly, Maloney et al.[146] reported that osteolytic lesions resolved in one-third of 40 hips treated with isolated liner exchange; in the remaining two-thirds of hips, the lesions reduced in size at a mean of 3.5 years following isolated liner exchange. Engh et al.[62] either changed out the polyethylene or performed removal of screws, curettage, and polyethylene exchange. They reported good results, with no tibial defects progressing and no development of new lesions.

If the components are grossly loose, revision of the components is in order. Because the defects are always larger in situ than they appear on film, a full armamentarium of revision instruments should be ready. In most cases, allografts and the full complement of modular augments should be available. In Engh et al.'s series,[62] in which the components were revised and structural allografts were used, four of five patients had excellent fixation interfaces at 2 years. There were no lucencies and no graft resorption. One patient with rheumatoid arthritis had a 1- to 2-mm radiolucency beneath the tibial plateau without any change in component alignment. The patient was pain-free at 6 years. Robinson et al.[196] reported on 17 revisions performed for osteolysis. The original method of component fixation was a mixture of hybrid fixation, including both cemented and cementless implants. The average time interval from the index surgery to radiographic evidence of osteolysis was 56 months. The prostheses used in the treatment of these 17 revisions were PS implants in 65% of cases and a constrained implant in 30%. Osteolytic defects were reconstructed with cement only in 47%, allograft in 30%, and metallic wedges in 35%. No follow-up or outcome data were available from this series. Kim et al.[122] reported the prevalence of osteolysis after simultaneous bilateral fixed-bearing and mobile-bearing TKAs in young patients. Osteolysis was identified in radiographs and CT scans in 6 knees (10%) in the anatomic molecular knee fixed-bearing prosthesis (DePuy Orthopaedics, Warsaw, IN) group and 4 knees (7%) in the low contact stress mobile meniscal bearing prosthesis (DePuy Orthopaedics, Warsaw, IN) group. Kim and Kim[120] also studied 62 patients who underwent simultaneous bilateral TKAs, with a unidirectional prosthesis implanted in one knee and a multidirectional prosthesis in the other. No differences in preoperative and postoperative knee and functional scores were seen. No patients had detectable tibial polyethylene liner wear or osteolysis.

Component Breakage

Breakage of components is rare[24,57,110] and usually restricted to hinges and linked designs.[112] Breakage is manifested by instability, pain, and deformity, but does not always call for immediate revision. Historically, one of our patients had a fracture of the femoral stem associated with an episode of transient pain 3 years after the arthroplasty. Although some instability was present, this patient functioned at a high level with little or no pain for another 5 years before revision became necessary for an increasing varus deformity.

Mechanical failure in surface replacement is rare. We encountered three fractured femoral components in the early version of the unicondylar and duocondylar prostheses. In these, the femoral runner was made of considerably thinner metal than that used on subsequent designs, and it is not expected that similar fatigue failure will be seen in current models. Fracture of unicondylar metal components also has been reported.[24] Whiteside et al.[230] examined fracture of femoral components in cementless TKAs. They compared 6172 Ortholoc II femoral components (Wright Medical Technology, Arlington, TN) with double-bead layers with 16,230 Ortholoc II femoral components with single-bead layers for fracture of components. They found a total of 32 fractured femoral components, of which 31 were in the double-bead layers. The overall minimum rate of failure for the double-bead layers was 0.42, whereas for

the single-bead layer, it was 0.006. They found that all the failures occurred at the junction between one of the level surfaces and the distal surface of the implant.

Fracture of the metallic tibial tray has been reported on isolated occasions.[57,139] Subsequently, in these designs, the metal tray was strengthened, particularly in the region of the posterior cruciate cutout. We have not seen a metal tray fracture in a cruciate-substituting design.

Polyethylene fractures are generally wear-related, as with late catastrophic failure of the tibial inserts of modular components. However, catastrophic fractures of the tibial post in posterior PS and constrained designs have been reported. Although these failures seem to occur predominantly in designs that do not provide adequate anterior clearances, which results in anterior post impingement in hyperextension, they have been reported in newer designs as well.[113,136,140] They also may occur as a result of overflexion of the femoral component or inadequate posterior slope of the tibial component. Thus, the importance of surgical technique relative to component positioning cannot be overemphasized. Even neutral intraoperative sagittal positioning of components is biased toward clinical hyperextension. This is because the combination of the anterior bow of the femur and the anterior-posterior slope of the tibial resection results in approximately 10 degrees of relative component hyperextension when the knee is placed in full extension.[10] As the femoral component moves from flexion to hyperextension, the intercondylar notch may contact the anterior region of the tibial eminence or tibial post, depending on the design of the implant (ie, PCL-retaining vs. PCL-substituting). If impingement occurs, fracture, significant polyethylene wear, or both may follow.[23,105,143]

Factors inherent to the polyethylene may also predispose it to fracture. Ionizing radiation improves the adhesive and abrasive wear resistance of polyethylene by producing cross linkages,[193] and a recent retrospective study has demonstrated that highly cross-linked polyethylene is safe for use in TKA.[89] However, in an oxygen environment, ionizing radiation can create free radicals that embrittle polyethylene through oxidation. Modern techniques such as vacuum processing, heat annealing, and remelting have been devised to avoid or eliminate these free radicals. However, it is interesting to note that if oxidation has occurred prior to implantation, it is likely to continue in vivo as the polyethylene implant is exposed to oxygen-containing body fluids.[132] In THA, the clinical effects of in vivo oxidation have been negligible, presumably because the ball and socket interface affords a degree of protection to most of the polyethylene component. In these cases, in vivo oxidation is most severe at the rim of the liner. For TKA, the implications are more severe because the tibial eminence or post is constantly bathed in synovial fluid. This may account for the high rate of early postoperative tibial post breakage reported by Bal et al.[9] for polyethylene implants sterilized with gamma radiation in an oxygen environment.

Component Wear

Retrieval analysis of removed total joint implants consistently has revealed polyethylene particles in the synovium.[30,79,80,156,182] In addition, acrylic debris and occasionally metallic particles have been seen. Inspection of the removed components often reveals embedded cement particles in the polyethylene component, with scratching, pitting, and burnishing of the articular surface. Distortion of the polyethylene and gross deformation

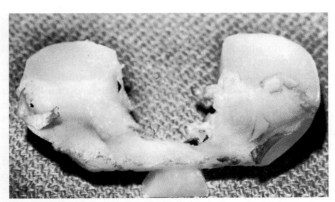

FIG 169.20 Retrieved geometric tibial component showing severe wear.

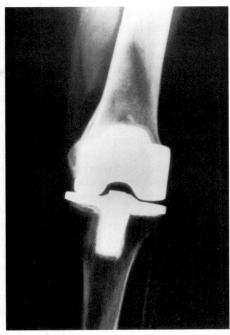

FIG 169.21 Radiograph of a Kinematic prosthesis 5 years postoperatively showing wear-through of the medial tibia.

of the component as a result of cold flow (Fig. 169.20) also may occur; this is particularly likely when the tibial polyethylene component is thin. Some earlier designs had a component that was deliberately made thin to minimize bone removal and often had a cruciate cutout. This combination sometimes led to gross distortion and deformation, which contributed to loosening of the component (the early UCI design was prone to this type of failure). It is now considered that unless the component is reinforced with a metal tray, a minimum thickness of 8 mm is desirable.

Metal femoral components may be observed to have scratches in the highly polished articular surface in more than 50% of retrieved specimens. It is believed that some of the debris is generated from free cement particles that have become trapped between the articular surfaces. Careful surgical technique can lessen cement entrapment; however, even in the absence of evidence of cement or body wear, polyethylene failure at the articular surface may be observed. This failure is manifested by pitting, scratching, burnishing, and abrasion of the surface. The amount of surface failure is highly correlated with the level of patient activity, body weight, and length of implantation, and seems to be more than that noted in retrieval analysis of total hip implants.[92]

The type of motion occurring in the articulation is also important. Sliding as opposed to rolling movements causes much greater wear, especially of the delamination type. The kinematic conditions in the joint seem to be of paramount importance.[22] Unconforming flat surfaces, together with lax ligaments, predispose to various sliding motions.

The durability of a spherically convex polyethylene patellar implant may be questioned in that this shape theoretically causes more wear. Retrieval analysis at the Hospital for Special Surgery of 20 patellar buttons[91] did not indicate that the rate of wear is greater than that of the tibial plateau. However, there was some deformation of the polyethylene, usually with elongation in the long axis and some flattening of the convex shape where it articulates with the femoral component. Figgie[69] has examined all-polyethylene dome patellar components and found a positive correlation between the amount of polyethylene damage and the ROM achieved postoperatively.

Metal backing of patellar components did not improve the wear performance characteristics but rather led to an increase in wear-related complications.[12,13,143,197,216] Up to 10 times serum levels of titanium, aluminum, and vanadium were measured in

patients with metal on metal contact after metal-backed patellar failure.[217] These extreme levels of debris have been associated with extensive osteolysis and periarticular soft tissue cysts and masses.[35]

Hsu and Walker[97] more recently studied wear patterns in patellar components. They found that wear occurred regardless of the design shape, although wear was most rapid in dome-shaped patellae with metal inlays. A dome-shaped patella is only in line contact with the femur until approximately 70 degrees of flexion, after which the patella contacts peripherally with the condylar runners. Contouring the shape of the patella (central convexity and peripheral concavity) greatly improved the wear characteristics, which was better still when the component was metal-backed. Even with optimal shape and metal backing, however, wear-through was ultimately predicted because of design constraints on the thickness of the polyethylene (approximately 3 mm). It was concluded that onset patellar replacements with metal backing should not be used at this time. Inlaying the patellar component allows a thicker layer of plastic, which may be an improvement from the wear point of view but does not allow polyethylene resurfacing at the margins of the patella, the regions that are subject to the greatest contact pressures when the knee is flexed. There has been a general return to cemented all-polyethylene patellar components, although agreement on this point is not uniform.[46]

Tibial polyethylene wear has emerged as a major clinical problem,[45,62,78,142] particularly with designs having flat tibial surfaces and thin polyethylene.[36] Isolated cases of wear-through initially were reported for the porous-coated anatomic prosthesis[61] and the variable axis prosthesis. In the cases described, the medial polyethylene wore through to the metal baseplate (Fig. 169.21). The original thickness of the components was about 5 mm. These were treated by replacing the polyethylene insert with a thicker one. Posterior wear-through to metal has been seen on the Robert Brigham unicondylar design on 6-mm components[128,129] and on the posterior polyethylene of Kinematic components, in which it was judged that excessive femoral rollback had occurred.

Wear damage to polyethylene is influenced by clinical and design factors.[194] Studies performed on tibial components of a single design have shown significant correlation between the amount of polyethylene damage to the articulating surface and patient weight and the length of implantation of the component.[240] Greater wear damage also has been found in patients who achieved better ambulatory status postoperatively.

Other factors also influence the wear characteristics of polyethylene. Polyethylene inserts are currently manufactured by compression molding of resin or machining of ram-extruded bars. Of these two processes, compression molding seems to provide greater resistance to articular[237] and backside wear,[141] although data are limited. Polyethylene has traditionally been sterilized with gamma radiation or gas plasma. Postproduction irradiation of polyethylene was serendipitously found to induce cross linking, which imparts statistically lower wear rates than conventional non–cross-linked polyethylene. In laboratory trials, this benefit is maintained across different rotating and fixed-bearing total knee designs.[222] However, the free radicals formed by irradiation in air can adversely affect the polyethylene through oxidation. In an in vivo wear analysis performed at the Anderson Orthopaedic Research Institute, wear rates were significantly greater for polyethylene components radiation-sterilized in air versus those sterilized in inert gas.[42] These findings have been confirmed by a recent survivorship analysis as well. Griffin et al.[83] compared the incidence of wear-related failure between two cohorts of patients who had received identical modular tibial trays and polyethylene sterilized by different methods. The polyethylene implants sterilized in air demonstrated an 87% 10-year survivorship, whereas those sterilized in an oxygen-free environment demonstrated a 97% 10-year survivorship. The locking mechanism for modular designs is also a factor in reducing wear. A recent retrieval analysis of three different total knee designs at the Hospital for Special Surgery found a lower incidence of backside wear for polyethylene components that were locked to the tibial baseplate with a peripheral capture mechanism, as opposed to partial dovetailing or pinning.[107] Finally, shelf life longer than 1.5 years is another independent variable that negatively influences wear.[41]

With the increased modularity afforded by metal tibial trays, undersurface or backside wear has become a recognized entity.[170] This problem is caused by micromotion between the polyethylene insert and the tray (usually made of titanium), causing particulate polyethylene debris to accumulate. In uncemented trays, the debris can filter down the screw holes, initiating osteolysis. Studies have documented that under physiologic loading, modular designs have motion between the tray and polyethylene insert, regardless of the locking mechanism.[169] Wasielewski et al.[228] examined 67 polyethylene tibial inserts from cementless TKAs retrieved at autopsy or revision surgery. The mean implantation time was 62.8 months. Polyethylene cold flow and abrasive wear on the monoarticulating insert surface (undersurface) were assigned a wear severity score (grades 0 to 4). The investigators found that severe grade 4 wear of the tibial insert undersurface was associated with tibial metaphyseal osteolysis or osteolysis around fixation screws. Time in situ was statistically related to grade 4 undersurface wear and tibial metaphyseal osteolysis.

Lessons learned from the polished undersurface of the mobile-bearing designs are being applied to fixed platform designs. Polishing the tibial baseplate may help lessen the extent of backside wear for fixed-bearing designs as well. In a laboratory trial, material and surface factors were found to influence backside wear. In fixed-bearing designs, polished titanium has slightly better wear characteristics than polished Co-Cr in decreasing the polyethylene wear, but both polished surfaces provide substantial benefits over their traditional nonpolished counterparts.[20]

Much attention has been placed on the development of mobile bearing designs. Despite theoretical benefits, an in vitro wear study comparing mobile- and fixed-bearing options of the same implant at over 6 million cycles failed to demonstrate statistically significant improvement.[88] Although previous retrieval analysis of mobile-bearing designs has not shown excessive wear of the back insert surface or tibial metaphyseal osteolysis,[28] more recent analysis has demonstrated that the articular surface of mobile-bearing designs remains vulnerable to wear, in addition to the independent inferior surface.[74] When compared with fixed-bearing designs, mobile-bearing knees seem to trade improved articular-sided wear characteristics for more serious backside wear.[145] On close inspection of retrieved implants, mobile-bearing designs are more susceptible to burnishing and scratching of the undersurface than fixed-bearing designs, and a higher incidence of burnishing is also noted on the articular surface.[63]

Meniscal-bearing designs, such as the Oxford and low contact stress (LCS), are theoretically the least liable to wear, but the possibility of dislocation of the bearings offsets the advantage to some extent.[15] Although backside wear seems decreased in these designs, it does occur and has been reported as a cause of bearing dislocation and catastrophic polyethylene failure.[98,99]

Landy and Walker[134] have examined 90 retrieved knee prostheses, with implant times of up to 10 years. Polyethylene wear was much greater than that seen in wear studies of acetabular components in total hip prostheses (Fig. 169.22). Abrasion, burnishing, and deformation were seen in approximately 90 of the components. Cement particles embedded in the surface were found in about half. Delamination, the most severe form of polyethylene degradation, was found in 37 prostheses. Eight flat unicondylar components, which had the longest mean implant times (7.8 years), showed the most severe delamination. Twelve dished unicondylar components (6.3-year implant time) showed less delamination. Six one-piece tibial components, with a mean wear time of 4.3 years, showed much less delamination, almost entirely restricted to the central margin. There was considerable variation in the range of molecular weights between manufacturers and even between different components from the same manufacturer; the wear score for compression-molded components was higher than for other components.

The widespread adoption of metal-backed tibial components reduces deformation (Fig. 169.23), but the extra thickness of the metal is obtained at the expense of greater tibial resection or thinner polyethylene. Apel et al.[5] have found that thicker (>10 mm) all-polyethylene components behaved similarly to metal-backed components. For this and economic reasons, we believe there may be some interest in returning to all-polyethylene components or monoblock metal-back tibial augments; however, based on high failure rates of flat on flat, all-polyethylene components, all-polyethylene components are

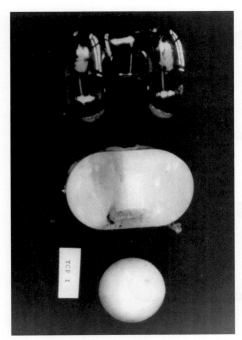

FIG 169.22 Retrieved total condylar prosthesis removed because of infection after having been implanted for 7 years in an active patient. The appearance of the tibial component shows some burnishing and a few small pits. The patellar component shows slight flattening in one area. There is no other evidence of cold flow, delamination, or cracking of the polyethylene.

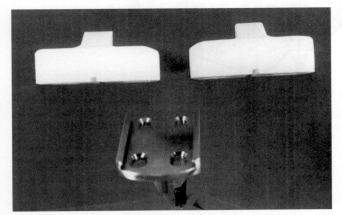

FIG 169.23 Metal tray support of the polyethylene prevents deformation.

extremely design sensitive. They should be used only after long-term clinical data accumulation.[137]

PATELLAR COMPLICATIONS

Subluxation and Dislocation

Various technical and design factors may contribute to subluxation and dislocation of the patella (Fig. 169.24).[‡]

‡References 18, 26, 81, 125, 142, 153, and 186.

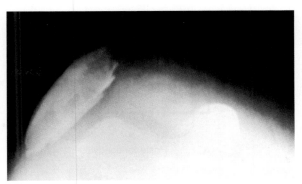

FIG 169.24 Gross rotary malposition of the tibial component leads to patellar dislocation.

Depth of the Femoral Trochlea. The design of the femoral sulcus is a compromise. A shallow sulcus predisposes the patella to instability, but an overly deep sulcus offers excessive constraint to the patella, which may lead to patellar component loosening and patellar fracture.

Position of the Femoral Component. Placement of the femoral component in internal rotation increases the lateral soft tissue tension as the knee is flexed.[191] As noted, some degree of external rotation is preferred (Fig. 169.25). We use the epicondylar axis to set the femoral rotation.

Malrotation of the Tibial Component. Internal rotation of the tibial component gives an external placement of the tibial tubercle, increasing the quadriceps angle and contributing to patellar instability. Malrotation of the tibial component is often the result of inadequate exposure. Sufficient dissection around the tibia to displace the tibial surface anteriorly provides the best visualization of the various landmarks for tibial component placement (Fig. 169.26).

Overall Valgus Alignment. Excessive valgus position increases the quadriceps angle. Reports have suggested that patellar instability often occurs in knees that were originally valgus.

Tight Lateral Retinaculum. A tight lateral retinaculum can contribute to patellar dislocation. Patellar tracking problems after TKA have been reported to occur with an incidence of 29%.[108] Subluxation is more common than dislocation.[18] Patients usually complain of anterior knee pain or gross subluxation or dislocation. The treatment of this complication depends on its cause. A patient with mild subluxation and a weak vastus medialis would benefit from intense physical therapy. The components could be malpositioned or malaligned, which could be determined preoperatively with a CT scan (Fig. 169.27). If this is the cause, a revision would be appropriate. In most cases, the treatment is a lateral retinaculum release, sometimes in conjunction with a proximal realignment. We do not recommend a tibial tubercle transposition because of its high complication rate.

Results of surgical treatment for patellar instability are good for combined lateral release and proximal realignment procedures. Grace and Rand[81] studied 25 knees with symptomatic lateral patellar instability after TKA. The knees were treated by one of three methods—proximal realignment, combined

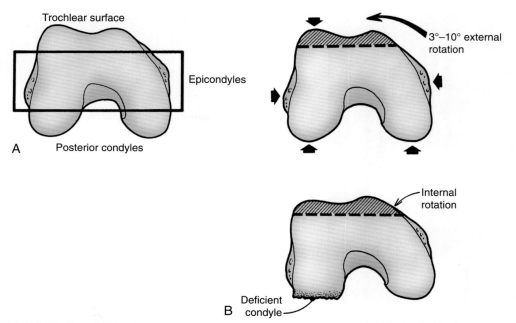

FIG 169.25 (A and B) Internal rotation of the femoral component is a cause of patellar dislocation. The component always should be in slight external rotation.

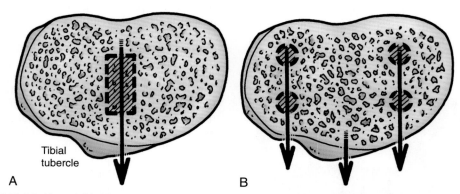

FIG 169.26 (A and B) Alignment of the tibial component is projected at a point slightly medial to the tibial tubercle. Alignment of a symmetrical component with the posterior margin of the tibial plateau usually results in some internal rotation of the tibial component. One should err on the side of external rotation.

proximal and distal realignment, or component revision. At a 50-month follow-up, 20 knees had normal patellar tracking and 5 had recurrent instability. Two of nine patients who had a combined realignment had patellar tendon rupture. The authors recommended proximal realignment alone in the absence of component malposition. If the component is malpositioned, component revision should be performed.

Merkow et al.[153] have reported their experience at the Hospital for Special Surgery. Between 1974 and 1982, 12 dislocations occurred in 11 patients. Trauma was the cause of dislocation in three knees, incorrect tracking of the patella in six, and malrotation of the tibial component in three. Many of the knees were in valgus preoperatively. Dislocations occurred in four different prosthetic designs, suggesting that in this series, design was not a factor. Unrestrained tibial rotation has been described as predisposing to patellar dislocation by others. Whiteside et al.[231] have

maintained that the degree of tibial rotation is determined by the ligaments, provided that the ligaments are correctly tensioned during surgery. They noted that rotational constraint in the prosthesis is unnecessary and may predispose to loosening. We believe, however, that knees with initial external rotation deformities of the tibia are managed more easily by a design with rotational constraint, and this feature is useful in managing a patellar dislocation that has already occurred. Altering the rotational position of the tibial component in a design with some constraint is the equivalent to transferring the tibial tubercle.

In Merkow et al.,[153] the patellar dislocation was managed by proximal realignment in 10 cases, lateral release in 1 case, and proximal realignment and revision of the tibial component into a more desirable externally rotated position in 1 case. None of the dislocations recurred, and transposition of the tibial tubercle was required in none. We agree with Rand and Bryan[188] that tibial tubercle transposition is inadvisable after TKA because the bone quality is often poor, and the proportion of complications is high. Wolff et al.[236] and Whiteside and Ohl[232] have claimed that tibial tubercle transposition is effective with good technique. They recommended taking a relatively large fragment of the tibial tubercle so that secure fixation with screws is attainable.

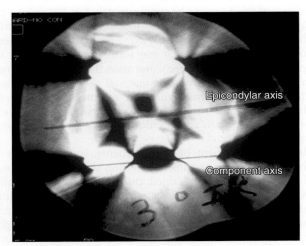

FIG 169.27 CT scan demonstrating 3 degrees of internal rotation of the femoral component compared with reference line through the epicondylar axis.

Soft Tissue Impingement. In 1982, we described a case in which a fibrous nodule was excised from the suprapatellar region of the quadriceps tendon. This nodule gave rise to what has become known as the patellar clunk syndrome (Fig. 169.28),[15,94,220,224] most commonly associated with the use of a PS prosthesis.

The deeper flexion provided by the initial Insall-Burstein (IB) stabilized design enabled the quadriceps tendon to extend beyond the trochlear groove of the femoral component. If the anterior edge of the femoral component terminates abruptly, synovium or scar residing on the tendon falls into the intercondylar groove. If this has occurred, the same tissue must ride up out of the intercondylar area and jump back up onto the femoral trochlea as the patient extends her or his knee. Within a few months after the arthroplasty, the offending (or offended) tissue hypertrophies and becomes rubbery. This creates the painful and noisy complication that has been described as patellar clunk. Historically, a case of patellar catching was mentioned by Insall in his original report on the PS knee. However, Hozack and colleagues appeared to be the first to define the term *patellar clunk syndrome*.[94] They described a prominent fibrous nodule at the junction of the proximal patellar pole and quadriceps tendon. They believed that during flexion, this fibrous nodule would enter the femoral component's intercondylar notch but not restrict flexion. However, as the knee extended, the nodule would remain within the notch while the rest of the extensor mechanism slid proximally. At 30 to 45 degrees of flexion, the tension on the fibrous nodule would be sufficient to cause the nodule to jerk out of the notch as it returned to its

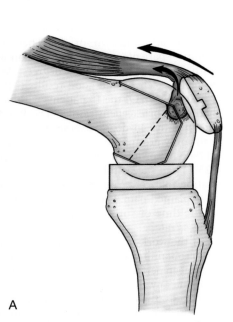
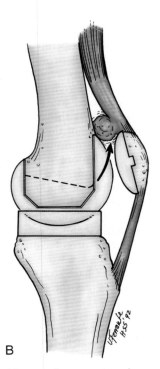

A   B

FIG 169.28 (A and B) Patellar clunk syndrome. The cause of this peculiar symptom is a suprapatellar mass of synovium and fibrous tissue that forms a nodule, which is caught between the patella and femoral component. This nodule typically forms at between 60 and 45 degrees of flexion and can result in locking of the knee in this position. As the knee is brought into terminal extension, the patella can be seen to pop, and the nodule is released from its entrapped position. The symptom can be cured by arthroscopic removal of the fibrous nodule.

normal position. This sudden displacement would cause the audible and palpable clunk found with this entity.

Synovial entrapment or hyperplasia is a similar entity but a less well-described syndrome.[179] It is caused by similar hypertrophy of soft tissue in the same location, but without a discrete nodule. Rather than a clunk or catch, the patient experiences pain and crepitus, typically with active knee extension from a 90-degree flexed position. This typically occurs during stair climbing or rising from a chair.

The original IB design had a high incidence of patellar clunk—up to 21%. This is likely related to the femorotrochlear geometry, a short trochlea with a sharp transition into the intercondylar notch.[2,38] Changes to the sagittal geometry of the femoral component in the IB II reduced the incidence to approximately 3% to 8% but did not eliminate the problem. Finally, with the introduction of the NexGen Legacy prosthesis (Zimmer, Warsaw, IN) in 1997, one of the main areas of focus was the patellofemoral articulation and the reduction of patellofemoral complications. The side-specific components with anatomically oriented trochlear grooves, lengthening and deepening of the femoral trochlea, and an increase in the number of femoral sizes, all helped reduce the incidence of patellar entrapment syndromes. In 238 knees reconstructed with the NexGen Legacy prosthesis, no cases of patellar clunk or synovial entrapment were seen with 24- to 72-month follow-up.

Treatment recommendations for patellar clunk syndrome and synovial entrapment have included physical therapy, surgical removal of the nodule, patellar prosthesis revision, open resection through a limited lateral incision, and arthroscopic débridement.[15,94,154,224] Pollock et al.[179] have reviewed the prevalence of synovial entrapment with three different cam-post designs. Those with proximally positioned or wide femoral boxes were more likely to have a higher prevalence of this problem.

Beight et al.[15] have reported on 14 operative procedures (11 arthroscopic débridements and 3 patellar component revisions) performed in 12 patients. As in other reports, they found a suprapatellar fibrous nodule that wedged into the intercondylar notch during flexion and dislodged as the knee extended, causing the clunk. It was found that the symptoms resolved after nodule excision. However, four of the knees treated with arthroscopic débridement had recurrence of symptoms. None of the knees that underwent arthrotomy and patellar button revisions had recurrence. The recommended treatment protocol commenced with a short course of nonoperative physical therapy, although it was acknowledged that these results were disappointing. Arthroscopic débridement was suggested for knees without radiographic component abnormalities. Arthrotomy was suggested for recurrent clunks or malpositioned or loose components.

Researchers at the Mayo Clinic have recently reported on a series of 25 patients who underwent arthroscopic treatment of patellar clunk syndrome (15 knees) or patellofemoral synovial hyperplasia (10 knees).[53] After surgery, patients reported knee pain and crepitus, but Knee Society knee and function scores improved in both groups. It was concluded that arthroscopic débridement of symptomatic patellofemoral synovium after TKA is a safe and effective procedure.

UNEXPLAINED PAIN

A certain proportion of patients continue to complain of pain for which there is no apparent explanation. Sometimes the arthroplasty is objectively functioning well and has a good ROM. The pain may be present continuously or mainly at rest. For example, one of our patients was able to walk considerable distances and climb stairs normally without difficulty. He complained of severe pain when sitting, and because his occupation involved frequent flying, this was a considerable problem for him. Complaints of pain may be associated with lack of motion or flexion contracture, although the components appeared to be well seated and well positioned. We estimate the incidence of these cases to be approximately 1 in 300 arthroplasties. The cause is usually difficult to show. There is an overlap with reflex sympathetic dystrophy,[117] particularly in patients who have restricted motion. It may seem, in retrospect, that the preoperative symptoms were worse than the pathologic condition of the knee. Some type of material allergy has been suspected but never proved, although in one of our patients with a loose metal on metal hinge prosthesis, we were able to show a skin allergy to cobalt chloride. Low-grade infection is always a possibility.

In the management of these patients, infection must be excluded as much as possible. Aspiration should be attempted, and if sufficient fluid is obtained, cultures can be quite reliable; 90% of our infected knees have been diagnosed by culture of the aspirate. Bone scintigraphy[90,115,181] also may be useful, although technetium-99m scanning after TKA yields highly variable results[204] in that asymptomatic knees may continue to have abnormal scans indefinitely. Indium scanning[187] was found to be 85% reliable in 18 infected knees. In a group of 20 knees with aseptic loosening, however, the scan results were not given.

When reflex sympathetic dystrophy is suspected, sympathetic block should be tried. If the response is good, a lumbar sympathectomy should be considered.

A 1996 study[159] examined the role of exploratory surgery in unexplained pain in TKA. In this study, 27 patients underwent exploration of their TKA secondary to severe debilitating pain of an unknown origin. They were divided into two groups—patients with ROM less than 80 degrees and patients with ROM greater than 80 degrees. At final follow-up, there were 11 excellent and good results (41%) and 16 fair or poor results (59%). Of the 15 patients with decreased ROM, 9 (60%) had good or excellent results. The ROM arc improved from a preoperative 43-degree average to an 81-degree average. For the pain-only group, there were only two excellent or good results (17%). If a problem was identified at surgery, only 3 of 12 knees (25%) had successful outcomes. This study highlights the frustration that can arise from performing surgery on patients for unexplained pain. Even when the authors identified a problem at the time of surgery and corrected it, they only had a 25% success rate.

If the work-up of a painful TKA is negative, one must consider obtaining fluoroscopically assisted radiographs. In this way, near-perfect perpendicular radiographs can be obtained to evaluate any radiolucencies, especially under the tibial tray. In one study that examined painful TKA without explanation,[68] fluoroscopic evaluation was used to study the knees. The authors had 20 patients referred to them for pain and disability after TKA, with normal-appearing radiographs. All 20 patients had fluoroscopic radiographs obtained. In 14 of 20 patients, the diagnosis of aseptic loosening was made with the new radiographs. Each of the patients considered to have a loose component at fluoroscopy did have a loose component at revision.

Each patient improved after revision, with an increase in Hospital for Special Surgery score of 26 points.

Great caution is recommended when deciding to revise a knee without good explanation of the pain, and in most cases, the condition of the patient is unimproved or is worse after revision, unless a convincing intraoperative cause is found. Sometimes overgrown soft tissues or an interposed meniscal fragment is found. Because these conditions can be managed without arthrotomy, an arthroscopic examination is recommended before revision is attempted.

Nonarticular causes of knee pain, including referred pain, should also be kept in mind when performing the clinical examination. Hip and lumbar spine pathology must be ruled out as the underlying cause of pain. Less recognized causes are patellar clunk, lateral patellar facet irritation, irritation from retained osteophytes, extruded bone cement, popliteus tendon dysfunction, and collateral ligament irritation caused by medial tibial displacement. Hypertrophic pulmonary osteoarthropathy as an unusual cause of late pain and effusion has been reported.[151]

Primary malignant neoplasms and metastatic disease have been described in association with total joint arthroplasty.[3] Cases of patients with periprosthetic non-Hodgkin's lymphoma, bronchogenic carcinoma, gastric carcinoma, and squamous cell carcinoma of the lung have been described in relation to THA.[32,151] Fehring and Hamilton[67] have reported a case of a 73-year-old patient with continued severe pain following TKA. Synovial biopsy revealed metastatic adenocarcinoma from colon. Therefore, a thorough history and physical examination should be done to identify the nature and cause of the pain. It is important that this phenomenon be considered in older patients when other causes have been ruled out.

KEY REFERENCES

7. Ayers DC, Dennis DA, Johanson NA, et al: Instructional course lectures: the American Academy of Orthopaedic Surgeons—common complications of total knee arthroplasty. *J Bone Joint Surg Am* 79:278, 1997.

19. Berry DJ: Recognizing and identifying osteolysis around total knee arthroplasty. *Instr Course Lect* 53:261, 2004.

25. Brassard MF, Insall JN, Scuderi GR, et al: Complications of total knee arthroplasty. In Scott WN, editor: *Insall & Scott surgery of the knee*, vol 2, ed 4, Philadelphia, 2006, Churchill Livingstone-Elsevier, pp 1716–1760.

37. Clarke HD, Fuchs R, Scuderi GR, et al: Clinical results in valgus total knee arthroplasty with the "pie crust" technique of lateral soft tissue releases. *J Arthroplasty* 20:1010, 2005.

50. Cushner FD: Transfusion avoidance in orthopedic surgery. *J Cardiothorac Vasc Anesth* 18(Suppl 4):29S, 2004.

146. Maloney WJ, Paprosky W, Engh CA, et al: Surgical treatment of pelvic osteolysis. *Clin Orthop Relat Res* 393:78, 2001.

150. Meding JB, Keating EM, Ritter MA, et al: Genu recurvatum in total knee replacement. *Clin Orthop Relat Res* 416:64, 2003.

159. Mont MA, Serna FK, Krackow KA, et al: Exploration of radiographically normal total knee replacements for unexplained pain. *Clin Orthop* 331:216, 1996.

168. Pagnano MW, Hanssen AD, Lewallen DG, et al: Flexion instability after primary posterior cruciate retaining total knee arthroplasty. *Clin Orthop Relat Res* 356:39, 1998.

187. Rand JA, Brown ML: The value of indium 111 leukocyte scanning in the evaluation of painful or infected total knee arthroplasties. *Clin Orthop* 259:179, 1990.

208. Scuderi GR: Revision total knee arthroplasty: how much constraint is enough? *Clin Orthop Relat Res* 392:300, 2001.

232. Whiteside LA, Ohl MD: Tibial tubercle osteotomy for exposure of the difficult total knee arthroplasty. *Clin Orthop Relat Res* 260:6, 1990.

The references for this chapter can also be found on www.expertconsult.com.

170

Extensile Exposures for Revision Total Knee Replacement

Nicholas J. Lash, Donald S. Garbuz, Bassam A. Masri

INTRODUCTION

With increasing rates of implantation of total knee replacements (TKR), revision knee replacement surgery is also increasing. A multifaceted approach to revision knee replacement is required to achieve the desired results.

Surgical exposure during revision TKR is the very beginning of the reconstruction, and without adequate exposure, achieving an adequate reconstruction can be challenging. Gaining exposure should be considered the first and one of the most important objectives in revision TKR surgery. There are a number of surgical techniques that will allow added access to the knee. These can be thought of as increasingly more powerful in allowing exposure of the knee joint.

This chapter will outline the surgical maneuvers available to increase exposure of the knee and will review the regional anatomy and the results of such maneuvers that can be considered while performing these techniques.

OBJECTIVES OF SURGICAL EXPOSURE IN REVISION TOTAL KNEE REPLACEMENT

The goals of any exposure of the knee for revision TKR are to achieve adequate and safe visualization of the knee to facilitate removal of the in situ TKR without creating additional bone loss, address the bone defects that exist, and allow implantation of an appropriately aligned and stable reconstruction. While performing this, the surgeon must avoid skin necrosis and wound healing issues and protect the extensor mechanism, collateral ligaments, and relevant neurovascular structures.

REGIONAL ANATOMY

To achieve the objectives of a good reconstruction, most aims include protection of anatomical structures. Knowledge of the regional anatomy of the knee is required to protect such structures. Breaking down the anatomy into layers, the knee is approached anteriorly through a series of layers that will be discussed, including particular issues that should be considered as the surgeon passes through the layers to access the knee joint.

Skin

In revision TKR, the incision through skin often uses previous surgical scars. When deciding to use the previous scar or place a new incision, several factors should be considered. The blood supply to the skin over the anterior aspect of the knee joint has been well described in cadaveric studies by Haertsch[17] and supported by Colombel et al.[7] Their findings showed that the blood supply to skin comes predominantly from the medial aspect of the knee (Fig. 170.1). The saphenous artery and descending geniculate artery supply perforating arteries that originate medially and create a medial to lateral blood flow. The location of the perforating arteries and their anastomoses lie just superficial to the deep fascia.

When a single previous incision is encountered, this should be used for exposure. If there are multiple incisions, the lateral most skin incision should be used because of the medial to lateral direction of blood flow. When past incisions run obliquely to the longitudinal axis of the limb, new incisions should cross at less acute angles, greater than 60 degrees, to avoid pointed skin flaps that may undergo tip necrosis. Past transverse skin incisions (traumatic, or used for patellectomy or tibial osteotomy) may be crossed at right angles (Windsor et al.[48]).

Once the location and orientation of the skin incision has been planned and performed, the depth of the incision should be full thickness down to the deep fascia. The location of the anastomosis of the perforating arteries is just superficial to the deep fascia, and keeping dissection as deep as possible will make injury to the dermal vessels supplying the skin less likely. In addition to making dissection straight down to the deep fascia, minimizing the width of subcutaneous flaps will also reduce the chance of skin necrosis.

There are two specific areas around the anterior aspect of the knee where resulting skin ischemia and necrosis pose particular problems. Directly over the anterior aspect of the patella, the skin remains thin and there is often a lack of soft tissue coverage. With previous midline incisions, the tissues may be atrophic, and the superficial prepatellar bursa, devoid of traversing blood vessels, means blood supply is also reduced. The other particular area of concern is the soft tissue coverage over the anteromedial tibial plateau. This area is lacking in underlying muscle and soft tissues. The pretibial area is extremely thin, with the anteromedial tibia easily palpable in most patients. The soft tissues that are in this area are relatively avascular tissues, including the pes anserinus insertion and superficial medial collateral ligament. When skin necrosis does occur, split skin grafting is seldom successful because of the lack of underlying vascular tissue upon which the skin graft can be placed and incorporated. Soft tissue coverage is often required in the form of a medial gastrocnemius muscle flap, which has been well

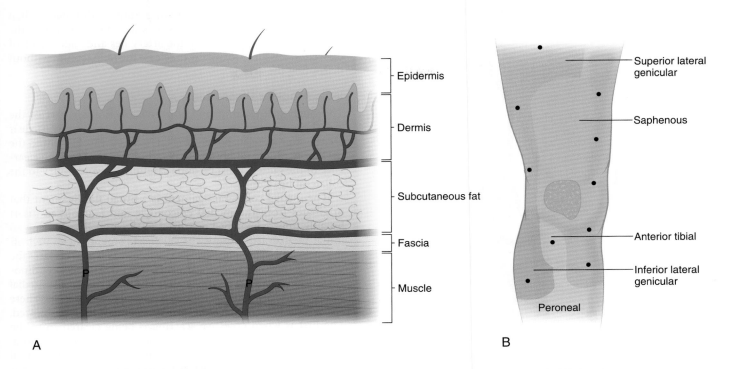

FIG 170.1 (A) Microvascular supply to the skin around the knee. Perforating vessels (*P*) deep to the fascia supply the subcutaneous tissue, where little communication occurs. (B) Areas of skin supplied by perforating vessels (*solid circles*). Most of the supply comes from the medial aspect, and therefore medial incisions carry increased risk of ischemia. (From Younger AS, Duncan CP, Masri BA: Surgical exposures in revision total knee arthroplasty. *J Am Acad Orthop Surg* 6:55–64, 1998).

documented as a successful option for dealing with medial skin and underlying tissue defects.* The medial gastrocnemius flap is favored for its relative ease, adjacent location, and not requiring vascular anastomoses required in other flaps. Other methods for addressing soft tissue defects include soft tissue expanders,[15,24,33,39] or free vascularized tissue flap reconstruction.[25,32]

Deep Tissues

The deep tissues include the deep fascia and the extensor mechanism, which consists of the quadriceps tendon, patella, patella tendon, and the expansions of the parapatella retinaculum. Proximally the vastus lateralis muscle and vastus medialis run either side of the extensor mechanism. These have been described as the four leashes,[10] with the lateral and medial leashes (lateral and medial vasti) being referred to as minor leashes, and the proximal (quadriceps tendon) and distal (patellar tendon) leashes referred to as major leashes. The minor leashes, typically medially, are released with any approach—often the only release required—combined with thorough synovectomy and scar excision.[10] When the exposure is inadequate with minor leash release and synovectomy has been performed, then release of one of the major leashes will be required to enhance the exposure.

Under the deep fascia is the joint capsule that may or may not be intact depending on the previous surgery. Often the

capsule will be replaced with dense scar tissue lying between the deep fascial layer and the joint synovium. Scar tissue can also be deposited within the joint as old hematoma undergoes fibrous metaplasia.

To access the joint, the medial parapatellar arthrotomy is used as a veritable workhorse for exposing the knee. The medial arthrotomy is familiar for most surgeons, and performing a medial arthrotomy and through intra-articular clearance of synovium and scar will be sufficient for exposure in most revision TKR cases.[10,42]

Another advantage is the easy addition or conversion of a medially based arthrotomy to a more extensile exposure, which will be discussed in extensile maneuvers. A standard arthrotomy is performed from the apex of the quadriceps tendon at the medial edge of the tendon passing distally along the medial patellar border, down to the medial aspect of the tibial tuberosity. A medial tissue release is performed, elevating the superficial medial collateral ligament and pes anserinus off the medial tibia as a composite sleeve, as required based on the deformity. With less severe varus deformities, less release is required, and the pes anserinus may be preserved. This tissue is elevated off the tibia as far posterior as the semimembranous tendon insertion at the posteromedial tibial corner.

When performing the arthrotomy, the surgeon should consider previous arthrotomy location. If previous lateral arthrotomy or lateral release has been performed, then medial arthrotomy may create a situation where the patella may lose critical blood supply. The blood supply to the patella comes

---

*References 1, 5, 25, 26, 28, 32, 34, 37, and 36.

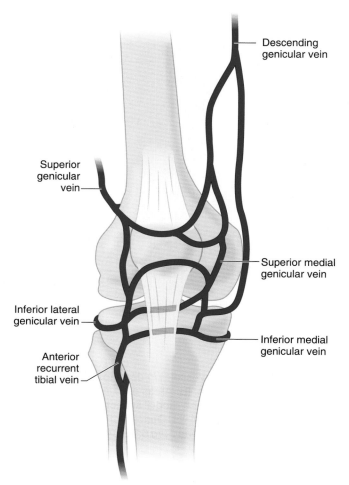

FIG 170.2 Blood Supply to the Patella. There are three blood vessels supplying each side of the patella. Use of previous arthrotomy is recommended to avoid disrupting the remaining blood supply to the patella. Lateral release carries risk of injury to the lateral blood supply. (From Younger AS, Duncan CP, Masri BA: Surgical exposures in revision total knee arthroplasty. *J Am Acad Orthop Surg* 6:55–64, 1998).

from the superior and inferior, lateral and medial geniculate arteries, and descending geniculate artery[21,22,40] (Fig. 170.2). In addition, the patella receives blood supply via the anterior tibial recurrent artery and infrapatellar and oblique prepatellar arteries. These vessels form a plexus that circumferentially supplies the patella, with the distal pole having direct blood supply and the remaining patella gaining supply through its anterior middle third. When one side of the patella has had its blood supply disrupted with previous lateral arthrotomy, lateral release, or with lateral menisectomy (lateral inferior geniculate), and infrapatellar fat pad resection (recurrent anterior tibial artery), performing arthrotomy on the remaining side comes with risk of osteonecrosis.[38] Even when a lateral release has not previously been performed, knowledge of the course of the superior lateral geniculate artery is valuable, should a lateral release be needed during revision TKR. The superior lateral geniculate artery runs horizontally at the distal end of the vastus lateralis muscle belly. For this reason, when performing lateral release, an intra-articular release is favored, as it avoids large subcutaneous flap

elevation to access the lateral retinaculum. Additionally, when the release starts distally, it is possible to undermine the synovium and capsule where the artery lies and slide a pair of dissection scissors proximally to release the retinaculum without disrupting the artery.

Intra-Articular Dissection

Thorough synovectomy and scar excision is a key part of the initial exposure of the in situ TKR. The key locations to clear are the suprapatellar pouch (Figs. 170.3 and 170.4), behind the patellar tendon, and both lateral and medial gutters. The clearance of the gutters must be done carefully to avoid injury to the collateral ligaments.

The medial collateral ligament is a broad flat ligament that originates from the medial epicondyle and fans out to insert broadly, approximately 3 cm distal to the joint line. During an initial medial arthrotomy, the medial ligament is elevated off the medial tibia in a subperiosteal fashion. This also elevates the pes anserinus insertion of sartorius, gracilis, and semitendinosus tendon insertion in some cases. The deep part of the medial ligament attaches at the joint line to the medial meniscus. There are several places where the medial ligament may be injured. The first is when excessive scarring is being cleared from the medial gutter and overzealous resection may injure the femoral origin at the medial epicondyle. The second is at the distal extent of the superficial part of the ligament, when elevation is performed. If the dissection strays out of plane from the subperiosteal region, then transection can occur. Lastly, the midsubstance of the ligament is at risk during medial meniscal resection (in the case of a primary knee replacement) or when performing a cut of the tibial plateau with a surgical bone saw in either primary or revision knee replacement.

The lateral collateral ligament morphology is different from its medial counterpart. It is a cord-like structure that runs from the lateral epicondyle of the femur and runs posterolaterally to insert on the fibular head along with the biceps femoris tendon. The lateral collateral ligament courses superficially to the popliteus tendon, and like the medial ligament, it is at risk with lateral gutter clearance. It may also be injured with lateral release of the iliotibial band and capsule if midsubstance release strays too far posterior.

Cruciate ligaments may or may not be present during revision TKR. Most modern prostheses will require the resection of the anterior cruciate ligament during the index operation. The posterior cruciate ligament (PCL) may still be present when a posterior cruciate retaining implant has been used. The PCL originates from the intercondylar notch on the medial condyle. It runs posteriorly to insert on the posterior aspect of the tibial plateau just lateral to its central posterior surface. The PCL remains directly anterior to the posterior capsule, and during resection, care must be taken to avoid penetrating posteriorly where the main neurovascular bundle runs. The safest place to perform resection is at its femoral origin, which is its most anterior aspect.

The popliteal artery is the major artery running in the popliteal fossa. Its course runs from the subsartorial canal in the distal medial thigh as the artery becomes the popliteal artery proper, and courses medially thorough the popliteal fossa in close proximity to the joint capsule. It gives off geniculate branches that tether it to the capsule, during its rather convex path, passing slightly laterally, after which it travels distally to exit through the soleal arch. The structures in close proximity,

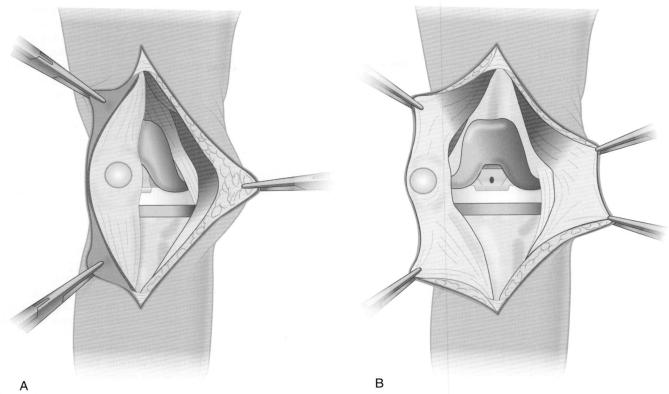

A   B

FIG 170.3 Intra-articular Dissection. (A) Initial arthrotomy reveals a tethered patella and limited exposure. (B) With clearance of the suprapatellar pouch, gutters, and retropatellar tendon areas, the exposure is improved. The femur is exposed to its periosteum and the undersurface of the quadriceps and patellar tendons are cleared of scarring. (From Younger AS, Duncan CP, Masri BA: Surgical exposures in revision total knee arthroplasty. *J Am Acad Orthop Surg* 6:55–64, 1998).

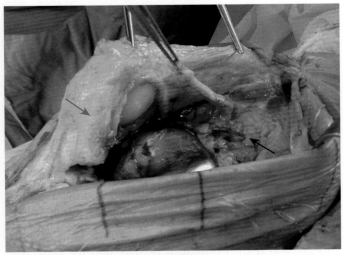

FIG 170.4 Intraoperative Adhesiolysis. Thickened scarring is present on the undersurface of the quadriceps and patellar tendon (*red arrow*). The suprapatellar pouch contains scar and adhesions connecting to the quadriceps tendon (*black arrow*).

anterior to the artery, from proximal to distal are the proximal femur, the oblique popliteal ligament, and the posterior horn of the lateral meniscus. Because of its central location, any posterior capsular release should avoid central release from either the femur or tibia and preferentially be released laterally and medially.

The tibial nerve becomes a separate branch of the sciatic nerve at the apex of the diamond shaped popliteal fossa. The tibial nerve travels directly straight down the popliteal fossa. Proximally it is lateral to the artery then crosses over the artery (as the artery deviates slightly laterally), so that at the joint line it is posterior to the artery. This makes the tibial nerve less likely to be injured, when compared to the artery, which remains closer to the joint capsule. The popliteal vein, the artery's counterpart, runs between the artery and nerve throughout their course.

The common peroneal nerve, the other terminating branch of the sciatic nerve, comes off high in the popliteal fossa and courses laterally along the lateral border of the diamond shaped fossa. It runs behind the biceps femoris muscle belly and tendon, lying over the plantaris, lateral gastrocnemius muscle belly, and curves anteriorly to pass around the fibular neck. It is easily palpated in slim patients at this point, where it enters the peroneus longus muscle and the lateral compartment of the leg. This nerve may be injured during errant retractor placement, aggressive lateral dissection, correction of valgus deformity, correction of severe flexion deformity, and in patients with previous neuropathy.

PATIENT ASSESSMENT

The review of the patient will aid the surgeon in being prepared for issues that may aid or hinder the achievement of the objectives of the surgery. As with any medical issue, assessment starts with history taking and physical examination, and proceeds with radiologic and blood tests.

History

History taking remains an essential part of patient assessment. Age, occupation, cigarette smoking, and drug use should be ascertained in the social history, with the later two factors being modifiable, in the patient's best interest to minimize wound complications.

With relevance to the topic of extensile exposures during revision knee replacement is the presence of stiffness. Stiffness may develop with ongoing failure in a TKR, or may be present in early on from primary TKR when malrotation of components exists. Stiffness is a major indication for a revision knee replacement. Also, the patient needs to be asked about weakness in the knee and his need for strong quadriceps function postoperatively, because some extensile exposures may lead to permanent quadriceps weakness and extensor lag.

Medications that may lower immunity, particularly in rheumatoid patients, and any anticoagulant medications the patient is on should be identified and held when appropriate. Often during reconstruction, antibiotic cement is used as a method of fixation or in staged surgeries for infection. An allergy history should be obtained, particularly for antibiotic allergy.

Physical Examination

Examination begins with inspection of the limb. Alignment, scar location, swelling, and abnormal kinematics during gait should be observed.

Scar appearance should be carefully examined for thinning of the skin, poor capillary return, or hemosiderin deposition that may indicate previous healing issues. Palpation of the knee should reveal increased temperature suggestive of inflammation, quadriceps bulk, and location of specifically painful areas. Range of motion should be assessed to ascertain stiffness, and to detect active motion and integrity of the extensor mechanism. Severe stiffness carries the risk of poor visualization of the joint and patellar tendon avulsion,[16] and its presence will give the surgeon an indication of whether an extensile maneuver will be required. Ligament stress tests are performed for varus/valgus stability. Anterior-posterior stress in flexion is performed to assess the integrity of the PCL (when present), or the polyethylene post (in PCL sacrificing devices).

Distal neurologic and vascular assessments are routinely performed, as are assessment of the hip joint and spine to detect pathology that may be causing referred pain.

Investigations

Routine anteroposterior (AP), posteroanterior (PA), lateral radiographs are obtained. Plain radiographs should help identify the implant type, fixation method, polyethylene liner type, lucencies, and their location. Lucent lines between the cement implant and cement bone interfaces should be observed. Oblique x-rays at 45 degrees can give a view of the posterior condyles to observe bone lysis. The alignment of the femoral prosthesis relative to the tibial component may highlight polyethylene wear and potential metal on metal wear. The lateral x-ray will show the station of the patella relative to the femur and tibia. Patella alta may indicate patellar tendon rupture; conversely, patella baja may indicate quadriceps tendon rupture or, more commonly, severe scarring. Where proximal or distal deformity is suspected from examination, standing long limb alignment radiographs will identify overall mechanical axis, defects, and any obstructions to instrumentation. In revision surgery, potential obstructions are broken hardware, screws, and cement columns.

Initial Exposure

As mentioned in the review of the relevant anatomy, most revision exposure begins with a medial arthrotomy and clearance of scar tissue for the suprapatellar pouch and lateral and medial gutters (see Figs. 170.3 and 170.4). This will be sufficient for most revision TKR cases.[10] Medial arthrotomy proceeds as for a primary case, with division of the quadriceps tendon proximally. This is done longitudinally, aiming to leave a small "cuff" of tendon attached to the vastus medius for repair at the end of the surgery. The longitudinal division proceeds distally around the medial border of the patella, continuing into the medial retinaculum to the level of the medial aspect of the tibial tuberosity. As with primary exposure, the deep medial collateral ligament is released from the medial plateau. This can be extended distally, elevating the fibers of the superficial medial ligament, in a subperiosteal fashion, from the medial tibia. This can be performed only as far as the distal extent of the superficial ligament before instability becomes a possible issue. To facilitate medial release, the proximal tibia can be flexed and externally rotated to deliver the posteromedial tibia, where the semimembranosus tendon can be divided for further release as required, in cases with severe varus deformity; however, this is not common in the revision TKR setting. Resection of adherent scar tissue posterior to the patellar tendon should also be performed to allow for safe lateral subluxation of the patella. The recess between the anterior proximal tibia (above the level of the tibial tuberosity) needs to be cleared of scarring also to allow mobility of the patella. Once a plane has been created between the native patellar tendon (longitudinal fiber orientation) and the retropatellar scar/remnant fat pad, proximal dissection can be performed up to the inferior pole of the patella. This will aid subluxation of the patella. It is our preference to only sublux the patella to avoid placing excessive force on the tendon's insertion at the tibial tuberosity. We strongly recommend against patellar eversion, as routine patellar eversion may lead to an increased need for extensile exposures.

A similar technique is then performed for the quadriceps tendon, with resection of supra-patellar scar on the undersurface of the tendon. Starting at the proximal pole of the patella, a plane between scar and tendon (longitudinal fibers) is identified and then extended proximally as far as the scar tissue exists. This excision is then continued laterally into the gutter and finally into the medial gutter. We aim to excise scarring but leave the periosteum remaining on the distal femur. This will aid in limiting blood loss and heterotopic bone formation. Lastly, removal of the polyethylene component (when modular) is performed to allow the removal of the necessary components, and the revision surgery to proceed. Once both proximal dissection and distal dissection has been completed, the knee can be flexed and the patella subluxed laterally.

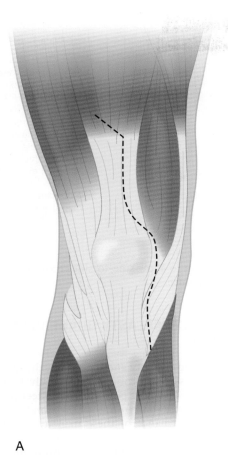

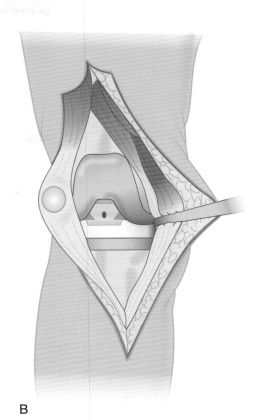

A   B

FIG 170.5 Quadriceps Snip. (A) The medial arthrotomy is extended proximally and laterally at an oblique angle. (B) With enhanced exposure by extending the snip laterally. A more distal and transverse snip will create more exposure. (From Younger AS, Duncan CP, Masri BA: Surgical exposures in revision total knee arthroplasty. *J Am Acad Orthop Surg* 6:55–64, 1998).

EXTENSILE EXPOSURES

When the standard initial exposure is performed but access to the knee joint remains difficult, proceeding to an extensile maneuver is required. The techniques to be described are grouped into proximal and distal techniques.

PROXIMAL TECHNIQUES

Rectus Snip

Regarded as a first line maneuver to enhance exposure, the rectus snip aims to relieve tension on the patella, allowing further subluxation and further exposure of the distal femur (Fig. 170.5).

The technique has been attributed to Insall[20] and is described as performing a medial arthrotomy, with the addition of a supplementary incision at the proximal extent of the arthrotomy. The incision in the quadriceps tendon turns at a 45 degree angle, travelling from distal and medial, to course to a point proximal and lateral. The finishing point will be at the proximal aspect of the quadriceps tendon, where the tendon meets the vastus lateralis muscle belly (Fig. 170.6). It is important to maintain some connection between the quadriceps tendon and the vastus lateralis muscle distally; otherwise the muscle will become defunctioned, no longer having a distal attachment to

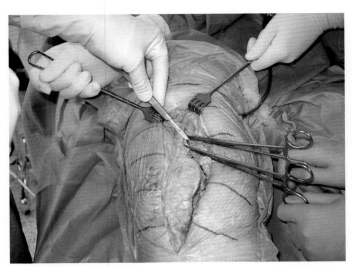

FIG 170.6 Intraoperative view of quadriceps snip. Note the oblique angle and location of extension of a medial arthrotomy.

TABLE 170.1   Results of Quadriceps Snip

Author (s)	No. of Patients	No. of Procedures	Mean Age (Years)	Follow-Up (Months)	Results
Garvin et al.[14]	16	16	65 (50-73)	30 (24-48)	HSS score: 10 excellent, 6 good (mean score: 87) 5 patients had FFD < 10°
Meek et al.[27]	107	50	—	40.5	WOMAC total: mean 64.4 Oxford score: mean 60.6 HSS score: mean 75 No comparable difference to medial arthrotomy
Barrack et al.[2]	131	31	—	30 (24-48)	KSS score: mean 134 Arc ROM: 104°, extensor lag 0.9° No comparable difference to medial arthrotomy

HSS, Hospital for Special Surgery; *FFD*, fixed-flexion deformity; *WOMAC*, Western Ontario and McMaster; *KSS*, Knee Society Score.

act on. Performing the "snip" at an oblique 45-degree angle allows for closure of the arthrotomy in a side-to-side fashion, whereas a transverse snip will create a situation where the repair will be end to end, and failure at this junction may lead to an extensor mechanism disruption or extensor lag.

The results of performing a rectus snip for revision TKR are encouraging, and in general postoperative therapy can continue as for standard arthrotomy. The literature available suggests good to excellent outcomes and low rates of complications.

The outcomes for rectus snip involved as exposure for revision TKR are summarized in Table 170.1.

Garvin et al.[14] reported on 16 patients that underwent rectus snip for exposure during revision TKR. In this small series, there were no complications—that is, failure of the extensor mechanism—and although no specific mention of extensor lag was made, there were five cases of fixed-flexion deformity (FFD). The average FFD was 7 degrees, and all were less than 10 degrees. When Cybex testing was performed, there was no difference between the operated and nonoperated side when comparing power and work. Fourteen patients had an increase in range of motion, to a mean of 38 degrees.

Meek et al.[27] have reviewed 107 patients in an age-, sex-, comorbidity-matched comparison study. Fifty-seven patients had revision TKR using a medial parapatellar approach and 50 patients using a rectus snip. A retrospective follow-up outcome questionnaire was used to gather outcomes data at a mean of 40.5 months. Comparing the two groups, no identifiable difference was found in the outcomes when using WOMAC subsets (pain, stiffness, function), Oxford Hip Score, Hospital for Special Surgery (HSS) scores, and SF-12 measurements.

Barrack et al.[2] outlined a subset of patients who underwent revision TKR using a rectus snip. In a review of 131 patients having revision TKR, 31 had a rectus snip for exposure. At an average of 30 months following surgery, the group of patients that had a rectus snip (*n* = 31) had no clinical difference when compared to a medial parapatellar arthrotomy (*n* = 63). The Knee Society score, arc range of motion, and extensor lag were allegedly the same, and at this point, the rectus snip and medial arthrotomy were combined together as a comparison group, against which tibial tubercle osteotomy (TTO) and quadriceps turndown were analyzed.

Overall, the literature suggests that a rectus snip performed for revision TKR has low complication rates and equivocal clinical results compared to the standard medial arthrotomy. However, as a technical point, it is still recommended to perform an oblique snip to allow side-to-side repair and avoid extensor mechanism failure.

V-Y QUADRICEPSPLASTY/QUADRICEPS TURNDOWN

The V-Y quadricepsplasty and its variant, the quadriceps turndown, are the second group of proximally based exposures. They are regarded as more powerful than a rectus snip; however, because of the separation from their proximal soft tissue attachments, the performance of these maneuvers comes with the possibility of generating an extensor lag. Because of the enhanced exposure these approaches afford, they may be considered when faced with a severely stiff TKR and are particularly useful when faced with a contracted quadriceps mechanism.

As with a rectus snip, an initial medial parapatellar approach is performed. At the apex of the medial incision, a contiguous incision is made that descends distally toward the lateral aspect of the superior pole of the patella, at an angle of 45 degrees (Fig. 170.7 and 170.8). This passes through the lateral retinaculum and is extended distally to the level of the tibia.[19] The triangular proximal flap of quadriceps tendon is then turned down to allow exposure of the knee joint. It may be repaired back to its original origin, or a V-Y advancement can be performed, where the inverted V is repaired at a more distal location and the remaining defect proximally is repaired in a side-to-side fashion, creating an inverted Y; hence its name. This maneuver allows for an easier closure, and hopefully greater knee flexion, but comes at the risk of generating an extensor lag, as the extensor mechanism has been effectively lengthened. Another option is to leave the lateral retinaculum division unrepaired, allowing a lateral release that can address other soft tissue restraints which may cause altered knee and patellar kinematics.

Aside from potential extensor lag, because of lateral and medial parapatellar soft tissue dissection, potential risk to damage of the blood supply to the patella exists. It has been suggested that blood supply is maintained via the superior lateral geniculate artery and vessels within the retropatellar fat pad.[19] However, in revision TKR, either of these blood supplies may have be previously transgressed. Scott and Siliski[41] has recommended a division of the lateral tissue closer to the tendinous insertion of the vastus lateralis, rather than further laterally through the retinaculum, in an effort to protect the superior lateral geniculate artery and its supply to the patella.

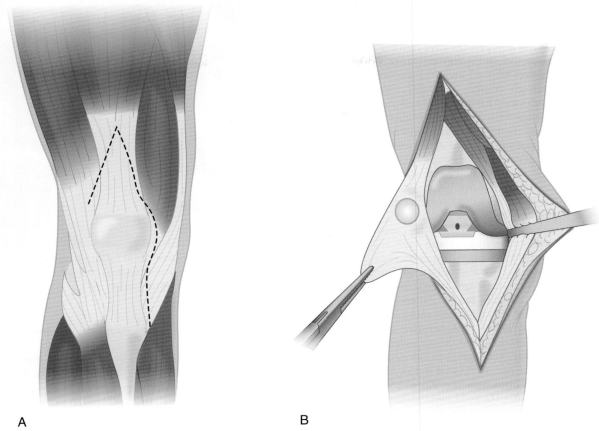

A   B

FIG 170.7 V-Y Quadricepsplasty/Turndown. (A) Medial arthrotomy and oblique incision extending laterally and distally forming an inverted V. (B) The exposure obtained by the turndown. Advancing the patellar tendon distally, Y shaped repair will allow lengthening of a shortened quadriceps tendon. (From Younger AS, Duncan CP, Masri BA: Surgical exposures in revision total knee arthroplasty. *J Am Acad Orthop Surg* 6:55–64, 1998).

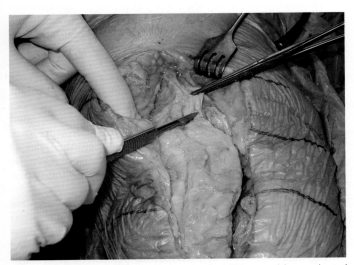

FIG 170.8 Intraoperative view of V-Y quadricepsplasty/turndown. An oblique proximal to distal incision is performed.

Postoperative management for such approaches may require a diversion from usual management. Recommendations differ, but varying authors have suggested no active extension for 6 weeks[11] and no flexion for the first 2 weeks to allow initial healing of the extensor mechanism.[19] Despite this approach being a less commonly used approach for exposure, when used at our institution, we recommend that the patient be allowed to flex the knee to the flexion limit that does not apply any tension on the repair, as noted intraoperatively. The patient needs to use assistive devices for walking initially until adequate quadriceps power has returned. This may take up to 6 weeks.

The result of using a quadricepsplasty/turndown in exposure in revision TKR has been studied by numerous authors. Trousdale et al.[43] reported on a series of 16 cases of quadricepsplasty/V-Y turndown in 14 patients. In their described technique, a standard medial arthrotomy, medial tibial release, and gutter clearance is performed. If exposure is still hampered, then an oblique incision in the quadriceps tendon from proximal-medial to distal-lateral is performed. A routine lateral release has already been performed 1 inch from the lateral border of the patella, and the oblique quadriceps incision is connected to this preexisting lateral release. The inverted V can be advanced to form an inverted Y at closure—it was not stated how many had a V-Y advancement, however, and for the remaining transcript, the operative knees were referred to as V-Y. When the cases where quadricepsplasty was used for primary TKR were removed, 11 cases in 10 patients were observed. The mean follow-up was 30 months, and preoperative motion was 4.7 to 69 degrees and increased to 5 to 89 degrees (range, 0 to 15, on average). Mean HSS scores were 41 and 70 preoperatively and postoperatively, respectively (range, 23 to 88). Cybex biomechanical testing was performed for strength measurements. The operative knee was significantly weaker at higher speeds and when the unaffected knee (comparison side) was normal. When the opposite knee was not normal and at slower speeds, there was no difference. The recommendation by these authors was that V-Y quadricepsplasty was useful for exposure and rendered minimal range of motion limitations. Weakness of the quadriceps was seen under certain circumstances, but overall results justified the use of such exposures.

Barrack et al.,[2] as previously mentioned, reviewed 123 cases of revision TKR based on the surgical approach required for exposure. Of this cohort, 14 cases used a quadriceps turndown for access. When compared to a standard group (where a medial parapatellar arthrotomy ± quadriceps snip was used), there were significant differences found. Patients who underwent turndown had lower mean postoperative Knee Society scores (117 vs. 134) and lower postoperative arc range of motion (93 degrees vs. 104 degrees). Mean extensor lag was larger in turndown patients (4.5 degrees vs. 0.9 degrees). When compared to patients that had a TTO (n = 15), there was no significant difference in outcomes for Knee Society scores (KSS), range of motion, but TTO had lower extensor lag (mean 1.5 degrees). However, when patient satisfaction was measured, turndown patients fared similarly to standard patients, while TTO patients had greater dissatisfaction, despite a smaller mean extensor lag.

Scott and Siliski[41] also reported on seven patients with stiffness, requiring a modified quadricepsplasty to gain access for revision TKR. This group had a mean gain in flexion of 49 degrees, however, at a cost of a mean extensor lag of 8 degrees.

Tibial Tubercle Osteotomy

The TTO is the distal procedure available to the knee surgeon to allow access without disturbance of the proximal soft tissues. It is used in conjunction with a medial parapatellar arthrotomy and is a powerful maneuver to increase exposure. The TTO is useful in cases of severe patella baja and when a previously implanted stemmed tibial component requires removal (Fig. 170.9). The modern technique, as popularized by Whiteside and Ohl,[46] has evolved from the original description by Dolin.[12] The principle of TTO is to allow a rotating bone fragment (tibial tubercle) that externally rotates around its long access, which allows the patellar tendon to move laterally to allow access to the anterior and lateral knee joint (Fig. 170.10). The osteotomy is made from medially to laterally, maintaining the lateral fascia/epimysium of the muscles of the anterior compartment of the leg, which enhances stability of the tubercle when fixed. An oscillating saw can be used initially; we recommend completing the osteotomy by cracking the lateral cortex with an osteotome, to aid in maintaining the lateral soft tissue attachment. If all soft tissues are released from the bone fragment, proximal retraction can be performed. This can be prevented by making a transverse cut with a reciprocating saw blade just proximal to the patellar tendon insertion into the tibial tubercle to create a bony shelf,

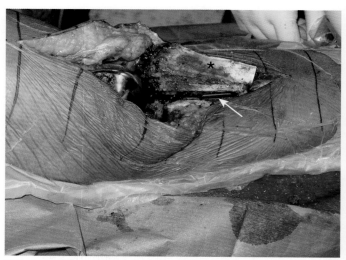

FIG 170.9 Intraoperative tibial tubercle osteotomy. The tibial tubercle (*star*) is osteotomized and hinged laterally to expose an in situ tibial stem (*white arrow*).

proximal to the osteotomy fragment, to prevent proximal migration.

The osteotomy should render a fragment that is approximately 2 cm wide, 1 cm thick, and 8 to 10 cm long, leaving sufficient bone stock and surface area for bone-to-bone healing (Fig. 170.11A). Distally, the osteotomy may be tapered to prevent a stress riser effect (Fig. 170.12B). The original description by Dolin used screw fixation; however, Whiteside recommended cerclage wires. When used, cerclage wires are placed around the lateral aspect of the osteotomy fragment and into the tibial canal, posteriorly behind the tibial stem (best done prior to inserting the tibial component and attached stem as seen in Fig. 170.11B). When the wires are placed around the tibial stem, this creates a secure post, upon which the wires can be tensioned, and having the wires passing in an intraosseous passage negates the risk of injury to posterior structures in the calf. If passed at an oblique angle from proximal-lateral to distal-medial, then the wire will also create a force vector to resist proximal migration of the bone fragment. Other authors have described a variety of fixation methods with generally good fixation and low levels of failure.[8,9] Finally, it is important to ensure the length of the tibial stem is greater than the osteotomy length to avoid a situation where stress is concentrated at an osteotomized location, whereupon tibial fracture may occur (see Fig. 170.12A). With such techniques, minimal deviation from standard mobilization postoperatively may be allowed. The patient may freely flex the knee as able and can be allowed to fully weight bear.[46]

Complications that may be encountered with TTO include fragmentation of the osteotomy fragment, proximal migration of the osteotomy fragment (generating an extensor lag), nonunion of the osteotomy, injury to posterior structures in the leg during fixation (screw or extraosseous placement of cerclage wires), tibial fracture, and metalware prominence causing soft tissue irritation requiring removal.

The results of TTO have been reported by Whiteside and Ohl.[46] In this review, 71 knees were exposed using a TTO, for primary (n = 17) and revision TKR (n = 54). Age ranged from 43 to 76, and follow-up was from between 1 and 5 years. Each

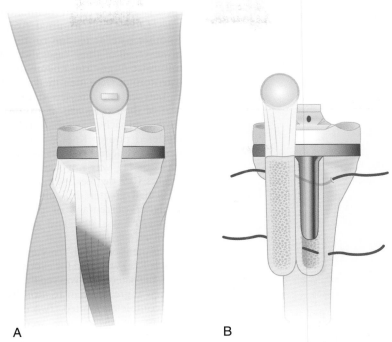

A   B

FIG 170.10 Tibial Tubercle Osteotomy. (A) Osteotomy location. (B) Exposure with rotation of the tuberosity fragment laterally. Access is afforded to the tibial canal and repair is made with wires passed. Lateral drill holes are proximal to the medial drill holes, pulling the tuberosity distal. (From Younger AS, Duncan CP, Masri BA: Surgical exposures in revision total knee arthroplasty. *J Am Acad Orthop Surg* 6:55–64, 1998).

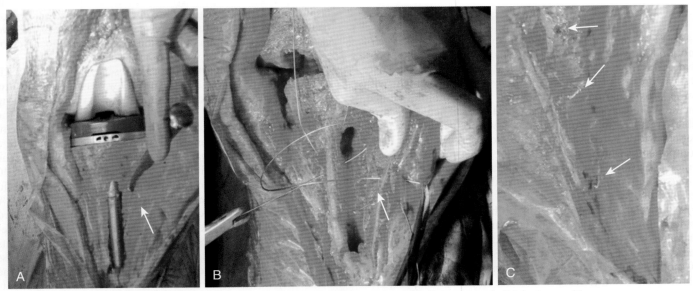

FIG 170.11 Intraoperative Tibial Tubercle Osteotomy. (A) Exposure of tibial stem with an osteotomized tubercle (*white arrows*) rotated laterally. (B) Wires are placed prior to stem insertion. Lateral drill holes are proximal; medial drill holes are distal to draw the tubercle distally. (C) Repaired tubercle fragment with wires securing osteotomy (*white arrows*).

knee underwent a TTO, as described previously, with cerclage fixation. Postoperative results showed a mean range of motion from 2.5 degrees to 97 degrees. The only complication was one case of proximal migration of the tubercle fragment by 1 cm. This had no flow on effect, with no extensor lag and flexion

possible to 115 degrees. All osteotomies united, and no hardware required removal.

Whiteside[45] reviewed this cohort again in an expanded group of cases totaling 136. There were 91 revision or repeated revision cases, 26 primary, and 19 infected cases. Age ranged from

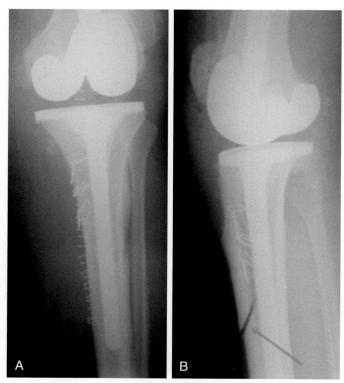

FIG 170.12 Postoperative Radiographs of Tibial Tubercle Osteotomy. (A) Tibial stem passes distal to the extent of the tubercle osteotomy. (B) The distal aspect of the osteotomy is tapered to avoid a stress concentration (*black arrow*).

34 to 88 years of age, and follow-up was at 2 years. Range of motion following surgery was a mean of 93 degrees. There were two cases of extensor lag that existed prior to surgery. There were two cases of fracturing of the osteotomy fragment with some proximal migration. However, all osteotomies united, including those performed in infected cases. There were three tibial fractures following surgery. Two occurred in a single patient with Charcot arthropathy, below short stemmed tibial components, which were revised to longer stems, achieving union. The other case occurred after a manipulation for poor range of motion; this case was treated in cast immobilization successfully.

Wolff et al.[49] reviewed 26 tibial tubercle osteotomies in 24 patients undergoing TKR. This accounted for 3% of all TKR primary or revision cases during a 4.5 year time period. The mean age was 61 years (range, 36 to 86). Mean follow-up was 40 months (range, 24 to 48). Seven cases used TTO in the setting of revision TKR; these cases had severe stiffness, with preoperative range of motion being 27 degrees flexion (range, 0 to 95). The technique of the TTO was performed in a variable fashion, with length of the osteotomy being between 3 and 9 cm long. The lateral soft tissue hinge was maintained and the TTO was fixed with screws (4.5 cortical or malleolar) or staples. Active extension was delayed until the 6-week mark, but active flexion was allowed soon after surgery. Mean flexion increased from 48 degrees to 77 degrees. There were a significant number of complications, with nine (35%) of the TTO cases having a complication. Four patients had an extensor lag (mean, 24 degrees) following extensor mechanism disruption. Three of

these cases occurred in rheumatoid patients with small osteotomies (3 cm) and minimal fixation (single screw or staple). Another patellar tendon rupture occurred in a fourth patient; however, all of these cases did not use a step cut osteotomy to minimize migration. Rheumatoid bone and small, nonstep cut osteotomies were identified as risk factors for failure of TTO.

Barrack et al.[2] reviewed 15 tibial tubercle osteotomies as a part of their comparison groups. When compared to 97 standard approaches (medial arthrotomy/quadriceps snip), TTO rendered poorer Knee Society scores (117 vs. 134), and less flexion (81 degrees vs. 104 degrees) following surgery. The mean extensor lag was not significantly different between the two groups (0.9 degrees vs. 1.5 degrees). Patients who underwent TTO had greater difficulty with kneeling and stooping, and a higher percentage of patients had unsuccessfully treated pain (20% vs. 7%) and return to activities of daily living (27% vs. 6%).

Zonnenberg et al.[51] reviewed 23 cases of revision TKR in which TTO was used for exposure. At the end of the reconstruction, the osteotomy was repaired with Vicryl 1.0 suture material. Review at greater than 16 months showed that 20 of the 22 cases had completely united. Two cases had partial union on radiographs; however, there were no symptoms regarding the incomplete union at this site. Clinically the mean range of motion and clinical outcome scores significantly improved. One osteotomy fractured before the 6-week mark; however, this went on to heal uneventfully. There were no cases of proximal migration of the osteotomy fragment.

Van den Broek et al.[44] reviewed the use of TTO in 39 cases of revision TKR. Their experience revealed two cases of proximal migration of the osteotomy as a result of inadequate fashioning of the step cut. All except one case used screws for fixation. The one case using cerclage wires was one of the two cases that had proximal migration. There were no cases of extensor lag.

Mendes et al.[29] reported on a large series of revision TKR cases in 67 knees where a step cut TTO was used for exposure. This series differed in technique in the way that cerclage wiring was through the intact proximal tibial bone adjacent to the osteotomy, as opposed to through the osteotomized fragment. If the proximal tibial bone stock was insufficient to perform a step cut, the fragment was engaged on the undersurface of the anterior aspect of the tibial implant. Mean follow-up was 30 months and the results of the group were good to excellent in 87% of cases, with a mean KSS of 86 points. There was a 7% complication rate related to the osteotomy itself. It was noted 13 patients had migration of the osteotomy, or had the osteotomy fixed with less than 2 cm proximal migration from its original location. In these patients, no extensor lag or weakness of extension was noticed. A symptomatic nonunion of the osteotomy was noticed in two patients (3%), and two patients had an extensor lag following migration of the osteotomy; the lag was tolerable and no further treatment was indicated.

Bruce et al.[4] reported on a small series of TTO. They found no complications in a series of ten patients. Mean range of motion improved from 59 to 78 degrees, and mean HSS scores improved from 47 to 79 postoperatively. These authors noted a difference in union time regarding different parts of the osteotomy. The proximal end healed faster at a mean of 8 weeks compared to the distal aspect of the osteotomy, mean 24 weeks. This can be accounted for by the difference in bone type, with the more cancellous proximal bone healing faster.

Young et al.[50] performed a longer-term follow-up of 42 cases of TTO used in revision TKR. The mean follow-up was 8 years, and review was performed to review surgical outcomes and complications. Mean postoperative range of motion was 4 degrees to 91 degrees, with the Knee Society score improving from 73 points to 124. Seventy-five percent of cases had an extensor lag that resolved in 66% of cases by the 6-month mark. In four of the six patients that had persistent extensor lag, it was noted that concomitant lateral release had been performed. Mean union time was 14 weeks.

Piedade et al.[35] have reviewed 126 cases of TTO for access in primary TKR. This group does not have any revision cases, but the principles apply. Both medial TTO and lateral TTO were performed, with 18 and 103 cases, respectively (group B). Because of primary procedures, no tibial stem was used and therefore screw fixation was used. Full weight bearing was allowed and flexion limited to 95 degrees for 2 months. The osteotomy group was compared with all other primary TKR (n = 1348) not using a TTO in the same defined period (group A).

There were no significant differences in mean range of motion, extensor lag, Knee Society scores, or postoperative pain. When complication was analyzed, it was found that there were no significant differences in complications except for tibial plateau fissures (nondisplaced cancellous bone fracturing) and skin necrosis. Despite a higher rate of these complications in TTO cases, this did not correlate with any higher rates of TKR component loosening or deep infections. It is important to note the predominance of lateral approach and TTO in this case series.

When faced with revision TKR, it is conceivable that a TTO has been previously used for access in the prior surgery. Chalidis and Ries[6] reported on a series of patients that had revision TKR in whom prior TTO had been performed, specifically analyzing union rates. Additionally, this case series also looked at whether an intramedullary osteotomy, opening the tibial medulla for removal of components or cement, created a setting of delayed or impaired healing. Eighty-seven cases with a mean age of 60 years were reviewed. Fifty-seven cases were extramedullary (cancellous bone bed), and 30 cases were intramedullary osteotomies. Healing of the TTO occurred in all cases. The median time to union for the extramedullary group was 12 weeks (6 to 47) and 21 weeks (7 to 38) for intramedullary osteotomies. Five cases of osteotomy migration were observed, three in the extra medullary and two in the intramedullary group. When migration was noticed, flexion was limited to 100 degrees, and quadriceps exercises are delayed for 3 months. As stated, no nonunions occurred, even in the five cases of migration and altered postoperative management.

Epicondylar Osteotomy

Epicondylar osteotomies can be performed for both the medial and lateral epicondyles. The medial epicondylar osteotomy was first described by Engh.[13] Its use has become a valuable technique to increase exposure when proximal or distal extensile approaches have already been made or are unsuccessful. The principle is that the release of the medial superficial collateral ligament is elevated, with the epicondyle attached to the medial sleeve of tissue (Fig. 170.13). Performing the osteotomy should be made carefully to ensure the fragment of bone is thick enough to repair, ideally more than 1 cm, and inclusion of the adductor tubercle allows a larger surface area for repair and increased stability of the fragment. An oscillating or reciprocating saw

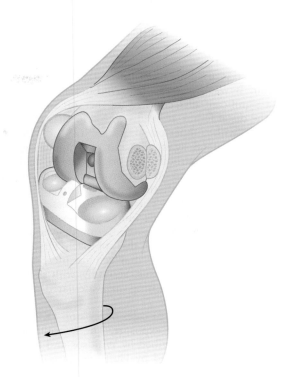

FIG 170.13 Medial Epicondylar Osteotomy. The medial epicondyle is osteotomized and reflected with a sleeve of tissue proximal and distal to the epicondyle. Dissection is extended posteriorly around the femur and tibia; external rotation aids in exposure. (From Younger AS, Duncan CP, Masri BA: Surgical exposures in revision total knee arthroplasty. *J Am Acad Orthop Surg* 6:55–64, 1998).

can be used to make the osteotomy. Engh originally described a $4 \times 4 \times 1$ cm^3 osteotomy performed with an osteotome. Standard release of the gutters and medial arthrotomy are also performed. With the medial epicondylar osteotomy, the tibia is externally rotated and placed into valgus to facilitate further exposure of the knee for implant removal and reconstruction. The medial soft tissue sleeve is left attached proximally and distally, so as not to cause valgus instability. The osteotomy fragment is secured back to its original location with a screw for fixation, although staples and suture repair has also been described, with the original series using the latter. However, this has been shown to have a relatively high rate of fibrous or nonunion of 43%.

Mihalko et al.[30] investigated comparison of soft tissue medial release versus medial epicondylar osteotomy in a cadaveric model. Valgus laxity testing showed in extension and levels of flexion less than 30 degrees that there was no difference in laxity. However, at levels of flexion of 60 degrees and greater, it was found that the epicondylar osteotomy group had significantly greater valgus laxity. A clinical series reported by the same authors revealed significantly improved ranges of motion and clinical outcome scores.

A lateral epicondylar osteotomy is also a procedure that can facilitate revision TKR. Admittedly the use of such osteotomies are usually performed in the setting of severe primary valgus gonarthrosis for soft tissue balancing and deformity correction[3,31]; the principles apply to revision TKR also and can be used when required, but this is extremely uncommon.

The Femoral Peel

This maneuver is used for circumferential exposure of the distal femur. It was described by Windsor and Insall[47] and involves a significant dissection of all the soft tissue attachments to the distal femur. It begins with a medial arthrotomy and proceeds with subperiosteal release of the synovium, capsule, both collateral ligaments, and any remaining cruciate ligaments, ± the gastrocnemius origins. In particular, the posterior capsule is released off bone from the femur and, with the remaining extensive soft tissue releases, creates excellent exposure of the distal femur. This may be necessary for excision of distal femoral neoplastic lesions; however, in revision TKR it allows for attending to severe flexion deformities. Two issues are potentially created with this approach. Firstly, a large flexion gap is created, and this may require increased levels of constraint to manage this issue. Secondly, with such extensive soft tissue dissection, creating an avascular distal femur may occur.

Lavernia et al.[23] reviewed 101 cases of revision TKR in which a femoral peel was used for exposure. The femoral peel was performed as originally described by Windsor and Insall, and its modification was suggested by Huff and Russell,[18] with a small modification where once the medial ligament was elevated off the bone (with cautery), an oscillating saw was used to run gently over the boney origin in a "brush-like" fashion to facilitate healing of the ligament back to its origin/insertion. In all cases, the minimum level of constraint was a constrained condylar knee design in 61 cases, and 32 cases required a hinged knee prosthesis for reconstruction.

Preoperative range of motion improved from a mean of 6 to 90 degrees to a mean of 1 to 100 degrees postoperatively. Mean postoperative extensor lag was 3 degrees, and mean flexion contracture was 1 degree. Mean WOMAC, Knee Society, and Hospital for Special Surgery scores improved from preoperative values of 54; 48; 56 to 13; 107; and 80, respectively.

There were 12 major surgical complications and 3 minor surgical complications.

SUMMARY

Revision TKR is a challenging surgery to perform. Being able to overcome difficult exposure by using extensile techniques will serve to help achieve the desired goals of revision knee replacement.

Extensile techniques have evolved over the last 30 years and have been shown to render good to excellent results in most studies. Low complications rates are now seen when the knee surgeon pays attention to certain issues faced with each extensile option.

KEY REFERENCES

2. Barrack RL, Smith P, Munn B, et al: The Ranawat Award. Comparison of surgical approaches in total knee arthroplasty. *Clin Orthop* 356:16–21, 1998.
12. Dolin MG: Osteotomy of the tibial tubercle in total knee replacement. A technical note. *J Bone Joint Surg Am* 65:704–706, 1983.
13. Engh GA, McCauley JP: Joint line restoration and flexion-extension balance with revision total knee arthroplasty. In Engh GA, Rorabeck CH, editors: *Revision total knee arthroplasty*, Philadelphia, 1997, Williams & Wilkins, pp 235–251.
14. Garvin KL, Scuderi G, Insall JN: Evolution of the quadriceps snip. *Clin Orthop* 321:131–137, 1995.
27. Meek RMD, Greidanus NV, McGraw RW, et al: The extensile rectus snip exposure in revision of total knee arthroplasty. *J Bone Joint Surg Br* 85-B:1120–1122, 2003.
41. Scott RD, Siliski JM: The use of a modified V-Y quadricepsplasty during total knee replacement to gain exposure and improve flexion in the ankylosed knee. *Orthopedics* 8:45–48, 1985.
46. Whiteside LA, Ohl MD: Tibial tubercle osteotomy for exposure of the difficult total knee arthroplasty. *Clin Orthop* 260:6–9, 1990.
45. Whiteside LA: Exposure in difficult total knee arthroplasty using tibial tubercle osteotomy. *Clin Orthop* 321:32–35, 1995.
47. Windsor RE, Insall JN: Exposure in revision total knee arthroplasty: the femoral peel. *Tech Orthop* 3(2):1988.
49. Wolff AM, Hungerford DS, Krackow KA, et al: Osteotomy of the tibial tubercle during total knee replacement. A report of twenty-six cases. *J Bone Joint Surg Am* 71:848–852, 1989.

The references for this chapter can also be found on www.expertconsult.com.

171

Revision of Aseptic Failed Total Knee Arthroplasty

Michael P. Nett, Giles R. Scuderi

Although the durability of total knee arthroplasty (TKA) with current techniques and implants is well established, failure still occurs as a result of instability, stiffness, component loosening or malposition, periprosthetic fracture, component breakage, polyethylene wear, and osteolysis. The number of primary total knee arthroplasties performed annually continues to rise rapidly.[38] With a much larger population of patients having undergone primary TKA, the number of patients requiring revision arthroplasty will also rise, despite improvements in technique, implant design, and biomaterials.[38] When failure occurs and revision is contemplated, the surgeon must recognize that revision TKA is a complex procedure that requires skill and meticulous technique to restore a predictable outcome. Preoperative evaluation should identify cause of failure to improve the likelihood of a successful outcome.[34,47] Once cause of failure has been identified, revision surgery is performed expediently. Consideration must be given to the incision and approach, management of soft tissues, techniques of implant removal, balancing of ligaments and flexion/extension gaps, management of bone loss, tensioning and alignment of the extensor mechanism, and choice of the appropriate revision implant. The objective of revision arthroplasty is similar to that of primary surgery: to have a well-aligned limb with a stable and securely fixed implant that allows restoration of function and reduces pain.

INDICATIONS FOR REVISION

Mechanical Failure

Indications for revision arthroplasty include mechanical failure, malalignment, stiffness, fracture, and infection. Mechanical failure is often because of technical error at the time of primary arthroplasty.[34] Mechanical failure includes aseptic loosening, polyethylene wear, osteolysis, instability, and extensor mechanism dysfunction.[73] If the components are loose or have shifted position, failure is inevitable and revision surgery should be performed expediently.[34] Similarly, revision is imperative with polyethylene wear-through of the tibia insert or a metal-backed patellar component. Delay will only result in additional metallic debris and massive metallic synovitis.

Osteolysis is one of the leading causes of late reoperation in patients who undergo TKA. The extent of osteolysis is often underappreciated with routine radiographs. Computed tomography (CT) or magnetic resonance imaging (MRI) can be obtained to more accurately image the osteolytic lesion and to determine the extent of bone loss.[58] Small, asymptomatic osteolytic lesions warrant close observation and possibly medical management with bisphosphonates and calcium supplementation.[27] Large, progressive, or symptomatic lesions are addressed with revision arthroplasty, ranging from simple polyethylene insert exchange to full component revision with structural bone graft or porous metal augments, depending on polyethylene availability, specific implant reliability, and extent of bone loss.[44]

Instability is another common cause of mechanical failure of TKA. The direction of instability at the tibiofemoral articulation can occur in the coronal (varus/valgus) plane, in the sagittal (anteroposterior [AP]) plane, or as a combination of planes. Early instability may result from malalignment of the components, failure to restore the mechanical axis of the limb, or imbalance of the flexion/extension space, as is often the case with midflexion instability.[49] Other common causes of early instability include intraoperative or postoperative rupture of the medial collateral ligament (MCL) or posterior cruciate ligament (PCL) with cruciate-retaining designs. Commonly, late instability occurs secondary to polyethylene wear. Asymmetrical polyethylene wear related to malalignment can result in relative lengthening of the collateral ligament on the involved side and subsequent coronal instability. In patients with cruciate-retaining knees, it is not uncommon for the PCL to elongate or attenuate. This can lead to progressive polyethylene wear and late sagittal plane instability.[40] However, late sagittal plane instability is seen not only with cruciate-retaining designs. Significant wear or fracture of the tibial polyethylene post in posterior stabilized knees may result in late sagittal plane instability.[55] Nonoperative management plays a small role in managing instability in TKA. Stability can often be achieved with a revision arthroplasty using a posterior stabilized design. A constrained condylar design may be necessary to address collateral insufficiency or flexion and extension gap imbalance. Occasionally, a hinged design may be indicated and should be readily available.[62]

Extensor mechanism dysfunction remains a cause of failure in TKA. Extensor mechanism dysfunction consists of maltracking, instability, polyethylene wear, and prosthetic loosening. Unfavorable prosthetic design and error in surgical technique lead to patellar maltracking, which may result in tilt, wear, loosening, subluxation, frank instability, or patellar fracture.[31] With improved prosthetic design and a better understanding of appropriate component position, the percentage of TKA failures related to extensor mechanism dysfunction is likely less than historical figures. Extensor mechanism failure responds poorly to nonoperative management and requires isolated component revision, extensor mechanism realignment, or complete component revision, depending on the cause of failure.

Stiffness

Stiffness is a disabling problem following TKA. Stiffness is often associated with a decrease in functional capacity and increased pain. Before revision arthroplasty is performed for stiffness, the cause should be determined and the extrinsic sources addressed. Extrinsic sources include but are not limited to osteoarthritis of the ipsilateral hip, muscle rigidity secondary to neurologic injury, and heterotopic ossification. After exclusion of an extrinsic source, the intrinsic origin should be determined. Intrinsic causes include infection, overstuffing of the patellofemoral joint, an oversized femoral component, an excessively tight flexion or extension gap, component malposition or malrotation, a tight PCL, and arthrofibrosis. If an intrinsic cause is identified and infection is ruled out, revision arthroplasty can be performed. The role of isolated arthrolysis and polyethylene component downsizing in patients with a stiff arthroplasty and well-fixed, well-aligned components remains unclear. Poor results with a high complication rate and no significant improvement in range of motion or pain were demonstrated with this approach in seven carefully selected patients with 4-year average follow-up.[2] Single-component revision may be successful in the stiff total knee with an oversized femoral prosthesis or a single malpositioned component.[29,41] However, revision of both components is usually necessary.[29] Full component revision is likely to provide improved results, but improvement in range of motion and level of pain has been shown to be modest in the hands of experienced surgeons despite meticulous patient selection.[29,51]

Periprosthetic Fracture

Periprosthetic fracture remains a problematic complication following arthroplasty. It is estimated that 0.3% to 2.5% of patients will sustain a periprosthetic fracture as a complication of TKA.[17] Patient-specific factors, including rheumatoid arthritis, osteopenic bone, and osteolysis, along with technique-specific factors such as anterior femoral cortical notching, have been implicated as potential causes of periprosthetic fracture. Frequently, fractures occur in the supracondylar area above a well-fixed implant.[33] Fractures of the tibia are much less common and frequently are associated with implant loosening.[20] In general, patients with fractures around loose implants are best treated with revision TKA, whereas those with fractures around well-fixed implants should be considered for open reduction and internal fixation.[17]

Infection

Deep infection remains one of the most devastating and challenging complications of TKA. It is estimated that by 2030, 65.5% of all revisions will be performed secondary to infection.[38] Currently, the risk of postoperative infection after total knee replacement (TKR) is 0.4% to 2.0%.[32] Appropriate treatment for acute infection remains debatable and depends on organism virulence, host factors, and time from onset to surgical intervention.[61,66] Chronic infection is treated most appropriately with two-stage reimplantation, including removal of components, débridement, and placement of a cement spacer, followed by 6 to 8 weeks of intravenous antibiotics and reimplantation once the infection has been eradicated[32] (Fig. 171.1). Complete discussion of the management of periprosthetic infection is beyond the scope of this chapter.

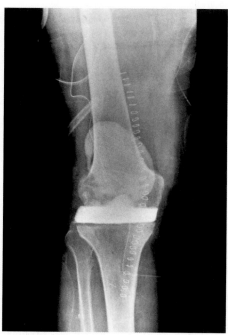

FIG 171.1 Radiograph showing antibiotic-impregnated cement spacers used after removal of an infected implant. The use of spacers contributes to eradicating infection and enhancing patient comfort and makes reimplantation technically easier. Routinely, 3 to 4 g each of vancomycin and tobramycin is used per batch of cement for creation of the spacer. Placement of intramedullary "dowels" should be considered.

PREOPERATIVE ASSESSMENT

History and Physical Examination

It is important to use a systematic diagnostic approach when evaluating the patient with a painful TKA. A thorough history and physical examination is an essential part of the preoperative evaluation and often can alert the surgeon to the possible cause of failure. An appropriately directed history may reveal critical issues that suggest infection, including delayed wound healing; prolonged drainage; fever; chills; night sweats; remote sources for hematogenous infection, such as urinary tract infection; or a recent invasive procedure, including dental work. It is also valuable to assess the pain pattern. An arthroplasty that was never pain free may lead the clinician to suspect nonarticular sources of pain, infection, or instability. A history of initial functional improvement followed by late onset of pain or dysfunction may suggest component loosening, late instability, or a hematogenously based infection. A history of start-up pain can suggest mechanical failure and implant loosening; persistent pain despite inactivity may suggest infection, regional pain syndrome, or tumor.

The wound and skin should be carefully evaluated for evidence of local infection or peripheral vascular disease. Meticulous palpation for point tenderness can lead to a diagnosis of tendinitis, bursitis, or cutaneous neuroma.[13] Physical examination of the hip and spine can reveal sources of referred pain, including ipsilateral hip arthritis or radiculopathy. Evaluation of the knee with regard to range of motion, stability, alignment, patellar tracking, and the presence of an effusion may provide additional evidence of local infection, malalignment, instability, stiffness, or extensor mechanism dysfunction.

Laboratory Evaluation

All patients presenting with a painful TKA should have a complete blood count with differential (CBC), erythrocyte sedimentation rate (ESR), and C-reactive protein (CRP). The CBC is often normal, even in the presence of infection. Any elevation in laboratory values should raise the clinician's suspicion for infection. Routine use of additional laboratory tests, including serum interleukin-6, procalcitonin, and tumor necrosis factor-alpha, in diagnosing infection has yet to be implemented, but may play a role in the near future.[6]

Aspiration is advisable whenever joint fluid is present.[13] The aspirate should be examined for signs of purulence, bleeding, metallic or polyethylene debris, or change in viscosity. The fluid is then sent for cell count, gram stain, and aerobic, anaerobic, and fungal culture. A synovial fluid leukocyte differential of greater than 65% neutrophils has a sensitivity of 97% and a specificity of 98% for diagnosing prosthetic joint infection; a leukocyte count greater than $1.7 \times 10^3/\mu L$ has a sensitivity of 94% and a specificity of 88%.[67] Ghanem et al.[23] reported similar results and recommend a cutoff of greater than 64% neutrophils and a leukocyte count greater than $1.1 \times 10^3/\mu L$, which demonstrated a combined positive predictive value of 98.6%.[23]

Radiographic Evaluation

Routine standing AP and lateral radiographs should be obtained and evaluated for component position, fixation, and sizing. Any evidence of osteolysis, polyethylene wear, component failure, loosening, or migration is noted. The most recent radiographs are compared with initial postoperative films to address concerns of subtle component migration, progressive radiolucent lines, or progressive osteolysis. A Merchant view is also essential in evaluating the patellofemoral articulation and extensor mechanism tracking. Obtaining a full-length hip-to-ankle film has several advantages. This film can be evaluated for sources of referred pain from the ipsilateral hip, including degenerative joint disease and stress fracture. It allows more accurate assessment of alignment of the involved limb and can detect distant osseous problems such as malunion, tumor, stress fracture, orthopedic hardware, or an adjacent joint arthroplasty that may be the source of pain or may interfere with a planned revision.[13] Additional radiographic views may be warranted in specific scenarios. Fluoroscopically positioned radiographs can be used to image the implant fixation interface tangentially and allow the diagnosis of subtle component loosening.[18] Oblique radiographs have been shown to enhance visualization of the periprosthetic bone and to facilitate diagnosis of early osteolysis, especially with posterior stabilized implants.[48] Stress radiographs are not routinely needed but may assist in diagnosing subtle ligamentous instability or PCL deficiency.[14]

Advanced Imaging

CT is used to more accurately diagnose and size periprosthetic osteolysis related to polyethylene wear. This can facilitate preoperative planning with regard to the management of bone loss during revision arthroplasty. Reish et al.[58] demonstrated that standard radiographs detected 17% of osteolytic lesions diagnosed by multidetector CT in 31 patients. CT is an effective and accurate way to measure tibial and femoral component rotation.[58] This may be most appropriate in the preoperative

evaluation of patients with extensor mechanism complications, including patellofemoral pain, excessive tilt, maltracking, subluxation, or dislocation.

Recent modifications of MRI pulse sequence parameters have permitted imaging of arthroplasty with significantly less artifact. MRI allows imaging of the surrounding soft tissue envelope, including nerves, tendons, and ligaments. In addition, MRI can be a useful tool to detect and quantify particle disease, osteolysis, synovitis, and prosthetic infection.[54] The exact role of MRI in evaluating the painful TKA has not yet been determined; however, it is likely that MRI will play a larger role in the future as imaging abilities continue to improve.

Nuclear medicine scans play an undefined role in evaluating the painful or failed TKA. Commonly used scans include the technetium-99m (Tc-99m)–labeled bone scan, the indium-111 or gallium-67 scan, the indium-labeled white blood cell scan, and the sulfur colloid bone marrow scan. Positive scans indicate loosening, stress fracture, infection, or complex regional pain syndrome. Nuclear scans typically provide high sensitivity but variable specificity. A Tc-99m–labeled bone scan may be positive up to 2 years following a successful arthroplasty, which may limit its role in evaluation of the recently postoperative patient. Smith et al.[64] reviewed the use of Tc-99m–methylene diphosphonate in evaluating 80 painful TKAs. They demonstrated low specificity (75.9%) and a positive predictive value (64.9%). Specifically, 33% of patients with an abnormal scan had a normal TKA with further follow-up. However, a negative bone scintigram has proved reassuring. In Smith's study, the sensitivity and negative predictive value were 92.3% and 95.0%, respectively. In-111–labeled white blood cell scans are used most often in evaluation for infection. Rand and Brown[57] evaluated 18 infected and 20 noninfected TKAs with In-111 scan. They demonstrated a sensitivity and specificity of 83% and 85%, respectively, along with a diagnostic accuracy of 84%. Similarly, Scher et al.[60] observed 84% accuracy and a 95% negative predictive value for the prediction of infection in 143 arthroplasty patients evaluated with In-111 leukocyte scan. As demonstrated, a positive In-111 scan is by itself nonspecific and can be positive because of marrow redistribution around a prosthesis. Therefore, the In-111 scan has been combined with a Tc-99m sulfur colloid scan to scan bone marrow. Incongruent uptake of the two is highly suggestive of infection.[64] Palestro et al.[52] demonstrated greater diagnostic accuracy (95%) with combined labeled leukocyte and sulfur colloid marrow imaging, compared with that of labeled leukocyte scintigraphy alone (78%).

Preoperative Planning

Preoperative planning is essential for successful revision surgery. The exact mode for failure of the prior arthroplasty must be identified.[34,73] The diagnosis of infection in the vast majority of cases is established prior to the procedure, so intraoperative "surprises" are rare.[73] The original operative report is obtained and reviewed whenever possible. This provides information regarding the previous approach; prior soft tissue management, including releases; and implant-specific information, including manufacturer, design, and size. This is particularly important if single-component revision is being entertained. Thought is given to the type of prosthesis and the amount of constraint that will be required for revision.[62] Any special components must be ordered in advance. The surgeon attempts to quantify the extent of bone loss and osteolysis present with the knowledge that it is often underestimated. The need for structural bone graft, augments, wedges, porous metal metaphyseal cones, and stems is anticipated, and they are made readily available during the revision. Preoperative templating for selected revision components can be helpful. This is essential in cases where extra-articular deformity or osseous pathology is present that may require osteotomy or may interfere with stem fixation. Revision components should be modular to allow intraoperative attachment of augments, wedges, and stems. The revision proceeds more predictably when the cruciate ligaments are excised and both posterior stabilized and constrained condylar designs are available. Ligament stability and integrity of the extensor mechanism are assessed. If ligament stability is compromised, at the time of revision, a hinged prosthesis is kept readily available. A compromised soft tissue envelope because of impaired skin viability or previous incision may warrant a plastic surgery consultation; occasionally, soft tissue expansion or a soft tissue flap will be required.[25,45]

SURGICAL TECHNIQUE

Exposure

The surgical approach most often uses the previous surgical incision. In cases with multiple longitudinal prior incisions, the most lateral and anterior incision is used to preserve the blood supply to the medial aspect of the lateral skin flap.[36] Attempts to maintain a minimum skin bridge of 6 cm between parallel incisions are recommended. Previous transverse incisions that cannot be avoided are crossed at 90 degrees if possible, but certainly at no less than 60 degrees. Soft tissue expanders can be considered in cases with multiple crossing incisions or densely adherent soft tissue.[45] Subcutaneous dissection is carried out in a limited manner, and flaps are kept as thick as possible to avoid ischemia. A medial parapatellar arthrotomy is performed. Synovial fluid is obtained as the first intraoperative culture. In revision arthroplasty with good preoperative motion, a medial subperiosteal exposure that allows the tibia to be externally rotated and anteriorly subluxed is usually sufficient for exposure. This is incorporated into a medial release if needed for soft tissue release and balancing. In revision for infection or arthrofibrosis, or during two stage reimplantation, a quadriceps snip may be anticipated and is performed early to prevent injury to the tibial tubercle and extensor mechanism[63] (Fig. 171.2). The quadriceps snip is a versatile exposure that is used in most revisions requiring extensile exposure; it does not require alteration of the postoperative weight-bearing protocol. When quadriceps snip does not allow adequate exposure, tibial tubercle osteotomy or a "banana peel" release of the patellar tendon can be considered[39,71] (Fig. 171.3). A long osteotomy as described by Whiteside and Ohl[71] is particularly useful in patients with marked patella baja, or to assist with removal of long cemented stems and well-fixed ingrowth components. A "step-cut" is performed at the most proximal aspect of the osteotomy. This allows more secure fixation and helps prevent proximal escape of the fragment. Care is taken to maintain the lateral soft tissue attachments to the osteotomized bone and to hinge the osteotomy open. This facilitates closure and maintains fragment vascularity. The fragment is repaired using cerclage wires or two screws.[71] With secure fixation, the postoperative weight-bearing protocol does not have to be altered. An alternative technique for additional exposure is V-Y quadricepsplasty.[1,63] V-Y quadricepsplasty provides excellent exposure and allows lengthening of the extensor mechanism if needed.

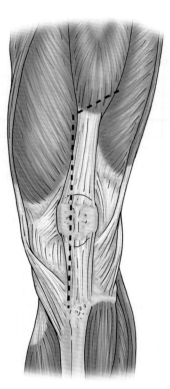

FIG 171.2 A quadriceps snip is a versatile technique used to provide expansile exposure without requiring a change in the postoperative protocol.

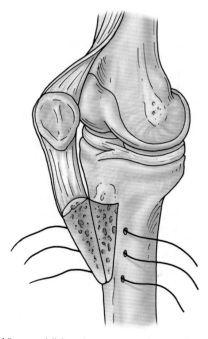

FIG 171.3 When additional exposure is needed, or in cases with severe patella baja or a stemmed cemented tibial component, a tibial tubercle osteotomy may be beneficial.

Quadricepsplasty necessitates postoperative immobilization in extension and may result in extensor lag. For patients with rigid deformity and arthrofibrosis, a femoral peel may be necessary. Because this procedure involves complete release of the medial and lateral supporting structures, use of a constrained design will be necessary.

Fixed angular deformities are often encountered during revision arthroplasty and are addressed during the exposure. A fixed varus deformity is corrected with subperiosteal release of deep and superficial portions of the MCL and the pes anserine insertion.[37] The distal insertion of the superficial MCL is elevated subperiosteally in an incremental fashion with a straight osteotome. Finally, while the tibia is externally rotated, the semimembranosus and posterior capsule are released off the posteromedial aspect of the tibia.[37] This results in skeletonization of the proximal medial tibia. A fixed valgus deformity is less common in the revision setting, but if encountered, it must be addressed. Mild valgus deformity of less than 20 degrees may be addressed with the lateral "pie-crust" technique.[10] Severe valgus deformities of greater than 20 degrees necessitate complete release of the lateral supporting structures from the femoral condyle with a subperiosteal peel or a lateral epicondylar osteotomy.

Débridement

Débridement of the suprapatellar and parapatellar regions is performed routinely. The medial and lateral gutters are re-created and cleared of all fibrous tissue. This facilitates exposure and removes debris of polyethylene, polymethylmethacrylate, and bone fragments. If the synovium is hypertrophic from reaction to intra-articular polyethylene and metal debris, a complete synovectomy is performed. The synovectomy also facilitates exposure of the joint.

Removal of Components

When operative inspection reveals granulation tissue, necrotic tissue, or other evidence of infection, the components should be removed, thorough débridement performed, and frozen section tissue examined. Evidence of acute inflammation is a reason for aborting the procedure until microbacterial cultures are available. Closing the wound over an antibiotic-impregnated polymethylmethacrylate spacer makes subsequent reentry of the knee easier in the event that cultures prove negative.

Revision operations are being performed increasingly for reasons other than loosening. Removal of well-fixed components can be difficult, especially if they are porous coated or have long cemented stems. Initially, all soft tissue is cleared from the bone/cement/prosthesis interface. Special instruments can facilitate component removal. If a modular tibial component is present, the polyethylene insert is removed first to open both flexion and extension spaces. This aids in obtaining additional exposure. The polyethylene insert is removed using manufacturer-specific tools for extraction, or by passing a straight osteotome between the insert and the tibial component. The femoral component is subsequently removed. A microsagittal saw blade is placed along the cement/prosthesis interface and is moved parallel to the component to avoid cutting into the bone (Fig. 171.4). Thin flexible osteotomes are then passed around the periphery of the component to separate the component at the cement/prosthesis interface and leave the underlying bone intact (Fig. 171.5A and B). Once the adhesion between component and cement is broken, a femoral component extraction tool is used to gently remove the femoral prosthesis (Fig. 171.6). If the procedure is performed properly, the cement is left behind still attached to the bone, with minimal bone loss from implant removal. The cement is then removed by cracking it with a small osteotome in a mosaic pattern.

The tibial component is addressed next. All polyethylene components are separated from the tibial surface with a microsagittal saw that cuts across any polyethylene pegs or stems that are subsequently removed. Metal-backed tibial components are approached in a similar manner as the femoral component. The

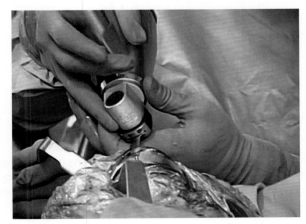

FIG 171.4 A flexible saw blade is placed along the cement/prosthesis interface and is moved parallel to the component to avoid cutting into the bone.

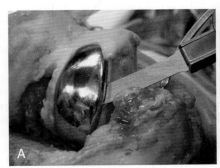
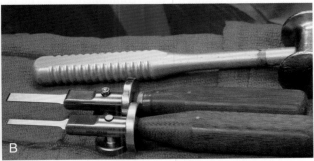

FIG 171.5 (A and B) Flexible osteotomes are passed parallel to the femoral component at the cement/prosthesis interface. These flexible osteotomes are much less likely to crush the underlying host bone, minimizing iatrogenic bone loss.

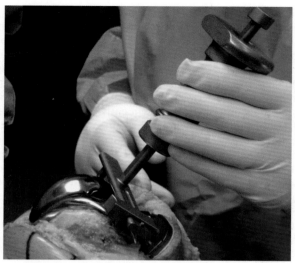

FIG 171.6 A sliding hammer is used to extract the femoral component once the bond at the cement/prosthesis interface is loosened.

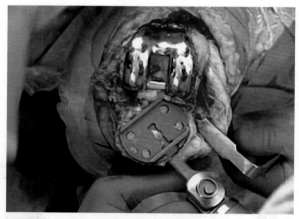

FIG 171.7 The microsagittal saw is passed beneath and parallel to the tibial component. Caution should be used to avoid digging into the tibial bone and causing unnecessary iatrogenic bone loss.

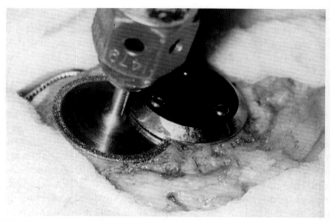

FIG 171.8 Removal of a well-fixed metal-backed patellar component with a diamond-edged saw blade.

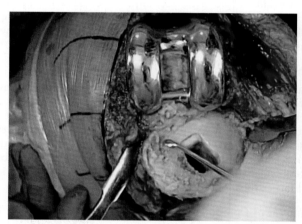

FIG 171.9 After removal of the components, retained cement and debris are removed with curettes, osteotomes, and a rongeur.

microsagittal saw is passed beneath and parallel to the tibial component (Fig. 171.7). Caution should be used to avoid digging into the tibial bone and causing unnecessary iatrogenic bone loss. Because of exposure, separating the tibial component from the cement mantle is most difficult on the posterolateral aspect of the tibia. Tibial exposure is improved by external rotation of the tibia and release of the semimembranosus and posterior capsule. The posterolateral aspect of the component is then reached by passing the microsagittal saw and thin flexible osteotomes under the posteromedial aspect of the tray to the posterolateral side. Once the bond is broken between the cement and the component, a manufacturer-specific extractor or the femoral component extractor is used to gently lift the component from the tibia. An osteotome is used to crack the remaining cement in a mosaic pattern.

A well-fixed, compatible patellar component that tracks well is left in place.[3,28] All polyethylene patellar components are removed by cutting between the cement/component interface

with an oscillating saw. The saw cuts across the pegs, which are subsequently removed with a small burr or drill bit. Metal-backed patellar components are more difficult to remove. A high-speed diamond-edged saw may be necessary to remove a well-fixed uncemented metal-backed patellar component[12] (Fig. 171.8).

After the components are removed, the bone surfaces are cleaned of cement, debris, and granulation tissue (Fig. 171.9). The bone ends are "freshened-up" in preparation for cement fixation of the revision component. In the revision setting in which infection has been ruled out, well-fixed cement in the canals that does not impact component stem placement can be left in place to avoid unnecessary iatrogenic bone loss or perforation of the canal. Removal of a cemented porous-coated prosthesis can be a difficult task, especially with stems designed for bone ingrowth. It may be necessary in this scenario to disassemble the components to gain access to the stems (Fig. 171.10).

Reconstruction

After removal of the components and thorough débridement comes time to rebuild the knee. The basic principle of revision arthroplasty involves creating a kinematically stable arthroplasty that is well fixed and well aligned. The key is to create equal

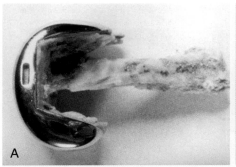
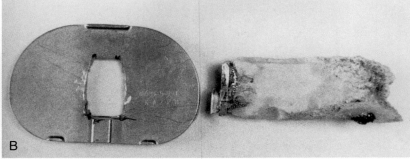

FIG 171.10 Photograph shows porous cemented components that were removed because of infection. This task was very difficult and resulted in some bone loss on the posterior surface of both the femur and the tibia. The tibial component could not be extracted until the central peg had been cut from the baseplate with a diamond-tipped saw.

flexion and extension gaps. Often this is not readily achieved, and adjustments need to be made. The surgeon must understand that adjustments made on the femoral side can affect the knee in flexion or extension, whereas adjustments on the tibial side will affect both. Reconstruction is approached using a three-step method: (1) re-create the flat tibial surface, (2) re-create the femur and rebuild the flexion space, and (3) rebuild the extension space.[8]

Re-Create the Tibia. The tibia is the foundation of the revision arthroplasty and is addressed first to establish the platform on which the subsequent arthroplasty is built.[8] Because the tibia affects the knee in both extension and flexion, a flat surface that is perpendicular to the mechanical axis must be created. If stems on the tibial component are to be used, the intramedullary canal often provides an excellent guide to re-creating a flat, perpendicular surface. Augmentation is used to re-create the proximal tibia to support the perpendicular, flat tibial surface as close to the original height of the tibia as possible. This will provide the surgeon with more options for choosing the appropriate polyethylene insert to balance flexion and extension gaps. Modular augments, wedges, blocks, or structural allograft may be needed (Fig. 171.11). In knees with severe tibial bone loss, modular tibial cones or sleeves are used to reconstruct the proximal end of the tibia[1] (Fig. 171.12). Care is taken to position the tibial component in the proper rotation using the tibial tubercle and the anteromedial aspect of the tibia as reference points.

Re-Create the Femur

Size the femur. Choosing the correct size of components is an essential step. Femoral component sizing specifically influences the flexion space by restoring the AP dimensions and the posterior condylar offset of the femur. It is helpful to preoperatively procure the operative notes from the previous procedure. Another useful preoperative step is to template the opposite side to obtain a relative idea of the size. Look at the size of the femoral component that is being removed, and determine whether it is appropriate. The remaining bone should be templated in the AP plane. Posterior bone loss usually occurs, so templating intraoperatively runs the risk of undersizing the femoral component (Fig. 171.13). The epicondylar width of the femur can also be helpful in selecting the appropriate femoral size.

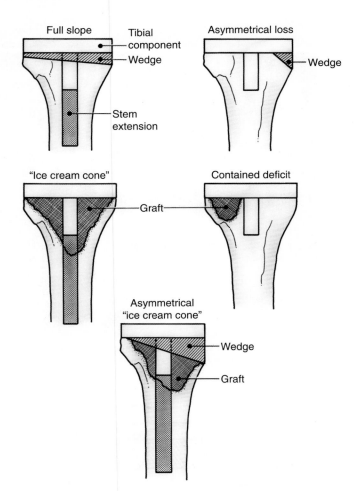

FIG 171.11 Reconstruction of Tibial Defects Symmetrical tibial deficiency can be compensated for by thicker tibial polyethylene. Stem extension is usually advisable.

The danger in selecting an excessively small femoral component is that this will fail to restore posterior femoral offset and will compromise flexion stability. It is better to select a larger femoral component and augment the posterior condyles to restore the AP dimension. Bone loss usually is most significant in the posterior femoral condyle area, but anterior femoral bone

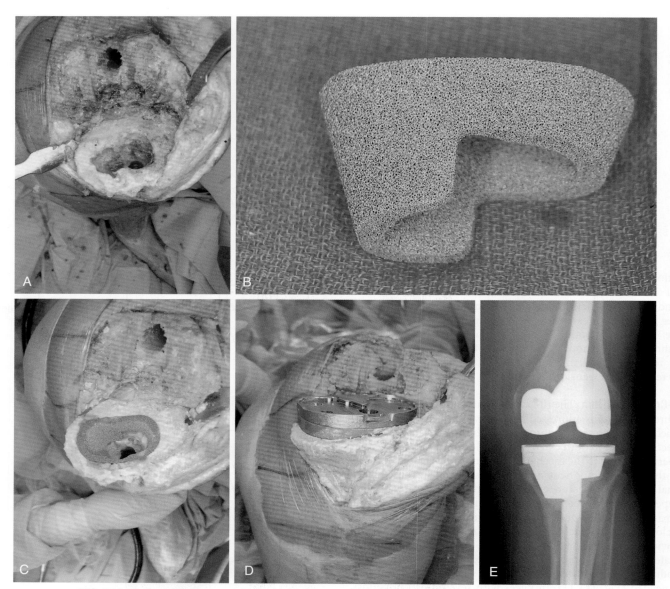

FIG 171.12 A trabecular metal cone is used to manage severe bone loss of the proximal tibia in revision total knee arthroplasty.

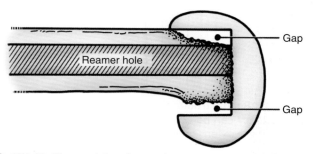

FIG 171.13 The revision femoral component must be sized from measurements of the opposite knee or estimated from the removed components. Typically, gaps will be noted anteriorly and posteriorly.

loss can occur and can influence sizing, especially sizing of the femoral component in the sagittal position (Fig. 171.14).

Femoral component rotation. Correct rotation of the femoral component is vital to knee kinematics and patellar tracking. The best way to determine rotation is to identify the medial and lateral epicondyles and establish the epicondylar axis. Rotational adjustments should be made to the residual distal femur, with shaving of bone from the anterolateral and posteromedial aspects of the femur usually required if the previous component was rotated internally. To ensure correct femoral component rotation, the posterolateral condyle generally has to be augmented. If a posterior stabilized or similar prosthesis is used, the intercondylar notch is prepared 90 degrees to the epicondylar axis. In cases of severe bone loss, the epicondyles may not be available. The tibial platform is then used as a reference for femoral component rotation with the knee at 90 degrees of flexion.

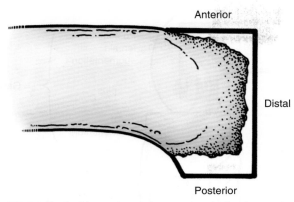

FIG 171.14 Typical bone loss after removal of a femoral component. Distal, anterior, and posterior bone deficiencies are illustrated.

Distal femur position. The key to this step is restoring the distance from the joint line, distally and posteriorly. The epicondyles are a useful landmark from which to determine the joint line, which on average is 25 mm from the lateral epicondyle and 30 mm from the medial epicondyle. Because the tibial cut is established at 90 degrees to the tibial mechanical axis, the joint line of a prosthetic knee of average size is 30 mm from both epicondyles.

After the appropriate joint line has been determined, the femoral component can be set provisionally to reestablish the distal joint line. Symmetrical distal femoral augments are used on both medial and lateral sides if there is symmetrical bone loss, or if the joint line has been previously elevated (Fig. 171.15). Unilateral distal augmentation or asymmetrical augmentation is used to accommodate asymmetrical femoral bone loss. Treatment of femoral bone loss depends on the severity of the deficiency and consists of cement, metal augmentation, modular cones, structural allograft, and distal femoral replacement[16,56] (Fig. 171.16). The distance from the epicondyles to the posterior joint line is similar to that of the distal joint line and is helpful in confirming the correct femoral component size.

Because this step is provisional, no bone should be resected to fit the augments until the final position and size of the femoral component have been determined. Additional adjustments to the position and size of the femoral component may be needed as the flexion and extension gaps are balanced.

Rebuild the Flexion Space

Balance the flexion space. This step requires choosing the correct tibial polyethylene articulation. With the provisional femoral component in place, the thickest tibial polyethylene surface that fills the flexion space is inserted on the provisional tibial tray (Fig. 171.17).

Rebuild the Extension Space. The knee is brought into extension with the tibial insert in place. If the knee can be fully extended and the gaps are equal and stable, the polyethylene insert is correctly sized and the femoral augments are finalized. Minor adjustments can be made to the polyethylene insert to achieve this goal. When an imbalance in the flexion and extension gaps is present, additional adjustments are required. Several possible basic scenarios[8] are detailed next and in Table 171.1:

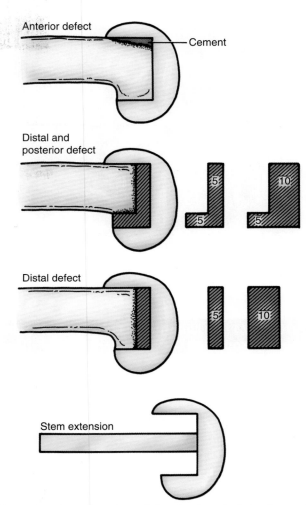

FIG 171.15 Augmentation of the distal end of the femur. The revision femoral component should have a stem extension; usually, both distal and posterior augments are required, although the amount of augmentation at each site may differ. Thus, 5 mm may be sufficient posteriorly, although distal augmentation of 10 mm could be required. This can be judged by considering the spacers needed in flexion and extension and the amount of distal augmentation necessary to restore the joint line.

1. If the knee is too tight in both flexion and extension, reducing the thickness of the tibial component may be sufficient to balance the knee.
2. If the knee is tight in flexion but acceptable in extension, there are two options:
   a. Check the sagittal position of the femoral component. If it is positioned too posteriorly, consider using an offset femoral stem extension. This will move the femoral component more anteriorly. Be careful to avoid overstuffing the patellofemoral joint because this will adversely affect motion and patellofemoral tracking.
   b. Downsize the femoral component.
3. If the knee is tight in flexion and loose in extension, consider the following three options:
   a. Check the sagittal position of the femoral component as in point 2, and consider using a thicker tibial component.

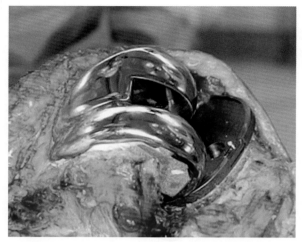

FIG 171.16 Final revision components demonstrating distal and femoral augmentation to restore the joint line and fill the flexion gap.

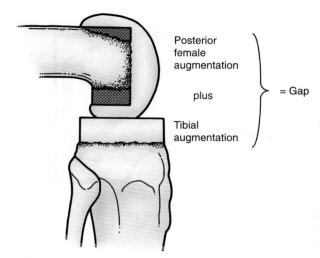

FIG 171.17 During reconstruction, the flexion gap is restored by a combination of posterior femoral and tibial augmentation.

TABLE 171.1 Nine-Point Grid for Balancing Flexion and Extension Gaps in Revision Total Knee Arthroplasty

		EXTENSION SPACE		
		Tight	**OK**	**Loose**
FLEXION SPACE	**TIGHT**	• Reduce the thickness of the tibial insert. • Remove symmetrical tibial augments if present.	• Downsize the femoral component. • Use an offset stem to adjust the sagittal position of the femoral component more anteriorly.	• Add distal femoral augmentation. • Downsize the femoral component, and use a thicker insert. • If possible, use an offset stem to adjust the sagittal position of the femoral component more anteriorly, and use a thicker tibial insert.
	OK	• Mild flexion contracture: • Subperiosteal posterior capsule release • Severe contracture: • Reduce the distal femoral augmentation. *or* • Resect additional distal femur.	• Balanced gaps — — — —	• Add additional distal femoral augmentation. — — — —
	LOOSE	• First, address the distal position of the femoral component. • Remove distal augmentation. • Resect additional distal femur. • Next, adjust the sagittal position of the femoral component. If possible, use an offset stem to move the component posteriorly. • If the femoral component is undersized, increase the size of the femoral component.	• Adjust the sagittal position of the femoral component. If possible, use an offset stem to move the component posteriorly. • If the femoral component is undersized, increase the size of the femoral component. — — —	• Increase the thickness of the tibial insert. • Add symmetrical tibial augmentation. — — —

b. Downsize the femoral component, and use a thicker tibial component.

c. If the femoral component is the correct size, increase the distal femoral augmentation until the extension gap is equal to the flexion gap. A thinner tibial component may be required to balance the knee. Be careful to not move the joint line too far distally, because this will adversely affect patellar tracking.

4. If the knee is acceptable in flexion but tight in extension, there are two options:

a. Reduce the distal femoral augmentation or resect more distal femoral bone. This will move the femoral component more proximally and increase the extension space.

b. If a preoperative flexion contracture is present, release the posterior capsule, preferably from the femur.

5. If flexion and extension gaps are equal, no further adjustments are necessary.

6. If the knee is acceptable in flexion and loose in extension, the solution is to augment the distal end of the femur so that

the extension gap requires the same amount of tibial polyethylene as the flexion gap.

7. The most common problem is that the flexion space is larger than the extension space. If the knee is loose in flexion and tight in extension, the solution is to go through a series of checks and adjustments.

   a. Check the sagittal position of the femoral component. If it is positioned too anteriorly, consider using an offset femoral stem extension. This will move the femoral component more posteriorly and reduce the flexion space.

   b. Check the distal position of the femoral component. Consider reducing the distal augmentation or resecting more distal femoral bone.

   c. Check the femoral component size. If it appears to be too small, consider choosing the next larger size, but be careful to not oversize the femur.

   d. If the previous maneuvers fail to balance the gaps, a constrained condylar knee (CCK) articulation may be needed.

   e. Depending on the experience of the surgeon, collateral ligament advancement and reconstruction may be considered.

8. If the knee is loose in flexion and acceptable in extension, moving the femoral component proximally and using a thicker tibial component may solve the problem. If this does not balance the knee, the options in point 7 should be considered.

9. If the knee is symmetrically loose in flexion and extension, a thicker tibial component will solve the problem.

Management of Bone Loss

Bone loss is frequently encountered during revision arthroplasty. Even unicompartmental replacements can leave substantial asymmetrical bone deficiencies (Fig. 171.18). Osteolysis is often more expansive than anticipated. The keys to management of intraoperative bone loss are anticipation and preoperative preparation. At the time of revision, all materials for reconstruction, including wedges, blocks, allografts, metaphyseal cones, and special components, are available.

Bone defects have been classified in numerous ways.[16,27,59] They can be classified as contained, uncontained, or a combination (Figs. 171.19 and 171.20). Contained defects have an intact cortical rim, while uncontained defects involve segmental bone loss with no remaining cortex. Treatment for bone loss depends largely on two factors: (1) whether the defect is contained or uncontained, and (2) the size of the defect. Small (<5 mm) contained defects are easily managed with cement or morselized bone graft. Small uncontained defects often are not large enough to adversely affect component stability. They have been managed historically with cement and screws but can be managed well with cement alone.[9] Large (>10 mm) contained cavitary defects can be managed with autogenous or allogenic bone graft. If the contained defect is large enough to compromise support of the implant, then impaction grafting, structural allograft, or metaphyseal cones should be considered.[56] Intermediate (5 to 10 mm) uncontained defects are managed well with modular wedges. Large uncontained defects often affect component stability and are best managed with modular augments, structural allograft, or metaphyseal filling cones.[56] The Anderson Orthopaedic Research Institute (AORI) classification scheme is useful and descriptive, and allows independent classification of

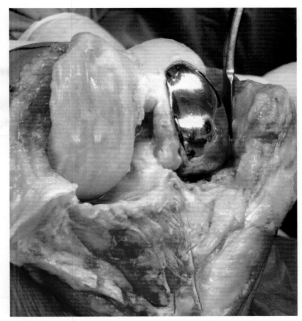

FIG 171.18 The most common reason for failure of unicondylar replacement is progressive arthritis of unreplaced compartments of the knee. Free or embedded particles of acrylic cement are frequently found.

the femoral and tibial sides.[59] Management of the bone defect based on the AORI scheme is detailed in Fig. 171.21.

Type 1 defects have healthy cancellous bone with an undamaged metaphyseal segment and no evidence of component subsidence or osteolysis. Type 1 defects most often are managed using cement or occasionally metal augments. Type 2 defects may or may not have a healthy cancellous bed of bone; the metaphyseal flare is shortened, and mild to moderate evidence of component subsidence and osteolysis is found. Type 2 defects are managed with cement, metal augments, or morselized and structural allograft, depending on intraoperative assessment. Typically, type 2 defects are ideal for modular metal augmentation.[28] Type 3 defects have a deficient metaphyseal segment at or above the levels of the epicondyles on the femur and at or below the level of the tubercle on the tibia. Considerable component subsidence and osteolysis are noted with type 3 defects. Type 3 defects typically are managed with metal augmentation, impaction grafting, structural allograft, and constrained condylar prostheses. Rarely, alternative components including allograft/prosthetic composite or a hinged prosthesis may be required, depending on the involvement of the epicondyles and the status of the collateral ligaments. In the AORI scheme, each type is subdivided into "A" for one condyle or one side of the tibial plateau involved, and "B" for bicondylar or total plateau involvement. The classification of bone loss should be performed intraoperatively after component removal.

Metal augmentation as part of modern modular revision systems is an effective and convenient modality to manage bone loss; however, it is not used without concern. Brooks et al. compared five different techniques in the treatment of wedge-shaped proximal tibial defects. They concluded that a metal wedge was an acceptable alternative to a custom-made component for reconstruction of tibial bone stock defects.[9] Brand et al.[7] reported good results with use of a metal wedge for

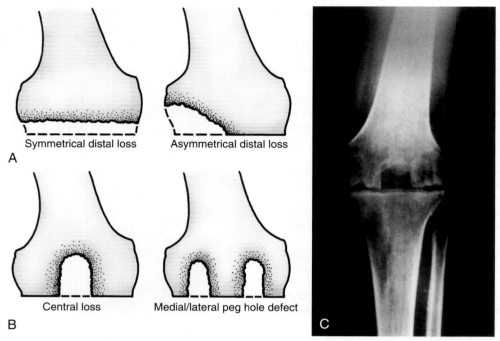

FIG 171.19 (A) In the coronal plane, distal femoral bone loss may be symmetrical or asymmetrical. (B) Contained defects may be created by central or peripheral fixation lugs. (C) Radiograph shows defects left after removal of the prosthesis, with a central box on the femur and a central stem on the tibia. Note the good preservation of medial and lateral bone.

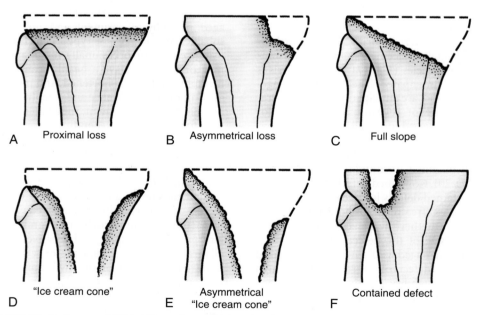

FIG 171.20 Patterns of Tibial Bone Loss (A) Proximal loss, (B) asymmetrical loss, (C) full slope, (D) "ice cream cone," (E) asymmetrical "ice cream cone," and (F) contained defect.

proximal tibial defects. In their series, 22 knees (in 20 patients) were monitored for an average of 37 months. No failures and no loosening of tibial components were reported. However, a 27% incidence of nonprogressive radiolucent lines was described. None of these patients required revision surgery, and all but one patient was pain free. Although the literature currently does not support these concerns, with reported 84% to 98% good or excellent results, theoretical disadvantages include undersurface wear between the augment and the component and dissociation of the augments.[28]

The use of morselized allograft to manage bone loss remains a viable option and has several advantages. Advantages include allow the surgeon to create intraoperatively constructs of any size or shape to fill the defect. These provide excellent initial support for the revision implant and, with biologic integration with host bone, will provide long-term support and will restore bone stock for future revision arthroplasty. Specific disadvantages of structural allografts include prolonged operative time required to shape the graft, limited availability of large allografts, nonunion, delayed union, graft resorption or collapse, and graft infection or disease transmission.[11] Dennis and Little[15] reported encouraging early clinical results and a high allograft/host union rate with use of structural allograft composite in revision knee arthroplasty. Unfortunately, midterm follow-up is not as promising. A recent study of 70 allografts demonstrated revision-free survival of 80% and 75% at 5 and 10 years, respectively.[4] Allograft failures (8 of 16) and infection (5 of 16) were responsible for 13 of 16 revisions during the follow-up period.

Impaction grafting is well established in revision total hip arthroplasty. Theoretically, impaction of morselized graft allows more rapid and complete revascularization compared with large structural allograft. Based on success in revision hip arthroplasty, surgeons have used impaction grafting to manage contained and uncontained defects in revision knee arthroplasty.[43] Although impaction grafting alone can be used in contained defects, uncontained defects usually require wire mesh to contain the graft. Advantages of impaction grafting include cost-effectiveness, restoration of bone stock, and the ability to accommodate defects of varying shapes and sizes. Disadvantages include technical difficulty, graft resorption, intraoperative fracture, disease transmission, and prolonged operative time spent fashioning mesh and impacting graft. Lotke et al.[43] reported no mechanical failures with impaction grafting in 42 patients with 2- to 7-year (average, 3.8-year) follow-up. Two infections and two late periprosthetic fractures were reported. All radiographs demonstrated incorporation and remodeling of the bone graft. Because of these encouraging results, the authors continue to use impaction grafting as their procedure of choice for managing large bone defects in revision knee arthroplasty.

More severe type 2 and most type 3 defects typically require more support than is offered by traditional wedge or block augments. Porous metaphyseal filling cone augments not only have the potential for long-term biologic fixation but can be used to fill large defects and to provide additional structural support without some of the concerns associated with structural allograft[1] (see Fig. 171.20). Modularity of cone augments allows accommodation for defects of various shapes and sizes without the added time and complexity associated with impaction grafting or shaping of structural allografts. In addition, issues of graft resorption, disease transmission, and graft fracture or failure are avoided. Early reports demonstrate excellent short-term follow-up with evidence of osseointegration and no mechanical failure in a combined 25 patients with 12- to 47-month follow-up.[46,56] Long and Scuderi[42] reported the results of 16 revision TKAs with tibial cones used to manage severe type 2 and 3 tibial bone defects. With minimum and average follow-up of 24 and 31 months, respectively, no mechanical failures occurred, and all radiographs demonstrated stable osseointegration into the cones. Larger studies with longer follow-up are needed, but these augments appear to provide a viable alternative to structural allograft and impaction grafting.

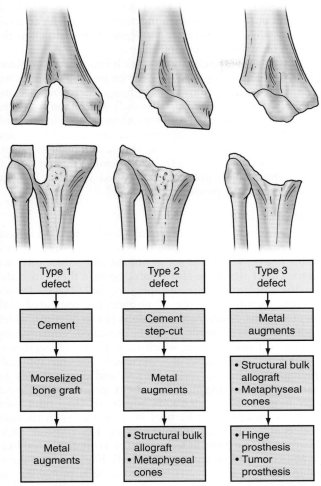

Type 1 defect	Type 2 defect	Type 3 defect
Cement	Cement step-cut	Metal augments
Morselized bone graft	Metal augments	• Structural bulk allograft • Metaphyseal cones
Metal augments	• Structural bulk allograft • Metaphyseal cones	• Hinge prosthesis • Tumor prosthesis

FIG 171.21 Managing bone loss in revision in total knee arthroplasty.

biocompatibility, versatility, cost-effectiveness, and restoration of bone stock. However, some disadvantages are known, including graft availability, late resorption, infection, and risk of disease transmission.[7] An absolute contraindication to allograft is infection; relative contraindications include immunosuppression, metabolic bone disorders, neuropathic arthropathy, and a deficient extensor mechanism. The use of allograft to manage bony defects has had some encouraging results for small and large defects. Whiteside[70] used morselized allograft for localized areas of bone defects in 56 cementless revisions. All 56 knees demonstrated increased density in the grafted zone. For larger defects, Wilde et al.[72] reported their results on 12 knees. Five of the knees had contained defects and seven had an uncontained defect; all were treated with structural allograft. Radiographs demonstrated complete incorporation of the graft in 11 of 12 knees at an average of 23 months after surgery. Single-photon emission CT scans showed uniform activity in the area of the graft in four of the five knees that were studied.

For more extensive bone loss, including AORI type 2B and three bone defects, structural allografts, impaction grafting, and metallic prosthetic augments are frequently used. Structural allografts, which have been used for decades in revision TKA,

MANAGEMENT OF THE PATELLA

After insertion of the trial components for a final check, patellar tracking is assessed. Lateral patellar release and balancing may be necessary, but proper femoral and tibial component rotation should be confirmed before it is assumed that a release is necessary. If augments have been chosen appropriately and the joint line restored, the patellar position will be in the "neutral zone." If the patella is out of the "neutral zone," then alteration or redistribution of the augments may be necessary (Fig. 171.22). Awareness of preoperative patellar position is essential. If patella baja was present preoperatively secondary to patellar tendon shortening, the patellar position will be difficult to alter. Here, patella baja may have to be accepted. Occasionally, patella baja is so severe that the patellar component articulates with the tibial insert. Attempts to lengthen the patellar tendon or to advance the tubercle should be avoided. One alternative is to remove the patellar prosthesis and reduce the size of the remaining patellar bone.[8]

Frequently, the patellar component is retained during revision arthroplasty.[28] If the patellar component is well fixed, compatible with the design of the prosthesis to be reimplanted, and tracks well, it may remain in place.[3,28] If the patellar component necessitates removal, the decision to implant a new prosthetic patella component depends on the patellar position and the remaining bone stock. In most cases, a new three-peg cemented component can be implanted. Consider omitting the patellar prosthesis when the patellar bone is insufficient

(<12 mm thick), or when the remaining bone quality is extremely poor. Trim the remaining patellar bone with an oscillating saw while performing a *patelloplasty*; this will allow the patella to fit well in the femoral sulcus.[8]

If the remaining patellar bone stock is insufficient for placement of a patellar component, aside from patelloplasty, alternative reconstruction options exist. Hanssen[30] described packing bone graft in the remaining patellar shell, which then is covered with a local soft tissue sleeve. This technique appears to result in bone graft remodeling, appropriate patellar tracking, and restoration of patellar bone stock. Trabecular metal augments are also available (Fig. 171.23). If a remaining shell of bone is present, these augments may be sutured in place and can support a cemented patellar component.[50]

Use of Stem Extensions

Stem extensions are almost universally used in revision arthroplasty. Femoral and tibial bone quality is compromised to a variable degree, and stems act to offload and reduce interface stresses. Offset stems are also helpful because they can better align the implant on the metaphysis (Fig. 171.24). Debate continues regarding the use of uncemented compared with cemented stems. Short-stem extensions (25 to 30 mm), which do not engage the diaphysis, should be cemented. Similarly, long and narrow-diameter stems, which are not canal filling, should be cemented. Fehring et al.[19] reviewed 202 metaphyseal-engaging stems in 113 revision TKAs and demonstrated an advantage of cementing metaphyseal-engaging stems. However, longer modular stem extensions, which are canal filling and diaphyseal engaging, can be used in a tight press-fit manner. Wood et al.[74] published their results of 135 revision TKAs performed using a press-fit technique (press-fit diaphyseal fixation and cemented metaphyseal fixation). Kaplan-Meier survivorship analysis at 12 years revealed a 98% probability of survival free of revision for aseptic loosening. This involves cementing the core prosthesis and inserting diaphyseal-engaging stem extensions in a tight press-fit manner, allowing establishment of limb alignment, offloading interface stresses, and easier removal, while long-term fixation is attained by cementing the core prosthesis.

Constraint in Revision Arthroplasty

It is most desirable to use the least amount of constraint necessary (Fig. 171.25).[62] This will minimize forces on bone/cement/prosthesis interfaces and theoretically will minimize the rate of aseptic loosening. Therefore, in most revisions, a posterior stabilized articulation is used.

When additional constraint is needed over a posterior stabilized prosthesis, a nonlinked CCK design is used. Concern over accelerated component loosening and wear related to increased constraint has not been supported by the available literature. Font-Rodriguez et al.[21] reported a 7-year survivorship of 98% in a cohort of 64 knees. Similarly, Trousdale et al.[68] reported 80% survivorship at 15.3 years following revision TKA in 20 patients using an earlier design of the CCK. Although every effort is made to minimize constraint during revision TKA, when necessary, a nonlinked CCK design can be used with apparently little detriment to long-term survival.

At times, even a constrained implant will not provide adequate stability. In these cases, a hinged implant should be kept available during revision surgery. Hinged implants are indicated in patients with global instability, a deficient extensor

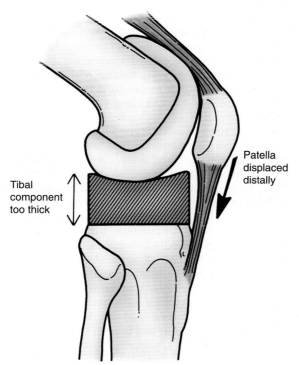

Tibal component too thick

Patella displaced distally

FIG 171.22 If an extra-thick tibial component is needed to stabilize the knee, the patella is displaced distally, thereby causing patella infera. Undersizing of the femoral component in the sagittal plane and anterior malpositioning are possible causes. Excessive distal resection of the femur in which the joint line is moved proximally is another cause.

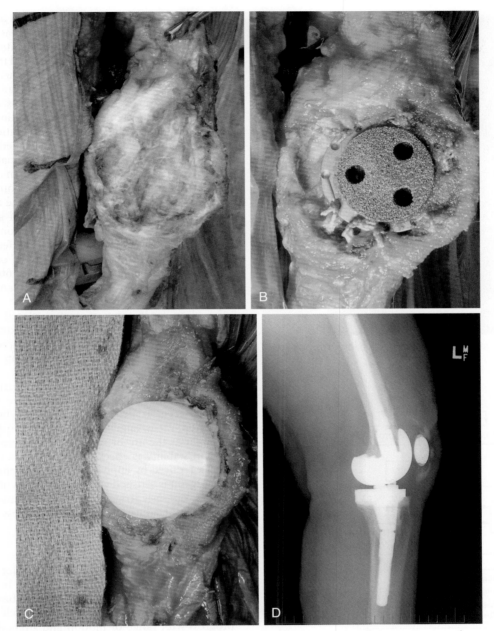

FIG 171.23 A trabecular metal patella is used to reconstruct the patellar component when only a shell of patellar bone remains.

mechanism, or severe bone loss after fracture or during tumor reconstruction.[62]

Final Preparation

The bone surfaces are cleaned with pulsatile lavage. Note that in most revision cases, even with considerable bone loss, the margins of the defect will consist of sclerotic bone or irregular contours. This bone is the strongest available and should not be removed or drilled, and no attempt should be made to obtain a cancellous surface. Even when this is possible, the quality of the bone may be poor and inadequate for providing proper prosthetic support.

The final components are assembled, selected modular augments and wedges are fixed with screws or cement according to the designer's intention, and intramedullary stems are attached. It is recommended that these stems be 1 mm larger than stems used for the trial reduction to get the firmest possible fit.

Cementing

Cementing the interface and the core prosthesis ensures that the prosthesis will fit perfectly on the inherently irregular surface. Cement serves to level the bone ends and causes even loading beneath the prosthesis. Implant fixation is provided by the shape of the component and the press-fit intramedullary stems. If metaphyseal cones are used, they are impacted prior to cementation. The interface of the cone is grafted and protected from cement extrusion.

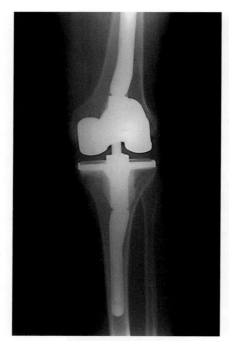

FIG 171.24 Offset stem extensions in revision arthroplasty.

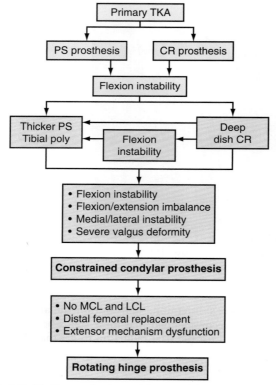

FIG 171.25 Constraint in revision total knee arthroplasty.

Two batches of cement are used for each component during standard revision TKA. Commercially prepared antibiotic-impregnated cement is used. Alternatively, 1 g of tobramycin powder may be added per bag of cement. With high-viscosity cement in the "doughy" phase, the surface of the tibia and the undersurface of the core tibial prosthesis are coated. Handling the cement in the "doughy" phase allows easy cement manipulation and avoids leakage of the cement into the intramedullary canal. Coating the surface of the bone and the implant produces a cement/cement interface during the curing process. Cement is prevented from entering the tibial canal. The component is gradually impacted into place. Excess cement is removed periodically to allow excellent visualization to ensure proper component rotation and depth. The rotational position of the trial tibial component is marked with methylene blue to serve as a reference during impaction of the final component.

Cement for the femoral side is then mixed. If the final femoral component is going to "float" on cement, it may be useful to mark the desired position of the anterior flange with the trial components in place. This will serve as a reference during impaction of the final femoral component. Cement is applied again to the surface of the distal femur and the underside of the core prosthesis in a "doughy" condition. The prosthesis is inserted and is gently impacted into the bone. Cement is prevented from entering the femoral canal. Excess cement is removed.

A clean laparotomy sponge is placed in the joint space between the final implants. The knee is extended, and attention is turned to the patella. The patellar component, when used, is cemented and held in place with a clamp until the cement is cured.

Once the cement is cured, the tourniquet is let down. Meticulous hemostasis is obtained. The previously selected tibial insert is trialed. The knee should be able to reach full extension. Varus/valgus stability is checked at full extension and throughout the arc of motion. Patellar tracking is reassessed. Flexion stability is checked at 90 degrees of flexion, with the patella reduced by applying an anterior and posterior draw. If the surgeon is satisfied with the thickness of the trial insert, the knee is copiously irrigated and the final insert is impacted into place. Minor adjustments to the thickness of the tibial insert can be made at this time, if necessary.

Aftercare

Aftercare for revision surgery does not differ from that indicated for primary cases, except with extensive bone grafting, which would require some protection in weight bearing. Even with the use of a quadriceps snip or a tibial tubercle osteotomy, we still progress with range-of-motion and strengthening exercises. If any question arises regarding fixation of the tibial tubercle osteotomy, motion and quadriceps exercises are limited for 6 to 8 weeks, or until the osteotomy is healed.

RESULTS OF REVISION SURGERY

Historical Results

Techniques for revision arthroplasty continue to evolve. Most available long-term results involve cases in which techniques were used that are not applicable today. As customized implants, metal augments, wedges, stems, and allograft techniques are refined, long-term results should continue to improve.

Bertin et al.[5] were the first to report results of revision TKA with the use of uncemented stems. A total of 24 revision arthroplasties performed using the Imperial College of London Hospital (ICLH) prosthesis with a mean follow-up of 18 months showed no radiographic evidence of subsidence or failure and 91% satisfactory relief of preoperative pain. These results, if anything, were better than those reported with primary arthroplasty. This experience led Freeman (personal communication) to use similar stems for all of his replacements.

The Hospital for Special Surgery published results using custom implants, augments, wedges, and stems.[69] This group reported an infection rate of 5% and an overall mechanical loosening rate of 3%. It is interesting to note that all mechanical failures occurred in knees reconstructed with short, cemented stems, and no knees reconstructed with long uncemented stems loosened. Of the noncemented stems, 96% showed a sclerotic halo around the stem and, in most cases, cortical reaction at the distal tip of the stem. This study highlighted the difficulty of accurate preoperative templating based on radiographs. Problems of sizing and fit occurred intraoperatively with the custom prosthesis. This, in part, led to the newer concept of modular design.

In 1982, Insall and Dethmers[34] reported 89% good to excellent results in 72 cemented revision TKAs with a minimum of 2 years of follow-up. This was the earliest report in which results of revision arthroplasty approached those of primary arthroplasty. Fewer excellent and more good results were described than in a primary arthroplasty series. Compared with primary knee arthroplasty, the authors noted a much higher incidence of radiolucent lines and a greater number of postoperative extensor mechanism problems. The short follow-up and high incidence of radiolucent lines were matters of concern regarding the longevity of the revision arthroplasties.

Goldberg et al.[26] reported the results of 65 consecutive revision TKAs performed for mechanical failure. The types of implants used included total condylar, posterior stabilized, total condylar III, and a kinematic rotating-hinge prosthesis. In this series, 46% of the knees were considered excellent or good, and 42% were poor or failures. The infection rate was 4.5%, and multiple revisions did poorly.

Jacobs et al. reviewed 24 patients with 28 failed TKAs replaced with porous-coated anatomic components.[35] Good and excellent results were achieved in 68%, along with three failures. Patients who underwent revision operations for severe pain or who had no clearly definable problem were not improved. Friedman et al.[22] presented the results of 137 revision total knees at the Brigham and Women's Hospital in Boston. Function instability, motion, and pain all improved after revision, but improvements were significantly less than those seen after primary TKR. A third of the patients still walked with crutches, with a walker, or not at all. Loosening was the most common reason for failure. The clinical success rate was 63% for a single revision, and the failure rate at 5 years was 5.8%.

Contemporary Results With Uncemented Stems

The results of our own experience with CCK components and uncemented stems have been examined.[28] A total of 68 revision operations were reported, and follow-up ranged from 2 to 10 years. Excellent and good results were obtained in 56 knees, with 11 poor results. Further revision was performed on six knees, all because of infection. A posterior stabilized tibial insert was used in 49 knees, 43 (88%) of which achieved excellent and good results, with 4 additional revisions. The CCK tibial insert was needed to give greater stability in 18 knees, and 13 (72%) knees were rated excellent and good, with 2 additional revisions. The overall infection rate was high (9%), which confirms the wisdom of avoiding intramedullary cement. Survivorship analysis of this group of patients was calculated to be 80% at

10 years—a figure less satisfactory than in a similar analysis performed on total condylar and posterior stabilized prostheses (90% and 94%, respectively). Thus, even with so-called modern techniques, the results of revision surgery are understandably less satisfactory than those of primary arthroplasty.

In 2002, Gofton et al.[24] reported results using uncemented stem fixation for 89 revisions. With an average of 5.9 years (range, 4.1 to 8.6 years) of follow-up, they demonstrated a Kaplan-Meier survivorship of 93.5% at 8.6 years. Four poor outcomes were reported, and five patients required subsequent revision for aseptic loosening (two), infection (one), arthrofibrosis (one), and instability (one).

In 2005, Peters et al.[53] reported on 50 consecutive revisions in 47 patients with uncemented stems. At an average of 36 months (range, 24 to 96 months) of follow-up, 88% good to excellent results were described. No patients demonstrated aseptic loosening. One patient had a poor outcome requiring an above-knee amputation for diabetic ulcers. Four patients (9%) developed deep infection, again highlighting the advantage of easier component removal with uncemented rather than cemented stem extensions.

As previously mentioned, Wood et al.[74] published results on 135 revisions with uncemented stems. Minimum follow-up was 2 years (mean, 5 years; range, 2 to 12 years). A total of 36 knees in 31 patients were lost to follow-up because of patient death. Of the remaining patients, six required subsequent revision for infection (two), instability secondary to MCL rupture (two), and aseptic loosening (two). Kaplan-Meier survivorship free of re-revision was 87% at 12 years. Kaplan-Meier survivorship free of re-revision or radiographic loosening was 82% at 12 years. It is impressive that Kaplan-Meier survivorship with aseptic loosening as an indication for re-revision was 98% at 12 years.

The point made by Jacobs et al.[35] about poor results of revision surgery performed for pain, without clear definition of the reason, is well taken and cannot be overemphasized. Our own experience confirms this, although we understand how difficult it is to manage a patient with a painful arthroplasty. The temptation to "give it a go" is sometimes irresistible, but the result most likely will be failure.

CUSTOM COMPONENTS

Since the introduction of modularity, custom components have a limited role in revision knee arthroplasty. A custom prosthesis can be considered if one of the following conditions prevails:

1. The bone is so oversized or undersized that standard components will not fit.
2. Stems are needed to enhance fixation, but bone shapes preclude the use of standard devices (e.g., when a fracture malunion occurs adjacent to the prosthesis [Fig. 171.26] or an offset stem is needed because of peculiarities in intramedullary alignment [Fig. 171.27]; shorter modular stem extensions and offset stems also provide a solution to this problem [Fig. 171.28]).
3. The size or location of bone loss cannot be accommodated by standard augments.

Otherwise, custom components should be avoided for the following reasons:

1. No instruments have been designed for implanting custom components.
2. Use of a custom component does not provide sizing options intraoperatively.

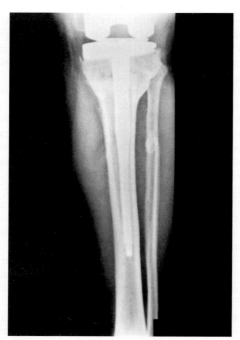

FIG 171.26 A long-stemmed tibial component is used during reconstruction following nonunion of an upper tibial osteotomy.

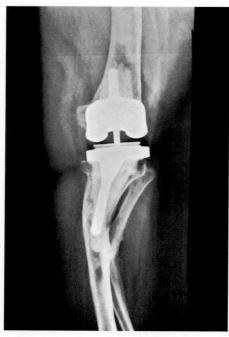

FIG 171.27 Severe proximal tibia deformity precludes the use of standard stems for tibial reconstruction. A custom, angulated tibial stem is used to eliminate the need for a corrective tibial osteotomy.

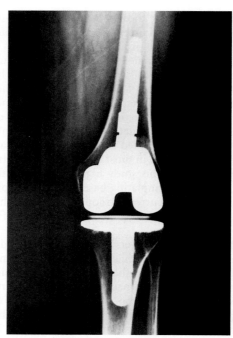

FIG 171.28 Radiograph of a "stubby" stem extension on the tibial component. The "stubby" stem impinges against the lateral cortex of the tibia. If a longer stem extension had been used, the tibial component would have tilted into valgus. Alternatively, the whole component could be medialized, but this would result in medial overhang of the prosthesis. In this case, an offset stem is required.

Generally, the high degree of modularity available with today's knee systems has obviated what little need there is for custom components.

SUMMARY

Revision TKA is not straightforward and is not technically easy. Instruments and guides are not as useful as they are for primary surgery. The surgeon needs to develop a good understanding of the principles of revision arthroplasty, and thorough preoperative planning is necessary. Even in the hands of experienced, well-prepared surgeons, complications and failures may occur.

Suarez et al.[65] asked the question, "Why do revision knee arthroplasties fail?" In their retrospective review of 566 revision knee arthroplasties, 12% failed at an average of 40.1 months. Predominant reasons for failure included infection (46%), aseptic loosening (19%), and instability (13%). Knees revised for infection had a fourfold higher re-revision rate (21%) compared with those revised for aseptic loosening (4.3%).

Use of a systematic approach to revision TKA can minimize failure. The surgeon must identify the reason for implant failure, rule out infection, and develop a preoperative plan. Optimal exposure, meticulous management of soft tissues, and knowledge of the techniques are essential. Minimizing bone loss, managing bone defects, and reconstructing the gaps while balancing soft tissues are the critical steps. Finally, adequate fixation is attained and the appropriate amount of constraint is used. Adhering to these steps will help the clinician achieve a well-aligned limb with a stable and securely fixed implant that allows restoration of function.

KEY REFERENCES

8. Brassard MF, Insall JN, Scuderi GR: Revision of aseptic failed total knee arthroplasty. In Scott WN, editor: *Surgery of the knee*, ed 4, Philadelphia, 2006, Churchill Livingstone Elsevier, pp 1761–1781.

13. Dennis DA: Evaluation of the painful total knee arthroplasty. *J Arthroplasty* 19(4 Suppl 1):35–40, 2004.

17. Engh GA, Ammeen DJ: Periprosthetic fractures adjacent to total knee implants: treatment and clinical results. *Instr Course Lect* 47:437–448, 1998.

18. Fehring TK, McAvoy G: Fluoroscopic evaluation of the painful total knee arthroplasty. *Clin Orthop Relat Res* 331:226–233, 1996.

19. Fehring TK, Odum S, Olekson C, et al: Stem fixation in revision total knee arthroplasty: a comparative analysis. *Clin Orthop Relat Res* 416:217–224, 2003.

28. Haas SB, Insall JN, Montgomery W, III, et al: Revision total knee arthroplasty with use of modular components with stems inserted without cement. *J Bone Joint Surg Am* 77:1700–1707, 1995.

29. Haidukewych GJ, Jacofsky DJ, Pagnano MW, et al: Functional results after revision of well-fixed components for stiffness after primary total knee arthroplasty. *J Arthroplasty* 20:133–138, 2005.

31. Hanssen AH, Pagnano MW: Revision of failed patellar components. *Instr Course Lect* 53:201–206, 2004.

32. Hanssen AD, Rand JD: Evaluation and treatment of infection at the site of a total hip or knee arthroplasty. *Instr Course Lect* 48:111–122, 1999.

42. Long WJ, Scuderi GR: Porous tantalum cones for large metaphyseal tibial defects in revision total knee arthroplasty: a minimum 2 year follow-up. *J Arthroplasty* 24:1086–1092, 2009.

44. Lucey SD, Scuderi GR, Kelly MA, et al: A practical approach to dealing with bone loss in revision total knee arthroplasty. *Orthopedics* 23:1036–1041, 2000.

46. Meneghini RM, Lewallen DG, Hanssen AD: Use of porous tantalum metaphyseal cones for severe tibial bone loss during revision total knee replacement. *J Bone Joint Surg Am* 90:78–84, 2008.

47. Mont MA, Serna FK, Krackow KA, et al: Exploration of radiographically normal total knee replacements for unexplained pain. *Clin Orthop Relat Res* 331:216–219, 1996.

62. Scuderi GR: Revision total knee arthroplasty: how much constraint is enough? *Clin Orthop Relat Res* 392:300–305, 2001.

63. Scuderi GR, Insall JN: Revision total knee arthroplasty with cemented fixation. *Tech Orthop* 7:96–105, 1993.

71. Whiteside LA, Ohl MD: Tibial tubercle osteotomy for exposure of the difficult total knee arthroplasty. *Clin Orthop Relat Res* 206:6–9, 1990.

The references for this chapter can also be found on www.expertconsult.com.

172

The Infected Total Knee Replacement

Erik P. Severson, Kevin I. Perry, Arlen D. Hanssen

INTRODUCTION

Periprosthetic joint infection (PJI) remains a challenging complication and is a leading reason for failure following total knee replacement (TKR). The economic burden of PJI exceeds $1 billion annually in the United States alone.[78] The difficulty in confirming a diagnosis combined with the complexity and duration of treatment options often overwhelm patients and their treating physicians.[80] It has been suggested that the demand for primary TKR is expected to grow by 673% in the year 2030.[52] As such, an associated increase in the number of infected knee arthroplasties is also likely.

Efforts at infection prevention have recently intensified, largely because of initiatives led by institutions that are increasingly responsible for the financial burden associated with infection treatment. Prevention relies on augmentation of the host response, optimizing the wound environment, and reduction of bacterial contamination in the preoperative, intraoperative, and postoperative time periods (Table 172.1).[37] Additionally, understanding the principles of proper diagnosis and treatment of the infected TKR are essential to patient outcome.

The treatment of PJI has become increasingly standardized over the past several decades. This includes a thorough débridement, the use of high-dose local antibiotics, intravenous (IV) antibiotic therapy, and an appropriate delay prior to TKA reimplantation.

INCIDENCE, RISK FACTORS, AND PREVENTION

The exact incidence of PJI varies throughout the literature and is highly dependent on patient, surgeon, and hospital factors. Despite the variability, most arthroplasty surgeons report an incidence of PJI of 1% to 2% after primary TKA.[51,82]

There are many inherent patient risk factors that are known to predispose toward postoperative deep infection. Host factors include a diagnosis of rheumatoid arthritis,[10,47,107] skin ulcers,[107] diabetes mellitus,[28,72] history of malignancy,[6] obesity,[28,72,92,101] a history of smoking,[72] renal or liver transplantation,[90] HIV-positive status,[71,96] prior open knee surgery or periarticular fractures,[47] and prior septic arthritis or adjacent osteomyelitis.[48] Every effort should be made preoperatively to optimize medical conditions and minimize these risk factors. For example, patients on immunosuppressive therapy often benefit from stopping certain medications in the perioperative time period (Table 172.2).[45] Additionally, preoperative *Staphylococcus aureus* screening and decolonization have proven to be cost-effective methods of reducing surgical site infections.[16]

There has been an interest in identifying preoperative nutritional factors that may influence the rate of PJI. In their series, Nelson et al. demonstrated that a low serum albumin increased the risk of PJI more than obesity.[67] Patients should be assessed preoperatively for risk factors and should be optimized medically to reduce their risk of PJI. Other factors that have been shown to increase the risk of PJI include an increased international normalized ratio (INR) in the postoperative period,[63] recent intra-articular injection of corticosteroids,[70] and prolonged operative times.[6,73]

Proper use of antibiotic prophylaxis remains the single-most effective method of reducing infection in total joint arthroplasty.[42] The use of low-dose antibiotic-loaded bone cement (ABLC) has become commonplace for reduction of infection in high-risk patients undergoing primary and revision TKA.[47] Thorough wound irrigation, meticulous surgical technique, and careful wound closure are all important variables that the surgeon can control that aid in preventing PJI.

Acute hematogenous infection after TKR remains a persistent problem in arthroplasty patients. The rate of bacteremia after invasive procedures appears to be highest with dental procedures,[100] followed by genitourinary manipulation and lowest in association with gastrointestinal procedures.[27] As such, invasive procedures that are known to cause bacteremia should be avoided in the first 3 to 6 months after TKR, if possible.

Currently, the American Academy of Orthopaedic Surgeons (AAOS) no longer has published guidelines for the use of prophylactic antibiotics for high-risk patients undergoing a high-risk procedure. Still, it is the authors' preference to provide patients with prophylactic antibiotics prior to high-risk procedures for at least the first year after TKR.

MICROBIOLOGY AND DIAGNOSIS

Although the precise diagnosis of PJI remains controversial, the Musculoskeletal Infection Society (MSIS) has recently provided criteria to consistently establish a diagnosis of infection[82]:

1. There is a sinus tract communicating with the prosthesis (Fig. 172.1); or
2. A pathogen is isolated by culture from at least two separate tissue or fluid samples obtained from the affected prosthetic joint; or
3. Four of the following six criteria exist:
   a. Elevated serum erythrocyte sedimentation rate (ESR) and serum C-reactive protein (CRP) concentration
   b. Elevated synovial leukocyte count

TABLE 172.1	**Prevention of Deep Prosthetic Infection**		
	Preoperative Period	**Operative Period**	**Postoperative Period**
Host	Altered immune system	Anesthetic agents	Rheumatoid arthritis
	Immunosuppressive medications	Transfusions	Altered immune system
	Diabetes mellitus	—	—
	Rheumatoid arthritis		
	Advanced age		
	Malnutrition		
	Anesthetic risk		
Bacteria	Urinary tract infection	Instrument sterilization	Antibiotic prophylaxis
	Skin ulcers	Operating room traffic	Urinary tract management
	Poor dental hygiene	Personnel ("dispersers")	Invasive procedures
	Preoperative shaving	—	Remote sites of infection
	Preoperative showers	Facemasks/hoods	Clean dental procedures
	Prolonged hospitalization	Exhaust suits	—
		Laminar airflow	
		Ultraviolet light	
		Prophylactic antibiotics	
		Antibiotic impregnated PMMA	
		Skin preparation	
		Gloves	
		Drapes/gowns	
		Wound irrigants	
		Sucker tips	
		Splash basins	
Wound	Extensive scarring	Duration of procedure	Postoperative hematoma
	Prior surgery	Surgical technique	Wound drainage
	Prior infection	Sutures	Skin necrosis
	Obesity	Implant selection	Reoperation
	Vascular disease	Antibiotic impregnated PMMA	Loose prosthesis
	Anatomic site	Bone graft	Particulate debris
	Condition of skin	Surgical drains	—
		Wound closure	

PMMA, Polymethylmethacrylate cement.
From Morrey BF: *An K-N: Joint replacement arthroplasty,* Philadelphia, 2003, Churchill Livingstone, p 1192, with permission from Mayo Foundation for Medical Education and Research; Hanssen AD, Osmon DR, Nelson CL: Prevention of deep periprosthetic joint infection. *Instr Course Lect* 46:555–567, 1997.

TABLE 172.2	**Perioperative Anti-rheumatoid Medication Recommendations**[a]	
Medication	**Important Drug Interactions**	**Comments**
Corticosteroids	Corticosteroid use with fluoroquinolones increases the risk of tendon rupture. Antifungal agents and clarithromycin may increase levels of corticosteroids.	Perioperative use depends on level of potential surgical stress.
Methotrexate	Methotrexate along with intravenous penicillins may lead to neutropenia.	Continue perioperatively for all procedures. Consider withholding 1 to 2 doses of methotrexate for patients with poorly controlled diabetes; the elderly; and those with liver, kidney, or lung disease who are undergoing moderate or intensive procedures.
Leflunomide	Leflunomide may elevate levels of warfarin and rifampin.	Continue for minor procedures. Withhold 1-2 days before moderate and intensive procedures and restart 1-2 weeks later.
Sulfasalazine	May increase INR in patients on warfarin.	Continue for all procedures.
Hydroxychloroquine	None	Continue for all procedures.
TNF antagonists	Avoid live vaccines in patients taking these agents; otherwise, no significant perioperative drug-drug interactions.	Continue for minor procedures. For moderate to intensive procedures, withhold etanercept for 1 week, and plan surgery for the end of the dosing interval for adalumimab and infliximab. Restart 10-14 days postoperatively.
IL-1 antagonist	None	Continue for minor procedures. Withhold 1-2 days before surgery and restart 10 days postoperatively for moderate to intensive procedures.

[a]American Academy of Orthopaedic Surgeons (2006).
IL, Interleukin; *INR,* international normalized ratio; *NSAIDs,* nonsteroidal anti-inflammatory drugs; *TNF,* tumor necrosis factor.
From Howe CR, Gardner GC, Kadel NJ: Perioperative medication management for the patient with rheumatoid arthritis. *J Am Acad Orthop Surg* 14:544–551, 2006.

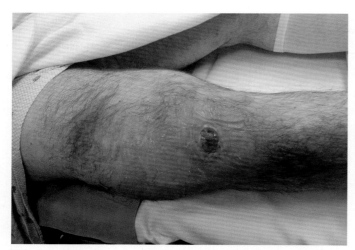

FIG 172.1 Photograph of a chronic sinus tract over the antero-lateral aspect of the knee joint in a patient with a chronically infected TKR.

c. Elevated synovial neutrophil percentage (polymorpho-nuclear [PMN]%)
d. Presence of purulence in the affected joint
e. Isolation of a microorganism in one culture of periprosthetic tissue or fluid
f. Greater than five neutrophils per high-power field in five high-power fields observed from histologic analysis of periprosthetic tissue at 9400 magnification

Optimal treatment outcomes are achieved by accurately identifying the offending microorganism(s), if possible, and providing treatment based on the microorganism and its susceptibilities.[72] Various features of individual bacteria complicate the clinician's ability to identify them with tissue or synovial fluid cultures. These features include their paucity in joint fluid, fastidious growth, the presence of a biofilm, and the previous antibiotic therapy. In most series, gram-positive bacteria are the most common offending organism*; however, polymicrobial infections are also common and represent approximately 9% of infected TKR.[72] Polymicrobial infections can be difficult to treat and are often associated with a reduced cure rate compared to monomicrobial infection.[108]

The identification of biofilm-creating organisms via traditional culture methods has lacked optimal sensitivity and specificity.[94] Culture-independent molecular methods have been developed to improve the diagnosis of prosthetic joint. Detection of 16S ribosomal deoxyribonucleic acid by polymerase chain reaction is one example of this technology.[58] Still, these techniques are in their infancy and need further research and testing prior to universal implementation by clinicians.

More recently, the detection of biomarkers identified in synovial fluid taken from TKRs has shown promise, in being both sensitive and specific.[21] Five biomarkers have emerged as 100% sensitive and 100% specific in the diagnosis of PJI. These biomarkers are human alpha-defensin, neutrophil elastase-2 (ELA-2), bactericidal/permeability-increasing protein (BPI), neutrophil gelatinase-associated lipocalin (NGAL), and lactoferrin.[21] Commercially made kits are now available for their clinical use.

The use of an alpha defensin immunoassay, in particular, has increased significantly since the last edition of this chapter.[†] Alpha-defensin protein is an antimicrobial peptide released by the body's neutrophils when responding to a pathogen in the synovial fluid.[23] This test is now widely available and has been shown to provide consistent results regardless of the organism type, Gram type, species, or virulence of the organism.[23] Further study is still needed to test its efficacy in the immediate postoperative setting as well as in the immunocompromised.

Sonication of implants to dislodge and culture adherent bacteria is another useful method to identify microorganisms. This technique involves low frequency ultrasound waves passed through liquid surrounding the prosthesis. Once bacteria are liberated from the prosthesis, the fluid can then be accurately cultured. It has been demonstrated to be an effective method to disrupt the biofilm and provides culture results more sensitive than conventional periprosthetic tissue culture in patients who have received antibiotics within 14 days of surgery.[95] This technique is now widely used in the authors' institution to improve the detection of organisms causing PJI.

A thorough history, physical examination, plain radiographs (Fig. 172.2), arthrocentesis, and assessment of inflammatory markers (ESR and CRP) are the cornerstones of the work-up for infection.

The timing of the clinical presentation is a critical factor in the identification and implementation of the correct treatment strategy. The various clinical presentations have been characterized and classified and can be a useful guide for treatment of the infected TKR (Table 172.3).[81] Postoperative infections diagnosed by positive intraoperative cultures after revision arthroplasty are generally low virulence organisms such coagulase-negative staphylococci and *Propionibacterium* spp. and are best treated by organism specific antibiotic suppression.[57]

In the early postoperative period, the diagnosis of acute infection can be difficult. The diagnosis is typically confirmed by joint arthrocentesis, as the ESR and CRP levels are nonspecific in the early postoperative period.[8,53,105] Persistent wound drainage is strongly suggestive of infection and should be treated with early irrigation and débridement.[104] Cultures of serous wound drainage are difficult to interpret and potentially misleading and are therefore discouraged. Empiric antibiotic use for persistent wound drainage should be avoided, as this suppresses the clinical symptoms of infection and potentially delays diagnosis and eliminates the possibility of implant salvage.

Acute hematogenous infections typically present with the sudden onset of pain in a previously well-functioning arthroplasty.[4] These patients often present with an elevated ESR and CRP, but the cornerstone for diagnosis is arthrocentesis. The synovial fluid should be analyzed for quantitative leukocyte count, cell differential, and culture for aerobic and anaerobic bacteria. Empiric antibiotics for the unexplained painful prosthesis, without attempt at definitive diagnosis, should not be practiced.

The vast majority of patients with an infected total knee arthroplasty are diagnosed in the subacute or chronic setting. Persistent pain after TKR, prolonged postoperative wound drainage (see Fig. 172.1), and TKR stiffness can all be indicative

---

*References 21, 58, 72, 75, 86, 87, and 94.

†References 8, 9, 20, 22, 23, 57, 75, 81, 83, 86, 87, and 95.

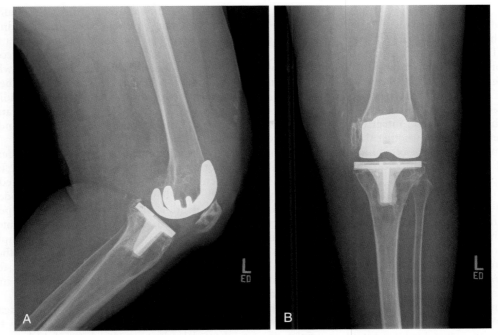

FIG 172.2 (A) Anteroposterior and (B) lateral radiographs of a patient with a chronically infected total knee arthroplasty. Radiolucencies at the bone-cement interface, which are typically late findings in periprosthetic infection, can be seen inferior to the tibial component on both views.

TABLE 172.3   Classification System of Prosthetic Joint Infection: Time to Onset of Infection Dictates Treatment

	Type 1	Type 2	Type 3	Type 4
Timing of diagnosis	Positive intraoperative cultures	Early postoperative infection	Acute hematogenous infection	Late (chronic) infection
Definition	Two or more positive cultures at surgery	Infection occurs within first month after surgery	Hematogenous seeding of previously well functioning arthroplasty	Chronic indolent clinical course; infection present for more than 1 month
Treatment	Appropriate antibiotics	Attempt at débridement with prosthesis salvage	Attempt at débridement with prosthesis salvage or prosthesis removal	Prosthesis removal

of PJI. Plain radiographs may reveal radiolucencies, focal osteopenia or osteolysis of subchondral bone, and periosteal new bone formation when infection is present.[65] All patients with suspected infection should be evaluated with a CRP, ESR, and arthrocentesis of the TKR. Some centers advocate for the use interleukin-6 (IL-6) to diagnose PJI. The advantage of IL-6 is that it quickly returns to normal after surgery with a mean half-life of only 15 hours.[89] Further study is needed, however, before its routine use becomes a standard of care.

Arthrocentesis is paramount to the work-up and evaluation of PJI. Synovial fluid analysis and culture facilitates identification of offending microorganisms. In addition, the synovial fluid quantitative leukocyte count and differential can be indicative of infection when a microorganism cannot be identified. Although the quantitative leukocyte count and differential may resemble a native joint infection in the acute hematogenous infection (neutrophil differential >90% and total nucleated cell counts >50,000/μL), most chronic TKR infections are associated with much lower values.[31,59,93] Although various cutoffs have been proposed, the authors have found a synovial fluid leukocyte differential of greater than 65% neutrophils (or a leukocyte count of >1.7 × 10₃/μL) to be both sensitive and specific for the diagnosis of PJI in patients without inflammatory arthropathy.[93] Patients should have all antibiotics discontinued several weeks prior to aspiration, as failure to do so can make microorganism identification difficult.[3] The use of radioisotope scans to diagnose PJI should be used judiciously.

Intraoperative evaluation of surgical tissue specimens can be used to help confirm the diagnosis of PJI. Gram stain and microscopic evaluation of frozen tissue samples are the two most commonly used intraoperative measures. Although commonly used across North America, the Gram stain is often unreliable, with both low sensitivity and specificity.[2,25] Microscopic evaluation of frozen tissue samples has been used with variable results.[24,30,55,66,68] This variability can be accounted for by differences in technique to retrieve tissue samples, pathologist experience, and the definition used to identify acute inflammation. Microscopic analysis of an intraoperative frozen section is most effective when an experienced pathologist evaluates the tissue samples.

TREATMENT

Several variables should be considered prior to initiating treatment of PJI. These variables include: (1) determining whether the infection is superficial or deep, (2) the duration of symptoms (and timing of index arthroplasty), (3) identification and optimization of host factors that may adversely affect the treatment of the infection, (4) appraisal of the soft tissue envelope surrounding the knee, (5) the integrity of the extensor mechanism, (6) determination of whether the implant is loose or well fixed, (7) identification of the offending microorganism, and (8) transfer of patient care to the definitive treatment center.

Treatment goals of the infected total knee arthroplasty include eradication of infection, alleviation of pain, and maintenance of a functional extremity. When treating PJI, six options exist. These include (1) antibiotic suppression, (2) open débridement and polyethylene exchange, (3) two-stage reimplantation, (4) arthrodesis, (5) resection arthroplasty, and (6) amputation. The proper implementation of these treatment options depend on host factors, microorganism virulence and sensitivities, and bone quantity/quality around the knee. With the exception of chronic antibiotic suppression, which does not eliminate infection, the cornerstone treatment principles of these treatment options include thorough surgical débridement, combined with the appropriate use of antibiotics and optimization of the host response.

Antibiotic Suppression

Antibiotic suppression alone does not eliminate deep periprosthetic infection. Nevertheless, this strategy can be used for treatment when the following criteria are met: (1) prosthesis removal is not feasible (usually because of medical co-morbidities, which preclude an operation), (2) the microorganism has low virulence, (3) the microorganism is susceptible to an oral antibiotic, (4) the antibiotic can be tolerated without serious toxicity, and (5) the prosthesis is not loose.[98] The presence of other joint arthroplasties or a cardiac valvular prosthesis are relative contraindications to this treatment approach.

The reported success rates with antibiotic suppression alone are low, ranging from 18% to 25%.[5,38] Nevertheless, when implementing this strategy, combination therapy tends to be more successful than use of a single antibiotic alone. Given its low success rate and the strict criteria for its use, judicious use of antibiotic suppression alone is recommended.

Débridement With Prosthesis Retention

Open irrigation and débridement is indicated for the acute infection in the early postoperative period (type II) and for the acute hematogenous infection (type III) of a previously well-functioning prosthesis. Specifically, this treatment strategy should only used when the following criteria are met: (1) the patient has been experiencing symptoms of infection for less than 4 weeks, (2) the microorganism identified is a susceptible gram-positive organisms, (3) the patient has not had prolonged postoperative drainage or a draining sinus tract, and (4) there is no evidence of prosthetic loosening.[12] Arthroscopic irrigation and débridement should never be attempted, because of inferior results as compared with open débridement.[64]

The results of open irrigation and débridement with polyethylene exchange are difficult to interpret because of differences in microbiology and subsequent antibiotic management,

variability in the time to treatment, the quality of the surrounding soft tissue envelope, the variability in débridement, the status of implant fixation, and the criteria used for success in each report. Kim et al.[50] reported a success rate of 60.7% with irrigation and débridement (with or without polyethylene exchange) for the acutely infected TKR. They identified several variables that improved outcomes, including a shorter time out from the index TKR, a lower preoperative ESR, identification of a susceptible microorganism, and exchange of the polyethylene.

The timing of the irrigation and débridement in relation to the onset of symptoms is critical.[12,64,79,81,91] In their study of 24 infected TKRs, Mont et al.[64] demonstrated a success rate of 100% in patients treated with open débridement and component retention in the early postoperative period and a success rate of 71% in patients with acute hematogenous infections treated within 30 days. These authors emphasized their strict patient selection criteria, attempting prosthesis salvage only in patients demonstrating infection for less than 30 days. Prosthetic retention should not be considered in patients with late, chronic infections.

Early treatment of specific microorganisms can affect treatment outcomes. This is particularly true for *S. aureus,* where delay in treatment beyond 48 hours after the onset of symptoms results in poorer outcomes.[54] Similarly, *S. aureus* PJI is associated with the lowest success rate following irrigation and débridement compared to other offending microorganisms.[19,79,107] In contrast, the penicillin-susceptible *streptococcal* species, if treated within 10 days of symptom onset, results in successful prosthetic retention in 90% of patients.[62] Early irrigation and débridement and polyethylene exchange should be used in healthy hosts with susceptible microorganisms, as failure of prior irrigation and débridement can compromise outcomes of the two-stage exchange protocol.[84]

Resection Arthroplasty

Resection arthroplasty is defined by implant removal with no subsequent knee reconstruction. Although the indications for this treatment strategy are rare, the ideal candidate is a patient with limited ambulatory demands, as resection arthroplasty allows the patient to sit more readily than a knee arthrodesis.

The technique for resection arthroplasty is straightforward and consists of an initial débridement and removal of all infected tissue and foreign material, temporary femoral-tibial fixation with pins or sutures to maintain alignment and apposition of the tibia and femur, and cast immobilization for at least six months. Resection arthroplasty is an effective treatment of infection, but most patients experience some pain, instability, and have limited ambulatory capacity. As such, current use of resection arthroplasty is limited.

Arthrodesis

Traditionally, arthrodesis was considered the standard treatment option for an infected TKR because of excellent infection eradication, pain alleviation, and providing reasonable function. The disadvantage of this technique is the elimination of knee motion, which can make sitting and other activities cumbersome. Currently, the functional limitations of an arthrodesis are poorly tolerated by most patients. When considering an arthrodesis, the surgeon should have a detailed discussion with the patient regarding the physical limitations and functional restrictions of knee arthrodesis. Indications for knee arthrodesis for an infected TKR are narrowing and include extensor mechanism disruption in young individuals with high functional demand jobs or patients with a poor soft-tissue envelope requiring extensive soft tissue reconstruction.[38] Relative contraindications to arthrodesis include (1) bilateral knee disease, (2) ipsilateral ankle or hip disease, (3) severe segmental bone loss, and (4) contralateral extremity amputation.

The fixation techniques most commonly used for knee arthrodesis include external fixation and internal fixation with either an intramedullary (IM) nail or dual plate fixation. The type of the prior knee implant, extent of bone deficiency, and the arthrodesis technique all affect the success of knee arthrodesis.[16,26,38]

Complications of knee arthrodesis following TKR are numerous and include nonunion (most common), malunion, recurrent infection, and ipsilateral limb fracture. Complications specific to external fixation include neurovascular injury during pin insertion, pin site infection, and fracture through pin sites.

In their report on 85 consecutive patients who underwent knee arthrodesis for an infected TKR, Mabry et al.[56] demonstrated successful fusion in 41 of 61 patients treated with external fixation, with an associated infection rate of 4.9%. In patients treated with IM nailing, successful fusion was achieved in 23 of 24 patients, with an associated infection rate of 8.3%. The authors concluded that knee arthrodesis remains a reasonable alternative for difficult to treat TKR patients. Still, they argued, one must consider the risks of both nonunion and infection when choosing the fixation method in this difficult patient population. From this report, IM nailing appears to have a higher trend toward successful union but is associated with a higher risk of recurrent infection compared to external fixation.

Amputation

Amputation is rarely indicated in the setting of TKR infection. The only true indications for amputation are life-threatening systemic sepsis that cannot be controlled with local débridement or massive bone loss that precludes reconstruction or arthrodesis in a patient that cannot tolerate resection arthroplasty. The frequency of amputation is estimated to occur in less than 5% of patients who are treated for an infected TKR.[38]

Amputation should occur at a level that maximizes function yet facilitates the eradication of the infection. Many patients have a cavernous bone defect of the distal femur, and local muscle transposition can be extremely helpful for dead space management as well as optimizing the soft tissue envelope of the amputation stump. Following amputation, many elderly patients become limited ambulators or become nonambulatory because of the increased energy expenditure required for walking.

In their series of 23 patients treated with above-the-knee amputation (AKA) for a failed TKR, Pring et al.[76] demonstrated that only seven patients were able to ambulate regularly. Similarly, 20 of the 23 used a wheelchair part of the day and 12 (55%) were confined to the wheelchair. The authors concluded that functional outcomes after AKA are quite poor in this difficult patient population. Fedorka et al.[29] similarly demonstrated functional outcomes following AKAs used for treatment of PJI were very poor. In this study, only half of the patients were able to ambulate postoperatively, and the patients that did ambulate demonstrated a very low overall functional ability.

Two-Stage Reimplantation

Although some authors advocated for a single-stage exchange,[85] the two-stage reimplantation protocol is currently of the gold-standard treatment of patients with a chronic, late infection after TKR.[13] This technique consists of two stages, as its name implies. The first stage consists of performing a resection arthroplasty, thorough débridement of all foreign and infected material and insertion of an antibiotic spacer. The patient is then treated with a 6-week course of IV antibiotics and a period of time off of antibiotics prior the second stage reimplantation of a TKR. Contraindications to this technique are medical conditions that prevent multiple reconstructive procedures, extensor mechanism disruption, and a soft tissue envelope about the knee joint that precludes reconstruction.[38] Contraindication to reimplantation is persistent infection. Occasionally, patients may be referred to another institution between the first and second stage of their reimplantation with an antibiotic spacer and débridement performed by somewhere other than the definitive treatment center. The authors strongly recommend performing a redébridement on these patients, as unpublished data out of the Mayo Clinic demonstrated retained cement is found in approximately 50% of knees and positive cultures are obtained in over 40% of patients at the time of redébridement. Using inflammatory markers to assess the eradication of infection in these patients has proven unreliable.

A six-week course of IV antibiotic administration prior to reimplantation has provided excellent success rates and is the current practice of most North American surgeons.[32,46,109] Nevertheless, the duration of antibiotic therapy can be individualized for each patient based on the virulence and number of offending microorganisms and patient co-morbidities.

Success with a modern, two-stage protocol for the treatment of the infected TKR ranges from 85% to 95% depending on the duration of follow-up.[‡] The precise duration of time between the first and second stages has not been established. Initially, a poor success rate (57%) was reported, treating 14 patients with insertion of a new prosthesis within several weeks after removal of the infected knee prosthesis.[77] In contrast, the two-stage reimplantation protocol proposed by Insall et al.[46] has been a highly effective method of treatment. This protocol includes soft tissue débridement, removal of the infected prosthesis and cement followed by 6 weeks of IV antibiotics, and subsequent reimplantation 6 weeks later. The success of this protocol was confirmed in a follow-up report of 64 infected TKR.[32] Modern two-stage exchange protocols follow many of the principals first introduced by Insall, but the addition of antibiotic-loaded cement (ABLC) in the form of spacers or for prosthetic fixation has proved a useful adjunct.

In addition to the ABLC spacers used during the first stage of a two-stage exchange, the use of antibiotic-loaded cement for prosthesis fixation at reimplantation has proved effective.[36,38] In their series of 89 infected TKR treated by two-stage reimplantation, Hanssen and Osmon[36] demonstrated that the use of ABLC for prosthesis fixation at the time of reimplantation was associated with a significant decrease in the rate of reinfection. Specifically, the authors demonstrated 7 (28%) of the 25 knees without the use of ABLC developed reinfection, compared with only 3 (4.7%) of 64 knees in which ABLC was used for prosthesis

---

‡References 7, 33, 34, 54, 81, and 97.

fixation. Low dose ABLC (<2 g antibiotic/40 g cement) is the recommended dosage for prophylaxis in reimplantation or in primary TKAs in high-risk patients or for prosthesis fixation at reimplantation.[35]

Antibiotic Cement Spacers

After TKR resection and débridement, local antibiotic delivery can be facilitated via static or articulating antibiotic spacers. Historically, many authors advocated for antibiotic ratios of only 1 g of antibiotic per 40 g batch of bone cement in the ABLC.[37,38,107] Currently, most investigators are using much higher ratios (4 to 6 g of antibiotics per 40 g batch of bone cement).[33,40,74] It is important to remember that these higher dosage ratios of antibiotic cement should be reserved only for the treatment of active infection, as greater than 4.5 g of antibiotic powder substantially diminishes the mechanical strength of bone cement and should not be used for prosthesis fixation.[41]

Antibiotic elution is highly dependent on the bone cement porosity. Mixing high doses of powdered antibiotics fortuitously creates considerable cement porosity, facilitating increased antibiotic elution for at least 4 weeks postoperatively.[40] Additionally, combining two antibiotics in bone cement improves elution of both antibiotics. The two most commonly used antibiotics in clinical practice currently are vancomycin and tobramycin.[38] The use of at least 3.6 g of tobramycin and 1 g of vancomycin per package of bone cement is recommended to obtain effective elution levels.[60,74] The local levels of antibiotic elution typically far exceed the levels observed in the serum during parenteral antibiotic administration and has been proven to be safe.[40,88] Up to 12 g of antibiotics per 40 g batch of bone cement may be added without prohibiting cement polymerization.[1] The authors currently use a ratio of 3 g of vancomycin, 3.6 g of tobramycin, and 150 mg of amphotericin per 40 g batch of cement for spacers used in the treatment of the infected TKR.

Antibiotic spacers function primarily to deliver local antimicrobial agents and maintain collateral ligament length.[11] Potential disadvantages of antibiotic block spacers include the presence of a foreign body and bone loss incurred (when using a static antibiotic spacer) while awaiting reimplantation.[14] There are several different types of antibiotic spacers that have been described. These include a simple tibiofemoral block, the molded arthrodesis block, articulating mobile spacers, and medullary dowels.

The simple tibiofemoral block was the original spacer block and was preformed and then inserted into the tibiofemoral space after the cement had polymerized. These blocks were shaped as either simple "hockey pucks" or "L-shaped" spacers, inserted into the tibiofemoral space. Additional antibiotic beads or thin discs were often placed into the suprapatellar pouch or lateral gutters to maximize antibiotic delivery. Disadvantages of this spacer include the inability to match the surfaces of the block with the irregular surfaces of the distal femur and proximal tibia, subluxation of the bony surfaces off of the spacer surface, risk of extensor mechanism necrosis, wound breakdown, and progressive bone loss.[14]

The molded arthrodesis block avoided some of the difficulties encountered with preformed spacer blocks.[40] These spacers are fabricated so that the cement is placed within the knee in a doughy state and polymerized within the knee so that the cement can conform to the irregular contour of the femur and

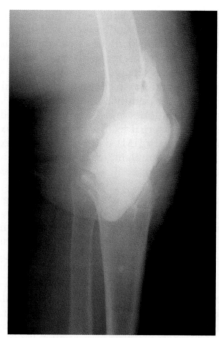

FIG 172.3 Lateral radiograph of a static antibiotic cement spacer, molded to conform to the femoral and tibial osseous surfaces with extension into the suprapatellar pouch to prevent scarring and adhesion of the extensor mechanism to the anterior femur.

tibia (Fig. 172.3). This macrointerdigitation of the cement into bony defects, the intercondylar notch, and extension into the medullary canals and suprapatellar pouch enhances the stability of the knee joint. In turn, patients are more comfortable during treatment, and less bone loss occurs between the first and second stages. Despite the interdigitation of cement into bone, these spacers are easy to remove at the time of reimplantation by splitting the block into several large pieces with an osteotome.

The mobile articulating spacer technique allows the patient to place the knee through a range of motion during the period following prosthesis removal and insertion of the new prosthesis.[33,44] In addition, this technique allows for easier exposure at the time of reimplantation. These spacers were originally facsimiles of shaped antibiotic-impregnated cement into femoral and tibial components.[33] Eventually, a system of molds was developed to incorporate small metal runners and polyethylene tibial trays so that cement surfaces were not articulating against each other.[33] Similarly, the use of a real femoral component coupled with a polyethylene insert cemented into place has become commonplace.[44] Still, theoretical advantages of the articulating antibiotic have yet to be proven.[39] The final functional result appears to be more dependent on the patient's overall medical and musculoskeletal functional status.[102]

The authors are strong proponents of using a real femoral component coupled with a polyethylene insert, as the cement-on-cement articulation seems to create a large amount of cement debris and scar formation at the time of reimplantation. In this chapter, we describe a technique for implanting a mobile spacer without the premolded, cement mobile spacers. Regardless of whether a static or mobile articulating antibiotic-loaded spacer is used, strong consideration should be given to insertion of antibiotic cement dowels into the canals.[40] There is extension of the infectious process into the medullary canals of the femur or tibia in roughly one-third of infected knee replacements without stems.[61] Insertion of antibiotic-impregnated medullary dowels is preferable to insertion of ABLC beads, as beads can be extremely difficult to remove at the time of reimplantation. A tapered cement dowel fashioned from the nozzle of a cement gun provides an excellent size and shape to be inserted into, and subsequently removed from, the medullary canal.[40]

Block spacers should be supplemented by external immobilization, such as a brace or cast, as the patient awaits the reimplantation. Patients with mobile articulating spacers are encouraged to participate with range of motion exercises and are allowed up to 50% partial weight bearing.[33] Further study is needed to assess the potential functional ability with a well-fixed mobile spacer.

Time Period Between Resection and Reimplantation.

Patients undergoing two-stage reimplantation are typically anemic, and 88% require allogeneic blood transfusions, particularly because the two surgeries are temporally close.[69] The presence of infection precludes traditional alternatives such as reinfusion or autologous blood donation; thus novel blood management practices are required in this patient population. A study of 39 consecutive two-stage reimplantations was enrolled in a prospective study to determine whether the use of recombinant human erythropoietin could lower allogeneic transfusion requirements.[18] When compared with a group of 81 patients not receiving recombinant human erythropoietin, the requirement for transfusion was significantly lowered ($p < 0.001$). In patients receiving recombinant human erythropoietin, 52% avoided transfusion for the entire time period, encompassing both stages of reimplantation.[18]

Although the precise time period between the first and second stage of the two-stage protocol has yet to be defined, most surgeons base this decision on evidence that the infection has been eradicated. Serially following the ESR and CRP can be important factors when considering reimplantation. In just 4 or 6 weeks, the ESR is not expected to normalize, however; the ESR should begin to trend down, especially relative to preoperative levels.[38] The CRP levels typically normalize by the 21st day after surgery, and if the levels remain elevated, persistence of infection should be considered.[8,38,105] Aspiration or open biopsy of the knee can be considered in select patients, although it has been the experience of the authors that preoperative aspiration prior to reimplantation lacks both specificity and sensitivity. If there is concern about the presence of persistent infection, it is prudent to perform another débridement, insert new ABLC spacers, close the wound, and await culture and sensitivity testing.

Results of Reimplantation

Mid- to long-term results of two-stage reimplantation have been quite favorable, with reported success rates between 85% to 95%.[32,34] A recent report by Volin et al.[99] demonstrated a 93.5% success rate in 46 infected TKRs, using the two-stage approach at average 5-year follow-up. The authors demonstrated no difference in failure rates between methicillin-sensitive and methicillin-resistant organisms. The authors concluded that two-stage protocol is the treatment of choice for infections involving resistant and virulent organisms, with a modest rate of reinfection. These results suggest a high likelihood of success after two-stage reimplantation for infected TKA that is maintained through the long-term follow up. Despite these promising results using a two-stage protocol, it is clear that morbid obesity, persistent elevation of inflammatory markers, and multiple patient comorbidities predispose patients to higher failure rates.[15,103]

Reinfection is more likely when treating an infected revision TKR, compared to an infected primary TKR.[43] This is intuitive, as revision patients typically have more bone loss and compromise of the soft tissue envelope. Although two-stage reimplantation remains the gold standard for PJI, reinfection following reimplantation can be devastating. In a series of 24 knees treated for reinfection after reimplantation,[41] 10 patients were treated with a successful knee arthrodesis, 5 were treated with infected prostheses maintained on suppressive oral antibiotics, 4 with AKAs, 3 with persistent pseudoarthroses, 1 with resection arthroplasty, and only 1 patient was infection free.

Staged Reimplantation Surgical Technique: Static Spacer

A thorough and complete débridement is paramount to ensure treatment success in a staged reimplantation of an infected TKR. Careful placement of the skin incision is critical, and when multiple prior incisions are present, the most lateral, longitudinal incision that can safely access the knee is recommended. Excision of heavily scarred tissue back to healthy tissue is advised, as well as excision of all sinus tracts. Subcutaneous tissue flap elevation during the approach should be minimized. A formal arthrotomy is preferred through a standard median parapatellar arthrotomy (Fig. 172.4). Subperiosteal release of

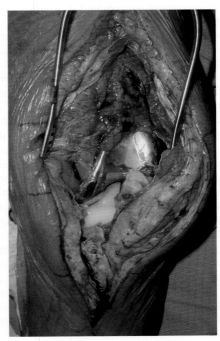

FIG 172.4 Medial parapatellar arthrotomy in a patient undergoing resection of an infected total knee arthroplasty. Gross purulent material and prominent synovial proliferation is visualized throughout the knee.

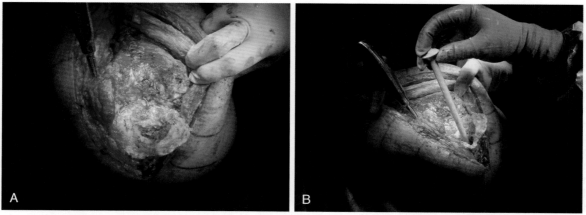

FIG 172.5 (A) Intraoperative picture of infected total knee arthroplasty after initial resection of the prosthetic components, demonstrating grossly purulent material lining the synovium and bone surfaces. (B) Proximal tibia after thorough débridement of purulent debris and necrotic bone, revealing a clean viable bony surface and insertion of an ABLC medullary dowel.

the deep medial collateral ligament allows external rotation of the tibia necessary for adequate exposure. Removal of the tibial polyethylene is performed at this point to reduce the tension on the extensor mechanism.

Eversion of the patella can be extremely difficult and dangerous during the exposure of the infected TKR, and subluxation of the patella is typically all that can be achieved. Adequate external rotation of the tibia allows lateral translation and subluxation of the extensor mechanism, minimizes the need for lateral retinacular release, and avoids undue tension on the patellar tendon insertion. If additional exposure is necessary, a quadriceps snip may be used, as a formal V-Y turndown and tibial tubercle osteotomy are avoided if at all possible because of the potential for extensor mechanism necrosis in this setting.

The femoral, tibial, and patellar components are carefully removed to preserve as much bone stock as possible. Particular attention should be paid to meticulous removal of all cement particles and debris, as well as débridement of any osteolytic defects and nonviable bone (Fig. 172.5). The tibial and femoral IM canals are thoroughly débrided when implants with stems are removed; however, it is not uncommon for the infectious process to extend into the medullary canals, even in the absence of medullary stems. The final step in the débridement process is the synovectomy and scar excision of the suprapatellar pouch, medial and lateral gutters, and posterior capsular region. Synovectomy at this stage facilitates cement and particulate debris removal that may have fallen into the synovium areas during removal of the prosthetic components. These fragments are easily identified and removed, along with the synovium and scar tissue during the synovectomy. It is critical to perform a meticulous and thorough débridement and synovial excision to viable bone and soft tissue. It is also imperative to obtain access and thoroughly débride the posterior aspect of the knee, as this represents a frequent location for missed cement particles and foreign material. Three to five tissue samples are routinely sent for culture and sensitivity testing.

The knee joint is copiously irrigated, and preparation is made for placement of the ABLC spacer. The antibiotic cement is mixed and placed into the tibiofemoral space in the final stages of polymerization to prevent solid interdigitation into

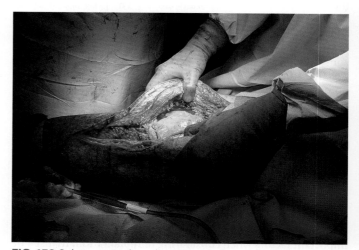

FIG 172.6 Intraoperative photograph of a static molded antibiotic cement spacer inserted after resection of an infected total knee arthroplasty. Notice the extension into the suprapatellar region to prevent adhesion of the extensor mechanism to the anterior femur.

the bone and rather is gently molded to the contour of the distal femur and proximal tibia. Intramedullary antibiotic cement dowels should be inserted prior to insertion of the tibiofemoral spacer. The cement from the tibiofemoral spacer is extended into the suprapatellar space to maintain the length of the extensor mechanism and minimize scarring and contracture against the anterior femur (Fig. 172.6). The wound is then closed over drains. Capsular closure is accomplished with a large absorbable monofilament suture and the skin closed with large monofilament retention sutures and smaller interrupted skin sutures. The importance of perfect epidermal apposition cannot be overemphasized, as this facilitates primary wound healing.

Mobile Spacer Technique

The technique for implanting an articulating antibiotic spacer uses similar principles to any revision TKR. Once the

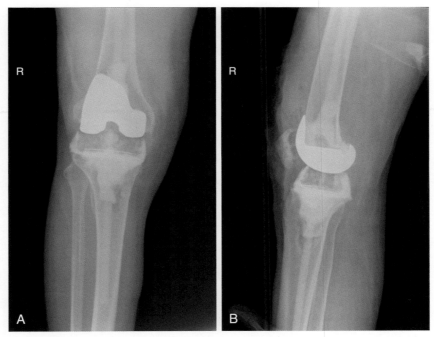

FIG 172.7 Anteroposterior and lateral radiograph of an articulating spacer with ABLC medullary cement dowels extending into the femoral and tibial canals.

débridement of the knee has been completed, attention is first turned to the femur. The femoral component should be sized to fit the remaining distal femur in the sagittal plane. This is critical, as choosing a component that is too small will necessitate further bone removal from the anterior or posterior femur (or both). Nevertheless, a perfect fit of the femoral component is not needed, as any gaps between host bone and the femoral component can be filled with ABLC. Next, the tibia should be sized and pulmonary embolism (PE) inserts trialed. If the existing flexion/extension gaps allow reasonable sagittal and coronal plane stability of the knee with the PE inserts available, the components can be opened, and preparation for cementation of the implants can commence. Occasionally, however, there is a large flexion/extension space that cannot be adequately filled with even the largest PE insert available. When this is encountered, augmentation of the proximal tibia with ABLC can facilitate closure of the flexion/extension gap. Texturing the proximal surface of any cement used to augment the proximal tibia helps facilitate fixation of the polyethylene at the time of prosthesis insertion. Once the cement on the proximal tibia has hardened, PE liners can once again be trialed, and the appropriate PE thickness chosen.

When the femoral component and PE insert sizes have been chosen, the surgeon should prepare to cement the implants. Two ALBC medullary dowels should be placed into the medullary canals of the femur and tibia prior to cementation. Prior to cementing the PE insert, small holes can be made in the undersurface of the PE insert to facilitate interdigitation of cement to the PE insert. Cement should be mixed on the back table in the ratio of 3 g of vancomycin, 3.6 g of tobramycin, and 150 mg of amphotericin powder per 40 g batch of methylmethacrylate (MMA) used. The femoral component should be

cemented first, followed by the PE insert. Once the cement has hardened, the knee is brought out into full extension and the wound is closed in layers. The patient should be placed into a sterile dressing and taken to the survey room for postoperative x-rays (Fig. 172.7).

The surgical approach at reimplantation is typically more difficult than at the time of implant removal. An extensive subperiosteal release of the deep medial collateral ligament from the tibia facilitates anterolateral subluxation of the tibia and lateral translation of the patella and extensor mechanism. If removal of the antibiotic spacer as a block segment cannot be achieved, the cement can be removed in pieces with an osteotome and a mallet. Forcible removal of the antibiotic spacer is not recommended, as this can result in a periprosthetic fracture of the femur or tibia. A thorough débridement is performed prior to reconstruction of the knee. Although the use of uncemented implants has been recommended for the use of reimplantation, the benefit of antibiotic cement for prosthesis fixation should be strongly considered in the setting of previous periprosthetic infection (Fig. 172.8).[37,106]

CONCLUSION

Two-stage reimplantation remains the gold standard for treatment of chronically infected knee arthroplasty in North America. Use of high dose ABLC spacers has allowed success (85% to 95%) in most patients, despite an increasing severity of drug resistant organisms and widened indications for reimplantation in the modern era. Efforts on prevention methods and improvement of an accurate diagnosis will facilitate the success and care of these patients.

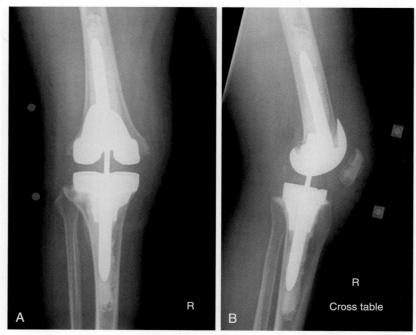

FIG 172.8 (A) Anteroposterior and (B) lateral radiographs of a reimplantation total knee arthroplasty using a semiconstrained prosthetic design. The femoral and tibial stems were cemented with low-dose ABLC using gentamicin and vancomycin.

KEY REFERENCES

6. Berbari EF, Hanssen AD, Duffy MC, et al: Risk factors for prosthetic joint infection: case-control study. *Clin Infect Dis* 27:1247–1254, 1998.

13. Burnett RS, Kelly MA, Hanssen AD, et al: Technique and timing of two-stage exchange for infection in TKA. *Clin Orthop* 464:164–178, 2007.

28. England SP, Stern SH, Insall JN, et al: Total knee arthroplasty in diabetes mellitus. *Clin Orthop* 260:130–134, 1990.

37. Hanssen AD, Osmon DR, Nelson CL: Prevention of deep periprosthetic joint infection. *Instr Course Lect* 46:555–567, 1997.

38. Hanssen AD, Rand JA: Evaluation and treatment of infection at the site of a total hip or knee arthroplasty. *Instr Course Lect* 48:111–122, 1999.

46. Insall JN, Thompson FM, Brause BD: Two-stage reimplantation for the salvage of infected total knee arthroplasty. *J Bone Joint Surg Am* 65:1087–1098, 1983.

50. Kim JG, Bae JH, Lee SY, et al: The parameters affecting the success of irrigation and debridement with component retention in the treatment of acutely infected total knee arthroplasty. *Clin Orthop Surg* 7:69–76, 2015.

57. Marculescu CE, Berbari EF, Hanssen AD, et al: Prosthetic joint infection diagnosed postoperatively by intraoperative culture. *Clin Orthop* 439:38–42, 2005.

58. Mariani BD, Martin DS, Levine MJ, et al: The Coventry Award. Polymerase chain reaction detection of bacterial infection in total knee arthroplasty. *Clin Orthop* 331:11–22, 1996.

70. Papavasiliou AV, Isaac DL, Marimuthu R, et al: Infection in knee replacements after previous injection of intra-articular steroid. *J Bone Joint Surg Br* 88:321–323, 2006.

78. Rezapoor M, Parvizi J: Prevention of periprosthetic joint infection. *J Arthroplasty* 30:902–907, 2015.

86. Springer BD: The diagnosis of periprosthetic joint infection. *J Arthroplasty* 30:908–911, 2015.

93. Trampuz A, Hanssen AD, Osmon DR, et al: Synovial fluid leukocyte count and differential for the diagnosis of prosthetic knee infection. *Am J Med* 117:556–562, 2004.

The references for this chapter can also be found on www.expertconsult.com.

173

Instability in Total Knee Arthroplasty

James A. Browne, Sebastien Parratte, Mark W. Pagnano

Ensuring that the knee is well balanced ligamentously in both flexion and extension has long been recognized as important in determining the durability of total knee arthroplasty (TKA). Among the major modes of failure of TKA, instability ranks near the top of every list for early, intermediate, and late failures that require revision surgery. In the early period within a year of index TKA, infection and instability each account for approximately 25% of all revisions; in the intermediate period of 1 to 5 years, malalignment and instability each again account for 25%; and late failures beyond 5 years are attributable to aseptic loosening and instability (35% and 20%, respectively).* Early failure in the first 5 years following the index arthroplasty is common when stability is not achieved,[7] and instability and infection are the cause of most revision TKA surgery done less than 2 years after the index operation.[36]

The clinical presentation of instability is variable and may include pain, swelling, frank giving way, a vague sense that something is not right, or delays in achieving the expected functional milestones during the recovery phase. Delineating whether the symptoms became apparent immediately after the index arthroplasty or manifested late is sometimes helpful in determining the underlying cause of instability. It has been noted that the patient's subjective report of "instability" does not make the diagnosis.[38] Buckling and giving way can have many causes, including pain, fixed flexion contracture of the knee, quadriceps weakness, hip arthritis, lumbar radiculopathy, and patellar dislocation.[38] Whereas gross instability may present with frank dislocation, subtle mechanical instability often presents with vague complaints of anterior knee pain, recurrent effusions, soft tissue tenderness to palpation, and above average range of motion.[30] Patients with subtle instability may also note difficulty in initiating ambulation after being seated.

An accurate history is important in determining the factors that led to failure. The examining surgeon should obtain information on the original diagnosis that precipitated the knee replacement, any preoperative deformity or contracture, previous knee procedures, type of prosthesis, the specifics of the operative technique for knee replacement, the postoperative rehabilitation program, and any trauma to the knee after surgery.[38,44,45] Extra-articular deformity, neuromuscular pathology, and large surgical corrections with ligament releases all have been cited as risk factors that predispose to postoperative instability.[38] Obesity has also been reported as a risk factor for intraoperative collateral ligament injury and complicates both intraoperative and postoperative assessment of soft tissue balance.[43]

The patient's complaints must be carefully reconciled with objective physical examination findings. The physical examination requires assessment of generalized ligamentous laxity and muscle strength. Observation of gait may reveal a varus or valgus thrust and may suggest coronal plane instability. The knee should be examined for anteroposterior and varus/valgus stability and symmetry in extension, 30 degrees of flexion, and 90 degrees of flexion. Subtle instability may be challenging to appreciate if the patient is guarding. Flexion laxity is often most evident when an anterior or posterior drawer test is performed with the patient sitting and the knee flexed to 90 degrees.[30] The precise amount of laxity and translation that is considered pathologic has not been defined. However, reproduction of a patient's symptoms during laxity testing is at least suggestive of a pathologic link. An above average range of motion may be observed commonly in an unstable knee replacement.[30] The integrity of the extensor mechanism should be assessed as a potential cause of global instability. Aspiration of synovial fluid from the knee may reveal hemarthrosis with elevated red blood cell counts.[33]

A complete set of radiographs, including full-length weight-bearing views, should be obtained. The size and position of the components should be assessed and the mechanical and anatomic axes determined. Weight-bearing views may stress and accentuate the instability (Fig. 173.1). Apparent instability may be readily explained by component wear or loosening, implant breakage, fracture, and bone loss (Fig. 173.2).[38] A large modular tibial insert often suggests problems with intraoperative balancing. Ligament attenuation may have occurred as the result of component overhang. Stress radiographs may provide an objective way to diagnose prosthetic knee instability, although they are rarely used in our clinical practice.

True mechanical instability may be the result of improper surgical technique, poor prosthesis selection, incorrect positioning of the implants, or overall limb-alignment problems. Historically, instability has been categorized into three types: extension instability, flexion instability, and genu recurvatum or hyperextension deformity. Extension and flexion instability can be further subdivided into asymmetrical or symmetrical. The exact nature of the instability should be determined before revision surgery is performed.

EXTENSION INSTABILITY: SYMMETRICAL

Symmetrical extension instability occurs when medial and lateral collateral ligament tensions are lax in extension. In this relatively rare situation, the combined thickness of the components is not sufficient to restore physiologic tension to

---

*References 4, 8, 15, 16, 37, 44, and 45.

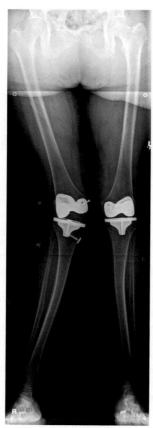

FIG 173.1 Full-length weight-bearing view of a patient with instability of the right knee secondary to medial collateral ligament insufficiency. The patient failed an attempt at allograft reconstruction and required revision to a constrained implant.

the ligaments in extension only; this has been termed *instability resulting from excessive bone resection.*[44,45] Excessive bone removal from the femur will selectively increase the extension gap without altering the flexion gap; this is termed *gap inequality.*[18]

Management of isolated symmetrical extension instability caused by excessive femoral bone loss can be challenging. A thicker tibial insert will not solve the problem. Increasing the tibial insert thickness will elevate the joint line and excessively tighten the flexion space (Fig. 173.3).[38,45] Elevation of the joint line can adversely affect knee kinematics (particularly the patellofemoral joint) and lead to worse clinical outcomes.[32] Distal femoral augments should be used to move the joint line distally. Such augments are available in most contemporary revision total knee systems.

EXTENSION INSTABILITY: ASYMMETRICAL

Asymmetrical extension instability is much more common than symmetrical extension instability.[31] This situation is typically related to preoperative angular deformity of the knee and is caused by persistent or iatrogenic ligamentous asymmetry after the knee is replaced (Fig. 173.4).[30,31,38,45] Fear of creating iatrogenic ligamentous instability in the opposite direction is a frequent reason for incomplete ligament balancing and undercorrection of deformity.

In the case of a varus knee, concerns about overreleasing the medial collateral ligament can leave the knee tight on the medial side—a situation exacerbated by leaving the limb alignment in varus.[30,38,45] Excessive medial collateral ligament tension and varus malalignment can result in medial overload with polyethylene wear and further stretching out of the lateral ligaments.[30,38,45] Recurrence of deformity may occur postoperatively. An appropriate medial release as originally described by Insall and associates should be performed when necessary.[15] A thicker tibial insert may be required following medial release to restore tension in the collateral ligaments. Lateral collateral ligament advancement can be considered if complete medial release fails to balance the knee.[19]

Asymmetrical extension instability may result from undercorrection of a valgus knee deformity. Failure to appropriately release contracted lateral tissues will leave laxity or redundancy in the medial collateral ligament. The medial collateral ligament has no ability to tighten over time, and the valgus deformity will recur.[38,44] Minimal laxity of the medial collateral ligament should therefore be accepted. Sequential lateral ligament release approaches[13,15] have been associated with frequent overrelease of the lateral soft tissues.[28] As a result, the "pie-crust" multiple puncture technique has gained widespread use.[5,28] To check for an overreleased lateral side, the trials can be inserted and the knee placed in a "figure-of-four" position (90 degrees of knee flexion while the surgeon holds the foot and allows the hip and knee to maximally externally rotate). If the post of a posterior stabilized insert subluxates from the femoral housing, a thicker or more constrained tibial insert should be used.[5]

Complete correction of severe valgus deformity incurs the risk of peroneal nerve stretch.[6] Satisfactory results have been reported with intentional deformity undercorrection and the use of a varus/valgus constrained implant to compensate for residual medial collateral ligament laxity.[6] This approach carries the theoretical concern that a constrained implant will impart additional stresses to the implant and fixation interfaces and should be reserved for older, lower demand patients.

Intraoperative iatrogenic collateral ligament injury can occur, most commonly when the proximal tibia is cut. Vigorous attempts to assess stability intraoperatively can lead to ligament stretch or rupture, typically of the medial collateral ligament. Surgical reapproximation of the ligament is the recommended approach.[22] The hamstring tendons may be used to augment the repair, and a condylar constrained implant may be used to enhance stability.[6,22] Postoperative bracing may help reduce stresses on the healing ligament.[22]

FLEXION INSTABILITY: SYMMETRICAL

Symmetrical flexion instability is likely underreported, since the diagnosis can be elusive. This distinct clinical entity can occur with both posterior stabilized and cruciate retaining designs and is characterized by painful subluxation of the tibia on the femur. This situation is often seen in patients in whom the total knee prosthesis is well aligned axially and well fixed.[30] Manifestations of flexion instability differ depending on the cause of the problem and the implant design.

A large flexion gap may result from inadequate filling with the implant, often as a result of underresection of the distal femur in an attempt to avoid elevating the joint line. In this scenario, the surgeon will typically preferentially balance the resulting tight extension gap at the expense of a loose flexion

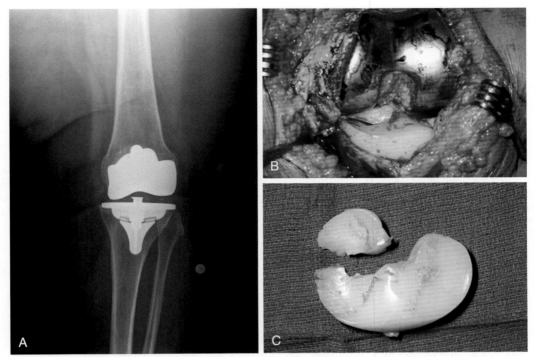

FIG 173.2 (A) Anteroposterior radiograph of an obese patient with an unstable left TKA. Note varus positioning of the components and lack of parallelism between the distal femoral component and tibial tray. (B and C) Intraoperative photographs at the time of revision demonstrating medial overload with wear and catastrophic failure of the polyethylene.

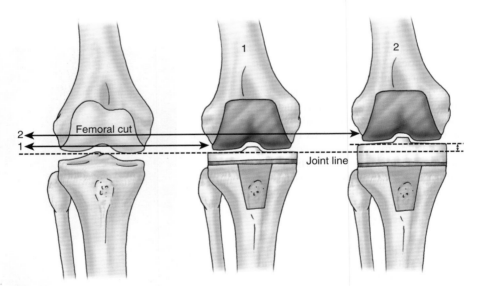

FIG 173.3 Excessive bone removal from the distal part of the femur cannot be managed with the use of a thicker tibial insert, which will elevate the joint line and excessively tighten the flexion space. (Reprinted with permission from Vail TP, Lang JE: Surgical techniques and instrumentation in total knee arthroplasty. In Insall JN, Scott WN (eds): *Surgery of the knee*, ed 4, vol 2, Baltimore, 2006, Churchill Livingstone, pp 1455–1521.)

gap. With trials in place, the tibia should have less than 5 mm of anteroposterior translation when the knee is tested intraoperatively at 90 degrees of flexion with the patella reduced.[31] The "figure-of-four" position, as described earlier, can be used to establish that the knee will not dislocate.

Dislocation of a posterior stabilized TKA is rare but dramatic, with a reported incidence between 0% and 0.5%.[10,17,23] If the flexion gap is large enough, the cam mechanism may jump over the post, resulting in posterior dislocation of the tibia on the femur. Dislocation typically occurs with marked knee

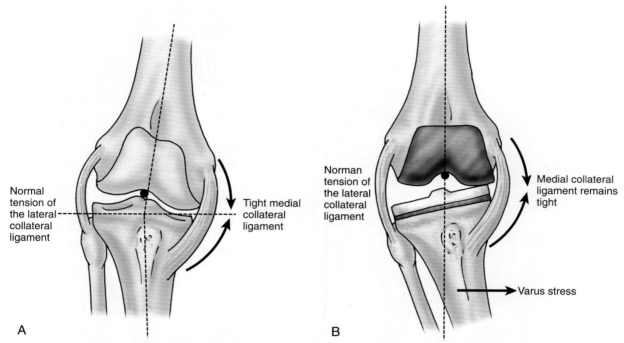

FIG 173.4 (A) Example of a varus knee with a contracted medial collateral ligament that has been incompletely released. (B) The medial collateral ligament remains tight, and the lateral collateral ligament is subsequently lax. (Reprinted with permission from Vail TP, Lang JE: Surgical techniques and instrumentation in TKA. In Insall JN, Scott WN (eds): *Surgery of the knee*, ed 4, vol 2, Baltimore, 2006, Churchill Livingstone, pp 1455–1521.)

flexion plus a valgus or varus stress (such as occurs when crossing the legs to put on socks or shoes).[9] At-risk patients include those who had correction of a large valgus deformity, particularly if they quickly regained knee flexion postoperatively.[35] First-time dislocations should be treated with closed reduction, a trial of bracing, and avoidance of the activity that induced the dislocation, although severe laxity will often lead to repeated dislocations. Mobile-bearing designs may require open reduction.[14] Recurrent dislocation may require revision with thicker polyethylene (if the extension space permits). A constrained condylar implant may be helpful but will not prevent repeat dislocation in the setting of continued gap imbalance (Fig. 173.5). The "figure-of-four" maneuver can be used to assess correction of the instability.

Posterior stabilized total knee replacements can be symptomatically unstable in flexion without dislocating. Schwab and colleagues described a typical constellation of symptoms and physical findings, including a sense of instability without giving way, recurrent knee effusions, multiple areas of soft tissue tenderness about the knee, and substantial anterior tibial translation at 90 degrees of flexion.[35] They reported reliable results in alleviating pain, improving stability, and improving patient satisfaction in 10 patients following revision, usually with a larger femoral component and posterior femoral augmentation.

Flexion instability after cruciate retaining TKA has been well described but likely remains underdiagnosed.[30] The clinical presentation is similar to that described previously for posterior stabilized knee designs. Typically, this occurs in knees with

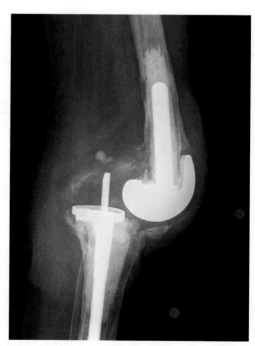

FIG 173.5 Revision to a constrained posterior stabilized implant can result in dislocation if the flexion gap is not balanced.

well-fixed, well-positioned implants.[30] A posterior sag or drawer sign is often observed (Fig. 173.6). Visible anterior translation of the tibia on the femur while the leg is extended from a seated, 90-degree flexed position may be present.[41] The knee is usually stable to varus and valgus stress in extension. Multiple causes of flexion instability after cruciate retaining TKA are possible (Table 173.1). A tibial liner with a flat sagittal plane contour offers little resistance to anteroposterior translation and may contribute to flexion instability.

Early flexion instability is often the result of technical error. Undersizing the femoral component in the anteroposterior dimension will decrease the posterior offset and selectively increase the flexion gap. Postoperative lateral radiographs may suggest overresection of the posterior condyles, compared with preoperative views. Excessive tibial slope will lead to a total knee that is well balanced in extension but loose in flexion (Fig. 173.7). This scenario puts the posterior cruciate ligament at risk for iatrogenic injury. In these cases, revision surgery should focus on rebalancing the knee; converting to a posterior-stabilized implant design is typically the most reliable approach.

Injury to the posterior cruciate ligament can manifest as early or late flexion instability. Direct iatrogenic injury at the time of knee replacement may lead to early failure. Leaving the flexion space excessively tight can lead to early indirect iatrogenic failure of the posterior cruciate ligament. Patients with a tight knee in flexion may work aggressively to regain motion in the postoperative period and rupture the posterior cruciate ligament. These patients often recall a specific event when a pop or snap occurs in concert with a sudden increase in motion. Late instability may be observed when the posterior cruciate ligament deteriorates from age-related changes or following reactivation of inflammatory disease (Fig. 173.8).[29] Posterior instability with incapacitating anterior knee pain and swelling has been reported in 8% of patients following cruciate retaining knees.[41] In patients with rheumatoid arthritis, late instability has been reported in 2% to 15% of knees at long-term follow-up using cruciate retaining implants.[2,11,27,29]

Initial treatment options include quadriceps strengthening and local modalities for tenderness and swelling. Bracing may afford some symptomatic relief. However, nonoperative

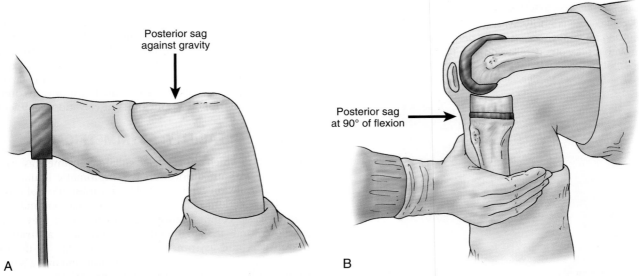

FIG 173.6 (A) A posterior sag at 90 degrees of flexion is typically observed with flexion instability. (B) A posterior drawer sign is also commonly observed. On a lateral radiograph, the tibia can be subluxated posteriorly beyond the anterior lip of the tibial insert. (Reproduced with permission from Pagnano MW, Hanssen AD, Lewallen DA, Stuart MJ: Flexion instability after primary posterior cruciate retaining TKA. *Clin Orthop* 356:39–46, 1998.)

TABLE 173.1   Causes of Flexion Instability After Cruciate Retaining Total Knee Arthroplasty

Cause of Flexion Instability	Presentation of Clinical Symptoms	Considerations	Revision Solution
Undersized femoral component	Early	Encouraged by anterior referencing	Use larger femoral components, posterior augments.
Excessive tibial slope	Early	Puts PCL at risk for iatrogenic damage	Recut tibia and rebalance; convert to PS implant.
Acute rupture of PCL	Variable	Flexion space too tight after TKA	Rebalance and convert to PS implant.
Attritional rupture of PCL	Late	Attrition of PCL or reactivation of inflammatory arthritis	Revise to PS implant.
Posteromedial polyethylene wear	Late	Functionally increases the flexion space, synovitis	Perform isolated polyethylene exchange or complete revision.

PCL, Posterior cruciate ligament; *PS*, posterior stabilized; *TKA*, total knee arthroplasty.

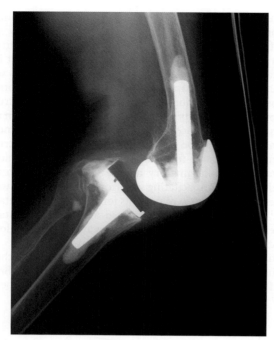

FIG 173.7 Flexion instability with posterior translation of the tibia occurring several years after revision knee replacement in a patient with a previous patellectomy. A flat polyethylene liner has exacerbated the instability.

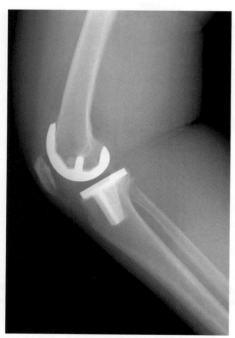

FIG 173.8 Excessive posterior slope (16 degrees in this example) can lead to symptomatic flexion instability.

treatment generally has not been successful in our experience. Operative management is often required for patients with incapacitating symptoms and marked disability.[2,27,30]

Operative management with isolated tibial polyethylene exchange is inherently appealing because it minimizes blood loss, bone loss, and operative time. However, this approach should be used with caution. Upsizing the liner does not address the underlying imbalance between flexion and extension gaps and therefore is not recommended. A high rate of failure has been reported with revision operations that included only insertion of a thicker tibial polyethylene.[2,30] One exception may occur when posteromedial polyethylene liner wear has functionally increased the flexion space, resulting in instability.

Conversion to a posterior stabilized design or a constrained condylar design is the preferred approach when a cruciate retaining implant is revised for flexion instability; it facilitates balancing of flexion and extension spaces. Careful attention must be directed toward gap balancing, as converting to a posterior stabilized prosthesis alone is likely to fail. In an initial series from our institution, 19 of 22 knees revised in this manner were satisfactorily improved.[30] Subsequently, Abdel et al.[1] comprehensively examined the midterm results of 60 patients who underwent revision TKA for flexion instability at Mayo Clinic between the years 2001 and 2010. In that series, there was a marked improvement in Knee Society pain and function scores postoperatively, and no patient had required further surgery for instability at midterm follow-up. Those authors identified a stepwise systematic approach to the surgical correction of flexion instability that involved (1) eliminating any posterior tibial slope (mean correction 5 degrees), (2) correcting component alignment and/or rotation on both the tibial and femoral sides, (3) increasing posterior condylar offset with a larger femoral component and/or femoral stem that allows posterior offset, and (4) elevating the femoral joint line until stability in both extension and flexion is obtained (the mean combined increase in posterior offset and joint line elevation was 9.5 mm).[1]

FLEXION INSTABILITY: ASYMMETRICAL

The extent to which mild isolated collateral ligament asymmetry in flexion without dislocation is symptomatic is unclear.[18] A rectangular flexion gap is created by a combination of posterior condylar resection, femoral component rotation, and/or ligament release. Femoral component malrotation may result in patellofemoral malalignment, an asymmetrical trapezoidal flexion gap, and asymmetrical collateral laxity in flexion.[21,34] Appropriate femoral component rotation remains a source of some debate, with so-called gap balancing surgeons advocating rotation of the femur to create a rectangular gap via bone cuts, and other surgeons favoring femoral rotation set to anatomic landmarks (often the transepicondylar axis) with rectangular gap symmetry subsequently created by selective ligament release.

The clinical implications of asymmetrical flexion instability are unclear. Whiteside, Krakow, and others have advocated setting femoral component rotation with bony landmarks and accepting slight soft tissue asymmetry.[18,42] However, Laskin found increased range of flexion and less medial tibial pain with a rectangular flexion space compared with an asymmetrical trapezoidal gap.[21] Large medial release with a resultant grossly asymmetrical flexion gap may lead to dislocation of the tibial component but may otherwise be asymptomatic.

MIDFLEXION INSTABILITY

The concept of midflexion instability is contentious, and the condition remains to be fully defined as a distinct clinical entity. When surgeons and researchers begin any discussion of midflexion instability, the first order of business is to determine the plane of instability that is being evaluated. Some major misunderstandings will emerge if one group is talking about coronal plane instability (varus-valgus) in midflexion while the other group is talking about sagittal plane instability (anterior-posterior) in midflexion. Coronal plane instability resulting from collateral ligament imbalance may be masked by tightness of the posterior capsule in full extension and may be experienced by the patient in early flexion. Patients may also experience true flexion instability earlier in the flexion arc.

In a cadaveric study, Martin and Whiteside found a significant increase in varus/valgus laxity during midflexion when the femoral component was positioned 5 mm proximally and 5 mm anteriorly.[24] Although collateral ligament tension appeared appropriate in full extension and 90 degrees of flexion, alteration in position of the joint line (either distally or posteriorly) appeared to alter ligament tension at intermediate angles. The authors suggested that this midrange laxity may lead to progressive stretching of secondary restraints and increased instability over time. Accelerated polyethylene wear can also occur as a result.[3]

Femoral component sagittal plane design may play a role in collateral ligament isometry in midflexion. In response to the traditional view that multiple instantaneous centers of flexion and extension rotation exist in the knee, femoral components have been traditionally designed with multiple radii of rotation. However, as our understanding of knee kinematics has changed, some systems have been designed with a single radius of rotation. The shift from a longer to a shorter radius within a multiple-radius design has been reported to cause temporary varus/valgus instability during knee flexion between 30 degrees and 45 degrees.[39] Corresponding functional performance differences have been reported,[40] although additional studies are required to determine the clinical significance of this finding. Other implant designs have moved to incorporate a constantly changing radius of curvature such that transition zones between one radius and the next are infinitely small. Some researchers have speculated that it is the transition zone that can result in some degree of anteroposterior translation that can be interpreted as midflexion instability.

Despite various descriptions of midflexion instability following primary TKA, no studies have been performed to evaluate approaches to treatment. Although this has not been proven, extrapolation from flexion instability would suggest that nonoperative management is likely to be unsuccessful in the patient with significant symptoms. No data are available on the outcomes of revision TKA for midflexion instability. Subsequent reports should delineate whether the primary perceived problem was midflexion instability in the coronal plane or the sagittal plane and include descriptions of the fundamental design features of the implants that were revised (single radius, multi-radius, constantly changing radius, etc.).

Midflexion instability has been described in revision TKA as rotational instability with combined external rotation and valgus stress in a knee flexed between 45 degrees and 90 degrees.[25] Anterior medial collateral ligament attenuation, femoral-tibial articular geometry, and tibial postfemoral box geometry were reported to contribute to this instability.

RECURVATUM OR HYPEREXTENSION DEFORMITY

Preoperative recurvatum in the primary TKA setting is rare and most commonly occurs in patients with neuromuscular

disease.[20,26] Patients with true quadriceps weakness, such as those with polio, will compensate by ambulating with the knee locked in hyperextension (the so-called back knee gait). Patients with a fixed valgus deformity and an isolated iliotibial band contracture may demonstrate recurvatum. This is a classic contraindication to TKA,[38] and surgery should be approached with caution. Postoperatively, the patient with marked quadriceps weakness will continue to force the knee into hyperextension to stabilize the joint during stance, resulting in progressive recurvatum. Consideration should be given to underresection or augmentation of the distal femur to move the joint line distally, with the knee left with a slight flexion contracture at the conclusion of the procedure (Fig. 173.9). Alternatively, the femoral origins of the collateral ligaments may be moved proximally and posteriorly to re-create normal tightening action during full extension of the knee.[20] The cam action of

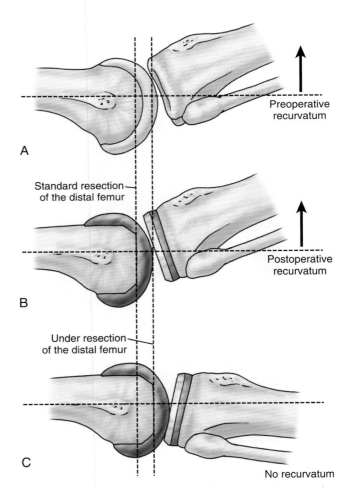

FIG 173.9 Consideration should be given to underresection of the distal femur at the time of TKA in the patient with (A) hyperextension, because (B) standard resection will leave the patient with a postoperative recurvatum deformity. It is reasonable to leave the knee with (C) a slight flexion contracture at the conclusion of the procedure. (Reprinted with permission from Vail TP, Lang JE: Surgical techniques and instrumentation in total knee arthroplasty. In Insall JN, Scott WN (eds): *Surgery of the knee*, ed 4, vol 2, Baltimore, 2006, Churchill Livingstone, pp 1455–1521.)

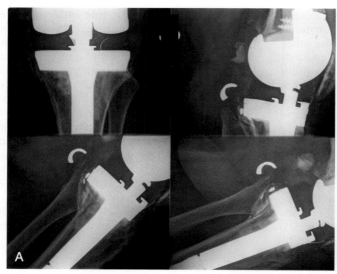
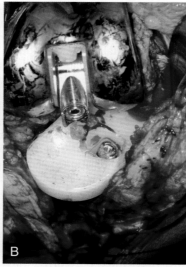

FIG 173.10 (A) Radiographs of a broken hinged revision TKA secondary to hyperextension. Note the metallic density in the posterior aspect of the knee. The patient was morbidly obese. (B) Intraoperative photograph shows the fractured hinge, necessitating complete femoral revision with distalization of the joint line.

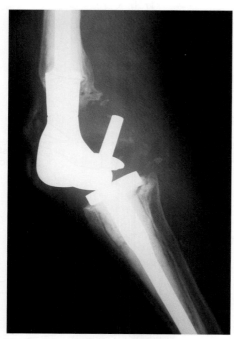

FIG 173.11 A dislocated hinged revision TKA. The hinge mechanism became disassociated from the tibial component in deep knee flexion.

the prosthesis with a curved insert combined with collateral ligament transfer can prevent recurvatum.

Once established, a recurvatum deformity following primary TKA is difficult to treat. A rotating-hinge total knee prosthesis with an extension stop has been advocated in patients with failed implants or quadriceps lacking antigravity strength.[12] Although this can provide a satisfactory solution, continued

hyperextension may lead to mechanical failure of the hinge, particularly in obese patients (Fig. 173.10). With some designs, persistently lax soft tissues in flexion may allow the hinge mechanism to dislocate from the tibial component (Fig. 173.11).

KEY REFERENCES

1. Abdel MP, Pulido L, Severson EP, et al: Stepwise surgical correction of instability in flexion after total knee replacement. *Bone Joint J* 96-B(12):1644–1648, 2014.

4. Callaghan JJ, O'Rourke MR, Saleh KJ: Why knees fail: lessons learned. *J Arthroplasty* 19(4 Suppl 1):31–34, 2004.

5. Clarke HD, Fuchs R, Scuderi GR, et al: Clinical results in valgus total knee arthroplasty with the "pie crust" technique of lateral soft tissue releases. *J Arthroplasty* 20:1010–1014, 2005.

6. Easley ME, Insall JN, Scuderi GR, et al: Primary constrained condylar knee arthroplasty for the arthritic valgus knee. *Clin Orthop* 380:58–64, 2000.

12. Giori NJ, Lewallen DG: Total knee arthroplasty in limbs affected by poliomyelitis. *J Bone Joint Surg Am* 84:1157–1161, 2002.

15. Insall JN, Binazzi R, Soudry M, et al: Total knee arthroplasty. *Clin Orthop* 192:13–22, 1985.

20. Krackow KA, Weiss AP: Recurvatum deformity complicating performance of total knee arthroplasty: a brief note. *J Bone Joint Surg Am* 72:268–271, 1990.

21. Laskin RS: Flexion space configuration in total knee arthroplasty. *J Arthroplasty* 10:657–660, 1995.

22. Leopold SS, McStay C, Klafeta K, et al: Primary repair of intraoperative disruption of the medial collateral ligament during total knee arthroplasty. *J Bone Joint Surg Am* 83:86–91, 2001.

30. Pagnano MW, Hanssen AD, Lewallen DG, et al: Flexion instability after primary posterior cruciate retaining total knee arthroplasty. *Clin Orthop* 356:39–46, 1998.

31. Parratte S, Pagnano MW: Instability after total knee arthroplasty. *J Bone Joint Surg Am* 90:184–194, 2008.

33. Raab GE, Fehring TK, Odum SM, et al: Aspiration as an aid to the diagnosis of prosthetic knee instability. *Orthopedics* 32:318, 2009.

35. Schwab JH, Haidukewych GJ, Hanssen AD, et al: Flexion instability without dislocation after posterior stabilized total knees. *Clin Orthop* 440:96–100, 2005.

36. Sharkey PF, Hozack WJ, Rothman RH, et al: Insall Award paper. Why are total knee arthroplasties failing today? *Clin Orthop* 404:7–13, 2002.

38. Vince KG, Abdeen A, Sugimori T: The unstable total knee arthroplasty: causes and cures. *J Arthroplasty* 21(4 Suppl 1):44–49, 2006.

43. Winiarsky R, Barth P, Lotke P: Total knee arthroplasty in morbidly obese patients. *J Bone Joint Surg Am* 80:1770–1774, 1998.

Full references for this chapter can be found on www.expertconsult.com.

174

Management of Bone Defects in Revision Total Knee Arthroplasty: Augments, Structural and Impaction Graft, and Cones

R. Michael Meneghini, Arlen D. Hanssen

BACKGROUND

Reconstruction of large bony defects in the femur and tibia during revision knee replacement remains a challenging clinical problem. Smaller bone defects have been traditionally and effectively treated with limited amounts of morselized cancellous bone graft,[5,36] cement augmented with screw fixation,[1,15,37,38] or the use of modular augments attached to revision prosthetic implants.[6,18] Large or massive bone defects require more extensive reconstructive efforts and have been traditionally managed with the use of large structural allografts,* impaction bone grafting techniques with or without mesh augmentation,[25,41,42,46] fabrication of custom prosthetic components,[11] or the use of specialized hinged knee components.[21] In the past decade, large metaphyseal defects have been effectively managed with partially porous metal stepped "sleeves" or porous tantalum metaphyseal cones, both of which have excellent early term results.† Finally, newly developed porous titanium metaphyseal cones have become available and offer an expedited bone preparation process.[27] Despite the multitude of treatment methods used, the best reconstructive technique for bone defects during revision knee replacement has not been clearly determined.[11]

PREOPERATIVE PLANNING

In revision knee arthroplasties with bone deficiency, it is helpful to determine several important variables to establish the requirements of reconstruction. Good-quality anteroposterior, lateral, and patellar views are usually sufficient for assessment of bone loss in the large majority of cases; however, tomograms are occasionally helpful. It is often stated that the magnitude of bone loss observed on preoperative radiographs vastly underestimates the true magnitude of bone loss discovered intraoperatively. This tenet is particularly true of bone loss associated with osteolysis secondary to wear debris. If a lateral radiograph of the knee obtained prior to the original arthroplasty is unavailable, a lateral radiograph of the opposite knee is valuable to determine the appropriate anteroposterior dimension of the knee. A true lateral radiograph, obtained with fluoroscopic

positioning, may occasionally be useful for accurate assessment of the anteroposterior dimensions of the femur.

Assessment of bone loss in the four primary areas of bone loss should be systematically assessed and noted. The severity and location of bone loss and quality of remaining bone should be assessed. The location of the joint line is marked and noted. The optimal joint line position is roughly 2 cm below the origin of the medial collateral ligament (MCL) and 2.5 cm below the prominence of the lateral epicondyle. In some knees, particularly those with "flexion instability," the prosthetic joint line may actually be lower than the anatomic joint line, which usually suggests that additional distal femoral resection will be required during the revision procedure to balance the flexion and extension spaces.

BONE LOSS ASSESSMENT AND CLASSIFICATION

The critical step in determining the appropriate reconstruction method in revision total knee replacement is to accurately determine the quantity, location, and extent of the bone loss. This is done after meticulous removal of the failed tibial and femoral implants, with careful attention to existing bone preservation. Once the components are removed, it is important to determine whether the defects are contained or uncontained (segmental). In addition, the location of supportive bone that surrounds the bone loss is essential, and will dictate the type and size of the augmentation that is required. Smaller contained defects can be treated with either cement fill with screw augmentation or morselized allograft fill, particularly in older patients. However, larger uncontained defects typically require larger reconstructive measures such as modular block augments, bulk allograft, or highly porous metal metaphyseal cones.

The Anderson Orthopaedic Research Institute Bone Defect classification is a common system of categorizing bone defects in revision knee arthroplasty.[11] This system permits communication and comparison of knees among different institutions and also allows preoperative and postoperative classification and management recommendations for specific bone defect severities. In this bone defect classification, type I defects describe only minor and contained cancellous bony defects within either tibial plateau, type 2A defects include moderate to severe cancellous and/or cortical bone defects of only one

---

*References 10, 12, 13, 17, 18, 30-32, 40, and 43.
†References 14, 19, 22-24, 28, 29, 34, and 45.

tibial plateau, type 2B defects include moderate to severe cancellous bone defects of both tibial plateaus and/or segmental cortical defects of one tibial plateau, and type 3 defects describe combined cavitary and segmental bone loss of both tibial plateaus.

RECONSTRUCTION WITH CEMENT AND SCREWS

The use of cement as a reconstructive augment has the attraction of being simple, inexpensive, and efficient because the revision knee arthroplasty already uses the material for fixation in most instances. This reconstruction method is typically indicated for smaller contained defects less than 5 mm in depth,[1,15] although some authors have advocated its use in larger defects with excellent clinical results.[37,38] When cement is used for defects in revision knee arthroplasty, augmentation with bone screws is typically recommended to enhance the biomechanical properties of the construct (Fig. 174.1). In addition, if the patient is young and active, it may be more advantageous to use morselized allograft to restore bone stock in these types of defects.

Surgical Technique

The surgical technique begins with the tibial or femoral provisional or freshening cuts. Once these are performed, a more accurate assessment of the defect is possible. A meticulous débridement of the defect is performed with removal of all fibrous tissue, which would impede adequate interdigitation of the cement and create suboptimal fixation. Sclerotic bone surfaces are frequently encountered in revision surgeries and these must be roughened with a small drill or a burr. Once the defect is clearly delineated and prepared, the location of remaining bone is identified for adequate screw fixation. Sloping surfaces are converted to step-shaped surfaces to minimize the amount of shear forces acting on the cement, as cement is known to be much more biomechanically stable and supportive in compression. If the defect is of minimal depth, it may be filled with

cement alone during cementation of the standard revision tibial or femoral components. If the defects are larger or the surgeon is uncertain, reinforcement with screw augmentation is recommended. Once the bone defect is adequately prepared for cement, titanium self-tapping cancellous bone screws are placed into the host metaphyseal bone and advanced so that the heads are positioned below the level of the eventual tibial tray or femoral component. Titanium screws are typically used to prevent galvanic corrosion that occurs with dissimilar metals, since the majority of tibial baseplates are composed of titanium. Once the screw is in position, the trial components are inserted to ensure there is no contact of the screw head with the prosthesis. Once the cement is mixed and in a doughy state, it is placed into the defect and around the screw heads and pressurized by hand. The final prosthesis is then placed and cement allowed to cure with removal of excess.

Clinical Results

Satisfactory mid-term results have been reported with the use of screws and cement for bone defects in total knee arthroplasty (TKA). Ritter reported on 57 total knee replacements with large (9 ± 5 mm) medial tibial defects reconstructed with screws and cement at an average of 6.1 years follow-up.[37] Although nonprogressive radiolucent lines were common and seen in 27%, there were no reported cases of tibial component loosening, component failure, or cement failure. In a subsequent report by the same authors, 125 TKAs that used screws and cement to fill large medial tibial defects secondary to severe varus deformities were reported at a mean of 7.9 years follow-up.[38] The authors reported two failures that occurred because of medial tibial collapse at 5 and 10 years, respectively, but there were no other failures or loosening observed in the remainder of the cohort. However, this was a series of primary knee arthroplasties without the typical stem extensions used in revision knee arthroplasty to augment fixation and prevent medial collapse in the setting of bone deficiency and suboptimal bone quality. Therefore, in smaller and contained defects that are encountered

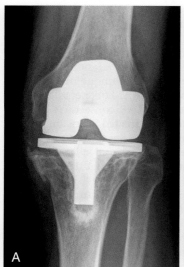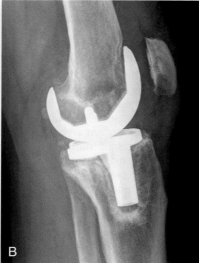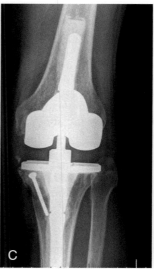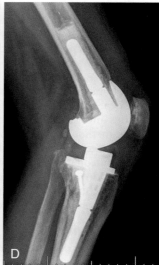

FIG 174.1 (A) AP and (B) lateral radiograph of contained medial tibial bone defect secondary to osteolysis. (C) AP and (D) lateral radiograph of the reconstruction using cement fill with screw augmentation at 12 months follow-up. Note the screw head well below and without contact with the tibial tray.

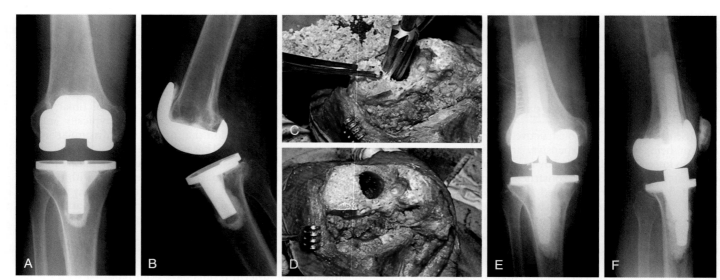

FIG 174.2 (A) AP and (B) lateral radiograph of a failed TKR with severe femoral bone loss in the lateral condyle secondary to osteolysis. (C) Intraoperative picture of impaction grafting using the intramedullary reamer to facilitate compaction of morselized allograft into the defect. (D) Removal of the reamer after morselized allograft compaction demonstrating complete fill and reconstitution of the contained defect. (E) AP and (F) lateral radiograph of the revision TKR in (A) and (B) demonstrating the reconstituted lateral femoral defect bypassed with an intramedullary stem.

in revision knee arthroplasty, particularly in older or less-active patients, the use of screws and cement is a viable and successful method of reconstruction that is inexpensive, relatively simple, and efficient.

RECONSTRUCTION WITH MORSELIZED ALLOGRAFT

Bone loss in revision knee arthroplasty can be treated reliably and successfully with morselized cancellous allograft and has an established clinical track record.[‡] This method is typically reserved for contained defects (Fig. 174.2) and is particularly attractive for younger patients in whom restoration of deficient bone stock is a priority given the potential for future reconstructive surgeries. Biologically, morselized cancellous allograft appears to incorporate similarly to cancellous autograft, albeit at a much slower rate. It is also beneficial to have a well-vascularized recipient bed to facilitate incorporation of the allograft bone and if a highly sclerotic defect is encountered, it may be beneficial to burr away the sclerotic bone to underlying cancellous and vascular bone or conversely use another reconstruction method such as a block augment. Furthermore, if the defect is large and segmental, although some authors have reported adequate results with impaction allografting,[25,26] reconstruction with more robust structural augments, such as metal blocks, bulk allograft, or metaphyseal porous metal cones, will typically produce more biomechanically stable constructs.

Surgical Technique

As with all the reconstructive techniques, the surgical technique of using morselized allograft to fill contained defects requires the meticulous débridement of the defect with careful attention

to removal of all fibrous tissue. Careful attention is paid to preparation of a vascular bed for allograft incorporation to host bone and long-term bone reconstitution. Once the defect is adequately débrided, prepared, and confirmed to be contained with supporting peripheral structure, the morselized allograft can be inserted into the defect. It is also preferential to grind up any larger pieces into a fine morselized consistency to facilitate both biologic and structural properties. It is helpful to place an adequately sized reamer or trial stem into the medullary canal and impact the morselized allograft material around the reamer, which facilitates compaction of the graft to optimize its ability to provide structural support (see Fig. 174-2C and D). Once this is complete, the reamer is removed and the final implant is inserted with an intramedullary stem for supplemental support.

Clinical Results

Midterm results are available for the technique of impaction allograft reconstruction in revision TKA. Lotke et al. prospectively studied the midterm results of 48 consecutive revision TKAs with substantial bone loss treated with impaction allograft.[26] At an average follow-up of 3.8 years, no mechanical failures of the revisions were reported and all radiographs demonstrated incorporation and remodeling of the bone graft. There were six complications out of the 42 revisions available for follow-up (14%); two periprosthetic fractures, one early infection salvaged with irrigation and antibiotics, one late infection resulting in fusion, and two patellar clunk syndromes. Although the authors concede that the technique is time consuming and technically demanding, they advocate impaction grafting for bone loss in revision TKA.[26] Whiteside et al. reported on 63 patients who had revision knee arthroplasty using morselized cancellous allograft to fill large femoral and/or tibial defects.[47] Firm seating of the components on a rim of viable bone and rigid fixation with a medullary stem were achieved in

---

[‡]References 7, 25, 26, 39, 44, and 47.

all cases. Fourteen reoperations occurred and a biopsy specimen was taken from the central portion of the allograft, which revealed evidence of active new bone formation. Evidence of healing, bone maturation, and formation of trabeculae were observed on all radiographs at 1-year follow-up. Two patients in this series required revision surgery for aseptic loosening and the authors felt both had greatly improved bone stock, so new implants could be applied with minor additional grafting.[47]

RECONSTRUCTION WITH BULK ALLOGRAFT

Bulk allograft has frequently been used to reconstruct large bone defects with the intention of providing mechanical support and reconstituting bone, which are certainly considered advantages of this technique. Bulk allograft is typically indicated for defects that are larger than 1.5 cm in depth and exceed the dimensions of typical metal block augments that accompany most revision total knee systems (Fig. 174.3). The advantage of bulk allograft is the potential for bone reconstitution, particularly in young patients for whom this goal is of great

importance with the likelihood of multiple future surgeries and reconstructions. The potential drawbacks are the potential for graft resorption, collapse, and graft-host nonunion. Patient factors that include health status, physiologic age, bone quality, and activity must be weighed heavily when considering using this reconstructive technique over other reconstruction strategies such as porous metal cones.

Surgical Technique

The technique involves shaping the defect to accept a bulk allograft, most commonly a femoral head. The shaping can be done with a high-speed bur or acetabular reamers. As with the morselized allograft, it is beneficial to ensure that the allograft bone is in contact with vascularized host bone, as opposed to the dense and frequently avascular sclerotic bone encountered in many revision knee defects. Once in place, the graft is secured to the host bone with threaded Steinman pins or screws (see Fig. 174.3C). It is advantageous to countersink the screw heads to avoid metal-metal contact with the prosthesis and the subsequent galvanic corrosion that can occur. The tibial (or

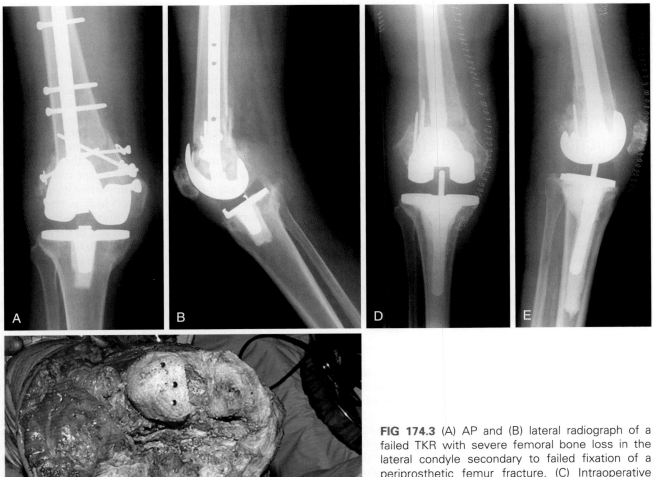

FIG 174.3 (A) AP and (B) lateral radiograph of a failed TKR with severe femoral bone loss in the lateral condyle secondary to failed fixation of a periprosthetic femur fracture. (C) Intraoperative picture of bulk femoral head allograft secured with three threaded Steinman pins. (D) AP and (E) lateral radiograph of the revision TKR in (A) and (B) demonstrating the lateral femoral condyle bulk allograft bypasses and supplemented with an intramedullary stem.

femoral) surface is then shaped accordingly, either free hand or with the knee revision system alignment cutting guides, and supplemental stem fixation with or without cement is used to bypass the reconstructed defect (see Fig. 174.3D and E).

Clinical Results

Recently, Engh and Ammeen reported on a series of 46 revision total knee replacements (TKRs) with reconstruction of massive tibial defects using bulk allograft.[12] The authors reported only four failures, two for infection, at a mean of 95 months follow-up with no evidence of graft collapse and recommend using bulk allograft for large tibial defects.[12] However, resorption and collapse of the allograft has been a concern from other authors.[7,22] In a series of 52 revision TKRs with bulk allograft followed prospectively, Clatworthy et al. reported that 13 knee replacements failed, yielding a 75% success rate at 97 months follow-up. Five knees had graft resorption, resulting in implant loosening, and two knees had nonunion between the host bone and the allograft. The survival rate of the allografts was 72% at 10 years.[10] In a 2009 retrospective study from the Mayo Clinic, authors reviewed 65 knees that underwent revision knee arthroplasty with bulk allograft for large bone defects and reported a 10-year revision-free survivorship of 76%. Sixteen patients (22.8%) had failed reconstructions and underwent additional surgery with 8 of 16 because of allograft failure and 3 because of failure of a component unsupported by allograft.[4] These reports support the use of bulk allograft for severe tibial or femoral bone defects in revision knee arthroplasty, yet also highlight the need for a more durable reconstruction method to facilitate long-term success and avoid the complications inherent with allografts, namely graft nonunion and resorption.

RECONSTRUCTION WITH MODULAR BLOCKS OR WEDGES

Modular blocks and wedges are indicated in small to moderate segmental tibial and femoral defects (Figs. 174.4 and 174.5). The modular metal blocks are advantageous because they are versatile, relatively technically straightforward, and do not require osseointegration. They are therefore particularly useful in older and less-active patients, but have the disadvantage of not restoring bone stock. The majority of revision total knee systems have numerous shapes and sizes of augments for both the tibia and femur, which facilitates restoration of the joint line and proper balancing of the knee in a relatively efficient manner as well.

Surgical Technique

The surgical technique of using modular metal blocks or wedges is relatively straightforward. Once the location and extent of the defects have been determined, the size and shape of the augment that best fits that defect is selected. In the tibia, wedges or blocks may be used and the majority of knee revision systems have alignment and cutting guides that prepare the bone for a nearly exact fit with the prosthesis. Although modular tibial wedges were designed to accommodate the frequently encountered defect seen in varus collapse of the medial tibia, there is legitimate concern that wedges subject the interface cement to shear forces, which are not favorable in the long term with cement. Therefore, many surgeons will remove a bit more bone and convert a wedge-shaped defect into one that will accept a block augment so that the cement interface is subjected to

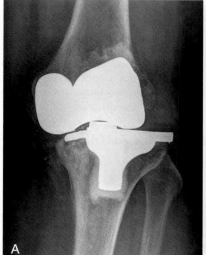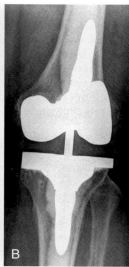

FIG 174.4 (A) AP radiograph of a failed TKR secondary to medial tibial collapse with a broken tibial baseplate creating a moderate medial tibial defect. (B) AP radiograph of the revision TKR reconstruction with a block augment and cemented stem extension.

predominantly compressive loads, which are much more favorable to cement in the long term. Furthermore, it has been shown that block augments are superior to wedges biomechanically in creating an overall more stable and rigid tibial construct.[9] It is helpful to use intramedullary instrumentation to align the tibial cut perpendicular to the mechanical axis of the tibia and the associated cutting guide will guide the 1- to 2-mm "skim" or "freshening" cut on each plateau to enact the least amount of bone removal, and remove bone to accept the exact size and shape of the augment. It is also important to determine the proper tibial component rotation, which is typically aligned with the medial one-third of the tibial tubercle, so that the sagittal cut of the block augment will seat in the corresponding correct rotational position (see Fig. 174.5D). Once the cuts are made, sclerotic bone is roughened to facilitate cement interdigitation and the final tibial component with stem extension is placed.

There are several factors that are unique to the femoral component preparation for modular block augments. First, the majority of augments are block shaped and come in a variety of sizes distally and posteriorly to accommodate the most common areas of bone loss encountered in revision knee arthroplasty. Once the tibial platform is reconstructed, as is typically the initial step in performing a revision TKA, the thickness of these augments can be altered to correctly position the femoral component with regard to balancing the flexion and extension gaps. For example, if the extension space is larger than the flexion space, distal augmentation may be used to balance the knee. This emphasizes the importance of determining the correct balance of the knee prior to making any femoral augment cuts, which may compromise the surgeon's ability to properly balance the knee. Conversely, if the flexion gap is larger than the extension gap, which is the more commonly encountered scenario, upsizing the femoral component and using thicker posterior augments to maintain bone contact and fixation will facilitate proper knee balancing. As with the

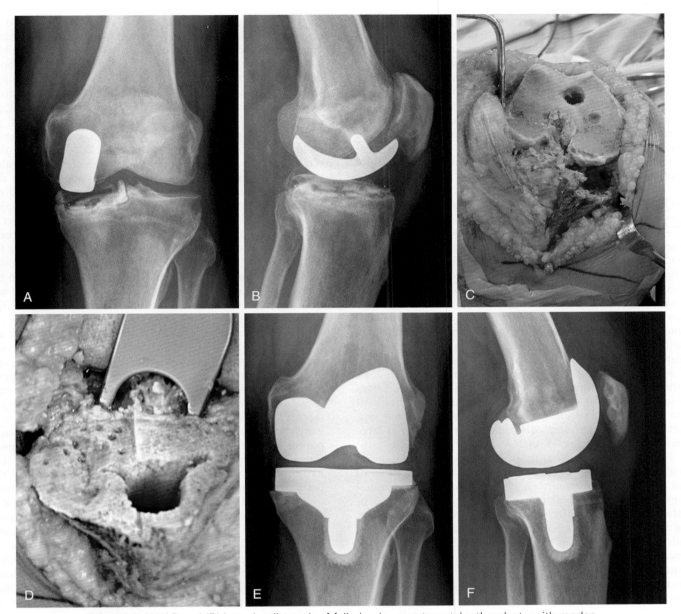

FIG 174.5 (A) AP and (B) lateral radiograph of failed unicompartmental arthroplasty with moderate tibial bone loss. (C) Intraoperative picture of moderate tibial defect. (D) Intraoperative picture demonstrating the correct alignment of the sagittal step cut for the block augment to correctly align the tibial component rotation with the tibial tubercle. (E) AP and (F) lateral radiograph of the revision TKR in (A) and (B) demonstrating the reconstruction with a cemented block augment and small cemented stem extension.

tibia, the correct alignment of the distal femoral cuts should typically be determined with intramedullary alignment guides, which also have cutting guides for correct placement and sizing of augments. The final and critical step in femoral component positioning is determining the correct femoral component rotation, which should align the implant with the transepicondylar axis as determined by the medial and lateral epicondyles. Frequently a larger posterior augment will be required laterally compared to the medial side to avoid placement of the femoral component in relative internal rotation, which is deleterious for patellar tracking and overall knee balance. Again, once the bone

preparation is complete, the final modular augments are applied to the femoral component and implanted with cement to bony surfaces that have been adequately prepared to facilitate cement interlock.

Clinical Results

Several studies have reported successful midterm results with modular metal augments in revision knee arthroplasty.[16,33,35] Patel et al. reported a prospective study of the 5- to 10-year results of 102 revision knee arthroplasties in patients with type 2 defects treated with augments and stems.[33] Average follow-up was 7 years (5 to 11) and nonprogressive radiolucent lines were observed around the augment in 14% of knees, but were not associated with decreased survivorship or increased failure of the implants. The overall survivorship of the components was 92% at 11 years.[33] Rand prospectively studied 41 consecutive revision TKAs with modular augmentation.[35] Modular augments were used for the distal femur alone in 2 knees, posterior condyles of the femur alone in 16 knees, and both distally and posteriorly in 12 knees. Tibial augmentation was used in 13 knees. At a mean of 3 years follow-up, 96% of the knees demonstrated good to excellent results and there were no cases of aseptic loosening.[35]

RECONSTRUCTION WITH POROUS METAL METAPHYSEAL CONES

Recently, highly porous metal metaphyseal cones were developed and used for large tibial and femoral defects and were designed to avoid the incidence of nonunion and resorption associated with bulk allograft reconstructions. Highly porous metals, particularly porous tantalum and titanium, are biomaterials that offer several potential advantages over traditional materials and include low stiffness, high porosity, and a high coefficient of friction. The design intent for these porous tantalum metaphyseal cones was to address the variable patterns of severe tibial bone loss encountered during revision knee arthroplasty, in addition to providing mechanical support with biologic integration and avoid allograft nonunion and resorption. Short- and medium-term evidence now exists that supports the use of these implants in the reconstruction of large tibial defects in revision TKA.[§]

The indications for the use of highly porous metaphyseal cones are similar to those traditionally used for bulk allograft and include large contained or uncontained tibial or femoral bony defects in a failed total knee replacement because of instability, osteolysis, infection, or aseptic loosening. The size of the defect is typically larger than is appropriately reconstructed with traditional modular blocks or wedges. The defects can be classified with the Anderson Orthopaedic Research Institute Bone Defect classification and the porous metaphyseal cones are typically indicated for types 2 and 3 defects, which are characterized by moderate to severe cancellous and/or cortical defects. The surgeon should keep in mind, however, that contained defects with a substantial supportive cortical rim may be more appropriate for impaction grafting, particularly in younger patients, and that small uncontained defects that are less than 5 to 10 mm in depth and isolated to one tibial plateau will likely be more amenable to standard metal blocks.

Alternatively, reconstruction of large tibial or femoral defects in young patients may be more appropriately performed with bulk allograft in an attempt to reconstitute bone stock for future revision surgery. Furthermore, large defects in patients with insufficient bone support or potential for osseointegration may be amenable to reconstruction with custom prostheses or tumor mega-prostheses.

Surgical Technique

The quantity and location of remaining cortical and cancellous bone must be noted and considered in the final assessment of

whether porous metal metaphyseal cones are indicated to augment the reconstruction. The most common tibial scenario appropriate for the porous metaphyseal cones is typically a severe contained or uncontained medial tibial plateau bony defect with varying amounts of lateral tibial plateau remaining for structural support (Fig. 174.6). The most common femoral defect appropriate for porous metal cones is a severe medial and lateral condyle cancellous bone deficiency with an intact, yet minimally supportive, cortical rim. The assessment should include the anticipated size and shape of the porous metaphyseal cone that will be appropriate, with respect to its fit within the tibial or femoral metaphysis and its tentative location and placement required to reconstitute the proximal tibial or distal femoral supporting surface. Visual inspection of the metaphyseal region and associated defect is performed with respect to the fit of the porous tantalum cone trial and a high-speed burr is used to contour the metaphyseal bone to accommodate the TM cone trial with the maximal bone contact and stability possible. The surgeon should not be overly concerned with the stability of the smooth plastic trials, as the actual implant will have a greater interference fit and stability because of the frictional resistance of the porous tantalum surface.

The appropriate porous tantalum cone size and shape are chosen and the final implant is impacted in the tibial or femoral metaphysis carefully with size-specific impactors. To minimize the chance of intraoperative periprosthetic fracture, the surgeon should avoid overly aggressive impaction of the final implant. Tibial and femoral metaphyseal bone in the revision setting is typically sclerotic, damaged, mechanically weak, and prone to inadvertent fracture. The frictional coefficient of the actual porous tantalum implant will create greater resistance to insertion and subsequent stability. Once the porous metal cone is in its final and stable position, any areas or voids between the periphery of the porous tantalum cone and the adjacent bone of the proximal tibia are filled with morselized cancellous bone or putty to prevent any egress of bone cement between the cone and host bone during cementation of the stemmed component (see Fig. 174.6C). The surgeon should also be aware that the rotation of the final implant is not dependent on the final rotation of the femoral or tibial components, as the porous metal cones are designed to fit within the defect to reconstitute the metaphyseal platform. There is typically sufficient room within the porous metal cone to allow rotation of the tibial and femoral components into correct position to optimize stability and patellofemoral mechanics, but this rotational freedom varies among implant systems.

The tibial and/or femoral revision prosthetic component is inserted through the cone using either cementless or cemented stem extensions. With either type of stem fixation, polymethylmethacrylate is placed between the porous cone and the tray and the proximal keel of the tibial component and/or between the box and augments of the femoral component. It is advantageous to contour and smooth the curing cement around the exterior of any exposed porous tantalum material, such as occurs in the area of uncontained defects, particularly in the vicinity of the MCL. This helps minimize the postoperative medial knee pain that can occur because of local irritation of soft tissues that are intended to be mobile, such as the MCL, against the high frictional surface of porous tantalum. Once the cement has hardened, the remainder of the surgical procedure is carried out in standard fashion with insertion of the appropriate polyethylene insert and meticulous wound closure.

[§]References 19, 22-24, 28, 29, and 45.

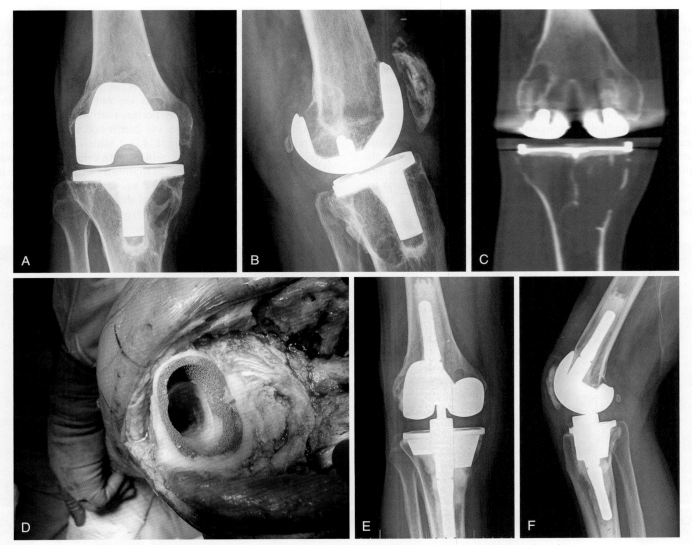

FIG 174.6 (A) AP and (B) lateral radiograph of a failed TKR with severe tibial bone loss because of medial tibial osteolysis. (C) CT scan demonstrating significant osteolytic defect in the medial tibia with cortical disruption. (D) Intraoperative picture of a severe tibial defect containing the highly porous tantalum metaphyseal cone implanted into the tibial defect with allograft bone putty impacted around the periphery between the surrounding tibial metaphysis. (E) AP and (F) lateral radiograph of the revision TKR in (A) and (B) demonstrating the porous metal metaphyseal cone and its intimate contact with the surrounding tibial bone while supporting the tibial component at 14 months follow-up.

The postoperative care of revision knee arthroplasty patients who have reconstructions using porous tantalum metaphyseal cones is no different than for those undergoing a standard revision TKA. Patients are allowed to bear weight as tolerated based on the implant stability and quality of reconstruction. If the surgeon achieves an inherently stable porous metaphyseal cone and final implant construct, the patient is allowed to bear weight as tolerated. If it is suspected that the mechanical stability of the construct is tenuous, the patient is kept partial weight bearing for 6 weeks and radiographs are obtained at that follow-up interval. If there is no evidence of implant or construct migration, the patients are then allowed to progress to weight bearing as tolerated.

Clinical Results

Early outcomes with highly porous metaphyseal cones used in large tibial defects for revision TKA have been reported by multiple authors.[24,28] Meneghini et al. reported a series of 15 revision knee arthroplasties that were performed with a porous metal metaphyseal tibial cone and were followed for a minimum of 2 years. All tibial cones were found to be osseointegrated radiographically and clinically at final follow-up with no reported failures in this initial series.[28] In a series of 16 revision TKAs with severe tibial defects, Long and Scuderi reported good results with osseointegration of the porous tantalum cone in 14 of 16 cases at a minimum 2-year follow-up. Two metaphyseal cones required removal for recurrent sepsis and were found to be well-fixed at surgery.[24] Similar results have been reported in the femoral version of the porous tantalum metaphyseal cones.[19,23,45] Howard et al. reported on 24 femoral porous tantalum cones in complex revision TKA and found no radiographic failure or loosening at a minimum of 2 years follow-up.[19]

Longer-term results are now available with highly porous tantalum metaphyseal tibial cones, and have demonstrated continued good results.[22] Kamath et al. recently reported on 66 highly porous tibial metaphyseal cones used in types 2 and 3 Anderson Orthopaedic Research Institute Bone Defect classification tibial defects. At a minimum 5-year follow-up, the authors report one revision for aseptic loosening and one radiograph with progressive radiolucencies concerning for fibrous ingrowth with a greater than 95% revision-free survivorship at latest follow-up.[22]

RECONSTRUCTION WITH NOVEL POROUS TITANIUM CONES

Recently, an alternative to porous tantalum metaphyseal cones was developed to optimize the surgical efficiency when addressing these large metaphyseal defects in revision TKA (Fig. 174.7A-G).[27] While clinical results are not yet available, the design premise of these highly porous titanium cones centers around the bone preparation via controlled reaming over a central reamer handle (see Fig. 174.7C), which facilitates more precise and intimate fit of the implant with optimized preparation efficiency. The highly porous titanium tibial cones come in a symmetrical and centrally based version as well as a lobed version for medial or lateral tibial defects. There is a single tapered reamer placed to the appropriate depth to ensure

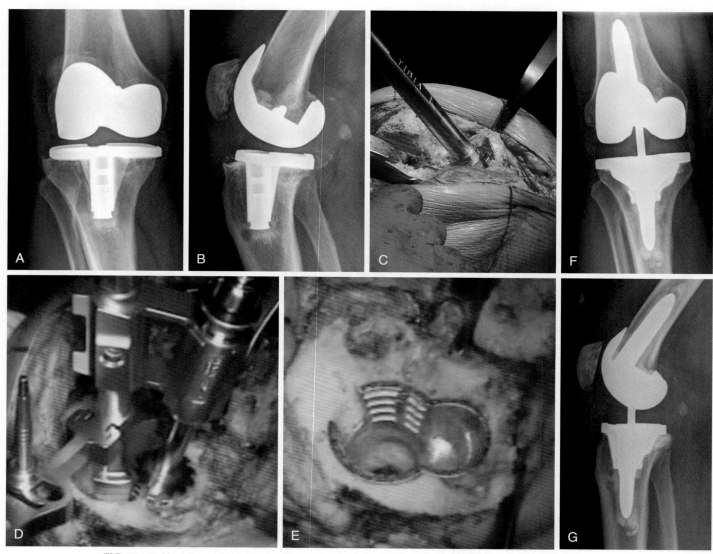

FIG 174.7 (A) AP and (B) lateral radiograph of a failed TKA with varus and posterior tibial collapse. (C) Central tapered reamer buried to the appropriate depth for a porous titanium cone and (D) additional single adjacent reamer to prepare for the (E) lobed tibial cone used to fill the medial tibial defect. (F) AP and (G) lateral postoperative radiograph showing the asymmetrical lobed tibial cone used in conjunction with a revision TKA with short cemented stems.

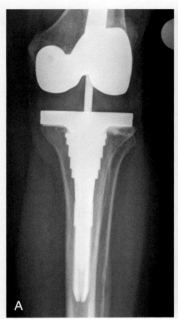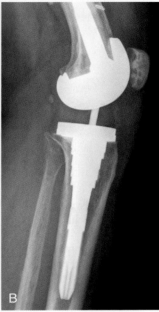

FIG 174.8 (A) AP and (B) lateral radiograph of a tapered titanium metaphyseal partially porous coated sleeve used to fill a central tibial defect and obtain adjuvant stability. Notice that the cemented tibial baseplate is in direct contact with the tibial bone and the sleeve is used for adjuvant fixation within the tibial metaphysis along with a cementless stem extension.

intimate bone contact and stability for a particular cone and defect size (see Fig. 174.7C). A lobed cone is an option for medial or lateral tibial defects and is prepared with one additional reaming step as shown in Fig. 174.7D. The reaming method of bone preparation facilitates an intimate press-fit of the final implant, which enhances mechanical stability and bone contact (see Fig. 174.7E-G). Long-term outcomes of these porous titanium cones will need to be evaluated to compare their clinical effectiveness to porous tantalum cones and tapered titanium sleeves, which both have successful early outcomes in revision TKA.

RECONSTRUCTION WITH METAPHYSEAL TITANIUM TAPERED SLEEVES

Cementless partially porous titanium tapered sleeves have emerged to treat larger metaphyseal tibial and femoral defects in revision TKA (Fig. 174.8A and B). The indications for these titanium sleeves are similar to those for the metaphyseal porous metal cones discussed in the previous section. The advantages of these implants are the ease of insertion with an aggressive and accurate broaching system, and a robust modular taper connecting the sleeve to the tibial and femoral components, which obviates the need for cement to unite the sleeve and bearing implant.

Excellent clinical results of the cementless partially porous titanium sleeves have been reported and demonstrate success in the early term.[2,3,8,14,20] A prospective study of 121 patients with 193 titanium sleeves that included 119 tibial and 74 femoral sleeves were followed for a mean of 3.6 months.[14] The authors

reported that 14 patients underwent revision; 3 of the 14 were for infection, leaving 11 revisions for loosening, instability of mechanical failure.[14] In another series, 35 revision TKAs in 34 patients were reported at a minimum of 2 years clinical and radiographic follow-up.[8] The authors used stem extensions in only a portion of the procedures in which the bone loss was more severe. In the remainder of revision TKAs with mild or moderate bone loss, the authors report using only the sleeve and cemented tibial tray or femoral component for fixation without the use of a stem extension and reported only one re-revision for a femoral cone failure at 3 years postoperatively.[8] In a series of 40 revision TKAs using a tibial porous coated titanium sleeve for Anderson Orthopaedic Research Institute Bone Defect classification type 2B or 3 defects, Alexander et al. reported 10 patients lost to follow-up and no mechanical failures related to the tibial cone at a minimum of 2 years.[2]

Interestingly, the methods of surgical technique described by the various authors discussed previously are varied and include allowing the tibial baseplate to sit proximal to the tibial metaphyseal bone surface as long as the titanium sleeve is rotational and axially stable, and allowing the sleeve to be implanted without stem extensions in cases of adequate sleeve mechanical stability.[2,8,14] However, caution should be exercised with respect to these practices because of the short-term follow-up of these reports and the unknown clinical consequences of surgical techniques that place large stresses and forces at the taper junction of the sleeve and the tibial or femoral component via unsupported implants or lack of stem extensions that engage the femoral or tibial diaphysis. In fact, one series reported two cases of implant failure because of mechanical breakage at the stem-sleeve junction, likely secondary to fatigue failure.[14] Therefore, the authors of this chapter recommend using stem extensions and carefully optimizing the tibial and femoral component cementation technique to ensure interdigitation with the host bone at the joint level to avoid large cyclic in vivo loads at the modular taper junction interfaces into the longer term.

KEY REFERENCES

 3. Barnett SL, Mayer RR, Gondusky JS, et al: Use of stepped porous titanium metaphyseal sleeves for tibial defects in revision total knee arthroplasty: short term results. *J Arthroplasty* 29(6):1219–1224, 2014.
 4. Bauman RD, Lewallen DG, Hanssen AD: Limitations of structural allograft in revision total knee arthroplasty. *Clin Orthop Relat Res* 467(3):818–824, 2009.
22. Kamath AF, Lewallen DG, Hanssen AD: Porous tantalum metaphyseal cones for severe tibial bone loss in revision knee arthroplasty: a five to nine-year follow-up. *J Bone Joint Surg Am* 97(3):216–223, 2015.
23. Lachiewicz PF, Bolognesi MP, Henderson RA, et al: Can tantalum cones provide fixation in complex revision knee arthroplasty? *Clin Orthop Relat Res* 470(1):199–204, 2012.
27. Meneghini RM, Harwin SF, Bowmik-Stoker M, Kirk AE: *Stability of Novel Porous Metal Metaphyseal Tibial Cones Designed for Surgical Efficiency Is Comparable to Traditional Cones.* American Association of Hip and Knee Surgeons, Dallas, TX, November 2015.
28. Meneghini RM, Lewallen DG, Hanssen AD: Use of porous tantalum metaphyseal cones for severe tibial bone loss during revision total knee replacement. *J Bone Joint Surg Am* 90(1):78–84, 2008.

The references for this chapter can also be found on www.expertconsult.com.

175

Patellar Revision

James A. Browne, Mark W. Pagnano

As the utilization of primary total knee increases, so too does the burden of revision surgery. Recent years have seen innovations in technology and technique that have undoubtedly improved a surgeon's ability to address many of the challenges inherent in revision procedures. Bone defects of the tibia and femur are well addressed with the stems, augments, cones, and wedges available in contemporary knee revision systems. However, management of the patella at the time of revision knee arthroplasty remains challenging with unsolved problems, a situation that is particularly problematic given that deficiencies of the patellar bone stock are commonly encountered. Many approaches have been advocated depending on a host of factors, including the design, wear, and fixation status of the existing component, along with the quantity and quality of the remaining patellar bone stock. Treatment can be particularly difficult if the patellar component is loose, malpositioned, or damaged.

The reasons for compromised patellar bone at the time of revision are numerous, with iatrogenic etiologies being common. Overresection or asymmetrical resection of the patella can compromise the residual bone stock and limit reconstructive options. Excessive medial malpositioning of the patellar component with osseous impingement and lateral subluxation of the remaining patella on the femoral component can lead to bony erosion or cause implant loosening and migration.[4,33] Bone fragmentation and compromise of fixation can also be caused by disruption of the vascular supply to the patella from extensive lateral dissection or retinacular release.[4] Loose patellar components can also lead to bony erosion.[4]

Osteolysis is another cause of patellar bone loss. Wear debris is most commonly generated from the tibiofemoral articulation but can also come from the patellofemoral articulation. Increased wear of the patellar polyethylene implant is seen in cases of high contact loading, with low conformity of the patellar and trochlear geometries.[20] Maltracking of the patella may also create high contact loading forces and lead to wear.[13] Polyethylene patellar components sterilized with gamma irradiation in air have been associated with failure because of wear,[30] as have metal-backed patellar implants.[3]

Finally, and perhaps increasingly so, the patella is damaged because of the necessity of removing a well-fixed implant in the face of infection. Removal of implant pegs and the interdigitated cement mantle can leave the patella severely compromised. Antibiotic-laden cement spacers can also further erode the patella and compromise future reconstruction.

Whether the patellar revision is for an isolated problem or part of revision where other components are being revised, a number of treatment options exist. An algorithm to direct management is presented in Fig. 175.1 and will be discussed further in this chapter.

THE WELL-FIXED PATELLA

The patellar component is often well fixed at the time of revision knee arthroplasty, and retention of this component is an attractive option when certain criteria are met. This approach is simple and avoids the potential morbidity of removal of a well-fixed implant and catastrophic compromise of the extensor mechanism.[26] Patellar component retention is feasible in many cases of aseptic revision total knee arthroplasty. In contrast, the patellar component should always be removed at the time of one-stage or two-stage revision done for deep prosthetic infection.

A well-fixed patellar component must be compatible with the prosthetic design of the rest of the knee to consider retention. The surgeon is often faced with the dilemma of leaving a patellar component that is mismatched with the implants used for revision of the femur and tibia. Patellar tracking can be used to gauge the appropriateness of leaving the patellar implant. Proper tracking ensures that the patellar component geometry is reasonably compatible with the femoral trochlear design, has been implanted in an appropriate position, and the overall patellar height is acceptable. Care must be taken to ensure that lateral subluxation of the patellar component has not resulted from an internally rotated femoral component, likely the greatest iatrogenic cause of maltracking in the revision setting.[26] A patellar component that is technically poor, from the asymmetrical resection of bone or overstuffing of the patellofemoral articulation, indicates that removal should occur.

Concerns about subtle mismatches in geometry and conformity between patellar and femoral components from different manufacturers have not been shown to lead to deleterious clinical results.[30] Looking at 73 total knee revisions, Barrack et al. reported that retaining a well-fixed patellar component gives equivalent short-term clinical results and patient satisfaction, compared with those obtained by successfully reimplanting a new patellar component.[2] Lonner et al. reported similar positive results with retention of a well-positioned, stable all-polyethylene patellar component in 202 revisions, provided that the polyethylene was not oxidized.[30]

Catastrophic wear and/or substantial surface damage of the patellar implant are clear indications for revision. However, minimal wear may be acceptable. Quantifying the exact amount of acceptable wear or deformation for component retention is impossible; the surgeon may consider patient age, activity level, bone quality, and the potential morbidity of the patellar component revision in that decision. Given that the forces generated at the prosthetic patellofemoral joint are often greater than the yield strength of polyethylene,[34] there is likely to be some wear or deformation of most patellar implants, and mild damage should not be an indication to revise all components.[26] Late failures because of wear from retained patellar components have been reported when the polyethylene was sterilized with gamma irradiation in air, and revision should be considered in the presence of obvious oxidation.[30]

Many authors have stated that presence of a metal-backed patellar implant is an indication for revision because of the poor track record and high rate of failure of many of these designs.[3,15,29,42] A review of metal-backed patellar components suggested that most large series reported a failure rate of approximately 6% to 8%, with late failures seen commonly at 6 or 8 years secondary to polyethylene wear and exposure of the metal backing.[42] However, others have argued that a well-fixed undamaged metal-backed component can be left in place with a reasonable expectation of success.[2] Some mobile-bearing metal-backed patellae have a good track record and may allow for isolated patella polyethylene exchange in selected cases.

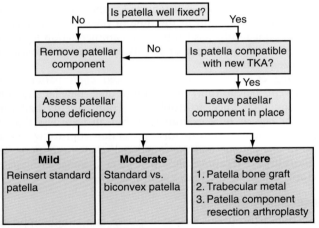

FIG 175.1 Algorithm to guide management of the patella at the time of revision knee arthroplasty. See the text for details.

Certain metal-backed patellae are extremely difficult to remove, and doing so risks the removal of significant bone and fracture. The surgeon must assess the potential risk of future failure because of a retained metal-backed component against the morbidity associated with patellar revision. It seems reasonable to retain a metal-backed patellar component when other criteria for component retention are met, particularly when the remaining bone stock is poor.[19]

PATELLAR COMPONENT REMOVAL

A malpositioned, damaged, or significantly worn patellar component will require revision. The grossly loose component presents little challenge. However, removal of a well-fixed implant must be performed with caution to minimize bone loss and avoid catastrophic extensor mechanism compromise.

Removal of an all-polyethylene component can be performed by separating the implant from the cement base with an osteotome or saw. Alternatively, a burr may be used to section the polyethylene, with subsequent piecemeal removal of the implant. Any residual cement can be removed in standard fashion by recutting the patella or using osteotomes, a burr, or a reamer.

A well-fixed metal-backed implant can be difficult to remove and risks bone loss or fracture if performed haphazardly. A diamond wheel cutting tool is often useful in separating the baseplate from the underlying host bone (Fig. 175.2).[12] If the metal-backed design includes lugs, they are typically well ingrown and can be removed with a fine tipped high-speed burr after removal of the baseplate. Alternatively, it is reasonable to consider leaving well-fixed lugs and covering them with the new patellar implant during aseptic revision. This can be accomplished by varying lug design (eg, by using a central peg design when revising a three-pegged component) or slightly repositioning the lugs when the host patellar bone allows.

PATELLAR COMPONENT REVISION

It is usually technically feasible and reasonable to implant a revision patellar component when only mild or moderate bone loss is encountered. Although the exact thickness of bone

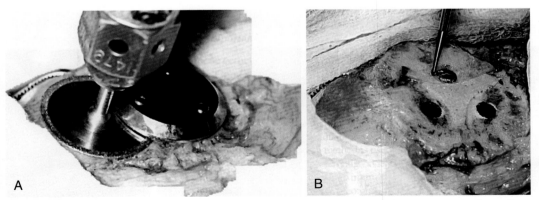

FIG 175.2 (A) A diamond wheel cutting tool can be used to separate a metal-backed patellar component from the underlying host bone. (B) If the metal-backed design includes lugs, they are typically well ingrown and can be removed with a fine tipped high-speed burr after removal of the baseplate.

required for an onlay all-polyethylene patellar component has not been precisely defined, a uniform thickness of 10 to 12 mm has been described as adequate.[40] A traditional onlay component may be used by preparing a flat surface and drilling new lug holes in the remnant bone. Meticulous removal of fibrous tissue and good cementation technique is important. Prior defects from lug holes and areas of cavitary bone loss can be filled with cement. An implant that matches the design of femoral component should be used.

When a patellar implant fails, isolated patellar revision has been associated with disappointing results and a relatively high rate of recurrent failure.[5,28] This is likely because of an incomplete understanding of the mechanism of patellar failure, which is often multifactorial and includes component rotation, relative "overstuffing" of the anterior compartment, lateral placement of the patellar component, and residual tightness of the lateral retinacular structures.[28]

Berry and Rand reported on 42 knees that underwent isolated revision of the patellar implant.[5] A relatively high complication rate was seen, including five late patellar fractures and a 19% reoperation rate directly related to the extensor mechanism. Adequate vascularity and thickness of the residual bone stock were felt to be important factors in a durable outcome. Other studies have also reported worse outcomes following isolated patellar procedures, compared with those who had concomitant femoral revision.[38]

An inset biconvex patella may be used when an intact rim of bone remains but there is too much central cavitary bone loss to provide support for a traditional onlay button (Fig. 175.3). Restoration of the composite thickness of the patella may be achieved with a thick but small diameter button.[19] The biconvex design allows for successful implantation in the patella with as little as 5 mm of central bone, although residual thickness less than 6 mm has been associated with fracture and implant failure.[14,21] The published clinical results of this technique have generally been good, with few complications at midterm follow-up.[21,31] In a recent report of 89 revision biconvex patellar implants, two cases of aseptic loosening and fracture were seen in association with avascular necrosis, to give an 98% survival rate at 10 years and 86% at 14 years.[14] Absence of a supportive rim of bone was thought to be a risk factor for radiographic loosening. The authors concluded that the presence of vascular bone was an important determinant in the satisfactory outcome of revision with a biconvex component.

SEVERE BONE LOSS

Severe bone loss is defined as residual bone stock insufficient for reimplantation of a prosthesis and has been reported to occur in 10% of revision total knees.[18] Most authors consider an absolute thickness less than 8 to 10 mm to be an contraindication to patellar revision,[42] although satisfactory results with a biconvex patella have been reported with central bone stock as little as 2 mm.[21] The typical patellar remnant consists of a thin bony shell with an intact anterior cortex and variable amounts of patellar rim.[18] Little cancellous bone usually remains.

A number of options exist for the management of severe bone loss. The traditional approaches in this setting have been either patellectomy or resection arthroplasty (patelloplasty).[18] Recently, alternative techniques including bone grafting and porous metal augmentation have been described in an attempt to improve clinical results. The respective advantages, disadvantages, and outcomes of these techniques will be reviewed.

Patellectomy

Patellectomy has been generally condemned for poor clinical results in revision total knee arthroplasty.[19] Inferior outcomes following primary total knee arthroplasty in patients with prior patellectomy have been well reported,[22] and although data are lacking for patellectomy at the time of revision, extrapolation of these poor results has led to the recommendation to restore or augment the deficient or absent patella in an attempt to optimize function.

Chang et al. retrospectively reviewed eight patients who underwent patellectomy for comminuted patellar fractures following total knee arthroplasty.[10] Four patients had mild extensor lags at final examination, but all were less than 10 degrees. Instability and quadriceps tendon rupture were each seen in one patient, and the functional results were poor. The authors urge that caution should be taken in considering patellectomy following total knee arthroplasty.

Resection Arthroplasty

Resection arthroplasty, or patelloplasty, is a simple approach where the patellar bone remnant is left unresurfaced. Unlike patellectomy, this approach maintains a fulcrum for knee extension. The remnant bone should be reshaped to remove sharp edges and rebalanced to optimize tracking. Avoiding additional attempts to resurface a compromised patella is appealing in that

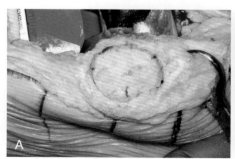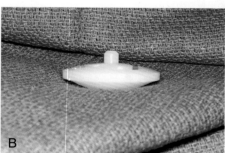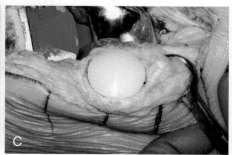

FIG 175.3 (A) Intraoperative photograph following removal of a loose patellar component. The peripheral rim of bone (outlined) is intact with a central cavitary defect. (B) A biconvex patella with a single central peg was used in this case to fill the defect and restore patellar height. (C) The final construct is shown.

it eliminates the risk of iatrogenic fracture and component loosening. However, the benefits of this approach, which also include ease of technique and low cost, must be weighed against the potential morbidity of postoperative fracture, maltracking, osteonecrosis, stiffness, extensor lag, and knee pain.[37]

Pagnano et al. reviewed 34 knees that were treated with patelloplasty when the patellar thickness was less than 10 mm and the bone stock precluded adequate implant fixation.[37] The clinical results were modest. Twenty-six patients were satisfied with the results of their revision operations, and five were dissatisfied. However, mild or moderate anterior knee pain persisted in one-third of these patients. Complications included fracture, recurvatum, extensor lag, flexion contracture, and stiffness. Fragmentation and lateral subluxation of the patellar remnant are common findings (Fig. 175.4). While the clinical results are somewhat unpredictable, Lavernia et al. reported that this technique does appear to avoid the untoward associations with patellectomy, such as quadriceps lag and extension weakness, and should be considered an acceptable strategy.[27]

A number of studies have attempted to retrospectively compare the results of resection arthroplasty to patellar component revision. Barrack et al. reported that the 21 cases treated with patelloplasty had a higher percentage of worse clinical outcomes and dissatisfaction compared to 92 cases treated with reimplantation of a patellar component.[1] However, a selection bias was clearly present, with the resection group having a significantly lower preoperative knee score. The authors acknowledge that patelloplasty may be an indicator of a more complicated and complex revision, and thus a lower quality result may be expected compared to patellar reimplantation.

More recent reports have not found patelloplasty to be inferior to resurfacing. Masri et al., in a retrospective matched cohort study, found that presence or absence of a patellar implant did not appear to affect pain, function, or satisfaction outcomes after revision total knee arthroplasty, suggesting that other variables are more important in determining outcome.[32] Similar results were reported more recently by Patil et al.[39] who also reported no differences in the improvement of Knee Society Scores, Short-Form 36 Scores, and satisfaction between patients managed with patelloplasty compared to retention of the patellar component or patellar resurfacing. Finally, Dalury and Adams reported satisfactory outcomes in 26 patients treated with patelloplasty with at least 6 years of follow-up.[11] Importantly, no patellar fractures or extensor mechanism complications were reported and no patients required additional surgery, suggesting patelloplasty may avoid many of the complication associated with other treatment options.

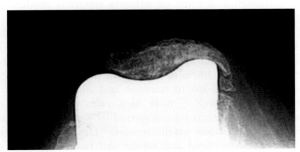

FIG 175.4 The remnant bone often remodels to the lateral condyle of the femoral component following resection arthroplasty.

Patellar resurfacing may be particularly challenging in the setting of a two-stage revision for infection, and patelloplasty may be the safest approach in many of these patients. Removal of the patellar component along with cement and necrotic tissue can leave the residual patella severely compromised, even when care is taken to avoid bone damage. The cement spacer may also migrate and further erode the patellar bone stock. Glynn et al. recently reported their experience with patellar management in the setting of two-stage revision and reported inferior results in clinical and functional outcomes when the patella could not be resurfaced.[16] Although the retrospective nature of this study and small numbers of heterogeneous patients makes definitive conclusions impossible, the authors recommend attempts be made to minimize bone loss at the first stage of resection arthroplasty to allow for patellar resurfacing during reimplantation.

One variation of patelloplasty involves a midline sagittal osteotomy of the patella to improve contour and tracking.[45] The so-called gull-wing greenstick osteotomy is performed by creating medial and lateral "wings" to form a convex patellar surface to articulate with the concavity of the femoral trochlear groove. This gives a V-shaped appearance on the patellar radiographic view. Successful early results of this technique have been reported in two small series, with acceptable patellar tracking and function with radiographic healing in most osteotomies.[24] Radiographic complications including avascular necrosis, lateral subluxation of the patella, and fibrous nonunion have all been reported with this technique, although function of the extensor mechanism may still be acceptable despite such findings.[24]

Bone Grafting

Techniques to bone graft the severely deficient patella have been developed in an attempt to address some of the disadvantages of resection arthroplasty. Potential restoration of bone stock is distinct advantage of these approaches. Two major categories of bone grafting exist: structural bone grafting and cancellous bone augmentation.

Structural autogenous bone grafting was first described by Buechel to address patients with prior patellectomy.[7] The technique involves harvesting iliac crest autograft, fashioning it in the shape of a patella, and sewing it into a subsynovial pouch for stabilization at the previous anatomic position of the patella. In cases where a patellar shell remains, autologous monocortical iliac crest graft can be shaped, opposed to the patellar remnant, and secured with screws.[43] Donor site morbidity is a clear disadvantage to autogenous bone grafting, and limited clinical reports make the outcome of these procedures uncertain.

The use of structural allograft has also been reported. Clinical results have been poor, with the use of patellar autografts in the setting of total knee arthroplasty and prior patellectomy.[8] A high rate of complications, including graft resorption, does not justify the routine use of this procedure.

Hanssen has reported the use of cancellous bone grafting of the deficient patella.[18] Building upon earlier work by Cave and Rowe,[9] this straightforward procedure involves the use of a soft tissue flap to contain morcellized autograft within the residual patellar bone shell (Fig. 175.5). The tissue flap functions as an interposition arthroplasty against the femoral trochlea and allows the contained bone graft to undergo molding and compression during range of motion.[19] Following preparation of the

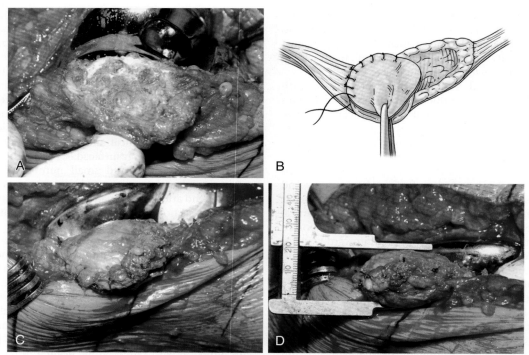

FIG 175.5 (A) Intraoperative photograph of a severely deficient patella without adequate bone to support an implant. (B) This patella was treated with Hanssen's bone grafting technique, in which a soft tissue graft is sutured to the remnant bony rim and peripatellar tissue to act as a pouch for bone grafting. (C) Photograph following graft impaction and closure of the pouch with sutures. (D) This technique allows for restoration of patellar height.

patellar shell, the peripatellar fibrotic tissue on the undersurface of the quadriceps tendon is elevated, turned down, and secured to the periphery of the patella using multiple nonabsorbable sutures. Fascia lata or Achilles tendon allograft may also be used for the flap if needed.[6] This creates a pouch into which the bone graft is inserted through a small purse-string opening. Tight impaction of the graft is performed to restore the patellar height (typically between 20 and 25 mm), and the small opening in the flap is closed.

Early clinical results of this technique are promising. Hanssen reported significant improvements in pain and function knee scores in nine patients at a mean follow-up of 3 years.[18] Patellar height ranged from 7 to 9 mm at the time of bone grafting. Minimal loss in patellar height was observed following the procedure (mean 22 mm on the immediate postoperative radiograph, compared to 19.7 mm at the time of most recent follow-up). Both cancellous autograft and allograft were seen to work successfully. Although one patient in this series had no evidence of revascularization at a subsequent operation, we have observed incorporation and gross bleeding of the graft using this technique (Fig. 175.6). With successful reconstitution of bone stock, the potential for future resurfacing exists.

Trabecular Metal Baseplate

Trabecular metal, a biomaterial fabricated from porous tantalum, has been used to fabricate an implant to address severe bone deficiency of the patella (Fig. 175.7). The design concept is analogous to the structural bone graft previously described.[19] The implant allows augmentation of patellar height by filling the central defect with metal. The flat articular sided surface of the patella has three holes to accept cementation of an all-polyethylene component. The patellar shell is prepared for the augment with domed reamers, and the augment is subsequently secured with sutures through a peripheral titanium ring.

Several series using this trabecular metal patellar implant have now been published.[25,26,35,41,44] The importance of adequate residual bone stock for fixation has been recognized by multiple authors. When 50% or more of the patellar implant is covered, the results have been good with stable fixation and good patient satisfaction.[35,41] These reports suggest that when fixation is possible, this option may compare favorably with patellar resection arthroplasty in the short term. Longer-term results are now beginning to be reported, and it appears that a reliable and durable result may be obtained with sufficient bone contact. Kamath et al. reported an 83% survivorship at a mean of 5 years, although one-third of patients reported moderate to severe anterior knee pain.[23]

However, when soft tissue (quadriceps tendon) is used for fixation of the implant, results have been consistently poor (Fig. 175.8). Ries et al. reported loosening and early migration of the patellar implant in 100% of cases, with no host bone contact, two of which went on to necrosis and discontinuity of the extensor mechanism.[41] Similar high rates of loosening and universally poor results were reported by Kwong and Desai in patients with previous patellectomies.[25] Despite experimental studies suggesting rapid and robust soft tissue ingrowth into porous tantalum,[17] this implant does not appear to provide predictable stability or clinical results when applied directly to tendon alone.

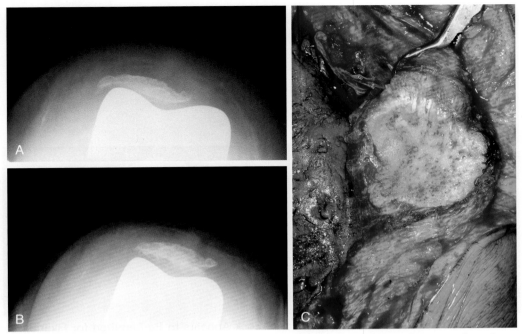

FIG 175.6 (A) Preoperative and (B) postoperative radiograph 18 months after cancellous bone grafting of the patella showing restoration and maintenance of patellar height. This patient subsequently developed a deep infection that required a two-stage revision. (C) An intraoperative radiograph at the time of resection arthroplasty revealed viable bleeding bone with reconstitution of patellar bone stock measuring 14 mm in thickness.

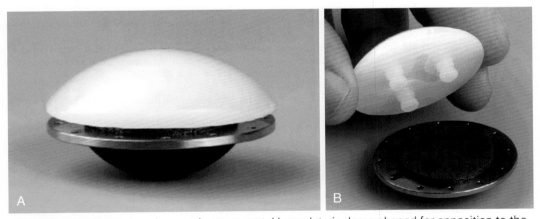

FIG 175.7 (A) The trabecular metal porous metal baseplate is dome shaped for apposition to the patellar shell. (B) The opposite surface has lugholes for cementation of the all-polyethylene component. (Reproduced with permission from Hanssen AD, Pagnano MW: Revision of failed patellar components. In Greene WB ed: Instructional Course Lectures, vol. 53, Rosemont, IL, 2004, American Academy of Orthopaedic Surgeons.)

CONCLUSION

Most revision total knee arthroplasties will be best served with retention of a well-fixed, compatible patellar component. When the patellar component requires removal, assessment of bone deficiency is crucial in guiding the subsequent treatment options. The multiple different approaches to address severe bone loss attest to the complexity and difficulty of this situation. Several techniques have been described to try to improve on patelloplasty, including the gull-wing osteotomy, cancellous bone grafting, and the trabecular metal implant. Early results of these procedures are encouraging in this challenging situation. Midterm outcomes of these approaches are now being reported and should improve our understanding of the value of these techniques. The underlying principle for any patellar revision is to ensure proper patellar tracking and avoid iatrogenic morbidity.

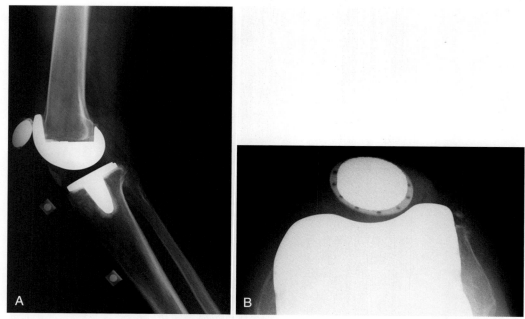

FIG 175.8 Some Amount of Residual Bone Stock Appears to Be Required for Fixation of the Trabecular Metal Implant. (A) Lateral and (B) patellar radiographs demonstrating migration of a trabecular metal patella that was sutured into the quadriceps tendon in a patient with prior patellectomy.

KEY REFERENCES

2. Barrack RL, Rorabeck C, Partington P, et al: The results of retaining a well-fixed patellar component in revision total knee arthroplasty. *J Arthroplasty* 15:413–417, 2000.
4. Berend ME, Ritter MA, Keating EM, et al: The failure of all-polyethylene patellar components in total knee replacement. *Clin Orthop* 388:105–111, 2001.
5. Berry DJ, Rand JA: Isolated patellar component revision of total knee arthroplasty. *Clin Orthop* 286:110–115, 1993.
18. Hanssen AD: Bone-grafting for severe patellar bone loss during revision knee arthroplasty. *J Bone Joint Surg Am* 83:171–176, 2001.
28. Leopold SS, Silverton CD, Barden RM, et al: Isolated revision of the patellar component in total knee arthroplasty. *J Bone Joint Surg Am* 85:41–47, 2003.
41. Ries MD, Cabalo A, Bozic KJ, et al: Porous tantalum patellar augmentation: the importance of residual bone stock. *Clin Orthop* 452:166–170, 2006.

The references for this chapter can also be found on www.expertconsult.com.

Patellar Fractures in Total Knee Arthroplasty

Daniel J. Berry

Extensor mechanism problems frequently have been cited as among the most common reasons for failure after total knee arthroplasty (TKA).[24,23,29] This may have changed as surgeons have learned more about the importance of tibial and femoral rotational alignment,[1] patellar component and trochlear groove design, and optimal patellar resurfacing techniques. Data from most national joint registries do not report the frequency of patellar problems separately, making a full accounting of the current burden of patellar-related problems challenging. Nevertheless, patellar fractures still occur after TKA.[2,3] About half of patellar fractures heal without major consequence; unfortunately, those that do not are often associated with serious problems.[17] Patellar fracture after TKA occurs far more commonly in resurfaced than in nonresurfaced patellae. A large proportion of fractures occur in the absence of a clear traumatic event. This chapter reviews risk factors for fracture, fracture classification, fracture results, and techniques of fracture management.

PREVALENCE AND RISK FACTORS FOR PATELLAR FRACTURE

The prevalence of patellar fracture varies in different series, with most reports describing between 0.5% and 6% for resurfaced patellae.* Ollivier et al. reported the largest series of patella fractures: 256 fractures that occurred after 32,754 primary TKA. The cumulative probability of a postoperative patella fracture at 20 years was 1.5% in this cohort, almost all of which had a resurfaced patella.[33] The prevalence is higher after revision TKA.[2] Prevalence probably varies according to many factors, including patient demographics, implant design, and surgical technique. The reported prevalence also undoubtedly varies in part due to deficiencies in completeness of follow-up for this complication. As surgeons and implant designers have become more aware of what causes extensor mechanism problems and how to prevent them, there is reason to believe that the incidence of patellar fracture has declined.

The strongest risk fracture for patellar fracture is resurfacing of the patella.[16,42] Grace and Sim[16] reported that the risk of fracture of nonresurfaced patellae was only 0.05%. Gender is a risk factor for fracture, and unlike most periprosthetic fractures, men are at higher risk for fracture than women. In the series of Ortiguera and Berry,[34] the overall prevalence of fracture in 12,246 consecutive TKAs was 0.68%. The prevalence was 0.40%

in women but 1.01% in men. One possible reason for the higher incidence in men could be the capability to generate greater quadriceps forces. Analysis of large patient groups by Meding et al.[31] from Indiana and Tamachote et al.[46] from the Mayo Clinic has demonstrated that increased body mass index (BMI) is a risk factor for fracture. In the large recent Mayo Clinic series, male gender (hazard ratio = 2.2) and BMI greater than 30 (hazard ratio = 1.3) were associated with higher risk of failure. Diagnosis leading to TKA and age at TKA have not yet been demonstrated to be major risk factors for patellar fracture.

Most patellar fractures are not associated with a substantial traumatic event. In the series of Ortiguera and Berry,[34] 11 of 78 fractures were associated with a blow to the knee, 6 occurred as the patient stood from sitting, 5 spontaneously while walking, 3 with knee hyperflexion, and 2 in patients with previous patellar subluxation; notably, in 48 patients, no clear event leading to fracture was recognized.

Technical and design factors also probably affect risk of fracture. In the recent large series reported by Ollivier et al.,[33] use of an uncemented patellar component was associated with higher risk of postoperative patella fractures (hazard ratio = 2.3), compared to cemented patellar components. Revision arthroplasty patients are at higher risk than primary TKA patients. The thickness of the patella probably affects risk, and both very thin and very thick resurfaced patellae are at increased risk. Thin patellae are likely at risk because of bone weakness. Erak et al.[13] reported that fractures were more common in revision TKA with an inset "biconvex" patellar component when the patellar remnant measured less than 6 mm in thickness. A recent article found a 1.5% risk of patellar fracture in 329 TKA in patients with rheumatoid arthritis, all of whom had been treated with patellar resurfacing. Thin residual patellar thickness was identified and associated with fracture risk.[21]

Patellar fractures are not uncommon after patellofemoral arthroplasty, a circumstance in which altered extensor mechanism dynamics and patellar anatomy have been present on a chronic basis in many patients. King et al.[25] reported a 9.1% patellar fracture rate in a contemporary series, with positive correlates of fracture risk, including change in patellar thickness (pre- to postoperatively), amount of patellar bone resection, large trochlear size, and in distinction to TKA, lower patient BMI.

Some patellar fractures clearly appear to occur in the presence of patellar osteonecrosis, but a clear link between lateral retinacular release and patellar fracture has not been established, and papers have been published both for and against an association.[28,37-39,43] Lateral retinacular release has been shown by scintigraphy methods[36] to produce transient

*References 2, 6, 7, 10, 18, 29, 31, and 50.

patellar hypovascularity. However, Kusuma et al.[26] evaluated 1108 consecutive TKAs, of which 314 had a lateral retinacular release and reported no cases of patellar fracture. An interesting study by Hempfing et al. studied intraoperative patellar blood flow during TKA with laser Doppler flowmetry.[19] After standard medial patellar arthrotomy and completion of the procedure, they did not identify major changes in patellar blood flow in 10 patients. They concluded the study did not support "the theory of postoperative patellar ischemia as a cause of anterior knee pain or patellofemoral problems." However, the possibility that postoperative patellar blood flow reduction may be an etiology of patellar fracture in some patients, possibly those with anatomic variations requiring larger soft tissue releases, remains unresolved by this study.

Malalignment of the limb and of tibial and femoral implants clearly has been shown to increase patellar fracture risk.[14] In Ortiguera's series,[34] 76% of patients had a major limb or implant axial malalignment and 6% a minor malalignment by Figge's criteria.[14] Seventeen of 18 patients in Tria's series[48] had a minor malalignment. Seo et al. reported a case control series of 88 patellar fractures occurring in 7866 consecutive TKAs from 1998 to 2009. They found fracture incidence was associated with the number of previous knee operations, greater mechanical malalignment preoperatively, lower postoperative patellar tendon length and Insall-Salvati ratio, and lower residual patellar thickness.[44] An excellent report by Meding et al. evaluated operative and patient factors associated with patellar fractures in 8530 posterior cruciate retaining TKAs treated from 1983 to 2003.[31] Patella fractures were identified in 5.2% of knees and correlated positively with male gender and preoperative knee alignment of more than 5 degrees of varus.

In recent years, the strong relationship between malrotation of tibial and femoral implants and extensor mechanism complications, including patellar fractures, has increasingly been demonstrated.[1] Certain femoral component designs with a boxy configuration on lateral projection may have been associated with higher patellar fracture risk. Patellae of certain designs,[51] including some components with a large central peg (as opposed to a three-anchoring-peg design), also may be associated with increased fracture risk.[27]

Little has been written about the chronology of patellar fractures after TKA, but they seem to occur most often in the first several years after TKA.[9] Ortiguera and Berry[34] reported that 82% of fractures occurred in the first 3 years after TKA, with 46% recognized in the first year. In the series of 18 fractures reported by Tria et al.,[48] fractures occurred from 3 to 22 months postoperatively, with a mean at 11 months postoperatively. In the series of 88 fractures reported by Seo et al.,[44] the mean time to recognition of fracture was 13.4 months (a range of 2 to 84 months). In the large unpublished series from the Mayo Clinic, Ollivier et al.[33] reported 0.01% of TKA sustained a patella fracture in the first 30 days after operation, 0.2% during the first year, 0.3% between year 1 and 5, and 0.2% between years 5 and 20.

Intraoperative patellar fractures can occur, but are rare, although they may be more common in revision than primary TKA. Ollivier et al.[33] reported an incidence of 0.02% in 32,754 primary TKA. Five of 8 fractures occurred during drilling of peg holes and were nondisplaced cracks.

CLASSIFICATION

Several different classification schemes for patellar fractures around TKA have been proposed[41] (Figs. 176.1 and 176.2). The classification of Goldberg et al.[15] considers fracture pattern, extensor mechanism disruption, and patellar subluxation. Type I fractures do not have disruptions of the extensor mechanism or implant fixation; type II fractures do have disruption of the extensor mechanism or implant fixation; type IIIa fractures have a disrupted extensor mechanism with an inferior patellar pole fracture; type IIIb fractures have the same characteristics as IIIa but with an intact extensor mechanism; and type IV fractures are patellar fracture dislocations. Hozack et al.[20] used

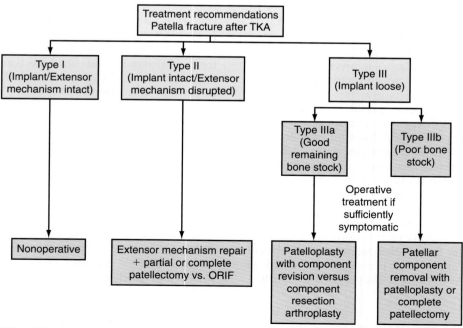

FIG 176.1 Classification and treatment algorithm proposed by Ortiguera and Berry.[34]

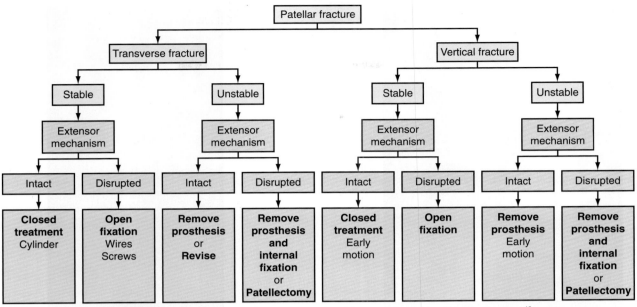

FIG 176.2 Classification and treatment algorithm proposed by Rorabeck et al.[40]

TABLE 176.1	**Classification of Periprosthetic Patellar Tracking According to Ortiguera**
Type I	Extensor mechanism intact; patellar implant well fixed
Type II	Extensor mechanism disrupted
Type IIIa	Patellar implant loose; patellar bone stock allows revision
Type IIIb	Patellar implant loose; patellar bone stock does not allow revision

From Ortiguera CJ, Berry DJ: Patellar fracture after total knee arthroplasty. *J Bone Joint Surg Am* 84:532–540, 2002.

a classification that included fracture displacement, presence or absence of extensor lag, fracture location, and failure of previous treatment.

The classification of Ortiguera and Berry[34] (Table 176.1) focuses on three main factors: integrity of the extensor mechanism, fixation status of the patellar implant, and remaining patellar bone stock. Type I fractures have an intact extensor mechanism Fig. 176.3 and a fixed patellar component; type II fractures have a functionally disrupted extensor mechanism (Fig. 176.4); and type III fractures have a loose implant but an intact extensor mechanism. Type III fractures are further subdivided as IIIa (Fig. 176.5) (satisfactory remaining bone stock for patellar component revision) and IIIb (unsatisfactory remaining bone stock for patellar component revision) (Fig. 176.6).

Recently Duncan et al.[49] introduced a Unified Classification System for periprosthetic fractures of all bones around joint arthroplasties. While not expressly devised for patellar fractures, the classification scheme provides valuable descriptive information, and interobserver reliability was found to be good and intraobserver reliability excellent.

RESULTS

Minimally displaced or nondisplaced fractures with an intact extensor mechanism commonly are successfully treated nonoperatively with satisfactory results. Ortiguera and Berry[34] reported

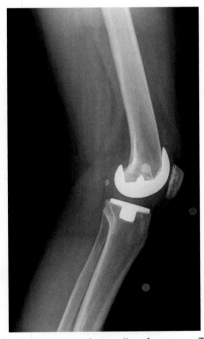

FIG 176.3 Ortiguera type I patellar fracture. The extensor mechanism is intact.

that all but 1 of 38 such fractures were treated successfully without operation. In the series of Parvizi et al.,[35] six of seven patients with such fractures had good results with nonoperative (cast or brace) treatment. In Goldberg's series,[15] good results of treatment also were seen in 16 patients with an intact extensor mechanism.

Fractures associated with a disrupted extensor mechanism have had the poorest results. In the series of Ortiguera and Berry,[34] 11 of 12 patients with this type of fracture were treated operatively, and complications occurred in 6 of these patients. Only one of six patients treated with open reduction and

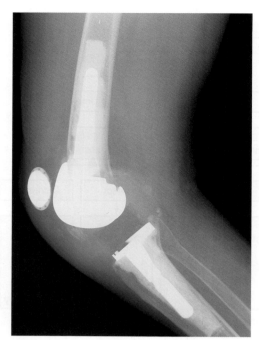

FIG 176.4 Ortiguera type II patellar fracture. The extensor mechanism continuity is disrupted.

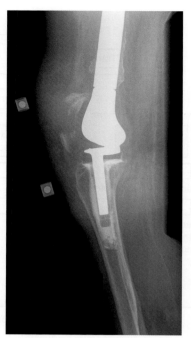

FIG 176.6 Ortiguera type IIIb patellar fracture. The patellar component is loose and patellar bone stock is severely deficient.

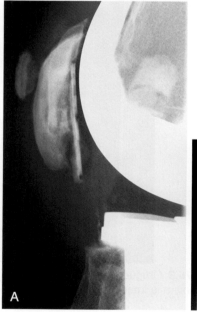

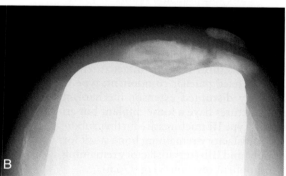

FIG 176.5 (A and B) Ortiguera type IIIa patellar fracture. The patellar component is loose but patellar bone stock remains.

internal fixation went on to bone-to-bone healing of the patella, and three of four patients treated with fragment excision and tendon advancement to bone had complications necessitating reoperation. Seven of the 12 patients had residual pain, weakness, or extensor mechanism instability. In the series of Goldberg et al.,[15] five of eight patients with an inferior pole fracture and a disrupted extensor mechanism had poor results. Keating et al.[22] reported on 17 patients with a disrupted extensor

mechanism: two were treated with open reduction and internal fixation, and neither healed.

For fractures associated with a loose patellar component, results vary considerably. In the series of Ortiguera and Berry,[34] a few patients with sufficient bone stock for patellar component revision (2 of 28 fractures with a loose implant) did well, as did many patients with sufficiently fewer symptoms to allow nonoperative treatment of this fracture type. When patients required resection arthroplasty and partial or complete patellectomy, the results were less satisfying: six of eight knees treated with resection arthroplasty and partial patellectomy remained symptomatic, and two of three knees treated with patellectomy remained symptomatic. Goldberg et al.[15] reported poor results in four of six patients with a loose patellar component. Keating et al.[22] reported that infection developed in four of nine patients treated with patellar component excision for an extruded patellar component in association with patellar fracture. Chang et al.[8] reported on 9 knees treated with patellectomy for comminuted patellar fracture after TKA: 2 of 9 patients had a complication of extensor mechanism disruption, 2 were unable to use stairs, and 4 patients had some mild extensor lag (less than 10 degrees). They concluded that patellectomy often provided satisfactory pain relief, but that functional results were often poor.

Treatment

A number of different fracture treatment algorithms have been proposed based on different fracture classification methods.[4,5,40] The Ortiguera classification method may be used as a framework for treatment of periprosthetic patellar fractures. This algorithm management strategy is similar to one proposed recently by a combined group of authors from the Mayo Clinic and Hospital for Special Surgery.[32]

Type I Fractures. A great majority of type I fractures may be treated nonoperatively, with a good likelihood of a favorable result (Fig. 176.7). At the time of presentation, the orthopedist should attempt to understand the time frame during which the fracture occurred. In many patients, these fractures occur spontaneously and are asymptomatic, and the first time they are found is on a routine follow-up radiograph. If it appears that the fracture is not acute and that it occurred at an indeterminate time in the past, discussion of the finding with the patient followed by observation alone is appropriate for most asymptomatic or minimally symptomatic patients. For acute fractures, the goal is to prevent notable displacement that could lead to functional extensor mechanism disruption. In most cases, this means protection or immobilization with a knee immobilizer or a cast for about 6 weeks. Depending on the clinical course and serial radiographic findings, the patient may progress to gentle passive motion of the knee at some point during the first 6 weeks of treatment in selected cases. The more at risk for displacement the fracture, the more cautious the orthopedist should be in progression of range of motion and active quadriceps activities. Many fractures will go on to bony healing, others to fibrous healing with an intact extensor mechanism; most eventually will be asymptomatic.

Type II Fractures. As discussed in the "Results" section of this chapter (earlier), type II fractures with a disrupted extensor mechanism are associated with a high rate of treatment-related complications. This finding likely relates in part to the difficulty of gaining good internal fixation and union of the thin, sometimes dysvascular, resurfaced patella, and to the risk of infection or other complications when operation is pursued. In some cases, despite a widely displaced patellar fracture, patients may have reasonable extensor mechanism power and little extensor lag because of intact medial and lateral retinacular soft tissues, through which the quadriceps can transmit force (Fig. 176.8). In some such patients, after careful discussion of the pros and cons with the patient, nonoperative management may be elected.[12] Nonoperative management also may be chosen in some very low-demand elderly patients and patients with other very serious medical problems, even when the extensor

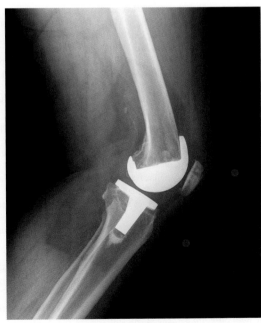

FIG 176.7 Nondisplaced patellar fracture (Ortiguera type I) that occurred 2 years following TKA. The patient was treated nonoperatively with a good result.

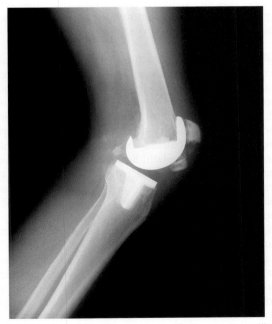

FIG 176.8 Displaced patellar fracture (Ortiguera type II) 1 year following TKA. The patient had a surprisingly modest extension lag (15 degrees) and because of multiple comorbidities was treated nonoperatively.

mechanism is notably functionally deficient; however, this decision should not be taken lightly because of the substantial long-term functional deficit that is likely to occur.

Most surgeons prefer to treat many patients with a type II fracture operatively in an attempt to restore extensor mechanism continuity.[3,45] When large fracture fragments with satisfactory vascularity are present, internal fixation using tension band wiring methods (often with addition of stabilizing adjunctive K-wires or cannulated screws) may be considered. When only a small fragment of the proximal or distal pole of the patella is present may the surgeon choose tendon advancement methods and fixation of the tendon to patellar bone with nonabsorbable sutures passed through small-diameter longitudinal drill holes in the patella, using Krackow-style stitches in the advanced tendon. Suture anchors also may be used when repair by suture fixation is contemplated.[30] A temporary protective wire or suture passed over the superior patella and through a drill hole in the tibial tubercle may be considered for patients with patellar tendon advancements. Whether the displaced patellar fracture is treated with internal fixation or tendon advancement, the surgeon should be aware that fixation and healing failure represent a serious threat to successful surgical outcome, and generous postoperative protection is justified, even at the risk of loss of some knee motion. Infection remains an ever-present risk when operative management of patellar fractures is employed, and all efforts to minimize infection risk, with appropriate antibiotic use, careful soft tissue handling, and maintenance of tissue vascularity, are recommended.

Some type II fractures present as chronic problems with long-standing extensor mechanism disruption.[47] In cases for which operative management is chosen, whole extensor mechanism allograft replacement or augmentation techniques (with quadriceps-patella-patellar tendon–tibial tubercle bone block or Achilles tendon with bone block) may be considered. Although technically challenging, such reconstructions can successfully restore extensor mechanism function to very disabled patients. Details of this method of reconstruction are discussed elsewhere in this textbook.

Type III Fractures. Many fractures of this type are minimally displaced and can be treated initially with nonoperative measures, as described earlier for type I fractures. If nonoperative measures fail because of ongoing pain and/or dysfunction related to the fracture or the loose implant, then operative treatment may be considered. For most Ortiguera type IIIa fractures, this involves patellar component revision to solve the problem of the loose implant. So long as the extensor mechanism remains intact (ie, the fracture has not become a type II fracture), nonessential fragments of the patella may be ignored, debrided, or excised, depending on their location and their value to extensor mechanism continuity.

Ortiguera type IIIb fractures often occur in the setting of a previously revised patella or osteonecrosis of the patella. Fortunately, some are insufficiently symptomatic to require reoperation, and in consultation with the patient, nonoperative measures and observations may be elected. The main options for more symptomatic patients include patellar component resection arthroplasty, patellar component resection arthroplasty with reshaping or excision of some patellar fracture fragments, or patellectomy. In most cases, one of the first two methods will be chosen as initial treatment, with patellectomy (discussed later) reserved for failure of one of these two methods. At operation, the surgeon should remove not only the loose patellar component but also the loose bone fragments and any cement retained on the posterior patellar surface. Patellectomy after TKA is usually considered a treatment method of last resort, but it can be successful in highly selected circumstances, such as persistent pain with a dysvascular, highly fragmented, chronic patellar fracture. The extensor mechanism tube method of Compere et al.[11] is favored because it provides a strong residual extensor mechanism, helps with extensor mechanism tracking, and provides extensor mechanism bulk, which helps restore the quadriceps lever arm and creates a cosmetically more normal appearing knee contour.

At the time of operation for any type III fracture, the surgeon should be prepared to perform a polyethylene insert exchange (for modular implants), because loosening of the patella often leads to third body debris damage to the polyethylene. The surgeon must strive to optimize extensor mechanism tracking. It is important to note that the surgeon should evaluate whether notable tibial or femoral implant malposition or malrotation is present as an underlying and predisposing condition for the fracture and should consider whether tibial/femoral component revision is warranted.

KEY REFERENCES

1. Berger RA, Crossett LS, Jacobs JJ, et al: Malrotation causing patellofemoral complications after total knee arthroplasty. *Clin Orthop* 356:144–153, 1998.
2. Berry DJ: Epidemiology: hip and knee. *Orthop Clin North Am* 30:183–190, 1999.
5. Burnett RS, Bourne RB: Periprosthetic fractures of the tibia and patella in total knee arthroplasty. *Instr Course Lect* 53:217–235, 2004.
11. Compere CL, Hill JA, Lewinnek GE, et al: A new method of patellectomy for patellofemoral arthritis. *J Bone Joint Surg Am* 61:714–718, 1979.
12. Dennis DA: Periprosthetic fractures following total knee arthroplasty. *Instr Course Lect* 50:379–389, 2001.
14. Figgie HE, III, Goldberg VM, Figgie MP, et al: The effect of alignment of the implant on fractures of the patella after condylar total knee arthroplasty. *J Bone Joint Surg Am* 71:1031–1039, 1989.
15. Goldberg VM, Figgie HE, III, Inglis AE, et al: Patellar fracture type and prognosis in condylar total knee arthroplasty. *Clin Orthop* 236:115–122, 1988.
22. Keating EM, Haas G, Meding JB: Patella fracture after post total knee replacements. *Clin Orthop* 416:93–97, 2003.
24. Kelly M: Extensor mechanism complications in total knee arthroplasty. *Instr Course Lect* 53:193–199, 2004.
31. Meding JB, Fish MD, Berend ME, et al: Predicting patellar failure after total knee arthroplasty. *Clin Orthop* 466:2769–2774, 2008.
34. Ortiguera CJ, Berry DJ: Patellar fracture after total knee arthroplasty. *J Bone Joint Surg Am* 84:532–540, 2002.
35. Parvizi J, Kim KI, Oliashirazi A, et al: Periprosthetic patellar fractures. *Clin Orthop* 446:161–166, 2006.
39. Ritter MA, Pierce MJ, Zhou HL, et al: Patellar complications (total knee arthroplasty): effect of lateral release and thickness. *Clin Orthop* 367:149–157, 1999.
41. Rorabeck CH, Taylor JW: Classification of periprosthetic fractures complicating total knee arthroplasty. *Orthop Clin North Am* 30:209–214, 1999.
45. Sheth NP, Pedowitz DI, Lonner JH: Periprosthetic patellar fractures. *J Bone Joint Surg Am* 89:2285–2296, 2007.

The references for this chapter can also be found on www.expertconsult.com.

177

Extensor Mechanism Disruption After Total Knee Arthroplasty

Matthew P. Abdel, Kelly L. Scott, Arlen D. Hanssen

INTRODUCTION

Extensor mechanism disruptions are one of the most challenging complications of total knee arthroplasty (TKA). The incidence of extensor mechanism complications after TKA varies, with estimates ranging from 1% to 12%.[52] The causes for disruption are often multifactorial and include, but are not limited to, preoperative risk factors, intraoperative technique, and postoperative management. The relative contribution of each cause varies, yet all can lead to disruption at any level of the extensor mechanism. Inadequate management will invariably lead to significant functional deficits. In the past, primary repair was attempted, but poor outcomes led to the clear emergence of reconstructive techniques as the superior method of management.[5,21,41,55]

This chapter focuses exclusively on disruptions of the quadriceps tendon and patellar tendon, with emphasis on accurate assessment and successful management of each type of complication.

ANATOMY

The extensor mechanism is composed of the quadriceps tendon, patellar bone, and patellar tendon. The quadriceps tendon is the confluence of the quadriceps muscle complex, which includes the rectus femoris (superficial layer), vastus medialis and lateralis (middle layer), and vastus intermedius (deep layer).[38,57,74] The tendon is approximately 8 mm thick at the superior pole of the patella,[63] having originated proximally as a narrow and thin tendon, often less than a few millimeters in width and depth at its most proximal portion. The quadriceps tendon coalesces into the patellar tendon at the inferior-dorsal surface of the patella. This patellar tendon inserts into the tibial tubercle. Proximally, the thickness of the patellar tendon ranges from 4 to 7 mm and as it proceeds distally, the width can be 20 to 30 mm[45,51] and the length approximately 35 to 55 mm.[57]

The vascularization of the extensor mechanism is vast and includes a network of anastomoses. The quadriceps tendon is perfused by the descending branches of the lateral femoral circumflex, the descending genicular, and the medial and lateral superior genicular arteries.[62] Of note, a watershed area exists approximately 1 to 2 cm from the superior pole of the patella.[54,64,73] The patellar tendon is perfused mainly by the inferior medial and lateral genicular arteries, with some of the blood supply provided by the recurrent anterior tibial artery.[66]

The patella acts as a fulcrum to increase the lever arm of the quadriceps,[39] almost doubling the efficiency of the extensor mechanism.[56] Walking generates forces of approximately 0.5 times body weight, stair-climbing is responsible for a force of 3.1 times body weight, and squatting generates the largest force, equivalent to 7 times body weight.[6,58]

PREOPERATIVE ASSESSMENT AND PLANNING

Patients with extensor mechanism disruptions usually present with pain, swelling, and loss of extension power. Additional symptoms particular to the level of the disruption are often present and provide insight into the mechanism of failure and the resulting defect.

Patients who present with symptoms that are suggestive of an extensor mechanism disruption should have a thorough history and physical examination. As with any potential complication, it is of utmost importance to rule out infection by obtaining erythrocyte sedimentation rate (ESR) and C-reactive protein (CRP) levels. If infection is suspected, a preoperative knee aspiration should be performed to assess cell count, differential, and cultures.

Radiographic images should consist of standing anteroposterior (AP) films, as well as lateral and patellar views of both knees. The lateral view is usually diagnostic of complete disruption of the extensor mechanism. Complete quadriceps tendon ruptures will result in patella baja, whereas complete patellar tendon ruptures will result in patella alta (Fig. 177.1A and B). Ultrasound (US) or magnetic resonance imaging (MRI) may be helpful in further classifying the defect.

QUADRICEPS TENDON RUPTURES

Incidence, Prevention, and Risk Factors

In a series of 23,800 TKAs performed at the Mayo Clinic between 1976 and 2002, Dobbs et al.[19] reported the incidence of a partial or complete quadriceps tendon disruption in less than 1% of patients. Partial ruptures, identified by an extensor lag, were twice as common as complete ruptures (23 partial vs. 11 complete). Current estimates of the incidence of quadriceps tendon ruptures range from 0.1% to 1.1%.[2,19,41] Patient factors that increase the risk for quadriceps tendon disruptions include systemic diseases such as rheumatoid arthritis, diabetes mellitus, and chronic kidney disease, as well as multiple prior knee surgeries.[19,22,41,52]

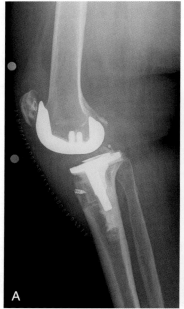
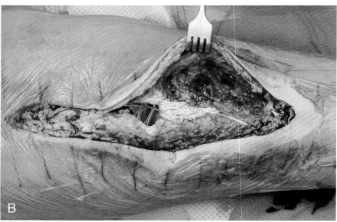

FIG 177.1 (A) Lateral radiograph of a 64-year-old woman who had a failed primary repair of a patellar tendon rupture at an outside institution, as evidenced by the patella alta. (B) Intraoperatively, there was near complete disruption of the patella tendon.

There are also intraoperative risk factors that may increase the risk of later quadriceps disruptions. For example, patients requiring a patellectomy during a TKA are at a higher risk of quadriceps dysfunction as a result of excessive bone removal that weakens the overlying quadriceps tissue. Chang et al.[15] reported that two of the nine patients (22%) with a patellectomy sustained a quadriceps tendon rupture. In a matched study of 50 patients, Yao et al.[72] also illustrated that patellectomized patients do not do as well as patients who retain the patella fulcrum, as assessed by the Short Form (SF)-12, Western Ontario and McMaster Universities Osteoarthritis Index (WOMAC), and Knee Society scores (KSSs).

The approach in a TKA can also adversely affect the integrity of the quadriceps tendon. For example, a quadriceps snip[3,4,24,47] is effective at obtaining an extensile exposure during a difficult revision TKA. Specifically, the quadriceps snip is a proximal extension of the medial parapatellar arthrotomy. The arthrotomy is in line with the tendon, which diminishes in width as it extends proximally. In performing a snip, the surgeon must not transect the tendon but rather extend the arthrotomy into the muscle parallel to the tendon fibers. Unfortunately, there have been modifications to this approach that potentially jeopardize the integrity of the tendon, increasing the risk for an extensor lag and/or complete rupture.[31]

Management

An extensor lag, which may be evidence of an insufficient extensor mechanism, is very difficult to fully correct. In fact, most situations are addressed nonoperatively with strengthening exercises. All too often, however, the patient may still require appropriate bracing. Partial ruptures of the quadriceps or patellar tendon can be managed in a standard nonoperative manner (ie, knee in extension for 4 to 6 weeks with protected weight bearing).

Complete ruptures of the quadriceps tendon typically require surgery. Unfortunately, unlike success in the nonarthroplasty patient, primary repairs in TKA patients are not successful. In the Dobbs et al. series,[19] complications included chronic recurvatum, knee instability, rerupture, and infection, with a rerupture rate of 40% and an overall complication rate of 55%.

Thus, many arthroplasty surgeons have abandoned primary repairs in favor of reconstruction techniques with autografts, allografts, and synthetic meshes.

PATELLAR TENDON RUPTURES AND AVULSIONS

Incidence, Prevention, and Risk Factors

Patellar tendon disruptions, including ruptures and avulsions, occur at an incidence ranging from 0.17% to 1.4% after TKA.[9,13,29,41,55] Patients with complete patellar tendon ruptures present with an inability to extend their knee from a flexed or extended position. A patellar tendon defect may be palpable with complete ruptures or avulsions, and a lateral radiograph will usually reveal patella alta.

Patient factors that increase the risk for patellar tendon ruptures include systemic diseases such as rheumatoid arthritis, diabetes mellitus, and chronic kidney disease.[19,22,30,65,69] Scarring and stiffness preoperatively place the patient at a higher intraoperative risk of sustaining an avulsion. In addition, history of multiple knee surgeries, previous patellar realignment surgeries, and previous high tibial osteotomies all pose a threat.*

Intraoperatively, ruptures may occur secondary to the surgical approach and subsequent exposure. There has been concern expressed that eversion of the patella during primary TKA puts excessive stress on the tendon insertion at the tubercle.[23,26,27,37,61]

*References 14, 41, 42, 46, 48, and 55.

While this is a concern, there is rarely enough stress in the primary setting to cause an avulsion, especially after the bony resections. Extensive exposures are often necessary during revision procedures, and safe alternative techniques such as the quadriceps snip or tibial tubercle osteotomy (TTO) can be used.[3,4,18,24,47] As previously noted, the quadriceps snip obliquely divides the apex of the quadriceps in the longitudinal line of the tendon at a 45-degree angle into the vastus lateralis. This diminishes the stress at the tibial tubercle. With an appropriately completed quadriceps snip, postoperative complications are minimal. Occasionally, a TTO is needed to obviate the potential for an intraoperative avulsion of the tendon. Of note, there have been reports of complications with tibial tubercle osteotomies (eg, fracture and nonunion of the site).[35,59,68]

Postoperative patellar tendon injuries can be traumatic or atraumatic. Traumatic causes include a fall on a hyperflexed knee, whereas repetitive contact or impingement of the tendon can lead to atraumatic ruptures.[52]

Treatment

Historically, attempts to treat patellar tendon ruptures by primary repair without augmentation have been less than optimal. In 1989, Rand et al.[55] performed primary repairs, including suture and staple fixation, without augmentation in 13 knees and repair with augmentation in 3 knees, for patients with rupture of the patellar tendon after TKA. At follow-up, the authors found 11 of 13 (85%) knees undergoing primary repair had failed. Of the three knees with augmentation, two had successful repair with xenograft, and the one with a semitendinosus reconstruction had failed.

In the presence of poor tissue quality or chronic tears, augmentation techniques should assist direct repair. Autograft (eg, semitendinosus, gracilis, gastrocnemius rotational flap), fresh-frozen or freeze-dried allograft (eg, Achilles tendon bone block or extensor mechanism allograft), or synthetic meshes (eg, Marlex mesh; CR Bard Inc., Murray Hill, NJ) are viable options when augmentation is needed and have shown promising results.[9,13,67]

SURGICAL MANAGEMENT OF EXTENSOR MECHANISM DYSFUNCTION

Because of the rarity of extensor mechanism disruptions, large series are rather scarce. In fact, most data is limited (Table 177.1). While some autografts have been used to reconstruct the extensor mechanism, they have been abandoned as a result of the use of more predictable allografts and synthetic materials. Until recently, whole extensor mechanism allografts or Achilles tendon allografts have been the workhorse of reconstructions. Today, the fresh-frozen, rather than the freeze-dried, allograft seems to be the most accepted.

In 1994, Emerson et al.[21] looked at 15 knees in which extensor mechanism allografts were used to treat patellar tendon ruptures. Nine grafts were freeze-dried, and six were fresh-frozen. Two complications were reported involving knees with the freeze-dried allograft, and the authors concluded that the results of this study called into question the strength of the freeze-dried material.

In 1999, Leopold et al.[40] evaluated the results of seven extensor mechanism reconstructions using fresh-frozen

TABLE 177.1 Results of Extensor Mechanism Reconstruction

Study (Year)	No. of Patients in Study	Technique	MEAN (RANGE) Age (Years)	MEAN (RANGE) Follow-Up (Months)	Patellectomy	INDICATIONS (%) Patellar Tendon Rupture, Avulsion	INDICATIONS (%) Patellar Fracture	INDICATIONS (%) Quad Tendon Rupture	INDICATIONS (%) Convert Fusion, Patella
Emerson et al. (1990)[20]	13	Extensor allograft	74 (36-81)	10 (6-57)	30.8	69.2	0	0	0
Emerson et al (1994)[21]	9	Extensor allograft	69 (36-81)	49 (28-96)	26.7	73.3	0	0	0
Nazarian and Booth (1999)[50]	40	Extensor allograft	71 (NA)	43 (21-120)	15	55	10	20	0
Leopold et al. (1999)[40]	7	Extensor allograft	73 (62-82)	39 (6-115)	0	85.7	14.3	0	0
Burnett et al. (2004)[10]	13	Extensor allograft	64 (51-77)	37 (27-46)	23.1	53.8	0	15.4	7.7
Barrack et al. (2003)[5]	14	Extensor allograft	61 (NA)	42 (24-60)	0	71.4	28.6	0	0
Burnett et al. (2006)[11]	19	Extensor allograft and Achilles tendon allograft	66 (51-81)	56 (24-96)	0	68.4	26.3	0	7.7
Bedard and Vince (2009)[7]	24	Extensor allograft	67.2 (48-79)	28.5	33	29	33	4	0
Crossett et al. (2002)[17]	9	Achilles tendon allograft	70 (57-81)	28 (16-36)	0	100	0	0	0
Browne and Hanssen (2011)[9]	13	Synthetic (Marlex) mesh	60 (37-77)	42 (11-118)	0	23	0	0	—

bone-tendon-bone allografts. They noted 100% clinical failure, as defined by persistent or recurrent extensor lag of more than 30 degrees. Four of the reconstructions were revised (57%). At the time of revision, attenuation was seen in two quadriceps tendon allografts (29%) and two patellar ligament allografts (14%), while one patellar ligament allograft had ruptured (14%). The authors attributed the failures to inadequate tensioning of the graft at the time of implantation. Also in 1999, Nazarian and Booth[50] assessed the outcomes of 36 extensor mechanism reconstructions using fresh-frozen bone-tendon-bone allograft. Extensor lag (mean, 13 degrees) was noted in 15 patients (42%). Eight (22%) of the reconstructions were deemed failures: six (17%) failed at the quadriceps junction, while two (6%) failed at the tibial tubercle junction. Each failure was treated with a repeat allograft, which was successful in all but two cases (two quadriceps tendon allografts reruptured; 6%).

Similarly, regarding the tension of the allograft, Burnett et al.[10] described a comparison of two techniques that encompass the essence of the extensor mechanism reconstruction using an allograft made of the tibial tubercle, patellar tendon, patella, and quadriceps tendon. The authors performed 20 reconstructive TKAs on two groups of patients. Group 1 consisted of 7 patients with a minimally tensioned allograft, while group 2 consisted of 13 patients with a tightly tensioned (in full extension) allograft. The results showed that all of the reconstructions in group 1 were clinical failures (mean postoperative extensor lag of 59 degrees and mean postoperative Hospital for Special Surgery [HSS] score of 52 points). All of the reconstructions in group 2 were considered clinical successes (mean postoperative extensor lag of 4.3 degrees and mean postoperative HSS score of 88 points). In terms of graft complications, five of the seven knees (71%) in group 1 required repeat surgery because of graft disruption: three had attenuation at the quadriceps or patellar tendon anastomoses, one patellar tendon allograft ruptured, and one failed at the patellar tendon insertion. During revision, care was taken to tightly tension the grafts. In group 2, one of the 13 (8%) knees required repeat surgery owing to the development of a nontraumatic, symptomatic partial tear of the quadriceps tendon anastomosis. The authors concluded that an extensor mechanism graft will only be successful if the graft is initially tensioned tightly in full extension.

Vince and Bédard[70] described a modification using an extensor mechanism allograft with an implanted tibial tubercle when concurrent arthroplasty is indicated. After the patellar height is set, a high-speed burr is used to prepare the anterior portion of the proximal tibial canal, deep to the tubercle, to receive the allograft bone block. Once the allograft is in its final position, a trial reduction is performed to make sure that the tibial component will seat. The graft sits in the medullary canal with its anterior surface against the endosteal side of the host tubercle and offset intramedullary stem extensions are used to supplement fixation. Bone cement is applied to the proximal cut bone surface and a prosthetic stem extension is positioned in the canal and held proud by 3 to 4 cm. The proximal portion of the canal and the anterior surface of the tibial keel are filled with cement; the stem extension prohibits cement from going down the canal. The component is driven into final position with a mallet and impactor. The allograft tubercle is implanted with the tibial component and the proximal tendinous junction is secured using the standard technique. There is usually good tissue to close over the top of the graft and the patient's own extensor mechanism is not disrupted.

Historically, the gastrocnemius flap technique, originally described by Malawer and Price[43,44] in the 1980s, was found to be reliable when used with an autologous bone graft to reinforce the reattachment of the patellar tendon to the prosthesis.[8] Kollender et al.[36] used a gastrocnemius flap to provide additional augmentation to the extensor mechanism in patients with bony tumors requiring proximal tibial endoprosthetic arthroplasty. All patients had good to excellent outcomes.

Gastrocnemius flaps that include a portion of the Achilles tendon have been used to reconstruct the patellar and quadriceps tendons.[12] In 1997, Jaureguito et al.[33] described six patients whose ruptured extensor mechanisms were reconstructed in this way. Specifically, the medial gastrocnemius was divided at its distal insertion into the Achilles tendon up to the level of the tibial condyles. The muscle was then transposed anteriorly and sutured to the residual patellar or quadriceps tendon. At follow-up assessment, all patients who were previously dependent on a walker were able to ambulate with or without a cane, and all patients who were previously dependent on a wheelchair were able to walk with the assistance of a walker. One of the coauthors of the original report collaborated on a more recent review of the technique,[25] illustrating the reliability of a medial or an extended medial gastrocnemius flap to reconstruct a ruptured extensor mechanism after TKA. The lateral gastrocnemius has also been used.[16] Restoration of the patellar fulcrum is not part of this procedure unless the flap is combined with an allograft.

Later, Busfield et al.[12] reported a similar experience for nine patients with chronic extensor mechanism disruptions reconstructed with an extended medial gastrocnemius rotational flap. Seven patients had a prior TKA, and two patients had chronic infections of their native knees. Of note, the patient cohort consisted of patients with poor soft tissue coverage, previous infection, or compromised immune system. At final follow-up (mean, 21 months), the mean extensor lag was 14 degrees and the mean range of motion was 2 to 93 degrees. All patients were able to regain sufficient extensor mechanism strength to return to independent ambulation. Complications after surgery included death (1), elective above-knee amputation (1), patient with reflex sympathetic dystrophy (1), and wound problems requiring a free flap (1).

In 2008, Roidis and associates[60] published a case report illustrating a modified biologic technique for extensor mechanism reconstruction. Specifically, the authors used a medial gastrocnemius flap in combination with a semitendinosus tendon autograft. Postoperatively, the patient, who was previously dependent on a walker, was able to walk without a cane.

SYNTHETIC MESH RECONSTRUCTION

It is our contemporary preference to use a synthetic mesh reconstruction for subacute and chronic extensor mechanism deficiencies. Synthetic mesh has been used in surgery for more than a century, primarily making its mark in hernia repair surgery. Its use in orthopedic surgery is relatively new. Advantages of synthetic mesh over other augmentation techniques include reliability, a technically straightforward operative technique, and low cost.[9]

This plastic mesh is porous, enabling it to act as a scaffold for tissue ingrowth, and its high tensile strength allows for solid support.[34,53,71] In 1978, Marlex mesh was used in the knees of dogs to replace ligamentous structures.[71] By four weeks, the graft demonstrated early collagen formation, numerous capillaries, and a mild inflammatory reaction. By 12 weeks, the graft had fibrous infiltration and the inflammatory response subsided. This histologic finding has been further replicated in orthopedic surgery, specifically in relation to the ruptured extensor mechanism. In 2015, Hohman et al.[32] published a histological case report on Marlex mesh used in a 56-year-old patient who underwent revision TKA with mesh reconstruction of his quadriceps tendon. Four months after implantation, the authors found infiltrating fibroblasts, neovascularity, and collagen deposition. Since 1995, Marlex mesh has been used in patellar and quadriceps tendon disruptions associated with TKA.

Surgical Technique

The surgical technique for reconstruction of patellar tendon disruptions has previously been described by the senior author (ADH).[1,9,28,49] The knitted, monofilament polypropylene graft is fashioned by folding a 10 × 14-inch heavy-weight mesh sheet onto itself until it is roughly 8 to 10 layers thick (Fig. 177.2). This creates a tubular graft, which is subsequently secured with heavy, nonabsorbable sutures.

If the existing components are appropriately rotated and well fixed, a portal between the tibial tubercle and the existing tibial implant is created with a burr to obtain anteromedial intramedullary access (a tibial trough) (Fig. 177.3). About 3 to 4 cm of the end of the graft is predipped in polymethylmethacrylate (PMMA) cement and inserted into the trough, which is also filled with cement. A transfixation hole is created beneath the medial or lateral plateau, just beneath the tray of the implant, and a cancellous lag screw, typically 40 to 60 mm, is inserted to transfix the cement, the cement within the mesh, and the mesh itself (Fig. 177.4). The screw travels to the posterior aspect of the tibia and often must be directed medially or laterally to avoid the tibial keel and/or stem. If concurrent revision of components is necessary, there is no need to create a portal. Instead, the graft can be placed directly into the cement-filled canal in front of the implant.

When a portal is used, it is created in the inferolateral aspect of the soft tissues to allow delivery of the graft from deep to superficial (Fig. 177.5A and B). The vastus lateralis is mobilized distally to restore appropriate patellar height and suture is used to tack down and secure the graft to the lateral retinaculum and the ventral surface of the vastus lateralis (Fig. 177.6). The vastus medialis, usually retracted well proximal, is then aggressively mobilized distally and laterally to ideally overlap the underlying graft and vastus lateralis (Fig. 177.7). The final construct,

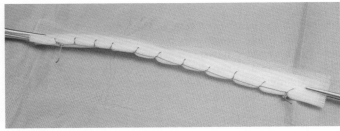

FIG 177.2 Intraoperative image depicting tubularization of the 10× 14-inch sheet of mesh and unitization with a heavy nonabsorable suture.

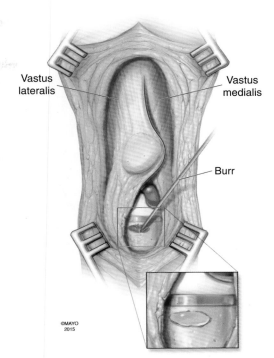

FIG 177.3 Illustration depicting a portal between the tibial tubercle and existing tibial implant that is created with a burr to form a tibial trough for the synthetic mesh.

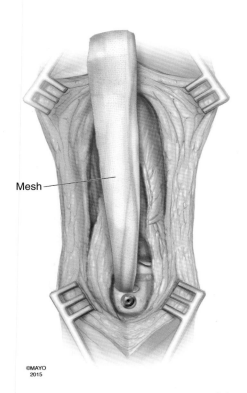

FIG 177.4 A transfixation hole is then created beneath the medial or lateral plateau, just beneath the tray of the implant, and a cancellous lag screw, typically 40 to 60 mm, is inserted to transfix the cement, the cement within the mesh, and the mesh itself.

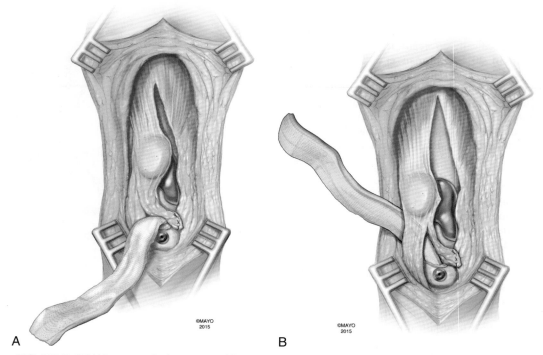

FIG 177.5 (A) When a soft tissue portal is needed, it is created in the inferolateral aspect of the soft tissues. (B) This allows delivery of the graft from deep to superficial.

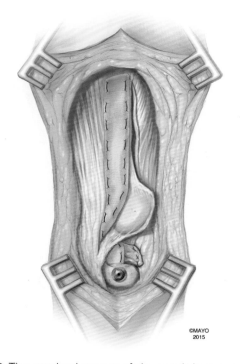

FIG 177.6 The proximal aspect of the mesh is secured to the ventral surface of the mobilized vastus lateralis with heavy, nonabsorbable sutures.

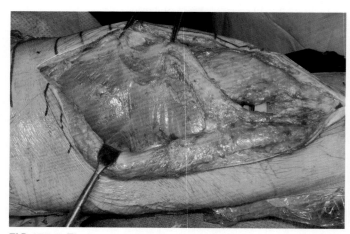

FIG 177.7 The vastus medialis is aggressively mobilized distally and laterally to ideally overlap the underlying graft and vastus lateralis.

referred to as "pants over vest" advancement, is secured into place with heavy nonabsorbable sutures (Fig. 177.8). It is important to note that intraoperatively, the knee cannot be flexed more than 30 to 40 degrees. The distal arthrotomy is closed tightly (Fig. 177.9) with complete coverage of the graft with host soft tissue (Fig. 177.10).

Postoperative Rehabilitation

After surgery, the patient is placed in a long leg cast for 10 to 12 weeks. For the following 12 weeks, the patient is placed in a restricted flexion brace with progressive range of motion and

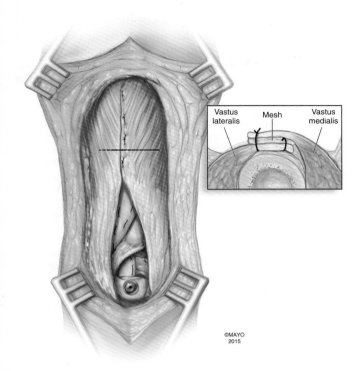

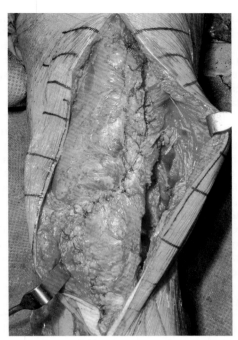

FIG 177.10 It is essential to have the mesh fully incorporated in host tissue with the use of heavy nonabsorbable sutures.

FIG 177.8 The final construct, referred to as "pants-over-vest" advancement, is secured into place with heavy nonabsorbable sutures.

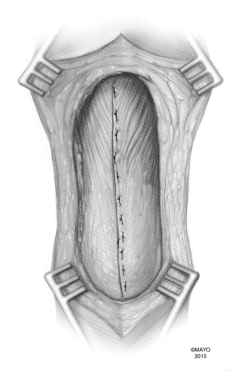

FIG 177.9 The distal arthrotomy is closed tightly, with complete coverage of the graft with host soft tissue.

partial weight bearing. The specific protocol includes flexion from 0 to 45 degrees for month one, 0 to 60 degrees for month two, 0 to 75 degrees for month three, and 0 to 90 degrees for month four.

Results

In 2011, Browne and Hanssen[9] published the first study to assess the outcomes of synthetic mesh (Marlex mesh) used in patellar tendon reconstructions. The authors first identified 43 patients who underwent extensor mechanism reconstruction with synthetic mesh between January 1995 and February 2008. Thirteen of these patients (eight females, five males) underwent reconstruction with synthetic mesh specifically for subacute or chronic patellar tendon disruption following TKA and comprised the study cohort. Eight patients had a prior revision TKA, and five patients had already been treated unsuccessfully with an allograft for an extensor mechanism disruption. At final follow-up (mean, 42 months), four patients suffered complications, including failure of the graft reconstruction (3) and recurrent infection (1). All four of these patients had a history of prior failed extensor mechanism surgery. Range of motion improved in all patients: 36-degree mean extensor lag preoperatively (all patients had an extensor lag) to 10-degree mean extensor lag postoperatively. It should be noted that when excluding the four patients who suffered complications, the mean postoperative extensor lag was 2.8 degrees. All patients maintained knee flexion (mean, 103 degrees preoperatively to 107 degrees postoperatively). KSSs for pain and function showed improvement (pain: 36 preoperatively to 75 postoperatively; function: 20 preoperatively to 50 postoperatively).

In a recent report from the Mayo Clinic (Rochester, MN), two of the authors (MPA and ADH) assessed the results of Marlex mesh used to repair acute quadriceps tendon ruptures in patients without an arthroplasty.[48a] Specifically, the authors retrospectively reviewed eight knees (seven patients; mean age, 69 years; all male) operated on using the surgical technique described by the senior author (ADH). While this is a small, retrospective series, these patients were included because they had an elevated body mass index (BMI) and other significant comorbidities. All patients had a palpable quadriceps defect and extensor lag requiring revision surgery. There were no intraoperative or immediate postoperative complications. At final follow-up, no patients had clinical evidence of failure. In fact, clinical outcomes were excellent. The mean flexion was 100 degrees, and seven of the eight knees had no extensor lag. One knee had developed a 10-degree extensor lag 9 years after the index procedure, probably secondary to the development of Parkinson's disease. Prior to this neurologic diagnosis, this patient had no extensor lag. The authors concluded that the use of Marlex mesh augmentation of acute quadriceps tendon ruptures has promising and durable clinical results and a feasible operative technique (low cost and reasonable operating room time).

SUMMARY

Extensor mechanism disruptions during and after TKA pose a serious and complex threat. Appropriate management, including prevention, meticulous surgical technique, and adequate postoperative care, can substantially reduce the risk. The literature clearly shows that primary repair is no longer an appropriate method of treatment for chronic ruptures. Rather, reconstructive techniques using autograft, allograft, and synthetic materials are mandatory, with synthetic meshes demonstrating the most promising results.

KEY REFERENCES

1. Abdel MP, Hanssen AD: Complex extensor mechanism reconstructions in total knee arthroplasties. *Curr Adv Total Knee Arthroplast* 80–89, 2014.
9. Browne JA, Hanssen AD: Reconstruction of patellar tendon disruption after total knee arthroplasty: results of a new technique utilizing synthetic mesh. *J Bone Joint Surg Am* 93(12):1137–1143, 2011.
48a. Morrey MC, Barlow JD, Abdel MP, et al: Synthetic mesh augmentation of acute and subacute quadriceps tendon repair. *Orthopedics* 39(1):e9–e13, 2016.
49. Nam D, Abdel MP, Cross MB, et al: The management of extensor mechanism complications in total knee arthroplasty. AAOS exhibit selection. *J Bone Joint Surg Am* 96(6):e47, 2014.

The references for this chapter can also be found on www.expertconsult.com.

Total Knee Arthroplasty Perioperative Management Issues

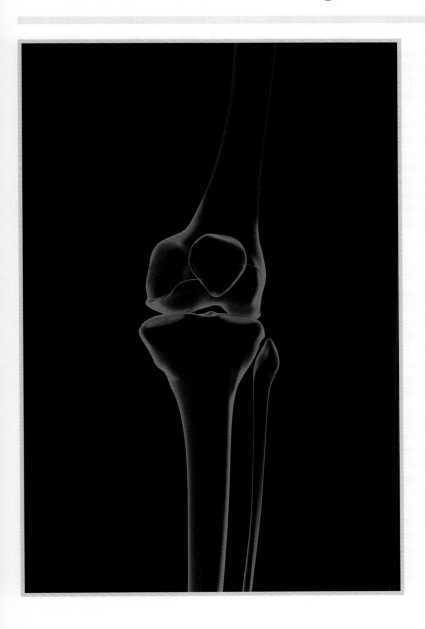

178

Obesity: Risks of Intervention, Benefits of Optimization

William A. Jiranek, Andrew Waligora, Shane Hess, Gregory Golladay

The body mass index (BMI) concept was developed in an effort to correlate a patient's weight with their overall size. It is calculated by dividing the patient's weight in kilograms, by their height in meters squared. It is an imperfect measure because there are nonobese individuals with high BMIs (one example commonly used is professional basketball player LeBron James). In addition, a BMI does not designate the location of the obese tissue. (Does someone who has predominantly truncal obesity have the same risk as another who has extremity obesity?) Nonetheless, the World Health Organization classifies weight status as follows: BMI greater than 30, overweight; BMI greater than 35, obese; BMI greater than 40, morbidly obese; BMI greater than 50, super obese. A practitioner should calculate the BMI of any patient who presents with knee pain, because increased BMI is certainly implicated in many knee problems. When counselling a patient with a high BMI, the practitioner should provide information on the effect of BMI on load across the knee joint, and the effect of each pound decrease on this load.

EPIDEMIOLOGY

The prevalence of obesity in the United States[18] and other countries[16] has continued to increase over the last 20 years. The rate of obesity in adults increased by 37% between 1998 and 2006 (18.3% to 25.1%).[17] According to the United States Centers for Disease Control and Prevention, 34.9% of adults and 17% of children and adolescents between 2 and 19 years of age are now classified as being obese. Furthermore, data demonstrates that 66% of adults between the ages of 65 and 74 are classified as overweight or obese.[89]

Obesity is a risk factor for the development of osteoarthritis.* This fact combined with the high prevalence of overweight and obese adults during the most common decades for arthroplasty[7,20] leads to the logical conclusion that the number of obese patients seeking arthroplasty will continue to increase. Furthermore, the rate of total knee arthroplasty (TKA) has far exceeded that of total hip arthroplasty (THA). In 2006, 10.3% and 4.2% of patients receiving a TKA and 2.9% and 7.1% of those receiving THAs were diagnosed as being obese and morbidly obese, respectively.[50] The use of TKA in patients with a BMI greater than 25 kg/m² was responsible for 95% of the differential increase.[22] More recent estimates demonstrate that 55% of patients undergoing TKA in the United States are obese.[68]

Is Obesity Related to Complications and Poorer Outcomes in Total Knee Arthroplasty?

The evidence of a causal association between arthritis and obesity is confused by comorbidities such as diabetes (the most common comorbidity), tobacco use, malnutrition, renal disease, and metabolic syndrome. Nonetheless, there is a large body of literature describing an increased degree of complications related to obesity and surgery.

There are many reports of increased difficulty with anesthesia, transfer and positioning, exposure, intraoperative fracture and nerve palsy, and closure.

Liabaud et al. demonstrated a direct linear relationship between BMI and surgical time.[56] They also noted that the higher the BMI, the higher the incidence of early postoperative complications in their series of 273 TKA patients. Numerous other surgical disciplines have noted an increased complication rate associated with longer operative times.†

In an analysis of TKA and THA, the Association for Academic Surgery studied the National Surgical Quality Improvement Program (NSQIP) database from 2005 to 2007 and found an association between obesity and infectious complications only in patients with BMIs greater than 40, Obese Class 3, [odds ratio (OR), 1.5].[88] This study found an increased OR for renal complications in patients with BMI greater than 35, Obese Class 2, (OR, 1.84) and, in patients with BMI greater than 40 (OR, 1.72), and found an OR of 2.42 for systemic complications in Obese Class 3 patients (BMI >40).

A workgroup convened by the Evidence Based Medicine Committee of the American Association of Hip and Knee Surgeons (AAHKS) reviewed the recent literature concerning obesity and TKA[99] and concluded, "There is a clear increase in wound healing complications and deep infection in reports examining joint replacement surgery in the obese." They cited one study of 7181 patients with primary hip and knee replacement where the incidence of deep periprosthetic infection was 67% in patients with normal BMI, and ranged to 4.66% in the morbidly obese.[47] In a recent study by the British National Joint Registry in 13.673 patients, the incidence of infection was significantly higher (17%) in patients who had a BMI between 40% and 60%.[10]

There have been many studies that have shown an increased risk of peri- and postoperative complications in obese patients who receive a TKA.[25,62,175a] After TKA, obese patients are 1.5

---

*References 33, 36, 39, 45, 58, 66, 79 and 87.

†References 14, 15, 51, 63, 76 and 77.

times more likely to have an in-hospital complication and more likely to suffer urinary tract infections.[1] Ward et al.[93] showed that a BMI greater than 40 kg/m^2 was an independent predictor of complications including increased risk of acute kidney injury, cardiac arrest, reintubation, reoperation, superficial infection, and death within 1 year. This finding is further supported by D'Apuzzo et al.,[21] who also showed that morbid obesity is an independent risk factor after TKA for in-hospital mortality with a risk of 0.08%. One study showed that for every 5-U increase in BMI, there was a statistically significant increased risk of complications involving the in-hospital and outpatient settings, readmission, and length of stay.[81] Others dispute that there is no significant increase in perioperative complication rates.[88] Odum et al.[71] found that 30% of obese patients had at least three comorbidities compared to only 7% of nonobese patients with the same number of comorbidities. An increased number of comorbidities in the obese population is further supported in the literature.[69]

Other studies of patients with high BMIs indicate similar findings. Schwarzkopf et al.[81] reported 8.44 higher odds of postoperative complications while in the hospital and 1.61 higher odds of having complications within the first year. Baker et al.[10] showed that patients with a BMI greater than 40 kg/m^2 had a statistically significant increase in postoperative wound complications compared to those who were simply overweight, 17% versus 9%, respectively. Namba et al.[69] demonstrated a 6.7 times higher risk for infection in patients with a BMI greater than 35 kg/m^2. Morbidly obese patients have been shown to have significantly higher rates of early wound complications.[53] In a review of the literature, Samson et al.[80] showed that patients with a BMI greater than 40 kg/m^2 were 3.3 to 9.0 times more likely to develop a deep periprosthetic joint infection. These individuals also had a significantly higher incidence of wound complications. The OR of infection can jump to 21.3 in those with a BMI greater than 50 kg/m^2.[1,61]

Super obese patients (BMI >50 kg/m^2) have up to 3.1 times higher odds of complications compared to nonobese patients.[70] Werner et al.[95] found that the rate of local complications within 90 days after TKA in the superobese was 8.8%, compared to 4.3% in the morbidly obese and 6.2% in the revision patients. Super-obese patients have a statistically significant increase in surgical blood loss as well as longer surgical and anesthesia times when compared to nonobese patients.[70] Venous thromboembolism (VTE) rates are 5 times higher in the super obese compared to the nonobese.[95]

In 2013, a workgroup of the AAHKS reviewed the literature on obesity and TKA[90] and found that all obese patients are at increased risk for perioperative complications. Most of these complications dramatically increase at a BMI greater than 40 kg/m^2. The consensus of the group was that elective surgical intervention should be delayed until the patient's BMI is less than 40 kg/m^2.

Intraoperative Considerations: Obesity

Intraoperative considerations related to knee surgery on obese patients include factors such as anesthetic choice, intravenous access, medication dosing, positioning, preparation and draping, incision placement, instrumentation, implant choices, implant positioning, fixation, and wound closure techniques. In addition, surgical case planning should include additional time for the procedure and room time in obese patients.[60] In particular, the suprapatellar index can be predictive of surgical time.[59]

Obesity correlates with obstructive sleep apnea (OSA), and screening for OSA should be included in routine preoperative evaluation of patients undergoing TKA.[41] OSA increases the risk for preoperative morbidity and mortality.[21] Though regional anesthesia is typically preferred for most arthroplasty procedures, proper airway management is also important. Neuraxial anesthesia may be more difficult because of a lack of reliable superficial anatomy and landmarks. Even an experienced anesthetist can have trouble identifying landmarks for administration of neuraxial anesthesia. In addition, dose effect may be prolonged in patients with a higher BMI, so dose reduction should be considered in obese patients to avoid extended anesthesia duration.[34] Weight-based prophylactic antibiotic administration should be used so that adequate tissue levels of antibiotic are present prior to incision. There is a larger volume of distribution for all medications and medication should be dosed accordingly. Establishment of intravenous access can be more difficult[32,83] and may be facilitated with use of ultrasound imaging (Sonosite; FUJIFILM Inc, Bothell, WA). In some cases, central intravenous access may be preferred.[3] If general anesthesia is chosen, the airway may be more difficult to visualize owing to a short neck. Endoscopic and image guidance should be available.

Positioning of obese patients for knee surgery should allow appropriate support of the limb and the upper and contralateral lower extremities should be properly secured. A lateral support post can be helpful to support the thigh and decrease the tendency for external rotation of the limb during flexion and extension. A larger tourniquet should be used and a tapered tourniquet may also improve suspension of the tourniquet and maintenance of hemostasis. When applying the tourniquet, traction is applied to the soft tissues of the thigh to improve suspension.[52] Higher tourniquet pressures are commonly necessary to minimize venous congestion or bleed-through.

The mobility of the fat layer is an important determinant of incision length. In general, the incision will need to be longer. Full-thickness flaps should be raised to minimize wound tension and necrosis. The tissue flaps should be handled atraumatically. A full-thickness flap laterally facilitates patellar subluxation or eversion[12] and the patellar clamp can be used to help hold the patella in an everted position during knee flexion.[85]

Bony landmarks can be more difficult to assess for proper implant alignment. Intraoperative imaging or computer assistance may be helpful to minimize malalignment.[49] Both intramedullary and extramedullary tibial instrumentation can provide satisfactory alignment, and extramedullary instruments may reduce surgical time.[59]

Tibial exposure can be facilitated by external rotation of the tibia. Longer retractors are also helpful to provide appropriate leverage. Protection of the patellar tendon insertion with placement of a pin in the tubercle can help avoid inadvertent avulsion. Standard instrumentation is otherwise typically adequate, provided that exposure is sufficient. There is a tendency to cut the tibia in varus because of pressure from the medial fat layer against the extramedullary guide.

Cement fixation is used in most knee replacements. Cementless fixation may be preferred in certain cases and can have good results, provided that the bony preparation is precise. Because of the added stress on the articulation related to weight-bearing load, the least constraint necessary for adequate balance and stability should be chosen.

Proper hemostasis is paramount to minimize wound complications and hematoma. Intravenous or topical administration of tranexamic acid or other topical hemostatic agents can be helpful, with either agent appearing to be equally efficacious.[37] Thorough wound irrigation may decrease postoperative infection risk, and some authors have advocated use of a dilute betadine irrigation to reduce infection.[13] Multilayer hemostatic wound closure helps minimize dead space and hematoma formation. Wound drains can be used at the surgeon's preference. Although studies have shown no benefit of routine use of drains and an increased transfusion risk with drained wounds[55,72,100]; selective wound drainage may be helpful for larger wounds with larger soft tissue dissection. Morbidly obese patients are at risk for prolonged wound drainage,[74] which can lead to infection. Use of an incisional vacuum-assisted closure device can be considered in larger patients, in whom wounds can be prone to prolonged drainage.

Postoperative Considerations

Rehabilitation After Total Knee Arthroplasty.
The literature is inconclusive regarding the functional outcomes of obese patients after TKA. BMI can have an inverse relationship when it comes to quality of life and physical function.[57] One study suggests that functional recovery is slower during the first 3 years after TKA in those with a BMI greater than 35 kg/m^2 and that obesity may be an independent risk factor for recovery.[48] Rajgopal et al.[78] showed that morbidly obese patients showed greater improvement in function compared to patients who were not morbidly obese, however morbidly obese patients did have statistically significant worse 1-year outcomes. Samson et al.[80] found that those with a BMI greater than 40 kg/m^2 have improvements in the clinical Knee Society Score but not as dramatic improvements in the functional Knee Society Score. Super-obese patients (BMI >50 kg/m^2) have statistically significant lower postoperative Knee Society functional scores when compared to nonobese patients, however there appear to be no differences in the Knee Society objective scores.[70] Others suggest that there is no difference.[42]

Pain relief is one of the most common reasons for desiring TKA. Although some may be concerned with increased weight, studies suggest that there is no difference when it comes to pain relief between obese and nonobese patients after TKA.[4,24,42,84] Singh et al.[84] reported on a large cohort of TKA patients observed for patient-reported pain outcomes and found that obesity was not associated with worse pain outcomes. They also found that higher comorbidity predicted a worse pain outcome after primary TKA along with female gender and younger age. Comorbidities have been shown to be associated with poorer outcomes in patients after TKA.[29]

Despite the inconclusiveness of the literature, it appears that the overall gains obese patients experience are less efficient and come at an increased cost.[92] Morbidly obese patients tend to have poor hamstring and quadriceps conditioning after TKA.[24] One study suggested that morbidly obese individuals might have a tendency to fall more often.[53] Obese patients are more likely to be discharged to rehabilitation facilities,[1] at rates as high as 10% in the morbidly obese.[21] This may become an important point of consideration with the changes in healthcare reimbursement. It is reported that the cost of treating obesity-related diseases is $117 billion per year.[27] D'Apuzzo et al.[21] showed that resource consumption, length of stay, and total hospital costs were higher in the morbidly obese.

Outcomes. Obesity increases the risk of a poorer quality of life after TKA.[57] Obese and morbidly obese patients tend to be less satisfied with nearly 30% not wishing to have the operation again.[9] BMI is a significant independent predictor of age at TKA with patients who have a BMI greater than 35 kg/m^2 being, on average, 7.9 years younger than those with a BMI less than 25 kg/m^2.[35] However, the ultimate influence of obesity on the outcomes of TKA remains controversial in the literature. Several studies have shown a poorer outcome in the obese population after TKA.[26,30,75,78] Dowsey et al. prospectively looked at 529 consecutive patients and found at 12 months that 21% of obese patients had gained weight, Knee Society Scores were lower, and there was a statistically significant increase in adverse events when compared to the nonobese patients.[26] However, there are other studies which do not correlate poorer outcomes with obesity.[‡]

When looking at BMI, patients with a BMI greater than 40 kg/m^2 have increased risks, increased complications, and decreased implant survivorship.[31] In a prospective, matched study, it was found that patients with a BMI greater than 40 kg/m^2 had inferior function scores, a higher incidence of radiolucent lines, a higher rate of complications, and inferior implant survivorship compared to nonobese patients at less than 4 years.[4] The outcomes of those with a BMI between 30 and 40 kg/m^2 are controversial. Collins et al. prospectively followed 445 consecutive primary TKAs and found no difference in complication rates and implant survivorship between nonobese (BMI <30 kg/m^2), mildly obese (BMI 30 to 35 kg/m^2) and highly obese (BMI >35 kg/m^2) patients.[19] One study suggested that obesity had a negative effect on the outcome of TKA notably in the time frame of 60 to 80 months with a statistically significant difference, compared to nonobese patients, when it came to survivorship and functional scores.[30] Obese patients tend to have lower functional scores at longer-term follow-up compared to nonobese patients.[19] Other studies support increased failure of TKA in the obese population.[91]

Weight Change After Total Knee Arthroplasty.
Interestingly, only 15% of obese patients considered themselves obese, but weight loss is a common point of discussion.[27] Specifically, patients generally relate their issues with weight management to the fact that their arthritic joint limits their mobility. If they had increased mobility and decreased pain, they would be able to be more active and therefore lose weight. It is well known that there is a relationship between increased weight and osteoarthritis.[6,28,35,94] Mokdad et al.[64] reported an increased prevalence of arthritis of 38% in overweight patients, 200% in obese patients, and 400% in morbidly obese patients. Obese men have a fourfold risk and obese women have a fivefold risk in the development of osteoarthritis.[6]

Weight loss finds a place in the management scheme in all aspects of care. There are associations with high preoperative weight and postoperative complications.[5,30,75,96] This has led some to advocate weight loss prior to surgical intervention including discussion of bariatric surgery in those under age 65 who have a BMI greater than 40 kg/m^2.[80] Bariatric surgery, however, may lead to increased rates of perioperative complications regardless of timing between the bariatric surgery and the TKA.[82]

---

‡References 5, 19, 23, 24, 53 and 65.

The literature is mixed when it comes to the results of weight or BMI change after TKA. Some advocate that females and patients with higher preoperative BMI are more likely to lose weight after TKA.[8] The underlying theme, however, is that there is no change in BMI or perhaps an increase in BMI from preoperative values. Woodruff and Stone found little or no effect on a patients weight 1 year after TKA.[98] Heisel et al. prospectively followed 100 patients who received a successful total hip or total knee replacement and found that all patients gained weight after surgery.[44] Another study found that 24% of morbidly obese women gained weight after TKA following counseling from a dietician and advice from a physician.[75] Lachiewicz and Lachiewicz found that overweight and obese patients experienced an increase in BMI 2 years after TKA despite being physically active.[54] These findings are important when discussing postoperative expectations with the presurgical patient and warrant the consideration of obesity as a factor independent of physical activity. However, one must remember that BMI takes into account the height of the individual and may not necessarily provide a true representation of total body fat. One study showed that over a 2-year period, almost 40% of patients had an average height loss of 1.27 cm.[45]

Wear. Patellofemoral symptoms are commonly reported by morbidly obese patients after TKA.[38,53a,86] Physiologic load across the patellofemoral joint can reach 2 to 3 times body weight and increased body weight increases the stress across the joint.[43] Dewan et al.[24] identified patients with a BMI greater than 40 kg/m² to be 5.4 times more likely to develop patellar radiolucencies.

If patellar radiolucencies developed, these patients had a significantly higher failure rate (40%) when compared to patients without patellar radiolucencies.

Naziri et al.[70] looked at a matched cohort of patients with a BMI greater than 50 kg/m² and found no significant differences in implant survivorship using aseptic loosening as the end point at a mean of 62 months. There was also no difference in survivorship for reoperation for any reason. Other studies have shown that at longer-term follow up, overall complications and implant survival showed no difference between obese and nonobese patients.[19] However, one study found that obese men, younger than 60 years, have a 10-year implant survival rate of only 35.7% when compared to nonobese individuals.[91] Increased body weight increases mechanical stresses and loads borne by the surrounding bone of the knee.[67] Foran et al.[31] followed a matched cohort of patients for 15 years and found that obese patients had lower knee scores and higher failure rates, and a trend toward influencing the rate of aseptic loosening compared to nonobese patients. Abdel et al.[2] found that patients with a BMI greater than 35 kg/m² had a twofold increase in aseptic tibial loosening within 7 years regardless of age or coronal alignment. Berend et al.[11] found that in patients with a BMI greater than 33.7 kg/m², varus tibial alignment led to a 168-fold increase in failure. The effect of moderate obesity on prosthetic alignment is controversial; some say that obesity does not affect prosthetic alignment and others feel there is a tendency for excess varus.[40]

The references for this chapter can also be found on www.expertconsult.com.

179

Pain Catastrophizers: A Subgroup at Risk for Poor Outcome After Total Knee Arthroplasty

John J. Mercuri, Daniel L. Riddle, James D. Slover

INTRODUCTION

Many patients with knee disorders state that they have difficulty coping with their pain, or they exhibit behaviors that are suggestive of coping difficulty. These verbal and nonverbal responses are reported to physicians in a variety of ways, in words and in behaviors such as protective movements and posturing. Some patients report that they cannot stop thinking about their pain. Others display pain-related behaviors such as distressed facial expressions or an intense focus on protecting the involved limb. Still others indicate that they are unable to accomplish even simple daily life activities because of their pain, and some insist that their pain indicates a more serious problem than physical findings suggest. These types of patients are also likely to report pain in other regions of the body, and some may report widespread pain, defined as pain in both right and left extremities and axial pain above and below the waist.[35]

The focus of this chapter is the construct of pain catastrophizing and how catastrophizing impacts outcomes after total knee arthroplasty. Patients who catastrophize about their pain have a tendency to magnify or exaggerate the threat value or seriousness of their pain sensations (eg, "I wonder whether something serious may happen."), they ruminate about the pain (eg, "I can't stop thinking about the pain."), and they tend to feel helpless when experiencing pain (eg, "There's nothing I can do to stop the pain.").[28] Understanding pain catastrophizing is crucially important because pain catastrophizers are a subgroup at high risk for poor results after total knee arthroplasty.

PAIN AND TOTAL KNEE ARTHROPLASTY

Pain and perioperative pain management are significant areas of focus in patients undergoing total knee arthroplasty. Pain after total knee arthroplasty has multiple causes including nociceptive, inflammatory, ischemic, neuropathic causes, mechanical, functional, and psychological.[9,20,22] On a cellular level, trauma during a total knee arthroplasty produces a peripheral noxious stimulus that traumatizes nerves and generates a secondary inflammatory response.[4] Local cell injury and inflammation may lower pain thresholds at the surgical site and in the surrounding tissues. In this way, prolonged acute pain can become chronic in nature with peripheral and central nervous system sensitization.[9] Some persons are likely to be predisposed to more severe pain because their central nervous system is more vulnerable to pain.[21] Failure to control

postoperative pain has a variety of effects including increased postoperative morbidity, hindered ability to perform needed physiotherapy, increased patient anxiety, disrupted sleep patterns, decreased patient satisfaction, and slowed postoperative recovery.[4]

It is important to recognize that pain after total knee arthroplasty is a complicated phenomenon with wide-ranging and inter-related causes. Some causes of pain after total knee arthroplasty can be determined by appropriate evaluation of the patient. These causes include mechanical issues such as loosening or instability, and biologic causes such as synovitis or infection. However, not all pain after total knee arthroplasty has a clear mechanical or biologic cause that may lend itself to a clear surgical or medical solution. After ruling out these traditional causes of pain, surgeons should consider nontraditional causes.

Persistent knee pain after total knee arthroplasty often has a psychological or central pain processing contribution that can differ widely among patients. Preoperative recognition of the risk factors for severe and persistent postoperative pain may allow for advanced perioperative management in the psychological, mechanical, and functional realms.[9] Patient responses to multimodal pain management strategies are variable, and a patient's level of perceived pain may not correlate with the noxious stimulus.[4] Patients with higher depression and anxiety scores, and those with poor coping skills, typically report higher levels of pain as compared to patients without these stressors. In older adults, associated depression can affect pain control after total knee arthroplasty, and psychological therapies may be beneficial.[18]

Many studies indicate that psychological factors may have a significant impact on clinical outcomes after total knee arthroplasty. For example, Noiseux et al. investigated preoperative predictors of pain following total knee arthroplasty.[19] The authors prospectively analyzed 215 patients with a variety of examination procedures. Patients with severe pain during knee range-of-motion testing before their total knee arthroplasty were 10 times more likely to still have moderate to severe pain 6 months after arthroplasty. These results suggest that a simple test of preoperative pain intensity with active flexion and extension can provide insight into risks for prolonged postoperative pain.

Brummett et al. investigated variance in pain after total knee and hip arthroplasty.[2] The authors performed a prospective, observation cohort study of 519 patients who underwent total joint arthroplasty. Those patients with higher postoperative opioid consumption tended to be younger, had more severe knee pain at baseline, and had a high preoperative fibromyalgia survey score. Similar to range-of-motion testing, the administration of a fibromyalgia screening tool may represent a simple way to predict postoperative pain and opiate requirements in arthroplasty patients.[2] Ideally, screening tools might be developed to identify psychological factors that influence perioperative pain for arthroplasty patients, thereby enabling an intervention to lessen the patient's pain and improve the patient's outcome.

DEFINING THE CONSTRUCT OF PAIN CATASTROPHIZING

The focus of this section is to acquaint the reader with the construct of pain catastrophizing. It will certainly assist in care planning to quantify pain catastrophizing when a patient exhibits behaviors or describes symptoms that suggest they may have difficulty coping with pain. Patients who catastrophize about their pain have a tendency to magnify or exaggerate the threat value or seriousness of the pain sensations, ruminate about the pain, and tend to feel helpless when experiencing pain.[28]

Pain catastrophizing involves a complex set of behavioral, cognitive, and neurophysiological pathways and systems. Patients who catastrophize when experiencing pain may exhibit enhanced central nervous system pain processing (ie, their pain processing is abnormal such that pain intensity will be greater and sensitivity to pain will be heightened). They also may have a limited ability to use adaptive thoughts in the face of pain and resort to maladaptive behaviors, such as over-reliance on family members for completing daily activities. These types of thoughts and behaviors are maladaptive because they may lead to continued pain and deconditioning, as well as impaired social interactions with friends, family, and the community. Depression and anxiety, two additional important sources of psychological distress, are moderately correlated to pain catastrophizing. Depression and anxiety can increase pain intensity. When combined with catastrophizing, depression and anxiety increase the risk of maladaptive thoughts and behaviors. Patients who catastrophize about their pain will likely manifest a variety of psychological, cognitive, behavioral, and neurophysiological issues, each of which may warrant treatment.

Traditionally, a patient who catastrophizes about his or her pain is extremely challenging to treat, not only because of the pain complaints but also because the cause(s) of these pain complaints are a diagnostic and therapeutic challenge to most physicians. Traditionally, pain was thought of as a purely sensory experience—the greater the tissue damage, the greater the pain intensity. We now know that the pain experience is influenced by a multitude of psychological, social, and genetic factors beyond the damaged tissue. Pain catastrophizing is one factor, and potentially the most important factor, that is associated with persistent pain following total knee arthroplasty.

For patients who seem to fit the catastrophizing profile, one can question whether pain catastrophizing is an enduring part of a person's makeup, much like personality (ie, a trait), or whether pain catastrophizing is only intermittently present and varies depending on the patient's current situation (ie, their state). Evidence suggests that both scenarios are likely true. Persons who catastrophize when encountering pain are likely to routinely catastrophize, and when pain increases, the severity of catastrophizing is likely to increase.[33] When a person is not experiencing pain, the level of pain catastrophizing is likely diminished relative to periods when pain is perceived. Interventions designed to reduce pain catastrophizing during painful episodes is the goal of cognitive behavioral therapies designed to improve pain coping skills.[12,13,25]

There are two main instruments available to quantify the extent of pain catastrophizing. The more commonly used instrument is the Pain Catastrophizing Scale (PCS).[28] The PCS was developed in 1995 by Michael Sullivan, a psychologist and researcher, along with his colleagues at the University Centre for Research on Pain and Disability at McGill University. The researchers were interested in the study of mechanisms in which catastrophizing impacts the pain experience. The researchers relied on prior experimental and clinical research evidence to identify items for the PCS. Factor analytic approaches have been applied to the PCS by many research teams, and these analyses have consistently indicated that catastrophizing is a multidimensional construct. The three dimensions have been labeled as rumination (eg, "I keep thinking about how much it hurts."), helplessness (eg, "It's awful and I feel that it overwhelms me."), and magnification (eg, "I become afraid that the pain will get worse.").

The scale includes 13 items, and patients respond to each item by indicating where they place themselves along the continuum from "not at all" (scored as a 0 for each item) to "all the time" and (scored as a 4 for each item). The PCS is depicted in Fig. 179.1. Scores obtained from the scale are summed to provide an overall score. It is this overall score that is most commonly reported in the literature and used to guide potential interventions to improve pain coping strategies. The PCS total score ranges from 0 (no catastrophizing) to 52 (very high catastrophizing). Subscale scores for rumination (items 8 to 11), helplessness (items 6, 7, and 13), and magnification (items 1 to 5, 12) can also be calculated by summing the respective items, but these are infrequently reported.

There is extensive evidence suggesting that high scores on the PCS are associated with an increased risk of poor outcome for a variety of conditions.[5] It is important to remember that pain catastrophizing occurs along a continuum from no catastrophizing to very high catastrophizing. From a practical standpoint, interpretation of scores is typically driven by a cut-point that separates scores into clinically important and clinically unimportant levels of catastrophizing. In this case, physicians are interested in identifying scores on the PCS that best identify persons who are at increased risk of a poor outcome following treatment because of their pain catastrophizing. To address this limitation in the evidence, Riddle and colleagues dichotomized the PCS by using the highest tertile of scores from a sample of 140 patients preparing to undergo total knee replacement surgery. Patients scoring in the highest tertile (ie, a PCS score of 16 or higher) were considered to have high pain catastrophizing, whereas patients who scored less than this cut-point were considered to have low pain catastrophizing.[26]

The second instrument designed to quantify the extent of pain catastrophizing is the two-item Pain Catastrophizing Subscale from the Coping Strategies Questionnaire (CSQ).[11] The two-item scale was derived from the original Pain Catastrophizing Subscale of the CSQ and developed in 1983. The two-item subscale was developed for quick and efficient clinical use. However, as would be expected, the use of an efficient two-item instrument leads to greater error in assessment when compared

Instructions: Please reflect on past painful experiences and place a checkmark (√) on the answer that indicates the degree to which you experience each of the thirteen thoughts or feelings when experiencing pain.

		Not at all	A little of the time	About half the time	Most of the time	All of the time
1.	I worry about whether the pain will end.	O	O	O	O	O
2.	I feel I can't go on.	O	O	O	O	O
3.	It's terrible and I think it's never going to get any better.	O	O	O	O	O
4.	It's awful and I feel that it overwhelms me.	O	O	O	O	O
5.	I feel I can't stand it anymore.	O	O	O	O	O
6.	I become afraid that the pain may get worse.	O	O	O	O	O
7.	I think of other painful experiences.	O	O	O	O	O
8.	I anxiously want the pain to go away.	O	O	O	O	O
9.	I can't seem to keep it out of my mind.	O	O	O	O	O
10.	I keep thinking about how much it hurts.	O	O	O	O	O
11.	I keep thinking about how badly I want the pain to stop.	O	O	O	O	O
12.	There is nothing I can do to reduce the intensity of the pain.	O	O	O	O	O
13.	I wonder whether something serious may happen.	O	O	O	O	O

FIG 179.1 The Pain Catastrophizing Scale.

to longer instruments. The two-item Pain Catastrophizing Subscale of the CSQ is depicted in Fig. 179.2.

Pain catastrophizing is a clinically important biopsychosocial construct that warrants attention from practitioners treating patients with chronic knee pain. The most commonly used instrument for quantifying the extent of pain catastrophizing is the PCS. Although the scale provides a continuous measure of catastrophizing, it appears that scores of approximately 16 or higher may be useful in identifying persons with clinically important maladaptive pain coping strategies that could adversely influence outcome following knee replacement surgery.

PAIN CATASTROPHIZING AND TOTAL KNEE ARTHROPLASTY

There is growing interest in the contribution of pain catastrophizing to postoperative pain and poor function following total knee arthroplasty. Multiple research studies over the past decade have reported on pain catastrophizing and total knee arthroplasty outcomes (Table 179.1). Additionally, recent review articles have helped bring the concept into the mainstream by summarizing new findings about the importance of catastrophizing following arthroplasty.[1] Identifying patients who catastrophize about their pain will enable surgeons to set realistic expectations for postoperative recovery and pain relief. Furthermore, research may elucidate interventions that can address pain catastrophizing, thereby improving pain and outcomes.

Instructions: Individuals who experience pain have developed a number of ways to cope, or deal with their pain. These include saying things to themselves when they experience pain or engaging in different activities. Below is a list of things that people have reported doing when they feel pain. For each activity, please indicate, using the scale below, how much you engage in that activity when you feel pain, where a 0 indicates you never do that when you are experiencing pain, a 3 indicates you sometimes do that when you are experiencing pain, and a 6 indicates you always do it when you are experiencing pain. Remember, you can use any point along the scale.

1.	It is terrible and I feel it is never going to get any better.	1 2 3 4 5 6
2.	I feel I can't stand it anymore.	1 2 3 4 5 6

FIG 179.2 The two-item Pain Catastrophizing Subscale of the Coping Strategies Questionnaire.

Pain Catastrophizing and Outcomes

Most of these research studies examine the presence of pain catastrophizing in the immediate perioperative period, including two studies that included only a preoperative assessment of total knee arthroplasty patients. Tonelli et al. investigated differences in pain, function, and physical activity between women and men scheduled to undergo total knee arthroplasty.[31] The results failed to show any differences in preoperative pain catastrophizing between men and women. Feldman et al. examined associations between socioeconomic status, pain,

TABLE 179.1   Pain Catastrophizing and Outcomes

Study	Patients	Investigated Characteristics	Results
Tonelli et al.[31]	208	Psychosocial measures at a preoperative visit, including the PCS.	Failed to show any differences in preoperative pain catastrophizing between men (n =70) and women (n =138).
Feldman et al.[7]	316	Preoperative pain and function status scores, along with PCS scores. Educational achievement and a US Census index score were used as surrogates to determine socioeconomic status. The results were adjusted for age, gender, and body mass index.	Higher socioeconomic status was associated with lower PCS scores in the cohort indicating less pain catastrophizing.
Roth et al.[27]	68	A variety of psychosocial metrics, including the PCS, both preoperatively and for the first 3 days postoperatively	Statistical analysis revealed the PCS scores predicted preoperative pain and pain on the second postoperative day, and catastrophizing was also found to correlate with negative mood in the perioperative period.
Witvrouw et al.[34]	43	Patients were administered the PCS.	Statistical analysis found that higher pain catastrophizing and older age predicted a longer hospital stay.
Lunn et al.[16]	97	Patients were exposed to preoperative tonic heat stimuli and their pain scores were recorded on a visual analogue scale. Eight other preoperative variables were recorded including the PCS score. The primary outcome was postoperative pain during walking 6 to 24 hours after surgery, with secondary outcomes of pain during walking on postoperative days 1-7, and pain during walking on postoperative days 14-30.	Catastrophizing, anxiety, and preoperative pain scores were found to correlate significantly with a patient's postoperative walking pain.
Sullivan et al.[30]	75	Various self-reported instruments including the PCS. Patients repeated the self-reports 6 weeks following surgery.	Pain catastrophizing was a unique predictor of higher postoperative pain as measured by the Western Ontario and McMaster University Osteoarthritis Index.
Hirakawa et al.[10]	90	The PCS was one tool used to assess the psychological realm in 90 patients at both 3 weeks and 6 weeks.	The results showed that PCS scores were significantly associated with higher postoperative pain at both time points.
Riddle et al.[25]	63	Compared 18 patients who received eight sessions of psychologist-directed pain coping skills training with 45 historical patients who received usual care. All patients had a score of 16 or higher on the PCS. The coping skills group was assessed prior to surgery and 2 months afterward	Patients who received the coping skills training had significantly greater reductions in pain severity and pain catastrophizing, as well as greater improvements in function compared with the control group.
Masselin-Dubois et al.[17]	189	89 patients undergoing total knee arthroplasty were compared to 100 patients undergoing breast cancer surgery. The PCS was used to assess pain catastrophizing preoperatively, and 2 days and 3 months postoperatively.	Statistical analysis demonstrated that preoperative pain magnification, one of the three dimensions of pain catastrophizing measured by the PCS, predicted postoperative chronic pain intensity in both total knee arthroplasty and breast cancer surgery up to 3 months postoperatively.
Riddle et al.[26]	140	Patients were followed for 6 months, and multiple psychological and health-related beliefs were evaluated. The PCS was used to evaluate catastrophizing.	After adjusting for confounding variables, pain catastrophizing was found to be the only predictor of poor pain outcomes in this cohort.
Edwards et al.[6]	43	Patients were evaluated for pain catastrophizing and depression as predictive factors in the development of pain. The authors utilized the catastrophizing subscale of the CSQ as their catastrophizing metric. Global pain ratings and pain at night were assessed both preoperatively and up to 12 months postoperatively.	Pain catastrophizing was found to be a unique predictor of only pain at night.
Sullivan et al.[29]	120	One week prior to surgery, and then again at 12 months after surgery, patients were evaluated for several predictors of pain severity and functional limitation, including pain catastrophizing.	Results demonstrated that high scores on the PCS were significant in predicting higher pain and lower function at follow-up, and this relationship remained significant after controlling for outcome expectations and preoperative pain intensity.
Yakobov et al.[36]	116	Perceived injustice was defined as a patient's appraisal of their illness in terms of unfairness, blame, and the severity and irreparability of losses. The authors also investigated the PCS scores of the patients. Patients were assessed before surgery, and measures of pain and disability were taken 1 year after surgery.	Statistical analysis after controlling for other variables revealed that pain catastrophizing predicted disability at 1 year, whereas perceived injustice predicted pain severity.
Forsythe et al.[8]	55	Comorbidities, preoperative pain, and preoperative pain catastrophizing as measured by the PCS were studied as potential predictors of long-term postoperative pain up to 24 months after surgery. Patient response rate was 84%.	PCS scores did not change over time; however, statistical analysis demonstrated that the preoperative PCS score and the rumination subscale score predicted the presence of pain at 24 months postoperatively.

CSQ, Coping Strategies Questionnaire; *PCS*, Pain Catastrophizing Scale.

function, and pain catastrophizing in patients who presented for total knee arthroplsty.[7] Higher socioeconomic status was associated with lower PCS scores in the cohort indicating less pain catastrophizing.

Pain catastrophizing and its effect on outcomes have been studied within the first postoperative week. Roth et al. focused on demographic and psychosocial predictors of acute perioperative pain following total knee arthroplasty.[27] Statistical analysis revealed that the PCS scores predicted preoperative pain and pain on the second postoperative day, and catastrophizing was also found to correlate with negative mood in the perioperative period. Witvrouw et al. investigated whether pain catastrophizing is associated with hospital length of stay after total knee arthroplasty.[34] Statistical analysis found that higher pain catastrophizing and older age predicted a longer hospital stay. Lunn et al. conducted a prospective, observational study to determine whether preoperative pain in response to heat stimulation was predictive of postoperative pain during the first month following total knee arthroplasty.[16] Catastrophizing, anxiety, and preoperative pain scores were found to correlate significantly with a patient's postoperative walking pain.

At 6 weeks postoperatively, Sullivan et al. examined psychological determinants of problematic outcomes following total knee arthroplasty.[30] Pain catastrophizing was a unique predictor of higher postoperative pain as measured by the Western Ontario and McMaster University Osteoarthritis Index. Hirakawa et al. investigated the prevalence and association of neglect-like symptoms and psychological factors on chronic pain after total knee arthroplasty.[10] The results showed that PCS scores were significantly associated with higher postoperative pain at both time points.

Pain catastrophizing has been shown to be a modifiable risk factor on poor total knee arthroplasty outcomes up to 2 months postoperatively. Riddle et al. investigated pain coping skills training for patients with high levels of pain catastrophizing who were scheduled for total knee arthroplasty.[25] Patients who received the coping skills training had significantly greater reductions in pain severity and pain catastrophizing, and greater improvements in function compared with the control group. Masselin-Dubois et al. studied whether psychological predictors of postsurgical pain were dependent on the type of surgery performed.[17] Statistical analysis demonstrated that preoperative pain magnification, one of the three dimensions of pain catastrophizing measured by the PCS, predicted postoperative chronic pain intensity in total knee arthroplasty and breast cancer surgery up to 3 months postoperatively. Riddle et al. also investigated pain catastrophizing and pain outcomes after total knee arthroplasty at the 6-month follow-up appointment.[26] After adjusting for confounding variables, pain catastrophizing was found to be the only predictor of poor pain outcomes in this cohort.

Three studies have followed total knee arthroplasty patients up to 1 year postoperatively and evaluated the impact of pain catastrophizing on patient outcomes. Edwards et al. investigated pain catastrophizing and depressive symptoms as predictors of outcomes following total knee arthroplasty.[6] Pain catastrophizing was found to be a unique predictor of only pain at night. Sullivan et al. examined presurgical expectations as predictors of pain and function 12 months following total knee arthroplasty.[29] Results demonstrated that high scores on the PCS were significant in predicting higher pain and lower function at follow-up, and this relationship remained significant

TABLE 179.2		Systematic Reviews of Pain Catastrophizing	
Study	Included Studies	Inclusion Criteria	Results
Vissers et al.[32]	17	Studies were identified with a minimum of 6 weeks of follow-up.	Patients with high levels of pain catastrophizing had more postoperative pain following total knee arthroplasty only.
Burns et al.[3]	6	Pain catastrophizing exposure, total knee arthroplasty patient population, chronic pain assessed postoperatively, prospective and longitudinal study design, original paper, and English language.	Moderate-level evidence for pain catastrophizing as an independent predictor of chronic pain following total knee arthroplasty.

after controlling for outcome expectations and preoperative pain intensity. Yakobov et al. studied the relationship between perceived injustice and pain after total knee arthroplasty.[36] Statistical analysis after controlling for other variables revealed that pain catastrophizing predicted disability at 1 year, whereas perceived injustice predicted pain severity.

One study followed total knee arthroplasty patients beyond the first postoperative year. Forsythe et al. sought to determine whether a prospective relationship existed between pain catastrophizing and chronic pain following total knee arthroplasty.[8] PCS scores did not change over time; however, statistical analysis demonstrated that the preoperative PCS score and the rumination subscale score predicted the presence of pain at 24 months postoperatively.

Systematic Reviews of Pain Catastrophizing

Two systematic reviews have been conducted examining the impact of pain catastrophizing among other psychologically based predictors on postoperative total knee arthroplasty outcomes (Table 179.2). Vissers et al. published a systematic review in 2012 of general psychological factors that influence the outcomes of total knee arthroplasty and total hip arthroplasty.[32] In the 17 studies with less than 1 year of follow-up, patients with high levels of pain catastrophizing had more postoperative pain following total knee arthroplasty only. Burns et al. published a systematic review in 2015 of pain catastrophizing as a risk factor for chronic pain after total knee arthroplasty.[3] Six included studies were rated for methodological quality.* Quantitative meta-analysis was not possible owing to the heterogeneity among the studies. Despite the variability, the authors found moderate-level evidence for pain catastrophizing as an independent predictor of chronic pain following total knee arthroplasty.

---

*References 6, 8, 17, 19, 26, and 29.

TABLE 179.3   Interventions and Pain Catastrophizing After Total Knee Arthroplasty

Study	Design	Participants	Intervention	Significant Results
Lunn et al.[15]	Prospective, double-blind, randomized, placebo controlled	120 patients with a preoperative PCS score over 21	10 mg of escitalopram	Less pain upon ambulation and less pain at rest on postoperative days 2 through 6 in the escitalopram group
Rakel et al.[23]	Prospective, randomized, intention-to-treat analysis	317 preoperative patients	TENS	Less pain with range of motion in TENS-group patients who had low PCS scores compared to TENS-group patients with high PCS scores

PCS, Pain Catastrophizing Scale; TENS, transcutaneous electrical nerve stimulation.

Interventions and Pain Catastrophizing

There has been limited research on interventions that might directly or indirectly influence catastrophizing patients in the perioperative period (Table 179.3). Lunn et al. studied the effect of escitalopram, a selective serotonin reuptake inhibitor, on reducing postoperative pain in total knee arthroplasty patients with high PCS scores.[15] This prospective, double-blind, placebo-controlled trial included 120 patients with preoperative PSC scores over 21. Patients were randomized to receive placebo or 10 mg of escitalopram from preanesthesia through postoperative day 6 following total knee arthroplasty. Pain with ambulation 24 hours after surgery was the primary outcome. Secondary outcomes included overall pain during ambulation up to 6 days postoperatively, as well as morphine equivalents, anxiety, depression, and side effects. There was no significant difference in pain upon ambulation at 24 hours between the two groups. However, pain upon ambulation and at rest was lower in the escitalopram group on postoperative days 2 through 6. Side effects were not significant.

Rakel et al. evaluated the efficacy of transcutaneous electrical nerve stimulation (TENS) in reducing pain and hyperalgesia, and increasing function after total knee arthroplasty.[23] They hypothesized that changes in pain with range of motion would differ based on psychological characteristics such as pain catastrophizing. A prospective, intention-to-treat analysis was conducted on 317 patients after primary total knee arthroplasty. Patients were randomized into TENS and non-TENS groups, and the PCS was administered among other metrics. Results demonstrated that TENS-group patients with low PCS scores had a greater reduction in pain with range of motion at 6 weeks compared to TENS-group patients with high PCS scores.

Future Interventional Studies

Future interventional studies are underway. Losina et al. reported the commencement of a motivational interview-based telephone intervention that focused on improving patient outcomes and satisfaction following total knee arthroplasty.[14] Among other variables, pain catastrophizing was assessed in patients over the first 6 months postoperatively. Riddle et al. have reported a protocol for a three-arm trial to determine if a pain skills training program delivered prior to total knee arthroplasty reduces function-limiting pain in patients with high levels of pain catastrophizing.[24] A total of 402 patients with high levels of pain catastrophizing on the PCS (great than 16) will be randomly assigned to a pain coping skills training arm, an arthritis education arm, or a usual care arm. The primary outcome will evaluate pain 12 months following surgery. The pain coping skills will be delivered by physical therapists trained to deliver pain coping skills over the telephone.

CONCLUSION

Research conducted to date on pain catastrophizing and total knee arthroplasty, though hampered by limited sample sizes and follow-up data, offers several conclusions. Preoperative pain catastrophizing is one of several psychological factors that may be predictive of chronic pain following total knee arthroplasty, and it may influence patient recovery. Pain catastrophizing may be one of the most important psychological risk factors for chronic postsurgical pain regardless of the type of surgery performed, and it is not static but rather a dynamic construct that varies depending on pain intensity. Several targeted interventions for total knee arthroplasty patients with elevated levels of pain catastrophizing have been investigated, including cognitive-behavioral techniques, patient education programs, and oral psychotropic medications. Although research is needed to determine which interventions will be cost effective and lead to improved outcomes for patients with total knee arthroplasty, we encourage surgeons to quantify the extent of pain catastrophizing in their patients and to consider psychologically based treatment in the more severe cases.

KEY REFERENCES

6. Edwards RR, Haythornthwaite JA, Smith MT, et al: Catastrophizing and depressive symptoms as prospective predictors of outcomes following total knee replacement. *Pain Res Manag* 14(4):307–311, 2009.

7. Feldman CH, Dong Y, Katz JN, et al: Association between socioeconomic status and pain, function and pain catastrophizing at presentation for total knee arthroplasty. *BMC Musculoskelet Disord* 16:18, 2015. doi: 10.1186/s12891-015-0475-8.

8. Forsythe ME, Dunbar MJ, Hennigar AW, et al: Prospective relation between catastrophizing and residual pain following knee arthroplasty: two-year follow-up. *Pain Res Manag* 13(4):335–341, 2008.

11. Jensen MP, Keefe FJ, Lefebvre JC, et al: One- and two-item measures of pain beliefs and coping strategies. *Pain* 104(3):453–469, 2003. doi: 10.1016/S0304-3959(03)00076-9.

15. Lunn TH, Frokjaer VG, Hansen TB, et al: Analgesic effect of perioperative escitalopram in high pain catastrophizing patients after total knee arthroplasty: a randomized, double-blind, placebo-controlled trial. *Anesthesiology* 122(4):884–894, 2015. doi: 10.1097/ALN.0000000000000597.

16. Lunn TH, Gaarn-Larsen L, Kehlet H: Prediction of postoperative pain by preoperative pain response to heat stimulation in total knee arthroplasty. *Pain* 154(9):1878–1885, 2013. doi: 10.1016/j.pain.2013.06.008.

23. Rakel BA, Zimmerman MB, Geasland K, et al: Transcutaneous electrical nerve stimulation for the control of pain during rehabilitation after total knee arthroplasty: a randomized, blinded, placebo-controlled trial. *Pain* 155(12):2599–2611, 2014. doi: 10.1016/j.pain.2014.09.025.

25. Riddle DL, Keefe FJ, Nay WT, et al: Pain coping skills training for patients with elevated pain catastrophizing who are scheduled for knee

arthroplasty: a quasi-experimental study. *Arch Phys Med Rehabil* 92(6):859–865, 2011. doi: 10.1016/j.apmr.2011.01.003.

26. Riddle DL, Wade JB, Jiranek WA, et al: Preoperative pain catastrophizing predicts pain outcome after knee arthroplasty. *Clin Orthop Relat Res* 468(3):798–806, 2010. doi: 10.1007/s11999-009-0963-y.

28. Sullivan M, Bishop SR, Pivik J: The pain catastrophizing scale: development and validation. *Psychol Assess* 7:524–532, 1995.

29. Sullivan M, Tanzer M, Reardon G, et al: The role of presurgical expectancies in predicting pain and function one year following total knee arthroplasty. *Pain* 152(10):2287–2293, 2011. doi: 10.1016/j.pain.2011.06.014.

30. Sullivan M, Tanzer M, Stanish W, et al: Psychological determinants of problematic outcomes following total knee arthroplasty. *Pain* 143(1–2):123–129, 2009. doi: 10.1016/j.pain.2009.02.011.

33. Wade JB, Riddle DL, Thacker LR: Is pain catastrophizing a stable trait or dynamic state in patients scheduled for knee arthroplasty? *Clin J Pain* 28(2):122–128, 2012. doi: 10.1097/AJP.0b013e318226c3e2.

34. Witvrouw E, Pattyn E, Almqvist KF, et al: Catastrophic thinking about pain as a predictor of length of hospital stay after total knee arthroplasty: a prospective study. *Knee Surg Sports Traumatol Arthrosc* 17(10):1189–1194, 2009. doi: 10.1007/s00167-009-0817-x.

36. Yakobov E, Scott W, Stanish W, et al: The role of perceived injustice in the prediction of pain and function after total knee arthroplasty. *Pain* 155(10):2040–2046, 2014. doi: 10.1016/j.pain.2014.07.007.

The references for this chapter can also be found on www.expertconsult.com.

180

Medical Optimization of Patients With Atherosclerotic Cardiovascular Disease and Cardiovascular Risk Factors

Nathaniel R. Smilowitz, Jeffrey S. Berger

PERIOPERATIVE CARDIOVASCULAR EVENTS

Perioperative cardiovascular complications are a frequent cause of morbidity and mortality among patients who undergo noncardiac surgery.[13,14,20,33] Although major orthopedic procedures have historically been designated as intermediate risk noncardiac surgery, cardiovascular events are not infrequent. Perioperative myocardial injury and/or myocardial infarction (MI) complicate 1% to 17% of orthopedic surgeries, depending on the population.* Risks are highest for older patients with cardiovascular risk factors or known atherosclerotic cardiovascular disease.[33] For these complex patients, thoughtful preoperative medical optimization is essential to reduce the burden of perioperative cardiovascular complications.

CARDIOVASCULAR RISK STRATIFICATION AND CORONARY ARTERY DISEASE

Modern clinical practice guidelines recommend systematic evaluation of patients for cardiovascular risk prior to noncardiac surgery.[16] The 1977 Goldman Index of Cardiac Risk was the first widely adopted risk prediction model for noncardiac surgery.[19] In recent years more accurate models have been developed to provide improved quantitative estimates of risk, including the 1999 Revised Cardiac Risk Index (RCRI), the National Surgical Quality Improvement Program (NSQIP) Perioperative MI and Cardiac Arrest (MICA) Risk Calculator, and the NSQIP Universal Surgical Risk Calculators.[8,21,27] All patients, but especially those with elevated cardiovascular risk, require medical optimization of cardiovascular risk factors prior to elective noncardiac surgery. In addition, patients with limited functional capacity or concerning symptoms may warrant noninvasive risk stratification to evaluate for evidence of myocardial ischemia because abnormal preoperative stress echocardiography and myocardial perfusion imaging are well-validated predictors of postoperative cardiovascular events.[16] However, routine coronary angiography and/or prophylactic revascularization is not recommended prior to noncardiac surgery, because of an absence of benefit.[16] In the Coronary Artery Revascularization Prophylaxis (CARP) trial 510 patients with significant coronary artery disease (CAD) who were scheduled to undergo nonurgent vascular surgery were randomly assigned to either coronary revascularization (with either percutaneous coronary intervention [PCI] or coronary artery bypass grafting) or medical management.[30] The median delay to noncardiac surgery was 54 days in patients assigned to revascularization and 18 days in the group assigned to medical therapy. After 2.7 years of follow-up, no differences in 30-day (3.1% vs. 3.4%, $p = 0.87$) or long-term (22% vs. 23%, $p = 0.92$) mortality were observed. Based on the results of this landmark trial, most patients with stable coronary disease appear unlikely to benefit from routine preoperative revascularization. Because subjects with left main disease were excluded from the CARP trial, it remains unknown whether routine preoperative revascularization would be beneficial in that group.[18]

MEDICAL THERAPY FOR CARDIOVASCULAR RISK FACTOR OPTIMIZATION

Aspirin

Aspirin is an irreversible cyclooxygenase-1 (COX-1) inhibitor that inhibits thromboxane A2 production and platelet aggregation and consequently reduces thrombotic risks, albeit with an increased risk of bleeding. Although aspirin is widely used for the secondary prevention of cardiovascular disease, the risks and benefits of aspirin therapy are uncertain in patients undergoing major orthopedic surgery. Early data from the Pulmonary Embolism Prevention (PEP) trial, which randomly assigned 13,356 inpatients undergoing hip surgery to 35 days of aspirin 160 mg or placebo (with at least one preoperative dose of study drug), demonstrated that perioperative aspirin therapy reduced the incidence of postoperative venous thrombosis but was not associated with reductions in perioperative MI (0.54% vs. 0.34%, $p = 0.12$; hazard ratio [HR], 1.57; confidence interval [CI,] 0.93 to 2.65) or vascular death (3.5% vs. 3.8%, $p = 0.46$; HR, 0.93; CI, 0.78 to 1.11).[34] The second Perioperative Ischemic Evaluation (POISE-2) trial also studied the efficacy and safety of perioperative aspirin in noncardiac surgery. In POISE-2, 10,010 patients at risk for cardiovascular complications were randomly assigned to either aspirin or placebo prior to surgery. Patients were stratified according to whether or not they had been taking aspirin prior to enrollment in the study. Among those enrolled, 3844 (38%) patients underwent orthopedic surgery.[14] No difference in death or nonfatal MI was observed at 30 days (7.0% vs. 7.1%, $p = 0.92$), and aspirin was associated with excess major bleeding (4.6% vs. 3.8%, $p = 0.04$). Surprisingly, aspirin did not confer any benefit in prespecified subgroups, regardless of aspirin use prior to randomization or the

---

*References 1, 4, 5, 10, 15, 23, 24, 26, 32, 41, and 43.

preoperative RCRI score.[14] Although the results of POISE-2 suggest that aspirin should not be routinely administered in the perioperative period, the benefit of aspirin remains uncertain for the subgroups of patients with the highest cardiovascular risks. Fewer than 25% of patients in POISE-2 had a history of CAD, only 4.7% had a history of PCI, and 1.2% had drug-eluting stents (DESs). Therefore most patients in POISE-2 may have lacked sufficient perioperative risk to derive a benefit from perioperative aspirin. Furthermore, there is insufficient evidence to conclude whether or not cessation of aspirin prior to surgery is safe in patients with a history of coronary stents. Thus for certain high-risk groups a multidisciplinary treatment team should consider individualized risks of thrombotic complications and perioperative bleeding prior to orthopedic surgery.

Lipid-Lowering Therapy and Statins

Lipid lowering with statin therapy prior to surgery is a promising approach to reduce perioperative cardiovascular events, although high-quality evidence to support this practice is currently limited. In a large propensity-matched analysis of 204,885 patients who underwent noncardiac surgery, those who were prescribed lipid-lowering agents early in their surgical hospitalization had substantially lower in-hospital mortality (adjusted odds ratio [OR], 0.62; 95% CI, 0.58 to 0.67).[28] A meta-analysis of observational studies and randomized controlled trials (RCTs) in noncardiac vascular surgery reported that statin use was associated with a reduction in a composite of MI, stroke, and death (OR, 0.45; 95% CI, 0.29 to 0.70).[3] Complicating matters, this meta-analysis included the controversial DECREASE III trial that reported a remarkable 53% reduction in death or MI with perioperative fluvastatin.[37] Since the publication of DECREASE III, the principal investigator, Don Poldermanns, has been accused of scientific misconduct and fabricated data, and his work has been largely discredited by the scientific community. A 2013 Cochrane review of RCTs of statins in noncardiac surgery excluding studies by Poldermanns reported insufficient evidence to conclude that statins reduce perioperative adverse cardiovascular events.[35] Based on the clinical trial data available to date, statins that are clinically indicated should be continued in the perioperative period of orthopedic surgery. Initiation of statin therapy prior to surgery may be considered for patients with indications for lipid-lowering therapy and elevated surgical risks.[16] Clinical trials to investigate the benefits of high-intensity statin therapy in patients undergoing noncardiac and orthopedic surgery are currently underway.[†]

Beta-Blockers

Beta-blockers blunt tachycardia, prolong diastole, enhance coronary perfusion, and decrease inotropy, contractility, and myocardial wall stress. These properties mitigate mismatch in myocardial oxygen supply and demand that can predispose patients to MI. Given these favorable attributes, beta-blockers were routinely used in the perioperative setting until the 2008 publication of the landmark POISE trial. POISE randomly assigned 8351 patients to metoprolol succinate 100 mg or placebo immediately prior to surgery, with continuation of the study drug for 30 days.[20] Orthopedic surgery was performed in 21% of patients. Overall, fewer patients receiving metoprolol had MI, cardiac arrest, or cardiovascular death (5.8% vs. 6.9%, $p = 0.039$), but beta-blockers were associated with increased all-cause mortality (3.1% vs. 2.3%, $p = 0.032$) and stroke (1.0% vs. 0.5%, $p = 0.0053$), raising significant safety concerns.[20] Critics of the POISE trial raise a number of valid issues. All subjects enrolled in the POISE trial began the study drug within 1 day of surgery, but studies suggest that longer, but not shorter, durations of preoperative beta-blocker administration are associated with improved perioperative outcomes.[17] The relatively high starting dose of metoprolol succinate was another important concern. Finally, in retrospective studies of patients undergoing noncardiac surgery, perioperative beta-blockers were only associated with reduced in-hospital mortality in the highest risk patients defined by preoperative RCRI scores greater than or equal to 2.[29]

Consequently, the usefulness of perioperative beta-blocker therapy remains questionable. Patients who normally receive beta-blockers as an outpatient should continue this therapy in the perioperative period, in the absence of bradycardia or hypotension.[16] Patients with ischemic heart disease or those with multiple RCRI risk factors may warrant initiation of beta-blockers prior to surgery, a decision that should be determined well in advance of surgery by a specialist in cardiovascular disease. However, based on available trial data, beta-blocker therapy should not be started on the day of surgery.[16] The optimal timing of initiation and dosing of perioperative beta-blockade remains uncertain, and additional prospective investigation is necessary. Consequently, cardiovascular specialists should guide the initiation of beta-blocker therapy in high-risk patients. When indicated, beta-blockers should be administered for a minimum of 1 week prior to orthopedic surgery to determine safety and tolerability.

Angiotensin-Converting Enzyme Inhibitors

Data to support continuation or cessation of angiotensin-converting enzyme (ACE) inhibitors or angiotensin receptor blocker (ARB) therapy in the perioperative period of noncardiac surgery are limited. Theoretical risks of perioperative ACE inhibitor or ARB administration include postinduction hypotension, increased need for vasoactive drugs, and worsening renal function. A large retrospective propensity-matched analysis of patients undergoing noncardiac surgery with and without chronic ACE inhibitor or ARB exposure revealed no significant differences in postoperative MI or worsening renal function, although ACE inhibitor or ARB combined with diuretic therapy was associated with increased rates of perioperative hypotension.[25] A smaller observational study also reported that ACE inhibitor or ARB therapy was associated with increased odds for moderate hypotension but with no differences in perioperative cardiovascular events.[11] In a retrospective cohort study of 237,208 patients undergoing major elective surgery, preoperative ACE inhibitor or ARB use was associated with lower rates of postoperative acute kidney injury treated with dialysis (adjusted relative risk [RR], 0.83; 95% CI, 0.71 to 0.98) and lower all-cause mortality (adjusted RR, 0.91; 95% CI, 0.87 to 0.95).[38] In contrast, in a separate observational analysis of 79,228 patients undergoing noncardiac surgery, ACE inhibitor use was not associated with in-hospital complications or mortality at 30 days.[42]

[†]Lowering the risk of operative complications using atorvastatin loading dose (LOAD), NCT01543555, and optimization of presurgical testing with an intensive multifactorial intervention to minimize cardiovascular events in orthopedic surgery (OPTMIZE-OS), NCT01837069.

Few RCTs of perioperative renin-angiotensin system blockade during noncardiac surgery have been conducted. In a small study of 51 patients chronically treated for hypertension with an ACE inhibitors and undergoing vascular surgery, cessation of ACE inhibitors therapy within 12 to 24 hours prior to surgery was associated with significantly less induction-induced hypotension than continuation of therapy.[12] In a separate randomized trial of 37 patients on chronic ACE inhibitor therapy undergoing vascular surgery, continuation of ACE inhibitor on the morning of surgery was associated with increased incidence of severe induction-associated hypotension and an increased need for vasoactive drugs.[7]

In light of the limited available evidence, current clinical practice guidelines recommend that continuation of ACE inhibitors or ARBs in the perioperative period of noncardiac surgery is reasonable.[16] If these agents are discontinued in the perioperative period, they should be resumed postoperatively as soon as clinically feasible.

CHALLENGING PATIENT POPULATIONS

Patients With Diabetes Mellitus

Diabetes mellitus afflicts nearly 285 million adults worldwide and nearly 13% of adults in the United States and independently confers a twofold excess risk of coronary heart disease (CHD) and stroke.[36,39] Patients with diabetes mellitus undergoing orthopedic surgery represent an important subgroup at elevated risk for perioperative complications. In a retrospective analysis of 15,321 individuals who underwent primary total knee arthroplasty, diabetes (OR, 2.99, 95% CI, 1.35 to 6.62) was a strong independent predictor of 30-day mortality.[6] Furthermore, poor glycemic control reduces healing of bones, soft tissues, ligaments, and tendons and in joint surgery is associated with deep surgical site infectious complications.[31,40]

The optimal management of diabetes mellitus in the perioperative setting can be challenging. The primary goal of glycemic control in the perioperative period is to prevent marked hyperglycemia without precipitating hypoglycemia. Although the American Diabetes Association (ADA) has proposed fasting glucose targets less than 140 mg/dL in hospitalized patients and random glucose targets less than 180 mg/dL, ideal perioperative glycemic targets are uncertain.[2] In a recent Cochrane meta-analysis of 12 randomized trials enrolling 1403 patients with diabetes undergoing surgery, intensive perioperative glycemic control was not associated with a reduction in postoperative infectious complications, adverse cardiovascular events, or mortality in comparison with conventional glycemic management but was associated with increased risk of hypoglycemia.[9] Consequently, individualized assessment of patients' risk of hypoglycemia is necessary prior to orthopedic surgery, followed by careful titration of insulin and oral diabetic agents to achieve appropriate perioperative glycemic targets.

Patients With Prior Percutaneous Coronary Intervention

Patients planned for orthopedic surgery who have revascularized CAD require careful preoperative evaluation. Even when other medical comorbidities have been optimized, the timing of elective noncardiac surgery among patients with recent PCI remains controversial. Noncardiac surgery following coronary stent placement has been associated with increased adverse cardiac events, often attributed to the inflammatory and prothrombotic effects of surgery combined with premature cessation of antiplatelet therapies. Surgery performed within 4 to 6 weeks of a coronary intervention is associated with the greatest risk. Consequently, modern clinical practice guidelines recommend that elective surgery should be delayed by at least 30 days following placement of a bare metal state (BMS) or a minimum of 1 year for DES.[46] A large, retrospective study of patients undergoing noncardiac surgery at Veterans Affairs hospitals within 2 years of implantation of a coronary stent demonstrated stable rates of cardiovascular events for surgeries that were delayed at least 6 months after PCI.[22] Based on these and other data,[22,45] elective noncardiac surgery may be considered 180 days after elective PCI with DES, provided that the risks of further surgical delay outweigh the risk of perioperative ischemic complications.[16] Additional prospective studies are necessary to validate this approach and to determine the optimal management of patients with recent DES who need elective noncardiac surgery but cannot wait the guideline recommended minimum 1-year delay.

Management of antiplatelet therapy following PCI is another major challenge, particularly for patients who must undergo surgery in which surgical site bleeding poses significant risks. In most cases, current guidelines recommend continuation of antiplatelet monotherapy with aspirin in the perioperative period. However, a cardiovascular disease specialist should guide the timing of withdrawal of $P2Y_{12}$ inhibitor therapy. In most cases clopidogrel and ticagrelor should be discontinued greater than or equal to 5 days prior to surgery, and prasugrel should be held for greater than or equal to 7 days preoperatively, based on the pharmacokinetic and pharmacodynamic properties of each drug. In rare circumstances continuation of dual antiplatelet therapy may be considered for patients who are at the highest risk of thrombotic events. However, dual antiplatelet therapy with aspirin and a $P2Y_{12}$ inhibitor has been associated with a substantial increase in postoperative moderate and severe bleeding and consequently is not frequently recommended in the perioperative period.[44]

CONCLUSIONS

All patients planned for orthopedic surgery warrant preoperative medical optimization and management of risk factors to mitigate adverse cardiovascular events in the perioperative period. A multidisciplinary team of anesthesiologists, cardiologists, and orthopedic surgeons should perform a thorough assessment of cardiovascular disease burden and determine surgery-specific thrombotic and bleeding risks. Only after the initiation of medical therapy and optimization of cardiovascular risk factors should a patient proceed to the operating room for orthopedic surgery.

KEY REFERENCES

2. American Diabetes Association: Standards of medical care in diabetes—2014. *Diabetes Care* 37(Suppl 1):S14–S80, 2014.
13. Devereaux PJ, Chan MT, Alonso-Coello P, et al: Association between postoperative troponin levels and 30-day mortality among patients undergoing noncardiac surgery. *JAMA* 307:2295–2304, 2012.
14. Devereaux PJ, Mrkobrada M, Sessler DI, et al: Aspirin in patients undergoing noncardiac surgery. *N Engl J Med* 370(16):1494–1503, 2014.
15. Fleisher LA, Beckman JA, Brown KA, et al: ACC/AHA 2007 guidelines on perioperative cardiovascular evaluation and care for noncardiac surgery: a report of the American College of Cardiology/American Heart Association Task Force on Practice Guidelines (Writing Committee to

Revise the 2002 Guidelines on Perioperative Cardiovascular Evaluation for Noncardiac Surgery) developed in collaboration with the American Society of Echocardiography, American Society of Nuclear Cardiology, Heart Rhythm Society, Society of Cardiovascular Anesthesiologists, Society for Cardiovascular Angiography and Interventions, Society for Vascular Medicine and Biology, and Society for Vascular Surgery. *J Am Coll Cardiol* 50(17):e159–e241, 2007.

16. Fleisher LA, Fleischmann KE, Auerbach AD, et al: 2014 ACC/AHA guideline on perioperative cardiovascular evaluation and management of patients undergoing noncardiac surgery: a report of the American College of Cardiology/American Heart Association Task Force on Practice Guidelines. *J Am Coll Cardiol* 64:e77–e137, 2014.

20. Group PS, Devereaux PJ, Yang H, et al: Effects of extended-release metoprolol succinate in patients undergoing non-cardiac surgery (POISE trial): a randomised controlled trial. *Lancet* 371(9627):1839–1847, 2008.

21. Gupta PK, Gupta H, Sundaram A, et al: Development and validation of a risk calculator for prediction of cardiac risk after surgery. *Circulation* 124:381–387, 2011.

22. Hawn MT, Graham LA, Richman JS, et al: Risk of major adverse cardiac events following noncardiac surgery in patients with coronary stents. *JAMA* 310(14):1462–1472, 2013.

27. Lee TH, Marcantonio ER, Mangione CM, et al: Derivation and prospective validation of a simple index for prediction of cardiac risk of major noncardiac surgery. *Circulation* 100(10):1043–1049, 1999.

29. Lindenauer PK, Pekow P, Wang K, et al: Perioperative beta-blocker therapy and mortality after major noncardiac surgery. *N Engl J Med* 353(4):349–361, 2005.

30. McFalls EO, Ward HB, Moritz TE, et al: Coronary-artery revascularization before elective major vascular surgery. *N Engl J Med* 351(27):2795–2804, 2004.

34. Prevention of pulmonary embolism and deep vein thrombosis with low dose aspirin: pulmonary embolism prevention (PEP) trial. *Lancet* 355(9212):1295–1302, 2000.

35. Sanders RD, Nicholson A, Lewis SR, et al: Perioperative statin therapy for improving outcomes during and after noncardiac vascular surgery. *Cochrane Database Syst Rev* (7):CD009971, 2013.

41. Thygesen K, Alpert JS, Jaffe AS, et al: Third universal definition of myocardial infarction. *J Am Coll Cardiol* 60(16):1581–1598, 2012.

The references for this chapter can also be found on www.expertconsult.com.

181

Decreasing the Risk of Surgical Site Infections Following Total Knee Arthroplasty

Joseph A. Bosco III, Jarrett D. Williams

EPIDEMIOLOGY AND FINANCIAL IMPLICATIONS

Surgical site infections (SSIs) following total knee arthroplasty (TKA) result in increased morbidity, increased cost, and inferior outcomes. Despite efforts to decrease or eliminate SSIs, the incidence continues to range between 0.5% and 1.6%.[11,46,53,86] This "small" percentage of infected TKAs adds a significant cost burden to the health care system. Patients who develop SSIs after TKA have longer hospital stays, more hospital readmissions, and accrue costs more than four times ($116,383 vs. $28,240) that of patients without deep surgical infections.[48] By 2030, the number of TKAs is expected to increase by more than 600% to 3.48 million procedures. Additionally, by 2030, the proportion of revisions caused by deep SSIs is expected to increase from 16.8% to 65.5%.[55,56] The cost of treating SSIs following TKA was $566 million in 2009 and is expected to reach $1.6 billion by 2020.[54] Thus any significant change in SSI rates will have a profound effect on health care costs.

The evolution from the traditional volume-based fee for service to quality-based total joint reimbursement strategies will exacerbate the financial consequences of SSIs. In 2015 Medicare announced a mandatory value-based purchasing plan called the Comprehensive Care for Joint Replacement (CJR) payment model for acute care hospitals furnishing lower extremity joint replacement services.[90] The government will randomly select one third of hospitals performing joint replacements to participate in the program. This is a bundled care arrangement, where the initial target reimbursement will be 98% of the individual hospital's last 2-year average of costs for all the care provided in the bundle time period. Any costs above this target price will not be reimbursed.[90] In a bundled payment arrangement, the health care providers (hospitals and physicians) assume the financial risk and responsibility for any costs associated with complications such as SSIs. Thus, the financial implications associated with SSIs are becoming even more severe for providers.

The purpose of this chapter is to present evidence-based strategies and interventions that reduce the likelihood of developing an SSI following TKA. For ease of presentation and clarity, we organized the chapter by time periods surrounding TKA. These time periods are preoperative, intraoperative, and postoperative. Most of the SSI reduction methods we will discuss are used during one of these three time periods. We have included only those interventions whose efficacy is supported by evidence-based medicine.

Preoperative

Evidence-based interventions during the preoperative period include: (1) a *Staphylococcus aureus* nasal screening and decolonizing program, (2) a patient-based SSI risk identification and risk modification program, and (3) an institution-wide robust antibiotic stewardship program (ASP). All three of these interventions must be implemented long before the patient enters the operating room or, in the case of an SSI identification and risk reduction program, before the patient is considered a surgical candidate.

Antibiotic Stewardship Program. An ASP refers to a multidisciplinary hospital program geared at selecting optimal drug use that will result in the best clinical outcomes for the prevention and/or treatment of infection, with minimal toxicity to the patient and minimal development of resistance.[63] Members of the team include infectious disease specialists, hospital epidemiologists, surgeons, microbiology lab leaders, and anesthesiologists. All antibiotic use, including the restriction of certain antibiotics and the proper use of recommended antimicrobials, is reviewed by the stewardship team.[15]

Nowak et al. implemented an ASP in 2007 and found significant improvements in antibiotic use without significant changes in patient length of stay, 30-day readmission rates, and clinical outcomes for pneumonia and abdominal sepsis.[75] They used data-mining software to create reports that included key pharmacy, clinical, and microbiologic data on all adult hospital patients receiving antibiotics. Based on the analysis of the file, recommendations were made to providers highlighting changes to improve their care management. Although physicians' judgment had priority over ASP recommendations, four out of five recommendations were accepted and used by providers. Implementation of the ASP saved $1.7 million dollars. In addition, the use of many antibiotics decreased, whereas survival among patients did not significantly change as compared to the period before implementation of the ASP.[75]

S. aureus species are the most common pathogens associated with SSI following TKA.[66,101] *Staphylococcus* species pathogenicity is a result of its ability to adhere to tissues and foreign bodies (joint prosthesis) and to secrete a biofilm. *S. aureus* has adhesive proteins on its surface that enhance its adherence to human tissue, such as the interior nose; these proteins are called *microbial surface components recognizing adhesive matrix molecules* (MSCRAMMs).[32,36] These molecules also enable *Staphylococcus* species to secrete a biofilm coating that blocks the access of antibiotics to the organisms, making infections in orthopedic procedures difficult to treat.[25] Many *S. aureus* species also have an external capsule that helps them elude opsonization by host phagocytic cells. In addition to capsular protection, *Staphylococcus* can also inactivate host complement factors, avoid the bactericidal effects of lysozyme, and survive within neutrophil phagosomes.[7,24,37]

The nasal mucosa serves as an *S. aureus* reservoir and a source of potential transmission to the knee.[48,51,55] Methicillin-sensitive *S. aureus* (MSSA) nasal colonization is present consistently in 20% of the population and is intermittently present in as much as 60%. Additionally, methicillin-resistant *S. aureus* (MRSA) is found in 2% to 3% of patients undergoing TKA.[51] As a result, patient nasal colonization prior to surgery is a known risk factor for SSI following TKA.[22] To address this issue, patients require nasal screening and decolonization prior to entering the operating room.

As in any intervention occurring within a complex hospital organization, a program of nasal screening and decolonization requires the cooperation of multiple stakeholders. These stakeholders include nurses, surgeons, microbiology lab staff, and anesthesiologists. Decolonization programs usually start with preadmission testing. In preadmission testing, patients are examined prior to surgery and have their anterior nares swabbed to identify if colonization is present. Regardless of the results, some programs prescribe intranasal mupirocin ointment to all patients twice daily for 5 days prior to surgery.[85] If the patient is found to be colonized with MSSA, they are prescribed a first-generation cephalosporin, such as cefazolin (2 g delivered 0.5 to 1 hour prior to surgery followed by 1 g every 8 hours for the next 24 hours on the day of surgery), whereas if they are colonized with MRSA, they are prescribed weight-based vancomycin[18,85,93]

Decolonization programs are effective in reducing SSIs following TKA. Recent studies report that mupirocin and preoperative antimicrobial prophylaxis reduces SSI by up to 40%.[9,38,50,85] Research has also shown that after implementation of a decolonization program, subspecialty orthopedic hospitals will experience a reduction in all infections caused by MRSA, including urinary tract infections (UTIs) and pneumonias.[71] Although mupirocin has been shown to be effective at eradicating *Staphylococcus* from the anterior nares, it is not effective at combating extra-nasal sites. This is done using wipes and baths with chlorhexidine. Chlorhexidine has been proven to effectively reduce SSI following surgical procedures by eradicating pathogens on the skin near surgical sites.[27,103]

In addition to mupirocin, another option for nasal decolonization is povidone-iodine (PI). One study found that patients receiving PI had significantly less adverse effect compared to patients receiving prophylactic mupirocin.[3] Additionally, the financial benefits of nasal PI, with its lower cost ($15), would favor increased patient compliance. Mupirocin can cost as much as $115 for some patients, leading to as many as 13% describing financial difficulties with using mupirocin before surgery.[84] Unlike mupirocin ointment, which requires a twice-daily 5-day application prior before surgery, nasal PI can simply be applied twice on the day of surgery.[80] This shortened application period does not decrease the efficacy of antimicrobial therapy; one study showed that patient use of nasal PI had similar rates of SSI following surgery compared to those using mupirocin.[80] PI was also found to cause less adverse reactions and cost less than mupirocin ointment, leading to increased health care value with the use of nasal PI.[70,81]

The process of obtaining nasal cultures prior to surgery and communicating the results to providers is cumbersome. This situation has led to the increased use of polymerase chain reaction (PCR) for detecting MRSA colonization.[38,50] PCR does not "culture" the organisms, but it detects the presence of an organism's DNA. Numerous studies have documented the accuracy and cost effectiveness of PCR in detecting MSSA and MRSA.*

IDENTIFICATION AND MODIFICATION OF RISK FACTORS PRIOR TO TOTAL KNEE ARTHROPLASTY

Risk Factors

Many risk factors exist for SSI following TKA. Several of these risk factors can potentially be modified prior to TKA, thus potentially decreasing the risk of SSI. For example, patients with inflammatory arthritis, sickle cell disease, diabetes, renal failure, and human immune deficiency virus have been shown to have increased infection rates with joint replacement. Although these risk factors cannot be completely eliminated, surgeons can ensure that the risks associated with these procedures are minimized. For example, preoperative consultation with a patient's rheumatologist should include a plan for discontinuing highly immunosuppressive medications perioperatively. Patients with sickle cell disease should be screened prior to joint replacement for skin ulcerations or potential sources of osteomyelitis, which can cause seeding of a prosthetic joint.

Tobacco use, poorly controlled diabetes, obesity, and *S. aureus* nasal colonization are patient risk factors that are amenable to perioperative interventions designed to decrease SSI risk. Singh et al. reported that patients using tobacco in the perioperative period had a 1.4 times greater risk of developing an SSI than those who did not use tobacco.[92] Sorensen demonstrated a 1.8 times increased risk of SSI in tobacco users. More importantly, they found that smoking cessation significantly decreased the risk of SSI.[94] Other authors have found that smoking cessation at least 4 weeks prior to total joint arthroplasty (TJA) can lead to fewer wound-related complications and fewer total complications.[49,61,72,98] Poorly controlled diabetes is generally associated with infection and poor wound healing. Improved diabetes management may reduce a patient's infection risk. Marchant et al. reviewed over one million primary and revision lower limb arthroplasty cases and found poorly controlled diabetes to be an independent risk factor for infection leading to a twofold increase in infection rates.[69] A recent study by Maradit et al. reported higher SSI rates for diabetic patients and for those with preoperative hyperglycemia, but found no specific association between hemoglobin A1c values and SSI rates.[68] Chrastil et al. similarly found an association between SSI and diabetes, but no association with SSI and increased levels of hemoglobin A1c.[21] Obesity is a risk factor for SSI following TKA.[74,89] Schwarzkopf et al. reported that patients with a body mass index (BMI) greater than 45 had an 8.44 times higher risk of developing inpatient complications than normal weight patients.[89] These complications include acute renal failure, respiratory failure, infection, venous thromboembolic disease, anemia requiring intensive care unit (ICU) transfer, UTI, and increased wound drainage. These complications increase in a linear fashion for each 5 kg/m² increase in BMI.†

The question of whether to proceed with TKA surgery in the face of these modifiable risk factors is a difficult one. A shared decision-making model is the best method for addressing these

---

*References 38, 50, 62, 67, 71, 84, and 91.
†References 8, 45, 47, 74, 83, and 89.

modifiable risk factors with the patient. The focus should not be on avoiding surgery for all high-risk patients, but on identifying those patients that carry some level of unacceptable but potentially modifiable risk. Once these patients are identified, the surgeon should make every effort to modify these risks prior to performing these elective surgeries. The concepts of patient autonomy (allowing the patient to decide what is best for them) and nonmaleficence (do no harm to the patient) must be balanced. The surgeon who delays a TKA to allow a patient to modify certain SSI risk factors is acting within acceptable ethical standards.

Intraoperative Interventions to Reduce Surgical Site Infections

These interventions include surgical hand asepsis, operative site skin preparation, maximizing operating room air quality, use of antibiotic cement, betadine lavage, vancomycin powder wound application, use of powderless gloves, antibiotic-coated sutures, and elimination of flash sterilization.

The object of a preoperative hand scrub is to leave as few as possible live bacteria on the hands of the surgeon. Aqueous scrub solutions comprised of water-based solutions of chlorhexidine gluconate (CHG) or PI were classically used. A recent Cochrane review[97] found alcohol-based rubs containing ethanol, isopropanol, or n-propanol as effective as aqueous solutions in preventing SSIs in patients. Hajipour et al.[39] reported that alcohol rubs were more effective than CHG or iodine-based scrubs in reducing bacterial colony forming units (CFUs) on the hands of surgeons. Other investigators reported that the use of scrub brushes had no positive effect on asepsis and may actually increase infections as a result of skin damage.[34] Based on this evidence, the recommended procedure for preoperative surgical hand asepsis is as follows: Preceding the first scrub of the day or when the hands are grossly contaminated, wash with soap and water, use a nail pick to clean under the nails, and dry with paper towels. Then use an alcohol-based rub for 3 minutes.[102] Use the alcohol-based rub for each subsequent case. The use of scrub brushes is not recommended.

Surgical Site Preparation

CHG-based solutions are the most effective means of eliminating bacteria from the skin of patients immediately prior to surgery and have largely supplanted the use of alcohol and iodine-based solutions. Ostrander et al.[78] examined the residual amounts of bacteria remaining on feet prepped with CHG, iodine/isopropyl alcohol, or chloroxylenol scrub. They found that CHG was superior to the other two prep solutions in reducing or eliminating bacteria from the feet prior to surgery. CHG skin prep is superior to 70% alcohol or iodine in decreasing infection associated with the placement of central venous catheters and the drawing of blood cultures.[2,5] Thus, the current evidence-based recommendation and best practices call for the use of a CHG-based solution for surgical site preparation and central venous catheter placement.

The use of *flash sterilization* increases the risk of SSI and should be eliminated whenever possible. Flash sterilization is a procedure used by operating room staff to sterilize instruments or implants with steam on an as-needed basis. Flashing is not equivalent to sterilization in central processing.[16,59] In central sterile processing, instruments are properly cleaned and all lumens are inspected, the contents are completely dried, and are delivered in closed sterile containers; most importantly, the

process is performed by trained, focused professionals. The entire process takes 3 to 4 hours. The proper indications for flash sterilization are dropped instruments, an emergent or unplanned procedure, and a test cycle failure. Proper presurgical planning will decrease the need for flash sterilization.

To reduce the incidence of flash sterilization, we recommend the following procedures: increase physician awareness about the inadequacy of flash sterilization; improve the accuracy of surgical booking; mandate cooperation from vendors to ensure timely delivery of equipment, including financial penalties for late delivery; identify the purchase of frequently flashed items; initiate surgical scheduling to accommodate and mitigate equipment shortages; and, finally, generate incidence reports when a flashed implant is used in a patient.[43] Adopting these policies and procedures leads to a decrease in the incidence of flash sterilization.[42]

Powderless Gloves

The use of powderless gloves reduces the overall risk of SSI. Traditionally, surgical gloves contained powder to aid in the manufacturing process and to allow for ease in donning. The powder was comprised of talc or lycopodium spores. Because of concerns with granuloma formation and adhesions associated with the use of these substances, cornstarch is now the powder of choice.[23] However, cornstarch is not benign. Cornstarch has been shown to cause foreign body granuloma formation, result in delayed wound healing, and can lower the amount of bacteria required to cause a clinically apparent infection.[44] Additionally, powder results in hypersensitivity reactions in those who use them frequently, leading to increased risk of bacterial shedding and time lost from work. Although powderless gloves are 25% more expensive than their powdered counterparts, they have been shown to be cost effective, by decreasing staff absenteeism.[52]

The risk of SSI is decreased by using antibiotic-coated sutures. In an in vitro SSI model, triclosan-coated sutures inhibited bacterial growth.[26] A recent randomized controlled trial comparing the SSI rate in cerebral spinal fluid shunt surgery with and without the use of antibiotic-coated sutures demonstrated significant reduction in SSI rates in the treatment group.[87] These sutures cost 7% to 10% more than their uncoated counterparts. To date, no cost-effectiveness analysis has been published; however, the use of these sutures in high-risk patients may be justified.

Operating Room Air Quality

Maximizing the quality of the operating room air is essential to decreasing the risk of SSI. The air in any closed environment such as an operating room contains bacteria-laden skin squames, lint, respiratory droplets, and dust. To minimize this contamination, the operating room air must be positively pressured with a minimum of 20 air exchanges per hour. Humidity and temperature should be controlled.[64] Additionally, airflow should be unidirectional and downward. Adequate unidirectional airflow does not require the use of expensive laminar flow systems. The only study that reported a decrease in SSI rates with the use of laminar flow reported that this decrease was only observed in patients if they did not receive prophylactic antibiotics. In the patients who received prophylactic antibiotics, the rates of SSI were not affected by the use of laminar flow.[60] More recent reviews have failed to demonstrate any reduction in SSI risk associated with the use of laminar airflow.[31,35] Thus the expense of laminar airflow units is not supported by any demonstrated SSI reduction and is not considered a useful intervention in preventing SSI.

There is a direct relationship between operating room traffic and SSI risk. Bedard et al.[6] observed the number of times a person entered and exited the operating room in 100 consecutive TJA cases. They reported that the mean number of door openings during primary TJA was 71.1 (range 35 to 176) with a mean operative time of 111.9 (range 53 to 220) minutes, for an average of 0.64 (range 0.36 to 1.05) door openings/minute. In a study of spine surgery, Olsen et al. reported that two or more residents scrubbed in a case was an independent variable for SSIs.[76] Babkin et al. found that SSI rates for left knee replacements were 6.7 times higher than for right knee replacements performed during the same time period and in the same operating rooms.[4] When the operating room door on the left side of the operating room was locked, preventing ingress or egress, the SSI rate of the left-sided knee replacements rapidly decreased to that of the right-sided knee replacements, demonstrating the importance of limiting operating room traffic. Thus, surgeons must limit the operating room traffic through increased awareness of the ill effects of door openings and better operative planning and communication.

Antibiotic-Loaded Bone Cement

The use of antibiotic-loaded bone cement in knee and hip primary arthroplasty has been well studied. Several large European registry studies established the efficacy of antibiotic cement in total hip arthroplasty (THA). The Norwegian registry data demonstrated significantly lower revision rates in patients receiving antibiotic cement for primary THA.[28,30] Similarly, analysis of the Swedish nation joint registry database demonstrated significantly decreased rates of revision for deep infection with the use of gentamicin-containing cement.[65] A recent Canadian registry study by Bohm et al. analyzed a sample of 36,681 TKAs, 45% of which used antibiotic cement. No significant difference was found in 2-year revision rates between the two groups for infection or for all causes of revision.[10] Two recent randomized controlled trials have attempted to prospectively address this efficacy question. In 2002, Chiu et al. randomized 341 TKA patients to cefuroxime-impregnated versus standard cement and found a significant difference in infection rate, with zero infections in the antibiotic cement group (0/178, 0%) versus five infections in the standard cement group (5/162, 3.1%, $p < .05$).[20] A 2013 trial by Hinarejos et al., in which they prospectively randomized 2948 TKA patients to standard cement versus erythromycin- or cilastin-containing cement, found the opposite result. Their cohort had comparable rates of deep infection, at 1.4% in the antibiotic group versus 1.35% in the standard-cement group ($p = .96$).[40] The literature supporting the use of antibiotic cement for TKA is not as robust as that supporting its use in THA.

Additionally, the average cost of premixed antibiotic in polymethylmethacrylate (PMMA) is approximately $300 per bag. Thus the routine use of antibiotic cement on every TKA would add a significant expense to the health care system without demonstrating value. Based on the available literature and expert consensus opinion, the 2013 Proceedings of the International Consensus on Prosthetic Joint Infection recommended that antibiotic-laden PMMA reduces infection and should be used in elective arthroplasty in high-risk patients.[79] These risk factors included diabetes, morbid obesity, and inflammatory arthritis, use of steroids, and previous history of joint infection.

Local Antibiotic Powder at Wound Closure and Povidone-Iodine

The use of vancomycin powder applied directly into a wound at the time of closure reduces the incidence of SSI in patients undergoing spine surgery.[13,77,95] However, currently there are no studies demonstrating efficacy of intrawound vancomycin powder in the TJA literature. The use of topically applied vancomycin powder is not associated with a systemic increase in serum vancomycin levels.[57] Additionally, Qadir et al. reported that addition of vancomycin powder to a total joint construct caused no difference in wear rates of the ultra-high molecular weight polyethylene liner.[82] Vancomycin is available in generic formulations that cost approximately $10. Thus its use does not add a significant expense to the procedure. Given the lack of data on efficacy in arthroplasty, and the potential for development of resistance, the use of topical vancomycin powder should be restricted to high-risk patients.

The efficacy of applying a dilute PI lavage just prior to capsule closure in reducing SSIs following TKA and THA has been investigated. The protocol consisted of applying a dilute PI lavage solution (0.35%) for 3 minutes to the open wound after the implants are placed and immediately prior to closure. Brown et al.[14] compared the SSI rates of 1862 consecutive cases (630 THA and 1232 TKA) done prior to the initiation of the PI protocol to 688 consecutive cases (274 THA and 414 TKA) after the initiation of the PI lavage. All cases were performed by the same surgeon at the same institution. Eighteen early postoperative infections were identified before the use of dilute PI lavage, and only one since the use of PI lavage began (0.97% and 0.15%, respectively; $p = .04$). Cheng et al.[19] reported similar results in a group of patients undergoing spinal fusion surgery. Neither author reported any complications associated with the use of this protocol. It is now suggested that PI solution in sterile packets be substituted for betadine because of the ability to obtain a sterile solution.

Postoperative Interventions

These interventions include establishing an evidence-based protocol for wound management consisting of the use of impregnated dressings and the adoption of an institution-wide strategy for blood management to decrease the need for allogeneic transfusions. In addition, each patient must be assessed for their risk of venous thromboembolism (VTE), followed by use of the VTE prophylaxis that has the best risk-benefit profile for each patient.

Postoperative Wound Management

The management of wounds in the perioperative period should be standardized using evidence-based guidelines. The basic concept of infection prevention is to keep the wound clean and dry. Therefore, soiled or blood-soaked dressings should be removed immediately, rather than reinforcing them. Silver-impregnated antimicrobial dressings have been shown to decrease the incidence of SSI following cardiac surgery[41] and lumbar fusion.[29] Other compounds such as polyhexamethylene biguanide (PHMB) have shown promise in small studies.[58,73] PHMB-containing dressings have an advantage in looking and feeling similar to traditional gauze dressings, and they are much less expensive than silver-containing dressings. The cost of a

PHMB-containing 4 × 4 sponge is roughly twice the cost of a regular 4 × 4 gauze, which is probably the least expensive antimicrobial dressing. Although no cost effectiveness studies exist, most people with expertise in wound care feel that the increased cost of these dressings is offset by the potential decrease in the incidence of SSI.

One cannot underestimate the importance of aggressive management of patients with persistent wound drainage. Any patient with persistent wound drainage should be returned to the operating room for irrigation and drainage with possible liner exchange. The use of oral antibiotics to "treat" wound drainage is not recommended. A frequent cause of wound drainage and postoperative bleeding is the anticoagulants used to prevent VTE events. Not all thromboprophylactic agents have the same risk of postoperative bleeding.[1] Similarly, not all TKA patients have the same risk of developing VTEs. Thus, to minimize the risk of bleeding, the choice of VTE prophylaxis agents should be customized to each patient based on their individual risk factors. This requires that each patient be evaluated for VTE risk preoperatively and that a formal institutionalized VTE prophylaxis protocol and order set be used.

Blood Management

An evidence-based universally applied protocol for the management of blood loss after TKA is essential to minimizing the risk of SSI. The use of allogeneic blood transfusions is associated with increased length of stay[88,100] and induces immunomodulation that can lead to increased risk for infection at the surgical site.[99] Talbot et al. reported a 3.2-fold increase of post-sternotomy infection among transfused patients, compared with those who were not transfused.[96] Bower et al. reported infections following cardiac surgery in almost twice as many transfused patients, compared with similar non-transfused patients.[12] In a study of 12,000 patients undergoing total hip or knee replacements, Friedman et al.[33] reported that patients who received allogeneic blood transfusion had a significantly greater rate of wound inflammation or infection compared to those who received autologous blood transfusion or no blood transfusion. They also reported that the rates of any infection, lower or upper respiratory tract and lung infection, were significantly increased in their patient population. Thus it is clear that allogeneic blood transfusion is associated with an increased risk of SSI.

We must understand the risks of not transfusing patients to make informed decisions as to the risk-benefit ratio of blood transfusion. An essential component of this decision is determining the hemoglobin threshold at which postoperative red-cell transfusion is indicated. Carson et al. conducted a multicenter, randomized control trial analyzing the outcomes of patients who sustained hip fracture surgery.[17] They randomized the cohort into two groups: (1) those who received transfusions for a hemoglobin level of 10 g/dL (liberal group) and (2) those who received transfusions for a hemoglobin level of less than 8 g/dL or who had symptoms of anemia (more restrictive group). The primary outcomes were death or an inability to walk across a room without human assistance on 60-day follow-up. They found no difference in the functional outcomes or mortality rates between the groups. They concluded that the more restrictive transfusion policy was safe in patients undergoing hip fracture surgery. Thus for asymptomatic patients with a hemoglobin of 8 g/dL or greater, the increased risk of SSI associated with allogeneic blood transfusion is not offset by any benefit in outcomes.

CONCLUSION

The purpose of this chapter was to present an evidence-based approach to minimizing the risk of SSI following TKA. The interventions are grouped according to the period in which they are used. Preoperative interventions include patient risk factor identification and modification, nasal decolonization protocols, and prophylactic antibiotic choice. Intraoperative interventions include the use of antibiotic cement, maintenance of operating room air quality, hand asepsis, surgical site preparation, the use of topical vancomycin, and the use of betadine lavage. Postoperative strategies include matching VTE prophylaxis to patient risk factors, wound care techniques, and blood management strategies. We have included only those interventions whose efficacy is supported by evidence-based medicine. Although we can never hope to completely eliminate SSIs following TKA, by using the discussed techniques, we can minimize the likelihood of SSIs occurring.

KEY REFERENCES

6. Bedard M, Pelletier-Roy R, Angers-Goulet M, et al: Traffic in the operating room during joint replacement is a multidisciplinary problem. *Can J Surg* 58(4):232–236, 2015.

9. Bode LG, Kluytmans JA, Wertheim HF, et al: Preventing surgical-site infections in nasal carriers of *Staphylococcus aureus*. *N Engl J Med* 362(1):9–17, 2010.

15. Campbell KA, Stein S, Looze C, et al: Antibiotic stewardship in orthopaedic surgery: principles and practice. *J Am Acad Orthop Surg* 22(12):772–781, 2014.

17. Carson JL, Terrin ML, Noveck H, et al: Liberal or restrictive transfusion in high-risk patients after hip surgery. *N Engl J Med* 365(26):2453–2462, 2011.

18. Catanzano A, Phillips M, Dubrovskaya Y, et al: The standard one gram dose of vancomycin is not adequate prophylaxis for MRSA. *Iowa Orthop J* 34:111–117, 2014.

22. Crowe B, Payne A, Evangelista PJ, et al: Risk factors for infection following total knee arthroplasty: a series of 3836 cases from one institution. *J Arthroplasty* 30:2275–2278, 2015.

35. Gastmeier P, Breier AC, Brandt C: Influence of laminar airflow on prosthetic joint infections: a systematic review. *J Hosp Infect* 81(2):73–78, 2012.

48. Kapadia BH, McElroy MJ, Issa K, et al: The economic impact of periprosthetic infections following total knee arthroplasty at a specialized tertiary-care center. *J Arthroplasty* 29(5):929–932, 2014.

54. Kurtz SM, Lau E, Watson H, et al: Economic burden of periprosthetic joint infection in the United States. *J Arthroplasty* 27(8 Suppl):61–65, e1, 2012.

67. Maoz G, Phillips M, Bosco J, et al: The Otto Aufranc Award: Modifiable versus nonmodifiable risk factors for infection after hip arthroplasty. *Clin Orthop* 473(2):453–459, 2015.

71. Mehta S, Hadley S, Hutzler L, et al: Impact of preoperative MRSA screening and decolonization on hospital-acquired MRSA burden. *Clin Orthop* 471(7):2367–2371, 2013.

74. Namba RS, Inacio MC, Paxton EW: Risk factors associated with deep surgical site infections after primary total knee arthroplasty: an analysis of 56,216 knees. *J Bone Joint Surg Am* 95(9):775–782, 2013.

79. Parvizi J, Gehrke T, Chen A: Proceedings of the international consensus on periprosthetic joint infection. *Bone Joint J* 95(11):1450–1452, 2013.

80. Phillips M, Rosenberg A, Shopsin B, et al: Preventing surgical site infections: a randomized, open-label trial of nasal mupirocin ointment and nasal povidone-iodine solution. *Infect Control Hosp Epidemiol* 35(7):826–832, 2014.

97. Tanner J, Swarbrook S, Stuart J: Surgical hand antisepsis to reduce surgical site infection. *Cochrane Database Syst Rev* (1):CD004288, 2008.

The references for this chapter can also be found on www.expertconsult.com.

182

Effects of Prehabilitation, Falls, and Musculoskeletal Comorbidity on Total Knee Arthroplasty Outcomes

Daniel L. Riddle

This chapter explores several issues that can increase or decrease the risk of a poor outcome following total knee arthroplasty (TKA). Outcome in the context of TKA can be conceptualized in several ways and outcome measures come in many forms. The outcome of most serious concern following TKA is death, but there are many other outcomes of interest. This chapter focuses on the three issues that affect TKA outcomes: (1) the effects of prehabilitation (or pre-rehabilitation) and a review of the evidence that explores the potential impact of prehabilitation on TKA outcomes; (2) whether fall risk, an infrequently discussed outcome, is changed following TKA in the short term and long term and whether interventions designed to reduce fall risk are effective in this population; and (3) the impact of musculoskeletal comorbidities on TKA outcomes.

Before we consider these issues, the concept of outcome in the context of TKA surgery needs to be defined. Table 182.1 provides a reasonably comprehensive list of potential outcomes of interest in TKA. In essence, outcomes are assumed to be a consequence of an intervention, although this is not always the case. Some outcomes are desirable (eg, reduced pain and improved function) and others are not (eg, prosthetic loosening or postoperative complications). The three main topics of this chapter—TKA prehabilitation, fall risk associated with TKA, and the role of orthopedic and neuromuscular comorbidity—can potentially influence all of the outcomes presented in Table 182.1.

EVIDENCE OF THE IMPACT OF PREHABILITATION ON TOTAL KNEE ARTHROPLASTY RECOVERY AND OUTCOME

Prehabilitation has traditionally been focused on the improvement of physical function and lower extremity strength, and reduction of pain prior to TKA. The concept of prehabilitation is an approach that, if successful at improving preoperative muscle strength, pain, or mobility, would theoretically improve postoperative outcome (Fig. 182.1). If a patient's preoperative pain or functional status can be improved, it is reasonable to conclude that postoperative function and pain status would be better, as compared to the outcome without prehabilitation. Topp et al. provided a nice illustrative figure to demonstrate this theory-based concept.[48] As the figure shows, patients with better preoperative status, as would occur if prehabilitation was successful at improving function or reducing pain (ie, the dashed line in the figure), would have better postoperative outcomes as compared to patients who did not have prehabilitation (ie, the

solid line in the figure). Evidence-based support for this theoretical model is substantial and shows that the higher (better) the functional status and the lower (less intense) the pain prior to TKA, the better the postoperative outcome.[15,16,28] In other words, preoperative status is one of the most potent predictors of postoperative pain and functional outcome. It is therefore somewhat surprising that the evidence base for prehabilitation is weak, particularly when considering intermediate or longer-term pain and functional outcome.

Although multipronged preoperative in-person and telephone-based educational interventions combined with multimodal analgesia and accelerated inpatient rehabilitation have been shown to reduce length of stay following TKA (from 6 days to 4) in observational design studies,[31] these interventions are difficult to study in randomized designs given their multifaceted nature and they can be costly and time consuming. Given more rapid discharge from the hospital in the current healthcare environment, the impact of these interventions in current practice is unclear.

For the traditional prehabilitation approaches focused primarily on improving preoperative physical function and pain intensity, the available studies examining the effects of these interventions involve small patient samples,[7,8,14,46,48] a systematic review,[42] and a narrative review.[19]

Santa et al. conducted a systematic review of all randomized trials and observational studies of prehabilitation on postoperative outcome for several surgical procedures, of which 22 studies met the inclusion criteria and 11 were studies of TKA or total hip arthroplasty (THA).[42] Overall, the authors found that in four of five studies on patients with joint replacement, prehabilitation had no effect on length of stay in the hospital. Regarding other postoperative outcomes, the evidence suggested some potential benefit in physical performance and self-reported pain and function in some but not all studies. Because of the lack of consistency in temporal characteristics of postoperative measurement across studies, no meta-analytic procedures were used. For example, 3 of 5 trials found that pain was improved between 4 and 26 weeks following surgery. In addition, the overall quality of the studies was rated as low to moderate and included a moderate risk of bias, so these conclusions are only preliminary and not strongly supported because of the design weaknesses and small sample sizes in the studies.

Several small-sample pilot randomized clinical trials[7,8,32,46,48] with sample sizes ranging from 11 to 36 persons per treatment arm have been conducted on persons preparing for TKA. With sample sizes this small, stable estimates of treatment effects, if any, are not available. Because strong randomized studies of the effects of prehabilitation are not available, there is essentially no evidence to support the use of prehabilitation despite a strong theoretical rationale.

In spite of this weak evidence, it is worth identifying descriptions from the literature that best illustrate an approach one could use for prehabilitation. Perhaps the most comprehensive description of a prehabilitation program was provided by Desmeules et al.[14] The authors describe a staging approach for prehabilitation that allowed a patient's preoperative status and abilities to guide the extent of prehabilitation. For example, for patients who could safely ambulate, had no reported falls over the prior 6 months, and whose functional status was rated as good based on self-report scores and physical performance–based tests, prehabilitation was minimal. These patients had a single visit to a physiotherapist for home exercise program training and education, and were provided with a list of community resources to increase activity. For patients at the other

extreme, with a history of repeated falls, poor physical performance or self-reported function, and a lack of support at home, the intervention was more substantial. These patients attended individual or group-level comprehensive strength, balance, and endurance exercise sessions three times per week over a 6- to 12-week period, and received occupational therapy, nutritional training, and nursing if needed.

In summary, the evidence for the use of prehabilitation can be characterized as weak and inconclusive. Studies examining the effects of prehabilitation have been small-sample pilot studies, and although some results from these pilot trials have been encouraging, the evidence is not strong enough to justify a comprehensive prehabilitation program. Although the theoretical justification for prehabilitation is strong, the amount of exercise needed to induce a meaningful improvement in pain or function prior to surgery has not been established. The staging approach described by Desmeules appears to have potential but more study is required before this approach should be adopted. This conclusion is supported by a recently published systematic review of 11 randomized controlled trials (RCTs) comparing patient outcomes following prehabilitation designed to reduce pain and improve lower extremity strength and function.[24] Kwok et al. concluded that there was no substantial evidence to support prehabilitation approaches and that the trials examining the role of prehabilitation are of poor quality and underpowered.

FALL RISK AND RISK PREVENTION FOR TOTAL KNEE ARTHROPLASTY

Falls are typically defined as an unintentional coming to rest on the floor or some lower level.[30] Causes of falls are numerous and are typically considered as caused by an obstacle (eg, icy surface or a throw rug) or owing to unknown or unconfirmed causes. Falls can be injurious or noninjurious, and although some falls are of no consequence in terms of downstream pain or functional status, it is generally agreed that falls should be avoided because of the risk of injury. In addition, falling can lead to fear of falling again, and this fear can result in reduced activity,

TABLE 182.1	**List of Potential Outcomes of Interest in Total Knee Arthroplasty**
Outcome	**Example(s)**
Mortality	
Morbidity	Infection, thromboembolism
Prosthetic performance	Prosthetic loosening
Physical impairment	Quadriceps strength, knee range of motion
Physical performance	Stair climbing test, 6-min walk test, walking test
Disease specific self-report questionnaire	KOOS scale, Oxford knee score
Generic self-report questionnaire	SF-36
Cost effectiveness	EQ-5D, direct medical costs
Patient satisfaction	Patient acceptable symptom state scale
Clinician assessment	Nonstandardized questions, for example, "How are you doing?"

KOOS, Knee Injury and Osteoarthritis Outcome Score.

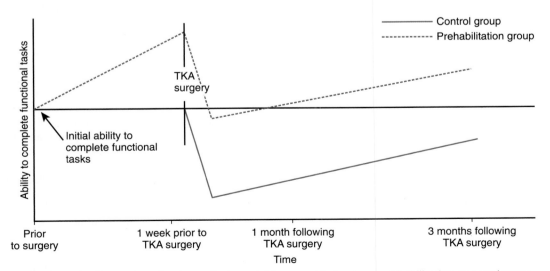

FIG 182.1 An illustration of a theoretical model for considering how prehabilitation may enhance outcome following TKA. (Reprinted from Topp R, Swank AM, Quesada PM, et al: The effect of prehabilitation exercise on strength and functioning after total knee arthroplasty. *Phys Med Rehab* 1(8):729-735, 2009.)

avoidance of weight-bearing activities, and a cycle of reduced health and activity avoidance.[49] Falls are avoidable most of the time, and research that identifies factors associated with increased fall risk can be helpful when attempting to reduce the risk of injury from falling.

Falls associated with TKA have been examined from various perspectives. First, work has been done to determine if persons who are planning to undergo TKA are at increased fall risk. Second, researchers have examined whether persons who underwent TKA are at risk for falls during the period of hospitalization. Third, some have examined fall risk after discharge home and in some cases, during the years following TKA. Finally, others have proposed strategies for reducing fall risk and associated adverse outcomes. Each of these issues will be explored.

ARE PERSONS WHO PLAN TO UNDERGO TOTAL KNEE ARTHROPLASTY AT INCREASED RISK FOR FALLS?

Patients preparing for TKA have several risk factors that predispose them to falling. The presence of severe pain combined with compromised mobility, likely weakness of the lower extremities, and general deconditioning are common, particularly among older adult patients, and predispose them to falling. The annual prevalence of falls among women 65 years and older with musculoskeletal pain is reported as 39%. These women were also at greater risk for injurious falls with fracture the most common injury.[26] Evidence also indicates that older adult persons with painful knees are at greater risk for falls relative to similarly aged persons without painful knees, and the greater the pain, the greater the risk. Only one study was found that examined fall rates specifically in persons prior to TKA.[4] Swinkels et al. studied a group of 99 patients scheduled for TKA in the United Kingdom. Patients completed monthly falls diaries preoperatively and up to 1 year postoperatively.[47] A total of 24.2% of persons reported a fall during the 3 months prior to TKA and fall rates decreased to 11.8% during each of the 3-month periods up to 1 year postoperatively. A total of 24.2% of persons reported at least one fall over the entire 1-year postoperative period. The strongest predictors of postoperative falls were more severe depressive symptoms and a history of preoperative falls.

In summary, although evidence on fall risk prior to TKA is not substantial, there is evidence to suggest that falls in persons with severe and painful knee osteoarthritis (OA), those who are most often candidates for TKA, are common and are higher than for persons without knee OA. Up to 25% of persons preparing for TKA will fall during the 3 months prior to surgery. Consequences of these falls are not clearly detailed in the literature, but a fairly substantial proportion of these falls result in important injury, usually a fracture.

FALL RISK AND RISK PREVENTION STRATEGIES FOR PATIENTS WITH TOTAL KNEE ARTHROPLASTY WHILE IN THE HOSPITAL

Because persons who undergo TKA have severely restricted mobility while recovering in the hospital, their risk of falling is increased. Falls during inpatient care are a substantial problem, not only with TKA, but also for several procedures and disorders. Some have suggested that the use of procedures like peripheral nerve blocks may increase the risk of falls for persons undergoing TKA and other surgical procedures because of the compromised immediate postoperative lower extremity function associated with this procedure.[21] Memtsoudis et al. determined the incidence of inpatient falls following TKA and predictive factors for increased fall risk.[33] Using an inpatient database, a total of 3042 of 191,570 persons (1.6% of the sample) reported a fall during hospitalization following TKA. Persons who fell while an inpatient in the hospital were older (68.9 vs. 66.3 years), had a greater burden of comorbidity, and had a greater number of major complications associated with their TKA. Persons who had neuraxial anesthesia had lower adjusted odds of falls as compared to persons who underwent general anesthesia. Peripheral nerve blocks were not found to be associated with falls while confined in the hospital.

In a related study, Pelt et al. examined the potential impact of the use of femoral nerve catheters as part of a multimodal analgesia protocol on fall incidence in the hospital and following TKA.[35] In addition, all patients participated in a fall prevention program including an educational program and approximately midway through the study, a "fall prevention contract" was instituted to improve uptake. Patients wore a knee immobilizer during ambulation for the first 3 days following surgery. The inpatient fall rate was 2.7% among the 707 patients who participated. The mean time to a fall was 1.6 days postsurgery and there was no association between falls and age, gender, or American Society of Anesthesiologists (ASA) score. Patients who participated in the fall prevention contract program had no difference in risk of falling as compared to persons who did not participate. The more common activities reported during a fall were getting out of bed and walking to the bathroom without assistance. Five patients fell while walking with assistance. A total of 68% of the patients who fell required additional medical care, most commonly imaging to rule out injury and three (15%) required reoperation.

Cui et al. also used a quasi-experimental design to examine the potential impact of knee immobilizer use on fall risk in a large university hospital setting.[12] Using a similar approach to Pelt et al.,[35] the authors conducted a retrospective chart review and chose a time period for study that did and did not include the adoption of a fall prevention approach, in this case a knee immobilizer following surgery. From 2008 to January 2010 a knee immobilizer was not used following TKA and beginning in January 2010, the knee immobilizer was required for all patients undergoing TKA. The authors compared fall rates and circumstances for the two time periods. Over the entire study, a total of 1102 patients underwent TKA and 30 patients (2.7%) reportedly had a fall. A total of 3.7% of persons fell prior to instituting the knee immobilizer policy and 1.6% fell after the knee immobilizer policy was started. This difference was statistically significant. Much like the study of Pelt et al.,[35] approximately 70% of falls required additional radiologic diagnosis or treatment. Mandl et al. used retrospective data to describe the proportion of TKA patients who fell over a 10-year period from 2000 to 2009 while in the Hospital for Special Surgery in New York City.[29] A total of 1.2% of TKA cases had a fall during hospitalization.

Wasserstein et al. conducted a retrospective chart review study of 2197 persons who had TKA at one institution over a 7-year period.[50] The authors were interested in identifying risk factors for falls among these persons. A total of 60 falls (2.7% of the sample) were documented and factors associated with increased fall risk were advanced age, body mass index (BMI) greater than 30, and continuous femoral nerve block. A single-dose femoral nerve block did not increase the risk of falling, whereas multiple doses increased the fall risk. Risk factors are cumulative; older adult patients with a BMI greater than 30 and with multiple doses of continuous femoral nerve block are at much great risk for falls as compared to patients with only one risk factor.

Johnson et al. used retrospective data from the Mayo Clinic to examine inpatient fall incidence following TKA and determined associations between falls and several fall prevention strategies that were implemented at various time points over a 10-year period from 2003 to 2012.[20] A total of 15,189 TKAs were conducted and the fall incidence rate was 1.5%. Risk factors for falls were older age, and surprisingly, the risk of falling was lower for patients undergoing revision TKA versus those undergoing primary TKA. Perhaps prior experience with TKA recovery helps to reduce fall risk. A total of 72% of falls occurred in the patient's room, and of these, 59% occurred while going to or from the bathroom or bedside commode. Most patients who fell (ie, 60%) were not rated as being at high risk for falling based on scores from the Hendrich II Fall Risk Model.[18] A total of 23% of falls were associated with additional morbidity. Interventions that were potentially associated with a slight drop in fall incidence were provider and patient education, use of fall-assessment tools, fall-alert signs, bed alarms, and the use of patient lifts. Little data were provided on the detailed implementation and adherence to these interventions, so the meaningfulness of these slight changes cannot be determined.

Evidence regarding inpatient fall risk[12,33,35,44,50] is surprisingly consistent; 1.5% to 3% of persons undergoing TKA are reported to fall and the consequences of these falls are substantial for most of these falls. The strength of evidence is somewhat weak because the papers reviewed are all retrospective in nature and rely on chart review in lieu of prospective approaches that would likely result in data of higher quality. Details on the implementation of fall prevention strategies were generally absent. Fall rates are very low, which only adds to the challenge of conducting prospective studies of the problem of falls following TKA. With a low incidence, many cases would need to be recruited in a prospective design to improve the current state of the evidence. With this said, the consequence of falls are substantial in most cases, so additional prospective research would likely provide valuable information regarding inpatient falls following TKA.

Consistently identified risk factors for falls are advanced age, BMI greater than 30, and continuous femoral nerve block; single-dose femoral nerve block does not appear to increase the risk of inpatient falls. Although intervention evidence is very weak because of the nature of the research, the preliminary evidence suggests that knee immobilizers, fall education and awareness programs, and multipronged approaches addressing several patient- and clinician-driven strategies may have mild preventive effects.

ARE PERSONS WHO UNDERWENT TOTAL KNEE ARTHROPLASTY AT RISK FOR FALLS FOLLOWING POSTSURGICAL RECOVERY?

The literature examining in-hospital risks and consequences of falls immediately following TKA is more substantial as compared to posthospitalization research. However, because falls are more common and time periods are generally much longer for pre- and posthospitalization studies as compared to inpatient studies, estimates are less prone to problems associated with the study of events that have very low incidence/prevalence. No studies were found that reported fall prevention strategies for reducing posthospitalization fall risk.

Swinkels et al. found a 1-year posthospitalization fall rate of 24.2% of persons falling at least once during the year following TKA.[47] A potentially useful predictor of 1-year postoperative fall risk is preoperative falls because 45% of persons who fell prior to surgery also fell after surgery. Of the 87 falls among the 24 persons who fell during the year following TKA, 40 falls resulted in cuts or bruises with 15 falls requiring medical care. Six falls resulted in upper extremity fractures.

In one of the few prospective studies examining fall incidence and fall risk, Matsumoto et al. studied 74 persons 60 years and older to determine fall rates up to 1 year following TKA and associations between physical function and falls.[30] Falls were assessed monthly for a 6-month period after surgery by use of prestamped mailed postcards that patients completed and sent back to the investigators. A total of 32% of the patients fell over the 6-month period. Persons who fell had more limited postoperative knee flexion and ankle plantarflexion motion as compared to persons who did not fall.

Jorgensen and Kehlet examined the incidence of falls following fast-track TKA or THA from patients in the Danish National Patient Registry. The purpose of the study was to identify characteristics of falls resulting in hospital admission within 90 days of discharge for fast track THA or TKA. The authors characterized the length of time from the surgery to the fall, the circumstances of the fall, and the types of injuries incurred. A total of 83 (1.6%) of 5145 persons undergoing total joint arthroplasty (TJA) were treated in a hospital following a fall that was judged to be related to surgery. Of the 83 patients, 43 were treated in the emergency room and did not require hospital admission. According to the medical chart review, 61 (73.5%) falls were classified as surgery-related falls, 12 (14.5%) were attributed to extrinsic factors, and 10 (12.0%) were related to physical activity. The authors used well-defined criteria to describe the extent of injury and the likely causes of the falls. The following was the classification system used for extent of injury: no injury, minor injury (minor cuts, minor bleeding from abrasions, swelling, and minor contusions), moderate injury (bleeding requiring cauterization, lacerations requiring suturing, temporary loss of consciousness, and soft tissue trauma), or severe injury (fractures, dislocation, major head trauma, injury requiring additional surgery, cardiac arrest, and death). The authors also used the following classification system to characterize fall circumstances: surgery-related falls (eg, falls because of sudden muscle weakness or indisposition and any fall during normal daily activities such as walking, going to the bathroom), falls related to more substantial physical activity (eg, ladder climbing, strenuous exercise, bicycling), and falls related to extrinsic factors (eg, slippery surfaces, being pushed by a closing door, alcohol intoxication).

Not surprisingly, patients who fell were more likely to be older, living alone, and using walking aids. Falls occurred most frequently during the first postoperative month (51.8%). Approximately half of falls (50.6%) were associated with major injuries, regardless of the circumstances leading to the falls.

Moderate injuries were associated with 9.6% of falls and minor injuries occurred in 21.7% of falls.

In summary, the state of the evidence related to fall risk, prevention, and mechanism for persons with TKA can be characterized as weak. The bulk of the evidence is retrospective in nature and vulnerable to biases and gaps related to chart review and routine medical chart reporting. With this said, this evidence can help to inform clinicians regarding risks for falls and strategies to reduce their incidence and consequences. Generally, a multipronged inpatient approach is better than a single strategy; the more individuals are made aware of fall risks, particularly in the hospital, and the more reminders of safe activity, particularly in patient rooms, the better. Evidence for fall risk reduction prior to or after TKA hospitalization is clearly lacking. Falls are relatively common prior to surgery and likely less common following hospitalization but still prevalent. The study by Jorgensen et al.[22] clearly characterized the consequences of these falls and although hospital or emergency room (ER) care is needed only rarely after TJA (ie, only 1.6% of cases), the consequences of these falls result in major injury most of the time. Reducing the rare but substantial adverse events should be a target of preventive care and research.

MUSCULOSKELETAL COMORBIDITY AND TOTAL KNEE ARTHROPLASTY OUTCOMES

This section focuses specifically on evidence that has explored the influence of musculoskeletal comorbidities on outcomes following TKA. This issue is important because if there are important comorbidities of the musculoskeletal system that are easily quantified during a preoperative evaluation, the patient's prognosis can be more clearly estimated and patient expectations can be adjusted depending on whether musculoskeletal comorbidities are present. Second, if musculoskeletal comorbidities are modifiable, they can theoretically be addressed preoperatively to reduce postoperative risk.

The presence of additional musculoskeletal comorbidity (beyond the affected knee) among persons seeking TKA is well known.[5] For example, among 1606 persons with unilateral or bilateral knee pain in the Osteoarthritis Initiative study,[25] more than 80% reported back or neck pain and up to 75% reported pain in other lower and upper extremity joints.[39] For patients undergoing total knee replacement (TKR) or total hip replacement (THR), approximately 50% had an additional joint replacement on another hip or knee 10 or more years following the original arthroplasty.[43] In addition, up to 50% of patients with knee OA and scheduled for primary TKA[36] or TKA revision surgery[34] report back or neck pain prior to surgery. Although there is substantial variation in these estimates across studies, these data indicate that musculoskeletal comorbidity in persons with TKA is very common and if these comorbidities influence outcome, they should be considered when discussing surgery and expected outcome with the patient.

Research on the impact of musculoskeletal comorbidity has taken the approach of examining the effect of pain in a single site (eg, the presence of low back pain) or counting the number of sites in which pain was reported (ie, a count of painful joints) and determining the effects on outcome. Ultimately, any study that examines prognostic effects of musculoskeletal comorbidity on outcome should consider all other important potential comorbidities as well to reduce the risk of confounding. Estimates of the magnitude of effects attributable to a specific prognostic factor (eg, presence of back pain) will likely be biased if other potentially important prognostic indicators are not also included in the statistical modeling procedures. For example, if a hypothetical study examines the effects of low back pain on 1-year TKA pain outcome, but the study does not account for baseline knee pain severity, estimates of the effects of low back pain will be biased because an important confounder, baseline knee pain, was not accounted for in the statistical modeling.

Another important issue to consider when reading studies of the prognostic effects of musculoskeletal comorbidity on outcomes following TKA is to consider the definitions of the comorbidities, how the comorbidities were measured, and whether chronicity of the comorbidity was taken into account. A substantial literature clearly indicates that chronic low back pain, for example, has a much greater prognostic impact than acute low back pain.[11,13] One limitation of the TKA prognostic literature is the lack of granularity in defining musculoskeletal comorbidities of interest. Typically, little detail is provided in these papers for how each comorbidity is defined, whether chronicity is considered, and whether pain severity in the joint of interest is accounted for when assessing the prognostic significance of the comorbidity.

BACK PAIN COMORBIDITY AND ASSOCIATIONS WITH OUTCOME

Clement et al. examined the prognostic effects of back pain on self-reported pain, function, and surgical satisfaction from a sample of 829 patients with TKA, 35% of whom reported back pain prior to surgery.[10] After adjusting for multiple potential confounders including comorbidity, preoperative outcome score, mental health, and gender, the authors found the presence of back pain was associated with a 2.4 point worsening in Oxford knee scores, 1 year following TKA. In addition, patients with back pain were one-third less likely to be satisfied with their TKA as compared to persons without back pain. Similar limitations apply as discussed earlier because the authors did not ask patients about the intensity or duration of the back pain. With this said, simply asking patients if they have back pain still provides useful prognostic information. Similar findings were reported by Boyle et al. for persons reporting low back pain.[6]

Chang et al. provided somewhat greater fidelity in defining low back pain symptoms in their study of 225 persons undergoing primary TKA, of which 51% reported at least one moderate or severe lumbar spine symptom.[9] The best predictor of poor outcome up to 2 years following TKA was the presence of more severe lumbar spine symptoms and severe radiating pain during activity.

Novicoff et al. assessed the prognostic effect of back pain on 6-month to 24-month self-reported pain and function outcome following TKA revision surgery conducted on 308 patients.[34] Whereas baseline pain and function scores were worse for persons with back pain versus those with no back pain, the follow-up data indicated a worse outcome for patients with back pain over all time periods except at 24 months. A weakness of the study is that back pain was not defined and the intensity or duration of the back pain reported by the patients was not reported. In spite of the somewhat blunt approach to measuring back pain, there was an important effect on outcome. A second limitation is the lack of adjustment for other variables (eg, psychological distress, other comorbidity) known to influence outcome beyond the baseline outcome score.

PAINFUL JOINT COUNTS AND ASSOCIATIONS WITH OUTCOME

One of the better papers on this topic is a paper by Perruccio et al. that examined the effects of multiple joint involvement on TKA outcomes. The authors followed 494 persons with TKA over a period of 1 year and found that as additional joints are affected by painful OA, a greater prognostic effect on 1-year postoperative pain and function occurred. To identify the number of painful OA joints, patients were instructed to complete a body diagram and mark all joints that were painful and affected by arthritis. Pain intensity or duration was not determined. A total of 45% of the sample reported four or more joints, not including the surgical joint. A total of 10% identified three joints, 12.8% identified two joints, and 16.6% identified one additional painful OA joint. The contralateral knee was the most common painful OA joint (57.1% of the time). Data suggested that pain in multiple joints, particularly in the lower extremity, led to worse pain and function outcomes after adjusting for common potential confounders and baseline outcome scores. Peter et al.[37] conducted a cross-sectional study of 521 persons between 7 and 21 months following hip ($n = 281$) or knee ($n = 240$) arthroplasty and found that approximately 20% of TKA patients reported severe back pain, 21% reported severe neck or shoulder pain, and 18% reported severe elbow, wrist, or hand pain. In the TKA group, the variables associated with a worse Knee Injury and Osteoarthritis Outcome Score (KOOS)[41] were elbow, wrist, and hand pain, a history of falling, and vision impairments. Surprisingly, severe neck or shoulder pain and severe low back pain did not affect KOOS outcome scores. However, this is a cross-sectional study that, at best, provides prevalence estimates for several musculoskeletal disorders in patients following TKA. Prognostically important predictors can only be derived from longitudinal studies like the one conducted by Perruccio et al.

In a systematic review and meta-analysis published in 2015, Lewis et al. identified predictors of persistent pain following TKA.[27] A total of 32 papers with a total of approximately 30,000 patients were included in the analyses. These studies defined the significant predictors of persistent pain in several ways depending on the pain scale used in the selected studies. Most commonly this was the Western Ontario and McMaster (WOMAC) Universities Osteoarthritis Index pain scale or a visual analogue pain scale. Each study defined persistent pain differently, but the persistent pain had to be present at least 3 months following surgery. A lack of standardization of outcome measures is a well-known limitation of this literature and use of various measures and cut-points to quantify persistent pain is a limitation of this paper and the TKA literature, generally.[40] The number of pain sites beyond the surgical knee was significant in univariate analyses, but when combined with other variables in a multivariate analysis, the "other pain sites" variable dropped out and the key predictors of persistent pain were pain catastrophizing, extent of comorbidities, poor mental health, and preoperative severity of pain in the surgical knee. Surgeons should be aware of these predictors because, in combination, they contribute in an additive way to a poor outcome. For example, patients who report very severe knee pain at baseline, and who are pain catastrophizers with multiple other comorbidities and

poor mental health are most likely to continue to report persistent pain following TKA.

In summary, there is evidence to suggest that musculoskeletal comorbidity is prognostic of poor outcome, but when considering psychological distress variables and preoperative knee pain intensity, musculoskeletal comorbidity becomes less important.

INFLAMMATORY ARTHRITIS VERSUS OSTEOARTHRITIS AND OUTCOME

Hawker et al. examined the effects of various preoperative variables, including the presence of inflammatory arthritis, on outcome as measured with the WOMAC Pain and Function subscales.[17] A good outcome indicating treatment success was defined using various approaches related to the minimally important difference.[1-3] Persons who had inflammatory arthritis were approximately one third as likely to have a good outcome as persons with knee OA, although only 14 persons with inflammatory arthritis were included in the sample of 202 persons. A strength of this study is the use of a large number of predictor variables including most importantly, the preoperative score for each outcome measure. Although persons with inflammatory arthritis do not appear to be at increased risk for mortality or perioperative adverse events (with the exception of infection[38]) as compared to patients with OA, there is additional evidence to suggest that pain and function self-reported outcomes are worse.[23,45] In summary, one can expect improved pain and function following TKA for persons with inflammatory arthritis, but the literature indicates that pain and functional improvement are not as substantial for persons with inflammatory arthritis compared to persons with OA. In addition, patients with rheumatoid arthritis (RA) are at greater risk for joint infection.

SUMMARY

Although relatively substantial with at least 11 trials, evidence related to prehabilitation is weak and inconclusive. Most of these trials are pilot studies and are underpowered. Evidence on fall risk is more substantial than prehabilitation evidence, but there are still limitations. Fall risk evidence provides guidance on prognostic factors associated with increased fall risk in the hospital and following hospitalization. Musculoskeletal comorbidity is an important factor to consider when evaluating potential candidates for TKA. However, after accounting for preoperative knee pain intensity and psychological distress, musculoskeletal disorders of the nonindex knee become less prognostically important.

KEY REFERENCES

7.   Brown K, Loprinzi PD, Brosky JA, et al: Prehabilitation influences exercise-related psychological constructs such as self-efficacy and outcome expectations to exercise. *J Strength Cond Res* 28(1):201–209, 2014.

10. Clement ND, MacDonald D, Simpson AH, et al: Total knee replacement in patients with concomitant back pain results in a worse functional outcome and a lower rate of satisfaction. *Bone Joint J* 95-B(12):1632–1639, 2013.

12. Cui Q, Schapiro LH, Kinney MC, et al: Reducing costly falls of total knee replacement patients. *Am J Med Qual* 28(4):335–338, 2013.

14. Desmeules F, Hall J, Woodhouse LJ: Prehabilitation improves physical function of individuals with severe disability from hip or knee osteoarthritis. *Physiother Can* 65(2):116–124, 2013.

17. Hawker GA, Badley EM, Borkhoff CM, et al: Which patients are most likely to benefit from total joint arthroplasty? *Arthritis Rheum* 65(5):1243–1252, 2013.

24. Kwok IH, Paton B, Haddad FS: Does pre-operative physiotherapy improve outcomes in primary total knee arthroplasty? A systematic review. *J Arthroplasty* 30:1657–1663, 2015.

30. Matsumoto H, Okuno M, Nakamura T, et al: Fall incidence and risk factors in patients after total knee arthroplasty. *Arch Orthop Trauma Surg* 132(4):555–563, 2012.

36. Perruccio AV, Power JD, Evans HM, et al: Multiple joint involvement in total knee replacement for osteoarthritis: effects on patient-reported outcomes. *Arthritis Care Res (Hoboken)* 64(6):838–846, 2012.

The references for this chapter can also be found on www.expertconsult.com.

183

Intra-articular and Periarticular Injections

Nima Eftekhary, Jonathan M. Vigdorchik

BACKGROUND

Forty-six million people in the United States (almost 22% of the adult population) are affected by knee arthritis.[14] Osteoarthritis (OA), the most common form of knee arthritis, can affect greater than 10% of the population worldwide. The disease progresses slowly, and in its late stages can cause debilitating pain and disability. It is among the top 10 causes of disability worldwide.[45] The treatment of osteoarthritis is a global issue with significant impact upon productivity and economic implications.

In addition, rheumatoid arthritis (RA) and juvenile rheumatoid arthritis (JRA, also known as juvenile idiopathic arthritis [JIA] or Still disease) are common and affect millions more.[14] The mainstay of treatment is with disease-modifying antirheumatic drugs (DMARDs). However, conservative management of RA of the knee overlaps greatly with treatment of knee OA.

Nonpharmacologic treatments include weight loss, activity modification, patient education, physical and occupational therapy exercises, topically applied creams, and braces and ambulation assist devices.[62] Oral pharmacologic therapies are broad and include acetaminophen, nonselective cyclooxygenase (COX) inhibitors, selective COX-2 inhibitors, glucosamine, and chondroitin sulfate. Once nonpharmacologic and oral medications have been exhausted, intra-articular injections are the last nonoperative treatment modality in the physician's armamentarium.[45]

Intra-articular injections are a mainstay of treatment of OA and RA variants that affect the knee. Thus, the treatment of knee arthritis with intra-articular injection is relevant and commonplace in many different medical specialties.[14]

Broadly, the pharmacologic composition of intra-articular injection into the knee can be grouped into four main categories: corticosteroids, hyaluronic acid, platelet-rich plasma, and stem cells.[12] The techniques for intra-articular administration of these injections, along with further detail on the background, mechanism of action, and use of each type of injection are described in this chapter.

TECHNIQUES

Intra-articular knee injections are commonplace and relatively simple procedures. In the hands of an experienced physician, they can accurately, effectively, and safely be performed in the office. Once the intra-articular agent of choice is selected, the physician can prepare for injection. The authors recommend diligent attention to anatomic structures, patient positioning, and obtaining necessary materials prior to injection. This ensures a successful injection and a more pleasant experience for the physician and patient.

For intra-articular injections in the knee, the authors recommend the no-touch technique. Key points include utmost attention to sterility, outlining anatomic structures, positioning, and preparation. The approach portals to the knee are varied and have been studied for their accuracy in intra-articular placement, with slight differences based on the knee pathology being addressed. These methods are accurate overall, but can be augmented with ultrasound to confirm intra-articular placement.

As with any procedure, the no-touch technique for knee injection begins with confirmation of the patient, injection site, and procedure side, along with obtaining informed consent. The physician should obtain supplies, which include one 5-mL or 10-mL syringe, one 1.5-inch 18-gauge needle, one 1.5-inch 22-gauge needle, the solution to be injected, sterile and nonsterile gloves, antiseptic solution (betadine or chlorhexidine swabs), gauze, an adhesive bandage, and a marking pen (optional).

The physician first puts on the nonsterile gloves and draws up the solution to be injected in the presence of the patient using an 18-gauge needle and syringe. The needle is switched to the 22-gauge needle for injection. The patient is positioned at a comfortable height for the examiner, supine or seated based on the approach portal used. Anatomic structures are palpated and can be marked out if desired. The approach portal of choice is marked with a marking pen or with the cap of the needle, pressing gently with the blunt cap to make an indentation at the approach portal site. The knee is cleaned with the antiseptic solution of choice and the physician switches to sterile gloves, ensuring that sterility of one hand is maintained. The injection is administered at the previously marked approach portal, taking care not to touch the disinfected area. Although this is a no-touch technique, maintaining sterility of one hand allows the physician to again palpate anatomic structures if difficulty is encountered when attempting to access the knee joint. The physician pulls back on the syringe to determine if synovial fluid is present and that a blood vessel has not been entered, and injects the solution into the knee. There should be minimal resistance. The needle is withdrawn from the knee, with all sharps placed into an appropriately marked sharps container. An adhesive bandage is applied. The patient should be counseled on after-procedure care and signs of complications.[15,22]

Multiple approach portals have been described, with various documented success rates and indications. These portals include the lateral and medial midpatellar, superolateral, superomedial, anterolateral, and anteromedial (Fig. 183.1).[35]

The lateral or medial midpatellar approaches have a success rate documented between 55% and 93%.[2,35,44] The approach may be uncomfortable or painful for the patient, and accuracy has been described as being proportional to the amount of knee arthritis. This technique accesses the patellofemoral joint. The physician pulls the patella medially or laterally and a needle is advanced under the patella. In the lateral midpatellar approach, the needle is directed at a 45-degree angle toward the medial aspect of the joint. In the medial midpatellar approach, the needle enters under the midpole of the patella and directed toward the lateral midpole.[35]

The superolateral approach has a documented accuracy of 91%, but this approach may be painful if the needle collides with the superior pole of the patella.[52] The superomedial approach has a 93% documented accuracy rate, but can damage the chondral cartilage of the patella. These approaches are particularly useful if there is a large effusion in the suprapatellar bursa. This approach is performed with the patient in the supine position with the knee in extension, and aims for the

suprapatellar pouch, with the needle passing underneath the patella.[35]

The anterolateral approach has a 71% to 85% accuracy rate, and is particularly useful when the knee cannot be fully extended. The anteromedial approach has between 55% and 75% accuracy and causes little pain or discomfort, but may be difficult for aspirating a knee effusion.[2,35,44] These are the same portals used in arthroscopy. With the knee flexed, the needle is inserted medial or lateral to the patella tendon, directed toward the femoral notch. These methods cross only the Hoffa fat pad to enter the joint, and avoid the extensor mechanism and blood vessels.[22,35]

STEROIDS

Background

Evidence supports the use of intra-articular steroid injections for knee arthritis in the conditions listed previously. The primary benefit is improvement in pain, with secondary improvement in functionality, lasting for months up to 1 year.[14] One systematic review of Level 1 studies noted a 22% greater reduction in pain within the first week after injection than placebo, with a statistically significant decrease in visual analog scale (VAS) pain scores by an average of 35 points. Currently, only a handful of corticosteroids have been approved by the U.S. Food and Drug Administration (FDA) for intra-articular injection into the knee.[45] These are dexamethasone, methylprednisolone (acetate), triamcinolone (acetate and hexacetonide), and betamethasone (acetate and sodium phosphate).[45] Although the anti-inflammatory potency of various corticosteroids has been published elsewhere, in general, intra-articular corticosteroid formulations tend to have similar potency when indications, dosing, timing, and administration are similar.[46] However, one review article suggested that triamcinolone hexacetonide offers superior efficacy over triamcinolone acetate, particularly in treatment of JRA (grade 2B evidence), and should be the intra-articular corticosteroid of choice (Table 183.1).[14]

Mechanism of Action

Corticosteroids act upon the painful knee through their anti-inflammatory and immunosuppressive properties. They directly act upon nuclear steroid factors to alter transcription and suppress the inflammatory response at multiple levels in the inflammatory cascade. Downstream, this modulation leads to decreased accumulation of inflammatory cells and inhibition of production of neutrophil superoxide and metalloproteinase. In addition, pro-inflammatory mediators such as leukotrienes and prostaglandins are inhibited.[8] The clinical response to these

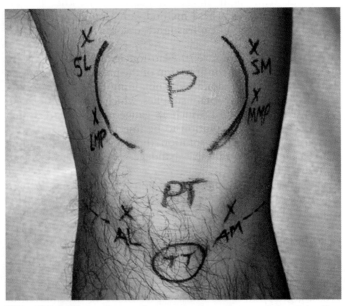

FIG 183.1 Right knee demonstrating the various injection portals and surface anatomy. *AL*, Anterolateral; *AM*, anteromedial; *LMP*, lateral midpatellar; *MMP*, medial midpatellar; *P*, patella; *PT*, patella tendon; *SL*, superolateral; *SM*, superomedial; *TT*, tibial tubercle; *dotted lines*, tibial plateau.

TABLE 183.1 Generic Names, Solubilities, and Joint Doses of Various Intra-articular Corticosteroids[6]

Generic Name	Solubility	Effect Onset	Large-Joint Dose (mg)	Small-Joint Dose (mg)
Triamcinolone acetonide	Somewhat insoluble	Variable	5-40	2.5-5
Triamcinolone hexacetonide	Somewhat insoluble	Variable	10-40	2-6
Methylprednisolone acetate	Slightly soluble	Very slow	20-80	4-10
Triamcinolone diacetate	Slightly soluble	Variable	20-40	2-5
Dexamethasone sodium phosphate	Soluble	Rapid	2-4	0.8-1
Betamethasone sodium phosphate and betamethasone acetate	Mixed	Rapid	6-12	1.5-3

changes manifests as decreased erythema, swelling, warmth, and pain.

Use

Steroid injections are the most common intra-articular knee injections used to treat acute and chronic inflammatory conditions.[57] In particular, in OA, its short-term benefit and effectiveness in addressing pain has been demonstrated across multiple studies, notably a 2005 Cochrane review that showed a significant improvement in pain, albeit short-lived (up to 4 weeks).[34] However, this review failed to find any significant evidence for efficacy in improvement of functionality, with no significant evidence for improvement in stiffness, walking distance, or quality of life. The American College of Rheumatology subcommittee on OA recommends intra-articular corticosteroids as an effective means of decreasing pain.[18] A recent review article on evidence-based intra-articular knee injections found evidence in support of intra-articular corticosteroid injections for the knee in RA (evidence level 1A), OA (evidence level 1A), and JRA (evidence level 2C).[14] However, the American Academy of Orthopedic Surgeons deemed the evidence inconclusive for intra-articular steroid injection and was unable to recommend for or against its use in symptomatic knee osteoarthritis.[51]

There may be patient-specific factors that portend a better outcome and improved response to intra-articular corticosteroid injection into the knee. Multiple studies have examined these factors. One study in particular concluded that joint effusion and successful aspiration of synovial fluid at time of injection were factors that may predict improved response to corticosteroid injection.[59] Another study suggested that the presence of effusion and decreased radiographic severity of degenerative changes predicted a better outcome.[31] Effusion may suggest an underlying inflammatory process, which could explain the improved response to corticosteroids. In addition, the ability to aspirate synovial fluid prior to injection confirms the intra-articular location of the injection. However, a recent systematic review found no consistent predictor of response to this treatment.[21] Further research is warranted.

Of particular interest to the orthopedic surgeon is the effect of prior intra-articular corticosteroid injection on rates of prosthetic joint infection following total knee arthroplasty (TKA). Many recent studies have addressed this concern. One systematic review concluded that there was a significant increase in infection within 3 months (odds ratio of 2) and 6 months (odds ratio of 1.5) of TKA if intra-articular corticosteroid had been administered less than 90 days prior to TKA.[55] There was no significant increase in infection risk if intra-articular corticosteroid was administered more than 3 months prior to TKA. Other studies have concluded that intra-articular steroid injection prior to TKA has no effect on infection rates, regardless of timing.[16,58] Further research is clearly warranted.

Intra-articular corticosteroid injection has rare side effects, with infrequent reactive flares lasting 6 to 12 hours. Local irritation and postinjection pain are other side effects.[45] One study noted no loss in knee joint space following multiple intra-articular steroid injections for OA, and no increase in loss of cartilage or bone after an intra-articular knee injection for RA.[20] The rate of septic arthritis is extremely low and has been cited at about 1 in 10,000. Other rare complications include cutaneous depigmentation, avascular necrosis, synovitis, and tendinopathy.[14,20]

HYALURONIC ACID

Background

Hyaluronic acid (HA) is a polysaccharide containing glucosamine and glucuronic acid, and is a major component in synovial fluid. HA also helps form a 1- to 2-micron layer on the surface of articular cartilage.[14] It was first used in cataract surgery in the 1970s. Its use abroad was approved in countries such as Japan, Canada, and Italy as early as 1987.[54] It was approved for intra-articular use in the United States in 1997.[12] Commercially available hyaluronic acid products approved by the FDA include sodium hyaluronate, Hylan G-F 20, and high–molecular weight hyaluronan, and can be divided into low–molecular weight (Orthovisc, Hyalgan) and high-molecular-weight (Synvisc) formulations (Table 183.2).

Mechanism of Action

HA is a natural component of synovial fluid. As a glycosaminoglycan, it contributes to elasticity and viscosity of synovial fluid.[47] Synovial cells, fibroblasts, and chondrocytes produce HA and secrete it into synovial fluid. Synovial fluid has viscoelastic properties. During slow joint movement, it acts as a viscous lubricant, and during rapid joint movement, it has elastic shock-absorbing properties.[45] These characteristics are altered in the synovial fluid of an osteoarthritic knee, which is less viscous and less concentrated than in healthy counterparts.[27] Multiple mechanisms have been proposed for the potential benefit of HA in intra-articular knee injection. In addition to restoring the viscoelastic properties of synovial fluid, viscosupplementation can potentially lead to decreased degradation of cartilage, inhibition of inflammatory mediators, and synthesis of a cartilaginous matrix. In addition, it may insulate pain

TABLE 183.2 Trade Names, Molecular Weights, and Sources of Various Hyaluronic Acid Products[48]			
Trade Name	**Molecular Weight (kDa)**	**Source**	**Mg/ml**
Hyalgan	500-730	HA extracted from rooster combs	20 mg/2 mL
Hyalubrix	1500	Fermentative HA	30 mg/2 mL
Artz (Supartz)	800-1170	HA extracted from rooster combs	25 mg/2.5 mL
Synovial (Jointex)	800-1200	Fermentative HA	16 mg/mL
Synvisc	6000	HA extracted from rooster combs	16 mg/2 mL
Durolane	9000	Synthetic HA	20 mg/3 mL
Euflexxa	2.400-3.600	Fermentative HA	20 mg/2 mL

HA, Hyaluronic acid.

fibers in the synovium and simultaneously increase natural synthesis of HA.[12]

Use

Injection schedules vary between one and five injections, and patients with a positive response are generally encouraged to repeat treatment within 6 months.[45] A series of randomized clinical trials have investigated the effect of HA injections in populations with OA. In a review of 13 randomized control trials that were mostly double-blind in design, most showed significant improvement in pain scores at varying postintervention intervals, but more consistent results were found from high-molecular-weight studies, with efficacy of the high–molecular weight formulation favored in multiple studies.[12,45] In a series of meta-analyses, two reported an overall beneficial effect, four reported a small benefit, and two reported no benefit to hyaluronic injection.* Injection regimens included five total injections of low– or high–molecular weight HA, with follow-up between 6 and 52 weeks. Outcomes included pain as measured on the VAS as a primary measure, and others also included function.

There are varied reports of efficacy and pain improvement in the literature. The National Health Service in Wales and England (NHS) perhaps best summarized the myriad of literature published on the topic. They conclude that although the evidence does suggest a benefit of intra-articular HA, the treatment is not a cost-effective option.[36,45] The American College of Rheumatology has no recommendations on hyaluronic acid injected intra-articularly, and the American Academy of Orthopedic Surgeons' consensus is that the evidence is strong against the use of HA in OA, with a high quality of evidence.[18,51] A double-blind randomized controlled trial (RCT) on HA in osteoarthritic knees noted that less than 50% of knees achieved satisfactory improvement in pain, with only 35% reporting increased functionality. Almost 30% went on to surgery within 7 months of injection. Patients with bone loss or complete collapse of joint space responded poorly to intra-articular HA. The authors concluded by recommending HA only for patients with significant risk factors precluding surgery, or those with mild radiographic disease that had failed conservative management.[50]

Side effects are generally minor and self-limited and include local irritation at the injection site (most common) and back pain.[12] Contraindications to HA injection reflect the contraindications to any injection and include overlying soft tissue infection or skin disease over the portal site. In addition, those with allergies to eggs or chicken should not receive injection with poultry derivatives.

PLATELET-RICH PLASMA

Background

Platelet-rich plasma (PRP) is obtained from autologous blood that is centrifuged down to obtain a dense concentrate of platelets. The concentration of platelets is 4 to 8 times the platelet levels found in whole blood.[10] In addition, the plasma layer, the acellular portion of the mixture, is isolated. Platelets undergo degranulation and release growth factors, notably platelet-derived growth factor (PDGF). The isolated plasma contains cytokines, thrombin, and other growth factors.

There are multiple preparations of PRP obtained by different methods of centrifugation. Three methods have been described. The double-spinning method yields a platelet concentration 4 to 8 times that found in whole blood and the resulting PRP also contains leukocytes. The single-spinning method increases platelet levels to 1 to 3 times that in whole blood. Selective blood filtration has also been described. These preparations are classified by their leukocyte and fibrin content: pure PRP, leukocyte-rich PRP, pure platelet-rich fibrin, and leukocyte- and platelet-rich fibrin.[3] Although some data suggests that leukocyte-depleted formulations may be more effective, the benefit of one formulation over another has not yet been proven.[5,45]

Mechanism of Action

The platelet-rich concentrate is prepared with calcium chloride, which activates the platelets. Activated platelets release various growth factors and biologically active molecules. The growth factors released include insulin-like growth factor (IGF), PDGF, and transforming growth factor beta 1 (TGFB-1). Activated platelets also release cytokines, chemokines, arachidonic acid metabolites, and nucleotides.[56] These factors are delivered to the injured area of interest.

The proposed benefits of these growth and biologically active factors include chondrogenesis, anti-inflammatory properties, cell differentiation, angiogenesis and proliferation, and remodeling of bone.[7,23] Experimental animal models on the effect of platelet-rich plasma on OA have suggested decreased chondrocyte cell death, greater proteoglycans in articular cartilage, and a decreased rate of OA progression.[4,29,28,45]

Use

PRP allows delivery of a plethora of known biological factors in a minimally invasive and simple way. However, the exact mechanism of the effect of PRP in OA in humans is still unknown.[5] Platelets contain over 300 growth factors and active factors, and it is unclear which of these are most important to the proposed healing mechanisms.[5] In delivering these factors to the knee, autologous blood is first collected from the patient. A platelet-rich formulation can be obtained via centrifugation or filtration as described earlier, activated with calcium chloride, and injected into the knee.

Multiple studies have evaluated the effect of PRP in intra-articular knee injections to address cartilage injuries or OA. Information on the first described PRP injection, an intra-articular knee injection to address an articular cartilage avulsion injury, was published in 2003.[42] Next, a series of studies on PRP in osteoarthritic knees noted a significant improvement in most patients at a series of time points, from 6 months to 1 year. A follow-up to one of these studies with 2 years of data showed that although there was an overall worsening of results from the earlier time points, that patients were still reporting an improved quality of life. The study concluded that PRP was best indicated for younger patients with mild OA, and that the median duration of action of the injection was 9 months.[6,11,60,61] Newer studies have confirmed many of these findings.†

The American Academy of Orthopedic Surgeons has interpreted the evidence as inconclusive regarding the effect of PRP in intra-articular injection, and was unable to recommend for or against the use of PRP in intra-articular knee injection in

---

*References 1, 25, 26, 34, 38, and 45.

†References 13, 24, 37, 41, 53, and 63.

patients with symptomatic OA of the knee.[51] Complications are minor and self-limited, with moderate pain, swelling, or effusion being the most common.[‡]

COMPARISONS

Comparisons between viscosupplementation (HA) and intra-articular steroid injection suggest that HA may have a longer period of benefit, with similar improvement in pain, although onset is slower and there is greater risk of local soft tissue adverse reactions. Both injections have a significant placebo effect.[60,61] In a Cochrane review comparing HA with steroids in knee injections for OA, there was no significant difference at the 4-week time point, however HA was shown to be more effective at 5 to 13 weeks after the index injection.[34]

PRP and HA have been similarly studied on a head-to-head basis. In one recent study, PRP had an increased benefit in pain reduction and function up to 6 months, particularly for younger patients with cartilage lesions or early OA. Benefit was similar in older patients (>50 years) with more advanced OA.[60,61] Another recent study noted improvements in pain and functionality with PRP superior to HA at 3- and 6-month time points.[39] Finally, in two recent Level 1 randomized clinical trials with HA controls, PRP decreased pain and improved function better than HA.[32,63]

A NOTE ON STEM CELLS, CYTOKINES, AND GROWTH HORMONE

Mesenchymal stem cells (MSCs) are of particular novel interest in the treatment of chronic knee pathology. MSCs have the potential to differentiate into various lineages, are minimally immunogenic, and can have immunosuppressive activity.[48] In addition, they are relatively easy to grow in culture. They are found in all human tissue, and have the capacity to differentiate into bone and cartilage precursors. MSCs are isolated from adipose tissue, muscle, or bone marrow aspirate and are being actively investigated as an autologous injectable treatment for chronic degenerative conditions of the knee. MSCs can be selected from bone marrow, adipose, or muscle, and cultured in the laboratory prior to injection into the knee. In addition, bone marrow aspirate can be directly injected (without first culturing) into the knee.[30,48]

A recent review investigated the impact of intra-articular knee injection of MSCs for OA in pain and function. Seven randomized clinical trials were included. The review found that the application of MSCs had no significant impact on pain. However, when low-quality studies were excluded, MSCs resulted in a significant decrease in pain. In addition, the review noted that MSCs led to a significant improvement in function compared to the control groups at all time points from 3 months to 2 years.[48]

In addition to MSCs, there are a group of biologically active proteins called growth factors that are released by cells in the body for various anabolic functions, including cellular division, growth, and differentiation.[40] Many of these growth factors work together in the development and regulation of articular cartilage throughout life, thus offering a promising outlook in the regeneration of cartilage.[40,43] As these growth factors have a wide variety of implications within the joint, the effects on cartilage, synovium, ligaments, menisci, subchondral bone, and MSCs all need to be considered. The ideal growth factor in restoring damaged articular cartilage would be pro-anabolic and anti-catabolic in restoring cartilage, would have no negative effects on the surrounding structures within the knee, and would demonstrate benefit regardless of patient's age or presence of osteoarthritis.[40]

TGFB-1 is one growth factor that stimulates cartilage synthesis and decreases catabolic activity of interleukin-1 (IL-1).[33] In vitro, it has been shown to stimulate chondrogenesis of MSCs.[9] However, certain animal studies have demonstrated negative effects of TGFB-1 supplementation, including synovial proliferation, fibrosis, and osteophyte formation.[19,33,40]

Insulin-like growth factor 1 (IGF-1) is a growth factor that reaches articular cartilage through synovial fluid, and plays an important role in homeostasis of cartilage by balancing synthesis and breakdown of proteoglycans. In fact, it is the main anabolic growth factor in articular cartilage.[40] Multiple studies have suggested that a decrease in available IGF-1 in addition to a decreased intra-articular response to IGF-1 can lead to cartilage with impaired structural and functional integrity.[40] The therapeutic benefit of IGF-1 has yet to be conclusively demonstrated.

PDGF is synthesized by a variety of mesenchymal cells and macrophages and stored in platelets. It is paramount in the wound healing cascade, leading to differentiation and chemotaxis in a variety of mesenchymal cells (fibroblasts, osteoblasts, and chondrocytes). Thus, it may play a significant role in tissue regeneration and repair. This particular repair mechanism is of importance in microfracture surgery, in which microperforations into the subchondral bone stimulate a release of growth factors, including PDGF, which provide a favorable microenvironment for wound healing and tissue formation.[40]

Finally, growth hormone is a centrally produced regulator of long bone growth and bone mineral density. In addition, it stimulates cartilage production, likely through involvement in IGF-1 production and direct stimulation of chondrocyte proliferation.[40] Certain animal studies have demonstrated that intra-articular growth hormone may enhance proliferation, synthesis of matrix, and differentiation of bone and cartilage cells.[17,49] However, few studies have investigated the use of intra-articular growth hormone in humans.

Although stem cells may have exciting potential, particularly in their ability to differentiate into precursors of bone and cartilage, further trials are needed. In addition, although growth factors are clearly paramount in the regulation and development of articular cartilage, potential therapy targeting these factors must consider the harmony required between these factors to achieve their intended goals. There is a shortage of adequately powered double-blinded randomized control trials on MSCs, cytokines, and intra-articular growth hormone with long-term follow up. Future studies will preferably include not only a placebo as control, but corticosteroid, hyaluronic acid, and platelet-rich plasma injections as well. Further research is warranted.

AUTHOR REMARKS

The literature on intra-articular injection for knee arthritis is expansive and includes thousands of studies. The potential

[‡]References 6, 11, 13, 41, 60, and 61.

benefit of steroid injections, HA, platelet-rich plasma, and stem cells is great, although physicians cannot reliably predict the magnitude and duration of the response to these agents. In addition, the side effect and risk profiles of each should be considered, along with the cost of each therapeutic agent.

No blanket statement can advise for or against the use of these agents in knee arthritis. Each patient's disease process, severity, and predicted response should be assessed on a case-by-case basis. In general, evidence indicates that patients with mild radiographic knee arthritis who have failed conservative measures (weight loss, physical therapy, oral medications) will be the best responders to intra-articular knee injections.

Because of underlying inflammatory pathology, patients with variants of RA will likely benefit from intra-articular steroid injection, and this is echoed in various literature reports including guidelines from the American College of Rheumatology.

The evidence for or against HA is mixed, and critics have pointed to the high cost-benefit profile of this treatment modality. However, multiple studies have demonstrated comparable results to intra-articular steroid injection in the appropriately selected patient.

Finally, platelet-rich plasma, stem cells, and growth factors are relatively novel therapies with potential for promising results. The physician trusted with the care of the patient with knee arthritis should expect to be well-versed in these potential treatment modalities in the years to come.

KEY REFERENCES

6. Baker K, O'Rourke KS, Deodhar A: Joint aspiration and injection: a look at the basics Rheumatol Network <http://www.rheumatologynetwork.com/articles/joint-aspiration-and-injection-look-basics>, June 7, 2011.

8. Bellamy N, Campbell J, Robinson V, et al: Intraarticular corticosteroid for treatment of osteoarthritis of the knee. *Cochrane Database Syst Rev* (2):CD005328, 2005.

9. Cancienne JM, Werner BC, Luetkemeyer LM, et al: Does timing of previous intra-articular steroid injection affect the post-operative rate of

12. infection in total knee arthroplasty? *J Arthroplasty* 30(11):1879–1882, 2015.

12. Cheng OT, Souzdalnitski D, Vrooman B, et al: Evidence-based knee injections for the management of arthritis. *Pain Med* 13:740–753, 2012.

13. Conaghan PG, Dickson J, Grant RL: Guideline Development Group, Care and management of osteoarthritis in adults: summary of NICE guidance. *BMJ* 336(7642):502–503, 2008.

16. Douglas RJ: Aspiration and injection of the knee joint: approach portal. *Knee Surg Relat Res* 26:1–6, 2014.

30. Halpern B, Chaudhury S, Rodeo SA, et al: Clinical and MRI outcomes after platelet-rich plasma treatment for knee osteoarthritis. *Clin J Sports Med* 23:238–239, 2013.

31. Hepper CT, Halvorson JJ, Duncan ST, et al: The efficacy and duration of intra-articular corticosteroid injection for knee osteoarthritis: a systematic review of level I studies. *J Am Acad Orthop Surg* 17:638–646, 2009.

33. Hochberg MC, Altman RD, April KT, et al: American College of Rheumatology 2012 recommendations for the use of nonpharmacologic and pharmacologic therapies in osteoarthritis of the hand, hip, and knee. *Arthritis Care Res* 64:465–474, 2011.

35. Jevsevar DS, Brown GA, Jones DL, et al: The American Academy of Orthopaedic Surgeons evidence-based guideline on: treatment of osteoarthritis of the knee, 2nd edition. *J Bone Joint Surg Am* 95(20):1885–1886, 2013.

37. Kon E, Buda R, Filardo G, et al: Platelet-rich plasma: intra-articular knee injections produced favorable results on degenerative cartilage lesions. *Knee Surg Sports Traumatol Arthrosc* 18:472–479, 2010.

43. Lo GH, LaValley M, McAlindon T, et al: Intra-articular hyaluronic acid in treatment of knee osteoarthritis: a meta-analysis. *JAMA* 290(23):3115–3121, 2003.

52. Pourcho AM, Smith J, Wisniewski SJ, et al: Intraarticular platelet-rich plasma injection in the treatment of knee osteoarthritis. *Am J Phys Med Rehabil* 93:S108–S121, 2013.

55. Schumacher HR, Chen LX: Injectable corticosteroids in treatment of arthritis of the knee. *Am J Med* 118(11):1208–1214, 2005.

63. Xia P, Wang X, Lin Q, et al: Efficacy of mesenchymal stem cells injection for the management of knee osteoarthritis: a systematic review and meta-analysis. *Int Orthop* 39:2363–2372, 2015.

The references for this chapter can also be found on www.expertconsult.com.

184

Techniques and Eligibility for Same Day/Next Day Discharge of Total Knee Arthroplasty

David A. Crawford, Keith R. Berend, Adolph V. Lombardi

INTRODUCTION

Total knee arthroplasty (TKA) is one of the most successful orthopedic surgeries performed; however it is also one of the most expensive. Surgeons and hospitals continue to look for ways to decrease the costs associated with high-volume surgeries while emphasizing patient safety and successful outcomes. Two strategies for reducing the cost of TKA are to shorten the length of the hospital stay and minimize perioperative and postoperative complications. Reducing readmissions and perioperative complications becomes increasingly important with the push toward outcomes-based reimbursement.

Historically, TKA has been performed as an inpatient to mitigate the risks of perioperative complications, decreased mobility, and difficulty controlling pain.[6] Length of stay (LOS) after TKA continues to decline[30] and over the past decade, studies have shown that a decreased LOS does not increase short-term complications, and may even decrease complications in some cases.* Vital to successfully decreasing LOS is the implementation of rapid recovery pathways. These pathways focus on patient education, perioperative medical management, aggressive pain control, and close coordination of postoperative care (Table 184.1). Overall, implementation of clinical pathways has contributed to the widespread reduction in LOS after TKA.[18] This chapter focuses on ways to successfully implement a same-day or next-day discharge after TKA.

SURGICAL SETTING

Where should you perform outpatient TKA? In the hospital or surgery center? Although it may be tempting to jump right into an outpatient surgery center, there are some advantages in beginning this transition in a hospital. First, the hospital setting is familiar to the surgeon. You know the staff, equipment, and may have multiple implants including revision components available. Second, you have the safety of being in a hospital if any complications arise. Medical consultants and intensive care unit (ICU) capabilities are available. The hospital poses unique challenges because the surgeon must work with hospital administration, deal with operating room (OR) competition with other surgical services, and often the surgeon has

no direct line of supervision of the perioperative staff. In a surgery center, the surgeon is more likely to have some management authority over staff and the potential to increase operating room efficiency.[14,46]

Our group bridged this transition with the development of a specialty hospital. We implemented a rapid recovery pathway in which all staff were involved. From admission nurses to discharge destination (ie home vs. SNF), everyone worked together with a common goal of patient directed care, reducing pain, complications, and in turn, LOS. In the years following the implementation of this hospital, an increasing number of patients were discharged on postoperative day 1 with the average LOS decreasing to 1.5 days. We found that there were many patients whom we believed did not need an inpatient stay at all and began moving toward same-day discharge. This shift was first done at the specialty hospital, and later transitioned to the outpatient surgery center.

Although we are advocates of using a surgery center for outpatient arthroplasty, we encourage a surgeon starting out to begin this transition in the hospital setting. The surgeon can move to an outpatient surgery center once the surgeon and staff have created a reproducible pathway that works well in the community.

PATIENT SELECTION

Any patient who is a candidate for a TKA can be considered for same-day or next-day discharge. Attention to detail is imperative throughout the entire preoperative, perioperative, and postoperative periods.

Preoperatively identifying and treating medical comorbidities can mitigate much of the risk of perioperative complication. In one study, preoperative medical evaluation uncovered a remarkable number of new diagnoses and 2.5% of the patients were deemed unacceptable as surgical candidates.[43] It is essential that a medicine physician evaluates all patients and treats any underlying conditions such as coronary artery disease (CAD) that may require revascularization prior to surgery.

Initial studies of the success and feasibility of same-day discharge after arthroplasty have selectively chosen patients.[7,8,30] Criteria considered were age, body mass index (BMI), medical comorbidities, and family support. Berger et al. later demonstrated in an unselected group of patients that same-day discharge after TKA and unicondylar knee arthroplasty (UKA) can be successful.[6]

---

*References 12, 26, 29, 30, 38, 45, and 51.

TABLE 184.1 Perioperative Regimen for Outpatient Knee Arthroplasty

Preoperatively

Orthopedic assessment
Medical assessment
Evaluation and instruction by physical therapist
Preoperative education class and/or video (DVD)
Educational booklet
Celecoxib 400 mg PO if no significant cardiac history
  ± pregabalin or gabapentin 600 mg PO (300 mg if >65 years old)
Acetaminophen 1 g PO
Dexamethasone 10 mg IV
Metoclopramide 10 mg IV
Consider scopolamine patch if no benign prostatic hypertrophy or
  glaucoma
Perioperative antibiotic
Tranexamic acid 1 g IV within 1 hr prior to incision
Start crystalloid for resuscitation/hydration

Intraoperatively

Adductor canal block: 15 mL 0.5% bupivacaine
Sciatic nerve block: low concentration 15 mL 0.1% ropivacaine
Light general anesthesia: propofol for short-acting sedation, ±
  short-acting inhalants; minimize narcotics (titrated as needed);
  ketamine 0.5 mg/kg IV prior to incision
Crystalloid 2 L IV for resuscitation/hydration
Periarticular injection: 50 mL 0.5% ropivacaine, 0.5 mL 1:1000
  epinephrine, and if renal function is normal 1 mL 30 mg ketorolac
Ondansetron 4 mg IV

Postoperatively

Tranexamic acid 1 g IV 3 hr after initial dose
Minimum 1 additional liter of crystalloid for resuscitation/hydration
Ondansetron 4 mg IV PRN
Phenergan 6.25 mg IV PRN
Hydrocodone/acetaminophen 5/325 1-2 tabs PO q 4 hr PRN
Oxycodone 5-10 mg PO q 4 h PRN
Acetaminophen 1 g PO scheduled prior to discharge
Dilaudid 0.5 mg IV q 10 min PRN
Urecholine 20 mg to minimize risk of urinary retention in male
  patients receiving spinal or having history of BPH
Celecoxib 200 mg PO qd continued for 2 weeks postoperative
Aspirin 325 mg PO bid for 6 weeks and portable, battery-powered
  intermittent pneumatic compression ambulatory calf pumps
Cryotherapy motorized unit
Predischarge instruction by nurse
Telephone call at 24 hr postoperative by nurse or medical assistant
Office evaluation at 6 weeks

BPH, Benign prostatic hyperplasia; *IV*, intravenously; *PO*, by mouth; *PRN*, as needed; *qd*, daily.

Patients with medical comorbidities, however, are at increased risk of complications after TKA.[15] Obesity, diabetes, smoking, and cardiac and pulmonary disease have been shown to increase complications after TKA.[15,19,40,53] To better identify patients who may not be great candidates for short stay after arthroplasty, Courtney et al. evaluated 1012 patients who underwent total hip or knee arthroplasty and evaluated risk factors for perioperative complication.[15] Overall, 6.9% of patients experienced a perioperative complication with 84% of these complications occurring after 24 hours postoperatively. Risk factors found to have a statistical correlation with perioperative risk were chronic obstructive pulmonary disease (COPD), congestive heart failure (CHF), CAD, and liver cirrhosis. With none of these risk factors, patients had a 3.1% risk of perioperative complication. Patients with just one risk factor had a 10% risk of perioperative complication, which increased with each additional risk factor.[15]

Although some institutions have had success with same-day discharge TKA in all patients regardless of medical and social status, it may be advisable to start on patients with low perioperative risk and stable social support.

PREOPERATIVE EDUCATION

The surgeon is only one part of the medical team that guides and treats patients through the process of short-stay arthroplasty. It is essential that the surgeon be surrounded by other individuals of a similar mindset. Everyone who comes in contact with the patient, such as office staff, medical assistants, physician assistants, perioperative nurses, and physical therapists, must be vested in the reality of outpatient arthroplasty. The education and planning from everyone on the team will have far more to do with the success of same-day arthroplasty than surgical technique and incision size. Less-invasive surgical techniques will decrease pain, but patient anxiety about dealing with that pain and social concerns at home may be the greatest issue to overcome for same-day discharge.

Establishing a standardized clinical pathway with a multidisciplinary approach is the best way to minimize patient anxiety and have reproducible clinical results. Rapid recovery pathways decrease errors and waste, and improve the patient's experience. In a randomized study, Dowsey et al. evaluated 163 patients divided into a clinical pathway group and a control group.[18] They found that clinical pathways resulted in a significant reduction in hospital LOS, earlier ambulatory ability, reduction in the readmission rate, and importantly, more accurate matching of the patient discharge destination (ie home vs. SNF) as determined by preoperative education. Patient anxiety can also be reduced by using a multidisciplinary health care team conducted a small group program.[32]

Comprehensive educational materials can answer most common questions and provide a description of the surgery process, although it may be helpful to have a nurse or medical assistant available to go into more detail if needed. During "joint camps" or multidisciplinary meetings, patients can meet many of the personnel involved in their care. Physical therapists can address medical equipment needs, teach patients how to adapt to activities of daily living, and prepare the patient's caregivers for the early postoperative period. Nurses can educate the patient on common complications and wound care management. When patients are aware of what to expect functionally in their immediate postoperative phase, there is a considerable decrease in the level of fear and anxiety.[5,34,36] To be successful with outpatient TKA, the patient must believe that same-day surgery can be performed safely with adequate at-home pain control and your team must work together to set those expectations.

PERIOPERATIVE PAIN MANAGEMENT

With the increasing popularity of short-stay arthroplasty, many high-volume centers have developed clinical pathways coupled with multimodal pain management protocols to accelerate the early recovery of patients and reduce their LOS.[†] The purpose

---

[†]References 4, 5, 9, 11, 34, 36, 42, and 48.

of these protocols is to minimize the risks and side effects in the perioperative period by combining minimally invasive surgical techniques with an effective anesthetic program. This approach reduces pain, nausea, and sedation, and enables patients to quickly mobilize and safely discharge to home on the same day as the surgery or the next day.

Ultimately, the quality of pain relief after TKA will affect the ability to perform this surgery as an outpatient. Any surgery is associated with some level of pain. To treat surgical pain it is important to understand the basic principles of pain signal transmission. Peripheral pain can be separated into neurogenic pain and pain as a result of inflammation.[56] Surgical trauma produces neurogenic pain, and inflammatory pain is secondary to a cascade of events that involve cytokines, prostaglandins, and several other chemical mediators.[56] Traditional postoperative management of pain does not reduce or block the immediate surgical stimulus that causes the neurogenic and inflammatory aspects of postsurgical pain. At this point, the painful stimulus of surgery has already triggered an inflammatory cascade.

Perioperative multimodal pain management involves preemptive analgesia that minimizes the inflammatory and neurogenic pain from the surgical trauma, ultimately reducing the perception of pain from reaching the central nervous system. Safe and effective postoperative pain management can be achieved with a combination of pre- and postoperative anti-inflammatory medication, antiemetics, regional anesthetics, and intra-articular injections. The aim is to minimize narcotic use, which will reduce postoperative sedation, hypoventilation, and subsequently allow the patient to discharge home on the day of surgery.

The first step is to block the inflammatory source of surgical pain, which can be achieved with anti-inflammatories. In a study evaluating the effect of adding a cyclooxygenase-2 (COX-2)-inhibiting nonsteroidal medication for patients who underwent THA and TKA with spinal or epidural anesthesia, Mallory and Lombardi found that patients who had the addition of COX-2 had a significant reduction in postoperative pain control issues.[39] Additionally, those patients had less postoperative confusion and less postoperative nausea than without COX-2.[39]

Gabapentin and pregabalin are non-narcotic medications that can be used in the perioperative period to reduce pain and the need for narcotics. Buvanendran et al. conducted a randomized double-blind study of 240 patients undergoing TKA.[10] One group was treated with 300 mg of pregabalin on the day of surgery and for 14 days following surgery. The other group received a placebo. The incidence of neuropathic pain at 3 and 6 months was significantly less in the pregabalin group. Patients in the pregabalin group also used less epidural opioids, required less oral opioid pain medication while hospitalized, and had greater active knee flexion over the first 30 postoperative days.[10]

Epidural anesthesia is effective as another way to block the pain signal pathway from reaching the brain. The use of intraoperative and postoperative epidural anesthesia is effective in decreasing postoperative narcotic use.[17] In addition, a randomized prospective study demonstrated that epidural anesthesia allowed more rapid achievement of in-hospital postoperative rehabilitation goals compared to general anesthesia.[54]

In patients undergoing spinal or epidural anesthesia, avoiding narcotics in the intrathecal space can help minimize potential postoperative sedation, nausea, and pruritus. Other medications can be used to minimize nausea including dexamethasone, metoclopramide, and scopolamine patches. To prevent postoperative nausea it is also important that the patient be well hydrated, which can be accomplished via 1000 mL of crystalloid prior to the operation and appropriate fluid management during surgery.

Regional anesthetics can reduce the side effects of parenteral narcotics, improve pain control, allow earlier functional recovery, and reduce LOS.[2] Lovald et al. found that patients undergoing TKA who had a femoral nerve block had a lower risk of readmission.[37] Proximal femoral nerve blocks, however, produce quadriceps weakness, which can increase fall risk.[2,49] Moving to a distal femoral block in the adductor canal can mitigate the quadriceps weakness and risk of falls. In a double-blind randomized study, Jaeger et al. found that quadriceps strength as a percentage of baseline was significantly higher in the adductor canal block group compared with the femoral nerve block group.[27] The adductor canal block can be performed with 12 to 15 mL of 0.5% ropivacaine under ultrasound guidance aimed at inducing a sensory-only block.

Direct injection of local anesthetics into periarticular tissue helps block immediate transmission of pain signals and provides prolonged postoperative pain control after epidural removal. The addition of intra-articular injection of 0.25% bupivacaine with epinephrine and a long-acting narcotic was shown to significantly reduce the need for a breakthrough narcotic on the day of surgery, reduce postoperative confusion, and allowed patients to achieve greater knee range of motion after TKA.[35]

Exparel (Pacira Pharmaceuticals, Inc.; Parsippany, NJ) is a newer long-acting local anesthetic that has been shown to be safe and reduce postoperative pain in a number of surgical procedures.[13,23,41] Exparel is liposomal-bound bupivacaine and can provide up to 72 hours of local anesthetic effect. Barrington studied the effect of local injection of Exparel in hip and knee arthroplasties.[1] This study evaluated more than 2000 joint replacements, with the first half of the patients treated using a periarticular injection of bupivacaine, ketorolac, and morphine. The second group of 1124 hip and knee arthroplasty patients was treated with the addition of liposomal bupivacaine in the periarticular injection. Patients in the liposomal bupivacaine group had significantly lower visual analogue scale (VAS) pain scores.[1] There was also a significantly higher percentage of patients in the liposomal bupivacaine group who reported having no pain.

The multimodal approach uses pretreatment of pain and nausea with anti-inflammatories, anti-emetics, and hydration. Epidural anesthesia, along with peripheral nerve blocks and periarticular injections, slows pain signal transmission to the central nervous system. Combining these treatment modalities allows outpatient discharge after TKA, provides patients with good pain control, and minimizes side effects.

SURGICAL APPROACH

Minimally invasive surgical techniques reduce soft tissue trauma and allow a more rapid recovery after TKA. A number of approaches have been described to gain access to the knee joint, with the standard approach being the medial parapatellar. In this approach, the quadriceps tendon is incised adjacent to the vastus medialis and continued distally into a medial parapatellar arthrotomy. More recent techniques have been developed in

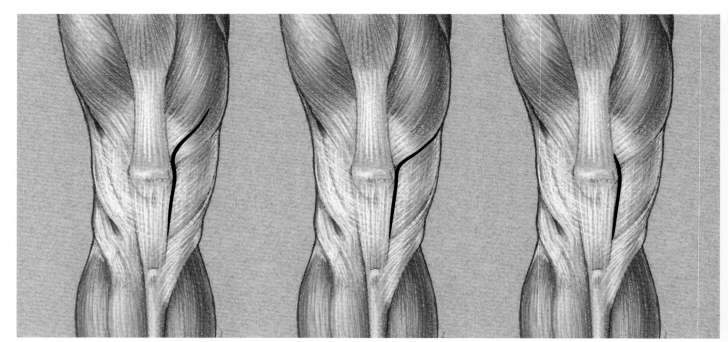

FIG 184.1 Minimally invasive surgical approaches to the knee reduce soft tissue trauma and allow faster recovery after TKA. Techniques that attempt to "spare" the quadriceps tendon include, from left to right, the midvastus, the subvastus, and the complete quadriceps-sparing technique. (Reproduced courtesy Joint Implant Surgeons, Inc., New Albany, OH.)

an attempt to "spare" the quadriceps tendon. These techniques include the subvastus, midvastus, and complete quadriceps-sparing technique described by Berger et al. (Fig. 184.1).[8]

In the subvastus approach, the entire vastus medialis is dissected off the medial intermuscular septum with the exposure carried distal into the medial parapatellar arthrotomy. The midvastus approach dissects through the muscle fibers of the vastus medialis, again with distal joint exposure with a medial parapatellar arthrotomy. Berger described a complete quadriceps-sparing approach with the arthrotomy stops at the superior pole of the patella and all cuts are made in situ without knee dislocation.[8] Some studies have shown a decrease in postoperative pain and improved function with quadriceps-sparing techniques,[16,33] whereas other randomized control trials have found no difference in outcomes.[24,52] Whichever approach is chosen, the surgeon should minimize the extent of exposure but ensure that all structures are properly protected. Without appropriate retractor placement, structures such as the medial collateral ligament (MCL), patellar tendon, or popliteal vessels could be at risk for injury.[3]

BLOOD MANAGEMENT

Aside from pain management concerns, another reason that surgeons may be wary of performing TKA in the outpatient setting is the possibility of the patient needing a blood transfusion. This is especially true if the surgery is being done at a surgery center, where blood storage may not be available and where it may not be feasible to monitor the patient following a transfusion. One important step in minimizing the need for transfusion is to preoperatively identify patients who are at high

risk for requiring a transfusion. A patient's preoperative hemoglobin level is one of the best predictors of postoperative hemoglobin levels.[47] If a patient's preoperative hemoglobin is greater than 13 g/dL, the transfusion rate drops close to zero.[25] If you identify at-risk patients preoperatively, you may choose to do their surgery in a hospital setting or take steps to increase their hemoglobin prior to surgery.

Other steps that can be taken to minimize transfusion risk are to perform regional anesthesia, which has been shown to reduce overall blood loss and transfusion rates,[28,44] and maintain hypotensive anesthesia with mean arterial pressures at or below 60 mm Hg.[21,50]

A newer and very effective way to minimize blood loss is the use of tranexamic acid (TXA). TXA reduces the rate of clot breakdown without increasing the rate of clot formation.[20] A number of studies have shown that blood loss can be significantly reduced with the use of TXA.[31,55] TXA can be dosed intravenously (IV) or topically. Both routes of administration are effective in reducing blood loss.[22,31,55] Dosing of TXA IV is typically done with 1 g prior to incision and a second 1 g dose at the end of surgery or in the recovery room. Topical application of TXA is done by mixing 2 to 3 g in 50 to 100 mL of saline and typically given at the time of wound closure. Studies have repeatedly shown that TXA reduces blood loss and lowers transfusion rates without increasing the rate of thrombotic events.[22,31,55]

IMMEDIATE POSTOPERATIVE CARE

The immediate postoperative protocol, recovery room nursing staff, and at-facility physical therapists are the next crucial components for successful same-day discharge after TKA. At this point, the multimodal protocol used in the perioperative period has hopefully minimized the need for postoperative narcotics and patient sedation and reduced nausea. The goal is for patients to be alert and able to participate in therapy.

The epidural catheter, if used, is typically pulled 1 to 4 hours post operation and the Foley catheter removed 2 hours post operation. Oral narcotics, acetaminophen, and anti-inflammatories are used to manage pain if needed. Physical therapy is initiated within 5 to 6 hours from the end of surgery. To discharge home, patients must demonstrate the ability to independently move from a supine to a standing position and to return from a standing position to a supine position. They must also be able to independently transfer to and from a chair and to a standing position.

After these initial criteria are met, patients must be able to ambulate at least 100 feet and ascend and descend a full flight of stairs. Other standard discharge criteria include stable vital signs and the ability to tolerate a regular diet. Prior to discharge, the staff again ensures that the patient has adequate pain control on oral medications to minimize readmission for pain control issues.

POSTOPERATIVE MANAGEMENT

Prior to surgery, arrangements must be made to ensure that the patient has support at home and a plan for postoperative therapy and monitoring of any early complications. Typically, in-home physical therapy is used initially to reduce the need for patient travel. This can be transitioned to outpatient therapy a few weeks after surgery.

Home health nurses can monitor any signs of surgical site infection, deep venous thrombosis (DVT), and assist in management of pain control. Other methods for early surveillance are to have a clinic nurse call the patient every few days and have the patient return to the office within the first week after surgery.

OUTCOMES

Studies of the success of short-stay TKA have been ongoing for the past decade. Berger first described his outcomes of outpatient TKA in a group of 50 selected patients.[8] Patients selected for that study were between the ages of 50 and 80. Exclusion criteria were a history within 1 year of myocardial infarction, pulmonary embolism, or anticoagulation therapy. Patients with a BMI greater than 40 kg/m^2 or more than three medical comorbidities were also excluded. All included patients had their surgery done as the first TKA of the day. The mean patient age was 68 years and BMI was 29.2 kg/m^2. Of the 50 patients, 96% were able to discharge home the same day. There were three readmissions. One patient was readmitted 8 days after surgery for gastric bleeding, one at 21 days for subcutaneous infection, and one at 9 weeks for a manipulation under anesthesia.[8]

Berger et al. performed a follow-on study in 2006 with 50 more patients with the same selection criteria. None of those patients required overnight stay, bringing the success of same-day discharge of these selected 100 patients to 98%.[7]

In another study examining the success of outpatient arthroplasty in selected patients, Kolisek et al. evaluated 150 patients undergoing TKA.[30] To be included in the same-day discharge treatment arm, patients had to live within 1 hour travel time of the office and have an adult at home to help. Patients were excluded from outpatient discharge if they had any history of diabetes, myocardial infarction, stroke, CHF, venous thromboembolism, cardiac arrhythmia, respiratory failure, or chronic pain requiring regular opioid medications. Of the 150 patients, 64 met the inclusion criteria. These 64 patients were matched by age, gender, BMI, and length of follow-up to a cohort of 64 patients who underwent TKAs during the same time period by the same surgeons, but had a conventional inpatient stay of 2 to 4 days. They defined outpatient discharge as discharge within 23 hours of surgery, and all patients in the outpatient cohort were discharged within 23 hours. They reported no readmission for any reason related to the TKA. At 24 months' follow-up they found no difference between the groups in Knee Society Knee Scores or knee range of motion.[30]

Given the success of selected patients, Berger examined the feasibility of outpatient arthroplasty in an unselected group of patients.[6] This study included TKA and UKA with the only exclusion criteria being surgery after 12 PM. In this study, 104 of 111 patients (94%) were discharged home on the day of surgery, three patients were discharged the following day, and four patients remained in the hospital because of pain control issues. In the first 3 months after surgery there were a total of eight patients (7.2%) readmitted, all of whom had a TKA. Four patients (3.6%) were readmitted for medical complications within the first week. Two of the four readmissions were for symptomatic anemia requiring a blood transfusion, one for gastrointestinal bleeding, and one for DVT. Between week 1 and 3 months after surgery, there were four (3.6%) additional readmissions. Two of the four readmissions were for wound complications, one for manipulation under anesthesia for stiffness, and one for a gastrointestinal bleed. Of importance for selection criteria, they found no differences in patients who required an overnight stay and those treated as an outpatient with regard to average age, body weight, BMI, or medical comorbidities.

CONCLUSION

Same-day or next-day TKA can be accomplished with a rapid recovery protocol and multimodal pain management in appropriately selected patients. It is probably best to start the transition to outpatient arthroplasty in a hospital setting and move to a surgery center later if desired. Patient education from a multidisciplinary team and pain management are the cornerstones of success. The surgeon must identify patients at risk for medical complications, including transfusion, and appropriately optimize these patients preoperatively. Using the steps outlined in this chapter, TKA can be performed safely with good results in the outpatient setting.

KEY REFERENCES

5. Berend KR, Lombardi AV, Jr, Mallory TH: Rapid recovery protocol for peri-operative care of total hip and total knee arthroplasty patients. *Surg Technol Int* 13:239–247, 2004.

6. Berger RA, Kusuma SK, Sanders S, et al: The feasibility and perioperative complications of outpatient knee arthroplasty. *Clin Orthop Relat Res* 467(6):1443–1449, 2009.

8. Berger RA, Sanders S, Gerlinger T, et al: Outpatient total knee arthroplasty with a minimally invasive technique. *J Arthroplasty* 20(7):33–38, 2005.

22. Gilbody J, Dhotar HS, Perruccio AV, et al: Topical tranexamic acid reduces transfusion rates in total hip and knee arthroplasty. *J Arthroplasty* 29(4):681–684, 2014.

27. Jaeger P, Nielsen ZJ, Henningsen MH, et al: Adductor canal block versus femoral nerve block and quadriceps strength: a randomized, double-blind, placebo-controlled, crossover study in healthy volunteers. *Anesthesiology* 118(2):409–415, 2013.

30. Kolisek FR, McGrath MS, Jessup NM, et al: Comparison of outpatient versus inpatient total knee arthroplasty. *Clin Orthop Relat Res* 467(6):1438–1442, 2009.

34. Lombardi AV, Berend KR, Adams JB: A rapid recovery program: early home and pain free. *Orthopedics* 33(9):656, 2010.

The references for this chapter can also be found on www.expertconsult.com.

185

Pain Management After Total Knee Arthroplasty Patients Leave the Hospital

Adam C. Young, Craig J. Della Valle, Asokumar Buvanendran

INTRODUCTION

The term *acute pain* encompasses the first initial phase of pain following surgery. Acute postoperative pain is a predictable response to the surgical stimulus of joint replacement. From the time of surgery until full recovery, the patient's pain medication needs will change dramatically. This chapter describes ideal pain management for patients from the time of surgery through recovery. In addition, it offers a guideline for weaning patients from medications in a safe and deliberate manner, and explains some of the nuances of the transition from acute to chronic pain.

MEDICAL MANAGEMENT OF ACUTE PAIN

Medical management of acute pain can be accomplished in a variety of ways. Recent evidence has supported the use of a perioperative multimodal analgesia (MMA) strategy because it has been shown to demonstrate superior efficacy and patient satisfaction. It is critical to realize that pain management with an MMA should begin early, preferably before surgical incision, and continue into the postoperative recovery phase even after patients leave the hospital. In fact, as patients undergo physical therapy at home, the MMA should be the mainstay of treatment and opioids should be weaned or stopped.

MMA is the method of combining analgesics with differing mechanisms of action, resulting in additive or synergistic analgesia, to achieve an analgesic effect superior to any single agent. Opioids have long been the mainstay of postoperative analgesia; the addition of non-opioid medications permits the use of lower doses of opioids while addressing postoperative pain by alternative mechanisms. These adjuvants enhance analgesia and reduce potential adverse effects of opioids. The following sections discuss some of the different analgesics that can be used for MMA.

NONSTEROIDAL ANTIINFLAMMATORY DRUGS AND ACETAMINOPHEN

Administration of cyclooxygenase-2 (COX-2) inhibitors in the perioperative period has consistently demonstrated decreased opioid consumption postoperatively, reduced pain scores, and improved range of motion following total joint replacement. It is ideal to continue the COX-2 inhibitor after major surgery for a period of at least 2 weeks coinciding with the duration of the surgical inflammatory process, although longer administration may have benefits and should be considered if the medication is well tolerated. Preoperative administration is ideal to obtain effective plasma and cerebrospinal fluid (CSF) levels of nonsteroidal antiinflammatory drugs (NSAIDs). Beginning on postoperative day 1, dosing should continue as twice-a-day dosing. A typical regimen would include celecoxib 400 mg administered preoperatively on the day of surgery followed by 200 mg every 12 hours postoperatively for a minimum of 2 weeks. Alternative regimens could include meloxicam 30 mg on the day of surgery followed by 15 mg every 12 hours for 12 weeks postoperatively or ibuprofen 800 mg on the day of surgery followed by 800 mg every 8 hours for 2 weeks postoperatively.

Considering the pain associated with physical therapy, it would be reasonable to continue NSAIDs until therapy has been completed to maximize functional outcome. Celecoxib and other NSAIDs do not need to be weaned or tapered; they may be stopped without the concern of precipitating withdrawal.

Nonselective NSAIDs and COX-2 specific inhibitors have demonstrated no increase in major bleed events following total hip and knee arthroplasties. Therefore, patients may continue to take these medications following surgery without an increased risk of hemorrhage, including patients on anticoagulation for deep venous thrombosis prophylaxis. Contraindications to celecoxib include allergy to aspirin, other NSAIDs, and sulfonamides. Patients with renal insufficiency or renal failure should be not given NSAIDs unless the benefits of analgesia without respiratory depression outweigh the potential for inducing acute or acute on chronic renal failure. In patients older than 70 years, the dose of these medications should be reduced by half. The risk of developing renal insufficiency or gastroduodenal ulcer appears to correlate with length of treatment with NSAIDs. They should be stopped or used less frequently once patients are through the acute phase of recovery.

The US Food and Drug Administration (FDA) recently strengthened its warning regarding non-aspirin NSAIDs. The FDA has stated that over-the-counter and prescription NSAIDs can increase the risk of myocardial ischemia (MI) and stroke. As part of their warning, the FDA states that MI or stroke can occur as early as the first weeks following initiation of an NSAID and that extended use may increase patients' risk. Additional risk factors for development of MI or stroke with NSAID use included higher doses of NSAID, presence of heart disease, or risk factors for heart disease. There are no specific NSAIDs implicated as being safer than another and no suggested dosages other than that "high" doses may confer greater risk.

Acetaminophen is believed to produce its analgesic effect by inhibiting central prostaglandin synthesis, although the exact mechanism of action is truly not known. Acetaminophen differs from NSAIDs because it has a relatively weak anti-inflammatory effect, it inhibits COX poorly in the presence of high concentrations of peroxides (such as those found at sites of inflammation), and it has no effect on platelet function or the gastric mucosa. It may produce analgesia by modulating the descending pain pathways; there is speculation that receptor activity other than prostaglandins may be involved. Systematic reviews have demonstrated that acetaminophen has similar effects in reducing postoperative pain after orthopedic procedures compared to traditional NSAIDs. Further, the combination of the two has been shown to confer superior analgesia than either drug alone, which highlights the likelihood of different mechanisms or sites of action.

Use of acetaminophen has become increasingly popular, as intravenous forms have gained acceptance and use in perioperative MMA for inpatients who cannot take oral medications. Despite decreased bioavailability, oral acetaminophen can be successfully used in outpatients as long as the prescribing physician takes into account the total daily dose a patient is consuming. It is quite common for acetaminophen to be used in combination with short-acting opioids (eg, hydrocodone/acetaminophen, oxycodone/acetaminophen), headache medications (eg, aspirin/caffeine/acetaminophen), and common cold medications (dextromethorphan/phenylephrine/acetaminophen). The FDA recently reduced the maximum daily dose to 3000 mg per day. As such, we recommend scheduled dosing of 1000 mg every 8 hours for patients following discharge as long as patients are not consuming acetaminophen from another source such as a combination opioid. Compared to 650-mg dosages of acetaminophen, 1000 mg has improved analgesia and fewer patients consumed rescue analgesics.

Following total knee arthroplasty (TKA), acetaminophen should be continued based on the patient's improvement in pain symptoms. Using the same rationale as continuing NSAIDs, it would be reasonable to continue acetaminophen until physical therapy is complete. Contraindications for acetaminophen include active liver disease or known allergy. Like NSAIDs, there is no need to taper or wean acetaminophen and it can be stopped abruptly without concerns of withdrawal.

ANTICONVULSANTS (GABAPENTINOIDS)

Among the anticonvulsants in the perioperative period, pregabalin has a noticeable advantage as it is more potent than gabapentin and unsurprisingly, achieves its efficacy at lower doses.

Perioperative use of pregabalin has been shown to decrease the incidence of chronic pain after TKA. This study used a dose of 300 mg, which led to a higher incidence of sedation in the study group. Randomized controlled trials have determined that lower doses of pregabalin are more useful, providing analgesia and avoiding excessive sedation, particularly in older adults.

Preoperatively, patients should be given a single dose of 150 mg pregabalin, followed by 75 mg every 12 hours (or 50 mg every 8 hours) for 2 weeks postoperatively. Studies of perioperative gabapentin use have been more heterogeneous and there

has been a lack of uniformity in dosing. A more recent study showed limited usefulness of gabapentin following TKA. This is likely because of the previously mentioned limitations of variable bioavailability and blood levels of the drug. We recommend a single 900-mg dose of gabapentin preoperatively followed by 300 mg every 8 hours postoperatively for 2 weeks. Anticonvulsants may be continued, and in all likelihood should be continued, if the patient experiences continued pain following their TKA. Contraindications for anticonvulsants include allergy to the compound itself or other medications in the same class. Doses should be reduced in patients with reduced renal function and in older adults. Caution is advised when prescribing anticonvulsants to patients with mental illness because these drugs have the potential to alter mood.

Gabapentin and pregabalin should be weaned. Generally, reducing the patient's pill burden by one tablet per day would constitute responsible weaning. As an example, a patient taking pregabalin 50 mg three times per day would reduce their dose to 50 mg twice per day, then to 50 mg once daily prior to stopping the drug altogether. Should a patient experience withdrawal, they may experience mood swings, anxiety, irritability, headaches, dizziness, difficulty sleeping, or muscle spasms. However, with such low doses given for limited periods of time, these symptoms are unlikely to manifest.

LOCAL ANESTHETICS

Following TKA, some patients experience peri-incisional sensitivity and burning. This symptom can be particularly bothersome but easily treated with transdermal lidocaine (Table 185.1). It is supplied as a 5% patch that can be cut and placed peri-incisionally or placed directly on the incision. Transdermal lidocaine is absorbed locally and acts on the cutaneous nerve endings to provide analgesia.

A lidocaine 5% transdermal patch can be placed on the skin for up to 12 hours. Between patch applications, it is recommended that 12 hours elapse, so that dosing typically consists of a "12 hours on/12 hours off" regimen. These patches should be avoided in patients with a history of allergic reaction to lidocaine or amide local anesthetics, or sensitivity to adhesive. Generally, they are well tolerated and can augment an MMA strategy.

N-METHYL D-ASPARTATE RECEPTOR ANTAGONISTS

Ketamine and memantine are N-methyl-D-aspartate (NMDA) receptor antagonists that can be used in the perioperative period for acute pain. The NMDA receptor has been indicated as a key target for researchers aiming to reduce chronic pain following surgery. The NMDA receptor may be responsible for the phenomena of wind-up, central sensitization, and potentiation of pain. The use of ketamine may be limited for outpatients given that it is traditionally administered as an anesthesia adjunct.

TABLE 185.1	**Properties of Commonly Used Local Anesthetics**			
Local Anesthetic	**Speed of Onset**	**Duration of Action**	**Cardiovascular Toxicity**	**Neurotoxicity**
Lidocaine	Rapid	Medium	+	+
Bupivacaine	Slow	Long	++	+
Ropivacaine	Slow	Long	—	+

Oral formulations of ketamine do exist, but have yet to be studied as a part of an MMA regimen following TKA. There is also little evidence to suggest that memantine might be a beneficial adjunct following surgery. However, there is a single study that explored the use of memantine perioperatively to reduce the incidence of phantom limb pain following lower extremity amputation. In that study memantine, in conjunction with a peripheral nerve infusion of local anesthetic, was able to reduce pain scores in the acute and subacute phase of postoperative pain, but had no long-term effect on the incidence of chronic pain.

Unfortunately, oral dosing of ketamine has not been investigated thoroughly and there is a paucity of evidence for NMDA receptor antagonist use in the TKA population. As more is accomplished in the realm of NMDA receptor antagonists as part of MMA, we may have an additional agent to blunt the mechanisms at play in the development of chronic pain.

OPIOIDS

Opioids exist in two formulations, long-acting and short-acting versions. This is important to note as pharmacodynamics vary substantially between the two and have the potential for causing respiratory depression and death. TKA is considered to be a quite painful procedure. As a result, long-acting opioids have been used by some orthopedic surgeons. Long-acting opioids are given on a scheduled basis and provide a steady low level of opioids in the patient's serum. Typically a patient would receive their first dose preoperatively on the day of the surgery and have that medication continue throughout the first 2 weeks following surgery. As an example, one could administer oxycodone extended-release (Oxycontin, Purdue Pharma) 10 mg preoperatively and continue the medication every 12 hours postoperatively for 1 week. Similarly, one could administer an extended release version of morphine (MS Contin, Purdue Pharma) in a similar fashion, MS Contin 15 mg preoperatively followed by dosing every 12 hours for 1 week. Great care needs to be taken to assure that patients with a history of obstructive sleep apnea (OSA) do not receive extended release formulations of opioids. A simple screening tool (STOP-BANG questionnaire) can be used to determine if patients are likely to have OSA (Table 185.2). The same caution should be exercised in patients older than 65 years because their metabolism may be altered and their ability to excrete metabolic by-products impaired leading to potential adverse events.

Short-acting opioids have been the most commonly prescribed medications for acute postoperative pain. These medications include tramadol and the combination products hydrocodone/acetaminophen and oxycodone/acetaminophen (Table 185.3). One of the drawbacks to using combination products is the addition of acetaminophen to the opioid, which impacts the total daily dose of acetaminophen consumed. Unfortunately, there is no immediate-release version of hydrocodone only. Oxycodone does come in an immediate-release version without acetaminophen. Oxycodone is considered to be approximately 20% stronger than hydrocodone. Patients can be prescribed oxycodone immediate-release 5 mg or 10 mg every 4 to 6 hours on an as-needed basis for breakthrough pain. We encourage patients to take this medication 1 hour prior to physical therapy or anticipated activity to maximize mobility with as little pain as possible. This amount of time will allow patients to have an effective blood level of the drug at the time of activity.

Weaning opioids should be done in a systematic manner. If a long-acting opioid is prescribed, it should be the first opioid weaned and stopped. After 1 to 2 weeks of dosing every 12 hours, a low-dose opioid may be stopped without the consequences of withdrawal. Short-acting opioids are prescribed to be taken on an intermittent, or as-needed, basis. This requires the patient to consume the medication only when they have pain or prior to an activity that is anticipated to produce significant pain (such as physical therapy). After 4 weeks, patients are considered to be through the acute pain phase of postsurgical recovery. Weaning at this point is done on an individual patient basis. During the subacute phase of postsurgical pain, weeks 4 to 12, patients should be weaned to the lowest effective dose of short-acting opioids.

This means that patients are taking the lowest cumulative dose of opioids per day necessary to participate in physical therapy and to perform the same activities of daily living they were performing prior to surgery. As an example, a patient consuming hydrocodone/acetaminophen 10/325 mg four times

TABLE 185.2	STOP-BANG Questionnaire		
Do you SNORE loudly (louder than talking or loud enough to be heard through closed doors)?		YES	NO
Do you often feel TIRED, fatigued, or sleepy during daytime?		YES	NO
Has anyone OBSERVED you stop breathing during your sleep?		YES	NO
Do you have or are you being treated for high blood PRESSURE?		YES	NO
Body mass index >35 kg/m^2?		YES	NO
AGE over 50 years old?		YES	NO
NECK circumference >16 inches (40 cm)?		YES	NO
GENDER: Male?		YES	NO

High risk of OSA: 5-8.
Intermediate risk of OSA: 3-4.
Low risk of OSA: 0-2.

TABLE 185.3	Properties of Common Immediate-Release Opioids				
Opioid	Onset of Analgesia (min)	Analgesia Duration (h)	Relative Potency	Typical Dosage (mg)	Dosing Interval (h)
Codeine	30-60	2-4	0.1-0.2	15-60	4-6
Morphine	30	2-4	1	15-30	4-6
Hydrocodone	30-60	3-6	5	5-20	4-6
Oxycodone	30-60	3-4	6	5-20	4-6
Hydromorphone	30-60	3-4	4	2-4	4-6

per day for the first month after TKA could be weaned to hydrocodone/acetaminophen 5/325 mg three times per day beginning week 5 post-op, reducing her total daily dose of hydrocodone from 40 to 15 mg. In this example, using short-acting opioids for breakthrough pain or as needed should be reinforced. By weaning opioids in this fashion, keeping in mind the lowest effective dose, the transition off opioids will be much smoother. Short-acting opioids are often continued until a satisfactory functional outcome has been obtained and physical therapy has been completed.

Opioid withdrawal is an uncomfortable experience that occurs when opioids are abruptly stopped or reduced in patients consuming high doses or in patients with prolonged use. Withdrawal typically begins 24 hours after cessation. Early opioid withdrawal symptoms include agitation, anxiety, myalgias, insomnia, rhinorrhea, or diaphoresis. The symptoms of withdrawal can continue for weeks, although this is uncommon with opioid use for acute postoperative pain. Late symptoms include nausea, vomiting, abdominal pain, diarrhea, mydriasis, hypertension, tachycardia, and formication. Oral and transdermal clonidine have been used to combat the early effects of withdrawal because it provides anxiolysis and blunts the increase in sympathetic activity. Anti-diarrheal and anti-nausea agents are often prescribed for patient comfort.

The liver carries out conversion of opioids to water-soluble metabolites; in turn, these substances (many biologically active) are excreted by the kidneys. Any degree of renal insufficiency results in their accumulation, and many of these metabolites are responsible for unwanted effects from opioids. As mentioned before, caution should be exercised when prescribing opioids to patients with a history of OSA and in older adults.

Prescription opioid overdose and death has become a concern among those prescribing these medications and the governing bodies that oversee opioid prescribing. This has led to consensus statements that recommend doses of no more than 50 mg morphine equivalent dose for acute postoperative pain. As a caveat to interpreting this statement, there is no differentiation between surgical procedures, surgical technique, anesthesia technique, or use of multimodal perioperative analgesia approach. Individual risk factors associated with adverse effects and death from opioids include concurrent use of benzodiazepines, marijuana, tobacco, alcohol, presence of psychiatric disorder (depression/anxiety), coronary artery disease, arrhythmia, history of substance abuse or aberrant medication-taking behaviors, or impulse control problems. In fact, the Centers for Disease Control (CDC) has new recommendations regarding opioid prescribing for acute pain that challenges traditional practices. Prescription opioids are often prescribed as a 30-day supply after surgery. The CDC highly discourages this and suggests that appropriate prescription doses of opioids need to be decided on discharge based on the individual patient and an exact amount prescribed to bridge the patient to their postoperative follow-up visit (Table 185.4).

CRYOTHERAPY

The application of ice packs or cold water to a surgical site is known as cryotherapy. Aside from inducing vasoconstriction, reducing blood flow, and slowing enzymatic function, cryotherapy has been suggested to diminish conduction of nerve signals. Despite theoretical benefits of reduced acute pain, this has not been reliably produced in research studies. Several

studies were included in a meta-analysis concluding that cryotherapy is a safe and effective means to reduce blood loss in TKA. Regarding pain, cryotherapy was able to reduce pain scores on postoperative day 2 only. The use of cryotherapy appears to be safe, however its ability to reduce acute pain may be limited.

EXTENDED REGIONAL ANESTHESIA

Regional anesthesia is a popular method of providing anesthesia and analgesia for TKA. Examples include spinal anesthesia, epidural anesthesia, and peripheral nerve blocks. These modalities are quite popular in the perioperative arena but have limited use once patients leave the hospital.

Epidural Infusions

Tunneled epidural infusions are not routinely used for patients undergoing TKA. The placement and maintenance of a tunneled epidural catheter requires a close working relationship between an interventional pain physician experienced in prolonged epidural infusion management and the orthopedic surgeon. There are subsets of patients who surgeons and pain physicians identify as candidates for this perioperative analgesia modality. This includes patients with a poor functional outcome with a prior TKA, patients who are unable to tolerate oral opioids, patients with a history of a chronic pain syndrome affecting the extremity to be operated on, and those on high-dose preoperative opioids. Prolonged infusions (up to 6 weeks) have been shown to improve functional outcomes in patients with knee stiffness following primary TKA who subsequently underwent lysis of adhesions and manipulation under anesthesia.

Prior to joint replacement, a pain physician can place an epidural catheter and tunnel a portion of the catheter under the skin to allow for a continuous epidural infusion. Additionally, the epidural catheter may be used to provide anesthesia for the surgical case. Following discharge from the hospital, patients with epidural catheters must be monitored on a weekly basis to assure absence of infection, absence of significant side effects, and adequacy of analgesia. Patients are not allowed to submerge the epidural dressing in water while the catheter is in place and are asked to take prophylactic antibiotics to cover skin flora. At weekly appointments, the epidural dressing is replaced in sterile fashion. Once an acceptable endpoint has been reached (functional recovery following surgery, significant side effects from the infusion, or completion of 6 weeks) the catheter is removed and transition to oral analgesics is made.

Medications typically used in epidural infusions include opioids, local anesthetics, and alpha-blocking agents. The concentration of these substances and rates of infusion are frequently altered throughout the postoperative phase to provide analgesia and minimize side effects. If opioids are used in the epidural infusion, no long- or short-acting opioids should be provided to the patient. The risk of respiratory depression increases substantially with concomitant administration of opioids via separate routes (eg, oral and epidural). Weakness is an important side effect to note. In the small study published on this technique, approximately 25% of patients experienced lower extremity numbness and/or weakness. Typically this is caused by the local anesthetic in the infusion and can be mitigated by titrating the concentration of the solution or reducing the rate of infusion. Of note, there were no falls reported in the referenced article.

Transition from epidural to oral analgesics can be a challenging task. Oral medications have approximately 1/30th the

TABLE 185.4   Example of Postoperative Oral Pain Regimen and Weaning Schedule

Drug	DAY OF SURGERY AM	PM	QHS	POD 1-8 AM	PM	QHS
Oxycodone ER 10 mg	X	X		X	X	
Oxycodone IR 5-10 mg	PRN every 4 h	PRN every 4 h	PRN every 4 h	PRN every 4 h	PRN every 4 h	PRN every 4 h
Acetaminophen 1000 mg		X	X	X	X	X
Celecoxib 200 mg	XX* (2 Tabs)			X	X	
Pregabalin 50 mg	XXX** (3 Tabs)			X	X	X

Drug	POD 9 AM	PM	QHS	POD 10-13 AM	PM	QHS
Oxycodone ER 10 mg		X				
Oxycodone IR 5-10 mg	PRN every 4 h	PRN every 4 h	PRN every 4 h	PRN every 4 h	PRN every 4 h	PRN every 4 h
Acetaminophen 1000 mg	X	X	X	X	X	X
Celecoxib 200 mg	X	X		X	X	
Pregabalin 50 mg	X	X	X	X	X	X

Drug	POD 14 AM	PM	QHS	2-6 WEEKS POST-OP AM	PM	QHS
Lidocaine 5% Topical Patch	X	OFF		X (Daily PRN)	OFF	
Oxycodone IR 5 mg	PRN every 6 h	PRN every 6 h	PRN every 6 h	PRN every 6-8 h	PRN every 6-8 h	PRN every 6-8 h
Acetaminophen 1000 mg	X	X	X	X (TID PRN)	X (TID PRN)	X (TID PRN)
Celecoxib 200 mg	X			X (Daily PRN)		
Pregabalin 50 mg	X	X	X† (Stop on POD 15)			

Drug	AFTER 6 WEEKS POST-OP AM	PM	QHS
Lidocaine 5% Topical Patch	X (Daily PRN)	OFF	
Acetaminophen 1000 mg	X (TID PRN)	X (TID PRN)	X (TID PRN)
Celecoxib 200 mg	X (Daily PRN)		

ER, Extended release; *IR,* immediate release; *POD,* postoperative day; *PRN,* as needed; *TID,* three times a day.

potency of epidurally administered medications. As such, it is often necessary to taper or wean the total daily dose of medications that can precipitate withdrawal. This includes alpha-blocking agents (eg, clonidine) and opioids. Withdrawal from opioids was mentioned previously in this chapter and will not be covered in this section. Alpha-blocking agent withdrawal can range from uncomfortable sensations of nervousness, agitation, headache, and tremor, to more serious situations such as elevated blood pressure and heart rate. In rare circumstances, hypertensive encephalopathy and stroke can occur. Withdrawal can be prevented by gradually decreasing the dose of the epidurally administered alpha-blocking agent and providing the patient with oral clonidine to be taken as needed for these symptoms.

Infection is a serious concern when considering placement of a tunneled epidural catheter for prolonged infusion. A small case series demonstrated that this can be mitigated when patients are monitored closely and postoperative care of the catheter insertion site is adhered to diligently. The epidural catheter insertion site is examined directly at the time of dressing changes and the patient queried as to worrisome symptoms of infection. Fevers, chills, and sweats along with malaise and back pain are warning signs that require intervention. This can include stopping the infusion, removing the epidural catheter, and obtaining contrast-enhanced imaging of the lumbar spine.

Peripheral Nerve Catheters

Continuous nerve blocks involving the femoral and sciatic nerve have been studied extensively for patients undergoing TKA. Few studies exist regarding maintenance of a continuous infusion following discharge from the hospital or ambulatory surgery center. One study demonstrated that continuous femoral nerve blocks for up to 4 days postoperatively made no significant difference in pain, joint stiffness, or functional disability. It is worthwhile to note that in this study, there was an increase in incidence of falls, albeit statistically insignificant. At this time, there is no data to suggest that continuous peripheral nerve infusions offer any superiority over an MMA oral regimen following discharge from the acute care setting.

Catheter placement in subcutaneous tissue to provide a similar type of slow, continuous infusion following surgery, has been shown in other types of surgery to provide short-term analgesia, while the infusion is running (typically 3 to 5 days). The surgical procedures studied involve soft tissue disruption of muscular tissue or fascial planes. It is not likely that such a technique would provide significant analgesia following TKA using modern surgical technique.

THE IMPORTANCE OF ADEQUATE ANALGESIA AND THE TRANSITION FROM ACUTE TO CHRONIC PAIN

Poorly controlled acute pain can have a number of detrimental consequences on patients following TKA. Functional outcome, measured by range of motion of the knee, can be significantly impaired by poorly controlled pain. Poor functional outcomes can lead to progressive loss of function, pain, and disability.

Chronic postsurgical pain (CPSP) affects up to 20% of patients who undergo TKA. CPSP is a term used to describe pain that persists beyond 3 months following the initial surgery.

In general, chronic pain is a significant problem that leads to loss of function, disability, and increased health care expenses. The transition from acute to chronic pain is a complex process that involves the central and peripheral nervous system, along with psychologic factors.

Among the risk factors for developing CPSP following TKA are those that can be modified and those that cannot. Although younger age and female gender are associated with CPSP following TKA, we will focus on modifiable risk factors. The strongest indicators appear to be a greater number of pain locations preoperatively and the irrational thought process referred to as *catastrophizing*. The latter is evidence that the manner in which a patient adjusts or interprets their pain is important. Catastrophizing is a complicated concept that involves pain magnification, rumination, and feelings of helplessness. Pain magnification may be conscious or unconscious exaggeration of one's symptoms of pain. Rumination is a persistent worrying about anticipated pain and an inability to control the fear associated with it. Helplessness stems from a feeling of a lack of control over one's pain experience. Depression, anxiety, higher levels of preoperative knee pain, and worse levels of preoperative function contribute to the development of chronic pain following TKA.

Armed with this information, it would seem prudent to assess mental health in patients preoperatively. Should they have a history of depression, anxiety, or demonstrate features of catastrophizing, referral to a psychiatrist or psychologist may be necessary. Simply addressing patient fears can be beneficial. However some patients require more intensive treatment preoperatively. This could include graded exposure or cognitive behavioral therapy.

Multiple locations of pain and increased preoperative pain may indicate referral to a pain specialist. By involving a pain specialist preoperatively, a comprehensive perioperative pain management plan can be put into place and patient concerns with regard to postoperative pain can be addressed. Poor preoperative function is the result of multiple factors, which may include lack of pain control, and may be best treated with involvement of a pain specialist and referral to physical therapy preoperatively.

Chronic pain following TKA is an interesting topic for which several risk factors have been elucidated. Preoperative management of these known entities will likely improve outcomes, but studies to validate this assumption are lacking. A comprehensive perioperative plan involving pain specialists, psychologists, and physical therapists may benefit patients at risk for developing CPSP following TKA.

For patients demonstrating an unexpected increase in analgesic requirement, those with persistent pain following TKA, or poor functional recovery, a referral to a pain physician with training to perform interventional and medical management seems prudent. Postoperative pain can be neuropathic or nociceptive; pain specialists can help differentiate between the two and use appropriate medications and/or suggest interventional techniques to treat the patient. MMA should be used beyond the initial acute postoperative phase in patients with CPSP to minimize the use of opioids and maximize functional outcomes following TKA. This is especially important in light of a recent study that demonstrated an alarming finding in patients following TKA—increased opioid consumption 1 year following surgery.

CONCLUSION

Pain is a predictable response to a surgical stimulus that can be modified through a number of different pathways. Using a multimodal perioperative analgesic strategy improves overall pain control while minimizing serious side effects from opioids. More advanced regional anesthesia techniques may emerge that will augment our ability to control pain and improve functional recovery following TKA. It is important to identify patients at risk of developing CPSP and appropriate referrals made as necessary.

KEY REFERENCES

4. Buvanendran A, Kroin JS, Della Valle CJ, et al: Perioperative oral pregabalin reduces chronic pain after total knee arthroplasty: a prospective, randomized, controlled trial. *Anesth Analg* 37:415–422, 2012.
8. Draft CDC Guidelines for Prescribing Opioids for Chronic Pain. <http://www.cdc.gov/drugoverdose/prescribing/guideline.html>, (Accessed 23.11.15.)
9. FDA strengthens warning that non-aspirin nonsteroidal anti-inflammatory drugs (NSAIDs) can cause heart attacks or strokes. FDA Drug Safety Communication. July 9, 2015.
11. Fuzier R, Serres I, Bourrel R, et al: Analgesic drug consumption increases after knee arthroplasty: a pharmacoepidemiological study investigating postoperative pain. *Pain* 155:1339–1345, 2014.
13. Gross JB, Apfelbaum JL, Caplan RA, et al: Practice guidelines for the perioperative management of patients with obstructive sleep apnea: an updated report by the American society of Anesthesiologists task force on perioperative management of patients with obstructive sleep apnea. *Anesthesiology* 120:1–19, 2014.
14. Hegmann KT, Weiss MS, Bowden K, et al: ACOEM practice guidelines: opioids for treatment of acute, subacute, chronic, and postoperative pain. *J Occup Environ Med* 56:143–159, 2014.
16. Kehlet H, Dahl JB: The value of "multimodal" or "balanced analgesia" in postoperative pain treatment. *Anesth Analg* 77:1048–1056, 1993.
20. Lamplot JD, Wagner ER, Manning DW: Multimodal pain management in total knee arthroplasty: a prospective randomized controlled trial. *J Arthroplasty* 29:329–334, 2014.
22. Lewis GN, Rice DA, McNair PJ, et al: Predictors of persistent pain after total knee arthroplasty: a systematic review and meta-analysis. *Br J Anaesth* 114:551–561, 2015.
23. Liu SS, Buvanendran A, Rathmell JP, et al: A cross-sectional survey on prevalence and risk factors for persistent postsurgical pain 1 year after total hip and knee replacement. *Reg Anesth Pain Med* 37:415–422, 2012.
25. Ong CK, Seymour RA, Lirk P, et al: Combining paracetamol (acetaminophen) with nonsteroidal anti-inflammatory drugs: a qualitative systematic review of analgesic efficacy for acute postoperative pain. *Anesth Analg* 110:1170–1179, 2010.
27. Saltzman BM, Dave A, Young A, et al: Prolonged epidural infusion improves functional outcomes following knee arthroscopy in patients with arthrofibrosis after total knee arthroplasty: a retrospective evaluation. *J Knee Surg* 29(1):40–46, 2016.
28. Schley M, Topfner S, Wiech K, et al: Continuous brachial plexus blockade in combination with the NMDA receptor antagonist memantine prevents phantom pain in acute traumatic upper limb amputees. *Eur J Pain* 11:299–308, 2007.

The references for this chapter can also be found on www.expertconsult.com.

PART I

Hospital Management
of TKA Patients

186

Continuous Passive Motion: Pros and Cons

Edward M. DelSole, Claudette Lajam, Parthiv A. Rathod, Ajit J. Deshmukh

INTRODUCTION

Stiffness following total knee arthroplasty (TKA) is a rare but debilitating complication with a prevalence of 1.3%.[21] Knee stiffness can be caused by extrinsic factors including ipsilateral hip osteoarthritis, neurologic compromise, excessively tight quadriceps or hamstrings, and heterotopic ossification. Intrinsic causes of knee stiffness include overstuffing of the patellofemoral articulation, tight flexion/extension gaps, a tight posterior cruciate ligament, component malrotation, arthrofibrosis, unresected posterior osteophytes, or anterior tibial slope.[4,21]

Assuming that intraoperative examination demonstrated full range of motion (ROM), the final postoperative motion obtained by the patient is a function of extrinsic factors and the prevention of arthrofibrosis. These potentially modifiable factors must be optimized through patient education, pain control, and physical rehabilitation protocols.

Rehabilitation strategies have evolved since the advent of TKA. The goals, however, remain the same—to optimize knee ROM, quadriceps strength, function, and minimize pain. Much work has been done to optimize motion and prevent fixed flexion deformity (FFD). Early postoperative leg position and motion protocols have continuously evolved to achieve this goal. There are four schools of thought for early management: extension splinting, flexion splinting, continuous passive motion (CPM) by means of a CPM machine, and early active mobilization without the use of CPM. The evidence for the use of CPM is reviewed in this chapter. Splinting will be reviewed in another chapter.

EARLY KNEE MOTION

Continuous Passive Motion: Theory and Principles

The concept of early motion after TKA began with the work of Salter after he observed that prolonged immobilization of synovial joints yielded persistent stiffness, pain, muscle atrophy, disuse osteopenia, and subsequent degenerative arthritis. Salter hypothesized that CPM could augment articular cartilage nutrition, stimulate mesenchymal cell differentiation into articular cartilage, and accelerate the healing of periarticular tissues. Subsequent work published by Salter demonstrated that CPM improved tendon healing, decreased the time of hemarthrosis clearance from a joint, enhanced surgical wound healing, decreased patient surgical pain, and more.[26]

Modern CPM consists of an electrically powered device upon which the operative leg rests and is taken through a ROM that is determined by the user, at a speed that can be modulated by the user as well (Fig. 186.1). Salter's original human protocol was 23 hours per day of CPM for 1 to 4 weeks.[27] Although not designed specifically for the postarthroplasty population, the effect of CPM on ROM and outcomes after TKA have been extensively studied.

Effect of Continuous Passive Motion on Range of Motion. Early support for CPM was generated by research that demonstrated its use was associated with significantly decreased duration of hospital stay and earlier achievement of functional ROM.* Some data suggested that CPM was more cost-effective and as effective as physical therapy in the hospital and at home after discharge.[19,30] Some data has suggested decreases in postoperative analgesia requirements and decreased postoperative wound complications.[6]

Insall and his group also contributed to the early body of literature supporting CPM. The group studied 42 patients using CPM after TKA compared to 20 controls who did not use CPM. Their data demonstrated that patients using CPM achieved 90 degrees of flexion more rapidly than those who did not, and that these patients were subsequently discharged from the hospital more rapidly than those not using CPM. At that time, achieving 90 degrees of motion was a requirement for hospital discharge. In this study, use of CPM was associated with a 30% decrease in the incidence of postoperative venous thromboembolic events (VTE). The authors did report that the ultimate ROM at time of discharge was not different between the groups, suggesting that CPM use increased the rate of motion gain, but not necessarily the final motion range.[28]

More support came from Coutts et al. who studied 82 patients undergoing TKA. Thirty of these patients were immobilized in plaster splints for 3 days postoperatively and thereafter mobilized, whereas the remaining patients were placed in a CPM device immediately following surgery and received CPM therapy for 20 hours per day. Coutts found that patients using CPM achieved 102 degrees of flexion by time of discharge, whereas those who were immediately immobilized achieved only 80 degrees of flexion at time of discharge. They found this trend was maintained at 1 year postoperatively with CPM patients achieving 115 degrees of flexion compared to 100 degrees in the control group.[7]

Wasilewski et al. performed a matched cohort comparison of patients who underwent TKA followed by postoperative immobilization for 3 days or immediate CPM. The patients in their CPM group had lower rates of wound healing complication and thromboembolic disease, had lower analgesic

---

*References 7, 8, 11, 17, 19, and 25.

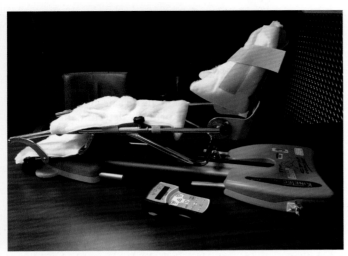

FIG 186.1 Modern Continuous Passive Motion Machine

requirements, and achieved straight-leg raise earlier.[29] Both groups had similar final ROM after surgery.

Despite this early support, several authors believed that the magnitude of benefit from CPM was questionable and potentially dose dependent. Two early retrospective studies found that postoperative CPM use was not associated with any appreciable clinical benefit in the hospital or in the posthospital rehabilitation setting.[20,22] Subsequently, a number of randomized prospective trials were performed that evaluate CPM versus no CPM after TKA.[†]

Pope et al. performed a prospective, randomized controlled trial (RCT) comparing postoperative extension splinting and regular physical therapy (PT) with immediate postoperative CPM application for 20 out of 24 hours per day during the hospital stay. They found that CPM yielded a significant increase in flexion and total ROM at 1 week postoperatively, but this difference had disappeared by 1 year. They found that CPM patients had a significant increase in analgesia requirement and an increase in surgical site drainage postoperatively.[23]

Bennett et al. studied the effect of CPM protocols on postoperative ROM after TKA. They prospectively randomized 147 patients to three different CPM protocols, including no CPM. They found that patients on an "early flexion" protocol of 90 to 50 degrees with gradual progression to full extension had significantly greater range of active and passive flexion than other groups at postoperative day 5, but this advantage normalized at the 3-month and 1-year time points. They found no difference between groups in patient length of stay, postoperative pain scores, wound healing time, Knee Society Clinical Rating System scores, and perceived health status according to the short form 12-item survey (SF-12). There were no significant differences in groups at 3-, 6-, and 12-month follow-up.[2]

Bruun-Olsen et al. conducted an RCT of 63 primary TKA patients who were randomized in two groups; the first group had active exercises with no CPM and the second group had active exercises with CPM. At 3-month follow up, they found no significant differences between treatment groups for postoperative ROM, visual analogue scale (VAS) scores, timed

up-and-go test, timed 40-minute walking distance, and timed stair climbing.[5]

Alkire and Swank looked at the use of CPM following computer-assisted (CA) primary TKA and evaluated the effect of CPM versus no CPM on postoperative ROM, wound drainage, functional ability, and pain. Their randomized prospective study of 65 patients found that the cohorts had statistically equivalent ROM and VAS pain scores at 2-week, 6-week, and 3-month follow-up.[1]

Maniar et al. prospectively evaluated CPM in 84 patients who were randomized to receive no CPM, 1 day of CPM, or 3 days of CPM and compared their clinical and functional outcomes based on the timed up-and-go test, the Western Ontario and McMaster Universities (WOMAC) score, SF-12 status, ROM, knee and calf swelling, and wound healing. They found no significant difference among patients on postoperative days 3, 5, 14, 42, and 90. The authors subsequently discontinued the use of CPM at their institution.[18]

Nadler et al. studied the usefulness of CPM use on patients admitted to an inpatient rehabilitation unit after hospital discharge. They retrospectively reviewed the charts of 29 patients who used CPM for 3 to 4 hours per day as an adjunct to physical therapy and 32 patients who had physical therapy alone. They reported no difference in knee motion or length of stay between groups, suggesting that the usefulness of CPM after hospital discharge is limited.[20]

Kumar et al. performed an RCT comparing the use of CPM after TKA with patients who underwent a flexed-knee arthrotomy closure in the operating room followed by an early 90-degree passive flexion protocol—aptly termed *drop and dangle* because of the mechanism of passive flexion (patients sat in a chair on postoperative day 1 and dangled the leg at 90 degrees). The authors found that drop and dangle allowed earlier discharge and statistically better knee extension at 6-month follow-up. The drop-and-dangle protocol was also associated with less wound drainage. The authors concluded that flexed-knee arthrotomy closure allowed improved early passive motion that surpassed extended-knee closures with CPM.[13]

MacDonald et al. performed a randomized controlled trial of 120 patients who underwent TKA. Patients were randomly assigned to one of three groups—no CPM, CPM from 0 to 50 with increases as tolerated, and CPM from 70 to 110. They found no differences in pain scores or analgesia requirements between groups. They found no difference in motion between groups at discharge, 6 weeks, 12 weeks, 26 weeks, and 52 weeks postoperatively. They concluded that CPM was not a useful postoperative tool.[16]

Lau et al. randomized 26 TKAs to CPM versus immobilization for the first postoperative week. The authors found that early active motion was improved in the CPM patients, but by day 28 the motion improvement had disappeared and the groups were similar. The authors also performed the same study on 17 patients who underwent one-stage bilateral TKA, with the first knee being treated with CPM and the second knee acting as an internal control. The same results were found. There were no differences in knee ROM found at 4 weeks postoperatively. The authors concluded that early CPM does not guarantee—and immobilization does not preclude—good knee ROM.[14]

Boese et al. performed an RCT of 160 patients who underwent TKA, randomized into three immediate postoperative

CPM protocols: no CPM, CPM applied with active knee motion, CPM applied with the knee fixed to 90 degrees flexion. They found no difference between the groups with respect to any outcome measure including knee ROM, VAS pain scores, perioperative hemoglobin drop, or change in knee girth. They concluded that CPM offered no benefit and was an unwarranted increase in perioperative cost.[3]

Most recently, Joshi et al. randomized 109 patients undergoing unilateral TKA to receive CPM or no CPM in addition to a standard physical therapy protocol. They found no difference in knee flexion at 6 weeks and 3 months postoperatively. They also found that patients who used CPM had significantly longer hospital stays, and the use of CPM during the hospital stay was $235.50 per TKA.[12]

Harvey et al. provided the highest level of evidence for post-TKA CPM through the Cochrane Foundation in a Cochrane Review. This group performed a systematic review and meta-analysis of available literature to determine the efficacy of CPM after TKA. They evaluated 24 RCTs including 1445 patients who underwent TKA. The review found that there was moderate-quality evidence that CPM did provide short-term benefits on knee ROM, knee function, and patient quality of life. There was low-quality evidence that CPM had any effect on postoperative pain control, rate of future need for manipulation under anesthesia, or risk of perioperative adverse events. They also reported insufficient evidence to comment on patient perceptions of CPM use on their rehabilitation.[9]

Effect of Continuous Passive Motion on Postoperative Venous Thrombotic Events. Some authors have suggested that postoperative CPM may decrease the incidence of VTE following TKA.[28] The theoretical basis for this is in the prevention of postoperative venous stasis, a component of the Virchow triad of venous thrombosis.

Lynch et al. sought to evaluate the effect of CPM in preventing deep venous thrombosis (DVT) in post-TKA patients. They studied 75 patients who used CPM and 75 patients who did not and found that CPM use did not decrease the risk of DVT after TKA.[15] Similar results were found in the previously cited study by Vince et al.[28] This prospective study found a 45% rate of thrombophlebitis after TKA with CPM use compared with a rate of 75% without. The authors thought that CPM was protective against thromboembolism in these patients.

In contrast, several studies have suggested that CPM has no influence on the incidence of postoperative thromboembolic events. The previously referenced study by Wasilewski et al. and McInnes et al. found no significant difference between CPM and no CPM groups with respect to the incidence of DVT.[19,29] In fact, the only DVT in the McInnes study occurred in the CPM group. Similarly, the previously referenced study by Kumar et al. found no difference in the incidence of DVT among patients receiving CPM compared to those who did not.[13]

Many more studies have been performed on this subject. In 2014, He et al., in conjunction with the Cochrane Group, performed a systematic review and meta-analysis of the available literature regarding the use of CPM and its effect on VTE after TKA. They evaluated 11 trials with 808 patients and concluded that the level of evidence is low and that most studies evaluated did not report the variables of interest. The authors concluded that sufficient evidence does not exist to support the use of CPM for prevention of VTE after TKA.[10]

SUMMARY

It seems that no consensus has been reached regarding a "most effective" postoperative mobilization protocol. Current practice includes a combination of early postoperative CPM, active motion, weight bearing, and multimodal analgesia. In today's era of managed care, the focus on safe and cost-effective delivery of care has become the primary determinant of hospital discharge. Patients are discharged typically as soon as they are medically stable and their pain is controlled. The use of modern knee arthroplasty techniques, components, and postoperative rehabilitation and discharge protocols make the early literature less relevant. Salter, in his early work, recommended a protocol involving at least 20 hours of CPM daily to achieve improved motion.[26] The dose dependence of CPM has been corroborated by some authors.[7,22] Such prolonged maintenance of CPM, however, is antithetical to many aspects of modern rehabilitation and early hospital discharge, and should not supersede early active motion exercises performed with physical therapists. The advantages of CPM seen in the early days of TKA appear to be offset by modern techniques and analgesia protocols.

The authors cannot currently endorse routine use of CPM as a mechanism of improving patient early or late ROM, function of the knee, or to alter the incidence of VTE after TKA. This conclusion is in accord with the highest level of evidence presented in Cochrane Database systematic reviews. Although CPM does not appear to cause any adverse effects, there is certainly some additional cost associated with its use.

On the other hand, patient satisfaction with CPM is a contentious issue. This has not been well studied and its effects are unknown. It is conceivable, however, that patient perceptions of rehabilitation may be affected by CPM use, and that use of the device may provide patients with reassurance and confidence in their progress. Additionally, in hospitals where multiple surgeons operate, if some surgeons use CPM and others do not, patients may wonder why their surgeon is not recommending CPM use. In such situations, the use of CPM should be determined by the individual surgeon.

Ranawat et al. have suggested that most TKA patients will obtain good postoperative motion and function regardless of the specific postoperative protocol used.[24] However, they do acknowledge a subset of patients who require more intensive efforts at rehabilitation, which frequently involves prolonged analgesia, physical therapy, social services, and occasionally manipulation. We feel that this statement accurately describes the current state of affairs.

The available evidence for a standard postoperative protocol in the context of a modern total joint arthroplasty pathway continues to evolve, and more research is needed to determine how to optimize outcomes in all patients. We suspect that postoperative motion protocols may need to be patient specific to truly optimize outcomes. A one-size-fits-all approach may not be the best strategy in our modern health care structure.

KEY REFERENCES

3. Boese CK, Weis M, Phillips T, et al: The efficacy of continuous passive motion after total knee arthroplasty: a comparison of three protocols. *J Arthroplasty* 29(6):1158–1162, 2014. doi: 10.1016/j.arth.2013.12.005.
5. Bruun-Olsen V, Heiberg KE, Mengshoel AM: Continuous passive motion as an adjunct to active exercises in early rehabilitation following total

knee arthroplasty—a randomized controlled trial. *Disabil Rehabil* 31(4):277–283, 2009. doi: 10.1080/09638280801931204.

6. Colwell CW, Morris BA: The influence of continuous passive motion on the results of total knee arthroplasty. *Clin Orthop Relat Res* 276(276):225–228, 1992.

7. Coutts RD, Toth C, Kaita JH: The role of continuous passive motion in the rehabilitation of the total knee patient. In Hungerford DS, Krakow KA, Kenna RV, editors: *Total knee arthroplasty: a comprehensive approach*, Baltimore, 1984, pp 126–132.

9. Harvey LA, Brosseau L, Herbert RD: Continuous passive motion following total knee arthroplasty in people with arthritis. *Cochrane Database Syst Rev* (2):CD004260, 2014. doi: 10.1002/14651858. CD004260.pub3.

11. Johnson DP, Eastwood DM: Beneficial effects of continuous passive motion after total condylar knee arthroplasty. *Ann R Coll Surg Engl* 74(6):412–416, 1992.

12. Joshi RN, White PB, Murray-Weir M, et al: Prospective randomized trial of the efficacy of continuous passive motion post total knee arthroplasty: experience of the hospital for special surgery. *J Arthroplasty* 30(12):2364–2369, 2015. doi: 10.1016/j.arth.2015.06.006.

16. MacDonald SJ, Bourne RB, Rorabeck CH, et al: Prospective randomized clinical trial of continuous passive motion after total knee arthroplasty. *Clin Orthop Relat Res* 380:30–35, 2000.

18. Maniar RN, Baviskar JV, Singhi T, et al: To use or not to use continuous passive motion post-total knee arthroplasty presenting functional assessment results in early recovery. *J Arthroplasty* 27(2):193–200, e1, 2012. doi: 10.1016/j.arth.2011.04.009.

19. McInnes J, Larson M, Daltroy LH, et al: A controlled evaluation of continuous passive motion in patients undergoing total knee arthroplasty. *JAMA* 268(11):1423–1428, 1992.

21. Nelson CL, Kim J, Lotke PA: Stiffness after total knee arthroplasty. *J Bone Joint Surg Am* 87(Suppl 1 Pt 2):264–270, 2005. doi: 10.2106/JBJS.E-00345.

22. Nielsen PT, Rechnagel K, Nielsen SE: No effect of continuous passive motion after arthroplasty of the knee. *Acta Orthop Scand* 59(5):580–581, 1988.

23. Pope RO, Corcoran S, McCaul K, et al: Continuous passive motion after primary total knee arthroplasty. Does it offer any benefits? *J Bone Joint Surg Br* 79(6):914–917, 1997.

24. Ranawat CS, Ranawat AS, Mehta A: Total knee arthroplasty rehabilitation protocol: what makes the difference? *J Arthroplasty* 18(3 Suppl 1):27–30, 2003. doi: 10.1054/arth.2003.50080.

26. Salter RB: The biologic concept of continuous passive motion of synovial joints. The first 18 years of basic research and its clinical application. *Clin Orthop Relat Res* 242:12–25, 1989.

27. Salter RB: Continuous passive motion: from origination to research to clinical applications. *J Rheumatol* 31(11):2104–2105, 2004.

The references for this chapter can also be found on www.expertconsult.com.

187

Cryotherapy After Total Knee Arthroplasty

Edward M. DelSole, Vinay K. Aggarwal, Parthiv A. Rathod, Ajit J. Deshmukh

INTRODUCTION

Cryotherapy is defined as the local use of low temperatures to treat a variety of medical conditions, with the goals of decreased inflammation, improved pain control, promotion of vasoconstriction, and prevention of muscle soreness and spasm.[10] The practice has been described in medical use as early as the 17th century and has long been an accepted method for treatment of musculoskeletal pain complaints and control of posttraumatic swelling.[5] When used near a superficial joint such as the knee, cryotherapy has also been shown to decrease the intra-articular temperature, which in conjunction with decreased nerve conduction velocities may provide a theoretical decrease in pain and blood flow to the joint.[1,7]

Cryotherapy can take many forms, ranging from the simple to the highly complex. First-generation therapy methods include basic ice packs affixed to the body with elastic bandages or cuffs. Second-generation products include commercially marketed continuous-flow cold sleeves, which may be enhanced via built-in pneumatic compression devices (Fig. 187.1). Finally, the newest version of cryotherapy may include computer-assisted cooling methods with controlled temperature modulation.[10]

In total knee arthroplasty (TKA), postoperative swelling and pain control have remained a significant obstacle for surgeons and patients alike. Despite the use of a variety of anesthetic protocols, including nerve blocks, indwelling catheters, and regional anesthesia, cryotherapy is heavily used around the country to adjunctively treat postoperative pain. The generally accepted theory is that cold therapy can help control swelling and thus improve wound healing, reduce drainage, enhance pain control, and ultimately lead to better rehabilitation outcomes after TKA surgery.

EARLY TRIALS

Healy et al. provide some of the earliest literature on use of specialized compressive cold cuff devices after TKA.[4] They prospectively randomized 50 patients to receive a compressive cold device, the Cryocuff (Aircast, Summit, New Jersey), and 55 patients to receive a simple ice pack therapy; they evaluated the two groups with regard to pain control, range of motion (ROM), knee/thigh swelling, and wound drainage. The study found no significant clinical difference between these groups in any of their outcome measures evaluated and was unable to recommend the Cryocuff over simple ice packs.

Although Healy's group did not compare cryotherapy to TKAs treated without any cold therapy, Morsi undertook a prospective study to evaluate the net benefit of cryotherapy in a cohort of 30 patients who underwent staged bilateral TKA.[8] The first TKA was treated postoperatively with a self-made noncommercial continuous-flow cold therapy device. The second TKA was performed 6 weeks later and received no cryotherapy. Morsi observed that patients treated with cryotherapy had significantly lower visual analog scale pain scores (VAS), lower narcotic consumption, lower hemovac output, lower total blood loss, and improved ROM at 1 and 2 weeks. The ROM difference between groups ultimately did normalize by the sixth postoperative week. This paper, which used an inherent control group via the same patient's contralateral TKA, suggested that cryotherapy carried significant analgesic and vasoconstrictive benefits compared to standard narcotic use alone without any cryotherapy.

Kullenberg et al. compared outcomes in 86 patients after TKA, randomized to using either 3 days of cold compression therapy or epidural anesthesia.[6] The authors hypothesized that it was not only the cold therapy that was vital in improving pain control and mobilization after TKA but the synergistic effects of compression as well. The results of the study were that the cold compression group (Cryocuff, Aircast, Summit, New Jersey) had significantly improved pain control measured on visual analog scores, better ROM at discharge, and even a significantly shorter hospital length of stay by 1.4 days.

In all the aforementioned studies, the authors reported no direct complications arising from the use of cryotherapy. However, in a case report by Dundon et al., the authors describe two patients who experienced total loss of skin over the patella after use of cryotherapy following TKA.[3] Both cases had necrotic skin tissue débrided and treated with wound care and plastic surgery teams to successfully assist healing via a variety of advanced wound management techniques.

ICE OR DEVICE?

One controversy in the use of cryotherapy is the concept of using standard ice packs or using "advanced therapy" consisting of iced cuffs or cryopneumatic compression devices, which deliver a dynamic compression and cooling to the surgical extremity. There are obvious cost implications of both treatment modalities; however, outcome studies are somewhat limited. As mentioned previously, the 1994 study by Healy et al. found no difference in ice pack therapy and the Cryocuff.

A more recent study in 2012 by Su et al. performed a blinded multicenter randomized control trial on the effect of a cryopneumatic cuff (GameReady device, Coolsystems, Inc., San Diego, California) versus static ice therapy after TKA.[9] The

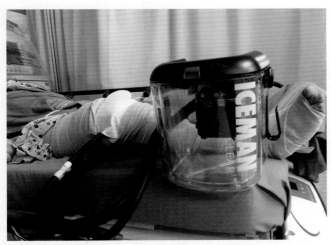

FIG 187.1 A Current Example of a Continuous Cold-Flow Cryotherapy Device The container in the foreground is filled with water and ice. A cuff is wrapped around the surgical extremity, connected to the ice water reservoir by a rubber conduit. The power source is applied, which cycles cold water through the cuff at designated intervals to provide cooling to the surgical site.

authors evaluated 280 patients across 11 hospitals randomized to each intervention and looked at outcome measures based on ROM, knee girth, 6-minute walk test (6MWT), timed up-and-go test (TUG), visual analog pain scores, and narcotic consumption. Cryotherapy in both arms of the study was worn for 2 hours on, 1 hour off for four daily cycles while in the hospital. After discharge the duration was changed to 1 hour on and 30 minutes off. The authors found that at 2 weeks postoperatively, there was no difference between groups in ROM, 6MWT, TUG, or knee girth. There was a significant decrease in narcotic consumption in the treatment group at 2 weeks but not at 6 weeks. Interestingly, this study commented on patient satisfaction scores with cooling therapy and found patients using the cryopneumatic cuff experienced significantly higher satisfaction than those with just ice packs.

Another randomized control trial comparing a cooling device to ice packs after TKA performed in Canada by Bech et al. showed similar results.[2] They found no difference in primary or secondary outcomes of numerical pain rating scale, ROM, opioid use, blood loss, or length of stay. However, they did report increased patient satisfaction scores in the device intervention group.

In 2014 Thienpont also investigated the role of an advanced cryotherapy device on postoperative pain control compared to a traditional ice pack protocol.[10] Both the device and ice pack groups contained 50 patients randomized to each group. Primary outcomes included visual analog pain scores and analgesic use. The results demonstrated no significant pain reduction or difference in analgesic use between groups. However, the authors do report that in the cryotherapy treatment group, there was a decrease in active flexion of 6 degrees (120 vs. 114 degrees) at 6 weeks postoperatively, which they found to be statistically significant. They attributed this to immobilization of the knee in extension during prolonged cryotherapy sessions.

Once again no consistent conclusions can be drawn regarding advantages or disadvantages of advanced cryotherapy devices compared to ice packs, based on the often conflicting results of current randomized trials in the literature.

PUTTING THE EVIDENCE TOGETHER

Although several independent studies with conflicting conclusions exist regarding the use of cryotherapy in knee arthroplasty outcomes, Adie et al. synthesized the results of the literature in a systematic review and meta-analysis in 2010 of all available randomized controlled trials available. The meta-analysis included 11 studies with 793 TKAs. Within the 11 studies, there was substantial heterogeneity in study design and cryotherapy protocol. The results of this study suggested that cryotherapy provides some mild improvement in postoperative blood loss and ROM at discharge. However, there were no identifiable improvements in pain control, analgesia requirement, swelling, length of hospital stay, and knee motion after discharge. The results of the meta-analysis yielded no perceivable benefits of cryotherapy use in the long term.

Adie et al. followed up on this study in 2012 with their Cochrane Database Systematic Review article, which included 12 trials with 809 total patients. They reported that all studies had low to very low quality of evidence, with small improvements on postoperative blood loss, VAS pain score, ROM, and transfusion rate. The clinical significance of these mild improvements was low and thus called into question the actual impact of cryotherapy on final outcomes after TKA. In this study, the authors concluded that the benefits of cryotherapy might be too small to justify the inconvenience and cost of its use.

CONCLUSION

Based upon the best available evidence at this time, we cannot recommend standard postoperative use of cryotherapy after TKA. Aside from isolated case reports, most literature does not note any major evidence of harm in using postoperative cryotherapy other than costs associated with advanced manufactured devices. The best available evidence suggests its use may decrease early post-TKA pain scores and analgesic requirements; however, this has not been uniformly proven in all studies and may ultimately not be clinically meaningful. Cryotherapy appears safe to use, although it has been associated with decreased active flexion at 6 weeks. The long-term effects of post-TKA cryotherapy at this time are unknown. The effects of cryotherapy on knee function, quality of life, and activity level are unknown. We could not identify any cost-effectiveness studies to date concerning cryotherapy after TKA.

The references for this chapter can also be found on www.expertconsult.com.

188

Immediate Motion versus Splinting After Total Knee Arthroplasty

Edward M. DelSole, David P. Taormina, Claudette Lajam, Ajit J. Deshmukh

The debate between early range of motion (ROM) versus splinting after total knee arthroplasty (TKA) has been waged for decades. The basis for early ROM is to protect patients against the risk of arthrofibrosis and postoperative knee stiffness. Splinting in extension or flexion has been thought to minimize the risk of flexion contracture or lack of flexion, respectively. Given that TKA is intended to be a function-restoring surgery and, in most cases, an ROM-restoring procedure, common practice includes early ROM after TKA.

Nonetheless, there are advantages and disadvantages associated with early ROM versus splinting after surgery. The disadvantages include blood loss, wound healing issues, pain control, diversion of patient and health care system resources, and potential effects on hospital length of stay (which may be confounded by other factors). Modern TKA protocols with emphasis on early and safe discharge from the hospital warrant a scientific basis for postoperative practices. This chapter addresses the use of postoperative splinting (extension vs flexion) and early ROM after TKA.

EARLY KNEE SPLINTING

Extension Splinting

Early semirigid extension splinting of the knee after TKA has been advocated. In early protocols, splints were applied intraoperatively to the extremity and maintained for up to 10 days with the aims to prevent postoperative fixed flexion deformity, keep dressings in place, minimize wound complications, and optimize postoperative pain control. Flexion contracture after TKA is a debilitating complication that is difficult to correct. The clinical manifestation of this entity is a partially flexed knee on which the quadriceps must continually contract to prevent buckling with applied loads. This ultimately leads to fatigue, decreased walking velocity, alteration of global truncal alignment, and overload of the contralateral leg.[12]

Routine prolonged splinting has generally fallen out of favor after studies suggesting minimal benefit to the practice.[5,14] Horton and colleagues[5] performed a randomized controlled trial of post-TKA patients undergoing early postoperative extension splinting for 48 hours versus no splinting. After 48 hours of splinting, flexion contracture was no different than in patients without splinting. At 3 months of follow-up, there continued to be no measurable effect of splinting on ROM or knee extension.

Zenios and coworkers[14] performed a randomized controlled trial of 48 hours of postoperative extension splinting versus no splinting. They found no difference in knee extension at 5 days or 6 weeks postoperatively. Patients who underwent splinting had significantly less flexion at 5 days and 6 weeks. Patients who underwent splinting had significantly less perioperative wound drainage than patients who did not undergo splinting; however, there was no difference in postoperative wound complications (dehiscence or infection) between groups.

Flexion Splinting

Some authors have advocated the use of flexion splinting after TKA.[4,9] Surgeons have theorized that flexion splinting could improve postoperative ROM, decrease wound drainage, and decrease blood transfusion requirement. It was thought that aggressive rehabilitation after flexion splinting would obviate the need for extension splinting to prevent fixed flexion deformity.

Ong and Taylor[9] presented early support for flexion splinting in a prospective trial of patients randomly assigned to three groups after TKA: (1) knee extended on the bed, (2) hip flexed to 35 degrees with knee flexed to 70 degrees, and (3) hip flexed to 35 degrees with knee fully extended. Patients with flexion splinting were splinted for the first 6 hours postoperatively and then taken down from this position. There was no difference in postoperative motion arc between groups, with all patients obtaining a mean motion arc of 80 degrees by postoperative day six. At 48 hours, both the 70 degrees flexion group and the 35 degrees hip flexion/knee extension group had 25% less decrease in hemoglobin compared with the group with the knee extended on the bed; however transfusion rates were no different.

Ma and associates[8] performed a randomized controlled study comparing 24 hours of fixed 70 degrees flexion splinting with fixed full extension splinting. They analyzed the groups for postoperative flexion, extension, drain output, hemoglobin decrease, blood transfusion needs, length of stay, and 6-week ROM and found there was no difference among any of these variables. The authors did not endorse flexion splinting.

Hewitt and Shakespeare[4] performed a prospective trial comparing postoperative static flexion with active extension protocols. Patients in the flexion group were held at 90 degrees flexion during the first postoperative night and then progressed to alternating 90 degrees static flexion and active physical rehabilitation exercises. Patients in the flexion group had shorter length of hospital stay (discharged 1 day sooner) and had a greater total ROM at 6 weeks. There was no difference in fixed flexion deformity between groups.

A prospective study by Li and colleagues[7] randomly assigned 110 patients to postoperative flexion or extension with leg elevation at 30 degrees. The patients in the flexion group kept their knees at 30 degrees flexion during the first 72 hours postoperatively, and the patients in the extension group had their knees maintained at 0 degree. Blood loss, hidden blood loss, swelling, ROM, and flexion deformity were analyzed at 6 weeks after surgery. Hidden blood loss was approximated by weighing dressings postoperatively. In the first week after surgery, patients in flexion had less blood loss, less swelling, and greater knee flexion. At 6 weeks follow-up, the groups averaged 98 degrees and 96 degrees of flexion, respectively, and there was no statistical difference.

In their systematic review, Faldini and associates[3] analyzed postoperative protocols of seven studies to determine the significance of flexion versus extension splinting and effect on blood loss and ROM. Overall, they found that a 48- to 72-hour postoperative period including a flexion protocol was an easy and cost-effective means for reducing blood loss and increasing ROM after TKA. Although the general protocols differed between the studies reviewed, there was a general trend toward early postoperative benefits (during the first week after surgery) of flexion versus extension protocols. However, these findings were generally insignificant at greater than 6 weeks of follow-up.

In a prospective randomized controlled study, Yang and colleagues[13] enrolled 46 patients who were assigned to a flexion or an extension group. The flexion group was maintained at 60 degrees with elevation at the hip of 60 degrees, whereas the extension group maintained full extension of the knee for 48 hours postoperatively. After 6 weeks, the flexion group had significantly better ROM. At 6 months, the difference was lost. One other finding was that hospital stay was decreased by 1.9 days in the flexion group. There was no difference in wound complications, infection, or deep vein thrombosis rates.

EARLY KNEE MOTION

The concept of early motion after TKA began with the work of Salter,[10,11] who reported that prolonged immobilization of synovial joints resulted in persistent stiffness, pain, muscle atrophy, disuse osteopenia, and subsequent degenerative arthritis. Early motion could be provided with the help of a continuous passive motion (CPM) device as well as active ROM and physical therapy protocols. Many researchers have studied the effects of CPM therapy after TKA. CPM is discussed in detail in Chapter 186. CPM does not appear to have any significant advantage in terms of achieving ROM and desired knee function after TKA compared with active ROM and physical therapy protocols.[1,6]

Some authors have compared the results of splinting with results of CPM. Coutts and colleagues[2] studied 82 patients undergoing TKA. Of these patients, 30 were immobilized in plaster splints for 3 days postoperatively and then mobilized, and the remaining patients were placed in a CPM device immediately after surgery and received CPM therapy for 20 hours per day. The authors found that patients receiving CPM therapy achieved 102 degrees of flexion by the time of discharge, whereas patients who were immediately immobilized achieved only 80 degrees of flexion by discharge. This trend was maintained at 1 year postoperatively, with patients in the CPM group achieving 115 degrees of flexion compared with 100 degrees in the control group.[2] This study suggests that CPM is superior to early extension splinting in terms of achievement of final ROM after TKA.

SUMMARY

No consensus has been reached regarding the most effective postoperative mobilization protocol after TKA. Current practice includes a combination of early active ROM with or without early postoperative CPM, weight bearing, and multimodal analgesia. In the present era of managed care, the focus on safe and cost-effective delivery of care has become the primary determinant of hospital discharge. Patients are discharged typically as soon as they are medically stable and their pain is controlled. The use of modern knee arthroplasty techniques and components and postoperative rehabilitation and discharge protocols makes early literature less relevant. Prior reports showing decreased length of hospital stay may no longer be applicable because of the changes in present discharge criteria.

There is evidence to recommend against routine postoperative splinting after primary TKA. There may be a role for extension splinting in revision procedures or in selected cases after correction of substantial flexion contracture in primary TKA; however, this has not been well studied.

Compared with splinting, early active and passive ROM does not significantly alter measurable and hidden blood loss, wound healing, and postoperative pain after primary TKA and is associated with better ROM. Therefore, common practice after primary TKA includes early ROM after surgery with a general avoidance of postoperative splinting. Early motion, whether achieved through physical therapy or CPM, appears to be important to long-term functional outcome.

KEY REFERENCES

5. Horton T, et al: Is routine splintage following primary total knee replacement necessary? A prospective randomised trial. *Knee* 9:229–231, 2002.
8. Ma T, et al: Effect of flexion/extension splintage post total knee arthroplasty on blood loss and range of motion—a randomised controlled trial. *Knee* 15:15–19, 2008.
14. Zenios M, et al: The use of knee splints after total knee replacements. *Knee* 9:225–228, 2002.

The references for this chapter can also be found on www.expertconsult.com.

189

Internet-Based versus In-Person Physical Therapy After Total Knee Arthroplasty

Vincent M. Moretti, Nayoung Kim, Peter F. Sharkey

Annual total knee arthroplasty (TKA) volume in the United States is projected to grow to more than 3.5 million by 2030.[19] Much of the popularity and increasing demand for TKA undoubtedly stems from its excellent outcomes, including significant improvement in quality of life and relatively high patient satisfaction.[2,30,31] However, these results are not immediate. In the early postoperative period, TKA has a profound detrimental effect on muscle function, muscle strength, gait, and activities of daily living.[12,15,21,24,25,32,33] This detrimental effect is presumably a direct consequence of the surgery, with the resultant pain and swelling leading to neuromuscular inhibition, decreased mobility, and muscle atrophy.[25,32] Postoperative physical therapy is almost universally recommended after TKA to help reverse these early musculoskeletal declines and optimize long-term outcomes.[20,23]

Physical therapy has traditionally been thought of as a service of care provided under the direction and supervision of a trained and certified physical therapist. After TKA, physical therapy has historically been delivered in several settings, including inpatient rehabilitation facilities, home-based physical therapist visits, and outpatient physical therapy facilities.[20,23] A common protocol after TKA involves 6 to 12 weeks of physical therapy under the guidance of a physical therapist in a sequential combination of all three settings. Immediately after surgery, patients typically remain at the hospital for at least 1 to 2 days for monitored recovery. During this time, physical therapists mobilize the patient while practicing range of motion, muscle strengthening, gait training, and activities of daily living. Patients able to be discharged to home often next receive 1 to 2 weeks of home physical therapy with a visiting physical therapist followed by an additional 5 to 10 weeks of sessions at an outpatient physical therapy facility.

Although a combination of inpatient, home-based, and outpatient physical therapy has been the standard of care after TKA for many years, there is a growing interest in Internet-based physical therapy programs (Fig. 189.1).* The Internet provides an alternative medium for patients and physical therapists to interact with one another in a convenient and potentially cost-effective manner. Internet-based physical therapy programs have been effectively used to help improve physical activity in patients with a variety of medical conditions, including diabetes, multiple sclerosis, heart failure, osteoarthritis, and other chronic diseases.[3,4,6,10,22,34,40] Programs specifically designed for patients after TKA have also been developed.[7,18,26-29,36,37] These Internet programs can come in many forms, but they all use up-to-date information and communication technologies to provide patients with remote access to rehabilitation services.

EXAMPLES OF INTERNET-BASED PHYSICAL THERAPY

Telerehabilitation

Telerehabilitation is a real-time form of physical therapy that can be delivered over Internet-based communication networks.[37] Most telerehabilitation programs use webcams and either a television or a computer screen to allow a patient to have real-time videoconference sessions with a physical therapist over the Internet.[7,18,26-29,36,37] The patient is able to see the physical therapist demonstrate exercises, ask questions, and report concerns. Likewise, the physical therapist is able to observe the patient completing the exercises, offer feedback, provide education, and track progression.

Several studies have investigated this form of telerehabilitation, demonstrating statistically and clinically significant improvements in physical and functional measurements from pretreatment to posttreatment assessment periods.[7,18,26-29,36,37] Patient and physical therapist satisfaction with telerehabilitation has also been evaluated and found to be high.[17,27,35] In direct comparisons with conventional physical therapy, multiple randomized controlled trials have shown equivalent outcomes with telerehabilitation for active knee flexion, active knee extension, hamstring length, knee swelling, visual analog pain scores, and conventional physical therapy.[18,26,28,29,36] Some of these randomized controlled trials have demonstrated significantly better results for telerehabilitation compared with conventional physical therapy in measures such as quadriceps strength and 36-Item Short Form Health Survey scores.[18,26,28,29]

Website-Based or Software-Based Rehabilitation

Website-based or software-based rehabilitation is another version of Internet-based physical therapy. This mode of rehabilitation is fairly new and takes advantage of the growing popularity and comfort with computer, tablet, and smartphone app technology.[6,40] After TKA, health care providers can offer their patients downloadable software or applications for their computer or mobile devices. Through these program interfaces, the patient can watch prerecorded videos and simulations demonstrating standard postoperative exercises. Reading material and other educational content can also be provided. The specific set of exercises and rehabilitation protocols can be personally created and uniquely assigned to each patient, depending on the patient's activity tolerance, goals, or needs.

---

*References 1, 3-7, 10, 18, 22, 26-29, 34, 36, 37, and 40.

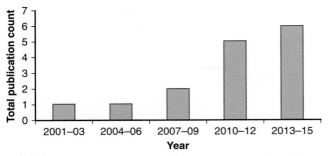

FIG 189.1 The annual number of publications in PubMed on topics related to Internet-based physical therapy for total knee arthroplasty has increased over the past 15 years. Data based on a systematic keyword search for "total knee," "knee replacement," or "knee arthroplasty" combined with "telerehabilitation," "teletherapy," "telemedicine," "Internet-based therapy," or "web-based therapy."

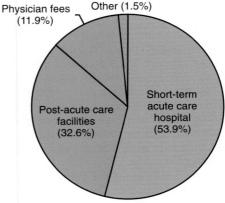

FIG 189.2 Percent of Medicare payments in the United States by setting for lower extremity joint replacement for 30-day fixed-length episodes between 2007 and 2009. (Data from Dobson A, et al: Medicare payment bundling: insights from claims data and policy implications. American Hospital Association and Association of American Medical Colleges. 2012.)

Through this platform, patients report their success or difficulty in performing each task, which helps health care providers regularly track each patient's compliance, outcomes, and subjective findings. These programs are predominantly self-driven by the patient, with minimal professional supervision. However, most programs allow and encourage frequent contact with the physical therapist or health care provider through electronic mail.

Data in the literature on the adequacy or outcomes of website-based or software-based physical therapy programs for TKA appear to be sparse. However, a few studies have used similarly designed physical therapy programs for patients with osteoarthritis, demonstrating effective clinical improvement with high patient satisfaction scores.[6,40] A randomized controlled trial by Urbani and colleagues[38] compared a group of patients after total hip arthroplasty who received outpatient physical therapy versus a group prescribed unsupervised home-based exercises. Primary outcomes in this study were the Harris hip score, Western Ontario and McMaster Universities Osteoarthritis Index, and 36-Item Short Form Health Survey. No significant difference was found between the groups in any of these outcome scores, suggesting that self-driven unsupervised rehabilitation can potentially be done in patients with total joint arthroplasty.

ADVANTAGES OF INTERNET-BASED PHYSICAL THERAPY

Internet-based physical therapy allows patients to have increased access to rehabilitation services. This is particularly beneficial for patients who live in rural or remote areas where outpatient physical therapy centers may be inconvenient or inaccessible. Additionally, in some health care systems and insurance plans, patients living in urban environments may have physical access to rehabilitation services, but there may be inadequate availability. For example, in Canada, it was reported that available rehabilitation resources will not meet the needs of their growing volume of patients with TKA.[37] This deficit was blamed on a lack of accessible services and a lack of health care professionals. Restrictive insurance carriers can similarly decrease availability by limiting patients to certain physical therapists covered by the insurance plan. This situation can potentially lead to excessive patient volumes per physical therapist and scheduling delays.

Internet-based physical therapy can benefit this patient population by allowing each individual physical therapist to work with and monitor a larger volume of patients, particularly with website-based or software-based programs. These automated patient-driven programs do not require constant or immediate input from the health care professional. Improved efficiency in physical therapist utilization offers the potential to immediately increase rehabilitation availability without any significant burden on the health care system.

Besides access and availability, Internet-based physical therapy can also offer a more convenient rehabilitation experience. With many website-based or software-based programs, patients can access their rehabilitation plan online 24 hours a day. No longer restricted to a physical therapist's appointment schedule or a facility's hours of operation, patients can complete their exercises on any day and at any time that is most convenient for them, such as on holidays, while away on vacation, late at night, or early in the morning. These features can be especially appealing for individuals who want to work in their own environment and in their own time.

The greatest advantage of Internet-based physical therapy over traditional in-person physical therapy is potentially the cost difference. Direct and indirect expenditures may be significantly lower for both the patient and the health care system. The patient's time and money spent traveling to and waiting at an outpatient physical therapy facility can be decreased, if not completely eliminated, with Internet-based programs. Additionally, the health care system as a whole can potentially reap significant savings by increasing the utilization of Internet-based physical therapy after TKA. At the present time, nearly one-third of the health care system's direct costs for a total joint arthroplasty go toward physical therapy and other post–acute care services (Fig. 189.2).[8] For Medicare patients in the United States, the annual cost for physical therapy after total joint replacement totaled more than $645 million in 2015.[23] Internet-based physical therapy has demonstrated lower costs compared with traditional physical therapy in the treatment of patients with medical conditions and has been suggested to offer cost savings of 18% to 123% in patients with TKA.[9,11,16,37]

DISADVANTAGES OF INTERNET-BASED PHYSICAL THERAPY

Internet-based physical therapy after TKA has several disadvantages. One major concern is the decreased direct contact from health care providers, which may risk safety. Without frequent in-person interactions, subtle signs or symptoms of a potentially severe problem, such as an infection, could be missed.[39] Patients may also misrepresent or misinterpret their progress in the self-driven website-based or software-based programs. This could potentially lead to complications and poor outcomes for a subset of patients.

The access and reliability of the Internet-based technology have also been questioned. Not all patients have a computer or Internet connection. Approximately 73.5% of Europeans and 87.9% of North Americans have Internet access.[13] Although these percentages are increasing nearly every year, the elderly subset of the population consistently has the lowest rates of Internet access, and this is the same population that comprises most patients with TKA.[13,14] For patients without the technologic equipment, additional costs will be required to provide it, which will have to be borne by either the patient or the healthcare system. Training will also be required on how to use this technologic equipment. Similarly, the exercise equipment available at most physical therapy centers is far different from equipment that is available in most homes. Internet-based rehabilitation protocols have to be altered to account for this deficiency. Some exercises can be completed with a creative repurposing of common household items. Others will require specialized exercise equipment to be provided for home use, but this is yet another potential cost to the patient or system.

Another disadvantage of Internet-based physical therapy programs is that they are not ideal for every patient. This type of rehabilitation relies heavily on the self-application and self-motivation of patients. Patients need a certain level of education and technologic understanding to succeed in these models.[14,38] As demonstrated by the study by Urbani and colleagues,[38] older patients with joint arthroplasty may be especially prone to unsupervised physical therapy failures.

CONCLUSION AND FUTURE DIRECTIONS

Internet-based physical therapy has the potential to revolutionize TKA rehabilitation. These interactive programs offer patients an accommodating and economical alternative to traditional physical therapy. They have the potential to increase access, availability, and convenience of rehabilitation services, while lowering the costs and health care burden. However Internet-based physical therapy remains a developing field. As information and communication technologies continue to evolve, further improvements in Internet-based physical therapy are sure to follow. Additional research is needed to confirm the clinical equivalence of Internet-based physical therapy to traditional in-person programs and to determine which patents are best suited for each option.

KEY REFERENCES

6. Brooks MA, et al: Web-based therapeutic exercise resource center as a treatment for knee osteoarthritis: a prospective cohort pilot study. *BMC Musculoskelet Disord* 15:158, 2014.

7. Cabana F, et al: Interrater agreement between telerehabilitation and face-to-face clinical outcome measurements for total knee arthroplasty. *Telemed J E Health* 16:293–298, 2010.

14. Jenkins PJ, et al: Socioeconomic deprivation and age are barriers to the online collection of patient reported outcome measures in orthopaedic patients. *Ann R Coll Surg Engl* 98:40–44, 2016.

17. Kairy D, et al: The patient's perspective of in-home telerehabilitation physiotherapy services following total knee arthroplasty. *Int J Environ Res Public Health* 10:3998–4011, 2013.

18. Kramer JF, et al: Comparison of clinic- and home-based rehabilitation programs after total knee arthroplasty. *Clin Orthop Relat Res* 410:225–234, 2003.

20. Lingard EA, et al: Management and care of patients undergoing total knee arthroplasty: variations across different health care settings. *Arthritis Care Res* 13:129–136, 2000.

23. Ong KL, et al: Prevalence and costs of rehabilitation and physical therapy after primary TJA. *J Arthroplasty* 30:1121–1126, 2015.

26. Piqueras M, et al: Effectiveness of an interactive virtual telerehabilitation system in patients after total knee arthroplasty: a randomized controlled trial. *J Rehabil Med* 45:392–396, 2013.

27. Russell TG, et al: Rehabilitation after total knee replacement via low-bandwidth telemedicine: the patient and therapist experience. *J Telemed Telecare* 10(Suppl 1):85–87, 2004.

28. Russell TG, et al: Internet-based outpatient telerehabilitation for patients following total knee arthroplasty: a randomized controlled trial. *J Bone Joint Surg Am* 93:113–120, 2011.

29. Shukla H, et al: Role of telerehabilitation in patients following total knee arthroplasty: evidence from a systematic literature review and meta-analysis. *J Telemed Telecare* 2016.

35. Tousignant M, et al: Patients' satisfaction of healthcare services and perception with in-home telerehabilitation and physiotherapists' satisfaction toward technology for post-knee arthroplasty: an embedded study in a randomized trial. *Telemed J E Health* 17:376–382, 2011.

36. Tousignant M, et al: A randomized controlled trial of home telerehabilitation for post-knee arthroplasty. *J Telemed Telecare* 17:195–198, 2011.

37. Tousignant M, et al: Cost analysis of in-home telerehabilitation for post-knee arthroplasty. *J Med Internet Res* 17:e83, 2015.

38. Urbani BT, et al: Formal physical therapy after primary total hip arthroplasty may not be necessary. Abstract presented at AAHKS Annual Meeting. 2015 Nov.

40. Williams QI, et al: Physical therapy vs. internet-based exercise training (PATH-IN) for patients with knee osteoarthritis: study protocol of a randomized controlled trial. *BMC Musculoskelet Disord* 16:264, 2015.

The references for this chapter can also be found on www.expertconsult.com.

190

Venous Thromboembolic Disease: Etiology and Risk Factors After Total Knee Arthroplasty

Vincent D. Pellegrini, Jr.

In 1984, Insall[13] suggested that "prevention of thrombophlebitis and pulmonary embolism should be a major goal of every orthopaedic surgeon who performs total knee arthroplasty." Stulberg and colleagues[38] reported venographic evidence of deep venous thrombosis (DVT) in 84% of patients undergoing total knee arthroplasty (TKA) in the absence of any thromboembolism prophylaxis; there were no fatal pulmonary emboli and clinically evident pulmonary embolism (PE) occurred in 1.7% of patients. Stulberg and colleagues[38] concluded that "the positive venogram, although not itself associated with local symptoms, is of clinical significance."

The NIH Consensus Conference on Total Knee Replacement[21] concluded 20 years later that "the effectiveness of anticoagulation for the prevention of PE is unclear" and noted that prophylaxis recommendations were based "primarily on the reduction of deep venous thrombosis (DVT) detected by venography following TKR [total knee replacement] … and the available data indicate that DVT prophylaxis does not alter the occurrence of symptomatic DVTs or PE, although no individual study was large enough to statistically assess effects on the occurrence of PE." The authors concluded that "a randomized, placebo-controlled trial of prophylactic anticoagulation that assesses the outcomes of PE, bleeding, wound complications, and death seems warranted."[21]

In the 3 decades that followed Insall's initial warning, many advances contributed to the refinement of the technical procedure, but understanding and prevention of venous thromboembolism (VTE) after TKA would progress much less definitively. TKA and total hip arthroplasty (THA) together are the most commonly performed elective operations paid for by the Centers for Medicare and Medicaid Services in the United States. TKA procedures alone approach 750,000 annually and continue to increase in number as a result of the aging of the baby boomer generation. Venous thromboembolic disease (VTED) is the most common life-threatening complication for these patients and is responsible for readmission in approximately 1.7% of patients in the 90 days following the procedure. Fatal PE occurs in 0.1% to 0.5% of patients, accounting for more than 1000 deaths each year.[24,33] DVT may also be responsible for morbidity related to chronic venous insufficiency. Analysis of patients with venogram-confirmed asymptomatic DVT showed 67% to have signs and symptoms of postthrombotic syndrome 5 years postoperatively compared with only 32% who had negative postoperative venograms. However, postthrombotic morbidity is more common after "idiopathic" than after postoperative DVT, probably owing to the fact that most postoperative thrombosis is nonocclusive in nature, and flow past the thrombus is maintained.

Considerable effort has been directed at identifying the optimal method to prevent VTE after joint replacement. Despite advances in anticoagulation therapy and the adoption of prophylaxis as the standard of care, postoperative PE and DVT remain a considerable threat to the well-being of patients with joint replacements. VTED after TKA has been more resistant to anticoagulant prophylaxis than VTED after THA, and TKA accounts for more cases of in-hospital PE than THA. This situation has attracted considerable attention just as enthusiasm for performing TKA as an outpatient procedure is gaining momentum. However, use of potent anticoagulants to mitigate activation of thrombogenesis after TKA must necessarily be tempered by consideration of the bleeding risk after these procedures where hemostasis from exposed bony surfaces is imperfect and the skin envelope is intolerant of hematoma formation.[25] VTE after TKA is an important and unsolved clinical problem that warrants the attention of practitioners, researchers, and patients.

ETIOLOGY AND PATHOPHYSIOLOGY OF VENOUS THROMBOEMBOLISM

The underlying pathophysiology of VTED after total joint replacement depends on the intrusion of fatty tissue and bone marrow elements into the venous sinusoids of the intramedullary canal and into the systemic vascular tree. This intravasation of fat is a potent activator of the clotting cascade and incites a systemic condition of hypercoagulability after disruption of the intramedullary canal of long bones, no matter whether it is the result of traumatic injury or elective instrumentation during a total joint replacement procedure. The lung acts as a filter in clearing this embolic material, including both marrow elements and thrombus, from the bloodstream. The differences in embolic material, determined by the size and aggregate volume of fat, marrow elements, or clot, determine the nature of the response of the lung to the embolic insult. In fat embolism syndrome, this material consists primarily of fat globules and marrow elements enmeshed in platelets, whereas in the setting of PE, the embolic load is primarily clotted blood. Considering that musculoskeletal injury, disease, and related operative procedures frequently involve disruption of the marrow contents and associated fat, it is not surprising that both VTE and fat embolism syndrome are clinical conditions with a strong propensity to uniquely complicate the course of orthopedic patients.

Disruption of the intramedullary canal during TKA, with intravasation of marrow fat resulting from use of intramedullary alignment guides as well as canal preparation and pressurization during stem cementation, is a very potent stimulus of the clotting cascade. As such, it is essential that the orthopedic surgeon have a clear understanding of the pathophysiology and treatment of these conditions. This understanding is necessary not only to effectively care for and communicate about the patient, but also to place treatment of these complications in the context of the patient's overall medical management. Appropriate prophylaxis of VTED after TKA cannot be thoughtfully prescribed without balanced consideration of the predilection for thrombosis as well as the perioperative bleeding risk inherent to the arthroplasty procedure.

The components of Virchow triad—stasis, intimal injury, and hypercoagulability—have not changed since their original description and remain relevant today. In the setting of THA and TKA, a systemic clotting diathesis is evident; bilateral venogram endpoint trials have revealed a 10% to 15% prevalence of DVT in the contralateral nonoperative limb after each procedure. An awareness of the intense activation of the clotting cascade, which occurs during surgery and persists for longer than 24 hours, underscores the importance of initiation of thromboprophylaxis during, or soon after, surgery. It has been observed that activation of the clotting cascade occurs during instrumentation of the medullary canal during THA; elevation in prothrombin activation fragment F1.2, thrombin-antithrombin complexes, fibrinopeptide A, and D-dimer was most pronounced during insertion of a cemented femoral component and continued to increase for 1 hour postoperatively.[35] One might logically expect a similar phenomenon with intramedullary instrumentation of the distal femur and cementation of a tibial stem during TKA. On release of the tourniquet during TKA, transesophageal echocardiography has demonstrated "noise" in the echo pattern from embolic material; marrow elements, fat, and thrombi have been recovered from aspirated femoral vein blood samples during the procedure.[2] Such is the evidence base for the practice of sequential, rather than simultaneous, bilateral TKA procedures when performed under the same anesthetic, in an effort to monitor and limit the embolic load by deferring the second procedure if oxygen desaturation is evident after release of the tourniquet following TKA on the first side. Most convincing of the intraoperative activation of the clotting cascade is the observation in one study that 70% of patients who ultimately developed DVT after TKA had positive contrast venography within 24 hours after surgery.[18] The problem is compounded by stasis in the lower extremity caused by obstruction of the popliteal vein and venous outflow from hyperflexion of the knee necessary for component implantation during the procedure. It is unclear whether use of a tourniquet during TKA aggravates this clotting propensity by causing stasis in the leg or whether the known stimulation of endothelial cell–mediated fibrinolysis mitigates this effect and results in a lower prevalence of thrombosis than might be observed without a tourniquet.[1] Moreover, kinking of the femoral or popliteal veins can produce endothelial intimal injury that provides a nidus for the formation and propagation of clots, particularly in an environment where stasis is substantial.

It is unclear whether stasis or intimal injury plays the major incremental role in local thrombogenesis following TKA after intravasation of marrow fat creates a systemic hypercoagulable state. In the era before routine use of chemoprophylaxis, proximal DVT accounted for 50% to 60% of all observed thrombi after THA. Conversely, 90% of DVT originated distally, primarily in the calf veins, after TKA. Proximal DVT, defined as involving the popliteal vein or more proximally, occurs only infrequently after TKA and accounts for less than 10% of all thrombi. When present, proximal thrombi are nearly always contiguous with more distal clot in the calf and rarely extend above the popliteal vein. It is logical to assume that most DVT after TKA originates in the calf. This distinctive regional distribution of DVT after TKA, with a predilection for distal clots, has remained unchanged despite the influence of modern antithrombotic agents. It is plausible that either intimal damage or venous stasis, both of which may occur with abrupt folding of the popliteal vein during the procedure, could be operative in producing the observed distribution of DVT after TKA. With use of contemporary chemoprophylaxis after THA, more than 90% of deep thrombi now occur in the calf with only rare appearance of primary proximal clots. Proximal thrombi after THA are segmental in nature and appear in the femoral vein near the region of the lesser trochanter. The reduction of these proximal thrombi, where the femoral vein is subject to considerable torsion during femoral canal access and preparation, with regular use of anticoagulants is consistent with the known efficacy of these pharmacologic agents in preventing thrombosis associated with intimal damage in the vessel wall. Conversely, the lesser reduction in overall clot occurrence as well as the persistent prevalence of distal clots after TKA despite the regular use of potent anticoagulants suggests that stasis rather than intimal injury may be a stronger local stimulus to thrombosis after TKA. Given that most thrombi after TKA occur distal to the trifurcation and that the pattern of thrombosis has not changed with the pervasive use of perioperative anticoagulant prophylaxis, it seems likely that stasis is a more potent factor than intimal vessel damage in producing venous thrombosis after TKA.

The natural propensity for distal thrombi after TKA and proximal thrombi after THA may be explained by the predominance of different components of Virchow triad after each procedure. Proximal clots are likely the result of intimal injury to the femoral vein, which is twisted during positioning of the lower limb for femoral preparation and component insertion regardless of the surgical approach[4]; such intimal injury is best mitigated by potent anticoagulants, which have markedly decreased the prevalence of proximal thrombi after THA. Conversely, the prevalence of distal thrombi after TKA may be more likely the result of stasis secondary to folding and occlusion of the popliteal vein during shotgun exposure of the knee.[38] This clot distribution after TKA has been historically unaffected by either use or avoidance of the tourniquet. Distal thrombi more likely resulting from stasis might be reasonably predicted to be more refractory to prophylaxis with potent anticoagulants alone. Furthermore, distal DVT after TKA has been shown to be uniquely preventable by solitary use of intermittent pneumatic compression devices or regional anesthetic techniques that mitigate the effects of stasis on the lower limb.[37,39,40] In contrast, pneumatic compression devices alone have been associated with reduction in only calf thrombosis after THA, with persistence or even increase in the prevalence of proximal thrombosis in the femoral vein.[8,12,22] Although substantially improved from the 80% to 90% rates observed before routine prophylaxis, the residual thrombosis after TKA has proven relatively refractory to solitary use of highly specific anticoagulants. Most surgeons favor use of intermittent pneumatic compression devices alone or in combination with chemoprophylaxis after TKA.

Two caveats regarding the differential pathogenesis and management of thromboembolic disease around the knee and hip warrant special discussion. Calf thrombosis is generally a less feared complication than proximal DVT because of an implied lower risk of direct embolization. However, longitudinal surveillance studies have demonstrated that 17% to 23% of these distal thrombi extend to the more proximal veins of the thigh where they acquire considerable embolic potential.[16,28] The relationship between these asymptomatic nonocclusive calf clots and late postthrombotic syndrome manifesting as chronic venous insufficiency is less clear; nevertheless, postoperative calf thrombi require continued anticoagulant therapy with extended prophylaxis for several weeks after operation to avoid risk of PE. There is much greater risk of proximal extension and embolization of calf clots in this setting than seen in ambulatory medical patients. Finally, with respect to bleeding related to anticoagulant prophylaxis, the skin envelope surrounding the knee is much less forgiving than the skin envelope around the hip. Accordingly, a wound hematoma is less well tolerated after TKA compared with THA.

Finally, the relative prevalence of clinically important PE has been historically greater after THA than after TKA.[33] This observation follows the distribution of proximal clots, which have been noted to be far more common after THA compared with TKA, as proximal thrombi are generally larger, are more likely to become emboli, and have greater hemodynamic consequences when they reach the lung. In one series of 1638 joint replacement procedures in patients receiving warfarin prophylaxis, readmission for symptomatic venous thromboembolic events after THA (1.8%; 19 of 1079) occurred more than three times as frequently as after TKA (0.54%; 3 of 559; $P = .04$).[26,27] However, observations of the prevalence of VTED after THA and TKA suggest that these patterns have changed under the influence of contemporary clinical practice and current prophylaxis regimens. One meta-analysis of 47 published reports of symptomatic VTED after nearly 45,000 THA and TKA procedures between 1996 and 2011 suggested that in-hospital events were twice as common after TKA compared with THA.[15] All patients in these studies received prophylaxis with either low-molecular-weight heparin or a direct thrombin or factor Xa inhibitor. The overall rate of symptomatic VTE before hospital discharge after TKA was 1.09% compared with 0.53% after THA. Likewise, DVT (0.63% vs 0.26%) and PE (0.27% vs 0.14%) were twice as common after TKA compared with THA.[15] When considering the significance of these data, it is important to keep in mind that most VTE events have a delayed presentation—6 to 12 weeks after hospital discharge. The 3-month cumulative prevalence of symptomatic VTE and PE after THA is 2.5% to 3.4% and 1.1%, respectively, compared with 1.8% to 2.4% and 0.8% after TKA.[10,41] More recent data from the Danish Knee Arthroplasty Registry, in which 83% of 37,223 patients with primary TKA received fractionated heparin or fondaparinux prophylaxis for a "short" perioperative period, demonstrate a 90-day readmission rate of 1.2% (441 of 37,223) at a median of 15 days after operation, with DVT accounting for 0.9% and PE accounting for 0.3% of events.[23]

Nevertheless, this meta-analysis portrays a picture considerably changed from the early decades of total joint replacement in the United States, when THA was associated with much greater morbidity and mortality from VTED and PE than TKA. The cause of this shift in the epidemiologic profile of VTED after TKA is uncertain. It might logically be attributed to a combination of the effectiveness of new potent anticoagulants in specifically preventing thrombi resulting from intimal damage, the predilection of intimal vessel injury to occur more commonly after THA than TKA, and the prolonged period of stasis that results from maintaining the knee in a hyperflexed position with folding and occlusion of the popliteal vein during the TKA procedure. Regardless of the cause, VTED has become a relatively more visible complication after TKA than after THA in the last decade and demands increasing attention from physicians and surgeons in the perioperative care of these patients. The combined impact of greater efficacy of chemoprophylaxis in preventing thrombosis after THA compared with TKA, along with the two to three times greater frequency of TKA performed each year, makes TKA responsible for most of the clinical VTE events that the average orthopedic surgeon will see in practice.

RISK FACTORS FOR VENOUS THROMBOEMBOLISM AND THEIR MODIFICATION

As suggested in the preceding discussion, TKA or THA represents greatest risk factor for VTED incurred by a patient undergoing one of these procedures. Accordingly, the Surgical Care Improvement Project considers all patients undergoing THA and TKA, by definition, to be in the highest risk category for VTED and warranting routine anticoagulant prophylaxis in the absence of a specific contraindication. There are other risk factors to be considered with the intent of modifying some to mitigate the overall risk of VTED.

Thrombogenesis After Musculoskeletal Injury and Orthopedic Surgery

It has long been recognized that orthopedic VTED is more refractory to standard prophylaxis than VTED occurring after general surgical procedures. This was first evidenced by the failure of subcutaneous heparin to prevent DVT after THA, despite successful use of subcutaneous heparin after major abdominal and chest surgery. This refractoriness has subsequently been shown to be due to a decline in circulating antithrombin III, which is a necessary binding intermediary for clinical effectiveness of the heparins, along with several other acute-phase reactants consumed after skeletal injury or manipulation of the medullary canal as occurs during total joint arthroplasty. This perturbation in the delicate balance of normal physiologic clot formation and dissolution forms the pathophysiologic basis for the strong predilection of orthopedic patients to develop VTED after TKA. There is a wealth of data to endorse the potency of the thrombogenic stimulus of long bone fracture in the polytrauma patient compared with the relatively modest effect of head, chest, and abdominal injury.[9]

Familial Thrombophilia

Familial thrombophilia, the heritable tendency to develop severe and recurrent VTED, often spontaneously, has been inadequately explained by any deficiency of circulating anticoagulants; levels of protein C, protein S, and antithrombin III were rarely found to be low in these patients. Similarly, mutations in genetic material encoding protein C, protein S, and antithrombin III were found in aggregate to account for less than 5% of all cases of familial thrombophilia.[6,7] In 1994, a single amino acid substitution of glutamine for arginine in the protein C cleavage region of factor V was reported to occur in

50% of familial thrombophilia cases compared with only 3% to 7% of the general population.[3] This single nucleotide substitution, known as factor V Leiden, is responsible for resistance of activated factor V to cleavage inactivation by protein C, which provides a physiologic checkrein on the clotting cascade.

Variable phenotypic expression of factor V Leiden has been shown to be associated with a host of clinical disease states related to thrombosis. More than half of all people with factor V Leiden develop DVT in the presence of a single additional risk factor, such as long bone fracture or total joint arthroplasty. The Physicians' Health Study followed almost 15,000 men for cardiovascular events and observed a similar 4% to 6% prevalence of factor V Leiden among individuals experiencing no events, myocardial infarction, or stroke; in contrast, factor V Leiden was found in 11.6% of individuals with PE or DVT for a relative risk of 3.5 times.[30] Similarly, among men older than age 60 presenting with primary spontaneous DVT, the prevalence of factor V Leiden was 26%. The risk of recurrent DVT was four to five times greater in men heterozygous for factor V Leiden compared with genetically unaffected men.[31] In regard to postoperative orthopedic VTED, in two preliminary studies of patients with THA and TKA, there was no correlation between factor V Leiden, or depletion of any of the other circulating anticoagulants, and the occurrence of VTED.[32,43] This negative observation may be explained by a thrombogenic stimulus associated with violation of the medullary canal during total joint arthroplasty that is so intense that it overshadows any heritable predisposition to thrombosis that factor V Leiden might impart. In short, the presence of factor V Leiden increases the risk of VTED after TKA, but it does not explain the occurrence of VTED in most patients undergoing TKA. Therefore, it is an inadequate screening tool to identify patients at risk for VTED complications after TKA.

General Versus Regional Anesthesia

Neuraxial anesthesia has beneficial influences on thrombogenesis after total joint replacement and VTED prophylaxis. The mechanism of reduction of VTE with spinal or epidural anesthesia/analgesia has been the subject of much conjecture. Inhibition of platelet and leukocyte adhesion and stimulation of endothelial fibrinolysis have been proposed, but controlled studies have not substantiated these as valid mechanisms.[36] Rather, the sympathectomy effect of epidural blockade resulting in increased lower extremity blood flow is likely responsible for the reduction in venous thrombosis by mitigating the adverse effects of stasis.[20] Fatal PE is likewise reduced by epidural anesthesia. A retrospective review of THA and TKA by Sharrock and colleagues[34] reported an in-hospital fatal PE rate of 0.12% (7 of 5874) with general anesthesia between 1981 and 1986 compared with 0.02% (2 of 9685; $P = .03$) with epidural anesthesia between 1987 and 1991. In several randomized clinical trials of THA, spinal or epidural anesthesia consistently reduced venographic DVT by approximately 50% compared with general anesthesia regardless of the type of anticoagulant prophylaxis employed.[19] The data are slightly less compelling after TKA; extended epidural anesthesia has been shown to reduce proximal thrombosis rates by 50% and calf clots by 20%.[37,42] The mechanism of action is thought to be related to an augmentation of venous return as a result of vasodilation secondary to the sympathectomy effect. There is no evidence for any direct influence of regional anesthesia on intraoperative thrombogenesis, but intimal stimulation of fibrinolysis may be enhanced by vasodilation. In general, regional neuraxial anesthetic techniques are preferred for TKA for many reasons, one of which is a clear beneficial effect on the reduction of DVT. There are no compelling data about the effects of regional peripheral nerve blocks on VTED after TKA, but the absence of profound sympathectomy with these more peripheral and local techniques suggests they would not be expected to have a profound effect on thrombogenesis.

Notwithstanding these advantages of regional anesthesia, when combined with potent anticoagulants for thromboembolism prophylaxis after TKA, such as fractionated heparins, there have been reports of bleeding complications at the spinal puncture site. Effective anticoagulation should not be present at the time of institution of neuraxial anesthesia, and catheter removal should be performed with care in between dosing intervals of anticoagulants or only with an international normalized ratio less than 1.5 in the setting of warfarin use.[11]

Venous Stasis and Pneumatic Compression

Intermittent pneumatic compression devices, in the form of plantar foot pumps, calf sleeves, or sequential compression sleeves for the entire lower limb, have gained great popularity in the orthopedic arena of VTE prophylaxis on the basis of their lack of associated bleeding complications. The intent of these devices is to substitute for the normal physiologic muscle pump during ambulation, and their mechanism of action is largely via enhancement of venous return from the capacitance vessels of the lower extremity, mitigating the effects of stasis in Virchow triad. Mechanical compression further augments the venous flow enhancement of regional anesthesia, and some authors have suggested a synergistic effect with combined use of these two modalities. Moreover, there is a theoretical basis for mechanical stimulation of the fibrinolytic activity of the vessel intima, which may further potentiate the effects of pneumatic compression devices.[5,14,17]

In contrast to after THA, where pneumatic compression alone has been associated with a decrease in calf thrombi accompanied by a reciprocal increase in segmental proximal thrombi,[8,22] intermittent pneumatic compression devices have been shown to reduce both proximal and distal thrombosis after TKA. In one study in which all patients received regional anesthesia for TKA, the addition of plantar foot pumps to standard aspirin prophylaxis resulted in more than a 50% reduction in overall thrombi from 59% (49 of 83) to 27% (22 of 81; $P < .001$).[40] In this study, there were no proximal clots in any patient using pneumatic compression compared with 14% (12 of 83; $P < .0003$) proximal thrombosis in patients receiving aspirin prophylaxis alone. Similarly, in a meta-analysis involving TKA, intermittent pneumatic compression and fractionated heparin were comparable in reducing DVT (17% and 29%, respectively) and significantly better than warfarin or aspirin.[39] However, in one TKA trial comparing warfarin and pneumatic compression boots, the use of a general rather than a regional anesthetic was the strongest predictor of proximal thrombosis and had a greater influence than either method of prophylaxis.[29] One might reasonably conclude that after TKA, the combination of mechanical compression and chemical anticoagulant appears to be superior to the isolated use of either method alone, but the optimal combination remains to be determined, and the anesthetic technique is just as important as the method of prophylaxis.

Other Risk Factors

Although convincing data are sparse to quantify different levels of VTE risk associated with other comorbid conditions after total knee replacement, many practitioners would intuitively assign a greater risk to certain medical conditions. These include a past personal history of PE after joint replacement despite appropriate anticoagulation prophylaxis, active estrogen replacement therapy, morbid obesity, smoking, and a concurrent diagnosis of metastatic cancer. Each of these conditions warrants consideration of alteration of the "routine" prophylaxis, especially if the standard regimen does not include an anticoagulant drug.

KEY REFERENCES

3. Bertina R, et al: Mutation in blood coagulation factor V associated with resistance to activated protein C. *Nature* 369:64–67, 1994.
10. Heit JA: Estimating the incidence of symptomatic postoperative venous thromboembolism: the importance of perspective. *JAMA* 307:306–307, 2012.
11. Horlocker TT, et al: Regional anesthesia in the anticoagulated patient: defining the risks (the second ASRA Consensus Conference on Neuraxial Anesthesia and Anticoagulation). *Reg Anesth Pain Med* 28:172–197, 2003.
13. Insall JN: *Surgery of the knee*, New York, 1984, Churchill Livingstone, pp 646–647.
15. Januel J-M, et al: Symptomatic in-hospital deep vein thrombosis and pulmonary embolism following hip or knee arthroplasty among patients receiving recommended prophylaxis: a systematic review. *JAMA* 307:294–303, 2012.
21. NIH Consensus Statement on Total Knee Replacement. NIH Consensus and State-of-the-Science Statements. US Department of Health and Human Services, Bethesda, MD. Volume 20, Number 1, December 8-10, 2003.
23. Pedersen AB, et al: Venous thromboembolism in patients having knee replacement and receiving thromboprophylaxis: a Danish population-based follow-up study. *J Bone Joint Surg Am* 93:1281–1287, 2011.
35. Sharrock NE, et al: Changes in mortality after total hip and knee arthroplasty over a ten-year period. *Anesth Analg* 80:242–248, 1995.
43. Williams-Russo P, et al: Randomized trial of epidural versus general anesthesia: outcomes after primary total knee replacement. *Clin Orthop Relat Res* 331:199–208, 1996.

The references for this chapter can also be found on www.expertconsult.com.

191

ACCP, SCIP, and AAOS Guidelines for Venous Thromboembolism Prophylaxis After Total Knee Arthroplasty

Paul F. Lachiewicz

Clinical guidelines in medicine have been devised to standardize and improve patient care for a variety of disorders. A clinical guideline addresses key clinical problems or questions and has a defined evidence base and strength of recommendations. These recommendations are reached by a review of available medical literature and, when no such data exist, through a consensus process of experts in the field. A clinical guideline should also encourage and guide future clinical research in the field. A clinical guideline is an educational tool, not a predefined protocol that is incapable of changing; also, it is not a substitute for sound clinical judgment. There are three clinical practice guidelines dealing with thromboembolism prophylaxis that affect orthopedic surgeons in the United States who perform total knee arthroplasty (TKA). These are the guidelines of the American College of Chest Physicians (ACCP), Surgical Care Improvement Project (SCIP), and American Academy of Orthopaedic Surgeons (AAOS). In the previous edition of this textbook, there was great disagreement among the recommendations of these three guidelines. However, as a result of major changes in one of the major specialty guidelines in 2012, there is now close agreement among these guidelines. This chapter describes the current clinical practice guidelines for the prevention of venous thromboembolism (VTE) after lower extremity total joint arthroplasty.

BACKGROUND

Orthopedic surgeons who perform TKA were greatly affected by the ACCP guidelines for the prevention of deep vein thrombosis (DVT). The ACCP is an organization of more than 16,500 members who provide clinical respiratory, sleep, critical care, and cardiothoracic patient care. Their VTE guidelines first appeared in 1986, and the most recent 9th edition was published in June 2012.[9] Before the most recent (9th edition) version, DVT, detected by venography or ultrasonography, was the primary outcome measure in the development of these guidelines. The strongest (1 A) recommendations in the 8th edition were based on a review of only prospective, randomized studies, with most of these comparing the efficacy of one pharmacologic agent with another or with a placebo. Surgical patients were grouped as "low," "medium," or "high" risk, but all patients undergoing TKA were considered "high" risk, despite patient age, activity level, or comorbidities. Several orthopedic surgeons voiced concerns with those guidelines that emphasized prophylaxis with aggressive pharmacologic agents.[3] Asymptomatic thrombi, detected by venography or ultrasonography, were considered as important an outcome as symptomatic thromboembolism. However, studies reported a low correlation between the occurrence of DVT (as detected by ultrasonography) and pulmonary embolism (PE; as detected by spiral computed tomography scan) and the occurrence of DVT after TKA and postphlebitic syndrome.[14,17] The definition of major bleeding in those guidelines did not include persistent wound drainage, wound bleeding, or joint hematoma, which may affect the overall clinical outcome of TKA for the patient. Finally, the members of the guideline panel had numerous potential conflicts of interest with pharmaceutical companies.[3]

CURRENT ACCP GUIDELINES

The most recent (9th) edition of the ACCP clinical practice guidelines on prevention of VTE, published in 2012, differed greatly from previous documents.[9] The panel members were new and, for the most part, had no relevant potential conflicts of interest related to the subject. The most recent guideline also focused on clinical events, symptomatic DVT and PE, rather than asymptomatic events. This guideline introduced the concept of "disutility," in which a major postoperative bleeding event for the patient was considered as serious as a symptomatic thromboembolic event. The current guidelines, with grade of evidence, are listed in Table 191.1.

The ACCP guidelines now recommend that patients undergoing TKA (and total hip arthroplasty) receive one of nine possible prophylactic regimens for 10 to 14 days postoperatively. For the first time, aspirin was included as one of the acceptable pharmacologic agents. The ACCP decided to review and reanalyze the older published data related to aspirin prophylaxis for VTE related to lower extremity joint arthroplasty and hip fracture.[2,18] Specifically, the Pulmonary Embolism Prevention trial included more than 17,000 patients, compared 180 mg aspirin with placebo, and reported a 22% reduction in symptomatic PE and a 28% reduction in symptomatic VTE.[18] There have also been two more recent studies of low-dose aspirin for preventing recurrence of VTE. In the WARFASA study, a multicenter, double-blinded study, patients with a first unprovoked VTE who had completed at least 6 months of oral anticoagulation were randomly assigned to aspirin 100 mg daily or placebo for 2 years.[4] The primary outcome was recurrence of VTE, and major bleeding was the primary safety outcome. VTE recurred in 28 of 205 patients (6.6%) taking aspirin and in 43 of 197

TABLE 191.1   Current ACCP Clinical Practice Guidelines for Prevention of VTE After THA/TKA

Recommendation	Grade
1. One of the following agents should be used for a minimum of 10–14 days rather than no antithrombotic prophylaxis:	
LMWH	1 B
Fondaparinux	1 B
Apixaban	1 B
Dabigatran	1 B
Rivaroxaban	1 B
Low-dose unfractionated heparin	1 B
Adjusted-dose vitamin K antagonist	1 B
Aspirin	1 C
IPCD	1 B
For THA, TKA, hip fracture, and receiving LMWH as prophylaxis, the agent should be started either ≥12 h preoperatively or ≥12 h postoperatively.	
2. Regardless of use of IPCD or length of treatment, LMWH should be used in preference to the following alternative agents:	
Fondaparinux	2 B
Apixaban	2 B
Dabigatran	2 B
Rivaroxaban	2 B
Low-dose unfractionated heparin	2 B
Adjusted-dose vitamin K antagonist	2 C
Aspirin	2 C
3. VTE prophylaxis should be extended in the outpatient period for up to 35 days from the day of surgery rather than for only 10–14 days.	2 B
4. Dual prophylaxis with an antithrombotic agent and IPCD during the hospital stay is recommended.	2 C
5. In patients with increased risk of bleeding, IPCD or no prophylaxis is recommended over pharmacologic treatment.	2 C
6. In patients who decline or are uncooperative with injections or IPCD, apixaban or dabigatran should be used (alternatively, rivaroxaban or adjusted-dose vitamin K antagonist should be used if apixaban and dabigatran are unavailable) rather than other forms of prophylaxis.	1 B
7. It is not recommended to use an inferior vena cava filter for primary prevention over no VTE prophylaxis in patients with an increased risk or contraindications to both pharmacologic and mechanical VTE prophylaxis.	2 C
8. Asymptomatic patients do not need ultrasound screening before hospital discharge.	1 B

ACCP, American College of Chest Physicians; *IPCD*, intermittent pneumatic compression device; *LMWH*, low-molecular-weight heparin; *THA*, total hip arthroplasty; *TKA*, total knee arthroplasty; *VTE*, venous thromboembolism.

patients (11.2%) taking placebo (hazard ratio, 0.58; 95% confidence interval, 0.36 to 0.93). One patient in each group had a major bleeding episode. This study concluded that aspirin reduced the risk of recurrent VTE.[4] In the ASPIRE study, 822 patients were randomly assigned to aspirin 100 mg daily or placebo for up to 4 years.[5] Aspirin reduced the rate of the two secondary composite outcomes, VTE, and myocardial infarction, stroke, or any cardiovascular death, by 33%.

The ACCP guidelines also specifically recommended the use of a mobile intermittent compression device with capability of monitoring hours of use or patient compliance.[9] At the time of the ACCP literature review, there was only one mobile mechanical device available that had published efficacy data.[6,7]

However, several other mobile devices are now available, and these devices, with alternative compression technology, are acceptable.

Routine screening for venous thrombosis with ultrasonography before hospital discharge was not recommended. Low-molecular-weight heparin (LMWH) was the most recommended prophylactic agent. However, when used, LMWH should be started either 12 hours or more preoperatively or 12 hours or more postoperatively because of concerns about local or operative joint bleeding. The recent ACCP guidelines included rivaroxaban and apixaban as acceptable prophylactic agents. However, a systematic review found that these agents were not more efficacious than LMWH, but had higher rates of bleeding.[1]

For the first time, the 9th edition ACCP guidelines discussed the risk factors for bleeding after total hip arthroplasty and TKA. These included nonsurgical factors, specifically previous major bleeding, severe renal failure, and concomitant use of antiplatelet drugs. The surgical factors mentioned were revision surgery, extensive surgical dissection, and surgical bleeding that is difficult to control during the index procedure. In these situations, a mechanical prophylaxis device or no prophylaxis is recommended over pharmacologic treatment. There was no mention in these guidelines of the use of tranexamic acid and its relationship to thromboembolism.[8]

SCIP GUIDELINES

SCIP was formed as a national organization partnership (including AAOS, American College of Surgeons, and others) with the goals of improving the quality of inpatient surgical care and reduction of postoperative complications. In collaboration with The Joint Commission and the Centers for Medicare and Medicaid Services (CMS), numerous SCIP "measures" (or guidelines or requirements) have been created, with the most relevant to surgeons who perform TKA being surgical site infection prophylaxis and VTE prophylaxis. These SCIP guidelines are now directly related to CMS payment programs, and hospitals that report data demonstrating compliance with these measures may qualify for "bonus" payments. The SCIP measures for VTE prophylaxis are called SCIP VTE-2 guidelines, and the initial version closely followed the 8th ACCP guidelines published in 2008. As a result, many orthopedic surgeons were compelled by their hospital staffs to use LMWH as their primary prophylaxis for lower extremity joint arthroplasty.

A new, or second, set of SCIP measures (guidelines) were created after the release of the 2012 9th edition of the ACCP guidelines and took effect on January 1, 2014.[16] The SCIP VTE-2 quality measure now requires that all patients receive (some type of) VTE prophylaxis *within 24 hours preoperatively to 24 hours postoperatively*. SCIP measures now include the following agents or devices for appropriate VTE prophylaxis for patients undergoing elective TKA or total hip arthroplasty: LMWH, factor Xa inhibitor, oral factor Xa inhibitor, vitamin K antagonist (warfarin), low-dose unfractionated heparin, aspirin (dose not specified), intermittent pneumatic compression devices (type not specified), and venous foot pump. These measures reflect the new ACCP guidelines but do not follow them exactly. For the first time, the SCIP guidelines include aspirin as an acceptable pharmacologic agent, and as a result, many hospitals have changed their computerized postoperative order sets to include this.

AAOS GUIDELINES

Rationale and Background

The primary concerns of orthopedic surgeons after TKA are the prevention of fatal and nonfatal symptomatic PE and minimizing serious joint bleeding and wound drainage that adversely affects the patient's outcome. The AAOS formed a work group in 2006 to develop a consensus guideline for the prevention of symptomatic PE after total hip arthroplasty and TKA, and the first AAOS guidelines were listed online in 2007 and published in 2009.[10,11] The work group, composed of eight members of the AAOS with known expertise in the field, consulted with an evidence review team from the Center for Clinical Evidence Synthesis at Tufts–New England Medical Center. The evidence base, determined by a consensus of the working group, was a review of the literature since 1996 that met certain strict criteria.

The first AAOS guidelines were derived from both the consensus process and the literature review and analysis process. All aspects of the guideline were to be followed, rather than selective implementation. A crucial recommendation was the preoperative evaluation of the patient by the orthopedic surgeon to assess the risk of PE and the risk of bleeding complications. Another recommendation was that the patient and surgeon consider (in consultation with the anesthesiologist) the use of regional anesthesia. The surgeon should consider using mechanical prophylaxis intraoperatively or immediately postoperatively with continuation until discharge.[10,11]

The first AAOS guideline recommendations for postoperative medication were derived from the literature review and analysis and stratified into four groups. Patients at "standard risk" of PE and major bleeding should be considered for aspirin, LMWH, synthetic pentasaccharides, or warfarin (international normalized ratio [INR] goal ≤2.0). Patients at "elevated risk" of PE and at standard risk of major bleeding should be considered for LMWH, synthetic pentasaccharides, or warfarin (INR goal ≤2.0). Patients at "standard risk" of PE and "elevated risk" of major bleeding should be considered for aspirin, warfarin (INR goal ≤2.0), or no medication. Patients at "elevated risk" of both PE and major bleeding should also be considered for aspirin, warfarin (INR goal ≤2.0), or no medication.

These first AAOS guidelines were evaluated by Lewis and colleagues[12] in 2014 in a prospective analysis of 3289 consecutive patients at a single institution. This study reported that the "first-generation" AAOS guidelines resulted in a low incidence of clinically important thromboembolic events in patients undergoing total hip arthroplasty and TKA. When properly used, the guidelines to minimize adverse outcomes were executable and effective. However, the first AAOS guidelines were not accepted by CMS or SCIP while they were extant.

Current AAOS Guidelines

In accordance with the standards of the National Guideline Clearinghouse, requiring updating or withdrawal of guidelines in 5 years, the AAOS updated and published their clinical practice guideline in December 2011. This guideline, "Preventing Venous Thromboembolic Disease in Patients Undergoing Elective Hip and Knee Arthroplasty," supersedes the prior guideline from 2007.[15] A committee of new members, without potential conflicts of interest, worked only with AAOS research staff and performed a systematic review of the highest available evidence since 1970. Statistical analysis included network meta-analysis, and all recommendations were based on a rigorous, standardized process. The current AAOS guidelines include 10 recommendations with grade of evidence (Table 191.2). Patients who are not at elevated risk of venous thromboembolic disease or bleeding should receive pharmacologic prophylaxis (aspirin included) and mechanical compressive devices for the prevention of venous thromboembolic disease. Patients are considered "high risk" if they have had a prior symptomatic PE or DVT. No other "high risk" factors were specified. Based on the available evidence, the AAOS group did not recommend any specific pharmacologic agent or mechanical devices. It was not possible to determine a difference in efficacy between the prophylactic agents with respect to symptomatic events. There was also insufficient evidence to make a recommendation regarding duration of prophylaxis. Many orthopedic surgeons were disappointed with the lack of

---

TABLE 191.2 Current AAOS Clinical Practice Guidelines for Prevention of VTE After Total Joint Arthroplasty

Recommendation	Grade
1. Against routine postoperative duplex ultrasonography screening	Strong
2. Assessing risk of VTE by history of previous VTE events should be considered	Weak
3. Patients should be assessed for known bleeding disorder (such as hemophilia) and for the presence of active liver disease, which increases risk for bleeding and bleeding-associated complications	Inconclusive
4. Discontinuation of antiplatelet agents (aspirin, clopidogrel) suggested before undergoing elective surgery	Moderate
5. Use pharmacologic agent and/or mechanical compression device for VTE prevention	Moderate
6. Cannot recommend for or against specific prophylactic regimen	Inconclusive
7. In the absence of reliable evidence, physicians and surgeons should discuss duration of prophylaxis	Consensus
8. In the absence of reliable evidence, patients who have also had a previous VTE should receive pharmacologic prophylaxis and use mechanical compression devices	Consensus
9. In the absence of reliable evidence, patients who also have a known bleeding disorder and/or active liver disease should use mechanical compression devices	Consensus
10. In the absence of reliable evidence, patients should undergo early mobilization after elective surgery	Consensus
11. Use of neuraxial anesthesia for patients is recommended to help limit blood loss, although evidence suggests that neuraxial anesthesia does not affect occurrence of VTE	Moderate
12. Cannot recommend for or against use of inferior vena cava filters because current evidence does not provide clear guidance about whether inferior vena cava filters prevent pulmonary embolus in patients who also have chemoprophylaxis and/or known residual VTE	Inconclusive

AAOS, American Academy of Orthopaedic Surgeons; *VTE,* venous thromboembolism.

recommendation of a specific prophylactic regimen.[13] However, this new AAOS guideline does not require orthopedic surgeons to change their present prophylaxis regimen, and it is compatible with the SCIP measures. Finally, this guideline noted 10 specific areas that are targeted for further research, including risk assessment, multimodal regimens, timing and duration of prophylaxis, and clinical trials in revision arthroplasty.[15] The AAOS plans a new working group to review the guideline at regular intervals in the future.

KEY REFERENCES

1. Adam SS, et al: Comparative effectiveness of new oral anticoagulants and standard thromboprophylaxis in patients having total hip or knee replacement. *Ann Intern Med* 159:275–284, 2013.
2. Antiplatelet Trialists' Collaboration: Collaborative overview of randomized trials of antiplatelet therapy-III: reduction in venous thrombosis and pulmonary embolism by antiplatelet prophylaxis among surgical and medical patients. *BMJ* 308:235–246, 1994.
4. Becattini C, et al, for the WARFASA Investigators: Aspirin for preventing the recurrence of venous thromboembolism. *N Engl J Med* 366:1959–1967, 2012.
5. Brighton TA, et al, for the ASPIRE Investigators: Low-dose aspirin for preventing recurrent venous thromboembolism. *N Engl J Med* 367:1979–1987, 2012.
6. Colwell CW, et al: A mobile compression device for thrombosis prevention in hip and knee arthroplasty. *J Bone Joint Surg Am* 96:177–183, 2014.
8. Duncan CM, et al: Venous thromboembolism and mortality associated with tranexamic acid use during total hip and knee arthroplasty. *J Arthroplasty* 2014.
9. Falck-Ytter Y, et al: Prevention of VTE in orthopedic surgery patients: antithrombotic therapy and prevention of thrombosis, 9th edition: American College of Chest Physicians Evidence-Based Clinical Practice Guidelines. *Chest* 141:278S–325S, 2012.
11. Lachiewicz PF: Prevention of symptomatic pulmonary embolism in patients undergoing total hip and knee arthroplasty: clinical guideline of the American Academy of Orthopaedic Surgeons. In Azar F, O'Connor M, editors: *AAOS Instructional Course Lectures, Volume 58:795-804,* Rosemont, IL, 2009, American Academy of Orthopaedic Surgeons.
12. Lewis CG, et al: Evaluation of the first-generation AAOS clinical guidelines on the prophylaxis of venous thromboembolic events in patients undergoing total joint arthroplasty. *J Bone Joint Surg Am* 96:1327–1332, 2014.
15. Mont MA, et al: American Academy of Orthopaedic Surgeons clinical practice guideline summary: preventing venous thromboembolic disease in patients undergoing elective hip and knee arthroplasty. *J Am Acad Orthop Surg* 19:768–776, 2011.
18. Pulmonary Embolism Prevention (PEP) Trial Collaborative Group: Prevention of pulmonary embolism and deep vein thrombosis with low dose aspirin: Pulmonary Embolism Prevention (PEP) trial. *Lancet* 355:1295–1302, 2000.

The references for this chapter can also be found on www.expertconsult.com.

192

Aspirin and Sequential Pneumatic Compression Devices: Strengths and Limitations

Javad Parvizi, Timothy Lang Tan

Venous thromboembolism (VTE), particularly symptomatic pulmonary embolism, is a concerning postoperative complication of total joint arthroplasty (TJA). Thus, there is universal agreement that a form of VTE prophylaxis is required in patients undergoing TJA. In the past decade, numerous prophylactic options for prevention of VTE have been introduced. However, there is no consensus on a specific, universally accepted agent for VTE prevention after TJA. All modalities have advantages and disadvantages and present a different risk-to-benefit ratio (Table 192.1). More recently, the orthopedic community and related clinical guidelines have shifted attention to symptomatic rather than asymptomatic VTE, which has little clinical significance and is detected through imaging. Furthermore, because of the relatively low incidence of symptomatic VTE and the transition toward earlier mobilization and the use of regional anesthesia, it has become crucial for the surgeon to balance the efficacy of prophylaxis with the potential for bleeding complications. Thus individualizing the type of VTE prophylaxis based on the patient's risk profile has been increasingly accepted by the orthopedic community. Because of their safety profile, aspirin and mechanical prophylaxis have become increasingly attractive options for most patients who are at low or medium risk of developing VTE. This chapter provides a guide to the use of aspirin and compression devices as VTE prophylaxis in patients undergoing TJA.

ASPIRIN

Background

The use of aspirin for prevention of VTE after TJA has increased in the past decade.[1,11,30] Aspirin is inexpensive, requires no monitoring, has an immediate effect on platelet aggregation (in contrast to other agents such as warfarin, which takes several days to be effective), and is better tolerated with fewer wound complications than other therapeutic agents.[27,30] Furthermore, as the focus of VTE has shifted to symptomatic VTE rather than asymptomatic events, several current guidelines have changed their stance on aspirin.[15,22,25,26] Because these guidelines provide surgeons with the freedom to choose prophylaxis based on the patient's individual risk, it is crucial for the surgeon to be aware of available options.[15,22]

Pathophysiology

Aspirin irreversibly inhibits the cyclooxygenase (COX) enzyme, which ultimately blocks production of a potent platelet aggregator, thromboxane A_2.[47] The COX enzyme has two variants: COX-1 is antithrombotic, and COX-2 exhibits antiinflammatory

effects.[3,39] Because aspirin preferentially inhibits COX-1, several studies have demonstrated that low-dose aspirin (eg, 75 to 150 mg/day) is sufficient to maximize the antithrombotic effects of aspirin, whereas higher doses are needed to achieve the antiinflammatory effects.[39] There is a consensus among chest physicians that the optimal dose range is 75 to 160 mg/day for preventing cardiovascular events and stroke and related death.[14] However, many authors report using 325 mg of aspirin twice a day in their clinical practice. Most published studies related to the use of aspirin for prevention of VTE, including the seminal Pulmonary Embolism Prevention trial, used low-dose aspirin.[41] A study from our institution has also demonstrated that low-dose aspirin (81 mg twice a day) is as effective as higher dose aspirin (325 mg twice a day) in prevention of VTE after TJA and has fewer gastrointestinal side effects.[36]

History of Aspirin for Venous Thromboembolism Prevention

In 1985 aspirin was the most frequently used VTE prophylactic agent for arthroplasties. However, a 1986 meeting by the National Institutes of Health ruled that aspirin "has not been shown to be beneficial" and instead recommended heparin, compressive devices, dextran, and warfarin.[46] This National Institutes of Health consensus statement, along with opposition from thrombosis experts, severely reduced use of aspirin by orthopedic surgeons. However, because of an increase in bleeding complications observed with other prophylactic methods, aspirin gained a resurgence in popularity because of its favorable safety profile, in contrast to other, more aggressive anticoagulants.[10,28,29,41]

With the introduction of newer anticoagulants in the last decade, a wide variety of therapeutic agents became available, which may have prevented aspirin from achieving more widespread use. Furthermore, between 1986 and 2008, the American College of Chest Physicians (AACP), reiterated that aspirin was insufficient VTE prophylaxis after TJA.[16,17,46] The ACCP guidelines were not embraced by the orthopedic community mostly because of lack of relevance of the endpoint (venographically proven distal deep vein thrombosis [DVT]) that the guidelines had used to reach the recommendations. Orthopedic surgeons insisted that fatal and nonfatal symptomatic pulmonary embolism (PE) should be the clinical endpoint to measure the efficacy of any modality. Thus in 2007 the American Academy of Orthopaedic Surgeons (AAOS) formed a work group and developed guidelines using PE as an endpoint, which was then modified to all symptomatic VTE in their 2011 guidelines.[22,25] In contrast to the ACCP guidelines, the AAOS recommended that aspirin could be used for patients with a standard risk of PE or for any patient with an elevated bleeding risk. However, the AAOS did not recommend a preferred chemoprophylaxis.

During this time period (2007–2012), the AAOS and ACCP guidelines on aspirin remained discordant. Orthopedic surgeons raised concerns that the ACCP valued efficacy more than safety. It was not until 2012 that the ACCP adopted fatal and symptomatic PE and VTE as the endpoint.[15] At that point, all publications related to the efficacy of aspirin in prevention of VTE were evaluated by the ACCP, leading to the most recent guidelines that endorse aspirin and mechanical compression devices as an effective modality for prevention of VTE after TJA (Table 192.2). In 2014 the Surgical Care Improvement Project endorsed the new ACCP guidelines, accepting aspirin as an effective VTE prophylaxis agent for patients undergoing TJA.[45]

Thus there has been a marked adoption of aspirin in North America as the most preferred method of chemoprophylaxis after TJA. In an unpublished survey of attendees of the American Association of Hip and Knee Surgeons, more than 60% of respondents preferred to use aspirin as the main modality for prevention of VTE after TJA.

Clinical Studies

Given the favorable safety profile of aspirin, many clinical studies evaluating its efficacy have been performed in the last decade.* The decision to include aspirin as appropriate prophylaxis was largely based on the Pulmonary Embolism Prevention trial.[41] This was a prospective, randomized controlled trial of 13,356 patients undergoing surgery for hip fracture and 4088 patients undergoing elective arthroplasty. The trial detected no difference in the rate of symptomatic DVT with aspirin compared with placebo for elective THA (1.1% vs 1.3%). However, a reduction was found in the hip fracture group for PE ($P = .03$) and DVT ($P = .02$) along with no difference in the bleeding rates between 160 mg aspirin daily and placebo (0.4% in each group). In recent years there have been further reports on the efficacy of aspirin in prevention of VTE after TJA. A prospective randomized study proved the efficacy of aspirin for prevention of VTE after total knee arthroplasty.[24] In this study the use of aspirin combined with mechanical prophylaxis resulted in a similar rate of DVT detected by duplex ultrasound as low-molecular-weight heparin with mechanical prophylaxis. The paucity of randomized, placebo-controlled clinical trials evaluating the efficacy of aspirin is likely due to a lack of sponsorship and economic incentive.

Although level 1 studies evaluating aspirin are scarce, there are many retrospective studies in the literature that have defined the role of aspirin for VTE prevention, demonstrating a risk reduction between 20% and 50%.[†] Several meta-analyses for total hip arthroplasty and total knee arthroplasty have demonstrated that aspirin can achieve comparable results to other anticoagulants.[6,7,13,49] Additionally, large-scale studies have

---

*References 2, 5, 18, 19, 21, 24, 29, 33, 35, 38, 41, 43, and 48.
†References 2, 5, 18, 19, 24, 29, 33, 35, 38, 41, and 48.

TABLE 192.1   Strengths and Limitations of Aspirin and Sequential Compressive Devices

Strengths	Limitations
Aspirin	
Low risk of bleeding complications	Gastrointestinal upset
Does not require monitoring	May be inadequate for high-risk patients
Lower risk of periprosthetic joint infection	VTE risk stratification unclear
Cost-effective	Few level 1 studies supporting efficacy in arthroplasty
Well tolerated/good patient compliance	
May reduce ischemic events (eg, myocardial infarction, stroke)	
Immediate effect on platelet aggregation	
Sequential Compressive Devices	
Low risk of bleeding complications	Lower compliance
Does not require monitoring	Uncomfortable
Ease of use as an adjunct	Not all have equal efficacy
	May be inadequate for high-risk patients

VTE, Venous thromboembolism.

TABLE 192.2   Brief Summary of Clinical Practice Guidelines

	ACCP	AAOS
Sequential Compressive devices	Recommended over no prophylaxis (1C)* Recommended with chemoprophylaxis during hospital stay (2C)	No recommendation for preferred prophylaxis (inconclusive)
Compression stockings	No recommendation	No recommendation for preferred prophylaxis (inconclusive)
Aspirin	Recommended over no prophylaxis (1B)	No recommendation for preferred prophylaxis (inconclusive) Discontinue antiplatelets before TJA (moderate)
LMWH	Recommended over no prophylaxis (1B) Recommended over other agents (2B and 2C) Start 12 h preoperatively or postoperatively (1B)	No recommendation for preferred prophylaxis (inconclusive)
Warfarin	Recommended over no prophylaxis (1B)	No recommendation for preferred prophylaxis (inconclusive)
Fondaparinux	Recommended over no prophylaxis (1B)	No recommendation for preferred prophylaxis (inconclusive)
Apixaban	Recommended over no prophylaxis (1B)	No recommendation for preferred prophylaxis (inconclusive)
Dabigatran	Recommended over no prophylaxis (1B)	No recommendation for preferred prophylaxis (inconclusive)
Rivaroxaban	Recommended over no prophylaxis (1B)	No recommendation for preferred prophylaxis (inconclusive)
LDUH	Recommended over no prophylaxis (1B)	No recommendation for preferred prophylaxis (inconclusive)

AAOS, American Academy of Orthopaedic Surgeons; ACCP, American College of Chest Physicians; LDUH, low-dose unfractionated heparin; LMWH, low-molecular-weight heparin; TJA, total joint arthroplasty; VTE, venous thromboembolism.
*Only portable, battery-powered intermittent pneumatic compression devices that can report daily compliance of at least 18 hours in both inpatients and outpatients are recommended.

resulted in similar findings, most notably the United Kingdom National Joint Registry, which demonstrated no difference in regard to PE or DVT in 22,942 TJAs.[23] Furthermore, in a large database study of 93,840 patients who underwent primary total knee arthroplasty, Bozic and colleagues[5] determined that aspirin prophylaxis demonstrated a lower VTE rate than warfarin but a similar VTE rate to injectable agents. Despite several studies demonstrating comparable efficacy between aspirin and other anticoagulants, not all studies revealed consistent findings. In a prospective study of 696 consecutive TJAs, the Intermountain Joint Replacement Center Writing Committee found that patients with a standard risk of VTE receiving aspirin had a higher rate of symptomatic PE (4.6% vs 0.7%) and VTE (7.9% vs 1.2%) than patients receiving warfarin.[21] The authors found that most embolic events (88.8%) occurred in total knee arthroplasties.

The literature supports that aspirin is a safer prophylactic agent than warfarin and injectable agents with regard to bleeding complications and hematoma.[2,38] However, a study has suggested that aspirin may reduce the risk of periprosthetic joint infection compared with warfarin.[20] There are numerous explanations for this finding, the most important being that patients receiving aspirin have a lower incidence of wound-related complications and hematoma formation, complications that are known to predispose patients to infection. In the study by Huang and coworkers[20] evaluating 3156 patients undergoing TJA, the incidence of periprosthetic joint infection in patients receiving aspirin at 0.4% was statistically significantly lower than 1.5% in the warfarin group ($P < .001$), even when controlling for other risk factors for periprosthetic joint infection.

Furthermore, although the AAOS recommends a risk stratification approach, few studies have elucidated the risk factors for VTE among patients with TJA, which makes stratification a subjective process.[37] The AAOS guidelines gave only a "limited" rating to assessing patients for their risk of VTE other than patients with a history of prior VTE. Thus the efficacy of aspirin in high-risk patients, such as patients with a prior history of VTE or comorbidities predisposing to development of VTE, remains relatively unknown. However, the few studies that have employed risk stratification in their selection of chemoprophylaxis have achieved promising results.[20,35,37] A study evaluating a large number of patients in the National Inpatient Sampling database developed a risk stratification model using the nomogram approach. The identification of the risk factors for VTE with their relative weight has allowed the investigators to develop and launch an iOS app that can identify patients at higher risk of developing VTE.[37,43]

MECHANICAL PROPHYLAXIS

Many forms of intermittent pneumatic compression devices, including calf sleeves, sequential compression devices, and plantar foot pumps, have gained popularity among arthroplasty surgeons. Similar to aspirin, the lack of bleeding complications and the relatively low cost of these devices has made mechanical prophylaxis an attractive option alone or in conjunction with chemoprophylaxis. However, patient compliance with using these devices remains a challenge, particularly when the devices are used in the outpatient setting. The compliance risk has been mitigated with the development of newer battery-powered portable compressive devices that can monitor patient compliance.[27]

Pathophysiology

Mechanical compression devices provide efficacy for formation of VTE by reducing venous stasis and congestion. Mechanical compression devices demonstrate efficacy for prevention of VTE by reducing venous stasis and congestion.

History and Guidelines

Many orthopedic surgeons use the AAOS and ACCP guidelines when determining which VTE prophylaxis to use. The current guidelines differ from previous guidelines in regard to mechanical compression.[15,22] Previously, the 2009 ACCP[16] and 2008 AAOS[25] guidelines considered mechanical compression an adjunctive measure for inpatient prophylaxis in favor of chemoprophylaxis as the standard of care. However, with technologic developments that improve utilization of mechanical compression in the outpatient setting and increased concerns of bleeding risk,[26,27] mechanical compressive devices have become increasingly utilized.

Current guidelines from both the AAOS and the ACCP consider mechanical compression as appropriate prophylaxis for prevention of VTE after TJA.[15,22] However, the AAOS does not recommend a preferred prophylactic modality, whereas the ACCP recommends the use of low-molecular-weight heparin in preference to the other agents. Additionally, the ACCP recommends combining mechanical compression with chemoprophylaxis in the inpatient setting and distinguishes between the types of available mechanical compression devices. Specifically, the ACCP guidelines endorse portable, battery-powered intermittent pneumatic compression devices that can report daily compliance.[15]

Types of Mechanical Prophylaxis

There are several types of mechanical devices, which can be separated into four categories: compression stockings, above-the-knee compressive devices, below-the-knee devices, and foot pumps. Compression stockings provide constant pressure and are not currently recommended by the ACCP.[15] Although the application of constant pressure is supposed to reduce venous stasis, one prospective study demonstrated that 98% of compressive stockings failed to produce a sufficient gradient, and 54% produced a reverse gradient.[4] Furthermore, multiple studies have demonstrated that compression stockings are not effective for VTE prophylaxis alone compared with chemoprophyaxis[9,44] and are associated with a fourfold increase in skin complications.[15]

Although studies on above-the-knee devices have been performed for total hip arthroplasty, there is a paucity of studies for total knee arthroplasty. However, several studies have suggested that above-the-knee devices may not be as effective as foot pumps or below-the-knee devices.[42,50] Foot pumps theoretically can provide only one-third the venous return compared with the calf device because of a reduced venous volume. Additionally, although the results have been generally promising, problems with patient compliance owing to disturbed sleep and difficulty ambulating limit their utility.[8,40]

Below-the-knee devices can be further categorized into sequential symmetric intermittent compression, rapid asymmetric mobile compression, and mobile venous phasic flow-regulated compression devices. Sequential symmetric devices work in circumferential compressions in a peristaltic manner, whereas rapid asymmetric devices compress only the back of the foot to achieve higher venous velocities. To increase utilization in the outpatient setting, mobile compressive devices were developed so that the device could function during ambulation. Most importantly, mobile compressive devices have been associated with increased patient compliance.[12,31,34] Additionally, more recent developments have allowed contractions to be synchronized with respiratory venous flow signals to increase venous return.[32] Overall, comparative studies between compression devices and chemoprophylaxis have demonstrated variable results, with several studies suggesting comparable efficacy, particularly when aspirin and mechanical compression were combined.[31,34]

CONCLUSION

Aspirin and sequential pneumatic compressive devices are both attractive options as monoprophylaxis or as adjuncts for prevention of VTE in patients at low risk for developing this complication. Compared with chemoprophylaxis, both options have become increasingly attractive in recent years because of the lack of bleeding complications. With new guidelines that now accept aspirin as acceptable prophylaxis, the literature regarding the efficacy of aspirin as VTE prophylaxis will continue to expand. Furthermore, although the use of mechanical compressive devices has been limited owing to patient compliance, more recent technologic developments have increased its appeal.

KEY REFERENCES

5. Bozic KJ, et al: Does aspirin have a role in venous thromboembolism prophylaxis in total knee arthroplasty patients? *J Arthroplasty* 25:1053–1060, 2010.

14. Eikelboom JW, et al: Antiplatelet drugs: Antithrombotic Therapy and Prevention of Thrombosis, 9th ed: American College of Chest Physicians Evidence-Based Clinical Practice Guidelines. *Chest* 141(2 Suppl):e89S–119S, 2012.

15. Falck-Ytter Y, et al: Prevention of VTE in orthopedic surgery patients: Antithrombotic Therapy and Prevention of Thrombosis, 9th ed: American College of Chest Physicians Evidence-Based Clinical Practice Guidelines. *Chest* 141(2 Suppl):e278S–325S, 2012.

20. Huang R, et al: Administration of aspirin as a prophylaxis agent against venous thromboembolism results in lower incidence of periprosthetic joint infection. *J Arthroplasty* 30(9):39–41, 2015.

21. Intermountain Joint Replacement Center Writing Committee: A prospective comparison of warfarin to aspirin for thromboprophylaxis in total hip and total knee arthroplasty. *J Arthroplasty* 27:1–9.e2, 2012.

22. Jacobs JJ, et al: American Academy of Orthopaedic Surgeons clinical practice guideline on: preventing venous thromboembolic disease in patients undergoing elective hip and knee arthroplasty. *J Bone Joint Surg Am* 94:746–747, 2012.

25. Johanson NA, et al: Prevention of symptomatic pulmonary embolism in patients undergoing total hip or knee arthroplasty. *J Am Acad Orthop Surg* 17:183–196, 2009.

29. Lotke PA, et al: Aspirin and warfarin for thromboembolic disease after total joint arthroplasty. *Clin Orthop Relat Res* 324:251–258, 1996.

31. McAsey CJ, et al: Patient satisfaction with mobile compression devices following total hip arthroplasty. *Orthopedics* 37:e673–e677, 2014.

37. Parvizi J, et al: Symptomatic pulmonary embolus after joint arthroplasty: stratification of risk factors. *Clin Orthop Relat Res* 472:903–912, 2014.

41. Prevention of pulmonary embolism and deep vein thrombosis with low dose aspirin: Pulmonary Embolism Prevention (PEP) trial. *Lancet* 355:1295–1302, 2000.

43. Raphael IJ, et al: Aspirin: an alternative for pulmonary embolism prophylaxis after arthroplasty? *Clin Orthop Relat Res* 472:482–488, 2014.

45. SCIP VTE measures changing in 2014. Available from: <http://www.aaos.org/news/aaosnow/nov13/cover2.asp>. (Accessed 19.08.15.)

49. Westrich GH, et al: Meta-analysis of thromboembolic prophylaxis after total knee arthroplasty. *J Bone Joint Surg Br* 82:795–800, 2000.

The references for this chapter can also be found on www.expertconsult.com.

193

Venous Thromboembolic Disease Stratification of Risk: Who Needs Aggressive Anticoagulation

Cory Messerschmidt, Seth Bowman, Jonathan Katz, Richard J. Friedman

The risk of venous thromboembolism (VTE) after major orthopedic surgery has decreased significantly in recent decades. The use of chemoprophylaxis has contributed much to this decreased risk. Low-molecular-weight heparins (LMWHs), warfarin, and fondaparinux have reduced the cumulative incidence of symptomatic VTE within 3 months of total knee arthroplasty (TKA) to approximately 2% from 41% to 85% without prophylaxis.[64] Perioperative management of patients has dramatically improved in the past 20 years. Many centers are mobilizing patients with physical therapy on the day of surgery. More patients are having TKA done under neuraxial anesthesia, which has been associated with decreased rates of deep vein thrombosis (DVT) and pulmonary embolism (PE) in total hip arthroplasty.[46] The average length of stay has decreased from 9 days to 3 days in 75% of patients, and many centers perform outpatient TKA or TKA with overnight stays.[21,34,37,43]

Another changing dynamic in TKA is the timing of most VTE events and prophylaxis. As the length of stay continues to decrease, the incidence of VTE events occurring after discharge continues to increase, making this mainly an outpatient issue. Data obtained from the Global Orthopaedic Registry illustrated a mean time to symptomatic VTE for TKA of 9.7 days, which occurred after discharge in 57% of patients who underwent TKA (Fig. 193.1).[64] As the length of hospitalization approaches 2 days or less, most symptomatic events will occur after the patient leaves the hospital, and VTE prophylaxis will be managed largely on an outpatient basis.

OPTIONS FOR THROMBOPROPHYLAXIS IN KNEE SURGERY

Methods of thromboprophylaxis for patients undergoing TKA include mechanical interventions, pharmacologic interventions, and a combination approach. Ideally, pharmacologic prophylactic agents should be efficacious and cost-effective, should require minimal monitoring, and should have minimal to no side effects of complications.

Mechanical Prophylaxis

Mechanical options for prevention of DVT include compression stockings, intermittent pneumatic compression (IPC) devices, and venous foot pumps. These devices act by increasing the speed of venous blood flow and the volume of blood returned from the extremities to the heart. IPC devices have been found to be effective in many small studies involving TKA.[8,29,33,47] However, patients must wear the devices 17 to 20 h/day.[24] This can be challenging with frequent postoperative physical therapy sessions, transfers to the bathroom, and patient compliance. Decreased hospital stays also make the continued use of IPCs difficult. However, new mobile battery-operated IPC devices, called continuous enhanced circulation therapy, have been developed. They have been compared with LMWHs for the prevention of VTE; continuous enhanced circulation therapy used in combination with LMWH significantly reduced the incidence of DVT compared with LMWH alone for TKA (6.6% vs 19.5%, $P = .018$).[20] In addition, in one study, patients using continuous enhanced circulation therapy devices had increased compliance compared with patients using traditional IPC devices.[26]

The potential effects of venous foot pumps are based on the large blood volume in the foot coupled with the beneficial effects of active muscle contraction foot pumps.[61] Two small trials have shown venous foot pumps to be effective in patients undergoing TKA; however, other studies have shown them to be less effective compared with LMWHs.[5,50,66,69] Venous foot pumps are likely a good adjunct to chemoprophylaxis but should not be used as the sole method of thromboprophylaxis.[24] Data on the use of graduated compression stockings in patients undergoing TKA are limited. However, the available data suggest that graduated compression stockings used alone or in combination likely have little effect on VTE prophylaxis in patients undergoing TKA.[32,42]

For best patient efficacy in VTE prophylaxis using mechanical means, devices should be applied during or immediately after surgery. Devices are most effective when worn up to 18 h/day.[24] Compliance can be difficult in the inpatient setting and often unrealistic in the outpatient setting. Interest has increased in combining multiple mechanical means of prophylaxis with chemoprophylaxis, such as graduated compression stockings, IPCs, and pharmacologic prophylaxis.[15]

Pharmacologic Prophylaxis

Anticoagulants used for thromboprophylaxis in orthopedic surgery patients act on various sites in the coagulation cascade (Fig. 193.2). The most commonly available and accepted agents are warfarin, LMWHs, direct factor Xa inhibitors (rivaroxaban and apixaban), direct thrombin inhibitors (dabigatran), and aspirin (Table 193.1).

Warfarin

Although warfarin offers the convenience of oral administration, many clinical limitations exist. Warfarin has a slow onset and offset of action. It also has a narrow therapeutic window (international normalized ratio 2 to 3) with considerable interindividual variability in dose-response relationship (Fig. 193.3). Complex pharmacodynamics requires frequent coagulation

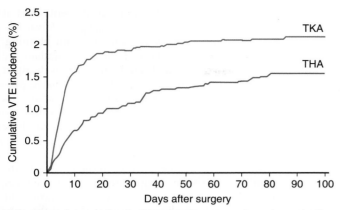

FIG 193.1 Cumulative incidence of venous thromboembolism *(VTE)* after total hip or knee arthroplasty. *THA*, Total hip arthroplasty; *TKA*, total knee arthroplasty. (From Warwick D, et al: Insufficient duration of venous thromboembolism prophylaxis after total hip or knee replacement when compared with the time course of thromboembolic events: findings from the Global Orthopaedic Registry. *J Bone Joint Surg Br* 89:799–807, 2007.)

monitoring and dose adjustment to achieve therapeutic levels. Additionally, there is a propensity for interaction with other drugs and various foods based on their vitamin K content, and metabolism is vulnerable to numerous genetic polymorphisms. Compliance reflects these difficulties associated with warfarin administration and monitoring, with only 33% of patients taking the recommended dose and 58% of patients outside the recommended international normalized ratio after hospital discharge.[11,25,58]

Low-Molecular-Weight Heparins

Extensive data have demonstrated that LMWHs are efficacious and safe for thromboprophylaxis after TKA. Numerous randomized trials have compared the efficacy of LMWHs and warfarin after TKA. Six of these randomized studies comparing LMWHs with warfarin showed a lower incidence of DVT with LMWH.[27] Superior efficacy of LMWH over warfarin has been demonstrated in numerous meta-analyses as well.[8,31] LMWH appears to be more effective in reducing overall asymptomatic DVT formation, with no difference in symptomatic VTE between groups and a higher bleeding rate compared with warfarin.

SIMPLIFIED COAGULATION CASCADE: ALL SITES

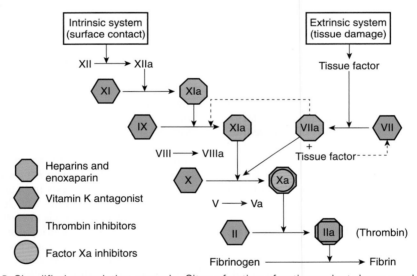

FIG 193.2 Simplified coagulation cascade. Sites of action of anticoagulant drugs used in thromboprophylaxis. Aspirin works outside the coagulation cascade.

TABLE 193.1 Old and Current Anticoagulants: Overview of Action and Administration

	Warfarin	LMWH	Dabigatran	Rivaroxaban/Apixaban	Aspirin
Dosing route	Oral[a]	SC[b]	Oral[a]	Oral[a]	Oral[a]
Fixed dose	No[b]	Yes[a]	Yes[a]	Yes[a]	Yes[a]
Inhibits clot-bound thrombin	No[b]	No[b]	Yes[b]	No[b]	No[b]
Extended use	Yes[a]	Yes[a]	Yes[a]	Yes[a]	Yes[a]
Risk for HIT	No[a]	Yes[b]	No[a]	No[a]	No[a]
Monitoring necessary	Yes[b]	No[a]	No[a]	No[a]	No[a]
Rapid onset/offset	No[b]	Yes[a]	Yes[a]	Yes[a]	No[b]
Drug-drug interactions	Yes[b]	No[a]	Minimal[a]	Minimal[a]	No[a]
Drug-food interactions	Yes[b]	No[a]	No[a]	No[a]	No[a]

[a]An advantage.
[b]A disadvantage.
HIT, Heparin-induced thrombocytopenia; *LMWH*, low-molecular-weight heparin; *SC*, subcutaneous.

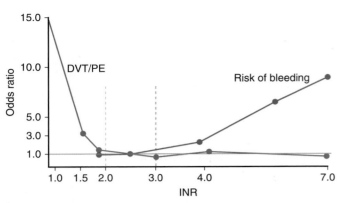

FIG 193.3 Narrow therapeutic range of warfarin. *DVT,* Deep vein thrombosis; *INR,* international normalized ratio; *PE,* pulmonary embolism.

Direct Factor Xa Inhibitors

The enzyme factor X is an attractive target for inhibition, as it occupies a critical junction between the intrinsic and extrinsic coagulation cascade.[40] Factor X is an enzyme that is essential for the conversion of prothrombin to thrombin, which leads to thrombus formation.[44] In response to vascular injury, factor X is activated to factor Xa, which combines with its cofactor factor Va to form the prothrombinase complex.[40] This complex then converts prothrombin to thrombin, which leads to increased generation of thrombin. Thus, direct factor Xa inhibitors block the conversion of prothrombin to thrombin to exert their antithrombotic effect.

Direct factor Xa inhibitors possess some advantages over indirect factor Xa inhibitors such as fondaparinux. Direct factor Xa inhibitors bind directly to factor Xa and do not require antithrombin to exert their effects, which prevents subsequent reactions leading to thrombin generation.[65] Additionally, they inhibit both free and platelet-bound factor Xa bound to the prothrombinase complex.[65] The two most notable direct factor Xa inhibitors are orally administered rivaroxaban and apixaban, and both are currently approved by the US Food and Drug Administration (FDA) for the prevention of VTE in adult patients undergoing elective hip or knee arthroplasty.[7,35]

Rivaroxaban. Current treatment recommendations for rivaroxaban for anticoagulation after TKA are 10 mg orally once daily for 12 days after surgery, with the initial dose taken 6 to 10 hours after surgery, provided that hemostasis has been established.[35] However, in clinical practice, most physicians delay initial dosing for 12 to 24 hours, as is done with LMWH, for hemostasis.

Apixaban. Apixaban is another potent oral direct factor Xa inhibitor similar to rivaroxaban. Apixaban has received FDA approval for patients undergoing TKA in the United States. Current recommendations for apixaban after TKA is 2.5 mg orally twice daily for 12 days after surgery, with the initial dose taken 12 to 24 hours after surgery.

Special Considerations for New Oral Anticoagulants
Reversal Agents. The FDA has approved idarucizumab, the first reversal agent for dabigatran that is indicated for emergency reversal of its anticoagulant effects. No reversal agents exist at the present time for any of the other new oral agents (rivaroxaban, apixaban). For most cases of clinically relevant bleeding, supportive care and discontinuation of the anticoagulant are recommended and often sufficient, given their relatively short half-lives.[36] Prothrombin complex concentrates, activated prothrombin complex concentrates, and recombinant factor VIIa all have been evaluated in multiple animal studies and in vitro human studies.[4,41] However, human clinical studies of these factor concentrates are lacking.

Perioperative Dosing Management. Doses of the new oral anticoagulants should be held before surgery or invasive procedures, although they have a quicker clearance time than warfarin. The usual empirical approach involves discontinuation of the anticoagulant before surgery, with the timing of discontinuation dependent on the specific half-life of the drug, the patient's renal function (creatinine clearance, with prolonged drug half-life as creatinine clearance decreases), and surgical risk of bleeding.[63] There is no universal consensus about timing of discontinuation, but a general recommendation is for discontinuation at least 24 hours before low-risk surgery (approximately two to three half-lives) and 2 to 4 days before high-risk surgery (approximately five half-lives) in patients with appropriate renal function (longer with renal impairment).[59,63] Similarly, timing of resumption of medications takes into account the same considerations of half-life, renal function, and bleeding risk, with a general recommendation for resumption of medications 24 hours after low-risk surgery and 48 to 72 hours after high-risk surgery (again, longer with renal impairment).[59,63]

Aspirin
The perioperative management of patients undergoing total joint arthroplasty (TJA) has changed significantly in the past 20 years. At the present time, emphasis is placed on early mobilization, use of regional anesthesia, regional pain blocks, concomitant use of pneumatic compression devices, and early discharge from the hospital.[16] Aspirin is now gaining increased attention for use in VTE prophylaxis in patients undergoing TJA. Large retrospective cohort studies have looked at aspirin and found favorable results with trends toward lower bleeding and wound complication rates.[6,56] Additional studies have looked at the use of aspirin in a risk stratification model, with "low-risk" patients receiving aspirin with favorable results noninferior to control prophylaxis and with fewer bleeding complications.[28,38]

In addition to the lack of quality randomized controlled studies available in the literature, the optimal dose of aspirin is unknown. Studies across the literature have evaluated dose of aspirin ranging from 81 mg once daily to 650 mg twice daily, with no current consensus on the optimal dose. With the acceptance of aspirin in guidelines from the American College of Chest Physicians (ACCP), American Academy of Orthopaedic Surgeons, and Surgical Care Improvement Project with no dosing recommendation, quality prospective research is necessary to determine its true efficacy and optimal dosing.

THROMBOPROPHYLAXIS IN KNEE ARTHROSCOPY

Arthroscopic procedures of the knee are among the most commonly performed orthopedic procedures, often done as an outpatient procedure in younger patients.[24] Traditionally, knee arthroscopy has been considered a low-risk procedure, and routine thromboprophylaxis is not considered standard of care. The overall incidence of venographic DVT after knee arthroscopy has been shown to be 18% in the absence of thromboprophylaxis.[18,22,60] Furthermore risk of DVT in patients undergoing arthroscopy is increased in patients with certain risk factors, including previous history of thrombosis (relative risk, 8.2; $P <$ .005) or two or more risk factors for VTE (relative risk, 2.94; $P < .05$).[17] Operative arthroscopy also appears to be associated with higher risk than diagnostic arthroscopy, related to longer surgical time and longer tourniquet time.

Reported DVT incidence after arthroscopic knee surgery without thromboprophylaxis has ranged from 1.5% to 41.2%.[45,49] A systematic review looked at the use of LMWH versus no thromboprophylaxis after arthroscopic knee surgery and found only 23 events with only 5 symptomatic DVTs and 1 symptomatic PE and no major bleeding.[55] In contrast, a large, randomized controlled trial looking at LMWH versus compression stockings significantly favored LMWH, with no difference in major or clinically relevant bleeding events between the groups.[10]

As the overall risk of VTE after arthroscopic knee surgery is low relative to other orthopedic procedures, the 9th edition ACCP guidelines suggest no thromboprophylaxis rather than prophylaxis for patients with no history of prior VTE (grade 2B).[43] However, the ACCP guidelines also state that stratification is necessary to identify "higher risk" patients, particularly patients with a history of prior VTE. In these patients, thromboprophylaxis with LMWH is recommended (grade 1B).[24]

THROMBOPROPHYLAXIS IN TRAUMA SURGERY BELOW THE KNEE

Lower limb injuries below the knee are also quite common and comprise a heterogeneous mix including fractures below the knee, tendon ruptures, and cartilage injuries of the knee and ankle. There is less evidence about the incidence of VTE events associated with these injuries compared with other major orthopedic procedures. Randomized controlled trials have shown the rate of VTE on venography to be 4% to 40% in patients with lower limb immobilization in the absence of thromboprophylaxis.[23,62] Risk factors for VTE in these patients include advanced age, fractures, and obesity, but it is unknown if surgical management is itself a risk factor.[30,39] Additionally, risk of DVT increases with proximity of the fracture to the knee (tibial plateau > tibial shaft > ankle).[1]

Efficacy of LMWH in prevention of VTE in patients with immobilized isolated lower leg injuries was evaluated in a meta-analysis of six randomized controlled trials involving patients requiring lower leg immobilization for at least 1 week.[23] The pooled estimate from all six trials showed a highly significant reduction in the risk of VTE from 17% with placebo to 9.6% with LMWH, without a significant increase in bleeding.[23] A Cochrane systematic review of the same six randomized controlled trials showed the use of LMWH significantly reduced the incidence of VTE on venography (incidence, 0% to 37%) compared with placebo or no prophylaxis (incidence, 4% to 40%).[62]

Given these data among patients with below-the-knee injuries, thromboprophylaxis with LMWH likely reduces frequency of asymptomatic DVT and thus in some countries is considered the standard of care.[2] However, data are limited regarding whether thromboprophylaxis reduces clinically relevant VTE

events and is cost-effective. For this reason, current ACCP guidelines suggest no prophylaxis rather than pharmacologic thromboprophylaxis in patients with isolated lower leg injuries requiring leg immobilization (grade 2C).[24] However, results from higher risk populations may be reasonably extrapolated to patients at higher risk of DVT (who were excluded from these studies), particularly patients with prior VTE.

VENOUS THROMBOEMBOLISM STRATIFICATION OF RISK AND WHO NEEDS AGGRESSIVE ANTICOAGULATION

VTE prophylaxis after TKA remains controversial. There is currently no consensus on the optimal strategy for prevention of VTE after TKA. With the increasing scrutiny and penalties imposed on surgeons by health care regulatory bodies in the United States for various "quality metric" considerations related to readmissions and reoperations, including VTE prevention and its complications, the notion of using anticoagulant agents that are not only effective but also less harmful is gaining momentum and greater endorsement.[16] Aggressive anticoagulants are associated with the highest number of adverse effects, including mortality.[48]

VTE prophylaxis presents a clinical dilemma of balancing postoperative thrombotic risk along with anticoagulation-related risk of bleeding, hematoma, and infection. In the most recent ACCP guidelines on prevention of VTE in orthopedic surgery patients, they stated that surgeon choice of VTE prophylaxis should be based on a balance between safety and efficacy of a particular anticoagulant, with risk stratification used to identify patients at standard risk or high risk of VTE or bleeding or both.[24] The challenge is determining which patients are at an increased risk of VTE and in need of more aggressive anticoagulants.

There are older and newer risk models to help with this decision. However, risk stratification can be difficult. Multiple risk factors determine the risk for VTE in a given patient. They may be grouped into inherited risk factors such as thrombophilias and clinical risk factors such as age, obesity, previous VTE, and duration and type of surgery.[12] Other commonly cited risk factors include oral contraceptive use or hormone replacement therapy, prolonged postoperative immobility, marked venous stasis, history of cardiovascular disease, varicose veins, long-term steroid use, and history of malignancy. The presence of multiple risk factors has a cumulative effect, leading to a high overall level of risk.[3,57,67]

Parvizi and colleagues[54] identified the preoperative comorbidities associated with an increased risk of symptomatic PE after TJA in a large group of patients. The authors concluded that patients with obesity, chronic obstructive pulmonary disease, atrial fibrillation, anemia, depression, or postoperative DVT as well as patients with a high Charlson comorbidity index are at an increased risk of having postoperative PE. They also concluded that greater than 90% of patients undergoing TJA can safely receive aspirin as anticoagulation prophylaxis, whereas a validated risk profile can be used to detect patients at a higher risk for VTE and in need of more aggressive agents.[54]

Numerous risk assessment models have been developed to predict the level of risk in a given patient. The 2012 ACCP Consensus Guidelines on VTE Prevention recommend the use of an individualized risk stratification tool to understand VTE risk, noting that existing tools are cumbersome and labor intensive.[24] One such model developed by Caprini and associates[12] assigns patients a score based on the presence of predefined risk factors within the 24 hours preceding surgery. It is based on expert opinion from more than 20 years ago but has subsequently become validated. "Reduced" models with fewer risk factors have been shown to predict risk similarly to full models.[51] The addition of more risk factors to existing risk models may impede, not improve, risk stratification.[52]

More recently, Pannucci and colleagues[53] used prospective data from a statewide clinical registry that included VTE-specific risk factors to create a validated risk-prediction tool for 90-day VTE in surgical patients. Seven risk factors were incorporated into a weighted risk index: personal history of VTE, current cancer, sepsis/septic shock/systemic inflammatory response syndrome, age 60 years or older, body mass index 40 kg/m^2 or greater, male sex, and family history of VTE. The observed 90-day VTE rates were similar between cohorts at each risk level. This model allows the identification of a specific high-risk group of patients who would benefit from more aggressive or extended-duration chemoprophylaxis.[53]

Risk assessment models targeted selectively for TJA have not been well defined. A prospective, randomized study by Kulshrestha and Kumar[38] investigating routine anticoagulation versus a risk screening approach for DVT prophylaxis after TKA developed a DVT scoring chart based on American Academy of Orthopaedic Surgeons guidelines and modified using additional inputs from cardiac and vascular society recommendations (Fig. 193.4). This chart was used to stratify patients into a standard-risk or high-risk group. The study concluded that symptomatic DVT rates after TKA were similar whether patients were routinely anticoagulated or selectively anticoagulated after risk screening, but rates of wound complications were significantly higher (8.4%, $P = .014$) after routine anticoagulation.[38] Patients receiving LMWH were eight times more likely to experience wound complications compared with patients taking aspirin.[9,19,28,38] Other studies regarding risk assessment also showed similar rates of VTE between groups with significantly higher rates of wound complications and bleeding in patients receiving aggressive chemoprophylaxis.[19,28]

The optimal duration of thromboprophylaxis after elective TKA is controversial. Prolonged anticoagulation therapy is associated with a perceived risk of increased bleeding episodes as well as wound complications. In a review of data from 24,059 patients undergoing primary TKA, the incidence of symptomatic VTE at 3 months was 2.1%, the median time to diagnosis was 7 days, and VTE was diagnosed after discharge from the hospital in 47% of cases.[68] A more recent study from a total joint registry found that the cumulative incidence of VTE within 3 months was 2.3% in patients who had undergone TKA (n = 8236).[64] The mean time to VTE was 9.7 days, and VTE occurred after the median time to discharge in 57% of patients who

RISK STRATIFICATION FOR DVT PROPHYLAXIS

Complete this form to stratify the patient for risk of DVT and bleeding and follow the chart given to institute DVT prophylaxis

1. Check all statements that apply.
2. Add up the number of points shown for each of the checked statements to get the DVT risk factor score.

Add 3 points for each of the following statements if true

    a) Age >75   b) H/O DVT or pulmonary embolism (PE) c) Family H/O thrombosis

    d) Family H/O blood-clotting disorders

Add 2 points for each of the following if true

    a) Age 60–74 yr   b) Cancer (current or previous)

    c) Recent (06 wks) major surgery lasting >45 minutes

    b) Recent (06 wks) confinement to bed for more than 72 hours

    c) Plaster immobilization lower limb in the past 6 wks   d) Central venous access

Add 1 point for each of the following if true

    a) Age 41–60 years   b) Varicose veins   c) Major surgery within the past month
    d) History of inflammatory bowel disease (IBD)   e) Legs are currently swollen
    f) Overweight or obese g) H/O recent MI   h) Congestive heart failure
    j) Serious infection (for example, pneumonia)   k) COPD   l) IDDM
    m) Currently on bed rest or restricted mobility   n) HRT
    o) Pregnant/had a baby within the past month   p) Smoker

ADD TOTAL SCORE: [ ]   HIGH RISK (>2); STANDARD RISK (0–2)

FIG 193.4 Deep vein thrombosis *(DVT)* risk scoring chart. *COPD,* Chronic obstructive pulmonary disease; *H/O,* history of; *HRT,* hormone replacement therapy; *IDDM,* insulin-dependent diabetes mellitus; *MI,* myocardial infarction. (From Kulshrestha V, Kumar S: DVT prophylaxis after TKA: routine anticoagulation vs risk screening approach—a randomized study. *J Arthroplasty* 28:1868–1873, 2013.)

developed VTE. These findings confirm that patients undergoing TKA are at increased risk of VTE after the usual period of hospitalization, with the risk peaking at approximately 7 to 10 days postoperatively and remaining until day 28.

Compared with total hip arthroplasty, less evidence supports extended thromboprophylaxis in patients undergoing TKA; therefore a strong recommendation has been lacking. A meta-analysis of six randomized trials comparing extended (4 to 5 weeks) and conventional (7 to 15 days) thromboprophylaxis with LMWH in patients undergoing hip or knee arthroplasty showed that the risk for clinical VTE was reduced by 50% in patients receiving extended thromboprophylaxis ($P = .009$).[13] However, five of the six studies were based on total hip arthroplasty populations. In a study done by Comp and colleagues[14] looking at extended prophylaxis in TKAs, the total VTE risk seen in 438 patients undergoing TKA who received enoxaparin (30 mg every 12 hours for 7 to 10 days followed by 40 mg once daily for 3 weeks) was 17.5% versus 21% in patients who received placebo, indicating no clinical benefit of extended enoxaparin prophylaxis after TKA.

Previous thromboembolic studies with various agents demonstrated that 10 to 14 days of prophylaxis should be adequate for most patients. Risk stratification can help determine which patients may benefit from extended prophylaxis out of 28 to 35 days. For patients undergoing TKA, current ACCP guidelines recommend thromboprophylaxis with the recommended options for at least 10 days (grade 1B) and suggest extending this for up to 35 days after surgery (grade 2B).[24]

CONCLUSION

The awareness of the risk of VTE in lower extremity TJA has increased significantly over the years, and almost all orthopedic surgeons now provide some form of prophylaxis. Mechanical prophylaxis and the numerous oral and injectable pharmacologic agents that have been developed over the years provide many options for surgeons. Although all patients are at significant risk, there is now a growing trend to risk stratify and choose an agent that best fits the patient's risk profile, while minimizing potential complications. The goal is to provide adequate prophylaxis, while minimizing the risks of bleeding.

The references for this chapter can also be found on www.expertconsult.com.

194

Bleeding and Infection Risk With Aggressive Anticoagulation: How to Minimize Suboptimal Outcomes

Charles L. Nelson, John M. Hardcastle

Appropriate anticoagulation after total knee arthroplasty (TKA) is a balance between preventing serious venous thromboembolism (VTE)–associated complications and minimizing the risk of bleeding. Both ends of the spectrum can have dire consequences for the patient. Multiple studies, many of which were industry funded, have evaluated the role of thromboembolism prophylaxis in the prevalence of VTE, symptomatic pulmonary embolism (PE), and death secondary to PE.[4,6-9,11-15,18,21-23] However, in the setting of TKA, there is no evidence demonstrating that deep vein thrombosis (DVT) is a surrogate for symptomatic or fatal PE.[4,5] Furthermore, the mortality rate secondary to PE in contemporary studies is generally 0.1% or less with various perioperative strategies including no prophylaxis, mechanical prophylaxis alone, aspirin, warfarin, low-molecular-weight heparins (LMWHs), fondaparinux, and newer oral factor Xa or direct thrombin inhibitors.[4-9,11-15,18,21-23]

There is no evidence that any of these regimens is associated with a decrease in mortality resulting from PE,[4,21] whereas there is evidence that aggressive anticoagulation leads to higher rates of bleeding complications.[1,16,24] Therefore it is important that decisions to initiate anticoagulation to decrease thromboembolic complications also consider the risks of adverse bleeding complications with aggressive anticoagulation for patients undergoing TKA.

In a study of 30,020 patients undergoing TKA in an integrated large community-based captured joint registry, Khatod and colleagues[21] evaluated the impact of mechanical or pharmacologic prophylaxis and anesthetic technique on incidence of PE, fatal PE, and death in a "real-world" setting. The overall incidence of PE and of confirmed fatal PE was 0.45% and 0.01%, respectively. The overall mortality rate was 0.31%. Even if all deaths of unknown cause were attributed as deaths related to PE, the fatal PE rate would increase to only 0.13%. The authors compared patients receiving mechanical prophylaxis alone, aspirin with or without mechanical prophylaxis, warfarin, LMWH, antiinflammatory agents, and combination anticoagulation. There were no differences in mortality, PE, or fatal PE in any of the groups. The only differences noted were a lower rate of overall PE in the warfarin group compared with the mechanical prophylaxis–only group and a lower rate of PE with regional versus general anesthesia.

Postoperative bleeding is associated with several important adverse events. In many studies, major bleeding has been defined as fatal bleeding, any intracranial bleeding, and non–surgical site bleeding of 2 g hemoglobin or greater or requiring 2 or more units of packed red blood cell transfusion (generally intra-abdominal or retroperitoneal bleeding).[4] Some studies also include epidural bleeding in the major bleed category and surgical site bleeding requiring a return to the operating room.[8,13,14] Major bleeding can have dire consequences including death, development of permanent neurologic deficits secondary to hemorrhagic stroke, or spinal cord compression following epidural hematoma. However, increased surgical site bleeding, generally not characterized as major bleeding in most studies, can also have serious consequences to patients, including higher rates of both deep and superficial infection, prolonged wound drainage, prolonged hospitalization, and increased medical costs.[1,16,24]

Aggressive anticoagulation can be defined as any pharmacologically mediated inhibition of coagulation associated with more bleeding than standard accepted VTE prophylaxis standards. This includes therapeutic doses of newer oral anti–factor Xa agents or LMWHs, therapeutic doses of unfractionated heparin, or warfarin therapy with an international normalized ratio greater than 3.0. Indications for aggressive anticoagulation can be broken down into preexisting conditions and events related to the surgery itself. Preexisting conditions for which more aggressive anticoagulation may be indicated include mechanical heart valves, atrial fibrillation, recent myocardial infarction, and recent thromboembolic stroke. In addition, more aggressive anticoagulation may be indicated for patients with thrombophilia, hypofibrinolysis, or a known history of or prior PE. Careful preoperative evaluation should assess these and other risk factors and help the patient and surgical team make an informed choice regarding the risk-benefit ratio of surgical intervention. If it is decided that the patient is an appropriate surgical candidate, proper management in the preoperative, intraoperative, and postoperative period is crucial in minimizing complications related to both thromboembolic phenomena and bleeding.

The other subset of patients often treated with aggressive anticoagulation are patients who develop perioperative thrombosis, with or without embolic events. The appropriateness of more aggressive anticoagulation depends on the relative risks of major thromboembolic events versus the risk of important bleeding complications. Even standard prophylactic warfarin therapy was shown in one large study to be associated with an increased risk of infection compared with use of aspirin, a less aggressive anticoagulant.[17]

LONG-TERM ANTICOAGULATION

Several studies have reported on the poor outcomes associated with patients undergoing arthroplasty who received long-term anticoagulation preoperatively and for whom more aggressive anticoagulation was either indicated or performed. Aggarwal and colleagues[1] performed a retrospective study on patients undergoing arthroplasty who received long-term anticoagulation for atrial fibrillation. Length of stay was 6.3 days versus 3.4 days compared with patients not receiving long-term anticoagulation. Postoperative hemoglobin levels did not show any difference; however, patients receiving long-term anticoagulation had a fourfold increase in transfusion requirements. Additionally, and perhaps most clinically significant, patients receiving long-term anticoagulation had a nearly 10-fold increased risk of developing infection. Haighton and coworkers[16] examined patients undergoing total joint arthroplasty who required bridging therapy perioperatively. They found significantly more blood loss in the bridged group. Half of the patients who were bridged with a therapeutic heparin drip had bleeding complications requiring return to the operating room. Most of these patients who returned to the operating room experienced catastrophic complications. Among the patients returning to the operating room for bleeding complications, 43% developed a neurologic deficit secondary to a hematoma, and 29% died. Despite this group of patients being at high risk for a thrombosis, there were no thromboembolic events.

Leijtens and colleagues[24] similarly reported on patients undergoing arthroplasty who were managed with bridging anticoagulation. Of 13 patients, 12 experienced bleeding-related complications. Return to the operating room to treat bleeding-related complications was required in 69% of patients. Periprosthetic infection developed in 15% of patients. None of these patients experienced a thromboembolic event. These studies highlight an important finding. Even in patients at high risk of thrombosis, aggressive anticoagulation may result in more bleeding-related complications than thromboembolic complications.[1,16,24] More studies are needed to determine the optimal management for patients who were anticoagulated before surgery or indicated for bridging therapy.

PREOPERATIVE FACTORS

Preoperative testing of patients on anticoagulation regimens should include laboratory work, particularly coagulation profiles. For most patients, it is appropriate to discontinue anticoagulation preoperatively at a time point that allows normal coagulation at the time of surgery. If the patient's condition requires bridging, short-acting anticoagulation, short-acting LMWH, or weight-based dosing of fractionated heparin can be used and then held several hours before surgery with acceptable results. The most appropriate anticoagulation is best assessed with a team-based approach with medical and surgical expertise regarding the patient-specific thromboembolic risks as well as the bleeding-associated risks to determine the best approach.

For patients who are either on or expected to require more aggressive anticoagulation regimens, it is important to start in the preoperative period to minimize the risk of bleeding-related complications. When appropriate, hemoglobin should be optimized preoperatively. Erythropoietin has been shown to be beneficial in patients with starting hemoglobin less than 13 g/dL in reducing the rate of transfusion.[27] Oral or intravenous iron supplementation is also helpful in increasing hemoglobin level preoperatively for most patients.

Antiplatelet agents such as aspirin, nonsteroidal anti-inflammatory drugs, or clopidogrel should be stopped at least 1 week before surgery unless otherwise contraindicated. For patients with congenital bleeding disorders such as hemophilia, von Willebrand disease, or other rare bleeding disorders, preoperative hematologic evaluation is important. In general, pharmacologic anticoagulation is not advisable for patients with hemophilia or other serious bleeding disorders; instead, these patients normally require correction using appropriate factor replacement preoperatively and perioperatively. Other medical conditions known to contribute to bleeding risk, such as cirrhosis, should be optimized before surgery if possible, and the decision for anticoagulation should take into consideration the risks of thromboembolism as well as the risks of bleeding complications. Some physicians recommend using agents with low risk of bleeding or avoiding anticoagulation altogether in patients with advanced liver disease.

INTRAOPERATIVE FACTORS

As discussed elsewhere in this text, intraoperative blood management and hemostasis are important in decreasing the rates of intraoperative complications. Bipolar sealers, topical fibrin sealants, intravenous or topical tranexamic acid, blood pressure control, meticulous hemostasis, and decreased operative times all can assist in reducing intraoperative blood loss. Meticulous hemostasis is even more critical for patients expected to be on aggressive anticoagulation regimens postoperatively. Antibiotic prophylaxis is always indicated, as is particular attention to sterility.

POSTOPERATIVE FACTORS

Postoperatively, the keys to minimizing bleeding-related complications from aggressive anticoagulation include avoiding unnecessary aggressive anticoagulation and expeditious correction of anticoagulation when serious bleeding concerns are encountered. Avoiding more aggressive anticoagulation must be weighed against avoiding serious thromboembolic related complications. When risks of serious bleeding complications and catastrophic thromboembolic complications are both high, alternative strategies may be indicated. For example, in the presence of a recent intracranial bleed with a concomitant large proximal femoral or pelvic deep vein thrombus in a patient with a history of PE, use of a removable vena cava filter may be indicated to allow less aggressive anticoagulation with a lower risk of PE in the acute setting.[3,20] When life-threatening or limb-threatening bleeding develops postoperatively, expeditious normalization of coagulation is generally advisable with careful consideration of thromboembolic risks.

Many traditional anticoagulants have antidotes that promote normalization of coagulation. Warfarin may be corrected with vitamin K and more rapidly with fresh-frozen plasma or cryoprecipitate. Unfractionated heparin and LMWHs can be reversed with protamine if rapid correction is indicated. Agents such as fondaparinux and many of the newer oral anti–factor Xa anticoagulants do not have specific antidotes. Strategies for reversal of these agents include many of the strategies used in the setting of congenital bleeding disorders such as prothrombin complex concentrate; fresh-frozen plasma; activated recombinant factor VII; activated prothrombin complex concentrate; and adjuncts of charcoal, hemodialysis, and antifibrinolytics.[28]

The timing of initiation of anticoagulation postoperatively depends on the onset of action of the agent, the risk of serious thromboembolic complications, and the risk of important bleeding complications. We limit our discussion to patients for whom more aggressive anticoagulation may be indicated. In patients identified preoperatively to receive more aggressive anticoagulation, the anticoagulation is generally initiated with an agent that has a rapid onset of action between 6 and 24 hours after surgery depending on the agent. For example, the recommendation for initiation of enoxaparin therapy is 12 to 24 hours after surgery.[13] Other patients receiving more aggressive anticoagulation include patients in whom presumed thromboembolic complications have developed postoperatively. In these patients, more aggressive anticoagulation is usually initiated when the presumed thromboembolic event has been diagnosed.

There is high morbidity associated with aggressive anticoagulation less than 7 days after TKA.[26] One way to decrease the risk of bleeding complications and infection related to aggressive anticoagulation after TKA is to avoid unnecessary aggressive anticoagulation of patients following TKA. It is important to establish a credible thromboembolic event or risk before starting aggressive anticoagulation. Detection of small distal DVT is not an indication for aggressive anticoagulation in the setting of a patient who was not preoperatively determined to be at high risk. The presence of DVT has never been established as a surrogate for fatal PE.[4,5] Hypoxia before 24 hours postoperatively is more likely to be due to fat embolism syndrome than PE.[2] Therefore respiratory support and close monitoring may be a better option than aggressive anticoagulation for certain patients with early postoperative hypoxia.

Even when aggressive anticoagulation is indicated, some patients develop serious bleeding-related complications. When ongoing blood loss is confirmed, identification of the site of bleeding is important. For bleeding outside the knee joint, involvement of appropriate specialists for nonsurgical, procedural, or surgical management is indicated. Surgical site bleeding or hematoma may be managed nonsurgically if bleeding has ceased, there is no wound drainage, and the patient is progressing appropriately. However, in the presence of new-onset or persistent wound drainage that is not improving, many surgeons would favor early return to the operating room for incision and drainage and evacuation of the hematoma. Studies have demonstrated an association between postoperative knee hematoma and wound drainage and both deep and superficial infection.[1,16,17,24] Furthermore, studies have demonstrated an increased rate of infection when return to the operating room is delayed for patients with persistent wound drainage.[25] A growing body of evidence suggests that postoperative factors including prolonged wound healing and drainage is associated with a higher incidence of infection owing to the ability of pathogens to gain access to the surgical space through the wound.[25]

When return to the operating room becomes necessary as a result of bleeding complications in the setting of aggressive anticoagulation, meticulous hemostasis following release of the tourniquet (if used) is important. Use of adjuvant local procoagulant agents or instruments such as topical tranexamic acid, topical fibrin sealants, and bipolar sealers may diminish

postoperative bleeding and complications following a return to the operating room. Although controversial after TKA, use of a postoperative drain after return to the operating room may be useful both to monitor ongoing bleeding and to decrease the likelihood of recurrence of a hematoma.

Another important consideration when using aggressive anticoagulation after TKA involves appropriate transfusion of blood products when indicated. Although transfusion of blood products is associated with an increase in complications after total joint arthroplasty, and avoidance of unnecessary transfusion is advisable when appropriate, transfusion of blood products, platelets, fresh-frozen plasma, or other procoagulant factors is critical is some cases to prevent mortality secondary to excessive blood loss. Blood transfusion is often necessary when aggressive anticoagulation is employed.

POSTOPERATIVE THROMBOTIC EVENTS REQUIRING AGGRESSIVE ANTICOAGULATION

Even with appropriate prophylaxis, some patients develop a postoperative thromboembolic event. When considering the rate of VTE after TKA, it is important to understand that DVT alone has not been demonstrated to be a surrogate for PE after TKA. Nevertheless, in the setting where the risk of major thromboembolic consequences exceeds the risk of major bleeding complications, more aggressive anticoagulation may be indicated. With careful initiation of therapeutic anticoagulation without use of a bolus dose, some studies have demonstrated reasonable safety when more aggressive anticoagulation becomes necessary. Della Valle and colleagues[10] compared the complication rate of patients undergoing arthroplasty and receiving intravenous heparin treatment for a postoperative thromboembolic event and a matched control group treated with a prophylactic dose of LMWH. Besides length of stay and transfusion requirements, there was no significant difference in the rate of bleeding complications.[10]

CONCLUSION

Choosing appropriate anticoagulation after TKA is a balance between the risks of major thromboembolic complications and the risks of serious bleeding-related complications. The main goal of pharmacologic anticoagulation after TKA is to prevent death secondary to PE. The rates of DVT range from 1% to 84%.[4] However, the incidence of fatal PE ranges from 0.0% to 0.3% in contemporary studies using many different anticoagulation regimens including use of no pharmacologic anticoagulation; anticoagulation with aspirin or low-dose warfarin; or more aggressive anticoagulation with higher dose warfarin, LMWHs, unfractionated heparin, fondaparinux, or newer oral anti–factor Xa or antithrombin anticoagulants.[4,6-9,11-15,18,21-23] Nevertheless, to date, despite extensive study, there is no evidence that more aggressive anticoagulation is associated with a lower rate of mortality secondary to PE.[4,6-9,11-15,18,21-23]

There is convincing evidence that there is an increase in serious bleeding complications with more aggressive anticoagulation.[1,16,24] Therefore it is important that physicians balance the risks of serious thromboembolic complications and serious bleeding events when prescribing more aggressive anticoagulation for patients undergoing TKA. Excess bleeding associated with TKA, especially in the at-risk group that requires aggressive anticoagulation, has many downsides. Besides the clinical manifestations of low hemoglobin, there are risks associated with blood transfusions. Transfusions can lead to infection, prolonged hospital stay, and increased medical costs.

Recognizing factors that can help mitigate bleeding is crucial to improving patient outcomes. These factors include preoperative, intraoperative, and postoperative factors. Preoperatively, when practical, patients should be optimized medically. Intraoperatively, blood conservation techniques should be used liberally including surgical precision and efficiency, meticulous hemostasis, neuraxial anesthesia, and perioperative hypotension. When appropriate and available, bipolar sealers, fibrin sealants, and topical or systemic tranexamic acid should be considered.[19] Postoperatively, avoidance of premature or overly aggressive anticoagulation when not indicated is helpful to minimize bleeding-related complications. When serious non–surgical site postoperative bleeding occurs, expeditious evaluation and management by specialists with expertise in the region of bleeding and correction of anticoagulation are indicated. When major surgical site bleeding occurs, in addition to correction of anticoagulation, prompt surgical management with irrigation and drainage of the hematoma and expeditious management of the surgical wound often may decrease the risk of wound complications and infection.[25]

KEY REFERENCES

4. Brookenthal KR, et al: A meta-analysis of thromboembolic prophylaxis in total knee arthroplasty. *J Arthroplasty* 16:293–300, 2001.

7. Colwell CW, Jr, et al: Flexibility in administration of fondaparinux for prevention of symptomatic venous thromboembolism in orthopaedic surgery. *J Arthroplasty* 21:36–45, 2006.

8. Colwell CW, Jr, et al: Efficacy and safety of enoxaparin versus unfractionated heparin for prevention of deep venous thrombosis after elective knee arthroplasty. Enoxaparin Clinical Trial Group. *Clin Orthop Relat Res* 321:19–27, 1995.

13. Fitzgerald RH, Jr, et al: Prevention of venous thromboembolic disease following primary total knee arthroplasty. A randomized, multicenter, open-label, parallel-group comparison of enoxaparin and warfarin. *J Bone Joint Surg Am* 83:900–906, 2001.

14. Freedman KB, et al: A meta-analysis of thromboembolic prophylaxis following elective total hip arthroplasty. *J Bone Joint Surg Am* 82:929–938, 2000.

21. Khatod M, et al: Pulmonary embolism prophylaxis in more than 30,000 total knee arthroplasty patients: is there a best choice? *J Arthroplasty* 27:167–172, 2012.

The references for this chapter can also be found on www.expertconsult.com.

PART II

Economics, Quality, and Payment Paradigms for Total Knee Arthroplasty

195

Total Joint Arthroplasty—Historical Perspective: Declining Reimbursement, Rising Costs

Amun Makani, William L. Healy

Total joint arthroplasty (TJA) is one of the most successful surgical advances of the last century.[9,15,16] TJA has had a success rate in relieving pain and allowing return to function better than most other medical and surgical interventions. The increasing demand for TJA is a result of its successful clinical results, an aging population, and a desire of baby boomers to stay active as they age.[15,20] The increased volume of TJA cases may also be associated with increased obesity rates throughout the United States.[1,14] In 2013, more than 480,000 hip replacement procedures and more than 760,000 knee replacement procedures were performed in the United States.[17,20] The fastest growing segment of joint reconstruction surgery has been revision knee arthroplasty, which in the United States increased 5.6% from 2012–2103 with more than 75,000 procedures performed in 2013.[17] As technology advances and indications expand for TJA to include younger and more active patients, the need and demand for this procedure will surely continue to increase.

TJA is currently one of the largest expenses for the Medicare program, and this cost center is expanding.[23] To control expenses, the Centers for Medicare and Medicaid Services (CMS) implemented reductions in professional payment for TJA and limited increases in payments to hospitals for TJA at a rate below inflation.[23] Additional alternative payment methodologies and risk-sharing paradigms have been implemented on an experimental basis to control cost and improve quality. It will take some time to validate efficacy. The goals of this chapter are to review current economic issues related to TJA and provide strategies to preserve hospital revenues by reducing costs.

EPIDEMIOLOGY

Health care costs are rising and are a significant expenditure in the United States. In 2013, health care expenditure accounted for approximately 17.1% of the gross domestic product, much higher than most industrial countries.[24] In 2008, annual health care expenditures were estimated at $2.4 trillion in the United States; however, that number rose to approximately $3.8 trillion just 6 years later.[2] It is projected that by 2022, health care costs will increase to more than $5 trillion.[3]

In 2000, 156,025 total knee arthroplasties (TKAs) and 18,031 revision arthroplasty procedures were performed in the Medicare population.[1] By 2011, those numbers had increased to 255,063 and 29,137, respectively.[1] The total number of primary TKA cases performed in the United States in 2013 was estimated at 762,400, which represented a 3.8% increase from the previous year.[19] By 2030, demand for primary TKA is expected to reach 3.48 million procedures per year.[15]

HOSPITAL REIMBURSEMENTS

As the demand for TKA has increased, so have its costs to the health care system. At the present time, TJA is the largest diagnosis related group (DRG) expenditure for the CMS.[5,25] In 2013, major joint replacement topped the list of Medicare hospitalization costs with nearly $7 billion awarded to hospitals.[22] Medicare is the primary payer for greater than 60% of TJAs performed in the United States annually.[21] Between 2000 and 2011, there was a 63.5% increase in utilization of TKA and 61.6% increase in utilization of revision knee arthroplasty cases in the Medicare population. Over this same time period, the Medicare population grew by 20.8%.[1]

Based on increased volume of cases and increased cost for care, TJA is a target for cost control by the CMS. Additionally, many private insurance providers set their reimbursement rates relative to Medicare rates. Thus, cost-control strategies used by the CMS impact the health care system at large. In 2015, the Medicare Sustainable Growth Rate formula was repealed by Congress and signed into law by President Barack Obama. This action prevented a 21% cut in professional reimbursement. Although this is positive news for all physicians, including adult reconstructive surgeons, it is clear that TJA has been and will be a target of increased focus of cost control for all payers.

Medicare is administratively divided into several parts. Parts A and B are most applicable to TKA. Part A payments are made to hospitals to cover inpatient expenses including postoperative care at a skilled nursing facility. It also covers the cost of the joint implants and surgical supplies. Part B payments are made to physicians such as orthopedic surgeons and anesthesiologists and include payments for outpatient postoperative follow-up care for the first 90 days after surgery.

In 2008, the CMS changed the hospital reimbursement methodology for TJA procedures. The case payment DRG system was replaced by the medical severity DRG (MS DRG) system.[20] The MS DRG system does not differentiate between hip and knee arthroplasty but does allow one to include information such as case complexity and primary or revision status.

Between 2008 and 2011, Medicare reimbursement rates to hospitals for primary and revision joint arthroplasty in uncomplicated patients without comorbid conditions declined by 0.7% and 0.6%, respectively, when adjusted for inflation.[1] However, for patients with major comorbidities, Medicare reimbursements to hospitals for primary TJA increased 5.3% when adjusted for inflation.[1]

Hospitals have been forced to deal with declining reimbursements, which may become even more pronounced as Medicare pursues bundled care payment plans for a specific care episode.

In that model of reimbursement, Medicare will provide a specific amount of payment for a particular episode of health care.[4] For example, in TJA, this would include payment for preoperative, perioperative, and postoperative care including readmission. Although this model provides an opportunity to align health care providers and hospitals around a common goal of increasing quality and cost-efficiency, this system also asks hospitals and providers to assume the responsibility for costs of the episode of care.[4,6] Although insurance companies exist to manage risk, physicians and hospitals are being forced to manage the economic risk of their operations.

PHYSICIAN REIMBURSEMENTS

Physician reimbursement for TJA has continued to decrease over time. Between 1991 and 2008, Medicare physician reimbursement for joint replacement decreased between 36% and 39%. During the same interval, the consumer price index increased 49.5%.[23]

Between 2000 and 2011, Medicare physician reimbursement rates for primary TKA decreased from $1350 to $1315, which represented a 2.4% decrease when adjusted for inflation.[1] During this same time period, physician reimbursement rates decreased 2.5% for primary total hip arthroplasty when adjusting for inflation from $1284 to $1218.[1] Although the CMS has made adjustments in reimbursements to hospitals based on the patient's medical comorbidities, there have been no such adjustments to reimbursements in this regard for physicians.

One study looked at the hypothetical financial impact of declining Medicare reimbursement on an adult reconstructive surgeon.[25] The authors created a model based on a scenario in which a total joint reconstructive surgeon treated only Medicare patients and performed 300 total joint reconstructive cases per year, of which 15% were revision surgeries, and 3000 outpatient visits were included. Compensation was based on 2012 Medicare reimbursement rates (1000 level III new outpatient visits and 2000 level III follow-up visits). They used the Medical Group Management Association (MGMA) cost survey from 2013 to obtain average practice expenses. They estimated annual physician compensation of approximately $72,502 after accounting for these expenses. Based on their findings, the authors concluded that an adult reconstructive orthopedic surgeon would be unable to sustain his or her current salary level with a Medicare-only population and that this disparity would continue to worsen with further decreases in Part B reimbursement.

These trends represent an increasingly challenging environment for joint reconstructive surgeons, which may have implications for patient access at a time when demand for these procedures continues to increase. This may result in fewer orthopedic surgeons specializing in adult reconstruction.[13] Gain sharing through bundled payment demonstration projects is allowed to incentivize surgeons by increasing reimbursement if quality and cost targets are realized. It remains to be seen if these programs will be attractive to adult reconstruction orthopedic surgeons.

IMPLANT COSTS

Implant costs vary by company and provide an opportunity to reduce hospital expense and increase profit margins. Implant companies in the United States enjoyed revenue of approximately $7.0 billion for hip and knee implants alone, which

represented a 3.9% increase from the prior year.[18] The average list price for an uncoated total knee implant in 2000 was $4664; that price increased to $11,582 by 2011.[18] This represented an annual 5.6% increase after adjusting for inflation. In addition to implant-related expenses, newer innovations in technology used during the surgical procedure will likely continue to lead to expanding costs.

However, the average cost of a hip and knee implant for a US hospital has decreased as increasing focus is placed on cost control strategies for TJA. The average selling price for a total hip implant in 2013 was $3193, which decreased 4.9% from 2012.[18] Primary and revision knee implants during this time frame decreased in selling price 2.9% and 1.8% from $5157 to $5006, and $9850 to $9677, respectively. These costs must be balanced with patient outcomes and hospital resources.

HOSPITAL COST CONTAINMENT

As a result of the increasing demands for use of newer technologies, services, and products within the current market, hospital expenses have continued to rise. Hospitals have implemented methods to control costs while still providing high-quality TKA operations and good outcomes. Multiple strategies have been used by hospitals for cost containment.[7-9,11,20] They mainly fall into the two general categories of utilization review and cost control and implant cost control.

UTILIZATION REVIEW AND COST CONTROL

Through the process of utilization review, hospitals have been able to control costs by implementing standardized best practice techniques in routine processes. This minimizes variation in the care of delivery and improves the quality of care experienced by patients. Some hospitals have created clinical pathways for procedures such as TKA. These pathways use a multimodality approach in which preoperative discharge planning, early ambulation, and preemptive pain and nausea management are routinely used. These clinical pathways have decreased the use of hospital resources by reducing the length of stay and have helped hospitals contain costs.[7] In the 1980s, the average length of stay following a knee replacement was approximately 20 days, which decreased to 9 days in the 1990s. By 2008, the average length of stay had decreased to approximately 3 to 4 days.[21] There has been increased interest in discharging selected patients with minimal medical comorbidities to home the day of surgery. As hospital stays continue to decrease in length, a team approach involving the patient, clinician, nurses, physical therapists, and discharge planners will be crucial. Clinicians have also become increasingly conscientious about ordering laboratory testing, pathologic review, and radiologic imaging throughout the perioperative phase.

A study aimed to address opportunities for quality improvement and cost reduction in hospitals considering accepting bundled payment and demonstrated that postdischarge care represented 36% of total costs for the complete episode of care and unexpected readmissions accounted for 11% of total costs.[4] These costs cannot be contained by the surgeon alone and must be addressed by collaboration between all members of the health care team. Utilization review and control when combined with vender cost control at the Lahey Clinic during 1991 and 2008 led to expenses for TKA being decreased by an additional 42% in inflation-adjusted dollars.[9]

IMPLANT COST CONTROL

Studies have demonstrated that implant cost has the highest contribution to hospital expense in TJA.[7,23] Thus, there is a good opportunity to decrease total expenses by controlling vendor costs. Several strategies for reducing vendor cost are described here. Lahey Clinic has published its experience with implant cost controls in the past.[11,12,21] The techniques that are discussed are vendor discounting, implant matching, price capping, competitive bid purchasing, and single price/case price purchasing programs. The single price/case price purchasing program developed by Lahey Clinic was most effective at reducing implant cost.[9]

Vendor discounting is the process by which hospitals negotiate directly with specific vendors for discounts on their implant supplies. With this strategy, surgeons in the hospital may use multiple vendors. However, if a surgeon insists on using a particular implant vendor, potential leverage is lost by the hospital in negotiating a discount.

Implant matching, or implant standardization, is the process by which the hospital restricts implant type for a given type of surgery, while maintaining options with regard to vendor. An example of this would be standardization to all-polyethylene tibial components in TKA, which has a cost savings compared with traditional uncoated modular tibial implants. This strategy requires a "buy-in" by all surgeons involved. Implant matching is controversial and has not been as effective as other cost control strategies.

Price capping is a process by which the hospital restricts implant cost by choosing a ceiling price, which all vendors have the opportunity to accept or reject. Surgeons have the freedom to choose any vendor who is able to provide the implant at or below the price set by the hospital. For the strategy to be successful, all surgeons must be willing to forgo loyalty to any specific vendor who is unable to accept the price cap. Without this understanding, this strategy is ineffective.

In competitive bid pricing, all implant vendors submit a bid for their implants with the most competitive offer accepted by the hospital. In accepting the bid, all surgeons agree to use that particular vendor's implants in all future cases. This strategy has advantages in that there is a potential decrease for surgical inventory as well as a negotiated cost savings for the hospital. Additionally, all members of the operating room staff can be trained to use a single vendor's instrumentation, which leads to potential increase in efficiency. Similar to some of the other strategies mentioned earlier, this strategy requires the cooperation of all the surgeons to use a particular vendor, regardless of their previous preferences.

The single price/case price purchasing program involves a bidding process by which the lowest price offer for all implants involved in a particular case is accepted by the hospital. In this model, the winning vendor would receive a fixed amount of payment for all implants involved in a TKA regardless of the implant choice. This strategy, when compared with the others mentioned, provided the greatest implant cost reduction for the Lahey Clinic.

In the Lahey Clinic experience, vendor discounting led to a 4% decrease in implant costs in TJA, whereas implant matching led to a 5% decrease in costs.[10,20] The Lahey Clinic realized a 35% decrease in implant cost with the competitive bidding program in 1995. In 1997, they used the single price/case price purchasing program to further decrease their knee implant prices by 23% without changing their current vendors. By using all these strategies between 1991 and 2008, they were able to convert a net loss for hospital per joint replacement to a profit.[10,20]

CONCLUSION

TKA is one of the most significant surgical advances of the last century and continues to provide durable long-term outcomes in patients by improving pain and function. The prevalence and need of TKA are projected to continue to increase to nearly 3.5 million procedures per year by 2030. As health care expenditures continue to occupy a bigger percentage of the gross domestic product, cost cutting in health care will remain a focus for payers. Professional reimbursements have decreased annually, and hospital reimbursement rates have not matched pace with inflation. For orthopedic programs to remain financially viable especially in the era of bundled payments, there must be a coordinated and concerted effort among all members of the health care team to reduce expenses associated with the procedure, while continuing to maintain a high level of quality. Additionally, regulation of implant cost will remain critical to controlling these expenditures.

KEY REFERENCES

1. Belatti DA, Pugely AJ, Phisitkul P, et al: Total joint arthroplasty: trends in medicare reimbursement and implant prices. *J Arthroplasty* 29(8):1539–1544, 2014.
4. Bozic KJ, Ward L, Vail TP, et al: Bundled payments in total joint arthroplasty: targeting opportunities for quality improvement and cost reduction. *Clin Orthop Relat Res* 472(1):188–193, 2014.
5. Fehring TK, Odum SM, Troyer JL, et al: Joint replacement access in 2016: a supply side crisis. *J Arthroplasty* 25(8):1175–1181, 2010.
6. Froimson MI, Rana A, White RE, Jr, et al: Bundled payments for care improvement initiative: the next evolution of payment formulations: AAHKS Bundled Payment Task Force. *J Arthroplasty* 28(8 Suppl):157–165, 2013.
7. Healy WL, Finn D: The hospital cost and the cost of the implant for total knee arthroplasty. A comparison between 1983 and 1991 for one hospital. *J Bone Joint Surg Am* 76(6):801–806, 1994.
8. Healy WL, Iorio R, Ko J, et al: Impact of cost reduction programs on short-term patient outcome and hospital cost of total knee arthroplasty. *J Bone Joint Surg Am* 84-A(3):348–353, 2002.
9. Healy WL, Iorio R, Lemos MJ, et al: Single Price/Case Price Purchasing in orthopaedic surgery: experience at the Lahey Clinic. *J Bone Joint Surg Am* 82(5):607–612, 2000.
10. Healy WL, Rana AJ, Iorio R: Hospital economics of primary total knee arthroplasty at a teaching hospital. *Clin Orthop Relat Res* 469(1):87–94, 2011.
11. Healy WL, Iorio R, Richards JA, et al: Opportunities for control of hospital costs for total joint arthroplasty after initial cost containment. *J Arthroplasty* 13(5):504–507, 1998.
12. Iorio R, Healy WL, Richards JA: Comparison of the hospital cost of primary and revision total knee arthroplasty after cost containment. *Orthopedics* 22(2):195–199, 1999.
13. Iorio R, Robb WJ, Healy WL, et al: Orthopaedic surgeon workforce and volume assessment for total hip and knee replacement in the United States: preparing for an epidemic. *J Bone Joint Surg Am* 90(7):1598–1605, 2008.
14. Kim S: Changes in surgical loads and economic burden of hip and knee replacements in the US: 1997-2004. *Arthritis Rheum* 59(4):481–488, 2008.

21. Rana AHW: Economics of Total Knee Arthroplasty. In Scott Ia, editor: *Surgery of the Knee*, 2008.

23. Scott WN, Booth RE, Jr, Dalury DF, et al: Efficiency and economics in joint arthroplasty. *J Bone Joint Surg Am* 91(Suppl 5):33–36, 2009.

25. Zuckerman JD, Koli EN, Inneh I, et al: Can a hip and knee adult reconstruction orthopaedic surgeon sustain a practice comprised entirely of Medicare patients? *J Arthroplasty* 29(9 Suppl):132–134, 2014.

The references for this chapter can also be found on www.expertconsult.com.

196

Payment Paradigms

Shaleen Vira, Jay Patel, Adam Rana

The demand for total joint arthroplasty is expected to increase in the coming decades[45] independent of fluctuating economic conditions.[21] The prevalence of total hip arthroplasty is expected to double by 2026.[20] Total hip arthroplasty has been determined to be more cost-effective than medical treatment of hypertension, coronary artery bypass surgery, hemodialysis, and liver transplantation.[18] Despite these contributions of arthroplasty to health in the United States, osteoarthritis is the most expensive condition among Medicare beneficiaries who do not belong to a health maintenance organization, with costs exceeding $7 billion that derive from episodes of elective hip or knee replacement.[8] Concomitantly, $700 billion a year accounts for health care services delivered in the United States that do not improve health outcomes.[1]

There is a widespread belief held among policymakers and legislators that controlling these rising health care expenditures requires changing the reimbursement structure of physicians.[38] This chapter discusses the traditional payment paradigms that are thought to have fueled these soaring costs and provides an overview of the novel payment paradigms that have been implemented to address these previously uncontrollable costs. Understanding these payment mechanisms is especially pertinent for arthroplasty surgeons, who face rising costs and declining reimbursements as detailed in prior chapters. Moreover, to retain reimbursements and market share in the community, arthroplasty surgeons must demonstrate that their practices provide superior "value" to patients, a concept that is relatively new in the history of medicine.

HISTORICAL PERSPECTIVE AND THE "VALUE" PROPOSITION

The origination and development of procedures such as total joint arthroplasty were not initially subject to questions of cost-effectiveness. Novel implant types, which continue to be introduced to the market at a rapid pace, have been a major contributor to increased costs of total joint arthroplasty.[18] By the advent of the 21st century, as policymakers and legislators attempted to contain costs, orthopedic surgeons experienced a disappearing margin for their services, driven by unfavorable hospital payment trends, new expensive innovations, trends from outpatient surgery to ambulatory surgery centers, increased utilization of premium joint implants, and uncontrolled increases in joint implant prices.[18]

These market forces have been channeled into developing better payment mechanisms to encourage the delivery of "high-value" arthroplasty care. Value is defined as health outcomes achieved per dollar spent over the episode of care for a specific health condition, or, more simply, outcomes divided by costs.[32] The term *outcome* refers to disease-specific, long-term measurements that cover specific interventions and the full cycle of care, including hospitalization, complications, rehabilitation, and recurrences.[44] The following sections examine each paradigm from the lens of this value proposition.

FEE FOR SERVICE

In a fee-for-service (FFS) payment structure, each procedure, treatment, or service provided generates revenue for the provider, and depending on the costs of delivering those services, providers may make or lose money. The individual physician is the residual claimant.[24] The modest variable costs involved (e.g., supplies) are overshadowed by substantial fixed costs, including rent and depreciation as well as malpractice insurance, office staff, and operations. High fixed costs mean additional services rendered are likely to be profitable even if on average the revenue received is less than the average costs. In other words, the marginal revenue exceeds marginal costs; this is the basis of why FFS incentivizes provision of more services.[24]

In the FFS payment structure, time spent doing procedures is rewarded more highly than time spent with patients or coordinating care.[24] Laugesen and Glied[22] demonstrated the association between higher incomes with higher fees between US orthopedic surgeons and foreign counterparts, concluding that volume of services was a driver of higher US spending, particularly in orthopedics. Similarly, Medicare and Medicaid use monopsony power to administer prices, which has the effect of driving hospitals to aggressively pursue some types of procedures that are highly profitable and shun unprofitable activities. Furthermore, this behavior results in cross-subsidization across service lines: orthopedic profits subsidize other less profitable parts of a hospital with concomitant underinvesting in divisions that fail to generate profits in this monopsonist regime.[7]

The FFS structure offers no economic incentives for clinicians to efficiently organize the care delivered by other providers.[24] There is nothing in the simple incentives of FFS payment that drives the overall process to become more efficient. For example, the instruments and approach a particular surgeon prefers may be optimal for him or her, but if each surgeon uses a different approach, the operating room team does not have the opportunity to standardize the procedures to reduce waste and errors.[24] Furthermore, traditional FFS rewards readmissions and complications by accepting the provider's charges for more services rendered. Conversely, efforts to reduce these adverse events come at a financial detriment to providers.[27]

Orthopedic services exhibit what is known as preference-sensitive care.[29] Preference-sensitive care is defined as situations in which more than one generally accepted treatment option is available, and thus choice should depend on the severity of pathology and patient preferences.[29] An important problem inherent in FFS is that it promotes, or does nothing to curtail, large variations in spending among providers.[35,41] With respect to geography, Medicare spending per beneficiary is 52% higher in regions that spend the most money compared with regions that spend the least money.[46] However, patients in higher spending regions do not get better-quality care than patients in lower spending regions,[12] and in many instances their outcomes and satisfaction were worse.[11]

Differences in health care resource utilization can also be traced down to the level of individual clinicians making individual health care decisions.[29,31] Orthopedic services, in addition to preference-sensitive care, also exhibit supply-sensitive care, which is the concept that the number of providers in a given region influence the overall rates of services rendered. A region that has a large concentration of arthroplasty surgeons will have a higher incidence of total joint arthroplasties, and this is one physician-derived source of cost variations.[10]

FFS is not organized around value for patients because it rewards health care providers who shift costs, bargain away or capture someone else's revenues, and bill for more services or procedures as opposed to delivering better value.[33] The roles of health plans have been defined by the zero-sum mentality of cost shifting and by the misguided assumption that health care services could be treated as a commodity whose cost should be minimized.[34] Micromanaging health care delivery by reviewing or specifying provider activities is a deep flaw in attempts to rein in FFS care. For example, Highmark, a Blue Cross Blue Shield affiliate, attempted to steer tests to high-volume facilities to avoid duplication of equipment by refusing to cover diagnostic imaging at any clinic that did not offer a broad line of services and that did not have at least one full-time accredited radiologist on staff. Instead, these rules created the incentive for every imaging provider to perform every kind of scan, leading to more duplication of investment.[13,17,34] This phenomenon can also result in a further increase in administrative costs associated with billing each additional service, magnifying the problem. Another example is the case of Aetna, which hired radiologists to review requests for expensive magnetic resonance imaging and other scans and second-guessing the physicians ordering the scans rather than measuring and comparing health outcomes.[26,34]

Based on these experiences, alternative models of payment were sought to provide quality care at affordable costs. The National Commission on Physician Payment Reform recommended that the transition to payment systems based on quality and value should start with testing new models of care. It also acknowledges that FFS will remain important into the future, and thus iterative recalibration of payments is necessary.[38]

CAPITATION

The introduction of provider risk via capitation was intended to provide a motivation to improve efficiency and care pathways that can potentially reduce spiraling costs. The success of capitation depends on many factors including the specific methods used to try to mold physicians' behavior, the form of delivery system or payment paradigm, and local/cultural norms.[2]

Capitation ostensibly gives providers an incentive to develop disruptive business models within integrated provider organizations, in that using lower cost venues of care and lower cost caregivers such as nurse practitioners and physician assistants drives greater surplus.[7] In arthroplasty care, controlling costs through improved care pathways can include inventory control, implant matching, minimizing acquisition cost, physician education on best practices, guidelines, and discharge planning to reduce length of stays.[36]

Although capitation was deemed a failure of policymakers and payers to reduce costs in a manner that is safe to patient care, several lessons were learned. First, individual physicians are poorly equipped to manage risk, and the risks of withholding needed care are highest when financial risk depends directly and immediately on a single physician.[2] Risk pools in capitated arrangements should be larger than individual physicians' practices. Second, the magnitude of risk must not be so great as to induce a physician to make clinically imprudent choices.[2] Third, although the aim of capitation was to encourage peers to exchange information and to increase cooperation that can lead to better programs of care, fragmentation of care by specialty and profession limits the ability to integrate and provide higher value care.[2] Capitation works only in integrated provider systems, which account for less than 10% of people with health insurance in the United States.[7] When capitation is attempted in a nonintegrated system, it places independent businesspeople in a zero-sum game, where one physician's gain becomes another's loss. Fourth, the services covered in a capitation should be what the risk-bearing entity (physicians) can make relevant prudent choices about, not services that the risk-bearing entity cannot influence. Finally, risk contracting should cross existing institutional boundaries but should not require formal mergers and acquisitions as a prerequisite to integrated care.[2] Some of these lessons were incorporated in the novel payment paradigms that are discussed subsequently.

GLOBAL PROVIDER BUDGETS

Global provider budgets are attractive to payers because annual spending is predictable and the payer has control over health care spending growth. Many countries use this model including the Department of Veterans Affairs system in the United States. In 2009, seven provider organizations in Massachusetts entered the Blue Cross Blue Shield Alternative Quality Contract, followed by four more organizations in 2010. This contract, based on a global budget and pay-for-performance for achieving certain quality benchmarks, places providers at risk for excessive spending and rewards them for quality. This participation over 2 years led to a savings of 3.3% compared with spending in groups not participating in the contract with improvements in quality of care, specifically for long-term care management, adult preventive care, and pediatric care.[41]

Blue Shield of California created a partnership with health care providers to use an annual global budget for total expected spending and to share risk and savings among partners for providing health care. Launched in 2010, the 2-year results showed that costs increased at less than half the rate at which premiums rose; savings stemmed from declines in inpatient lengths of stay and 30-day readmission rates.[25]

However, despite these examples of modest gains, several limitations exist in the long term. First, the provider's revenue is disconnected from the volume, mix, and complexity of conditions the provider treats. This leads to rationing with long wait times to cope with demand that exceeds supply. Second, providers prioritize urgent or acute care over preventive services and long-term care. Third, if a provider has lower than expected demand, there is no incentive to generate more business resulting in unused capacity. This represents a rise in overall costs. Finally, when global provider budgets are independent of outcomes achieved, providers underinvest in skills and technology that offer the potential for better outcomes because they must absorb all the costs of new technology and innovation but do not share in the benefit.[28] These factors all undermine value, and thus novel payment paradigms are required.

BUNDLED PAYMENT

The history of bundled payment can be traced back to 1984 when the Texas Heart Institute developed a pricing plan for cardiovascular surgery without adversely affecting quality.[9] This concept of reducing costs without affecting outcomes, or improving outcomes without increasing costs, is the goal of efforts to improve value based on the concept that value is outcomes divided by costs. A bundled payment paradigm, also known as episode-based payment, consists of a single payment to the provider for treating a patient with a specific medical condition across a full cycle of care. This includes care for common complications and comorbidities but not unrelated medical conditions.[24] For a total joint arthroplasty, the bundled payment covers the initial visit, preoperative education, acute surgical care episode, and 90-day postoperative therapy and visits. The payment is contingent on risk-adjusted outcomes including care guarantees, and payment amount is based on the cost of efficient and effective care as opposed to past charges as done in an FFS system.

Based on the experience from capitation, several features must be in place for bundled payment to work. First, the payment should be above the actual cost incurred and be contingent on achieving good patient outcomes. As discussed in prior chapters, arbitrarily reducing reimbursements can work against this goal. Second, payments should be risk stratified and include stop loss provisions to protect against catastrophic cases. Thus in the bundled payment model, the risk for unexpected costs is borne by the provider. In contrast, in other paradigms, methods exist to control and contain this risk. Reinsurance policies that protect against risk of unusually expensive cases can be covered by the bundled payment and may avoid providing strong incentives to physicians to withhold needed care. Reinsurers will have an interest keeping down such costs and can help providers manage this risk.[24]

Additionally, the price received from a bundled payment should be stable over a specified period to allow providers to capture benefits from outcomes and process improvements. In other words, the financial incentives must be in place long enough for them to be realized by providers. These gain-sharing techniques may help align the incentives of hospitals and surgeons to make headway in reducing the total bill for a total joint arthroplasty that have previously been formidable obstacles to cost reduction attempts.[42] For example, the single price/case price purchasing program at the Lahey Clinic allowed for surgeons to agree on common implants to reduce the overall cost of implants.[18,19]

The Affordable Care Act (ACA) contends that providing financial incentives for physicians to improve quality and aggregating fee-for-service reimbursement into payments for broader bundles of care will lead to greater efficiency in the provision of care and thus lower costs.[8] Support for this theory comes from economic analyses such as the one by Cutler and Ghosh,[8] who calculated that episode-based bundled payments have the potential to reduce costs by encouraging efficiency in treating the conditions on which spending is high, regardless of whether the region as a whole is low cost. The ACA provides that 1% of Medicare payments be redistributed to health care providers and institutions that performed well on a variety of cost and quality measures. By 2017, a total of 2% of Medicare payments will be redistributed under the program. On the physician side, the incentive program began in 2015 with large group practices on a voluntary basis and is progressing to a mandatory program that will include smaller and solo practices by 2017. In 2011, the Centers for Medicare and Medicaid Services initiated a new Bundled Payment for Care Improvement initiative with the goal of introducing a payment model that would lead to higher quality, more coordinated care at a lower cost to Medicare.[6,19] Almost 7000 hospitals, physician organizations, and post–acute care providers have signed up to participate in bundled payment initiatives created under the ACA.[3]

Several challenges remain with the design and implementation of bundled payments. First, legislation must continue to alter and refine existing gain-sharing regulations such that providers who attempt to integrate vertically and horizontally are not accused of conflicts of interest. Second, when attributing a readmission within a 90-day time frame, the reason for readmission must be ascertained. In some instances, a readmission is clearly a complication of care such as a wound infection. In other cases, the readmission is unrelated, such as a postdischarge motor vehicle accident. However, most readmissions have less clear causes and can be intermingled with comorbidities over which arthroplasty surgeons may not have full control.[24] Third, although one physician may "manage" the clinical aspects of an episode of care, he or she may find it challenging for specialists in other fields such as anesthesiology, radiology, and pathology who work in an academic system entrenched in professional silos to agree on a practice approach or otherwise coordinate activities. The accountable care organization system developed with the ACA may not work well for independent practitioners who are not highly integrated within a health care system and therefore have little means to coordinate episodes of care.[16] Again, various laws and regulations have historically precluded such financial interconnections.[24] Finally, physician leadership will be the key to success of bundled payments: Patients will look to their physician for reassurance that practice redesign is driven by an effort to improve the patient experience and quality of care and not simply another cost reduction tactic.[15]

CONTRARIAN VIEWPOINT AND ALTERNATIVE PATIENT-BASED FINANCIAL MECHANISMS

An inherent assumption to transitioning from volume-based to value-based care is that financial incentives for providers will result in meaningful improvements in unnecessary hospital costs and procedures performed. The bearing of risk by orthopedic providers has stimulated studies on understanding the costs of a particular procedure.[43] Setting payments based on what it takes to achieve superior outcomes will incentivize physicians to improve risk adjustment techniques that account for comorbidities, fostering innovation that will increase quality.[24]

In 2008, Medicare introduced a policy that reduced payments for hospital-acquired infections.[37] Some states responded to this no pay for poor performance measure aggressively and slashed hospital-acquired infection rates.[5] However, a 2012 study found that overall the policy had no measurable effect on the rates of central catheter–associated bloodstream infections and urinary tract infections across US hospitals.[23] In 2011, the Cochrane group published two systematic reviews that failed to show convincing evidence that financial incentives can improve patient outcomes.[14,39] Another study showed that payer type has little effect on the rate of operative treatment and the orthopedic surgeon's work intensity.[4] Taken together, it appears that pay for performance programs are helpful in catalyzing, but not sustaining, meaningful change.[30] The study of economic incentives is truly complex, and perhaps the current policies remain "blunt" instruments to affect change in a way that improves patient outcomes.

Based on these findings, perhaps providing financial incentives for patients, as opposed to providers, may help curtail costs. One identified factor that has contributed to waste with respect to the design of health plans is that combining coverage for low-priced, predictable recurrent health care events (e.g., routine vision checkups) with low probability but financially disastrous events (e.g., polytrauma) destroys economic value.[7] Unbundling these disparate types of expenditures into a high-deductible insurance plan and a health savings account (HSA) may provide control to the individual patient and reduce administrative overhead of large costly comprehensive plans. HSAs were enabled by the Medicare Prescription Drug, Improvement, and Modernization Act in 2003 and allow a tax-free portable savings vehicle to help people pay for low-cost, relatively predictable, and recurrent medical expenses. These savings accounts are offered with a high-deductible insurance policy that, ideally, covers costs when they are over and above what HSAs can cover.[7]

These mechanisms are gaining in popularity by employers and employees, but their effects on overall costs are unclear at the present time. The rate of adoption has been modest because HSAs are offered as one option among many health plans and represent the option that carries risk to the patient: There exists an out-of-pocket-gap between what HSAs cover and when the high-deductible plan contributes coverage. Patients opt to stick with conventional comprehensive coverage to avoid bearing risk. Additionally, HSAs are offered in isolation of truly disruptive business model innovations, which limits the desirability of using one's "own" health care dollars to patronize what remains a very inefficient health care system.[7]

CONCLUSION

There is no one payment paradigm that can address all the challenges associated with the complex health care system in the United States. The key methodology to evaluate any current or future mechanism that an arthroplasty surgeon may face for his or her practice is by examining the effects of that mechanism on value for patients. In other words, does the plan reduce costs without damaging quality or improve quality without increasing costs? The effects of recent legislation and market-based payment innovations on value have yet to be determined but may represent a first step toward providing affordable health care for all Americans.

KEY REFERENCES

3. Blumenthal D, Abrams M, Nuzum R: The Affordable Care Act at 5 Years. *N Engl J Med* 372:2451–2458, 2015. doi: 10.1056/NEJMhpr1503614.

14. Flodgren G, Eccles MP, Shepperd S, et al: An overview of reviews evaluating the effectiveness of financial incentives in changing healthcare professional behaviours and patient outcomes. *Cochrane Database Syst Rev* (7):CD009255, 2011. doi: 10.1002/14651858.CD009255.

15. Froimson M: Perioperative Management Strategies to Improve Outcomes and Reduce Cost during an Episode of Care. *J Arthroplasty* 30:346–348, 2015. doi: 10.1016/j.arth.2014.12.030.

16. Froimson MI, Rana A, White RE, et al: Bundled payments for care improvement initiative: the next evolution of payment formulations: AAHKS bundled payment task force. *J Arthroplasty* 28:157–165, 2013. doi: 10.1016/j.arth.2013.07.012.

18. Healy WL, Iorio R: Implant selection and cost for total joint arthroplasty: conflict between surgeons and hospitals. *Clin Orthop Relat Res* 457:57–63, 2007. doi: 10.1097/BLO.0b013e31803372e0.

19. Iorio R: Strategies and tactics for successful implementation of bundled payments: bundled payment for care improvement at a large, urban, academic medical center. *J Arthroplasty* 30:349–350, 2015. doi: 10.1016/j.arth.2014.12.031.

25. Markovich P: A global budget pilot project among provider partners and Blue Shield of California led to savings in first two years. *Health Aff* 31:1969–1976, 2012. doi: 10.1377/hlthaff.2012.0358.

28. Miller HD: From volume to value: better ways to pay for health care. *Health Aff* 28:1418–1428, 2009. doi: 10.1377/hlthaff.28.5.1418.

32. Porter ME: What is value in health care? *N Engl J Med* 363:2477–2481, 2010. doi: 10.1056/NEJMp1011024.

35. Rettenmaier AJ, Wang Z: Regional variations in medical spending and utilization: a longitudinal analysis of US Medicare population. *Health Econ* 21:67–82, 2012. doi: 10.1002/hec.1700.

42. Taylor B, Fankhauser RA, Fowler T: Financial impact of a capitation matrix system on total knee and total hip arthroplasty. *J Arthroplasty* 24:783–788, 2009. doi: 10.1016/j.arth.2008.03.005.

43. Virani NA, Williams CD, Clark R, et al: Preparing for the bundled-payment initiative: The cost and clinical outcomes of reverse shoulder arthroplasty for the surgical treatment of advanced rotator cuff deficiency at an average 4-year follow-up. *J Shoulder Elbow Surg* 22:1612–1622, 2013. doi: 10.1016/j.jse.2013.01.003.

44. Wei D, Hawker G, Jevsevar D, et al: Improving value in musculoskeletal care delivery: AOA critical issues. *J Bone Joint Surg Am* 97:769–774, 2015.

The references for this chapter can also be found on www.expertconsult.com.

197

Physician-Hospital Partnerships

Mark Pinto, Paul Woods, Gary Lawera, Dawn Pedinelli, Mark Froimson

In an era of growing discontent regarding the structure and function of the health care system in the United States, physicians and health systems are being challenged to adopt new models of care delivery. In addition, the passage of the Patient Protection and Affordable Care Act (ACA) in 2010 has provided fundamental changes in payment and incentives that have spurred transformational change in all clinical, financial, and operational aspects of US health care. As a result, physicians and hospital systems are collaborating, consolidating, and strategizing both independently and together as they contemplate how to best position themselves to be successful in meeting these challenges for the future. As new model partnerships are being evaluated and embraced, there are advantages afforded to both physicians and the health system as well as pitfalls that are material and substantial. To that end, new business and health care delivery models are being developed and traditional models are being modified to promote efficient, high-quality care. Outcomes verified by validated metrics are now expected by all stakeholders including patients, payers, and purchasers.

Inherent in these new ventures is the goal to create a cost-conscious system that encourages health promotion and disease prevention. An equally important goal is to reimburse only interventions that verifiably improve health and well-being or improve health outcomes for both procedures and chronic disease states—the often referred to goal of shifting from volume to value. To be successful, new payment models, relationships, and partnerships must align provider behavior with these goals by rewarding participating providers for their part in the management and delivery of efficient, high-quality health care.

The provisions of the ACA, along with resulting payment models in the commercial payer sector, require care delivery organizations to provide integrated and coordinated care in a cost-conscious way. This often involves fixed funding envelopes, associated with either an acute episode of care (eg, hospitalization for an arthroplasty), in which the provider organization and professionals receive a single bundled payment for all services associated with the episode, or a "total cost of care" methodology, in which a patient's care over a period of time is paid for in a risk-adjusted capitation model, or as a percent of premium.

In addition, these organizations need to demonstrate performance against prespecified quality and cost metrics that must be shared with payers in a fully transparent manner. Given the fact that a single payment covers the entire episode of care, this new payment system places care organizations at risk for both the quality and the cost of care delivered. This new reality will force more intentional interaction between physicians, nonphysician providers, and administrators across the continuum of care to facilitate new directions and collaboration. The lack of correlation between clinical quality and the associated cost of care are just beginning to be realized; simply put, you don't get better care for more money spent. Furthermore, as increasing responsibility for the cost of care is shifted from payers to patients through higher deductibles and copayments, excellence in a cost- and quality-transparent world will be critical to having a competitive advantage. As a result, productive and progressive physician–health system relationships will be critical to success in the new risk-based health care market, and both physicians and health systems will need to identify mutually beneficial ways to work together to enhance their ability to compete in this rapidly changing environment.

Forward-thinking health care systems are now recognizing the categorical imperative that success depends on their ability to deliver the Triple Aim goals simultaneously: better health, better care, and lower per capita cost. As a result, going forward, systems with high quality at lower cost will be preferred providers for payers and patient consumers. Payers prefer such systems because their customers are receiving high-quality care (better clinical outcomes, better experience, less complications) at a lower cost. Providers can succeed in a competitive market by delivering the highest value care, and by assuming risk through alternative payment contracts, they can see that value accrue to them, reaping financial gains. Proactive health systems that are confident in their ability to create value are actively pursuing "at risk" contracts. The business model is that if quality metrics are met while services are provided at lower total cost, the cost savings (arbitrage) will be "shared" by the payer and system through incentive payments. Significant challenges, including establishment of meaningful metrics and accurate cost and expense benchmarks that can be monitored and improved on, drive both lower costs and superior quality in "at risk" contracts. These aggressive goals can be accomplished only through collaboration among physicians, other health care team members, and health systems.

Physicians in this milieu are increasingly interested in models that decrease the personal financial risk that is inherent in maintaining a practice and that provide greater work-life balance. In this environment, new and different physician–health system partnerships will be created to satisfy the interests of health systems, physicians, and other stakeholders. Hospitals and health systems will need to partner with physicians who stand uniquely qualified to determine what constitutes meaningful adjudication of quality and to step forward in a new way to lead health care teams to meet these new quality measures. The various partnerships each offer some inherent advantages and challenges and should be viewed by the participants as vehicles to accomplish mutually agreed-on goals.

These affiliations are presented empirically in order of increasing level of alignment and resulting decreasing level of business autonomy. Although physicians have historically sought autonomy and the ability to run their business in the manner that they wish, new models provide counterbalancing features that may be more highly valued by physicians facing certain market conditions.

TRADITIONAL PARTNERSHIP

The most common partnership involves physicians in private practice with privileges at one or more hospitals. In essence, hospitals provide the equipment, physical plant, and staff to perform procedures and care for patients beyond the scope that can be performed in a physician's office. The physicians voluntarily participate in call coverage, leadership, and committees to help manage the hospital and the health care it delivers. Until more recently, this traditional setup that relies on private practice physicians contributing in this way was the predominant relationship. It allows physicians to have direct control over their income with a traditional fee-for-service payment model. Voluntary participation in hospital and health system affairs provides the opportunity for physicians who refer their patients and procedures to the institution to have a voice in operations and clinical and administrative policy development and management. Health systems similarly benefit from such arrangements. This model encourages meaningful engagement of voluntary/affiliated physicians to maintain the hospital-physician relationship at little or no cost to the hospital system. Furthermore, it allows hospitals to build alignment of a broad spectrum of physicians across many specialties. By providing the "shop," the hospital can be the common unifying body for the local medical community, allowing multiple groups and independent physicians their platform for much of their high-value, fee-for-service interventions.

Despite the historical preference for this model, private practice is clearly on the decline. Given the volatile changes accompanying the ACA, physicians, especially primary care disciplines but surgeons as well, are seeking employed tracks and are deferring to hospitalists for inpatient care. As both experienced and new physicians seek better work-life balance and income security, they are showing less interest and obligation to "give back" to the hospital through voluntary activities. Consequently, the prevalence of the traditional model is rapidly diminishing. Hospitals are finding that they can no longer rely on this presumed obligation for physicians on staff to serve on committees or fulfill call schedules. This, in many cases, has created a crisis that has been highlighted with voids in call schedules for health systems, as they have little control or influence on physicians' availability for clinical work or where they direct the care of their patients.

Essentially, with the traditional model, there is no financial alignment between the health system and physicians. Given that physician practices are usually organized at a local level, they have limited resources and few incentives to engage in larger scale planning for the health system. There is often a lack of structure and rigor at the individual physician practice level to act on initiatives, if they exist. Finally, unless the physician practice is part of a clinically integrated network/accountable care organization, there is a limited ability to influence clinical

and administrative decisions and processes beyond the participation in committees.

MEDICAL DIRECTORSHIP

Another partnership that may be advantageous to physicians is the creation of a formal medical director position. This leadership position, with compensation, requires a physician or group to provide leadership for a designated service line or hospital service. The physician is paid a fair market value, which may need to be validated through third-party valuation, for managing a service. The payment is usually structured based on a traditional fee-for-service model, where the fair market value payment is made for the administrative time committed to this position. However, depending on the productivity of the physician, the administrative compensation model may represent a lower payment than would be earned in clinical activities. That being said, physicians have the ability to contribute and leverage clinical expertise that may result in efficiencies, care improvement, and quality of hospital practice that otherwise would have been more difficult to influence. In addition, it offers the physician an opportunity to develop administrative skills while gaining exposure to broader health care strategic planning and operations within a health system. This position also allows the physician to have increased control over quality of work life, through protected administrative time compared with voluntary roles.

Through use of medical directorships, the health system can align with key physicians who are able to provide subject matter expertise and contribute to strategic decisions. In addition, the hospital or health system is able to define the scope of the management responsibilities that the medical director will have, and, in so doing, the system can better control and predict physician leadership expenses, particularly for budget planning purposes.

As previously mentioned, this setup helps the system to work with physicians who are in a variety of compensation models that sometimes create conflicting incentives and motivations. As a result, the system must navigate many stakeholders and economic partners to be truly successful.

SERVICE LINE PRIORITIZATION

With service line prioritization, the health system prioritizes a service line or particular service offered. The system creates a separate entity or "center" with a designated space, staff, and physician leadership to increase market share and quality in a very specific area. The physicians are often motivated to participate given the professional satisfaction and recognition gained from the system. With this arrangement, the physician or group is given the opportunity to work in an environment that supports increased specialization of skills and provides a dedicated team of personnel with similar talents. As a result, the system and physicians can realize higher quality outcomes. Beyond the system recognition, the physicians are often recognized as being associated with an elite institution with potential for regional or national recognition as a center of excellence. By creating a high-quality clinical environment, the physicians are given access to equipment and technology that supports cutting edge clinical practice to drive the outcomes sought. Indirectly, the physicians often have the opportunity for an ownership stake in the real estate associated with a separate entity or other economic participation in models that present passive income streams.

The hospital system, by creating a separate entity, has the ability to market to the local and broader region that it is providing high-quality, specialized care to patient populations that otherwise might be unavailable from other health systems or physician groups in the service area. As such, these ventures often create a strategic and competitive advantage that may be difficult to replicate by other competitors. By developing a center of clinical expertise that results in higher quality, the system is able to realize increased retention of specialists who benefit from the association. In addition, as payers move from pay for performance to pay for outcomes, this type of center of excellence will be attractive to insurers and narrow networks and may directly affect patient flow patterns.

Service line management of partnership requires significant due diligence in its design and implementation. First, the system must determine which physicians will be chosen to participate. Second, this type of arrangement may require an exclusive commitment. As a result, the system needs to carefully navigate a complex compliance and regulatory environment. In addition, the system must be mindful of the perception of preferential treatment of physicians who are involved in the separate entity, both within that specialty and in the broader physician community. The system may inadvertently lead physicians not involved in the entity to question whether the commitment of the health system to other specialty areas has been diluted.

MANAGEMENT SERVICE ORGANIZATION

A management service organization is a vehicle for a health system to sell practice management and other administrative services to individual physicians or a physician group. When structured appropriately, the physicians directly see a decrease in administrative burden as the management services organization takes on the global responsibility of general support and management of key functions such as information technology, billing, human resources, marketing, contracting support, and other ancillary practice necessities. Beyond the readily recognized advantages, physicians have access to practice management expertise in an increasingly complex health care regulatory environment. Given that the health systems generally have more robust management and business intelligence support tools, overhead expenses and business trends can be more effectively managed than with what is usually available in private practice. The combination of all these offerings can support physicians to have more productive and better quality clinical and personal time.

The health system benefits through the obvious further alignment between the system and physicians. The system also can develop efficiencies that benefit both parties by establishing standardization and consistency of support functions that can be offered to other groups. The health system, through specialized professional management in collaboration with physicians, can gain easier access to data and its ability to track details that can be used to improve the quality and cost of care. As the management services organization provides and aggregates core clinical and business metrics, such as experience of care, both physicians and the health system can obtain a composite view of key clinical care indicators. The shared goals, supported with closer alignment and quality control, are that both the system and the physicians can make meaningful improvements

that will lead to consistent quality and outcomes. The management service organization can provide the infrastructure and services to support these goals.

High quality is the goal, and the challenges of how to optimize the efficiency of physician practice processes and where to concentrate limited resources can be difficult to ascertain. Beyond which processes to focus on, the health system must invest in physician practice expertise and tools to offer high-quality services and flexibility and to make the transition to a management service organization seamless. The challenge related to practice management is a cultural and business adjustment, and the transition may be more difficult than anticipated.

MANAGEMENT SERVICE AGREEMENT

A management service agreement capitalizes on the content expertise of physicians within a health system. It sets up a management relationship to provide oversight of a particular service or initiative within the health system (as opposed to a management service organization that focuses on the physician practice) in which the participating physicians are actively involved in the management of quality, efficiency, and patient satisfaction and experience of care. With a management services agreement model, both employed and affiliated physicians can participate. As a result, there is opportunity for broader extension of leadership roles across the entire medical staff. If structured properly, physicians may participate in shared savings, another opportunity for additional revenue. Furthermore, opportunity for broader physician leadership contributes to a shared "voice" in the decision making and enhances the ability of physicians to form a strong and meaningful partnership with the health system. Management service agreements delineate specific responsibilities, roles, and outcomes expected for investments made and often require significant commitment of time to design or redesign systems of care management within the scope of the agreement.

The health system also benefits from the increased accountability of key physician stakeholders for outcomes. The inherent "buy in" that such designs can engender can have a broader positive effect with the medical staff at large. This model gives the system the ability to pool expertise and benefit from "best practice" work by engaging physicians in both economic and clinical integration. As such, properly structured, this model becomes a vehicle to bring together both the employed and the affiliated physicians with the goal of meeting quality and cost metrics that otherwise might not have been realized without this type of integrative design.

With this model, physicians may be taking on financial risk. In contrast to the traditional fee-for-service models, redesigned care models focusing on value-based payments and improvement of population health may place traditional compensation at risk depending on the achievement of certain utilization and quality metrics and objectives. That being said, all payers are shifting risk to health systems and providers. Systems that are more progressive and willing to embrace this new compensation and care model will clearly be at a competitive advantage.

JOINT PAYER CONTRACTING RELATIONSHIP

To help balance the influence of third-party payers, health systems and physicians may create an entity that contracts with third-party payers on behalf of both physicians and hospitals. For physicians, this structure allows for the optimization of payment rates without the risk of collusion. Beyond the monetary advantages, joint contracting arrangements can create large, high-quality networks without necessarily any infringement on the independence of the physician practice. In addition, physicians, by becoming part of a large network, are given access to a larger patient pool compared with independent contracting.

The health system can generate a broad care delivery network and alignment with physicians with this type of engagement, while creating customer (payer and patient) loyalty. By ensuring prudent criteria for inclusion in the network as well as mechanisms for quality and cost control, the health system can realize better physician alignment through joint cost-containment efforts, coupled with quality measures to improve outcomes.

Inclusion criteria and other limits of such a network can create a need for a finite number of specialists. As a result, such arrangements may alienate nonparticipating or excluded physicians or groups. Physicians may then be loyal to one system or another but lose leverage if one system is "saturated" with that type of specialty.

JOINT VENTURE

A joint venture is another arrangement with which most physicians are familiar, particularly specialists. A joint venture is a collaboration that creates a legal entity that is owned by physicians, health systems, and potentially other investors. Typical joint ventures revolve around revenue-generating activities and structures such as outpatient surgery centers, stand-alone diagnostic centers, or professional office buildings. Most importantly to physicians, this type of relationship provides access to facility and technical fee revenue streams beyond the revenue stream from personally performed clinical activities. In addition, the burden of the administrative management of the entity usually falls to the health system or other partner, while the physicians often manage clinical areas to optimize care and clinical effectiveness. As a result, synergies are realized as the health system and the physicians contribute their own areas of expertise.

Health systems have entered into joint ventures, often reluctantly, to maintain the continued alignment of physicians with their system. More importantly, joint ventures can increase revenue opportunities the hospital might have otherwise lost to a venture without the health system involvement. Beyond these obvious realized advantages, the system is given a platform to experiment with designs, refine efficiencies, and lower costs that can be translated to hospitals, especially as health care shifts more to outpatient care.

Overall, for health systems, participation is frequently a defensive strategy to avoid revenue loss and maintain physician alignment. However, it can be embraced as a key component of a plan to obtain a partnership with physicians as the system attempts to increase market share and market penetration. Although the expectation is for joint ventures to contribute to a lower cost of care that includes overhead, it is not guaranteed to succeed. Joint ventures require significant commitment to efficiency by all parties, given the amount and structure of facility and technical fees paid to these facilities (eg, ambulatory surgery centers).

Beyond these concerns, due diligence must determine whether payers recognize the joint venture facility to maximize patient access and maximize appropriate use of the facility. Furthermore, the nature of joint ventures is such that their value must be considered over a longer time horizon with the inherent risk of a changing market landscape causing the attractiveness of the venture to change over time. Parties must weigh their desire to protect their long-term interests with the concern of being locked into a relationship that may be at risk of outlasting its attractiveness, especially as each party develops new relationships with additional entities.

PROFESSIONAL SERVICES AGREEMENT

A hybrid of the employed and traditional models is a professional services agreement, sometimes referred to as a purchased service agreement. In this arrangement, the hospital or health system assumes some or all of the risk of the physician practice including billing and collection via a contractual agreement for professional services, office staff, and facilities while the group continues to operate as an independent entity. This model is a competitive alternative to the full employment model. It provides both physicians and hospitals the ability to implement this type of agreement in varying degrees, which provides flexibility that can be tailored to the physicians, while the hospital is afforded better vertical integration with their services. Perhaps most importantly, it preserves the autonomy of physicians, which may be critical as they transition away from a traditional model. Additionally, it allows physicians to maintain business ownership and benefits that may be unavailable in an employed model.

The health system is potentially able to maintain lower overhead charges by avoiding significant benefits costs. Furthermore, this hybrid model can be a pathway to a full employment model, which may be more amenable for younger physician partners. It can also be undone amicably, but not always easily, if needed, should the physicians and health system choose to return to a traditional model or move to full employment.

For the health system, this type of partnership may have implications for accreditation and compliance standards in regard to federal and state laws as well as regulatory bodies such as The Joint Commission. Therefore, a fair amount of due diligence is required to ensure the components of the program are legal and compliant. Finally, the health system may have less control than desired over operations and decisions given financial and legal risks they have assumed with this type of agreement.

PHYSICIAN EMPLOYMENT

The final partnership described in this chapter involves physicians who are employed by the hospital or health system through formal employment agreements. With the ever-changing health care environment, this type of agreement is rapidly on the rise. It gives physicians greater security with better predictability in income, benefits, and defined work schedules and hours. With employment, physicians have greatly reduced administrative burdens compared with private practice, as these responsibilities are shifted to the health system. Finally, employment allows physicians greater access to system capital, equipment, technology, and the potential for better third-party contracts than could be achieved independently.

The hospitals and health systems also realize an advantage through the employed model compared with the traditional model of physician alignment and commitment. In the employed scenario, the health system has a ready portfolio of providers linked to its system, which facilitates and leverages the negotiation of value-based contracts. This provides for vertical integration, which allows the health system and providers to have a competitive business advantage in rapidly changing markets. This alignment supports patient loyalty and minimizes leakage to other health care entities. It increases vertical integration, with the goals of controlling costs and improving quality. These goals are met through the judicious use of ancillary services offered by the system such as laboratory, imaging, and physical therapy. Finally, such alignment allows the system to employ key physician leaders and, perhaps more importantly, specialty physicians, who are critical to the mission, vision, and strategy of the health system.

An important issue for the health system is whether it is able to, or desires to, employ every physician who seeks employment. Employment of physicians may decrease the loyalty and commitment of the health system's affiliated physicians. The hospital system also runs the risk of creating overcapacity and bearing the risk of possibly employing too many physicians for a given market. Health systems tend to remain loyal to physicians and have little experience or appetite for severing relationships, even when market conditions suggest an overcapacity exists. In addition, maintaining the physician's sense of ownership of his or her practice can be challenging when a physician is treated as an employee rather than a partner. Successful physician employment models attempt to foster a collegial, partnership culture that incentivizes productivity and rewards innovation and clinical improvement activities. When fostering of this culture is done well, physicians can often find that their sense of autonomy seems paradoxically higher than they had been experiencing in the waning days of their attempts to remain in a stressful private practice.

CONCLUSION

As the pace of health care reform has increased, physicians and other providers have seen a steady move of compensation models from pay for performance of individual services to pay for value, with an attendant shift of risk to patients, purchasers of health services, health systems, and the physicians who work within the health systems and partner with them. These new reimbursement models will require innovative designs that will modify the traditional physician–health system relationship. Physicians are interested in models that decrease the personal financial risk that is inherent in maintaining a private practice and provide greater work-life balance. The traditional model of the on-staff physician, who volunteers for committees and call at a hospital, is rapidly declining. With the transformation of health care, physicians are seeking more security and concomitantly better work-life balance. The various designs discussed in this chapter can help to achieve physicians' individual professional and life goals in this regard. In some cases, the employed model may provide an ideal answer in the current turbulent environment, and indeed it is rapidly on the rise. Current trends suggest that physicians are choosing to be employed or engaged in a hybrid format through professional service agreements. For physicians who choose not to participate in these models, consolidation into very large, specialized private practices, or multispecialty groups, may be necessary to leverage economies of scale and facilitate achievement of cost and clinical outcomes. These models have become requisite to keep pace with the ever-changing health care environment. As a result, well-designed physician–health system partnerships will be a critical element to the success of both physicians and health systems in the new and very dynamic health care environment.

The references for this chapter can also be found on www.expertconsult.com.

198

Value-Based Purchasing

Lorraine H. Hutzler, Joseph A. Bosco III

VALUE IN HEALTH CARE

Porter and Lee[18] defined health care value as patient outcomes divided by the cost of achieving those outcomes. Value is created by either improving outcomes of patients with a particular condition over an entire cycle of care for groups of patients with similar needs or by decreasing the cost of care provided. It is measured and managed only in terms of a defined need that is being met so that outcomes can be clearly defined and costs compared.[17] As the federal government is the largest purchaser of health care, the new Medicare payment strategies that shift reimbursement from volume based to value based have altered the way providers deliver medical services. Because of the shift of payment from volume to value, hospitals must change how they provide care if they are to remain financially solvent.

The goal of value-based purchasing (VBP) is to transform Medicare from a passive payer of claims to an active purchaser of care.[14] In the past, health care organizations were profitable as long as they received patients.[18] For decades, health care systems have responded to incentives that rewarded volume regardless of quality. VBP is an effort to change the focus of how care is paid for: In essence, the government wants *value*—not just quantity—for the money that it spends. Kathleen Sebelius, the former Secretary of Health and Human Services, explained the goals of VBP: "Under this initiative, Medicare will reward hospitals that provide high-quality care and keep their patients healthy. As hospitals work to improve their performance on these measures, all patients, not just Medicare patients, will benefit."[9] VBP creates a model in which hospitals that perform well are rewarded and hospitals that perform poorly are penalized. Beginning in fiscal year 2013, incentive payments for VBP were funded by a 1% cut in reimbursements for diagnosis-related group payments (which will increase to 2% beginning in fiscal year 2017). The government will redistribute the money saved by these payment reductions to institutions that demonstrate high-quality care. The quality of care is determined based on performance on 13 metrics divided between two domains of care measures: clinical process and patient experience.[14]

PAY FOR PERFORMANCE

Pay for performance is an umbrella term for initiatives (ie, VBP) designed to financially reward health care providers for improvements in quality, efficiency, and overall value of health care they provide. These arrangements provide financial incentives to hospitals, physicians, and health care providers to carry out improvements and achieve optimal patient outcomes. Pay for performance has become popular among policy makers as well as private and public payers including Medicare and Medicaid. The typical pay for performance program provides a bonus to health care providers if they meet or exceed agreed-on quality or performance measures; however, the program can also impose financial penalties on providers that fail to achieve specified goals or cost savings. The quality metrics used in pay for performance fall into the following four categories: process, outcome, patient experience, and structure measures. Process measures assess the performance of activities demonstrated to contribute to positive health outcomes for patients. Outcome measures refer to the effects care had on patients. Patient experience measures assess patients' perception of the quality of care they have received and their satisfaction with the care experience. Lastly, structure measures relate to facilities, personnel, and equipment used to treat patients.[12]

CENTERS FOR MEDICARE AND MEDICAID SERVICES VALUE-BASED PROGRAMS

Hospital Inpatient Quality Reporting Program

The Hospital Inpatient Quality Reporting Program was implemented by Section 501(b) of the Medicare Prescription Drug, Improvement, and Modernization Act of 2003. The program gave the Centers for Medicare and Medicaid Services (CMS) permission to pay hospitals that properly reported specific quality measures at higher rates compared with hospitals that did not. Hospitals that improperly reported these data saw a 0.4% reduction in the annual market basket update. After 2005, this reduction was increased to 2.0%. Quality measures include domains ranging from readmission rates to surgical care improvement projects.[5] Under this program, hospitals are rewarded for reporting outcomes and are not penalized or rewarded for the outcomes themselves.

Hospital Outpatient Quality Reporting Program

The Hospital Outpatient Quality Reporting Program was developed by the CMS in 2006, similar to the inpatient program. According to the CMS, hospital outpatient departments need to meet administrative, data collection and submission, validation, and publication requirements. Similar to the inpatient program, if measures are not met, hospitals see a 2% decrease in their annual payment from the CMS.[6]

Physician Quality Reporting System

The Physician Quality Reporting System was developed by the CMS to encourage health professionals and group practices to report the quality of patient care to the CMS. Starting in 2015, Medicare began to apply reimbursement cuts to providers and group practices based on 2013 data. Providers and group practices that did not satisfactorily report data on patient care quality measures for Medicare Part B Physician Fee schedule covered services in 2013 saw a 1.5% cut for these services in 2015. In 2016, providers and group practices were expected to see the reimbursement decrease by 2% based on data from 2 years prior—2014 data for 2016, 2015 data for 2017, and so on.[2,7] This program currently applies to physician group practices of 100 or more.[2]

CONTROLLING COSTS AND QUALITY OF CARE

Both public and private payer payment policies place increased responsibility on health care providers for improving care and controlling costs. In the United States, in specialties such as oncology and solid organ transplantation, in which registries have been mandated, outcomes have improved, and provider variation has decreased over time. In other countries where the government is the single payer of health care, such as Sweden, government (payer) registries have long been used in orthopedics, and similar improvements in outcomes have been seen. However, in the United States, outcomes reporting has historically been variable at the individual provider level, preventing its widespread acceptance and use. Although many US institutions (eg, the Mayo Clinic and Kaiser Permanente) have orthopedic registries, the establishment of national orthopedic registries has been slow to develop. Several strong, multi-institutional registries have been established, and the American Academy of Orthopaedic Surgeons has rejuvenated its efforts to establish a national joint replacement registry through the implementation of the American Joint Replacement Registry. These registries hold great hope for the realization of the measurement and reporting of outcomes that is fundamental to value.

There are promising steps toward encouraging patients and providers to be more value conscious. Medicare payments for surgeons and hospitals have begun to incorporate value measures through their hospital and physician quality programs. In addition, private insurers have Centers of Excellence programs that require surgeons and hospitals to collect and report on quality measures to qualify for inclusions in networks. For example, our facility NYU Hospital for Joint Diseases is a part of the Aetna Institutes of Quality Orthopaedic Surgery Program. Aetna makes information about the quality of cost of health care services available to its members to help them make informed decisions about their health care needs. The CMS is increasing transparency of hospital costs and outcomes through their Hospital Compare website. This site is designed to help patients compare hospital performance through musculoskeletal-specific quality measures including perioperative antibiotic administration, venous thromboembolism prophylaxis, readmission rates, mortality rates, frequency of hospital-acquired conditions, patient experiences (Hospital Consumer Assessment of Healthcare Providers and Systems [HCAHPS] scores), Medicare volume, and Medicare payment per beneficiary. Although these data are risk-adjusted for patient-specific factors (ie, sex, age, severity of illness scores), social factors such as low socioeconomic status, living situation, race, and social support are not risk-adjusted and are believed to impact these quality measures.[3]

QUALITY AND METRICS

Internal Metrics

Improving internal metrics involves detecting and correcting errors. It is vital to identify where improvements can and should be made in the process of care delivery. The objective nature of internal metrics simplifies their measurement and allows straightforward calculations regarding improvement. Improving internal metrics places importance on conformance to well-designed standards and consistency in their execution. The application of quality management principles is vital to reduce defects, the standard by which clinical process domain improvement is measured.

External Metrics

In the patient care domain, outcomes are governed by patient preferences, attributes, expectations, and perceptions. These factors are difficult to measure and vary from person to person and among populations. Satisfaction cannot be assessed until each episode of care delivery has been completed. This is assessed through HCAHPS scores, which can provide a challenge in regard to standardization of patients' desired delivery models.[14]

Financial Incentives and Penalties

The financial consequences of VBP will be substantial. Hospitals earn financial bonuses on the basis of levels of performance and quality improvement relative to specified benchmarks. Up to 2% of an institution's revenue from diagnosis-related group payments is at risk. Immediate effects on bottom lines of hospitals must be carefully monitored, particularly among safety net hospitals, which operate on exceptionally small margins.[18]

Patient Experience

The patient's perceptions of the medical care received from both individual providers and health care institutions are assuming greater importance in determining the quality of care provided and ultimately the reimbursement for that care. The HCAHPS is a national, standardized survey of patient perceptions of hospital care. It was publicly developed by the CMS and the Agency for Healthcare Research and Quality (AHRQ), and its results are publicly reported. Public reporting of care metrics via HCAHPS and other means has generated a significant amount of quality improvement initiatives. HCAHPS results also play an important role in the VBP program. VBP ties a portion of hospital revenues via the Inpatient Prospective Payment System to performance on certain quality measures in a Clinical Process Domain (70% of total score) and in a Patient Experience Domain (30% of total score) that combine to form a Total Performance Score. The results of HCAHPS are the basis of the Patient Experience Domain score. Therefore, patient experiences of quality of care will directly affect hospital revenues via VBP.[8]

Patient Outcomes

Quality of care can also be measured by complication rates. The CMS has targeted a select group of complications that it has designated hospital-acquired conditions (HACs). The formation of this list of complications was mandated by the Deficit Reduction Act of 2005 in an attempt to curb Medicare and Medicaid expenditures and prevent their financial insolvency. Medicare and Medicaid comprised 21% and 15% of national health expenditure in 2011. National health expenditure was $8680 per person in 2011, or 17.9% of gross domestic product.[16] HACs are thought to represent a costly quality gap for Medicare beneficiaries. As such, HACs are defined as occurrences that are (1) high cost or high volume, (2) result in assignment of a case to a Medicare Severity Diagnosis-Related Group that has a higher payment when listed as a secondary diagnosis, and (3) "could reasonably have been prevented through the application of evidence-based guidelines."[4] For discharges after October 1, 2008, the CMS Inpatient Prospective Payment System began to pay for these cases as if the secondary diagnosis were not present (ie, stopped reimbursing hospitals for additional costs of treating HACs). HACs are an objective measure of the technical quality of patient care. Their prevention is an area of ongoing quality improvement efforts. Since the 2008 cessation of reimbursement for cost of treating HACs, most studies have examined the effect of the policy on rates of reimbursement or patterns of coding or documentation. Although strategies for reducing HACs may differ, there is general agreement that minimizing their occurrence is an appropriate goal. Professional guidelines are available to aid in formation of prevention strategies.[8]

PERCENTILE BREAKDOWN OF QUALITY MEASURES AND FEE STRUCTURE

In the context of health care delivery, VBP allows payers to hold health care providers accountable for controlling costs and quality of care. Through a system of financial incentives and penalties, VBP leverages patient outcomes and patient experience data to improve the quality of care and reduce inappropriate care. At the present time, the CMS measures the quality of patient care based on 45% process of care measures such as Surgical Care Improvement Project measures, 30% patient experience measures, and 25% clinical outcomes. Starting in 2017, clinical process measures will be reduced to 5%, patient experience measures graded by HCAHPS will constitute 25%, safety will constitute 20% (which will include methicillin-resistant *Staphylococcus aureus* and *Clostridium difficile* rates for 2017 and looking forward to 2019 hospital-level risk-standardized complication rates following elective primary total hip and total knee arthroplasty), clinical outcomes will constitute 25%, and efficiency will constitute 25% (Fig. 198.1). Although the initial changes were expected to go into effect in 2016, data collection occurred before this. Medical providers can increase value by improving costs through consistent use of evidence-based medicine and clinical practice guidelines, minimizing complications, and eliminating disparity of care. The overriding goal is to improve quality and reduce costs by offering physicians meaningful incentives for achieving standard, recognized, and attainable measures.[10]

DOMAIN WEIGHTS

Hospital payments are based on their performance in four domains that reflect hospital quality: clinical process of care domain, patient experience of care domain, outcome domain, and efficiency domain (Fig. 198.2). The total performance score comprises all four domains: 20% clinical process of care (comprising acute myocardial infarction, heart failure, pneumonia, surgical care improvement scores, and hospital-associated infections), 30% patient experience of care (comprising HCAHPS survey questions regarding communication with

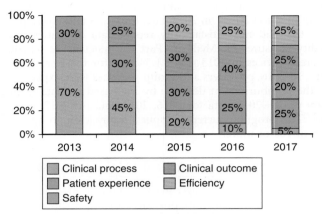

HOSPITAL VALUE BASED PURCHASING DOMAIN WEIGHTS

FIG 198.1 Hospital value-based purchasing program domain weights.

nurses, communication with physicians, responsiveness of hospital staff, pain management, cleanliness and quietness of hospital environment, communication about medicines, discharge information, and overall rating of hospital), 30% outcome (30-day mortality rates for acute myocardial infarction, heart failure, pneumonia, and central line–associated bloodstream infections, all AHRQ Patient Safety Selected Indicators), and 20% efficiency (measure of efficiency based on assessment of payment for services provided to a beneficiary during a spending-per-beneficiary episode that spans from 3 days before an inpatient hospital admission through 30 days after discharge). Each data set comprises a measure score representing the higher of either the achievement or the improvement points; an achievement score, which is awarded to a hospital that achieves certain levels of performance compared with other facilities; an improvement score, which is awarded to a hospital showing whether the hospital improved over its own baseline performance period; and a condition score, which is the sum of measures for a specific condition or procedure.[11]

MEDICARE SPENDING MODELS

Medicare is changing the way it pays hospitals for services provided to its beneficiaries. Instead of paying only for the number of services a hospital provides, Medicare is also paying facilities for providing high-quality services. Medicare links quality to payment in the following three VBP programs: Hospital Readmissions Reduction Program (HRRP), Hospital VBP Program, and HAC Reduction Program.

Hospital Readmissions Reduction Program

The Affordable Care Act (ACA) authorizes Medicare to reduce payments to acute care hospitals with excessive readmissions that are paid under the CMS Inpatient Prospective Payment System, which began on October 1, 2012. The program initially focused on patients who were readmitted for selected high-cost or high-volume conditions (acute myocardial infarction, heart failure, pneumonia). High rates of readmission can result from numerous factors including complications from treatments during the initial hospital stay, inadequate treatment, inadequate care coordination, and worsening of illness after hospital discharge.

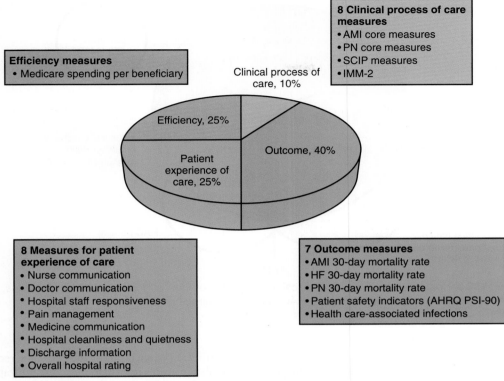

Efficiency measures
• Medicare spending per beneficiary

8 Clinical process of care measures
• AMI core measures
• PN core measures
• SCIP measures
• IMM-2

Clinical process of care, 10%

Efficiency, 25%

Outcome, 40%

Patient experience of care, 25%

8 Measures for patient experience of care
• Nurse communication
• Doctor communication
• Hospital staff responsiveness
• Pain management
• Medicine communication
• Hospital cleanliness and quietness
• Discharge information
• Overall hospital rating

7 Outcome measures
• AMI 30-day mortality rate
• HF 30-day mortality rate
• PN 30-day mortality rate
• Patient safety indicators (AHRQ PSI-90)
• Health care-associated infections

FIG 198.2 The 2016 value-based purchasing redistribution was expected to increase to 1.75% of Medicare payments. *AHRQ,* Agency for Healthcare Research and Quality; *AMI,* acute myocardial infarction; *HF,* heart failure; *IMM-2,* Influenza Immunization Measure; *PN,* pneumonia; *PSI-90,* Patient Safety Indicators 90; *SCIP,* Surgical Care Improvement Project.

Hospital Value-Based Purchasing Program

The Hospital VBP Program, established by the ACA, implements a pay-for-performance approach to the payment system that accounts for the largest share of Medicare spending affecting payment for inpatient stays in approximately 3000 hospitals across the United States. Under the Hospital VBP Program, which began in fiscal year 2013, Medicare adjusts a portion of payments to hospitals beginning based on either how well they perform on each measure compared with other facilities or how much they improve their own performance on each measure compared with their performance during a prior baseline period. The goal of this program is to improve clinical outcomes for hospitalized patients and improve their experience of care during their hospital stay.

Hospital-Acquired Condition Reduction Program

The ACA authorized Medicare to reduce payments to hospitals ranking in the worst performing quartile of hospitals with respect to HACs. The worst performing quartile is identified by calculating a total HAC score that is based on the hospital's performance on risk-adjusted quality measures. Hospitals with a total HAC score above the 75th percentile of the total HAC score distribution were subject to payment reductions beginning on October 1, 2014 (Fig. 198.3).[15]

HOW HOSPITALS FARED ON THE FIRST ROUND

The Hospital VBP Program redistributed approximately $126 million in hospital payments for fiscal year 2015. Of 3089

hospitals receiving a Hospital VBP Program payment adjustment, 44.5% (1375 hospitals) were penalized. For these hospitals the Hospital VBP Program payment adjustment was less than 1.5% of base operating payments, the amount that each hospital contributed to the Hospital VBP Program payment pool. Among penalized hospitals, the mean penalty was approximately 0.2% of total operating payments, or $92,000, and for nearly half of them, the penalty totaled less than $50,000. Among the 55.5% of hospitals receiving a bonus from the Hospital VBP Program, the mean bonus was approximately 0.4%, or $73,000. Of these hospitals, 10% accounted for approximately 46% of the total bonuses from the Hospital VBP Program; for 60% of hospitals awarded a Hospital VBP Program bonus, that bonus totaled less than $50,000.

In contrast to the Hospital VBP Program, the HRRP is not budget-neutral, and it has greater effects on hospital payments. In fiscal year 2015, approximately three-quarters of the 3478 hospitals for which an HRRP adjustment was reported by the CMS were penalized under the HRRP. The average HRRP penalty for this group was 0.5% of total operating payments, or $161,000, and aggregated losses totaled $424 million. The effects of the program are concentrated: 10% of hospitals accounted for nearly half of the HRRP penalties. For most other penalized hospitals, losses were modest, totaling less than $50,000 for 44% of hospitals.

The HAC Reduction Program payment adjustments for fiscal year 2015 showed major teaching hospitals to be disproportionately penalized. Of the hospitals receiving a HAC Reduction Program penalty, 56.5% were major teaching hospitals. In

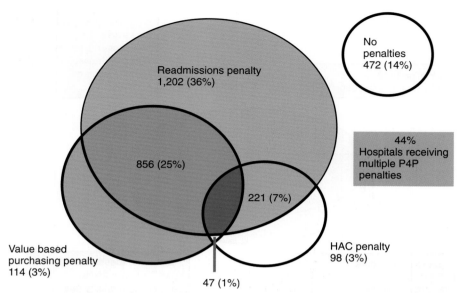

FIG 198.3 Hospitals receiving final fiscal year 2015 pay for performance (P4P) penalties. *DSH,* Disproportionate share hospital; *HAC,* hospital-acquired condition.

contrast, less than 10% of the nonteaching hospitals in the HAC penalty group had a Medicare DSH patient percentage greater than 50% (Fig. 198.4).[13]

PUBLICLY AVAILABLE DATA

Demonstrating quality, value, and patient safety in health care remains an industry focus, and the types of quality and performance metrics available to the public and providers continue to increase. Both public and private organizations collect and provide quality and performance measures data to consumers. Facility and provider participation in these initiatives is voluntary unless mandated by legislation. Organizations may choose to participate in voluntary initiatives for reasons such as financial incentives or public perception. Each facility or provider externally reports the data to a third party, which presents the data in a report card. Some of the most well-known performance organizations include the following:

The Leapfrog Group provides a consumer and a hospital view of its data, allowing for ease in comparing and selecting health care providers. Participation in reporting information is voluntary.

HealthGrades is an independent organization that offers consumers ratings of physicians, hospitals, and nursing homes based on data from the most current 3-year data set available from the CMS, several individual states (where available), publicly available directories, and telephone surveys. The information is free, with more detailed reports available for purchase. HealthGrades also offers educational information to providers on how it determines the ratings.

The Joint Commission provides certification and accreditation information to patients and health care providers. The information is based on information provided from facilities accredited by The Joint Commission.

Hospital Compare is a CMS-sponsored site that provides consumers with information on hospital performance and recommended patient treatments. The site offers perceptions of Medicare beneficiaries of the care they received at a facility. It also provides information on the utilization of facilities in regard to the median Medicare payment and number of Medicare patients treated for specific conditions.

AHRQ provides information regarding quality and performance measures as well as a searchable compendium of health care report cards. The reports in the compendium are designed for consumers. The compendium includes comparative data on quality for health care organizations and provider type.[1]

FUTURE CHANGES AND IMPLICATIONS

The National Quality Forum submitted recommendations in January 2015 on 199 performance measures for Health and Human Services to consider in 20 federal programs. Many of the proposals seek to better align measures among various programs and replace narrow process-oriented metrics. Numerous physicians question whether these measures can accurately measure quality, and there is little agreement on what measures matter most or are more likely to produce value. As of 2014, 33 federal programs asked providers to submit data on 1675 quality measures, according to a government count. State, local, and private health plans use hundreds more. In 2015, many of the federal pay-for-performance programs financial penalties went into full effect. Collectively, HAC, VBP, and readmissions place 5.5% of Medicare inpatient reimbursement at risk in fiscal year 2015; this will increase to 5.75% in fiscal year 2016 and 6% in fiscal year 2017. Hospitals and physicians may lose millions of dollars in Medicare payments for missing filing deadlines or improvement benchmarks in programs that track hospital-acquired infections, readmissions, and electronic record use. At the present time, approximately 80% of traditional Medicare spending is already tied to pay-for-performance programs, but the agency wants that to increase to 90% by 2018. The CMS would also like to have 50% of Medicare spending in alternative payment models, in which providers are accountable for quality and the cost of care for groups of patients. According to a CMS

	Hospital-acquired condition (HAC) reduction program	Hospital value-based purchasing (VBP) program		Hospital readmissions reduction program (HRRP)
	% of hospitals with penalty	% of hospitals with penalty	% of hospitals with bonus	% of hospitals with penalty
Total	21.9	44.5	55.5	75.8
Ownership				
Government	23.2	44.3	55.8	77.1
Investor	17.5	48.7	51.3	73.5
Tax exempt	22.7	43.2	56.8	78.1
Urban/rural				
Rural	13.3	33.4	66.7	78.5
Other urban	22.9	45.1	54.9	71.8
Large urban	26.6	50.7	49.3	80.2
Teaching status				
Non teaching	17.1	38.7	61.3	74.8
Other teaching	25.5	53.6	46.4	78
Major teaching	56.5	66.4	33.6	93.9
Number of beds				
<100 beds	13.8	26.8	73.2	64.8
100–399 beds	23.9	52.6	47.4	84.3
400 or more beds	40.9	59.8	40.2	86
Medicare disproportionate-share hospital patient percentage				
0–25%	19.5	36	64	70.7
26–50%	22.2	49.7	50.3	83.6
51–65%	35	65.2	34.8	80
>65%	30.7	65.2	34.8	80

FIG 198.4 Penalties under Medicare's pay for performance programs by hospital type fiscal year 2015.

report, more than 2600 hospitals will see their Medicare payments cut between 1% and 3% in 2015 for a total of $428 million for not reducing 30-day readmissions sufficiently. Many of the current quality metrics are available to the public on websites such as the CMS Hospital Compare and Physician Compare websites. Metrics that would allow patients to compare an individual physician's complication rates are not yet available but are something to expect in the future.[10]

The references for this chapter can also be found on www.expertconsult.com.

199

Quality Measures and Payment for Total Knee Replacement

Brian J. McGrory, David A. Halsey

INTRODUCTION

Health care spending management is crucial for society, and at the same time most Americans want to maintain or improve the quality of their care. Some argue that our historical fee-for-service payment model incentivizes health professionals to concentrate on quantity, not quality, of care. In recent years there has been an increased emphasis to "pay-for-performance" as a way to achieve high-quality care at a lower cost. There are multiple programs from both private and public payers focusing on efficiencies so as to increase health care value.[6,7] Differential reimbursement has been used to encourage participation in alternative payment models for individual physicians. Such a strategy uses one or more measures representing quality to affect payment to health care providers in an attempt to encourage health systems to maintain or improve quality in some way. Because of the high burden of arthritis for both patients and also for health care spending, it is no wonder that payers are using arthritis treatment as one model for these new payment strategies. Total knee arthroplasty (TKA), the most frequently performed inpatient procedure among patients aged 45 years and older,[20] is one such operation that is being assessed in this way.

A recent AMA-RAND study evaluating the impact of various payment models on physician practices, their professional lives, and on the delivery of patient care found that physicians wanted to embrace these new payment methods.[8] They understood the potential value that models like pay-for-performance could bring, but also noted that infrastructure changes were needed to make these innovations maintainable. For example, streamlining and standardizing quality metrics were high on the list of physician concerns. They were apprehensive about the variability and imprecision in the large array of quality measures being promoted by commercial and public payers.

This chapter will outline the more common strategies that are used in pay-for-performance and highlight the quality measures both currently being used and those in development for knee arthroplasty. This will help knee surgeons understand the way that we are currently being evaluated and reimbursed, and also highlight some of the challenges ahead.

EXAMPLES OF PAY-FOR-PERFORMANCE MODELS

Numerous programs and pilots from both public and private payment sources have used a variation of the pay-for-performance model. One such private payment reform initiative introduced by Blue Cross Blue Shield of Massachusetts, Alternative Quality Contract (AQC), provides financial incentives based on performance.[18] The three performance measurement categories that this program focuses on are process, outcome, and patient experience. Surgical process measures include infection prevention participation; outcome measures include postoperative complications, hospital-acquired infections, and condition-specific mortality; patient experience includes discharge quality, staff responsiveness, and physician and nurse communication.

Nationally, the Centers for Medicare and Medicaid Services (CMS) has a number of pay-for-performance programs including the Hospital Acquired Conditions (HAC) payment provision of the Inpatient Prospective Payment System (IPPS), the Hospital Readmissions Reduction Program (HRRP), Hospital Value Based Purchasing (VBP), Value-Based Payment Modifier Program (VPMP), Merit-Based Incentive Program (MIP), and Bundled Payments for Care Improvement (BPCI).

Under IPPS, cases are categorized into diagnosis-related groups (DRGs), and payment weights are allotted. The HAC payment provision stipulates that CMS will not reimburse for the higher cost of care resulting from a hospital-acquired condition that could have been practically prevented through use of evidence-based care. One of the fourteen HAC categories is deep vein thrombosis and pulmonary embolism after total knee replacement. The poorest performing hospitals with regard to HAC will be penalized 1% of their total Medicare payment.

The HRRP requires CMS to reduce payments to IPPS hospitals with greater than expected readmissions after five conditions, one of which is elective joint replacement. The maximum penalty has been recently increased from 2% to 3% of all Medicare payments based on readmissions of these five conditions. Recent analysis has demonstrated that this program has led to a significant decrease in readmissions, particularly among 65- to 84-year-old patients.[15]

VBP applies to hospital payments for inpatient stays, and the program went into effect on October 1, 2012. The program is a so-called zero-sum program, funded by withholding a percentage of participating (IPPS contracted) hospitals' DRG payments and paying higher performing hospitals. Payments are based on both how well a hospital performs and also how much it improves. The maximum penalty or payout will be reached in 2017 and is capped at 2% of all Medicare payments.

Initially, the VBP program quality measures were broken into "process" and "patient experience" categories. The process measure was adherence to Surgical Care Improvement Project (SCIP) recommendations for prevention of surgical infection.

The patient experience score was based on the hospital's Hospital Consumer Assessment of Healthcare Providers and Systems (HCAHPS) survey (Appendix 199.1). Of note, authors have reported that this measure is process based, and does not correlate with care quality effectiveness or validated patient reported outcomes.[9,16] Individual questions ask whether the hospital room was clean and quiet at night, and composite scores focus on the patient's experience with physician and nurse communication, pain management, new medication communication, and responsiveness to the their needs.[10] An outcome score focusing on 30-day mortality and hospital acquired infections (HAI) was added in 2014 and an efficiency score in 2015. The outcomes score provides for a 1% penalty for those hospitals with the highest percentage of medical errors. The efficiency score is based on the cost to Medicare per beneficiary, for a specific episode of care. In 2016, the total performance score will be based on efficiency (25%), outcomes (40%), patient experience of care (25%), and clinical process (10%).

The BPCI initiative is a voluntary program composed of four broadly defined models of care, which associate payments for the multiple services beneficiaries receive during an episode of care. Hip and knee replacement is one of the 48 clinical episodes a hospital can choose to target (under models 2, 3, and 4). With this initiative, organizations enter into payment arrangements that include financial and performance accountability for episodes of care. The quality measures followed include unplanned readmission rate, emergency department use without readmission, and mortality. These models are ostensibly designed to achieve a higher quality and more coordinated care, at a lower cost to Medicare.

In 2015, the Medicare Access and Children's Health Insurance Program (CHIP) Reauthorization Act repealed the sustainable growth rate (SGR) formula and pushed participation in alternative payment models for individual physicians. One such rule adopted by CMS in 2016 is the VPMP, in which physicians can receive payment incentives for providing "high-quality, efficient care." Underperformers are subject to payment adjustments. The VPMP provides for differential imbursement to a physician or group of physicians under the Medicare Physician Fee Schedule (PFS), based upon the quality of care furnished compared to the cost of care during a performance period. One quality measure with this program is all-cause hospital readmission after surgery. This program is set to expire in 2018, and the MIP begins in calendar year 2019.

CMS has guidelines that require each specialty to have a number of performance measures in place so that their members can participate in programs like VBPM and Physician Quality Reporting Systems (PQRS). CMS plans on using data from quality reporting programs to institute MIP. The MIP System will replace meaningful use, PQRS, and VBPM.

Quality Outcome Data work group and the NIH initiative Patient Reporting Outcomes Measure Information System (PROMIS) may ultimately be used as quality measure benchmarks. On August 31, 2015, the American Association of Hip and Knee Surgeons (AAHKS) convened a "Patient Reported Outcome Summit for Total Joint Arthroplasty" in Baltimore, Maryland, and reached consensus recommendations regarding patient reported outcomes (PRO) and risk variables suitable for arthroplasty performance measures.[11] Representatives from orthopedics organizations (AAHKS, the American Academy of Orthopaedics Surgery [AAOS], The Hip Society, The Knee Society, and American Joint Replacement Registry [AJRR]), CMS, Yale–New Haven Health Services Corporation Center for Outcomes Research and Evaluation (Yale/CORE); private payers; and other stakeholders participated in the summit.[1,13,14]

The group proposed that CMS require the use of only one general health questionnaire for the proposed reported outcome measure, either the VR-12[17] or the PROMISE-10-Global instrument.[2,4] For a disease-specific instrument for total knee replacement, the seven-question KOOS, JR. questionnaire[12] was recommended (Appendix 199.2). Lastly, the consensus of the summit was to recommend a staged approach of the candidate risk variables because some variables are more clinically relevant and are easier to collect at the present time. The group proposed a priority list of variables (including body mass index (BMI),[21] ethnicity, smoking status, preoperative use of narcotics, health status, and pain in a nonoperative joint of the lower extremity or back); a future desired list of three risk variables (socioeconomic status, literacy, and marital status); and a list of three risk variables that should not be included (mode of collection, American Society of Anesthesiologists [ASA] score,[3] and range of motion).[13]

SURGICAL DATA CURRENTLY BEING EVALUATED

The most transparent data collection system currently being used is from the United States government, through the Hospital Inpatient Quality Reporting (IQR) program. CMS has been analyzing data collected on surgical complications and readmissions for knee replacement patients since January 1, 2013. The inclusions for the risk-standardized complication rate following elective primary TKA includes acute myocardial infarction, sepsis, or septicemia within 7 days of admission; surgical site bleeding, pulmonary embolism, and death within 30 days of admission; and mechanical complication, periprosthetic joint infection, or wound infection within 90 days of admission. For a 30-day all cause risk-standardized readmission rate following elective primary arthroplasty, the patient must be readmitted to an inpatient unit; if the patient happens to be readmitted more than once, the readmission will only be counted once for this measure; planned readmissions are not counted. This data has been recently reformulated and a portion re-reported in relation to individual surgeons on the website of the nonprofit corporation ProPublica (a self-described independent newsroom that produces investigative journalism in the public interest).[19]

CMS measures adjust for each hospital's case mix (patient age and comorbidities), so presumably hospitals that care for older, sicker patients are on a "level playing field" with hospitals serving healthier patients. Ongoing work will be necessary to accurately predict risk because this is still a challenge, even with current risk calculators.[5]

PROPOSED COMPREHENSIVE CARE FOR JOINT REPLACEMENT

On July 9, 2015, CMS released a proposed rule to establish a new payment model for primary hip and knee replacements performed in hospital inpatient settings. Hospitals under this mandatory initiative designed by the Center for Medicare and Medicaid Innovation (CMMI) would be accountable for all costs associated with the episode of care from surgery until 90 days after hospital discharge, and the retrospective bundled payment would cover all Part A and Part B services. Although the model only applies to hospitals, they are responsible for reconciling expenses, including physician's fees and postacute payments. This model will be tested at hospitals in 75 randomly selected geographic areas (Medicare Service Areas, Massachusetts) over the next 5 years, and would affect more than 800 hospitals and 100,000 Medicare beneficiaries. This represents approximately 25% of Medicare and Medicaid hip and knee replacement discharges.

One goal of this payment model is to hold hospitals financially accountable for both the cost and quality of an episode of care. Concern over achieving this goal while taking into account patient values, appropriate and valid risk-adjustment, and transparent and evidence-based quality measures has been raised in the orthopedics community and voiced by AAOS President Davis D. Teuscher, MD.[7]

To qualify for payment or avoid penalty measured against historic and expected spending with this model, hospitals must meet quality performance thresholds on three "quality measures": hospital-level risk-standardized complication rate, hospital-level 30-day all-cause risk-standardized readmission rate, and responses to the HCAHPS survey (see Appendix 199.1). The goal of these measures is to encourage orthopedic programs to create and implement processes and procedures to ensure patients are optimized for surgery, risks and complications are reduced, and discharge planning is included in the care plan. The HCAHPS survey attempts to measure the patient's experience, but is not an outcome measure, per se.[9,16]

Of note, there are currently no specific TKA quality measures in this program. The Quality Measurement Program, Yale-New Haven Health Services Corporation/CORE, is acting as CMS contractor and currently developing risk-adjusted hospital-based patient reported outcome-based performance measures (PRO-PMs) for patients undergoing knee arthroplasty. Their work and recommendations from the Technical Expert Panel (TEP) have influenced the proposed PRO-PM data collection requirement for the CCJR. AAHKS has made recommendations for both improving the specificity of risk stratification, as well as proposed outcome measures.[13]

Even before this new program is implemented, the HRRP continues to affect hospital payments by penalizing hospitals with a high number of 30-day Medicare readmissions. This program was created under the Affordable Care Act, which required CMS to reduce payments to hospitals with excess readmissions of patients originally in the hospital for one of five conditions, including hip or knee replacement. To determine the penalty levied, CMS uses a formula based on the expected readmission rate from patient mix and national performance; the maximum penalty in 2015 was a 3% reduction in Medicare payments.

TOTAL KNEE PERFORMANCE MEASURE SET

The American Medical Association–convened Physician Consortium for Performance Improvement (PCPI) is a driving force in evidence-based clinical performance measurement. An AAHKS project co-chaired by David R. Mauerhan, MD, and Jay R. Lieberman, MD, culminated in the development of a total knee replacement performance measurement set, approved by the PCPI in January 2013. Further approval by the National Quality Forum (NQF) is in process. The performance set is shown in Table 199.1.

TABLE 199.1 **Total Knee Replacement Performance Measurement Set, Approved by the Physician Consortium for Performance Improvement in January 2013**

Measure	Measure Description
1a*	Percentage of patients undergoing a total knee replacement who had a history completed within 1 year prior to the procedure that included all of the following: onset and duration of symptoms, location and severity of pain, activity limitations (eg, walking distance, use of assistive devices, difficulty with stairs)
1b*	Percentage of patients undergoing a total knee replacement who had a physical examination completed within 1 year prior to the procedure that included all of the following: gait, knee range of motion, presence or absence of deformity of the knee, stability of the knee, neurologic status (sensory and motor function), vascular status (peripheral pulses), skin, height, and weight
1c*	Percentage of patients undergoing a total knee replacement with radiographic evidence of arthritis within 1 year prior to the procedure
2	Percentage of patients undergoing a total knee replacement with documented shared decision making, including discussion of conservative (nonsurgical) therapy (eg, NSAIDs, analgesics, exercise, injections) prior to the procedure
3	Percentage of patients undergoing a total knee replacement who are evaluated for the presence or absence of cardiovascular risk factors within 30 days prior to the procedure including history of DVT, PE, MI, arrhythmia, and stroke
4	Percentage of patients undergoing a total knee replacement who had the prophylactic antibiotic completely infused prior to the inflation of the proximal tourniquet
5	Percentage of patients undergoing total knee replacement whose operative report identifies the prosthetic implant specifications, including the prosthetic implant manufacturer, the brand name of the prosthetic implant, and the size of the prosthetic implant

*Measures 1a, 1b, and 1c are a composite measure and must be used together. ©2012. American Association of Hip and Knee Surgeons. All Rights Reserved. CPT Copyright 2011 American Medical Association.
DVT, Deep venous thrombosis; *MI,* myocardial infarction; *PE,* pulmonary embolism.

SUCCESS

Successful practice under a pay-for-performance system depends on understanding the evaluation process. Cooperation between the knee surgeon and the hospital is paramount because many of the pay-for-performance parameters are linked to specific programs and rely on process improvements as well as documentation. Patient selection, risk mitigation (patient optimization), education, and appropriate discharge planning as well as execution of excellent surgery are all important for a successful outcome.

SUMMARY

TKA is the most frequently performed inpatient procedure among patients aged 45 years and older in the United States,[20] and is under scrutiny from both private and public payers concentrating on efficiencies so as to increase health care value. In recent years there has been an increased emphasis on so-called pay-for-performance programs as a way to achieve high quality care at a lower cost. Such a strategy uses one or more measures representing quality to affect payment to health care providers in an attempt to encourage health systems to maintain or improve quality in some way. This chapter outlines the ever-changing landscape of the measures currently in use and highlights several proposed measures that a knee arthroplasty surgeon may use for patient care in the future.

KEY REFERENCES

5. Edelstein A, Kwasny M, Suleiman L, et al: Can the American College of Surgeons Risk Calculator predict 30-day complications after knee and hip arthroplasty? *J Arthroplasty* 30(9 Suppl):5–10, 2015.

12. Lyman S Abbreviated knee injury and osteoarthritis outcome score (KOOS, Jr.) validation. Paper presented at 4th International Congress of Arthroplasty Registries, Gothenburg, Sweden, 2015.

15. Purvis L, Carter E, Morin P: *Impact of the medicare hospital readmission reduction program on hospital readmissions following joint replacement surgery*, 2015, AARP Public Policy Institute, pp 1–8.

The references for this chapter can also be found on www.expertconsult.com.

APPENDIX 199.1.

Hospital Consumer Assessment of Healthcare Providers and Systems (HCAHPS) survey. This survey is used for various Centers for Medicare and Medicaid services (CMS) programs to monitor patient experience.

HCAHPS Survey

Survey Instructions

You should only fill out this survey if you were the patient during the hospital stay named in the cover letter. Do not fill out this survey if you were not the patient.

Answer <u>all</u> the questions by completely filling in the circle to the left of your answer.

You are sometimes told to skip over some questions in this survey. When this happens you will see an arrow with a note that tells you what question to answer next, like this:

Yes

No   *If No, Go to Question 1*

You may notice a number on the survey. This number is used to let us know if you returned your survey so we don't have to send you reminders.

Please note: Questions 1-25 in this survey are part of a national initiative to measure the quality of care in hospitals. OMB #0938-0981

Please answer the questions in this survey about your stay at the hospital named on the cover letter. Do not include any other hospital stays in your answers.

YOUR CARE FROM NURSES

1. **During this hospital stay, how often did nurses treat you with <u>courtesy and respect</u>?**
   1. Never
   2. Sometimes
   3. Usually
   4. Always

2. **During this hospital stay, how often did nurses <u>listen carefully to you</u>?**
   1. Never
   2. Sometimes
   3. Usually
   4. Always

3. **During this hospital stay, how often did nurses <u>explain things</u> in a way you could understand?**
   1. Never
   2. Sometimes
   3. Usually
   4. Always

4. **During this hospital stay, after you pressed the call button, how often did you get help as soon as you wanted it?**
   1. Never
   2. Sometimes
   3. Usually
   4. Always
   5. I never pressed the call button

YOUR CARE FROM DOCTORS

5. **During this hospital stay, how often did doctors treat you with <u>courtesy</u> <u>and respect</u>?**
   1. Never
   2. Sometimes
   3. Usually
   4. Always

6. **During this hospital stay, how often did doctors <u>listen carefully to you</u>?**
   1. Never
   2. Sometimes
   3. Usually
   4. Always

7. **During this hospital stay, how often did doctors <u>explain things</u> in a way you could understand?**
   1. Never
   2. Sometimes
   3. Usually
   4. Always

THE HOSPITAL ENVIRONMENT

8. **During this hospital stay, how often were your room and bathroom kept clean?**
   1. Never
   2. Sometimes
   3. Usually
   4. Always

9. **During this hospital stay, how often was the area around your room quiet at night?**
   1. Never
   2. Sometimes
   3. Usually
   4. Always

YOUR EXPERIENCES IN THIS HOSPITAL

10. **During this hospital stay, did you need help from nurses or other hospital staff in getting to the bathroom or in using a bedpan?**
    1 Yes
    2 No   If No, Go to Question 12

11. **How often did you get help in getting to the bathroom or in using a bedpan as soon as you wanted?**
    1 Never
    2 Sometimes
    3 Usually
    4 Always

12. **During this hospital stay, did you need medicine for pain?**
    1 Yes
    2 No   If No, Go to Question 15

13. **During this hospital stay, how often was your pain well controlled?**
    1 Never
    2 Sometimes
    3 Usually
    4 Always

14. **During this hospital stay, how often did the hospital staff do everything they could to help you with your pain?**
    1 Never
    2 Sometimes
    3 Usually
    4 Always

15. **During this hospital stay, were you given any medicine that you had not taken before?**
    1 Yes
    2 No   If No, Go to Question 18

16. **Before giving you any new medicine, how often did hospital staff tell you what the medicine was for?**
    1 Never
    2 Sometimes
    3 Usually
    4 Always

17. **Before giving you any new medicine, how often did hospital staff describe possible side effects in a way you could understand?**
    1 Never
    2 Sometimes
    3 Usually
    4 Always

WHEN YOU LEFT THE HOSPITAL

18. **After you left the hospital, did you go directly to your own home, to someone else's home, or to another health facility?**
    1 Own home
    2 Someone else's home
    3 Another health facility If Another, Go to Question 21

19. **During this hospital stay, did doctors, nurses or other hospital staff talk with you about whether you would have the help you needed when you left the hospital?**
    1 Yes
    2 No

20. **During this hospital stay, did you get information in writing about what symptoms or health problems to look out for after you left the hospital?**
    1 Yes
    2 No

OVERALL RATING OF HOSPITAL

Please answer the following questions about your stay at the hospital named on the cover letter. Do not include any other hospital stays in your answers.

21. **Using any number from 0 to 10, where 0 is the worst hospital possible and 10 is the best hospital possible, what number would you use to rate this hospital during your stay?**
0	0	Worst hospital possible
1	1	
2	2	
3	3	
4	4	
5	5	
6	6	
7	7	
8	8	
9	9	
10	10	Best hospital possible

22. **Would you recommend this hospital to your friends and family?**
    1 Definitely no
    2 Probably no
    3 Probably yes
    4 Definitely yes

UNDERSTANDING YOUR CARE WHEN YOU LEFT THE HOSPITAL

23. **During this hospital stay, staff took my preferences and those of my family or caregiver into account in deciding what my health care needs would be when I left.**
    1 Strongly disagree
    2 Disagree
    3 Agree
    4 Strongly agree

24. **When I left the hospital, I had a good understanding of the things I was responsible for in managing my health.**
    1 Strongly disagree
    2 Disagree
    3 Agree
    4 Strongly agree

25. **When I left the hospital, I clearly understood the purpose for taking each of my medications.**
    1 Strongly disagree
    2 Disagree
    3 Agree
    4 Strongly agree
    5 I was not given any medication when I left the hospital

ABOUT YOU

There are only a few remaining items left.

26. **During this hospital stay, were you admitted to this hospital through the Emergency Room?**
    1 Yes
    2 No

27. **In general, how would you rate your overall health?**
    1 Excellent
    2 Very good
    3 Good
    4 Fair
    5 Poor

28. **In general, how would you rate your overall <u>mental or emotional health</u>?**
    1 Excellent
    2 Very good
    3 Good
    4 Fair
    5 Poor

29. **What is the highest grade or level of school that you have <u>completed</u>?**
    1 8th grade or less
    2 Some high school, but did not graduate
    3 High school graduate or GED
    4 Some college or 2-year degree
    5 4-year college graduate
    6 More than 4-year college degree

30. **Are you of Spanish, Hispanic or Latino origin or descent?**
    1 No, not Spanish/Hispanic/Latino
    2 Yes, Puerto Rican
    3 Yes, Mexican, Mexican American, Chicano
    4 Yes, Cuban
    5 Yes, other Spanish/Hispanic/Latino

31. **What is your race? Please choose one or more.**
    1 White
    2 Black or African American
    3 Asian
    4 Native Hawaiian or other Pacific Islander
    5 American Indian or Alaska Native

32. **What language do you <u>mainly</u> speak at home?**
    1 English
    2 Spanish
    3 Chinese
    4 Russian
    5 Vietnamese
    6 Portuguese
    7 Some other language (please print):
    _____

THANK YOU

Please return the completed survey in the postage-paid envelope.

[NAME OF SURVEY VENDOR OR SELF-ADMINISTER-ING HOSPITAL] [RETURN ADDRESS OF SURVEY VENDOR OR SELF-ADMINISTERING HOSPITAL]

Questions 1-22 and 26-32 are part of the HCAHPS Survey and are works of the U.S. Government. These HCAHPS questions are in the public domain and therefore are NOT subject to U.S. copyright laws. The three Care Transitions Measure® questions (Questions 23-25) are copyright of The Care Transitions Program® (www.caretransitions.org).

Sample Initial Cover Letter for the HCAHPS Survey

[HOSPITAL LETTERHEAD]

[SAMPLED PATIENT NAME]
[ADDRESS]
[CITY, STATE ZIP]

Dear [SAMPLED PATIENT NAME]:

Our records show that you were recently a patient at [NAME OF HOSPITAL] and discharged on [DATE OF DISCHARGE]. Because you had a recent hospital stay, we are asking for your help. This survey is part of an ongoing national effort to understand how patients view their hospital experience. Hospital results will be publicly reported and made available on the Internet at www.medicare.gov/hospitalcompare. These results will help consumers make important choices about their hospital care, and will help hospitals improve the care they provide.

Questions 1-25 in the enclosed survey are part of a national initiative sponsored by the United States Department of Health and Human Services to measure the quality of care in hospitals. Your participation is voluntary and will not affect your health benefits.

We hope that you will take the time to complete the survey. Your participation is greatly appreciated. After you have completed the survey, please return it in the prepaid envelope. Your answers may be shared with the hospital for purposes of quality improvement. [OPTIONAL: You may notice a number on the survey. This number is used to let us know if you returned your survey so we don't have to send you reminders.]

If you have any questions about the enclosed survey, please call the toll-free number 1-800-xxxxxxx. Thank you for helping to improve health care for all consumers.

Sincerely,

[HOSPITAL ADMINISTRATOR]
[HOSPITAL NAME]

Note: The OMB Paperwork Reduction Act language must be included in the mailing. This language can be either on the front or back of the cover letter or questionnaire, but cannot be a separate mailing. The exact OMB Paperwork Reduction Act language is included in this appendix. Please refer to the Mail Only, and Mixed Mode sections, for specific letter guidelines.

Sample Follow-up Cover Letter for the HCAHPS Survey

[HOSPITAL LETTERHEAD]

[SAMPLED PATIENT NAME]
[ADDRESS]
[CITY, STATE ZIP]

Dear [SAMPLED PATIENT NAME]:

Our records show that you were recently a patient at [NAME OF HOSPITAL] and discharged on [DATE OF DISCHARGE]. Approximately three weeks ago we sent you a survey regarding your hospitalization. If you have already returned the survey to us, please accept our thanks and disregard this letter. However, if you have not yet completed the survey, please take a few minutes and complete it now.

Because you had a recent hospital stay, we are asking for your help. This survey is part of an ongoing national effort to understand how patients view their hospital experience. Hospital resultswill be publicly reported and made available on the Internet at www.medicare.gov/hospitalcompare. These results will help consumers make important choices about their hospital care, and will help hospitals improve the care they provide.

Questions 1-25 in the enclosed survey are part of a national initiative sponsored by the United States Department of Health and Human Services to measure the quality of care in hospitals. Your participation is voluntary and will not affect your health benefits. Please take a few minutes and complete the enclosed survey. After you have completed the survey, please return it in the prepaid envelope. Your answers may be shared with the hospital for purposes of quality improvement. [*OPTIONAL*: You may notice a number on the survey. This number is used to let us know if you returned your survey so we don't have to send you reminders.]

If you have any questions about the enclosed survey, please call the toll-free number 1-800-xxxxxxx. Thank you again for helping to improve health care for all consumers.

Sincerely,

[HOSPITAL ADMINISTRATOR]
[HOSPITAL NAME]

Note: The OMB Paperwork Reduction Act language must be included in the mailing. This language can be either on the front or back of the cover letter or questionnaire, but cannot be a separate mailing. The exact OMB Paperwork Reduction Act language is included in this appendix. Please refer to the Mail Only, and Mixed Mode sections, for specific letter guidelines.

OMB Paperwork Reduction Act Language

The OMB Paperwork Reduction Act language must be included in the survey mailing. This language can be either on the front or back of the cover letter or questionnaire, but cannot be a separate mailing. The following is the language that must be used:

English Version

"According to the Paperwork Reduction Act of 1995, no persons are required to respond to a collection of information unless it displays a valid OMB control number. The valid OMB control number for this information collection is 0938-0981. The time required to complete this information collected is estimated to average 8 minutes for questions 1-25 on the survey, including the time to review instructions, search existing data resources, gather the data needed, and complete and review the information collection. If you have any comments concerning the accuracy of the time estimate(s) or suggestions for improving this form, please write to: Centers for Medicare & Medicaid Services, 7500 Security Boulevard, C1-25-05, Baltimore, MD 212441850."

APPENDIX 199.2.

Seven question knee injury and Osteoarthritis Outcome Score (KOOS, JR.) questionnaire.[15] This was recommended as a patient reported outcome (PRO) by consensus at an August 31, 2015, American Association of Hip and Knee Surgeons (AAHKS), convened "Patient Reported Outcome Summit for Total Joint Arthroplasty" in Baltimore, Maryland.

KOOS, JR. KNEE SURVEY

INSTRUCTIONS: This survey asks for your view about your knee. This information will help us keep track of how you feel about your knee and how well you are able to do your usual activities. Answer every question by ticking the appropriate box, *only* one box for each question. If you are unsure about how to answer a question, please give the best answer you can.

Stiffness
The following question concerns the amount of joint stiffness you have experienced during the last week in your knee. Stiffness is a sensation of restriction or slowness in the ease with which you move your knee joint.

1. How severe is your knee stiffness after first wakening in the morning?

    None   Mild   Moderate   Severe   Extreme

Pain
What amount of pain have you experienced the **last week** during the following activities?

2. Twisting/pivoting on your knee

    None   Mild   Moderate   Severe   Extreme

3. Straightening knee fully

    None   Mild   Moderate   Severe   Extreme

4. Going up or down stairs

    None   Mild   Moderate   Severe   Extreme

5. Standing upright

    None   Mild   Moderate   Severe   Extreme

Function, daily living
The following questions concern your physical function. By this we mean your ability to move around and to look out for yourself. For each of the following activities please indicate the degree of difficulty you have experienced in the **last week** due to your knees.

6. Rising from sitting

    None   Mild   Moderate   Severe   Extreme

7. Bending to floor/pick up an object

    None   Mild   Moderate   Severe   Extreme

Tumors About the Knee

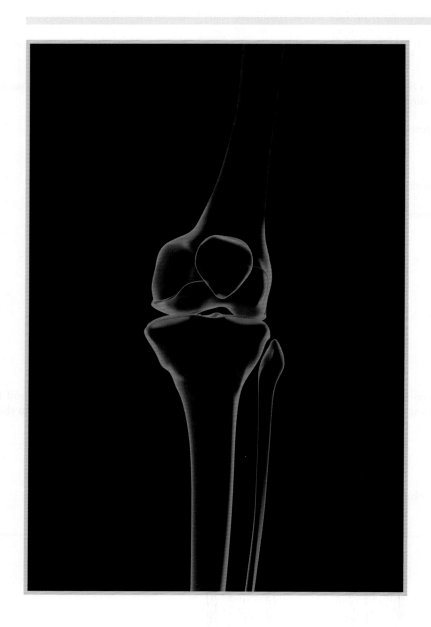

200

Evaluation of the Patient With a Bone Lesion About the Knee

Ginger E. Holt, Robert J. Wilson II

Evaluation of a patient with a bone lesion about the knee requires a thorough history and physical examination, imaging studies, and sometimes associated laboratory studies to formulate a differential diagnosis, make a diagnosis, and provide appropriate treatment. The differential diagnosis then determines the need for further investigation (eg, biopsy).

HISTORY

Symptoms

Bone tumors about the knee are brought to clinical attention for a variety of reasons. Common presenting symptoms include pain, a mass, decreased range of motion, and a finding incidental to the presenting symptoms. Bone lesions may be painful for primary or secondary reasons. Primary bone pain results from rapid intraosseous and soft tissue pressure caused by tumor expansion and malignant tumor cell proliferation. Secondary pain results from mechanical instability and is caused by the tumor destroying cortical bone. It is exacerbated by weight bearing. A pathologic fracture is the extreme form of mechanical instability.

A soft tissue mass may arise from direct tumor extension through cortical bone or may be the result of extension through the haversian canal system, as in the case of Ewing sarcoma. The resulting soft tissue mass may be the presenting symptom noted by the patient or may be the cause of diminished range of motion secondary to a mechanical block. A characteristic nocturnal pain pattern relieved by aspirin or nonsteroidal anti-inflammatory drugs in association with characteristic findings on plain x-ray or computed tomography (CT) scan is diagnostic for an osteoid osteoma.[14]

As important as presenting symptoms are to defining the nature of a bone lesion about the knee, lack of symptoms can be just as important. A benign bone tumor may be discovered as a result of a radiographic finding that is incidental to the presenting symptoms.

Patient Age

Although many bone tumors may have a similar appearance and presentation, patient age can narrow the differential diagnosis, with certain conditions being more likely to occur in a specific age range (Fig. 200.1).[21] For example, a lytic epiphyseal lesion in a skeletally immature patient is more likely a chondroblastoma, and consideration must be given to a giant cell tumor of bone in a skeletally mature patient.[22]

Activity Level

Assessment of activity level, participation in contact sports, or a recent history of trauma may be helpful in determining the cause of a bone lesion. Patients who have had a sudden increase in activity level may be at risk for a stress fracture, particularly in the proximal tibia. A patient who has had direct trauma to the thigh or calf may present with an apparent bone tumor that is actually heterotopic ossification.

Past Medical History

Past medical history can be helpful in uncovering significant diagnostic information. A personal history of cancer may lead to several diagnostic possibilities. A lytic bone lesion in a patient with a personal history of cancer is metastatic disease until proven otherwise.[1] A patient with a medical history of metastatic carcinoma treated with radiation therapy may have a postradiation sarcoma or a radiation-related insufficiency fracture, and patients who have undergone chemotherapy or radiation treatment may have osteonecrosis.[8] A past medical history of local or systemic infection should be evaluated for potential osteomyelitis. Patients with a history of chronic obstructive pulmonary disease, asthma, or conditions commonly treated with steroids should be questioned regarding their steroid history, and consideration should be given to osteonecrosis.[9]

A family history should be obtained for benign familial osteochondromatosis.[17] Li-Fraumeni syndrome is a well-known example of an inherited predisposition for cancer. Germline mutations of the *p53* gene predispose patients to many cancers, including osteosarcoma.[3]

PHYSICAL EXAMINATION

Patients with a bone lesion about the knee require an in-depth physical examination to elucidate potential clues as to the diagnosis. Examination of the integumentary system may provide diagnostic details in narrowing down a differential diagnosis. Café au lait spots may be indicative of neurofibromatosis, and cutaneous angiomas are associated with Maffucci syndrome. Previous skin incisions or draining sinuses should be evaluated to determine whether previous trauma or surgery may reveal underlying osteomyelitis. A long-standing draining sinus may be indicative of a Marjolin ulcer, suggesting underlying squamous cell carcinoma. Other skin lesions associated with an underlying bone tumor may suggest a bacterial infection as well as a fungal infection such as blastomycosis.

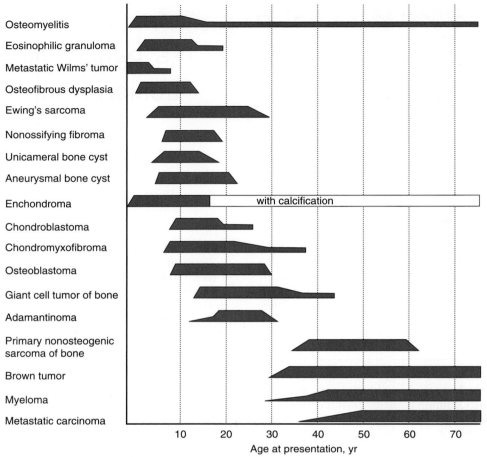

FIG 200.1 Range of patient ages at presentation for various radiolucent lesions. (From Springfield DS: Radiolucent lesions of the extremities. *J Am Acad Orthop Surg* 2:306–316, 1994.)

A complete physical examination includes a lymph node survey. An underlying bone lesion with enlarged lymph nodes may be diagnostic of lymphoma. A patient with a suspected metastatic bone lesion should undergo a directed examination of the thyroid, prostate, or breasts, as a primary tumor may be found.

IMAGING

Local

Plain radiography is the most specific noninvasive means of establishing a differential diagnosis for primary bone tumors. When evaluating a bone tumor about the knee, the initial imaging study should include plain radiographs in two perpendicular planes. Commonly, the benign or malignant nature of a tumor can be determined on plain radiographic evaluation. Enneking's four questions should be asked of any bone tumor to formulate a differential diagnosis.[4,5] These questions include (1) where the tumor is located, (2) what the tumor is doing to the bone, (3) what the bone is doing to the tumor, and (4) whether underlying matrix is present. Tumors may have diaphyseal, metaphyseal, or epiphyseal locations or may be surface tumors. If the diagnosis is not clear after plain radiographic evaluation, a more specific examination may be warranted. The next test obtained is based on the question being asked.

CT is the best tool with which to evaluate endosteal cortical bone, skeleton erosion, and lesion mineralization.[6] Magnetic resonance imaging (MRI) provides information on anatomy including bone and soft tissue as well as definitive tumor margins.[24] MRI can give specific information as to the matrix of the tumor. An expansile bone lesion that is multiloculated with multiple fluid-fluid levels is suggestive of an aneurysmal bone cyst. A lesion that is dark on both T1-weighted and T2-weighted sequences is suggestive of a fibrous lesion such as an extra-abdominal desmoid, and a tumor that is bright on both T1-weighted and T2-weighted images is suggestive of a lesion high in water content such as a myxoma.

Systemic Imaging

Systemic staging includes evaluation for multifocal disease, metastatic disease from a primary bone tumor, or the source of metastatic disease causing a secondary bone tumor. A whole-body technetium-99m–labeled methylene diphosphonate bone lesion scan is useful in evaluating multifocal skeletal disease.[15] Although this may assist in determining an alternative biopsy site if the underlying diagnosis is unknown, it rarely aids in narrowing the differential diagnosis.

A CT scan of the chest, abdomen, and pelvis determines the origin of metastatic disease in approximately 85% of cases.[16] These scans serve as systemic staging for primary malignant bone tumors as well.[13]

[^{18F}]2-Fluoro-2-deoxy-D-glucose positron emission tomography (FDG-PET) uses the glucose metabolism of tumors to detect tumor activity.[18] This mechanism of systemic staging is most useful for melanoma, adenocarcinoma, and lymphoma. Combining CT imaging (chest, abdomen, and pelvis) with FDG-PET improves decision making in greater than 80% of cases; therefore, when an FDG-PET scan is considered, it should be performed concomitantly with a CT scan.[25]

LABORATORY EVALUATION

Serum and urine tests for the most part are nonspecific and should be ordered selectively. Elevated white blood count, erythrocyte sedimentation rate, and C-reactive protein suggest infection, although all may be elevated in many malignant tumors. Prostate-specific antigen should be ordered in men with lytic bone lesions to evaluate for prostate cancer. Serum protein electrophoresis and urine protein electrophoresis are useful in evaluating multiple myeloma. Alkaline phosphatase may be elevated in primary bone tumors (osteosarcoma) and Paget disease. Serum calcium and parathyroid hormone levels are increased in brown tumors of hyperparathyroidism. Serum lactate dehydrogenase and alkaline phosphatase have been shown to have prognostic significance, and patients with elevated levels have shorter survival times compared with patients who present with normal values.[15] Calcium levels should be checked in patients with a bone tumor, especially patients undergoing surgery, as these patients often present with hypercalcemia. Urine tests of *N*-telopeptide and hydroxyproline may be helpful in evaluating bone turnover in patients with Paget disease or osteoporosis.

DIFFERENTIAL DIAGNOSIS

See Table 200.1 and Fig. 200.2.

TABLE 200.1 Differential Diagnosis by Tumor Location

Not Tumor	Benign	Malignant
Diaphyseal		
Infection	Osteoid osteoma	Osteosarcoma
Stress fracture	Osteoblastoma	Ewing sarcoma
	Osteofibrous dysplasia	Adamantinoma
	Fibrous dysplasia	Lymphoma
		Histiocytosis
		Myeloma
Metaphyseal		
Infection	Osteoblastoma	Osteosarcoma
Brown tumor	Aneurysmal bone cyst	Chondrosarcoma
Bone infarct	Unicameral bone cyst	Lymphoma
Paget disease	Giant cell tumor	Metastatic disease
	Enchondroma	
	Chondromyxoid fibroma	
	Nonossifying fibroma	
Epiphyseal		
Infection	Chondroblastoma (skeletally immature)	Osteosarcoma
Osteochondral defect	Giant cell tumor (skeletally mature)	Clear cell chondrosarcoma

BIOPSY

General Considerations

Biopsy is the final procedure in the assessment of a bone lesion. Biopsy of a bone lesion involves complex cognitive skills. A biopsy must be well planned and executed to maximize treatment and minimize risks. Poorly planned incisions, soft tissue contamination, and performing surgery without a tissue diagnosis can negate limb salvage surgery (Figs. 200.3 and 200.4). Mankin and colleagues[11,12] determined that patients were adversely affected when biopsy of a skeletal sarcoma was performed musculoskeletal oncologists without training for performing bone biopsy. The recommendation of these studies was that lesions suspected to be malignant should be referred before biopsy to a specialist in the care of malignant bone tumors.

Needle versus Open Biopsy

The decision to perform a needle versus an open biopsy is based on many factors. The comfort of the treating pathologist in making a diagnosis from a limited tissue source such as a needle biopsy versus an open biopsy is a consideration. This decision may also depend on the availability of operative time in performing a biopsy. The lesion itself may not be amenable to a needle biopsy. Less solid tumors, such as Ewing sarcoma or myeloma, may have a low yield with a needle biopsy and may require an open biopsy. Lesions that appear to have a large necrotic center or that have a large associated hematoma may be poorly represented on a needle biopsy. These lesions should be considered for an open biopsy. The ability to obtain an adequate amount of tissue for future treatment, including genetic evaluation, may be another determining factor as to whether needle versus open biopsy should be performed. The more information the orthopedist can provide to the pathologist, the more accurate the diagnosis.

In addition, the surgeon must determine how experienced the treating pathologist is in evaluating musculoskeletal pathology. Obtaining a correct diagnosis for musculoskeletal pathology may be challenging. One study of 262 bone tumors in children found only 60% of initial pathologic diagnoses were correct, and 22% of malignant tumors were misdiagnosed as benign.[23] Even experts in musculoskeletal pathology may have difficulty obtaining a correct diagnosis. A study of eight musculoskeletal pathologists reviewing 12 cases of osteosarcoma found that they agreed on a diagnosis of osteosarcoma for only 58% (7 of 12) of the cases.[10] Another study of a combined review of cartilaginous tumors by musculoskeletal pathologists and musculoskeletal radiologists found low reliability in differentiating benign from malignant lesions and low-grade from high-grade malignant lesions.[20] A well-executed biopsy with ample tissue obtained can be for naught if the pathologist does not have adequate experience diagnosing musculoskeletal pathology.

Biopsy Technique

Several general factors go into the technique of an open biopsy as outlined in Table 200.2. An initial consideration is holding parenteral antibiotics until cultures are obtained. Once intraoperative cultures have been obtained, antibiotics may be administered. Some specific techniques regarding anatomic sites may be considered. When a biopsy of the distal femur is performed, the biopsy itself should avoid the quadriceps tendon, and the specimen should be taken just medial or lateral to this.

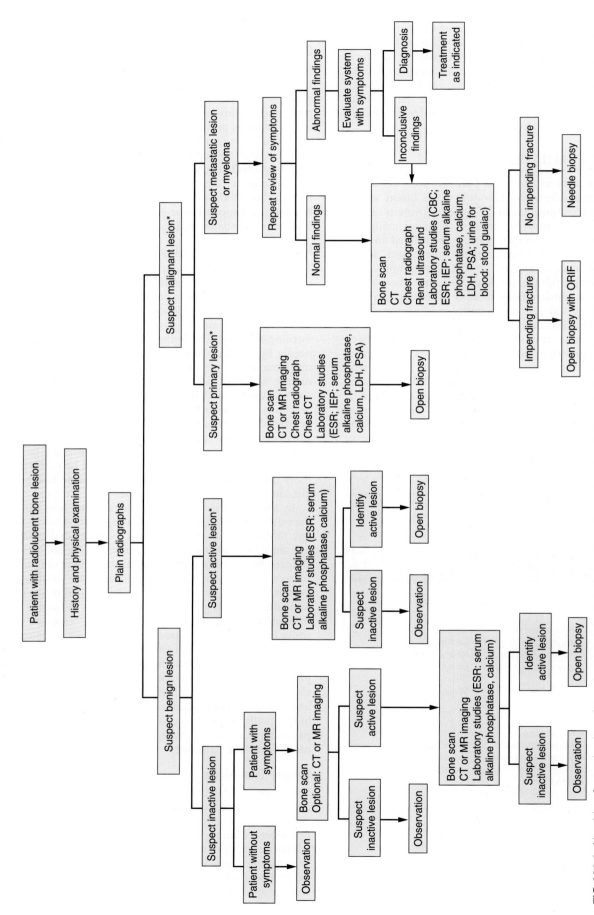

FIG 200.2 Algorithm for evaluation of a patient with a radiolucent lesion of an extremity. *Asterisk* indicates the point at which referral is indicated if the evaluating physician is not prepared to treat the patient. *CBC,* Complete blood cell count; *LDH,* lactate dehydrogenase; *ORIF,* open reduction and internal fixation; *PSA,* prostate-specific antigen. (From Springfield DS: Radiolucent lesions of the extremities. *J Am Acad Orthop Surg* 2:306–316, 1994.)

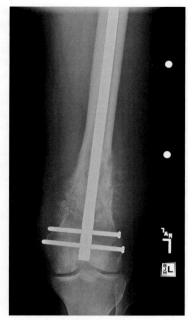

FIG 200.3 Distal femur osteosarcoma with pathologic fracture inappropriately stabilized without a preoperative tissue diagnosis.

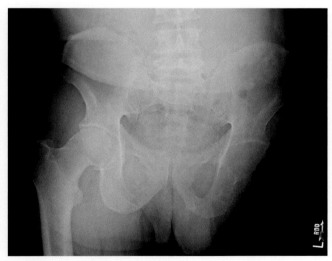

FIG 200.4 Postoperative radiograph after hip disarticulation in the same patient shown in Fig. 200.3.

In returning for definitive resection, this spares the quadriceps tendon from resection. Biopsy of the proximal tibia must avoid the patellar tendon. An attempt should be made to perform the biopsy where any potential hematoma would be contained by muscle tissue within the anterolateral proximal lower leg, as opposed to biopsy over the subcutaneous tibia, which may result in continued drainage and infection. Biopsy of the proximal fibula is best performed anteriorly, avoiding contamination or potential damage to the peroneal nerve. When a biopsy of the popliteal fossa is performed, a short oblique biopsy may be appropriate, as the definitive procedure likely will require a "lazy S"–shaped incision.[19]

TABLE 200.2   Principles of Musculoskeletal Biopsy

Principle	Rationale
Perform longitudinal incision in line with future resection	Longitudinal incision is extensile
	Biopsy tract can be excised with final resection
Avoid critical structures, ie, neurovascular bundles	Contamination of critical structures precludes limb salvage
Obtain biopsy specimen from soft tissue component when present	Bone is weakened when its cortex is disrupted
Maintain strict hemostasis	Avoid increased contamination outside of biopsy tract by iatrogenic tumor spread

STAGING OF BONE TUMORS

Following a complete history and physical examination, local and systemic imaging evaluation, and diagnosis of tumor type and grade, the bone tumor may be staged. Systems exist for both benign and malignant bone tumors. In general, staging allows prediction of the risk metastatic disease and determination of appropriate treatment.

Benign bone tumors may be staged by the Campanacci system[2] or the surgical staging system (SSS) developed by Enneking and associates.[5] The Campanacci system is based on plain radiographs. Latent lesions (stage A) are contained within the bone. Active lesions (stage B) remain within the bone but have a responsive cortical reaction. Aggressive lesions (stage C) breach the cortex. The SSS is based on compartmental anatomy. In the SSS system, a benign bone tumor is stage 0. Malignant bone tumor staging consists of the SSS or the American Joint Commission on Cancer (AJCC) system.[7] In the SSS system, malignant bone tumors are graded by histology and compartment status.

Histologically, tumors are graded as low or high, and compartment status is evaluated by confining the tumor to a compartment (intracompartmental) or not (extracompartmental). Histologically, stage I tumors are low-grade lesions, and stage II tumors are high-grade lesions. Compartmental status is determined as stage A when the tumor remains within the bony compartment; stage B represents an extracompartmental tumor. Stage III defines low-grade or high-grade metastatic tumors. Most malignant tumors are high grade and extracompartmental (stage IIB) lesions. The SSS does not apply to Ewing sarcoma or rhabdomyosarcoma.

The AJCC staging system uses the tumor-node-metastasis (TNM) classification scheme. It determines prognosis based on tumor size (T_1 ≤8 cm, T_2 >8 cm), grade (grade 1 and 2 = low; grade 3 and 4 = high), lymph nodes (±), and metastases (±). See Campanacci and colleagues,[2] Enneking and associates,[5] and Greene and colleagues.[7] For a complete overview of the Campanacci, SSS and AJCC staging systems, see Campanacci and colleagues,[2] Enneking and associates,[5] and Greene and colleagues.[7]

CONCLUSION

The most critical aspect in evaluating a patient with a bone lesion about the knee is making a diagnosis. Arriving at this vital juncture requires a thorough history, physical examination, imaging studies, appropriate differential diagnosis, and ultimately an appropriately executed biopsy. Staging follows the diagnosis of a malignant tumor to aid in prognosis and treatment. Once accurate diagnosis and staging are complete, treatment can follow.

KEY REFERENCES

1. Biermann JS, et al: An approach to the management of the patient with metastatic bone disease. *J Bone Joint Surg Am* 91:1518–1530, 2009.
5. Enneking WF, et al: A system for the surgical staging of musculoskeletal sarcoma. *Clin Orthop Relat Res* 153:106–120, 1980.
8. Holt GE, et al: Fractures following radiotherapy and limb-salvage surgery for lower extremity soft tissue sarcomas: a comparison of high dose versus low dose radiotherapy. *J Bone Joint Surg Am* 87:315–319, 2005.
9. Kerachian MA, et al: Glucocorticoids in osteonecrosis of the femoral head: a new understanding of the mechanisms of action. *J Steroid Biochem Mol Biol* 114:121–128, 2009.
11. Mankin HJ, et al: The hazards of biopsy in patients with malignant primary bone and soft-tissue tumors. *J Bone Joint Surg Am* 64:1121–1127, 1982.
12. Mankin HJ, et al: The hazards of the biopsy, revisited. Members of the Musculoskeletal Tumor Society. *J Bone Joint Surg Am* 78:656–663, 1996.
14. Papathanassiou ZG, et al: Osteoid osteoma: diagnosis and treatment. *Orthopedics* 31:1118, 2008.
17. Sandell LJ: Multiple hereditary exostosis, EXT genes, and skeletal development. *J Bone Joint Surg Am* 91(Suppl 4):58–62, 2009.
21. Springfield DS: Radiolucent lesions of the extremities. *J Am Acad Orthop Surg* 2:306–316, 1994.
25. Worsley DF, et al: Impact of F-18 fluorodeoxyglucose positron emission tomography–computed tomography on oncologic patient management: first 2 years' experience at a single Canadian cancer center. *Can Assoc Radiol J* 61:13–18, 2010.

The references for this chapter can also be found on www.expertconsult.com.

201

Surgical Treatment of Benign Bone Lesions

Matthew G. Cable, Nicholas P. Webber, R. Lor Randall

Benign bone lesions around the knee are relatively common entities. These lesions can be a cause of pain, deformity, and emotional distress. Oen, the treatment of these lesions is straightforward, with little associated morbidity.[11,92] The knee is an extremely common location for most benign bone tumors. They present in a variety of ways, from incidental findings on radiographs to pain and deformity. A thorough clinical and radiographic evaluation of the patient with a bone lesion is critical (see Chapter 204). This chapter focuses on the surgical treatment of common benign bone lesions around the knee for the general orthopedic surgeon and the musculoskeletal oncologist.

STAGING OF BENIGN BONE TUMORS

Led by Dr. William Enneking, staging systems were developed for benign and malignant bone tumors.[29] The three-stage system for the staging of benign bone tumors is widely used to describe, and more importantly, to guide treatment of benign bone tumors.[28,31] The system is based on the biologic behavior of these tumors determined by examination of the radiographic findings.[49,77]

Stage 1 lesions are considered latent. They are generally asymptomatic and are usually found incidentally on radiographic studies ordered for reasons unrelated to the tumor. These lesions are typically well demarcated in their radiographic appearance. They can progress in size and symptomatology in rare situations, although they usually resolve. Initially, these lesions should be observed.

Stage 2 lesions are considered active. They tend not to resolve spontaneously and are less well demarcated in their radiographic appearance in contrast to stage 1 lesions. Frequently they require surgical intervention with aggressive treatment. Recurrence is not infrequent.

Stage 3 lesions are considered locally aggressive lesions and they often demonstrate extensive local extracompartmental destruction. Treatment often requires wide en bloc resection. Some stage 3 lesions can undergo malignant transformation and should be followed closely after surgical treatment.

TREATMENT OF SPECIFIC BENIGN CONDITIONS

The treatment of benign neoplasms of bone around the knee is based on the resultant symptomatology. Most benign bone lesions around the knee can be observed if they do not cause pain, deformity, cosmetic concern, functional disability, or increased risk of pathologic fracture. Mechanical irritation outside of the joint itself is a common cause for elective surgical treatment of tumors in this location. Benign bone lesions rarely cause internal derangement of the knee, with the rare exception of chondroblastomas and osteoid osteomas. This section describes the presentation, natural history, and treatment of the most common types of benign bone tumors around the knee.

Benign Bone-Forming Tumors

Osteoid Osteoma. The most common benign bone-forming tumor is the osteoid osteoma, accounting for 10% of all benign bone tumors. It is more common in males than in females, with the peak incidence in the second decade of life. With regard to the knee, the proximal femur is the most common location, although it can also arise in the distal femur, proximal tibia, and fibula. Dull aching pain is the most frequent symptom. Previously, some investigators believed that an osteoid osteoma was an inflammatory process such as a Brodie abscess, which has a somewhat similar clinical and radiographic appearance.[89] Currently, it is accepted that an osteoid osteoma is a true osteoid-forming neoplasm, without histologic evidence of lymphocytes or plasma cells. Histologically, the nidus demonstrates aggressive but benign woven bone formation, with large numbers of osteoblasts and osteoclasts in a vascular fibrous stroma. No chondroid areas are seen.

The characteristic radiographic feature of an osteoid osteoma is a central lytic nidus that can measure up to 1 cm in diameter. In the common cortical lesion (Fig. 201.1), there will be an extensive reactive sclerosis creating a fusiform bulge on the bone surface. If the nidus is more centrally located in metaphyseal bone, less sclerosis is seen and the radiographic appearance is less diagnostic. Technetium bone scans are invariably positive. A computed tomography (CT) scan is helpful to better locate the lesion anatomically for improved preoperative planning.[24] Magnetic resonance imaging (MRI) may miss the nidus, making establishment of the diagnosis more difficult.[35]

Osteoid osteomas have been attributed to otherwise unexplainable knee pain.[2,15,20] If the nidus is close to a joint or within the joint, which can occur in approximately 10% to 12% of cases,[40,57] inflammatory synovitis may result. This synovitis may inappropriately suggest the diagnosis of pyarthrosis, subacute osteomyelitis, or rheumatoid arthritis.[89,93] If the bony reaction is focal and intense, the lesion can take on the appearance of an exostosis.[67] Furthermore, an osteoid osteoma can mimic pes anserinus syndrome, when the lesion is located medially in the proximal tibia.[84]

Generally, symptoms are relieved with nonsteroidal anti-inflammatory drugs (NSAIDs) secondary to a high concentration of prostaglandins in the nidus.[21,41,72,102] Osteoid osteomas

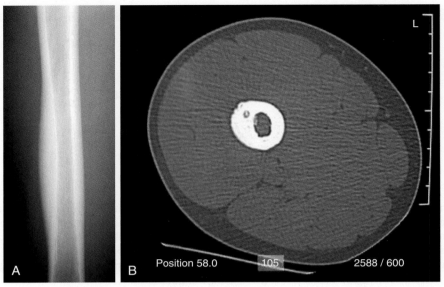

FIG 201.1 **Osteoid Osteoma of the Femur** (A) Anteroposterior (AP) radiograph demonstrates dense bone formation with a nidus that is difficult to appreciate. (B) CT scan reveals the nidus.

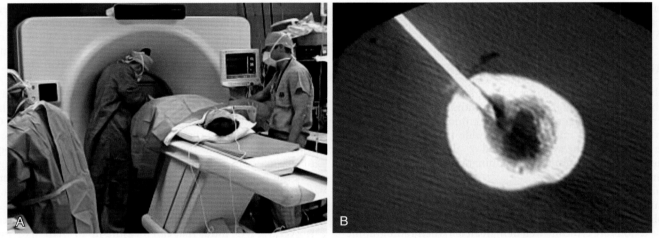

FIG 201.2 (A and B) CT-guided radiofrequency ablation of a femoral osteoid osteoma.

may also have a unique pathogenic nerve supply, a finding that may be common among bone tumors.[65,75]

Most cases of osteoid osteomas are stage 1 lesions because they resolve spontaneously. They can be treated symptomatically with aspirin or NSAIDs.[37] If the patient fails nonsurgical treatment, surgical intervention is usually successful. If surgery is elected, it is important to eradicate the entire symptomatic nidus. Removal of a large amount of the surrounding sclerotic bone should be avoided because it can severely weaken the bone and may result in an iatrogenic pathologic fracture. For open techniques concerning cortical lesions, adequate exposure is required to enable the surgeon to visualize the bulging cortex. Intralesional resection via the burr-down technique is generally preferred over en bloc resection. The nidus can be identified visually by the hyperemic pink color in the adjacent reactive bone. It is imperative to carry out curettage on the nidus followed by high-speed burring to advance the margin another 2 to 3 mm. If the lesion is not visible on the surface, which is usually the case in medullary lesions, radiographic markers

should be placed intraoperatively prior to making the cortical window. Percutaneous thermal ablation using radiofrequency or interstitial laser ablation is another less invasive method of treating osteoid osteoma (Fig. 201.2). This technique continues to gain wide acceptance as a preferable management modality.[5,27,55,81,82] Depending on location, CT guidance or surgical navigation may be necessary, and is often extremely helpful to obtain successful eradication of the lesion.[19] In cases in which there is an intra-articular lesion, arthroscopic treatment has been used successfully in adults and children.[2,34,57,70]

Osteoblastoma. An osteoblastoma is a large osteoid osteoma. According to the World Health Organization, the nidus of a true osteoblastoma is larger than 2 cm.[106] Its incidence around the knee is less than osteoid osteoma and accounts for 1% of all bone tumors overall. Osteoblastomas arise more commonly in males than in females and occur in the same age group as osteoid osteomas.[96] Infrequently, osteoblastomas are found in the metaphyses of the distal femur, which should raise the suspicion for more ominous diagnoses. The most common presenting symptom is pain, and the lesion can be latent to locally aggressive.[6]

Radiographically, an osteoblastoma has a more lytic and destructive appearance than an osteoid osteoma. Its larger nidus has less sclerotic reactive bone at the periphery and may take on the appearance of an aneurysmal bone cyst. Histologically, the nidus of the osteoblastoma is almost identical to that of the osteoid osteoma but can show excessive osteoblastic activity, osteoid formation, and vascularity with numerous giant cells in a vascular fibrous stroma.

The treatment modalities for osteoblastomas are similar to those used to treat osteoid osteomas. Treatment usually consists of a vigorous curettage of the lesion, which may require a bone graft if instability results because of the relative size of the lesion after mechanical or thermal expansion of the margin. Radiofrequency ablation may also prove useful in the management of this lesion and is currently being used at many centers.[81,82,101]

Osteofibrous Dysplasia. Osteofibrous dysplasia is a rare condition that is seen almost exclusively in the tibia of children younger than 10 years. It is more common in boys than in girls and is frequently asymptomatic. It commonly affects the diaphysis and results in anterior cortical bowing. However, it can occur in the fibula and can be seen bilaterally in rare cases. True involvement of the knee is equally rare.

Radiographically, the lytic changes seen in the anterior tibial cortex are surrounded by sclerotic margins, creating a soap-bubble appearance similar to the radiographic picture of fibrous dysplasia and adamantinoma.[10] Some studies have suggested that osteofibrous dysplasia may be a precursor to adamantinoma, with the recently described entity *osteofibrous dysplasia-like adamantinoma* existing somewhere in the middle.[36,42,43] Histologically, the lytic lesion shows a benign, trabecular, alphabet soup pattern in a fibrous stroma. The histologic findings are similar to those in fibrous dysplasia, although the lesions of fibrous dysplasia lack the prominent surface layer of rimming osteoblasts seen in osteofibrous dysplasia. The two can be distinguished by a variety of clinical, immunohistochemical,[64,88] and molecular markers.[63,87] These lesions are usually latent or active and, rarely, locally aggressive, because there is a relatively wide spectrum of disease.

Surgical treatment in osteofibrous dysplasia should be reserved for patients in whom the disease is poorly controlled with conservative treatment or those who have a high possibility of impending fracture and progression of their deformity.[38,71] Early attempts at surgical curettage and grafting may result in a high failure rate because of recurrence. It is generally suggested that if intervention is necessary, it should be deferred until the patient reaches adolescence, when there is an improved chance that the disease may be arrested following surgery or spontaneously resolve.[33]

Benign Cartilage-Forming Tumors

Enchondroma. An enchondroma refers to a centrally located benign cartilage neoplasm of medullary bone.[61] These tumors are relatively common lesions, accounting for more than 10% of all benign bone tumors. Approximately 50% of cases arise in the small tubular bone of the hands and feet, with the next most common locations being the proximal humerus and distal femur. An enchondroma develops in a growing bone as a hamartomatous process. It is frequently asymptomatic and may

avoid detection until the patient reaches adulthood. The lesion is usually discovered as an incidental finding on a routine radiographic examination, MRI for arthrographic examination or, more rarely, in association with a pathologic fracture.

Radiographs of enchondromas show geographic lysis of normal trabecular bone, with sharp margination and central stippled calcification (Fig. 201.3). Infrequently, there is associated pain, cortical scalloping, and dilation of the bone by a large tumor. When such features are present, one must be concerned about the possibility of a chondrosarcoma. Enchondromas are latent or active lesions.[61] If a lesion is considered to be locally aggressive, it is much more likely to be chondrosarcoma, and referral for treatment is universally warranted.

Enchondromatosis, or Ollier disease, is a rare nonfamilial dysplasia with multiple enchondromas that is typically seen on half of the body and may be similar to fibrous dysplasia. When it is bilateral, one side tends to be more involved than the other. This condition can be extensive, with significant involvement of metaphyseal areas, resulting in bowing and shortening of the long bones (Fig. 201.4). Such dramatic changes are rarely seen in cases of a solitary enchondroma. Varus deformities can be severe and may be managed by a variety of techniques.[62]

A large solitary enchondroma in a large bone will convert to a low-grade chondrosarcoma in fewer than 5% of cases.[4] If malignant transformation does occur, it will invariably take place during adulthood, and is very rarely in the short bones of the hands and feet. A secondary chondrosarcoma in enchondromatosis can arise in 20% to 40% of cases and may be related to inactivation of particular tumor suppressor genes.[12,99]

Patients with solitary enchondromas are treated symptomatically. If the patient has a pathologic fracture, it is usually best to allow the fracture to heal and perform a simple curettage and bone grafting procedure at a later date. This usually results in good function and a low chance of recurrence. Patients with Ollier disease or Maffucci disease (enchondromatosis

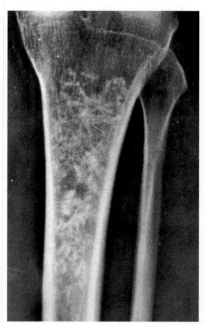

FIG 201.3 AP radiograph of the proximal tibia demonstrates loss of the normal bone trabecular pattern with central calcification. There is no endosteal scalloping or dilation.

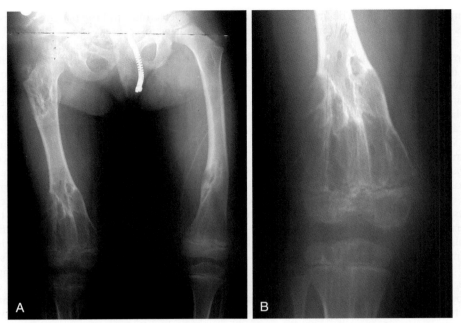

FIG 201.4 (A) Full-length lower extremity AP radiograph demonstrates the windswept deformity caused by Ollier disease. (B) AP radiograph of the patient's right knee.

associated with soft tissue hemangiomas) must be followed carefully because of the increased risk of malignant degeneration. This transformation usually occurs over a period of decades, and is more common in the long bones and pelvis.[12,99]

Periosteal Chondroma. A periosteal chondroma, also called a juxtacortical or cortical chondroma, is a rare benign cartilage lesion seen on the surface of a bone. Patients may have multiple lesions, with the most common location being on the proximal humerus. The distal femur is a relatively common site, and intra-articular involvement has been reported.[83,107] Radiographically, periosteal chondromas often have a thin shell of bone and appear to lie on the exterior cortical surface. There is no periosteal reaction, and MRI shows a soft tissue lesion with lobulated margins often with evidence of pressure erosion of the underlying cortical bone (Fig. 201.5). These lesions are latent or active, and should be treated with observation. Periosteal chondromas can grow to be relatively large. A lesion larger than 4 cm suggests a peripheral primary chondrosarcoma and should be referred to a tumor specialist.

Management of periosteal chondromas consists of observation at regular intervals to ensure that it does not enlarge as the patient reaches adulthood. In cases in which simple local resection without bone graft is indicated, the procedure is associated with a low morbidity and low recurrence rate.

Osteochondroma. Solitary osteochondromas are the second most common benign tumor of bone after nonossifying fibromas. However, they are usually more symptomatic than nonossifying fibromas because of their location and morphology. For this reason, they are the most common benign tumor around the knee presenting to orthopedic surgeons and primary care physicians. Similar to an enchondroma, an osteochondroma is a developmental or hamartomatous process that arises from a defect in the outer edge of the metaphyseal side of the growth plate. This results in an exostosis that is directed opposite to the

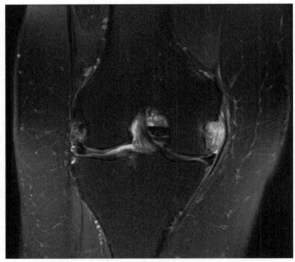

FIG 201.5 Coronal T2 MRI of the knee shows a periosteal chondroma of the anteromedial distal femur.

joint of origin as the lesion advances away from the growth plate during the growing years.

The three components of an osteochondroma include the cartilage cap, perichondrium, and bony stalk or base.[86] The bony stalk of an osteochondroma is in direct communication with the medullary canal of the bone from which it arises, which is an essential component of correctly diagnosing these lesions. Osteochondromas can be pedunculated (narrow base), as is commonly seen around the knee (Fig. 201.6), or can be sessile (broad base). An associated cartilaginous cap on the bony base is required to make the diagnosis of osteochondroma. This cap has the histologic features of a normal growth plate during the growing years and is the only neoplastic portion of the osteochondroma. Osteochondroma growth plate activity

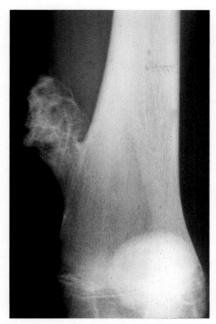

FIG 201.6 AP radiograph of the knee demonstrates a typical pedunculated osteochondroma.

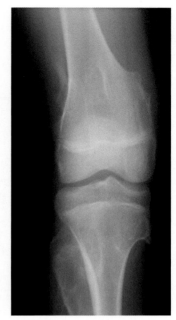

FIG 201.7 AP radiograph of the knee demonstrates the typical metaphyseal flaring and numerous osteochondromas seen in multiple hereditary exostoses.

subsides at the same time as the activity in the larger plate from which the osteochondroma arose.

A familial form of osteochondroma, multiple hereditary exostoses (MHE), is an autosomal dominant disorder that is 10% as common as a solitary osteochondroma, affecting 1 in 50,000 individuals.[23] Three genetic loci have been determined to be involved with MHE involving the EXT gene, the most common being EXT1 and EXT2.[78] This condition can vary from mild to extensive and may involve symmetrical limb shortening and deformity in all extremities. Valgus knee deformity has been reported to be a common manifestation that may require corrective osteotomy.[90] The metaphyseal portions of long bones are often deformed and widened (Fig. 201.7). The histologic findings in multiple exostoses are similar to those in solitary osteochondromas.

Conversion of a solitary osteochondroma to a chondrosarcoma occurs only during adulthood in less than 1% of cases. In MHE, there is a 1% to 5% chance of malignant conversion to secondary chondrosarcoma, especially in the larger, more proximal lesions (Fig. 201.8). However, this conversion rate is highly variable based on many years of literature reports.[23,39]

Solitary osteochondromas are latent lesions. Symptoms are caused secondary to mechanical effects on surrounding structures. Most children and adults with solitary osteochondromas are asymptomatic and therefore do not require surgical treatment. In some cases, the lesion may be palpable and irritating, as well as cosmetically unsettling.[90] Surgical removal is appropriate in these cases to address the symptoms. Removal of the tumor as a prophylaxis for chondrosarcomatous degeneration is not recommended. Symptomatic lesions in patients with MHE are also addressed surgically as needed. Corrective osteotomy is occasionally required because of angulatory deformity around the knee—and loss of pronosupination of the forearm should be examined closely in children.

In adults with a solitary osteochondroma or with multiple exostoses, a previously quiescent lesion that begins to enlarge

should be evaluated for potential sarcomatous degeneration with MRI. Attention is directed to the cartilaginous cap on imaging because this is where malignant degeneration can occur.

Chondroblastoma. A chondroblastoma is an epiphyseal lesion of childhood that has a histologic appearance typical of the benign metaphyseal-epiphyseal giant cell tumor of young adulthood. However, chondroblastomas are about 20% as common as giant cell tumors. They differ from other bone tumors in that they are almost always associated with epiphyseal or apophyseal bone. Most cases arise in the second decade of life. Males are affected more often than females.[86] The most common location is the peripheral proximal humeral epiphysis. Other common locations are the distal femoral and proximal tibial epiphyses. Because of their proximity to joints, chondroblastomas may present with symptomatic joint effusions.

Radiographically, chondroblastomas present as a lytic lesion with a sharp sclerotic margin and central stippled or flocculated calcification in the chondroid portion of the tumor. As the growth plate closes, the tumor can expand gradually into the metaphyseal area and may become aneurysmal. Chondroblastomas have the histologic appearance of a giant cell tumor, with numerous macrophages usually seen in areas of hemorrhage. The stromal cells of the chondroblastoma are polyhedral, like those of a giant cell tumor, with associated halos that give the chondroblastoma a chicken wire appearance. Although chondroid metaplasia in chondroblastoma is not always readily apparent, it must be present to firmly establish the diagnosis. Most chondroblastomas are active lesions, but may become locally aggressive.[95]

Surgical treatment of a chondroblastoma is often recommended because of the potential danger to the periarticular area in young children. Treatment for a chondroblastoma consists of aggressive intralesional resection with curettage and

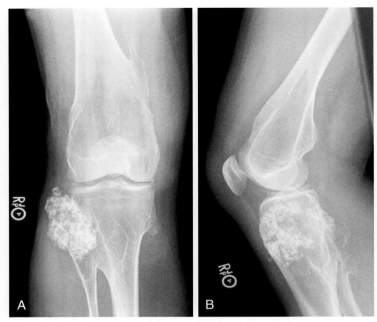

FIG 201.8 (A and B) Malignant degeneration of a proximal fibular osteochondroma that enlarged rapidly and became painful in a 70-year-old patient with multiple hereditary exostoses. Note the aggressive appearance compared with Fig. 201.7.

reconstruction with bone graft or polymethylmethacrylate (PMMA). Local recurrence with this technique is 5%.[105] Osteochondral allograft can be used in rare cases when the articular surface has been breached.[32] With recurrent disease, more aggressive marginal or wide resection may be necessary. Many major centers treat chondroblastomas with radiofrequency ablation.[104]

The spontaneous conversion of chondroblastoma to a malignant tumor is extremely rare. As with the case of giant cell tumors, conversion to sarcoma can occur following radiation treatment. Although chondroblastomas are considered benign, they have been reported to metastasize to the lung in rare cases.[60] Consequently, it is imperative to follow these lesions locally and with chest radiography. Nevertheless, the diagnosis of chondroblastoma carries an excellent prognosis.

Benign Fibrous Tumors of Bone

Fibrous Cortical Defect. Fibrous cortical defects (FCDs) or cortical desmoids are extremely common small hamartomatous fibromas seen almost exclusively in the metaphyseal areas of the lower extremities of growing children. The distal femur is the most common site, followed by the tibial metaphyses. They can involve multiple sites, and as many as 25% of normal children will have an asymptomatic lesion at 5 years of age. The lesions tend to disappear as the result of bone remodeling before skeletal maturity. If excessive stress is placed across the lesions, the lesions may become symptomatic and result in stress fracture.[56]

Microscopic studies of FCDs show benign-appearing fibroblasts with occasional areas of histiocytes, foam cells, and benign giant cells. The radiographic appearance is characteristic of this entity, with the lesion located eccentrically in the bone with a sharp margin and surrounding sclerosis[11] (Fig. 201.9). A biopsy is usually not necessary. These are latent lesions and can

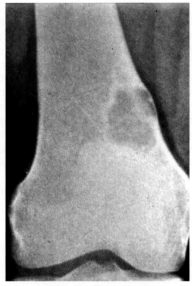

FIG 201.9 AP radiograph of the distal femur demonstrates a large FCD, which could also be called an NOF.

generally be observed, with the exception of those at risk for pathologic fracture.

Nonossifying Fibroma. A nonossifying fibroma (NOF) is considered a larger form of FCD, just as an osteoblastoma is considered to be a larger or more extensive form of osteoid osteoma. It is typically seen in the lower extremity of children. Because of its size, an NOF may not entirely resolve by skeletal maturity and can persist into adult life. If the lesion is large, approaching 50% of the diameter of the bone, pathologic fracture may ensue.

The fracture healing process may facilitate resolution of the lesion. Careful consideration of fracture prophylaxis should be reserved for large lesions and those in high-stress areas.[11] NOFs are latent lesions.

As with FCDs, NOFs do not require biopsy because their radiographic appearance is diagnostic. Large lesions that place the bone at risk of pathologic fracture may be treated with curettage and bone grafting. Similar to their smaller counterpart, there may be multiple sites of NOFs that take on the appearance of fibrous dysplasia. This should be distinguished from the rarely encountered Jaffe-Campanacci syndrome, with multiple NOF lesions associated with café au lait skin patches and other cutaneous manifestations of neurofibromatosis.[66]

Fibrous Dysplasia. Fibrous dysplasia of bone is a genetic, noninherited disease caused by activating mutations of the GNAS1 gene, encoding the alpha subunit of the stimulatory G protein, Gs.[47,87,94] Fibrous dysplasia is a dysplastic anomaly of bone-forming mesenchymal tissue with an inability to produce mature lamellar bone. Accordingly, the bone is arrested in the woven state with a resultant proliferation of spindle cell fibroblasts.

Fibrous dysplasia can present in a variety of ways, including monostotic or polyostotic, and may be seen in association with a number of syndromes.[73] Most cases are diagnosed within the first 3 decades of life and have a distinct female predilection. The monostotic presentation (70% to 80%) is more common than polyostotic (20% to 30%). The polyostotic form tends to be unilateral, with multiple foci on that side. Nevertheless, it can involve any bone of the body. The most common location is the proximal femur, where it results in the so-called shepherd's crook deformity (Fig. 201.10). Other areas frequently involved include the tibia, pelvis, humerus, radius, and ribs. It is unusual for monostotic involvement of the knee. If a patient presents

with knee pain with a history of fibrous dysplasia, it is very important to obtain hip and pelvis radiographs to rule out the perilous shepherd's crook deformity.

In addition to bony involvement, patients can demonstrate café au lait skin pigmentation. These patches usually have a rough border (coast of Maine), in contrast to the smooth border of those seen in neurofibromatosis (coast of California). Patients with fibrous dysplasia may have associated endocrine problems. Of patients with the polyostotic form of fibrous dysplasia, 5% will also exhibit precocious puberty (McCune-Albright syndrome). Other associated endocrine abnormalities include hyperthyroidism, acromegaly, Cushing disease, and hypophosphatemic osteomalacia. Polyostotic fibrous dysplasia with soft tissue myxomas is known as Mazabrand syndrome. Fibrous dysplasia can also involve the skull and jaw bones, mimicking ossifying fibroma of the jaw.

In fibrous dysplasia, microscopic findings include an alphabet soup pattern of metaplastic woven bone scattered through a benign fibrous tissue stroma. This woven stroma has an absence of osteoblastic rimming, a key difference from osteofibrous dysplasia. Foam cells, giant cells, and cholesterol deposits can be seen. Large cystic areas and even areas of cartilage formation are commonly present.

Studies have implicated an activating mutation in the Gsα proteins involved in Wnt/β-catenin signaling, which suppresses osteoblast maturation and inhibits bone formation.[80] The Gsα mutation also results in increased expression of the c-Fos oncoprotein.[51] Fibrous dysplasia tends to be active during the growing years and fades away in adult life. Less than 1% of lesions will convert to osteosarcoma, fibrosarcoma, or chondrosarcoma.[45] If there is conversion, it almost always occurs during adulthood.

In pediatric patients with active disease, curettage and grafting should be avoided because of high recurrence rates. The goals in managing pediatric patients should be the prevention and treatment of deformity, especially in the lower extremity. Most cases should become quiescent with skeletal maturity. If not, the best surgical management in adults consists of rigid fixation, preferably with an intramedullary implant, and realignment osteotomies as needed.[48,54] This treatment has a higher success rate in the adult group than in the pediatric group. Medical management with bisphosphonates was initially advocated because of prominent osteoclastogenesis seen in histology, and although treatment has been shown to be of benefit in some cases,[17] recent studies show no benefit in pain scores or functional parameters.[13] Irradiation is contraindicated, because it may lead to irradiation-induced sarcoma at a later date.[46]

Benign Cystic Lesions of Bone

Simple Bone Cyst. A simple bone cyst, also known as a unicameral bone cyst, is a common pseudotumor of bone and is the most frequent cause of pathologic fractures in children. Bone cysts typically affect patients between 5 and 15 years of age and occur more often in boys than in girls. They are found in the proximal humerus in 50% of cases but can also be seen in the proximal tibia (Fig. 201.11) and distal femur. Patients are asymptomatic until a pathologic fracture occurs, and generally present with hesitation to use the affected arm.[11] Fractures usually arise from the central metaphyseal side of an epiphyseal or apophyseal growth plate. The cystic process continues to grow away from the physis. When it remains in contact with the

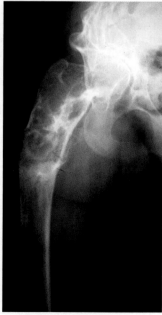

FIG 201.10 AP radiograph of the proximal femur demonstrates the typical shepherd's crook deformity of the proximal femur. Early hip symptoms may present as knee pain.

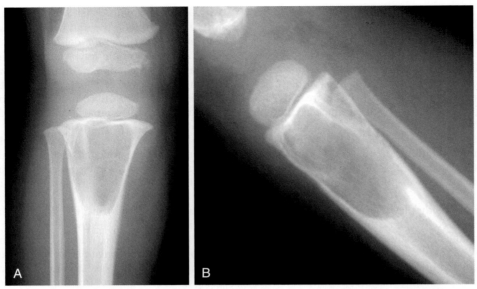

FIG 201.11 (A) AP and lateral radiographs (B) of a child with a simple bone cyst of the proximal tibia. These are generally asymptomatic until a fracture occurs.

physis, it is termed *active;* when it separates from the physis, it is termed *inactive.*

Radiographs typically show a solitary cyst that is centrally located in the metaphyseal area and has marked thinning of the adjacent cortical bone and a pseudoloculated appearance without reactive sclerosis (see Fig. 201.11). The bone cyst is filled with bloody or straw-colored serous fluid and there is increased pressure during the active phase. Although the fact that this pressure gradually decreases as the cyst becomes inactive suggests a hydrodynamic mechanism, the cause is a matter of debate.[22] In the presence of a pathologic fracture, a fragment of cortex present within the cyst is termed the "fallen leaf" sign, but may also be present in any pathologic fracture through a cystic lesion.

The cyst cavity is lined with a fibrinous membrane that contains giant cells, foam cells, and a slight osteoid formation, and is similar to the fibrous tissues seen in other fibrous bone lesions, including fibrous dysplasia. The periosteal covering in the area of a cyst is normal and pathologic fractures heal normally, in most cases without the need for surgery. Unfortunately, the cyst will usually persist after fracture union and may require further treatment. Bone-resorbing factors, such as matrix metalloproteinases, prostaglandins, interleukin-1, interleukin-6, tumor necrosis factor-alpha and oxygen-free radicals, have all been reported in the cyst fluid,[53] but the cyst fluid also supports osteoblastic growth and differentiation.[1] Elevated nitrate and nitrite levels have also been noted to be higher in the cyst fluid than in serum.[52]

Historically, the standard treatment for a solitary bone cyst was aggressive curettage or resection followed by bone grafting.[79] In patients with active disease, the recurrence rate was 30% to 50% and repeated grafting was frequently necessary.[26] In patients with inactive disease, particularly those older than 15 years, the surgical results were much better and the recurrence rate was lower, although the necessity of treatment in this age group is debatable.

Currently, treatment is a function of location and symptomatology. In weight-bearing bones, such as the proximal tibia and proximal femur, lesions should be treated aggressively with curettage, bone grafting, and often internal fixation. The decision to prophylactically treat a peritrochanteric cyst with a flexible intramedullary nail remains controversial.[14] Surgical management of lesions not at risk of adverse consequences (eg, those posed by peritrochanteric lesions) usually involves aspiration or injection with bone marrow or corticosteroid. The injections are carried out with bone biopsy needles and are repeated three to five times at intervals of 2 to 3 months, depending on the radiographic response. The best results are when the patient is between 5 and 15 years old, at which time the disease is active and macrophage activity is greatest in the cyst lining. The Simple Bone Cyst Trial Group recently conducted a multicenter randomized clinical trial[103] in which the rates of healing of simple bone cysts were compared based on the method of treatment. It was found that patients treated with intralesional injections of methylprednisolone had superior radiographic evidence of healing when compared with those treated with intralesional injection of bone marrow.

Curettage and bone grafting may also be an effective modality. Indirect limited curettage through a small bone window using a flexible nail to break up septations, followed by percutaneous bone grafting, is used at some referral centers, with promising early results. For realized fractures in preadolescents, flexible nails are an acceptable internal fixation device.[25]

Surgeons should note that sarcomas can take on the radiographic appearance of a solitary bone cyst. For this reason, if needle aspiration does not reveal cystic fluid or if it is not possible to inject contrast material and obtain radiologic confirmation of a cystic lesion, referral should be made to a tertiary center.

Aneurysmal Bone Cyst. An aneurysmal bone cyst is a hemorrhagic lesion that has many characteristics of a giant cell tumor but is only half as frequent. Giant cell tumors are rare in patients younger than 20 years and with open physes, and 75% of the cases of aneurysmal bone cyst occur in patients 10 to 20 years old. Aneurysmal bone cysts and giant cell tumors are more common in females than in males. The distal femur is the most frequently affected site, followed by the proximal tibia. Consequently, knee surgeons are likely to encounter these entities (Fig. 201.12).

Radiographically, aneurysmal bone cysts appear as aggressive osteolytic lesions with extensive permeative cortical destruction that may give the initial impression of a malignant process, such as Ewing sarcoma or telangiectatic osteosarcoma. A large aneurysmal bulge may occur outside the bone, with a thin reactive shell of bone forming at the outer edge (Fig. 201.13). Less soap bubble–type pseudoseptation is seen in aneurysmal bone cysts than in solitary cysts.

At the time of biopsy, the aneurysmal bone lesion may demonstrate large hemorrhagic cysts, but bleeding is typically modest. The hemorrhagic cysts are broken up by thick spongy fibrous septae that histologically contain great numbers of large giant cells and have thin osteoid seams. Even if a few mitotic figures are seen, the diagnosis of a benign lesion can reasonably be retained. A carefully placed biopsy with multiple samples is needed to rule out other well-known skeletal tumors that may demonstrate an aneurysmal component. These include giant cell tumor, chondromyxoid fibroma, and most perilous, telangiectatic osteosarcoma. Aneurysmal bone cysts may arise secondarily as a variant of some other underlying neoplastic process.[68] Like the solitary bone cyst, this cyst may have a hydraulic pressure origin that is secondary to hemorrhage and could be traumatically induced. Several translocations have recently been described in primary aneurysmal bone cysts, with t(16;17) being the most common, however there is no consensus on the cause of this tumor.[76] All identified translocations result in upregulation of the USP6 gene on chromosome 17p13. USP6 induces expression of matrix metalloproteinases and inhibits pre-osteoblast differentiation. USP6 rearrangement is also absent in giant cell tumors and telangiectatic osteosarcoma, and may be a useful diagnostic tool.[94]

An aneurysmal bone cyst is usually active or locally aggressive. Left untreated, aneurysmal bone cysts may involute spontaneously, during which time they will develop a heavy shell of reactive bone at the periphery. However, the typical treatment of aneurysmal bone cysts is with extended surgical curettage and bone grafting. Using this modality, the tumor can be eradicated from its metaphyseal location and more mechanically stable bone graft or cement can be left in its place (see video on the website). Radiation is no longer recommended. Another option for treating extremely large lesions is repeated embolization to reduce the rate of hemorrhagic expansion.[100] Aneurysmal bone cysts are associated with a relatively high rate of recurrence and have been proposed to recur most commonly at the juxtaphyseal locations, where they are often found.[58] It is imperative to use appropriate techniques of eradicating the tumor with extended surgical curettage and adjuvant techniques while preserving the chondral and physeal surfaces.

Giant Cell Tumor of Bone

Of all benign bone tumors, 5% to 10% are true giant cell tumors, occurring most frequently in the third decade of life. They are more frequently found in women than in men. In about half of the cases, the tumor is found around the knee and

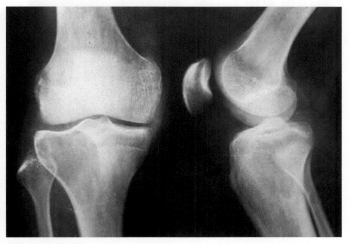

FIG 201.12 AP and lateral radiographs of the knee demonstrate an eccentric radiolucent mass consistent with an aneurysmal bone cyst.

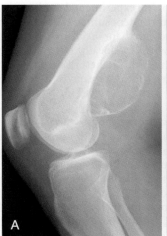
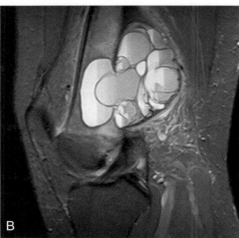
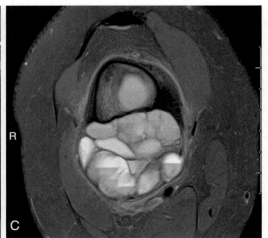

FIG 201.13 (A) Lateral radiograph of the distal femur reveals an aggressive process that was of concern for a telangiectatic osteosarcoma, which was actually an aneurysmal bone cyst. (B and C) MRI scans showing characteristic fluid levels of an aneurysmal bone cyst.

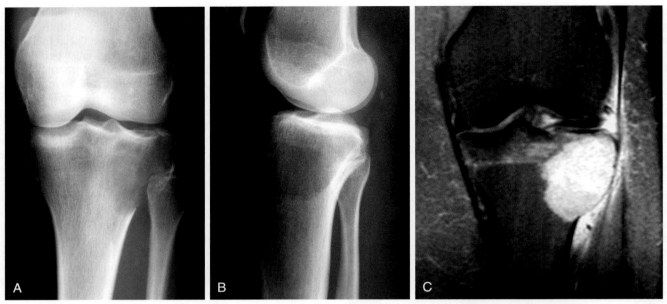

FIG 201.14 AP (A) and lateral (B) radiographs of the knee demonstrating a lytic lesion of the proximal tibia concerning for giant cell tumor. (C) Coronal MRI scan demonstrates the typical proximity to the joint.

can arise in the patella.[3] The tumor is usually painful for several months prior to diagnosis and can cause a pathologic fracture. It can also cause a painful effusion because of its juxtaposition to a major joint. Radiographically, the lesion appears lytic in nature and is located in the epiphyseal-metaphyseal end of a long bone (Fig. 201.14). The lesion grows toward the joint surface and frequently comes into contact within 1 cm of the articular cartilage but rarely breaks into the joint.

Numerous tumors contain histologic evidence of giant cells, but not all are true giant cell tumors. Most of the giant cell tumor variants are seen in children and include aneurysmal bone cysts, chondroblastomas, simple bone cysts, osteoid osteomas, and osteoblastomas. Hemorrhagic (telangiectatic) osteosarcoma is the most malignant of the variants; it is difficult to distinguish this from an aggressive benign giant cell tumor. The brown tumor of hyperparathyroidism is a non-neoplastic variant seen in primary and secondary hyperparathyroidism.

Like chondroblastoma, a benign giant cell tumor can metastasize to the lung. A recent case series of 167 patients reported a 6.6% chance of metastasizing to the lung, with recurrent tumors having a 13.0% chance of metastasis.[16] Accordingly, pulmonary staging is an important component in the initial evaluation and follow-up of giant cell tumors. The prognosis for survival with this complication is favorable, and the tumors may resolve spontaneously. Rarely, benign giant cell tumors can convert to a malignant condition such as an osteosarcoma or leiomyosarcoma[50] and may be related to older radiation therapy techniques.[85] This has come into question with newer radiation therapy modalities.[91,97]

Currently, most surgeons elect an aggressive curettage followed by the use of adjuvant therapy such as a high-speed burr, phenol, hydrogen peroxide, liquid nitrogen, or argon beam. The resulting void is packed with PMMA or bone graft. With this approach, the recurrence rate is 12% to 27%, but decreases to 0% to 12% with en block resection.[8,30,97] Regarding giant cell tumors around the knee, risk of recurrence and development of osteoarthritis are increased if more than 70% of subchondral bone is involved or if tumor-cartilage distance is 3 mm or less.[98] Treatment of recurrent giant cell tumors around the knee generally consists of another attempt at curettage, mechanical marginal expansion with a high-speed burr, and local adjuvant therapy, or resection of the involved area and reconstruction with a large osteoarticular allograft, endoprosthesis, or excisional arthrodesis. When giant cell tumor involves an expendable bone, such as the proximal fibula or ilium, primary resection is a reasonable treatment option. En bloc resection continues to be used for multiple recurrent tumors, intensive soft tissue involvement, or massively destructive cases. Embolization may also prove palliative and/or curative in unresectable cases. For advanced, multiply recurrent, or aggressive metastatic cases, investigators are developing experimental medical protocols that use serial embolization or denosumab systemic therapy, although this is generally reserved for axial or unresectable disease.[18,44,59,74,97] Close follow-up for locally recurrent disease and pulmonary involvement is critical. Chest radiography every 6 to 12 months for the first 2 to 3 years is a reasonable consideration.

Intraosseous Lipoma. Intraosseous lipomas are a very rare subset of benign bone tumors formed by the proliferation of mature lipocytes.[69] In fact, some consider them to be the rarest of all benign bone neoplasms.[7] They are usually located in the calcaneus and very rarely seen in the distal femur and proximal tibia, often being misdiagnosed as other benign neoplasms. They are often found to involute spontaneously through a process involving infarction, calcification, and cyst formation and have been classified based on this process. Intraosseous lipomas around the knee are rarely, if ever, symptomatic. Truly symptomatic lesions can be treated with curettage and bone grafting.

CONCLUSION

The knee surgeon must be familiar with the basic clinical aspects of benign bone lesions because the knee is a common site for a variety of lesions. Distinguishing benign from malignant conditions is of paramount importance. In most cases, history and physical examination and plain radiography are adequate to diagnose these common conditions appropriately. Consultation with an experienced orthopedic oncologist is always encouraged if there are any questions or concerns about a more aggressive process.

KEY REFERENCES

6. Atesok I, Alman A, Schemitsch H, et al: Osteoid osteoma and osteoblastoma. *J Am Acad Orthop Surg* 19(11):678–689, 2011.

11. Biermann JS: Common benign lesions of bone in children and adolescents. *J Pediatr Orthop* 22:268–273, 2002.

14. Cha SM, Shin HD, Kim KC, et al: Does fracture affect the healing time or frequency or recurrence in a simple bone cyst of the proximal femur? *Clin Orthop* 472(10):3166–3176, 2014.

16. Chan CM, Adler Z, Reith JD, et al: Risk factors for pulmonary metastasis from giant cell tumor of bone. *J Bone Joint Surg Am* 97(5):420–428, 2015.

23. Czajka M, DiCaprio R: What is the proportion of patients with multiple hereditary exostoses who undergo malignant degeneration? *Clin Orthop* 473(7):2355–2361, 2015.

26. Dormans JP, Hanna BG, Johnston DR, et al: Surgical treatment and recurrence rate of aneurysmal bone cysts in children. *Clin Orthop* 421:205–211, 2004.

30. Errani C, Ruggieri P, Asenzio MA, et al: Giant cell tumor of the extremity: a review of 349 cases from a single institution. *Cancer Treat Rev* 36:1–7, 2010.

55. Lanza E, Thouvenin Y, Viala P, et al: Osteoid osteoma treated by percutaneous thermal ablation: when do we fail? A systematic review and guidelines for future reporting. *Cardiovasc Intervent Radiol* 37(6):1530–1539, 2014.

60. Lin PP, Thenappan A, Deavers MT, et al: Treatment and prognosis of chondroblastoma. *Clin Orthop* 438:103–109, 2005.

73. Muthusamy S, Subhawong T, Conway SA, et al: Locally aggressive fibrous dysplasia mimicking malignancy: a report of four cases and review of the literature. *Clin Orthop* 473(2):742–750, 2015.

92. Steffner R: Benign bone tumors. *Cancer Treat Res* 162:31–63, 2014.

94. Szuhai K, Cleton-Jansen AM, Hogendoorn PC, et al: Molecular pathology and its diagnostic use in bone tumors. *Cancer Genet* 205(5):193–204, 2012.

97. van der Heijden L, Dijkstra PD, van de Sande MA, et al: The clinical approach towards giant cell tumor of bone. *Oncologist* 19(5):550–561, 2014.

99. Verdegaal H, Bovée V, Pansuriya C, et al: Incidence, predictive factors, and prognosis of chondrosarcoma in patients with Ollier disease and Maffucci syndrome: an international multicenter study of 161 patients. *Oncologist* 16(12):1771–1779, 2011.

105. Xu H, Nugent D, Monforte L, et al: Chondroblastoma of bone in the extremities: a multicenter retrospective study. *J Bone Joint Surg Am* 97(11):925–931, 2015.

The references for this chapter can also be found on www.expertconsult.com.

202

Surgical Management of Malignant Bone Tumors Around the Knee

Michael D. Neel

The surgical management of malignant tumors around the knee requires a basic understanding of tumor biology, knowledge of common tumors, and their clinical and radiographic behavior. To treat malignant tumors successfully, it is essential to understand general principles of sarcoma surgery, including staging of a bone tumor, appropriate biopsy techniques, patient selection for limb salvage surgery versus amputation, and methods of resection and reconstruction. These topics will be discussed in this chapter. Initial workup, including staging and biopsy of a bone tumor, are covered elsewhere in this text. Reconstructive options that will be reviewed include arthrodesis, allograft reconstruction, and rotationplasty. Reconstruction with a megaprosthesis or allograft-prosthetic composite is discussed elsewhere. Common malignant bone tumors around the knee include osteosarcoma, chondrosarcoma, Ewing sarcoma, and lymphoma of bone, and these will also be reviewed.

TUMOR BIOLOGY

Primary malignant tumors have the capacity to metastasize to distant sites. They are also locally aggressive, destroy bone, and involve adjacent soft tissue structures. Malignant tumors are typically subclassified as low, intermediate, or high grade based on the histologic grade. Grade is a feature of the amount of cellular activity, cellular pleomorphism, mitotic activity, and tumor necrosis. It is reflective of the tumor's aggressiveness.

Malignant bone tumors spread locally by centrifugal tumor expansion. As the tumor cells divide and the mass grows, normal tissue is compressed. Microscopic pseudopods of tumor invade normal surrounding tissue. In an effort to control the tumor, an inflammatory response is established adjacent to the tumor. This reactive zone consists of inflammatory cells, edematous tissue, and neovascularity feeding the advancing tumor. The compressed normal tissue produces a pseudocapsule about the mass. Thus, the surrounding soft tissue around the malignant tumor is slowly invaded by satellites of advancing tumor. To remove the tumor completely, the resection must be well beyond the reactive zone and into normal adjacent soft tissue of bone, thus avoiding leaving satellites behind.[12] Unfortunately, current imaging modalities such as magnetic resonance imaging (MRI), positron emission tomography (PET) scan, and bone scanning cannot identify microscopic tumor extension adequately. Often, the edematous tissue can be well identified, but this really provides no clear information regarding the presence or absence of microscopic tumor satellites.

This aggressive local spread of tumor is frequently halted by anatomic barriers, such as cortical bone, periosteum, cartilage, synovium, and fascia. These barriers are relative and do not offer an absolute stopping point for tumor growth. They can be breached with tumor extension beyond their confines. However, they do serve to force tumor growth into a longitudinal pattern. Tumors can extend for great distances along bone and soft tissue planes and attain a large bulky size before being detected. Tumors that remain within the confined bone or soft tissue compartment are termed *intracompartmental*.[2] Tumors that extend beyond the compartment of origin and involve adjacent structures are termed *extracompartmental*. As the tumor spreads, it frequently displaces rather than encases neurovascular structures. Occasionally, these structures can be circumferentially engulfed by tumor but tend to remain patent and functional unless significantly compressed by a large mass. Destruction of bone and presence of a soft tissue mass can lead to pain, the most common presenting symptom of malignant tumors of bone. The subcutaneous nature of the distal femur and proximal tibia lead to early detection of a soft tissue mass associated with a bone tumor.

PRINCIPLES OF SURGICAL MANAGEMENT

On completion of appropriate staging and the determination of an accurate diagnosis, attention is now turned toward treatment. Cure of malignant tumors requires local control of the tumor as well as control of systemic disease. Surgical management of malignant bone tumors is often the foundation for local control. The principles of surgical management are outlined here. Adjuvant treatments for common malignant tumors are found elsewhere in this text in discussions of each of the common bone malignancies.

Surgical Margins

In collecting, analyzing, and reporting surgical data, it is imperative to use a language that is common among surgeons as to which surgical procedure has been performed. The relationship between the surgical plane of resection of the tumor and surrounding tissue is known as the surgical margin. Enneking and Shirley[3] have established a nomenclature to describe oncologic surgical procedures in terms of four surgical margins. The margin can be achieved by amputation or a limb salvage procedure.

Intralesional margins are achieved if the surgical plane of dissection is through the tumor, leaving behind gross residual disease. This typically occurs when a biopsy is done but also with curettage or a debulking procedure. Tumor is obviously left behind and the procedure is not curative for malignant bone tumors. This margin is appropriate only in the palliative

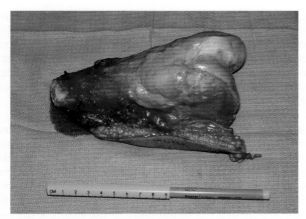

FIG 202.1 Surgical specimen demonstrating wide margins following resection of distal femur. Note cuff of normal tissue surrounding the tumor and inclusion of a biopsy track.

setting or for very low-grade lesions amenable to local control with curettage alone.

Marginal margins are achieved when the plane of dissection is the pseudocapsule itself. The main body of the tumor easily peels away from the surrounding pseudocapsule. This leads the surgeon to inadvertently perform a shell-out procedure. Failure to recognize the real potential for microscopic foci of the tumor within and beyond the pseudocapsule results in an inadequate margin. Several studies have demonstrated the high rate of tumor cells in this reactive zone after a shell-out or gross total resection. Even after adjuvant therapies, local recurrence is high with a marginal margin. Consequently, tumor bed re-excisions are often recommended after gross total resections or shell-out procedures are performed. In tumors treated preoperatively with chemotherapy or radiation, a marginal margin can be accepted only adjacent to vital structures such as a neurovascular bundle. In this situation, the preoperative treatment would have (hopefully) sterilized any microscopic satellite lesions in these areas.

Wide margins are the most commonly achieved margins when dealing with bone malignancies. The resection plane is beyond the pseudocapsule and reactive zone. It results in a cuff of normal tissue surrounding the tumor. The specimen contains the biopsy tract (skin and underlying soft tissue), body of the tumor, pseudocapsule, reactive zone, and a cuff of normal tissue. The appropriate thickness of that cuff is subject to study and debate. The key principle is that the cuff is wide enough to be beyond any satellite or skip lesions that may be present. A wide margin is the goal of surgical treatment in bone and soft tissue sarcomas to minimize the risk of local tumor recurrence[12] (Fig. 202.1).

Radical margins are achieved when the involved bone and soft tissue component are resected in their entirety. An extra-compartmental resection is thus achieved. When managing tumors that are extracompartmental, the entire involved bone and involved adjacent musculature must be excised to be considered a radial resection. Radical margins are typically unnecessary for bone sarcomas.

Patient Selection for Limb Salvage versus Amputation

In this modern age of treatment, most patients are candidates for limb-sparing resections. Several factors play a role in determining which patients should or should not undergo a limb salvage procedure. Local anatomic extent, involvement of major neurovascular structures, adjacent soft tissue attachments, and reconstructive options all play a role in determining the most appropriate procedure. Additionally, response to chemotherapy may render a previously unresectable lesion resectable. Adjuvant therapies can influence the decision of limb salvage or amputation. The decision to attempt limb salvage versus an amputation lies with the surgeon's ability to achieve an appropriate oncologic margin. If the appropriate oncologic margin can be obtained, it must be determined whether the reconstruction will provide a stable construct to support the limb. The functional result of a limb-sparing procedure must be as good as or better than an amputation.

Principles of Tumor Resection

Once a patient is considered a candidate for limb salvage, careful preoperative planning of the resection and reconstruction is essential to achieving a successful outcome. Review of initial and interval imaging studies during the course of treatments allows the surgeon to plan the definitive surgery. Bone resection is determined by initial tumor imaging and is typically done with a 3- to 5-cm resection of bone to achieve a wide surgical margin. In some cases, this margin may be as close as 1 cm. The subchondral bone provides an excellent barrier to tumor extension. Even when the tumor extends into the epiphyseal bone, it is rare for the tumor to extend into the joint. This allows for tumor resection of the proximal tibia or distal femur in an intra-articular fashion. Tumors that involve the proximal tibia often require removal of the proximal fibula through the proximal tibia–fibula joint if the joint is in danger of tumor penetration or in close proximity to the tumor. Tumors of the proximal fibula are usually treated with resection of the fibula alone but may require removal of the proximal tibia/fibula joint in an extra-articular fashion, removing a small portion of the adjacent tibia. Large tumors or tumors with an intra-articular extent require resection in an extra-articular fashion. If there has been tumor extension into the knee joint or contamination from a previous ill-planned biopsy, the joint must be removed en bloc by resection beyond the capsular attachments at the proximal tibial and distal femoral levels. The patella and extensor mechanisms are resected along with the joint. The resection must include any skip metastases in the bone or soft tissues.

Special consideration is also given for the skeletally immature child who has significant growth remaining. Resection of the distal femoral and proximal tibial physis can result in a significant limb length inequality. Special reconstruction options must be considered for these growing children. Amputation, rotationplasty, and an expandable prosthesis are reconstructive options for this group of patients. Resection level may be influenced by the desire to save the physis, but always the best oncologic margin is what determines the resection level.

Once the bone margins are determined, consideration is given to the soft tissue resection. Most tumors of the distal femur are adequately covered by deep layers of soft tissue. Frequently, an adequate amount of quadriceps mechanism may be spared to provide appropriate soft tissue coverage of the reconstruction and satisfactory functional result. Usually, only a small portion of the vastus medialis oblique or vastus lateralis is removed with resection of the biopsy track. The remainder of the quadriceps, patella, and patellar tendon can be spared. Typically, the deep soft tissue margin (providing coverage over the tumor) is provided by the vastus intermedius. In large bulky tumors, more extensive quadriceps resection may be required. This may have an effect on function and should be considered when deciding on amputation versus limb salvage. The neurovascular bundle may be displaced by the sarcoma but is usually not encased by tumor and can be spared. The cruciate ligaments, collateral insertions, and gastrocnemius insertions are all removed from the distal femur, requiring a constrained design if arthroplasty is the method of skeletal reconstruction. The adductors are divided as well.

The pes anserine and hamstring insertions on the tibia and fibula are usually left intact when performing distal femoral resections. Resection of ligamentous insertions is always done with a short cuff of tissue to ensure adequate margins. Typically, the resection is performed by first dissecting through soft tissues, which allows the biopsy tract to be removed with the specimen, performing the arthrotomy, continuing with the soft tissue dissection, and then osteotomizing the femur. Often, the posterior soft tissues are more easily approached after the femoral osteotomy has been performed. The specimen is removed and inspected by the surgeon and pathologist for margins. Attention is then turned toward reconstruction.

On the tibial side, tumors frequently involve the tibial tubercle. This requires division of the patella tendon, which must be reconstructed to provide an adequate extensor mechanism. The pes anserine and hamstring insertions are divided near the bone with a cuff of normal tissue. On the femoral side, the gastrocnemius and adductor insertions are spared. The cruciate and collateral attachments are also removed from the proximal tibia when resecting the proximal tibial lesion.

PRINCIPLES OF RECONSTRUCTION

When choosing the optimal reconstruction, the surgeon must consider the patient's age and functional demands as well as the anticipated bone and soft tissue deficits. Bone loss must be reconstructed with local grafts, allografts, endoprosthetic replacements, or a combination of these. Soft tissue defects, such as the extensor mechanism, can be reconstructed with local advancement flaps or allograft reconstruction. In the case of extensive bone and soft tissue loss, an arthrodesis may be the appropriate reconstructive method. In a young child, rotationplasty affords the ability to resect the tumor and reconstruct the knee in a semiamputated fashion. These techniques will be reviewed. Megaprosthesis and allograft-prosthetic composites are the two most commonly used reconstructions and are discussed elsewhere. Osteoarticular allografts may still be considered for reconstruction in young patients to avoid resurfacing of the uninvolved articulation. No one option is good for all patients.

Arthrodesis

Before the availability of endoprosthetic joints, resection followed by arthrodesis was the only viable option for surgical reconstruction for limb salvage procedures. With the advent of the successful modular oncology megaprosthesis, fewer patients receive arthrodesis. Arthrodesis is typically accomplished with the use of local grafts from the opposite side of the resected joint or large bulk intercalary allografts. In either case, the fusion is held in place with intramedullary rods, and/or plates and screws. These provide stability to the construct and promote healing of the graft-host junction. The knee joint is fused in a position that allows easy swing-through of the extremity during the swing phase of normal gait. The desired position is 5 degrees of valgus, 10 to 15 degrees of knee flexion, and slight external rotation. The extremity is typically shortened by 1 cm to maximize gait mechanics.[12] Once healed, the arthrodesis provides a durable, stable reconstruction. Unfortunately, the lack of knee motion is a functional deficit that most patients dislike.

Local Autografts. As described by Enneking,[2] the use of local autografts for knee arthrodesis can produce a durable reconstruction with reliable consolidation. The technique described uses a segment of adjacent bone and fibula to bridge the resection gap. Fixation is maintained with an intramedullary rod. Preoperative planning necessitates determining the resection length. Defects larger than one-third of the length of the bone require consideration of alternative methods of reconstruction because of the inability to achieve adequate stability. Radiographs in both planes help determine the most appropriate size and length of the rod. Most manufacturers can provide off-the-shelf interlocking fusion rods. For patients with small-diameter bones or unusually large femoral bows, a custom device may be required. After appropriate reaming, a guide rod is placed in a retrograde fashion through the proximal femur and out the piriformis fossa. A spacer made from polymethylmethacrylate is placed temporarily in the segmental defect to maintain the length while placing the rod. The rod should extend to within 3 to 4 cm of the ankle joint. The rod is then placed in an antegrade fashion down the femur, across the defect, and into the tibia.

Local grafts are now harvested. For distal femoral resections, a segment of anterior tibia is harvested. It consists of the anterior half of the bone. This is 2 cm longer than the resection segment because the graft will be keyed into the native bone on either side of the defect. The overall length of the leg will be planned to be 1 cm short. A bridge of bone measuring 3 cm should be left at the proximal tibia to provide structural support for the graft. For proximal tibial resections, the anterior cortex of the femur is harvested in a similar fashion. Next, the fibula is harvested. Care is taken to protect the peroneal nerve. The fibula is harvested long enough to span the defect. The fibula is then placed in the posterior aspect of the defect and fixed with screws or Steinmann pins. The proximal fibula is beveled to provide additional surface area for healing.

The spacer is now removed and the graft is placed into the defect. The graft is countersunk into the remaining bone. The segment is measured to ensure that the reconstructed defect is 1 cm shorter than the removed specimen to shorten the extremity by 1 cm overall. The graft is fixed to the bone proximally and distally. Additional graft is placed around the fusion areas to promote healing and consolidation. Proximal and distal interlocking screws are then applied. Local muscle flaps may be created, if needed, to provide soft tissue coverage. This also provides a vascular soft tissue to assist in fusion consolidation. The wound is closed over drains. Toe touch weight bearing is allowed until the graft consolidates at approximately 4 to 6 months.

Large Bulk Allograft. With the advent of bone and tissue banking, the use of bulk allograft for arthrodesis has been popularized. Bulk allografts have the advantage of reconstructing larger defects than can be done with local grafts. Fixation can be achieved with intramedullary rods or plates and screws, or in combination.

Preoperative measurements are used to order the appropriately sized allograft. Typically, a distal femoral graft is used. The length should be several centimeters longer than the anticipated resection length. This allows intraoperative flexibility. Following resection and inspection, the specimen is measured. The graft is then cut to match the defect minus 1 cm. Preparation for rodding is as detailed earlier, with the allograft reamed to 1 to 2 mm larger than the selected rod to ensure ease of rod insertion through the graft. The selected rod is inserted in an antegrade fashion into the femur, allograft, and then tibia. Short derotational and compression plates may be used at the proximal and distal junctions to provide stability and promote healing of the allograft to the host bone.

Alternatively, the allograft can be secured with plates and screws instead of an intramedullary rod with supplemental plates. Typically, two 4.5 large-fragment dynamic compression plates or locking plates are used. The graft is placed as described. Plates are placed on the anterior and anterolateral positions spanning the proximal and distal junctions. A few screws are placed in the graft. Multiple screws have been implicated in allograft fractures. Compression techniques are used to provide stability and promote fusion.

In either method of fixation, additional graft material can be applied at both junctions. A gastrocnemius muscle flap is recommended for soft tissue coverage. This also provides the junction with a covering of well-vascularized tissue. With either technique, the patient is allowed toe touch weight bearing until consolidation occurs at approximately 4 to 6 months.[14]

Rotationplasty

Rotationplasty is another method of reconstruction following resection of tumors around the knee and is commonly used for treatment of the skeletally immature patient. Tumors of the distal femur and proximal tibia can be reconstructed with this technique. Rotationplasty essentially uses the ankle joint as the knee joint. By rotating the foot 180 degrees, the plane of motion in the ankle is in the same plane as the knee joint (Fig. 202.2). After resection of the tumor, the foot and ankle are rotated and brought up to the level of the contralateral knee joint. The residual tibia is then fixed to the femur. In some patients, the circumference of the soft tissue envelope at the level of the distal femur resection will be significantly larger than that of the proximal tibial soft tissue circumference. A proximally based triangular incision has been successfully used in such patients.[7] Eventually, the extremity is fitted for a special prosthesis in which the foot fits into a special component. The reconstruction essentially functions as a below-knee amputation.[12] Without the restrictions given to patients with an endoprosthesis, the patient with a rotationplasty has few functional limitations. The durability of the reconstruction limits future surgery as compared with other reconstructions. Rotationplasty may also be considered for patients with extensive intra-articular involvement or large, associated soft tissue masses. This procedure provides the ability to perform an extra-articular resection of the knee and wide margin in large, extensive sarcomas.

One of the disadvantages of rotationplasty is the obvious cosmetic appearance of the extremity. However, in most cases, the rotated foot is contained within the special prosthesis in which it is fitted. With careful patient selection and preoperative counseling, patients have not demonstrated any significant increase in psychosocial disturbances compared with other types of reconstruction. Rotationplasty is an excellent alternative to

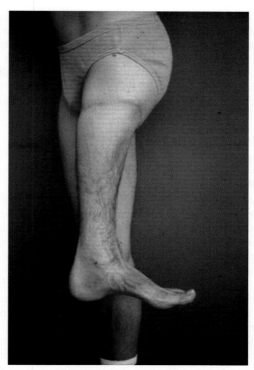

FIG 202.2 Clinical appearance of a patient with a Van Ness rotationplasty. (Courtesy Dr. N. Lindner.)

amputation in the properly selected patient.[6,12] Patients with larger tumors unresponsive to preoperative chemotherapy or those with preoperative pathologic fractures are at higher risk of complications, presumably related to compromise of the venous drainage of the leg.[11]

As with other reconstructions, extensive preoperative planning is essential for a successful outcome. Based on patient age and anticipated future growth of the contralateral extremity, the level of ankle placement is determined. To accommodate the resection and rotation, a unique circumferential skin incision is used. With some variations, it is essentially a modified rhomboid shape, with the long axis oriented along the anterior thigh.[4] Circumferential incisions along the thigh and calf are then connected with a posterior lateral incision. The level of the proximal circumferential incision for distal femoral resection is a few centimeters around the bone resection level. The tibial incision is just distal to the level of the tibia tubercle. The neurovascular bundle is exposed and protected in the same fashion as for resections around the knee. En bloc resection of the vessels with subsequent reanastomosis may be required for tumor involvement. Osteotomy is performed at the predetermined level. A Steinmann pin is placed proximal to the osteotomy and a second pin is placed in the tibia, perpendicular to the first. This provides a guide to rotation during fixation of the bones.

An intra-articular versus extra-articular resection is then performed, as required. This is followed by soft tissue resection in a transverse fashion above and below the tumor, with appropriate margins. As per preoperative planning, the tibia is divided at the proper level. The foot and ankle are rotated, brought up to the level of the resected femur, and fixed with plates and screws. The neurovascular bundle is typically coiled to prevent kinking. Wound closure is performed over drains. Postoperatively, the extremity is dressed with a compression dressing to avoid undue swelling. Early weight bearing is allowed via an ischial-bearing prosthesis. The limb is eventually fitted with a modified prosthesis in which weight bearing is through the foot, fitted into a special platform. Function is similar to a below-knee amputation.

COMMON MALIGNANT BONE TUMORS OF THE KNEE

Osteosarcoma

Osteosarcoma is a neoplastic process in which osteoid is produced by malignant cells. There are a variety of histologic subtypes producing a range of clinical entities. The subtypes have been organized into classic (conventional), parosteal, periosteal, high-grade surface, telangiectatic, low-grade central, and small cell osteogenic sarcoma. Osteosarcoma is further subclassified by whether it arises as a primary de novo lesion or as a secondary lesion. Secondary lesions can arise from Paget disease, osteogenesis perfecta, or multiple hereditary exostosis or as radiation-induced tumors.[15]

Osteosarcoma is the most common malignant bone tumor of childhood. Classic osteosarcoma is seen with a peak incidence in the second decade, with male predominance. Parosteal osteogenic sarcoma has a slightly older mean age group of 30 years of age. Secondary tumors and radiation-induced tumors have a much higher peak incidence between the ages of 35 and 45 years. Most osteosarcomas, approximately 80%, appear in the long tubular bones. The knee is a favored site with approximately 40% to 45% of osteosarcomas arising in the femur and 15% to 20% in the tibia. The tumor is typically metaphyseal. The parosteal variant is most commonly seen in the posterior aspect of the distal femur. Pain is the most common presenting complaint across all subtypes. The notable exception is a parosteal osteogenic sarcoma, which typically presents as a painless mass.

In these young active patients, pain is often attributed to injury, overuse, or growing pains commonly seen around the knee. The insidious constant nature of the pain steadily increasing in severity and duration usually is cause for alarm and referral to a clinician. Night pain and pain associated with weight bearing also typically herald the presence of a malignant process. The average duration of symptoms prior to presentation is approximately 3 months.[1] The serum alkaline phosphatase level will be increased in approximately 50% of patients.

Conventional osteosarcoma may have a lytic, blastic, or mixed mineralization pattern on plain radiographs. A parosteal lesion will appear as a lobulated ossified mass. A periosteal reaction, Codman triangle, cortical disruption, and soft tissue mass are seen in more than 90% of patients and are all features common to high-grade subtypes. MRI is performed to better evaluate the extent of bone and soft tissue involvement critical to surgical planning. Moreover, MRI is the most sensitive tool for identifying skip metastases. The prognostic factors that seem to influence outcome most significantly in patients with osteosarcoma are the extent of disease at presentation and the presence of a high-grade lesion. Tumors that are large or are located in an anatomic site that precludes appropriate wide margins have a poorer prognosis. Response to induction chemotherapy, as measured by tumor necrosis of the resected specimen, has been shown to be of prognostic value.[8]

Surgical removal of the primary tumor for local control and administration of chemotherapy for systemic control represent the foundation for modern treatment protocols for osteosarcoma. Radiation is reserved for unresectable lesions or metastatic disease, but has no significant role outside of the palliative setting.[9]

Chondrosarcoma

Chondrosarcoma is the second most common malignant bone tumor. It is characterized as a neoplastic process that produces cartilage from malignant cells; it is typically classified based on grade, anatomic location, or presentation of primary versus secondary lesions. Common clinical subtypes include conventional chondrosarcoma, secondary chondrosarcoma arising from osteochondroma, and mesenchymal, dedifferentiated, or clear cell chondrosarcoma. There is a 60% male predominance, with a peak incidence in the third to sixth decade. Treatment is often determined by the grade of the lesion more than by any other classification.[12] Fortunately, the knee is not commonly involved and most chondrosarcomas are low grade. Benign aggressive active lesions can be similar histologically to low-grade lesions. Prior to any biopsy being done, consultation should be obtained with an experienced radiologist and pathologist familiar with evaluating this difficult tumor.

Pain is the most common presenting symptom in over 75% to 95% of patients with chondrosarcomas.[1] By comparison, less than 5% of benign enchondromas produce pain. With the incidental finding of a painless enchondroma, the incidence of chondrosarcoma is less than 1%. Most chondrosarcomas present after a protracted clinical course of several months, consistent with the common low-grade nature of the lesion. Simon and Springfield[12] have recommended that lesions larger than 6 cm are at an increased risk of being a high-grade lesion and require careful observation and follow-up.

The radiographic appearance of chondrosarcoma corresponds to the subtype of tumor. Low-grade lesions exhibit features in common with benign aggressive lesions. Matrix calcification is an indication of low- to intermediate-grade lesions. High-grade lesions have a more aggressive radiographic appearance, as is expected. In the long bones, chondrosarcoma tends to occur in metadiaphyseal or diaphyseal locations, with epiphyseal lesions usually consistent with a clear cell subtype. More than 60% are calcified.[13] Endosteal scalloping is frequently seen in all cartilage tumors, regardless of grade. It is believed that endosteal scalloping involving more than 50% of the cortex is consistent with a more aggressive lesion. Periosteal reaction is not a common characteristic, except with very active enlarged lesions. Many lesions will have mixed areas of calcification and radiolucencies, suggestive of a malignant process. There is usually no crisp border or area containing reactive bone noted radiographically.

Secondary chondrosarcomas, especially those associated with osteochondromas, can be difficult to differentiate from their benign counterparts. Associated soft tissue masses and large cartilaginous caps larger than 2 cm and adjacent radiolucencies and cortical erosions are indicative of malignant transformation of these lesions. Adult patients with a cartilaginous cap more than 1 to 2 cm or children with cartilaginous caps larger than 2 to 3 cm should raise suspicion for possible malignant transformation of an osteochondroma.

Computed tomography (CT) is helpful in determining the amount of cortical disruption, periosteal reaction, soft tissue mass, and matrix calcification present within the lesion. MRI can be used to determine the thickness of the cartilage cap. Cross-sectional imaging is important in determining the local tumor extent and adjacent involved soft tissues, and in identifying aggressive features that will help with the diagnosis. This, together with the clinical presentation and plain film findings, are essential in determining the aggressiveness of a particular lesion. Review of these critical images with the pathologist is essential when a biopsy is indicated.

Treatment of chondrosarcoma is primarily surgical. Low-grade lesions that are readily resectable with wide margins typically require only surgery. High-grade and dedifferentiated lesions are frequently treated with neoadjuvant chemotherapy protocols because of the high risk of systemic spread despite lack of data to show improved long-term survival. Radiation therapy is only used in the palliative setting. The best prognosis for chondrosarcoma is based on the grade of the lesion.[5]

Ewing Sarcoma

Ewing sarcoma is a high-grade malignant tumor of bone and soft tissue consisting of small round blue cells. The cells produce scant osteoid matrix scattered throughout sheets of blue cells. These cells fill the trabeculae of the normal surrounding bone. It is the third most common bone tumor and the second most common malignant bone tumor in childhood. The commonly used term *Ewing sarcoma* is giving way to the more accurate term *primitive neural ectodermal tumor* or *Ewing sarcoma family of tumors* (ESFTs).[9] Turc-Carel et al.[13] have demonstrated that 80% to 90% of ESFTs have the distinct (11;22)(q24;q12) translocation. This cytogenetic abnormality helps in differentiating the lesion from neuroblastoma and other histologically similar lesions.[1]

ESFTs have a peak age incidence in the second decade of life, with a slight male predilection. The tumor most commonly occurs in long tubular bones; there is a 15% incidence of ESFTs occurring around the knee.[12,15] Pain and swelling are the most common presenting complaints. The presence of low-grade fever, elevated sedimentation rate, and increased white blood cell count is not uncommon. The presence of abnormal laboratory test results, soft tissue mass, and fever often leads to this tumor being confused with osteomyelitis with associated soft tissue abscess. Grossly, the tumor can appear with an almost liquid-like consistency. This can also cause confusion with chronic osteomyelitis.

On plain radiographs, the lesion appears within the metadiaphyseal or diaphyseal region of bone as a permeative lesion, with poorly defined margins and no reactive rim of bone. Areas of radiolucencies and radiodensities can be seen within the lesion itself. An associated soft tissue mass is frequently present. Onion skinning (layered, wavelike periosteal reaction) of the bone is a common feature. Soft tissue size and the extent of bony destruction are best evaluated with MRI and are essential for surgical planning.

Treatment consists of neoadjuvant chemotherapy followed by surgery, radiation therapy, or a combination thereof for local disease control and subsequent additional chemotherapy. The impact on survival of surgery is somewhat controversial. Because of the excellent response to chemotherapy and its radiosensitivity, ESFTs have traditionally used these modalities for local and systemic control. Initially, surgery was reserved for expendable bones, those that were easily resected with wide margins. There is now a growing trend toward managing these tumors more aggressively with surgery. More recent studies seem to indicate that surgery alone can yield acceptable rates of local control, avoiding the morbidity of radiotherapy.[10]

Lymphoma of Bone

Primary lymphoma of bone is a lymphoproliferative malignancy arising in bone. Lymphoma can be a single, solitary bone lesion or one of multiple bony sites, without any evidence of soft tissue involvement. It can also arise as a bone lesion in association with soft tissue (eg, lymph nodes, liver, spleen). Lymphoma can arise primarily in the bone or occur in the bone in a metastatic fashion. Histologically, lymphoma shows a diffuse proliferation of cells, with little matrix. Reticulum stains are positive. Immunohistochemistry and flow cytometry help diagnose and differentiate the lesion.[15] The peak age of incidence is in the sixth decade, with a male predominance. Lymphoma is rare in patients younger than 20 years. Lymphoma of bone tends to arise in the pelvis and proximal femur. Around the knee, approximately 8% occur in the distal femur and 4% in the proximal tibia. Within the bone itself, they tend to be diffuse within the metadiaphyseal region, involving the entire bone. Patients typically present with a complaint of progressive constant pain and a soft tissue mass. About 25% of patients will present with a pathologic fracture, usually with a history of minimal trauma. Occasionally, patients will present with only minimal complaints.

Lymphoma of bone typically presents as a permeative, destructive process on plain films. There are commonly areas of radiolucency adjacent to radiodense areas. A moth-eaten permeative appearance is common. Because of the rapid growth and tendency to percolate through the trabeculae, most lesions do not demonstrate any periosteal reaction. There will be little to no reactive bone and borders of the tumor are indistinct. The cortex may be thickened, giving an indication of a more indolent process. Presence of a soft tissue mass, often large, is frequently seen. MRI is helpful for determining the local extent of disease and subtle changes in the bone, such as localized bone marrow edema. The mainstay of treatment is chemotherapy and radiation therapy, with surgery limited to resection for extensive bone loss or fracture. The prognosis of patients with lymphoma of bone is 40% to 50% survival at 5 years.[1]

CONCLUSION

Surgical treatment of malignant tumors around the knee requires careful preoperative planning to achieve appropriate oncologic results. Skillful skeletal and soft tissue reconstruction is essential to achieving functional success. Such treatments should be performed by surgeons with appropriate experience. Rewarding results are often achievable with these patients.

KEY REFERENCES

2. Enneking WF: *Musculoskeletal tumor surgery*, New York, NY, 1983, Churchill Livingstone.

Malawar M, Sugarbaker PH, editors: *Musculoskeletal cancer surgery, treatment of sarcoma and allied diseases*, Dordrecht, The Netherlands, 2001, Kluwer Academic Publishers.

12. Simon M, Springfield D, editors: *Surgery for bone and soft tissue tumors*, Philadelphia, PA, 1998, Lippincott-Raven.

15. Wold L, McCleod R, Sim F, et al, editors: *Atlas of orthopedic pathology*, ed 2, Philadelphia, PA, 2002, WB Saunders.

The references for this chapter can also be found on www.expertconsult.com.

203

Allograft Prosthetic Composite Reconstruction of the Knee

Christopher P. Beauchamp, Ian D. Dickey

The goal of surgical management of musculoskeletal tumors about the knee is to obtain wide surgical margins and, if possible, preserve a functional mobile knee. In most cases, satisfactory results are obtained.[33] Reconstruction options for attaining a mobile knee include use of an osteoarticular allograft, oncology prosthesis, or allograft prosthetic composite (APC); the latter two approaches are used most commonly.[41,42] Each method of reconstruction has its advantages and disadvantages. The specific option that is chosen should be based on a multitude of factors because one method is not necessarily better than another.

An osteoarticular allograft has the advantage of offering a biologic solution to the problem; in the absence of complications, results can be good.[1-3] However, the disadvantages can be considerable. Fixation problems, nonunion, delayed weight bearing, fracture, graft dissolution, ligamentous instability, degenerative arthritis, extensor weakness, and disease transmission are only some of the problems associated with this method of reconstruction.[4,11,36,38]

Reconstruction with an endoprosthesis has the advantage of being predictable. These implants are modular, easily available, and easily implanted, and they deal with bone loss very well.[16,17] Fixation is often immediate, weight bearing can be started early, stability is built in,[28] and disease transmission is eliminated. However, two main concerns have arisen. The first involves the issue of soft tissue attachment, namely the extensor mechanism and the difficulty of obtaining secure, functional fixation. This usually results in an extensor lag. Current metallic prostheses do not provide an attachment surface that has an environment for stable, functional soft tissue ingrowth because they are nonbiologic constructs with metal coatings that are being used.

Research achieving effective soft tissue attachment to metal implants is currently underway using advanced metals with an internal structure similar to bone, termed trabecular metal. Tantalum and titanium are looking like promising materials for this purpose. However, attempts at ensuring soft tissue attachment to metal so far have not been clinically successful. Efforts to reconstitute the extensor mechanism have included securing the native tendon to transposed gastrocnemius fascia, or into the fibula. Incorporation and maintaining appropriate tension are difficult to achieve and are often inconsistent, resulting in compromised quadriceps strength. This is reflected in the persistent degree of extensor lag often found in this patient group. The other major issue involves the long-term durability of the device itself because these are often implanted in a young patient population.[45] This is further compounded by the long lever arms present at the points of weakness of these devices as a result of the large defects they must bridge.[27,28,49]

Allograft prosthetic reconstruction of the proximal tibia combines the benefits of osteoarticular allografts (soft tissue extensor reconstruction) with all of the advantages of prosthetic replacement; thus reconstruction of all or parts of the extensor mechanism from the quadriceps tendon to the tibial tubercle is possible by taking advantage of the secure allograft patellar tendon insertion[22] (Fig. 203.1). The combination of bulk allograft and metallic prosthesis provides a biologic construct to which tendons and ligaments can be attached and into which they can incorporate over time. Long-term durability remains an issue, but many of the major disadvantages of osteoarticular allografts are diminished or eliminated with the addition of a prosthesis. It must be acknowledged that with allograft prosthetic reconstruction, the cost, supplies needed, and operating room/anesthesia time can be greater because the procedure is technically more demanding and therefore has a potentially higher complication rate.[20,40,43,47] Allograft prosthetic reconstruction was first undertaken and continues to be performed in the belief that these risks are outweighed by the benefits of a more biologic reconstruction that leads to a better functioning limb, as the extensor mechanism is anatomically reconstructed.

In contrast, distal femoral APCs offer little if any advantage over endoprosthetic replacement.[9,10,31] The use of a bulk allograft has risks of complications that include delayed union, nonunion, dissolution, infection, fracture, disease transmission, and risk for postoperative wound complications.[5,12,37,39,43] In addition, if anything less than a fully constrained device is used, instability of the knee can be an issue.

Our experience with APC versus endoprosthetic reconstruction of the proximal tibia has supported superior performance of the APC with regard to extensor mechanism strength and subsequent function. Gilbert et al. demonstrated consistently good functional results with an acceptably low complication rate.[21] Donati et al. reported on a large series of 62 patients at the Rizzoli Institute and noted a Musculoskeletal Tumor Society score of satisfactory in 90.4% of patients, with a 5-year survival rate of 73.4%. Their reported survival rates were comparable with those of reconstruction with a modular prosthesis. Because of a high infection rate, not seen in other series, the authors advised not using this technique for patients receiving chemotherapy.[15] What has never been objectively determined is whether there is a clinically relevant difference between these two reconstructive options with respect to validated outcome scores and biomechanical function as determined by gait analysis.[6,40,47] The few studies published to date have looked at long-term survival of the reconstruction choice primarily and not at the functional difference between surviving reconstructive

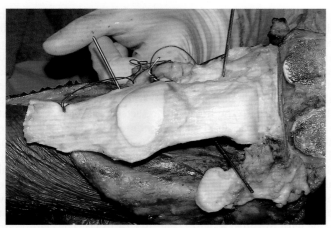

FIG 203.1 The advantage of an allograft prosthetic composite is the presence of soft tissue attachments. Here, the allograft is provisionally fixed to the host bone. The distal femur has already been prepared for the prosthesis. After the tibial component is cemented into the graft and host, the extensor mechanism can be sewn in a pants-over-vest fashion to the remaining host patellar ligament.

options. Most of these studies look at and compare outcome scores only, with no formal analysis of dynamic function.[6,47]

BASIC PRINCIPLES OF ALLOGRAFT PROSTHETIC RECONSTRUCTION

1. Fixation needs to span the graft.

   One of the major complications of using allografts is graft fracture. This problem is aggravated by graft dissolution. One of the advantages of using a prosthesis with an allograft is that the prosthesis can reconstruct the joint surface and can also provide graft fixation while maintaining the strength of the allograft. This is why it is important to span the entire length of the graft and extend into the host bone. Fixation by any means should not stop within the substance of the allograft.[23,24]

2. Allograft host fixation needs to be rigid.

   Until recently, options for press-fit fixation have been limited. Conventional primary components were fixed to segmental allografts, and allograft host fixation was accomplished with a rod or a plate. A locked intramedullary nail cannot provide adequate rigid fixation, hence the risk of nonunion is increased. Plate fixation provides good rigid fixation but brings with it increased risk of allograft fracture and fragmentation. In general, the use of plates with allografts should be avoided. If plate fixation must be used, screw fixation should be minimal, and consideration should be given to filling the allograft with bone cement to increase the strength of the allograft.

   Currently available prosthetics have a tremendous range of reconstructive capabilities. Options for stem fixation include long-stem cemented stems, smooth press-fit stems, fluted stems, locked stems, and fully porous coated stems. Thus far no studies have compared the various forms of fixation, but the basic principle is generally to fix the prosthesis to the allograft with cement and obtain a rigid press-fit to the host bone. Fully porous coated stems around the knee

are now available. In our experience, in the proximal femur the best results have been seen with cement in the allograft and a long, porous, coated femoral stem in the host bone. Donati et al. used a variety of techniques to fix the allograft to the host bone. Plate fixation, cement in the graft and press-fit into the host, and cement in the graft and host were used. When the prosthesis was cemented into the graft and fixed to the host bone with a plate, the rate of nonunion was higher. Best results in this study occurred with a press-fit stem, but this technique resulted in a delayed union rate of 12.9%, requiring additional surgery. Our experience with the proximal tibia has been to universally use cement fixation in both the allograft and the host bone. Cement fixation of the prosthesis is done in one step and will be described below.

3. Avoid gaps at the graft-host junction.

   Good contact between the host and the graft is critical to healing. Some authors have championed the need for or the desirability of a step cut. We have found it technically very difficult to achieve a satisfactory step cut that does not have significant gaps. This is more likely to be seen when a line-to-line press-fit stem is used. The ultimate fit of the step cut is determined by the final alignment ascertained by the fit within the host canal. We have found a simple butt joint easier to manage. To fine-tune the final fit, a small bevel is made prior to stem insertion on the endosteal side of the allograft at the end that matches the host. When the APC is almost seated, a thin high-speed burr can remove a small amount of bone to allow an exact fit without scoring the implant. A step cut or an oblique osteotomy increases the surface area of contact, also increasing the likelihood of healing, and provides additional stability. It is used ideally when the implant does not interfere with final fixation of the graft-host junction.

4. Cementing into host bone *is* okay.

   We believe a press-fit stem is ideal; unfortunately for tumor reconstruction, many patients receive chemotherapy that has a detrimental effect on bone ingrowth.[14,25,26] In addition, no good press-fit options for the tibia are available. Cementing the composite may be a better choice *if* certain conditions can be met. The major problem with cement in an APC reconstruction involves the cement technique itself. The usual method described is cementation in two steps: first, cementing the prosthesis to the graft and, second, cementing the composite to the host bone. This results in a poor cement technique in both instances. When the prosthesis is cemented to the allograft, it is difficult to contain the cement within the graft and keep it from running out both ends of the graft. When cementing into the host bone, it is difficult to keep the cement out of the graft-host junction, contributing to problems with healing. If cement is chosen as the method of fixation, we cement the stem into the allograft and the host at the same time with standard third-generation techniques. When the cemented stem is inserted into the host bone, the stem must not have any influence on the graft-host junction relationship; therefore rigid provisional fixation must be used to hold the graft and the host bone together, so they can be prepared and cemented in a single step.

5. Size does matter.

   Infection remains one of the leading causes of failure of APC reconstruction and is a significant concern any time bulk allografts are used.[37] Wound healing complications continue to be a major contributing factor to the development of infection. Management of the soft tissue envelope is the key to avoidance of soft tissue wound healing problems. One advantage of using an allograft with a prosthesis is the option of using a slightly smaller graft to allow for a relative increase in the soft tissue envelope. Accurate sizing of osteoarticular allografts is critical to their success, but this does not hold true for composite reconstructions. However, in the revision situation, canal diameter does come into play, and this may be the limiting factor in selection of the graft if a press-fit configuration is used. Most allografts are of relatively small diameter compared with those in older patients with failed implants, and to use a press-fit stem of sufficient diameter, a larger allograft may be necessary. Fortunately this does not apply to short distal femoral reconstructions because the metaphyseal region will permit a large-diameter stem.

6. Provide soft tissue coverage.

With all reconstructions around the knee, good reliable coverage of the implant and allograft is essential. The threshold for the use of local muscle flaps with skin graft should be very low, and if one must err, it is better to exercise this option than to deal with the consequences of infection.

7. Anticipate, anticipate.

Anything that can go wrong can and will go wrong. If you do not have the luxury of a large bone bank in your facility, consider the following scenarios. We have encountered all of these problems.

1. Have a plan if your graft becomes contaminated. Dropping the graft on the floor is a disaster. As soon as the graft is brought to the patient, we suture it to the patient with a single safety suture.
2. Are you sure it will fit? We check all grafts with a repeat in-house x-ray to make sure. Will the prosthesis you have chosen fit both the graft and the host?
3. Grafts can be mislabeled. If we are certain we will be using a graft, we try to thaw the graft before the procedure is begun. This is not possible if the graft may not be used.
4. Some grafts will come without soft tissue attachments. If soft tissue attachments are necessary for your reconstruction, first be certain they are there. We specify that the graft must have all of the soft tissues attached, including the quadriceps tendon.

Allograft Prosthetic Composite Reconstruction of the Tibia: Technique

This method of reconstruction has the advantage of allowing for numerous reconstructive options of the extensor mechanism. Any or all of the allograft extensor mechanisms can be replaced. We use osteoarticular allografts that are stored with all of the capsular and ligamentous soft tissues attached. The entire extensor mechanism, quadriceps tendon, patella, and patellar ligament are retained with the allograft. Ideally, up to 15 cm of quadriceps tendon can be retrieved with the allograft. The remaining host tissues determine the method of reconstruction to be used. The prosthetic chosen is typically a constrained rotating hinge device,[30] but a ligamentous reconstruction with a conventionally constrained implant can be chosen, although it carries the risk of ligament failure and subsequent instability. We use a constrained (rotating hinge) device in almost all cases because the ligamentous reconstruction required adds only more complexity to an already complex reconstruction.

Choose an allograft of appropriate length and diameter with the soft tissues attached, as described previously. The graft proximally should be no larger in circumference at the plateau, and in fact should be smaller, than the resected specimen to facilitate soft tissue coverage. Remove the capsule and ligaments that will not be used. Use a safety suture through tissue on the allograft, and sew it to the patient to protect against dropping the allograft onto the floor. The resected tibia is cut at a right angle; a butt joint is used for this method of reconstruction. The allograft is cut at the same distance as the resected specimen. The remaining host tibia is then prepared for the tibial stem by reaming to the appropriate size. The distal portion of the tibial allograft is similarly prepared. The allograft is attached to the host tibia provisionally. This is accomplished using two specially prepared bone clamps that are fixed to the allograft and host bone with threaded K-wires (Fig. 203.2A to D). The clamps are simply modified by drilling holes into the jaws of the bone clamp. These holes allow the wires to be driven into the cortex of the allograft and host bone to secure the clamps to the bone. This fixation permits compressive forces to be applied to the bone clamps.

Standard cerclage cables are passed under the jaws of the bone clamps, so that with application of tension through the cables to the clamps, the two clamps are drawn together, providing enough compression at the graft-host junction site that stable temporary fixation is attained. The K-wires must not penetrate into the intramedullary canal of the allograft or host bone; otherwise, they would interfere with reaming of the allograft host composite. The principle is similar to that of skull traction. At this point the allograft host construct is prepared in standard fashion to accept a stemmed tibial tray. Most implants are available in stem lengths of 180 mm and longer. After the proximal tibia is cut, a high-speed burr should be used to remove most of the proximal metaphyseal bone. The remaining allograft and host bone can be reamed together if necessary; the provisional fixation should be stable enough to allow for gentle reaming. The canal is then plugged, and the entire length of the tibial component is cemented (Fig. 203.3A and B).

Cement offers the advantage of allowing immediate weight bearing and predictable fixation with preservation of allograft-host junction compression. It also reduces the risk of nonunion. Allograft union is directly related to the rigidity of fixation. Cementing into the allograft and press-fitting distally is an option; the stem is inserted until it engages the host bone, and the cement is then injected into the prepared metaphyseal bone. Alternatively, the prosthesis can be fixed to the allograft on the back table, and the stem press-fitted into the host bone after the cement has set.

The practical issues and possible disadvantages of noncemented distal fixation are worth addressing. Currently, the leading fixed rotating-hinge designs that have the necessary requisite modular stems for the tibial component are press fit. These assembled implants rely on hoop stresses of the host tibia for fixation and the splines for rotational stability. These stems are designed to rely on cement fixation of the body of the implant in the allograft and press-fit stability of the stem; unlike a fully porous coated stem, they are not designed to achieve distal fixation. Although this may be a reasonable strategy with an intact tibia in the revision setting, relying on the proximal cement mantle in the APC setting in which there is a bony discontinuity does not seem prudent, given that immediate rigidity is the key to bony union at the allograft-host bone

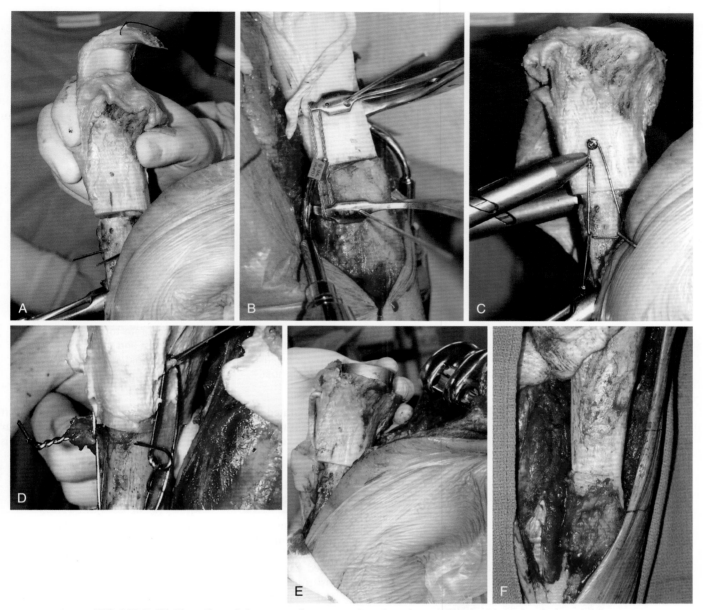

FIG 203.2 (A) The allograft is cut to the appropriate length and fitted with a simple butt joint. (B to D) The graft is fixed temporarily to the host bone. A variety of techniques are shown here. All methods are based on provisional fixation with unicortical wires or screws, and a compressive force is applied with wires or cables. Modified Verbrugge clamps and cables with a tensioning device is the current preferred technique. (E) After the stem is cemented into both the graft and host bone, the provisional fixation is removed. The graft is now securely and rigidly fixed. (F) The butt joint fit with this technique provides excellent cortical contact.

junction. In addition, the stem usually is highly polished and does not encourage the desired long-term stability via biologic fixation. A long fully porous coated ingrowth modular stem is in development by several of the major implant manufacturers and is available on a custom basis, but this option is very expensive, difficult to obtain, and certainly not available as an on-the-shelf item to provide realistic flexibility in the operating room. Thus our current preference in achieving reliable host-graft junction union is to cement the whole construct. As other ingrowth stems become available, this method of implant fixation merits reevaluation.

EXTENSOR MECHANISM REPAIR

The simplest reconstructive situation exists when the entire patellar ligament is present. The host ligament is sewn pants-over-vest[34] to the allograft ligament, with the allograft tissue placed deep to the host tissue. More tissue from the allograft can also be used. The allograft patella can be removed, leaving the periosteum intact and resulting in a long strip of tissue that can be split and passed around the host patella and woven into the quadriceps tendon of the host bone (Fig. 203.4). If necessary, the allograft patella and the quadriceps tendon can be

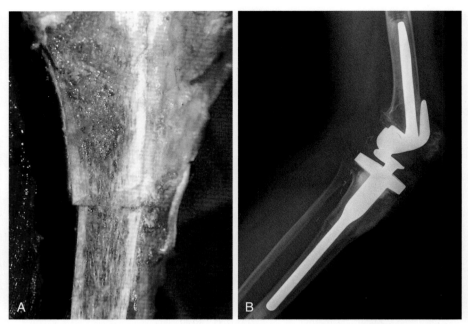

FIG 203.3 (A and B) The graft-host junction is a simple butt joint; this allows for accurate total contact and permits even compression. Fixation of the stem with cement into the host and the allograft at the same time does not disturb the provisional fixation because it is rigid. The radiograph demonstrates perfect fixation of the graft to the host.

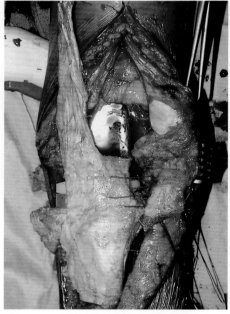

FIG 203.4 Our current method of reconstructing the extensor mechanism when the patient's entire extensor mechanism can be preserved. The patient's own patellar ligament is sewn over the top of the allograft patellar tendon. The allograft patella is removed, and the remaining allograft tendon complex is sewn around the medial aspect of the patella and is woven into the host quadriceps mechanism.

incorporated into the remaining host tissue. If the allograft patella is used, it can be resurfaced or left intact. It has been our preference to resurface, but we have no data to support this practice.

ALLOGRAFT PROSTHETIC COMPOSITE RECONSTRUCTION OF THE DISTAL FEMUR

For reasons outlined previously, we normally would reconstruct distal femoral defects with a prosthesis.[31] Authors have described the usefulness of an APC reconstruction in the situation of a failed endoprosthesis; in this case the allograft is valuable in assisting in issues of fixation caused by loosening, osteolysis, and ectasia of remaining host bone. Use of a distal femoral allograft may be a good choice if fixation options are limited in the host bone because of remaining available bone or preexisting implants.

Select an allograft of appropriate length and canal diameter that will allow for the fixation method you have chosen: press fit or cemented. As in the proximal femur, it is our preference to fix with a press-fit fully porous coated stem, with the prosthesis cemented into the allograft (Fig. 203.5). The graft is prepared on the back table in an allograft vise with standard arthroplasty instruments. Ligaments and soft tissues are removed or retained depending on the level of constraint of the implant the surgeon chooses. The osteotomy used to remove the tumor is a simple right-angle cut, and the allograft is fitted to the host bone with a butt joint if the entire stem is cemented. The provisional compression system is used as described previously. This method cannot be used if the stem is press-fitted, because the geometry of the stem will determine the fit of the butt joint. In this situation the stem is first cemented to the allograft on the back table. The portion of the stem that is press-fitted is first coated with a plastic film to prevent cement

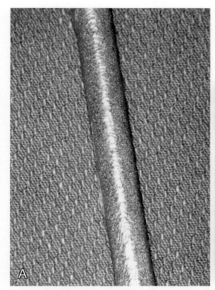 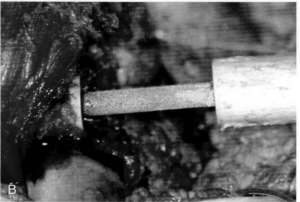

FIG 203.5 Reconstruction of the distal femur with an APC using a press-fit stem. (A) The stem is cemented into the femoral allograft. For its protection, the porous coated stem is first coated with a thin plastic adhesive that is removed after cementation. (B) The stem is then inserted into the host bone. Note the butt joint, rather than the technically more challenging step cut.

from coating it (see Fig. 203.5). The cement is injected into the graft and is pressurized as much as possible, the prosthesis is inserted, and the plastic coating is removed before the cement sets. The resulting composite is carefully driven into place, with adjustments made to the allograft-host interface with a high-speed burr or a small saw as the two surfaces are coming together. Supplemental fixation with a plate or onlay struts can provide additional fixation and rotational control. Plates are best avoided because they are associated with increased risk of graft fracture and resorption. Step cuts provide improved rotational control and an increased surface area for healing (Fig. 203.6), but the same problem of fit exists when a press-fit stem is used; it is the final insertion that determines the orientation of the osteotomy. It is technically challenging to achieve a tight junction. Soft tissues are repaired as determined by the level of constraint selected. A rotating-hinge implant requires no capsular or ligamentous repair.

ALLOGRAFT EXTENSOR MECHANISM TRANSPLANTATION

Absence of the extensor mechanism presents a very difficult problem to manage.[7,13,48] This occurs rarely in oncologic situations but is commonly a problem with primary or, more often, revision knee arthroplasty patients.[8,18,19,29,38] Most common are traumatic ruptures with and without a history of underlying inflammatory conditions.[32,35,44,46] Few options are available to repair this; extensor allograft reconstruction is one. Fortunately this problem is rare; consequently, few reports on the results of treatment have been published.

In general, attempts to repair this problem using local tissue have been unrewarding.[36] We use a variation of the technique described by Emerson et al.[19] If there is a major absence of the extensor mechanism involving the patellar ligament, we replace the quadriceps tendon, patella, patellar ligament, tibial tubercle, and anterior cortex of the tibia with an allograft (Fig. 203.7A to

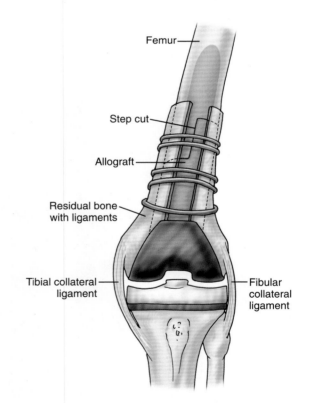

FIG 203.6 Diagram of the step cut osteotomy at the allograft-host bone junction, the stemmed component, and cerclage wire securing the residual host bone around the interface to reconstruct an uncontained circumferential defect of the distal aspect of the femur.

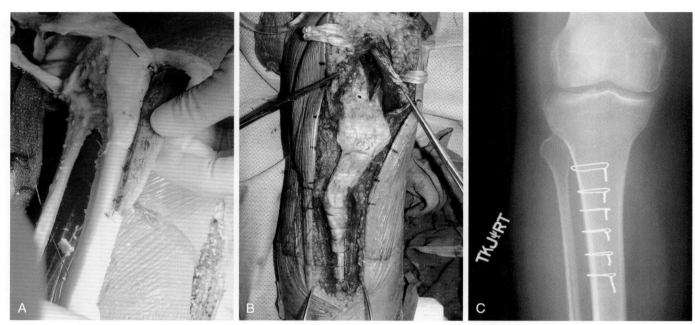

FIG 203.7 (A) Ten centimeters of anterior tibial cortex and tubercle is replaced with allograft in continuity with the extensor mechanism. Here, the host bone with an absent extensor mechanism is used to measure the allograft extensor mechanism before the graft is cut. (B) Fixation is made with numerous 18-gauge wires without penetrating the allograft bone. The extensor mechanism with unresurfaced patella is woven through the remaining extensor mechanism in a patient with a chronic extensor disruption following a revision total knee replacement. (C) Postoperative x-ray of the tibial tubercle reconstruction.

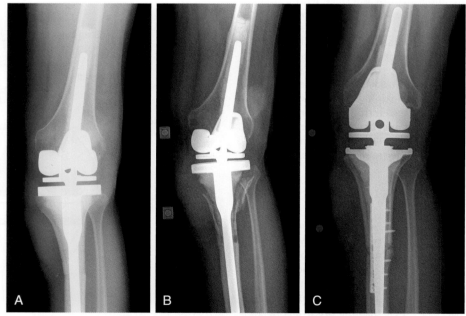

FIG 203.8 An illustrated failure 16 years after the index reconstruction.

C). Again as mentioned previously, the patella is variable with respect to the decision to resurface. Certainly in the patient without a prosthesis, we do not resurface. Approximately 10 cm of anterior tibial cortex is transplanted and fixed with wires. We try to avoid screw fixation in allografts to minimize resorption risks. Our experience with this technique has yielded promising early results.

Complications to Anticipate

APC reconstruction about the knee is a highly complex, technically demanding procedure and as such comes with a high complication rate. The major complications unique to this procedure are extensor mechanism failure, graft resorption, and wound issues. Surprisingly, nonunion has not been an issue.

Salvage options for APC failure remain the same as for the original defect. However, a deep infection almost always ends with an amputation. In the absence of infection, the APC can be repeated as long as the soft tissue envelope permits. Fig. 203.8A to C illustrates a failure 16 years after the index reconstruction.

KEY REFERENCES

4. Barrack RL, Lyons T: Proximal tibia–extensor mechanism composite allograft for revision TKA with chronic patellar tendon rupture. *Acta Orthop Scand* 71:419–421, 2000.

7. Burks RT, Edelson RH: Allograft reconstruction of the patellar ligament: a case report. *J Bone Joint Surg Am* 76:1077–1079, 1994.

18. Emerson RH, Jr, Head WC, Malinin TI: Reconstruction of patellar tendon rupture after total knee arthroplasty with an extensor mechanism allograft. *Clin Orthop* 260:154–161, 1990.

20. Ghazavi MT, Stockley I, Yee G, et al: Reconstruction of massive bone defects with allograft in revision total knee arthroplasty. *J Bone Joint Surg Am* 79:17–25, 1997.

22. Gitelis S, Piasecki P: Allograft prosthetic composite arthroplasty for osteosarcoma and other aggressive bone tumors. *Clin Orthop* 270:197–201, 1991.

23. Harris AI, Gitelis S, Sheinkop MB, et al: Allograft prosthetic composite reconstruction for limb salvage and severe deficiency of bone at the knee or hip. *Semin Arthroplasty* 5:85–94, 1994.

29. Hungerford DS: Management of extensor mechanism complications in total knee arthroplasty. *Orthopedics* 17:843–844, 1994.

35. Larsen E, Lund PM: Ruptures of the extensor mechanism of the knee joint: clinical results and patellofemoral articulation. *Clin Orthop* 213:150–153, 1986.

36. Leopold SS, Greidanus N, Paprosky WG, et al: High rate of failure of allograft reconstruction of the extensor mechanism after total knee arthroplasty. *J Bone Joint Surg Am* 81:1574–1579, 1999.

38. Lotke PA: Management of extensor mechanism complications. *Orthopedics* 21:1046–1047, 1998.

41. Sim FH, Beauchamp CP, Chao EY: Reconstruction of musculoskeletal defects about the knee for tumor. *Clin Orthop* 221:188–201, 1987.

47. Wunder JS, Leitch K, Griffin AM, et al: Comparison of two methods of reconstruction for primary malignant tumors at the knee: a sequential cohort study. *J Surg Oncol* 77:89–99, discussion 100, 2001.

48. Zanotti RM, Freiberg AA, Matthews LS: Use of patellar allograft to reconstruct a patellar tendon-deficient knee after total joint arthroplasty. *J Arthroplasty* 10:271–274, 1995.

The references for this chapter can also be found on www.expertconsult.com.

204

Megaprostheses for Reconstruction Following Tumor Resection About the Knee

Dieter Lindskog, Mary I. O'Connor

INTRODUCTION

Resection of the distal femur or proximal tibia for tumor necessitates reconstruction of the skeletal defect to restore limb function. This chapter will focus on the use of megaprostheses for reconstruction following resection of the distal femur or proximal tibia for treatment of neoplasm.

RATIONALE FOR USE OF MEGAPROSTHESES

Options for reconstruction following resection of the distal femur or proximal tibia include use of a megaprosthesis (implant designed to replace the resected large bone segment) or the combined use of a structural allograft with a revision-type arthroplasty implant (allograft-prosthetic composite). In the past, a perceived advantage of an allograft-prosthetic composite was the potential for bone stock restoration. However, long-term studies show that little of the structural allograft actually becomes remodeled to viable bone[9] and resorption of the allograft and fracture can occur over time.[2] Allograft-prosthetic composites do provide the potential for effective host tendon healing to allograft tendon, a critical advantage in reconstruction of the extensor mechanism following resection of the proximal tibia as discussed in the previous chapter. Although new implant materials (eg, trabecular metal) show potential for effective healing of host tissue and tendon to the actual metal prosthesis, results of such implants have yet to be reported.

Following resection of the distal femur for tumor, an allograft-prosthetic composite has no clear advantage over a megaprosthesis. In this setting, collateral and cruciate ligament function is best reconstructed by a constrained arthroplasty articulation. Furthermore, a megaprosthesis is appropriate for patients who will receive chemotherapy or radiation therapy after surgery, modalities that increase the risk of allograft infection and nonunion.

INDICATIONS

A segmental modular rotating-hinge megaprosthesis knee system is appropriate for reconstruction of the distal femur following tumor resection. Segmental modular systems allow for intraoperative determination of the implant size based on the extent of bone resection necessary for an appropriate oncologic resection. A rotating-hinge design allows motion in flexion-extension, rotation, and longitudinally along the axis of the extremity by permitting some distraction of an inner bearing component with its outer articulation and is favored over a fixed-hinge design. A rotating hinge will minimize stress transfer to the fixation interface and decrease the risk of aseptic loosening.

Following resection of the proximal tibia, a segmental modular rotating-hinge megaprosthesis knee system is appropriate for patients who require postoperative radiation or have an extensor mechanism that cannot be reconstructed with an allograft-prosthetic composite (Fig. 204.1). Although chemotherapy can retard bone healing at the allograft–host bone junction, the administration of postoperative chemotherapy is not an absolute contraindication to use of an allograft-prosthetic composite in the proximal tibia.

In skeletally immature patients, expandable implants can compensate for the loss of growth from resection of the involved physis. Noninvasive means of expansion have been developed that simplify the use of these implants and potentially decrease the complication rate.

METHODS OF FIXATION OF MEGAPROSTHESES

Fixation of the intramedullary stems of the femoral and tibial components may be achieved with various methods. Cemented and uncemented fixation have been effective.[5,11,12,15,27-29] Cement fixation should be considered for patients with poor-quality bone and those who will require postoperative radiotherapy. Some surgeons favor the use of a hydroxyapatite (HA) coating on the intramedullary stem component of megaprostheses to promote fixation of the uncemented stem.[4,22,27,28]

With press-fit or cement stems, implant systems typically have an option of a porous-coated collar on the intramedullary stem component (Fig. 204.2). This design feature encourages the formation of extracortical bone bridging between the host bone and the collared portion of the implant (Fig. 204.3). Bone graft material can be placed in this region prior to wound closure to promote bone bridging. Ward et al. postulated that extracortical bridging between the host bone and implant with bone or soft tissue may retard osteolysis by preventing implant debris–containing synovial fluid from contacting the bone-implant or bone-cement interface (Fig. 204.4).[37]

The degree of development of extracortical bone bridging has been variable. In the distal femur, extracortical bridging more commonly develops posteriorly[6,19,21] and along the compression side of the femur.[19] Chao et al. noted the total percentage of the length of the porous coated region that was covered with bone formation in the distal femur and knee to be 75 ± 31% in 15 implants with follow-up of 2 to 21 years.[6] The formation of this extracortical bone bridging stabilizes by 2 years following surgery. These authors also found that the prevalence

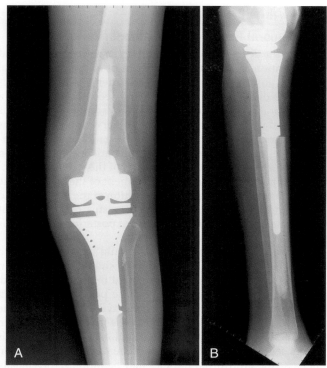

FIG 204.1 Proximal Tibial Replacement Knee Arthroplasty Following Sarcoma Resection (A) Anteroposterior view. Suture holes in the proximal tibial body to assist with extension mechanism reconstruction. (B) Lateral view.

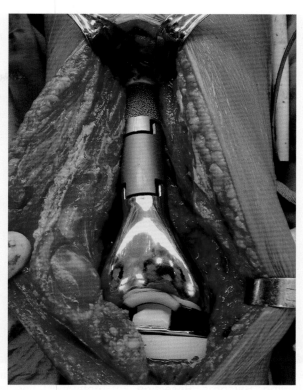

FIG 204.2 Intraoperative Photograph of Modular Distal Femoral Replacement Knee Arthroplasty The femoral component is composed of a distal articulating body, an intercalary segment to provide appropriate length, and a proximal intramedullary stem with a porous-coated collar. Bone graft has not yet been applied to the junction of the host bone and the porous-coated collar of the implant. The patella was not resurfaced.

of stem loosening was very low suggesting that extracortical bone bridging improved long-term fixation. Kawai et al. noted an association between extracortical bone bridging and higher limb function scores.[20]

Although clinical data suggest that the presence of extracortical bone bridging improves long-term success, this bone bridging may not actually grow into the porous coating of the implant. Lucent lines between the extracortical bone and porous surface may be observed.[19] Furthermore, histologic analysis of five retrieved tumor megaprostheses showed no bone ingrowth into the porous-coated segment of the implant, despite radiographs of these implants suggesting that there was bone ingrowth into the porous-coated segment.[31] Instead, transmitted light microscopy showed fibrous tissue between the extracortical bone and the porous coating. Nonetheless, the presence of this extracortical bone/fibrous tissue may increase prosthetic stability. With the application of new implant materials that more effectively promote the ingrowth of bone (eg, trabecular metal), true extracortical bone bridging of bone ingrowth into the porous surface may occur (Fig. 204.5).

A different method of achieving bone ingrowth fixation of a megaprosthesis is compressive osseointegration. Developed by James O. Johnston, MD, a porous-coated titanium surface with a conical section is mounted transverse to the axis of the femur. Compression of the implant against host bone occurs through Belleville spring washers tightened by a bolt over an intramedullary traction bar. Retrieval from 12 patients with Compress implants (Zimmer Biomet, Warsaw, IN) who underwent revision surgery for infection, periprosthetic fracture, or local tumor recurrence showed only two patients

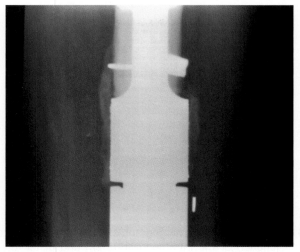

FIG 204.3 Close-up radiograph of host–bone implant junction illustrating extracortical bone bridging.

with infection-demonstrated loosening at the bone-prosthetic interface and no evidence of osteonecrosis at an average 3.3 years after implantation.[23] In a comparison of uncemented femoral megaprosthesis fixation, the prosthetic survival rates at 5 years were comparable among 50 patients with intramedullary

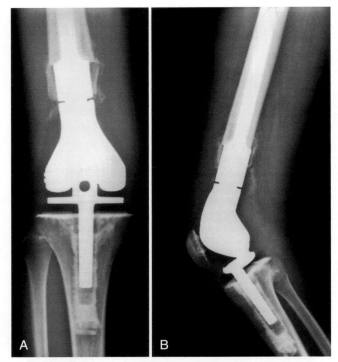

FIG 204.4 Distal Femoral Replacement Knee Arthroplasty Following Sarcoma Resection (A) Anteroposterior view showing all polyethylene tibial components. Metal inner bearing component allows some longitudinal distraction between the inner bearing and cemented tibial component. Polyethylene bushings, an axle, and a polyethylene extension bumper comprise the remainder of the articular portion. The femoral component, in this case, consists of only the articular body component and the stem. A bone graft has been placed to promote extracortical bone bridging. (B) Lateral view. The patella has been resurfaced on this patient.

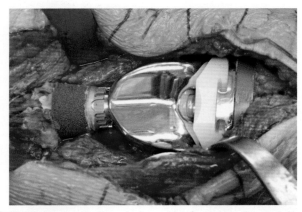

FIG 204.5 Intraoperative photograph of a trabecular metal collar at the junction of the intramedullary stem and distal femoral replacement component. A bone graft was applied to the region of the trabecular metal collar.

uncemented stem (85%) and 41 patients with Compress fixation (88%).[10] Another series Compress fixation duplicated this success rate.[26] Longer-term follow-up has shown durable success rates with 80% 10-year survival rate, equivalent to other bone fixation methods.[16]

SURGICAL TECHNIQUE

Distal Femoral Replacement Arthroplasty

Although the degree of bone and soft tissue resection is dictated by the location of the tumor, the extent of quadriceps removal influences postoperative function. In patients who had resection of the distal femur for tumor and reconstruction with a distal femoral replacement arthroplasty, resection of the vastus lateralis and vastus intermedius (and preservation of the vastus medialis) resulted in a more physiologic gait and more physiologic knee-loading pattern than seen in patients with resection of the vastus medialis (and preservation of the vastus lateralis).[1] The importance of this data is in placement of the biopsy: if the surgeon has a choice, the preferred position of the biopsy should be lateral to allow preservation of the vastus medialis. If not appropriate, the biopsy should be placed posterior in the vastus medialis to minimize muscle resection.

Primary distal femoral sarcomas should be resected with a wide margin. The entire lower extremity should be included in the sterile field to permit more proximal dissection if needed. A sterile tourniquet may be used. If the prior biopsy was an open procedure, the prior biopsy site is excised en bloc with the specimen. The superficial femoral vessels may be identified in the adductor canal prior to the femoral osteotomy if there is any concern regarding compromise of the vasculature by tumor. Otherwise the uninvolved muscles may be mobilized (typically the rectus femoris and the vastus lateralis or vastus medialis), leaving the vastus intermedius intact around the femur. The medial and lateral intermuscular septum are cut along the long axis of the femur leaving a cuff of tissue as a tumor margin. The anterior femoral and corresponding anterior tibial cortexes are marked with the knee in full extension to aid in placement of the distal femoral component in proper rotation. The level of the femoral osteotomy is marked and the vastus intermedius and any additional muscle to be transected at this level are cut. The underlying vessels are protected during the osteotomy. The marrow at the proximal osteotomy margin is sent for frozen section analysis to confirm a negative margin. The proximal aspect of the resection specimen (distal aspect of femoral osteotomy level) is retracted anteriorly, medially, or laterally to facilitate transection of the remaining soft tissues. The middle geniculate branch is identified and ligated. The popliteal vessels are easily identified and protected. The heads of the medial and lateral gastrocnemius muscles are detached, again leaving a cuff of tissue on the specimen. The knee capsule and the collateral and cruciate ligaments are transected; this may occur before or after the osteotomy to facility mobilization of the distal femur. Negative margins are confirmed on frozen section analysis. After resection of the distal femur, the proximal tibia is prepared with a perpendicular bone cut as in a standard knee arthroplasty. The proximal tibia is prepared for the stem portion of the tibial component. The femoral canal is prepared for a cemented, press-fit, or compression fixation application. The patella may or may not be resurfaced depending on the status of the articular cartilage.[7] Trial components are placed to assess for limb length, soft tissue tension, and proper patellar tracking. After the final implant is inserted, the prostheses should be completely covered with soft tissue. If inadequate muscle remains, a medial gastrocnemius muscle flap should be considered. The implant should not be left in a subcutaneous position. A deep drain should be placed and perioperative antibiotics administered. Wound healing takes priority over early knee motion. Most patients gain excellent flexion; active extension is dependent on the quality of the remaining quadriceps.

Proximal Tibial Replacement Arthroplasty

Sarcomas of the proximal tibia should be resected with a wide margin. A tourniquet may be placed high on the thigh; if there are any concerns regarding the potential for more proximal dissection, a sterile tourniquet is appropriate. If an open biopsy was performed, the biopsy site is included in the en bloc resection. In all possible areas, a margin of deep soft tissue should remain over the resected specimen. The patellar tendon is cut to permit a safe tumor margin and preserve as much length for subsequent repair as possible. The knee capsule, collaterals, and cruciates are cut at the level of the knee joint. The posterior tibial vessels and nerve are protected. Prior to specimen removal, rotation of the distal femur relative to the remaining tibia should be marked to assist in placement of the implant in proper rotation. The remaining proximal tibia is prepared to the intramedullary stem of the implant. The distal femur is resurfaced and fashioned to receive the hinged prosthesis. The patella may or may not be resurfaced.

The main challenge in resection of the proximal tibia is reconstruction of the extensor mechanism. With use of a megaprosthesis, a common reconstructive technique is rotation of the medial head of the gastrocnemius to cover the implant and provide a repair site for the patellar tendon.[25] The limb is initially protected in extension; gradual flexion is subsequently permitted. Others have described use of a trevira tube, which is fixed to the megaprosthesis by nonabsorbable sutures; the extensor tendon and gastrocnemius flap are sutured to the trevira tube. In retrieved specimens from various anatomic locations, histologic findings showed fibrous tissue ingrowth into the trevira tube without a foreign body or inflammatory reaction.[14] Megaprosthesis designs with a trabecular metal tubercle attachment allow for direct attachment and may simplify extensor mechanism reconstruction, but clinical results are not yet published.

CLINICAL RESULTS

There is little data on comparison of megaprostheses and allograft-prosthetic composites performed at the same institution. Wunder et al. reviewed their experience with use of irradiated allograft-implant composites or megaprostheses after sarcoma resection of the distal femur or proximal tibia.[39] Reconstructive failure occurred in 6 of 11 (55%) allograft-prosthetic composites compared to 10 of 64 (16%) megaprostheses. Statistically significant improvement in limb salvage was observed with megaprostheses (95%) as compared to allograft-prosthetic composites (64%). Functional outcomes were also significantly improved in patients with megaprostheses.[39] However, irradiation of the allografts used in this series may have contributed to the high rate of allograft fracture (36%) by decreasing the mechanical strength of the grafts. The smaller number of allograft-prosthetic composites and the relatively higher use of allografts in the proximal tibia may also have influenced these results because this location is known to have a higher rate of complications than the distal femur.

Distal Femur

The extent of bone resection appears to influence survival of distal femoral replacement implants. Cobb et al. reported 94%

survival of the implant at 10 years with distal resections of less than 40% of the femur compared to 49% survival with resection of more than 40%.[8] Kawai et al. studied patients who had resection of the distal femur and reconstruction with a Lane-Burstein semiconstrained hinge segmental knee prosthesis (Biomet, Warsaw, Indiana; 82 patients) or a Finn rotating-hinge segmental knee implant (Biomet; 31 patients).[21] Five- and 10-year Kaplan-Meier prosthetic survival rates were 71% and 50%. Univariant analysis showed patients with more than 40% resection of the distal femur and those with complete resection of the quadriceps had significantly worse prosthetic survival with aseptic loosening as the primary cause of late failure. Ward et al. used supplemental fixation of a cemented interlocking pin through the femoral stem and into the femoral head and neck in patients with extensive bone resection and less than 4 inches of retained diaphysis below the lesser trochanter.[35] Although the degree of bone resection performed is dictated by the extent of the tumor, only the amount of bone necessary to provide an adequate margin should be resected to promote implant longevity.

Prosthetic design may also influence implant survival data. Analysis of long-term follow-up of various Stanmore implant designs shows that the risk of aseptic loosening of endoprosthetic replacement of the distal femur at 10 years was 35% with a fixed-hinged implant, 24% with a rotating-hinge implant without an HA collar, and 0% for the rotating-hinge with an HA collar.[27] With the introduction of the rotating-hinge articulation, stress transmission to the bone-cement interface lessened and loosening rates decreased.

Cemented and uncemented fixation has proven successful. Using the Kinematic rotating-hinge (Howmedica, Mahwah, NJ) distal femoral replacement prosthesis with cement fixation, Choong et al. reported 90% implant survival at 2 to 7 years in 30 patients with 20 patients having good to excellent function and flexion of 120 degrees or more.[7,35] Sharma et al. reported 5-year implant survival of 84% and 10-year survival of 79% using the same implant with cement fixation.[29] Slightly better results were published by Bickels et al. with an overall prosthetic survivorship of 93% at 5 years and 88% at 10 years in 110 patients with custom, modular, or expandable distal femoral megaprostheses.[3] Using press-fit stems in most of the 25 distal femoral patients, Kawai et al. reported prosthetic survival at 5 years of 88% with the Finn rotating-hinge implant (Biomet Orthopedics, Warsaw, IN). In a more recent publication from some of the same authors, intramedullary uncemented femoral fixation had an 85% 5-year prosthetic survival and the Compress device showed an 88% implant survival at 5 years for femoral fixation and 80% at 10 years.[10,16]

Failures of cemented distal femoral replacements have primarily been a result of aseptic loosening, infection, or extensor mechanism dysfunction. Ward et al. found greater body weight and poorer range of knee motion as predictors of failure.[35] In another study from the same institution, failure from aseptic loosening was found more likely in men and in patients younger than 26 years of age at initial or revision surgery.[38] Choong et al. reported 9 complications in 7 of their 30 patients, including extensor mechanism problems (4 patients), posttraumatic periprosthetic femur fracture (2 patients), posttraumatic aseptic loosening (1 patient), wound infection (1 patient), and temporary peroneal nerve palsy (1 patent). Because of patellar complications encountered and the lack of functional difference between patients who had patellar resurfacing and those who did not, Choong et al. recommended only selective patellar resurfacing.[7] In a study of patients with cemented distal femoral implants who survived more than 5 years after their first procedure, 22 of 83 patients required 26 additional procedures for aseptic loosening ($n = 7$), component breakage ($n = 2$), and polyethylene wear ($n = 12$) with all patients but one (amputation for tumor recurrence) retaining a mobile knee joint.[12] In this cohort, the 5-, 10-, and 15-year survival rate for aseptic loosening was 86% from the time-zero point of 5 years after the first procedure.

In patients with uncemented femoral fixation, failure may more commonly result from infection or mechanical failure with a lower risk of aseptic loosening. Myers et al. reported no aseptic loosening in 15 HA-coated stems with an HA collar stem fracture at minimum 5-year follow-up.[27] Analyzing distal femoral and proximal tibial uncemented fixed-hinge endoprostheses, Griffin et al. identified 6 stem fractures, 10 infections, and only 2 cases of aseptic loosening in 99 patients at a median follow-up of 24 months.[15] Myers et al. expressed disappointment that failure because of infection and local recurrence has not improved with time, whereas in their experience, aseptic loosening has been improved with advances in the design of uncemented implants.[27]

Proximal Tibia

Megaprosthetic replacement of the proximal tibia has not been as successful as in the distal femur. Malawer and Chou reported less than 50% prosthetic survival at 4 years in 13 cases.[24] Kawai et al. reported a 5-year prosthetic survival rate of 58% in a small series of 7 patients, all with a rotating-hinge implant.[20]

Prosthetic advances appear to have improved these early dismal results. In an excellent longitudinal study of proximal tibia replacements, Myers et al. reported on their experience over 30 years with 194 patients who underwent a proximal tibial replacement using a Stanmore implant.[28] At mean follow-up of almost 15 years, 115 patients were alive and the risk of revision for any reason in the fixed-hinge group was 32% at 5 years, 61% at 10 years, and 75% at 15 and 20 years compared to the rotating-hinge group with 12% risk of revision at 5 years, 25% at 10 years, and 30% at 15 years. The most common reason for failure of the current rotating-hinge implant (cemented stem with HA collar) was infection with the risk of aseptic loosening decreased to 3% at 10 years. An early very high infection rate was reduced with the use of a medial gastrocnemius rotational flap to provide appropriate deep soft tissue coverage to the prosthesis.

Other encouraging results have been reported. In 44 patients treated with an uncemented proximal tibial endoprosthesis, early follow-up showed no cases of aseptic loosening (mean follow-up of 60 months, range, 9 to 152 months)[11] Complications still occurred in 12 patients (27%) including infection ($n = 7$), stem fracture ($n = 2$), rotational instability ($n = 1$), vascular compromise ($n = 2$), and local tumor recurrence ($n = 2$).

COMPLICATIONS

With prosthetic advances, the risk of aseptic loosening has declined. Complication of infection, mechanical failure, and fracture remain problematic. Further advances in prosthetic design may help lower the risk of infection. Silver coating of the Mutars megaprostheses (Implantcast, Buxtehude, Germany) showed reduced infection rates without toxicologic side effects

in a rabbit model.[13] This coating design has shown decreased infection rates early on but long-term studies are needed.

Mechanical problems related to hinge design can occur.[34,36] Ward et al. studied the association between the length and taper of the center rotational stem and stability of several different rotating-hinge implants.[36] Their results show that the Howmedica, Techmedica, Intermedics/Sulzer Medica, and Wright Medical Technology/Dow Corning Wright designs required at least 39 mm of distraction prior to dislocation. The S-ROM rotating-hinge design dislocated with only 26 mm of distraction and the Biomet knee dislocated at 33 or 44 mm of distraction depending on the thickness of the polyethylene tray used. The authors concluded that rotating-hinge designs with short, tapered central rotational stems without a mechanical stop to distraction may dislocate in patients in whom bone and soft tissue resection permit excessive distraction.

Rotatory laxity of the Kinematic rotating-hinge distal femoral prosthesis was studied by Kabo et al. and found to be greater than in the nonoperative knee at 2 and 3 years following surgery, with the peak at 2 years.[18] Residual soft tissues play an important role in preventing excessive in vivo axial rotation. The authors noted that their results implied that maturation of the periprosthetic scar strength may vary among individuals and may take 2 years.

Periprosthetic fracture has not been commonly reported in most series.[12,27-29] Rates of perioprosthetic fracture have been reported at 0.9% for the distal femur and 2% for the proximal tibia.[17] With the introduction of the Compress implant with its transverse fixation pins, some concern was raised regarding a higher risk of bone fracture. In a retrospective review of the incidence of periprosthetic fractures associated with use of a Compress device, 14 of 221 (6.3%) patients had ipsilateral limb fractures, periprosthetic fractures in 6 patients, and nonperiprosthetic fractures in 8 patients.[32] Although the risk of fracture may be higher with use of the Compress device, the authors note that if a fracture does occur, the Compress technology provides for a relatively straightforward revision.

REVISION OF FAILED HINGE MEGAPROSTHESES

Revision of failed hinge implants is challenging because of the loss of bone and functional soft tissues. Revision of a failed fixed-hinge implant to another fixed-hinge implant is not likely to be successful[30,33]; a rotating-hinge device should be considered.

Revision of a failed rotating-hinge megaprosthesis to another rotating-hinge megaprosthesis is often successful. Wirganowicz et al. reported second failures in 9 of 48 megaprosthesis revisions (most involved the distal femur).[38] Time from the index procedure to the first revision was similar to the time from the first revision to the second revision. In their total series of 64 failed megaprostheses (42 involving the distal femur and 7 the proximal tibia), the 7-year failure rate was 31% for primary reconstructions and 34% for revision procedures. Shin et al. reported a 5-year survival probability of revision megaprosthesis about the knee of 72% at 5 years and 38% at 10 years.[30] They concluded that reoperation for failed initial segmental replacement implants is feasible and effective.

SUMMARY

Megaprostheses for reconstruction of skeletal defects about the knee following tumor resection are successful in most patients.

The degree of bone and soft tissue resection is determined by the extent of the tumor. As much bone and soft tissue as possible should be spared. A rotating-hinge device is preferred to a fixed-hinge device. Cemented and uncemented fixation techniques provide good results, and advances in prosthetic design with uncemented implants may essentially eliminate the risk of aseptic loosening. Good muscular soft tissue coverage of the implant is important to minimize wound healing problems and infection. Patients should be counseled to avoid activities that are stressful to the limb. Although the reconstructed knee is not "normal," preservation of the limb in these patients is highly gratifying and provides a durable functional limb.

KEY REFERENCES

5. Bruns J, Delling G, Gruber H, et al: Cementless fixation of megaprostheses using a conical fluted stem in the treatment of bone tumours. *J Bone Joint Surg* 89-B:1084–1087, 2007.

10. Farfalli G, Boland P, Morris C, et al: Early equivalence of uncemented press-fit and compress® femoral fixation. *Clin Orthop* 467:2792–2799, 2009.

11. Flint M, Griffin A, Bell R, et al: Aseptic loosening is uncommon with uncemented proximal tibia tumor prostheses. *Clin Orthop* 450:52–59, 2006.

12. Frink S, Rutledge J, Lewis V, et al: Favorable long-term results of prosthetic arthroplasty of the knee for distal femur neoplasms. *Clin Orthop* 438:65–70, 2005.

13. Gosheger G, Hardes J, Ahrens H, et al: Silver-coated megaendoprostheses in a rabbit model—an analysis of the infection rate and toxicological side effects. *Biomaterials* 25:5547–5556, 2004.

15. Griffin A, Parson J, Davis A, et al: Uncemented tumor endoprostheses at the knee: root causes of failure. *Clin Orthop* 438:71–79, 2005.

17. Jeys LM, Kulkarni A, Grimer RJ, et al: Endoprosthetic reconstruction for the treatment of musculoskeletal tumors of the appendicular skeleton and pelvis. *J Bone Joint Surg Am* 90:1265–1271, 2008.

23. Kramer M, Tanner B, Horvai A, et al: Compressive osseointegration promotes viable bone at the endoprosthetic interface: retrieval study of Compress® implants. *Int Orthop* 32:567–571, 2008.

27. Myers G, Abudu A, Carter S, et al: Endoprosthetic replacement of the distal femur for bone tumours. *J Bone Joint Surg* 89-B:521–526, 2007.

28. Myers G, Abudu A, Carter S, et al: The long-term results of endoprosthetic replacement of the proximal tibia for bone tumours. *J Bone Joint Surg* 89-B:1632–1637, 2007.

29. Sharma S, Turcotte R, Isler M, et al: Cemented rotating hinge endoprosthesis for limb salvage of distal femur tumors. *Clin Orthop* 450:28–32, 2006.

31. Tanzer M, Turcotte R, Harvey E, et al: Extracortical bone bridging in tumor endoprostheses. Radiographic and histologic analysis. *J Bone Joint Surg Am* 85-A:2365–2370, 2003.

32. Tyler WK, Healey JH, Morris CD, et al: Compress periprosthetic fractures: interface stability and ease of revision. *Clin Orthop* 467:2800–2806, 2009.

36. Ward WG, Haight D, Ritchie P, et al: Dislocation of rotating hinge total knee prostheses. A biomechanical analysis. *J Bone Joint Surg Am* 85-A:448–453, 2003.

39. Wunder JS, Leitch K, Griffin AM, et al: Comparison of two methods of reconstruction for primary malignant tumors at the knee: a sequential cohort study. *J Surg Oncol* 77:89–99, discussion 100, 2001.

The references for this chapter can also be found on www.expertconsult.com.

205

Metastatic Disease About the Knee: Evaluation and Surgical Treatment

Timothy A. Damron

According to the latest cancer statistics, at least 1,658,370 new cancer cases are diagnosed annually in the United States.[3] Those cancers with a propensity for bone metastases rank among the most commonly diagnosed types of new cancers. Breast and prostate cancer rank first in numbers of new cases for women and men, respectively. Lung cancer ranks second for men and women, thyroid cancer ranks fourth among women, and kidney cancer ranks seventh among men. Although multiple myeloma is a less common cancer overall, as a bone marrow process, it involves bone in all full-blown cases.

Metastatic disease to bone occurs less commonly about the knee than it does in more proximal femoral sites, but the distal femur is not an uncommon site of metastatic lesions or pathologic fractures.[11] Metastatic disease is particularly rare distal to the knee joint, just as it is distal to the elbow in the upper extremity. In these acral sites, lung and kidney cancer are the most common primary sources. Metastatic disease to the tibia has been estimated to account for only 4% of pathologic fractures, although lesions in this location are probably more frequent.[14,17] Metastatic involvement in the patella is rare but has been reported.[18,24] In part, the less frequent involvement by metastatic disease in these sites has presented a challenge to its orthopedic management because of the paucity of literature available on which to base guidelines.

In addition, the relatively distal location in the extremity presents its own challenges for diagnosis and treatment. The distal femur and proximal tibia are comprised predominantly of cancellous metaphyseal bone, so lesions may become large before they are evident radiographically. The occurrence of metastatic disease to bone or synovium following total knee replacement is a rare occurrence but should be kept in mind as a potential source of pain after total knee replacement.[1,6,9,27]

Fixation is also a potential problem. Supracondylar femur and tibial plateau fractures in the older population most commonly affected by metastatic disease frequently occur in osteoporotic bone, making fixation difficult, even when there is no tumor involvement. The presence of a tumor increases the level of difficulty of internal fixation. Currently available fixation devices designed specifically for the distal femur do not allow the surgeon to accomplish the goal of protecting the entire femur, including the intertrochanteric region and femoral neck, from coexistent or subsequent development of other lesions, although very long plates may protect most of the femur. Plate-and-screw devices designed for the proximal tibia carry the same limitation below the knee, whereas intramedullary devices for the proximal tibia may be technically challenging in holding a reduction in the often compromised proximal metaphyseal bone.

Hence, metastatic disease around the knee is a topic of great interest to the orthopedic oncologist and general orthopedic surgeon alike. Comparatively little is known and much research is needed. This chapter will describe the general treatment principles of metastatic disease to bone, evaluation of the patient with suspected metastatic disease, prediction of pathologic fracture, and surgical management.

TREATMENT PRINCIPLES

Operative management of metastatic lesions to the distal femur or proximal tibia should follow the same principles of treatment as for metastatic lesions to any site. The most important principle is that a patient's recovery time from surgery should not outlast their expected survival. Even patients with a 4- to 6-week life expectancy are likely to benefit from improved quality of life if the operative intervention improves their overall function. Although the recovery time following an intramedullary rodding or plate fixation is relatively short, poor fixation, which requires a prolonged period of restricted weight bearing to allow healing, does not benefit the patient. Cement supplementation or prosthetic replacements that obviate the need for bone healing and allow full weight bearing immediately decrease the recovery time and benefit the patient. Hard and fast rules regarding minimum life expectancy to warrant operative intervention are less important than an individualized assessment of the patient in conjunction with the medical oncologist and family members. In general, a patient should be expected to survive the hospitalization and from 30 to 90 days postoperatively. A moribund, immediately preterminal patient is not considered a good operative candidate.

The corollary to the minimum survival rule is that the operation should result in a stable reconstruction that allows immediate weight bearing and durability for the patient's shortened life span. The improved function and pain relief provided by an immediately stable construct will translate into improved quality of life over the period of limited survival. Although a cemented endoprosthetic reconstruction following resection of the diseased segment of bone will usually reliably accomplish this goal, the same may often be achieved by internal fixation. In a fracture situation, supplementing internal fixation with bone cement will often allow immediate weight bearing, but fixation durability relies on fracture healing. If the patient survives long enough and the fracture fails to heal, the construct will likely fail.

The healing of pathologic fractures is slowed by local disease progression and by radiotherapy, but is also closely related to the underlying disease process and expected survival (Table 205.1).

TABLE 205.1   **Five-Year Relative Survival Rates at Diagnosis for Distant Metastatic Disease According to Primary Cancer (US SEER Data 2004–2010)**

Primary Cancer Source	Five-Year Survival Rate (%)
Breast (female)	**25**
Colon and rectum	13
Esophagus	4
Kidney	**12**
Larynx	35
Liver	35
Lung and bronchus	**4**
Melanoma of the skin	16
Multiple myeloma	29*
Oral cavity and pharynx	37
Ovary	27
Pancreas	2
Prostate	**28**
Stomach	4
Testis	73
Thyroid	**55**
Urinary bladder	6
Uterine cervix	16
Uterine corpus	18

*From American Cancer Society. Multiple Myeloma (www.cancer.org/acs/groups/cid/documents/webcontent/003121-pdf.pdf), 2014.
Source: Abstracted from table entitled, "Five-year Relative Survival Rates (%) by Stage at Diagnosis, US, 2004-2010" in American Cancer Society. Cancer Facts & Figures 2015. Atlanta: American Cancer Society, 2015.

Patients with metastatic lung cancer, for example, have a 1-year survival rate of 26%, so although their fractures rarely heal, it is usually of little consequence, because the fracture fixation usually outlives the patient. Metastatic renal cancer patients, particularly those with disseminated disease, also have a poor prognosis. However, although their survival is often relatively shortened, their lack of responsiveness to radiotherapy may lead to local disease progression and loss of fixation even over the short term. Some fractures in patients with breast and prostate carcinoma metastases will heal, given appropriate treatment, because many will live longer than 6 months, but because they survive longer, there is an increased potential for fixation failure if the fractures do not heal. Even the best reported healing rate for pathologic fractures, which occurred for multiple myeloma, was only 67%.[10]

The role of polymethylmethacrylate (PMMA) as an adjunct to the treatment of pathologic fractures is well established for internal fixation devices and for endoprostheses. As a supplement to internal fixation devices, bone cement improves pain relief and ambulation for lower extremity fixation devices more than internal fixation alone. This is particularly true in metaphyseal regions, such as those around the knee. In contrast, when metastatic lesions occur in diaphyseal locations, a number of series have demonstrated the success of intramedullary rodding without adjuvant bone cement. Even in diaphyseal locations, however, cement adds stability to the construct, so its use in addition to intramedullary rodding remains controversial. As the means of fixation for endoprostheses, bone cement obviates the need for healing by bony ingrowth into porous-coated implants, which can be hampered not only by the underlying disease process but also by radiotherapy.

A traditional axiom for orthopedic treatment of metastatic disease is the recommended protection of the entire bone proximal and distal to the lesion (Fig. 205.1). This is certainly crucial to address preexisting bone lesions that may progress to weaken the bone or cause fracture, but it is also classically recommended to prophylactically address new sites that may arise as the disease progresses. However, recent evidence has questioned the frequency with which the latter situation arises.[2]

A retrospective chart review of 96 patients with metastases, myeloma, or lymphoma who underwent stabilization or arthroplasty of impending or actual femoral or humeral pathologic fractures showed that only 1 patient of 96 developed a new bone lesion at a site independent of those originally recognized at the time of the index surgery. However, in the attempt to protect the entire bone by using predominately intramedullary fixation devices and long-stem arthroplasties, 12 (12.5%) patients experienced physiologic nonfatal complications potentially attributable to embolic phenomena from those long intramedullary implants.[2] Hence, the question has been raised as to whether the potential benefit of protecting the entire bone beyond the region initially recognized to have lesions outweighs the risks.

Having said that, most of the lesions in the described study were proximally situated in the femur or humerus.[2] For metastases involving the distal femur, the question is whether attempting to protect the entire proximal bone including the intertrochanteric region is worthwhile. This question remains unanswered because it has not been evaluated in any reported series. Furthermore, with the more frequent occurrence of metastases in the proximal femur, and with the increased stresses there, consideration should be given to protecting as far proximal as possible. Certainly, fixation should extend well proximal to any identifiable weakened areas in the bone. With fixation of the distal femur using a retrograde intramedullary nail or long-stemmed femoral total knee component, the intertrochanteric region and/or femoral neck remain unprotected. Failure to consider proximal femoral impending pathologic fractures may result in pathologic fracture proximal to an internal fixation or prosthetic device. Prior to operative intervention, radiographs of the entire affected bone should be reviewed to identify lesions that should be bypassed prophylactically. Although protection of the entire long bone involved for possible development of subsequent lesions remains controversial, certainly those lesions that are present should be identified and protected with the appropriate device (Fig. 205.2).[20]

Finally, radiotherapy should be used postoperatively to protect the entire instrumented region of the bone. When intramedullary reaming is done, the entire bone should receive irradiation. Failure to irradiate postoperatively leads to a higher rate of implant failure and lower functional benefit overall.[25] Consultation should be obtained with a radiation oncologist preoperatively or in the early postoperative course for this purpose. When incisions are laterally placed, they can often be avoided by anteroposterior-posteroanterior (AP-PA) radiation treatment, but incisions within the actual radiation field should usually be allowed to heal completely before initiating radiotherapy.

EVALUATION

Before treatment may be undertaken, the correct diagnosis must be established. The diagnosis of metastatic disease as the cause for a specific new bone lesion in any location should never be assumed unless the patient already has biopsy-proven

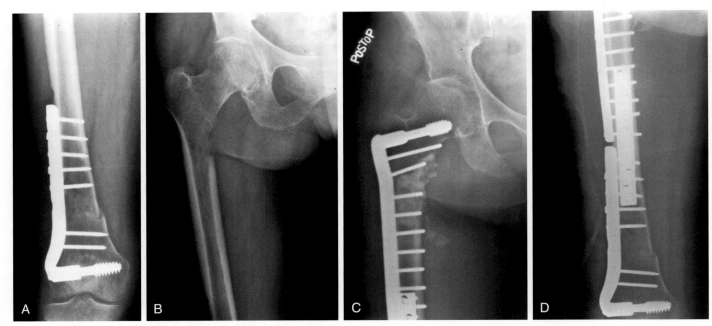

FIG 205.1 Importance of Imaging the Entire Affected Long Bone and Adjacent Joints Prior to Surgery (A) AP radiograph of the distal femur in a patient who underwent open reduction and internal fixation of a pathologic supracondylar femur fracture (open reduction internal fixation [ORIF]) with a DCS device. The patient complained of groin pain in the early postoperative period. (B) Subsequent right hip radiographs show a lytic lesion involving the subtrochanteric right femur. (C) Because of the impending fracture proximal to the already placed screw device, another DCS device was placed proximally. (D) To minimize the stress riser effect at the junction between the two lateral plates, the gap was spanned with a 90:90 anterior femoral plate.

metastatic disease. The danger lies in incorrectly treating a primary bone sarcoma as a metastatic lesion, with typically disastrous results for the patient and physician. In patients older than 40 years, sarcomas are rare compared with metastatic disease, multiple myeloma, and lymphoma, but they do occur. Furthermore, solitary metastatic lesions from renal cell or thyroid carcinoma may be treated by resection for cure rather than internal fixation, so this scenario should also be given due consideration. Even in a patient with a history of a malignancy with a propensity for bone involvement, the first bone metastasis usually should be proven by biopsy before proceeding with operative intervention. Beyond the consideration of mistreating a sarcoma, some lesions, such as those from metastatic renal carcinoma, myeloma, and thyroid carcinoma, are notorious for being highly vascular. Consideration should be given to preoperative embolization for these vascular lesions.

Primary malignancies with a propensity for bone involvement include breast, prostate, lung, kidney, and thyroid carcinoma, as well as multiple myeloma, although almost all primary cancers have been reported to involve bone. Most breast and prostate bone metastases will present in patients with an established diagnosis of the corresponding primary, whereas the most common sources for a bone metastasis without an established primary are lung and renal carcinomas.

For patients without an established diagnosis, a comprehensive history should seek knowledge of any prior biopsies or tumor excisions, however remote (Table 205.2). Physical

TABLE 205.2 Key Elements in Evaluation of Patient With Metastatic Disease of Unknown Primary	
Key Element	**Features of Metastatic Disease to Evaluate**
History	Carcinomas, biopsies; purpose of hysterectomy, TURP
Physical examination	Breast or prostate examination, thyroid, abdominal masses, lymphadenopathy
Laboratory evaluation	CBC, SPEP-UPEP, PSA, LDH, calcium levels
Radiographic evaluation	Chest radiograph, radiographs of entire affected bone Total skeleton ^{99}Tc bone scan CT scanning of chest, abdomen, pelvis

CBC, Complete blood count; *LDH,* lactate dehydrogenase; *PSA,* prostate-specific antigen; *SPEP,* serum protein electrophoresis; ^{99}*Tc,* technetium-99; *TURP,* transurethral resection of prostate; *UPEP,* urine protein electrophoresis.

examination should also be comprehensive, including evaluation of the breasts or prostate, abdomen, and thyroid and may be best performed by an internist or oncologist. Lymphadenopathy should also be evaluated by physical examination. Serologic examination, including serum and urine protein electrophoresis for multiple myeloma and prostate-specific antigen in men, should be done along with checking the serum calcium level to identify hypercalcemia. Radiographic evaluation, including chest radiography and mammography, when appropriate, should be done initially, followed by chest computed tomography (CT), and abdominal-pelvic evaluation by

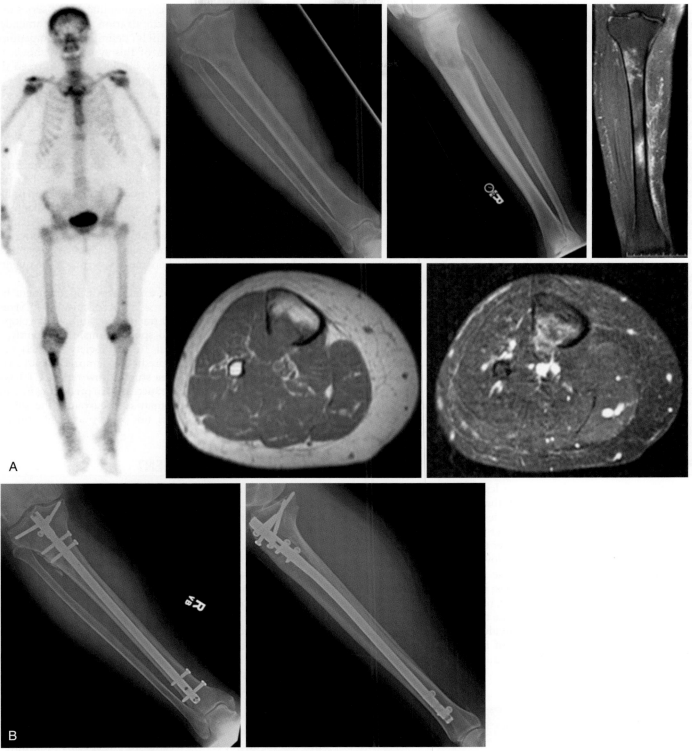

FIG 205.2 Importance of Prophylactic Fixation When Distal Lesions Are Identified (A) Despite what appears on plain AP and lateral radiographs of the tib-fib region to be a solitary proximal tibial metadiaphyseal lytic lesion, the bone scan and coronal short tau inversion recovery (STIR) magnetic resonance imaging (MRI) image also showed a more distal mid-diaphyseal lesion. Inset axial T1-weighted (T1W) and STIR MRI images through the more proximal lesion show the cortical disruption with soft tissue extension warranting concern regarding impending pathologic fracture. (B) Postoperative AP and lateral tib-fib radiographs show both lesions to be prophylactically fixed with a proximally and distally locked intramedullary nail.

CT or ultrasound. This approach will reveal the diagnosis in approximately 85% of patients.[23]

Submitting intramedullary reamings as biopsy material during placement of a retrograde nail for a distal femoral lesion is not appropriate when the diagnosis is in doubt. The same can be said for reamings obtained during placement of a tibial intramedullary nail for a proximal tibial lesion. If the patient is subsequently found to have a sarcoma, the entire knee joint, as well as the reamed portion of the femur or tibia, respectively, would have to be considered to be contaminated. Instead, a straight, longitudinal, laterally placed extracapsular incision is usually appropriate for lesions of the distal femur. However, when the distal femoral cortex is breached medially and there is soft tissue extension in that direction, a medial biopsy is preferred. The proximal tibia is more commonly biopsied anteromedially. When possible, the defect in the cortex in the distal femur or proximal tibia should be made through the thin metaphyseal bone to minimize the additional weakening that occurs when more structurally sound diaphyseal cortex is breached. When biopsy of a small metaphyseal or epiphyseal lesion establishes the diagnosis of metastatic disease, curettage and cementation of the region, with or without reinforcement pins, followed by postoperative irradiation, may suffice as treatment.

Although the surgical treatment principles for multiple myeloma are essentially the same as those for metastatic carcinoma, the diagnosis of multiple myeloma can usually be made based on the finding of a monoclonal spike on the serum protein electrophoresis or Bence-Jones proteins in the urine. Hence, biopsy is less frequently needed once the serologic diagnosis of multiple myeloma has been established.

PREDICTION OF IMPENDING FRACTURE

Prediction of fracture risk from bone lesions is an evolving field, but the classic guidelines suggest that prophylactic fixation should be entertained for any bone lesion that involves more than 50% of the cortical bone, is larger than 2.5 cm in maximal dimension, is accompanied by a lesser trochanteric fracture, or has failed radiotherapy treatment.[13] However, these are relatively insensitive guidelines that fail to take into account numerous other potentially important variables. Mirels' scale for prediction of pathologic fracture is based on four variables (Table 205.3).[19] Each variable is assigned one to three points based on relative risk of fracture for the individual lesion, and the total number of points defines the risk of fracture. In the original article, Mirels set the definition of an impending pathologic

fracture at a total of 9 points, corresponding in the series to a 33% risk of fracture. Prophylactic fixation was recommended for those lesions that met Mirels' definition of impending fracture. Prospective evaluation of this system has shown its reliability across experience levels, but has also confirmed the low specificity for prediction of fracture.[7]

The distal femur and proximal tibia are uncommon sites of pathologic fracture, in large part because of the rarity of occurrence of metastatic disease in these anatomic locations. According to Mirels' scale for the prediction of fracture risk in pathologic lesions, sites in the lower extremity other than the subtrochanteric region are weighted equally for fracture risk. Hence, distal femur and proximal tibial lesions carry the same risk implications as a diaphyseal femoral lesion. However, unlike devices available for the proximal femur and femoral diaphysis, apart from antegrade femoral nailing for distal femoral diaphyseal lesions, the devices and techniques used for prophylactic fixation of the distal femur do not allow prophylactic stabilization of the proximal femur, where metastases may subsequently develop.

More recently, the extent of axial cortical involvement has been found to predict fracture risk more specifically.[15,26] Structural rigidity analysis to predict fracture was initially developed using benign bone lesions and spine lesions, but recently, as the result of a Musculoskeletal Tumor Society (MSTS) prospective study, its validity in predicting femoral fracture risk has been established.[8,21,22] Three studies now report CT-based structural rigidity analysis to be successful in predicting fracture in the proximal femur. This analysis is currently the subject of a prospective study, but is not widely available outside of the trial.

ORTHOPEDIC MANAGEMENT

Nonoperative management is appropriate for many bone lesions caused by metastatic disease or multiple myeloma. Some patients require no treatment, but these are restricted to immediately preterminal patients and those whose medical comorbidities do not allow operative intervention. Some patients may be observed with only routine radiographic follow-up. These patients should be restricted to those with small asymptomatic lesions. In general, even small lesions, if symptomatic, should be considered for radiotherapy to achieve pain relief and to prevent progression. When nonoperative treatment is elected, bracing is an option, although it is often poorly tolerated. For distal femoral lesions, a knee-ankle-foot orthosis (KAFO) with drop-lock hinges may provide stability when standing. For proximal tibial lesions, a similar KAFO or a patellar tendon–bearing orthosis (PTBO) may be prescribed.

With the preceding exceptions, many patients with pathologic fractures or impending pathologic fractures around the knee will require operative treatment. The specific procedure is determined by the location and size of the lesion and by the presence or absence of a pathologic fracture.

Surgical treatment for metastatic disease of the distal femur includes prophylactic stabilization for impending fractures, open reduction and internal fixation of pathologic fractures, and resection with endoprosthetic reconstruction for large lesions or complicated pathologic fractures that preclude fixation (Table 205.4). Techniques for prosthetic reconstruction by the use of megaprostheses and alloprosthetic

TABLE 205.3 **Mirels' Scoring System for Pathologic Fracture Risk in Long Bones**			
	1SCORE		
Variable	**1**	**2**	**3**
Site	Upper limb	Lower limb	Peritrochanteric
Pain	Mild	Moderate	Functional
Lesion	Blastic	Mixed	Lytic
Size*	<⅓	⅓-⅔	>⅔

*Proportion of shaft diameter.
From Mirels H: Metastatic disease in long bones. A proposed scoring system for diagnosing impending pathologic fractures. *Clin Orthop* 249:256–264, 1989.

TABLE 205.4   Surgical Treatment Options for Distal Femoral Impending and Pathologic Fractures

Option	DISTAL FEMORAL ANATOMIC SITE			
	Distal Diaphysis	Metaphysis (Supracondylar)	Epiphysis (Condylar)	Metaepiphyseal Combination
Antegrade locked reconstruction intramedullary rodding	✓			
Retrograde locked intramedullary rodding				
Without cement	✓	X		
With cement augmentation	X	✓		
Plate fixation augmented with bone cement		✓	✓	
Curettage and cementation with or without pins*		✓	✓	X
Long-stemmed cemented total knee arthroplasty with augmentations		X	✓	X
Resection and distal femoral replacement endoprosthetic reconstruction		X	X	✓

*Generally reserved for small lesions or after biopsy for diagnosis alone.
✓, Viable option; X, limited indications.

composites in the distal femur and proximal tibia are discussed in Chapter 150.

Prophylactic stabilization of the distal femur may be divided into three areas—distal diaphysis, distal metaphysis, or epiphysis. In actuality, the metastatic lesion may affect more than one of these areas. In those cases, the most distal extent of the lesion often dictates the available options. For the distal femoral diaphysis, an antegrade reconstruction intramedullary nail is preferred when the tip of the nail will be two diaphyseal widths distal to the lesion and the distal interlocking screws are in uninvolved bone (Fig. 205.3). This is the only option that will provide adequate prophylactic protection of the proximal femur, including the femoral neck, from a pathologic fracture in a proximal bone lesion, should one be present or develop there. As mentioned before, the importance of such prophylactic stabilization has been questioned.[20] Cephalomedullary nails (antegrade femoral reconstruction nails with a tip of trochanter insertion site) are an excellent option here (Fig. 205.4).

When the distal femoral metaphysis (supracondylar femur) is involved by a lesion that is considered an impending fracture, an antegrade nail is usually not a viable alternative because the lesion extends to the end of the intramedullary canal. The options here include plate fixation supplemented by bone cement, retrograde intramedullary stabilization, and curettage and cementation, with or without pins. Options for plate fixation in the supracondylar femur continue to evolve. Traditionally, a dynamic condylar screw (DCS) has been used when 5 cm or more of distal bone is intact, a blade plate has been used when the distal bone is limited to 3 cm or less, and a condylar buttress plate has been used when the distal bone is even more severely compromised. The availability of locking plates has largely replaced those historical options because it combines the advantage of multiple potential points of distal fixation previously available only with a condylar buttress plate with the distal rigidity of a blade plate.[12] This is biomechanically superior to the condylar buttress plate in its initial stability, but technically easier to apply than a blade plate. Further studies are needed to define the precise role of locking condylar plates in the treatment of impending supracondylar femur fractures. In general, metaphyseal bone lesions large enough to warrant surgical treatment and treated by any means of

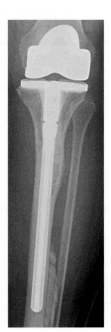

FIG 205.3 In isolated cases where concomitant total knee replacement is indicated or where epiphyseal lesions need to be bypassed, long total knee stems may be used to bypass the defect(s). In this case, a patient with metastatic breast cancer with a good prognosis who was to undergo total knee arthroplasty above a proximal tibial lytic lesion was treated with a very long stemmed tibial component to bypass the defect in the tibia and protect as much of the tibia as possible.

plate stabilization should usually be supplemented by the use of bone cement.

Retrograde intramedullary stabilization fails to protect the proximal femur and relies on adequate remaining distal bone to provide secure fixation for the interlocking screws. This technique is contraindicated when there is a proximal femoral impending fracture lesion already present, and care should be taken to allow room for proximal femoral fixation should such a lesion develop later. Supplementation with bone

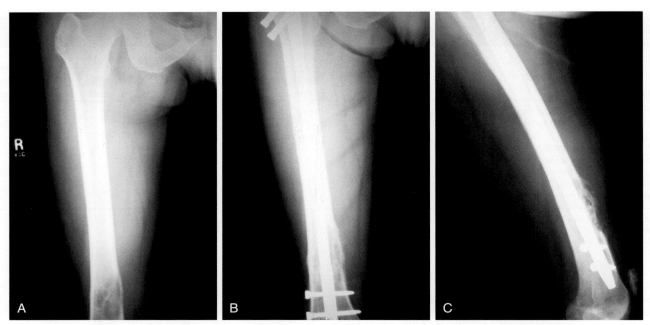

FIG 205.4 A Distal Diaphyseal Impending Pathologic Femur Fracture Is Best Treated With an Antegrade Locked Reconstruction Nail if There Is Adequate Distal Bone to Obtain Secure Fixation With the Distal Interlocking Screws (A) A mixed lytic and sclerotic distal femoral diaphyseal bone lesion in a patient with established non–small cell lung carcinoma is shown. (B) AP and lateral (C) radiographs show the postoperative appearance following antegrade reconstruction nailing. This nail protects the proximal femur and achieves fixation distal to the lesion, but if the lesion had been any further distal, another option might have been needed.

cement at the distal lesion may be needed if distal interlocking screw fixation is suspected. Nuts are available for the distal interlocking screws when bone quality in the region is poor.

Curettage and cementation alone or combined with intramedullary pins has been reserved for small lesions of the distal metaphysis. These techniques are especially appropriate when a small asymptomatic lesion must be approached for diagnostic purposes only and would otherwise not warrant surgical treatment as a true impending pathologic fracture. Aggressive curettage of the lesion should be carried out to allow the bone cement to interdigitate with intact bone trabecula. Preexisting cortical transgression should be used for intramedullary access, when feasible, to avoid further weakening of the intact bone. Fully threaded Steinman pins may be inserted into the femoral canal prior to introduction of the bone cement, similar to the technique used for giant cell tumors of bone. Alternatively, Rush rods or other similar relatively flexible pins have been inserted retrograde through the epicondyles and into the distal femoral diaphysis, followed by distal femoral cementing of the defect.[28] From a biomechanical perspective, these techniques are probably inferior to intramedullary rodding or plate stabilization. Furthermore, they fail to provide adequate prophylactic stabilization of the remaining femur. Hence, their use should be restricted and done with caution.

Epiphyseal lesions in the distal femur from metastatic disease are rare and fixation is problematic because there is no bone distally to allow internal fixation. For small lesions requiring access for diagnostic purposes, the curettage and cementing techniques discussed earlier may suffice. For larger but truly epiphyseal lesions, conventional long-stemmed total knee arthroplasty, supplemented with built-up cement or metal augments to address the distal defects, may suffice. Although these stems are needed to transfer the stresses well beyond the area of deficiency, they are rarely long enough to protect the entire remaining bone. For lesions that involve the epiphysis and supracondylar region, resection and reconstruction with megaprostheses should be considered.[5]

The indications for resection of the distal femur in the presence of only an impending pathologic fracture are twofold.[5] The first indication is when inadequate bone remains to allow secure fixation even when supplemented with bone cement (Fig. 205.5). The second indication is the solitary renal cell or thyroid metastasis, where resection for cure may be of benefit. These techniques are discussed in Chapter 150.

Internal fixation for pathologic fractures of the distal femur are similar to those used for impending fractures, but here the fixation device must provide rigid fixation if it is to achieve the goal of immediate stability. Therefore, curettage and cementation alone or supplemented with Steinmann pins or flexible nails is not an acceptable alternative in this situation. As for impending distal femoral diaphyseal lesions, an antegrade, distally locked intramedullary nail should be used whenever possible. However, many of these lesions are too distal to achieve adequate intramedullary nail length distal to the fracture. In those situations, a retrograde nail may be used, but with careful consideration of the lack of proximal femoral protection provided by this device. In the presence of proximal disease

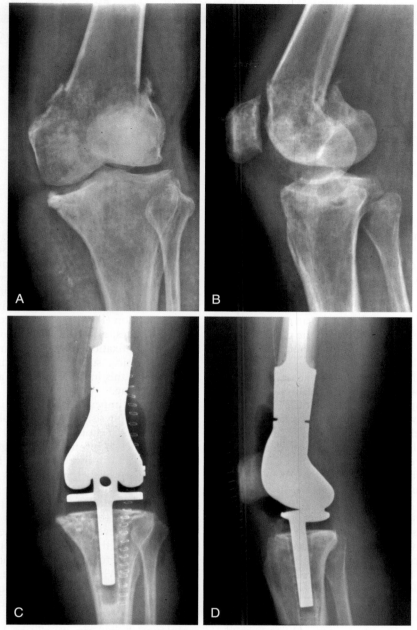

FIG 205.5 Distal Femoral Replacement Should Be Used for Very Limited Indications, Although in SOME Cases There is no Better Alternative (A) AP and lateral radiographs (B) of a pathologic supracondylar fracture of the distal femur. (C and D) Because of the extensive degree of distal destruction, the patient underwent resection of the distal femur with a distal femoral endoprosthetic cemented replacement.

combined with a distal fracture, a combination of devices must sometimes be used (eg, a dynamic hip screw device proximally and a retrograde rod distally, or a proximal endoprosthetic reconstruction or cephalomedullary nail combined with a plate-and-screw device distally). When two devices are being used to cover the entire femur, overlap of at least two diameters of the bone should be the goal—that is, a plate extends beyond the tip of an intramedullary device by at least two diameters of the bone. The screws in the region overlapping the rod may be

angled around the rod, or cerclage cables around or attached to the plate may be used instead. When the lesion is too extensive or too distally placed for even a retrograde intramedullary rod, a plate-and-screw device is often the best alternative. The options for plate-and-screw fixation of the distal femur were discussed earlier in the section on impending distal femur fractures. The advantage of these techniques, particularly when supplemented by bone cement, is that they have the potential to provide rigid fixation. However, they have the limitation of

TABLE 205.5   Surgical Treatment Options for Proximal Tibial Impending and Pathologic Fractures

Option	PROXIMAL TIBIAL ANATOMIC SITE			
	Metaepiphyseal Combination	Epiphysis	Metaphysis	Proximal Diaphysis
Resection and proximal tibial replacement with endoprosthetic reconstruction	✓	X		
Long-stemmed cemented total knee arthroplasty with augmentations	X	✓	X	
Curettage and cementation, with or without pins*		✓	X	
Plate fixation augmented with bone cement		✓	✓	X
Locked antegrade tibial intramedullary rodding		X	X	✓

*Generally reserved for small lesions or after biopsy for diagnosis alone.
✓, Viable option; X, limited indications.

not protecting the proximal femur, so the remaining bone should be carefully evaluated in advance.

The surgeon must have a lower threshold for resection following pathologic fractures of the distal femur, in comparison to the impending fracture situation, when adequate fixation cannot be obtained with the usual techniques. Resection for the solitary thyroid or renal cell metastasis remains an option, even in the setting of pathologic fracture, although the potential for soft tissue dissemination increases the likelihood of local recurrence.

Proximal tibial metastatic bone lesions may require operative intervention for the same reasons as the distal femur—prophylactic fixation of impending fractures, internal fixation of fractures, and resection with endoprosthetic reconstruction (Table 205.5). Paralleling the difficulties in the distal femur, epiphyseal and metaphyseal lesions are difficult to address in a fashion that protects the remainder of the bone. The added concern in the proximal tibia is the presence of the extensor mechanism, which must be maintained or reconstructed after resection.

There is very little literature regarding the surgical treatment of tibial bone metastases.[16] In a series of 16 patients published recently, lung was the most common primary, consistent with its being a common source of metastases distal to the knee. In that series, 11 of the 16 patients had proximal lesions. Impending pathologic fracture was believed to be prevalent among the patients in this series, because 15 of the 16 patients received operative treatment despite there being only one pathologic fracture. The most commonly performed procedure (nine patients) was curettage and cementation with or without internal fixation followed by resection and reconstruction with proximal tibial replacement (six patients). Surgical treatment was effective in this small series in decreasing the visual analog scale (VAS) scores and improving the MSTS functional scores.[16]

For proximal tibial epiphyseal lesions, as for those in the distal femoral epiphysis, curettage and cementing should be restricted to small lesions. Larger epiphyseal lesions that represent impending fractures may be resected and spanned with long-stemmed tibial components on a total knee replacement. Lesions extending into the epiphysis but more extensively involving the metaphysis may be treated by a combination of curettage, internal fixation using plate and screws, and cementing, or by resection and endoprosthetic reconstruction.[28,29]

For proximal tibial metaphyseal impending fractures, the options include antegrade locked tibial rodding and plate fixation. If adequate proximal bone remains to provide acceptable proximal interlocking screw fixation through an intramedullary nail, the goal of protecting the entire tibia can be achieved. However, when the extent or proximal location of the tibial metaphyseal lesion precludes adequate fixation using an intramedullary nail, plate fixation is the better internal fixation option (Fig. 205.6). More conventional proximal tibial buttress plates, as well as newer locking plates, are available for internal fixation of the proximal tibia. Regardless of the fixation choice, supplementary curettage and cementing is advisable in this location to allow adequate stability for early weight bearing.

When the impending proximal tibial lesion is located in the proximal diaphysis, antegrade tibial intramedullary nailing is the technique of choice (Fig. 205.7). The decision to use cement as an adjunct to intramedullary stabilization of long bones is controversial. The more distal the lesion and the smaller the lesion, the less likely that cement is needed, particularly in the impending fracture stabilization.

For pathologic fractures of the proximal tibia, the options are essentially the same as those described for impending fractures. However, cementing alone is not a viable alternative. For fractures of the proximal tibial epiphysis, resection or curettage of the fractured segment usually requires endoprosthetic replacement. Whether this can be accomplished with long-stemmed standard total knee components and build-up blocks or proximal tibial megaprosthesis replacement depends on the extent of the lesion.[4,14,29] Fractures through the rare isolated epiphyseal lesion can usually be handled with conventional components, but fractures through lesions extending into the metaphysis often require proximal tibial replacement, which is discussed in Chapter 150.

Fractures of the proximal tibial metaphysis are analogous to supracondylar femur fractures. Intramedullary stabilization here will rarely provide adequate proximal fixation, so plates and screws, supplemented with bone cement, usually represent the internal fixation of choice. Extensive involvement that precludes adequate internal fixation, however, requires resection and reconstruction. Proximal diaphyseal tibial fractures should be treated by intramedullary stabilization when enough proximal tibial bone remains to allow secure fixation of the proximal interlocking screws (Fig. 205.8). If not, plate stabilization should be chosen using the longest plates possible to protect as much of the bone as possible. Consideration should be given to supplementary cementing.

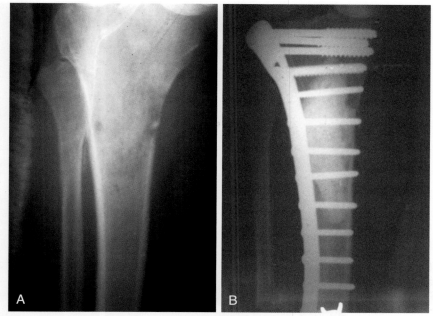

FIG 205.6 (A) This woman, with a metastatic uterine carcinoma to bone, had a painful lytic destructive lesion of the proximal tibial metaphysis with a probable nondisplaced pathologic fracture. (B) Appearance following curettage and cementation with lateral tibial buttress plate stabilization.

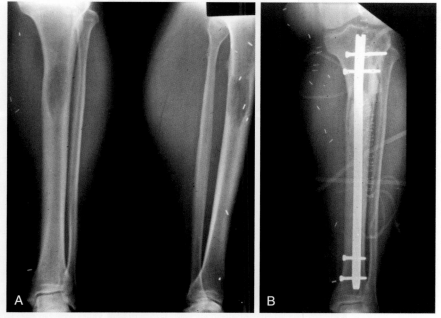

FIG 205.7 (A) Two-view radiographs of the tibia show a proximal tibial diaphyseal lytic lesion in a patient with multiple bone metastases from a renal primary. (B) Postoperative radiograph shows an antegrade intramedullary locked rod in place.

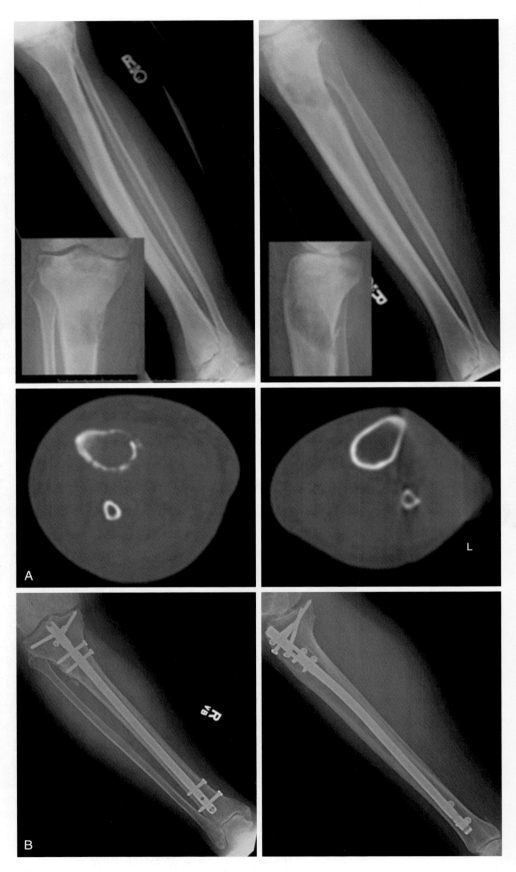

FIG 205.8 Proximal Tibial Diaphyseal and Metadiaphyseal Pathologic Fractures May Be Stabilized in Some Cases With Newer Locked Intramedullary Nails That Allow Internal Fixation With More Proximal Screws Than Nails of the Past (A) Anteroposterior and lateral tib-fib radiographs show a proximal tibial metadiaphyseal lytic lesion in a patient with biopsy-proven metastatic lung adenocarcinoma. *Inset* views show a nondisplaced tibial short oblique fracture. CT axial images of the right and left tibia at corresponding levels show the permeative cortical destruction seen on the right. (B) Postoperative AP and lateral radiographs show internal fixation of the fracture with three screws proximal to the fracture, a procedure done relatively percutaneously in this patient with limited survival.

KEY REFERENCES

1. Alden KJ, Weber KL, Hungerford MW: Periprosthetic thyroid metastasis after total knee arthroplasty: a report of two cases and review of the literature. *J Surg Orthop Adv* 16:148–152, 2007.
5. Camnasio F, Scotti C, Peretti GM, et al: Prosthetic joint replacement for long bone metastases: analysis of 154 cases. *Arch Orthop Trauma Surg* 128:787–793, 2008.
6. Currall VA, Dixon JH: Synovial metastasis: an unusual cause of pain after total knee arthroplasty. *J Arthroplasty* 23:631–636, 2008.
9. Fehring K, Hamilton W: Metastatic carcinoma as an unusual cause of knee pain after total knee arthroplasty. A case report. *J Bone Joint Surg Am* 91:693–695, 2009.
11. Getty PJ, Awan AM, Peabody TD: Metastatic disease of the distal femur. In Heiner JP, Kinsella TJ, Zdeblick TA, editors: *Management of metastatic disease to the musculoskeletal system*, St. Louis, MO, 2002, Quality Medical Publishing, pp 459–468.
14. Heiner JP: Metastatic disease of the tibia, foot, and ankle. In Heiner JP, Kinsella TJ, Zdeblick TA, editors: *Management of metastatic disease to the musculoskeletal system*, St. Louis, 2002, Quality Medical Publishing, pp 469–477.
19. Mirels H: Metastatic disease in long bones. A proposed scoring system for diagnosing impending pathologic fractures. *Clin Orthop* 249:256–264, 1989.
22. Nazarian A, Entezari V, Zurakowski D, et al: Treatment planning and fracture prediction in patients with skeletal metastasis with CT-based rigidity analysis. *Clin Cancer Res* 21(11):2514–2519, 2015.
24. Saglik Y, Yildiz Y, Basarir K, et al: Tumours and tumour-like lesions of the patella: a report of eight cases. *Acta Orthop Belg* 74:391–396, 2008.
27. Watson AJ, Cross MJ: Non-Hodgkin lymphoma as an unexpected diagnosis after elective total knee arthroplasty. *J Arthroplasty* 23:612–614, 2008.
29. Yasko AW, Lin PP, Rutledge J: Site-specific management of tibial metastases. Presented at the ISOLS/MSTS Combined Meeting, Boston, MA, September 23–26, 2009.

The references for this chapter can also be found on www.expertconsult.com.

206

Soft Tissue Tumors of the Knee

Kimberly Templeton

Soft tissue tumors about the knee reflect the same benign and malignant histologic features as those at other anatomic locations. However, when compared with other locations, the diagnosis of tumor at the knee may be delayed because of difficulty differentiating it from the more common sports injuries or degenerative changes in the knee. These more common diagnoses occur in patients in the same age range at which soft tissue tumors occur. In addition, patients frequently relate a history of trauma before the diagnosis of tumor.

CLINICAL FEATURES

Patients with tumors may have a painless mass but, especially with intra-articular neoplasms, may also complain of joint pain, loss of motion, locking, or effusion, further complicating the clinical picture. In a retrospective review of patients with benign or malignant bone or soft tissue tumors about the knee, Muscolo et al.[50] found that 3.7% of these patients had previously undergone an invasive diagnostic or therapeutic procedure for a presumptive diagnosis of a sports-related injury, such as meniscal lesions, patellofemoral subluxation, or anterior cruciate ligament rupture. These patients were re-examined, including evaluation by magnetic resonance imaging (MRI), because of lack of improvement after the initial procedure. More than half these patients ultimately underwent a more extensive oncologic procedure than would have been offered on the basis of the original studies as a result of soft tissue contamination during the initial procedure or progression of the tumor because of delay in diagnosis. Lewis and Reilley,[40] in a review of tumors originally misdiagnosed as sports-related injuries, found that half these tumors were soft tissue neoplasms, with synovial sarcoma being the most frequent diagnosis. Soft tissue tumors about the knee may arise from the surrounding soft tissue and have an incidence similar to that of benign and sarcomatous masses seen at other anatomic locations. Benign lesions include lipomas, extra-abdominal desmoids, and peripheral nerve sheath tumors. Malignant lesions include synovial sarcoma, rhabdomyosarcoma, pleomorphic sarcoma (malignant fibrous histiocytoma), lymphoma, and soft tissue metastases from remote carcinoma. Soft tissue masses may also originate from within the intra-articular space and include pigmented villonodular synovitis (PVNS), primary synovial chondromatosis, and lipomatous lesions. Cystic lesions, such as Baker cysts, meniscal cysts, and proximal tibiofibular cysts, may also be manifested as juxta-articular masses. Rarely, nonneoplastic entities, such as calcific hemorrhagic bursitis of the infrapatellar or prepatellar bursae[62] or gouty tophus,[7] have been described as mimicking soft tissue masses of the knee (Fig. 206.1).

The clinical features of soft tissue tumors about the knee vary, depending on whether the mass is intra-articular or in the surrounding soft tissue. Patients with tumors in the adjacent soft tissue typically have a mass that may have been present for months to years. The mass may or may not have been noted to enlarge. These masses are typically painless, unless there is erosion into the underlying bone or involvement of adjacent nerves. Lesions in the popliteal fossa may also lead to loss of motion, if of sufficient size. Lesions within the joint may produce such symptoms as effusion, locking, or pain (Fig. 206.2). In addition, PVNS may be associated with recurrent hemarthrosis. Cystic lesions, such as Baker or meniscal cysts, may also cause symptoms referable to underlying joint pathology. Patients with proximal tibiofibular cysts may have symptoms from compression of the peroneal nerve. Patients may relate an episode of trauma that initially drew attention to the mass.

The age of the patient may also help in the diagnosis, especially with the malignant neoplasms. Rhabdomyosarcoma is typically seen in younger patients, synovial sarcoma is more common in younger adults, and pleomorphic sarcoma is seen in older patients.

EVALUATION

Physical examination should be used to evaluate the location, whether superficial or deep, and the approximate size of the mass. Lesions greater than 5 cm in greatest dimension and deep are more likely to be malignant. However, approximately a third of soft tissue sarcomas arise from subcutaneous tissue. Change in character of the mass with position of the knee should also be evaluated. For example, Baker cysts typically become less tense with knee flexion and firmer with knee extension. Position relative to the joint should likewise be determined, although meniscal and Baker cysts may dissect away from the joint and true neoplasms may exist at the joint line. The presence of a knee effusion should also be evaluated. This may be useful in ruling in or out intra-articular pathology, such as PVNS or synovial chondromatosis, as well as degenerative changes potentially associated with juxta-articular cysts. Distal neurologic examination may reveal changes resulting from nerve compression, such as with a proximal tibiofibular cyst, or direct nerve involvement by a tumor. However, the latter is unusual. Proximal lymph node examination may reveal involvement by lymphoma.

Radiographic evaluation initially consists of plain films, which will help to confirm that the palpable mass is arising from the soft tissue and not the underlying bone or periosteum. In

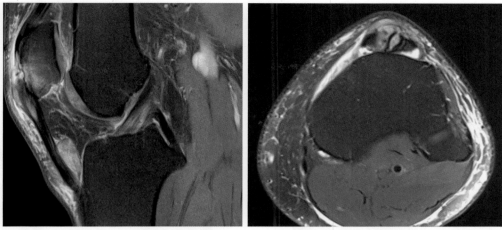

FIG 206.1 Sagittal and axial proton density weighted fat suppression (PD FS) images of a 69-year-old male who presented with a 1-year history of a painful, enlarging knee mass. The lesion was consistent with a gouty tophus involving the patella tendon.

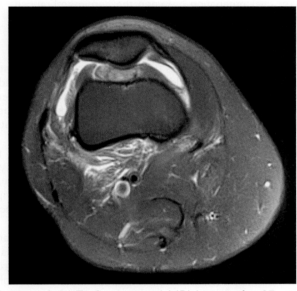

FIG 206.2 Axial T2 fat-saturated MRI image of a 37-year-old female with a history of anterior knee pain who presented with acute onset of a locked knee after a twisting episode. The MRI findings are nonspecific. Her pathology was consistent with localized PVNS.

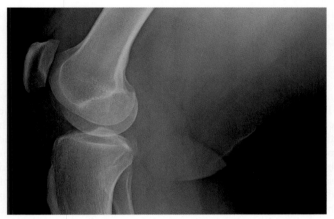

FIG 206.3 Lateral radiograph of a 37-year-old male with new onset of progressive knee pain and swelling with activity. Plain films are nonspecific, although there is a suggestion of a mass along the anterior aspect of her knee. MRI and operative findings were consistent with an early phase of synovial chondromatosis.

addition, secondary involvement of the bone can be determined. Subchondral cysts, especially if present on both sides of the joint, suggest intra-articular pathology, such as PVNS or synovial chondromatosis. Frequently, the masses are seen as only soft tissue shadows on the films (Fig. 206.3). Some lesions, such as synovial sarcoma, synovial chondromatosis, and mesenchymal chondrosarcoma, may exhibit mineralization within the lesion. Ultrasound can help to confirm the cystic nature of lesions, such as Baker cysts.

MRI can further help to delineate the location and composition of the lesion and can assist in the evaluation of lesions whose diagnosis cannot be determined from physical examination and other radiographic modalities (Fig. 206.4). MRI can confirm the cystic nature of Baker and meniscal cysts, as well

as identify any associated intra-articular pathology. These cysts are typically homogeneous, with high signal on T2-weighted images. However, there may be some heterogeneity because of hemorrhage or debris. If the image is not characteristic, especially if there is no associated intra-articular pathology, the diagnosis of meniscal or Baker cysts should be made with caution.[49] MRI may confirm the cartilaginous nature of synovial chondromatosis, which may or may not be mineralized and detected on plain films. MRI can also indicate the presence of hemosiderin within PVNS, as well indicating the extent of intra- or extra-articular involvement. Lipomas are easily detected with MRI; they should have the same appearance as subcutaneous tissue, especially on fat-suppressed sequences. Most other soft tissue masses do not have a characteristic appearance on MRI. Enhancement of the lesion with gadolinium helps to confirm the neoplastic nature of the lesion. Heterogeneity, as well as involvement of adjacent tissue, is suggestive but not diagnostic of malignancy.

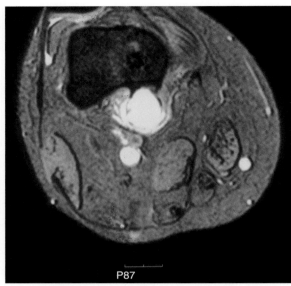

FIG 206.4 Sixteen-year-old patient with a palpable mass in the popliteal fossa. A T2-weighted axial view shows a lesion arising from the posterior aspect of the femur, consistent with a periosteal chondroma.

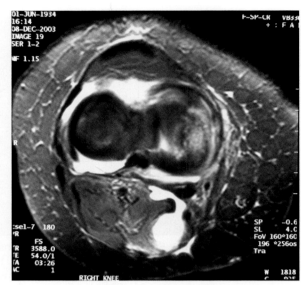

FIG 206.5 T2-weighted axial image of the knee demonstrating a Baker cyst emanating between the semimembranosus and medial head of the gastrocnemius.

When the diagnosis remains in question after MRI or malignancy is suspected, the histology should be confirmed by biopsy. The biopsy may be either needle or open, depending on the clinical situation, comfort of the pathologist in working with the small amount of tissue obtained with a needle biopsy, or the need for tissue for additional studies. Whichever method of biopsy is chosen, the location of the biopsy should be planned so that it is in an area that can be easily excised at the time of definitive surgery if the tumor proves to be malignant. For open biopsies, the incision should be longitudinal, and soft tissue flaps should not be developed to decrease the degree of surrounding soft tissue contamination.

DIFFERENTIAL DIAGNOSIS

Cystic Lesions

Cystic lesions adjacent to the knee may reflect involvement of the bursae related to the patella, pes anserinus, iliotibial band, or collateral ligaments.[45] However, symptomatic cysts are more commonly found in the popliteal space (Baker cyst), at the joint line (meniscal cysts), or within the joint (intra-articular ganglion cysts). The first two are typically associated with intra-articular pathology.

Baker cysts typically arise in adults between the tendons of the semimembranosus and medial head of the gastrocnemius (Fig. 206.5). The prevalence of Baker cysts increases with age. These cysts are filled with joint fluid and reflect intra-articular pathology, such as meniscal tears or degenerative joint disease. In patients with Baker's cysts, 82% are found on MRI to have an associated meniscal tear, most commonly medial, and 13% to have a tear of the anterior cruciate ligament.[28] Adult patients may complain of aching and a feeling of fullness in the posterior aspect of the knee, as well as symptoms from the associated knee pathology.[20] Rupture of the cysts can cause acute pain and swelling in the posterior aspect of the knee and leg. Treatment of cysts in adults is targeted at the underlying joint pathology. In

a follow-up study of patients treated arthroscopically for intra-articular lesions without addressing the popliteal cysts, chondral lesions were the most relevant prognostic factor for persistence of the cyst.[54] If the cyst persists and remains symptomatic, open excision, with suturing or cauterization of the stalk emanating from the joint, may be undertaken.

Unlike adults, popliteal cysts in pediatric patients are not usually associated with intra-articular pathology. Patients typically have a mass in the posterior medial aspect of the knee. In pediatric patients, these cysts are usually asymptomatic. Popliteal cysts in children generally resolve and do not require operative intervention.

Meniscal cysts are located more medial or lateral than a popliteal cyst. They are typically, but not exclusively associated with a meniscal tear. The diagnosis is more straightforward if the lesion is homogeneous on MRI. The lesions may be lobulated and septate.[61] Treatment is aimed at the underlying meniscal pathology.

Intra-articular ganglion cysts are not associated with other intra-articular pathology. They may be found in the infrapatellar fat pad, adjacent to the anterior cruciate ligament, or adjacent to the posterior cruciate ligament, with the latter being the most common in the series by Kim et al.[38] The clinical findings of intra-articular ganglion cysts vary according to the location of the cyst. Lesions in the infrapatellar fat pad may be characterized by a palpable mass. Patients with cysts in the intercondylar notch may have pain, especially in a squatting position.[38] Patients may also have symptoms of knee locking. MRI is typically diagnostic in these cases, with the cysts usually demonstrating homogeneous high signal on T2-weighted images. Symptomatic cysts may be removed via an open procedure or arthroscopically.

In a review of 654 MRI scans of the knee, the prevalence of proximal tibiofibular cysts was found to be 0.76%.[35] Only half of these cysts were symptomatic. When proximal tibiofibular joint cysts are symptomatic, an anterior soft tissue mass is typically present (Fig. 206.6). With time, these cysts may lead to

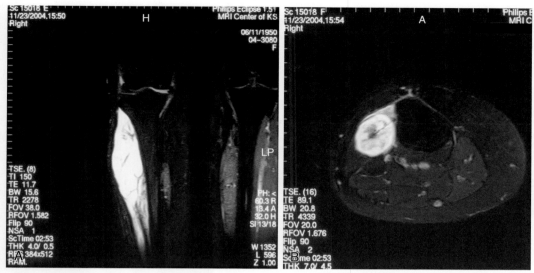

FIG 206.6 (A) Coronal T2-weighted image showing a cystic structure arising from the proximal tibiofibular joint. The patient had a painful anterior leg mass and foot drop. (B) Axial T2-weighted image of the proximal part of the leg showing the cyst in the anterior compartment compressing the deep peroneal nerve.

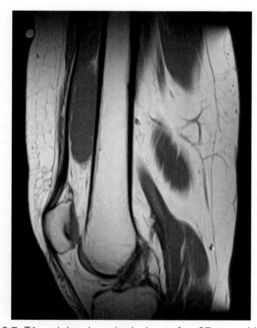

FIG 206.7 T1-weighted sagittal view of a 27-year-old female runner with new onset of anterior knee pain and giving way symptoms. The lesion was removed and was consistent with a neurofibroma.

compromise of peroneal nerve function. Removal of these cysts may require dissection of the cyst from the epineurium[21] but can lead to recovery of at least some degree of nerve function.

Intra-Articular Pathology

Intra-articular tumors of the knee can be difficult to diagnose because the presenting symptoms, as noted above, are non-specific, such as pain, loss of motion, and occasionally swelling or mechanical symptoms, and can be attributed to more common causes. These lesions are most commonly benign. A variety of lesions, such as fibromas, neurofibromas[37] (Fig. 206.7), and extra-abdominal desmoid tumors,[4,42] have been noted in case reports to occur within the knee. However, the most common pathologies are PVNS, synovial chondromatosis, hemangiomas, and lipomas.

PVNS is a condition of unknown etiology, with both inflammatory and neoplastic causes suggested. Its propensity for local recurrence, including recurrence in the subcutaneous tissue adjacent to arthroscopy portals,[43] as well as its monoclonality, may point toward a neoplastic origin. In addition, a variety of balanced chromosomal translocations, primarily involving chromosome 1p13, have been identified. Cupp et al.[19] have identified colony-stimulating factor 1 (CSF1) as the gene at the typical 1p13 breakpoint. Although only a minority of cells evaluated from PVNS resection specimens contained this translocation, the authors hypothesized that the aberrant CSG1 expression resulted in the accumulation of nonneoplastic macrophages and monocytes, forming the tumor mass. PVNS can affect any joint, with involvement of the knee being the most frequent, included reported involvement of the proximal tibiofibular joint.[39] It can also extend into and involve the surrounding soft tissues. PVNS occurs in a localized (nodular) or diffuse form (Fig. 206.8), with the latter being more common. Patients typically have recurrent knee swelling (hemarthrosis) and pain; they may also complain of locking and feelings of instability. This tendency for bleeding within the lesion may be related to the upregulation of genes involved with angiogenesis, as noted by Chiang et al.[13] Because of these nonspecific symptoms, the diagnosis can be difficult, with an average delay of longer than 4 years from the onset of symptoms.[27] Plain films do not demonstrate any mineralized lesions, which may help to distinguish PVNS from synovial chondromatosis, although the latter is not always mineralized. MRI in PVNS typically demonstrates a knee effusion. MRI either demonstrates a single intra-articular mass, in the localized form or, in the diffuse form, multiple intra-articular masses (Fig. 206.9); the latter may also demonstrate extension into the adjacent extra-articular soft tissues. These masses are low signal on T1- and T2-weighted

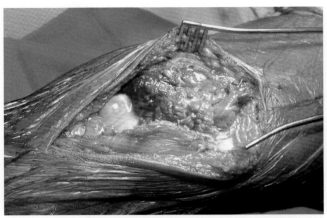

FIG 206.8 Intraoperative appearance of pigmented villonodular synovitis demonstrating extensive involvement of the knee.

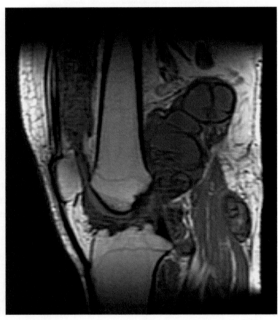

FIG 206.9 T2-weighted axial MRI appearance of diffuse PVNS of the knee. The patient was a 34-year-old male who had had open posterior synovectomy at another institution 5 years prior to presentation.

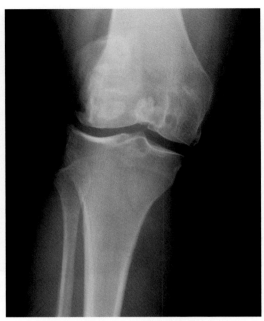

FIG 206.10 Anteroposterior radiograph of the knee in a 45-year-old woman with recurrent pigmented villonodular synovitis. Subchondral cysts and marginal osteophytes are seen on the femur and tibia.

images because of the presence of hemosiderin.[61] The presence of hemosiderin is also responsible for the so-called blooming artifact. The appearance of hemosiderin is considered diagnostic for PVNS. Other imaging modalities have been proven useful in the diagnosis of PVNS. In particular, these lesions can be hypermetabolic on positron emission tomography (PET) imaging and can be mistaken for malignancy.[3,8] Erosion into adjacent bone by PVNS may be seen on both plain films and MRI, although bone involvement is less common in the knee than in other joints, such as the hip. The presence of bone involvement is thought to be because of the presence of a narrow joint space (Fig. 206.10).[12] However, Uchibori et al.[65] found increased production of matrix metalloproteinases 1 and 9, thus suggesting an additional mechanism for bone and cartilage loss in PVNS. Geldyyev et al.[31] found significantly elevated

expression of HYPERLINK "http://www.ncbi.nlm.nih.gov/pmc/articles/PMC1892410/" receptor activator of nuclear factor κB ligand (RANKL), a key modulator of osteoclast differentiation and activation, in PVNS tissue, compared with synovial tissue of patients with osteoarthritis. RANKL was not expressed in normal synovial tissue. Although there were no differences demonstrated in RANKL activity between PVNS lesions that demonstrated adjacent boney erosion versus those that did not, the authors hypothesized that this increased expression of proteins involved in bone loss might facilitate intraosseous extension of PVNS. Taylor et al.[63] noted that PVNS-derived giant cells expressed an osteoclast phenotype and that zoledronate abolished bone resorption by these cells. However, Ota et al.[53] found that CSF1, a factor in osteoclast formation, was expressed in PVNS tissue and that higher positivity was significantly correlated with the presence of osteochondral lesions. RANKL was noted in all tumors; however, the degree of positivity was associated with osteochondral loss or local recurrence. Markers of bone and cartilage loss, as well as local recurrence, have not been clearly identified; this may prove an avenue for development of additional treatment options. Treatment of PVNS requires removal of the abnormal tissue, either a discrete mass and subtotal synovectomy in the localized form or total synovectomy in the more diffuse form. Removal may be accomplished through either open or arthroscopic procedures. Arthroscopy is less invasive, with more rapid rehabilitation and decreased risk of joint stiffness. However, in some cases it may not provide adequate exposure, especially with posterior localized or diffuse disease. Some patients may require both anterior and posterior approaches, particularly for lesions adjacent or posterior to the posterior cruciate ligament. Even with open synovectomies, residual disease can be noted on postoperative MRI[11]; however, the clinical significance of this is not known.

Localized or nodular PVNS is found most commonly in the suprapatellar pouch or femora notch; these may be removed via either an open or arthroscopic approach. In addition, this form tends to be less clinically aggressive. In a long-term follow-up study of 10 patients with localized PVNS treated arthroscopically, Dines et al.[26] noted no local recurrences. All patients had full range of motion at follow-up, without complaints of pain, swelling, or mechanical symptoms. In contrast, diffuse PVNS has a propensity for local recurrence. However, reported local recurrence rates have been variable, and the optimal treatment has not been clearly defined. Zvijac et al.[71] reported a 14% local recurrence rate after arthroscopic partial or total synovectomy, all of the recurrences occurring in patients with diffuse disease. In a review of patients with both localized and diffuse disease treated with open synovectomy and evaluated at an average of 6 years after the procedure, Sharma et al.[58] noted no local recurrences among those with localized disease and a 23% incidence of recurrence among those with diffuse disease. Sharma and Cheng[57] evaluated the outcomes of patients with both forms of the disease, treated either arthroscopically or with an open procedure. The goal of treatment was to remove all of the grossly involved tissue through either approach. They noted that diffuse disease and arthroscopic synovectomy were risk factors for local recurrence. In addition, they also noted that using the same indications for treatment of recurrent disease resulted in similar levels of local control, compared with treatment of primary lesions. In comparing all-arthroscopic to arthroscopic anterior and open posterior synovectomy to all open synovectomies of diffuse PVNS, Colman et al.[17] found the lowest recurrence rate in the second. This again demonstrates issues with removing diffuse disease only via arthroscope; there may have been a bias with patients having more extensive disease undergoing open anterior and posterior synovectomies. However, arthroscopic anterior and open posterior synovectomies remain a viable treatment option; Mollon et al.[46] noted improved postoperative range of motion, excellent Musculoskeletal Tumor Society Scores (MSTSs), and a 13% incidence of symptomatic local recurrence using this approach. Gu et al.[32] noted shorter operative time, less blood loss, better knee scores, and lower rate of local recurrence in patients with diffuse disease treated only arthroscopically versus open synovectomies. However, the authors noted the need for modified portals when attempting to address this condition only arthroscopically. Because of the risk for local recurrence, and additional risk for complications with additional surgery to treat these recurrences, adjuvant therapy, such as external beam radiotherapy or radiosynovectomy, has been suggested for the treatment of diffuse or recurrent PVNS. However, the role of radiation therapy in the treatment of PVNS is not clear. In a small series, Shabat et al.[56] found no complications with the use of yttrium 90 after synovectomy, and all patients achieved excellent results. de Visser et al.[25] reported an equal distribution of excellent and fair functional results after radiosynovectomy for recurrent disease. Ward et al.[67] noted a low local recurrence rate and excellent function results with the use of colloidal chromic P32 synoviorthesis after gross operative synovectomy. Horoschak et al.[34] noted improved local control with external beam radiotherapy used after synovectomy; however, they noted continued progression of lesions treated solely with radiotherapy. Wu et al.,[68] in a review of patients with extra-articular involvement, most likely indicative of an even more aggressive disease process, treated with anterior and posterior open synovectomies and external beam radiation therapy,

noted one, asymptomatic, local recurrence among nine patients treated and followed for a mean of 67 months. However, in a retrospective study of 40 patients with primary or recurrent diffuse PVNS treated by open synovectomy with or without adjuvant radiotherapy, Chin et al.[14] reported an 18% local recurrence rate. All recurrences in this series were in patients receiving radiosynovectomy or external beam radiation therapy. In a meta-analysis of articles published between 1981 and 2012 Mollon et al.[47] found that, based on low-quality evidence, local recurrence was less in patients treated with all open or combined open and arthroscopic procedures; however, adjunct radiotherapy decreased local recurrence only in those patients treated with an all open or all arthroscopic approach. The use of radiation therapy did not seem to increase the risk of stiffness or wound complications. Guidelines on the use of radiotherapy in the treatment of nonmalignant disorders provide a grade B level of recommendation on ranges of doses to be administered to the entire synovial space.[55] The concern regarding local recurrence of diffuse PVNS after surgical resection and, on occasion, radiotherapy, has led to continued interest in developing novel treatment modalities. Blay et al.[6] initially reported on the use of imatinib in a patient with relapsing PVNS of the elbow. The use of this chemotherapeutic agent was based on the presence of genetic alterations of CSF1, a ligand of the tyrosine kinase receptor. Since then, additional studies have indicated a potential role for this drug for lesions that are progressive or otherwise not responsive or amenable to surgical resection and/or radiotherapy. Chen et al.[10] noted in an in vitro study that imatinib inhibited the survival of PVNS fibroblast-like synoviocytes, through induction of apoptosis. In clinical studies of imatinib, Stacchiotti et al.[60] noted symptomatic and radiologic response in two patients with progressive PVNS of the knee; Cassier et al.[9] noted an overall response rate of 19% and stable disease in 74% of patients with locally advanced PVNS; 17 of the 29 patients in this latter study had PVNS of the knee. Although this treatment may be promising, the toxicities of this medication, especially if it would require long-term treatment, need to be considered. Primary synovial chondromatosis is a condition characterized by the metaplastic or neoplastic formation of cartilaginous nodules in the synovium (Fig. 206.11).[23] It is typically monoarticular and may arise anywhere with the joint, with occasional case reports of lesions noted along the synovium adjacent to the anterior cruciate ligament (ACL) or posterior cruciate ligament

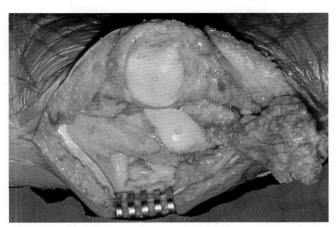

FIG   206.11 Intraoperative appearance of synovial chondromatosis.

(PCL). The etiology of primary synovial chondromatosis is unknown. Crawford et al.[18] found that cells cultured from primary synovial chondromatosis (PSC) demonstrated multiple potential lineages of differentiation, unlike normal synovium. The authors hypothesized that the development of primary synovial chondromatosis might be secondary to deregulation of intra-articular mesenchymal progenitor cells. Symptoms of primary synovial chondromatosis include joint pain, swelling, and occasional mechanical symptoms. This condition is distinct from secondary synovial chondromatosis, which is seen in patients with preexisting joint pathology. Primary synovial chondromatosis has been described as progressing through phases, initially with nonmineralized lesions within the synovium, to frank cartilaginous bodies; with time these bodies may undergo ossification. Depending upon the phase of maturation, the lesions may not be noted on plain radiographs or the radiographs may show nodules with stippled calcification within the joint (Fig. 206.12), along with occasional secondary degenerative changes. This radiographic calcification/ossification is seen in only two-thirds of cases. Plain radiographs may only demonstrate soft tissue swelling around the knee. The lesion can be isolated to the anterior aspect of the knee or may be diffuse, including involvement of the popliteal space.[59] Nodules that are more cellular histologically are less likely to be calcified or ossified. The cartilaginous nature of the lesions can be confirmed by MRI, especially lesions not well visualized on plain films, although early in the course of the disease, lesions may be nonspecific on MRI.[44] At this stage the diagnosis can be difficult to make, as the symptoms, especially any mechanical symptoms, can be attributed to other pathologies, such as meniscal tears.[41] Later in the course of the disease, it demonstrates heterogeneous high signal on T2-weighted images, with areas of signal void reflecting calcification/ossification (Fig. 206.13). Early diagnosis and treatment is recommended before

there is further articular cartilage damage from mechanical wear by the loose cartilaginous or osteocartilaginous bodies. Treatment consists of removing the loose bodies and/or partial synovectomy, either arthroscopically or open, depending on the extent of disease. Davis et al.[23] reported a 15% local recurrence rate, which they thought was because of inadequate removal of loose bodies and/or involved synovium. To address the issue of local recurrence, Chong et al.[15] used radiotherapy in a patient with multiple, rapid recurrences. The disease progression was halted at 5 years of follow-up. The authors' use of this modality was based on their hypothesis that PSC and heterotopic ossification shared similar etiologies. However, there is little additional evidence to support the use of this modality, and typical treatment involves only surgical resection.

Malignant degeneration of primary synovial chondromatosis to secondary chondrosarcoma is rare. Multiple recurrences or rapid deterioration, especially in long-standing disease, in symptoms may indicate malignant degeneration.[23] In addition, the diagnosis can be challenging clinically, radiographically, and histologically. Both synovial chondromatosis and synovial chondrosarcoma can demonstrate adjacent bone erosion.[70]

Other lesions reported in the knee include those composed of fat, both solitary intra-articular lipomas and the more diffuse lipoma arborescence. Intra-articular lipomas are much less common than those presenting in subcutaneous or intramuscular locations. However, the knee is the most common joint in which they occur. They are typically in the anterior aspect of the knee, usually in the region of the suprapatellar or infrapatellar fat pads (Fig. 206.14). Patients with intra-articular lipomas typically complain of a painless soft tissue mass, mild joint swelling, and pain.[69] These patients may also complain of pressure in their knee. Rarely, they may experience locking of the knee, especially if the mass is located within the intercondylar notch or deep to the extensor mechanism. These lesions are

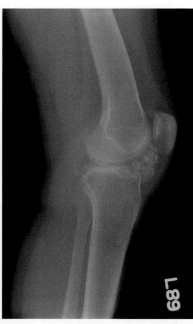

FIG 206.12 Lateral radiograph of a patient with synovial chondromatosis, demonstrating lobular mineralization, primarily within the anterior aspect of the joint.

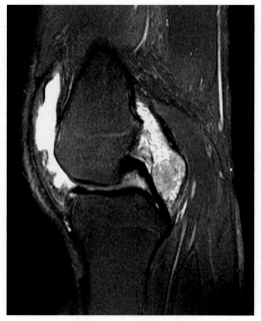

FIG 206.13 T2-weighted MRI of the knee in a 25-year-old woman with a 6-month history of pain, swelling, and locking. Lobular cartilaginous masses are noted, primarily posterior to the PCL.

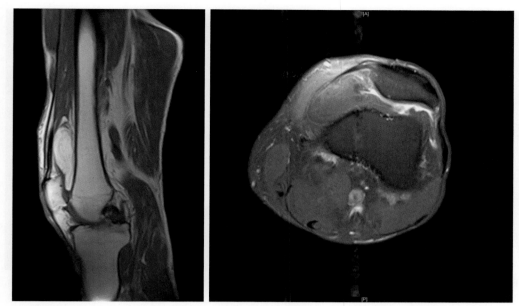

FIG 206.14 T1-weighted axial and T1 fat-saturated MRI images of a 67-year-old male who presented with a feeling of fullness in his knee and swelling. Pathology was consistent with an intra-articular lipoma.

uncommon in the intercondylar region and thought to arise from tissue adjacent to the cruciate ligaments. Lipoma arborescence is a more common condition but of unknown etiology. It is thought to be a reactive process associated with inflammatory, traumatic, or degenerative joint disease. Lipoma arborescence is characterized by replacement of subsynovial tissue by mature fat, which results in villous proliferation of the synovium.[66] This proliferation is most commonly found in the suprapatellar and lateral recesses of the knee. Patients typically have a slow-growing painless mass and intermittent joint effusion, and there have been occasional case reports of patients with bilateral knee lesions. Both of these entities are readily diagnosed by their MRI appearance. Intra-articular lipomas have the typically appearance of being hyperintense on T1 and hypointense on T2 or fat-suppressed images. Septations may be seen within the lesion. Lipoma arborescence can be differentiated from lipoma because it demonstrates areas of high signal intensity on both T1- and T2-weighted images and can be differentiated from PVNS by its high signal on T1-weighted images. Both lipomas and lipoma arborescence can be treated with either open or arthroscopic resection, depending on the size and location of the lesion. Malignant lesions within the knee are rare. In addition to intra-articular chondrosarcoma, discussed previously, there have been occasional reports of synovial liposarcoma and other rarer tumors, such as clear cell sarcoma[33] and epithelioid sarcoma[16] occurring within the knee. Although still rare, there have been more reports of intra-articular synovial sarcoma. Synovial sarcoma mostly commonly occurs in the lower extremity, especially around the knee. However, despite the confusing name, these lesions typically do not involve synovium. Most synovial involvement, when noted, is secondary. However, there have been case reports of synovial sarcoma originating within the knee. This can mimic more common knee conditions, including meniscal cysts.[36] Although MRI is the diagnostic imaging modality of choice, appearance of intra-articular synovial sarcoma is variable, especially in

lesions less than 5 cm.[30] These smaller lesions may be homogeneous and diffusely enhance, findings that are nonspecific. These lesions may be thought to represent benign lesions, most commonly localized PVNS or cysts, based on MRI (Fig. 206.15). In attempting to define MRI characteristics that could differentiate localized PVNS from intra-articular synovial sarcoma, Nordemar et al.[52] noted that the only difference was the presence of larger effusions in patients with the former lesion. Because these primary sarcomas tend to occur in the younger, athletic population, a clear diagnosis needs to be made prior to surgical intervention, such as arthroscopy, that may impact patient outcome. Biopsy of the lesions should not be performed arthroscopically. Treatment of these lesions, as with other sarcomas, includes wide resection. This is more challenging for intra-articular sarcomas because adequate resection would need to be extra-articular. In addition, metastatic lesions have been noted within the knee, although it is unclear if these are metastasis directly to the synovium or reflect secondary bone involvement from metastases to adjacent bones (Fig. 206.16). The most common primary site of origin is lung—especially adenocarcinoma, with gastrointestinal malignancies being second in frequency. Intra-articular metastases typically occur in patients with widespread malignancies. Patients present with knee pain and swelling in a single joint, helping to differentiate this from paraneoplastic polyarthritis.[5]

Benign Soft Tissue Neoplasms

Benign soft tissue masses may occur adjacent to the knee in a proportion similar to that in other anatomic locations. Lipomas, hemangiomas, extra-abdominal desmoid tumors, and schwannomas commonly occur in this area. The first two are typically superficial. However, they may arise from deeper structures originating in the thigh, whether intramuscular or intermuscular, with extension to the level of the knee. These masses are usually painless and exhibit gradual, if any, increase in size. Approximately one-eighth of extra-abdominal desmoids

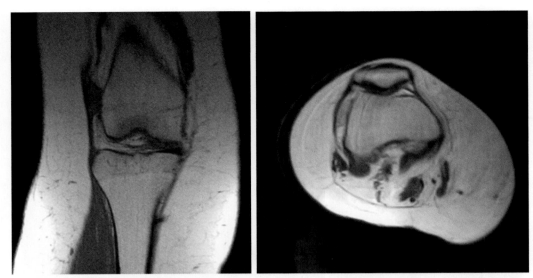

FIG 206.15 Coronal T1 and axial T2 MRI images in a 29-year-old female who presented with lateral knee pain and no swelling. Findings on her MRI were nonspecific but thought to be consistent with localized PVNS. Pathology at the time of open biopsy was consistent with intra-articular synovial sarcoma.

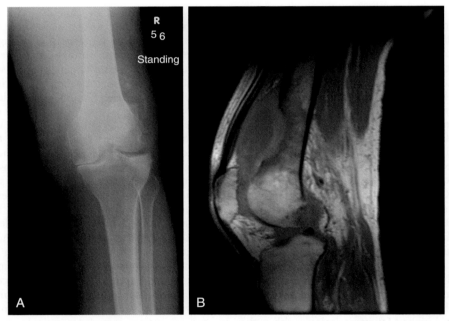

FIG 206.16 (A) AP radiograph of a 67-year-old male with rapidly progressive knee pain and swelling and a history of metastatic lung carcinoma. Cytology of synovial fluid from his knee was consistent with adenocarcinoma. There were no lesions noted with the adjacent bone, making this consistent with a synovial metastasis. (B) Sagittal T1-weighted image of a patient with metastatic non–small cell lung carcinoma who presented with a rapidly enlarging knee mass and pain. Synovial involvement within the knee was secondary to an adjacent bone metastasis.

occur in the thigh or popliteal fossa.[22] These tumors may slowly increase in size and are firm to palpation on initial evaluation. The tumors may result in distal neurologic or vascular compromise if they originate in the popliteal fossa. Schwannomas are typically slowly enlarging masses. Despite their location adjacent to nerves, they are usually painless, without demonstration of distal neurologic compromise. These may arise from large or small nerves.

Tumors may also arise in the Hoffa fat pad, although lesions seen in this area are more commonly the result of trauma. The fat pad is intracapsular but extrasynovial. In a retrospective review of 27 patients with tumors within the fat pad, Albergo

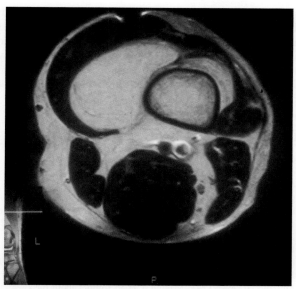

FIG 206.17 T1-weighted axial image of the distal part of the thigh showing a fatty lesion deep to the vastus medialis, consistent with lipoma.

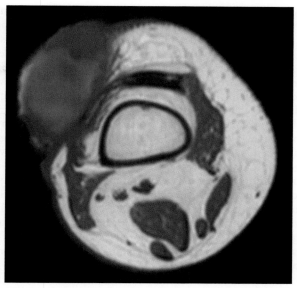

FIG 206.18 T1-weighted axial image of the distal part of the thigh showing a lateral, superficial, heterogeneous lesion. The pathologic diagnosis was consistent with undifferentiated pleomorphic sarcoma.

et al.[1] noted that pain, frequently anterior knee pain, and swelling were the more common presenting symptoms. Importantly, 85% of patients in this series reported no history of trauma, which should raise suspicion of spontaneous masses in this area being neoplastic in origin. The most common lesions noted in this series were PVNS and hemangiomas. However, other lesions, such as fibroma of tendon sheath, have also been described around the fat pad.[48] After the diagnosis is confirmed, benign symptomatic lesions can be successfully treated with arthrotomy and resection.[24]

MRI is useful in the evaluation of these tumors. Lipomas should be homogeneous high signal on T1 weighted images and uniformly low on fat-suppressed images (Fig. 206.17). If there are areas of high signal on fat suppressed images, the diagnosis of lipoma should be questioned. Extra-abdominal desmoids show low signal intensity on both T-1 and T-2 weight images. However, this appearance is not diagnostic and requires biopsy for confirmation. MRI may be suggestive of a schwannoma, when the mass is seen adjacent to a nerve. There may be cystic areas noted within the schwannoma, especially in larger lesions.

Treatment of benign soft tissue masses of the knee is identical to treatment in other locations. However, other confounding factors are potential involvement of the popliteal structures. If diagnosis of the lesion is confirmed by MRI, such as with a lipoma, and the lesion is asymptomatic and not enlarging, observation is warranted. If the diagnosis is confirmed but the lesion is symptomatic or enlarging, marginal resection is the treatment of choice, except in the case of desmoids, for which wide margins should be attempted. If the diagnosis is not certain, biopsy is recommended.

Malignant Soft Tissue Tumors

Malignant tumors reflect the histologic findings described in other locations. These tumors may arise from the adjacent muscle, such as rhabdomyosarcoma in children, synovial sarcoma in adolescents and young adults, and pleomorphic sarcoma (malignant fibrous histiocytoma) (Fig. 206.18) or liposarcoma in older adults. Occasionally, lesions may originate in the popliteal fossa, such as malignant peripheral nerve sheath tumors. Malignant lesions rarely arise from within the joint; tumors reported in this location have been synovial chondrosarcoma and synovial sarcoma.[51] The tumors are initially seen as enlarging masses. They are usually pain free, unless there is involvement of the adjacent neurovascular or bony structures. MRI of these lesions demonstrates heterogeneity, seen best on T2-weighted images. However, this appearance is not diagnostic. Staging studies to evaluate for potential metastatic disease are performed in patients with lesions that are worrisome for sarcoma. Specifically, computed tomography of the chest is performed because soft tissue sarcomas primarily metastasize via a hematogenous route. Histologic diagnosis is obtained after open or needle biopsy.

Options for treatment of soft tissue sarcoma include amputation and limb salvage. With adequate treatment, both have statistically equivalent rates of overall survival. If wide resection of the tumor would leave adequate tissue for limb function, limb-sparing resection is preferred. If only a marginal surgical margin can be obtained because of the proximity of neurovascular structures, limb salvage may still be appropriate if adjuvant radiotherapy can be administered. In addition, vascular bypass/reconstruction may be performed if a wide resection necessitates en bloc removal of a segment of blood vessel(s). Preoperative radiation therapy necessitates resection through an irradiated bed, with an increased risk for wound complications. Postoperative radiation therapy requires irradiation of the entire tumor bed exposed at the time of surgery, thereby resulting in a larger volume of irradiated tissue and increased risk for long-term complications, such as lymphedema. Chemotherapy is an additional modality to consider. However, the impact of chemotherapy on local recurrence or long-term survival has not been definitively elucidated. It may be considered in patients with large, deep-seated, high-grade tumors.

Additional factors must be considered when contemplating limb salvage for tumors around the knee. Lesions in the popliteal fossa are extracompartmental, therefore without the fascial boundaries seen in other anatomic areas that frequently serve as barriers to tumor spread. In addition, the proximity of the neurovascular structures in the popliteal fossa may make wide resection difficult, if not impossible. However, in a retrospective study of 18 patients with soft tissue sarcoma located in the popliteal fossa, Turcotte et al.[64] noted a 7% local recurrence rate, even though 11 patients had microscopically positive margins. Most patients in this series were treated with limb salvage surgery and radiation therapy.

In addition to potential vascular injury at the time of surgery, irradiation in this area can contribute to morbidity; it may lead to loss of nerve function, especially the peroneal nerve.[2] There may also be fibrosis of the joint capsule leading to decreased range of motion of the knee. Moreover, the proximity of the physes of the distal femur and proximal tibia in children may place them at risk of injury. Fletcher et al.[29] reported on the development of varus and valgus deformities of the knees in children treated for synovial sarcoma with brachytherapy or external beam radiation.

SUMMARY

Soft tissue tumors of the knee may present diagnostic challenges because typical symptoms, such as pain and swelling, may be attributed to more common conditions, such as intra-articular injury or arthritis. Symptoms out of proportion to a reported traumatic episode or that persist longer than anticipated warrant further evaluation. The presence of a palpable soft tissue mass, either at the joint itself or in adjacent soft tissue, should also lead to further diagnostic evaluation. Frequently, plain films may be diagnostic, such as in the case of synovial

chondromatosis. In some instances, other modalities, such as MRI, may be needed. Treatment of benign and malignant soft tissue masses is similar to that in other anatomic locations. However, in the case of malignant tumors, limb salvage may be complicated by the proximity of the vessels and nerves in the popliteal fossa, as well as the femoral and tibial physes in children.

KEY REFERENCES

11. Chen W-M, Wu P-K, Liu C-L: Simultaneous anterior and posterior synovectomies for treating diffuse pigmented villonodular synovitis. *Clin Orthop* 470:1755–1762, 2012.
32. Gu H-F, Zhang S-J, Zhao C, et al: A comparison of open and arthroscopic surgery for treatment of diffuse pigmented villonodular synovitis of the knee. *Knee Surg Sports Traumatol Arthrosc* 22:2830–2836, 2014.
34. Horoschak M, Tran PT, Bachireddy P, et al: External beam radiation therapy enhances local control in pigmented villonodular synovitis. *Int J Radiat Oncol Biol Phys* 75:183–187, 2009.
50. Muscolo DL, Ayerza MA, Makino A, et al: Tumors about the knee misdiagnosed as athletic injuries. *J Bone Joint Surg Am* 85:1209–1214, 2003.
54. Rupp S, Seil R, Jochum P, et al: Popliteal cysts in adults. Prevalence, associated intraarticular lesions, and results after arthroscopic treatment. *Am J Sports Med* 30:112–115, 2002.
57. Sharma V, Cheng EY: Outcomes after excision of pigmented villonodular synovitis of the knee. *Clin Orthop* 467:2852–2858, 2009.
61. Stacy GS, Heck RK, Peabody TD, et al: Neoplastic and tumor like lesions detected on MR imaging of the knee in patients with suspected internal derangement. *Am J Roentgenol* 178:595–599, 2002.
66. Vilanova JC, Barceló J, Villalón M, et al: MR imaging of lipoma arborescence and the associated lesions. *Skeletal Radiol* 32:504–509, 2003.

The references for this chapter can also be found on www.expertconsult.com.

207

Common Pitfalls in Tumors About the Knee: How to Recognize and Avoid

Courtney E. Sherman, Mary I. O'Connor

The knee is a common site for oncologic conditions. It is the most common site for the development of osteosarcoma. In other primary malignancies, such as Ewing sarcoma, the lower extremity is also a frequent site of disease, in addition to benign bone tumors and metastatic disease.[13] The knee is the most common site for many synovial disorders, such as pigmented villonodular synovitis (PVNS) or synovial chondromatosis. Over the past two decades, there has been a shift from amputation to limb-sparing surgery for primary bone malignancies.[2] This chapter focuses on common pitfalls to recognize and avoid when evaluating a patient with a potential orthopedic tumor about the knee.

HISTORY AND PHYSICAL EXAMINATION

Patients with a bone lesion or soft tissue tumor typically present with a clinical mass, which can be painful or painless. Patients can also present with a pathologic fracture. At times patients are referred for incidentally noted lesions on their clinical examination or routine radiographs obtained for another reason.

Details in their history that should be evaluated include how the patient noted the lesion, location, onset and duration of symptoms, timing of symptoms (rest pain, night pain, pain with palpation), alleviating and exacerbating factors, any changes in size over time/growth, weight loss, fevers, sweats, chills (constitutional symptoms), personal history of cancer, and family and medical history that could predispose them to tumor conditions (neurofibromatosis, multiple hereditary exostoses, Ollier disease, Gardner syndrome, or Li-Fraumeni syndrome).[3,12]

Age is an important factor for differential diagnosis of patients with orthopedic tumor conditions. Osteosarcoma is the third most common cancer in adolescence. Benign bone tumors, such as nonossifying fibroma, unicameral bone cysts, and aneurysmal bone cysts, are almost exclusively seen in children and adolescents. In patients older than 40 years of age, multiple myeloma and metastatic disease are the most common malignant bone lesions.

Please see Chapter 200 "Evaluation of the Patient With a Bone Lesion About the Knee," for details of the initial evaluation, age of presentation of different tumor conditions, and location.

Referred pain can be a pitfall in tumors around the knee. As in multiple types of knee conditions, referred pain from the hip can present as knee pain. In addition, fibular lesions or tibial lesions can present as knee pain. Fig. 207.1 demonstrates a giant cell tumor of the proximal fibula that presented as knee pain.

In general, if the patient has significant night pain, growth of a mass (especially if >5 cm), constitutional symptoms, history of a lesion in the knee region, and/or a physical examination that demonstrates a mass, further evaluation with radiographs and three-dimensional imaging is warranted.

IMAGING

All patients who present with a mass should have a plain radiograph as the first line imaging modality. Even if patients have had magnetic resonance imaging (MRI) as their first imaging that noted a lesion, the patients still need a plain radiograph to further evaluate the lesion. The correlation between plain radiograph and MRI is often essential for diagnosis. Plain radiographs can often help to narrow the diagnosis for benign versus malignant bone lesions. Worrisome features for malignant tumors are shown in Table 207.1. For soft tissue masses, plain radiographs help to evaluate if the soft tissue mass is from a bone lesion, if it has an effect on the bone, or if there is calcification or mineralization with in the mass. Multiple soft tissue masses/tumors have mineralization on plain radiographs, including tumoral calcinosis, heterotopic ossification, myositis ossificans, pleboliths in vascular lesions, and synovial chondromatosis (Fig. 207.2A to D).

If the radiograph and clinical examination do not give a definitive diagnosis or if the radiographs and history are concerning for a more aggressive lesion, then three-dimensional imaging is typically indicated. If possible, the imaging should be guided by an orthopedic oncologist and/or musculoskeletal radiologist to obtain optimal imaging of the lesion.[10]

Radiologic interpretation is a common pitfall of tumors around the knee. In orthopedic oncology, three-dimensional imaging, including computed tomography (CT) and MRI, has proven critical in promoting and improving the safety and efficacy of limb-sparing surgical resections of bone and soft tissue sarcomas. These studies and their ability to adequately evaluate the pathology and local anatomy and to provide a differential diagnosis and allow local staging of the musculoskeletal neoplasm is directly related to the quality of the study and the interpretation by the radiologist. Heck found that only 30 of 56 (54%) of the outside MRI reports listed the most likely diagnosis as such when 56 outside MRI studies were independently reviewed by a panel of three expert musculoskeletal radiologists. A wide range of nontumoral bone lesions and soft tissue lesions may be misinterpreted as sarcoma, including hematopoietic bone marrow, stress fractures, avulsion fractures, nonossifying fibromas, fibrous dysplasia, brown

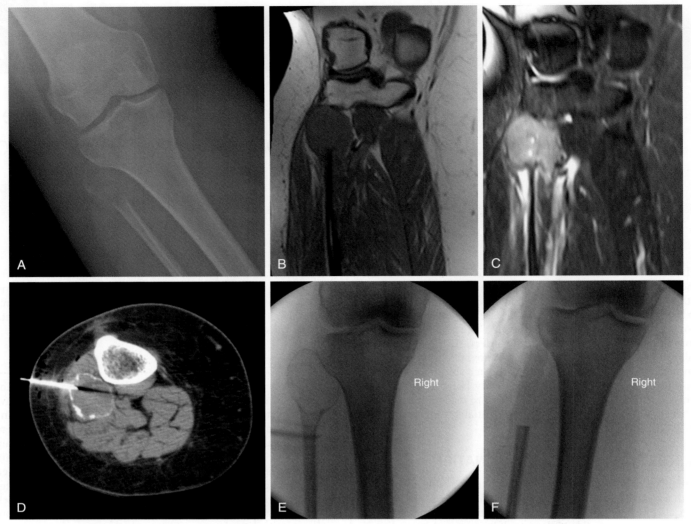

FIG 207.1 (A) Anteroposterior (AP) radiograph of a 39-year-old female who presented with lateral knee pain; radiograph demonstrates a proximal fibular lytic lesion. (B and C) MRI imaging demonstrates the proximal fibular epiphyseal lesion with soft tissue extension and thin cortices. The main differential is giant cell tumor; however, biopsy recommended to rule out metastasis or primary malignancy, such as clear cell chondrosarcoma. (D) CT-guided needle biopsy performed anteriorly to avoid contamination of the peroneal nerve and to rule out malignancy. Pathology confirmed giant cell tumor. (E and F) Intraoperative x-ray demonstrated surgical resection. The patient's lateral collateral ligament and biceps femoris were repaired with suture anchors to the right proximal tibia.

TABLE 207.1 Worrisome Features of Malignant Bone and Soft Tissue Tumors

Bone Tumors	Soft Tissue Tumors
Clinical History and Physical Examination	
Night pain/rest pain	>5 cm
Soft tissue component	Deep location
Weight loss	Firm or solid consistency
Enlarging in size	Enlarging in size
Increasing symptoms	Increasing symptoms
Imaging	
Cortical destruction	>5 cm
Permeative lesion/wide zone of destruction	Deep location
Soft tissue mass	Invasive lesion
Periosteal new bone formation	Heterogeneous
MRI—Low on T1, High on T2	MRI—Low on T1, High on T2

Reprinted with permission from Sherman CE, O'Connor MI: Lumps and bumps: initial evaluation and management of bone and soft tissue tumors. *Northeast Fla Med* 63:19–23, 2012.

TABLE 207.2 Key Information From Imaging Studies of Suspected Neoplasm for Orthopedic Oncologist[13]

Character of the Lesion
Benign, aggressive, malignant, indeterminate

Size and Location of the Lesion
The relationship to palpable or fluoroscopically identifiable anatomic landmarks should be included (e.g., greater trochanter, knee joint line)
Which compartments are and are not involved by the lesion

Extent of Lesion
Intra- versus extra-compartmental
Presence of skip metastases

Relationship of Lesion to
Neurovascular structures
Articular surface
Critical soft tissues (eg, patellar tendon)

Potential for Needle/Core Biopsy

Reprinted with permission from O'Connor MI: Musculoskeletal imaging: what information is important to the orthopedic oncologist? *Semin Musculoskelet Radiol* 11(3):273–278, 2007.

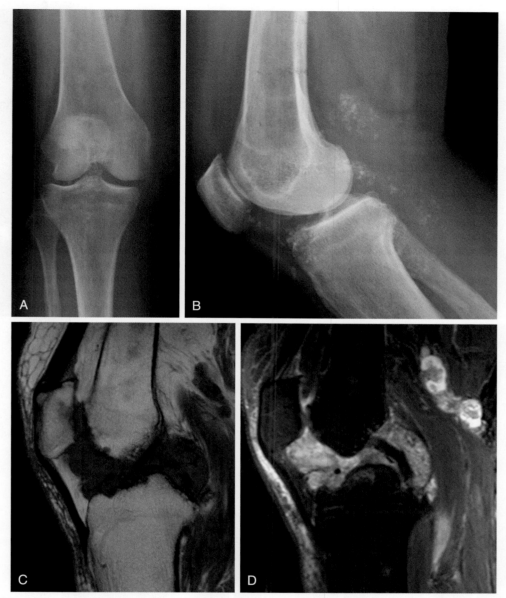

FIG 207.2 (A and B) Anteroposterior (AP) and lateral views of the knee in this 74-year-old female demonstrates evidence of synovial chondromatosis with multiple ossified loose bodies. Patient presented with knee swelling and mild pain. (C and D) MRI images confirm synovial chondromatosis and marginal erosions of the femoral condyles and tibial plateau.

tumors, pseudotumors, synovial herniation pits, Paget disease, eosinophilic granulomas, bone infarcts, geodes (subchondral cysts), hematoma, myositis ossificans, and tumoral calcinosis.[1,4] Therefore it is very important to review imaging with a well-training musculoskeletal radiologist and/or orthopedic oncologist when a musculoskeletal tumor is suspected. Table 207.2 demonstrates key information from imaging studies of suspected neoplasms that are important to an orthopedic oncologist.

Fig. 207.3 demonstrates a common pitfall of imaging. A knee protocol MRI was ordered of a patient with a bone lesion on x-ray that demonstrated only a portion of the lesion (osteosarcoma) and to adequately stage the patient a new MRI had to be obtained of the entire femur, which demonstrated a skip lesion that required surgical resection. If the imaging is directed by a musculoskeletal radiologist or oncologist, often they can adjust the protocol to only obtain one set of imaging of the patient.

MAKING THE DIAGNOSIS

As discussed in Chapter 204, for malignant conditions, staging and biopsy are required to make a final diagnosis and plan a treatment program for the patient. Biopsy planning is of utmost importance and is a common pitfall, which, if performed incorrectly, could lead to an amputation or more extensive surgery that may have not been required if the biopsy were performed/directed by an orthopedic oncologist/specialist. It should be stressed that lesions suspected of being malignant should be referred for a biopsy to be performed by the treating physician.[7,8]

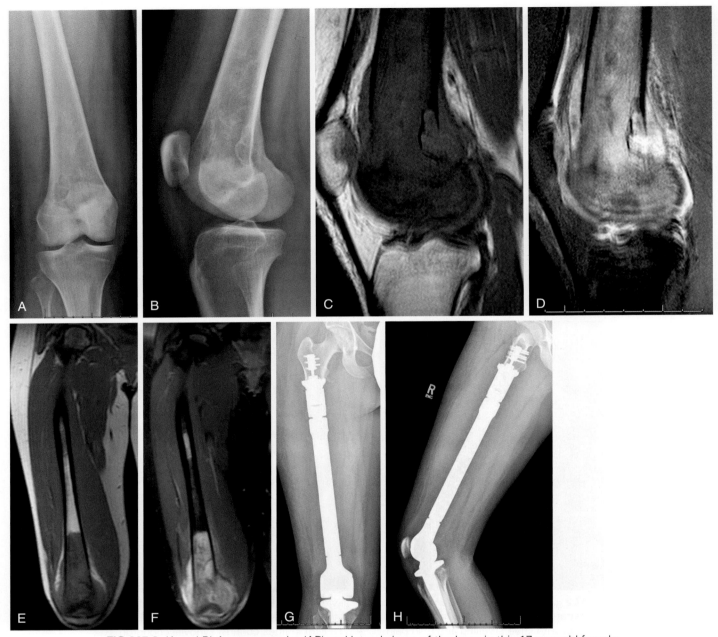

FIG 207.3 (A and B) Anteroposterior (AP) and lateral views of the knee in this 17-year-old female demonstrates an ill-defined mixed lytic and sclerotic heterogeneous lesion in the distal femoral metaphysis. Clinically the patient had severe pain with night pain and inability to bear weight. (C and D) Demonstrates the MRI knee protocol that was ordered, which does not demonstrate the extent of the lesion. It does demonstrate a destructive lesion with periosteal elevation and soft tissue mass all consistent with a primary bone malignancy, and needle biopsy demonstrated high-grade osteosarcoma. (E and F) Demonstrates the MRI ordered to evaluate the entire femur for adequate staging, which demonstrated a skip metastasis proximally. (G and H) AP and lateral femur x-rays after limb salvage surgery with resection of the primary lesion and skip metastasis.

For benign conditions, often the diagnosis can be made from clinical history and examination and imaging studies. The pathologic analysis for benign conditions can often be performed at the same time as surgical treatment. However, if the diagnosis of a benign condition is indeterminate on imaging studies, a biopsy should be performed to rule out a malignant lesion.

For suspected metastatic disease, the evaluation of skeletal metastases of unknown origin by Rougraff et al. is indicated to evaluate the patient.[11] This diagnostic strategy involves a history and physical examination; labs including multiphasic chemistry, serum protein electrophoresis (SPEP), urine protein electrophoresis (UPEP), and prostate-specific antigen (PSA) (for males); chest x-ray; CT of the chest, abdomen, and pelvis; and whole body bone scan. Using this strategy the primary site of malignancy is identified in 85% of cases.[11] This strategy helps to avoid the pitfall of assuming a lesion is a metastatic lesion when rarely it could be a primary sarcoma.

SPORTS TUMORS AROUND THE KNEE

There are many reports in the literature of patients presenting for "sports injuries" and their final diagnosis ends up being a tumor. The majority of these cases could have been accurately diagnosed with correct radiographs, three-dimensional imaging, and careful history and physical examination. Joyce and Mankin noted that extra-articular lesions of bone can simulate intra-articular pathology of the knee.[5] They noted

that errors included not obtaining presurgical radiographs, not obtaining radiographs close to the time of a planned arthroscopy, poor quality radiographs or the lesion was not recognized, lesion was ignored, and/or an arthroscopic biopsy was performed that contaminated the joint.[5] Lewis and Reilly noted 36 patients initially diagnosed as a sports-related injury but later diagnosed with a bone or soft tissue tumor or tumor-like condition.[6] Muscolo et al. noted 25 out of 667 patients (3.7%) with bone and soft tissue knee tumors were treated with an intra-articular procedure because of an erroneous diagnosis of an athletic injury.[9] Oncologic surgical treatment was affected in 15 of the 25 patients. Fig. 207.4 demonstrates a case of a misdiagnosed pathologic fracture that led to an eventual hip disarticulation.

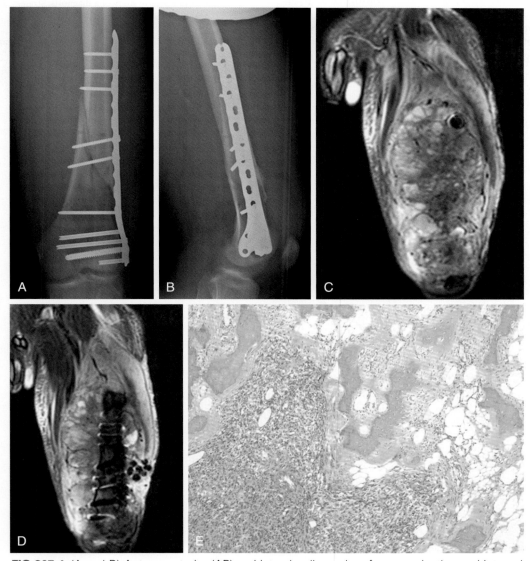

FIG 207.4 (A and B) Anteroposterior (AP) and lateral radiographs of open reduction and internal fixation of a fracture in a 19-year-old male sustained while bull riding. It was noted that the patient's thigh was significantly larger than his other side but was thought to be secondary to his fracture and swelling. Patient's thigh remained tense over multiple months and his incision began draining. He underwent multiple irrigations and débridements. Pathology was not obtained during irrigation and débridements. He was then transferred to a tertiary referral center with antibiotic beads in place for presumed infected nonunion. (C and D) MRI was obtained and demonstrated a large soft tissue mass. (E) An open biopsy was performed, which demonstrated a high-grade osteosarcoma. The patient eventually underwent a hip disarticulation.

SUMMARY PEARLS AND PITFALLS

- Have a high index of suspicion when patients present with worrisome features of bone and soft tissue tumors.
- Patient's age, location, and plain radiographs help to narrow the differential diagnosis.
- Three-dimensional imaging delineates the tumor or tumor-like condition and can help to narrow the differential diagnosis.
- Interpretation of radiologic imaging should be evaluated with an orthopedic oncologist and musculoskeletal radiologist trained in orthopedic tumors.
- Imaging should be directed by a musculoskeletal radiologist or orthopedic oncologist for appropriate local staging.
- Biopsies should be directed by the treating orthopedic oncologist.
- Thorough workup with the Rougraff diagnostic strategy for suspected metastatic disease is important to identify the primary malignancy and ensure a primary sarcoma is not missed.

- The knee is a common site for "sports tumors." It is important to have accurate, good-quality radiographs and three-dimensional imaging when indicated and to avoid performing biopsies of extra-articular lesions through an arthroscopic approach.

KEY REFERENCES

7. Mankin HJ, Lange TA, Spanier SS: The hazards of biopsy in patients with malignant primary bone and soft tissue tumors. *J Bone Joint Surg Am* 64:1121–1127, 1983.
10. O'Connor MI: Musculoskeletal imaging: what information is important to the orthopedic oncologist? *Semin Musculoskelet Radiol* 11(3):273–278, 2007.
11. Rougraff BT, Kneisl JS, Simon MA: Skeletal metastases of unknown origin. A prospective study of a diagnostic strategy. *J Bone Joint Surg Am* 75:1276–1281, 1993.

The references for this chapter can also be found on www.expertconsult.com.

Note: Page numbers followed by "f" refer to illustrations; page numbers followed by "t" refer to tables; page numbers followed by "b" refer to boxes.

Axial artery, 57
Axial engagement index, 866–867
Axial view
  description of, 87–89, 88f
  patellofemoral joint, 853, 854f–855f, 917–921,
    918f–921f
Azathioprine, 1050t

B

Bacillary angiomatosis, 1027
Back pain, 1992–1993
Backside wear, 361f–362f, 362–364, 364f
Baker's cyst, 167f, 187, 188f
  aspiration of, 291, 292f
  description of, 21, 2128, 2130
  imaging of, 109f
  magnetic resonance imaging of, 2130, 2130f
Balanced steady-state free precession, 195
Bare metal stents, 1037
Bartonella henselae, 1027
BCIS. See Bone cement implantation
    syndrome
Beals syndrome, 1238, 1240f
Beath pin, 613, 662–663, 943
Bereiter trochleoplasty, 874, 959–960
Besilesomab, 259
Beta-blockers, 1980
Betamethasone sodium phosphate/
    betamethasone acetate, 1996t
Biceps femoris
  anatomy of, 39–40, 41f
  anomalous attachment of, 56
Biceps femoris complex
  anatomy of, 205–210
  distal, 210
  injuries to, 205–206, 208f
  magnetic resonance imaging of, 207–210,
    208f–209f
Biceps femoris tendon
  anatomy of, 40f, 592–594, 594f
  long head of, 592–594
  short head of, 592–594
Biceps-capuslo-osseous iliotibial tract confluens,
    206–207, 208f, 212
Bicompartmental knee arthroplasty, 1405, 1407,
    1471–1475, 1472f–1475f. See also Knee
    arthroplasty
  activities of daily living limitations as reason
    for, 1478
  advances in, 1476
  arthroscopy before, 1479
  biomechanics of, 1480
  combinations for, 1476
  complications of, 1485
  definition of, 1476
  imaging for, 1479
  implant design for, 1476–1478
  indications for, 1423f, 1478
  instability treated with, 1478
  loosening of components, 1485
  modular
    design of, 1476–1477
    results of, 1485
  monolithic, 1477–1478
  nonmodular
    design of, 1477–1478
    results of, 1485
  Oxford meniscal bearing prosthesis for, 1476
  pain treated with, 1478
  patellofemoral, 1480
  patient selection for, 1478
  physical examination for, 1479
  radiologic criteria for, 1479
  results of, 1485
  stiffness treated with, 1478
  surgical techniques for, 1481–1484,
    1482f–1484f

Bicompartmental knee arthroplasty (Continued)
  technological advances, 1485–1486
  unicompartmental knee arthroplasty and
    contraindications for, 1480
    indications for, 1480
    rehabilitation after, 1482
    surgical technique for, 1481–1482,
      1482f
Bicondylar prostheses, 1383
Bicruciate-retaining total knee arthroplasty. See
    also Posterior cruciate ligament-retaining
    total knee arthroplasty
  advantages of, 1487
  benefits of, 1493–1494
  challenges associated with, 1492
  clinical outcomes of, 1489–1491
  Cloutier, 1487, 1488f–1489f
  fluoroscopic analysis of, 1488
  geometric knee prosthesis, 1487, 1488f
  Gunston polycentric knee, 1487, 1488f
  history of, 1487
  indications for, 1494–1496, 1494f–1495f
  kinematics of, 1487–1489, 1493–1494
  outcomes of, 1489–1491
  overview of, 1487
  proprioceptive benefits of, 1494
  prosthetic design for, 1494–1495
  results of, 1495–1496
  studies of, 1493
  surgical technique for, 1491–1492, 1494–
    1495, 1494f–1496f
Biepicondylar breadth, 300
Biglycan, 396
Biguanides, for diabetes mellitus, 1040
Bioabsorbable interference screws, for
    bone-patellar tendon-bone graft fixation,
    614–615, 617f, 628–629, 632, 688
BioCart, 460–461, 461f
Biologic adhesive and photopolymerized
    hydrogel with microfracture, 457
Biomet Sports Medicine drill guide, 803,
    804f
Biomet Sports Medicine knee ligament
    graft-tensioning boot, 805f
Biomet XP knee prosthesis, 1490f
Biopsy
  bone lesion evaluations, 2081–2083, 2083t
  musculoskeletal, 2083t
  needle, 2081
  open, 2081–2083
  principles of, 2083t
  soft tissue tumors, 2130
  ultrasound-guided, 292, 295f–296f
Bioresorbable interference screw, 1295f
Bioscaffolds. See Scaffolds
Bioseed C, 460
Bipartite patella, 855–856
  causes of, 122, 241
  description of, 51, 51f–52f, 1222
  displaced patellar fracture versus, 122
  incidence of, 122
  magnetic resonance imaging of, 241, 242f
  radiographic findings in, 90, 91f, 122, 124f,
    849
Blackburne-Peel index, 851–853, 853f, 911, 912f,
    1297, 1325f
Bleeding
  anticoagulation as cause of, 2045–2047
  after total knee arthroplasty, 2045–2047
Blood loss, 1078
  allowable, 1078
  blood transfusions for, 1078
  estimation of, 1078
  in total knee arthroplasty
    description of, 1056
    simultaneous bilateral, 1052
  tranexamic acid for prevention of, 1052,
    1074–1077, 1076f, 2004

Blood management, 1079
Blood products, 1079–1080
Blood transfusions
  blood loss treated with, 1078
  human immunodeficiency virus transmission
    through, 1021–1022
Blood vessels, 1065–1066
Bloodborne pathogens, 1022
Blue Shield of California, 2054
Blumensaat line, 86, 87f, 163–164, 169, 849, 910,
    1169f, 1197
Body mass index
  description of, 1968
  surgical time and, 1968
  total knee arthroplasty outcomes and,
    1971
Body temperature, 1157
Bohler test, 69, 72f
Bone. See also specific bone
  physiology of, 2
  properties of, 994
Bone atlas, 299, 299f
Bone cement, 1004
  acrylic, 1056
Bone cement embolism
  biologic model of, 1069
  embolic model of, 1069
  mechanisms of, 1069
  monomer-mediated model of, 1069
Bone cement implantation syndrome, 1056
  description of, 1069
  diagnosis of, 1069–1070
  severity classification of, 1069–1070
Bone contusions, 119f
Bone cysts
  aneurysmal, 2092–2093, 2093f
  simple, 2091–2092, 2092f
Bone grafts
  bone defects in total knee arthroplasty
    corrected with, 1713, 1713f–1715f
  human immunodeficiency virus transmission
    through, 1021–1022
  patellar bone loss managed with, 1949–1950,
    1950f–1951f
  for tibial plateau fractures, 1191–1192
  tibial plateau fractures treated with,
    1191–1192
Bone marrow
  contusion patterns of, 118–120, 162–163,
    162f
  edema of
    description of, 162f–163f, 266
    in psoriatic arthritis, 998
  lesions of, 994
Bone morphogenetic proteins, 82
Bone plugs
  for meniscal allograft transplantation,
    535–536, 535f–536f
  patellar tendon, 674–675
Bone scan, 481f
Bone scintigraphy, of total knee arthroplasty
    infection, 254, 256f
Bone tumors and lesions, 2140t. See also
    Osseous tumors
  age of patient and, 2079, 2080f
  algorithm of, 2082f
  amputation of, 2097
  anatomic barriers, 2096
  aneurysmal bone cysts. See Aneurysmal
    bone cysts
  benign
    description of, 2083
    staging of, 2085
  biology of, 2096
  bone cysts. See Bone cysts
  chondroblastoma, 2089–2090
  chondrosarcoma, 2100–2101
  computed tomography of, 2080

Cartilage (Continued)
  description of, 393
  disruption of, 398–399
  extracellular matrix, 394–396
    collagens in, 394–396, 455
    composition of, 394
    damage to, 398
    functions of, 394
    glycoproteins in, 396
    macromolecules of, 394–396
    noncollagenous proteins, 396
    proteoglycans in, 394, 395f, 396
    regions of, 396
    schematic diagram of, 395f
    tissue fluid in, 394
    zones of, 396–397
  freezing of, 442
  healing response of, 398–399
  homeostasis of, 399
  hyaline. See Hyaline cartilage
  imaging of, 11f, 19f
  injuries to. See Cartilage injuries
  loading responses by, 398
  magnetic resonance imaging of, 19f, 104,
    104f, 189–192, 190f, 195–196, 436–439,
    439f
  MOCART grading system for, 439
  nonsteroidal anti-inflammatory drugs effect
    on, 1314
  osteoarthritis effects on, 191
  patellar, 104
  "preosteoarthritis", 399
  preservation procedures for
    distal femoral osteotomy with, 1336
    high tibial osteotomy with, 1329–1330
    tibial tubercle osteotomy with, 1340–1341,
      1340f–1341f
  repair of. See Cartilage repair
  structure of, 393–397, 394f
Cartilage Autograft Implantation System, 424,
  459
Cartilage defects and lesions
  autologous chondrocyte implantation for,
    414–415, 415f
  full-thickness, 191f–192f
  "kissing lesion", 466, 467f
  magnetic resonance imaging of, 191f–192f
  Outerbridge classification scale for, 414–415,
    533, 533t
  pain associated with, 464
  partial-thickness, 191f
  physical examination for, 464
  shouldered, 415, 415f
  signs and symptoms of, 464
Cartilage grafts, for patellar cartilage lesions,
  1410
Cartilage injuries
  categories of, 398
  cell and matrix damage, 398
  healing response of, 398–399
  magnetic resonance imaging of, 189–192
  mechanism of, 189–190
  Outerbridge scale of, 190
  partial thickness disruption, 398–399
  subchondral bone disruption, 399
  with subchondral penetration, 399
Cartilage lesions. See Cartilage defects and
  lesions
Cartilage oligomeric matrix protein, 396
Cartilage registry report, 421
Cartilage repair
  autologous chondrocyte implantation for,
    462, 466f
  bioscaffolds for
    Agili-C, 458
    attributes of, 455t
    bioactivity of, 456
    biocompatibility of, 455–456

Cartilage repair (Continued)
  biologic adhesive and photopolymerized
    hydrogel with microfracture, 457
  biologic characteristics of, 455–456
  cartilage autograft implant system, 459
  Cell Replacement Technology, 459
  cell-delivery function of, 454
  with cells cultured on or within a scaffold,
    459–461
  characteristics of, 455–456
  Chondrotissue, 457
  ChonDux, 457
  composite bone allograft plug, 458–459,
    458f
  cord blood stem cells with hyaluronan,
    459
  CR-Plug, 458, 458f
  degradation of, 456
  GelrinC, 457, 457f
  history of, 456
  matrix-modulated marrow stimulation,
    457
  mechanical strength of, 455
  multiphase, 457–458
  physical characteristics of, 455
  polyglycolic acid, 457
  polymer, 458–459
  requirements, 454–455
  Revaflex, 459
  scientific basis, 454–456
  with seeded cells
    allogeneic, 459
    autologous, 459
  structure of, 455
  support structure function of, 454–455
  TRUFIT BGS plug, 457–458, 458f
  without cells at time of implantation,
    456–459
  failed
    autologous chondrocyte implantation, 462,
      466f, 467
    clinical evaluation of, 462–464
    early failure, 462, 463f
    history-taking, 464
    imaging of, 464, 465f
    late failure, 462
    microfracture as cause of, 462, 463f
    osteochondral allograft transplantation,
      462, 465f, 467
    overview of, 462
    physical examination for, 464
    rehabilitation after revision for, 467
    revision for, 464–467, 466f
    risk factors for, 462
    treatment of, 464–466, 466f
  meniscal allograft transplantation with,
    539
  requirements for, 454
Cartilaginous tumors
  chondroblastoma, 266, 267f
  enchondroma, 264–266, 266f
  osteochondroma, 264, 265f
  periosteal chondroma, 266, 267f
Cartipatch, 460
CartiPlug, 460
CASPAR, 1809, 1809t
Catastrophizing, 1134. See also Pain
  catastrophizing
Categorical data, 580
Catheter(s)
  adductor canal, 1113, 1113f–1114f
  sciatic, 1113–1114, 1114f
  subsartorial, 1113, 1113f–1114f, 1115
Catheter-associated bloodstream infections,
  2056
Caton method, 913f
Caton-Deschamps index, 851, 852f, 868f,
  1289–1290, 1325f, 1337

Cavovarus deformity, 1852
Cavus foot and ankle
  calcaneal osteotomy for, 1841–1843
  clinical evaluation of, 1837–1838, 1838f
  Coleman block test for, 1837, 1839f
  computed tomography of, 1840
  dorsal closing wedge osteotomy for, 1841
  forefoot-driven, 1841, 1841f
  gait in, 1837
  hindfoot-driven, 1841
  nonoperative management of, 1840–1841
  operative management of, 1841–1843,
    1841f–1842f
  orthotics for, 1840–1841
  pathomechanics of, 1837
  "peek-a-boo heel" sign associated with, 1837,
    1838f
  peroneus longus to peroneus brevis transfer
    for, 1841
  radiographic evaluation of, 1838–1840,
    1839f–1840f
  range of motion assessments, 1837
  sequelae of, 1837
  stability and strength assessments, 1837
  standing examination for, 1837, 1838f
  tenderness assessments, 1837, 1839f
  treatment of, 1840–1843
  varus deformity in, 1842
CD4+ T cells, 1020, 1024
CDAI. See Clinical Disease Activity Index
Ceiling effect, 1365–1366
Celecoxib, 1049, 1131, 2007, 2011t
Cell therapy, 492
Celsus, 1150
Cement
  acrylic bone, 1056
  antibiotic cement spacers, 1922–1923,
    1922f
  bone. See Bone cement
  knee wear affected by, 364, 366f–367f
Cemented total knee arthroplasty
  description of, 1696–1698
  failed, 1574–1575
  hybrid technique, 1574
  literature review of, 1573–1574
  results of, 1573, 1573f
  in young patients, 1573
Cementless fixation, of prostheses, 1392–1393,
  1392f–1393f, 1873
Cementless total knee arthroplasty
  advantages of, 1572
  alignment in, 1581
  Anatomic Graduated Component, 1578
  blood loss in, 1583
  clinical considerations for, 1583
  controversy regarding, 1576
  CR Ortholoc I, 1578
  early
    complications in, 1577–1578
    designs in, 1576–1578
    success with, 1578
  economic drivers of, 1576
  evolution of, 1572
  failed/failure of
    description of, 1576–1578, 1577f
    diagnosis of, 1574–1575, 1575f
    fixation-related, 1576, 1577f
  femoral components, 1576, 1577f, 1581,
    1582f
  femur in, 1581
  fixed-bearing, 1581
  follow-up for, 1583
  future of, 1580
  history of, 1576
  hybrid technique, 1574
  literature review of, 1573–1574
  long-term results of, 1578, 1578t
  Low Contact Stress design, 1578

Morphine, 1125, 1127, 2009
Morphing, 1684–1685
Mosaicplasty, 1259–1260
Motion, 562–563
Moving patella apprehension test, 906
Moxibustion, 1321
MSCRAMMs. *See* Microbial surface
   components recognizing adhesive matrix
   molecules
^{99m}Tc-besilesomab, 259
Multi-biomarker disease activity score, 1010
Multiligamentous knee injuries
   algorithm for, 822*f*
   definition of, 819
Multimodal analgesia, 2003, 2007
Multimodal pain management
   acetaminophen, 1131
   after arthroscopy, 1143
   interventional techniques, 1132
   nonsteroidal anti-inflammatory drugs,
     1131
   opioids, 1132
   periarticular injection, 1132
   protocol for, 1133*b*
Multiple hereditary exostoses, 2089, 2089*f*
Mu-opioid receptor, 1127, 1128*t*
Muscle
   abnormalities of, 56–57
     accessory muscles, 56–57
     anomalous attachments, 56
     hypertrophy, 56–57
     hypoplasia, 57
   pneumatic tourniquet effects on, 1064–1066
Muscle-derived stem cells, 82
Muscle/myocutaneous flaps, 1163–1166,
   1165*f*–1166*f*
Musculoskeletal Infection Society, 1916–1918
Mycobacterium tuberculosis, 1027
Myeloma, 270–271, 273*f*
Myositis ossificans, 296*f*
Myxoid-type liposarcoma, 284
Myxoma, 283, 284*f*

N

Namaz position, 374–375, 386*f*
Naproxcinod, 1319–1320
Nateglinide, 1040
National arthroplasty registers, 1630
National Quality Forum, 2066–2067
National Surgical Quality Improvement
   Program, 1968
Natural-Knee II, 1577
Nausea and vomiting
   epidural analgesia-related, 1124
   neuraxial opioids as cause of, 1126
   opioids as cause of, 1126–1127
   postoperative, 1058, 1128–1129, 1129*f*
Navigation. *See* Computer-assisted navigation
Navio PFS, 1814, 1814*f*–1815*f*
Necrosis, wound, 1160
Needlestick injuries, human immunodeficiency
   virus transmission through, 1022–1023
Negative likelihood ratio, 579*t*, 580
Negative predictive value, 579*t*
NeoCart, 460, 460*f*
Neoplasms, 1025
Neosporin, 1158
Nerve(s). *See also specific nerve*
   abnormalities of, 58
   anatomy of, 41–44
   pneumatic tourniquet effects on, 1064–1066
Nerve blocks
   continuous. *See* Continuous nerve blocks
   general anesthesia and, 1059
   knee arthroplasty using, 1060
   peripheral. *See* Peripheral nerve blocks
   saphenous, 1059

Nerve sheath tumors, 280–281, 281*f*, 295*f*
Neuraxial anesthesia
   anticoagulants/anticoagulation and, 1124,
     1147–1148, 1148*t*
   arthroscopy under, 1058, 1141–1143
   contraindications, 1059–1060
   definition of, 1125
   disadvantages of, 1142
   femoral nerve block versus, 1089
   general anesthesia versus, 1058–1059
   hemorrhagic complications associated with,
     1147
   hypotension caused by, 1083–1084
   knee arthroplasty using, 1059–1060
   moderate sedation with, 1058
   opioids used in
     intrathecal, 1125
     lipid solubility of, 1125
     mechanism of action, 1125
     postoperative analgesia using, 1125
     side effects of, 1125–1126
   risks associated with, 1059–1060
   spinal hematoma associated with, 1147
   thrombogenesis reductions using, 2028
   thromboprophylaxis and, 1147–1148
   total knee arthroplasty using, 1132
   urinary retention associated with, 1124,
     1142
Neurilemmoma. *See* Schwannoma
Neuroarthropathy, 1852–1854, 1855*f*
Neurofibroma, 280–281, 282*f*
Neurofibromatosis, 281, 2079
Neuropathy
   autonomic, 1043
   diabetic, 1043
Neurovascular sheath cannulation, 1147
Neutrophil gelatinase-associated lipocalin,
   1003–1004
Newton's second law, 323
NexGen Legacy prosthesis, 1530, 1530*f*, 1540
Next-day total knee arthroplasty
   blood management in, 2004
   minimally invasive, 2003–2004, 2004*f*
   outcomes of, 2005
   overview of, 2001
   pain management for, 2002–2003
   patient selection for, 2001–2002
   perioperative regimen for, 2002*t*
   postoperative care and management of,
     2004–2005
   preoperative education for, 2002
   summary of, 2005
   surgical approach for, 2003–2004, 2004*f*
   surgical setting for, 2001
Nickel allergy, 1004–1005
Nicotine, 1152
Nietosvaara technique, 1295*f*
Nitric oxide, 995
Nitric oxide synthase, 1066–1067
Nitrite oxide, 995
NMDA. *See* N-methyl-D-aspartate receptor
   antagonists
N-methyl-D-aspartate receptor antagonists,
   1131, 2008–2009
Nodular synovitis, 283, 284*f*
Noncardiac surgery, cardiac evaluation for,
   1034*f*, 1034*t*
Nonossifying fibroma, 266–268, 268*f*,
   2090–2091
Nonparametric statistical tests, 581
Nonsteroidal anti-inflammatory drugs
   cardiovascular risks associated with, 1131
   chondroprotective actions of, 1314
   contraindications, 1131
   gout managed with, 988–989
   nonselective, 1313
   osteoarthritis managed with, 996, 1313–1314,
     1314*t*

Nonsteroidal anti-inflammatory
   drugs *(Continued)*
   osteoid osteoma symptoms managed with,
     2085–2086
   pain management using, 1131, 2007–2008
   recommendations for, 1314
   rheumatoid arthritis treated with, 1010, 1049
   side effects of, 1313
   wound healing affected by, 1154
Nonunion
   distal femoral lateral opening wedge
     osteotomy, 1336
   of distal femur fractures, 1178–1179, 1178*f*
   after osteochondral allograft transplantation,
     452
   of patellar fractures, 1205–1206
   of tibial plateau fractures, 1194
   tibial tubercle osteotomy, 1341
Norman index, 913, 913*f*
Notchplasty, 169–170, 611–612, 612*f*
Novocart 3D, 460
NovoStitch, 527, 527*f*
Noyes and Grood rotatory instability model,
   566–567, 566*f*
NSAIDs. *See* Nonsteroidal anti-inflammatory
   drugs
Nuclear medicine, 107–110
   applications of, 107
   gallium-67 citrate scan, 110
   labeled white blood cell scan, 108
   radioisotopes, 107–108
   revision total knee arthroplasty uses of, 1899
   safety of, 110
   technetium 99m-methylene diphosphonate
     scan, 108, 109*f*
   technetium 99m-sulfur colloid scan, 108,
     109*f*
   technique of, 107–110
Nuclear scintigraphy
   osteoid osteoma evaluations, 269–270
   osteosarcoma, 273
Null point, 1527*f*
NuSurface Meniscal Implant, 552
Nutraceuticals, 1319
Nutrition, wound healing affected by, 1154

O

Obesity
   ambulatory surgery considerations, 1140
   distal femoral osteotomy and, 1330
   epidemiology of, 1968–1971
   intraoperative considerations for, 1969–1970
   medial unicompartmental knee arthroplasty
     and, 1436–1437
   obstructive sleep apnea and, 1140, 1969
   osteoarthritis risks secondary to, 993,
     1968–1969
   positioning considerations in, 1969
   tibial exposure affected by, 1969
   total hip arthroplasty in, 1968–1969
   total knee arthroplasty in
     description of, 1968
     intraoperative considerations, 1969–1970
     outcomes of, 1372, 1970
     postoperative considerations, 1970–1971
     rehabilitation considerations, 1970
     weight loss, 1970–1971
   unicompartmental knee arthroplasty and,
     1422
   wear secondary to, 1971
   wound healing affected by, 1968
Oblique intermeniscal ligaments, 56, 56*f*
Oblique osteotomy, 894, 895*f*
Oblique popliteal ligament
   anatomy of, 19–20, 39–40, 41*f*, 217*f*,
     219*f*–220*f*, 222, 223*f*
   injuries to, 226–227